CURRENT DIAGNOSIS 6

CURRENT
DIAGNOSIS
6 ▬▬▬▬▬▬▬▬▬▬

Edited by

HOWARD F. CONN, M.D.

REX B. CONN, Jr., M.D.

W. B. SAUNDERS COMPANY
PHILADELPHIA · LONDON · TORONTO

W. B. Saunders Company: West Washington Square
Philadelphia, PA   19105

1 St. Anne's Road
Eastbourne, East Sussex BN21 3UN, England

1 Goldthorne Avenue
Toronto, Ontario M8Z 5T9, Canada

Listed here are the latest translated editions of this book together
with the language of the translation and the publisher.

Spanish (1966–67 Edition) — Editorial Labor, Barcelona, Spain
Italian (1971 Edition) — Editrice Universo, No. 1, via G. B. Morgagni, Rome, Italy
Greek (1974 Edition) — Anglo-Hellenic Agency, Athens, Greece

Current Diagnosis–6

ISBN   0-7216-2707-2

Last digit is the print number: 9   8   7   6   5   4   3   2   1

CONTRIBUTORS

CLARENCE P. ALFREY, M.D., Ph.D.
Professor of Medicine, Baylor College of Medicine. Attending Physician, The Methodist, Ben Taub General, and Houston Veterans Administration Hospitals, Houston, Texas.
Acquired Hemolytic Anemia

J. RICHARD ALLISON, Jr, M.D.
Clinical Associate Professor of Dermatology, University of South Carolina School of Medicine and Medical University of South Carolina. Staff, Richland Memorial Hospital, Columbia; Consultant, U. S. Veterans Administration Hospital, South Carolina Department of Mental Health, Columbia, South Carolina.
Premalignant and Malignant Lesions of the Mouth

DAVID H. ALPERS, M.D.
Professor of Medicine, Washington University School of Medicine. Staff Physician, Barnes Hospital, St. Louis, Missouri.
Functional Disorders of the Gastrointestinal Tract

MURRAY N. ANDERSEN, M.D.
Professor of Surgery, State University of New York at Buffalo. Chief, Thoracic and Vascular Surgery, Erie County Medical Center, Buffalo, New York.
Lung Abscess

LARRY G. ANDERSON, M.D.
Associate Rheumatologist, Maine Medical Center, Portland, Maine.
Sjögren's Syndrome

MARION C. ANDERSON, M.D.
Professor of Surgery, Medical University of South Carolina, Columbia, South Carolina.
Acute and Chronic Pancreatitis

RONALD J. ANDERSON, M.D.
Assistant Professor of Medicine, Harvard Medical School. Staff Physician, Robert B. Brigham Hospital, Boston, Massachusetts.
Rheumatoid Arthritis

MASON C. ANDREWS, M.D.
Professor and Chairman, Department of Obstetrics and Gynecology, Eastern Virginia Medical School. Director, Obstetrics and Gynecology, Norfolk General Hospital, Norfolk, Virginia.
Endometriosis

CONSTANTINE ARVANITAKIS, M.D.
Associate Professor of Medicine, University of Kansas School of Medicine. Attending Gastroenterologist, Kansas University Medical Center, Kansas City, Kansas.
Intestinal Disaccharidase Deficiency

SANDA NOUSIA-ARVANITAKIS, M.D.
Associate Professor of Pediatrics, University of Kansas School of Medicine. Attending Pediatrician, Kansas University Medical Center, Kansas City, Kansas.
Intestinal Disaccharidase Deficiency

RUTH A. ATKINSON, M.D.
Assistant Professor of Neurology and Pediatrics, University of New Mexico School of Medicine. Attending Staff, Bernalillo County Medical Center; Consulting Staff, Presbyterian Hospital, Los Lunas Hospital and Training School, and Veterans Administration Hospital, Albuquerque, New Mexico.
The Unconscious Child

EDWARD AUSTIN, M.D.
Associate Staff, Cedars–Sinai Medical Center, Los Angeles, California.
The Acute Abdomen in Childhood

WILLIAM WARREN BABSON, M.D., F.A.C.S.
Surgeon Staff, Addison Gilbert Hospital, Gloucester, Massachusetts.
Acute Appendicitis

VICTOR G. BALBONI, M.D.
Senior Physician, Massachusetts General Hospital, Boston, Massachusetts.
Septic Arthritis

MARIO G. BALDINI, M.D.
Professor of Medical Science, Brown University. Chairman, Department of Medicine; Director, Division of Hematologic Research, Brown University at Memorial Hospital, Pawtucket, Rhode Island.
Purpura Due to Capillary and Platelet Disorders

GENE V. BALL, M.D.
Professor of Medicine, Division of Clinical Immunology and Rheumatology, Department of Medicine, University of Alabama at Birmingham, Birmingham, Alabama.
Back and Extremity Pain

WILLIAM E. BARRY, M.D.
Professor of Medicine, Temple University School of Medicine. Attending Physician, Temple University Hospital; Consultant in Hematology, Northeastern, St. Mary, and Frankford Hospitals, Philadelphia, and Phoenixville Hospital, Phoenixville, Pennsylvania.
Anemia Due to Inadequate Erythrocyte Production

JAMES W. BASS, M.D., Col, MC
Professor and Chairman, Department of Pediatrics, Uniformed Services University of the Health Sciences, Bethesda, Maryland and Walter Reed Army Medical Center, Washington, D.C.
Whooping Cough

LOFTY L. BASTA, M.D., M.R.C.P., M.R.C.P.E., F.A.C.P., F.A.C.C.
Clinical Professor of Medicine and Division Director of Cardiology, Tulsa Medical College. Clinical Director of Cardiology, St. John's Medical Center, Tulsa, Oklahoma.
Ischemic Heart Disease

CHARLES B. BEAL, M.D.
Division of Environmental Medicine, Palo Alto Medical Center; Associate Clinical Professor of International Health, University of California San Francisco; Associate Clinical Professor of Family, Community, and Occupational Medicine, Stanford University Medical School. Chief Attending Physician, Tropical Disease Outpatient Clinic, University of California San Francisco; Attending Physician, Stanford University Hospital, Stanford, California.
Parasitic Diseases of the Intestines

ARTHUR C. BEALL, Jr., M.D.
Professor of Surgery, Baylor College of Medicine, Houston, Texas.
Vascular Disease of the Mesentery

VICTORIA L. BECKETT, M.D.
Assistant Professor of Internal Medicine, Mayo Medical School. Consulting Rheumatologist, Mayo Clinic, Rochester Methodist Hospital and St. Marys Hospital, Rochester, Minnesota.
Scleroderma

WILLIAM BERENBERG, M.D.
Professor of Pediatrics, Harvard Medical School. Senior Physician, Children's Hospital Medical Center, Boston, Massachusetts.
Varicella (Chickenpox)

ARTHUR BERGNER, M.D.
Clinical Associate Professor of Medicine, University of Vermont College of Medicine. Attending in Medicine, Medical Center Hospital of Vermont, Burlington, Vermont.
The Asthmas in Adults

RENEE K. BERGNER, M.D.
Clinical Professor of Pediatrics, University of Vermont College of Medicine. Attending in Pediatrics, Medical Center Hospital of Vermont, Burlington, Vermont.
The Asthmas in Adults

BRAM H. BERNSTEIN, M.D., F.R.C.P.(C)
Associate Professor of Clinical Pediatrics, University of Southern California School of Medicine. Attending Physician, Division of Rheumatology and Rehabilitation, Children's Hospital of Los Angeles, Los Angeles, California.
Juvenile Rheumatoid Arthritis

JOHN W. BEST, M.D.
Chief Emeritus, Division of Urology, Department of Surgery, York Hospital, York, Pennsylvania.
Hydronephrosis

JOHN E. BETHUNE, M.D.
Professor of Medicine, Chairman, Department of Medicine, University of Southern California Medical School. Chairman, Department of Medicine, University of Southern California–Los Angeles County Medical Center, Los Angeles, California.
Chronic Adrenal Insufficiency

PAUL J. BILKA, M.D.
Clinical Professor, University of Minnesota. Attending Rheumatologist, Metropolitan Medical Center and Veterans Hospital, Minneapolis, Minnesota.
Ankylosing Spondylitis

CHARLES E. BIRD, M.D.C.M., Ph.D., F.R.C.P.(C), F.A.C.P.
Professor of Medicine, Queen's University at Kingston. Attending Staff Physician, Kingston General Hospital, Kingston, Ontario, Canada.
Acute Adrenocortical Insufficiency

WILLIAM BRADFORD BLANCHARD, M.D.
Assistant Professor, Department of Pediatrics, Division of Cardiology, University of Florida College of Medicine. Attending Cardiologist, Shands Teaching Hospital, Gainesville, Florida.
Congenital Heart Disease in Infants and Children

PHILIP M. BLATT, M.D.
Associate Professor of Medicine and Pathology, University of North Carolina School of Medicine. Associate Director, Clinical Coagulation Laboratory, North Carolina Memorial Hospital, Chapel Hill, North Carolina.
Hemophilia and Other Hereditary Defects of Coagulation

EDWIN B. BOLDREY, M.D.
Professor Emeritus of Neurological Surgery, University of California, San Francisco.
Brain Abscesses

ROBERT J. BOLT, M.D.
Professor of Medicine, University of California Davis, School of Medicine. University Medical Center, Sacramento; Consultant, Martinez Veterans Administration Hospital, Martinez, California.
Diseases of the Gallbladder and Biliary Tract

GREGORY C. BOLTON, M.D.
Assistant Professor, Department of Obstetrics and Gynecology, University of Pennsylvania School of Medicine. Associate Obstetrician and Gynecologist, Pennsylvania Hospital, Philadelphia, Pennsylvania.
Inflammation and Infection of the Female Genital Tract

HARISIOS BOUDOULAS, M.D.
Associate Professor of Medicine, Ohio State University College of Medicine. Attending Cardiologist, Ohio State University Hospitals, Columbus, Ohio.
Syncope

JERRY E. BOUQUOT, D.D.S.
Associate Professor of Pathology, West Virginia University School of Medicine; Associate Professor of Oral Pathology, West Virginia University School of Dentistry, Morgantown, West Virginia.
Non-neoplastic Lesions of the Oral Mucosa

JOHN M. BOWMAN, M.D.
Professor of Pediatrics and Director of the Rh Laboratory, University of Manitoba. Attending in Neonatology, Health Sciences Centre, Winnipeg, Manitoba, Canada.
Hemolytic Disease of the Newborn

PAUL F. BRENNER, M.D.
Associate Professor, Department of Obstetrics and Gynecology, University of Southern California School of Medicine. Staff, Womens Hospital, Los Angeles County–University of Southern Medical Center, Los Angeles, California.
Functional Menstrual Disorders

DAVID C. BREWSTER, M.D.
Assistant Professor of Surgery, Harvard Medical School. Assistant Surgeon, Massachusetts General Hospital, Boston, Massachusetts.
Aneurysms of the Aorta

PHILIP A. BROMBERG, M.D., F.A.C.P.
Professor of Internal Medicine; Chief, Division of Pulmonary Diseases, University of North Carolina School of Medicine. Attending Internist, North Carolina Memorial Hospital, Chapel Hill, North Carolina.
Atelectasis

PAUL BROWN, M.D.
Laboratory of Central Nervous System Studies, National Institute of Neurological and Communicative Disorders and Stroke, National Institutes of Health, Bethesda, Maryland.
Viral Encephalitis and Encephalopathy

LEONARD HATHAWAY BRUBAKER, M.D.
Professor of Medicine (Hematology–Oncology), Medical College of Georgia. Attending Physician, Talmadge Hospital; Consultant, Forest Hills Veteran's Hospital, Augusta, Georgia.
Neutropenia and Agranulocytosis

CAROLYN M. BRUNNER, M.D.
Associate Professor of Internal Medicine, University of Virginia School of Medicine, Charlottesville, Virginia
Systemic Lupus Erythematosus

THOMAS ROY BRYANT, M.D.
Clinical Assistant in Obstetrics and Gynecology, University of Oklahoma College of Medicine. Obstetrician and Gynecologist, Oklahoma City Clinic and Presbyterian Hospital, Oklahoma City, Oklahoma.
Benign Uterine Tumors

HERBERT J. BUCHSBAUM, M.D.
Professor of Obstetrics and Gynecology, Director, Division Gynecologic Oncology, University of Texas–Southwestern Medical School. Attending Physician, Parkland Memorial and St. Paul Hospitals, Dallas, Texas.
Ovarian Tumors

DAVID C. BUDSON, M.D.
Pulmonary Internist, Kaiser Foundation Hospital, Vallejo, California.
Atelectasis

GERARD N. BURROW, M.D.
Professor of Medicine and Obstetrics and Gynecology, University of Toronto. Director, Division of Endocrinology and Metabolism, Toronto General Hospital, Toronto, Ontario, Canada.
Hypothyroidism

HUGO CABRERA, Ph.D.
Hospital Epidemiologist and Director of Department of Microbiology, Mt. Carmel Medical Center, Columbus, Ohio.
Gas Gangrene and Similar Anaerobic Soft Tissue Infections

ERIC D. CAINE, M.D.
Assistant Professor of Psychiatry, Neurology, Pharmacology, and Toxicology, University of Rochester School of Medicine and Dentistry. Attending Psychiatrist, University of Rochester School of Medicine and Dentistry, Rochester, New York.
The Confused Elderly Patient

CRAIG J. CANFIELD, M.D., COL, MC
Director, Division of Experimental Therapeutics, Walter Reed Army Institute of Research, Washington, D.C.
Malaria

ERSKINE M. CAPERTON, M.D.
Clinical Associate Professor, University of Minnesota School of Medicine. Attending Rheumatologist, University of Minnesota Hospitals and Metropolitan Medical Center, Minneapolis, Minnesota.
Ankylosing Spondylitis

JOHN A. CARLSTON, M.D.
Associate Professor of Medicine (Allergy), Eastern Virginia Medical School. Active Staff, General Hospital of Virginia Beach; Consultant Staff, Medical Center Hospitals, Norfolk, Virginia.
Hay Fever, Alias Seasonal Allergic Rhinitis, Seasonal Pollinosis

THOMAS CASEY, M.D.
Associate Professor of Medicine, University of Rochester School of Medicine. Director of Medical Education, Rochester General Hospital, Rochester, New York.
Chronic Abdominal Pain

DONALD O. CASTELL, M.D.
Professor of Medicine and Chief, Digestive Disease Division, Uniformed Services University of the Health Sciences, Bethesda, Maryland.
Dysphagia

PRAN N. CHHUTTANI, M.D., D.T.M., F.A.Sc., F.A.M.S.
Professor Emeritus of Internal Medicine, Postgraduate Institute of Medical Education and Research, Chandigarh, and Nehru Hospital, Chandigarh, India.
Amebiasis

ARAM V. CHOBANIAN, M.D.
Director, Cardiovascular Institute and Professor of Medicine, Boston University School of Medicine. Head, Hypertension and Atherosclerosis Section and Visiting Physician, University Hospital, Boston, Massachusetts.
Hypertension

JOHN F. J. CLARK, M.D.
Professor of Obstetrics and Gynecology, Howard University College of Medicine. Obstetrician–Gynecologist and Chief of Gynecology, Howard University Hospital, Washington, D.C.
Postpartum Complications

C. G. CLOUGH, M.B., M.R.C.P.(U.K.)
Registrar in Neurology, Hull Royal Infirmary, Yorkshire, England.
Migraine and its Variants

RAY E. CLOUSE, M.D.
Instructor in Medicine, Washington University School of Medicine, St. Louis, Missouri.
Functional Disorders of the Gastrointestinal Tract

MARTIN H. COHEN, M.D.
Associate Professor, George Washington University School of Medicine and Health Sciences, Washington, D.C. Deputy Chief, National Cancer Institute–Veterans Administration Medical Oncology Branch, National Institutes of Health, Bethesda, Maryland.
Lung Cancer

ISIDORE COHN, JR., B.S., M.D., D.Sc. (Med)
Professor and Chairman, Department of Surgery, Louisiana State University School of Medicine. Senior Visiting Surgeon and Surgeon in Chief, Charity Hospital. Consultant, Veterans Administration Hospital, New Orleans, Louisiana.
Intestinal Obstruction

DAVID E. C. COLE, M.D.
MRC Research Fellow, McGill University, Montreal Children's Hospital, Montreal, Quebec, Canada.
Rickets

MORTON COLEMAN, M.D.
Associate Professor of Medicine, Cornell University Medical College. Associate Attending Physician, New York Hospital, New York, New York.
Multiple Myeloma

DAVID L. COLLINS, M.D.
Associate Clinical Professor of Surgery, University of California San Diego School of Medicine. Attending Surgeon, Children's Hospital Medical Center, San Diego, California.
Common Surgical Diseases of the Newborn

ROBERT W. COLMAN, M.D.
Professor of Medicine, Temple University School of Medicine. Head, Hematology/Oncology Section, Department of Medicine, Temple University Hospital, Philadelphia, Pennsylvania.
Hemorrhagic Diseases Due to Disseminated Intravascular Coagulation, Accelerated Fibrinolysis, and Circulating Anticoagulants

EDWARD J. COLWELL, M.D.
Attending Physician, Peninsula General Hospital, Salisbury, Maryland.
Malaria

DOYT L. CONN, M.D.
Associate Professor of Medicine, Mayo Medical School. Consulting Rheumatologist, Mayo Clinic,

Rochester Methodist and St. Marys Hospital, Rochester, Minnesota.
Scleroderma

WILLIAM E. CONNOR, M.D.
Professor of Medicine, University of Oregon Health Sciences Center. Director, Lipid Clinic; Director, Family Heart Study, University of Oregon Hospital, Portland, Oregon.
Hyperlipidemia

RICHARD A. COOPER, M.D.
Professor of Medicine, University of Pennsylvania School of Medicine. Chief, Hematology–Oncology Section, Hospital of the University of Pennsylvania, Philadelphia, Pennsylvania.
Diseases of the Spleen

AVRAM M. COOPERMAN, M.D.
Professor and Chief of General Surgery and Surgical Oncology, Columbia University College of Physicians and Surgeons, Columbia Presbyterian Medical Center, New York, New York.
Pancreatic Cysts and Neoplasms

STANLEY W. COULTHARD, M.D.
Associate Professor, Surgery, Chief, Section of Otorhinolaryngology, University of Arizona Health Sciences Center, Tucson, Arizona.
Neck Tumors

LARRY COUSINS, M.D.
Assistant Professor, Reproductive Medicine, University of California San Diego School of Medicine. University Hospital, University of California Medical Center, San Diego, California.
Vaginal Bleeding in Pregnancy

JOHN F. COYLE, M.D.
Clinical Instructor, Department of Medicine, Tulsa Medical College. Attending Cardiologist, St. John's Medical Center, Tulsa, Oklahoma.
Ischemic Heart Disease

JOHN J. CRANLEY, M.D.
Associate Clinical Professor of Surgery, University of Cincinnati Medical Center. Director of Medical Education, Director of Surgery, Director of Vascular Laboratory, Good Samaritan Hospital, Cincinnati, Ohio.
Peripheral Venous Disease

CLYDE E. CULP, M.D.
Assistant Professor of Proctology, Mayo Clinic and Mayo Medical School. Consultant, Section of Colon and Rectal Surgery, Mayo Clinic, Rochester, Minnesota.
Anorectal and Perianal Disorders

ANGELO E. DAGRADI, M.D.
Professor of Medicine, UCLA School of Medicine. Chief, Endoscopy Section, Harbor–UCLA Medical Center, Torrance, California.
Gastritis

CHARLES P. DARBY, M.D.
Professor of Pediatrics, Medical University of South Carolina, Charleston, South Carolina.
Measles

R. CLEMENT DARLING, M.D.
Associate Professor of Surgery, Harvard Medical School. Senior Vascular Surgeon and Chief of Vascular Clinic, Massachusetts General Hospital, Boston, Massachusetts.
Aneurysms of the Aorta

HARVEY D. DAVIS, M.D.
Assistant Professor Pediatrics (Allergy), Eastern Virginia Medical School. Active Staff, King's Daughters Hospital, Norfolk, Virginia.
Hay Fever, Alias Seasonal Allergic Rhinitis, Seasonal Pollinosis

JOHN S. DAVIS, IV, M.D.
Professor of Internal Medicine, University of Virginia School of Medicine, Charlottesville, Virginia.
Systemic Lupus Erythematosus

ROBERT P. DAVIS, M.D., F.A.C.S.
Associate, Department of Surgery, Northwestern University Medical School. Attending Surgeon, Columbus–Cuneo-Cabrini Medical Center and Veterans Administration Lakeside Hospital, Chicago, Illinois.
The Acute Abdomen in Adults

WALTER E. DAVIS, M.D.
Clinical Assistant Professor, Duke University School of Medicine. Chief, Hematology–Oncology, Durham County General Hospital, Durham, North Carolina.
Anemias due to Erythrocyte Enzyme Deficiencies

WILLIAM B. DEAL, M.D.
Professor of Medicine, Vice President for Health Affairs, and Dean, University of Florida College of Medicine. Attending Physician, Shands Teaching Hospital, University of Florida; Consultant, Veterans Administration Medical Center, Gainesville, Florida.
Relapsing Fever

FLOYD W. DENNY, M.D.
Professor and Chairman of Pediatrics, University of North Carolina School of Medicine. Attending Pediatrician, North Carolina Memorial Hospital, Chapel Hill, North Carolina.
Virus and Mycoplasma Pneumonias

VINCENT T. DeVITA, JR., M.D.
Director, Division of Cancer Treatment, National Cancer Institute, National Institutes of Health, Bethesda, Maryland.
Malignant Lymphomas

DAVID D. DeWEESE, M.D.
Professor Emeritus and Past Chairman, Department of Otolaryngology and Maxillofacial Surgery, University of Oregon Medical School. University

of Oregon Hospitals and St. Vincent Hospital, Portland, Oregon.
Episodic Vertigo

RAYMOND P. DiPHILLIPS, M.D.
Associate Professor, The Chicago Medical School. Director, Division of Pulmonary Diseases, Edgewater Hospital, Chicago, Illinois.
Chest Pain

BROWN M. DOBYNS, M.D. PH.D.
Professor of Surgery, Case Western Reserve University School of Medicine. Associate Director of Surgery, Cleveland Metropolitan General Hospital; Assistant Surgeon, University Hospital; Consultant Staff, Hillcrest Hospital, Cleveland, Ohio.
Thyroid Tumors

ADRIAN P. DOUGLAS, M.D.
Associate Professor of Medicine, University of Southern California School of Medicine. Attending Physician (Gastroenterologist), Head Physician, Division of Gastroenterology, Los Angeles County–University of Southern California Medical Center, Los Angeles, California.
Anorexia, Nausea and Vomiting

MICHAEL DULLIGAN, M.D.
Neurosurgeon, Holt Krock Clinic, Ft. Smith, Arkansas.
Acute Bacterial Meningitis

JOHN T. DUNN, M.D.
Professor of Medicine, Division of Endocrinology, University of Virginia School of Medicine, Charlottesville, Virginia.
Thyroiditis

EDWARD R. EICHNER, M.D.
Professor of Medicine, University of Oklahoma College of Medicine. Chief of Hematology-Oncology and Attending Physician, University Hospital and Veteran's Administration Hospital, Oklahoma City, Oklahoma.
The Sideroblastic Anemias

BENJAMIN HILLEL EIDELMAN, M.D., D. PHIL., M.R.C.P.
Assistant Professor, University of Pittsburgh School of Medicine. Attending Neurologist, Presbyterian–University Hospital, Pittsburgh, Pennsylvania.
Cerebrovascular Disease

GEORGE H. ELDER, M.D., M.R.C.PATH.
Professor of Medical Biochemistry, Welsh National School of Medicine. Cardiff, United Kingdom.
The Porphyrias

PETER A. EMERSON, M.D., F.R.C.P. F.A.C.P.(HON)
Consultant Physician, Westminster Medical School, University of London, London, England.
Disorders of the Pleura

RICHARD W. EMMONS, M.D., PH.D.
Chief, Viral and Rickettsial Disease Laboratory, State of California Department of Health Services, Berkeley, California.
Colorado Tick Fever

ALLAN D. ERICKSON, M.D.
Assistant Professor of Medicine, Brown University School of Medicine. Associate Chief, Pulmonary Disease Section, Veteran's Administration Medical Center, Providence, Rhode Island.
Hemoptysis

NORMAN H. ERTEL, M.D.
Professor of Medicine, College of Medicine and Dentistry of New Jersey–New Jersey Medical School, Newark. Chief, Medical Service, Veterans Administration Medical Center, East Orange, New Jersey.
Pheochromocytoma

ROBERTO F. ESCAMILLA, M.D.
Clinical Professor of Medicine, University of California School of Medicine, San Francisco, California.
Hypopituitarism

LUIS R. ESPINOZA, M.D.
Associate Professor of Medicine; Director, Rheumatology/Immunology Laboratory, University of South Florida College of Medicine. Staff, Tampa General Hospital and James A. Haley Veterans Administration Medical Center, Tampa, Florida.
Gout

STEPHEN A. ESTES, M.D.
Assistant Professor of Dermatology, University of Cincinnati College of Medicine. Attending Dermatologist, University of Cincinnati Medical Center Hospitals, General Division and Holmes Division; Cincinnati Children's Hospital Medical Center; Veterans Administration Hospital, Cincinnati, Ohio.
Dermatomyositis

DAVID N. F. FAIRBANKS, M.D.
Associate Clinical Professor Otolaryngology, George Washington University School of Medicine. Chairman, Division of Otolaryngology, George Washington University Hospital, Washington, D.C.
Otitis Media; Otitis Externa

JOHN FERNANDES, M.D.
Professor of Pediatrics, University of Groningen, Department of Pediatrics. University Hospital, Groningen, The Netherlands.
Errors of Carbohydrate Metabolism in Infants and Children

BRANCH T. FIELDS, JR., M.D.
Assistant Professor of Medicine, University of Arkansas College of Medicine. Chief, Infectious Diseases Section, Little Rock Veterans Administration Medical Center, and Staff Member, Uni-

versity of Arkansas Medical Sciences Campus Hospital, Little Rock, Arkansas.
Blastomycosis

FRANK A. FINNERTY, JR., M.D.
Clinical Professor of Medicine, George Washington University School of Medicine. Director of Hypertension Center, Washington, D.C.
Hypertensive States in Pregnancy

NICHOLAS J. FIUMARA, M.D., M.P.H.
Clinical Professor of Dermatology, Boston University School of Medicine. Associate Visiting Physician for Dermatology, Boston City Hospital, Boston, Massachusetts.
Gonorrhea

CHARLES A. FLOOD, M.D.
Professor Emeritus of Clinical Medicine, Columbia University College of Physicians and Surgeons. Consultant, Presbyterian Hospital, New York, New York.
Crohn's Disease

DENYS K. FORD, M.D.
Professor, Division of Rheumatology, University of British Columbia School of Medicine. Attending Rheumatologist, Vancouver General Hospital and the Arthritis Centre, Vancouver, British Columbia, Canada.
Reiter's Syndrome

J. PETER FORNEY, III, M.D.
Assistant Professor, Obstetrics and Gynecology, Associate Director, Division of Gynecologic Oncology, University of Texas, Southwestern Medical School. Attending Physician, Parkland Memorial and St. Paul Hospitals, Dallas, Texas.
Ovarian Tumors

GIRAUD VERNAM FOSTER, M.D., PH.D.
Associate Professor, Johns Hopkins University School of Medicine. Staff Physician, Johns Hopkins Hospital, Baltimore, Maryland.
Hyperparathyroidism

HJORDIS M. FOY, M.D., PH.D.
Professor of Epidemiology, School of Public Health and Community Medicine, University of Washington, Seattle, Washington.
Influenza

ROBERTO FRANCO-SAENZ, M.D.
Professor of Medicine and Attending Endocrinologist, Medical College of Ohio at Toledo, Ohio.
Cushing's Syndrome

ROBERT S. FRASER, M.D., F.R.C.P.(C)
Professor of Medicine, Faculty of Medicine, University of Alberta. Active Staff, University of Alberta Hospital; Consultant in Cardiology, Royal Alexandra, Charles Camsell and Misericordia Hospitals, Edmonton, Alberta, Canada.
Valvular Heart Disease

CHARLES F. FREY, M.D.
Professor and Vice Chairman, Department of Surgery, University of California Davis School of Medicine. Chief, Surgical Service, Veterans Administration Medical Center, Martinez, California.
Hepatic and Perihepatic Abscess

SIDNEY FRIEDLAENDER, M.D.
Clinical Professor of Medicine, Wayne State University School of Medicine. Chief, Allergy and Immunology Service, Sinai Hospital of Detroit, Michigan.
Drug Reactions

DANIEL ERIC FURSTE, M.D.
Assistant Professor of Medicine/Rheumatology, UCLA School of Medicine, Los Angeles, Calfornia.
Periarteritis Nodosa

WESLEY FURSTE, M.D., F.A.C.S.
Clinical Professor of Surgery, Ohio State University School of Medicine, Columbus, Ohio.
Tetanus

THOMAS G. GABUZDA, M.D.
Professor of Medicine, Jefferson Medical College, Thomas Jefferson University. Chief, Division of Hematology, Lankenau Hospital, Philadelphia, Pennsylvania.
Anemia

JOHN R. GAMBLE, M.D.
Chairman, Department of Medicine, Presbyterian Hospital of Pacific Medical Center, San Francisco, California.
Chronic Ulcerative Colitis

STEPHEN L. GANS, M.D., F.A.C.S. F.A.A.P.
Clinical Professor of Surgery, UCLA School of Medicine. Attending in Surgery and Chief, Division of Pediatric Surgery, Cedars–Sinai Medical Center, Los Angeles, California.
The Acute Abdomen in Children

PIERCE GARDNER, M.D.
Professor of Medicine and Pediatrics, University of Chicago, Pritzker School of Medicine. Director, Clinical Training Program in Infectious Diseases, Billings Hospital, University of Chicago Pritzker School of Medicine, Chicago, Illinois.
Psittacosis; Varicella (Chickenpox)

ROBERT A. GARRETT, M.D.
Professor, Indiana University School of Medicine. Staff, Indiana University Hospitals, Riley Hospital for Children, Wishard General Hospital, Indianapolis, Indiana.
Tumors of the Urinary Bladder

MICHAEL A. GERBER, M.D.
Assistant Professor of Pediatrics, University of Connecticut School of Medicine. Attending Pediatrician, Waterbury Regional Department of Pediatrics, Waterbury, Connecticut.
Infections of the Throat

BERNARD F. GERMAIN, M.D.
Assistant Professor of Medicine; Director, Division of Rheumatology, University of South Florida College of Medicine. Staff, Tampa General Hospital and James A. Haley Veterans Administration Medical Center, Tampa, Florida.
Gout

FRANCES McNIELL GILL, M.D.
Associate Professor of Pediatrics, University of Pennsylvania School of Medicine. Senior Physician and Associate Hematologist, the Children's Hospital of Philadelphia, Philadelphia, Pennsylvania.
Thalassemia

ROBERT H. GILMAN, M.D.
Assistant Professor of Medicine, Johns Hopkins University School of Medicine. Attending Physician, Baltimore City Hospital, Baltimore, Maryland.
Bacillary Dysentery

ALLEN L. GINSBERG, M.D.
Associate Professor of Medicine, George Washington University School of Medicine. Staff, George Washington University Hospital, Washington, D.C.
Hepatitis

RICHARD H. GLEW, M.D.
Associate Professor of Medicine and Microbiology, University of Massachusetts Medical School. Chief, Infectious Disease Service, The Memorial Hospital, Worcester, Massachusetts.
The Acute Infectious Disease Syndrome

ELLIOT GOLDSTEIN, M.D.
Professor of Medicine, University of California Davis School of Medicine, Davis, California.
Actinomycosis

ROBERT A. GOLDSTEIN, M.D., PH.D.
Chief, Allergy and Clinical Immunology Branch, IAIDT, National Institute of Allergy and Infectious Disease, Bethesda, Maryland.
Sarcoidosis

G. BROWNE GOODE, M.D.
Associate Clinical Professor of Neurology, University of California San Francisco School of Medicine. Staff Neurologist, Kaiser-Permanente Medical Center, San Francisco, California.
The Narcolepsy Syndrome

CLEON W. GOODWIN, M.D., MAJ., MC
Burn Study Branch, U.S. Army Institute of Surgical Research, Brooke Army Medical Center, Ft. Sam Houston, Texas.
Peritonitis and Intra-Abdominal Infection

BURGESS L. GORDON, M.D.
Visiting Professor of Medicine, Jefferson Medical College, Thomas Jefferson University, Philadelphia, Pennsylvania.
Chronic Bronchitis

GERALD GORDON, M.D.
Fellow in Infectious Diseases, University of Chicago Pritzker School of Medicine, Chicago, Illinois.
Psittacosis

COLUM A. GORMAN, M.B., B.CH., PH.D.
Associate Professor of Medicine, Mayo Clinic and Mayo Medical School. Consultant in Endocrinology and Metabolism and Internal Medicine, Mayo Clinic, Rochester, Minnesota.
Hyperthyroidism

HARRY GRABSTALD, M.D.
Professor of Urology and Director of Urologic Oncology, University of Florida College of Medicine. Chief, Urologic Oncology, Shands Teaching Hospital, University of Florida, Gainesville, Florida.
Prostatic Cancer

GREGORY M. GRAVES, M.D.
Fellow in Surgical Oncology, Department of Surgery, Memorial Sloan Kettering Cancer Institute, New York, New York.
Hepatic and Perihepatic Abscess

J. THOMAS GRAYSTON, M.D.
Professor of Epidemiology, School of Public Health and Community Medicine, and Vice President for Health Affairs, University of Washington, Seattle, Washington.
Influenza

ALEXANDER NICHOLS GUNN, II, M.D., F.A.C.S.
Assistant Chief of Surgery, Addison Gilbert Hospital, Gloucester. Surgical Staff, Beverly Hospital, Beverly, Massachusetts.
Acute Appendicitis

J. CAULIE GUNNELS, JR., M.D.
Professor of Medicine, Duke University School of Medicine. Attending Nephrologist, Duke Hospital, Durham, North Carolina.
Pyelonephritis

RICHARD A. GUTHRIE, M.D.
Professor and Chairman, Department of Pediatrics, University of Kansas School of Medicine. Staff, St. Francis Hospital and Wesley and St. Joseph Medical Centers, Wichita, Kansas.
Diabetes Mellitus

MICHAEL GUTKIN, M.D.
Clinical Associate Professor of Medicine, College of Medicine and Dentistry of New Jersey–New Jersey Medical School, Newark. Chief, Hypertension Division, Attending Physician, Renal Section, St. Barnabas Medical Center, Livingston, New Jersey.
Pheochromocytoma

DAVID R. HABURCHAK, M.D., LTC, MC
Assistant Clinical Professor of Medicine, Medical College of Georgia. Chief, Infectious Disease

Service, Dwight David Eisenhower Army Medical Center, Ft. Gordon, Georgia.
Rickettsial Disease

HENRY HAIMOVICI, M.D.
Clinical Professor Emeritus of Surgery, Albert Einstein College of Medicine. Chief Emeritus, Vascular Surgery, Montefiore Hospital and Medical Center, Bronx, New York.
Chronic Arterial Occlusive Disease of the Lower Extremity

MICHAEL V. HALBERSTAM, M.D.
Associate Clinical Professor of Medicine, George Washington Medical School, Washington, D.C.
Fatigue

JOHN W. HALLETT, JR., M.D.
Clinical and Research Fellow at Massachusetts General Hospital and Harvard Medical School; Vascular Fellow, Massachusetts General Hospital, Boston, Massachusetts.
Aneurysms of the Aorta

GEORGE W. HAMBRICK, JR., M.D.
Professor of Dermatology, University of Cincinnati College of Medicine. Attending Dermatologist, University of Cincinnati Medical Center Hospitals, General Division and Holmes Division; Cincinnati Children's Hospital Medical Center; Veterans Administration Hospital, Cincinnati, Ohio.
Dermatomyositis

JOHN W. G. HANNON, M.D., F.C.C.P., C.I.H.
Staff, Washington Hospital, Washington, Pennsylvania; West Penn Hospital, Pittsburgh, Pennsylvania.
Pneumoconiosis

HERBERT S. HARNED, JR., M.D.
Professor of Pediatrics, University of North Carolina School of Medicine. Attending Physician, North Carolina Memorial Hospital, Chapel Hill, North Carolina.
Innocent Heart Murmurs in Children

RICHARD N. HARNER, M.D.
Associate Professor of Neurology, University of Pennsylvania School of Medicine. Chairman, Department of Neurology and Medical Director, Community Epilepsy Center, Graduate Hospital, Philadelphia, Pennsylvania.
Convulsive Disorders in Adults

J. OCIE HARRIS, M.D.
Associate Professor of Medicine, University of Florida College of Medicine. Chief, Pulmonary Section, Veterans Administration Medical Center, Gainesville, Florida.
Hypersensitivity Pneumonitis

R. H. HARRISON, M.D.
Consulting Urologist, Texas A & M University Medical School and Medical Center. Consultant

Staff, Bryan and St. Joseph Hospitals, Bryan; and Caldwell General Hospital, Caldwell, Texas.
Benign Prostatic Hypertrophy

ROBERT C. HARTMANN, M.D.
Professor of Medicine, Division of Hematology, University of South Florida College of Medicine. Staff Hematologist, James A. Haley Veterans Administration Hospital; Staff Physician, Tampa General Hospital; Consultant Hematologist, St. Joseph's Hospital and University Community Hospital, Tampa, Florida.
Hereditary Spherocytosis; Hereditary Elliptocytosis (Ovalocytosis); Paroxysmal Nocturnal Hemoglobinuria

PAUL R. HASTINGS, M.D.
Assistant Professor, Surgery and Anesthesia, Louisiana State University Medical Center. Staff, Charity and Hotel Dieu Hospitals, New Orleans, Louisiana.
Intestinal Obstruction

ARTHUR HAUT, M.D.
Professor of Medicine, Division of Hematology and Oncology, University of Arkansas for Medical Sciences, College of Medicine. Attending Physician, University Hospital; Consultant in Hematology and Oncology, Veterans Administration Hospital, Little Rock, Arkansas.
Iron Deficiency Anemia

IAN D. HAY, M.B., PH.D., M.R.C.P.
Instructor in Medicine, Mayo Clinic and Mayo Medical School. Senior Clinical Fellow in Endocrinology, Mayo Clinic, Rochester, Minnesota.
Hyperthyroidism

HARLEY A. HAYNES, M.D.
Associate Professor of Dermatology, Harvard Medical School. Director, Dermatology Division, Peter Bent Brigham Hospital; Chief of Dermatology, West Roxbury Veterans' Administration Hospital; Consultant, Medical Oncology Division (Dermatology), Sidney Farber Cancer Institute, Boston, Massachusetts.
Mycosis Fungoides

ROBERT GALBRAITH HEATH, M.D., D.M.SCI.
Professor and Chairman, Department of Psychiatry and Neurology, Tulane University School of Medicine. Chief, Psychiatry and Neurology Services, Tulane University Hospital; Chief of Psychiatry and Neurology Services, Charity Hospital; Senior Consultant in Psychiatry and Neurology, Veterans Administration Hospital, New Orleans, Louisiana.
Schizophrenia

ERNEST M. HEIMLICH, M.D.
G. D. Searle, Skokie, Illinois (Regional Medical Director, Europe). Visiting Investigator, Allergy Laboratory, University of Geneva; Faculty of Medicine, Cantonal Hospital, Geneva, Switzerland.
Asthma in Childhood

FREDERICK W. HENDERSON, M.D.
Assistant Professor of Pediatrics, University of North Carolina School of Medicine. Attending Pediatrician, North Carolina Memorial Hospital, Chapel Hill, North Carolina.
Virus and Mycoplasma Pneumonias

LEO M. HENIKOFF, M.D.
Professor of Pediatrics and Medicine, Dean and Vice President for Medical Affairs, Temple University School of Medicine. Attending Physician, Temple University Hospital, Philadelphia, Pennsylvania. Visiting Physician, Rush–Presbyterian St. Luke's Medical Center, Chicago, Illinois.
Rheumatic Fever (Acute Rheumatic Fever, Acute Articular Rheumatism)

JANE E. HENNEY, M.D.
Special Assistant for Clinical Affairs, Division of Cancer Treatment, National Cancer Institute, National Institutes of Health, Bethesda, Maryland.
Malignant Lymphomas

ROBERT S. HEPLER, M.D.
Professor of Ophthalmology, Jules Stein Eye Institute, UCLA School of Medicine. Attending Neuro-ophthalmologist, UCLA Center for the Health Sciences and Wadsworth Veterans Administration Medical Center, Los Angeles, California.
Optic Neuritis

ROBERT E. HERMANN, M.D.
Head, Department of General Surgery, Cleveland Clinic, Cleveland, Ohio.
Pancreatic Cysts and Neoplasms

CHARLES E. HESS, M.D.
Associate Professor, Internal Medicine, Hematology-Oncology Division, University of Virginia School of Medicine. Attending Hematologist, University of Virginia Hospital, Charlottesville, Virginia.
Lymphadenopathy

MARGARET W. HILGARTNER, M.D.
Professor of Pediatrics, Cornell University Medical College. Attending in Pediatrics, New York Hospital, Hospital for Special Surgery, Memorial Hospital, New York, New York.
Bleeding Disorders in the Newborn

ROBERT J. HOAGLAND, M.D.
Chief, Department of Medicine, Fauquier Hospital, Warrenton, Virginia.
Infectious Mononucleosis

SHEPHEN F. HODGSON, M.D.
Assistant Professor of Medicine, Mayo Clinic and Mayo Medical School. Consultant, Endocrinology and Metabolism, Mayo Clinic; Attending Physician, Rochester Methodist Hospital and St. Marys Hospital, Rochester, Minnesota.
Empty Sella Syndrome

MARGARET M. HOEHN, M.D., F.R.C.P.(C), F.A.C.P., F.A.A.N.
Associate Clinical Professor, Department of Neurology, University of Colorado School of Medicine. Staff, Colorado General Hospital, Denver Veterans Administration, Hospital, Denver, Colorado.
Parkinson's Disease and Parkinsonian Syndromes

ERNEST LOYD HOPKINS, M.D.
Professor of Obstetrics and Gynecology, Howard University College of Medicine. Attending Obstetrician–Gynecologist, Howard University and Providence Hospitals, Washington, D.C.
Postpartum Complications

SIMON HORENSTEIN, M.D.
Professor and Chairman, Department of Neurology, St. Louis University. Director, Department of Neurology, St. Louis University Hospitals; Chief, Neurology Service, St. Louis Veterans Administration Hospital, St. Louis, Missouri.
Metabolic Encephalopathy

ALLEN L. HORWITZ, M.D., PH.D.
Assistant Professor of Pediatrics, University of Chicago Pritzker School of Medicine. Staff, The Joseph P. Kennedy, Jr. Mental Retardation Research Center; the Committee on Genetics, Wyler Children's Hospital, University of Chicago Hospitals and Clinics, Chicago, Illinois.
Mucopolysaccharidoses

TAH-HSIUNG HSU, M.D.
Associate Professor of Medicine, Johns Hopkins University School of Medicine. Staff Physician, Johns Hopkins Hospital, Baltimore, Maryland.
Hyperparathyroidism

RONALD LAWRIE HUCKSTEP, C.M.G., M.A., M.D., (CAMB.), F.R.C.S. (ED.), F.R.C.S. (ENG.), F.R.A.C.S.
Professor, Faculty of Medicine, University of New South Wales, Sydney, New South Wales, Australia, and lately Professor, Faculty of Medicine, Makerere University, Kampala, Uganda, East Africa. Consultant Surgeon, The Price of Wales/Prince Henry Hospitals Group, Royal South Sydney and Sutherland Hospitals, Sydney, Australia.
Typhoid Fever

DOUGLAS W. HUESTIS, M.D.
Professor of Pathology, University of Arizona School of Medicine. Chief, Immunohematology, University Hospital, Tucson, Arizona.
Acute Transfusion Reaction

GEORGE HUG, M.D.
Professor of Pediatrics, University of Cincinnati College of Medicine. Attending Pediatrician, Children's Hospital Medical Center, Cincinnati, Ohio.
Glycogen Storage Disease

JESSE D. IBARRA, JR., M.D., F.A.C.P.
Lecturer, Texas A & M College of Medicine. Director, Division of Endocrinology, Scott and White Clinic and Hospital, Temple, Texas.
Hypoglycemia

YASUO IKEDA, M.D.
Research Fellow, Brown University, Program in Medicine. Hematology Fellow, Division of Hematologic Research, The Memorial Hospital, Pawtucket, Rhode Island.
Purpura Due to Capillary and Platelet Disorders

HAROLD L. ISRAEL, M.D., M.P.H.
Honorary Professor of Medicine, Jefferson Medical College, Thomas Jefferson University. Attending Physician, Thomas Jefferson University Hospital, Philadelphia, Pennsylvania.
Sarcoidosis

CHARLES I. JAROWSKI, M.D.
Clinical Instructor in Medicine, Cornell University Medical College. Assistant Attending Physician, New York Hospital, New York, New York.
Multiple Myeloma

M. HUSAIN JAWADI, M.D.
Assistant Professor, Internal Medicine-Endocrinology, University of Kansas School of Medicine. Chief of Endocrinology, Veterans Administration Hospital, Wichita, Kansas.
Diabetes Mellitus

JOHN W. JENNE, M.S., M.D.
Professor of Medicine, Loyola University Stritch School of Medicine. Staff, Veterans Administration Medical Center, Hines, Illinois.
Bronchiectasis

ERNEST W. JOHNSON, M.D.
Professor and Chairman, Physical Medicine, Ohio State University College of Medicine. Attending Psychiatrist, Ohio State University Hospitals, Columbus, Ohio.
Anterior Horn Cell Disease of Infancy and Childhood and the Progressive Muscular Dystrophies

THOMAS W. JOHNSON, SR., B.S., M.S., M.D.
Professor, Division of Dermatology, Department of Internal Medicine, Meharry Medical College. Attending Staff, G. W. Hubbard Hospital; Consulting Staff, Riverside Hospital, Nashville, Tennessee.
Lymphogranuloma Venereum; Granuloma Inguinale

C. CONRAD JOHNSTON, JR., M.D.
Professor of Medicine, Indiana University School of Medicine. Director, Endocrinology and Metabolism Section, Indiana University Medical Center, Indianapolis, Indiana.
Osteoporosis

ROBERT F. JOHNSTON, M.D.
Professor of Medicine, Director of Division of Pulmonary Diseases, Department of Medicine,

Hahnemann Medical College and Hospital. Active Staff, Jeanes Hospital, Magee Memorial Rehabilitation Center, Philadelphia, Pennsylvania.
Chest Pain

CHRISTOPHER J. JOLLES, M.D.
Chief Resident, Gynecology, University of California Medical Center, San Diego. Chief Resident in Gynecology, University Hospital, University of California Medical Center, San Diego, California.
Vaginal Bleeding in Pregnancy

MELVIN C. KADESKY, M.D.
Clinical Associate Professor, The University of Texas Southwestern Medical School. Chief of Urology, Presbyterian Hospital of Dallas; Consultant, Baylor University Medical Center, Dallas, Texas.
Intrascrotal Masses and Tumors

JOHN T. KAEMMERLEN, M.D.
Associate Professor of Medicine, Brown University School of Medicine. Chief, Pulmonary Disease Section, Veteran's Administration Medical Center, Providence, Rhode Island.
Hemoptysis

RAJENDRA KAPILA, M.D.
Associate Professor of Internal Medicine, Division of Infectious Disease, College of Medicine and Dentistry of New Jersey – New Jersey Medical School. Staff, College Hospital, Newark, New Jersey.
Histoplasmosis

EDWARD L. KAPLAN, M.D.
Professor of Pediatrics, University of Minnesota School of Medicine. Attending Pediatrician, University of Minnesota Hospitals, Hennepin County Medical Center, St. Paul–Ramsey Medical Center, Minneapolis, Minnesota.
Infections of the Throat

LESTER KARAFIN, M.D., F.A.C.S., B.A.
M.Sc. (UROL)
Professor of Urology, Medical College of Pennsylvania. Chief, Section of Urology, Hospital of the Medical College of Pennsylvania; Attending, Temple University Hospital and St. Christopher's Hospital for Children, Philadelphia, Pennsylvania.
Pyuria

IRVIN A. KAUFMAN, M.D.
Assistant Adjunct Professor, Department of Pediatrics, University of California San Diego Medical School. Director, Pediatric Education, Children's Hospital and Health Center, San Diego, California.
Genetic Defects of Amino Acid Metabolism and Transport

B. H. KEAN, M.D.
Clinical Professor Emeritus of Tropical Medicine and Public Health, Cornell University Medical

College. Attending Physician, The New York Hospital, New York, New York.
Toxoplasmosis

A. PAUL KELLY, M.D.
Chief and Associate Professor of Dermatology, Assistant Dean of Graduate Medical Education, Charles R. Drew Postgraduate Medical School. Chief of Dermatology and Director of Graduate Medical Education, Martin Luther King, Jr. General Hospital, Los Angeles, California.
Syphilis

A. RICHARD KENDALL, M.D., F.A.C.S., B.A.
Professor of Urology, Temple University School of Medicine. Attending Urologist, Temple University Hospital and St. Christopher's Hospital for Children, Philadelphia, Pennsylvania.
Pyuria

SIDNEY KIBRICK, M.D., PH.D.
Professor of Pediatrics and Microbiology and Associate Professor of Medicine, Boston University School of Medicine. Visiting Physician for Pediatrics, Boston City Hospital; Consultant in Infectious Diseases, the Children's Hospital Medical Center, Boston, Massachusetts.
Coxsackie and Echo Viral Infections

JOSEPH H. KIEFER, M.D.
Professor Emeritus of Urology, University of Illinois Abraham Lincoln School of Medicine. Emeritus Staff, University of Illinois, St. Joseph, and Augustana Hospitals, Chicago, Illinois.
Urinary Infections

JAMES KIERAN, M.D.
Clinical Professor of Medicine, University of California School of Medicine, San Francisco, California.
Pulmonary Emphysema

THOMAS W. KIERNAN, M.D.
Clinical Assistant Professor of Medicine, College of Medicine and Dentistry of New Jersey – New Jersey Medical School. Chief, Liver and Nutrition Section, Medical Service, Veterans Administration Medical Center, East Orange; Associate Attending Physician, College Hospital, Newark, New Jersey.
Cirrhosis of the Liver

ANNE C. KIMBALL, PH.D.
Associate Professor of Microbiology (Retired), Cornell University Medical College, New York, New York.
Toxoplasmosis

MICHAEL W. KIMBALL, M.D., F.A.C.G.
Clinical Instructor, Department of Medicine, University of California San Diego School of Medicine. Senior Staff Gastroenterologist, Scripps Memorial Hospitals, La Jolla and Encinitas, California.
Diverticular Disease of the Colon

DAVID W. KINNE, M.D.
Assistant Professor of Surgery, Cornell University Medical College. Associate Attending Surgeon, Chief, Breast Service, Memorial Hospital, New York, New York.
Breast Lesions

DAVID G. KLINE, M.D.
Professor and Head of Neurosurgery, Louisiana State University School of Medicine. Staff, Charity, Ochsner Foundation, Southern Baptist, and Hotel Dieu Hospitals and Touro Infirmary, New Orleans, Louisiana.
Acute Bacterial Meningitis

DIANE M. KOMP, M.D.
Professor of Pediatrics, Yale University School of Medicine. Staff, Yale–New Haven Hospital, New Haven, Connecticut.
Histiocytosis X

RICHARD A. KOPHER, M.D.
Instructor, Obstetrics and Gynecology, University of Minnesota School of Medicine. Staff, University of Minnesota Hospitals, Minneapolis, Minnesota.
Pregnancy

OKSANA M. KORZENIOWSKI, M.D.
Associate Professor of Internal Medicine, Medical College of Pennsylvania. Attending, Infectious Diseases, Hospital of the Medical College of Pennsylvania and Veterans Administration Hospital, Philadelphia, Pennsylvania.
Infective Endocarditis

FREDERICK KOSTER, M.D.
Assistant Professor of Medicine, Johns Hopkins University School of Medicine. Staff Physician, Baltimore City Hospital, Baltimore, Maryland.
Bacillary Dysentery

D. DHODANAND KOWLESSAR, M.D.
Professor of Medicine, Director, Division of Gastroenterology, Jefferson Medical College, Thomas Jefferson University, Philadelphia, Pennsylvania.
Celiac Disease

GREGORY B. KROHEL, M.D.
Assistant Professor of Ophthalmology and Neurology, Albany Medical College of Union University. Attending Neuro-ophthalmologist, Albany Medical Center Hospital and Veterans Administration Medical Center, Albany, New York.
Optic Neuritis

KENNETH A. KROPP, M.D.
Professor of Surgery/Urology and Chairman, Division of Urology, Medical College of Ohio at Toledo, Toledo, Ohio.
Neoplasms and Cystic Disease of the Kidney

JOHN E. KURNICK, M.D., F.A.C.P.
Associate Clinical Professor of Medicine (Hematology/Oncology), University of California Irvine School of Medicine, Irvine, California.
Polycythemia Vera

JOHN F. KURTZKE, M.D.
Professor of Neurology and Community Medicine, Georgetown University School of Medicine. Chief of Neurology Service, Veterans Administration Medical Center, Washington, D.C.
Multiple Sclerosis

MONTAGUE LANE, M.D.
Professor of Pharmacology and Medicine, Baylor College of Medicine. Attending, Methodist Hospital and Ben Taub Hospital; Consultant, Veterans Administration Hospital, Houston, Texas.
Carcinoid Tumor and Carcinoid Syndrome

PAUL R. LEBERMAN, M.D.
Professor Emeritus of Urology, University of Pennsylvania School of Medicine, Philadelphia, Pennsylvania.
Prostatitis

KENNETH K. LEE, M.D.
Assistant Clinical Professor, University of California Davis School of Medicine, Davis, California. Full-time Staff, Section of Infectious Diseases, Department of Internal Medicine, Kaiser Hospital, Sacramento, California.
Actinomycosis

JOHN M. LEEDOM, M.D.
Hastings Professor of Medicine, University of Southern California Los Angeles School of Medicine. Head, Division of Infectious Diseases and Chief, First Medical Division, Los Angeles County, Los Angeles, California.
Poliomyelitis

GLEN A. LEHMAN, M.D.
Assistant Professor of Medicine, Indiana University School of Medicine. Attending Gastroenterologist, Indiana University, Wishard Memorial, and Veterans Administration Hospitals, Indianapolis, Indiana.
Tumors of the Small Intestine

THOMAS J. A. LEHMAN, M.D.
Head, Pediatric Rheumatology Branch, Naval Regional Medical Center. Consultant, Rheumatology, Childrens Hospital and Health Center, San Diego, California.
Juvenile Rheumatoid Arthritis

A. MARTIN LERNER, M.D.
Professor of Medicine, Chief, Division of Infectious Diseases, Wayne State University School of Medicine. Chief, Hutzel Hospital Medical Unit, Detroit, Michigan.
Septicemia

ERWIN LEVIN, M.A., M.D.
Assistant Clinical Professor in Medicine, Case Western Reserve University. Associate Physician, Mt. Sinai Hospital; Associate Visiting Physician, Cleveland Metropolitan Hospital; Consultant in Gastroneurology, Deaconess and Womens Hospitals, Cleveland, Ohio.
Gastrointestinal Bleeding

RICHARD P. LEWIS, M.D.
Professor of Medicine, Director, Division of Cardiology, Ohio State University College of Medicine. Attending Cardiologist and Director, Division of Cardiology, Ohio State University Hospitals, Columbus, Ohio.
Syncope

ROBERT D. LIBKE, M.D.
Assistant Clinical Professor of Medicine, University of California San Francisco School of Medicine. Assistant Chief of Medicine, Director of Infectious Disease, Valley Medical Center, Fresno, California.
Coccidioidomycosis

JOHN LINDENBAUM, M.D.
Professor of Medicine, Columbia University College of Physicians and Surgeons, Chief, Hematology, Harlem Hospital Center; Attending Physician, Columbia–Presbyterian Medical Center, New York, New York.
Pernicious Anemia and Other Megaloblastic Anemias

STEPHEN L. LISTON, F.R.A.C.S., F.R.C.S.
Assistant Professor of Otolaryngology, University of Minnesota. Staff, United and Childrens Hospitals, Bethesda Hospital, St. Paul, Minnesota.
Disorders of the Paranasal Sinuses

LINDA C. LONEY, M.D.
Instructor in Pediatrics, Washington University School of Medicine. Staff Pediatrician, St. Louis Children's Hospital, St. Louis, Missouri.
Nephrotic Syndrome

DONALD B. LOURIA, M.D.
Professor and Chairman, Department of Preventive Medicine and Community Health, College of Medicine and Dentistry of New Jersey – New Jersey Medical School, Newark, New Jersey.
Histoplasmosis

EDWARD C. LYNCH, M.D.
Professor of Medicine, Baylor College of Medicine. Attending Physician, The Methodist, Ben Taub General, and Houston Veterans Administration Hospitals, Houston, Texas.
Acquired Hemolytic Anemia

JOSEPH M. MALIN, JR., M.D.
Attending Urologist, Kadlec, Kennewick, and Our Lady of Lourdes Hospitals, Tri–Cities, Washington.
Acute Renal Failure

THOMAS C. MALVAR, M.D.
Assistant Clinical Professor, University of Illinois Abraham Lincoln School of Medicine. Assistant Clinical Professor, University of Illinois Hospital; Attending, St. Joseph and Augustana Hospitals; Consulting, West Side Veterans Administration Hospital; Associate Attending, St. Mary of Nazareth Hospital, Chicago, Illinois.
Urinary Infections

RICHARD A. MARCUCCI, M.D.
Associate Professor of Medicine, Loyola University Stritch School of Medicine. Staff, Veterans Administration Hospital, Hines, and Foster G. McGaw Hospital of Loyola University, Maywood, Illinois.
Bronchiectasis

S. MICHAEL MARCY, M.D.
Associate Clinical Professor of Pediatrics, University of Southern California School of Medicine. Consultant, Children's Hospital, Los Angeles; Staff Pediatrician, Kaiser Foundation Hospital, Panorama City, California.
Mumps

ROBERT L. MARTUZA, M.D.
Assistant in Neurosurgery, Massachusetts General Hospital, Harvard Medical School, Boston, Massachusetts.
Intracranial Neoplasms

ELMO F. MASUCCI, M.D.
Assistant Professor of Neurology, Georgetown University School of Medicine. Assistant Chief of Neurology, Veterans Administration Center, Washington, D.C.
Idiopathic Polynephritis

KENNETH L. MATTOX, M.D.
Associate Professor of Surgery, Baylor College of Medicine. Deputy Chief of Surgery and Director of Emergency Surgical Services, Ben Taub General Hospital, Houston, Texas.
Vascular Disease of the Mesentery

WILLIAM L. McGUFFIN, JR., M.D.
Assistant Professor of Medicine, University of Texas Health Science Center, Houston. Attending Nephrologist, Herman Hospital, Houston, Texas.
Pyelonephritis

DONALD M. McLEAN, M.D., F.R.C.P.(C)
Professor of Medical Microbiology, University of British Columbia. Consultant in Microbiology, University of British Columbia Health Sciences Centre Hospital, and Children's, St. Paul's, Shaughnessy, and Vancouver General Hospitals, Vancouver, British Columbia, Canada.
Aseptic Arthritis and Viral Meningitis

WILLIAM F. McMANUS, M.D., LtC, MC
Chief, Clinical Division, U.S. Army Institute of Surgical Research, Brooke Army Medical Center, Ft. Sam Houston, Texas.
Peritonitis and Intra-Abdominal Infection

GEORGE R. McSWAIN, M.D.
Attending Surgeon, Manatee Memorial and Blake Memorial Hospitals, Bradenton, Florida.
Acute and Chronic Pancreatitis

NANCY B. McWILLIAMS, M.D.
Associate Professor of Pediatrics, Medical College of Virginia. Consultant Pediatric Hematologist, St.

Mary's, Chippenham, and Richmond Memorial Hospitals, Richmond, Virginia.
Leukocytosis and Leukemoid Reaction

JERRY R. MENDELL, M.D.
Professor of Medicine, Ohio State University College of Medicine. Attending Neurologist, Ohio State University Hospitals and Children's Hospital, Columbus, Ohio.
Anterior Horn Cell Disease of Infancy and Childhood and the Progressive Muscular Dystrophies

FRANK J. MENOLASCINO, M.D.
Professor of Psychiatry and Pediatrics, University of Nebraska College of Medicine. Staff, University of Nebraska Hospital and Clinic and Nebraska Psychiatric Institute, Omaha, Nebraska.
Down's Syndrome

AARON E. MILLER, M.D.
Assistant Professor of Neurology, Albert Einstein College of Medicine. Attending Neurologist, Hospital of the Albert Einstein College of Medicine and Bronx Municipal Hospital Center, Bronx, New York.
Diseases of the Central Myelin (Other than Multiple Sclerosis)

DANIEL R. MISHELL, JR., M.D.
Professor and Chairman, Department of Obstetrics and Gynecology, University of Southern California School of Medicine. Staff, Women's Hospital, Los Angeles County–USC Medical Center, Los Angeles, California.
Functional Menstrual Disorders

GILLES R. G. MONIF, M.D.
Associate Professor of Obstetrics and Gynecology, University of Florida College of Medicine. Director, Laboratory of Infectious Diseases, Gainesville, Florida.
Rubella

M. BRITTAIN MOORE, JR., M.D.
Dermatologist, Watson Clinic; Consultant Staff, Lakeland General Hospital, Lakeland, Florida.
Chancroid

WILLIAM L. MOORE, JR., M.D., COL, MC
Professor of Medicine, Medical College of Georgia. Assistant Chief, Department of Medicine, Dwight David Eisenhower Army Medical Center, Ft. Gordon, Georgia.
Rickettsial Disease

KENNETH M. MOSER, M.D.
Professor of Medicine, University of California, San Diego School of Medicine. Director, Pulmonary Division, University of California San Diego, San Diego, California.
Pulmonary Embolism and Infarction

ARNOLD M. MOSES, M.D.
Professor of Medicine, State University of New York Upstate Medical Center College of Medicine.

Attending in Medicine and Director of Clinical Research Center, State University Hospital; Chief, Endocrinology Section, Veterans Administration Hospital, Syracuse, New York.
Diabetes Insipidus

PATRICK J. MULROW, M.D.
Professor of Medicine, Medical College of Ohio at Toledo. Attending Endocrinologist, Chief of Internal Medicine, Medical College of Ohio Hospital, Toledo, Ohio.
Cushing's Syndrome

THOMAS C. MYERS, M.D.
Clinical Assistant Professor, University of South Alabama College of Medicine, Mobile, Alabama.
Extremity and Back Pain

DAVID HAROLD NEUSTADT, M.D.
Clinical Professor of Medicine, University of Louisville School of Medicine. Attending Rheumatologist, Jewish Hospital; Consultant in Rheumatology, Veterans Administration Hospital, Louisville, Kentucky.
Bursitis and Tendinitis

WARD D. NOYES, M.D.
Professor of Medicine, University of Florida College of Medicine, Gainesville, Florida.
Iron Storage Diseases

WILLIAM L. NYHAN, M.D., Ph.D.
Professor of Pediatrics, University of California San Diego School of Medicine, San Diego, California.
Genetic Defects of Amino Acid Metabolism and Transport

RICHARD T. O'BRIEN, M.D.
Associate Professor of Pediatrics, University of Utah College of Medicine. Attending Pediatric Hematologist, Primary Children's Medical Center, Salt Lake City, Utah.
Hemoglobinopathies

ROBERT G. OJEMANN, M.D.
Professor of Surgery, Harvard Medical School. Visiting Neurosurgeon, Massachusetts General Hospital, Boston, Massachusetts.
Intracranial Neoplasms

JAMES A. O'LEARY, M.D.
Professor, University of South Alabama College of Medicine. Staff, University of South Alabama Medical Center, Mobile, Alabama.
Ectopic Pregnancy

SEAN O'REILLY, M.D., F.R.C.P. (EDIN.)
Professor of Neurology, George Washington University School of Medicine. Attending Neurologist; George Washington University Hospital; Active Staff, Children's Hospital and Medical Center of the District of Columbia; Consultant Neurologist, Clinical Center, National Institutes of Health, Bethesda, Maryland.
Hepatolenticular Degeneration (Wilson's Disease)

GEORGE W. PAULSON, M.D.
Clinical Professor of Neurology, Ohio State University College of Medicine. Senior Attending Staff, Riverside Methodist Hospital, Columbus, Ohio.
Tetanus

J. M. S. PEARCE, M.D., F.R.C.P.
Consultant Neurologist, Hull Royal Infirmary, Yorkshire, England.
Migraine and its Variants

CARL M. PEARSON, M.D., F.A.C.P.
Professor of Medicine and Director, Division of Rheumatology, UCLA School of Medicine. Consulting Staff, Wadsworth Veterans Administration and Sepulveda Veterans Administration Hospitals and Harbour-UCLA Medical Center, Los Angeles, California.
Polyarteritis Nodosa

EDWARD JOHN PERRINS, B.Sc., M.B., M.R.C.P.
Senior Registrar, Westminster Hospital, University of London, London, England.
Pericarditis

JAMES B. PETER, M.D., Ph.D.
Professor, UCLA School of Medicine. Director, Arthritis Treatment Center, Santa Monica, California.
Osteoarthritis

BRUCE H. PETERS, M.D.
Professor of Neurology, University of Texas Medical School at Galveston. Attending Physician, John Sealy Hospital; Consultant Physician, St. Marys Hospital, Galveston, Texas.
The Unconscious Adult

RAYMOND J. PIETRAS, M.D.
Professor of Internal Medicine, University of Illinois Abraham Lincoln School of Medicine. Attending Cardiologist, University of Illinois Hospital, Chicago, Illinois.
Cardiomyopathies

J. RAINER POLEY, M.D.
Professor of Pediatrics, Department of Pediatrics, Eastern Virginia Medical School, Norfolk, Virginia.
Chronic Diarrhea

MICHAEL POLLAY, B.S., M.S., M.D.
Professor of Neurosurgery, University of Oklahoma School of Medicine. Chief of Neurosurgery, University Hospital and Clinics, Oklahoma Children's Memorial Hospital, and Veterans Administration Medical Center, Oklahoma City, Oklahoma.
Expanding Intracranial Lesions

BASIL A. PRUITT, Jr., M.D. Col, MC
Commander and Director, U.S. Army Institute of Surgical Research, Brooke Army Medical Center, Ft. Sam Houston, Texas.
Peritonitis and Intra-Abdominal Infection

BARRY W. RAMO, M.D., F.A.C.P., F.A.C.C.
Clinical Associate Professor of Medicine, University of New Mexico School of Medicine. Director, Cardiac Care Unit, Presbyterian Hospital, Albuquerque, New Mexico.
Cardiac Arrhythmias

RAYMOND V. RANDALL, M.D., M.S. (MED.)
Professor of Medicine, Mayo Medical School. Senior Consultant, Endocrinology and Metabolism, Mayo Clinic; Attending Physician, Rochester Methodist and St. Marys Hospitals, Rochester, Minnesota.
Acromegaly; Hyperprolactinemia; Empty Sella Syndrome

ROBERT A. RANKIN, M.D.
Assistant Professor of Medicine, Indiana University School of Medicine. Attending Gastroenterologist, Indiana University, Wishard Memorial and Indianapolis Veterans Administration Hospitals, Indianapolis, Indiana.
Tumors of the Small Intestine

MORTON I. RAPOPORT, M.D.
Professor of Medicine, University of Maryland School of Medicine, Baltimore, Maryland.
Tularemia

JOHN T. REEVES, M.D.
Professor of Medicine, University of Colorado School of Medicine, Denver, Colorado.
Pulmonary Hypertension

OSCAR M. REINMUTH, M.D.
Professor and Chairman, Department of Neurology, University of Pittsburgh School of Medicine. Chief, Neurology Services, Hospitals of the University Health Center of Pittsburgh, Pennsylvania.
Cerebrovascular Disease

DONALD E. RICHARDSON, M.D., F.A.C.S.
Associate Clinical Professor, Neurological Surgery, Louisiana State University School of Medicine. Director of Pain Rehabilitation Unit, Hotel Dieu Hospital; Chief of Neurosurgery, Baptist Hospital, New Orleans, Louisiana.
Facial Pain

JOEL E. RICHTER, M.D.
Instructor in Medicine, Uniformed Services University of the Health Sciences. Staff Gastroenterologist, National Naval Medical Center, Bethesda, Maryland.
Dysphagia

JOSEPH ALFRED RIDER, M.D., PH.D., F.A.C.P.
Staff, Franklin Hospital; Staff (Courtesy), St. Mary's Hospital, San Francisco, California.
Aerophagia

STEPHEN I. RIFKIN, M.D.
Assistant Professor of Medicine, Division of Nephrology, Department of Internal Medicine,

University of South Florida College of Medicine. Attending Nephrologist, Tampa General Hospital; Assistant Chief, Nephrology Section, James A. Haley Veterans Administration Medical Center, Tampa, Florida.
Glomerulonephritis

HERBERT S. RIPLEY, M.D.
Professor Emeritus of Psychiatry and Behavioral Sciences, University of Washington School of Medicine. Attending Psychiatrist, University Hospital and Harborview Medical Center; Consultant, Veterans Administration Hospital, Seattle, Washington.
Hysterical Neurosis

GUY F. ROBBINS, M.D.
Clinical Associate Professor, Cornell University Medical College. Senior Attending Surgeon, Breast Service, Memorial Hospital, New York, New York.
Breast Lesions

HAROLD R. ROBERTS, M.D.
Professor of Medicine and Pathology, University of North Carolina School of Medicine. Director, Clinical Coagulation Laboratory, North Carolina Memorial Hospital, Chapel Hill, North Carolina.
Hemophilia and Other Hereditary Defects of Coagulation

NORMAN REID CLIFFORD ROBERTON, M.A., M.B., F.R.C.P.
Associate Lecturer in Paediatrics, University of Cambridge. Consultant Paediatrician, Cambridge Maternity Hospital, Cambridge, England.
Neonatal Pulmonary Disorders

ALAN M. ROBSON, M.D., M.R.C.P.
Professor of Pediatrics; Director, Division of Pediatric Nephrology, Washington University School of Medicine. Pediatrician, St. Louis Children's Hospital, St. Louis, Missouri.
Nephrotic Syndrome

GENE S. ROSENBERG, M.D.
Teaching Assistant in Urology, New York University Medical School. Chief Resident in Urology, Bellevue Hospital, New York, New York.
Prostatic Cancer

CHARLES R. ROST, M.D.
Fellow in Endocrinology and Metabolism, Naval Research Medical Center, Oakland, and University of California Clinical Study Center, San Francisco General Hospital, San Francisco, California.
Hyperaldosteronism

BENNETT E. ROTH, M.D.
Assistant Professor of Medicine, UCLA School of Medicine. Chief of Medicine, Sherman Oaks Community Hospital; Staff Gastroenterologist, St. Joseph Medical Center, Los Angeles, California.
Peptic Ulcer

RANDALL G. ROWLAND, M.D., PH.D.
Assistant Professor, Indiana University School of Medicine. Attending Staff, Indiana University Hospitals; Consulting Staff, Veterans Administration and St. Vincents Hospitals, Indianapolis, and Johnson County Memorial Hospital, Franklin, Indiana.
Tumors of Urinary Bladder

JACK E. ROZANCE, M.D.
Instructor of Medicine in Neurology, University of Rochester School of Medicine. Staff Neurologist, Department of Neurology, Permanente Medical Group, Sacramento, California.
The Confused Elderly Patient

RALPH W. RUCKER, M.D.
Associate Adjunct Professor, University of California Irvine College of Medicine. Director, Critical Care Units, Childrens Hospital of Orange County, Orange, California.
Cystic Fibrosis

WILLIAM W. H. RUDD, M.D., F.R.C.S.(C), F.A.C.S.
Founder and Director, Rudd Clinic for Surgery of the Colon and Rectum; Staff, Central Hospital, Toronto, Ontario, Canada.
Tumors of the Colon and Rectum

E. C. RUSSELL, M.D.
Assistant Professor of Pediatrics, Medical College of Virginia. Consultant, St. Mary's Hospital, Richmond, Virginia.
Leukocytosis and Leukemoid Reactions

HUSSAIN I. SABA, M.D., PH.D.
Associate Professor of Medicine; Director, Division of Hematology, University of South Florida College of Medicine. Staff Hematologist, James A. Haley Veterans Administration Medical Center; Staff Physician, Tampa General Hospital; Consultant Hematologist, University Community and St. Joseph Hospitals, Tampa, Florida.
Hereditary Spherocytosis; Hereditary Elliptocytosis (Ovalocytosis); Paroxysmal Nocturnal Hemoglobinuria

ARUN K. SAMANTA, M.D.
Assistant Professor of Medicine, College of Medicine and Dentistry of New Jersey – New Jersey Medical School. Staff Physician, Liver and Nutrition Section, Medical Service, Veterans Administration Medical Center, East Orange; Associate Attending Physician, College Hospital, Newark, New Jersey.
Cirrhosis of the Liver

MERLE A. SANDE, M.D.
Professor of Internal Medicine, University of Virginia School of Medicine. Attending in Infectious Diseases, University of Virginia Hospital, Charlottesville, Virginia.
Infective Endocarditis

W. EUGENE SANDERS, JR., M.D.
Professor and Chairman, Department of Medical Microbiology; Professor of Medicine, Creighton University School of Medicine. Attending Physician, St. Josephs and Veterans Administration Hospitals, Omaha, Nebraska.
Fever of Unknown Origin

MORRIS SCHAEFFER, M.S., PH.D., M.D.
Adjunct Professor of Medicine, New York University Medical Center. Bureau of Biologics, Food and Drug Administration, Bethesda, Maryland.
Rabies

MORRIS SCHAMBELAN, M.D.
Associate Professor of Medicine, University of California, San Francisco. Assistant Director, Clinical Study Center, San Francisco General Hospital, San Francisco, California.
Hyperaldosteronism

LABE SCHEINBERG, M.D.
Professor of Neurology, Albert Einstein College of Medicine. Attending Neurologist, Hospital of the Albert Einstein College of Medicine, Bronx Municipal Hospital Center, Bronx, New York.
Diseases of Central Myelin (Other Than Multiple Sclerosis)

C. DuWAYNE SCHMIDT, M.D., F.A.C.P., F.C.C.P.
Clinical Professor of Medicine, University of Utah College of Medicine. Chief, Division of Pulmonary Disease, LDS Hospital; Consultant, Pulmonary Medicine, Salt Lake Clinic, Salt Lake City, Utah.
Chronic Cough

CHARLES R. SCRIVER, M.D., F.R.S.C.
Professor of Pediatrics, Genetics and Biology, McGill University. Director, De Belle Laboratory for Biochemical Genetics, Montreal Children's Hospital, Montreal, Quebec, Canada.
Rickets

WILLIAM D. SEYBOLD, M.D.
Clinical Professor of Surgery, Baylor College of Medicine. Attending Surgeon, St. Luke's Episcopal Hospital, Houston, Texas.
Neoplasms of the Stomach

EDWARD B. SHAW, M.D., L.L.D. (HON.)
Professor Emeritus of Pediatrics, University of California, San Francisco, California.
Diphtheria

AMJAD I. SHEIKH, M.D.
Instructor in Medicine, University of Illinois Abraham Lincoln School of Medicine. Fellow in Cardiovascular Diseases, University of Illinois Hospital, Chicago, Illinois.
Cardiomyopathies

DANA L. SHIRES, JR., M.D.
Professor of Medicine, Director, Division of Nephrology, Department of Internal Medicine,

University of South Florida College of Medicine. Attending and Consulting Nephrologist, Director, Renal Transplantation Service, Tampa General Hospital, Tampa, Florida.
Glomerulonephritis

JAY D. H. SILVERBERG, M.D.
Lecturer, Department of Medicine, University of Toronto, Toronto, Ontario, Canada.
Hypothyroidism

MURRAY N. SILVERSTEIN, M.D., Ph.D.
Professor of Medicine, Mayo Medical School. Chairman, Division of Hematology, Mayo Clinic and Mayo Foundation; Rochester Methodist and St. Mary's Hospitals, Rochester, Minnesota.
Agnogenic Myeloid Metaplasia

ALICE FAYE SINGLETON, M.D., F.A.A.P., M.P.H.
Assistant Professor of Pediatrics, Charles R. Drew Postgraduate Medical School. Director, Ambulatory Pediatric Division and Director, Pediatric Health Services Research, Martin Luther King, Jr. General Hospital, Los Angeles, California.
Syphilis

DAVID B. SKINNER, M.D.
Dallas B. Phemister Professor of Surgery, University of Chicago Pritzker School of Medicine. Chairman, Department of Surgery, University of Chicago Medical Center, Chicago, Illinois.
Diaphragmatic Hernias

FRANK E. SMITH, M.D., F.A.C.P.
Associate Professor, Pharmacology and Medicine, Baylor College of Medicine. Attending Physician, Methodist, Ben Taub, and Veterans Administration Hospitals, Houston, Texas.
Carcinoid Tumor and Carcinoid Syndrome

IAN M. SMITH, M.D., F.R.C.P.(G), F.R.C.Path.
Professor, Internal Medicine, University of Iowa College of Medicine. University of Iowa Hospitals and Clinics, Iowa City, Iowa.
Brucellosis

JOHN PUNTENNEY SMITH, M.D.
Associate Professor, Ohio State University School of Medicine. Chief of Urology, Columbus Children's Hospital, Columbus, Ohio.
Lower Urinary Tract Obstruction in Children

KAIGHN SMITH, M.D.
Professor, Obstetrics and Gynecology, Jefferson Medical School, Thomas Jefferson University. Chairman, Department of Obstetrics and Gynecology, Lankenau Hospital, Philadelphia, Pennsylvania.
Abortion

STEPHEN PUNTENNEY SMITH, M.D.
Clinical Instructor, Ohio State University School of Medicine. Attending Pediatric Urologist, Columbus Children's Hospital, Columbus, Ohio.
Lower Urinary Tract Obstruction in Children

RUSSELL D. SNYDER, M.D.
Professor of Neurology and Pediatrics, University of New Mexico Medical Center. Attending Staff, Bernalillo County Medical Center; Consulting Staff, Presbyterian, St. Joseph and Veterans Administration Hospitals, Albuquerque, New Mexico.
The Unconscious Child

MAURICE SONES, M.D.
Clinical Professor of Medicine, Medical College of Pennsylvania. Director, Medical Outpatient Services, Hospital of the Medical College of Pennsylvania, Philadelphia, Pennsylvania.
Pulmonary Tuberculosis

DAVID H. P. STREETEN, M.B., D.Phil.
Professor of Medicine and Head, Section of Endocrinology, State University of New York Upstate Medical Center College of Medicine. Attending in Medicine, State University Hospital; Consultant in Medicine, Veterans Administration, Crouse-Irving Memorial and St. Joseph's Hospitals, Syracuse, New York.
Diabetes Insipidus

JOHN STUDD, M.D., M.R.C.O.G.
King's College Hospital, University of London, London, England.
The Menopause

ROBERT L. SUMMITT, M.D.
Professor of Pediatrics, Anatomy and Child Development, and Associate Dean for Academic Affairs, College of Medicine, University of Tennessee Center for the Health Sciences. Attending Pediatrician, Le Bonheur Children's and City of Memphis Hospitals; Consultant, Baptist Memorial, Methodist, and St. Joseph Hospitals and Naval Regional Medical Center, Memphis; Consultant, T. C. Thompson Children's Medical Center and Baroness Erlanger Hospital, Chattanooga, Tennessee.
The Noonan Syndrome and Abnormalities of the Sex Chromosomes

RICHARD SUTTON, M.B., M.R.C.P. F.A.C.C.
Recognised Teacher, Westminster Hospital Medical School, University of London. Consultant Cardiologist, Westminster Hospital, London, England.
Pericarditis

GEORGE E. TAGATZ, M.D.
Professor of Obstetrics and Gynecology, University of Minnesota School of Medicine. Staff, University of Minnesota Hospitals, Minneapolis, Minnesota.
Pregnancy

WALTER J. K. TANNENBERG, M.D.
Assistant Clinical Professor of Medicine, Tufts University School of Medicine. Associate Medical Staff, New England Medical Center Hospital and St. Elizabeth's Hospital, Boston, Massachusetts.
Disorders of Protein Metabolism

ALEXANDER TAYLOR, M.D.
Late Assistant Clinical Professor of Medicine, University of California School of Medicine San Francisco, San Francisco, California.
Hypopituitarism

RUSSELL V. TAYLOR, M.D.
Chief Resident, Medical College of Ohio at Toledo, Toledo, Ohio.
Neoplasms and Cystic Disease of the Kidney

JOHN M. TEW, JR., M.D.
Associate Professor (Anatomy), University of Cincinnati College of Medicine. Director of Neurosurgery, Mayfield Neurological Institute, Good Samaritan Hospital, Cincinnati, Ohio.
Painful Neuralgias of the Trigeminal, Glossopharyngeal, Vagus, and Geniculate Nerves

JAMES R. TILLOTSON, M.D.
Associate Professor of Medicine, Albany Medical College. Staff, Albany Medical Center Hospital and Albany Veterans Administration Hospital, Albany, New York.
Bacterial Pneumonias

FRANK B. VASEY, M.D.
Assistant Professor of Medicine, University of South Florida College of Medicine. Staff, Tampa General Hospital and James A. Haley Veterans Administration Medical Center, Tampa, Florida.
Gout

W. LANE VERLENDEN, M.D.
Resident in General Surgery, University of California Davis School of Medicine, Davis, California.
Hepatic and Perihepatic Abscess

BENJAMIN EDUARDO VICTORICA, M.D.
Associate Professor, Department of Pediatrics, Division of Cardiology, University of Florida, College of Medicine. Attending Cardiologist, Shands Teaching Hospital, University of Florida, Gainesville, Florida.
Congenital Heart Disease in Infants and Children

GALEN S. WAGNER, M.D.
Associate Professor of Medicine, Duke University School of Medicine. Director of Cardiology Fellowship Training Program, Director of Cardiac Care Unit, Duke University Medical Center, Durham, North Carolina.
Cardiac Arrhythmias

STANLEY WALLACH, M.D.
Professor of Medicine, Albany Medical College. Chief, Medical Service, Veterans Administration Medical Center; Attending Physician, Albany Medical Center Hospital, Albany, New York.
Hypoparathyroidism

ROBERT A. WAUGH, M.D.
Assistant Professor of Medicine, Duke University School of Medicine. Director of Cardiovascular Education Center and Teaching Scholar for American Heart Association, Duke University Medical Center, Durham, North Carolina.
Cardiac Arrhythmias

ALAN J. WEIN, M.D.
Associate Professor of Urology, University of Pennsylvania School of Medicine. Acting Chief, Division of Urology, Hospital of University of Pennsylvania, Philadelphia, Pennsylvania.
Prostatitis

LEWIS R. WEINTRAUB, M.D.
Professor of Medicine, Boston University School of Medicine. Chief of Hematology, University Hospital, Boston, Massachusetts.
The Leukemias

NANETTE K. WENGER, M.D.
Professor of Medicine (Cardiology), Emory University School of Medicine. Director, Cardiac Clinics, Grady Memorial Hospital, Atlanta, Georgia.
Congestive Heart Failure

T. FRANKLIN WILLIAMS, M.D.
Professor of Medicine, University of Rochester School of Medicine and Dentistry. Medical Director, Monroe Community Hospital; Attending Physician, Strong Memorial Hospital, Rochester, New York.
The Confused Elderly Patient

L. JAMES WILLMORE, M.D.
Associate Professor of Neurology, University of Florida College of Medicine. Director, EEG Laboratory, Veterans Administration Hospital, Gainesville, Florida.
Epilepsy and Other Convulsive Disorders

B. JOE WILDER, M.D.
Professor of Neurology, University of Florida College of Medicine. Chief, Neurology Service, Veterans Administration Hospital, Gainesville, Florida.
Epilepsy and Other Convulsive Disorders

WILLIAM P. WILSON, M.D.
Professor of Psychiatry, Duke University School of Medicine. Head, Division of Biological Psychiatry, Head, Division of Electroencephalography, Duke University Medical Center, Durham, North Carolina.
Depression

RONALD A. YOUMANS, M.D.
Clinical Associate Professor, Neurology, University of Kansas School of Medicine, University of Missouri at Kansas City School of Medicine. Clinical Director, Myasthenia Gravis Clinic, Menorah Medical Center; Chairman, Neurology Section, Baptist Memorial Hospital, Kansas City, Missouri.
Myasthenia Gravis

HERMAN ZAIMAN, M.D.
Mercy Hospital, Valley City, North Dakota.
Trichinosis

DONALD C. ZAVALA, M.D.
Professor of Medicine, University of Iowa School of Medicine. Director, Pulmonary Diagnostic Laboratories, University of Iowa Hospitals and Clinics, Iowa City, Iowa.
Hyperventilation Syndrome

KENNETH D. ZEITLER, M.D.
Fellow in Hematology, North Carolina Memorial Hospital, Chapel Hill, North Carolina.
Hemophilia and Other Hereditary Defects of Coagulation

ROBERT D. ZIPSER, M.D.
Assistant Professor of Medicine, University of Southern California-Los Angeles County Medical Center. Chief, Endocrine Clinics, University of Southern California Medical School, Los Angeles, California.
Chronic Adrenal Insufficiency

CLIFFORD W. ZWILLICH, M.D.
Associate Professor of Medicine, University of Colorado School of Medicine, Denver, Colorado.
Pulmonary Hypertension

PREFACE

This sixth edition of *Current Diagnosis* represents the fifth complete revision since the book first appeared in 1966. The necessity for six editions in this period of time reflects the rapid accumulation of new medical knowledge, as such advances as computed tomography, ultrasound, fetal monitoring, radioimmunoassay, immunologic testing and increased accuracy in technology now help the physician to make specific diagnoses more quickly. It also indicates that a single volume source of the best currently available information on medical diagnosis has been useful to a large group of practicing physicians.

The editors have carried out this revision with the same objective as for previous editions: to provide concise up-to-date summaries of the most effective diagnostic approaches to both common and uncommon clinical conditions. Thus the objective of the revised and rewritten *Current Diagnosis 6* is to present new information that has been developed since the last edition and to provide a new look at all of the available information, both new and previously published. A new group of contributors has been selected to present their concepts and to discuss their understanding of current diagnostic practices.

As in previous editions, the first part of the book is devoted to aspects of differential diagnosis that present unusual problems, and this is followed by sections covering specific disease entities. Each article includes a definition of the condition, a discussion of presenting signs and symptoms, and a description of physical findings. Diagnostic laboratory and radiologic studies that have proved useful are described, and the most important pitfalls that may lead to an erroneous diagnosis are discussed. The editors appreciate that the physician will use *Current Diagnosis* primarily when he has a diagnostic problem, and the authors were asked to go beyond the "textbook picture" to include information that will be helpful in studying patients with atypical and perhaps misleading manifestations. The most frequent diagnostic problem is one in which the physician suspects that the patient has a certain condition, and he must find the most direct and definitive methods for confirming his provisional diagnosis. The relevant article should assist him in doing this. The authors have been requested to avoid involved discussions of differential diagnosis and to focus instead on the information needed to diagnose the disease entity. To assist the physician when he must choose between an unknown number of possible diagnoses, we have incorporated numerous cross-references and an extensive index that lists the symptoms, signs, and findings mentioned in the various sections.

The present volume is a result of the combined efforts of over 300 leading medical authorities, both in the United States and abroad. The contributors were selected not only because they are familiar with current information on medical diagnosis but also because they are practicing physicians who apply this information in their daily patient care activities. The editors wish to express their sincere appreciation to these physicians for summarizing their accumulated experience. The editors also wish to thank Mr. C. F. Robinson for his valuable assistance and the members of the staff at the W. B. Saunders Company who have provided assistance, recommendations, and guidance in preparing *Current Diagnosis 6*.

HOWARD F. CONN, M.D.
REX B. CONN, M.D.

CONTENTS

Section 9
DISORDERS OF METABOLISM

Section 1

AIDS TO DIAGNOSIS

FEVER OF UNKNOWN ORIGIN

By W. EUGENE SANDERS, JR., M.D.
Omaha, Nebraska

Fever of unknown origin is arbitrarily defined as pyrexia for a period of at least 3 weeks without a readily apparent cause. Adherence to this definition is necessary to exclude patients with acute, self-limiting illnesses, such as most viral infections. The fever is often accompanied by a variety of nonspecific manifestations such as headache, malaise, diaphoresis, vague aching, anorexia, and weight loss. High fever may be associated with confusion, delirium, or convulsions. Fevers of unknown origin ultimately may be attributed to infection, malignant neoplasms, connective tissue diseases, and a variety of other miscellaneous causes. In some patients the cause is never identified.

A fever of unknown cause may be one of the most perplexing problems in diagnostic medicine. Few other clinical dilemmas demand such meticulous and often repetitive attention to detail to arrive at a precise diagnosis. On the other hand, one must resist the temptation to perform indiscriminately a vast array of diagnostic tests and procedures that are often expensive, painful, and occasionally more life-threatening than the underlying disease itself. In most instances a logical and orderly approach will lead to identification of the origin of the fever.

APPROACH TO DIFFERENTIAL DIAGNOSIS

History. It is imperative that the history be thorough. In difficult cases the history should be repeated to gain greater detail and to permit the patient to recall information that may have been forgotten or overlooked initially. Often additional insight may be gained by discreet questioning of the patient's family, friends, and employer. Past medical records, even those located at great distances, should be obtained promptly and reviewed meticulously. Careful attention should be given the history of travel, recreation, occupation, and possible exposure to toxins or known vectors of infectious disease. The family history should be extended to include all contacts of a more than casual nature. All drugs used should be identified. Over-the-counter medications, vitamins, and illicit drugs should not be overlooked. Finally, if the physical examination or diagnostic tests suggest disease within a specific organ or system, the relevant history should be repeated in detail.

Physical Examination. The physical examination should be no less meticulous than the history. No component, such as examination of genitalia or rectum, should be "deferred" because of the patient's anxiety or discomfort. Portions of the examination should be repeated daily until the cause of fever is identified. Repetitive inspections of skin and mucous membranes, auscultation of heart and lungs, ophthalmoscopy, and palpation of viscera are among the procedures most likely to provide clues to the diagnosis.

At least initially, the patient's temperature should be recorded frequently at regular intervals. Use of antipyretics should be avoided until the fever pattern is defined; patients with extremely high temperatures or those at risk from the hypermetabolism may be excepted. Characteristic patterns of fever historically have been associated with specific infectious diseases and other illnesses.

Sustained fever varies little more than 1 F in either direction during any 24-hour period. This pattern has been associated with pneumococcal pneumonia, typhoid and paratyphoid, scarlet fever, rickettsioses, tularemia, brucellosis, many central nervous system infections, psittacosis, enterococcal endocarditis, and fever due to drugs that are slowly eliminated from serum.

Remittent fever varies widely but does not return to normal. The fluctuations may accentuate the normal diurnal variation, as seen in mycoplasma pneumonia, many acute viral respiratory infections, rheumatic fever, rheumatoid arthritis, subacute infective endocarditis, falciparum malaria, and Legionnaire's disease. The fluctuations also may reverse the normal diurnal rhythm, as observed occasionally in tuberculosis, pseudomonas pneumonia, and salmonella bacteremia.

Intermittent fever is characterized by daily elevations in temperature with return to normal or subnormal in the interval between spikes. This has been associated with gram-negative bacteremia, disseminated tuberculosis, nonfalciparum malaria, pyogenic abscesses, acute infective endocarditis, and intermittent administration of antipyretics to patients with other patterns of fever. The occurrence of two temperature spikes daily is occasionally referred to as the "double quotidian fever of Notnagle." This pattern may result from severe quartan malaria, gonococcal endocarditis, visceral leishmaniasis, disseminated tuberculosis, or intermittent administration of aspirin for a sustained fever.

Relapsing or recurrent fever is characterized by bouts of pyrexia lasting several days interspersed with periods of normal temperature. Relapsing fever is associated with ascending cholangitis, brucellosis, chronic meningococcemia, malaria, extrapulmonary tuberculosis, rat bite fever, and relapsing fever due to *Borrelia recurrentis*. The Pel-Ebstein symptom (fever) of Hodgkin's disease is characteristically relapsing; however, other patterns of fever occur more commonly in this disease. Biphasic illnesses that may produce a camel-backed fever curve include poliomyelitis, leptospirosis, Colorado tick fever, yellow fever, dengue, infectious mononucleosis, and lymphocytic choriomeningitis.

Exceptions have been noted to nearly every one of the associations between defined fever patterns and specific diseases. Thus, in abstraction, fever patterns seldom provide useful diagnostic clues. However, in the context of other abnormalities in the physical examination and laboratory evaluation, they may be very helpful. For example, a sustained fever alone may be due to a vast array of infectious or noninfectious diseases and this pattern does little to lead one toward a diagnosis of typhoid fever. However, if a prostrate patient is found to have a sustained fever, constipation, and rose-colored spots on his trunk, typhoid fever should be placed at or near the top of the list of diagnoses to be differentiated.

The heart rate normally increases approximately 9 beats per minute per degree Fahrenheit of fever. Relative bradycardia often occurs in typhoid and paratyphoid fevers and in yellow fever. It may be encountered somewhat less frequently in psittacosis, tularemia, brucellosis, Colorado tick fever, infectious mononucleosis, mycoplasma pneumonia, and febrile central nervous system diseases, especially those with elevated cerebrospinal fluid pressure. Patients with myocarditis, hepatitis, and hepatic or cardiac decompensation may also have a relatively slow pulse.

Recording the absence or the presence and number of rigors may be useful in differential diagnosis. For example, shaking chills occur rarely in viral hepatitis, rheumatic carditis, and most nonbacterial pneumonias; however, they are observed in many patients with ascending cholangitis, acute bacterial endocarditis, and bacterial pneumonia. The occurrence of only one rigor should suggest pneumococcal pneumonia, soft tissue infection with streptococci, tularemia, plague, typhus, osteomyelitis, leptospirosis, and influenza. Repeated shaking chills occur primarily in those diseases associated with intermittent or relapsing fevers and in febrile patients who are given antipyretics intermittently.

Fever blisters (herpes labialis, herpes febrilis) occur commonly with pneumococcal, streptococcal, and rickettsial infections, and during malaria. They occur occasionally during salmonellosis but rarely in infections due to *Salmonella typhi* (typhoid fever). They are noted often with meningococcal meningitis and seldom with meningococcemia. Fever blisters are unusual with mycoplasma pneumonia, tuberculosis, and brucellosis.

Judicious Use of the Laboratory. One should resist the temptation to order immediately a vast array of laboratory tests to "cover" a myriad of diagnostic possibilities. In the absence of specific localizing signs or symptoms, it is prudent to order simple screening tests that might indicate involvement of certain organs, such as liver or kidney. Implicated organs then may be examined in more detail. Tests to identify the more common, potentially remediable causes of prolonged fever should be given priority. Unless clearly and urgently indicated, the more painful and expensive tests should be deferred until other approaches to the diagnosis have failed. It is often helpful to discuss personally the differential diagnosis and selection of tests with the pathologist, the microbiologist, and the radiologist in the laboratory.

Simple hematologic tests should be performed on every patient. Although seldom indicative of a precise cause of the fever, they may be useful in limiting the number of diagnoses to be differentiated. The white cell count and differential may distinguish pyogenic from nonpyogenic infections, or suggest presence of hematologic or reticuloendothelial malignancies. The nature and severity of anemia, if present, may aid in diagnosis and prognosis. Hemolytic anemia may accompany a relatively small number of the many causes of prolonged fever. A significant normochromic, normocytic anemia suggests that the underlying illness is severe and relatively long-standing in duration. A rapid erythrocyte sedimentation rate usually indicates more severe disease, while a slow rate indicates a good prognosis or the presence of factitious fever. Urinalysis and culture of urine should be performed routinely.

Blood should be obtained for culture from every patient over a period of 3 to 5 days. The laboratory should be advised to hold the cultures for at least 4 weeks in order to identify fastidious pathogens such as brucellae. Cultures of sputum, cerebrospinal fluid, superficial lesions, or other secretions should be ordered if indicated by signs, symptoms, or abnormalities in the screening laboratory examinations. For serologic tests, samples of sera should be drawn immediately, stored, and then paired with samples obtained 2 to 3 weeks later. Single serologic tests, such as febrile agglutinins, are more often confusing than helpful. Feces should be examined microscopically in most patients and cultured if the underlying disease appears to involve the gastrointestinal tract. Available skin tests for chronic infectious diseases should be applied. However, it should be emphasized that a positive skin test may reflect either recent or remote infection. Only a conversion from negative to positive indicates active infection. Anergy may result from overwhelming infection, debility, sarcoidosis, or reticuloendothelial diseases.

Radiographic examination can be valuable in localizing the underlying disease to specific organ systems. A chest roentgenogram and a flat plate of the abdomen should be performed on nearly all patients. Additional roentgenographic procedures should be selected on the basis of other evidence that suggests involvement of certain organ systems. Indiscriminate scanning of a variety of organs seldom provides useful information.

Invasive Diagnostic Procedures. Biopsy with culture, stains for microorganisms, and histopathology will often establish the diagnosis. However, substantial evidence for involvement of a given tissue should be obtained *before* the procedure. If several organs are implicated, the least hazardous biopsy should be performed. Biopsies or aspirations of soft tissue masses, liver, bone marrow, and lymph nodes may be especially helpful.

Exploratory celiotomy should be considered when fever is prolonged and the previously mentioned examinations have failed to yield a diagnosis. Specific indications include persistent abdominal symptoms, hepatic or other abdominal tenderness, palpable masses, abnormal tests of liver function, or pleural effusion in the absence of bronchopulmonary disease.

Therapeutic Trials. Trials of therapy with antimicrobial agents in the absence of a specific diagnosis are often more confusing and hazardous than helpful. Spontaneous remission of the fever, as seen in Hodgkin's disease, may be interpreted as a therapeutic response and the true underlying disease may progress without detection or appropriate therapy. A therapeutic trial may be warranted if there is reason to suspect infection and if the patient's life is imperiled.

SPECIFIC CAUSES OF PROLONGED FEVER

Infections. Infections are found ultimately to cause approximately one third of all cases of fever of unknown origin. In general, the longer the fever persists, the less likely infection will be proved responsible. Tuberculosis is the most commonly encountered infection. Miliary or disseminated tuberculosis may be especially difficult to diagnosis because pulmonary lesions may be absent, the skin test may be negative, and the disease may mimic other causes of prolonged fever such as reticuloendothelial malignancies, disseminated mycoses, and other granulomatous bacterial infections. Localized pyogenic infections or subacute infective endocarditis account for most of the remaining infectious causes. Less commonly encountered infections include brucellosis, chronic meningococcemia, gonococcemia, disseminated mycoses, toxoplasmosis, typhoid fever, and amebiasis. Even rarer causes of prolonged fever of undetermined origin are malaria, trichinosis, cytomegalovirus infection, and Q fever.

Malignant Neoplasms. Malignant neoplasms account for approximately 20 per cent of all cases of prolonged fever of uncertain cause. They are most common in patients over 40 years of age. Reticuloendothelial and hematologic malignancies often present with unexplained fever and account for a large proportion of these cases. Carcinomas of lung and abdominal viscera, especially with hepatic metastases, may present with fever; however, localizing signs or symptoms are usually detected with ease. Localization and diagnosis of hypernephroma or lymphoma confined to the retroperitoneal lymph nodes may be especially difficult. The diagnosis of hypernephroma in febrile patients may be suggested by subtle symptoms referrable to the flank, abnormalities in urinary sediment, or occasionally by erythrocytosis or a leukemoid reaction. Occasionally, elevated uric acid or alkaline phosphatase may be the only early clue to retroperitoneal lymphomas in febrile patients.

Connective Tissue Diseases. Connective tissue or collagen vascular diseases are implicated in 15 to 20 per cent of patients with fever of unknown origin. Almost all patients with systemic lupus erythematosus develop fever at one time or another. Other causes include rheumatoid arthritis, polyarteritis nodosa, rheumatic fever, Still's disease, polymyalgia rheumatica, temporal arteritis, and other vasculitides. Among all connective tissue diseases, scleroderma and dermatomyositis are least likely to present with prolonged fever.

Miscellaneous Diseases. A variety of miscellaneous diseases are responsible for approximately 5 to 15 per cent of cases. Examples include extrapulmonary sarcoidosis, granulomatous hepatitis, Wegener's granulomatosis, inflammatory bowel disease, familial Mediterranean fever, and thyroiditis.

Drug Fever. Persistent fevers due to drugs appear to be encountered with increasing frequency. Unfortunately, other signs and symptoms of allergy, such as itching, rash, or eosinophilia, are often absent. The only clues to drug fever may be sustained pyrexia in a patient who is not as ill as his temperature might indicate. The penicillins, sulfonamides, iodides, antituberculous agents, thiouracil, barbiturates, quinidine, and illicit drugs are most often implicated.

Factitious Fever. Factitious fever is more common among women and neurotic patients with a background in medicine or the health sciences. Clues include an otherwise healthy patient, erratic swings in temperature, lack of corresponding changes in pulse and respiratory rate, disproportionately cool skin, absence of sweating with presumed defervescence, and normal erythrocyte sedimentation rate. Patients suspected of this condition should be constantly observed each time the temperature is taken.

Unidentified Causes. In approximately 5 to 15 per cent of cases, the cause of the fever remains unidentified. Some patients with undiagnosed prolonged fevers recover spontaneously. Others succumb and the diagnosis may not be made after postmortem examination.

In summary, fever of unknown origin may present one of the most perplexing, challenging, and at times frustrating problems in diagnostic medicine. No single approach will yield the diagnosis in all, or even a majority, of patients. After a meticulous history, physical examination, and a few simple laboratory tests in every patient, further evaluation must be planned individually. Usually this process succeeds. If not, the entire history and physical examination should be repeated. More often than not, this simple repetition at the bedside succeeds when all else appears to have failed.

THE ACUTE INFECTIOUS DISEASE SYNDROME

By RICHARD H. GLEW, M.D.
Worcester, Massachusetts

The patient with an acute infectious disease may present with diverse complaints and physical signs, and it is critically important for the physician to recognize the varied clinical clues that suggest that an infection may be responsible for the patient's illness. Although the most common manifestation of infection is fever, many patients such as neonates, the aged, and patients with renal failure or those receiving corticosteroid therapy may not demonstrate fever during an acute infection. Moreover, fever commonly occurs in many noninfectious illnesses, including collagen vascular disease, allergic reactions (to drugs, blood products), neoplasia (e.g., lymphoma), hemorrhage (subarachnoid, retroperitoneal), gout, and pulmonary embolism. Nevertheless, it is prudent to consider that fever is due to infection until extensive diagnostic efforts have failed to document an infection. Most infectious diseases do not produce characteristic fever profiles. However, patients with malaria often exhibit regular febrile cycles, with chills and fevers occurring every third day counting the day of occurrence as the first day (tertian pattern, seen with *P. vivax, P. ovale,* and *P. falciparum*) or every 72 hours (quartan pattern, seen with *P. malariae*); however, most patients who reside in areas nonendemic for malaria and who acquire infection during travel manifest hectic, unremitting symptoms rather than classic periodicity. A biphasic, camel-backed fever course is commonly noted in patients with leptospirosis or dengue, but these illnesses are relatively uncommon in the United States and are usually seen in patients with a history of animal exposure (leptospirosis) or travel (dengue).

Chills may occur in patients experiencing abrupt, rapid temperature rises, but true bone-shaking, teeth-rattling chills (rigors) are strongly suggestive of an acute bacterial infection (although malaria commonly is associated with repeated, dramatic rigors as well). A single chill is commonly one of the earliest symptoms noted by patients with pneumococcal pneumonia, cellulitis, and erysipelas. Repeated chills in a patient with pneumonia should suggest the likelihood of necrotizing pneumonia involving *Staphylococcus aureus* or gram-negative bacilli such as Klebsiella. Recurrent chills and hectic fevers are common in patients with localized, pyogenic infections (abscesses, cholangitis).

HISTORY

The first priority in the evaluation of a patient suspected of harboring an infectious disease is to determine whether the patient's past history indicates a predisposition to infections that are likely to be fulminant or fatal. This predisposition may be due to the debilitating nature of the underlying disease (e.g., acute leukemia, obstructing lung carcinoma, and chronic renal, cardiac, or pulmonary insufficiency), the severity of the associated infection (e.g., *Staphylococcus aureus* bacteremia-endocarditis in the parenteral drug abuser, *Pneumocystis carinii* pneumonia in a patient with lymphoma), or the adverse interaction of host and parasite (e.g., *Streptococcus pneumoniae* bacteremia in asplenic patients, Salmonella infections in patients with hemoglobinopathies).

Epidemiology. Are there epidemiologic clues in the patient's history that may suggest specific infectious causes? The patient's geographic and ethnologic roots may reveal exposure to appropriate animals or animal products as a source of brucellosis, bovine tuberculosis, or ecchinococcosis. Recent exotic travel may have exposed the patient to malaria, dengue, typhoid fever, yellow fever, or leishmaniasis. However, even within the continental United States there are regional and seasonal variations in the distribution of infections: coccidioidomycosis in the Southwestern United States, histoplasmosis largely in the Mississippi and Ohio river valleys and plague from the Rocky Mountains westward. The various arbovirus encephalitides exhibit characteristic distribution as to locale and season (usually summer incidence in temperate areas). Occupational and avocational history may reveal exposure to sporotrichosis (gardeners), anthrax (handling of raw wool, hides or bones, especially products originating outside the United States), brucellosis (slaughterhouse workers), tularemia (hunters or trappers of rabbits, squirrels, muskrats, or other rodents), leptospirosis (exposure to rats, cattle, dogs), toxoplasmosis (cat owners, especially if involved in the handling of litter boxes), psittacosis (parrots, pigeons),

or salmonellosis (turtles). A history of animal-related trauma may suggest cat-scratch disease (typically via scratches or bites by young cats), *Pasturella multocida* cellulitis or osteomyelitis (penetrating bite of cat or dog), or rabies (skunks, bats, foxes, dogs, and cats).

Knowledge of any illness in members of the patient's household and community may be important. Many viral syndromes such as influenza and enterovirus infections exhibit seasonal clusterings with notable peaks of incidence in the community. Such viral illnesses as well as infections due to *Mycoplasma pneumoniae* and Group A Streptococcus tend to spread throughout families, often with widely varying manifestations in different family members. One should ask if any member of the household has ever had tuberculosis, or if anyone has recently been ill with hepatitis or dysentery.

In the case of a febrile patient recently hospitalized or otherwise under medical care, additional historical avenues must be explored. Recent anesthesia predisposes patients to pulmonary infections. A history of antecedent dental manipulation may provide a clue to the diagnosis of bacterial endocarditis. Administration of antibiotics may alter a patient's normal endogenous microbial flora, increasing susceptibility to colonization and infection by drug-resistant and often unusual organisms, including gram-negative bacteria and fungi. Corticosteroids produce broad, potent immunosuppression and may predispose the patient to opportunistic infections by a variety of organisms. Moreover, many chronic illnesses are commonly associated with a tendency to develop specific infectious problems: staphylococcal pyarthrosis in patients with rheumatoid arthritis, pneumococcal peritonitis in children with nephrotic syndrome, brain abscess in patients with cyanotic congenital heart disease, gram-negative peritonitis in patients with cirrhosis, and malignant external otitis (with *Pseudomonas aeruginosa*) in patients with diabetes mellitus.

Symptoms. Localization of the infection in a patient may be facilitated by a history of pain (headache, pleurisy, flank pain, joint or bone pain), organ dysfunction (altered consciousness, cough, symptoms of congestive heart failure, dysuria), or organ irritability (diarrhea, urinary frequency).

The temporal sequence of symptoms often provides guidance in determining the alacrity with which medical evaluation should be accomplished. A rapidly fulminant clinical course in a critically ill, febrile patient mandates a rapidly paced diagnostic evaluation and prompt therapeutic intervention, whereas a patient with a protracted, insidious history warrants a more studied, laborious approach. Moreover, the evolution of clinical events and the occurrence of seemingly unrelated symptoms may shed light on the patient's more obvious presenting complaint. For example, a prior history of otitis media or sinusitis may be recalled in the history of a patient subsequently brought to the physician with meningitis or brain abscess; the patient with staphylococcal pneumonia often relates a history of initial recovery from an earlier influenza syndrome, followed by the appearance of a productive cough, chest pain, fever, and chills; and the patient with monoarticular gonococcal pyarthrosis commonly describes recent migratory polyarthralgias, and papulopustular skin eruption.

PHYSICAL EXAMINATION

Examination of the skin and mucous membranes may provide a variety of diagnostic clues in the infected patient. A primary infection of the skin (cellulitis, lymphangitis) may be noted. There may be evidence of disseminated infection such as the pustular lesions of staphylococcal or gonococcal septicemia, the petechial rash of Rocky Mountain spotted fever or meningococcemia, the varied rashes of secondary syphilis, the papulovesicular lesions of varicella, and the many dermatologic manifestations (subungual or conjunctival splinter hemorrhages, Osler's nodes, Janeway lesions) of bacterial endocarditis. Cutaneous eruptions may reflect infection on the basis of toxin production (scarlet fever) or immunologic mechanisms (erythema nodosum). Finally, exanthems (often characteristic) may be seen in patients with noninfectious febrile illnesses such as drug reactions, sarcoidosis, juvenile rheumatoid arthritis, and systemic lupus erythematosus. The optic fundi should be examined for evidence of endocarditis (Roth spots), disseminated candidiasis (fungal endophthalmitis), or miliary tuberculosis (choroidal tubercles). Enlarged lymph nodes may indicate an infection in the region drained by the nodes or may be a manifestation of systemic disease (infectious mononucleosis, secondary syphilis, miliary tuberculosis, lymphoma). Moreover, there may be prominent regional lymph nodes draining the site of primary cutaneous inoculation with infectious agents that subsequently have produced disseminated infection: tularemia, plague, syphilis, lymphogranuloma venereum, cat-scratch disease.

Examination of the chest may demonstrate the presence of an effusion or pneumonia; however, in viral and mycoplasma pneumonia, physical findings may be minimal despite the demonstration of extensive pulmonary involvement by chest roentgenogram, and effusions, when present, are small. Auscultation of the heart may disclose a rub typical of pericarditis or murmurs suggestive of endocarditis. Examination of the abdomen may demonstrate diffuse tenderness and guarding suggestive of peritonitis or local findings related to cholecystitis, appendicitis or abscess. Occasionally, impressive abdominal findings (tenderness, diminished bowel sounds) can be seen in patients with extraperitoneal infections such as pyelonephritis or lower lobe pneumonia. Splenomegaly may be due to local disease (splenic abscess or infarction) but more commonly occurs as part of a systemic infection such as bacterial endocarditis, malaria, brucellosis, or typhoid fever as well as in noninfectious conditions such as lymphoma and various collagen vascular diseases. Examination of bones and joints for local tenderness or swelling, effusion, or restricted motion may suggest pyarthrosis, osteomyelitis, or systemic rheumatologic disease such as rheumatoid arthritis, systemic lupus erythematosus, or gout. Rectal and pelvic examination may demonstrate prostatic abscess, perirectal abscess, or pelvic inflammatory disease (including pelvic abscess). Abnormalities found on neurologic examination can suggest meningitis, encephalitis, brain abscess, or cerebral infarction secondary to septic emboli.

LABORATORY

The hematologic hallmarks of pyogenic bacterial infection are neutrophilic leukocytosis, increase in the number of immature granulocytes, and the presence within neutrophils of vacuolization and toxic granulation. However, severe and overwhelming infection due to bacterial septicemia or typhoid fever may be associated with neutropenia, and neutrophilic leukocytosis has been described in patients with several viral infections (influenza pneumonia) or granulomatous infections such as miliary tuberculosis. Eosinophilia can be seen in patients with trichinosis, drug reactions, and exfoliative skin disorders including scarlet fever. Red blood cell production may be suppressed by a variety of infections, but anemia (usually normochromatic and normocytic) is most likely to occur in chronic infections. Hemolysis with acute onset of anemia may be seen in bacteremia due tc *Clostridium perfringens*. Although the causative mechanisms are poorly understood, anemia in malaria may be moderately severe and out of proportion to the level of parasitemia.

A chest roentgenogram may reveal evidence of pneumonia, pulmonary infarction, lymphadenopathy, pericardial or pleural effusion, all of which can be inapparent on physical examination. An abdominal roentgenogram may reveal the presence of genitourinary stones, renal calcification due to tuberculosis, peritonitis, free intraperitoneal air indicative of rupture of a viscus, bowel displacement or spasm secondary to an adjacent abscess, or intraluminal air-fluid levels suggestive of functional or anatomic obstruction.

Examination of the urinary sediment may demonstrate pyuria suggestive of urinary tract infection. Microscopic hematuria is compatible with bacterial endocarditis, collagen vascular disease (systemic lupus erythematosus, polyarteritis nodosa, Wegener's granulomatosis), or renal tuberculosis but may also be seen with bacterial urinary tract infections, particularly cystitis.

Abnormal collections of fluid, including pleural effusions, ascites, joint effusions, and pericardial effusions, should be aspirated diagnostically (and often therapeutically for relief of pain or mechanical compromise) unless the procedure would be technically dangerous or the fluid collection is seemingly unrelated to an obvious focus elsewhere. A lumbar puncture to obtain cerebrospinal fluid must be performed immediately if there is any possibility of meningitis. It is important to remember that the diagnostic value of such fluids may be reduced after antibiotic therapy has been instituted. All such body fluids should be subjected to cell counts, Gram stain, and determination of sugar and protein concentrations. Special studies may be indicated, including polarizing microscopy of joint fluids for crystals, acid-fast stain of fluids in cases of possible tuberculosis, determination of rheumatoid factor titers, and serologic testing of cerebrospinal fluid (CSF) for syphilis reactivity. Gram or Wright stains of stool specimens may reveal the presence of polymorphonuclear neutrophils, suggestive of inflammatory diarrhea due to *Salmonella* or *Shigella*, pseudomembranous colitis, or inflammatory bowel disease.

The clinical microbiology laboratory is of tremendous value, since cultures of various body fluids can confirm the presence of an infectious disease and provide positive identification and indicate susceptibility of the invading organism to various antimicrobial agents. Specimens of blood (at least two samples from separate venipunctures) and urine (well-supervised clean-catch or catheterized specimen) should be routinely obtained. Any purulent drainage, easily aspirated collections of pus, abnormal body fluid collections (joint, pericardial or pleural fluid, ascites) and CSF (when central nervous system infection is suspected) should be cultured routinely for bacteria. Special handling and plating techniques to ensure survival of anaerobic organisms should be utilized when infection due to anaerobes is suspected (intra-abdominal or intrapelvic infections, foul odor, gas in tissues). Similarly, special media should be utilized if disease due to mycobacteria or fungi is suspected, although some fungi, including Candida species and *Cryptococcus neoformans,* are able to grow on routine bacterial media. Although viral diagnostic laboratories are not commonly available and their services are frequently expensive, the isolation of a significant viral pathogen (e.g., Cytomegalovirus) may enable the physician to make a definitive diagnosis and avoid further diagnostic evaluation.

Serologic tests are widely available and are often of more value than the virology laboratory in confirming the diagnosis of viral infection as well as infections due to other organisms (*Mycoplasma pneumoniae,* leptospira, and rickettsiae), which are difficult to isolate from patients. However, since a rising or falling (at least fourfold) serologic titer is more indicative of recent infection than a single positive titer, which may simply indicate prior infection, serologic tests usually provide only retrospective or confirmatory diagnostic information. Nevertheless, on admission, patients with an enigmatic clinical picture should have serum frozen and stored for possible later use in serologic testing. On the other hand, the presence of cryptococcal antigen in cerebrospinal fluid can be detected quickly by immunologic testing and is the most sensitive test available for diagnosing cryptococcal meningitis. Similarly, the presence of the heterophile antibody is indicative of infectious mononucleosis due to the Epstein-Barr virus. Several studies have suggested potential value in the rapid detection of bacterial or fungal antigens by counter-immunoelectrophoresis or chromatographic methods, but the clinical utility of these tests is not yet known.

Skin tests, particularly those of the delayed hypersensitivity type (e.g., tuberculin), may be of diagnostic value. However, a positive skin test simply indicates that exposure to the antigen has occurred in the past and does not signify active infection. Moreover, anergy is commonly seen in patients with lymphoma, sarcoidosis, terminal malignancy, or overwhelming infection such as miliary tuberculosis and may occur temporarily in patients with viral illnesses such as mumps, measles, and smallpox and may decline temporarily following immunization against these viruses.

Although abnormalities of blood chemistries may reflect nonspecific manifestations of severe infection, they may also indicate primary or predominant involvement of a specific organ. Abnormalities of liver function studies occur in patients with viral hepatitis, cholangitis, leptospirosis, infectious mononucleosis, or liver abscess (bacterial or amebic). Renal function abnormalities may occur in patients with bacterial septicemia and shock, acute pyelonephritis with bilateral papillary necrosis, disseminated candidiasis, leptospirosis, severe falciparum malaria, or fulminant vasculitis.

Infrequently, it may be necessary to obtain biopsy material for histopathologic examination and culture in order to establish a diagnosis. Caseating tubercles in pleura, bone marrow, lymph nodes, or liver are strongly suggestive of tuberculosis but can also be seen in patients with disseminated histoplasmosis and brucellosis, whereas non-caseating tubercles are characteristic of sarcoidosis. Muscle biopsy is often helpful in the diagnosis of trichinosis. Finally, lung biopsy (transbronchial via bronchoscopy or as an open surgical procedure) may be necessary for prompt diagnosis of opportunistic pulmonary infection in the immunocompromised host with fever and pulmonary infiltrates.

CHRONIC COUGH

By C. DUWAYNE SCHMIDT, M.D.
Salt Lake City, Utah

INTRODUCTION

Cough is the most common symptom in pulmonary disease. It is a forced expiratory maneuver during which the respiratory muscles perform work to remove airway secretions or foreign materials, or both. The cough reflex is an occasional event in almost everyone, but frequent or annoying coughing is abnormal. In the majority of persons, a cough is acute in onset, self-limiting, and is usually secondary to a minor viral or bacterial infection. When a cough persists and continues beyond 8 to 12 weeks, it can be considered chronic. The etiology may now be serious, and its proper investigation requires a detailed history, physical examination, and appropriate laboratory studies.

To help determine the cause of a cough, one should systematically consider the anatomic location of cough receptors and their associated afferent nervous pathways to the central nervous system. After a precise cause is established, definitive therapy can then be initiated. Symptomatic treatment should be considered only when the etiology of the cough remains unknown, when it performs no useful function, or when the cough presents hazards or serious discomfort to the patient.

COMPLICATIONS OF COUGH

Complications can occur from chronic and vigorous coughing. Intrathoracic pressures as high as 300 mm Hg have been recorded. In addition to fatigue, headache, insomnia, vomiting, and dyspnea, trauma to the muscular skeletal system can occur. This may range from asymptomatic elevation in the serum creatine phosphokinase (CPK), to more serious problems such as rupture of the rectus abdominal muscle, hernia, or hematoma of the abdominal wall. Rib fractures frequently occur in the lateral margins. They are more common when the patient has metastatic carcinoma, multiple myeloma, or severe metabolic disorders. Chronic irritation of the larynx and upper airways with coughing can cause hoarseness, substernal aching, or bronchospasms. On occasion, pneumothorax, pneumoperitoneum, or subcutaneous emphysema can occur.

Cardiovascular complications may include rupture of veins of the conjunctiva, nose, or anus. Associated increased vagal tone may lead to bradycardia or a degree of heart block. These arrhythmias are more serious in patients having preexisting cardiovascular problems. Loss of consciousness (cough syncope) is not uncommon. The pathophysiology of this phenomenon is thought to be related to cerebral vascular hypoperfusion secondary to high pressures within the thoracicoabdominal cavity. This pressure is transmitted to the prevertebral veins and then to the cerebral spinal fluid. Electroencephalographic studies during cough syncope reveal tracings similar to those seen in patients with cerebral contusion. A reduced cardiac output can also develop from impaired venous return to the right side of the heart, as seen with the Valsalva maneuver.

ETIOLOGY

Cough can develop via inflammatory, mechanical, chemical, or temperature stimulation of the cough receptors or merely by tactile pressure in the ear canal (Arnold's nerve reflex). One must search widely for the cause. Inflammation can be initiated by edema or hyperemia of the mucous membranes or both. Infectious causes may include aerobic and anaerobic bacteria, tuberculosis, filterable agents (e.g., viruses, mycoplasma, or rickettsiae), fungi, or protozoa. Other mechanisms include collagen-vascular or allergic disease, irradiation, drug reaction, or pneumoconiosis.

Mechanical and obstructive stimuli include inhaled dust and pressure and tension on airway walls. Lesions may be intramural or extramural and the forms may include bronchogenic carcinoma, bronchial adenomas, foreign bodies, and granulomatous endobronchial disease. Extramural pathology may include aortic aneurysm, granuloma, pulmonary neoplasm, and various mediastinal tumors. Disorders such as chronic interstitial pneumonitis, fibrosis, pulmonary edema or atelectasis or both cause coughing by tension upon the air passages and stretch receptors. This is associated with a reduced pulmonary compliance. Chemical stimuli include inhalation of irritant gases, fumes, or smoke. In certain patients, hot or cold air may also act as a cough stimulus.

DIAGNOSTIC EVALUATION

On taking the *medical history* one must remember that unfortunately a cough is a nonspecific symptom of pulmonary disease. Patients often deny its existence or adapt to its presence. For example, coughing is so common in cigarette smokers that it is frequently ignored or minimized. Female patients often swallow sputum rather than expectorate. This can lead to an incorrect conclusion that the cough is nonproductive or irritative in nature, or both. A family member or close friend in this situation is often a better historian than the patient.

The physician must be alert to any change in a chronic cough. This is important if one is to establish an early diagnosis of bronchogenic carcinoma or the addition of an acute infection to an already existing lung disease.

The character or quality of a cough may suggest the location of the pathology. For example, a "barking" cough suggests epiglottal disease. A "brassy" cough is associated with tracheal airway pathology. "Hacking" or "clearing of the throat" is often caused by a postnasal discharge. A "hoarseness" with coughing suggests laryngotracheal bronchitis or impaired function of the recurrent laryngeal nerve, as from aneurysm of the aorta, left atrial enlargement, or mediastinal malignancy. Inspiratory stridor suggests an upper airway obstruction, whereas a "wheezy" cough is usually associated with bronchospasm.

It is helpful to observe whether the patient's cough is dry or productive. The former is usually due to a viral infection, nervous habit, or an interstitial disease of the lung parenchyma. This type of cough can also be seen with tumors or from inhalation of respiratory irritants. This should not be confused with an "inadequate" cough, i.e., inability to adequately raise secretions within the major airways. This cough is weak but audible; coarse rhonchi are usually present. Etiologic factors may include debility, weakness, oversedation, pain, or poor motivation.

A chronic productive cough almost always indicates significant bronchopulmonary disease. It should never be ignored. When it is associated with large volumes of purulent sputum, the conditions of chronic bronchitis and of bronchiectasis or bacterial pneumonias, or both, are suggested. Other diagnostic possibilities include tuberculosis, fungal infections, alveolar cell carcinoma, or lung abscesses. Nonpurulent mucoid plugs with a wheezy cough are seen with bronchial asthma. Associated hemoptysis also raises the possibility of a malignant process, bronchiectasis, lung abscess, or chronic bronchitis.

Temporal factors supply further clues. A cough aggravated by recumbency often is associated with chronic sinusitis, bronchiectasis, or congestive heart failure. In contrast, an early morning cough and sputum production is seen with chronic bronchitis. Paroxysmal nocturnal coughing may be associated with bronchial asthma, left heart failure, or aspiration. Coughing following ingestion of food or fluids suggests neuromuscular disease of the upper airway, esophageal problems such as motility abnormalities, stricture, diverticuli, fistula, or hiatal hernia with an incompetent lower esophagogastric junction.

Physical examination may reveal signs such as carious teeth, infected gums, tonsillar disease, or sinusitis. These are often associated with bronchiectasis or lung abscess. An inspiratory stridor with wheezing means an upper airway obstruction from laryngeal pathology or a thyroid or tracheal tumor. The finding of a tracheostomy scar or the history of a previous prolonged period with ventilatory support via an endotracheal tube suggests a tracheal stricture. A low-pitched inspiratory-expiratory fixed wheeze in one location indicates the presence of a major airway obstructive lesion. In contrast, variable fine rhonchi heard principally during expiration are associated with a diffuse obstructive process such as chronic bronchitis or bronchial asthma. Coarse, late subcrepitant inspiratory crackles (rales) are characteristic of an interstitial fibrotic disease. They are frequently associated with signs of a restricted chest cage, clubbing, and cyanosis. Local persistent moist crackles repeatedly heard in the same area are present with bronchiectasis. Signs of consolidation point to a pneumonic process or atelectasis. The finding of pleural fluid or palpable nodes suggests other diagnostic possibilities, such as infection or malignancy. Neurologic signs accompanied by complaints of headache and drowsiness and coupled with papilledema are seen in patients with respiratory failure and hypercapnia.

A fresh *sputum examination* may be helpful in directing the clinician to the cause of a patient's cough. The sputum should be collected by the physician during his examination to make sure it is an adequate specimen. On occasion, a complete 24-hour collection can also be helpful. Sputum should be assessed as to volume, color, character, consistency, odor, and the presence of blood or foreign material.

Patients with chronic bronchitis usually produce small quantities of sputum daily. A specimen is usually mucoid but with infection becomes yellow or green and rarely may be bloody. Patients with advanced chronic bronchitis, and particularly those with bronchiectasis, produce daily copious sputum, often positional-related, purulent, and sometimes blood-streaked. Patients with pneumococcal pneumonia classically produce purulent, brown or rusty sputum, but with antibiotic therapy this may be aborted. Sputum with a foul or fetid odor is seen with infections from fusospirochetal or anaerobic organisms. This usually occurs in patients with aspiration or lung abscesses. Patients with bronchial asthma usually produce mucoid sputum and raise small bronchial casts of the bronchial tree from this inspissated mucus. Thick, viscous, mucopurulent sputum is commonly encountered in cystic fibrosis. Sputum from patients with pulmonary tuberculosis, pulmonary emphysema, or neoplasms usually tends to be mucoid, unless there is secondary infection. A few patients with alveolar cell carcinoma may expectorate copious amounts of mucoid or milky secretions. Frankly bloody or blood-streaked sputum suggests a pulmonary thromboembolism with infarction of the lung. This is also seen with pneumonias, bronchiectasis,

neoplasm, or pulmonary tuberculosis. The appearance of thin, sometimes frothy sputum with or without a pinkish tinge suggests pulmonary edema. Gross hemoptysis is potentially dangerous and invariably is associated with significant pulmonary disease. It is important to establish whether the blood originates from the upper or the lower respiratory tract.

Microscopic examination of sputum may be helpful. This simple and often neglected "wet preparation" may reveal numerous eosinophils, Charcot-Leyden crystals, and free eosinophilic granules. These findings suggest a potential allergic process. In contrast, multiple pus cells or foreign material such as oil or pigments suggests other etiologic processes. A Gram stain when properly prepared from a fresh adequate specimen frequently leads to the diagnosis of a specific infectious cause and is more useful than a culture except when fungi or tuberculosis is suspected. Special stains include those for acid-fast organisms, fungi, eosinophils, or protozoa.

Chest roentgenograms (posterior-anterior and lateral views) are essential in the work-up of any patient with a chronic cough. They may show the presence of a central or peripheral intrapulmonary mass, an alveolar filling process due to pneumonia, perhaps interstitial fibrosis, honeycombing, cyst formation, or hilar adenopathy. Additional roentgenographic views such as oblique projections may help clarify the character and location of a disease process. Laminograms may define the presence of cavitary disease or calcium within a focal lesion. Bronchography may be needed to prove the presence of bronchiectasis or on occasion may be helpful in delineating a tumor. A negative perfusion scan when properly performed can exclude acute pulmonary embolism. Pulmonary arteriograms may also be needed in evaluating for a possible pulmonary embolism or may help delineate a sequestration.

Pulmonary function studies are also helpful. Recent studies have shown that a chronic cough may be the sole presenting manifestation of early bronchial asthma. The presence of expiratory airflow obstruction may also assist in evaluating emphysema, chronic bronchitis, and asthma. An objective bronchodilator effect may be helpful in the diagnosis of the latter. Reduced lung volume with impaired oxygen transport or reduced diffusion capacity or both point to a restrictive disease process. These may be abnormal before the patient's x-ray becomes diagnostic.

Bronchoscopy should be considered in any patient in whom the cause of a chronic cough has not been determined. Modifying factors may include patient age, general condition, or the presence of other complicating factors such as a known malignancy. When appropriate, many clinicians prefer a short therapeutic trial of steroids and cough suppression to exclude "hidden asthma" before proceeding with bronchoscopy. New fiberoptic techniques allow excellent evaluation of the distal tracheobronchial tree. Local brushing, washing, aspiration of material, and when necessary endobronchial or transbronchial biopsies are all possible. The collection of postbronchoscopy sputum for appropriate bacteriologic and cytologic studies can be very helpful. The use of Carbowax in collecting sputum for cytology study is often recommended.

In summary, cough is an indispensable mechanism for clearing of excessive secretions or foreign material from the respiratory tract. Unfortunately, a wide variety of disease processes and problems are involved in its pathogenesis. When faced with the problem of a chronic cough and the possibility of serious disease, the clinician must perform a careful analysis of all clinical and laboratory data in order to establish a definite cause. Only then can an appropriate course of therapy be initiated.

HEMOPTYSIS

By JOHN T. KAEMMERLEN, M.D.,
and ALLAN D. ERICKSON, M.D.
Providence, Rhode Island

INTRODUCTION

"Spitting up" blood is an alarming symptom for which the patient invariably seeks prompt medical attention. Hemoptysis is often the first symptom of serious disease and may herald the approach of massive hemorrhage and sudden death. A history of known lung disease, the amount of blood produced, and the character of the sputum in which the blood is mixed may be helpful diagnostic clues, but it is essential to establish the exact cause of the bleeding or at least identify the site. In most clinical situations, there is little question that the patient is actually coughing up blood. On the other hand, malingerers and patients with Munchausen's syndrome may falsely complain of hemoptysis. Thus, it is important for the physician to examine a specimen that the patient has been seen to expectorate.

Although hemoptysis is usually defined as bleeding from below the glottis, upper respiratory and gastrointestinal tract hemorrhage must be considered. At times, this differentiation is difficult on the basis of history alone. Blood that "wells up in the throat" is usually thought to arise from the respiratory tract, but it may be from esophageal varices. Conversely, blood from the lower respiratory tract may be swallowed and subsequently vomited. In these difficult cases, a careful evaluation of the mouth, upper airway, and upper gastrointestinal tract is indicated if no pulmonary or cardiovascular cause can be readily identified.

When it is difficult to ascertain the origin of the blood, one should assume that it is coming from the lung. Today, the most common causes of hemoptysis are acute and chronic bronchitis, bronchogenic carcinoma, pulmonary tuberculosis, necrotizing pneumonia, and pulmonary infarction. The chest roentgenogram and bronchoscopy will be the most rewarding studies in establishing the diagnosis.

HISTORY

Since the differential diagnosis of hemoptysis is very complex and includes almost all pulmonary diseases as well as a number of cardiovascular and hematologic disorders (Table 1), a careful history is needed for proper orientation. Basic information such as a history of known pulmonary or cardiovascular disease, availability of previous chest roentgenograms, bleeding or telangiectatic disorders in patient or family, and medications the patient is taking must be elicited. Patients who have hemoptysis while receiving anticoagulants may actually have underlying pathology, and they deserve a complete evaluation. Diagnostic clues may be obtained by questions about the amount of blood expectorated, the appearance and odor of the sputum mixed with the blood, the acuteness or chronicity of the bleeding, the number of cigarettes smoked, and the presence of systemic symptoms such as fever, sweats, malaise, or weight loss. The patient who is coughing up mouthfuls of blood usually has pulmonary pathology nourished by bronchial artery circulation on the basis of neovascularization.

Table 1. *Abbreviated List of Causes of Hemoptysis*

Infections
Bronchitis
Pneumonia
  Bacterial
  Fungal
  Parasitic
Pulmonary tuberculosis
Bronchiectasis
Cystic fibrosis
Lung abscess

Neoplasm
Bronchogenic carcinoma
Bronchial adenoma
Metastatic cancer

Cardiovascular
Pulmonary infarction
Mitral stenosis
Congestive heart failure
Congenital heart disease
Arteriovenous fistula
Hereditary hemorrhagic telangiectasia

Trauma
Lung contusion
Penetrating foreign body
Tracheobronchial tear or fracture
Iatrogenic (lung biopsy, bronchoscopy, intravascular
  catheterization)

Clotting disorders

Miscellaneous
Cysts and bullae
Aspergilloma
Broncholithiasis
Goodpasture's syndrome
Idiopathic pulmonary hemosiderosis
Pulmonary endometriosis
Idiopathic

It is always important to consider the possibility of pulmonary emboli with infarction in the differential diagnosis since this clinical situation constitutes an emergency, and the usual hemoptysis evaluation is not indicated. Although fewer than one third of patients with pulmonary emboli have hemoptysis, any patient who experiences the sudden onset of dyspnea, pleuritic or substernal chest pain and who has a reason for venous stasis of the legs must be evaluated for this disorder. When purulent sputum is mixed with the blood, one suspects an infectious process such as chronic bronchitis, pneumonia, or bronchiectasis. Putrid sputum signifies the presence of anaerobic bacteria often associated with a necrotizing pneumonia or lung abscess. In a cigarette smoker, the symptoms of chronic bronchitis blend into the symptoms of bronchogenic car-

cinoma. Even in the absence of other symptoms suggesting cancer, hemoptysis should never be attributed to chronic bronchitis without a complete evaluation. The history of blunt trauma to the chest and other injuries may not be volunteered by the patient. Aspiration of a foreign body may have gone unnoticed. Fungal diseases such as coccidioidomycosis or histoplasmosis may not be considered until a travel history is obtained.

PHYSICAL EXAMINATION

As with the history, the physical examination may not demonstrate the exact cause of the hemoptysis, but it may be very useful. Tiny, reddish telangiectases of the lips, tongue, face, and palmar and plantar surfaces indicate the presence of hereditary hemorrhagic telangiectasia. Pulmonary arteriovenous fistula may be associated with this entity. Cutaneous ecchymoses or petechiae suggest a bleeding disorder. Clubbing of the fingernails is found in lung cancer, bronchiectasis, chronic lung abscess, and congenital cyanotic heart disease. If painful, tender wrists, knees, or ankles are found, the presence of hypertrophic pulmonary osteoarthropathy must be considered and appropriate roentgenograms obtained. If this periosteal lesion is found, bronchogenic carcinoma is the most likely diagnosis. Furthermore, lung cancer may be suspected when there is a localized wheeze, lymphadenopathy, or organomegaly suggesting metastases, or when paraneoplastic states such as Cushing's syndrome or dermatomyositis are present. Examination of the heart may reveal evidence of congenital heart disease or mitral stenosis. In the presence of pulmonary embolic disease, there may be a pleural friction rub or an accentuated second heart sound. A careful search of the chest wall for evidence of trauma may be rewarding on occasion. In most patients with hemoptysis, however, the precise cause of the bleeding will remain unproven until certain diagnostic studies are completed.

CHEST ROENTGENOGRAM

Before a detailed history is taken, we recommend that the physician carefully evaluate upright posteroanterior and lateral views of the chest. This deviation from the classic evaluation of a patient may save time and can furnish valuable diagnostic clues at the outset. In about 70 per cent of patients, the films will be abnormal. Abnormalities often include both the cause and result of pulmonary hemorrhage. One may see evidence of tuberculosis, bronchogenic carcinoma, necrotizing pneumonia, fungus ball, or localized basilar fibrosis and cystic disease suggesting bronchiectasis. Although patients with pulmonary emboli often have normal chest films, the presence of pleural effusion, elevated hemidiaphragm, or parenchymal infiltrates suggesting infarction can sometimes be detected. Cardiovascular abnormalities will be recognized. On the other hand, patients with acute and chronic bronchitis may have remarkably normal films. Bronchial adenomas are usually too central to appear on the chest roentgenogram. In Goodpasture's syndrome and idiopathic pulmonary hemosiderosis, the diffuse alveolar abnormality is caused by the accumulation of blood itself. Often, the chest roentgenogram will indicate which specific laboratory tests are appropriate.

LABORATORY STUDIES

Routine laboratory tests are rarely diagnostic but should be obtained in all patients. Anemia may be associated with the underlying disease, for example, tuberculosis or Wegener's granulomatosis, but only rarely is secondary to the pulmonary hemorrhage itself. Leukocytosis may be associated with many infections causing hemoptysis. Hematuria may suggest Goodpasture's syndrome or Wegener's granulomatosis and can be seen in patients with generalized and severe problems with hemostasis. Clotting studies are necessary to exclude a primary bleeding disorder and should also be obtained before bronchoscopy is contemplated. Other specific tests, such as aspergillus precipitins, serum anti-basement membrane antibody titers, and systemic lupus erythematosus preparations, are not screening tests and should be obtained only when clinically indicated.

Although a pigment produced by certain strains of *Serratia marcescens* can be interpreted falsely as bloody sputum, the presence of blood is easily documented by microscopic examination. Smear and culture of expectorated sputum for mycobacteria and fungi are important in the setting of an abnormal chest roentgenogram, and sputum cytology is an effective means of diagnosing a malignancy, although the presence of blood may render a cytologic evaluation more difficult. Several new and useful techniques for obtaining lower respiratory tract secretions are available, e.g., transtracheal aspiration and transbronchoscopic "contamination-free" catheterization, and in selected patients may be appropriate.

BRONCHOSCOPY

Most patients with hemoptysis undergo bronchoscopy. In patients with frank hemoptysis, this procedure is especially important to determine the laterality of the bleeding should surgical intervention become necessary. Although a bleeding site can be identified in 90 per cent of patients if they have bronchoscopy during active bleeding, bronchoscopy performed later reveals a source in only half of the patients. The flexible fiberoptic bronchoscope is the instrument of choice in almost all patients because of greater patient acceptance and better visualization of the bronchial tree, especially the upper lobes. In those patients in whom an upper airway source of bleeding is suspected, one can carefully examine the nasopharynx and hypopharynx. Central and more peripheral intrabronchial lesions can be brushed and biopsied, although most bronchoscopists are careful to avoid biopsy of suspected bronchial adenomas because of their rich vascularity. In the setting of massive pulmonary hemorrhage, the rigid bronchoscope is often used because of more efficient suction and ventilation capabilities. Similarly, when a foreign body lodged within the airway is found in the patient with hemoptysis, extraction through the rigid bronchoscope is the more practical approach.

ANGIOGRAPHY

In patients suspected of having pulmonary emboli and in whom the perfusion or ventilation-perfusion scan is not of "high probability," a pulmonary angiogram may be needed for diagnosis. The study is also useful in documenting the presence of arteriovenous anomalies. In those centers in which the technique is available, visualization of the bronchial artery circulation may produce excellent definition of the location and extent of the lesion causing hemoptysis. Many of the pathologic states causing hemoptysis are associated with hypervascularity of the bronchial circulation. Examples of these conditions include bronchiectasis, chronic parenchymal infection including tuberculosis and lung abscess, bronchogenic carcinoma, and cystic fibrosis. Bronchial arteriography is especially useful in patients with hemoptysis who have negative chest roentgenograms or bilateral pulmonary disease. As this technique becomes more generally available, the incidence of "idiopathic" hemoptysis may decrease.

BRONCHOGRAPHY

Even though it is reported that over 90 per cent of chest roentgenograms are abnormal in the presence of bronchiectasis, the abnormalities are nonspecific. Only in the case of cystic bronchiectasis is the roentgenographic diagnosis secure. In order to prove the location and extent of bronchiectasis, a bronchogram must be performed. This study is not without risk in the patient with significant pulmonary insufficiency. Bronchography should be delayed until the airways are cleared of blood and secretions to avoid false interpretation of the study.

OTHER SPECIAL STUDIES

Tomograms are usually performed to define more clearly parenchymal or mediastinal lesions and may be very helpful in certain situations. For example, a previously unsuspected broncholith may be found penetrating the airway. Echocardiography is an excellent method for establishing the presence of mitral stenosis and other cardiac abnormalities. The role of computerized axial tomography in the evaluation of the patient with hemoptysis has not yet been established.

MASSIVE PULMONARY HEMORRHAGE

Fortunately, life-threatening hemoptysis is not a common clinical event. Most authors define massive bleeding as the expectoration of at least 600 ml of blood in a 24-hour period. When this occurs, a medical emergency exists and prompt identification of the bleeding site outweighs other diagnostic considerations. Careful quantitation of blood loss is extremely important in this setting, and arterial blood gases should be routinely performed in these patients, since they usually die from asphyxiation rather than hemorrhagic shock. There is a 40 per cent mortality when the loss of 600 ml of blood occurs in a 48-hour period, and the mortality climbs to 75 per cent when the same volume of blood is lost in 16 hours.

The major causes of massive pulmonary hemorrhage are those diseases characterized by hypervascularity of the bronchial circulation (see preceding paragraphs). In patients with neoplastic or suppurative lung disease, the bronchial arteries enlarge and proliferate and numerous vascular anastomoses may ap-

pear. Because of the presence of a large network of vessels under systemic pressure, when bleeding occurs, it is often massive and life-threatening.

SUMMARY

Any patient who complains of hemoptysis and is proved to be "spitting up" blood requires a careful diagnostic evaluation. It is important to discover the cause of the bleeding in a rapid, expeditious manner. When an exact diagnosis is not established initially, it is necessary to demonstrate the anatomic source of the hemorrhage; therefore, the patient should have bronchoscopy during active bleeding. Knowledge of the site of hemorrhage enables the physician to focus special studies on a single anatomic area and may be life-saving information for the patient with massive bleeding. Chest roentgenography and bronchoscopy are the most useful tools for obtaining this information. In the 10 to 20 per cent of cases in which no cause or specific site for the bleeding is established, the patient should be reevaluated for at least one year.

CHEST PAIN

By RAYMOND DiPHILLIPS, M.D., and ROBERT F. JOHNSTON, M.D.
Philadelphia, Pennsylvania

One of the most frequent and at times most frustrating of differential diagnoses that a physician must make is that of chest pain. The specter of ischemic heart disease immediately arises to both the physician and the patient, but not all chest pain is caused by an ischemic myocardium or indeed has a cardiac origin. Many of the structures composing or encased by the thorax can give rise to pain and the physician must decide whether the pain is somatic or visceral; if the pain indicates serious or even life-threatening disease; which are the most appropriate laboratory tests to prove or disprove the clinical impression; and how the pain can be relieved. This chapter will consider the commoner causes of chest pain and the differentiation of those causes based on history, physical examination, and readily available laboratory studies.

CHEST WALL PAIN

Chest wall pain is for the most part localized, can be reproduced or aggravated by pressure applied to the affected area or with movement of the thorax or arms, and is usually sensed by the patient as superficial pain. Any of the structures that make up the thoracic cage—bone, cartilage, muscle, fat, nerves — can give rise to pain since these somatic structures are all well endowed with pain fibers. The afferent pain fibers enter the spinal cord via a dorsal nerve root at a single segmental level before synapsing onto ascending cortical tracts. This entrance of the pain impulse at a single spinal level accounts for the patient's precise localization of chest wall pain. The afferent fibers from the viscera, on the other hand, enter the spinal cord at several segmental levels before synapsing onto ascending neural tracts. The patient's appreciation of visceral pain is therefore not as well localized as the appreciation of chest wall pain. Thus, in general, chest wall pain is superficial, precisely localized, and reproducible with pressure or movement, whereas visceral pain is deeper, not well localized, and not reproducible with pressure.

Myalgia. The intercostals and the pectoralis muscle groups may be involved with general myositic processes such as trichinosis or dermatopolymyositis or may be the sole muscle group giving rise to pain. Trauma accounts for the most frequent intercostal myalgia and a history of trauma is usually easily obtained. However, occult trauma such as that which occurs during seizure activity or during the nocturnal thrashings of a patient with a sleep disorder may not be historically obvious. In a population that is becoming increasingly conscious of physical fitness, trauma to the pectoralis minor can occur during non-isometric exercise, particularly after weight lifting. Persistent, severe cough as with acute bronchitis or chronic obstructive lung disease can also give rise to intercostal muscle strain or hemorrhage. Any of these traumatic myositides can present without visible erythema or ecchymosis.

Chondro-Ostalgia. As is the case with myalgias, trauma is the most common cause of chest pain arising from the ribs and cartilages. The trauma can be sustained either in the community (e.g., steering wheel injuries in auto accidents) or in the hospital (e.g., cardiac resuscitation) and can include rib fractures, chondral dislocations, or periostitis without fractures. Severe coughing for whatever reason in a patient who is osteoporotic because of advanced age or corticosteroid use can give rise to spontaneous rib fractures. Tumor, particularly metastatic carcinoma, multiple myeloma, and sarcoma, can produce bone pain in the thorax. Myelocytic leukemia with proliferation of sternal marrow elements can cause anterior midline chest pain.

The chondral junctions can also give rise to pain. Relapsing polychondritis, which can occur as an isolated entity or be part of a systemic autoimmune disease such as rheumatoid arthritis or systemic lupus erythematosus, can present with fever, uveitis, chest wall chondral pain, and other sites of chondral inflammation such as the external ear or nasal septum. Isolated costochondritis without fever or other constitutional symptoms is known as Tietze's syndrome. It is an idiopathic disorder with no demonstrable microscopic pathology, which is usually treated symptomatically with salicylates or local injections of anesthetics or steroids. The importance of these chondral pain syndromes lies in their differentiation from pain of cardiac origin, since the localization of both cardiac and costochondral pain is in the same sternal area even though the characteristics of these pains are different.

Neuralgia. As was stated previously, pain sensation in the chest wall begins at the cutaneous nerves, travels along a particular intercostal nerve, and enters the spinal cord at the lateral aspect of the dorsal nerve root. The area supplied by this branching neural system is called a dermatome. Chest wall pain can be simulated by irritation of this neural pathway anywhere along its course. A common cause of chest wall pain of neural origin results from mechanical compression or stretching of the dorsal nerve root by thoracic spine disease.

The impingement on the dorsal nerve root can be caused by a variety of disorders. Degenerative disc disease, osteoarthritic bony spurs, vertebral body collapse secondary to senile or postmenopausal osteoporosis, and Paget's disease of bone are frequent causes of pain in patients of advanced age. Vertebral collapse is a well-known complication of corticosteroid use. Metastatic tumor — particularly from the breast and prostate — multiple myeloma, infection producing osteomyelitis, and paraspinal abscess can damage the vertebral bodies and ultimately cause vertebral collapse, resulting in irritation of the dorsal nerve root that produces pain in a dermatome distribution. Tumor, whether it be metastatic to the chest wall or locally invasive from the lung or posterior mediastinum, can directly invade a dorsal nerve root or an intercostal nerve and elicit pain without any bone involvement by the tumor. Blunt trauma to the thoracic spine that fractures or dislocates a transverse vertebral process can also irritate a dorsal nerve root.

Most of the spinal pathology mentioned can

be detected by four-view thoracic spine x-rays. Each view is designed to show a particular view of spinal anatomy, such as the posteroanterior view to evaluate the vertebral pedicles that are destroyed early by tumor or the lateral view to evaluate vertebral body height and demonstrate collapse if present. Frequently, however, pathology and symptoms can be present early before any obvious roentgenographic changes appear, in which case a pyrophosphate bone scan would be of greater value in detecting and localizing an early disease process.

A radiculitis (or pain along a dermatome) can also be provoked by herpes zoster infection of the chest wall nerves, a condition commonly known as shingles. The pain is sharp and severe, associated with fever, and usually precedes the typical vesicular eruption by several days. A prior episode of shingles may suggest the diagnosis to the patient. Often, however, the diagnosis is obscure until the typical rash appears. Postherpetic neuralgia can persist for weeks or even months after the eruption has resolved, so the patient should be questioned about prior shingles and the chest wall should be examined for typical scars in a dermatome distribution.

Pleuropulmonary Pain. The parietal pleura is well innervated with pain fibers. These fibers originate from inwardly branching intercostal nerves and as a result pleural pain is precisely localized to the anatomic area that is involved by the pathologic process. On the other hand, the visceral pleura and the pulmonary parenchyma have no pain fibers. Therefore, pleuritic pain necessarily means irritation or stretching of the parietal pleura. Pleuritic pain is usually described by the patient as a sharp, stabbing pain that characteristically increases with deep inspiration, cough, sneeze, hiccup, or laugh. It is therefore more accurate to describe this as inspiratory pain. It would seem that the pain increases because of the stretching of the inflamed parietal pleura when the intercostal space widens during inspiratory maneuvers, compounded by the visceral pleura rubbing against the outer pleural surface. It will be remembered, however, that chest wall pain may also increase during these same actions that require thoracic cage movement. As a result there can be at times a considerable diagnostic dilemma in deciding between chest wall pain and pain originating in the parietal pleura. Chest wall pain will increase with direct pressure on the area of tenderness and with sufficient movement of the arms to stretch the thoracic muscles. Pleuritic pain may also increase somewhat with pressure and movement but not to the same degree as pain originating in the outer chest wall.

Pleuritis is a general term for any inflammation of the pleural surface, whether the inflammation be infectious (bacterial, fungal, tubercular, or viral), traumatic, vascular, mitotic, or autoimmune. The patient will complain of pleuritic chest pain and depending on the cause may also complain of cough, hemoptysis, or dyspnea. Physical examination may reveal decreased movement of the involved hemithorax during inspiration and a pleural friction rub over the painful area. A rub is the hallmark of pleuritis. The rub is a harsh, scratchy sound that is usually present during both inspiration and expiration when the pleural surfaces chafe against one another. However, if a pleural effusion accompanies the pleuritis, the pleural surfaces are separated and as a result the rub is usually absent. Chest roentgenograms may be normal, may show localized pleural thickening or an effusion, or may demonstrate a peripheral infiltrate or a tumor adjacent to the pleura.

When pleuritis is caused by a contiguous pneumonia, the symptoms and signs of pneumonia are also found (e.g., fever, productive cough). Physical examination may show consolidation and the chest roentgenogram a "pneumonic" infiltrate. Pneumonias such as those accompanying mycoplasma infection, Legionnaire's disease, or psitticosis have milder symptoms than bacterial pneumonias, and pleuritis is much less common in these nonbacterial pneumonias. Tuberculosis rarely causes pleuritic chest pain, presumably because of the fibrinous quality of the pleural reaction, which produces adherence of the pleural surfaces and prevents their rubbing against one another.

Viral pleuritis is a difficult diagnosis to make and in many cases is really a diagnosis of exclusion. It is preceded by an upper respiratory infection or a generalized viral prodrome and presents with pleuritic chest pain of several days' duration, with or without a low-grade fever or a small pleural effusion. There are no routine laboratory findings other than the atypical lymphocytosis seen with any viral infection and no specific x-ray findings. The virus can at times be harvested from pleural fluid if an effusion is present. The diagnosis is usually made by the history of an antecedent viral infection and the resolution of all symptoms in a matter of days.

Pleuritis may also occur with connective tissue diseases and is most common with systemic lupus erythematosus, including drug-induced lupus (hydralazine, procainamide, isoniazid, etc.). Other symptoms of multisystem disease may be present and the diagnosis suggested by a positive antinuclear antibody study (ANA) or confirmed by the presence of lupus erythematosus (LE) cells in the serum or pleural fluid if an effusion is present. Postirradiation pleuritis can also be seen occasionally, especially after tangential radiation to the thorax for chest wall metastases.

Pneumothorax is another cause of inspiratory pain. The causes of pneumothorax are many, including interstitial lung disease, bullous emphysema, and asthma, but the cause may also be idiopathic with no demonstrable underlying lung disease. The pain is of sudden onset, may be sharply localized and classically pleuritic but at times is diffuse over the entire hemithorax and poorly characterized. The onset of the pain of pneumothorax sometimes follows strenuous exercise that requires repeated Valsalva maneuvers or deep inspirations but more commonly occurs at rest. Physical examination reveals increased percussion resonance, absent breath sounds, and tactile fremitus. Chest x-ray reveals a sharp pleural line, usually in the upper lung fields where the visceral pleura separates from the parietal pleura.

Pleuritic pain is understandably caused by pulmonary infarction but is also found in many patients with pulmonary embolism without detectable infarction. Predisposing factors such as obesity, immobilization, pelvic surgery, and use of birth control pills define the common clinical settings for pulmonary embolus. The patient complains of the sudden onset of pleuritic pain, usually at the base of the lung, accompanied by cough. Physical examination reveals a tachycardic, tachypneic patient who may or may not have evidence of deep vein thrombosis in the legs. Examination of the lungs may be normal or reveal a pleural friction rub or evidence of effusion in the area of the pain. An electrocardiogram (ECG) may demonstrate the new appearance of a rightward shift of the electrical axis or atrial fibrillation or both. Usually the ECG shows sinus tachycardia only. Chest x-ray may show a variety of nonspecific findings such as basilar linear atelectasis, small pleural effusions, or a new pulmonary infiltrate. A normal chest x-ray is still compatible with the diagnosis and indeed is the most common x-ray presentation of pulmonary embolus. The diagnosis can be excluded by a normal radionucleotide perfusion scan. Typical perfusion defects in a patient with no prior lung disease is convincing evidence for pulmonary embolism. If for any reason the scan is equivocal, pulmonary angiography is needed. The diagnosis is made by exhibiting filling defects in the pulmonary vasculature.

Tumors of the lung, whether they be primary or metastatic, can cause pain if they invade through the pulmonary parenchyma to the parietal pleura. This pain is usually constant rather than pleuritic and can be sharp or dull.

Mesothelioma is a primary malignant tumor of the pleura that may cause the same kind of constant boring pain as tumor metastatic to the pleura. However, mesothelioma is an uncommon tumor and particularly rare in patients who have no history of asbestos exposure.

VISCERAL PAIN

Cardiac. Ischemic heart disease can be thought of as a continuum starting with stable angina pectoris at one end, extending through unstable angina or coronary insufficiency, to acute myocardial infarction at the other end of the spectrum. The ischemia is produced when myocardial oxygen demands exceed oxygen delivery. This imbalance of demand exceeding delivery is usually the result of a blockage in the coronary vasculature by an atheromatous plaque that impedes distal circulation to a stressed myocardium. A septic coronary embolus from an infected left-sided valve or a murantic coronary embolus from a thrombus in a hypokinetic left ventricle can also produce a sudden drop in myocardial oxygen delivery and hence can produce ischemic cardiac pain. Recently it has been demonstrated that spasm of the coronary vasculature without atheromata can also produce the pain complex associated with myocardial ischemia.

Classically the patient complains of severe, vice-like, crushing pressure or tightness beneath the sternum. The patient sometimes tries to demonstrate the severity of the pressure by placing a clenched fist over the sternum. The pressure sensation may be confined to the retrosternal area or may radiate to the neck, up into but not beyond the area of the mandible to the shoulders, or down the left arm or both arms. In some cases the patient will complain only of recurrent left arm aching or jaw pain without the substernal discomfort, in which case the clinician may be sorely challenged to consider ischemic heart disease as a cause for the complaint. The chest pain may also be accompanied by other symptoms, such as diaphoresis (from increased sympathetic tone), dizziness (from falling cardiac output), palpitations (from arrhythmias), shoulder pain (from diaphragmatic irritation if the inferior or diaphragmatic surface of the heart is ischemic), and shortness of breath (if pump function of the left ventricle fails and pulmonary edema ensues). There is no pleuritic component to the pain.

Since the pain of ischemic heart disease occurs when oxygen demand exceeds delivery, patients usually experience pain during physical exertion or psychologic stress, when cardiac work increases. However, as disease progresses, less strenuous exertion is required to cause pain and the patient notes that a lesser amount of exercise produces more frequent or more prolonged pain. The pain of angina typically is relieved promptly by rest or nitroglycerin within 10 minutes; the pain of coronary insufficiency or acute myocardial infarction usually lasts longer, minutes to hours, and may be lessened though not completely relieved by rest or nitroglycerin.

Physical examination of a patient during an ischemic episode may reveal tachycardia with or without arrhythmia, tachypnea if cardiac failure is present, and a blood pressure that is normal, decreased if cardiac output is decreased, or increased if hypertension is a predisposing factor to the ischemic episode. There may be distended neck veins with acute right heart failure or crackles in the lung with acute left heart failure. Examination of the heart often reveals an atrial gallop (S4) and perhaps a murmur of mitral insufficiency if the papillary muscle is ischemic and dysfunctional, or a protodiastolic gallop (S3) if heart failure is present. Chest x-ray may be normal or may reveal an enlarged left ventricle with pulmonary hyperemia or edema. The electrocardiographic findings will vary according to where the patient is on the ischemic continuum. During an anginal attack there will be ST segment depression in those leads that reflect the particular ischemic segment of myocardium, but between attacks the ECG may be perfectly normal. An acute myocardial infarction has a variety of ECG manifestations but characteristically consists of ST segment elevation and T wave inversion followed eventually by the appearance of Q waves in those leads that reflect the infarcted segment of myocardium. The only blood studies of great value in the diagnosis of myocardial infarction are those of cardiac enzymes, serum glutamic oxaloacetic transaminase (SGOT), lactic dehydrogenase (LDH), and creatine phosphokinase (CPK) and its isoenzymes, which will rise in a predictable fashion with infarction. Enzyme elevations are not noted with attacks of stable angina or with coronary insufficiency, as there is no actual necrosis of myocardium with either of these two events.

The diagnosis of angina is ideally made from the history of exertional chest pain that is relieved by rest but there are many occasions when the physician's diagnostic suspicion must be confirmed by stress testing. The differentiation between coronary insufficiency and myocardial infarction is sometimes difficult when the initial ECG is not diagnostic and obliges the clinician to follow serial cardiograms and cardiac enzyme levels or even resort to radionucleotide studies of the myocardium to make a diagnosis accurately.

Other causes of chest pain of myocardial origin are myocarditis (rheumatic carditis, viral carditis, etc.) and cardiomyopathies. Two particular myocardopathies that have been widely acknowledged in the past decade should be mentioned. One is asymmetric septal hypertrophy, (ASH) or idiopathic hypertrophic subaortic stenosis (IHSS), an obstructive cardiomyopathy in which the left ventricular outflow tract to the aorta is narrowed by a hypertrophied interventricular septum. In some patients with this anomaly, the hypertrophied septum abuts against the anterior leaflet of the aortic valve during systole. This causes outflow obstruction and mimics aortic stenosis. There are clinical characteristics that can differentiate the two clinical conditions, among which is the upstroke of the carotid pulse; this is slowed in aortic stenosis and sharp and bisferious in ASH. These patients can present with a variety of cardiac complaints, among which is chest pain that may be vague or identical to the pain of ischemic heart disease. Diagnosis is suggested by the finding of a systolic ejection murmur with a brisk carotid upstroke, and confirmation of the diagnosis is made by echocardiographic examination of the ventricular septum.

The other cardiomyopathy to be mentioned that can also give rise to chest pain is the mid-systolic click murmur syndrome, which is now being found more frequently because of the wider use of echocardiography. This developmental anomaly consists of a mitral valve leaflet that is too large and redundant for the mitral valve orifice. As a result, during systole, when the mitral valve should be closed, this valve leaflet billows into the left atrium thereby causing the auscultatory phenomenon of a click, which is sometimes followed by the murmur of mitral regurgitation. These patients may also present with a variety of cardiac complaints that includes chest pain that can mimic angina. The pain is thought to be due to the stretching of the papillary muscle and chordae tendinae during systole.

An uncommon cause of visceral chest pain is primary pulmonary hypertension. The classic presentation is that of a young female who presents with increasing shortness of breath over months to years, perhaps accompanied by occasional syncopal episodes and who may have vague nondescript substernal chest pain or exertional chest pain that may mimic angina pectoris. Physical examination may be normal early in the course of this eventually fatal disorder, but with time examination will demonstrate evidence of pulmonary hypertension (distended neck veins with a prominent A wave, a right ventricular heave, loud pulmonary component of the second heart sound that is widely split and may even be palpable, and a right-sided third or fourth heart sound). Chest x-rays demonstrate right-sided cardiac enlargement and large distended pulmonary arteries that taper quickly so as to make the periphery of the lungs oligemic ("pruned tree" appearance). The diagnosis is made by a combination of cardiac catheterization to rule out cardiac causes of pulmonary hypertension, particularly silent mitral stenosis, and a pulmonary angiogram to rule out recurrent pulmonary emboli. This disorder is uniformly fatal to date and early diagnosis probably does not prolong the course of the disease.

The pericardium can also be a source of visceral pain. It is not completely understood how irritation of the pericardium produces the sensation of pain, since the pericardial surface, unlike the parietal pleural surface, contains no pain fibers. The pain of pericarditis is usually substernal, although on occasion it is parasternal or referred to either the subclavicular or epigastric areas. The pain is described as a feeling of fullness and vague discomfort or an aching pressure in the anterior midline chest. There may be a distinctly pleuritic component to the pain, which usually is not as well localized as chest wall pain or as severe as ischemic myocardial pain. Physical findings include distant heart sounds if a large pericardial effusion is present and a pericardial rub that is a loud, scratching sound with several components heard throughout the cardiac cycle. It may be difficult to distinguish a pericardial rub from a pleural rub, but the distinction can usually be made by having the patient hold his breath at end-expiration and listening for the rub to continue synchronous with the cardiac rhythm. A chest radiograph may be normal or reveal a cardiac silhouette enlarged by a pericardial effusion. Pericardial effusions in general — and small pericardial effusions in particular — are best demonstrated with echocardiography. The ECG findings of pericarditis consist of ST segment elevations and eventual T wave inversions present in multiple leads, especially across the chest leads V2 to V6. These findings are somewhat similar to those of acute myocardial infarction, in which the ST segment elevation is still present when the T waves invert, when there are reciprocal ST segment depressions, and when Q waves develop in those leads that reflect the myocardial wall undergoing necrosis. In pericarditis, the ECG findings are found in all leads, the T waves invert after the ST segments have become isoelectric, there are no reciprocal ST segment changes, and no Q waves develop.

There are many causes for pericarditis, including infectious (bacterial, tubercular, viral), tumor metastatic to the pericardium, autoimmune diseases including drug-induced syndromes, irradiation, trauma, and aftereffects of pericardiotomy. This differential is remarkably similar to the causes of pleuritis, as the pericardial inflammatory reaction represents the same kind of serosal response to a variety of insults.

Mediastinal. In the mediastinum, diseases of the esophagus, trachea, and aorta can give rise to substernal chest pain. Esophagitis is often caused by reflux of acid from the stomach into the esophagus through an incompetent lower esophageal sphincter. The patient complains of substernal or epigastric burning that may spread cephalad and result in sour-tasting, acid secretions in the hypopharynx. The symptoms are more common after a large meal and are aggravated by bending over or lying down or by the ingestion of coffee or fat or by smoking. The symptoms are relieved by antacids. When severe, however, the pain may closely resemble the pain of cardiac origin. Diagnosis is made by either fluoroscopic observation of reflux during a barium swallow or by the installation of a 0.1 N hydrochloric acid solution into the esophagus via a nasogastric tube, which should reproduce the patient's pain.

Other causes of esophagitis that can give rise to retrosternal pain include persistent vomiting either from viral gastroenteritis, staphylococcal food poisoning, or alcoholic gastritis, which may also present as "heartburn." Severe vomiting can produce a tear in the esophageal mucosa (Mallory-Weiss syndrome) and present as hematemesis with chest pain. A through-and-through rupture of the esophageal wall (Boerhaave syndrome), either from trauma or instrumentation or protracted vomiting, presents as mediastinitis and a hydropneumothorax due to perforation into a pleural space. At the time of the rupture the patient will complain of a tearing or burning pain in the chest, but these symptoms will quickly progress to a toxic, shock state. Both acid gastric contents and oropharyngeal material spill into the mediastinum and produce both chemical inflammation and a pyogenic infection. Clues on the chest radiograph suggesting ruptured esophagus and mediastinitis are air in the mediastinum and usually a left hydropneumothorax. The pleural fluid has an extremely low pH from the gastric acid and a high amylase content from the saliva.

Another cause of retrosternal pain is esophageal spasm, a motility disorder that may occur in diabetes, amyotrophic lateral sclerosis, or early achalasia. The patient complains of severe retrosternal or epigastric pain on swallowing a large bolus of food or cold liquids. This condition can be relieved somewhat by nitroglycerin so that at times its differentiation from angina pectoris is difficult. Diagnosis is made either by fluoroscopic observation of spasm during a barium meal or by esophageal manometry.

Dissection of the thoracic aorta from either blunt chest trauma or inflammatory or degenerative diseases presents as severe, tearing midline chest pain or posterior thoracic pain, depending on whether the ascending or descending thoracic aorta is involved in the dissection. Physical examination may reveal a difference in pulse pressures between the right and left arms or between the carotids and chest radiograph often shows a widened mediastinum. The diagnosis is confirmed by aortography.

Tracheobronchitis either from an acute viral infection or associated with prolonged cigarette smoking can present with substernal discomfort or burning. The pain is referred to the upper anterior chest, since the trachea is an anterior structure that bifurcates at the level of the fourth anterior rib. The pain is always associated with a persistent cough that may or may not be productive. Diagnosis is made from the history.

OTHER CAUSES OF CHEST PAIN

Referred abdominal pain from a hiatal hernia, peptic ulcer disease, or gallbladder disease can present as epigastric or lower retrosternal pain or burning that can easily be mistaken for cardiac disease. Palpation of the abdomen should localize the tender areas to the stomach or gallbladder. However, there are times when the patient will have no localized area of abdominal tenderness but only complains of chest pain. If the search for obvious causes of chest pain is fruitless, referred abdominal pain should always be kept in mind.

Chest pain may occur as part of the hyperventilation syndrome. The typical patient is a young female presenting with diaphoresis and respiratory distress. Rapid, deep respirations are usually present. There may also be retrosternal discomfort varying from a vague tightness to crushing, severe pain. The main differential diagnoses are acute myocardial infarction, pulmonary embolus, and pneumothorax. Diagnostic clues that indicate the patient is suffering from a hyperventilation syndrome are lack of history or objective findings of cardiopulmonary disease and concomitant paresthesias in the fingers and around the mouth caused by an acute respiratory alkalosis. An arterial blood gas will demonstrate a low PCO_2, a high pH with a normal bicarbonate level. The arterial PO_2 should also be above the normal range and the calculated alveolar-arterial oxygen gradient should be normal. If the degree of alkalosis is

severe enough, carpopedal spasm may occur; this is uncommon in other causes of hyperventilation. The cause of the syndrome is usually anxiety, although pulmonary embolism must be excluded.

The discovery of the cause of persistent chest pain is a challenge that often confronts physicians. The problem is often difficult but proper interpretation of a comprehensive history and physical examination, correlated with skillfully chosen laboratory tests, will usually yield the correct solution.

ANEMIA

By THOMAS G. GABUZDA, M.D.
Philadelphia, Pennsylvania

INTRODUCTION

While a normal blood count is no guarantee of health, finding that a patient is anemic is a sure sign that something is wrong. In many cases the problem is easily handled with minimal cost and few diagnostic tests. On the other hand, a low hemoglobin level may point toward associated disease that requires a major effort for accurate diagnosis and correct management. Common sense and good clinical judgment will direct the physician upon a proper course of action, and conversely, a lack of these good qualities leads to inadequate or excessive use of the laboratory and of special diagnostic procedures.

The only way to determine whether a patient is anemic or not is to check the blood counts. It may be that a physician who has known a patient for a long time can detect a changed appearance with significant pallor of the skin and mucous membranes. More often it is impossible to judge from the patient's appearance whether or not anemia is present. For example, patients with cirrhosis and profuse cutaneous blood flow may have an almost plethoric appearance while they are anemic, and on the other hand patients in peripheral vasoconstriction demonstrate intense pallor with normal hemoglobin concentration.

The symptoms that a patient may report are just as capricious as superficial appearance among patients. Some deny any symptoms despite the presence of severe anemia, while others report fatigue with even minimal degrees of anemia. No doubt a great deal of this variation is related to the patient's personality type, but even making allowance for this, there still is considerable variation in the symptoms produced by anemia. Perhaps some of the variation is explained by differences in the degree to which the whole blood oxygen affinity curve adapts to the presence of anemia. For example, patients with sickle cell anemia tolerate their anemic state very well, even with half the normal level of hemoglobin. Presumably one reason for this is the fact that the whole blood oxygen affinity curve is shifted considerably to the right as it generally is in anemic subjects. This adaptive shift means that a greater proportion of the oxygen bound to hemoglobin is yielded to the tissues at a given partial pressure of oxygen (Fig. 1). Thus the lowered level of hemoglobin may be partially compensated for by a process whereby it is forced to surrender a greater proportion of its bound oxygen.

Not infrequently, the major symptom is related to the impact of tissue hypoxia on the heart, which produces angina pectoris or congestive heart failure. Syncope and visual blurring may be symptoms of intracranial hypoxia, and intermittent claudication may be the result of hypoxia in the peripheral circulation. Increased cardiac output causes increased heart action and pulse pressure, systolic "hemic" murmurs, and a pulsatile rushing sound in the ears. The hypermetabolic state may evoke low-grade fever.

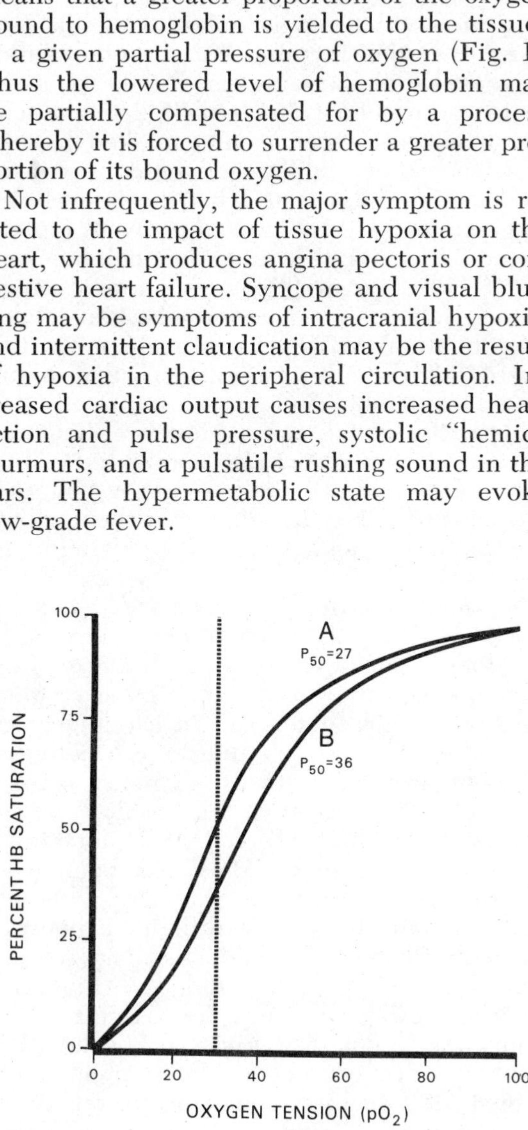

Figure 1. Oxygen dissociation curves of whole blood from a normal subject (A) and a patient with sickle cell anemia (B). At a pO_2 of 30 torr, normal blood loses 43 per cent of its oxygen. At the same pO_2, sickle cell anemia blood gives up 61 per cent of its oxygen.

Although chronic deficiency states of iron, vitamin B_{12}, or folates lead to a smooth tongue, it is unusual for the patient to report awareness of glossitis. Pica is a commonly overlooked symptom; patients will rarely volunteer information such as ice craving or starch eating unless it is specifically asked for. A positive response leads the physician to suspect iron deficiency. Reports of weakness or ataxia might be indicative of an associated neuropathy that warrants more careful attention to the neurologic examination. The same is true of paresthesias or changes in the mental status of the patient. Women are sometimes more concerned about brittle fingernails than they are about low hemoglobin concentrations, and the promise that their fingernails will be improved after 6 or more months of iron therapy can provide a greater incentive for them to take their iron pills than the assurance that the hemoglobin level will be raised. Patients with significant hemolytic anemia may show no clinical jaundice whatsoever, and if they do, it is usually slight. Intense jaundice always reflects some degree of hepatobiliary tree dysfunction, which may be intensified by an associated hemolytic process. All these comments notwithstanding, it appears likely that most cases of anemia are detected by the often random decision of the physician to order a blood count in a patient with any kind of complaint or even during the course of a routine check-up.

This brief overview of anemia will be limited to a discussion of normal values, the use and abuse of the laboratory in the diagnosis of anemia, and a few highlights about various categories of anemia covered in more detail in subsequent chapters (Table 1).

NORMAL VALUES

A standard table of normal values is the reference generally used in order to determine whether or not the patient is anemic (Table 2). However, it is worth reconsidering in some detail how anemia should be defined. A precise definition of the term anemia is a difficult if not impossible task. For example, the patient with adrenal insufficiency may have a normal level of hemoglobin together with a shrunken blood volume. In terms of the total mass of red cells, the patient is anemic, but the deficiency of red cells is masked by concomitant deficiency of plasma volume. To arrive at a determination that such a patient really is anemic requires determination of total red cell mass. A similar circumstance applies to the patient with anorexia nervosa, in which the anemia becomes manifest only

Table 1. *Pathophysiologic Classification of Anemia*

Relative anemia
Hemodilutional (e.g., pregnancy)

Absolute anemia
A. Decreased production
  1. Aregenerative (stem cell deficit):
      Aplastic anemia
      Pure red cell aplasia
      Anemia of chronic disease
      Anemia of uremia
      Endocrine lack anemia
      Leukemia
      Myelophthisic anemia (myelofibrosis, cancer)

  2. Impaired DNA synthesis (megaloblastic anemias):
      Vitamin B_{12} deficiency
      Folate deficiency
      Antimetabolite chemotherapy (e.g., methotrexate,
        6-mercaptopurine)
      Acquired myelodysplastic syndromes
      Rare hereditary defects

  3. Impaired hemoglobin synthesis (hypochromic
    anemias):
      Iron deficiency anemia
      Thalassemia
      Lead poisoning
      Sideroblastic anemias

B. Increased loss
  1. Blood loss anemia

  2. Hemolytic anemia:
      Intrinsic defects (inherited):
      Membrane (hereditary spherocytosis,
        elliptocytosis, stomatocytosis)
      Enzyme (G-6-PD, pyruvate kinase, other
        enzymopathies)
      Hemoglobin (sickle cell anemia, hemoglobin C
        disease and SC disease, unstable hemoglobin,
        other hemoglobinopathy)
      Intrinsic defects (acquired):
      Paroxysmal nocturnal hemoglobinuria
      Extrinsic defects (acquired):
      Chemical and oxidative hemolysis
      Physical (burn, drowning)
      Infections, (malaria, *Clostridium welchii*,
        Bartonellosis)
      Mechanical (cardiac, microangiopathic)
      Plasma lipid abnormality (spur cell anemia
        of cirrhosis)
      Autoimmune (warm antibody, cold agglutinin,
        cold hemolysin)
      "Hypersplenism"

---

when the patient starts to eat and enters the edematous phase of nutritional repletion. This is associated with a reexpansion of a previously contracted plasma volume and the appearance of anemia, that is, a decrease in the hemoglobin concentration, which is actually a sign that the patient is getting better. Expansion of plasma volume may cause dilutional anemia. This is seen normally during the course of pregnancy, in which red cell mass expands by about 20 per cent but plasma volume expands even more, causing a lowered hemoglobin level that is not really anemia in terms of the total volume of red cells in the circulation. A similar situation may apply to the plasma volume expansion in patients with congestive heart failure, liver disease, or massive splenomegaly.

How do we classify the patient who has a normal hemoglobin concentration but whose red cell indices are not normal? For example, a mean corpuscular volume (MCV) of 115 fl (see Table 2) is not normal, even if the hemoglobin concentration falls within the normal range. This circumstance may actually occur in patients with megaloblastic anemia and warrants further investigation. A patient with a hemoglobin of 15 grams per dl (100 ml) and a mean corpuscular volume of 65 fl might actually have polycythemia vera masked by iron deficiency. Such a patient would be considered anemic relative to what the hemoglobin level would be if the iron stores were replete. An MCV of 65 fl with a hemoglobin only about 1 to 2 grams below the normal range, especially if the mean corpuscular hemoglobin concentration (MCHC) is normal, points to a likelihood that the patient has thalassemia trait. Hemoglobin S-C disease frequently presents with not only normal levels of hemoglobin and hématocrit but also normal red cell indices. The red cell morphology is abnormal and should give the clue that hemoglobin electrophoresis and sickle cell preparation are indicated.

Not too many decades ago it was inconvenient to order a red cell count because it had to be done manually. Red cell indices were therefore not often available. However, today electronic cell counters are in use almost everywhere, and red cell indices are automatically provided on virtually all blood samples analyzed. Paradoxically, the results are not always thoroughly observed. It is not rare to find that an abnormal MCV has been overlooked.

Above and beyond the difference between the normal values for adult men and women, normal values also differ with age (Figs. 2 to 4). The newborn with a hemoglobin of 20 grams per dl is perfectly normal; a value of 15 grams per dl must be considered anemic. The normal MCV at birth is macrocytic relative to the normal adult range. The hemoglobin concentration falls during the first few months of life, with the nadir reaching a lower limit of about 10 grams per dl. Following this there is a slow continued increase of the normal range throughout childhood until adolescence is

Table 2. *Normal Adult Laboratory Values**

		Old System	New System
Red cell count	Men:	4.6–6.0 (5.1) $\times 10^6$/mm^3	$\times 10^{12}$/l
	Women:	4.1–4.8 (4.5) $\times 10^6$/mm^3	$\times 10^{12}$/l
Hemoglobin	Men:	14.5–16.7 g/100 ml	g/dl
	Women:	12.2–15.0 g/100 ml	g/dl
Packed cell volume	Men:	42–49%	.42–.49 l/l
	Women:	38–45%	.38–.45 l/l
Erythrocyte indices			
Mean corpuscular volume		82–$92\mu^3$	fl
Mean corpuscular hemoglobin		27–$32\mu\mu$g	pg
Mean corpuscular hemoglobin conc.		32–36 g/100 ml	g/dl
White cell count		5000–10,000/mm^3	5–10×10^9/l
Differential			
Neutrophils (segs)		54–62%	%
Neutrophils (bands)		5–10%	%
Absolute neutrophil count		3000–7000/mm^3	3–7×10^9/l
Eosinophils		0–3%	%
Basophils		0–1%	%
Lymphocytes		18–35%	%
Monocytes		3–7%	%
Platelet count	Men:	210,000–340,000/mm^3	210–340×10^9/l
	Women:	208,000–380,000/mm^3	208–380×10^9/l
Reticulocyte count		0.5–2.6%	%
Absolute reticulocyte count		25,000–125,000/mm^3	25–125×10^9/l
†Serum iron		80–180μg/100 ml	14–32μmol/l
†Total iron binding capacity		250–425μg/100 ml	45–76μmol/l
% Saturation		20–50 (35) %	%
†Serum ferritin	Men:	20–200 ng/ml	μg/l
	Women:	10–200 ng/ml	μg/l
†Serum B$_{12}$		200–1100 pg/ml	ng/l
†Serum folate		1.9–14 ng/ml	μg/l
†Schilling test	Stage I	10–40 (18) % of dose	%
	Stage II	10–42 (18) % of dose	%
Haptoglobin (hemoglobin binding capacity)		50–150 mg/100 ml	5–1.5 g/l
Bilirubin (total)		0.1–1.2 mg/100 ml	1–12 mg/l
Bilirubin (direct)		0–0.3 ng/100 ml	0–3 mg/l
Serum lactic dehydrogenase		100–225 mU/ml	0–90 IU/l 30 C
Hemoglobin A$_2$		1.8–3.3%	%
Hemoglobin F		<2.0%	%

*Data taken from Ersley, A. J., and Gabuzda, T. G.: Pathophysiology of Blood. Philadelphia, W. B. Saunders Co., 1979. Ranges given in terms of ±2 standard deviations. Mean values in parentheses.

†Normal values vary with technique used.

reached, at which point the difference between men and women appears. As mentioned earlier, during normal pregnancy the hemoglobin concentration also falls a little bit, with a lower range of normal of about 10 grams per dl. Values below this should be considered anemic.

In summary, there are a number of yardsticks to keep in mind when we ask ourselves the question, is this patient anemic? The physician who is careful to evaluate the laboratory results he obtains and interprets them in the light of the clinical picture will most often come to a correct judgment.

USE AND ABUSE OF THE LABORATORY

The technology base in medicine has become so broad and available that there is

temptation to peck away at it at random in the vaguely conceived hope that an answer will be generated without consideration of whether the effort is worth the cost involved. In this section of the discussion, I shall attempt to provide some framework for the sequence in which one should use the laboratory in the evaluation of the anemic patient, with the realization that an individual case may prove to be the exception to any given set of rules.

The effective performance of electronic counting devices has led to a well-justified faith in their overall accuracy and reliability. However, machines like humans are capable of making errors. Electronic counters directly measure hemoglobin concentration, count the number of particles per unit volume, and measure the mean size of these particles. From these three parameters, that is, the he-

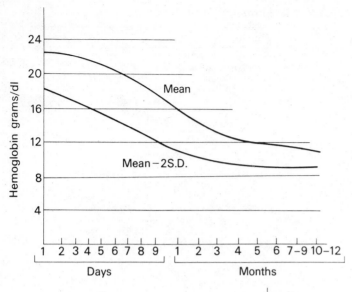

Figure 2. Normal values for hemoglobin level during infancy. The lower limit of normal is 2 standard deviations below the mean. (From Walsh, R. J., and Ward, H. K.: A Guide to Blood Transfusion. Australian Red Cross Society [N.S.W. Division], Blood Transfusion Service, Sydney, Appendix 1, 1957, as reprinted in deGruchy, G. C.: Clinical Haematology in Medical Practice. Oxford, Blackwell Scientific Publications, 4th ed., 1978.)

Figure 3. Normal childhood values for hemoglobin level. (Lower limit of normal and acknowledgment as in Figure 2.)

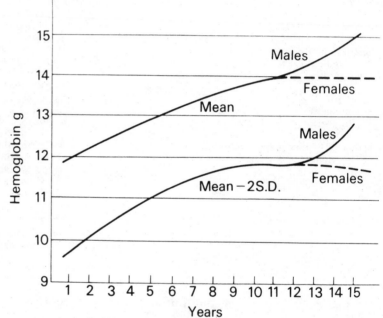

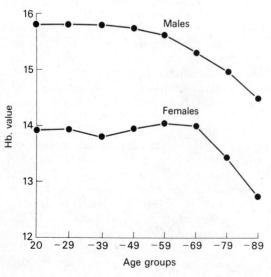

Figure 4. Normal mean adult values for hemoglobin level. (From Walsh, R. J., and Ward, H. K.: A Guide to Blood Transfusion. Australian Red Cross Society [N.S.W. Division], Blood Transfusion Service, Sydney, Appendix 1, 1957, as reprinted in deGruchy, G. C.: Clinical Haematology in Medical Practice. Oxford, Blackwell Scientific Publications, 4th ed., 1978.)

moglobin concentration, the hematocrit, and the mean corpuscular volume, the other indices are calculated. Errors may creep into any of the directly measured values. For example, the hemoglobin measurement might be speciously high if the solution is turbid from high lipid concentrations or abnormal serum proteins. Cold agglutinins cause red cell clumping with cell counts too low and mean corpuscular volumes too high. Excessively high white counts above 50,000 per cu mm cause erroneously high red cell counts, as might the presence of giant platelets. In particle counting, a "window" screens out particles outside the size range being counted, so excessively small red cells might be missed. These errors would be carried over into the calculated values. For example, a speciously high hemoglobin concentration would be reflected in a high MCH and MCHC. A speciously high red cell count would be reflected in an erroneously increased hematocrit, along with incorrectly low MCH and MCHC values.

The granulocytes and platelets share a common origin in the bone marrow with red cell precursors, and finding an abnormal hemoglobin level should provoke immediate interest in the white cell count, neutrophil percentage, and platelets as routinely assessed in the microscopic examination of the peripheral blood film made from an ethylenediamine tetraacetic acid (EDTA) anticoagulated whole blood tube. (The purpose of the EDTA is to achieve proper dispersion of the platelets so they are not clumped on the glass slide.) Depending on the circumstances, it is often necessary to perform a platelet count.

Similarly, the reticulocyte count does not need to be considered as a routine measurement for all anemic patients, but its determination should certainly be an early consideration. Reticulocyte counts should be interpreted in terms of absolute numbers (that is, the reticulocyte percentage multiplied by the red blood cell count) in considering the numbers present in the circulation (Table 2). An absolute reticulocyte count above 125,000 per cu mm usually indicates increased bone marrow production of red cells, but this is not always true. The allocation of reticulocytes between bone marrow and peripheral blood normally is approximately even, and circumstances that cause a shift of reticulocytes from the marrow into the peripheral blood might increase the absolute peripheral count without necessarily indicating increased production. This occurs in extramedullary hematopoiesis secondary to such conditions as myelofibrosis with myeloid metaplasia. When increased

bone marrow production is present, it usually is in response to blood loss or to hemolysis. However, it is well to bear in mind that an increased reticulocyte count is not always found in hemolytic states. For example, in acute hemolysis, there is insufficient time for the bone marrow to generate reticulocytes. This normally takes approximately 4 to 7 days. As another example, the patient with chronic hemolytic anemia in the midst of aplastic crisis will have a low reticulocyte count.

It has long been the fond wish of every hematologist that the examination of the peripheral blood film should be just as much a part of the physical examination as the auscultation of the heart. This wish will probably never become a reality, but it must be emphasized that morphologic examination of the peripheral blood requires a great deal of skill and experience. It should not be left to the subjective impressions of a laboratory technician operating within a routine. The skilled morphologist must know what to look for, and this important piece of information is denied to the technician involved in routine testing. Sometimes examination of the peripheral blood film is the only procedure that is necessary in order to give an accurate diagnosis of the cause of the anemia. Even finding that the red cell morphology is entirely normal is a vital piece of information that can be used to direct the continued work-up of a patient along correct lines. The situation is not helped by the fact that many clinical laboratories of lesser technological capability do not produce consistently satisfactory peripheral blood films. The procedure does involve certain tricks that depend on the climate and the batch of stain, not to mention constant laboratory supervision to see that a high level of quality is maintained. The subject of peripheral blood morphology will not be discussed in detail here, but one should remember that there are well-characterized alterations that point to a diagnosis of such conditions as iron deficiency anemia, megaloblastic anemia, hemolytic anemia of one kind or other, hemoglobinopathy, leukemia, or sideroblastic anemia.

Following evaluation of the blood cells, the testing for occult blood in stools is necessary in patients who have iron deficiency anemia, especially in any adult male or in females past the menopause. Indeed, it is being emphasized as a screening test for the normal adult population at risk for carcinoma of the colon, one of our major public health problems in which early detection is of vital importance in determining prognosis. Similarly, finding hemoglobinuria or hematuria calls attention to intravascular hemolysis of the urinary tract in the interpretation of the patient's anemia. Menorrhagia demands a thorough gynecologic examination, especially to rule out uterine cancer.

A printout of a series of chemistries done almost routinely these days might call attention to something relevant to the cause of the anemia. An elevated bilirubin, for example, suggests measurement of the conjugated and unconjugated fractions to determine whether a hemolytic state exists. An elevated lactic dehydrogenase (LDH) level (if we can be sure that it is not related to artifactual in vitro red cell lysis) might also suggest hemolysis. Low cholesterols are regularly found in any kind of anemia. Hypercalcemia might suggest an underlying malignancy; an elevated blood urea nitrogen, the anemia of uremia; and abnormal liver function tests, one of the anemias associated with liver disease.

At this point, the physician selects additional tests in a more discriminating manner. If the patient has a hypochromic microcytic anemia, serum iron and iron-binding capacity studies might be considered a logical next step. However, the diagnosis can often be made on the basis of the clinical context, the blood counts, and peripheral blood film alone. Conversely, when the diagnosis is in some doubt, knowing the serum iron and iron-binding capacity may not resolve the issue, especially in the evaluation of anemia of chronic disease and its distinction from iron deficiency anemia, both of which are characterized by low serum iron. In order to assist in this distinction, the measurement of serum ferritin concentration has come into some prominence in recent years, and a serum ferritin concentration below the normal range is probably the single most reliable test in the laboratory identification of iron deficiency anemia. However, when chronic disease states coexist with iron deficiency anemia, the serum ferritin concentration may not be reduced. Hemoglobin A_2 and F quantitation is used to confirm the presence of beta-thalassemia trait, but it must be recalled that these values are not increased in alpha-thalassemia trait. The latter diagnosis is difficult to establish by means of laboratory confirmation. An unexplained anemia of chronic disease warrants an erythrocyte sedimentation rate and possibly tests for autoimmune disorders, such as an antinuclear antibody, along with a search for hidden malignancy. Suspicion of endocrine insufficiency suggests thyroid function tests.

Perhaps the most overused laboratory tests are the measurement of serum B_{12} and folate concentrations. These are commonly done almost as a routine evaluation in the assessment of any anemic patient without much rhyme or reason. Their use should be limited to the accurate diagnosis of the patient with megaloblastic anemia. Indeed, recent reports have indicated that commercial kits provided for the measurement of B_{12} levels have resulted in overestimations in many patients, so much so that patients with pernicious anemia would have been missed if reliance had been placed only upon the measurement of serum B_{12} level. The Schilling test is also not without its disadvantage, especially since it depends on an adequate urine collection, normal renal function, and careful monitoring to make sure that stool has not contaminated the urine sample. It should also be pointed out that the ileal absorption of B_{12} might be temporarily impaired in classic pernicious anemia, leading to an abnormal Stage II (with intrinsic factor) as well as Stage I (without intrinsic factor) Schilling test until after several months of treatment. With these reservations, this procedure is useful in identifying the nature of B_{12} deficiency; in cases of treated pernicious anemia, it is the only readily available clinical test for determining whether or not the patient actually has pernicious anemia, since serum B_{12} levels as well as peripheral blood and bone marrow morphology would be normal in the treated state. A somewhat underused test in the evaluation of the patient with megaloblastic anemia is the measurement of gastric acidity after stimulation, the presence of which rules out classic pernicious anemia in the adult. An added dividend of gastric analysis is the opportunity to do a cytologic examination. Non-megaloblastic macrocytosis might be explained on the basis of abnormal liver function, biliary tract obstruction, or a rather significantly elevated reticulocyte count. The clinical picture of aplastic anemia might also explain macrocytic indices. High serum iron and low serum iron binding capacity with increased per cent saturation are found in ineffective erythropoiesis, so characteristic of the megaloblastic anemias, as well as in aplastic erythropoiesis.

In the laboratory evaluation of the patient suspected of having hemolytic anemia, chemistries may or may not have shown an increased serum bilirubin and LDH to highlight suspicion in this direction. LDH isozymes may indicate whether the elevation may be of erythrocytic origin (LDH–1, LDH–2). It should be noted, however, that the highest levels of LDH, with values often over 1000 units per dl, are found in the megaloblastic anemia states caused by intramedullary hemolysis. Perhaps the most sensitive test is the measurement of serum haptoglobin concentration, which may be absent in the presence of hemolysis. However, a sample drawn soon after the administration of a blood transfusion will likely show absent haptoglobin because of the small quantity of hemolyzed red cells present in the transfused blood. Haptoglobin is an acute phase reactant; its concentration increases in response to many neoplastic and inflammatory disease states. Thus, finding a normal or elevated level does not rule out the coexistence of a hemolytic state.

The clinical context might suggest whether one is dealing with an inherited or an acquired hemolytic condition. If the patient is young or belongs to an ethnic group with a high frequency of such disorders, inherited conditions should be thought of first. The screening test for glucose–6–phosphate dehydrogenase (G-6-PD) deficiency, a hemoglobin electrophoresis, and a sickle cell preparation for hemoglobinopathy yield reasonably high dividends in black patients. On the other hand, older adults, especially if they are white, are more likely to have acquired hemolytic conditions. There is a long list of causes of acquired hemolytic anemia, and sometimes the clinical context immediately provides the explanation. However, when this is not true, one should think of autoimmune hemolytic anemia and obtain a Coombs' test. The Coombs' test ordinarily is done with a broad-spectrum antiserum and is sensitive to the presence of both warm and cold antibodies; it will detect either IgG or complement on the red cell surface. A positive Coombs' test warrants further evaluation with a cold agglutinin test and possibly the use of narrow spectrum Coombs' sera to more precisely identify the character of the hemolytic anemia one is dealing with. It should also be emphasized that a Coombs' test may be positive in the absence of significant hemolysis. If the patient is on a medication that might cause oxidative hemolysis, such as a sulfonamide derivative, inspection of the peripheral blood film for the presence of "bitten out" cells, distorted spherocytes, Heinz bodies, and a methemoglobin level, and an assessment for deficient enzymes or unstable hemoglobin might be in order. If significant intravascular hemolysis is suspected, one observes the plasma for the presence of hemoglobin and the urine for both free hemoglobin and hemosiderin.

The decision whether or not to perform a bone marrow examination should be made at this stage of the evaluation and often should actually precede the consideration of the other laboratory tests. When the procedure is done skillfully, it is essentially without discomfort or risk to the patient. This is especially true since the posterior iliac crest has now become preferred for bone marrow aspiration rather than the sternum. The ease with which the procedure is done depends upon the skill of the operator, but with gentle cutaneous anesthesia and a reassured patient, the task can be accomplished with minimal patient complaint.

As with any other test, whether or not to proceed to a bone marrow aspiration is a matter of clinical judgment, but some ground rules might be laid. The test is apt to be more rewarding when the cause of the anemia is not clear after examination of the patient and of the initial peripheral blood counts and morphology. Macrocytosis, other peculiarities of red cell size and shape, and abnormal white cell or platelet counts favor doing this procedure. Suspicion of an underlying neoplastic condition, such as leukemia, multiple myeloma, or metastatic carcinoma involving the bone marrow, is a further indication. Staining the bone marrow aspirate for iron is a rapid and accurate way of ascertaining whether or not the patient is iron deficient. It is particularly useful in distinguishing the anemia of chronic disease from iron deficiency. On the other hand, the routine case of iron deficiency, the clearly explained chronic disease anemia, the patient with uncomplicated thalassemia trait or hemoglobinopathy, all represent situations in which the bone marrow examination is usually of no benefit. In almost every instance in which a bone marrow aspiration is done, it is worthwhile to submit a clotted specimen of the bone marrow to the pathology department for staining of the fixed clot with hematoxylin and eosin and other appropriate stains. When this is done, a patient with unsuspected non-Hodgkin's lymphoma, miliary tuberculosis, or cancer may be discovered. These are not always evident, in fact are frequently not evident, in the routine aspiration examined on stained marrow smears.

Percutaneous needle biopsy of the bone may be done in addition to aspiration. This is particularly useful in the staging of Hodgkin's disease, in the diagnosis of metastatic cancer, myelofibrosis, or aplastic anemia, or in the evaluation of any marrow aspirate yielding a "dry tap." We have recently observed several examples in which culture of the bone marrow aspirate confirmed the diagnosis of miliary tuberculosis in patients with fevers of unknown origin. In summary, the bone marrow evaluation is of use in the diagnosis of a wide variety of primary bone marrow disorders as well as of other conditions that secondarily affect this tissue. The decision whether or not to proceed with a bone marrow study should be made very early in the evaluation of the patient.

CLINICAL AXIOMS

Individual types of anemia will be discussed in detail in subsequent chapters, but at this point I should like to present a few useful guidelines to keep in mind in dealing with the anemic patient. First, iron deficiency anemia is never related to diet alone. True, dietary intake of iron may not be sufficient to keep up with the increased iron requirements posed by growth during infancy, adolescence, or pregnancy, or by increased blood loss in the urine, menses, or stools. Even though it may not always be easily possible to document significant blood loss in adults, this loss probably has been present, perhaps minimally over a period of many years and occurring on and off. While any adult male or postmenopausal female found to be iron deficient warrants a thorough evaluation of the entire gastrointestinal tract to identify the site of blood loss, it is not necessary routinely to submit the two-year-old, the adolescent, or the young adult woman with heavy menstrual flow or multiple pregnancies to the bother and cost of this evaluation, unless a suspicion arises that such study would be rewarding.

There is a common category of anemia that might be called "nonspectacular anemia," identified by the following criteria: normal or almost normal red cell morphology and red cell indices, exclusion of iron deficiency anemia by appropriate laboratory tests and possibly bone marrow examination stain for iron, and a lack of obvious explanation for the anemic state (Fig. 5). Nonspectacular anemia falls into two subclasses. The first is due to occult chronic disease, either neoplastic or inflammatory, and is characterized by low serum iron, a low iron-binding capacity, a reduced saturation in the range of 10 to 25 per cent, and usually an elevated sedimentation rate. Further studies might bring to light the presence of an occult neoplasm or a hitherto undiagnosed connective tissue disorder, such as systemic lupus erythematosus or polymyalgia rheumatica. The second type of nonspectacular anemia is characterized by a normal serum iron, normal iron-binding capacity, and normal per cent saturation of the iron-binding protein. Sedimentation rate is normal. These features are suggestive of the anemia of endocrine dysfunction, usually hypothyroidism. A significant percentage of hypothyroid patients are detected because they are found to have mild anemia.

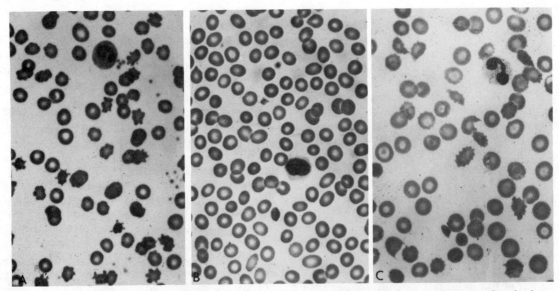

Figure 5. "Nonspectacular anemia" is illustrated in *B* by normal red cell indices and morphology. *A* and *C* also have normal red cell indices but do not qualify as "nonspectacular anemia." *A* shows the morphologic changes seen in anorexia nervosa and *C* those seen in microangiopathic hemolytic anemia.

The terms macrocytic and megaloblastic are often but incorrectly used interchangeably. Not all macrocytic anemias are megaloblastic. The features of megaloblastic anemia include anisocytosis, oval macrocytosis, hypersegmentation of polys, and characteristic megaloblastic changes in the bone marrow aspirate. Perhaps the most common cause of a mild increase in the mean corpuscular volume without megaloblastosis is chronic liver disease. Reticulocytosis also may be associated with an increased mean corpuscular volume. Acquired idiopathic sideroblastic anemia is usually macrocytic, even though the peripheral blood film characteristically shows a minor population of microcytic hypochromic erythrocytes. The bone marrow examination showing large numbers of ring sideroblasts gives the diagnosis and indicates the near certainty of refractoriness to treatment. Patients on chemotherapy for neoplastic states also commonly show an increased mean corpuscular volume as a result of the action of the chemotherapeutic agent on the bone marrow.

Refractory anemias are rather common in patients in the older age group. These comprise a variety of conditions that are usually macrocytic or normocytic, sometimes associated with a significant increase in bone marrow myeloblasts, ring sideroblasts, or myelomonocytic proliferation. These refractory anemias, previously referred to as "preleukemia," are now called myelodysplastic syndromes. Most of them remain stable or demonstrate progressive bone marrow failure rather than conversion to overt acute leukemia, which takes place only about 10 per cent of the time. For this reason use of the term preleukemia is discouraged. At any rate, the anemias found in this category of syndromes are notoriously refractory to treatment, sometimes requiring transfusional support. Others are stable and require no particular treatment.

In Figure 6 is a rich assortment of medicines yielded from the bathroom cabinet of an elderly woman who succumbed to aplastic anemia. In the medical history she reported taking only digitalis and a diuretic. If a peek into the bathroom cabinet were part of a physician's routine work-up, a number of similar surprises would no doubt be turned up. Today's polypharmacy being as vast, diverse, and potent as it is, physicians have a deeper responsibility than ever to limit promiscuous dissemination of medications. Every prescription should be preceded by a thought about its risk-to-benefit ratio. If the benefit is zero, the ratio is infinity. Aplastic anemia is fortunately a rare toxic reaction, but a fatal case occurring among the patients in one's own practice is a calamitous price for an iatrogenic complication, especially if the untoward reaction was to a medication given for a trivial reason.

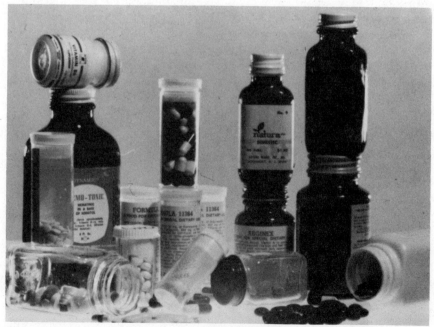

Figure 6. Polypharmacy from the bathroom cabinet of an elderly woman with aplastic anemia.

LYMPHADENOPATHY

By CHARLES E. HESS, M.D.

Charlottesville, Virginia

INTRODUCTION

From a diagnostic standpoint, lymphadenopathy presents one of the most challenging problems in all of clinical medicine. Not only are enlarged lymph nodes frequently missed on physical examination, but more importantly, a systematic approach is often not followed when these patients are evaluated. Too often a lymph node biopsy is either performed unnecessarily or not done when clearly indicated to establish a diagnosis.

DIAGNOSTIC APPROACH

The major decision in most patients is whether or not to perform a lymph node biopsy to rule out a malignant neoplastic process. If the lymphadenopathy is localized and is secondary to inflammation in the area drained by the enlarged lymph node or nodes, or if generalized and secondary to a well-defined systemic illness (e.g., viral infection, systemic lupus erythematosus), a lymph node biopsy is generally not indicated. When making this decision, there are several factors that are very helpful; these include: (1) age of patients, (2) clinical history, (3) physical examination, (4) anatomic location and extent of the lymphadenopathy, and (5) proper selection of laboratory investigations that may establish a diagnosis without the need for lymph node biopsy.

Age of Patient. Hypertrophy of lymph nodes and other lymphoid tissue (e.g., adenoids, tonsils) is often a normal physiologic process in infants and children. In addition, the occurrence and extent of lymphadenopathy in response to a variety of stimuli such as viral and bacterial infections and vaccinations is much greater in infants and children than in adults. This age difference is of such importance to warrant an almost totally different diagnostic approach to patients before and after puberty. In children with either localized or generalized lymphadenopathy, an infectious cause usually is easy to demonstrate, and lymph node biopsy is not indicated. Other than treatment of the underlying infection when indicated, follow-up to document resolution of the lymphadenopathy is all that is needed.

The strikingly enlarged lymph nodes that are seen in infectious mononucleosis in young adults should not be biopsied if the clinical history, physical findings, and more importantly, the serologic studies are consistent with that diagnosis. Not only is lymph node biopsy unnecessary to make a diagnosis, but histiopathologic interpretation of these lymph nodes presents a very difficult differential diagnostic problem, particularly when attempting to distinguish the changes from those found in non-Hodgkin's lymphomas, Waldenström's macroglobulinemia, and lymphocyte-predominant Hodgkin's disease. Other reactive processes (e.g., postvaccinal lymphadenitis, syphilis, toxoplasmosis, drug-induced lymphadenopathy) present similar problems with histiopathologic interpretation. Because of these problems, most hematopathologists will demand the results of a careful history and physical examination and a serologic test for syphilis, toxoplasmosis, and heterophile antibody before rendering a final interpretation in such cases.

Clinical History. A careful clinical history is invaluable in the evaluation of the patient with lymphadenopathy, and frequently leads one to a correct diagnosis without the need for lymph node biopsy. The mode of onset and the duration of the lymphadenopathy are very important factors. In addition, specific inquiries regarding drugs, allergies, animal exposure, and occupation should be made. Tender, painful lymph nodes that appear and progress over a period of a few days or weeks are often secondary to an inflammatory process in the area drained by the lymph nodes. The diagnosis in such patients may be obvious, as in a patient with unilateral cervical lymphadenopathy secondary to dental infection, or it may be very difficult, as in a patient with cat-scratch fever with lymphadenopathy involving the epitrochlear, axillary, and supraclavicular areas if a history of exposure to cats is not obtained.

Enlarged nontender lymph nodes in the epitrochlear, axillary, femoral, and inguinal areas are often seen in patients with certain occupations in which recurrent and usually minor injury to the extremities occurs. Generalized and usually asymptomatic lymphadenopathy also is found in patients with such chronic dermatologic disorders as eczema. The lymphadenopathy that occurs as a part of the hypersensitivity reaction to anticonvulsant drugs presents a particularly difficult clinical and histiopathologic diagnostic problem; the atypical hyperplasia in these lymph nodes may be very difficult and at times impossible to distinguish from Hodgkin's disease. If the lymphadenopathy does not regress after the drug is stopped, a repeat biopsy is recommended.

Physical Examination. The physical examination is equally important. One should become very familiar with the normal anatomy of the lymphatic system. In general, a lymph node that is larger than 1 cm in diameter should be considered enlarged. When palpating for enlarged lymph nodes, the physician must "take off the boxing gloves." Lymph nodes that are only minimally enlarged or fixed to underlying tissue may not be appreciated if one does not use a "gentle" approach; enlarged supraclavicular and axillary nodes are missed most frequently (a Valsalva maneuver may aid in detecting supraclavicular lymphadenopathy).

The size, shape, and consistency of lymph nodes are also very important when deciding whether to do lymph node biopsy or which lymph node to biopsy. Lymph nodes that are enlarged but flat, smooth, and relatively soft are usually normal or show only hyperplasia if biopsied. When the enlarged lymph node is irregular and has a rubbery or hard consistency, biopsy usually reveals involvement by a malignant neoplastic process such as lymphoma or carcinoma or by sarcoidosis.

Enlarged, tender lymph nodes are usually secondary to infection, either primary in the lymph node or in the area drained by the lymph node. One must keep in mind, however, that patients with lymphoma, particularly with Hodgkin's disease, may occasionally present with tender, painful lymphadenopathy. If the enlarged lymph node is fluctuant and is not secondary to an obvious distal site of infection, a needle aspiration for special stains and culture will often give a diagnosis and thus avoid the need for biopsy; a diagnosis of tuberculous lymphadenitis can often be made by aspiration alone. In lymphadenitis secondary to bacterial infection, the lymph node may become very large and fluctuant, particularly in children, and require incision and drainage as part of the treatment.

A careful examination for the presence of splenomegaly or hepatomegaly, or both, should be performed in all patients with lymphadenopathy. The presence of splenomegaly usually indicates a systemic process (e.g., infectious mononucleosis, chronic lymphocytic leukemia, lymphoma) and will often direct attention to investigative studies other than lymph node biopsy that will lead to the diagnosis.

Anatomic Location and Extent of Lymphadenopathy. When lymphadenopathy is confined to one lymph node region or involves two or more regions that are contiguous with each other, a thorough knowledge of disorders that are known to affect lymph nodes and other structures in that particular area is invaluable. An effort should be made to eliminate inflammatory disease before performing a diagnostic lymph node biopsy. Unilateral lymphadenopathy in the neck or in an extremity is often due to infection of structures drained by those lymph nodes (inguinal lymphadenopathy secondary to an infected wound of that extremity, an enlarged submental node secondary to tooth abscess).

There are situations in which an infectious cause, although highly suspected, cannot be established; in such instances treatment of the infection when indicated and close follow-up to document resolution of the lymphadenopathy is all that is required. In cat-scratch fever, the distribution of the lymphadenopathy (unilateral involvement of the epitrochlear, axillary, and supraclavicular lymph nodes) and the clinical course, if associated with a history of a cat scratch or just contact with a cat, is a good example of such a disorder. A similar clinical picture may be seen in rat-bite fever, bubonic plague, sporotrichosis, anthrax, rickettsial disease, or with any infective agent for which the portal of entry is the skin.

There are several nonmalignant disorders that show a predilection for certain lymph node regions; these include rubella, oculoglandular syndrome, sinus histiocytosis with massive lymphadenopathy, syphilis, sarcoidosis, pneumoconiosis, angiofollicular mediastinal lymph node hyperplasia, lymphogranuloma venereum, and acute mesenteric lymphadenitis. In *rubella,* enlarged posterior auricular, and less commonly, suboccipital and posterior cervical lymph nodes are very characteristic, and in certain instances, a diagnostic finding. *Oculoglandular syndrome* involves anterior auricular lymphadenopathy associated with a variety of inflammatory lesions of the eyelids and conjunctivae (e.g., rubella, trachoma, cat-scratch fever).

Sinus histiocytosis with massive lymphadenopathy is a benign disorder of unknown cause that occurs in children and young adults and is characterized by painless massive cervical lymphadenopathy, usually bilateral; fever; neutrophilia; and an elevated erythrocyte sedimentation rate (ESR). The lymphadenopathy progresses slowly over a period of a few weeks to several months and regresses after 6 months to several years. Histopathologically, there is marked histiocytic infiltration in the sinuses of the lymph node; a biopsy is necessary to rule out a malignant neoplastic process.

The bilateral epitrochlear lymphadenopathy

of *syphilis* has long been considered of diagnostic importance in secondary syphilis but is more commonly due to recurrent injury to the hands in people who do manual labor; lymph node biopsy generally is not indicated. Bilateral hilar lymphadenopathy in an asymptomatic patient or in association with erythema nodosum is so characteristic of *sarcoidosis* that a diagnosis usually can be made without biopsy confirmation. Close follow-up for several months is mandatory, however, to document resolution. In *pneumoconiosis,* the parenchymal lung involvement is frequently accompanied by bilateral hilar lymphadenopathy. *Angiofollicular mediastinal lymph node hyperplasia* is a disorder, usually of young adults, characterized by the presence of a large solitary mediastinal mass that may compress the bronchus. Biopsy of the mass reveals atypical hyperplasia, which may resemble a thymoma. The disorder is self-limiting, but a biopsy for documentation and close follow-up is necessary.

In *lymphogranuloma venereum,* unilateral inguinal lymph node enlargement is a characteristic finding. *Acute mesenteric lymphadenitis* is characterized by recurrent abdominal pain in children and young adults and often mimics acute appendicitis.

Lymphadenopathy that is confined to certain lymph node regions also has diagnostic importance in the evaluation of a patient for a suspected malignant neoplasm. Isolated supraclavicular lymphadenopathy is frequently due to either metastases from an intrathoracic or intra-abdominal malignant neoplasm or malignant lymphoma. Generally, isolated left supraclavicular lymphadenopathy is seen more with intra-abdominal malignant neoplasms, while isolated right supraclavicular lymph node involvement is seen more often with intrathoracic malignant lesions. Even in the absence of palpable lymphadenopathy, a scalene node or "fat-pad" biopsy may be very helpful in the evaluation of intrathoracic lesions.

Intra-abdominal or retroperitoneal lymphadenopathy, particularly if gross enough to be felt on physical examination of the abdomen, is usually due to a malignant process. Abdominal exploration and biopsy should be performed if necessary to establish a diagnosis. If a malignant lymphoma is found, a staging procedure (splenectomy, bone marrow biopsy, and multiple liver biopsies) should be done at the same time. Patients with moderate to marked enlargement of retroperitoneal lymph nodes often present with backache. If the back pain is associated with other findings (e.g.,

fever, weight loss, night sweats), a thorough search should be made for retroperitoneal lymphadenopathy. The bipedal lymphangiogram and, more recently, sonography and computerized tomography of the abdomen and pelvis have aided greatly in the diagnosis of intra-abdominal lymphadenopathy. If these tests are normal, intra-abdominal lymphadenopathy essentially is eliminated.

Generalized lymphadenopathy, defined as involvement of two or more noncontiguous lymph node regions, occurs in a variety of disorders. Not only is lymph node biopsy unnecessary in many instances, but if performed, it usually reveals only nonspecific histopathologic change. Disorders frequently associated with generalized lymphadenopathy include: viral infections, toxoplasmosis, dermatopathic lymphadenopathy, connective tissue disorders, chronic lymphocytic leukemia, malignant lymphomas, and sarcoidosis.

In *viral infections,* generalized lymphadenopathy occurs much more frequently in children and young adults with any viral illness than in older adults. In most of these infections the diagnosis can be made from the clinical course of the illness (e.g., rubella, rubeola). The diagnosis of infectious mononucleosis usually requires examination of a peripheral blood smear for presence of atypical lymphocytes and a serologic test for heterophil antibody. Diagnosis can be very difficult if the clinical findings suggest infectious mononucleosis and the test for heterophil antibody is negative. There are several viral infections that can produce this "seronegative infectious mononucleosis-like illness" (e.g., cytomegalovirus, viral hepatitis, adenovirus, influenza). A lymph node biopsy is not helpful except to rule out a malignant neoplastic process.

The acquired form of *toxoplasmosis* frequently presents with generalized lymphadenopathy. The clinical course may mimic infectious mononucleosis (approximately 10 per cent of seronegative infectious mononucleosis is due to toxoplasmosis). The diagnosis is established by demonstrating a rise and fall in antibody titer to the protozoan *Toxoplasma gondii* using the toxoplasmosis dye test; the titers may not start to rise for 3 weeks after onset of illness. A high titer that does not change with time may occasionally be found in lymphomas. A lymph node biopsy is usually performed in most patients because of the long course of the illness and the prominence of the lymphadenopathy, especially in the cervical area. Although the histopathologic findings are not pathognomonic (hyperplasia and aggregation of histiocytes in and around germinal centers), they are characteristic and should lead to other studies to establish the diagnosis. The cysts or organisms of *Toxoplasma gondii* are rarely seen in the sections.

Dermatopathic lymphadenopathy is seen most often with exfoliative dermatitis and mycosis fungoides. Lymph node biopsy is frequently necessary in patients with mycosis fungoides to evaluate for systemic spread of this lymphoma. Of the *connective tissue disorders*, generalized lymphadenopathy is most often seen in active rheumatoid arthritis and systemic lupus erythematosus. Unless an associated malignant neoplastic process is suspected, a lymph node biopsy is not indicated.

A cardinal feature of *chronic lymphocytic leukemia* is generalized lymphadenopathy. A lymph node biopsy is not indicated since the peripheral blood and bone marrow findings are diagnostic. With *malignant lymphomas*, generalized lymphadenopathy is much more common in non-Hodgkin's lymphomas, particularly in the more differentiated lymphocytic types. A lymph node biopsy and interpretation, preferably by a hematopathologist, is necessary for diagnosis.

Although generalized lymphadenopathy is one of the most characteristic clinical findings in *sarcoidosis*, a lymph node biopsy is indicated in most patients to confirm the diagnosis. Because of the increased incidence of nonspecific granulomatous reactions in lymph nodes and other organs in Hodgkin's disease, multiple lymph node biopsies may be indicated to eliminate Hodgkin's disease if the clinical course is atypical for sarcoidosis.

Other disorders such as bacterial infections, (brucellosis, secondary syphilis, leptospirosis), hypersensitivity drug reactions (anticonvulsant drugs), and hyperthyroidism may occasionally be associated with generalized lymphadenopathy.

Laboratory Investigation. A thorough knowledge of which laboratory studies to obtain on the basis of the clinical features of a particular patient is mandatory in order to arrive at a diagnosis promptly and avoid unnecessary lymph node biopsies. Most of these studies, and the clinical situations in which they should be performed, have been mentioned in this article. Generally, before a lymph node is biopsied, a white blood cell count and a careful inspection of a peripheral blood smear should be done. The selection of other studies before making a decision to do a lymph node biopsy must be individualized (e.g., a bone marrow biopsy and aspiration is preferred to lymph node biopsy if leukemia is suspected).

LYMPH NODE BIOPSY PROCEDURE

Once a decision is made to perform a lymph node biopsy, there are certain guidelines that must be followed in order to obtain the information necessary to make a diagnosis. The selection of which lymph node to biopsy is critical. Because of the chronic changes (such as scarring) that are frequently present in lymph nodes in the inguinal region, biopsy in this area should be avoided if possible. In general, the largest lymph node in the area selected for biopsy should be removed. All too often, smaller nodes are removed that show only reactive changes secondary to a malignant neoplastic process in a larger, adjacent lymph node; this is particularly true in Hodgkin's disease. Multiple lymph node biopsies are indicated in some patients to rule out a malignant neoplastic process. These repeat biopsies may be indicated during the initial work-up or on follow-up if the lymphadenopathy progresses.

Proper handling and processing of the lymph node also is very important. The specimen should be placed in formalin as soon as possible and fixed for 24 hours. Because of the slow penetration of the formalin, larger lymph nodes should be sectioned into smaller pieces prior to being placed in the formalin. If a frozen section is desired, only a portion of the lymph node should be submitted for this study, the rest being processed as just discussed. If lymph node imprints are obtained, the lymph node should be sectioned one or more times prior to being placed in formalin. Several "touch" preparations and smears should be made for Wright stain and other special stains (e.g., periodic acid–Schiff [PAS], nonspecific esterase) as indicated. These preparations are helpful in the subclassification of non-Hodgkin's lymphomas.

Other studies that are helpful in the differential diagnosis of malignant neoplastic disorders, but unfortunately are available only in certain centers at the present time, include electronmicroscopy and immunologic studies (e.g., immunofluorescent stains, lymphocyte typing). Lymph code cultures are not indicated routinely but are important studies to obtain if the clinical manifestations suggest an infectious process or if the lymph node reveals necrosis when sectioned.

ANOREXIA, NAUSEA, AND VOMITING

By ADRIAN P. DOUGLAS, M.D.

Los Angeles, California

ANOREXIA

Anorexia is loss of appetite. It is common as a temporary phenomenon when it is of little significance, but when persistent it is of great importance, since prolonged anorexia may lead to weight loss and consequent profound secondary disturbances of bodily function. Loss of appetite may be the result of emotional upset, a depressive state, anemia, disease of the gastrointestinal tract, any chronic disease process such as tuberculosis or heart failure, or drugs used to treat such processes. Some of these various etiologic conditions are listed in Table 1.

To understand anorexia, so that a logical approach to its differential diagnosis can be made, it is important to understand the factors associated with the desire to eat and their control. Hunger is the need for food; it is often accompanied by disagreeable sensations of abdominal discomfort (hunger pains) and irritability. Appetite is a desire to ingest food, is often independent of hunger, and is strongly influenced by numerous psychologic stimuli, including senses of taste and smell, willful choice, and conditioning. Loss of the desire to eat is usual after hunger has been satiated, but in anorexia the absence of a desire to eat persists despite the presence of the physiologic stimuli normally producing hunger.

Data from experimental animals and humans with diseases of the midbrain indicate that the hypothalamus plays a major role in regulating food intake. In its ventromedial nucleus is a "satiety center" that when stimulated inhibits feeding and whose destruction leads to hyperphagia. In the ventrolateral area of the hypothalamus is a "feeding center" whose stimulation leads to increased food ingestion. These centers apparently are affected by various stimuli in intact animals and man. Visual, auditory, tactile, olfactory, and enteroreceptive (vagally mediated) reflexes act on the feeding center; temperature, gastric and intestinal distension, food and intravenous glucose amino acids and fatty acids stimulate the satiety center. The centers themselves influence each other. The satiety center, not unreasonably, inhibits the feeding center and the feeding center, by increasing food intake, stimulates the satiety center. Overriding all these subcortical factors is the influence of psychologic factors, themselves influenced by genetic, environmental, cultural, and economic ones.

Anorexia is usually only transient and unassociated with significant metabolic changes. Prolonged anorexia and diminished calorie intake will lead to weight loss and the metabolic consequences of starvation, including amenorrhea, metabolic acidosis, ketosis, and hyperuricemia. It is unusual for prolonged anorexia to be the predominant symptom, since the underlying disease process will become more florid. Even in the psychologic syndrome anorexia nervosa, anorexia is rarely the predominant complaint (of either the patient or her mother). A careful history will usually indicate the probable cause with attention to five particular facts: whether the anorexia is for all or special foods, its duration, its degree, the presence of associated symptoms such as pain and vomiting, and the extent of weight loss. Inquiry should also be made regarding the senses of taste and smell because they influence appetite strongly; particularly in such chronic intestinal disease as Crohn's there is often profound loss of taste due to zinc deficiency. The history will usually suggest the particular areas of the physical examination that should be concentrated on. Psychologic factors should always be considered so that a firm diagnosis can usually be made with a minimum of special laboratory tests when the complaint is anorexia nervosa. Table 2 lists laboratory tests that may aid in diagnosis of anorexia, nausea, and vomiting.

NAUSEA AND VOMITING

Although both these symptoms may be influenced, like anorexia, by psychologic factors, their presence, particularly when persistent, is almost always indicative of serious illness.

Nausea is an unpleasant sensation in the throat or upper abdomen associated with a desire to vomit or a feeling that vomiting is imminent. Vomiting is the expulsion of gastric and intestinal contents through the mouth and involves relaxation of esophageal sphincters and reverse peristalsis in the stomach and esophagus. Nausea is not always followed by the act of vomiting; the influences of psychologic factors and "self-control" are important

Table 1. *Causes of Anorexia, Nausea, and Vomiting*

I. Infections
   A. Viral (epidemic vomiting)
   B. Bacterial
   C. Fungus
   D. Parasitic
II. Gastrointestinal
   A. Oral cavity
      1. Stomatitis
      2. Gingivitis
      3. Dental caries
      4. Neoplasms
   B. Esophagus
      1. Esophagitis
      2. Motility disturbances
      3. Neoplasms
      4. Strictures
   C. Stomach
      1. Gastritis
      2. Ulcer
      3. Neoplasms
      4. Gastric retention
   D. Duodenum and small bowel
      1. Ulcer (with or without pyloric
         stenosis)
      2. Regional enteritis
      3. Sprue
      4. Mesenteric vascular insufficiency
      5. Neoplasms
      6. Radiation injury
      7. Postgastrectomy
      8. Food allergy
      9. Intestinal obstruction
      10. Acute appendicitis
      11. Ascariasis and other infestations
   E. Pancreas
      1. Pancreatitis
      2. Neoplasms
   F. Liver
      1. Hepatitis
      2. Neoplasms
      3. Abscess
      4. Hepatic encephalopathy
   G. Gallbladder and bile ducts
      1. Cholecystitis and cholelithiasis
      2. Neoplasms
      3. Extrahepatic obstruction
   H. Colon and rectum
      1. Ulcerative colitis
      2. Granulomatous colitis
      3. Mesenteric vascular insufficiency
      4. Neoplasms
   I. Peritoneum and mesentery
      1. Peritonitis
      2. Mesenteritis

III. Neurologic
   A. Psychiatric diseases
      1. Anorexia nervosa
      2. Depression
      3. Schizophrenia
      4. Neuroses
      5. Acute psychoses
      6. Habit vomiting
   B. CNS diseases
      1. Neoplasms
      2. Abscess or meningitis
      3. Vascular insufficiency or
         infarction
      4. Degenerative diseases
      5. Migraine
      6. Meniere's disease
      7. Labyrinthitis
      8. Tabes
IV. Cardiovascular
   A. Congestive heart failure
   B. Coronary artery insufficiency
   C. Rheumatic heart disease
   D. Pericarditis
V. Pulmonary
   A. Pulmonary insufficiency
   B. Pneumonia
   C. Bronchitis and/or bronchiectasis
   D. Neoplasms
VI. Renal
   A. Renal insufficiency
   B. Chronic pyelonephritis
   C. Neoplasms
   D. Electrolyte imbalances (alkalosis,
      sodium deficiency)
VII. Endocrine
   A. Pituitary insufficiency
   B. Hypothyroidism
   C. Adrenal insufficiency
   D. Diabetic ketoacidosis
   E. Pregnancy
   F. Hyperparathyroidism
   G. Cyclic vomiting
VIII. Musculoskeletal
   A. Collagen vascular diseases
   B. Alcohol addiction
   C. Amphetamines
   D. Digitalis toxicity
   E. Emetics

here. Neither is vomiting always preceded by nausea. The absence of preceding nausea is often an indication that vomiting is due to posterior pharyngeal irritation, to a cerebral cause, to achalasia, or to habit vomiting.

Acute nausea is usually associated with an acute vomiting illness. Recurring episodes of nausea lasting a few days can be the only symptom of gastric or duodenal ulcer. Nausea as a persisting symptom, without vomiting, should raise the possibility of early tuberculosis, renal failure, anxiety states, or a salt deficiency state. Vomiting as an episode can be due to any acute illness, not necessarily gastrointestinal, or to a functional or nervous condition such as acute anxiety or migraine. The cause is usually indicated by the associated symptoms and signs. It is important to inquire

Table 2. *Laboratory Tests for Anorexia, Nausea, and Vomiting*

I. Infections
   A. Complete blood count (CBC)
   B. Cultures and sensitivity studies
   C. Radiographic studies
II. Gastrointestinal
   A. Radiographic studies
   B. Cytologic examination
   C. Histologic examination of biopsies
   D. Measurement of gastric acid or pancreatic secretion
   E. Endoscopic examination
   F. Angiographic studies
   G. Isotopic scans
   H. Liver function tests
III. Neurologic
   A. Examination of cerebrospinal fluid
   B. Electroencephalogram
   C. Radiographic studies (skull series, pneumoencephalogram, angiography)
   D. Isotopic scans
IV. Cardiovascular
   A. Electrocardiogram
   B. Radiographic studies
   C. Cardiac catheterization
V. Pulmonary
   A. Radiographic studies
   B. Pulmonary function tests
   C. Arterial gas studies
   D. Bacterial and fungal cultures
   E. Cytologic examination
   F. Skin tests
   G. Bronchoscopy
VI. Renal
   A. Urinalysis
   B. Renal function tests
   C. Cytologic radiographic studies
   D. Cytologic examination
   E. Serum electrolytes (including zinc)
VII. Endocrine
   A. Blood sugar
   B. Blood lactate
   C. Blood cortisol
   D. Thyroid, pituitary, and adrenal function tests
   E. Pregnancy test
VIII. Drugs
   A. Measurement of drug levels in serum

---

regarding other people with similar symptoms, the possibility of food poisoning, associated acute diarrhea, and psychologic influences. The acute episode of motion sickness is readily recognized.

Vomiting becomes a problem when it becomes persistent; then the majority of conditions listed in Table 1 may need to be considered. There are four questions that should be asked of the patient.

It is important to know the frequency and forcibility of the vomiting; the relationship of vomiting to meals and time of day; the presence of associated symptoms, particularly nausea and pain; and the quantity and nature of the vomitus. Some common causes of vomiting and their differentiation are listed in Table 3. It is important to remember that the strain of vomiting can easily induce blood streaking and even brisk bleeding (Mallory-Weiss syndrome).

Organic obstruction affecting the alimentary tract will naturally cause vomiting. A good general rule to remember is that vomiting occurs early with high obstruction and late with low obstruction. The absence of nausea may indicate an esophageal condition, but nausea may be absent also in the effortless vomiting of pyloric obstruction or low intestinal obstruction. Obstruction may be due to mechanical, vascular, or inflammatory cause. Peptic ulcer may be manifested with recurrent vomiting, sometimes without associated pain; when there is pain the patient may obtain relief by the induction of vomiting. Vomiting of bile without food is a feature of afferent-loop

Table 3. *Differential Features of Some Common Causes of Vomiting*

	Onset, Duration, and Character	Character of Vomitus	Associated Findings	Key Lab Data
GASTROINTESTINAL DISORDERS				
Pyloric obstruction	Long time after meals; often nocturnal; projectile in infants	Retained food from previous meals	Ulcer history; succussion splash	Large volume aspirate; hypochromic, hypokalemic alkalosis
Gastric cancer	Gradual onset; initially after heavy meals; free periods	Normal gastric contents, bile, blood or "coffee grounds"	Belching, early satiety; anemia; lymphadenopathy	X-ray and/or endoscopy
Alcoholic gastritis	Begins during or shortly after alcohol binge, lasts hours or days	Much mucus and bile; may be fresh blood	Signs of present and past alcohol abuse	Early endoscopy (usually unnecessary)
Intestinal obstruction	Sudden onset; persists till obstruction relieved	First food, then bile, then fecal-smelling material	Colicky pain, constipation, diffuse tenderness, increased bowel sounds, visible peristalsis	X-ray
Biliary colic	Sudden onset	Normal contents	Pain in RUQ radiating to back and shoulder; chills; cholangitis; jaundice	X-ray
Pancreatitis	Sudden	Normal contents	History of alcohol or biliary disease; severe pain; shock	Elevated amylase; peritoneal aspirate
CENTRAL NERVOUS SYSTEM DISORDERS				
Brain tumor	Sudden or gradual onset; no nausea	Normal contents	Headache; fits; neurologic signs	CT scan
Brain abscess	Same as for tumor	Normal contents	Headache; fever; ear problems; history of trauma	CT scan
Meniere's	Sudden onset	Normal contents	Tinnitus and hearing loss	Caloric tests and audiometry
Migraine	Gradual onset	Normal contents	Unilateral headache; sensory abnormalities	Relieved by parenteral ergotamine
Digitalis intoxication	Sudden onset	Normal contents	Cardiac findings; diarrhea	ECG abnormal
SYSTEMIC DISORDERS				
Diabetic acidosis	Gradual; increasing	Normal contents	Lassitude; polyuria, polydipsia; epigastric pain; acetone smell, Kussmaul breathing	Blood glucose, ketones high, and acidosis present
Uremia	Frequent and recurrent often before breakfast	Normal contents; blood terminally	Kussmaul breathing; lassitude; nocturia	Elevated BUN and creatinine

stasis in the postgastrectomy patient. Reflex ileus, with nausea and vomiting, can occur with any intra-abdominal inflammation, including pelvic inflammatory disease and pyelonephritis.

Metabolic causes of vomiting are easily overlooked if too much attention is given to the alimentary tract. All sodium deficiency states cause vomiting. These include diarrhea, chronic aspiration of intestinal contents, salt-losing renal disease, hypoadrenalism, and hypopituitarism. Potassium retention will also produce vomiting and is most commonly due to renal failure. Liver failure is often characterized early on by nausea and vomiting and in the preicteric phase of infectious hepatitis these may be the only symptoms.

Pregnancy is a cause of vomiting to be remembered during the reproductive period of life. It is not uncommon for the diagnosis to be made in the outpatient department of a hospital to which the patient has come because of her "gastric" symptoms.

Nervous or habit vomiting is a quite definite syndrome, usually occurring soon after eating but characteristically unassociated with weight loss. In some patients it is undoubtedly one manifestation of a hysterical personality but in others it seems to be a simple habit developed initially under some emotional strain. A form of nervous vomiting that responds readily to simple management is the early morning sickness associated with anxiety and preceded by bouts of coughing, during which air is swallowed, and introspective habits such as intensive tongue inspection and overly brisk teeth brushing.

GASTROINTESTINAL BLEEDING

By ERWIN LEVIN, M.A., M.D.
Cleveland, Ohio

INTRODUCTION

Massive hemorrhage or occult bleeding into the alimentary tract may be due to many different causes. Bleeding into the gastrointestinal tract, either occult or massive, should be investigated thoroughly, as it definitely reflects pathology. Fortunately, during the last decade testing methods for diagnosis of gastrointestinal bleeding have been so developed that the cause can be readily determined in the majority of patients. There still remains about 10 per cent of patients in whom no cause can be determined in spite of all diagnostic measures, including surgical exploration and even postmortem examination.

OCCULT BLEEDING OR GRADUAL BLEEDING

As a rule, patients are unaware that they are losing small amounts of blood in the gastrointestinal tract. Only after prolonged blood loss will they seek medical help for symptoms such as malaise and easy fatigability. Easy fatigability is present in the morning and increases as the day proceeds. Individuals with cardiovascular disease may complain of angina, palpitations, and dyspnea. As soon as the diagnosis of iron deficiency anemia is established, stools should be checked for occult blood by one of the various commercial methods available. If positive, especially if the patient is on a red meat–free diet, a careful gastrointestinal investigation should be undertaken. A history, however vague, may give an important clue as to the source. A history of dyspepsia, heartburn, recurrent upper epigastric distress relieved by food or milk, immediate postprandial substernal pain in recumbent position with no evidence of weight loss or decrease in appetite are all highly suggestive, but not conclusive, of benign disease of the upper gastrointestinal tract, such as peptic ulcer or hiatal hernia with reflux esophagitis. On the other hand, a history of the recent onset of dysphagia, pain aggravated by eating, loss of appetite, and weight loss are usually associated with tumors of the upper gastrointestinal tract. A careful history of drug ingestion such as aspirin-containing compounds or reserpine may explain the blood loss. Abdominal cramps, chronic diarrhea, weight loss, and recurrent low-grade fever can indicate inflammatory disease of the small intestine or colon. Patients with colonic tumors, especially those of the cecum, can present with iron deficiency anemia in the absence of bowel symptoms.

All patients with chronic secondary anemia should first have a digital rectal examination and proctosigmoidoscopic examination to eliminate the rectosigmoid area as the source of bleeding. Fifty to 67 per cent of colorectal cancers are within reach of the sigmoidoscope and 6 to 10 per cent of polyps are found with this procedure. If proctosigmoidoscopy is negative, barium enema with air contrast should be done and if this is negative, an upper gastrointestinal series with small bowel follow-through should be performed. If the barium studies do not reveal the source of bleeding, fiberoptic endoscopic examination is definitely indicated. The history and physical examination in these patients may indicate whether to examine the upper or lower gastrointestinal tract initially. Usually esophagogastroduodenoscopy is done first when no clue is obtained from the investigation to date. The procedure is relatively easy and safe when performed by an experienced endoscopist. Pathology that is difficult to detect by x-ray, such as reflux esophagitis, erosive gastritis, shallow erosions, or early carcinoma of the esophagus or stomach, may be frequently seen during endoscopic examination. Patients with gastric ulcers on a rigid medical program who persistently show occult blood in the stools should have upper gastrointestinal endoscopy with biopsy, as these ulcers may be malignant.

If the upper gastrointestinal tract is found to be normal after all of the tests mentioned, colonoscopy is indicated. It is reported to disclose the actual or probable bleeding source in 40 per cent of patients with unexplained rectal bleeding. The common sources are small cancers or polyps not disclosed by barium enema and benign-appearing diverticula. Patients who have jaundice that waxes and wanes with intermittent occult blood in the stools should be considered for endoscopic retrograde cholangiopancreatography (ERCP) because malignancy of the ampulla of Vater is strongly indicated.

On occasion, unsuspected cases of hereditary hemorrhagic telangiectasis, carcinoid, and Crohn's disease of stomach and cecum are discovered with endoscopy.

To date, there is no conclusive evidence that computerized axial tomography, selective angiography, or echography is of much aid in making a diagnosis of undetected occult bleeding.

ACUTE GASTROINTESTINAL BLEEDING

Acute bleeding is probably the most frequent critical emergency of the gastrointestinal tract confronting both internists and surgeons. The diagnosis of the source may be both demanding and complicated. Localizing the general area, as in differentiating between upper and lower gastrointestinal bleeding, can usually be determined by a good history and physical examination alone. During the past decade, techniques have been developed whereby it is possible to find not only the exact location but also the cause, in spite of the fact that there are 45 to 50 causes. The cause in the majority is intrinsic gastrointestinal disease. Hematemesis and melena as a rule indicate the source of bleeding originating above the ligament of Treitz. The description of the vomitus may be of some help. Vomiting of bright red blood or blood clots usually indicates active massive bleeding, while coffee-ground material may indicate a slower bleeding process or old blood in the stomach from a very recent hemorrhage. Melanotic stools are tarry stools, pitch black, caused by blood coming in contact with free hydrochloric acid secreted by parietal cells located in the fundus of the stomach. One also notes melanotic stools in patients bleeding from Meckel's diverticulum containing ectopic parietal cells. One should not mistake melanotic stools for the dark-gray stools noted after the ingestion of dark green vegetables, bismuth, or iron-containing compounds. Frequently the dark mahogany stool seen in lower gastrointestinal bleeding is described as "tarry or black." Here again if the latter is examined carefully a red sheen is seen or when placed on filter paper a red zone appears. Blood arising from the transverse colon and distally is almost always bright red and blood clots may be seen in the stool.

A careful history is essential. The knowledge of the presence of previous uncomplicated gastrointestinal disease such as peptic ulcer, hiatal hernia, cirrhosis of liver, inflammatory bowel disease, diverticuli, or ulcerative colitis is helpful. A history of previous gastrointestinal bleeding increases the possibility that the patient is bleeding from the same lesion. However, in certain instances this may be misleading. For example, alcoholics known to have bled previously from esophageal varices may present with bleeding from alcoholic gastritis or peptic ulcer.

The presence or absence of pain and the nature of the pain if present prior to the onset of bleeding may suggest the source of bleeding. Peptic ulceration may produce characteristic epigastric pain for several days or weeks prior to the onset of hemorrhage. Vomiting of food and severe retching prior to hematemesis may indicate a Mallory-Weiss tear.

A drug history such as ingestion of aspirin, corticosteroids, anticoagulants, antimetabolites, alcohol, and many others on a regular or irregular basis is frequently associated with erosive gastritis. Cancer patients receiving chemotherapy have an increased risk to bleeding from gastritis.

Significant findings on physical examination such as jaundice, hepatosplenomegaly, ecchymosis, ascites, and telangiectasia are signs of chronic liver disease; they suggest the presence of esophageal varices. Retinal angioid streaks, papular lesions in skin folds, telangiectasia of mucous membranes with history of recurrent hemorrhage may indicate blood loss from vascular malformation in the wall of the gastrointestinal tract.

A history of upper respiratory pulmonary disease should be ruled out, as hematemesis can occur following the swallowing of blood from these areas. Although many possibilities exist, it should be recognized that 70 to 80 per cent of all cases of upper gastrointestinal hemorrhage are caused by any one of four lesions, namely peptic ulcer, hemorrhagic gastritis, esophagogastric varices, or Mallory-Weiss syndrome. Each one of these carries a different prognosis and for this reason the specific bleeding site should be determined.

What were once considered less frequent causes of upper gastrointestinal hemorrhage are becoming more common because of prolongation of life of patients with various chronic illnesses such as uremia, blood dyscrasia, and malignancies treated with chemotherapy. Therefore, careful history not only from the patient but also from the family must be obtained.

In most institutions endoscopic examination is the method of choice and most accurate way to localize the source of upper gastrointestinal bleeding. The procedure should be carried out as soon as possible after the patient's condition has been stabilized and bleeding has substantially decreased or ceased. Prompt endoscopy usually indicates the source of bleeding in over 90 per cent of the patients. It is superior to routine x-ray because it can disclose superficial bleeding from gastritis, esophagitis, or tear, whereas x-rays usually will be negative. When there is brisk continued bleeding and the patient is facing imminent major surgery, it is important to perform an endoscopic examination as soon as possible, day or night, and not to wait until stabilization occurs and the bleeding diminishes. It should be pointed out that merely identifying either fresh or old blood in the gastric contents does not tell the specific source of bleeding but only indicates the general area. Endoscopy is indicated in patients who are admitted with history of melena or hematemesis but who show no signs of active bleeding on admission. Frequently a clot is seen at the site of the bleeding.

In about 10 to 15 per cent of cases of massive upper gastrointestinal hemorrhage endoscopy is unsuccessful owing to the presence of a large amount of clots and blood. In such cases selective and subselective celiac and superior mesenteric arteriography will disclose the bleeding site in a significant percentage of patients when performed during active bleeding of over 0.5 ml per minute. Extravasation of the contrast material from the vascular tree into the stomach or small bowel localizes the site of bleeding. In addition, angiographic changes may indicate evidence of unsuspected varices, arteriovenous malformations or other abnormalities that may be the source of bleeding. It is important that no barium is given prior to angiography, because it will obscure the findings. Angiography has the additional benefit of providing a means of controlling bleeding via an intra-arterial infusion of pressor agents.

After the active bleeding has stopped and endoscopic examination has been performed, barium studies of the gastrointestinal tract are indicated. A minor episode of bleeding with minimal blood loss rarely requires aggressive diagnostic measures. Endoscopy may be performed electively and will permit identification of lesions not readily seen by x-ray. Also, in such patients it is unreasonable to postpone a gastrointestinal series while awaiting elective endoscopy. Double or air contrast study of the upper gastrointestinal tract is now gaining popularity. Small amounts of highly concentrated barium and a source of gas or air such as effervescent drink or tablets through a nasogastric tube is used. Small superficial lesions and some signs of active bleeding have been reported in patients in whom routine barium meals have been negative.

Lower gastrointestinal bleeding is the passage per rectum of bright or dark red blood originating below the ligament of Treiz. In all instances evidence of upper gastrointestinal bleeding has been reasonably eliminated in diagnosis. Unfortunately, swift and precise diagnosis as is possible with upper gastrointestinal endoscopy is not generally possible when bleeding occurs from the lower tract.

Again, history is important; however, unlike upper gastrointestinal bleeding, the history seldom provides information to pinpoint a specific cause. Intermittent blood streaking on the surface of the stool suggests a local problem such as anal fissures, hemorrhoids, or neoplastic lesion in the rectum. Severe anemia may be present when the bleeding has continued over a prolonged period of time. Moderate bleeding suggests polyps and colonic malignancy. Colonic diverticula are the leading cause of massive hemorrhage. In young people and children, profuse bleeding suggests a Meckel's diverticulum. In the elderly, sudden massive bleeding accompanied by abdominal pain suggests ischemic colitis, mesenteric infarction, or an intussuscepting lesion. In the young, intermittent bleeding with diarrhea suggests ulcerative colitis or inflammatory bowel disease. Bleeding associated with weight loss or change in bowel habits is frequently indicative of carcinoma of the bowel. Ecchymosis of the skin and purpura may be the first clue to a bleeding diathesis or Henoch-Schönlein disease. A family history of gastrointestinal cancer, colonic polyposis, or Rendu-Osler-Weber syndrome is important. Unfortunately, the general physical examination does not as a rule prove to be very helpful. However, a diligent search for specific clues should be undertaken and may uncover rarer causes. For example, perioral and buccal melanin pigmentation is associated with Peutz-Jeghers syndrome. Ecchymosis or purpura may be indicative of bleeding disorders, Metastatic carcinoma of the colon is frequently associated with enlarged nodular liver. Abrupt onset of abdominal pain and hemorrhage is characteristic of mesenteric embolism secondary to atrial fibrillation. Rarely, an abdominal aneurysm will rupture into the bowel.

Because of the difficulties frequently encountered in pinpointing the exact location of the bleeding point, a systematic diagnostic approach should be followed. When rectal bleeding is significant, aspiration of the gastric contents is essential in order to rule out upper gastrointestinal bleeding. The aspiration should be continued until bile is obtained. Although a negative aspirate under these circumstances does not conclusively rule out upper bleeding, one can proceed to the lower bowel. However, if there still is any doubt, upper gastrointestinal endoscopy should be performed, as a significant percentage of bleeding duodenal ulcers will produce negative aspirates in the presence of massive rectal bleeding.

The rectal examination is an essential part of the immediate work-up and may give an immediate answer. Hemorrhoids, anal fissures, and other inflammatory lesions of the area will be detected.

Following rectal examination, sigmoidoscopy should be done in all patients. The success or failure of this examination depends on whether or not the bleeding has stopped and how rapid the bleeding is at the time. If the bleeding rate is greater than 1 ml per minute, the blood may obstruct vision and make detection of a lesion difficult. However, under ideal conditions, lesions such as rectal polyps, rectal carcinomas, and inflammatory bowel disease, especially ulcerative colitis, can be diagnosed immediately. If no diagnosis is made at this point, the next procedure depends upon the severity of the bleeding. If the hemorrhage has ceased, a barium enema should be obtained as soon as possible. Barium enema with air contrast is the procedure of choice. Colonic polyps, malignancies, ischemic colitis, ulcerative colitis, Crohn's disease, diverticulitis, and other colonic lesions can be detected with regularity.

If the hemorrhage is massive and life-threatening, barium enema will probably be unrevealing; therefore, arteriography should be considered, particularly when surgical intervention is being considered. Here again the procedure must be done while the patient is actively bleeding. In order to identify the bleeding site, the rate of bleeding must be more than 0.5 ml per minute. Aside from pinpointing the bleeding locale, this permits a precise surgical approach. The leading cause of massive rectal bleeding is diverticular disease. In contrast to barium enema, which only confirms the presence of diverticula with no proof that a specific diverticulum is the actual source of blood, arteriography permits localization to a precise region of the colon. Although bleeding will subside in most instances, a number of patients will either continue to bleed or have recurrent bleeding; thus precise localization of the bleeding site is important. In addition, arteriography is helpful in diagnosing bleeding from vascular tumors, arteriovenous malformations, angiodysplastic lesions, and in younger patients from Meckel's diverticulum. Arteriography has the additional advantage of permitting infusion of vasopressor agents directly through the catheter, which is in place. This has been successful in controlling both upper and lower gastrointestinal bleeding.

Colonoscopy can be used to examine the entire colon and should be considered as a necessary adjunct to barium enema. Whenever possible, it should be employed after digital rectal examination, sigmoidoscopy, barium enema, and when the patient's condition is stabilized and massive bleeding has ceased. Colonoscopy does not supplant good radiologic examination and arteriography. Colonoscopy is definitely indicated whenever the previously mentioned studies are negative. This is especially true when in the search for small bowel tumors these tests are followed by a negative upper gastrointestinal series, including a small bowel examination. Colonoscopy has been reported to disclose the probable bleeding source in approximately 30 to 40 per cent of patients having negative barium enemas.

The use of scanning with labeled technetium (^{99m}Tc) has been reported helpful in detecting Meckel's diverticulum. ^{99m}Tc is secreted by the ectopic gastric mucosa. Thus, if a bleeding Meckel's diverticulum is suspected, scanning with ^{99m}Tc offers a simple and safe diagnostic tool.

In a significant percentage of patients with lower gastrointestinal bleeding a specific diagnosis cannot be made in spite of advances in diagnostic techniques. In those patients in whom the bleeding persists, exploratory surgery may be required.

THE ACUTE ABDOMEN IN CHILDHOOD

By STEPHEN L. GANS, M.D., *and* EDWARD AUSTIN, M.D.

Los Angeles, California

A discussion of differential diagnosis of the acute abdomen in childhood is best carried out by considering the causes by age groups. Each period has its own group of problems quite different from the others.

THE NEONATE

In some conditions there is no differential diagnosis per se but the main problems are in their management. These shall be dealt with briefly.

The diagnosis of *omphalocele* or *gastroschisis* is made by inspection.

A neonate with respiratory distress and abdominal distension should be suspected of having *gastrointestinal perforation*. This diagnosis can be established rapidly by the demonstration of free air in the peritoneal cavity by means of a plain film in the upright position.

Necrotizing enterocolitis usually occurs in small and sick preterm infants who often have needed vigorous resuscitation and umbilical vessel cannulation. Peritoneal signs accompany intestinal necrosis, intramural air is seen in the intestines and sometimes in the portal system and intrahepatic portal veins, and finally perforation and free air may appear in the peritoneal cavity. Blood findings associated with disseminated intravascular coagulation are a frequent complication.

Any newborn presenting with vomiting of greenish material or an increased amount of green gastric aspirate, and with absent, scanty, or abnormal stools, must be suspected of an obstruction of some part of the intestinal tract. Abdominal distension may depend on the level of obstruction and the length of time it has existed. Differential diagnosis is an interesting but usually simple problem. It is initiated by getting a plain film of the infant in the upright position. This film will indicate the level of the obstruction and frequently its cause. Three groups of conditions are then considered according to this level.

The first group is duodenal obstructions. If the upright films show the characteristic "double-bubble," signifying air in the stomach and in the duodenum but no air beyond this point, the diagnosis is most likely to be *duodenal atresia*. If on the other hand there are a few bubbles of air beyond the duodenum, this signifies that the obstruction of the duodenum is incomplete. *Duodenal stenosis, annular pancreas, duodenal bands*, and *malrotation* with or without *midgut volvulus* must be considered. No further studies will delineate the first two; indeed, they may even coexist. However, the diagnosis of malrotation can be established or ruled out by barium enema. This is an important thing to do, because of all duodenal obstructions, this is the only one demanding urgent surgery, because vascular compromise of the intestine involved in an associated midgut volvulus may be present. Indeed, blood in the stools of an infant with duodenal obstruction may by itself indicate volvulus.

In the second group, when the upright film of the abdomen shows a few air-filled loops of intestine with air-fluid levels and no air beyond this, the diagnosis is *jejunoileal obstruction*, and the differential diagnosis is between *atresia, stenosis*, or obstruction caused by an abnormal band, usually connecting to the umbilicus. The level can be determined by counting the number of loops or air-fluid levels. There is no way to distinguish between these conditions short of surgical exploration.

The third group of neonatal intestinal obstructions occurs at the level of the distal ileum and the colon. In addition to atresia and stenosis, the other conditions are meconium ileus and aganglionic megacolon (Hirschsprung's disease). A plain film in the upright position will show many air-filled loops of intestine. If air-fluid levels are not present, the diagnosis will most likely be meconium ileus. A Gastrografin enema will demonstrate a microcolon and will often also be therapeutic in that it may wash out the obstructing plugs. If air-fluid levels are present, meconium ileus can usually be ruled out, but a Gastrografin enema is again indicated for further differential diagnosis. The findings of atresia and stenosis are self-evident. In aganglionic megacolon, it may be possible to demonstrate the characteristic narrow rectum and colon, opening up to a normal caliber proximally.

This method of differential diagnosis of intestinal obstruction in the newborn is based on the use of plain films in the upright position. The use of radiopaque material is limited to the specified indications and it is always introduced through the anus. The method is simple, logical, quite accurate, rapid, and safe.

Further differential points are associated with complications of these conditions. Calcified areas in the peritoneal cavity may be present if there has been an intrauterine perforation of the bowel and meconium peritonitis. In the newborn, failure to make a diagnosis and to initiate supportive measures and definitive treatment may result in dehydration, necrosis of bowel with perforation and peritonitis, with all of the associated symptoms and findings.

INFANCY

After the newborn period, those conditions incompatible with life without correction have been eliminated from consideration. Still held over are late-appearing necrotizing enterocolitis, aganglionic megacolon, and malrotation with or without volvulus. The signs and symptoms are similar to those in the neonate.

Appearing usually at 2 to 4 weeks of age is the gastric obstruction due to *hypertrophic pyloric stenosis.* The history is that of increasing vomiting, usually becoming projectile, ordinarily colorless or resembling a recent feeding, and occasionally blood-stained or coffee ground in appearance. The infant will become dehydrated, with a hypochloremic hypokale-

mic alkalosis developing in late stages if untreated. Observation of gastric waves, palpation of a pyloric tumor, and the characteristic appearance of an upper gastrointestinal study by x-ray will establish the diagnosis and rule out other conditions.

Rarely occuring in infancy are appendicitis and Meckel's diverticulitis. These are discussed in the section covered in the "childhood" period.

Intussusception occurs most commonly from 2 months to 2 years of age. It is characterized by crampy intermittent severe abdominal pain alternating with periods in which the infant appears quiet, listless, perhaps pale, and even "shocky." Blood may appear in the stools in any form and a mass may be palpated in the abdomen, usually in the right upper or mid abdomen. Barium enema is now indicated in most instances because frequently it is therapeutic as well as diagnostic when carried out properly. The diagnostic picture is that of a partial or complete obstruction with a "coiled spring" or "inverted goblet" appearance. The differential diagnosis is from crampy constipation or gastroenteritis; this will be settled by the plain film and barium enema when necessary.

Appearing in any age group, but quite frequently in this one, is the abdominal pain and sometimes vomiting associated with an incarcerated or strangulated inguinal, or rarely umbilical hernia. The appearance is obvious.

CHILDHOOD

The most common cause of the acute abdomen in children is appendicitis and this must be primary in making a diagnosis until another source is positively identified. Appendicitis is a much more serious disease in children because the rupture rate is higher, which in turn produces higher morbidity and mortality. Making an accurate diagnosis of acute appendicitis in children is more difficult because of the difficulty in obtaining an informative history and the variability of presenting signs and symptoms. Children with abdominal pain are frequently unable to communicate their distress to adults, who may delay in bringing the child to the physician. Children with appendicitis initially show symptoms of pain, irritability, listlessness, and anorexia, and almost always develop vomiting before medical help is obtained. At this point it is not uncommon for the appendix to have already ruptured or be nearly to that point.

When the child with abdominal pain is seen, it is important to ask about the duration and continuity of pain and if it alters his normal daytime behavior or stops him from play. A child with acute appendicitis frequently limps to avoid stretching the psoas muscle and has marked increase of pain when required to jump or hop.

Steady abdominal pain persisting for over 6 hours is not likely to be due to *gastroenteritis*, which is characterized by crampy abdominal pain and diarrhea. When diarrhea is a presenting complaint, it is important to know if any family members or friends have similar complaints.

Constipation may be a presenting symptom, but it is so common in children that its presence or absence does not contribute aid in making the diagnosis of appendicitis. A child may have abdominal pain without vomiting, a soft abdomen, and an x-ray that shows a colon filled with stool; the diagnosis of appendicitis is not likely in this case.

Examination of the child with appendicitis is a challenge. Localization of tenderness to the right lower quadrant may be elicited from the older child verbally. The younger child must be distracted and close assessment of his reactions to palpation is necessary. After gently listening for bowel sounds, deeper palpation with the head of the stethoscope may be helpful. Many children will become hysterical the minute the physician enters the room, and under such circumstances an adequate examination is impossible. A moderate dose of analgesic or sedative followed by sufficient time for it to take effect will aid immeasurably in assessing the acute abdomen and will not mask the findings of appendicitis.

Muscle rigidity or involuntary guarding in the right lower quadrant is a significant sign. If the appendix has ruptured and peritonitis is present, a generalized rigidity may be appreciated. A mass palpated in the right lower quadrant may indicate rupture and organization of a periappendiceal abscess. The constipated child may also present with a right lower quadrant abdominal mass that is less tender and is distinguishable on x-ray. Bowel sounds may be diminished in early appendicitis, especially when the patient is vomiting. Rectal examination without sedation in the young child is difficult and the findings usually are equivocal. The presence of a mass is significant when noted.

The temperature and pulse rate in a child with appendicitis are usually elevated slightly, although both may be normal in many cases. The white blood cell count may also be normal, but, appendicitis is unlikely if the temperature, pulse, and white blood cell count are all normal.

Acutely ill children with abdominal pain and equivocal abdominal findings should have a plain x-ray film taken of the abdomen. This study occasionally shows a fecalith lying within the area of the appendix, but more often the gas distribution and amount of stool may suggest an alternative diagnosis. At times, an intravenous pyelogram is helpful to rule out *genitourinary tract conditions* and may show medial displacement of the right ureter or a right pelvic mass that had not been palpable by either abdominal or rectal examination. Abdominal and pelvic ultrasound studies may also demonstrate a cystic or solid mass and do not expose the child to x-rays. *Ovarian cysts* and *tumors* are especially amenable to ultrasound diagnosis. In occasional circumstances when all diagnostic criteria are equivocal and an adequate period of observation has elapsed without improvement, laparoscopy has proved to be a useful tool for establishing the correct diagnosis.

Primary peritonitis has become a rare occurrence in children since the advent of antibiotics, except in patients with nephrosis. The pain can be extremely severe and the patient extremely ill with dehydration, high fever, and rapid pulse rate. The abdomen is boardlike and often distended. Except in known nephrotic patients, exploratory laparotomy or laparoscopy may be the only means by which primary peritonitis can be distinguished from a ruptured appendix.

Of the many nonsurgical conditions that must be differentiated from appendicitis, the most common are gastroenteritis and acute mesenteric adenitis. In *gastroenteritis* the clinical presentation is variable; the onset is apt to be slow, the pain crampy, and vomiting is more frequent and diarrhea more pronounced. Abdominal tenderness is usually diffuse and involuntary guarding is absent. If the tenderness does not resolve after a suitable period of observation and rehydration, usually 6 to 12 hours, an appendiceal perforation should be suspected.

Mesenteric adenitis is one of the most common causes of abdominal pain in childhood. Typically, the pain is preceded by an upper respiratory tract infection, begins in the right lower quadrant, and is not persistent, Vomiting is not severe. Temperature elevation, pulse rate, and leukocytosis are more pronounced in relation to the physical signs. Gradual improvement over a period of observation and hydration will differentiate this condition from appendicitis.

Acute pyelonephritis and *renal calculi* will present as acute abdominal pain on occasion.

Examination of the urine and intravenous pyelogram will help in diagnosing these conditions. A chest x-ray should be performed if the cause of pain is unclear, and may demonstrate *pneumonia* as the cause. *Sickle cell crisis* should be suspected in patients with a family history of this disease and may be documented by laboratory studies.

Acute cholecystitis is a rare condition during childhood. The pain and tenderness occur in the right upper abdomen and are exacerbated by eating. A tender mass may be palpated below the right costal margin. Elevation in serum bilirubin and liver enzymes points toward this diagnosis, which is confirmed by oral or intravenous cholecystogram or ultrasound examination.

The diagnosis of *regional ileitis* is very often made at the time of exploratory laparotomy. Children with repeated bouts of colicky abdominal pain, diarrhea, and unexplained fevers should have a small bowel study if this condition is considered, especially when there is a positive family history.

Blunt abdominal trauma is a frequent cause of the acute abdomen in children. History of injury is almost always available in the conscious adult, but a child will sometimes refuse to admit injury for fear of punishment or to protect a playmate who has been his assailant. Most children hospitalized for abdominal trauma will have sustained their injuries in pedestrian or automobile accidents, bicycle and skateboard incidents, or in a fall.

Abdominal contusion, without visceral injury, may be severe enough to cause abdominal pain, tenderness, rigidity, and even vomiting. The patient may have hypoactive or absent bowel sounds and even a transient leukocytosis. The only way abdominal contusion can be differentiated from more serious injury is by close observation and repeated evaluation.

The most commonly injured intra-abdominal organs are the spleen, liver, and kidneys. Hemorrhage from a tear in the spleen or liver will present initially as localized tenderness at the site of injury, progressing to generalized tenderness and rigidity. Continuous monitoring of the pulse rate, blood pressure, serum hemoglobin level, and serial examinations will indicate whether surgical intervention is required or not. Peritoneal tap or lavage may document the presence of intra-abdominal hemorrhage, but these findings are not absolute criteria for exploratory laparotomy. Diagnostic laparoscopy is a useful procedure in the patient with multiple injuries, especially when a depressed sensorium may obscure abdominal signs and symptoms.

Children with blunt abdominal trauma and hematuria should always have a cystogram and intravenous pyelogram to determine the severity of injury to the kidneys, ureters, and bladder. A retroperitoneal hematoma may also be demonstrated by displacement of the kidneys or ureters.

THE ACUTE ABDOMEN IN ADULTS

By ROBERT P. DAVIS, M.D.
Chicago, Illinois

INTRODUCTION

One of the most challenging clinical entities is the diagnosis and management of the acute abdomen in adults. Its diagnosis requires a thorough knowledge of anatomy, physiology, and pathology. When the signs and symptoms are classical, the diagnosis is made easily, but more often than not this is not the case and the full breadth of the clinician's knowledge and judgment must be utilized.

Initial evaluation generally elucidates the cause as secondary to inflammation, obstruction, hemorrhage, or trauma. Laboratory data, including a complete blood count (CBC), urinalysis, and appropriate roentgenographic studies, should be considered for substantiation of the diagnosis. In every instance, the ultimate decision reached must address the question of whether or not operative intervention is necessary. Depending on the nature of the abdominal process and the time interval involved, the timing of operative intervention may be critical. Occasionally, an exploratory laparotomy may be the only way to make the diagnosis. Therefore, at the very least, the responsible physician must be able to determine whether or not an abdominal surgical condition is present.

CLINICAL EVALUATION

The meticulous and complete historical evaluation of any patient presenting with an acute abdomen is mandatory. Almost invariably the presenting symptom is pain. The mode of onset of the pain is often most elucidating. The acute onset of pain in a patient with a perforated ulcer is exceedingly dramatic (the patient can often state the exact time that the pain began), while on the other extreme, the vague onset of mid abdominal discomfort associated with an acute appendicitis is less dramatic.

The character of the pain may provide additional information. Colicky pain is almost invariably related to the contraction of a hollow viscus against an obstruction, as in ureteral lithiasis, the colic of obstructed bowel, and the colic of an impacted gallstone. More constant pain is generally present in the inflammatory process associated with such entities as appendicitis or diverticulitis.

Probably the most important aspect of the patient's pain is its location. For practical purposes, the abdomen may be divided in half. Those conditions producing pain above the umbilicus are generally secondary to a pathologic process involving the upper abdomen, while pain below the umbilicus is almost invariably related to organs of the lower abdomen. Only occasionally may one be misled by the lower right quadrant pain caused by irritating material that has leaked through a perforated ulcer and run down the right gutter.

The anatomic distribution of the gastrointestinal tract intervention makes conditions involving these organs more understandable. The midgut from the stomach to the right half of the transverse colon carries the same autonomic intervention and visceral pain is therefore reflected into the mid abdomen; on the other hand, the hindgut from the left half of the transverse colon to the rectum is innervated by sacral nerves arising from the pelvis. Inflammation of the parietal peritoneum is carried via somatic fibers of the spinal cord and is better localized to a specific quadrant. The radiation of the pain further elucidates this concept. The initial pain of acute appendicitis is periumbilical; this inflammatory process is visceral and is mediated via the autonomic nerves of the midgut. As the parietal peritoneum becomes inflamed over the appendix, the pain begins to radiate to the right lower quadrant; this pain is somatic and is carried through nerve fibers of the spinal cord. Similarly, the pain of pancreatitis radiates to the back, while inflammatory processes or traumatic accidents of the right and left upper quadrants may radiate to the respective shoulders.

The associated symptoms often may be helpful. A change in bowel habits with significant weight loss may be present in a patient with an underlying malignancy that has presented with an acute bowel obstruction. Conversely, an antecedent history of diarrhea may make one suspect regional enteritis. Bloody diarrhea in a patient with excruciating abdominal pain may suggest an acute vascular accident. Clay-colored stools in a patient with right upper quadrant pathology is highly suggestive of choledocholithiasis and possible ascending cholangitis. In general, nausea and vomiting are less specific and are subsequently not often helpful in diagnosis.

The careful physical examination is an essential part of the clinical evaluation of a patient with an acute abdomen. Prior to palpation, the clinician should first inspect the abdomen, taking note of previous surgical incisions, and whether it is distended or scaphoid. Then auscultation should be performed. The knowledge of the presence or absence of bowel sounds is essential. If bowel sounds are present, their character must be known. Rushes and tinkles with a distended abdomen are diagnostic of obstruction. If bowel sounds are totally absent, the possibility of an ileus or frank peritonitis exists. Again, prior to palpation, the patient should be asked to point with one finger to the site of maximal tenderness and then palpation may be begun, generally in a quadrant removed from this point. In this way, knowledge of the remainder of the abdomen can be gained prior to accentuating the patient's pain by direct palpation. The presence of point tenderness and guarding or rebound, or both, should all be noted. This is particularly important in a patient in whom the diagnosis is unclear and subsequent examinations are to be employed. A rectal examination, and a pelvic examination in a female, should be performed even though the diagnosis may be obvious and not related to these structures. If the rectal examination in a female demonstrates an exquisitely painful cervix on manipulation, a pelvic examination is mandatory, for pelvic inflammatory disease is likely to be present. If the patient is to be operated upon, a repeat physical examination of the abdomen should always be performed following general anesthesia. This examination is often quite helpful in elucidating the presence of a mass previously undetected owing to the contraction of the abdominal musculature.

LABORATORY DATA

A complete blood count (CBC), urinalysis, and SMA–18 are generally a part of the routine admission blood test. Similarly, a roentgenogram of the chest and electrocardiogram should be a component of the routine admission work-up. In addition, a serum amylase value should be obtained in every patient with acute abdominal pain. If trauma is present or blood loss suspected, type and cross-match should be requested with the initial blood sample. In all women of childbearing age, pregnancy must be tested for.

An electrocardiogram should be obtained to eliminate myocardial disease as the cause of upper abdominal pain and to establish whether pre-existent myocardial disease is present.

Roentgenograms of the patient may be useful. An upright chest film is extremely valuable, for it eliminates the possibility of pneumonia mimicking an inflammatory process in the abdomen, but, more importantly, it is the best examination to locate free air under the diaphragm. Abdominal films are helpful in patients with bowel obstruction, for they often help delineate the level of obstruction. The presence of air-fluid levels provides additional information, while the presence of air throughout the gastrointestinal tract is more compatible with a paralytic ileus. Additional information can often be obtained, such as the presence of a fecalith, a ureteral calculus, or, in 10 per cent of patients, a calcified gallstone.

Further diagnostic information may be provided noninvasively by ultrasound examination of the abdomen. It may elucidate the presence of an undetected appendiceal abscess, an ovarian cyst that has undergone torsion, a pancreatic pseudocyst, or cholelithiasis.

Barium studies are not generally indicated in most patients with inflammatory disease. However, prior to any contemplated barium studies, the patient should have a proctoscope examination. Similarly, if pathology is thought to be present in the urinary tract, an intravenous pyelogram must be obtained. Gentle barium enemas may be useful to reveal the cause of large bowel obstruction but are not indicated in acute diverticulitis. Visualization of the appendix eliminates the possibility of acute appendicitis in most instances, and numerous clinicians have used this procedure in the atypical case. Further invasive procedures such as arteriography should be used only for selected patients. Colpocentesis is often useful in the patient with pelvic disease in which further information is to be gathered preoperatively. The computerized axial tomography (CT) scan is a diagnostic procedure rarely necessary in the patient with acute abdomen.

PYURIA

By LESTER KARAFIN, M.D.,
and A. RICHARD KENDALL, M.D.
Philadelphia, Pennsylvania

DEFINITION

By definition, pyuria is the presence of white blood cells in the urine. Significant numbers of leukocytes in the urine in a centrifuged specimen are usually more than 5 white blood cells (WBCs) per high power field in the male and 3 to 5 in the female.

A cloudy urine may be caused by crystals and does not necessarily signify pyuria. The finding of white blood cells in the urine cannot be considered pathognomonic of bacteriuria; however, it is suggestive. Clumps of these cells may indicate a more severe urinary tract infection.

METHOD OF COLLECTION OF URINE SPECIMENS

Urinalyses should be conducted by the physician himself or a reliable paramedic on a properly collected specimen without delay.

In the female, a midstream clean-catch specimen obtained after a thorough cleansing of the vagina and spreading of the labia during urination is sufficient. Suprapubic and needle aspiration or catheterization may be needed to rule out the source of the pyuria. Rather than labeling the condition a urinary tract infection merely because of pyuria or bacteriuria in a voided specimen, it is safer to catheterize the patient to establish exactly what is going on.

In the male, it is much easier to obtain a reliable specimen. The patient should be instructed to void into two separate glasses with a continuous flow into the second glass. Sometimes a third glass specimen is taken so that the area of the vesicle neck and prostate can be evaluated. The third glass specimen can be obtained after the prostate has been massaged. The first glass usually represents the urethral flora, the second glass consists of the bladder and kidney urine, while the third glass after prostatic massage contains the prostatic washes. Once again, it is important to have the specimen examined promptly and by the urologist or an experienced paramedic.

DIFFERENTIAL DIAGNOSIS OF THOSE CONDITIONS CAUSING PYURIA

Pyuria almost always indicates an infection or inflammation of the urogenital system. However, bacteria must be demonstrated by stain or culture in order to make a diagnosis of a urinary tract infection. Remember that pus in the urine of a female can be from contamination caused by vaginal disease and in the male from secretions around the foreskin. Pyuria can signify the presence of residual urine.

A special situation in which pyuria is found without bacteria in the urine (sterile pyuria) indicates a tuberculous infection; special cultures have to be done. Virus infections can produce pyuria as well as irritation secondary to trauma of instrumentation, a foreign body, or a silent calculus. Prostatitis can produce pus in the bladder that appears in the voided urine but is not part of the urinary tract infection. Another point is that antibacterial medication can eliminate the bacteria but pus will persist for a number of days.

Pyuria is usually associated with symptoms; however, it may not be. A chronic upper tract inflammatory disease such as in pyelonephritis can result in pyuria without symptoms. Any obstructive uropathy either of the upper tract or in the bladder will produce the same thing. An important point is that marked renal infections producing a great deal of pyuria may not show in the urine because of complete ureteral or ureteral-pelvic occlusion.

Another category of disease possibly producing a secondary inflammation of the bladder and subsequent pyuria is pelvic inflammatory disease, including ovarian abscess, seminal vesicle and prostatic abscesses, and appendiceal and intestinal disease. There may be fistulas between the bowel and the bladder that produce abnormal findings in the urine. Abnormalities in the bladder such as tumor, stone, or diverticulum can be associated with pyuria. Simple hypertrophy of the prostate with residual urine and pyuria can be present. The lower urinary tract when affected by conditions such as prostatitis and seminal vesiculitis and inflammation of Skene's, Cowper's, and Littre's glands is also a possibility.

As far as the upper tracts are concerned, any obstructing type of disease such as stones, tumor, and hydronephrosis may produce pyuria, as also may acute inflammatory disease such as pyelonephritis, pyonephrosis, and tuberculosis.

If these causes are not considered, they will not be differentiated. If cystoscopy is done, the source of the pyuria may have to be ascertained by passing a ureteral catheter and obtaining a specimen from each kidney. This will help in localizing the source of the infection. Recurrent attacks of pyuria in a female after intercourse can be related to the urethra and the actual manipulation that occurs during coitus. Voiding after intercourse and medical prophylaxis can be prescribed.

SUMMARY

Pyuria is a sign of urologic disease, either primary or secondary. Thorough evaluation for the presence or absence of bacteria is extremely important, and an anatomic abnormality should be sought. The method of obtaining the specimen is vital and will help in the differential diagnosis. A complete urologic examination and survey is indicated in anyone who has persistent pyuria.

FATIGUE

By MICHAEL J. HALBERSTAM, M.D.
Washington, D.C.

If you would like to know the epidemiology, differential diagnosis, and prognosis of fatigue as the presenting symptom in office practice, don't bother checking the standard medical literature. I have, and it's worthless. There is no more telling indictment of academic medicine and its separation from the real world of patient care than the articles listed under "Fatigue" in *Index Medicus*. Therein are listed for each year a host of articles on muscle physiology ("Aldolase activity during fatigue in isolated muscles of frog, *Rana hexadactyla*") and on clinical psychology ("Effect of fatigue and alcohol on observer perception"), but next to nothing on fatigue in clinical practice. During the years 1966 to 1978 not a single article appeared with any actual data on the outcome of tired patients. This article attempts to remedy this lack.

Fatigue is one of the most common presenting symptoms in a clinician's office. Variants of "I just don't seem to have any energy," "I'm tired all the time," and "I don't seem to be able to get out of bed," are extremely common as the spontaneously expressed chief complaint. Furthermore, many patients who present with symptoms ostensibly related to another system ("I think I have the flu") quickly sort themselves into the category of fatigue. (The "flu" turns out to be of 6 months' duration and characterized not by cough or fever, but by loss of energy.)

In an attempt to quantify the picture of fatigue in the office practice of internal medicine, I kept a running score sheet of new patients over a 2-month period. In addition, I asked two internist colleagues of mine, with separate practices and with different patient populations, to keep track of patients presenting with fatigue. They (and others) were asked to recall cases in which unexplained fatigue was eventually linked to organic disease.

From this study (which is continuing), certain facts emerged that should come as no surprise to the primary care physician, but that should be helpful in formulating a systematic approach to fatigue.

AN APPROACH TO DIAGNOSIS

1. In office practice, fatigue as the sole or major presenting symptom is overwhelmingly due to psychologic disarray, usually depression.

2. The history will indicate the correct diagnosis in over 90 per cent of the patients.

3. When the history is equivocal, the basic laboratory tests will establish the diagnosis in all but a handful of the remaining patients.

4. Despite the massive predominance of psychologic factors as the cause of primary fatigue, occasional cases are caused by unsuspected organic illness. Some of the more common of these rarities are discussed below.

Primary Causes. The clinician's empiric observation that most primary fatigue is caused by depression was borne out in my office study. Of 38 patients presenting with fatigue and its variants, only one had organic disease. My practice is an urban one, canted toward young-to-middle-aged patients, about 60:40 white and black, predominantly middle class with a smaller proportion of blue-collar workers. There are no active farmers, ranchers, or factory workers in the patient population. The practices of my two colleagues vary somewhat from mine in patient age and social background, but not in occupation. While figures are not available from their practices, their observations support the notion that depression is by far the commonest cause of fatigue. Simple overwork as a cause of fatigue is rare in my experience — most people enjoy hard work and recognize the physiologic fatigue that accompanies it. It is

the man who is underworked and bored who is more likely to bring his fatigue to a doctor's attention.

Importance of the History. The history usually makes the diagnosis. When "lack of energy" is the chief complaint, when it has been present over a month, when it is unaccompanied by weight loss, documented fever (not "I feel like I've got a low-grade temperature"), when there has been no persistent localized pain, when there has been no other dramatic change in the systems review, psychologic factors are almost surely the cause. Look for a recent loss or separation in the patient's life.

It is crucial in history-taking to make sure that you and the patient are talking about the same thing. In particular, the patient should be questioned specifically about whether "tiredness" means generalized fatigue or localized muscle aching. The other crucial distinction is between fatigue and shortness of breath. Of course, some patients with severe cardiorespiratory disease complain primarily of "breathlessness." This is often the equivalent of dyspnea at rest. Genuine fatigue of over a month's duration without any other evidence of systemic illness is rarely caused by organic disease. There are, however, instances in which the history can keep one pointed in the direction of somatic illness. These will be discussed.

Role of Laboratory Testing. While the history may strongly suggest depression and while the physical examination may be, and usually is, unrevealing, the patient presenting with persistent fatigue deserves an appropriate laboratory work-up. Anemia, hypocalcemia, hypokalemia, uremia, and hypothyroidism in their earlier or less severe forms may all be apparent on laboratory tests and not on physical examination. I have seen experienced clinicians examine a patient with a hematocrit of 30 ml per dl and fail to detect any physical evidence of anemia. I've done so myself, particularly with blacks and Orientals. Renal failure can creep up insidiously with no localizing signs or symptoms until a creatinine of 3.0 is detected on a "routine" scan. Significant adult-onset diabetes (not merely a 2-hour after meal glucose of 160, but 300 or 350) can present without polyuria, polydipsia, or weight loss. Besides a urinalysis, a chest x-ray can be unexpectedly helpful. Hodgkin's disease, sarcoid, and malignancies may all shout their presence from a chest x-ray in the total absence of any pulmonary symptoms.

These tests — complete blood count with sedimentation rate, sequential multiple analysis (SMA), electrolytes, urine, x-ray — are the basic minimum in laboratory testing for chronic, global fatigue. The cost-cutters and Medicare, indeed, may even quibble about the morality of doing electrolyte testing on a 24-year-old woman who has been tired for 2 years. They are correct in believing that it is unlikely that the test will be abnormal, but you are correct in ordering it. Anyone who has been tired for 2 years deserves a work-up for what is unlikely as well as for what is likely.

Further laboratory testing depends on the case, and particularly on the physician's intuition about whether the basic cause is somatic or psychologic (for the purposes of this discussion I will accept a total separation of the two, acknowledging that they are inseparable). Physician intuition is nothing mystical but rather a computer-like summation of past personal experience, the medical literature, and clues provided by the patient.

When the Cause Is Organic. Time after time I have seen interns and residents label patients as "crocks" because the patients did not arrive displaying gross manifestations of their disease. After all, hospitalized patients usually *do* present far-advanced evidence of illness or they would be treated or diagnosed on the outside. Confronted with a patient complaining of persistent fatigue (or persistent pain or persistent dizzy spells) and with no other abnormalities, the house officer and the inexperienced practitioner is likely to offer up a psychologic etiology and go on to "sicker" patients. There is no more grievous error. As foolish as it is to persist in laboratory testing on a patient with endogenous depression, it is worse to miss the only curable case of Addison's disease you are ever going to see. There are ways to minimize this risk.

Neurosis and depression rarely strike suddenly in middle age. Most of the time, but not always, there is a long history of hypochondriasis or of mild depression, the kind that brings 27-year-old lawyers into your office when they haven't been able to find the right sort of mate or the proper kind of job. But when a 45-year-old woman walks into your office complaining of recent onset of fatigue and has no past history and no present evidence of depression, watch out! Do not make the House Officer's Mistake — do not diagnose psychologic disease just because there is no immediate evidence of somatic disease. Depression is *not* a diagnosis of exclusion. In addition to fatigue, there are other confirmatory physical sensations that accompany it, and, most convincingly, the patient usually has psychologic evidence of depression. The depressed patient who presents to a family practitioner or internist (as opposed to a psychiatrist) may not immediately announce, "I'm depressed," but will on questioning say, "My job is just a job — I don't enjoy it any more" or "I don't know . . . it seems that my wife and I hardly talk any more."

The fatigued patient who steadfastly denies any problem besides fatigue and whose lifestyle data support this statistically deserves an extra-hard search for organic illness. (Be suspicious of the recently separated parent who says he or she feels "just great except I can't get out of bed in the morning.") If the blood tests were all normal 4 weeks ago and the patient still feels bad, repeat the tests. If everything is normal and the only symptom is a mild queasiness in the abdomen, don't forget about the early abdominal nodes in lymphoma. Thyroiditis can have absolutely no specific signs and symptoms; the only early clue may be an elevated sedimentation rate. If all the initial laboratory work is normal except for a white blood cell count of 6900 per cu mm with 85 per cent polys, it is not all normal. Something is going on. Find a toehold somewhere from which you can advance the diagnostic work-up. That vacation trip may have provided your patient with a low-grade infestation of giardia and the intestinal symptoms may have long since been masked by a slight, generalized, persistent malaise. The elevated mean corpuscular volume (MCV) may be the only evidence that your patient has been less than candid in giving you his drinking history. Remember that rheumatoid arthritis and, indeed, most of the autoimmune diseases can have as their harbinger only a sudden, profound fatigue. Look for abnormalities of the globulins and don't be afraid to order fluorescent antinuclear antibody test (FANA) in the absence of flagrant lupus. It is axiomatic that any medicine the patient is taking may be causing fatigue; "elimination pharmacology" is a logical first step.

In my own experience and that of my colleagues, infectious disease is rare today as the cause of primary fatigue, although low-grade salmonella infections can sometimes be overlooked, particularly in the elderly. The major disease seen today that presents as fatigue and fatigue alone is malignancy, particularly lymphoma. Here is an example in which the low-grade fever so typical of hypochondria ("My temperature got up to 99.2, but that's high for me. I usually run 97") may in fact be another early manifestation of tumor. Not every patient with persistent fatigue should or can have every laboratory test, and certainly few need to be hospitalized for a diagnostic work-up. Yet, if the clinical context suggests organic disease, if there is no positive evidence of depression, and if the clinician's suspicions remain strong enough, all the technology of modern medicine may be brought to bear on the problem. The third-party payers and the house officers may grumble, but the physician's job is to make the diagnosis in the hard cases as well as the easy ones. If one remembers that every disease must have its first symptoms and that the first symptom may be very vague and very mild, fewer large mistakes will be made. Symptoms are the early warning signal of disease. They will almost always appear before the physical examination becomes abnormal and often before laboratory results are out of line. A convincing history for organic disease is as significant as a hematocrit of 32, and needs to be studied just as thoughtfully.

SYNCOPE

By HARISIOS BOUDOULAS, M.D.,
and RICHARD P. LEWIS, M.D.

Columbus, Ohio

Syncope is defined as temporary loss of consciousness due to a reversible disturbance of cerebral function. Presyncope and near syncope are less well defined but probably represent lesser degrees of the same mechanisms. When syncope begins after middle age, organic disorders are the most likely causes. The basic mechanisms of syncope are shown in Figure 1. Syncope or presyncope or both can be the result of a generalized or localized reduction of cerebral blood flow or inadequate concentration of substances necessary for brain function. In many instances syncope is the result of more than one cause and occasionally no specific mechanism can be found.

A. *Generalized reduction of cerebral blood flow as cause of syncope*

Complete interruption of cerebral perfusion for 2 to 3 seconds results in a feeling of faintness, often described as dizziness, and for 10 seconds results in syncope. Since cerebral perfusion is directly pressure dependent, a sudden drop in systolic aortic pressure below 70 mm Hg usually produces syncope. Hypotension is more likely to occur in the upright posture position, where the brain is more sensitive to hypotension. This accounts for the frequent association of syncope with the standing position. Three pathophysiologic mechanisms produce a generalized reduction of cerebral blood flow: severe impairment of cardiac function (cardiac syncope), volume depletion or venous pooling or both, and decrease in peripheral arterial resistance.

1. *Cardiac syncope.* Either severe obstruction to cardiac output or disturbances of cardiac rhythm can produce syncope. Obstructive lesions and dysrhythmias frequently coexist and indeed one abnormality may precipitate the other. The diagnosis of lesions producing obstruction to flow can usually be made by physical examination. The recognition of dysrhythmias is more difficult because of their transient nature.

a. *Obstruction to cardiac output.* The most common obstructive cardiovascular lesions producing syncope are shown in Table 1. Syncope, particularly with effort, is a major symptom of aortic stenosis. The mechanisms are unclear, but studies suggest an apparent reflex fall in peripheral vascular resistance as the usual cause. However, a failure of the cardiac output to increase with exercise may also play a role. Finally, transient dysrhythmias may also precipitate syncope. Syncope associated with effort is also observed in patients with idiopathic hypertrophic subaortic stenosis but often occurs after exertion. Increased outflow obstruction due to the combination of increased contractility, a fall in peripheral resistance, and a decreased ventricular volume are probable explanations. Transient dysrhythmias also play a role in some cases.

Left atrial myxoma may obstruct left ventricular filling and leads to low cardiac output and syncope. This may be related to certain body positions. Mitral stenosis, prosthetic valve malfunction, and cardiac tamponade may produce syncope, particularly if tachycardia or other dysrhythmias are present.

Primary pulmonary hypertension or pulmonary hypertension secondary to congenital heart disease may be complicated by syncope, particularly with effort. The right ventricle cannot increase the cardiac output on demand. Syncope has been reported as the initial or the predominant symptom of pulmonary embolism.

In tetralogy of Fallot, the magnitude of the right-to-left shunt increases with effort because the right ventricular outflow obstruction is fixed while systemic resistance drops. The result is marked arterial hypoxia, which may result in syncope.

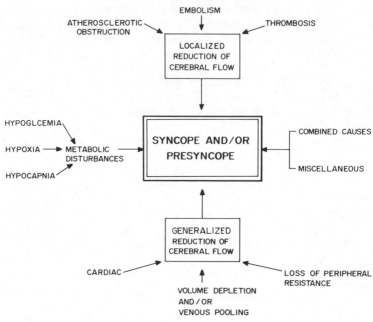

Figure 1. Basic mechanisms of syncope.

The procedures commonly used to establish the diagnosis in cases of syncope due to obstruction to cardiac output are shown in Table 2. The history and physical examination usually suggest the diagnosis but not always the severity of the disease. The next step is to perform appropriate noninvasive tests. Dense calcifications of the aortic or mitral valve or both usually indicate a severe stenotic lesion. Fluoroscopy is the simplest method to define valvular calcification. It is also useful to evaluate prosthetic valve function and abnormalities in the pulmonary vasculature. The echocardiogram is the method of choice for the diagnosis of mitral stenosis; pericardial effusion, which may lead to tamponade; idiopathic hypertrophic subaortic stenosis;

and left atrial myxoma. It is also useful for evaluation of prosthetic valve function and for the diagnosis of tetralogy of Fallot and pulmonary hypertension. A prolonged left ventricular ejection time is consistent with significant aortic stenosis or idiopathic hypertrophic subaortic stenosis and it is easily obtained from the systolic time intervals. The upstroke of the carotid pulse distinguishes between these two forms of aortic outflow obstruction. Radioisotopic techniques are useful for the diagnosis of pulmonary embolism. If the noninvasive tests are inconclusive, cardiac catheterization and angiography may be required.

b. *Dysrhythmias.* Either extremes of ventricular rate can depress cardiac output to a point of

Table 1.   *Cardiac Causes of Syncope*

Obstruction to Cardiac Output

LEFT HEART	RIGHT HEART
Aortic stenosis	Eisenmenger's syndrome
Idiopathic hypertrophic subaortic stenosis	Tetralogy of Fallot
Mitral stenosis	Pulmonary embolism
Prosthetic valve malfunction	Pulmonary hypertension
Tamponade	
Myxoma	

Dysrhythmias
Profound sinus bradycardia or sinoatrial exit block
Supraventricular tachycardia
High-grade atrioventricular block
Frequent premature ventricular beats (PVB's)
Repetitive pairs of PVB's
Ventricular tachycardia
Pacemaker malfunction
More than one dysrhythmia

Table 2. *Diagnosis of Cardiac Causes of Syncope*

Obstruction to Cardiac Output
History
Physical examination
Electrocardiogram
Fluoroscopy–chest x-ray
Echocardiogram
Systolic time intervals
Radioisotopic methods
Cardiac catheterization–angiography

Dysrhythmias
Electrocardiogram
Exercise testing
Ambulatory monitoring
Electrophysiologic studies

critical hypotension and syncope. Dysrhythmias are a common cause of syncope and must be considered in all patients unless the cause is obvious. The most common dysrhythmias producing syncope are shown in Table 1. More than 50 per cent of patients with rhythm disturbances leading to syncope or presyncope are not aware of their dysrhythmias.

Syncope due to dysrhythmias often depends on other factors. For example, patients with normal cardiac function can tolerate most of the dysrhythmias listed in Table 1. This is not true if there is obstruction to flow or severe myocardial failure. Symptoms also may be related to the patient's position, blood pressure, or blood volume. Thus, the same dysrhythmias may not always cause the same symptoms.

Methods used to study dysrhythmias are shown in Table 2. Because of the transient nature of most dysrhythmias, the routine electrocardiogram (ECG) is of limited value. The ECG may be useful to identify patients with Wolf-Parkinson-White syndrome and patients with prolonged QT interval, conditions known to be associated with dysrhythmias. While identification of second or third degree atrioventricular block is very useful, the presence of bundle branch block alone or in combination with hemiblock has not proved to be a reliable predictor of syncope.

Exercise testing is a method for directly provoking dysrhythmias and many clinical and physiologic studies support this approach. The chance of detecting transient and random dysrhythmias is increased by prolonged monitoring. Although this can be done in the hospital monitor unit, experience has shown ambulatory monitoring to be superior. A 24-hour period constitutes one complete diurnal wake-sleep cycle, but the optimal time for ambulatory monitoring is not clear. In some patients whose symptoms are intermittent, repetitive studies may be necessary until the abnormality is detected, or else the patient can be given a portable ECG transmission device.

Figure 2 shows the results of a study of 119 patients with syncope of no obvious cause. Both 24-hour ambulatory monitoring and treadmill exercise testing were performed. A significant dysrhythmia considered to be the cause of syncope or presyncope was found in 76 patients. Dysrhythmias were found in 63 patients with ambulatory monitoring alone, in 3 with exercise alone and in 10 with both methods. Exercise produced a low yield of supraventricular dysrhythmias but the yield increased for patients with malignant ventricular dysrhythmias.

Electrophysiologic studies employing intracardiac recordings have been used to evaluate patients with syncope in whom the standard methods have not yielded a clear-cut answer. Most of these patients are older and have diffuse conduction system disease. They usually fall into the "sick sinus syndrome" category.

Sinus node and atrial function is evaluated by measuring the sinoatrial recovery time, sinoatrial conduction time, and inter- and intra-atrial conduction times. In patients with syncope due to tachycardia, supraventricular or ventricular tachycardia can be reproduced in the catheterization laboratory by introduction of premature stimuli. This approach also allows definition of the mechanism of the tachycardia and evaluation of drug therapy.

Patients with a dysrhythmic basis for syncope usually have two or more electrophysiologic abnormalities, while patients without syncope have either no electrophysiologic abnormalities

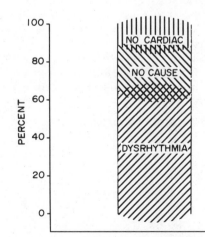

Figure 2. Cause of syncope in 119 patients with no obvious cause of symptoms. A significant dysrhythmia considered to be the cause of syncope or presyncope was found in 64 per cent of the patients. A noncardiac cause was found in 13 per cent, and in 23 per cent no cause was identified. (Reprinted with permission of J. Electrocardiology 12:103, 1979.)

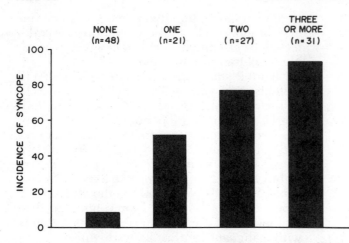

Figure 3. Relationship between the number of electrophysiologic abnormalities and the incidence of syncope. In 65 patients with no obvious cause of syncope and in another 62 with no history of syncope, electrophysiologic stress testing was performed to identify the cause of symptoms. The frequency of syncope is plotted against the electrophysiologic abnormalities. As the number of abnormalities increased, the incidence of syncope increased as well. (Reprinted with permission of J. Electrocardiology *11*:339, 1978.)

or only one abnormality. The incidence of syncope increases as the number of abnormalities increases (Fig. 3). Syncope is unlikely to be due to sinoatrial dysfunction or atrioventricular conduction defects if abnormalities are not detected by electrophysiologic stress testing.

The diagnostic approach to a patient with no obvious cause of syncope is shown in Figure 4. A 24-hour ambulatory monitoring is performed first, followed by exercise testing if the diagnosis is not established. In instances in which dysrhythmias are strongly suspected, prolonged ambulatory monitoring or electrophysiologic studies or both become necessary.

2. *Volume depletion or venous pooling.* Hypovolemia due to loss of blood, water or electrolytes, or all three, causes decreasing venous return, hypotension, and syncope (Table 3). Large varicose veins may be accompanied by syncope owing to decreased venous return under orthostatic stress. Pharmacologic agents, such as nitrates, that relax smooth muscle of capacitance vessels produce syncope by the same mechanism.

3. *Loss of peripheral resistance.* Atrial hypotension due primarily to a deficiency of peripheral arteriolar resistance is also responsible for

syncope. There are two major types of loss of peripheral resistance: active and passive.

Active loss of resistance, as in vasodepressor syncope (common faint), is characterized by a reflex dilatation of systemic arterioles. The stimuli precipitating faint include essentially all forms of physical and emotional stress, such as pain, venipuncture, and so forth. Predisposing factors include illness, fatigue, upright posture, hot weather, hunger, anxiety, and recent blood or fluid loss. Pallor, anxiety, and sweating are present. The pulse is weak and may be absent. The heart rate usually is normal or slow but occasionally is fast. Complete loss of consciousness is rare. Vasodepressor syncope is the single most common cause of syncope. Approximately 15 to 25 per cent of young men experience one or more episodes of vasodepressor syncope at some time during early adolescence. Syncope that is vasodepressor in origin almost always begins in early life and rarely occurs after 35 years of age. The clinical characteristics are usually diagnostic, but careful history and examination should be obtained to rule out organic causes. Active loss of peripheral resistance probably also constitutes one of the major factors for the syncope due to aortic steno-

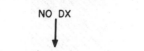

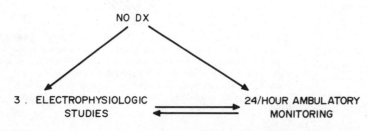

Figure 4. Diagnostic evaluation of patients with no obvious cause of syncope. A 24-hour ambulatory monitoring is performed first followed by exercise testing if the diagnosis is not established. In several instances in which dysrhythmias are strongly suspected, prolonged monitoring or electrophysiologic studies or both are necessary.

Table 3. *Volume Depletion or Venous Pooling as Cause of Syncope*

Dehydration
Excessive diuresis
Bleeding
Varicose veins
Adrenal insufficiency
Nitrates
Combined factors

sis and with acute inferior myocardial infarction.

Passive loss of peripheral resistance is secondary to physiologic disturbances, neurologic diseases, and use of pharmacologic agents. Physiologic disturbances include prolonged bed rest, prolonged standing, and pregnancy. The common neurologic disorders and pharmacologic agents responsible for orthostatic hypotension and syncope are shown in Table 4. Normally in the upright posture an increase in peripheral vascular resistance compensates for the fall in cardiac output due to the pooling of blood.

The syndrome of orthostatic hypotension may be identified at the bedside by the characteristic persistent fall in systolic and diastolic pressure in the upright position. A fall in blood pressure and a small rise in heart rate for the degree of hypotension are characteristics of idiopathic orthostatic hypotension. In idiopathic orthostatic hypotension, syncope occurs without sweating, tachycardia, or hyperpnea because adrenergic and cholinergic failure are present.

B. *Localized reduction of cerebral blood flow*

Reduction of cerebral blood flow by atherosclerotic obstruction or thrombus can result in a transient ischemic attack or stroke. Syncope is a prominent feature when the vertebral-basilar artery system is involved.

In some cases, the symptoms are due to embolism from atherosclerotic plaque or thrombus. Occasionally the embolic material originates from the heart (Table 5).

The internal carotids and the vertebrals may be mechanically compressed during certain movements of the head or neck. This is especially common if cervical arthritic or vertebral artery disease or both are present. Thus, attacks may follow turning of the head or hyperextension of the neck. This may mimic carotid sinus syncope. However, there is a lag between the time of head movement and occurrence of syncope, since several seconds of reduction in cerebral blood flow are necessary to produce syncope. Attacks may occur in any position and under any circumstances, but are more likely to occur when the patient is standing or when he suddenly assumes the standing position, or when he performs certain head movements. This occurrence may also suggest the syndrome of benign positional vertigo, but this condition is not associated with syncope.

The specific symptomatology of the transient ischemic attack is, of course, determined by the area of brain that is most deprived of its blood supply. The syndrome can be classified in terms of the areas of brain supplied by each of the major arteries, although this alone does not necessarily identify which arteries are involved, since collateral circulations are highly variable. The presence of the transient focal neurologic symptoms and the findings of carotid bruits or diminished carotid pulses will suggest the diagnosis. The diagnostic procedures used to evaluate a patient with syncope secondary to obstruction of cerebral blood flow are shown in Table 5.

C. *Metabolic causes*

Syncope can be the result of inadequate concentration of critical constituents in the blood perfusing the brain (Fig. 1). These mechanisms are unusual causes of syncope. The lapse of

Table 4. *Loss of Peripheral Resistance as Cause of Syncope*

Active	*Passive*
Vasodepressor syncope	Physiological disturbances
Aortic stenosis	Prolonged bed rest
Acute inferior myocardial infarction	Prolonged standing
	Pregnancy
	Peripheral neuropathy (diabetes)
	Spinal cord disease
	(Syringomyelia, tabes dorsalis)
	Idiopathic orthostatic hypotension
	(Shy-Drager syndrome)
	Pharmacologic agents
	Antihypertensives
	L-dopa
	Nitrates
	Phenothiazides, other tranquilizers

Table 5. *Localized Reduction of Cerebral Blood Flow as Cause of Syncope*
(Central nervous system diseases as cause of syncope)

Condition
  Atherosclerotic obstruction
  Thrombosis
    Carotid
    Vertebral
    Basilar
  Embolism
    Atherosclerotic plaque
    Endocarditis (bacterial–nonbacterial)
    Calcific valves
    Prosthetic valves
    Mitral valve prolapse
    Left atrial–left ventricular thrombus or mass

Diagnosis
  History
  Physical examination
  Ophthalmodynamometry
  Oculoplethysmography
  Skull, cervical spine, chest x-ray
  Doppler techniques
  Electroencephalogram
  Echoencephalogram
  Computerized axial tomography (CT) scan
  Cerebral angiography

---

consciousness caused by hypoxia or hypoglycemia usually persists much longer than the several seconds characteristic of syncope. Hyperventilation is another cause of syncope that may develop in the sitting or even in the recumbent position. The mechanism seems to be related to hypocapnia, which leads to a transient increase in cerebrovascular resistance with simultaneous peripheral vasodilation. Hyperventilation syndrome usually occurs in patients with anxiety or panic attacks and almost always begins early in life.

D. *Combined causes*

In many instances, particularly in the older age groups, several factors are responsible for syncope (Fig. 5). While each factor may be unable to produce syncope alone, the combination does.

E. *Miscellaneous conditions causing or mimicking syncope*

1. *Carotid sinus hypersensitivity.* Stimulation of the carotid sinus by pressure or massage can produce syncope of three types: (1) cardioinhibitory type, manifested by profound bradycardia, sinus standstill, or atrioventricular block and blocked by atropine; (2) vasodepressor type, manifested by a hypotensive response to carotid sinus stimulation without bradycardia and blocked by epinephrine but not by atropine; and (3) central type of syncope without

bradycardia or hypotension, which is blocked by neither atropine nor epinephrine.

Whether this very rare type of carotid sinus hypersensitivity is caused by a cerebral reflex or by obstruction in the carotid arteries has not been definitely established. Carotid sinus syncope should be diagnosed with caution. An exaggerated response to carotid sinus pressure, including syncope, does not necessarily indicate that a person's spontaneous attacks of syncope are due to a hypertensive carotid sinus. Carotid sinus syncope may be suspected if it is induced by tight collars, by sharp turning of the head, or by stretching of the neck.

2. *Aortic arch syndromes (pulseless disease, subclavian steal syndrome).* This is a rare syndrome, in which there is stenosis or obstruction of most of the major vessels arising from the aortic arch. Usually the common carotid, innominate, and subclavian arteries are involved, with consequent interference in flow to the internal carotids and vertebrals. The syncopal attacks characteristically occur with mild or moderate physical activity and with certain head movements and more readily in the erect position. The association of syncopal or visual symptoms with physical activity has led to use of the term "intermittent cerebral claudication." Pulsations on the neck and arm vessels are usually absent (pulseless disease).

In the subclavian steal syndrome, obstruction of one subclavian artery proximal to the origin of the vertebral artery leads to reversal of flow in the latter. With exercise of the involved arm, blood is diverted from the brain to the arm and syncope occurs. Such patients usually demonstrate a supraclavicular arterial bruit and a decreased brachial blood pressure (>20 mm systolic) on the affected side. In patients with subclavian steal syndrome, intracranial disease often is present. Syncope caused by the same mechanisms is occasionally seen after the Blalock-Taussig operation in patients with tetralogy of Fallot.

3. *Tussive syncope.* This refers to syncope that occurs during prolonged repetitive coughing. Multiple factors are involved. Extremely high intrathoracic pressure develops during the coughing and stops the venous return. In the brain there is very high cerebrospinal fluid

DYSRHYTHMIA
    +
VOLUME DEPLETION
    +
LOSS OF PERIPHERAL RESISTANCE
    +
OBSTRUCTION TO FLOW
    +
OBSTRUCTION TO CEREBRAL FLOW, ETC.

Figure 5. Combined causes of syncope.

pressure with compression of cerebral vessels and cerebral ischemia. Reflex cardiac standstill may also occur.

4. *Micturition syncope.* Occasionally, syncope occurs immediately preceding, during, or following micturition. It most often occurs when the patient arises from bed to void and may represent hypotension combined with a cardioinhibitive reflex mechanism from the bladder that causes bradycardia, cardiac standstill, or atrioventricular block.

5. *Swallow syncope, or glossopharyngeal neuralgia.* Episodes of syncope associated with swallowing or with glossopharyngeal neuralgia have been reported. The patient usually developed severe bradycardia, sinus standstill or atrioventricular block, or both, owing to pain associated with esophageal disease of glossopharyngeal neuralgia.

6. *Syncope due to brain tumor.* Syncope with brain tumor or other expanding lesions is uncommon. In many instances symptoms are vague and falling occurs with or without loss of consciousness. Such symptoms usually occur in relation in movement of the head or change in posture. These symptoms are due to compression of the brainstem or of the vessels supplying it.

7. *Cataplexy.* This is a syndrome in which the patient experiences a sudden loss of muscle tone and falls to the ground. This occurs most commonly during sudden emotional expression. Consciousness is not lost and muscle tone returns promptly. There may be some relationship between cataplexy and vasodepressor syncope (loss of arterial resistance).

8. *Seizure disorders.* These are usually associated with tonic clonic muscular activity but may occasionally appear as syncope, especially in minor seizures in children.

9. *Labyrinthitis.* Acute labyrinthitis may be associated with syncope, but severe vertigo, dizziness, and inability to stand or sit upright are associated symptoms. Nystagmus is a prominent finding.

10. *Hysterical syncope.* Attacks are usually frequent and may occur with an unvarying pattern over several years. Episodes occur in dramatic situations such as in a family gathering, at a party, or at the theater. The patient is rarely injured during a fall. Hysterical syncope almost always begins in early life. The diagnosis is based upon negative studies and the detection of a severe personality disorder.

In this review we have attempted to include all the conditions known to produce or mimic syncope. In clinical practice, many of these conditions are rare. In our experience the following are the most common causes of syncope: vasodepressor syncope (common faint), rhythm dis-

turbances, volume depletion, and aortic stenosis. However, a combination of mechanisms leading to syncope may well be the most common etiology, and by its very nature the most difficult to diagnose.

FACIAL PAIN

By D. E. RICHARDSON, M.D.
New Orleans, Louisiana

The differential diagnosis of facial pain is complicated by the multiplicity of descriptions and variations of the same clinical entity with rather minor or subtle differences. In an attempt to simplify and reduce this confusing mixture of pain problems, I have attempted to reduce the diagnosis to nine clinical groups that should be routinely considered:
1. Trigeminal neuralgia
2. Anesthesia dolorosa
3. Acute sinus disease
4. Acute dental disease
5. Atypical face pain
6. Malignancy of the head and face
7. Myofascial pain syndrome
8. Cluster headaches
9. Temporal arteritis

TRIGEMINAL NEURALGIA (TIC DOULOUREUX)

This is the classic face pain described in the middle ages as "the devil's grip" and is one of the best understood types of face pain since it responds to surgery on the fifth cranial nerve. It usually occurs in the elderly but may occur at any age, in rare cases even in the very young. The youngest patient in my series had the onset of pain at age 13.

Clinical Picture. The pain is usually described as lancinating, stabbing, sharp, pulsating, or similar to electrical radiation in character. It rarely awakens the patient from sleep. It is classically set off by stimulation of a trigger point that may be in the face, lips, nose, tongue, gums, or buccal mucosa. Very slight stimulation of this area of the face initiates an attack. Attacks often may be precipitated by eating, washing the face, talking, or even exposure to slight drafts of wind. The pain distribution is always larger than the trigger area, which is usually fairly small. Confusion with glossopharyngeal neuralgia is possible if the trigger point is deep within the mouth, a serious consideration if surgical intervention is contemplated. The disease is also characterized by spontaneous exacerbations and spontaneous remissions, but late in its course remissions become short or nonexistent. The pain may spread from one division of the fifth nerve to another, but rarely becomes bilateral. This is so rare that bilateral pain almost rules out tic as a possibility.

Diagnostic Tests. Temporary peripheral nerve block is helpful in the difficult diagnostic case. Lidocaine block of the area of the trigger point produces immediate and usually complete relief of the pain and this may outlast the expected duration of anesthesia. Blocking the supraorbital, infraorbital, mental, or mandibular nerve may clarify the difficult diagnostic problem easily and promptly. It must be remembered that the placebo effect of nerve blocks on psychogenic pain should be considered and repeat blocks, if adequate, will always relieve true tic pain.

Diagnostic Therapy. A trial on phenytoin (Dilantin) or carbamazepine (Tegretol) is usually a reliable test, since these drugs do not affect other types of face pain, except briefly from the placebo effect. (This use of phenytoin is not listed in the manufacturer's official directive.) Other drugs are of little diagnostic value and are nonspecific in their action.

ANESTHESIA DOLOROSA

This is a deafferentation pain syndrome occurring in patients who have sensory loss of the face following denervation from trauma, surgery, or destructive procedures reducing sensation of the face. It is characterized by pain in an area of decreased sensation and is usually described as a burning, aching pressure sensation, thickening, or woodiness in the area of sensory loss. Occasionally a sensation of a foreign body in the eye is described. The pain is persistent and rarely remits. It is not relieved by nerve block. In contrast to those with tic pain, these patients do become habituated to narcotics and tranquilizers.

ACUTE SINUS DISEASE

Sinusitis pain is usually persistent but may fluctuate in intensity. It usually is described as an aching, constant, focal discomfort and is often associated with local tenderness. It may be confused with dental pain and if from an allergic reaction rather than infection, may not be associated with elevation of temperature or white blood count. It is usually of short duration and may be associated with rhinitis or otitis. Tenderness over the affected sinus and mucosal thickening and fluid levels in the associated sinus on x-ray are diagnostic, except in the occasional patient with a malignancy or more than one disease.

ACUTE DENTAL DISEASE

At onset, acute dental disease may be referred to larger areas of the face but usually localizes with time to the affected area. Stimulation by heat, cold, or mechanical stimuli to the affected dental structure will usually exacerbate the pain; dental x-rays are usually diagnostic.

ATYPICAL FACE PAIN

This classification is a collection of a multiplicity of face pain that has been referred to as Sluder's neuralgia, histamine face pain, sphenopalatine neuralgia, lower-half headaches, and Horton's neuralgia. The clinical picture is usually persistent, unrelenting, deep-seated aching pain of the face, not related to trigger points, without lancination, and refractory to most therapy, except analgesics. It may be associated with evidence of parasympathetic overactivity such as tearing, rhinorrhea, erythema of the face, or unequal pupils. The pain does not respond to phenytoin (Dilantin) or carbamazepine (Tegretol), but usually does to analgesics or tricyclic antidepressants. Section of the trigeminal nerve and nerve blocks do not significantly affect the pain, and may indeed increase it.

MALIGNANCY OF THE HEAD AND FACE

Persistent or recurring pain that may be poorly localized, worse at night, and increasing in severity, with relief only by analgesics, may herald a malignant process. Fortunately, this is a rare cause of face pain but must be remembered in the patient with relatively short history of pain. Loss of function of the face, jaw, ear, or eye, or anatomic changes in structure on examination make this diagnosis a prime consideration.

MYOFASCIAL PAIN SYNDROME

Pain secondary to muscle spasm from tension, anxiety, teeth clinching, grimacing, and teeth grinding usually produces pain from spasm of the muscles of mastication; this can be a diagnostic dilemma unless muscle spasm can be palpated. Secondary or primary temporomandibular joint pain and tenderness may be demonstrated. Referred pain to the ear from external pterygoid spasm can be confused with ear infection or disease.

CLUSTER HEADACHES

While usually confined to the calvarium, this pain may extend to the face. The pain occurs in groups of attacks and each attack may be of very brief duration, lasting only 30 minutes, or it may be prolonged. The pain is usually of sudden onset, severe in nature, and is unrelated to activity, time of day, or emotional precipitation. It is almost always unilateral and involves structures outside the trigeminal nerve distribution. The pain is usually described as aching and severe. This is one of the few pain syndromes that awaken the patient from sleep. Therapeutic trials of ergot, methysergide, or propranolol may give a therapeutic diagnostic test, but negative results do not necessarily rule out this possibility.

TEMPORAL ARTERITIS

This is a disease of the elderly. Symptoms are usually severe and usually persistent pain in the temporal area and the eye are present. This disease is almost always unilateral and often associated with reduced vision in the ipsilateral eye. Sedimentation rate is usually elevated and differential diagnosis can be established by temporal artery biopsy or response to steroid therapy, which is good presumptive evidence for this rare condition.

BACK AND EXTREMITY PAIN

By THOMAS C. MYERS, M.D.
Mobile, Alabama

and GENE V. BALL, M.D.
Birmingham, Alabama

Pain is an unpleasant sensory experience that has its psychophysiologic basis in the reception of a stimulus, the neural conduction of electrochemical messages, and the integration of these messages at the cerebral level. Because of the limited number of neural pathways and integrative capabilities, similar pain perceptions may result from dissimilar pathologic processes. Thresholds for pain are comparable from patient to patient, but perception of quality and degree differ so that the pain of a serious disorder is minimized by the stoic and "trivial" pain is aggrandized into life-threatening proportions by the less stoic. These built-in vagaries make evaluation of pain difficult and interesting. In spite of these limitations, a careful analysis of its characteristics and concomitant symptoms and the physical findings can limit diagnostic possibilities. Once these are pared, laboratory, radiographic, and other diagnostic tests may be chosen parsimoniously.

THE HISTORY

Differential characteristics of pain include location, mode of onset, provoking and alleviating factors, duration, quality, severity, and the relationship of pain to other symptoms. Pain may be described as superficial or deep, well localized, segmental, or diffuse. Pain that is superficial and well localized is less likely to cause diagnostic difficulties than is deep and less well-localized pain. For example, the pain of superficial thrombophlebitis and extremity arthritis is well localized, whereas referral pain arising from the abdominal viscera or deep structures of the back is poorly localized. Approximate localization is important even in segmental or diffuse pain, since its source must reside in structures of the same sclerotome.

The mode of onset of pain may be a clue to its origin. For example, pain of abrupt onset related temporally to change in posture, lifting, or straining suggests that tearing, rupture, or collapse of a supporting tissue has occurred. Examples include aortic dissection, herniated nucleus pulposus, and acute lumbosacral strain. Relationships between pain and activity should be sought (e.g., actions that mimic the Valsalva maneuver are likely to induce the pain of nerve root compression). Provoking and alleviating factors offer important clues to suggest that pain originates from viscera. Classic illustrations of this point are exercise-induced arm pain in myocardial ischemia and alleviation of pancreatic pain by spinal flexion.

Inquiry as to the time of occurrence may uncover the late afternoon exacerbation characteristic of tension and posture-induced discomfort, the nocturnal exacerbation of dysesthesias in peripheral and entrapment neuropathies (especially carpal tunnel), or the early morning intensification of pain noted in inflammatory back and joint disorders. The quality and severity of pain are less useful than the other characteristics. An exception is the burning pain of nerve irritation and the excruciatingly severe pain of acute aortic dissection or ureteral colic. In analyzing pain of obscure origin, a careful review of systems may illumine the thoracic or abdominal viscera as the source of back or extremity pain or declare the pain a feature of multisystem disease.

SPECIFIC BODY AREAS

The Back. Evaluation begins with inspection of the disrobed standing patient. The back is viewed for levelness of shoulders and iliac crest, symmetry of the bony and soft tissues, and alignment of thoracic and lumbosacral spine. This simple maneuver may reveal several abnormalities capable of producing back pain: leg length discrepancy, kyphosis, scoliosis, and spondylolisthesis. Bony and soft tissue structures that are palpated gainfully include the spinous processes and interspinous ligaments, sacroiliac joints, coccyx and ischial tuberosities, and trapezius and paraspinal muscles. Crude ranges of spinal motion are estimated by stabilizing the pelvis and requesting full flexion, extension, lateral bending, and rotation. Motion at the costovertebral articulations is measured indirectly by chest expansion. Other important components of the examination in the back-pain patient are the straight leg raise test, the Valsalva maneuver, and evaluation of muscle strength and deep-tendon reflexes in the lower extremities.

In both lumbosacral strains and herniated disc, paraspinal muscle spasm and tenderness are prominent; but in the latter, the straight leg raise and Valsalva maneuver may exacerbate the pain. Later in the course of a herniated disc, muscles supplied by the compressed nerve(s) may exhibit weakness and diminished deep-tendon reflexes. For example, compression of the L4 spinal nerve results in weakness of dorsiflexion and inversion of the foot and a diminished knee jerk. Compression of L5 causes weakness of dorsiflexion of the great toe and S1 causes weakness of the gastrocnemius and diminished ankle jerk.

The fibrositis syndrome is characterized by exquisitely tender points in the upper border of the trapezius, interspinous ligaments, medial border of the scapula, and upper outer quadrant of the buttock. Several disorders are capable of producing pain and tenderness of the spinous processes of the vertebral column.

These include the metabolic bone diseases osteomalacia and osteoporosis, Paget's disease, infections of the disc, vertebrae or epidural space, and malignancy.

Physical examination is useful in patients with spondyloarthropathies such as ankylosing spondylitis, Reiter's syndrome, psoriatic arthritis, and inflammatory bowel disease. Inflammation of synovial joints and spinal ligaments results in sacroiliac joint tenderness, reduced painful range of motion, reduction of lumbar lordosis, accentuation of thoracic kyphosis and reduced chest expansion. Tenderness over bony points such as the greater trochanter, the iliac crests, the ischial tuberosities, and the heels is also typical of spondyloarthritis. Sacroiliitis resulting in piriformis muscle spasm with sciatic nerve compression can mimic nerve root pain, although loss of reflexes is seldom found in piriformis muscle spasm.

The Shoulder. Inspection of the shoulders for symmetry, contour of the deltoids, and arm position is followed by systematic palpation for tenderness or swelling of the sternoclavicular, acromioclavicular, and glenohumeral joints, the clavicle, the acromium and subacromial bursa, and the tendons of the biceps and rotator cuff. In bicipital tendinitis, maximal tenderness is found in the bicipital groove and exacerbation of pain occurs with active supination of the forearm against resistance (Yergason's sign).

Inflammation may also occur in any of the tendons that form the rotator cuff and when it does, the overlying subacromial bursa is similarly affected. The physical findings in rotator cuff tendinitis and subacromial bursitis are tenderness in the subacromial area and extreme pain on early abduction (0 to 45 degrees). Acute tendinitis may cause muscle inflammation by contiguity and may even elevate muscle enzymes.

Acromioclavicular arthritis is recognized by the location of tenderness or swelling and by the accentuation of pain with active shrugging of the shoulder against a resistance force applied to the arm. Involvement of this joint occurs frequently in rheumatoid arthritis and less often in spondyloarthropathies, septic and crystal-induced arthritis, and osteoarthritis.

The glenohumeral articulation is commonly involved in rheumatoid arthritis, adhesive capsulitis, amyloidosis, ankylosing spondylitis, pseudogout, and aseptic necrosis but uncommonly in gout. In adhesive capsulitis, decrease in range of motion may be extreme, while tenderness is minimal. Osteoarthritis is less usual in this location unless there has been previous trauma.

The Elbow. The elbow is inspected for carrying angle and swelling, extension being limited generally in systemic inflammatory arthritis, particularly rheumatoid arthritis. Osteoarthritis is a less common cause of elbow pain, it being often post-traumatic, while neuropathic arthritis ("Charcot joint"), which is seldom painful, may involve the elbow and produce gross deformity. Soft tissues should be palpated for swelling, nodules, synovial or bursal enlargement, and ulnar nerve tenderness. Acute bursal effusions denote gout or infection most often, illustrating the clinical similarities of these two entities and emphasizing the need for needle aspirations of most acute effusions and examination for crystals or bacteria. Nonchronic effusions are common in rheumatoid arthritis, and also occur in response to repeated trauma. Epitrochlear lymph nodes are uncommonly tender or painful. Nodules along the extensor surface of the forearm near the elbow are usually rheumatoid nodules or gouty tophi and less often are the nodules of systemic lupus erythematosus, rheumatic fever, or xanthomas. Rheumatoid nodules are at times "bony hard." These are all most often painless; painful nodules of erythema nodosum or nodular panniculitis occur on the arm or forearm much less frequently than on the lower extremity.

Tenderness of the lateral epicondyle and pain on forced flexion of the extended wrist are characteristics of "tennis elbow." Passive movement of the elbow in this condition is full, as it is in joints adjacent to other tenoperiosteal lesions such as inflammation of the insertions of biceps and flexor carpi ulnaris. The medial epicondyle is less frequently painful than is the lateral epicondyle. Entrapment of the ulnar nerve at the elbow may cause considerable forearm pain and numbness of the fourth and fifth fingers, at times intensified by percussion over the ulnar nerve. This is an occasional complication of trauma or less often arteritis, its pathogenesis reflecting inflammation of the vasa nervorum and pressure. Electrophysiologic diagnostic tests are of particular value in the differentiation of various causes of pain in the arm and forearm, particularly in peripheral entrapment syndromes, herniated cervical disc, thoracic outlet syndromes, superior sulcus syndromes, and brachial plexus injuries.

One must not overlook acute distal tendinitis as the cause of pain referred proximal to the tendinitis; carpal tunnel syndrome, de Quervain's disease, and palmar flexor tendinitis have all been observed as the cause of pain radiating proximally to the forearm, the arm, or the shoulder. Sparing of the elbow may be important in suggesting the cause of upper extremity pain, as in shoulder-hand syndrome.

The Wrist and Hand. While careful inspection and examination of the wrist are of great importance, a normal examination does not obviate a local disorder as the cause of pain. For example, hypertrophic osteoarthropathy involving the distal radius and ulna may be painful at times without visible or palpable swelling of the affected parts. Conversely, the firm and gross swelling of amyloidosis in the wrist may be painless, as are ganglia arising from the dorsum of the wrist.

Examination of the wrist is sometimes pivotal in the differentiation of various forms of arthritis. Rheumatoid arthritis involves the wrist far more frequently than does osteoarthritis, which is nevertheless often present in the first carpometacarpal joint. Pseudogout favors the wrist, and gonococcal tenosynovitis is a common cause of acute wrist pain in younger patients. Acute tenosynovitis of the abductor pollicus longus and extensor pollicus brevis (de Quervain's disease) causes pain at or near the radial styloid process, which is intensified when the patient's thumb is enclosed by his clenched fist and the examiner ulnar-deviates the wrist. While most often palmar and phalangeal, the discomfort of carpal tunnel syndrome may also be felt in the arm and shoulder. The evoked physical finding in this syndrome is the producing of paresthesia in the median nerve distribution either by percussion over the carpal tunnel or by prolonged hyperflexion of the wrist. Pain in the fingers is probably most often due to trauma, while various forms of arthritis and Raynaud's phenomenon account for most pain that is a component of systemic disease. Glomus tumors are found in nail beds as purplish-red spots and, despite their insignificant appearance, cause pain that is severe and lancinating. Neurologic causes for finger pain have been alluded to earlier; endocrine and neoplastic disorders rarely cause finger pain. Trigger fingers due to nodularities in the flexor tendons are sometimes distressingly painful.

The Hip. Gait is altered in most painful hip conditions. An antalgic gait indicates pain on weight bearing and is characterized by abbreviation of the stance phase, whereas the gluteal gait or limp is due to weakness or shortening of the gluteus medius muscle responsible for hip abduction and pelvis stabilization. This gait, seen in malunion of femoral neck fractures, gluteus medius atrophy, and also painful hip, is characterized by body tilt toward the weakened side during the stance phase. Long-standing painful hip conditions, disc disease, and rarely Leriche's syndrome cause atrophy of the gluteus maximus. Intra-articular inflammation results in hip adduction, flexion, and internal rotation at rest.

Palpation of the femoral triangle, inguinal area, ischial tuberosity, sciatic nerve, greater trochanter, and the anterior hip joint helps to localize pain. Tenderness in the femoral area occurs with femoral hernia, femoral vein thrombophlebitis, and iliopsoas strain. Femoral pulses are decreased and bruits present when buttock pain is due to ischemia. Hip pain occurring in the supine position at times denotes osteoid osteoma of the femur.

Inguinal hernias and inflamed lymph nodes are capable of producing pain in areas where hip pain is also felt. Ischial and trochanteric bursitis, which on physical examination are manifested as tenderness over the ischial tuberosity or greater femoral trochanter, most often are idiopathic or traumatic in origin.

Tenderness of the sciatic nerve at the midpoint between the ischial tuberosity and the greater trochanter with the hip flexed 90 degrees is an indication of sciatic nerve irritation. Hip joint tenderness and decreased range of motion are common findings in all diseases capable of producing intra-articular inflammation. These include rheumatoid, degenerative, and septic arthritis; aseptic necrosis; the spondyloarthropathies, especially ankylosing spondylitis; calcium pyrophosphate-induced synovitis; and in children acute transient synovitis, Legg-Calvé-Perthes disease, juvenile rheumatoid arthritis, and slipped epiphysis. "Hip pain" may in reality be meralgia paresthetica, an entrapment syndrome involving the lateral cutaneous branch of the femoral nerve.

An anteroposterior (AP) pelvis film is necessary to evaluate hip pain; tomograms of the area are sometimes indicated, as in early aseptic necrosis. Metastases to the pelvis occur rather frequently; one may even find oddities such as transient osteoporosis of the hip.

The Knee. A painful knee is another cause of antalgic gait, and if quadriceps weakness or knee joint instability is present, then the stance and swing phases occur with the knee in full extension ("back-kneeing").

Inspection may reveal the quadriceps atrophy of disuse, denervation, or myopathy; medial and suprapatellar joint effusion of arthritis; or the sometimes massive anterior swelling of prepatellar bursitis. It will also disclose alignment abnormalities such as genu valgum and varum, and flexion contracture. Palpation of the popliteal fossa may disclose the pulsatile painful mass of popliteal an-

eurysm or the smooth swelling of a popliteal cyst.

Several bursitis syndromes occur near the knee. Prepatellar bursitis, on the basis of trauma or infection, manifests as swelling and tenderness anterior to the patella, whereas anserine bursitis, common in obese women and in the fibrositis syndrome, is characterized by tenderness over the insertion of sartorius gracilis and semitendinosis into the proximal medial tibial metaphysis. In retropatellar tendon bursitis, tenderness is present on compression of the relaxed patellar ligament.

Tenderness of the infrapatellar fat pad may occur with direct trauma or with inflammation of the adjacent synovial membrane of the knee. Tenderness, synovial hypertrophy, and effusions of the knee joint occur in rheumatoid arthritis, osteoarthritis, joint infection, uric acid– and calcium pyrophosphate–induced synovitis, spondyloarthropathies, and a number of less common conditions. The pattern of other joint involvement, extra-articular features, radiographs, synovial analysis and culture, and laboratory tests will aid in the differentiation of these entities.

Monarticular knee inflammation or swelling is a common presentation of septic arthritis, gout, pseudogout, osteochondritis dissecans, pigmented villonodular synovitis, and trauma to the knee.

Traumatic effusions can be seen with patellar dislocation or with meniscal, cruciate, or ligamentous disruptions. Most patellar dislocations are transient but can be suspected on the basis of history and patient apprehension when the patella is laterally displaced by the examiner. Cruciate tears result in abnormal anterior and posterior motion of the tibia on the femoral condyles with the knee flexed 90 degrees (Drawer sign). Meniscal injuries may produce locking of the knee and pain or clicking with McMurray's maneuver.

Patellofemoral joint pain can accompany inflammatory conditions of the tibiofemoral joint or it may occur separately as an idiopathic condition, chondromalacia, or degenerative arthritis. In each of these, physical examination reveals crepitance and pain when the patella is pressed into the trochlear sulcus and moved in anterior-superior or medial-lateral directions.

Finally, it is well to remember that knee pain occurs with hip disease or nerve compression.

The Ankle and Foot. The first concern in evaluation of ankle and foot pain should be with whether pain is localized or is part of a more symmetrical, and hence systemic, process. Unilateral ankle or foot pain is frequently due to trauma, which may be as subtle as the overuse in an obese patient that culminates in the painful heel of plantar fasciitis. The cause of pain may be apparent on inspection, as in the painful nodularities of Kaposi's sarcoma or plantar warts. Except for the burning pain of peripheral neuropathy, pain in this area is usually worse on weight bearing. Not all burning pain can be sorted out as clear-cut peripheral neuropathy, since burning pain is also an early stage of causalgia at a time when x-ray films are normal and only joint scan will show changes. Later the foot becomes swollen, warm, and sweating, and later still patchy osteoporosis may be seen on x-ray film. Burning paresthesias may also be due to a systemic disease such as diabetes or a local problem such as tarsal tunnel syndrome, one of a number of nerve entrapment syndromes involving the foot. The latter produces symptoms distal to entrapment of the medial and plantar nerves along the medial malleolus. Tarsal tunnel syndrome is at times a phenomenon secondary to the tendinitis of rheumatoid arthritis. A more common form of tendinitis in the foot is Achilles tendinitis, seen in increasing frequency among joggers. What seems to be Achilles tendinitis may be a subtendon bursitis. Another frequent site for tendinitis in the foot is at the tarsal insertion of the anterior tibial muscle. Tumors, fractures, Kohler's disease, and Freiberg's infarctions are all detectable on x-ray films. Because of the complexity of the ankle and foot, films should be taken of both feet unless the radiologist or clinician has detailed knowledge of the normal anatomy of these structures.

Pain between the third and fourth toes may arise from an interdigital neuroma. Pain in the foot that is aggravated by activity but diminishes with cessation of activity despite continued weight bearing should suggest ischemic arterial disease. Apart from x-ray examinations, electrophysiologic diagnostic studies may be useful in defining the cause of foot pain.

Radiographic Examination

The x-ray is an indispensable tool in the evaluation of back and extremity pain. Its proper use requires an explicit differential diagnosis and a knowledge of sensitivity and specificity of the radiographic examination in that context.

Radiographs of the spine allow detection of congenital and developmental disorders such as spondylolisthesis and sacralization of the transverse process of L5. They also allow visualization of vertebral bodies for localized lytic lesions seen in many metastatic tumors; for the generalized osteopenia of osteomalacia, osteoporosis, and multiple myeloma; for local blastic lesions of prostatic carcinoma; for mixed blastic-lytic changes of Paget's disease; and for detection of compression fractures. The integrity of the pedicles, a favorite site for metastatic disease, is evaluated on AP films of the vertebral column.

Anterior and posterior osteophytes are noted, and, if symptoms warrant, oblique views are obtained to evaluate encroachment into the neural foramina.

Inspection of the end plates of the vertebral bodies and intervertebral disc height may give a clue to degenerative or septic disc disease. Calcification of the annulus fibrosus portion of the disc accounts for the syndesmophytes of ankylosing spondylitis, while large segments of the anterior longitudinal ligament may be calcified or ossified in diffuse idiopathic skeletal hyperostosis (DISH). The disc itself becomes calcified in ochronosis.

The synovial apophyseal joints of the spine are also examined. They are commonly involved in both degenerative and inflammatory arthropathies. Synovitis of the articulation of the odontoid and atlas may result in laxity and consequently in atlantoaxial subluxation.

Pain may arise from involvement of sacroiliac joints in spondyloarthropathies, sarcoid, hyperparathyroidism, infection, and rarely gout. Unilateral abnormality is the rule in infection, while bilateral but asymmetric involvement is common in Reiter's syndrome, psoriatic arthritis, and sarcoid. Symmetrical bilateral involvement occurs in ankylosing spondylitis and in inflammatory bowel disease.

Radiographic examination of the extremities may yield important information when the differential diagnosis includes diseases of bones or joints. Osteomyelitis, Brodie's abscess, bone tumors, and hypertrophic osteoarthropathy have characteristic radiographic findings.

In periarticular shoulder pain, calcification of ligaments of the rotator cuff may point to that as the origin of pain.

Radiographs are normal in most entrapment neuropathies that produce extremity pain, an exception to this being the occasional patient with thoracic outlet syndrome secondary to a cervical rib.

Radionuclide bone scans are capable of demonstrating areas of active bone turnover caused by fracture, some metastatic tumors, causalgia, osteomyelitis, osteomalacia, hyperparathyroidism, and Paget's disease. Bone scans may prove to be more sensitive than symptoms, phosphatase enzyme elevations, or routine bone radiographs. Exceptions to this generalization include multiple myeloma and thyroid and oat cell carcinoma.

Although radionuclide joint and sacroiliac scans are widely available, their ultimate usefulness is yet to be defined. Subclinical synovitis may be apparent on most scans, giving a pattern of synovitis not appreciated on physical examination. Similarly, scan sacroiliitis would favor certain diagnoses depending upon symmetry and bilaterality, as in the x-ray film.

THE LABORATORY

Laboratory tests in the evaluation of back and nonarthritis extremity pain are of considerably less importance than the history, physical examination, and radiographs. With their sensitivity and specificity in mind, tests are chosen so that the results will lend weight to one or more of the diagnostic possibilities. Laboratory testing is seldom revealing in periarticular inflammatory conditions, trauma, or congenital/developmental structural disorders.

The sedimentation rate is widely used as an indirect measurement of acute phase reactants. It is elevated in most patients with inflammatory disorders and markedly so in polymyalgia rheumatica and giant cell arteritis, multiple myeloma, and severe active rheumatoid arthritis. It is normal in osteoarthritis, fibrositis, and strain syndromes. Polyclonal increases in gamma globulin are common in chronic inflammatory conditions, whereas monoclonal increases are characteristically encountered in neoplasms of the B cell line of lymphocytes.

Rheumatoid factor is an immunoglobulin, usually IgM, with antibody activity against IgG immunoglobulin. It is detectable by a number of methods having quite different sensitivities and specificities, the most widely used of which is the latex fixation method. Slide tests for the detection of rheumatoid factor tend to be more sensitive and less specific than the tube detection latex fixation. Rheumatoid factor is detectable in 70 to 80 per cent of patients with definite or classic rheumatoid arthritis and in almost all patients with rheumatoid nodules. The detection of rheumatoid factor is a useful adjunct to the clinical diagnosis of rheumatoid arthritis but in itself is not sufficient to warrant that diagnosis. Low titer positivity is common in middle-aged and elderly people, as well as in patients with the chronic inflammatory, infectious, and autoimmune diseases.

Fluorescent antinuclear antibody tests are the most useful screening tool for systemic lupus erythematosus. Antinuclear antibodies (ANAs) are present in 98 per cent of patients with definite disease and rarely in normal controls. Intermediate percentages of positivity occur in patients with mixed connective tissue disease, progressive systemic sclerosis, and other autoimmune diseases including those of the liver. When the fluorescent antinuclear antibody is positive, clinical criteria must also be present before a disease can be diagnosed. The lupus erythematosus (LE) cell phenomenon parallels the fluorescent antinuclear antibody, but at a lesser sensitivity. The LE cell prep is no longer available in all laboratories, having been superseded by the ANA.

In younger patients with back pain or arthritis that is seronegative, asymmetrical, or predominantly lower extremity, positive tissue typing for HLA B27 enhances the probability of a spondyloarthropathy as the origin of the symptoms.

When synovial fluid is present in a patient with joint pain, it should be aspirated for examination. On the basis of white cell counts and protein content, synovial fluids are imperfectly separated into noninflammatory and inflammatory-septic groups. Because of considerable overlap, the slightest suspicion of infection should lead to culture of the effusion with special attention given to gonococcal culture media. Synovial fluid evaluation is incomplete without examination by polarized microscopy for the birefringent crystals of uric acid and calcium pyrophosphate. Similarly, effusions in bursae should be aspirated and subjected to the same scrutiny.

Back and extremity pain, secondary to metastatic disease, may result from bone involvement with or without radiographic changes. Bone fraction alkaline phosphatase is often elevated in this setting, but it too suffers from nonspecificity in that elevation occurs in osteomalacia, hypoparathyroidism, and Paget's disease.

THE CONFUSED ELDERLY PATIENT

By JACK E. ROZANCE, M.D.,
ERIC D. CAINE, M.D.,
and T. FRANKLIN WILLIAMS, M.D.
Rochester, New York

A number of anatomic and physiologic changes have been described with normal aging of the central nervous system, including reduction in brain weight, decrease in the number of neurons and nerve fibers, enlargement of ventricular volume, and decline in performance on standard cognitive function tests. These accepted changes of aging often lead to an uncritical acceptance of failing mental function in the aged.

Although population surveys suggest a prevalence of dementia (irreversible mental deterioration accompanied by pathologic changes) in almost 10 per cent of people over 65 years of age, most of the elderly remain unscathed by this process. When new changes in memory and behavior affect this latter group, every effort must be made to look for reversible causes of the mental deterioration. Even when the diagnosis of dementia has been established previously, an abrupt deterioration of function may be related to other, reversible illnesses whose recognition and treatment can lead to restoration of some function and relative independence. The features of these reversible causes of mental decline must be recognized and are emphasized in this chapter.

THE HISTORY

When considering the history and physical examination of the confused elderly patient, one would like to reliably distinguish between *dementia,* with its chronic course and often irreversible pathologic changes, and *delirium,* an acute, frequently reversible state usually unaccompanied by demonstrable pathologic changes in the brain. Although delirium can usually be distinguished from dementia during physical and mental status examination, the history may prove a critical element in separating these syndromes. An abrupt or rapid onset points to delirium, while dementing disorders are characterized by an insidious deterioration of cognitive function. The separation of these conditions is also complicated by the frequent occurrence of deliria in demented patients.

Patients with impaired intellectual functioning cannot provide the history necessary for evaluation of their condition. Other informants must be sought, including spouse, relatives, and friends. However, close relatives frequently have not appreciated the subtle initial changes of a dementing illness, including withdrawal from social contacts, trouble concentrating, constriction of interests, or difficulty carrying out tasks and achieving goals. These are often attributed to "growing old." The physician must try to ferret out information regarding the earliest onset of abnormal intellectual decline, often through more creative and individualized questions: Has the patient been unable to balance the checkbook, shop in the grocery store with or without a list, follow a recipe or project to completion, read a book, or follow the news? Does the patient get lost in the neighborhood or home? Are former manual and job skills no longer used or used incorrectly? Have these abilities been lost slowly or in a stepwise fashion? Has there been a subtle change of "personality" or inexplicable alteration of mood? The emphasis of questioning will shift when the physician is faced with a confused elderly patient who has been failing gradually for years, as opposed to one who has been without apparent problems until recently.

Other data must be routinely obtained. A complete history of medication use (both prescription and over-the-counter drugs) must be obtained from the patient or family and friends. This often involves having someone bring in all the medication bottles that are in the patient's home. A history of head injury, headache, nausea, emesis, gait difficulties, or incontinence raises the possibilities of subdural hematoma, tumor, or normal pressure hydrocephalus. A history of fever prompts a search for infection. If combined with headache and vomiting, it may suggest the possibility of meningitis.

Complaints or problems noted by the patient or family, combined with a routine review of systems, may elicit other data that suggest the presence of pulmonary, cardiac, hepatic, gastrointestinal, renal, or endocrine disease. Disorders in these systems frequently lead to sudden alteration of mental status function.

Finally, a careful dietary history should be sought, including an inquiry into the use of alcohol. Poor food intake or alcohol abuse or both are all-too-common contributory causes to dementia.

THE GENERAL PHYSICAL EXAMINATION

Important data can be gathered through observation and inspection. This is often more revealing than any individual part of the examination. In addition to signs of cranial or body trauma, stigmata of malnutrition should be elicited, including dermatitis, cheilosis, and wasting. The texture of skin and hair is noted. The overall level of alertness and cooperation can be assessed. Altered levels of consciousness seen as drowsiness, lethargy, or stupor, combined with physiologic alterations such as tremor, agitation, sweating, and tachycardia, are all the hallmarks of delirium and as such suggest a treatable, often reversible condition.

Vital signs including temperature, heart rate and rhythm, and respiratory pattern should be recorded. The presence of carotid bruits and nuchal rigidity must be interpreted in the light of the history and overall examination. Asymptomatic bruits and neck movement limited by osteoarthritis are often found in the elderly. A careful cardiac evaluation searching for evidence of valvular heart disease, arrhythmia, or dyskinetic ventricular wall segments may uncover sources of multiple cerebral emboli. The finding of fever prompts a thorough examination for sources of infection inside and outside the central nervous system.

THE NEUROLOGIC EXAMINATION

Mental status testing, a key component of the neurologic examination, should include assessment of orientation, memory, language skills including reading and writing, spatial perception, thought processes, affect, and judgment. Memory, often the most impaired function, should be tested by assessing immediate repetition (e.g., digits forward), new learning, and recall of distant and more recent events. Cranial nerve evaluation includes careful inspection of: (1) optic discs for papilledema, (2) eye movements for the symmetric nystagmus of sedative intoxication, (3) pupillary responses for a dissociation between light and accommodative reaction, and (4) assessment of visual and auditory acuity. Failure in these spheres has been mistaken occasionally for mental decline, particularly when the patient is not cognitively normal. Visual fields are best tested using simultaneous stimuli in the opposite parietal or occipital area.

Motor examination is often best done through functional testing. Pronation and flexion at the fingers, wrist, and elbow in an outstretched arm may reveal a subtle cortical paresis that may not be detected by individual muscle testing. Unilateral hyperreflexia or Babinski sign points to focal pathology in the opposite cerebral hemisphere and raises the possibility of subdural hematoma, tumor, or past cerebral infarction. Myoclonus (random, irregular muscle jerks), particularly with attempted movement, and asterixis (an irregular loss of posture in the outstretched hands, feet, or tongue) strongly suggest the presence of a metabolic delirium caused by drug intoxication, uremia, respiratory failure, or liver disease.

A number of signs found in the setting of disease of both frontal lobes have been called the frontal release signs. "Frontal release signs" including grasp, palmomental, snout, and suck reflexes are seen frequently in normal elderly patients and are not specific enough to unequivocally indicate frontal lobe disease. More reliable and specific signs of frontal disease include a positive glabellar response (persistent blinking with continued tapping on the forehead; the

normal or negative response is cessation of blinking), impersistence or inability to sustain tongue protrusion for 30 seconds or lateral gaze for 10 seconds, and an abnormal nuchocephalic response of head lag after brisk shoulder turning.

Gait apraxia, an inability to initiate or carry out walking despite adequate involuntary use of the legs, is seen with bifrontal diseases and normal pressure hydrocephalus. Paratonia is a failure of relaxation during passive movements of the limbs; the patient's resistance frequently increases as the examiner continues to move the limb (*Gegenhalten*). It results from bifrontal brain dysfunction, as well.

SITUATIONS SIMULATING DEMENTIA OR DELIRIUM

A number of other, specific neuropsychologic deficits may be confused with dementia syndromes. They require careful differential diagnostic consideration.

Aphasia. The syndrome of Wernicke's aphasia, with fluent speech output, impaired comprehension, and deficient repetition (also accompanied by problems with naming, reading, and writing) often leads to a picture of confusion and distress. Such fluent aphasias can develop abruptly after embolic strokes, or slowly due to a tumor or a subdural hematoma. Wernicke's aphasia may not be accompanied by obvious hemiparesis, although a hemianopic visual field deficit may be apparent. Careful assessment of comprehension to simple commands, repetition, naming, and writing, and listening for word distortions (paraphasias) or new words (neologisms) will detect the aphasia. Dementia syndromes can be dominated by marked language dysfunction. The history and presence of paratonia and other frontal release signs may help to distinguish dementia from aphasic disorders.

Transient Global Amnesia. This entity is characterized by the sudden appearance of confusion and amnesia for recent events. There is no apparent loss of personal identity or impaired recall of well-learned information. It usually lasts several hours. After recovery, amnesia for events during the episode remains. Theories regarding the etiology point toward a transient ischemic attack in one or both deep temporal lobes that triggers a localized seizure. During the amnesia, other cognitive functions are impaired variably.

Pseudodementia. Depression of the elderly can be difficult to distinguish from an early dementia; impairment of memory and poor intellectual performance can be seen in depression. Whenever there is a question about the diagnosis, treatment of depressive symptoms with antidepressants or electroconvulsive therapy is warranted. Furthermore, depression superimposed on well-defined organic dementia should be treated vigorously.

ETIOLOGIES OF DEMENTIA

Alzheimer's Dementia. "Senile dementia" (Alzheimer's dementia) is a progressive disruption of cortical neurons and their connections, accompanied by loss of cortical neurons and ventricular enlargement. Microscopic changes include neurofibrillary tangles in neurons and amyloid-containing senile plaques. The cause is unknown and the disease is identical pathologically whether it occurs before or after age 65.

Multi-infarct Dementia. Multi-infarct dementia is characterized by definable episodes leading to progressive deterioration of motor and cognitive function. Important predispositions include hypertension, with its large and small vessel (lacunar) occlusions, and recurrent cardiac emboli from atrial fibrillation, prosthetic heart valve, or ventricular wall aneurysms. Bilateral carotid disease with embolization and stenosis can present as a dementing illness, often with stepwise decrements in function. Although multi-infarct dementia is usually irreversible, it is reasonable to attempt to halt the underlying process, whether with antihypertensives, anticoagulants, or carotid surgery.

Trauma. Subdural hematoma is a notorious cause of confusion in the elderly. It can occur without focal signs, suggesting localized cerebral compression. The absence of a history of trauma does not exclude a subdural hematoma, as the cortical bridging veins to the superior sagittal sinus can rupture from insignificant trauma. This diagnosis must receive prime consideration in any confused elderly patient who has a fluctuating level of consciousness. Scalp bruises and unilateral skull percussion tenderness should serve to heighten suspicion. It is also notable that concussive head injury with cerebral contusion may produce confusional states lasting for days even without subdural hematoma formation.

Neoplasms. Brain tumors can masquerade as a dementing illness rather than the more common presentation of increasing focal signs. Slow-growing meningiomas can compress dominant hemispheric language centers and present with a slowly evolving aphasia. Centrally placed tumors that compress or invade both frontal lobes produce personality and cognitive changes that often give the impression of a dementing illness. A similar picture can develop from multiple cerebral metastases, carcinomatous meningitis, or a brainstem metastasis causing obstructive hydrocephalus. Patients with these disorders, however, usually have headache, nausea, emesis, and anorexia. They may have a past history of a primary tumor or one that is readily apparent on breast examination or chest x-ray. Therapy may provide substantial relief.

The following disorders command major attention because of potential reversibility. Prompt diagnosis and therapy are essential.

Drug Toxicity. The increased vulnerability of the elderly to adverse drug effects is not well understood but must be related in part to slower rates of metabolism and excretion, as well as an increased sensitivity of the aging nervous system. Besides sedatives and tranquilizers, which may produce paradoxical confusion and agitation, many commonly used compounds can lead to confusion, including antihypertensives, anticholinergics, antidepressants, antiparkinsonian agents, digitalis glycosides, narcotic and non-narcotic pain relievers such as propoxyphene and pentazocine, and anti-inflammatory drugs including aspirin. When toxic confusional states are considered, all administered drugs must be reviewed for their potential contributions. In the absence of compelling clinical reasons, it is wiser to discontinue their use.

Systematic and Central Nervous System Infections. Infections not directly involving the brain can produce a confused, encephalopathic state. Although bacterial and tuberculous meningitis must be considered in any febrile, confused elderly patient (even in the absence of nuchal rigidity), more often systematic infection outside the nervous system is found. Pneumonia, pyelonephritis, endocarditis, and intra-abdominal infection must be considered in any patient with a fever and leukocytosis.

Neurosyphilis. General paresis is a potentially treatable cause of progressive mental decline. It may be ushered in by seizure or punctuated by the abrupt appearance of focal signs. Tremors of the lips, tongue, and fingers during voluntary movements may be seen in association with a slow, slurred, tremulous speech, and ataxia. The Argyll Robertson pupil is seen in upwards of 90 per cent of all patients. Parenteral penicillin given daily over 3 weeks often leads to some improvement.

Myxedema. Hypothyroidism progresses slowly and can lead to systemic and neurologic symptoms and signs that are incorrectly attributed to other diseases or to "aging." The intellectual decline may be unaccompanied by the other clinical signs that usually point to the diagnosis; it is imperative to evaluate thyroid function in all patients with confusion. Cerebellar ataxia and distal paresthesias may be present concomitantly with confusion.

Vitamin Deficiencies. Vitamin B_{12} deficiency may cause mental deterioration, usually accompanied by a subacute combined degeneration of the spinal cord that is manifested by leg weakness with Babinski signs and impaired position sensation. However, confusion may be the sole symptom; typical megaloblastic anemia may not be present. Thiamine deficiency, usually related to alcohol abuse, is dominated by acute or chronic memory loss with signs of ataxia, neuropathy, nystagmus, and ocular palsies. Pellagra (with characteristic dermatitis in sun-exposed areas, diarrhea, and dementia) is quickly reversed by niacin treatment.

Metabolic. Primary diseases of kidney, liver, or lung can lead to confusional states through accumulation of unidentified toxins or chronic hypoxemia. Acute and chronic cardiac disease with low output states may also impair mentation.

Hypercalcemia and disorders of sodium balance must be considered in the confused patient. Dehydration may be detected by dry mucous membranes and postural blood pressure changes. A history of insulin or oral hypoglycemic agents raises the possibility of acute or chronic hypoglycemia.

Normal Pressure Hydrocephalus (NPH). NPH is suggested by the triad of incontinence, gait apraxia, and marked memory loss with apathy. In half the cases of NPH, the syndrome has been a late sequel to subarachnoid hemorrhage, head trauma, or meningitis. The radiologic criteria for diagnosis include enlarged ventricles on computerized axial tomography (CT) scanning and accumulation of lumbar-injected radioisotope within the cerebral ventricles. Cerebrospinal fluid shunting may benefit up to 40 per cent of patients with the clinical and radiologic syndrome.

Hypothermia. Accidental or alcohol-related hypothermia may cause acute confusional states that are reversible with rewarming. Elderly individuals with limited incomes and substandard housing are particularly vulnerable to this disease. A clinician must have a thermometer that records below 95 F (35 C) to confirm this diagnosis.

Complex Partial Seizures Status. Repetitive temporal lobe seizures without interictal clearing can occur in the elderly. This invariably produces a confusional state. This syndrome should be suspected when abrupt and transient alterations in the level of alertness are seen in association with darting nystagmoid eye movements, lip smacking, and other motor or behavioral automatisms. Anticonvulsant therapy may completely reverse the confusion. The underlying cause can be a small focus of temporal or frontal lobe infarction, and need not be a more ominous problem such as tumor.

LABORATORY EVALUATION

Confusion in an elderly patient requires thorough, prompt laboratory evaluation. Initial assessment should include:

1. Determination of complete blood count (CBC) with sedimentation rate, electrolytes, glucose, blood urea nitrogen (BUN), calcium, liver function tests, arterial blood gases, chest x-ray, and electrocardiogram (ECG).

2. Screening of the urine and serum for drugs and alcohol when there is a history of potential drug or toxin exposure.

3. A thorough search for infection in febrile patients. When no obvious source is found, a lumbar puncture is indicated to look for meningitis; however, lumbar puncture is contraindicated when there are signs suggesting a cerebral mass lesion.

4. Thyroid studies, fluorescent treponemal antibody absorbed (FTA-Abs), and vitamin B_{12} level are routine screening tests.

5. Skull x-rays are necessary to look for fractures or pineal shift.

CT scanning provides a sensitive, noninvasive means of delineating internal cerebral anatomy. Cortical and ventricular dimensions are readily apparent. Cerebral edema, displacement or midline shift, hemorrhage, and multiple infarcts are all seen readily. With contrast enhancement, most tumors and all meningiomas will become apparent. Ventricular enlargement, with or without prominent sulci, suggestive of normal pressure hydrocephalus, is apparent readily; postoperative return of the ventricles to normal size is one means of evaluating shunt function.

The brain scan may occasionally confirm the presence of a chronic subdural hematoma, when the CT scan may only indicate absent or less prominent cortical sulci on that side.

Cerebral angiography is essential when evaluating potential extracranial vascular disease.

The electroencephalogram (EEG) cannot match the CT scan for identifying structural lesions, but may be helpful when trying to separate pseudodementia from dementia or delirium. It may be diagnostic in cases of drug intoxification and is essential when a seizure disorder is suspected.

THE UNCONSCIOUS CHILD

By RUSSELL D. SNYDER, M.D.,
and RUTH A. ATKINSON, M.D.
Albuquerque, New Mexico

Unconsciousness is a symptom and not a specific disease entity. Unconsciousness in children* may be a symptom of diseases as diverse as Reye's syndrome and subdural hematoma. Because of the many potential causes of unconsciousness and because only limited time may be available before irreversible brain damage occurs, a planned systematic approach to diagnosis of the unconscious child becomes mandatory.

Unconsciousness implies a failure in functioning of the ascending reticular activating system or a failure in functioning of both cerebral hemispheres. The ascending reticular activating system, located in the brainstem and diencephalon, is that part of the brain that causes the "awake" situation and alerting. Small lesions in the reticular activating system can affect consciousness; large lesions elsewhere may not affect consciousness. Lesions restricted to one cerebral hemisphere do not usually produce unconsciousness.

In the pathophysiologic sense, three causes for unconsciousness occur.

1. *Supratentorial mass or destructive lesions.* Because of increasing volume these lesions indirectly produce dysfunction of the brainstem reticular activating system. Also, widespread destructive lesions may cause dysfunction of both hemispheres. Neoplasms of the hemispheres and subdural hematomas are examples of such lesions.

2. *Infratentorial mass or destructive lesions.* These lesions may directly compress or destroy the ascending reticular activating system and thus interfere with consciousness. Small brainstem hemorrhages from trauma are examples of such lesions.

3. *Toxic-metabolic encephalopathy.* Unconsciousness may be produced by interference with the metabolism of the cerebral hemispheres and the brainstem reticular activating system. This form of unconsciousness can be produced by an exogenous poison or by a metabolic problem such as anoxia.

---

*Unconsciousness as it occurs in the newborn and premature is not considered in this article.

MANAGEMENT OF THE UNCONSCIOUS CHILD

The human brain is delicate; aggressive management of any circumstance that threatens to upset its internal milieu is mandatory. Such circumstances include exposure to toxins, metabolic derangements, pressure, and abnormalities in the blood supply. The anatomic and physiologic substrate of neural mechanisms deteriorates with remarkable rapidity, making the brain extremely vulnerable to insults. Three of the central neurotransmitters provide an illustration of this vulnerability. Norepinephrine, dopamine, and serotonin exist as neurotransmitters in three independent systems of nerve cells, axons, and synapses. These neurotransmitters lose their in vivo characteristics within 1 hour of death and cannot be identified by fluorescent histochemical techniques when this amount of time has elapsed.

The first priorities in the management of the unconscious child are general medical measures. The diagnosis of most neurologic disorders can safely be deferred. If possible, irreversible brain damage must be prevented.

Emergency measures include: (1) assurance of adequate respiratory functioning. This may include use of suctioning, endotracheal tube, respirator, and blood gases. The brain is dependent upon an adequate supply of oxygen. (2) Maintenance of circulation. An intravenous line is mandatory. Blood volume loss should be treated by replacement and vasopressors should be given as indicated. Cardiac arrhythmias may need specific treatment. (3) Administration of glucose. The brain is an obligate user of glucose. Time should not be lost in attempting to establish the presence of hypoglycemia by laboratory test. Intravenous 50 per cent glucose will not damage the patient who is not hypoglycemic. (4) Lowering of increased intracranial pressure, if necessary. Hyperventilation, ventricular drainage and osmotic diuretics such as mannitol appear to be effective measures for reducing acute increased intracranial pressure. With subacute or chronic increased intracranial pressure, steroids, and pentobarbital may be considered. (5) Management of seizures. Repeated or prolonged seizures may damage the central nervous system. Diazepam is an effective and safe drug with which to treat seizures in the setting of depressed consciousness. (6) Control of body temperature. Either hyperthermia or hypothermia may exacerbate problems with cerebral metabolism. Hyperthermia increases cerebral metabolic demand. Cooling and warming blankets should be utilized appropriately. (7) Restoration of acid-base balance. Respiratory alkalosis and metabolic acidosis are particularly common with coma. Acid-base abnormalities can interfere with cerebral metabolism as well as produce problems with the cardiovascular system (Table 1).

GENERAL EXAMINATION

After the child's condition is stable, complete general and neurologic examinations may provide clues to the cause of the unconsciousness. Vital signs, inspection of the body surface, and examination of the heart, lungs, and abdomen are all parts of the initial examination. Evidence of injury to the head can establish head trauma as a cause, although head trauma may be a secondary event related to a fall such as during a seizure. Blood in the ears or nose is an additional confirmatory sign of head trauma. A stiff neck may be seen in meningitis, cerebellar tonsillar herniation, and in cervical injury. A temperature elevation suggests infection or a thalamic lesion. Hypothermia may occur with intoxication. Hypotension and slow, shallow respirations also suggest intoxication. Progressive neurologic deterioration is an indication for aggressive therapy in addition to supportive measures. Almost any cause of coma may be associated with convulsions. Convulsions occur more frequently in children than in adults and may be generalized, focal, multifocal, or myoclonic.

NEUROLOGIC EXAMINATION

The neurologic examination of the unconscious child is similar to the examination of the unconscious adult: pupillary reactivity; fundi, oculocephalic, and oculovestibular responses; corneal reflex; gag reflex; spontaneous movements of extremities; and response of extremities to passive movement and noxious stimulation. The fontanel provides a unique feature in the examination of the small child. Examination of this anatomic structure becomes a simple and immediate method for determining the presence of increased intracranial pressure. Fontanel pressure should be determined, if possible, with the child in the upright position.

Table 1.　*Emergency Measures in the Management of the Unconscious Child*

1. Assurance of adequate respiratory function
2. Maintenance of circulation
3. Administration of glucose
4. Lowering of increased intracranial pressure
5. Management of seizures
6. Control of body temperature
7. Restoration of acid-base balance

Papilledema is a rare occurrence in the acutely comatose child; retinal hemorrhage suggests head trauma.

Five aspects of the neurologic examination are particularly useful in assessing the unconscious child (Table 2).*

1. Level of Consciousness. Progressive decline in the level of consciousness may indicate clinical deterioration; improvement in the level of consciousness has the opposite clinical significance. Consciousness is evaluated by response to verbal and noxious stimuli. The terms used to describe the level of consciousness are, unfortunately, rather vague and imprecise:

Obtundation. Responses to verbal stimuli are present but slow and often inappropriate. Clouding of consciousness and disorientation may be associated findings.

Stupor. A state of unresponsiveness from which the patient can be aroused only by vigorous and repeated stimuli.

Coma. Unarousable unresponsiveness even to repeated vigorous stimulation.

2. Respiratory Pattern. The respiratory pattern may provide a useful indicator of brain function. With severe damage to both hemispheres, Cheyne-Stokes respirations may occur. Cheyne-Stokes respirations associated with stupor frequently indicate bilateral diencephalic disease and may be an early sign of impending serious brainstem compression. With damage to the upper brainstem, shallow hyperventilation occurs that has been referred to as "central neurogenic hyperventilation." Further progression leads to dysfunction of the pons or medulla, causing irregular respirations incapable of supporting life.

3. Pupillary Size and Reaction. A hand lens should be used in examining the pupils if necessary. Metabolic diseases, even in the situations in which deep coma occurs, usually produce small but reactive pupils. With supratentorial mass lesions, the pupils may be small and reactive early. As intracranial pressure increases, the pupils become unreactive and may dilate either unilaterally or bilaterally. However, a unilateral mass lesion must always be considered when pupillary asymmetry occurs. Structural disease of the upper brainstem of sufficient magnitude to produce unconsciousness is usually associated with midposition fixed pupils. Pinpoint, unreactive pupils may occur in structural disease of the pons. In poisoning, fixed dilated pupils are *not* necessarily supportive evidence for the irreversible ces-

---

*See Plum, F. and Posner, J. B.: The Diagnosis of Stupor and Coma, ed 2. Philadelphia, F. A. Davis Co., 1972.

Table 2. *The Neurologic Assessment of the Unconscious Child*

1. Level of consciousness
   a. Obtundation
   b. Stupor
   c. Coma
2. Respiratory pattern
3. Pupillary size and reaction
4. Eye movements
5. Motor responses

sation of brain function. Anoxia produces dilated pupils.

Great variability exists in pupillary responses. Mass lesions, as just noted, may cause dilated or constricted pupils, depending upon the location of the mass. Dilated or constricted pupils may be nonspecific signs of brainstem dysfunction secondary to increased intracranial pressure rather than indicators of structural lesions.

4. Eye Movements. In the normal child, the oculovestibular response tested by ice water against the tympanic membrane results in nystagmus with the quick component in the direction opposite to the ear being stimulated. As depression of neurologic functioning occurs, the oculovestibular response becomes tonic, with the eyes deviated toward the side of the ice water stimulus. With further depression of function, the oculovestibular response totally disappears, which implies severe brainstem damage or metabolic depression of vestibular function. The oculocephalic response (doll's eye movements), determined by passive movement of the head from side to side, should not be tested until cervical fracture has been absolutely excluded. Testing for the oculocephalic response in the child with a cervical lesion could be a catastrophic event. A full range of eye movements will occur on oculocephalic testing in the lightly depressed child who has intact brainstem functioning. The oculocephalic response disappears early with either metabolic depression or structural lesions of the brainstem. Abnormal movements such as skew deviation and internuclear ophthalmoplegia suggest structural brainstem disease.

5. Motor Responses. Loss of appropriate response to noxious stimuli and abnormal responses such as decorticate posturing occur with disease of the cerebral hemispheres. Decorticate posturing consists of flexion of the arms with extension of the legs and sometimes extension of the head and spine. Decerebrate posturing appears with diencephalic and midbrain problems. Decerebrate posturing is similar to decorticate posturing except that the arms are in extension with hyperpronation of the forearms; decerebrate posturing indicates more severe brain disease than does decorticate posturing. Either form of posturing may be asymmetric and present only intermittently, such as when the patient is disturbed in suctioning. Flaccidity follows the decerebrate state if the disease process progresses. With progressive deterioration, deep tendon reflexes initially become hyperactive and are then lost.

DIFFERENTIATION BETWEEN STRUCTURAL AND TOXIC-METABOLIC CONDITIONS

The clinical signs of toxic-metabolic encephalopathy may permit differentiation from structural central nervous system abnormalities. Normal oculovestibular response, preservation of pupillary light reflex with bright light and magnification, and the absence of focal deficits despite respiratory depression, decerebrate state, or flaccidity are all evidence against structural lesions. With toxic-metabolic encephalopathy, random conjugate movements of the eyes may occur rather than maintained lateral deviation or dysconjugate movements. In deep coma from a toxic-metabolic cause, all reflexes and conjugate movements of the eyes are lost and decerebrate posturing may occur. In severe toxic-metabolic encephalopathy with coma, cerebral edema, and brainstem depression, the patient may display the progressive neurologic deterioration of structural central nervous system disease (Table 3). During clinical improvement, these signs reappear in reverse sequence.

Hemiplegia (noted as a difference in tone between the two sides in the comatose patient), conjugate ocular deviations, and unequal pupils all suggest structural problems. Toxic-metabolic encephalopathy displays a more symmetrical examination. However, focal signs, usually transient and mild, may occur with toxic-metabolic encephalopathy. Small but reactive pupils and conjugate eye movements on caloric testing provide additional evidence for toxic-metabolic encephalopathy. Certain drugs, such as atropine, may cause confusion by producing dilated pupils. Anoxia also causes dilated pupils.

The differentiation between structural and toxic-metabolic conditions by examination is always imprecise.

LABORATORY EXAMINATION

Laboratory tests may be helpful in the diagnosis and management of the unconscious child. These tests include such studies as blood

Table 3.   *Signs of Neurologic Deterioration in the Unconscious Child**

	Normal	Intermediate Stages		Profound Loss of Neurologic Functioning
Level of consciousness	Normal	Obtundation	Stupor	Coma
Respiratory pattern	Normal	Cheyne-Stokes	Central neurogenic hyperventilation	Very irregular
Pupils	Midposition, reactive	Pinpoint, reactive	Fixed, midposition	Fixed, dilated, or midposition
Oculocephalic response	Absent	Present	Hyperactive	Absent
Caloric response	Normal	Nystagmus opposite stimulus	Tonic deviation toward side of stimulus	Absent
Motor response	Normal	Decorticate rigidity	Decerebrate rigidity	Flaccid
Tendon reflexes	Normal	Hyperactive		Absent

*Modified from Plum, F., and Posner, J. B.: The Diagnosis of Stupor and Coma, ed 2. Philadelphia, F. A. Davis Co., 1972, pp. 25–57.
†In a deteriorating patient, the listed signs may move from column to column, from left to right, and in an improving patient from right to left.

gases, blood sugar, electrolytes, toxicologic analyses, ammonia, serum glutamic oxaloacetic transaminase (SGOT), prothrombin time, blood urea nitrogen (BUN), skull films, cervical spine films, and computerized tomography of the brain (CT) with contrast enhancement and lumbar puncture (but see later discussion). The laboratory tests obtained will vary with the clinical situation and the age of the child.

Spread of sutures on a child's skull films is an indication of increased intracranial pressure. Since the advent of the CT scan, cerebral arteriography and pneumoencephalography are rarely indicated in the management of the acutely comatose child. Also, the information gained by the CT scan is generally much more useful than the information obtained by radioisotope brain scan or echoencephalography. Radioisotope brain scan and echoencephalography may be indicated in situations in which CT is not readily available.

Lumbar puncture is a procedure of some risk in children with depressed consciousness accompanied by increased intracranial pressure. Acute brain herniation can occur in children as well as adults. Lumbar puncture is necessary immediately in situations in which bacterial meningitis is a strong consideration; in other situations the test is best deferred until after its relative safety has been established by other examinations such as the CT scan. In the patient with depressed consciousness, an attempt to determine cerebrospinal fluid pressure is indicated.

The electroencephalogram (EEG) may occasionally be helpful. A specific EEG pattern may be seen with drug ingestions, encephalitis, and hepatic encephalopathy. An isoelectric EEG is an extremely unfavorable prognostic sign.

BRAIN DEATH

The problem of brain death is relevant to a discussion of depressed consciousness. The criteria for brain death have been developed for application to adults. These criteria are probably also applicable to children beyond the newborn period, although the specific applicability will be determined by future research.

Once brain death has occurred, a patient is no longer in coma. The traditional criteria of cessation of heart beat and circulation indicate death only when the cessation persists for a sufficient period of time for the brain to die. A person is not dead unless the brain is dead. When the clinical criteria for brain death are met, somatic death almost inevitably follows in the adult but may be significantly delayed or not occur at all in the child. At autopsy, in cases of brain death, nearly all cerebral, cerebellar, and brainstem structures have been destroyed.

The general criteria for brain death have achieved wide acceptance; disagreement may occur on certain relatively minor features. The criteria should be present on two clinical examinations performed several hours apart. An established cause is desirable but, at least in children, not always available. Intoxication must be excluded and, in children, this may mean the performance of a blood barbiturate level measurement, other appropriate toxicologic studies, and perhaps even a blood ethanol level measurement. Significant hypothermia should not be present. No spontaneous respiratory or muscular movements may occur and there must be no evidence of decerebrate or decorticate posturing or shivering. Certain cephalic reflexes must be absent, including absent pupillary response to light, absent corneal reflexes, unresponsiveness to intensely painful stimuli such as supraorbital pressure, absent response to upper and lower airway stimulations such as in suctioning, absent ocular response to head turning (oculocephalic response), and absent ocular response to irrigation of the ears with ice water (oculovestibular response). An isoelectric EEG is generally confirming evidence for the presence of cerebral death but not an essential feature for the diagnosis. However, an isoelectric EEG may be a reversible finding in barbiturate coma and hypothermia. The deep tendon reflexes, which are basically spinal reflexes, are occasionally preserved in brain death.

DIFFERENTIAL DIAGNOSIS

The causes of unconsciousness in children can be grouped into differential diagnostic categories as follows: Those causes related to (1) seizures, other paroxysmal disorders, or the postictal state; (2) intoxication or ingestion; (3) infection; (4) injury or tumor; and (5) extracranial or intracranial illness. These will be discussed separately but are not mutually exclusive (Table 4).

Causes of Unconsciousness Related to Seizures, Other Paroxysmal Disorders or the Postictal State. Almost any cause of depressed consciousness may be associated with seizures. The history of previous seizures in a child or his family leads the physician to suspect a seizure-related cause for coma, but intoxication, infection, injury, tumor, and metabolic disorders must also be considered. A seizure may lead to trauma if the patient falls. Major motor status epilepticus from whatever cause is usually obvious. Petit mal or temporal lobe status epilepticus is not so easily recognized, may be confused with psychiatric conditions or delirious states, and requires an EEG for identification.

Both short-lived seizures with little motor activity and major motor seizures may be followed by postictal state from which the patient cannot be aroused. Paroxysmal discharges on the EEG associated with diffuse slowing can help to identify the postictal nature of unconsciousness.

Table 4. *Differential Diagnosis of the Unconscious Child*

Paroxysmal Disorders
 Seizures and the postictal state
 Petit mal and psychomotor status
 Confusion migraine

Intoxication and Ingestion
 Salicylate
 Tricyclic antidepressant
 Atropine
 Sedative
 Iron
 Lead
 Mercury
 Thallium
 Hydrocarbon
 Ethyl alcohol
 Carbon monoxide
 Penicillin
 Propranolol
 Nose drops
 Phencyclidine

Infection
 Bacterial meningitis
 Brain abscess
 Rickettsia
 Viral encephalitis
 Protozoa
 Fungus
 Parainfectious encephalomyelitis
 Pertussis immunization encephalopathy

Injury or Tumor
 Shock
 Fat embolism
 Concussion
 Contusion
 Laceration
 Skull fracture
 Subdural hematoma
 Epidural hematoma
 Intracerebral hematoma
 Neoplasm

Extracranial or Intracranial Illness
 Hypoglycemia
 Hyperosmotic state
 Hyponatremia
 Hypertension
 Hypoxia
 Coagulopathy
 Aneurysm
 Collagen disease
 Reye's syndrome

Childhood migraine may present with confusional agitation resembling a toxic psychosis. This syndrome occurs in children of either sex between the ages of 5 and 16 years. The acute confusional state is the initial manifestation of migraine in some patients. Family history of migraine is an important clue. The attacks may be as brief as 10 minutes or last as long as 20 hours, and terminate with the child in a deep sleep. Upon awakening, the child appears normal. The mechanism is believed to be cerebral ischemia of one or both hemispheres.

Causes of Childhood Unconsciousness Related to Intoxication or Ingestion. Clinically significant childhood poisoning is common and depressed consciousness is a frequent mode of presentation. Almost any poisoning agent can be associated with convulsions.

Salicylates, because of their availability, are among the more common substances ingested in excess by preschoolers. Hyperventilation is a clue to the presence of salicylism. Tinnitus can be an early complaint in the older child. Excitability occurs, followed by depressed consciousness and convulsions. Respiratory alkalosis, present early, is replaced by metabolic acidosis. Blood salicylate levels correlate with clinical severity. Salicylates in the blood or urine produce a brown-to-purple color with ferric chloride, as do phenothiazines.

Coma and convulsions associated with cardiac arrhythmias are suggestive of tricyclic antidepressant toxicity. These substances are administered to children particularly for enuresis and are commonly used in adults. Blood levels for tricyclics are available in some laboratories.

Agitation, hallucinations, dilated pupils, beet-red color, dry skin, and fever are symptoms of poisoning with atropine or the atropine-like agents: Jimson weed, scopolamine, and lysergic acid diethylamide (LSD).

Depression of consciousness is common in narcotic, synthetic narcotic, barbiturate, antihistamine, and tranquilizer overdose. Intoxication with any of these agents may produce central nervous system excitement early in the course of the poisoning. Opiates and barbiturates produce slow respirations, pinpoint pupils, and coma.

The initial symptoms of iron intoxication are vomiting and bloody diarrhea followed by shock, convulsions, and coma. Radiographic examination of the abdomen may show the radiopaque tablets.

Children with acute lead poisoning usually present with an acute coma, which may be preceded by a variety of vague prodromal symptoms, such as loss of newly acquired skills, irritability, anorexia, nausea, vomiting, incoordination, abdominal pain, and constipation. Signs of the acute encephalopathy are those of increased intracranial pressure: projectile vomiting, depressed consciousness, convulsions, and papilledema. Cerebrospinal fluid pressure and protein content are raised and a moderate mononuclear leukocytosis (10 to 100 cells per cu mm) exists. Lumbar puncture in this situation can lead to brainstem herniation.

Lead can be detected in the blood, urine, and hair. Decreased erythrocyte delta-aminolevulinic acid dehydratase, increased free erythrocyte protoporphyrin, and increased urinary coproporphyrin are helpful in diagnosing lead poisoning. Lead lines appear on the gingiva of older children, and radiographic abnormalities may be found in the metaphyses of long bones.

The symptoms of organic mercury poisoning are confusion, depressed consciousness, ataxia, peripheral neuropathy, constriction of visual fields, chorea, and athetosis. A latent interval of weeks to months between ingestion and symptoms may occur. Mercury can be detected in the blood, urine, and hair.

The onset of symptoms of thallium poisoning may be gradual or rapid, depending upon the amount ingested. Initial symptoms are those of peripheral neuropathy: pain, flaccid paresis, areflexia, cranial nerve palsies, and optic neuritis. Miosis may exist. A temporary but complete loss of scalp hair occurs 2 to 4 weeks after ingestion, with sparing of axillary and pubic hair. Mees' lines (cross-banding of the nails) may be seen. Symptoms can progress rapidly to unconsciousness. Thallium is detectable in blood, urine, and hair.

Aspiration of volatile hydrocarbons is associated with dysequilibration, blurred vision, convulsions, and depressed consciousness. Aspiration pneumonia often occurs. Petroleum distillates can be found in the blood.

Symptoms of ethyl alcohol ingestion include nausea, ataxia, confusion, convulsions, and depressed consciousness. Hypoglycemia may occur. The characteristic alcohol odor to the breath is a useful clue. Blood alcohol levels correlate well with clinical symptoms in acute intoxication.

Mild toxicity from carbon monoxide causes headache, weakness, miosis, dyspnea, sweating, nausea, and vomiting. Severe intoxication results in disorientation, depression of consciousness, convulsions, retinal hemorrhages, and cardiac irregularities. The cherry-red skin has been overemphasized. Carbon monoxide poisoning can be detected by elevated blood carboxyhemoglobin.

Penicillin and carbenicillin toxicity may cause decreased levels of consciousness, myoclonic jerks, and seizures primarily in patients with impaired renal function.

The use of propranolol, a beta-adrenergic blocking agent, in children may be complicated by the development of significant hypoglycemia, loss of consciousness, and convulsions. This is most likely to occur after prolonged periods of reduced food intake.

Nose drops, such as naphazoline (Privine), tetrahydrozoline hydrochloride (Tyzine), oxymetazoline hydrochloride (Afrin), and xylometazoline hydrochloride (Otrivin), when used for infants under 1 year of age, may produce profound sedation and hypotonia lasting, for example, from 12 to 48 hours after a single instillation of a 0.1 per cent solution of tetrahydrozoline, but more commonly after repeated doses given over several days.

Phencyclidine hydrochloride (angel dust, PCP) has become popular in drug abuse. The agent can produce a euphoria similar to being drunk. Toxic symptoms include hallucinations, agitation, miosis, ataxia, convulsions, depressed consciousness, and respiratory depression. Symptoms may evolve over a period of many hours after exposure to the drug.

Infectious Causes of Unconsciousness. Bacterial infections of the nervous system and its coverings should be suspected in every comatose child. Examination of the cerebrospinal fluid (CSF) is the single most valuable diagnostic test when central nervous system infection is suspected. *Hemophilus influenzae* is a common cause for meningitis in children between 6 months and 3 years of age. Older children are likely to have meningococcal or pneumococcal meningitis. In tuberculous meningitis the onset is slow and other central nervous system manifestations are usually apparent prior to depressed consciousness. The depression of consciousness may be secondary to parenchymal brain damage or irritation, subdural collections, or the development of hydrocephalus.

Brain abscess can cause unconsciousness, usually preceded by headache and fever. Children with congenital heart disease and right-to-left shunts are particularly at risk. Focal neurologic symptoms may be present. Sudden onset of coma in a patient with preceding symptoms of brain abscess suggests that the abscess has ruptured into a ventricle. The diagnosis is best made by CT scan.

Coma may be seen in the more severe rickettsial infections of the nervous system. Usually the early manifestations of fever, headache, and skin rash suggest the diagnosis prior to onset of depressed consciousness.

Viral encephalitis occurs in children and may cause profound depression of consciousness followed by apparent complete recovery. Cases of encephalitis caused by arboviruses and enteroviruses tend to cluster geographically and seasonally. Herpes simplex encephalitis often presents as an intracranial mass lesion but may present as a psychiatric illness or delirium because of its predilection for the temporal lobes. The CSF in viral meningitis shows an initial polymorphonuclear pleocytosis that later becomes monocytic, mild elevation of protein, and normal sugar. Red blood cells may occasionally be found in the CSF. The responsible virus is presumptively identified by demonstration of significant titer rise in the serum. Absolute diagnosis requires isolation of the virus from nervous tissue.

Protozoa, such as malaria and ameba, are causes of meningitis in tropical and subtropical climates. In malarial meningitis, constitutional symptoms of malaria are present prior to the onset of coma. The parasites cause stasis in multiple small vessels of the brain. Amebic meningoencephalitis has a more subacute course and is one of the causes of so-called eosinophilic meningitis.

Fungal meningitis may occur after intense exposure to the organism, or in patients with a compromised immune state because of malignant disease or immunosuppressive drugs. Diagnosis depends upon identification of the organism in the CSF.

Pyogenic infections of the epidural or subdural spaces may lead to coma and can be suspected in the presence of focal neurologic signs and a compatible CT scan. Infection of the paranasal sinuses, middle ear, or mastoid may produce thrombosis of the cerebral veins or dural sinuses. Periorbital edema, scalp edema, and dilation of the collateral venous channels on the scalp and face are diagnostic clues.

Multifocal showers of septic emboli into the brain will cause sudden coma with resolution over the ensuing 24 to 48 hours. Usually, peripheral manifestations of embolization such as splinter hemorrhages, splenomegaly, and microscopic hematuria can be found.

Postinfectious or parainfectious encephalomyelitis may occur following common childhood viral infections and exanthems. Headache, fever, and alterations of consciousness follow the viral illness by several days. The spinal fluid is normal in about 20 per cent of these patients. Acute hemorrhagic leukoencephalopathy is similar to parainfectious encephalomyelitis except that a history of prior viral illness is frequently not present and the neurologic symptoms are more severe.

Pertussis immunization encephalopathy occurs most commonly in children between 3 and 8 months of age. Focal or generalized convulsions are seen 20 minutes to 72 hours after pertussis immunization without relationship to fever. This may be followed by severe neurologic deterioration with coma. Severe, prolonged, generalized major motor convulsions 7 to 10 days after smallpox vaccination occur in postvaccinal encephalomyelitis.

Any severe systemic infection (e.g., bacterial pneumonia, pyelonephritis, soft tissue abscess) can lead to depressed consciousness.

Causes of Unconsciousness Related to Injury or Tumor. Occasionally, unconsciousness can occur as a result of head injury without external evidence of trauma. History should be sought regarding the possibility of an injury. Scalp swelling in the temporal area suggests an underlying hematoma and fracture through the temporal bone. Retroauricular hematoma or ecchymosis (Battle's sign), periorbital ecchymosis, and hemorrhage behind the tympanic membrane are indications of basilar skull fracture, as are otorrhea or rhinorrhea. Clear fluid draining from the nose or ear is presumed to be CSF if the fluid contains glucose.

In younger children, hemorrhage from a fractured femur may be sufficient to cause hypovolemic shock and coma. Fat embolism from long bone fractures is less common in children than in adults but must be considered in the differential diagnosis of coma associated with trauma. When fat embolism is present, fat droplets may be seen in the urine with fat stain or with darkfield illumination.

If cervical vertebral fracture is suspected, the patient must be moved with the neck immobilized until cervical x-rays rule out that possibility.

Concussion is a term used to refer to a mild alteration in consciousness following blunt head trauma. The term implies absence of microscopic or gross neuropathology. If alterations of consciousness persist beyond an arbitrary limit of 24 hours, more severe injury to the brain is presumed. When this is the case, contusion of the brain is clinically considered with the implication of bruising, focal hemorrhages, and necrosis. Laceration of the brain is a still more serious injury.

Skull fractures assume immediate clinical importance if they are depressed or cross the middle meningeal artery groove. Depressed skull fractures are usually associated with laceration of the brain and dura and may lead to a fatal acute subdural hemorrhage regardless of surgical intervention. Fractures across the middle meningeal artery groove may tear the middle meningeal artery with epidural hemorrhage, a neurosurgical emergency. In epidural hemorrhage, depressed consciousness is present immediately following the injury and is then followed by a "lucid interval." As the hematoma enlarges, subacute depression in consciousness ensues, proceeding to death unless intervention occurs.

Acute subdural bleeding is often associated with contusions and lacerations of the brain and brainstem. When the clot is the main or sole lesion, surgical treatment may be most gratifying. Unconsciousness continuing from the time of injury or rapid deterioration of consciousness should arouse suspicion of acute subdural bleeding. Pupillary.dilation, loss of extraocular movements, retinal hemorrhages, and papilledema may be seen. Frequently, contralateral hemiparesis and focal or generalized seizures occur. Subdural hematomas occur with equal incidence in the presence and absence of skull fracture. Tearing of connecting veins between the cortical surface and dura is the most frequent cause of subdural hematoma; headache is followed in time by a gradual lapse into stupor, which may be mistaken for psychiatric dysfunction. Focal or vague neurologic signs may be present.

With intracerebral hematomas a lucid interval may occur with increasing headaches. Contralateral paresis may develop with progression to stupor and coma. Pupillary inequality is not as common as in subdural and extradural collections; papilledema is uncommon. One third of patients have no skull fracture and another third have a fracture contralateral to the hematoma. Intraparenchymatous hematomas of the cerebellum frequently produce a disturbed mental state with confusion, agitation, and psychotic behavior associated with stupor and lethargy. Localizing signs are usually absent; when present, they consist of ipsilateral hypotonia, dysmetria, dysdiadochokinesia, and nystagmus.

The diagnosis of intracranial bleeding and its site is best confirmed by CT scan. Cerebral angiography may be needed.

Neoplasms often present as intracranial mass lesions with the signs depending upon the location of the mass. Depression of consciousness is common, especially when the lesion obstructs CSF pathways resulting in hydrocephalus.

Electrocution and exposure to extremes of heat and cold or to rapid reduction in atmospheric pressure are other rare physical causes of unconsciousness in children.

Causes of Childhood Unconsciousness Related to Extracranial or Intracranial Illness. Most causes of childhood unconsciousness in this category can be grouped under the following headings: hypoglycemia, hyperosmotia, hyponatremia, hypertension, hypoxia, hemorrhage, and hepatic disorders (Reye's syndrome). A number of clinical features are shared by all metabolic encephalopathies. The earliest symptom is gradual impairment of consciousness. In infants this often presents as irritability, loss of appetite, and diminished alertness. Periodic hyperpnea may progress to Cheyne-Stokes respiration. Eye movements are random initially but ultimately become decreased and the eyes assume mid position.

Severe hypoglycemia is associated with generalized or focal seizures in almost all children. Blood glucose levels below 30 mg per dl are probably required to produce neurologic symptoms. Lesser degrees of hypoglycemia may trigger seizures in persons who are seizure-prone. Cortical function is involved early. The brainstem is last to be involved. The response to intravenous glucose is immediate in patients who have not sustained permanent neurologic damage. The causes of hypoglycemia in infants and children after the neonatal period are most often pharmacologic (e.g., related to insulin overdosage, accidental or surreptitious oral antidiabetic agents, or poisoning with ethanol, propoxyphene, or salicylates). Other causes include liver disease, insulin-producing pancreatic or extrapancreatic tumors, other endocrine abnormalities (hypothyroidism or hyperthyroidism, hypothalamic-pituitary dysfunction, adrenal cortical insufficiency), Reye's syndrome, glycogen storage diseases, prediabetic states, and leucine-sensitive hypoglycemia.

Hyperosmotic states are usually hypernatremic or hyperglycemic or both. Hypernatremic dehydration results in neurologic complications more often than hyponatremic dehydration in infants under 6 months of age, and enteric disease is the usual basis. Acute hypernatremia may occur with inadvertent salt overload given in infant feeding or in gastric washing. Hypernatremia has been known to occur after administration of radiologic contrast media. Clinically significant levels of serum sodium are above 155 to 160 mEq per liter. Convulsions and coma may be precipitated by too-rapid correction of the abnormality. Subdural hematoma is a rare complication. CSF protein is occasionally elevated. Transient diabetes insipidus and hypernatremia may occur with intracranial disorders. Diabetic ketoacidosis and hyperglycemia are other causes for the hyperosmotic state.

The clinical picture of hyponatremic dehydration is also nonspecific. Serum sodium levels below 115 to 120 mEq per liter are usually required before neurologic symptoms develop. Listlessness and fatigue progress to irritability, drowsiness, headache, coma, and convulsions. Hypotonic musculature and depressed stretch reflexes are found. Cerebral venous thrombosis is a rare but important complication of severe dehydration and shock. The thrombosis usually affects the sagittal sinus, resulting in bilateral hemiparesis and convulsions. The CSF may contain red blood cells and elevated protein. Hyponatremia may also result from overhydration.

Almost any acute and severe intracranial process may be associated with "inappropriate" antidiuretic hormone secretion. Causes include anesthetic agents, drugs, craniocerebral trauma, encephalitis, and meningitis. The symptoms are those of hyponatremia and the laboratory findings indicate hypervolemia, oliguria, and increased urinary osmolality.

Other causes of hyponatremia include excessive salt loss from the skin in burns and in cystic fibrosis, heat stress, salt-losing renal diseases, and adrenal insufficiency.

Hypertension in children may be caused by chronic or acute renal insufficiency. Acute glomerulonephritis may present with severe hypertension and depressed consciousness. Familial dysautonomia, pheochromocytoma, and ingestion of sympathomimetic agents are other conditions associated with hypertension in children. Hypertension may be present with increased intracranial pressure from any cause.

Hypoxia is frequently responsible for prolonged and, many times, irreversible unconsciousness in children following cardiopulmonary arrest; the diagnosis is made by exclusion of other metabolic causes for coma. This is a situation in which the question of brain death often arises. Hypoxic attacks, more common during the first 2 years of life, are seen in 12 to 15 per cent of patients with cyanotic congenital heart disease; the attacks may occur many times a day and are related to activity. Permanent neurologic sequelae sometimes result. Hypoxic damage may occur from smoke and carbon monoxide inhalation.

Hemorrhage related to deficiency of plasma clotting factors may occur in the subarachnoid space, subdural space, or intracerebrally. Subarachnoid hemorrhage in the child can occur from rupture of an aneurysm or an arteriovenous malformation. Clinical symptoms are similar to those in adults, though the child may not mention the severe headache prior to collapse and coma. Stiff neck is not found as consistently in children as in adults. The CSF is grossly bloody and does not clear as more fluid is removed. Location of the lesion is established by arteriography.

Polyarteritis, systemic lupus erythematosus, and granulomatous angitis predispose to intracerebral hemorrhage or thrombosis and may present with depression of consciousness. Lupus cerebritis can also cause depressed consciousness in children.

Liver failure associated with hepatic coma and elevated blood ammonia occasionally occurs in children. Reye's syndrome is an illness with fatty degeneration of the viscera, coma, and severe cerebral edema. Reye's syndrome begins approximately 1 week after a presumed viral illness. Severe vomiting and confusion progress rapidly to delirium. Signs of increased intracranial pressure may be present. The most useful laboratory test is an elevated serum glutamic oxaloacetic transaminase. Hyperammonemia and hypoglycemia may be present. The prognosis is grave and death is often due to cerebral herniation.

THE UNCONSCIOUS ADULT

By BRUCE H. PETERS, M.D.
Galveston, Texas

Caring for the unconscious patient represents a special challenge. A life is held in threat and a diagnosis must be quickly and accurately made and specific therapy begun. But the patient, whose complaints and history hold the diagnostic key, cannot communicate. The approach must be systematic and rapid. Jumping to conclusions based on insufficient evidence, and missing a secondary diagnosis when there is more than one cause for depressed consciousness, must be avoided. The physician must not hesitate to seek information from people who know the patient or from prior health records. The physical examination must be especially carefully performed; however, because the patient is unable to cooperate with testing of voluntary function, the relevant portion of the examination may be performed rather quickly. The physician must at all times be prepared to interrupt his diagnostic studies to give emergency supportive care.

CLASSIFICATION OF ALTERED CONSCIOUSNESS

Descriptions of consciousness range from deep coma through stupor, drowsiness, or delirium to normal wakefulness. Such terms are imprecise. An exact description of the state of awareness provides a basis for prognosis and for serial examination by other health care providers to ascertain whether the patient's status is changing. The description should include the intensity and type of stimulation used in attempting to arouse the patient to alertness and the kinds of purposeful actions that the patient can then perform. The Glasgow Responsiveness Scale is useful, as it provides the desired quantitation of consciousness. This scale measures the eye opening, best motor response, and verbal response to stimulation. The scale ranges from 3 in the deepest coma to a maximum of 15 in a fully conscious patient. Eye opening is given 4 points if done spontaneously, 3 if in response to speech, 2 if in response to pain, and 1 if nil. Best motor response is recorded as 6, if the patient obeys commands, 5 if he localizes to annoying stimulation, 4 if there is withdrawal of a limb from stimulation, 3 if there is abnormal flexion (decorticate posturing) of the arms, 2 if stimulation provokes extension and internal rotation of the arm (decerebrate posturing), and 1 if nil. Verbal response is scored as 5 points if the patient is oriented, 4 if able to converse but confused, 3 if conversation is inappropriate, 2 if speech is incomprehensible, and 1 if no verbal response. The scale values are easily recorded and understood by all members of the patient-care team.

INITIAL ASSESSMENT AND RESPONSE

The physician's primary duty is to ascertain that the airway, heart action, and blood pressure are adequate and any blood loss is controlled before proceeding with further examination. If there appears to be any reasonable possibility that the patient is hypoglycemic, give 25 to 50 ml of 50 per cent glucose intravenously. Blood glucose, electrolytes, blood urea nitrogen (BUN), liver enzymes, and arterial pH, PO_2, and PCO_2 should be drawn at this time if a metabolic problem is suspected. An intravenous line is left in place. If there is increased intracranial pressure, measures such as steroids (dexamethasone 10 mg intravenously followed by 4 mg each six hours parenterally), osmotic diuretics (mannitol, 50 grams of 20 per cent solution over 20 minutes in patients not in renal failure), and lowering the PCO_2 by hyperventilation can protect the swollen brain. Continuous or recurrent generalized seizure activity must be quickly treated. The appearance of a metabolic coma accompanied by pinpoint but reactive pupils suggests opiate intoxication. This is best treated with naloxone HCl 0.4 mg intravenously repeated every 5 minutes until consciousness is regained. The physician must be sure that the neck is not fractured. In cases of trauma, the neck must be assumed broken and any movement is done with the neck held in slight extension with traction until cervical spine films clarify the situation. If the neck is not fractured, passive neck flexion is done. If the neck is rigid when flexed but there are no focal neurologic abnormalities, subarachnoid hemorrhage, meningitis, or encephalitis is suggested. If there are coexistent focal signs, cerebral hemorrhage or subarachnoid hemorrhage is likely. In metabolic coma, the neck is often moderately and equally stiff in both flexion and rotation.

The patient's purse or billfold may hold an address so that relatives or neighbors can be contacted to provide information on the mode of onset of the illness, prior diagnosis and medications, and problems such as alcoholism, drug dependency, suicidal depression, convulsive disorders, hypertension, diabetes, or head injury.

The central issue is the specific cause of coma. The four major categories are: (1) supratentorial mass with brainstem compression or bihemispheral dysfunction, (2) infratentorial mass or destruction, (3) metabolic encephalopathy (which also includes cerebral toxins, infections, hypoxia, and inflammatory diseases, all of which may diffusely impair cerebral function), and (4) psychogenic unresponsiveness.

Wakefulness depends on an intact cortex and at least one cerebral hemisphere that is kept aroused by an intact brainstem reticular activating system. Therefore, unconsciousness, for which we will now use the general term coma, results only from bilateral hemispheral suppression or damage, impaired brainstem activation, or both. A strictly unilateral hemispheral disorder does not commonly result in coma unless there is seizure activity or unless single hemisphere disease results in brain swelling that compresses the brainstem or the opposite hemisphere. In metabolic coma, both hemispheres are suppressed and the brainstem becomes involved as the coma deepens. Structural diseases are associated with physical signs, which are usually focally persistent and often asymmetrical. In metabolic coma, the examination usually shows symmetric neurologic signs. In some metabolic disorders the neurologic signs will shift so that there may briefly appear to be a focal process. Repeated examination is mandatory, as only in structural disease will abnormalities be focally persistent.

EXAMINING THE COMATOSE PATIENT

Testing of sensory discrimination and volitional movement are impossible in the comatose patient and the examination must depend on meticulous observation of the patient's spontaneous and provoked motor activity, muscle tone, reflexes, posture, ocular movements, pupillary function, respiratory pattern, and optic fundi. Specific dysfunctions characterize each level of brain involvement, allowing localization of coma cause. Table 1 shows major examination features of coma types.

Spontaneous and Reflex Motor Activity and Tone. Random, diffuse, twitching movements (myoclonus) and asterixis, which is a myoclonic jerking movement produced by holding a part in extension, suggest metabolic coma. Rhythmic jerking of a single limb or body region (focal seizure) indicates a contralateral hemispheral lesion. Generalized seizures can result from spread of a focal, supratentorial, electrically discharging lesion, or metabolic disease. Focal cerebellar or brainstem disease can result in forceful tonic extensor spasms that may resemble the tonic phase of a generalized seizure. Careful observation of spontaneous limb movements and of movements in response to moderately noxious stimuli (tissue-damaging stimulation is unneeded) is made and appropriateness and asymmetry of motion noted. A paralyzed limb will fall flaccidly when dropped. A limp and unmoved limb that rests in an uncomfortable or externally rotated position is probably paretic. Paratonia is a condition in which the patient pushes or pulls involuntarily resisting limb movement and is seen in those with moderate metabolic encephalopathy and may occur contralateral to a frontal lobe focal lesion. Facial weakness is identified in the comatose by a flattened nasolabial fold, sagging jaw angle, or respiratory-synchronous puffing out of the buccal pouch. Sensory examination is limited to noting the response to pain. Abducting a part to stimulation usually indicates the movement is voluntary. Asymmetry of response to corneal touch indicates pontine structural disease. The muscle stretch reflexes and response to plantar stimulation are tested the same as in the awake patient and have the same meaning. Bilateral Babinski signs are sometimes seen in metabolic coma and do not necessarily indicate a structural corticospinal tract lesion.

POSTURE

Decorticate posture consists of adduction of the upper limbs with elbow and wrist flexion; the lower limbs are held extended and inwardly rotated. This posture indicates a lesion involving the pyramidal system at the midbrain level. In decerebrate rigidity there is neck and back hyperextension and extension of the legs with extension, adduction, and pronation of the arms. Decerebrate rigidity is seen with focal damage of the brainstem, as a late stage in the rostrocaudal deterioration that results in an expanding supratentorial process that compresses lower structures, and sometimes in profound

Table 1. *Major Features of Coma Types*

Etiology	*Posture*	*Motor Response*	*Pupils*
Metabolic	Symmetric motor impairment, flaccid	Loss and preservation of function at same level, variable and changing response, asterixis or myoclonus, reflexes usually symmetric	Usually small, equal and reactive; pinpoint and reactive with opiate intoxication, dilated and fixed with anticholinergic intoxication, mid position and fixed in glutethimide intoxication
Cerebral hemispheral disease	Focal abnormalities of tone on side opposite lesion	Paresis or paratonia, abnormal reflexes on side opposite to lesion	Small and reactive
Diencephalic disease	Symmetric or asymmetric impairment or decorticate posture	Paresis or decorticate posturing on stimulation	Small and reactive
Uncal herniation	Focal abnormality, usually on side opposite dilated pupil	Asymmetric reflexes, paresis, or paratonia	Unequal, dilated pupil on side of herniation
Midbrain disease	Asymmetric or symmetric impairment, decorticate or decerebrate posture	Decorticate or decerebrate movements to stimulation	4 to 6 mm bilaterally and fixed
Pontine disease	Symmetric or asymmetric decerebrate or lower limb flexion posture	Decerebration or lower limb flexion to stimulation, jaw may deviate on corneal stimulation (oculomandibular reflex)	Bilateral pinpoint, very sluggish light reaction
Isolated medullary lesion	Flaccid or lower limb flexion	None or lower limb flexion	Small and reactive
Psychogenic	No movement but normal tone	May be absent or normal, symmetric reflexes	Normal reaction and size

Table 1. *Major Features of Coma Types—Continued*

Spontaneous Eye Movements	Oculovestibular Response	Respiration
May be slightly divergent	Tonic conjugate deviation on doll's eye maneuver (oculocephalic response) and on caloric testing	Varies with specific causes, hyperventilation with metabolic acidosis and respiratory alkalosis
Tonic conjugate deviation toward side of lesion (unless seizure drives eyes contralaterally)	Conjugate deviation	Cheyne-Stokes respiration or sighing
Conjugate or binasal deviation	Tonic conjugate deviation	Cheyne-Stokes respiration or eupnea
Paresis of vertical and internal movement of eye ipsilateral to herniation	Tonic deviation with unilateral paresis of medial gaze of ipsilateral eye	Eupnea or central neurogenic hyperventilation
Limited or internuclear ophthalmoplegia	Sluggish or internuclear ophthalmoplegia	Cheyne-Stokes respiration or central neurogenic hyperventilation
Eyes deviate conjugately toward more paralyzed side	Symmetrically or asymmetrically absent caloric and oculocephalic response	Ataxic or apneustic
Full in isolated lesion, absent in rostrocaudal deterioration reaching medullary level	Normal unless higher brain levels also involved	Ataxic or apnea
Conjugate without sustained deviation	Normal ipsilateral deviation with contralateral nystagmus on cold caloric testing, absent oculocephalic response	Normal or hyperventilation

metabolic encephalopathy. Decerebrate and decorticate posture may be provoked by noxious stimulation if not spontaneously apparent.

Spontaneous and Provoked Ocular Movements. In the unconscious patient without an ocular movement mechanism lesion, the eyes are conjugate or slightly divergent. Conjugate deviation of the eyes toward the side of the lesion characterizes destructive anterior hemispheral disease, whereas the conjugate deviation is toward the side of the weakness in a pontine lesion. Downward, binasal eye deviation occurs in pretectal lesions (as in thalamic hemorrhage), but also may be seen in hepatic or other encephalopathies. If the eyes are vertically dysconjugate (skewed), one suspects a pontine lesion, or cerebellar lesion with secondary pontine pressure, on the side of the downward-pointing eye.

Ocular motility is tested by observing oculocephalic or oculovestibular reflexes. After making certain that the neck is not fractured, the examiner initiates the oculocephalic reflex (doll's eye maneuver) by quickly rotating the head from side to side. The awake patient's eyes will not of themselves rotate during head rotation unless the patient is purposefully fixating on a stationary object. When consciousness is impaired, the eyes move conjugately in a direction opposite that of head movement as a result of a brainstem vestibular-proprioceptive reflex that is inhibited in the awake person. When seen, this reflex demonstrates that the oculomotor nerves and brainstem ocular movement connections are intact. In extremely deep coma, even when nonstructural in cause, this reflex may be absent.

The oculovestibular reflex is elicited by positioning the head 30° above horizontal and then injecting a stream of ice water into the external auditory canal and against the tympanic membrane. The tympanic membranes are visualized before this test is done to be certain they are intact. In the conscious or psychogenically unresponsive patient, the eyes deviate toward the stimulated side; rapid corrective movements directed to the opposite side result in nystagmus. In depressed consciousness due to bilateral hemispheral or metabolic disorder, the tonic movement is seen, but the frontal cortex-mediated rapid corrective movement is absent and nystagmus is not seen.

Coma in which oculocephalic and oculovestibular responses are normal is not likely to be due to a focal brainstem lesion.

Pupillary Responses and Optic Fundi. Use a very bright light stimulus so that even minimal response can be appreciated. Herniation of the uncus of the temporal lobe results in an ipsilateral fixed and dilated pupil because of compression of the third (oculomotor) cranial nerve. Midposition but bilaterally fixed pupils develop as the midbrain is compressed from above (as in uncal herniation or a central herniation caused by increased supratentorial pressure with rostrocaudal deterioration). Pinpoint pupils, with minimal light reactivity, are seen in lesions of the pons. Glutethamide intoxication can result in pupils medium in size but unresponsive to light. In most metabolic or toxic encephalopathies the pupils are small or normal in size and react briskly to light even though other brainstem functions at the same, or even lower, levels are severely impaired. Severe degrees of anoxia, ischemia, hypothermia, or sedative intoxication can cause enlarged pupils.

Papilledema reflects increased intracranial pressure. Flat-topped globular collections of blood (preretinal hemorrhage) may be seen in subarachnoid bleeding. Yellow or white emboli may be seen at retinal arteriole branching points.

Respiratory Pattern. The respiratory rate, depth, and rhythm reflect the level of brain lesion. Bilateral cerebral hemisphere structural or metabolic disease results in Cheyne-Stokes respiration (apnea alternating with periods of hyperpnea). When the midbrain–upper pontine level of the brain becomes damaged, sustained deep rapid respiration (central neurogenic hyperventilation) intervenes. An appearance of central neurogenic hyperventilation can be seen in hypoxia and persists for hours after its correction. Inspiration followed by a prolonged pause (apneustic breathing) and then an irregular pattern of random shallow and deep breaths (ataxic breathing) follow as the mid and caudal portions of the pons, and then the medulla oblongata, are damaged. Apnea and death supervene as the medullary respiratory centers are fully suppressed and unresponsive to even extreme hypoxia and hypercapnea.

General Examination. Laceration of the scalp or face, or a palpable skull depression, suggests a traumatically induced coma. Basilar skull fracture is suspected when there is a localized ecchymosis over the mastoid region (Battle's sign) or blood or cerebral spinal fluid issuing from an ear. Nontraumatic skin ecchymoses suggest that meningococcal or pneumococcal meningitis, or a consumptive coagulopathy, be considered. A bullous eruption may indicate barbiturate intoxication. A brilliant cherry-red skin color accompanies carbon monoxide poisoning. Spider telangiectasis or jaundice necessitates consideration of hepatic dysfunction, or coma resulting from alcohol withdrawal. Needle tracks suggest possible drug abuse. A dry coarse skin accompanying hypothermia characterizes myxedema coma. Heart murmurs or cardiac arrhythmia gives clues about possible embolic disease. The patient's breath may have the characteristic odor of alcohol, but it is important to remember that trauma, subdural hematomas, seizures, and other causes of coma can coexist in the inebriated. The fruity odor of hepatic failure occasionally will be present even when hepatic destruction is so advanced that serum hepatic enzyme levels are normal; a uriniferous breath suggests azotemia. Check the tongue for evidence of biting; this suggests that a seizure may have occurred.

LABORATORY STUDIES

It is important not to ignore seeking a history and carefully examining the patient before turning to the laboratory for help. When the circumstances suggest a metabolic cause of coma, blood tests should include those for blood glucose, blood urea nitrogen (BUN), serum sodium, potassium and calcium, and liver function tests. If the examination or function tests indicate hepatic dysfunction, serum ammonia is measured. In any unknown metabolic coma, or when drug toxicity is suspected, both blood and urine are screened for drugs. Body fluids (blood, urine, vomitus or gastric aspirate) are preserved when poisoning is suspected. When there is possible organophosphate pesticide exposure (metabolic coma with tiny pupils and bradycardia), serum and erythrocyte acetylcholinesterase levels are measured. Hypoxia and hypercapnea can exist even when there is no obvious cyanosis or hypoventilation; this makes arterial PO_2 and PCO_2 important tests in obscure metabolic encephalopathies.

The electroencephalogram (EEG), a physiologic test, is very useful for screening the comatose patient. Metabolic dysfunction can cause specific patterns of EEG abnormality, all characterized by a diffuse slowing of electrocerebral activity. When the examination suggests a structural cause for coma, skull x-rays are done to exclude skull fracture. Plain skull x-rays are inadequate to determine structural brain disease. The radionuclide brain scan can help show cerebral infarctions or masses. A structural brain lesion can be inferred from focal slowing of the EEG. The advent of the computerized tomogram (CT scan) has revolutionized the localization of structural brain disease. This is a rapid, noninvasive, and, when appropriately used, cost-effective test that documents the presence of an intracerebral hematoma, mass obstructive hydrocephalus, brain infarction, or edema.

Remember that the CT scan does not, except by inference, reflect the brain's physiologic status, as does the EEG. Arteriography may serve to identify the same lesion as the CT scan, although often with less specificity and increased risk. In cases of subarachnoid hemorrhage, a ruptured aneurysm may not be identified except through arteriography.

It is important that a lumbar puncture *not* be done when there are signs of an expanding intracranial mass and especially when focal neurologic abnormalities are accompanied by fever and nuchal rigidity, indicating a possible brain abscess. Herniation of intracranial structures may follow a lumbar puncture in such circumstances. In patients with nuchal rigidity without focal features in whom meningitis, encephalitis, or subarachnoid hemorrhage is suspected, a lumbar puncture is indicated. It is important that the spinal fluid pressure be recorded and fluid taken for cell count, protein, glucose (along with blood glucose), and appropriate cultures. When there is diffuse cerebral disease, unassociated with a cerebral mass, the risk of lumbar puncture is relatively small, even when intracranial pressure is elevated. If it is suspected that a focal mass lesion exists, a CT scan or substitute procedure should precede the performance of a lumbar puncture.

SPECIFIC CAUSES OF COMA

Some causes of coma are shown in Table 2. The careful physician will also consider additional possibilities. The following conditions bear special consideration.

Epidural and Subdural Hematomas. An epidural hematoma may develop when trauma causes a temporal skull fracture resulting in delayed hemorrhage from a meningeal artery. Blood under arterial pressure rapidly collects between dura and skull and compresses the hemisphere. Depressed consciousness develops, then unresponsiveness with a dilated fixed pupil ipsilateral to the hemorrhage and contralateral (usually) hemiparesis. Death may result unless the pressure is immediately surgically relieved. A subdural hematoma may soon follow trauma or be delayed by weeks. In this condition venous blood collects, causing unilateral (and in 20 per cent of cases bilateral) hemispheral compression. Alcoholics, demented patients, those with a convulsive disorder, and combative patients have increased likelihood of sustaining trauma and may have some cerebral atrophy; this allows stretching of bridging cortical veins so that subdural hematomas more easily result from trauma.

Intracerebellar Hemorrhage. Rapid devel-

Table 2. *Causes of Coma*

I. Structural brain disease
   A. Supratentorial
      1. Neoplasm (usually subacute onset)
      2. Subdural hematoma
      3. Epidural hematoma
      4. Intracerebral hematoma
      5. Cerebral infarct (with cerebral edema causing bilateral involvement)
   B. Infratentorial
      1. Brainstem infarction, hemorrhage, or mass
      2. Cerebellar hemorrhage, with brainstem compression

II. Toxic (drug overdose)
   A. Sedative and hypnotics
   B. Antidepressants
   C. Alcohol

III. Metabolic
   A. Respiratory insufficiency (hypoxia, hypercarbia)
   B. Hypoglycemia
   C. Diabetic acidosis and nonketotic hyperglycemia
   D. Hyponatremia (inappropriate ADH secretion, water intoxication)
   E. Uremic encephalopathy
   F. Hepatic encephalopathy
   G. Myxedema coma

IV. CNS infections
   A. Meningitis
   B. Encephalitis
   C. Abscess (acts as focal lesion)

V. Central nervous system vasculitis

VI. Psychogenic unresponsiveness

VII. Other
   A. Cerebral concussion
   B. Subarachnoid hemorrhage
   C. Postictal state

opment of a hematoma in the cerebellum occurs in some hypertensive patients. The history is often of sudden headache and neck stiffness, sometimes with a brief interval of ataxia and slurred speech, then progression to coma. There is nuchal rigidity and dysconjugate eye movements and findings characteristic of brainstem compression. Lumbar puncture must be avoided lest cerebellar tonsil herniation through the foramen magnum occur. A timely CT scan or vertebral arteriogram assists diagnosis of this life-threatening and surgically treatable disorder.

Anticholinergic Intoxication. Overdosage of scopolamine (found in some proprietary sleeping medications) causes coma with fever, flushed, dry skin, tachycardia, and markedly dilated pupils with poor light response.

Locked-in Syndrome. In this human tragedy the patient is not comatose, but deafferented, so that he can make no voluntary movement other than vertical eye movement. The cause is often infarction of the pontine base so that cortical-spinal and cortical-bulbar tracts mediating limb, mouth, and horizontal eye movements are damaged. The reticular activating system, cerebral hemispheres, and optic and auditory systems are functional so that the patient remains aware of his environment.

Psychogenic Unresponsiveness. Persons of hysterical temperament can, when severely stressed, become unresponsive to their environment although their pupils remain equal and reactive. There is no oculocephalic response, normal nystagmus occurs with caloric stimulation, tone is normal, and there are no respiratory or reflex abnormalities.

CHRONIC ABDOMINAL PAIN

By THOMAS H. CASEY, M.D.
Rochester, New York

THE PROBLEM

Pain that has been present for weeks or months, often for years, and that the patient perceives to be somewhere within the area of the abdomen is one of the more common problems confronting the practicing physician. The pain may be persistent from day to day or intermittent with acute exacerbations. It may be consistent or variable in its quality, intensity, and location. The patient's physical and emotional well-being are frequently affected by the persistence of this problem, and it must be remembered that many conditions causing chronic pain are capable of acute life-threatening complications. Pain is a protective mechanism, a warning signal to the patient that something is not right. Perhaps the problem has become chronic because the insidious nature of its onset led the patient to minimize its significance until symptoms worsened, because the patient has tried various self-medications without permanent benefit, or because of an inability of the physician to ascertain the underlying cause of the problem and to institute appropriate therapy. At times the problem has been correctly identified, but complete relief of the pain has proved impossible and the patient continues to go from physician to physician seeking the unobtainable.

APPROACH TO THE PROBLEM

A thorough and detailed medical history is the single most valuable tool in the evaluation of any patient with chronic abdominal pain. The patient's description of the location, radiation, character, severity, mode of onset, and duration is sought. Factors that aggravate the pain as well as those that relieve it must be delineated. One must inquire about associated features such as nausea and vomiting, appetite, the patient's weight and any change therein, the effect of eating on the pain, how the pain is influenced by the quantity of food ingested as well as specific types of foods. Evidence of gastrointestinal blood loss as manifested by hematemesis, melena, or hematochezia should be sought, as well as a history of anemia. Careful assessment should be made of the act of swallowing and any influence this may have on the pain. Just as important is evaluation of the function of the lower end of the gastrointestinal tract in its relationship to the patient's pain, namely the act of defecation, the occurrence of diarrhea or constipation, and the passage of flatus.

Since we are dealing with a problem that has been occurring over a considerable period of time, it is important that an appreciation of the time course of the illness be developed. Have the symptoms been static or have they been progressive? Did the weight loss occur at the beginning of the illness or gradually over the entire course of the problem? Have associated features been present all along or have they developed as time passed? The past medical history will bring out information regarding previous operations, exposures to infectious diseases, and travel to areas where intestinal parasites might be encountered. A systemic review may disclose important information of problems in other organ systems that might have a profound relationship on the abdominal complaint. An inquiry must be made into the use of medications, particularly those that might be ulcerogenic. Drug allergies need to be recorded, as well as the patient's use of tobacco, alcohol, and caffeine-containing beverages. One must not overlook the family history because an important clue might be obtained here, particularly regarding such entities as peptic ulcer disease, pancreatitis, gallbladder disease, or inflammatory bowel disease.

After taking a careful and thorough history from the patient, even before the physical examination has been performed, the physician will be formulating ideas as to the mechanism of the pain. From the patient's localization of the pain one begins to think of the underlying organs and the possible pathology therein. Pain in the region of the subxiphoid area is often associated with lesions of the lower esophagus or cardia of the stomach, such as reflux esophagitis, esophageal or high gastric ulcer, or carcinoma. Inquiry should be made about pyrosis and dysphagia. Lesions in the fundus and upper part of the body of the stomach, such as a high gastric ulcer, tend to produce pain to the left of the midline in the upper abdomen. Disease in the lower body and antrum of the stomach as well as that near the pylorus, a not infrequent site for peptic ulcer disease, tends to produce pain in the mid epigastrium, while the usual duodenal ulcer arising in the first portion of the duodenum produces its discomfort in a similar location. A duodenal ulcer arising in the descending duodenum, whether associated with salicylate usage or as part of the Zollinger-Ellison syndrome, may cause pain in an area close to the umbilicus, as do other lesions arising in the more distal duodenum and jejunum.

Pain produced by lesions in the ileum will generally be felt above or about the umbilicus, namely in the mid abdomen. Pain arising from the bile ducts and pancreas will generally be felt in the upper abdomen, toward the midline, sometimes more to the right or to the left of the midline, depending on the exact site of origin. Pain arising from pancreatic disease often is felt through to the back, particularly to the left of the spine. Disease of the gallbladder and biliary tree often begins with midline epigastric pain before any pain is felt in the right upper quadrant of the abdomen. It is only when there is irritation of the peritoneum in the right upper quadrant—whether arising from the gallbladder, the hepatic flexure of the colon, the liver, or the duodenum— that the patient will complain of localizing pain in the right upper quadrant, often with appropriate physical findings in the area.

A rather common complaint is that of a dull pressure-like discomfort intermittently in the right upper quadrant of the abdomen in patients with no other associated features or physical findings. Such distress has been attributed to gas trapped in the splenic flexure of the colon. Lesions of the stomach, liver, biliary tract, colon, right kidney, duodenum, and mesentery must be excluded. Left upper quadrant abdominal pain raises questions about lesions in the body and tail of the pancreas, the transverse colon, splenic flexure, and upper descending colon as well as the spleen. Left lower quadrant discomfort focuses attention on the lower descending colon, rectosigmoid, and sigmoid colon. Diseases of the urinary tract and the left adnexa must be considered as well. Pain in the right lower quadrant raises consideration of disease in the terminal ileum, cecum, and ascending colon as well as the urinary tract on that side and right adnexa.

Pain in the back, as mentioned earlier, is often associated with pancreatic disease, either inflammatory or neoplastic, and this pain seems to penetrate directly through to the back from the left upper quadrant or from the mid epigastrium. Posterior penetration of a peptic ulcer regularly produces back pain. The patient with gallbladder disease may often have radiation of pain around the right costal margin to or near the angle of the right scapula. Otherwise uncomplicated disease in the gastrointestinal tract does not usually cause radiation of pain to the back unless the posterior parietal peritoneum or the mesenteric attachment of the bowel is involved. This may be seen with regional enteritis with extensive mesenteric involvement, as well as with lesions of the pancreas and kidney.

The patient's description of the character and degree of severity of the pain reveals much about its origin. Pain arising from the abdominal wall is usually sharper, well localized, and intense. Abnormalities of the abdominal wall itself are infrequently encountered and frequently forgotten. Small hernias certainly can generate considerable discomfort. Their detection, particularly in an obese patient, may not always be easy. A hematoma in the rectus sheath may result in a chronic problem and a history of trauma or anticoagulation therapy may underlie such difficulty. Primary tumors of the abdominal wall are particularly infrequently encountered. Metastatic carcinoma to the abdominal wall is somewhat more frequent.

Pain arising from visceral structures has a dull, aching quality. The patient with an active peptic ulcer complains of the familiar gnawing hunger sensation, a burning, or an ache. Colicky pain suggests intestinal spasm, while the so-called colic of biliary or renal origin is really not colicky but a pain that steadily becomes more intense, reaching a plateau of severity that lasts for a considerable period of time, waxing and waning but not having the brief rhythmic intermittency that is seen with true colic. With intestinal colicky pain the pa-

tient may also be aware of hyperperistalsis and borborygmy during the episodes of pain, or with temporary relief of the pain. As long as the process causing the pain is confined to the viscera, without involvement of the parietal peritoneum, there is a diffuseness of location with a general awareness of the pain toward the mid abdomen. With involvement of the parietal peritoneum, localization to the overlying area of the abdomen occurs and the pain generally is felt to be more intense just as if it were arising from the abdominal wall itself. However, pain may be felt in the skin or deeper tissues of the abdomen as a result of a more intense visceral stimulus without involvement of the parietal peritoneum. Such referred pain is sometimes felt between the scapulae or near the tip of the right scapula in patients with cholecystitis. Similarly, pain in the flank radiating to the testis in the male should suggest a ureteral origin. Pain arising in the lower esophagus is often felt as a burning sensation in the subxiphoid area but in approximately 1 patient in 10 such a sensation may be referred to the throat. As the stimulus for this pain becomes more intense, referred pain is felt in the middle of the back. The uterus is a hollow viscus and produces pain in response to distention, severe contraction, or obstruction. Such pain is felt in the low abdomen and the lower back. The ovary is an infrequent source of pain unless there is torsion and strangulation or rupture of a cyst.

The duration of the patient's complaint, its recurrence over time, and its relationship to physiologic functions or activities provide valuable clues to the origin of the problem. The most characteristic feature of peptic ulcer pain is its tendency to recur from 1 to 4 hours after the ingestion of food, day after day, week after week. This rhythmicity and periodicity are associated with no other abdominal disease. Ulcer pain is usually relieved by the ingestion of food or antacids. Pain of a more constant sort, lasting for weeks or months, is more suggestive of a low-grade inflammatory process or a mass lesion, either cystic or neoplastic. Pain occurring very shortly after the ingestion of food suggests a gastric origin and should be appropriately located in the epigastrium or left upper quadrant of the abdomen, or both. Gastritis or an infiltrating neoplasm of the stomach would produce such symptoms. Late postprandial pain occurring in the epigastrium and occurring in isolated episodes is suggestive of biliary tract disease or pylorospasm. Abdominal angina must be considered in the patient whose pain develops in a variable period after eating, tends to have a quantitative relationship to the amount of food ingested, and is invariably associated with weight loss. A fear of eating develops and may be quite striking despite an apparently normal appetite. Evidence of other manifestations of vascular disease such as angina pectoris or intermittent claudication as well as a history of diabetes mellitus or hypertension should be sought. These patients tend to be in the older age group but not exclusively so.

Inflammatory lesions of the intestine, such as Crohn's disease or nongranulomatous ulcerative jejunoileitis, regularly produce painful symptoms with the development of peristalsis. Such peristaltic activity follows the ingestion of food, and the intensity of pain may be greater with a larger quantity of roughage in the diet. Diarrhea is a prominent symptom in most instances. Partially obstructing lesions of the intestine, such as primary neoplasms or extrinsic adhesions, may be similarly symptomatic. Carcinoid tumors tend to produce partial small bowel obstruction with or without the carcinoid syndrome. Primary lymphoma of the small intestine may be focal, producing symptoms of partial obstruction due to intermittent intussusception, or diffuse with prominent symptoms of malabsorption along with pain. Lower abdominal pain relieved by defecation or the passage of flatus suggests a problem in the distal colon or rectum, either of an organic or functional nature.

One's understanding of potential abdominal involvement by diseases that are not generally thought of as having gastrointestinal manifestations must be recalled as the history is developed. Long-standing rheumatoid arthritis treated with corticosteroids has been associated with vascular lesions, bowel infarctions, perforation, peritonitis, and amyloidosis. Systemic amyloidosis has resulted in ulcerations of the stomach and colon and been associated with mesenteric ischemic attacks. Abdominal pain may be seen with scleroderma and with dermatomyositis, while systemic lupus erythematosus may produce pancreatitis, peritonitis, perisplenitis, or perihepatitis. Abdominal pain is a frequent complaint of patients with systemic mastocytosis; complaints of diarrhea, flushing, and a cutaneous eruption should suggest the diagnosis. The association of hyperparathyroidism with peptic ulcer disease and with pancreatitis is generally well known. Known pulmonary fibrosis and exposure to asbestos would suggest primary mesothelioma of the peritoneum or pleural cavity.

Recurrent episodes of fever with painful episodes suggest an inflammatory process, that is, possible infection with abscess formation; appendicitis and diverticulitis are high on the list of possible causes. However, more rare entities such as mesenteric panniculitis should not be forgotten. A palpable mass is usually felt in the majority of patients.

When the history reveals that the location, radiation, character, and severity of the pain are not consistent with established physiologic principles, a psychogenic origin for this problem must be considered. Here the patient's description of the difficulty is often somewhat vague, and one might note a discrepancy between the patient's description of the severity of the pain and his behavior. A relationship to periods of psychologic stress might be encountered. A history of other pain problems occurring concomitantly elsewhere in the body or on previous occasions is commonly noted. Thus a psychogenic origin for the patient's complaints can be strongly suspected from the history alone, particularly when information is developed about extensive laboratory, roentgenographic, and endoscopic procedures performed in the past that have not revealed abnormalities.

Despite the fact that the patient may have had previous unrevealing physical examinations, a complete examination with special attention to the abdomen is in order. As implied earlier, the physical examination is not as likely to reveal the underlying cause of the patient's pain problem as is a good medical history. A physical finding of diagnostic importance quite likely would have been found on previous examinations. Nevertheless, a careful examination may reveal just the clue to unravel the entire problem.

If abdominal distension is noted, care should be taken to determine whether this is due to intraluminal gas, ascites, enlarged abdominal organs, or a cyst or tumor. A conspicuous venous pattern over the abdominal wall might signal some degree of obstruction in the superior or inferior vena cava or the portal circulation, depending upon the particular area of venous prominence and the direction flow within the veins. Visible peristaltic waves might be noted and coincide with colicky pain, with increase in bowel sounds, or with an intermittently palpable mass. Findings of partial intermittent small bowel obstruction might not be noted if the examination is performed after the patient's food intake has been restricted but might be brought out if the patient has eaten a meal high in residue an hour or more before the examination. Pulsations of unusual force might be visible and suggest the possibility of an enlarged aorta or the transmitted pulsation of a mass in the area. The detection of a bruit is not particularly specific for an intravascular cause but is suggestive.

If the pain arises in close proximity to a scar of a previous operation, careful search should be made for an incisional hernia. A small defect may easily escape detection, just as a small epigastric hernia, a Richter's hernia, or a femoral or obturator hernia might. The latter possibility, though infrequently encountered, should be suspected in the elderly woman who has lost considerable weight and, in addition to her abdominal symptoms, complains of a dull, achy pain on the inner aspect of the thigh to the level of the knee (Howship-Romberg sign).

After careful inspection and auscultation of the abdomen, the entire abdomen is palpated lightly, then more firmly and deeply. When the patient's symptoms have suggested that the problem may lie in a particular area of the abdomen, this is the last region to be palpated. Any area of cutaneous hypersensitivity is noted. Deep palpation should be performed with the abdominal wall well relaxed and then again with the abdominal muscles made taut, by having the patient raise either his feet or his head from the table. If the tenderness elicited on deep palpation persists when the abdominal wall is taut, an abdominal wall source for the discomfort must be considered. Careful attention should be paid to any inequality in the resistance to the palpating hand on the two sides of the abdomen. Muscle guarding and rigidity may at times be marked, but at other times a very subtle difference in tone between the two rectus muscles may be the only clue to underlying pathology.

The colon can often be palpated in the left lower quadrant as a sausage-shaped, movable tube. The transverse colon is less frequently palpated, except in a very thin patient. The ascending colon often contains fluid and gas and can be compressed in the right side of the abdomen. Tumors are not often palpated in the left colon but, as carcinoma may reach considerable size in the cecum and ascending colon, they are much more frequently palpated there. Accordingly, extremely careful palpation should be carried out in the ileocecal region. Crohn's disease, too, may produce a palpable mass in this area particularly, as may tuberculosis of the bowel or amebiasis.

When the edge of the liver is palpated, its size and shape, the character of its surface and edge, any tenderness, and upper border of dullness should be noted. The latter, of course, is found by percussion. The spleen should be carefully sought, as it normally is not palpable. The finding of a palpable gall-bladder is most often encountered in association with obstructive jaundice owing to carcinoma of the head of the pancreas but may also be seen in the nonjaundiced patient when there is obstruction to the cystic duct with hydrops or empyema or when there is a mass arising from the wall of the gallbladder itself. The gallbladder may become calcified (porcelain gallbladder), and this is associated with the development of carcinoma at times.

While exerting pressure with one hand in the costal vertebral angle and palpating with the other hand high up in the corresponding upper quadrant of the abdomen, the examiner should attempt to palpate each kidney as the patient takes a deep breath. The lower pole of the right kidney is quite often felt in patients with an asthenic habitus. Any unusual degree of ptosis should be noted. Enlargement of the kidney, by hydronephrosis, cystic disease, infection, or tumor, should be recognized. Pseudocyst of the pancreas may be palpated.

Abnormalities arising from the uterus, fallopian tubes, or ovaries may be detected on abdominal examination but are most likely to be detected by a bimanual pelvic examination. The rectal examination, of course, is important in the female as well as the male to detect abnormalities within the pelvis and rectum. In the male the prostate, seminal vesicles, epididymis, and testes must be carefully evaluated.

LABORATORY STUDIES

Determination of the blood count, examination of the blood smear, a urinalysis, and an erythrocyte sedimentation rate are basic laboratory investigations. A platelet count is determined if any deviation from the norm is suggested by the blood smear. Occult blood in the stool should be tested for and, if indicated by circumstances, stool should be examined for ova and parasites. Any signs or symptoms of malabsorption or maldigestion would dictate a determination of fecal fat as well as a consideration of a D-xylose absorption test. Evaluation of the function of the liver, pancreas, and biliary system, as well as an indication of hemolysis, is obtained by a determination of the serum bilirubin, alkaline phosphatase, the amino transferases (SGOT and SGPT) gamma-glutamyltranspeptidase, albumin and globulin, amylase and lipase. A 2-hour urinary amylase determination should be obtained if pancreatic disease is suspected, while demonstration of increased urinary clearance of amylase relative to creatinine would make that diagnosis more definite. The blood urea nitrogen must always be determined and, if elevated, serum creatinine obtained. Serum sodium, potassium, chloride, and carbon dioxide content may give an indication of unsuspected metabolic derangements. Hypercalcemia is associated with pancreatitis or may be the product of an abdominal neoplasm, so serum calcium and phosphorus should be considered. In the patient shown to have hyperlipoproteinemia of types 1, 4, or 5, pancreatitis must be considered as a cause of abdominal pain.

The possibility of recurrent abdominal pain being due to crises of sickle cell anemia is likely when hemolytic anemia is associated with a positive sickling preparation and abnormal mobility of hemoglobin on electrophoresis. Pain owing to splenic infarction has been reported with other hemoglobinopathies such as sickle cell trait and sickle cell hemoglobin C disease, but only in circumstances of reduced arterial oxygen tension as in travel in unpressurized aircraft. Given a patient with such a history, appropriate hematologic studies should be obtained. Serologic tests for syphilis and cerebrospinal fluid examination are in order when the gastric or visceral crises of tabes dorsalis are suspected, but the history of lightning pains elsewhere and the physical findings (Argyll Robertson pupils, hypotonia, ataxia, decreased position and vibratory sensation, and Romberg's sign) should have made the diagnosis quite evident. Acute intermittent porphyria is infrequently encountered but regularly considered in the differential diagnosis of recurrent abdominal pain, and the diagnosis depends upon the demonstration of increased urinary excretion of delta-aminolevulinic acid and porphobilinogen. The qualitative test with Ehrlich's aldehyde reagent is usually satisfactory. Chronic lead intoxication may produce abdominal pain and neuropathy and increase delta-aminolevulinic acid in the urine, similar to acute intermittent porphyria, but the Ehrlich's reagent test is usually negative. Basophilic stippling of the red cell is nonspecific for chronic lead poisoning but is a clue; the diagnosis depends ultimately on finding elevated blood and urine lead content.

Other Investigations

For decades roentgenographic investigation of the abdomen has been the basis for evaluation of the patient with gastrointestinal complaints, particularly those with chronic pain. More recently the development of flexible fiberoptic instruments has permitted a more thorough evaluation of the stomach than earlier instruments permitted. In addition it has allowed entry into the duodenum, cannulation of the pancreatic and common bile ducts with opacification of these structures, and visualization of the entire colon, possibly even the terminal ileum at times, rather than merely the terminal 10-inch segment that the rigid sigmoidoscope was capable of examining. Endoscopy has pointed out the inadequacy of the traditional single contrast radiography techniques of showing luminal anatomy and has stimulated the development of double or air contrast techniques to show the finer mucosal structures of the gastrointestinal tract, particularly in the stomach and colon and in the hypotonic study of the duodenum.

Generally, a well-planned roentgenographic investigation of the patient's problem is in order as the initial step. When the patient has had numerous x-ray studies in the past, it is certainly well to review these films in detail and determine their quality, to decide whether or not they adequately demonstrate the areas that one has questions about, and then to repeat studies only when they are necessary. Discussion of the problems with the radiologist before the examination is always valuable in obtaining the maximum information.

Some x-ray studies have greater limitations than others. When the small bowel is involved by diffuse mucosal disease, a regional inflammatory process, or a partially obstructing lesion, a small bowel series may well be of great value. Focal lesions, however, are often missed by this determination. In the absence of a gallbladder removed in previous surgery, an intravenous cholangiogram is usually obtained to evaluate the biliary tract. If good visualization is obtained, a proper interpretation is possible; however, in a significant number of instances the visualization is less than optimal, particularly when abnormalities of hepatic function exist.

Plain films of the abdomen should not be neglected. Various calcifications that may suggest lesions might be obscured by contrast material. Milk of calcium bile in a decreased gallbladder can be interpreted as a normally functioning gallbladder during an oral cholecystogram if filming had not been done before the ingestion of the contrast agent. Plain films taken during episodes of pain may well show bowel gas patterns suggesting a cause for the pain. Definite or suspected abnormalities on the roentgenograms are followed up with endoscopic visualization of the area in question. When a strong suspicion exists of a possible abnormality in one area of the gastrointestinal tract despite negative roentgenographic findings in the area, one would logically proceed with endoscopic evaluation of the area.

Thus x-ray contrast studies and endoscopy have provided us with efficient means of investigating those areas of the gastrointestinal tract that develop the great majority of lesions. Contrary to this, the solid abdominal organs, particularly the pancreas, have tended to elude noninvasive imaging techniques until the development in recent years of ultrasound scanning and also computerized tomography (CT). Selenomethionine isotope scanning of the pancreas proved to be rather sensitive but to have poor specificity and has been essentially abandoned. The pancreas of thin patients, which lacks retroperitoneal fat, is usually well imaged by ultrasound, while the patient with normal amount of fatty tissue might be expected to have the pancreas better demonstrated by CT scan. Pseudocyst of the pancreas is ideally demonstrated by ultrasound scanning. With the development of real-time imaging, an ultrasonic "fluoroscopy," even more accurate demonstration of intraabdominal organs and lesions, is possible. Radioisotope imaging of the liver has been a standard procedure for many years but does not show anatomic detail. Changes in size and contour as well as "cold spots" within the substance of the liver are looked for. Functional abnormality may be evident by a decrease in hepatic accumulation of the radiocolloid as well as increase in uptake by the spleen and bone marrow. Ultrasound scanning of the liver is capable of demonstrating cystic and solid structures within the hepatic substance, as well as demonstrating gallstones and changes in the size of the extrahepatic or intrahepatic bile ducts.

In the jaundiced patient ultrasound scanning is a worthwhile initial examination to determine whether the problem is extrahepatic or intrahepatic, on the basis of the presence or absence of dilated bile ducts. The procedure is reported to be 97 per cent accurate in reaching this conclusion. Approximately half of patients with extrahepatic obstruction may have the site of obstruction demonstrated by ultrasound scanning. Percutaneous transhepatic cholangiography is used to demonstrate the site in the remaining patients. In patients without dilated ducts the problem would appear to be intrahepatic; for them, consideration is given to percutaneous hepatic biopsy. Endoscopic retrograde cholangiography may be considered in those patients with apparent extrahepatic biliary tract obstruction in whom percutaneous transhepatic cholangiography has not demonstrated the lesion. In the patient who has a nonfunctioning gallbladder shown by oral cholecystography, ultrasound scanning of the gallbladder may well be of value to disclose whether stones are present.

Endoscopic retrograde cholangiopancreatography provides a way to visualize the pancreatic ducts. Its limitation is largely that of the availability of personnel skilled in this variety of endoscopy. Arteriography to evaluate the vasculature of the pancreas in suspected pancreatic neoplasms is less frequently necessary today than in recent years.

Arteriography is a mandatory procedure in the patient who is suspected of having abdominal pain as a consequence of chronic ischemic vascular disease, abdominal angina. The potential for this condition to lead to acute bowel ischemia with infarction is well known. Mention has been made of the relative ineffectiveness of barium contrast examination in visualizing focal lesions of the small bowel. Tumors in this area may well be visualized by arteriographic means. Carcinoids of the small bowel are the most frequent malignancies encountered in this area and have a characteristic appearance by angiography. Carcinoma and metastatic tumors of the small bowel by their infiltration of arteries produce a picture similar to that seen and leiomyomas and leiomyosarcomas are quite vascular and therefore readily detected. Lymphomas are not particularly characteristic on angiography; fortunately they are often relatively easily demonstrated with barium contrast examination.

Laparoscopy should be considered in selected patients in whom other studies have not provided an answer but suspicion exists of disease that might be visualized on the parietal peritoneum of the abdominal wall, the surface of the liver, the pelvic organs, the mesentery, the anterior serosal surface of the stomach and proximal duodenum, and head of the pancreas. This procedure, long popular in Europe, is finding new acceptance among gastroenterologists and abdominal surgeons, somewhat because of success that gynecologists have reported with it and also because of improved equipment. Its use might be considered before laparotomy, but performed when pain is the only symptom and when physical findings and laboratory results are within normal limits, it is very likely to be unrewarding. When appropriate, biopsy of specific sites is carried out, either by percutaneous or endoscopic route or, if necessary, at laparotomy.

PROBLEM AREA

Frequently the patient is seen in a pain-free period and important points about symptoms or physical findings that would be present during periods of pain are not noted. If possible, the patient should be seen during a period of pain. Laboratory investigations also might be more rewarding during symptomatic periods.

If the patient shows evidence of depression, treatment should be directed actively toward that problem, and it should not be assumed that the depression is caused by the pain problem as the patient often insists.

It must not be assumed that previously normal roentgenographic studies are infallible. Pathologic processes change with time and may be demonstrable on repeat studies. Be alert to the finding of one lesion that does not explain the patient's symptoms but that has captivated the examiner's attention, causing a second lesion to be missed.

Determine the patient's response to specific therapeutic programs, such as intense antacid therapy, and his response to infiltration with lidocaine of a locally painful area of the abdominal wall, or to manipulation of the fat or roughage content of the diet. Be certain, though, that this response is not just a transient one.

CONVULSIVE DISORDERS IN ADULTS

By RICHARD N. HARNER, M.D.

Philadelphia, Pennsylvania

INTRODUCTION

Epileptic seizures in adults occur as a result of excessive, highly synchronized discharges of neurons and nerve terminals in the cerebral cortex or subcortical gray matter. Primary generalized seizures arise almost simultaneously in widely separated areas of the brain and result in immediate loss of consciousness, myoclonic jerks, or bilateral, tonic and clonic motor activity — the grand mal seizure. More often, however, seizures begin focally in one portion of the brain and then spread to adjacent areas of the cortex. If the rate of spread is slow, symptoms of focal brain disturbance may be noted by the patient before propagation of seizure activity to the rest of the brain results in loss of consciousness. Otherwise, subsequent tonic clonic motor activity is indistinguishable from that occurring in a primary generalized motor seizure. The fundamental distinction between focal and generalized mechanisms for convulsive seizures helps the clinician to begin the search for treatable causes of recurrent seizures and to distinguish epilepsy from disorders producing similar symptoms.

A second fundamental mechanism has to do with the seizure threshold of the brain. In the simplest case, when a normal threshold is exceeded by an intense stimulus, such as electroshock, a single nonrecurrent seizure may result. In patients with epilepsy, recurrent seizures result from persistent lowering of seizure threshold, whatever the cause. Still further lowering of the seizure threshold results in status epilepticus, during which seizures become continuous and are uninterrupted by periods of normal brain function.

SEIZURE CLASSIFICATION

The clinician will find it useful to classify seizures according to whether the predominant mechanism is primary generalized, focal (partial), or focal with secondary generalization. Each type of seizure may occur as an isolated event, as a recurrent process (epilepsy) or as an uninterrupted sequence of seizures — status epilepticus.

PRIMARY GENERALIZED SEIZURES

A primary generalized seizure may occur as an isolated event following an adequate stimulus to the brain. Hypoglycemia, hypoxia, drug withdrawal, and cardiac arrest are examples of systemic processes that may result in seizures. Characteristically, the neurologic examination is normal, as is the electroencephalogram. It is important to recognize that brief seizures may occur during the course of an otherwise benign process such as syncope. The clinician should also consider primary cardiac causes of an apparent seizure disorder when the electorencephalogram (EEG) and the neurologic examinations are normal.

Hypoglycemia may cause seizures that are usually nonfocal but sometimes contain focal components, surprisingly. A history of weight loss (or gain) occurrence of seizures after fasting, and relief by glucose intake are helpful but not obligatory clues to the diagnosis.

Recurrent primary generalized seizures in the absence of an external precipitating cause occur most often as a primary autosomal genetic disorder with variable penetrance.

Characteristically, a triad of generalized seizures occurs: absence (petit mal) attacks, myoclonic jerks, and grand mal seizures. Petit mal attacks are seen mainly in the first or second decade and may occur, 20 to 50 times per day with durations of 5 to 30 seconds. Each attack begins suddenly, without warning. Observation of the patient during the attack often shows blinking of the eyes 2 to 3 times per second, and purposeless movements may occur. These must be distinguished from temporal lobe seizures to be described under Focal Seizures.

Grand mal seizures often have their onset at about the time of puberty. Both petit mal and grand mal seizures may persist into adult life, but there is a tendency toward improvement in the third decade. Myoclonic seizures occur as random jerks involving the face and extremities, especially upon awakening, or when exposed to light. Since occurrence of myoclonic jerks of this type is almost pathognomonic for genetically determined, primary generalized epilepsy, specific questioning in this area will be very rewarding to the clinician.

Continuous primary generalized seizures occur in two forms, grand mal status and petit mal status, or spike-wave stupor. Grand mal status of primarily generalized origin cannot be distinguished from that which began focally in one portion of the brain until after the patient has been treated and comes out of the acute crisis. Several diagnostic points are important. First, hypoxia and hypoglycemia are the most serious precipitating causes of status epilepticus since brain damage can result if either is allowed to persist for more than a few minutes. Intravenous glucose should be given (after drawing blood for glucose and other studies) at the slightest suspicion of hypoglycemia. Second, the most common cause of generalized motor status is failure to take anticonvulsant drugs. Determination of serum anticonvulsant levels in the acute state should be followed by an incremental dose of one of the major anticonvulsant drugs that the patient had been receiving.

Petit mal status, or *spike-wave stupor*, occurs in children and adults up to 70 years of age. Prolonged spike-wave discharge in the electroencephalogram (EEG) is associated with a confusional state that may last hours or days without total loss of consciousness, as might be expected. Careful observation of the patient may reveal isolated myoclonic jerks or blinking of the eyes that belie the recurrence of spike-wave activity in the brain. Once recognized, petit mal status is usually responsive to intravenous diazepam (Valium).

FOCAL SEIZURES

When an *isolated focal seizure* occurs, there is an increased likelihood of recurrent seizures. This is true of febrile seizures occurring in the infant and of focal seizures following head trauma or an acute stroke in the adult. If there are persistent neurologic findings or focal irritative features (spikes, spike-wave activity) in the EEG, the likelihood of recurrent seizures is further increased.

Recurrent focal seizures in the adult are usually the sign of an underlying structural brain lesion. Fortunately, some of these structural lesions may represent scars that have existed for many years, particularly involving the medial aspects of the temporal lobes and related to birth injury or other early trauma. However, the possibility of a neoplasm, arteriovenous malformation or inflammatory process must also be considered and the possibility of cerebrovascular insufficiency is increasingly likely after the age of 60.

Clearly, focal symptoms may be of any type, depending on the locus of brain involvement. If there is focal motor activity, the hand and face are most often involved. Focal sensory involvement also is most common in the hands and face. Less often is the foot or leg the primary site of either motor or sensory seizures. Most common of all focal seizures are those that arise in the *temporal lobe*. Patients may present with simple loss of consciousness (absence attack) or with a remarkable sequence of symptoms, based on the complex functions of the temporal lobe and adjacent structures — complex partial seizures. Altered perceptions, frank sensory hallucinations, intense emotional feelings, speech arrest, early loss of consciousness and amnesia, and complex motor activity (automatisms) may occur in temporal lobe seizures that fail to become generalized.

In patients with recurrent focal seizures of adult onset, the neurologic examination is usually normal. An abnormal neurologic examination—facial asymmetry, hyperreflexia, hemiparesis, speech disturbance, and the like—confirms the presence of an underlying structural lesion and the· need for intensive diagnostic evaluation. In three out of four patients with recurrent focal seizures the EEG shows focal spikes, slow acitivity, or depression of normal EEG rhythms. The EEG may be normal when seizures are infrequent or when the primary area of involvement is in the inferior or medial aspect of the brain, distant from scalp electrodes.

Continuous focal seizures are sometimes termed "epilepsia partialis continua" and are commonly due to one of three causes. The first is accentuation of a pre-existing focal seizure disorder by failure to take anticonvulsant medication. The second cause is an acute cerebral infarction or hemorrhage, and the third is a cerebral tumor, usually malignant. Rarely, focal seizures of this type may be caused by a systemic metabolic disorder such as hypoglycemia or hyperosmolar coma.

In most instances epilepsia partialis continua is characterized by repetitive twitching of the contralateral arm and face at the rate of about one per seond, with varying intensity. Sometimes, a continuous focal seizure produces no external symptoms other than the loss of function. An EEG is required to show the ictal mechanism of such *deficit symptoms*.

FOCAL SEIZURES WITH SECONDARY GENERALIZATION

Focal seizures with secondary generalization rarely occur as isolated events. They usually occur in association with a structural lesion of the brain and the likelihood of recurrent seizures is high, especially when the neurologic examination is abnormal and the EEG shows corresponding irritative features. The problem of recurrent focal seizures with secondary generalization is very common and potentially confusing for the clinician. Even though the patient presents with a generalized seizure and the neurologic examination is normal, the underlying focal cause must be sought in order to determine the best therapy. In this instance, the EEG is particularly helpful. It is abnormal in more than 75 per cent of cases when performed with appropriate activation techniques and special electrodes and may provide the only indication of an underlying focal lesion. Focal abnormalities should be followed by further neurologic evaluation including skull x-rays, brain scan, and — most helpful if available — computerized tomography (CT) of the brain with contrast enhancement.

SEIZURES OF FUNCTIONAL ORIGIN

A surprising number of patients are referred to our epilepsy center for diagnosis and treatment of seizures that have no organic cause. Typically, such seizures occur in patients between the ages of 12 and 30 years and the incidence in females is more than 2 to 1. Injury may occur during the seizures. I recall a young woman who fractured her pelvis during one such episode. Most often, however, observation of the seizure reveals a bizarre pattern that does not correspond even to the complex patterns that are characteristic of temporal lobe seizures. Waving movements of the arms, thrusting movements of the pelvis, unexpected responsiveness to stimulation, and immediate recovery of consciousness following the seizure should suggest a nonorganic seizure. If the behavior and the EEG can be recorded concurrently on videotape, further improvement in diagnosis may occur. When the clinical seizure pattern is atypical, the lack of associated EEG abnormality during or after the seizure is further evidence against the presence of an organic disorder.

DIAGNOSTIC EVALUATION

The foregoing paragraphs indicate that clinical history and neurologic examination provide the most important diagnostic information for separation of focal from nonfocal seizures. The next highest yield is obtained from the *electroencephalogram*, a uniquely dynamic evaluation of regional brain function.

In order to be an effective tool, the EEG should be recorded for a minimum of 30 minutes but preferably for 1 hour while the patient is awake and asleep. Nasopharyngeal electrodes increase the yield of focal seizure disorders by about 10 per cent and should be requested routinely. Hyperventilation and photic stimulation should be included to provide maximum information about a possible seizure disorder in an EEG that records only a short segment of the patient's brain activity. Videotape recording of EEG and the patient's behavior can provide very useful clinical information, particularly when the pattern and origin of focal seizures are uncertain or when functional seizures are being considered. EEG recordings from *depth electrodes* are being used increasingly to provide improved localization of seizure foci prior to surgical removal in patients with focal recurrent seizures that are severe and unresponsive to appropriate anticonvulsant therapy.

The *CT scan* shows abnormalities in more than half of the patients with focal seizures but is almost always normal in patients with primary generalized epilepsy. Most of the focal lesions detected are atrophic, as evidenced by widening of the cortical sulci and enlargement of the underlying lateral ventricle. In patients with tumor or arteriovenous malformation, focal areas of increased density may be detected, particularly during contrast enhancement.

The *radionuclide brain scan* is helpful in detecting treatable disorders, particularly in concert with the EEG and when the CT scan is not available. While the EEG is quite sensitive to malignant tumors of the brain and to strokes, brain scan is more effective in detecting benign extrinsic tumors such as meningiomas.

Additional studies should be obtained in those patients whose epileptic mechanism remains obscure after these evaluations. Even though the yield is low, the therapeutic implications are high. Thus the patient should be screened for hypoglycemia, hypocalcemia, unsuspected renal failure, occult infection, and immunologic disorders. Fortunately, the cost of effective multiscreening laboratory studies is now low.

SUMMARY

Although the mechanism of seizure initiation in the cerebral cortex is unknown, our understanding of the distinction between primary generalized and focal mechanisms of epileptogenesis aids in evaluating patients suffering from one or more seizures. Recognition of the characteristic patterns of epileptic activation, particularly in temporal lobe epilepsy, aid in the distinction of epileptic behavior patterns from those of functional origin. Detection of focal symptoms, focal neurologic findings, or focal findings in the EEG leads to the increasing likelihood of a recurrent seizure disorder and an underlying structural lesion that may require further diagnostic and therapeutic efforts. The EEG may be viewed as an extension of neurologic examination in providing additional information about the location and mechanism of disturbed brain activity. While the brain scan serves to detect many treatable tumors causing epilepsy, CT represents a major advance in determining the nature of structural lesions causing seizure disorders that could only be presumed in the past.

Section 2

INFECTIOUS DISEASES

INFLUENZA

By HJORDIS M. FOY, M.D., Ph.D.,
and J. THOMAS GRAYSTON, M.D.
Seattle, Washington

SYNONYMS

Flu, la grippe.

DEFINITION

Influenza is an acute respiratory disease with systemic manifestations caused by influenza virus types A, B, and, very rarely, C. Typical disease is distinguished from other viral and respiratory infections by abrupt onset of shaking chills and head and muscle aches, followed by prostration. Influenza infection can be confused with a variety of other acute respiratory infections when presenting with milder symptoms and when the disease occurs during a nonepidemic period.

CAUSATIVE AGENT

Three types of influenza viruses are recognized, types A, B, and C. Types A and B cause typical influenza, whereas type C causes milder upper respiratory symptoms and is rarely recognized in the community. The type-specific genome of the virus consists of single-stranded RNA covered with a protein coat. The surrounding envelope has spikes of hemagglutinin and neuraminidase, which are the most important antigenic determinants. Influenza viruses are unique in their capacity to change these surface antigens, and thereby circumvent the acquired immunity in the population. An antigenic "shift" is defined as a major change in either the hemagglutinin or neuraminidase, whereas a "drift" consists of a minor mutation in either antigen. Shifts in the antigenic composition of influenza type A have been followed by pandemics such as in 1918–1919 (Spanish flu) and in 1957 (Asian flu) when presumably both the neuraminidase and hemagglutinin antigens changed, or in 1968 (Hong Kong flu) when only the hemagglutinin changed completely.

EPIDEMIOLOGY

In the United States, sharp epidemics of influenza usually occur in winter or spring, and are often signaled by high absentee rates in schools. Morbidity is characteristically high, mortality low. However, influenza A epidemics are followed within a couple of weeks by an increase in mortality of the elderly and those chronically ill. The epidemics spread rapidly, and usually last for only a month or two. Since the 1930s, influenza type A epidemics have tended to occur at 1- to 2-year intervals, whereas major pandemics associated with antigenic shifts have been recorded with about 11-year intervals. The 1918–1919 pandemic was unusual in generating a high mortality rate among young adults. Serologic evidence suggests that it was caused by an influenza strain identical with or similar to a strain endemic in herds of swine since the 1930s. It has been called "swine" strain. There is evidence that influenza viruses may recycle; serologic studies of persons born before 1900 suggest that Asian- and Hong Kong–like strains circulated in the 1890s. This had led to speculation that a swine-like influenza virus may cause the next major human pandemic. Thus, when spread of human infection with a swine virus strain was detected at Fort Dix, New Jersey, in 1976, a government campaign was mounted to vaccinate the entire United States population against this virus. The virus did not spread beyond Fort Dix and no pandemic materialized. However, the theory that influenza strains may recycle was confirmed by the reappearance in 1977 of the "Russian" virus, a strain prevalent also between 1947 and 1957. The threat of a reappearance of a highly pathogenic strain such as the swine strain was in 1918 will continue to exist.

Changes in the surface antigens of the influenza B virus have been less dramatic. Influenza B causes localized outbreaks of influenza at irregular and longer intervals; children have higher attack rates than adults.

PRESENTING SYMPTOMS AND SIGNS

Typical influenza begins with shaking chills, fever, and head and muscle aches, with an onset so abrupt that the patient may be able to tell the hour of the day it started. Respiratory symptoms, including sore throat, stuffy and runny nose, hoarseness, substernal soreness, and a shallow nonproductive cough, soon follow, or may precede onset. Dizziness and prostration are common complaints; the latter may linger. In some epidemics pain in the thigh muscles has been characteristic. Epistaxis may occur. However, some influenza infections may be asymptomatic, and others cause merely fever or common cold symptoms.

The incubation period in experimental infections may be as short as a day; in families the incubation is more commonly 1 to 5 days.

The patient may look flushed and perspiring. Eyelids may be swollen and conjunctivae injected; muscular movements of the eyeball may hurt, but photophobia is rare. Mucous membranes of the throat and nasal passages are usually injected and slightly edematous; watery discharge from the nose may be present. Moist, fine rales may be heard at the bases of the lungs despite lack of evidence of infiltrate on chest x-rays. Loss of appetite is common, but nausea, vomiting, and diarrhea are rare except in children.

COURSE

In mild cases and in children the illness may be over in 3 days. In the more severe cases symptoms linger, especially the cough, which may become debilitating and turn productive, sometimes with blood-tinged sputum. Complaints of fatigue, cough, and even mental depression lasting for a couple of months after influenza disease are not unusual. Influenza virus is capable of destroying the ciliary epithelium in the bronchial tree, which accounts for the prolonged cough and also allows superinfection with bacteria. A second fever peak is suggestive of secondary bacterial infection.

Symptomatology may vary with epidemic strain, and also a wide spectrum of manifestations may be seen within the same family. Children under the age of 2 may have croup, and a prolonged febrile illness. The symptoms are usually more severe in those over the age of 40, and especially among those with pre-existing heart and lung or other chronic diseases.

COMPLICATIONS

Only rarely does influenza per se lead to viral pneumonia and death. Patients with cardiac disease (especially mitral stenosis) or chronic pulmonary disease and pregnant women are at higher than average risk. Onset of viral pneumonia is characterized by dyspnea, tachycardia, and cyanosis. The pulmonary infiltrate is characteristically hemorrhagic, and the sputum is serosanguineous. The patient is in obvious respiratory distress, often in shock and with feeble pulse. Blood tests show elevated pH and hypoxia. Death from viral pneumonia may have been more common in the 1918–1919 epidemic of swine influenza, when heliotropic cyanosis was observed at onset of disease. The most common complications consist of laryngitis, tracheitis, bronchitis, bronchiolitis, and bacterial pneumonia. The pneumonia may be of pneumococcal, staphylococcal, and even meningococcal origin, or may be due to *Hemophilus*

influenzae, beta-hemolytic streptococci, gram-negative rods, or anaerobes. During the Asian influenza epidemics (1957–1958) staphylococcal pneumonia was a serious problem. This was a time when virulent staphylococcal phage types were prevalent in the community. A defervesence followed by a second rise in temperature, occasionally accompanied by one-sided chest pain or frank pleuritis, is an indication of secondary pneumonia. Depending on the offending organism, sputum may become purulent or otherwise reflect the bacterial invader.

Influenza viruses may cause exacerbations of chronic bronchitis with deterioration of pulmonary function. Electrocardiogram (EKG) may indicate mild myocarditis. Occasionally aseptic meningitis, encephalitis, or polyneuritis, including Guillain-Barré syndrome, occurs. Hemorrhagic myringitis occurs, especially in children; bacterial otitis and sinusitis may also follow.

Reye's syndrome is an acute encephalopathy of childhood with fatty degeneration of the viscera, particularly of the liver, associated with enzymatic changes. It is observed after viral infections; influenza type B has often been implicated.

LABORATORY DIAGNOSIS

Peripheral Blood. At onset of disease, leukocytosis up to 15,000 per cu mm may be observed, followed by leukopenia with relative lymphocytosis. Polymorphonuclear leukocytosis in excess of 15,000 per cu mm later in the course of illness suggests bacterial complications.

Urinalysis. Urinalysis is usually normal; however, intranuclear inclusions in cells have been described, and mild febrile albuminuria may occur.

Chest X-Ray. The chest x-ray is usually normal in uncomplicated influenza, despite findings of fine rales on auscultation.

Primary influenza pneumonia is characterized by bilateral infiltrates with an interstitial alveolar pattern that often fans out from the hilum. It may become coalescent and closely resemble pulmonary edema. Secondary bacterial pneumonia may have bronchial distribution, or may be localized. The characteristics of the secondary invader dominate. It may appear as a lobar dense infiltrate in classic pneumococcal pneumonia, or may show cavitation in severe staphylococcal pneumonia (see Bacterial Pneumonia, pp. 146 to 148).

SPECIFIC DIAGNOSIS

Definite proof of influenza infection is obtained by isolation of the virus from respiratory secretions or by serologic methods. The former method requires special laboratory facilities; the latter method necessitates collection of acute and convalescent sera. Immunofluorescent and immunoperoxidase techniques are useful for rapid diagnosis.

Isolation of the virus is necessary for characterization of the epidemic strain, whereas serology is most practical for routine diagnosis.

Isolation of the Virus. Isolation should be attempted within 3 days of onset of illness, because the virus gradually disappears from the upper respiratory tract within a week. The influenza viruses are grown in embryonated hen's egg or mammalian cell culture. Primary monkey kidney cells are preferred, but other cell lines are also susceptible. The success rate of isolation attempts varies with different epidemic strains. Influenza type A is often isolated more easily in eggs than in cell culture. Usually, the isolation rate is less than 50 per cent of influenza cases. Respiratory secretions for virus isolation must be attained in special collection medium, such as veal infusion broth with albumin or trypticase soy broth, and refrigerated during transport. The virus withstands freezing at −70 C if inoculation has to be postponed. Irrigation of the nose and having the patient gargle with the collection medium provide specimens that give the best virus yield. However, nasopharyngeal specimens, collected by rubbing a cotton swab on the tonsillar area and gently rotating a swab in the nose prior to immersion in collection media, are satisfactory.

Isolation of the virus takes a minimum of 3 to 5 days — longer if blind passages are necessary. An isolate can be identified as influenza A or B immediately, whereas determination of specific antigenic composition of the virus strain requires additional testing, using a battery of strain-specific antisera. Such identification is carried out in specialized reference laboratories, such as the one at the National Center for Disease Control in Atlanta, Georgia (WHO Influenza Center for the Americas).

Serologic Methods. The diagnosis of influenza can be confirmed by observing a rise (fourfold or greater) in antibody titer between serum collected in the "acute" stage of disease and a "convalescent" specimen taken as early as 10 days later, preferably 3 to 4 weeks later. Several test systems are available. Clinical laboratories prefer the complement fixation (CF) antibody test, utilizing soluble (S) group-specific antigen. The hemagglutination inhibition (HI) test is strain specific but is complicated by the need to remove naturally occurring non-

specific inhibitors from the serum. Neuraminidase (N) antibody can be measured by several test systems, but none of them are practical for routine diagnosis.

A multitude of new and promising antibody assays have been developed. In the single radial diffusion (SRD) test the diameter of antigen-antibody reaction around a well filled with serum is visualized and quantititatively related to antibody content without using cumbersome serum dilution methods. The test can be used to detect antibody both to specific hemagglutinin and to neuraminidase. It is simple and rapid.

Complement fixing antibodies decay faster than hemagglutinin antibody, and the presence of a high titer ($\geq$1:32) in a single convalescent serum is suggestive, but not diagnostic, of a recent infection. Hemagglutinin antibodies may persist almost for life. In an older person, the anamnestic response to the type of hemagglutinin first encountered as a child may be higher than for the hemagglutinin of a current infection — "the doctrine of original antigenic sin." Serum specimens can be transported refrigerated by mail. They should be stored at or below −20 C.

Response to influenza vaccine consists in a rise, especially in hemagglutinin and neuraminidase antibody (surface antigens). Killed whole-virus vaccines are relatively free from the nucleoprotein antigen, and minimal or no CF antibody response is elicited. Subvirion vaccines elicit CF antibody response, especially in children.

PITFALLS IN DIAGNOSIS

The terms influenza and flu are often used by laymen to describe a nonspecific gastrointestinal illness characterized by nausea and diarrhea — "intestinal flu." This is an unfortunate semantic ambiguity, and patients claiming to have or have had the "flu" should be questioned about their exact symptoms.

Influenza may easily be confused with a multitude of other acute febrile respiratory illnesses, such as those caused by parainfluenza and respiratory syncytial viruses (both common childhood infections). ARD (acute respiratory disease), a syndrome frequently observed in military recruit populations, is due to adenovirus and may mimic influenza; onset is less abrupt and sore throat more prominent. Q fever, histoplasmosis, coccidioidomycosis, psittacosis, and *Mycoplasma pneumoniae* infections may also resemble influenza. Rhinoviruses and coronaviruses usually cause afebrile common colds, and may be confused with mild cases of influenza. Bacterial pneumonia should be suspected in patients with high white blood cell counts, especially if the chest x-ray shows an infiltrate. During influenza epidemics, presumptive diagnosis of influenza may be made in patients with acute febrile respiratory disease. The diagnosis is likely to be overlooked during summer and early fall, when suspicion is not aroused.

In patients with chronic pulmonary or cardiac problems, the diagnosis may easily be overlooked, because the infection may manifest itself as an exacerbation of the underlying conditions. Elderly patients are at high risk of dying of influenza infection during epidemics, although they may not exhibit characteristic fever or other symptoms.

VIRUS AND MYCOPLASMA PNEUMONIAS

By FREDERICK W. HENDERSON, M.D., *and* FLOYD W. DENNY, M.D.

Chapel Hill, North Carolina

DEFINITION

The term pneumonia is usually used to indicate the presence of inflammatory disease of the pulmonary alveoli and suggests that bronchioles, bronchi, trachea, and larynx are not involved. Experience has shown, however, that although one area of the lung may be the primary site of infection, one or more adjacent areas may also be involved. Therefore many patients diagnosed as having pneumonia also have involvement of the conducting airways; similarly, patients diagnosed as having tracheobronchiolitis may also have an element of pneumonia present. This is particularly true of viral and mycoplasmal pneumonias, in which the airways are invariably affected.

SYNONYM: ATYPICAL PNEUMONIA

Historically, infections of the lung not typical of pneumococcal lobar pneumonia and associated with elevated cold hemagglutinins were called "atypical" pneumonia. This term is no longer adequate for describing lung infections and should be discarded. Classification by the

specific causative agent should be attempted in all instances of pneumonia.

PNEUMONIA

The incidence of pneumonia varies with age. The highest attack rate is in children less than 5 years old, in whom the incidence is approximately 40 episodes per 1000 children per year. In schoolage children and young adults the rate is about 5 episodes per 1000 persons per year. This rate is stable throughout life until age 60, when a gradual increase in frequency begins. In those persons over 70, the incidence of pneumonia is approximately 15 episodes per 1000 per year.

Establishing the cause of illness in the individual patient with pneumonia is difficult for several reasons: (1) pulmonary infections can be caused by a multitude of organisms of different classes, including bacteria, mycobacteria, fungi, viruses, rickettsia, protozoa, chlamydia, and *Mycoplasma pneumoniae;* (2) diagnostic microbiologic tests, including isolation and identification of agents and serologic confirmation of infection, are frequently difficult and time consuming or are not readily available; and (3) pulmonary tissue or secretions for culture are difficult to obtain without contamination with normal upper respiratory flora that frequently contain bacteria with the potential for pulmonary pathogenicity. All the pathogens just listed must be considered in one clinical-epidemiologic setting or another; however, the most frequent diagnostic dilemma for physicians evaluating community-acquired pneumonia in previously healthy children and adults is differentiating those patients with viral or mycoplasmal pneumonia from those who have disease caused by bacteria. Rapid, specific diagnostic procedures for viruses and *Mycoplasma pneumoniae* are rarely available, and, as stated, the interpretation of bacterial cultures of pulmonary secretions obtained by noninvasive methods is confusing because of the high rate of recovery of *Streptococcus pneumoniae* and *Hemophilus influenzae* in situations in which they have no pathogenic significance.

VIRUS AND MYCOPLASMA PNEUMONIAE PNEUMONIA

Epidemiologic studies of community-acquired pneumonia in previously healthy individuals have firmly established a viral or mycoplasmal cause for 50 per cent of childhood pneumonia and 35 per cent of adult disease. One should not assume that the remaining patients in these studies had bacterial pneumonia,

Table 1. *Viral Pneumonia in the Compromised Host*

Virus	Host	Syndrome
Cytomegalovirus, herpesvirus hominis, rubella	Newborn	Congenital pneumonia
Cytomegalovirus, herpesvirus hominis, rubeola, varicella	Immunologically compromised children and adults	Severe, progressive, frequently fatal pneumonia

for this was not established. It is our impression that the majority of those pneumonia patients without a defined cause also had disease caused by viruses or *Mycoplasma pneumoniae*.

Although discussion of community-acquired illness is the main theme of this article, two additional aspects of viral pneumonia require comment. Nosocomial acquisition of common respiratory viruses occurs, and these infections may be associated with pneumonia. Respiratory syncytial virus, parainfluenza viruses, and influenza A virus are prime offenders in children, and influenza A virus infections are of major significance in adults. Second, viruses that do not usually cause pneumonia in normal persons may do so in the immunologically compromised host. Table 1 lists these situations, which are not further discussed in the text.

Any of the viruses that regularly infect the respiratory tract of man may be associated with lower respiratory tract illness, including pneumonia. The epidemiologic studies just referred to have established the etiologic significance of respiratory syncytial virus, parainfluenza viruses, adenoviruses, and influenza A and B viruses in patients with pneumonia. *Mycoplasma pneumoniae* is the only human mycoplasma associated with respiratory disease, and it is a major cause of pneumonia in schoolage children and young adults. Rhinoviruses, enteroviruses, coronaviruses, and rubeola in unimmunized children are less frequent causative agents of pneumonia.

EPIDEMIOLOGY AND CLINICAL ILLNESS SYNDROMES

Because of the difficulty in rapid diagnosis of viral and mycoplasmal infections, the most important data base for defining the role of these agents in individual patients with pneumonia is an understanding of the clinical and epidemiological characteristics of these infections. The information to be collected includes the age and sex of the patient, season of the year, associated anatomic sites of involvement within the lower respiratory tract (bronchiolitis, tracheobronchitis, croup), and characteristics of illness occurring simultaneously in the community, the family, or other epidemiologic niches of which the patient is a member, such as day care center,

school, or place of employment. This type of information can assume major diagnostic importance because of the lack of epidemicity of bacterial pneumonias.

The clinical and epidemiologic features of respiratory syncytial virus, parainfluenza virus, adenovirus, and *Mycoplasma pneumoniae* disease are discussed in the following paragraphs. Influenza virus infection, a major cause of pneumonia in preschool and school children, is discussed on pages 99 to 102.

RESPIRATORY SYNCYTIAL VIRUS

Respiratory syncytial virus (RSV) is the most common cause of bronchiolitis and pneumonia in infancy and early childhood. Infections occur any time after birth, with little evidence of protection by maternal antibody. The majority of the cases of pneumonia caused by the RSV occur in the first 3 to 4 years of life, with occasional cases up to age 5 to 7 years. During the first 6 months of life bronchiolar obstruction and interstitial pneumonia may cause severe respiratory compromise with an occasional fatal outcome. Bronchiolitis and pneumonia caused by the RSV are more common in boys than in girls.

RSV disease occurs in yearly epidemics of 8 to 12 weeks' duration, almost exclusively in the winter and spring. When RSV infections occur in families, older children and adults will manifest mild upper respiratory symptoms if they become ill. When RSV is prevalent in the community, there will be an increase in patient visits to health care facilities because of bronchiolitis and pneumonia and increased hospitalizations of infants and young children with pneumonia. There will be no associated increase in pneumonia in schoolage children and normal adults. Adults with chronic obstructive lung disease may have exacerbations of lower respiratory difficulty associated with RSV infections. Recently, outbreaks of lower respiratory disease due to RSV have been described among elderly persons in nursing homes.

PARAINFLUENZA VIRUSES

Parainfluenza viruses types 1, 2, and 3 are responsible for the majority of human parainfluenza respiratory illness. Especially in children, illnesses caused by types 1 and 2 are clinically and epidemiologically distinct from type 3 disease.

The primary significance of parainfluenza virus type 1 and 2 infections in children is their etiologic association with croup. During periods of prevalence of parainfluenza virus croup, infants and young children with pneumonia caused by these agents will be seen occasionally. When this occurs, the clinical illness is indistinguishable from RSV or parainfluenza type 3 pneumonia. Parainfluenza type 1 and 2 epidemics are not usually associated with an increased incidence of pneumonia.

Parainfluenza type 1 and 2 infections occur both in endemic and epidemic patterns. Epidemics of infections with these agents have a marked predilection for occurring in the fall season.

Parainfluenza type 3 is the second most common cause of bronchiolitis and pneumonia in infants and children. As with RSV, there is little evidence of protection afforded by transplacentally acquired antibody. Pneumonia is most frequently a manifestation of infection during the first 3 years of life. Infants less than 6 months of age are at risk for severe respiratory compromise secondary to bronchiolar obstruction and interstitial pneumonia.

Although there is no basis for clinical distinction of RSV and parainfluenza virus type 3 disease, the two agents have different epidemiologic patterns of occurrence. Parainfluenza virus type 3 infections are endemic and occur throughout the year. There may be short periods of increased prevalence of this virus, but this agent is not commonly associated with community-wide epidemics and consequently is only occasionally associated with discrete periods of increased pneumonia incidence in infants and young children.

Parainfluenza virus infections in families usually result in mild upper respiratory illness in older children and adults; however, there is a low incidence of parainfluenza virus–associated pneumonia in normal adults, the risk being higher in the elderly.

ADENOVIRUSES

Adenoviruses types 1, 2, and 5 are endemic in the population, and there is a low incidence of bronchiolitis and pneumonia in infants and young children associated with infections by these serotypes. Adenovirus type 3, 7, 14, and 21 infections occur less frequently in infancy and early childhood; yet they account for the majority of severe episodes of bronchiolitis and

pneumonia, occurring primarily in children less than 2 years of age. Severe lower respiratory infections with these types have occurred both sporadically and in epidemics. Epidemics have been both institutional and community wide but have been few in number. All adenovirus infections increase in frequency in winter months.

Adenovirus epidemics caused by types 4, 7, and 21 occur regularly in military recruits, and pneumonia occurs in approximately 10 per cent of those infected. Except for this special epidemiologic situation, severe adenovirus lower respiratory disease is unusual in adults.

MYCOPLASMA PNEUMONIAE

Mycoplasma pneumoniae and influenza virus type A are the two most common causes of nonbacterial pneumonia in persons over age 5 years. While *M. pneumoniae* infections occur before the age of 5 years, it is unusual for these infections to be associated with illness, although occasional instances of mycoplasmal pneumonia are encountered in pre-school children. After 5 years of age mycoplasma infections are frequently symptomatic, with tracheobronchitis and pneumonia the most common pulmonary manifestations. The majority of *M. pneumoniae* pneumonias occur in the 5-to-30-year age group, with the highest incidence in 5-to-15-year-old children. During epidemic periods persons up to age 45 to 50 may be involved; however, mycoplasma-associated pneumonia after this age is infrequent.

M. pneumoniae infections are endemic in large communities. On this background of activity, prolonged smoldering epidemics occur at irregular intervals. These periods of increased prevalence usually begin in the fall and last 1 to 2 years. In small communities the endemic pattern of infection may be less apparent. During endemic periods approximately 20 per cent of adult pneumonias are caused by *M. pneumoniae*. During epidemic periods as much as 60 per cent of pneumonia in the 5-to-30-year age group may be due to this agent.

The major epidemiologic unit for *M. pneumoniae* infections is the family, and infection is usually introduced by the schoolage child. Secondary attack rate in family children is approximately 60 per cent and in family adults 30 to 40 per cent. Unlike illnesses caused by respiratory viruses, which have an incubation period of 1 to 4 days, the incubation period of *M. pneumoniae* infections is 2 to 3 weeks. In general, consecutive respiratory illnesses occurring in family members with a 2- to 4-day interval between cases are not due to *Mycoplasma pneumoniae*.

SIGNS AND SYMPTOMS

Virus and mycoplasma pneumonias are frequently associated with clinical findings of pathologic involvement throughout the lower respiratory tract. Cough and coarse rhonchi characteristic of tracheobronchitis are common, and evidence of bronchiolitis is not unusual. Likewise, upper respiratory symptoms are prominent, and extrarespiratory manifestations, including headache, malaise, and myalgia, are common in adult viral and mycoplasmal infections. Pleuritic chest pain, splinting respirations, and hemoptysis are not usually seen in virus and mycoplasma pneumonias. Temperatures greater than 102 F (39 C) occur with equal frequency in viral, mycoplasmal, and bacterial pneumonia. As has been stated, the degree of respiratory compromise in patients with viral pneumonia may be quite marked; consequently, illness severity alone is not a good differentiating clinical feature to include or exclude a bacterial cause.

CHEST X-RAY

Although the classic radiographic appearance of viral and mycoplasmal pneumonia is that of a patchy bronchopneumonia, lobar consolidation indistinguishable from pneumococcal lobar pneumonia occurs in 20 per cent of childhood and adult viral and mycoplasmal pneumonias. The presence of pleural fluid, pneumatoceles, abscesses, circular pneumonia, and lobar consolidation with evidence of volume expansion of the involved lobe should be considered inconsistent with viral or mycoplasmal disease, although small amounts of pleural fluid may be seen in occasional patients with viral or mycoplasmal pneumonia.

LABORATORY FINDINGS

Thirty per cent of patients with viral or mycoplasmal pneumonia have peripheral blood white cell counts greater than 10,000 per cu mm, but generally less than 10 per cent have white counts above 15,000 per cu mm. Patients with bacteremic pneumococcal pneumonia have white cell counts above 15,000 per cu mm 75 per cent of the time. Therefore a peripheral blood WBC less than 15,000 per cu mm is not helpful, whereas a white cell count greater than 15,000 per cu mm increases the likelihood of a bacterial cause.

Sputum from patients with *M. pneumoniae* pneumonia frequently demonstrates a predominance of polymorphonuclear leukocytes. Patients with viral pneumonia may also have purulent sputum. Thus the microscopic examination of sputum has limited value. Furthermore, sputum cultures are difficult to interpret, because sputum is frequently contaminated with pneumococci, which are commonly present in the upper respiratory tract of both healthy children (40 to 50 per cent) and adults (30 to 40 per cent).

Two noninvasive tests are of value in establishing the role of bacteria in patients with pneumonia. Blood cultures should be obtained in all patients with pneumonia in whom the diagnosis is in question. Whereas only 3 to 4 per cent of children with pneumonia have positive blood cultures, approximately 20 per cent of adults with acute labor pneumonia have blood cultures positive for pneumococci. Examination of sputum, serum, and urine by counter-current immunoelectrophoresis for the presence of bacterial antigens can detect pneumococcal polysaccharide antigen in approximately 60 per cent of adults presumed to have a pneumococcal pneumonia syndrome. This test has not been used to evaluate the entire scope of adult pneumonia; therefore the etiologic significance of bacteria in an unselected population of adult pneumonia remains to be determined. The usefulness of this test in pediatric patients remains to be elucidated.

Examination of serum for the presence of cold hemagglutinins is helpful in approximately 50 per cent of patients with *M. pneumoniae* disease. The median maximum cold agglutinin titer in those patients with positive tests is approximately 1:128. A cold agglutinin titer of 1:32 or less is not helpful in confirming or excluding this diagnosis.

Specific diagnosis of viral and mycoplasmal infections depends on isolation of the agent or detection of an antibody rise. For virus isolation, respiratory secretions should be obtained by performing a throat swab and a saline nasal washing. Anal swab cultures are confusing because of the prolonged rectal shedding of adenoviruses and enteroviruses, and these are not recommended. Sputum cultures are preferred for the isolation of *M. pneumoniae*. Acute-phase serum should be obtained on the day of diagnosis, and convalescent serum 10 days to 3 weeks later. Rapid virus diagnosis may be available in some centers by fluorescent antibody staining of exfoliated respiratory epithelial cells.

Although the specific diagnostic tests outlined may not reveal the etiologic diagnosis of an individual patient during the acute illness, the use of these services is frequently prudent. During periods of epidemic prevalence of lower respiratory disease, knowledge of the cause of illness in a few patients would make possible a reasonable estimate of the diagnosis in many patients.

PSITTACOSIS

By GERALD GORDON, M.D.,
and PIERCE GARDNER, M.D.
Chicago, Illinois

SYNONYMS

Parrot fever; ornithosis — same disease, reservoir in non-psittacine birds.

DEFINITION AND EPIDEMIOLOGY

Psittacosis (ornithosis) is a systemic infectious disease caused by *Chlamydia psittaci*, an obligate intracellular parasite that was once considered to be a large virus. Properties of chlamydiae that differentiate them from viruses include their mode of replication (binary fission of parental cell), nucleic acid content (both RNA and DNA), and susceptibility to antibiotics (e.g., tetracycline). Unlike bacteria, chlamydiae cannot be cultivated in artificial media but require living cells to supply growth factors (e.g., ATP and NADH).

With rare exceptions psittacosis is a zoonotic disease resulting from direct or indirect human exposure to birds harboring *C. psittaci*. Humans become infected primarily by inhaling aerosols from infected bird droppings or infected tissues. Avian infection may be asymptomatic or may be manifested by apathy, weight loss, diarrhea, and ruffled feathers. Infected birds may develop a sticky exudate around the nares. Psittacine birds, (including budgerigars and cockatiels), turkeys, and pigeons are the most common species associated with outbreaks of psittacosis, although *C. psittaci* has been isolated from members of nearly all avian species. Approximately 75 cases of human psittacosis are reported to the Center for Disease Control annually. The disease has only rarely been documented in children. Cases occur primarily among persons with a high vocational or avocational exposure to birds. Intimate contact with infected birds is not essential. Psittacosis has occurred following brief exposure to a room that previously had housed an infected bird, and at least one outbreak has been traced to pigeons living on a windowsill outside an office. In almost 20 per cent of serologically confirmed cases a history of bird exposure cannot be elicited.

Rare instances of human-to-human transmission of psittacosis (including nosocomial spread to hospital personnel) have been reported. Therefore patients with psittacosis should be considered contagious and respiratory precautions should be observed during the initial diagnosis and treatment period.

PRESENTING SYMPTOMS AND SIGNS

Psittacosis should be suspected when a person who has significant exposure to birds (veterinarian, poultry processing worker, bird owner, pet store owner, aviary worker, or bird fancier) develops a "flu-like" illness. The characteristic symptoms of psittacosis are fever (in some cases to 105 F [40.5 C] with rigors), dry nonproductive cough, severe diffuse headaches, malaise, dyspnea, lethargy, myalgias, and photophobia. Nausea and vomiting and less commonly hemoptysis, epistaxis, and abdominal pain may be present. Although the symptoms usually have a gradual onset over several days, the illness may begin abruptly and the patient may appear toxic without major respiratory symptoms early in the illness. A milder form of psittacosis that mimics other mild atypical pneumonias also occurs. This form is characterized by gradual onset of symptoms, fever that peaks at 5 to 7 days, and a dry nonproductive cough. In some cases fever may precede cough by a week or more. Subclinical infection may also occur. The incubation period of psittacosis is usually 6 to 15 days, although it may be as long as 39 days.

PHYSICAL FINDINGS

The clinical spectrum of psittacosis is varied. Fever is characteristic and in some cases a pulse-temperature dissociation (slow pulse relative to the level of temperature elevation) has been noted as is seen in classic typhoid fever, brucellosis, Legionnaires' disease, and other illnesses. The chest examination may show a spectrum of findings ranging from no abnormalities or fine sibilant localized rales to signs of frank lobar consolidation. Chest roentgenograms usually show abnormalities considerably worse than suggested by the physical examination. Hepatic and splenic enlargement are seen in a variable number of patients, although clinical jaundice is rare. Findings that have been occasionally noted include a transient erythematous rash (Horder's spots) similar to the rose spots seen in typhoid fever, pleural and pericardial friction rubs, and confusion and meningismus (seen in more severe cases).

COURSE

Complete recovery from psittacosis tends to be prolonged and relapses may occur, especially in patients receiving inadequate courses of tetracycline. Even with specific treatment, the acute "flu-like" illness may not respond for several days and the fact that the patient is not afebrile after 72 or 96 hours of tetracycline therapy should not be misconstrued as a treatment failure. Malaise may persist for protracted periods after acute symptoms such as headache, fever, and chills have resolved. Without specific antibiotic therapy the moderately ill patient characteristically has a 2 to 3 week illness that peaks at about 10 days with gradual resolution of fever and cough thereafter. Milder cases generally run a shorter course. Fatalities in treated cases are rare (<1 per cent), although in unrecognized cases mortality may reach 20 per cent.

COMMON COMPLICATIONS

Psittacosis is primarily a pulmonary infection with systemic symptoms. Extrapulmonary complications are uncommon. Focal hepatocellular necrosis and granulomatous hepatitis are occasionally seen. Rare complications include pericarditis, myocarditis, and endocarditis. Thrombophlebitis and pulmonary embolization may occur in the recovery phase of psittacosis. Myositis, meningitis, or encephalitis occasionally is seen in severe infections. Psittacosis is occasionally responsible for fever of unknown origin.

LABORATORY FINDINGS

General. The roentgenographic abnormalities in patients with psittacosis are variable. The characteristic x-ray findings are patchy interstitial infiltrates involving the basilar lung fields and extending to the hilum. Atelectasis and lobar consolidation are common. Extensive pulmonary infiltrates are seen occasionally. Typically, the white blood count is less than 13,000 per cu mm but in some patients it may be higher with a predominance of immature forms. The erythrocyte sedimentation rate is usually elevated. Urinalysis may show mild degrees of proteinuria. Moderate elevation of certain liver function tests, including serum glutamic oxaloacetic transaminase (SGOT), serum glutamic pyruvic transaminase (SGPT), and alkaline phosphatase, is a frequent finding, although bilirubin levels are rarely increased. The electrocardiogram, while typically normal, may show evidence of pericardial injury or prolongation of the QT interval and other changes consistent with myocarditis. The MM fraction of creatine phosphokinase (CPK) may be elevated. Sputum is usually scant but if present will contain polymorphonuclear leukocytes, alveo-

lar macrophages, and occasionally tracheal mucosal cells, and the Gram-stained smear will not show bacteria.

Specific. The serologic response to infection measured by complement fixation (CF) titer is the mainstay of the diagnosis of psittacosis in most laboratories. A fourfold rise in the group-specific complement fixation titer for Chlamydia species in paired sera taken 2 or more weeks apart is strongly suggestive of active chlamydial infection. In untreated patients, the majority develop significant titer rises by the third week of illness. Treatment may delay CF titer rises as long as 6 to 8 weeks. Occasionally, patients with clinically apparent psittacosis will not develop significant titer rises. CF titer of 1:32 may be seen in the normal population, presumably as a result of previous exposure to other chlamydia. Isolated CF titers of 1:64 or higher are suggestive of recent chlamydial infection. Because the CF test is a chlamydial group-specific test, patients who develop lymphogranulorum venereum and some with trachoma may have abnormal CF titers. False-positive titer rises are uncommon but have been reported in some patients with Legionnaires' disease (*Legionella pneumophilia*). The IgM response to chlamydial infection appears to be more specific for psittacosis.

Culture of *C. psittaci* in embryonated hen's eggs, in mice, or in tissue culture is possible, but this is rarely attempted in routine laboratories because of the hazard of laboratory-acquired disease.

Biopsy material from the lung (or on occasion sputum) may show intracytoplasmic inclusion bodies when stained with Giemsa or Machiavello stains. Specific immunofluorescent testing is possible but is generally unavailable. Microimmunofluorescent serologic titers are available in research laboratories and may prove to be helpful in confirming the diagnosis of psittacosis.

PITFALLS IN DIAGNOSIS

Failure to elicit a history of bird exposure in patients with pneumonia is the most frequent reason for not considering psittacosis in the differential diagnosis. Psittacosis is often missed, as it is a rare cause of "flu-like" illness and presents with protean symptoms. More common causes of these symptoms include viral pneumonias (especially influenza, parainfluenza, and adenoviruses), mycoplasma pneumonia, infectious mononucleosis, and viral hepatitis. Among the bacterial diseases that may produce a similar picture, typhoid fever, brucellosis, tularemia, tuberculosis, and Legionnaires' disease should be considered. Rickettsial (Q fever), fungal (cryptococcus, coccidioidomycosis, histoplasmosis, and aspergillosis) and protozoan (toxoplasmosis) etiologies also belong in the differential diagnosis.

Hypersensitivity reactions to inhalants (bird fancier's lung) or drugs (e.g., nitrofurantoin) must also be considered.

The serologic response of psittacosis is characteristically slow and may take several weeks to document. The initial diagnosis of psittacosis is therefore a clinical one. Consequently, the physician who has a high index of suspicion based on the epidemiology history and disease presentation should place the patient on respiratory isolation and initiate tetracycline therapy before confirmatory data become available.

LYMPHOGRANULOMA VENEREUM

By THOMAS W. JOHNSON, M.D.

Nashville, Tennessee

SYNONYMS

Lymphopathia venereum, lymphogranuloma inguinale, Durand-Nicholas-Favre disease, climatic bubo, tropical bubo, lymphogranulomatosis inguinalis, poradenitis.

DEFINITION

Lymphogranuloma venereum is an infectious disease that primarily involves the lymphatic system. The causative agent belongs to the genus Chlamydia and is known as *Miyagawanella lymphogranulomatosis*. The organisms are morphologically indistinguishable from other microorganisms in this group (also called PLT [psittacosis-lymphogranuloma-trachoma], Miyagawanella, and Bedsonia). They range from 0.2 to 1 μm in diameter, and are obligate, intracellular parasites that contain both DNA and RNA.

The disease is worldwide in its distribution, although there is a marked concentration of cases in tropical and subtropical areas. In the United States, the majority of cases are reported from the Southeastern states. Transmission of the infection occurs almost exclusively venereally, although the occurrence of cases in

laboratory workers and medical personnel tends to implicate other routes of infection. Cases are reported more frequently in the male than in the female, suggesting the possibility that subclinical infection is more prevalent in the female than in the male.

PRESENTING SIGNS AND SYMPTOMS

The incubation period of lymphogranuloma venereum may vary from 5 to 21 days. The primary lesion is frequently painless and inconspicuous and tends to heal rapidly. In many instances its presence is not noticed by males, and rarely is noticed by females. The lesion usually occurs on the genitalia and consists of a solitary papule, solitary vesicle, or small cluster of vesicles that may rupture, leaving a nonindurated, shallow erosion of 2 to 3 mm in diameter with an erythematous halo.

From 7 to 30 days after the appearance of the primary lesion, regional lymphadenopathy occurs as a result of lymphatic and hematogenous dissemination of the organisms from the site of initial entry. The enlarged nodes are initially firm, tender, and discrete. As the condition progresses, the nodes tend to become matted together, considerably enlarged, and adherent to the surrounding tissue. Frequently, they are bisected by a depression formed by the inelastic Poupart ligament, forming an upper and a lower portion. When this occurs, it is quite characteristic of lymphogranuloma venereum. Multilocular abscesses may form with eventual rupture onto the skin, forming multiple fistulous openings through which a seropurulent exudate may drain. Healing may occur slowly with the formation of puckered, retracted scars.

In the male, the primary lesion occurs most frequently on the glans penis, on the prepuce, and in or near the urethral meatus. In most instances lymphadenopathy is unilateral, but it may be bilateral.

In the female, the primary lesion usually occurs intravaginally, perivaginally, in or around the urethra, or on the cervix. Lymphadenopathy then involves the nodes found in the perirectal, rectosigmoidal, anorectal, sacral, and hypogastric chains. Signs and symptoms of the disease will occur late in the course of the infection.

In those instances in which primary infection occurs within the anal or rectal canals, initial symptoms may include a mucopurulosanguineous discharge from the rectum, obstipation, tenesmus, and pain.

Systemic signs and symptoms of the disease may include chills, fever, sweating, headache, weight loss, arthralgias, myalgias, and polyarthritis. Hepatosplenomegaly may occur. Urticarial, scarlatiniform, erythema multiforme-like, and papulopustular eruptions may occur.

COURSE

Evidence would suggest that in many instances infections with lymphogranuloma venereum may not progress beyond the occurrence of the primary lesion. This evidence is based upon the presence of complement-fixing antibodies for lymphogranuloma venereum in persons with no documented evidence of recent or remote presence of overt disease. Progression of the disease results from early dissemination from the initial site of entry by way of the lymphatic and blood systems, with subsequent disease manifestations restricted mainly to the lymphatic drainage of the site of initial invasion. Although the primary lesion tends to heal without scarring, the later stages of the disease may progress to scar formation with all the related consequences. Scarring sequelae are most marked in females, in whom any of the following could occur: (1) cicatricial stenosis of the urethra and vagina, (2) rectal strictures and fibrosis of the rectal wall, (3) perirectal and perianal abscess, (4) vaginovesical and vaginorectal fistulas, (5) elephantiasis of the genitalia, or (6) fibrous growth around the anus. The homosexual male may develop the rectal and anal complications.

Extragenital primary lesions are rare but can occur on the lip, tongue, and finger. Regional lymphadenitis may occur and may result in Parinaud's syndrome. Sclerokeratitis, uveitis, and iridocyclitis may also occur.

PHYSICAL EXAMINATION

The primary lesion of lymphogranuloma venereum is essentially asymptomatic and inconspicuous and regresses rapidly. Usually it is not a prominent feature as a sign of the disease. When noted, however, it initially occurs as a small papule, vesicle, or cluster of vesicles that rupture to leave a small, shallow erosion with a halo of erythema. The lesion may be located on the glans, on the prepuce, or within the urethral meatus in the male and on the vulva, urethra, vaginal vault, or cervix in females. When genitorectal contact occurs, the lesion may occur in the perianal or anal areas.

Prominent as a feature of the disease are the findings related to the lymph nodes. When the lymphatic drainage of the primary lesion dictates, the inguinal nodes, either unilaterally or bilaterally, are involved. Early nodes are enlarged, matted, and adherent to the overlying skin, which may become discolored. Discoloration may vary from a violaceous to a dusky hue, depending upon the basic pigmentation of the individual. Longitudinal cleavage of the enlarged, matted nodes by the inelastic Poupart ligament is characteristic of lymphogranuloma venereum. In some patients spontaneous resolution may occur at this stage, although in the majority of patients the enlarged node will develop multilocular abscesses with subsequent rupture and drainage of a seropurulent exudate from fistulous tracts. Subsequent healing by scar tissue formation results in a puckered cicatrix.

In the female, vulvar enlargement, ulceration, and subsequent scarring may occur. There may be progressive ulcerations of the labia, urethra, and vagina with eventual cicatricial stenosis of the urethra and vagina. Proctocolitis and anorectal strictures may occur: Such strictures are also seen in homosexual males and may be detected on rectal examination.

Systemic findings include chills, fever, sweating, headache, weight loss, arthralgias, myalgias, polyarthritis, hepatosplenomegaly and skin eruptions such as urticarial, scarlatiniform, erythema-like, and papulopustular eruptions. Generalized lymphadenopathy may also be present.

COMMON COMPLICATIONS

Pneumonitis, meningitis, meningoencephalitis, and cystitis can occur as complications of infections by the causative agent of lymphogranuloma venereum. Other complications may be seen in spite of adequate treatment of the disease. Strictures, which are the complication of greatest consequence, occur more frequently in females than in males. Strictures of the colon usually occur within 10 cm of the anal orifice and frequently within 5 cm. Ulcerative colitis–like syndromes with potential intestinal obstruction and/or perforation of the rectum and rectosigmoid areas may occur. Strictures of the urethra in females, along with fistulas and fenestrations of the clitoris and labia minora, may also occur. There may be elephantiasis of the genitalia secondary to lymphatic and lymph node scarring. Rectovaginal fistulas are seen in females, and pararectal abscesses and sinuses are seen in females and homosexual males. Squamous cell carcinomas of the penis, vulva, bladder, anus, and rectum are frequently associated with lymphogranuloma venereum.

LABORATORY FINDINGS

Peripheral Blood. Peripheral blood changes

are nonspecific with positive findings relating to systemic signs only.

The Frei Test. This is an intradermal test that detects a state of hypersensitivity to the causative agent of lymphogranuloma venereum. The antigen, known commercially as Lygranum C.F., is derived from the infected yolk sacs of chick embryos, and normal yolk sac material is utilized as a control.

The test is performed by injecting 0.1 ml of the antigen intradermally into the flexural surface of the forearm and 0.1 ml of the control material into a similar area of the opposite forearm. A positive test is reflected by the occurrence of an area of focal induration at least 5 mm or greater in diameter within 48 to 96 hours after injection with a control area of focal induration 5 mm or less in diameter. The severity of the skin test reaction, which can progress to the point of ulceration, does not correlate with the severity of the infection. The skin test becomes positive 12 to 40 days after the onset of adenitis and usually remains positive for life. Approximately 20 per cent false positive reactions may occur. A test that is negative in the early stages of the disease should be repeated at a later date; once the test is positive, repeated tests will not alter the degree of the response.

Complement Fixation Tests. A positive complement fixation test may precede a positive intradermal skin test (Frei test). The test utilizes an antigen specific for the chlamydial group of microorganisms, prepared from infected yolk sacs of chick embryos or infected mouse lung suspensions or extracts, which gives a complement fixation reaction when mixed with serum from patients infected with lymphogranuloma venereum. A titer of 1:40 or more is significant; typically, early in the disease, a titer of up to 1:160 will occur. Later higher titers (e.g., 1:640) may occur, and an increase in titer (fourfold or greater) in two successive tests is considered diagnostic. Cross-reactions occur in patients who have been infected with or have recovered from psittacosis, ornithosis, cat-scratch disease, and viral pneumonia, inasmuch as a species-specific antigen for lymphogranuloma venereum, although possible through specific extraction procedures of infected yolk sac material, is not stable enough for routine use.

The sensitivity of the complement fixation test for lymphogranuloma venereum renders it a more significant and useful test than the Frei Test.

Viral Cultural Techniques. Inoculation of either the yolk sacs of chick embryos or brains of mice with blood, purulent exudate, excised lymph nodes, or cerebrospinal fluid can result in isolation of the causative organism. These techniques are not done routinely in most laboratories, however.

PITFALLS IN DIAGNOSIS

Lymphogranuloma venereum must be differentiated from other sexually transmitted diseases such as herpes simplex, syphilis, chancroids, and granuloma inguinale. It must also be differentiated from such diseases as actinomycosis, tuberculosis, tularemia, plague, lymphomas, ulcerative colitis, and carcinoma.

The disease must be considered in a differential diagnosis when presenting signs and symptoms would tend to dictate. All positive confirmatory tests must be carefully interpreted, and negative tests should be repeated at appropriate intervals.

MEASLES

By C. P. DARBY, M.D.
Charleston, South Carolina

SYNONYMS

Rubeola, morbilli, red measles.

DEFINITION:

Measles is an acute generalized infection caused by an RNA-containing paramyxovirus, characterized by fever, conjunctivitis, cough, coryza, and an enanthem, with the eventual development of a generalized maculopapular rash. The disease is usually transmitted by airborne droplets from an infected person and the incubation period is 10 to 12 days. Following the incubation period, fever, conjunctivitis, coryza, and cough begin almost simultaneously. These symptoms continue to worsen until the fifth or sixth day when the rash appears.

On the third to fourth day the enanthem can usually be seen on the buccal mucosa opposite the molars.

PRESENTING SIGNS AND SYMPTOMS

Fever. Generally, the fever begins at a low grade and gradually climbs in a stepwise fashion; however, occasionally, it remains 103 to 105 F (39.4 to 40.5 C) during the entire febrile course of the illness. Without complications the temperature will rapidly return to normal 2 to 3 days after the rash appears.

Conjunctivitis. The bulbar and palpebral conjunctivae are both inflamed and there are often thick lacrimal secretions. The patient may experience photophobia.

Cough. The cough is a result of a inflammation of the air passages. It usually has an early onset, is nonproductive, and may last for 7 to 10 days after the fever subsides.

Koplick's Spots. These small lesions have come to be known as the pathognomonic lesions of measles. They are described as small red spots with a minute bluish-white speck in the center. They appear on the second or third day of fever along buccal mucosa opposite the molars. As the rash approaches, the Koplick's spots increase in number, coalescing to diffuse erythematous mucosa.

Rash. The rash generally develops on the third to fifth day of the illness, but may develop as early as the first day or as late as the seventh. The rash begins along the hairline and forehead, then progresses downward to cover the trunk and extremities.

Lymphadenopathy. Generalized hypertrophy of the lymph nodes may be palpated. The postauricular occipital and cervical nodes tend to be enlarged.

Measles may be modified when the child is passively immunized with gamma globulin. The incubation period may be prolonged and the illness shortened. Hemorrhagic measles, or "black measles," is a severe form of measles resulting in hyperpyrexia, convulsions, delirium, respiratory distress, and hemorrhagic eruption of the skin and mucous membranes.

PHYSICAL FINDINGS

The generalized maculopapular rash preceded by a fever, coryza, conjunctivitis, and cough, along with the characteristic Koplick's spots, should enable one to diagnose measles.

COMMON COMPLICATIONS

Bacterial otitis media is the most common complication of measles. Pneumonia may result from extension of the viral process, bacterial invasion, or a combination of both.

Acute encephalitis is the most serious complication. Central nervous system involvement may be noted between the second and sixth day of the rash. This usually begins with fever, headache, vomiting, convulsions, and coma. The cerebrospinal fluid generally has a pleocytosis with a predominance of lymphocytes. The course may be mild and brief, but many children suffer irreparable brain damage and often death.

Subacute sclerosing panencephalitis (SSPE) is considered by many to be a late complication of measles. The disease is characterized by a gradual progressive neurologic deterioration beginning several months or years after the initial infection. Appendicitis occasionally develops during an attack of measles, perhaps owing to the disturbance in normal host immunity.

LABORATORY FINDINGS

The virus has been isolated, but isolation is of little practical value in individual patient management. Complement fixing, hemagglutination, inhibition, and neutralizing antibodies generally rise and peak 2 to 4 weeks after the beginning of the infection. The disease is usually associated with a leukopenia.

PITFALLS IN DIAGNOSIS

There is always a serious responsibility for the physician to sort out the various exanthematous diseases. Scarlet fever, meningococcemia, rubella, typhus, toxoplasmosis, cytomegalovirus infection, roseola, enteroviral infections, infectious mononucleosis, toxic erythemas, mucocutaneous lymph node syndrome, Rocky Mountain spotted fever, and drug eruptions may be mistaken for measles. The careful assessment of the associated symptoms, the prodromal period, and the character distribution and duration of the rash will enable one to differentiate the diagnosis. Clinically it may be difficult to establish the diagnosis and laboratory diagnostic test may be helpful.

The widespread use of measles vaccine in this country has greatly reduced the incidence of the disease, but a number of cases continue to occur each year.

The disease occurs sporadically — this makes it more of a challenge for the physician to recognize.

RUBELLA

By GILLES R. G. MONIF, M.D.
Gainesville, Florida

SYNONYMS

German measles, three-day measles, red measles, röteln, rubeola notha.

DEFINITION

Rubella is an acute viral exanthema that, if acquired in utero, may have pronounced effects on organogenesis and somatic development. The disease is caused by a large encapsulated RNA virus. The spread is by aerosol dissemination with the nasopharynx and oropharynx constituting the primary portals of infection. The period of time between acquisition of infection and onset of rash is influenced by the intimacy of contact. The incubation period ranges from 11 to 14 days.

PRESENTING SIGNS AND SYMPTOMS

Rubella in the young child is a relatively innocuous disease with little significant morbidity or mortality. The prodrome, when present, is primarily seen in adolescents and adults and consists of malaise, myalgia, and headache. In young children there is no recognized prodrome or if it occurs it is very minimal.

The onset of prodrome usually corresponds with the development of postauricular lymphadenopathy, which often precedes the rash by as much as 6 or 7 days.

The rash of rubella usually begins on the upper thorax and spreads in a wavelike manner over a 3-day period to involve first the thorax and then the abdomen and finally the extremities. It is maculopapullary in character. Frequently the rash will be fully developed on the lower extremities while exhibiting evidence of fading on the thorax and abdomen.

Although rubella is extremely infectious and has a high attack rate, 50 to 60 per cent of all cases are subclinical in nature. Despite the failure of rash to appear, postauricular adenopathy (particularly in preadolescents) will appear at the time of anticipated or presumed rash. The postauricular lymphadenopathy will persist for up to 2 weeks. When a high hemagglutination-inhibiting (HAI) antibody titer and postauricular lymphadenopathy are present in a patient who had an antecedent rash, rubella should be suspected.

CLINICAL COURSE

The clinical course is of relatively short duration, lasting 2 to 4 days. Unlike rubeola (measles), bacterial superinfection is not a major clinical consideration. Arthralgia, if it develops, usually does so following the appearance of cutaneous lesions.

PHYSICAL EXAMINATION FINDINGS

Physical examination reveals a fine, discrete red rash. The individual areas are elevated, and the skin has a sandpaper texture to it. Unlike the rash of rubeola, it has no tendency to coalesce. The rash will fade centrally while being pronounced on the peripheral extremities. Frequently, patients will exhibit small, discrete macular areas on the soft palate, which may be punctuated or patchy in appearance. Systemic symptoms can occur in the absence of a discernable rash.

The postauricular adenopathy is commonly a concomitant finding, even in young adults. The combination of a characteristic rash of 2 to 3 day duration and the presence of postauricular adenopathy constitutes reasonable, circumstantial evidence for the presumptive diagnosis of rubella but is *not* diagnostic in a definitive sense.

COMMON COMPLICATIONS

The sequelae of rubella infection in children and adults are extremely limited. There is a propensity among adults, particularly young women, to develop arthralgia and, in extremely rare instances, arthritis. The incidence of arthralgia is influenced by the strain virulence. The attack rate may be as high as 20 per cent. The development of disseminated intravascular coagulopathy and thrombocytopenia has been described. In rare instances, this may be of sufficient magnitude to produce hemorrhages following minimal trauma. Extremely rare cases of myocarditis and encephalitis have been reported.

PATHOGENESIS

Congenital infection is usually the consequence of two separate events: a maternal viremia and a fetal viremia. Maternal viremia is responsible for virus replication within the trophoblastic cells. To effect a fetal viremia, virus replication must occur with fetal endothelial cells. Fetal viremia results in widespread organ involvement. Once the fetal tissues are colonized, successful virus replication within these tissues is extended well beyond the neonatal period. Approximately 90 per cent of children with congenital rubella syndrome can be shown to be excreting infectious virus in all their biological fluids, with the partial exception of blood.

The classic stigmata of congenital rubella syndrome, namely, ocular, cochlear, central nervous system, and cardiac pathology, are the consequences of continued virus–cell interaction in tissues with limited regenerative capacity. The mechanism by which rubella embryopathy is achieved is apparently twofold. One part involves direct cytopathic effect (CPE), and the other appears to be caused by the inhibition of mitosis, due to the effects of either double-stranded RNA or a specific inhibitory protein.

CLINICAL MANIFESTATIONS

The consequences of rubella infection during pregnancy present a wide spectrum, from spontaneous abortion, stillbirth, live birth with one or more fetal anomalies, to normal children.

Thrombocytopenia purpura is one of the most common manifestations of rubella embryopathy. These infants with overt infection often have hepatomegaly or hepatosplenomegaly and may exhibit jaundice in the first 24 hours. Retardation of intrauterine growth and development may result in a low-birth-weight-for-dates neonate. Growth development characteristics, as seen by weight gain, increase in head circumference and dentition, and significant linear growth, are delayed. This pattern is most prominent in infants who remain infected for months after birth. Microcephaly is a common residuum of rubella embryopathy. Central nervous system involvement is often multifaceted and includes microcephaly, mental or motor disabilities, and neurosensory impairment. While a wide spectrum of cardiac anomalies has been observed in congenital rubella infants, the most commonly associated lesions are patent ductus arteriosus (PDA) or pulmonary artery stenosis (PA) or both. Myocardial necrosis and myocarditis may be concomitantly present. The endarteritis-produced arterial stenosis may affect peripheral vessels.

The spectrum of ocular pathology is impressive. The cataracts caused by congenital rubella are of a unique sort. As first described by Gregg, they were

... dense, white opacities completely occupying the pupillary area... after dilation the opacities appeared densely white—sometimes quite pearly—in the central area with a small apparently clear zone between this and the pupillary border of the iris.... The cataractous process seemed to have involved all but the outermost layers of the lens, and was considered to have begun early in the life of the embryo....

The cataracts are generally bilateral and detectable at birth. Chorioretinitis, presenting as retinitis pigmentosa, can frequently be demonstrable. The latter is seen as focal aggregation of black pigment on fundoscopic examination. While both of these lesions appear to be the consequence of viral cytopathic effect (CPE), other ocular lesions, such as microphthalmia, iris hypoplasia, and glaucoma (resulting from incomplete development of the chamber angle), appear to be due to retardation of somatic growth.

Congenital rubella results in a panorganic involvement. Persistence of the virus and continued virus-cell interaction in utero can produce a wide spectrum of clinical disease in the neonatal period, including hemolytic anemia with extramedullary hematopoiesis, hepatitis, interstitial pneumonitis, myocarditis, myocardiopathy, interstitial nephritis, encephalitis, interstitial pancreatitis, and osteomyelitis. These manifestations of cellular dysfunction and necrobiosis have prompted the use of the term "the expanded congenital syndrome."

POSTNATAL PERSISTENCE

Approximately 90 per cent of all neonates with congenital rubella syndrome have virus in most of their extravascular biological fluids, e.g., cerebrospinal fluid (CSF), urine, tears, and swabbings of the conjunctiva and posterior part of the oropharynx. The virus present is infectious. Congenital rubella infants may be the instigators of small epidemics within the hospital community or the direct cause of the condition in infants with second-generation congenital rubella. In the community, there is a similar need for education concerning the infectiousness of the infant with rubella embryopathy. Any female of childbearing age in the immediate vicinity of such an infant should be screened and, if susceptible and not pregnant, vaccinated as an integral part of primary care.

LABORATORY FINDINGS

Maternal Diagnosis. Although rubella virus can be recovered in several tissue culture systems, the paucity of laboratories that can attempt viral isolation from oropharyngeal swabs limits the practicality of this approach. Rubella antibody first makes its appearance at the time of rash or presumed rash. Documentation of maternal rubella is almost invariably contingent on the demonstration of an eightfold or greater rise in specific HAI antibody titer obtained from serum specimens drawn on or before the rash and 7 to 10 days following its clinical appearance. The pre- and postconvalescent specimens must be quantitated under identical test circumstances in at least duplicate testing before the serologic diagnosis of rubella can be accepted.

When a patient is evaluated several days after the rash has cleared, advantage can be taken of the fact that complement-fixing (CF) antibodies develop later than HAI antibodies. For cases in which it may not be possible to demonstrate an eightfold or greater rise utilizing HAI antibodies, the diagnosis may be documented by analysis of CF antirubella antibodies.

DIAGNOSIS OF CONGENITAL RUBELLA

A presumptive diagnosis of congenital rubella can be inferred on purely clinical grounds; however, the absence of overt evidence of virus–cell interaction does not exclude the possibility of congenital rubella. The demonstration of an elevated cord IgM level by radial immunodiffusion may be construed as evidence favoring the probability of intrauterine infection. The only definitive means of documenting or excluding congenital involvement in the immediate neonatal period is isolation of the virus or the demonstration of IgM antirubella antibodies. African green monkey kidney cultures used with the enterovirus interference techniques constitute the most sensitive in vitro indicator system for the detection of rubella virus.

PITFALLS IN DIAGNOSIS

Postnatal Rubella. The diagnosis of postnatal rubella cannot be made on a purely clinical basis. Other viral agents are capable of producing an exanthematous rash that, in both character and duration, mimics that observed with rubella virus infection. Exanthemas comparable to that observed with rubella virus have been described with the echoviruses, Coxsackieviruses, and hepatitis type A viruses. Prior history of rubella without serologic documentation may or may not be accurate. The absence of a history of rubella, particularly in older children and adults, does not preclude immunity.

The rubella HAI test has many variables that may, in any given situation, result in at least a twofold variation. This degree of variability makes it difficult to interpret the significance of antibody titers of two separate samples obtained from different laboratories or even from the same laboratory. For the serologic diagnosis of rubella, the following criterion must be met: a greater than fourfold rise in titer must be established between two specimens run simultaneously, in, at least, duplicate, within the same test.

Congenital Rubella. As previously stated, the absence of overt evidence of rubella embryopathy does not exclude the possibility of congenital disease. A small but significant percentage of congenitally infected infants will be totally normal by all gross parameters in the immediate neonatal period and the first few months of life. Ultimately, such clinical signs as microcephaly, motor retardation, deafness, or chorioretinitis surface, which alert the pediatrician to the underlying diagnosis of congenital rubella.

RABIES

By MORRIS SCHAEFFER, M.D.
Bethesda, Maryland

SYNONYMS

Hydrophobia, rage, lyssa.

DEFINITION

Rabies is an acute viral encephalomyelitis, with lesions concentrated in those parts of the cerebrospinal axis that are in direct neural continuity with the site of the infection. Propagating along neuromuscular tissue, the virus travels cranially up the regional nerve trunks, eventually reaching the brain, there engendering a spotty or generalized inflammatory response with perivascular collections of lymphocytes and scattered accumulations of glial and Hortega cells. A variable number of neurons may be found to contain viral inclusion bodies known as Negri bodies, and these are pathognomonic.

EPIDEMIOLOGY

Rabies is most frequently transmitted by the saliva of infected animals. In the United States wild or domestic carnivores (skunks, foxes, raccoons, cats, and dogs) or insectivorous bats are the most common sources. The virus is usually inoculated by the bite of a rabid animal, or infrequently it may enter from the saliva through a skin lesion. Droplet infections from cave-dwelling bats have been described. Children are more frequently the victims of rabies than adults, because they spend more time outdoors and are eager to play with animals. Man-to-man transmission is possible by contact with infected saliva, particularly before the patient is isolated and after hospitalization during emergency care, such as the performance of a tracheostomy.

The incubation time in man is from 10 days to 2 years; usually, 1 to 3 months.

PRESENTING SIGNS AND SYMPTOMS

Onset is marked by 2 to 4 days of prodromal symptoms consisting of fever, headache, malaise, anorexia, nausea, and sore throat. Abnormal sensations about the site of wound, including pain, burning, sensation of cold, pruritus, tingling, or formication, may occur in about 80 per cent of the patients, and this is of diagnostic significance. In general, the early symptoms, resulting mainly from the stimulative action of the virus on the neurons, predominantly those of the sensory system, are manifested by hyperesthesia of the skin and extreme sensitivity to external stimuli.

The patient may complain of drafts and bedclothes, because they produce general stimulation of the skin. Bright lights or loud noises may further disturb the patient, who in the acute excitation phase displays a severe state of nervousness, anxiety, and apprehension. A sense of impending death is common. Nevertheless, there is a strong desire to be up, the patient indulging in aimless wandering and talking in disconnected sentences.

The body temperature varies but seldom exceeds 101.5 F (38 C). There is usually some nuchal rigidity. Dilated pupils, excessive perspiration, rhinorrhea, cutis anserina ("goose flesh"), chills, nausea, and vomiting are common.

COURSE

The course is usually short. The patient seldom survives longer than 1 week. Only a few instances have been recorded in which patients with fully developed symptoms recovered.

In most patients the state of hyperexcitability persists up to the time of death. However, in some instances depressive or paralytic symptoms may be predominant from the beginning or, more frequently, may supervene at any time after the onset of the excitement phase. The outstanding clinical symptom, appearing as the disease progresses, is related to the act of swallowing. When fluid comes in contact with the fauces, spasmodic contractions of the muscles of deglutition and of the accessory muscles of respiration are produced, causing a violent and painful expulsion of the fluid. This reflex irritability may be so intense that the sight of liquids or the mere suggestion of the act of swallowing may precipitate a spasm of the throat: hence the term "hydrophobia." Some patients exhibit no fear of water but have difficulty in swallowing and a sense of constriction in the throat. In avoiding the act of swallowing, the patient is apt to drool from the mouth and develop progressive dehydration. Choking, when attempting to swallow, may produce spasm of the respiratory muscles with prolonged apnea, cyanosis, and gasping respirations. Convulsive seizures may occur which, when severe, may lead to opisthotonos. Periods of intense excitement, unmanageability, and maniacal behavior may be interspersed with relatively quiet states in which the patient is well oriented and alert and responds intelligently. Many patients succumb in the excitement phase during a convulsion. In others, there ensues a paralytic phase as a result of a progressive degeneration of the motor neurons. Paralysis of the muscles of phonation becomes evident by hoarseness or loss of voice. Weakness of the facial and masseter muscles may be present, and there may follow a general flaccid paralysis with urinary retention and obstipation. Anxiety and excitement are replaced gradually by apathy, stupor, and coma.

PHYSICAL EXAMINATION

General. Most patients are so nervous, irritable, and anxious that they may be mistaken for severe psychoneurotics. Some may show marked depression or melancholia. Whether or not the history of an animal bite has been elicited, a healing or healed wound may be found on one of the extremities or elsewhere on the body. In cases with incubation period of several months' duration, the failure of a patient or his relatives to recollect a minor wound by an apparently healthy dog is not uncommon.

Head and Neck. The pupils may be dilated, constricted, or unequal and react poorly to light. The corneal reflex is decreased or absent, and the cornea may appear dry. Hippus, nystagmus, diplopia, strabismus, and vertigo may be present. Facial expressions may be overactive, or there may be facial palsy with attendant difficulty in the closing of the eyes or mouth and loss of facial expression.

Heart. The heart rate may be 100 to 120 per minute at bed rest, but this may shift to bradycardia with a rate of 40 to 60 per minute.

Respiration. Respiration tends to be shallow, and speech may be interrupted by sighing inspirations. Cheyne-Stokes respiration is observed in most patients.

Nervous System. The neurologic picture is that of a severe encephalomyelitis with profound dysfunction of the central nervous system. Early signs are referable to stimulation of the sympathetic nervous system, including dilation of the pupils, lacrimation, increased salivation, and excessive perspiration. There is usually stiffness of the neck, but Kernig's and Brudzinski's signs are not elicited. A Babinski sign may be obtained. At onset, there may be increased activity of the tendon reflexes and general increase in muscle tone. Muscle tics, vermiform and fibrillar muscular contractions, and general tremors may occur. As the disease progresses, incoordination and weakness of the extremities may occur, and this may be preceded by loss of tendon reflex. Local sensation to pinprick, heat, and cold is diminished.

COMMON COMPLICATIONS

Because few patients live longer than 3 to 4 days after the development of the acute excitement phase, the complications are few and inconsequential. Dehydration and incontinence are the chief problems in those with prolonged illness.

LABORATORY FINDINGS

Specific diagnosis by laboratory means during the course of illness is difficult, if not impossible, with currently available methods. The clinical diagnosis may be considered confirmed if the biting animal was captured and its brain tissue proved positive when examined for the presence of rabies virus particles. In absence of this information, attempts must be made to confirm the diagnosis by specific fluorescent antibody staining of corneal impressions, mucosal scrapings, frozen skin sections, or brain biopsy for presence of intracytoplasmic virus. Effort should also be made, by intracerebral mouse inoculation, to isolate the virus from the saliva or salivary gland of the patient or, more likely from the brain when obtained at autopsy. If a viral agent is isolated, it must subsequently be identified by animal inoculation, special staining procedures, and appropriate serologic tests. These involve complicated and time-consuming techniques that can be properly conducted only in a few specialized laboratories.

The red blood cell count is not altered except in the presence of dehydration, when the blood is concentrated. The white blood cell count is usually increased, reaching 20,000 to 30,000 cells per cu mm with a relative increase in polymorphonuclear and mononuclear cells. The urine may show an increase in albumin and positive sugar and acetone reactions. Hyaline casts may be found in the sediment. The spinal fluid is usually under moderately increased pressure. It appears consistently clear with a slight increase in protein and cell count. The cells, rarely more than 100 in number, are predominantly of the mononuclear type.

PITFALLS IN DIAGNOSIS

Other diseases transmitted by animal bites should be ruled out. These include pasteurella infections from cats and dogs, B-virus from monkeys, rat-bite fever, cat-scratch fever, and possibly tetanus.

B-virus infection caused by *Herpesvirus simiae* is a highly fatal ascending encephalomyelitis, occurring in veterinarians, laboratory workers, and others in close contact with monkey or monkey cell cultures. Encephalitis and encephalomyelitis caused by other viruses must also be considered.

Some persons not actually infected after the bite of an animal may display severe neurotic symptoms (hysteric phenomena). There may be anxiety, restlessness, insomnia, general irritability, and pain at the site of the bite; but irritability at the site of water and painful spasms of the deglutitory and respiratory muscles alternating with flaccid paralysis are generally absent. In this condition, therapeutic tests are successful and the symptoms tend to abate within a week, during which time rabies-induced phenomena would worsen.

In the Guillain-Barré syndrome, probably an immunologic disease, despite moderate damage to the axons and myelin sheaths of the involved nerves, the sensory disturbances are never severe. There is always an increase of protein, but not of cells, in the cerebrospinal fluid. Recovery from the flaccid motor paralysis, first of the legs and then of the arms, takes from 1 to 6 or more months, a period too long for the normal course of rabies.

Tetanus has been mistaken for rabies when the facial muscles are involved, but risus sardonicus and the lack of hydrophobia in tetanus may assist in the differential diagnosis.

MUMPS

By MICHAEL MARCY, M.D.
Panorama City, California

SYNONYMS

Epidemic parotitis, mumps (Dutch, *mompen:* to sulk).

DEFINITION

Mumps is an acute generalized infectious disease caused by a member of the paramyxovirus group. Although painful parotid enlargement is the characteristic clinical feature, mumps encompasses a spectrum ranging from inapparent infection to involvement of multiple organ systems. The propensity of the virus to invade glandular and nervous tissue often results in the widespread involvement of seemingly unrelated structures. Aseptic meningitis, epididymo-orchitis, and pancreatitis are the most commonly associated features.

EPIDEMIOLOGY

Mumps is predominantly a disease of young schoolage children, yet significant numbers of cases, approximately 10 per cent, occur in adolescents and young adults. The disease is endemic throughout the year, with a peak incidence during the winter and early spring. Epidemics occur in the general population in 2 to 4 year cycles.

Transmission of mumps to a susceptible host occurs through direct contact with infected air-suspended droplets, saliva, or contaminated fomites. Although mumps virus has been isolated from the saliva of infected persons from 7 days before to 9 days after onset of symptoms, the effective period of communicability is uncertain. Patients are generally considered capable of spreading the disease from 3 days before onset of clinical mumps until parotid swelling has subsided. Those with inapparent infection or with mumps sparing the salivary glands are equally effective sources of exposure. Transmission through an immune third party has not been documented.

PRESENTING SIGNS AND SYMPTOMS

The incubation period of mumps averages 18 days, with a range of 12 to 25 days. Approximately one third of infected persons will have negligible symptoms or no manifestations of disease. Diagnosis in such cases can be established only through viral isolation or serologic methods.

Clinical disease usually begins with prodromal symptoms of low-grade fever, myalgia, headache, malaise, or anorexia. In typical cases early parotid involvement becomes apparent within 1 or 2 days in the form of "earache" and tenderness on palpation over the angle of the jaw. Bilateral parotitis occurs in about 75 per cent of patients, with swelling of one gland usually preceding that of the other side by 1 to 5 days. Parotitis is the most common manifestation, but all possible combinations of multiple or single salivary gland infection have been described. Isolated submaxillary or sublingual gland involvement is, however, infrequent.

Swelling of the salivary glands generally increases for 24 to 72 hours, persists an equal length of time, and then subsides over the next week. As glandular enlargement progresses, the orifices of Wharton's and/or Stensen's ducts may become red and swollen. Obstruction of these ducts by inflammatory edema and cellular debris is responsible for the sharp intensification of pain produced by chewing or drinking sour liquids. Temperature usually remains around 101 to 102 F (38.3 to 38.9 C), but may on occasion be normal or exceed 104 F (40 C). Fever, pain, and constitutional symptoms usually subside after salivary gland swelling has reached its maximum.

Early or mild enlargement of the parotid glands is most readily detected as an asymmetry of the neck profile when the patient is viewed from behind. As swelling progresses there is an obliteration of the angle between the earlobe and the mandible, with upward and outward displacement of the earlobe. When observed from the side, swelling of the gland extends diffusely in an area above the angle of the jaw and is bisected by the long axis of the ear. Palpation of the gland presents a doughy and brawny edematous sensation fading into indistinct lateral borders. Drawing one's fingers over involved glands should express clear mucus from the ducts; purulent material is not seen. Presternal or laryngeal edema, probably on the basis of lymphatic obstruction, can occur with severe glandular swelling. Extensive sialadenitis may be confused with the bullneck swelling described in diphtheria or Ludwig's angina.

COMMONLY ASSOCIATED MANIFESTATIONS (Table 1)

Although sialadenitis is the hallmark of mumps infection, the ability of the virus to invade a wide range of host tissues often results in the involvement of organ systems far removed from the salivary glands. Such manifestations are more properly considered features of the natural disease rather than complications. *They may occur before, during, after, or in the absence of salivary gland involvement.*

Viral (Aseptic) Meningitis. This is the most common secondary manifestation of mumps. Over half of all patients will have an asymptomatic pleocytosis, and about 10 per cent evidence clinical signs or symptoms referable to the central nervous system (CNS).

Symptoms are identical to those seen in other benign viral meningitides: fever, headache, nausea, vomiting, and lethargy predominate. Nuchal rigidity is usually mild to moderate, and the signs of Kernig and Brudzinski are frequently absent. Fever and symptoms generally subside after 5 to 10 days. Persistent neurologic sequelae are extremely rare.

Mumps Encephalitis and Encephalomyelitis. Brain or spinal cord involvement or both are rare manifestations of mumps, occurring only once in each 6000 cases. On the basis of clinical and pathologic observations it has been suggested that CNS injury may be caused either by direct viral invasion alone (primary encephalomyelitis) or through an immune response of the host to breakdown of products of cells and

Table 1. *Systemic Manifestations of Mumps**

Glandular
  Sialadenitis (70%)
  Orchitis (20% of postpubertal males)
  Epididymitis (85% of cases of orchitis)
  Prostatitis
  Seminal vesiculitis
  Oophoritis (about 5% of postpubertal females)
  Bartholinitis
  Pancreatitis (about 5%)
  Mastitis
  Dacryoadenitis
  Thyroiditis
  Thymus enlargement
Nervous system
  Asymptomatic pleocytosis (about 50%)
  Symptomatic meningitis (about 10%)
  Meningoencephalitis†
  Postinfectious encephalitis†
  Myelitis
  Neuritis of cranial nerves II, III, VI, VII, VIII
  Polyneuritis (meningoradiculitis)
  Guillain-Barré syndrome
  ?Acquired aqueductal stenosis/hydrocephalus
Other manifestations
  Labyrinthitis
  Conjunctivitis/Keratitis/Iritis
  Myocarditis/pericarditis (ECG changes in 3 to 15%)†
  Nephritis†
  Thrombocytopenic purpura
  Splenomegaly
  Arthritis
  Fetal wastage
  ? Hepatitis
  ? Endocardial fibroelastosis (intrauterine mumps?)†
  ? Exanthem, maculopapular

---

*From Marcy, S. M., and Kibrick, S.: Mumps. *In* Hoeprich P. D., Infectious Diseases. Hagerstown, Md., Harper & Row Publishers, Inc., 1977.

†Has been associated with fatalities.

myelin (postinfectious demyelinating encephalomyelitis).

The clinical features suggesting cerebral involvement include convulsions, focal neurologic signs, movement disorders, or profound changes in sensorium. The signs and symptoms of meningitis are usually, but not invariably, also evident. If myelitis is present, segmental involvement of the spinal cord primarily in the lower thoracic and lumbar regions, or a paralytic poliomyelitis-like syndrome, may be seen.

Long-term sequelae of mumps encephalitis are infrequent; however, fatalities have been reported. Aqueductal stenosis and hydrocephalus have been described following encephalitis in several patients.

Epididymo-orchitis. Infection of the testis is quite rare before adolescence but has been reported in infants as young as 7 months of age. About 20 per cent of postpubertal males with mumps develop orchitis, preceded or accompanied by epididymitis in most instances. Gonadal involvement is bilateral in approximately 25 per cent of patients.

The initial period of rapid testicular swelling is usually accompanied by the abrupt onset of systemic symptoms consisting of high fever, chills, nausea, and vomiting. Rarely, testicular pain is first referred to the right lower quadrant and may mimic appendicitis. Pain and tenderness are often intense, and may increase progressively as the testicle enlarges, up to three or four times its original size in extreme cases. Pain, fever, and swelling generally begin to subside after 3 to 5 days; however, the residual glandular swelling and tenderness may last for several weeks.

Approximately 50 per cent of affected testicles will manifest some degree of atrophy. Sterility after mumps orchitis is rare, and no cases of true hypogonadism have been reported. Psychologic impotence may follow testicular atrophy.

Oophoritis. Evidence of ovarian involvement is found in approximately 5 per cent of postpubertal females. Abdominal pain is usually mild but can be severe and may closely mimic appendicitis when the right ovary is infected. An enlarged tender ovary may be palpated on pelvic examination. Mumps oophoritis has no effect on subsequent fertility.

Pancreatitis. Clinical evidence of pancreatitis occurs in about 5 per cent of patients with mumps. A rise in temperature, deep epigastric pain with tenderness on palpation, nausea, and persistent vomiting are the most common findings. Complete recovery takes place over 5 to 7 days but may be delayed for up to 2 weeks in severe cases of necrotizing pancreatitis. A relationship between mumps pancreatitis and subsequent diabetes has been postulated but never proved.

Deafness. By virtue of the large number of children who acquire mumps, this is one of the leading causes of unilateral neurosensory deafness in children and young adults. The incidence (about 1 in every 15,000 cases) is, however, low. Onset of hearing loss may be sudden or gradual, and is sometimes preceded by symptoms of acute Meniere's disease. Deafness is complete and permanent in most cases, but fortunately is bilateral in only about 25 per cent of patients. Loss of vestibular reactions may accompany the hearing loss.

Arthritis. This infrequent manifestation of mumps is seen most commonly in young adult males. Migratory polyarthritis, monoarticular arthritis, or arthralgias, chiefly affecting the larger joints, may occur. Symptoms persist for periods ranging from several days up to 3 months; however, resolution is spontaneous and complete, and residual joint damage has not been described.

Nephritis. The incidence of this manifestation in children is not known. In one carefully studied series of 20 young adult males all had transient abnormalities in renal function, frequently accompanied by microscopic hematuria and proteinuria. Recovery is almost always complete, although severe nephritis leading to death has been reported.

Myocarditis. Transient electrocardiographic changes compatible with myocarditis have been observed in from 3 to 15 per cent of adults with mumps. Pericarditis has also been described, though less frequently. Although symptomatic cardiac involvement is unusual, deaths have been reported.

LABORATORY FINDINGS

Peripheral blood leukocyte counts may be depressed, normal, or elevated, with or without a relative lymphocytosis; they are of little value in establishing a diagnosis. Lymphocytic leukemoid reactions have been described. Elevated sedimentation rates may occur with mumps arthritis and orchitis.

Urinalysis is normal in most cases of mumps. Microscopic hematuria, proteinuria, or the presence of red blood cell casts should suggest a diagnosis of mumps nephritis.

The cerebrospinal fluid (CSF) in mumps meningitis or meningoencephalitis usually contains fewer than 500 cells per cu mm, with only occasional cell counts exceeding 2000 per cu mm. In most cases the cells are almost exclusively mononuclear from the outset; polymorphonuclear leukocytes predominate for the first few days in only a small percentage of patients. Pleocytosis may continue for as long as 5 weeks. CSF protein concentrations are normal or slightly elevated, and the glucose concentration is usually normal. Rarely, depressed CSF glucose concentrations (less than 40 mg per 100 ml) may be present initially and persist for several days.

Serum amylase is increased during the period of swelling and for about 10 days thereafter in 90 per cent of patients with parotitis. Prolonged elevations lasting up to 3 weeks may be helpful in establishing a retrospective diagnosis of mumps. Occasionally, this enzyme is also increased in the serum of patients with subclinical parotitis. It may be normal when only nonparotid salivary glands are involved. Since high serum levels of parotid amylase preclude the use of this study for diagnosis of pancreatitis,

determination of serum lipase may be used as an alternative, though less reliable, method. The clinical value of measuring pancreatic versus parotid isoamylases has not as yet been established.

VIROLOGIC AND SEROLOGIC TESTS

Mumps virus has been recovered from the saliva, CSF, urine, blood, breast milk, and infected tissues of patients with mumps. Attempting viral isolation for diagnostic purposes is usually warranted only in special circumstances. Local state health departments should be consulted for appropriate methods for handling and preserving specimens.

Serologic confirmation is the most reliable and practical method for establishing a diagnosis of mumps. Measurement of complement-fixing (CF) antibodies against the S (soluble, internal ribonucleoprotein core) and V (viral, outer envelope) antigens is the most widely used serologic test. The S antibodies usually rise within the first week of illness, the V antibodies appearing 1 or 2 weeks later. A presumptive diagnosis of mumps virus infection can therefore be made when elevated S antibodies are found in the absence of V antibodies. A fourfold or greater rise in either of these antibodies 2 or 3 weeks later is confirmatory. S antibodies usually disappear after 6 to 12 months, whereas V antibodies persist at low levels for years. Thus an elevation of V antibodies in the absence of S antibodies suggests previous, but not current, mumps infection.

Hemagglutination-inhibiting (HAI) antibodies arise rapidly following infection and may reach maximum levels within 4 to 8 days, precluding demonstration of a diagnostic fourfold rise unless the acute serum is taken early. Measurement of HAI antibodies has not proved as reliable as the CF test. Neutralizing antibodies serve as the most reliable index of the immune status of a person following either natural disease or administration of the live attenuated virus vaccine. Unfortunately, their determination is currently impractical as a routine diagnostic procedure.

Heterotypic antibody responses frequently occur during infections with parainfluenza and mumps viruses, probably on the basis of shared antigenic components in the viral envelopes. Thus an antibody rise to mumps virus can occur following parainfluenza infection, and similarly, parainfluenza virus antibodies may rise after a mumps infection. Since infection with parainfluenza virus types 1 and 3 has been associated with disease clinically indistinguishable from mumps, serologic data must be carefully evaluated. Ultimately, viral isolation procedures might be necessary to determine a specific diagnosis.

The mumps skin test, which utilizes inactivated mumps virus, converts during convalescence and is therefore unreliable in attempting to establish a diagnosis during the acute infection. Furthermore, since skin-test antigen is identical with the killed vaccine, use of the skin test may itself recall mumps antibodies, thus interfering with the interpretation of serologic data. The value of the mumps skin test in establishing the immune status of an individual has been seriously questioned in recent years. It is no longer commercially available.

Rapid diagnosis of paramyxovirus infection has been made through electron microscopic examination of clinical specimens, including nasopharyngeal secretions and CSF. Immunofluorescent techniques have been used to identify mumps antigen within hours in CSF cells and within 1 or 2 days in experimentally inoculated cell cultures. These methods are not, at present, generally available but will probably become increasingly useful in future years.

PITFALLS IN DIAGNOSIS (Table 2)

A history of exposure within the preceding 2 or 3 weeks, together with clinical criteria, is generally sufficient to establish a diagnosis in typical mumps with parotitis. There are, however, a number of other conditions associated with parotid swelling that may, particularly when acute in onset, closely resemble epidemic parotitis. Some are characteristically unilateral (e.g., tumors, cysts, obstructive lesions), whereas others are bilateral (e.g., drug effects and metabolic diseases). Swelling caused by drugs and metabolic abnormalities is generally asymptomatic; infectious and obstructive lesions are most commonly associated with pain or discomfort. Many conditions causing parotid swelling are associated with, or even secondary to, an increase or decrease in the rate of salivary secretion.

A number of conditions affecting the anterior cervical lymph nodes, periauricular skin, or mandibular structures may appear to resemble parotid enlargement on casual observation. A careful physical examination followed by appropriate laboratory studies should serve to differentiate these illnesses from mumps.

Table 2. *Differential Diagnosis of Parotid Swelling*

I. Infectious
   Viral: mumps, parainfluenza types 1 and 3, Coxsackievirus A, echovirus, lymphocytic choriomeningitis, influenza A
   Bacterial: Acute suppurative parotitis (staphylococcal, pneumococcal, occasionally gram-negative bacilli), recurrent parotitis (primarily *Streptococcus viridans*), typical and atypical mycobacterial parotitis
   Other: trichinosis, actinomycosis

II. Obstructive
   Sialolithiasis
   Papillary trauma (including ill-fitting dentures)
   Foreign body in Stensen's duct
   Parotid–masseter hypertrophy–malocclusion syndrome
   Chronic sialectasis
   Tumor of duct

III. Tumors or cysts
   Benign and malignant parenchymal tumors
   Hemangiomas
   Lymphangiomas
   Cysts, congenital and acquired

IV. Drugs
   Iodides ("pyelography mumps")
   Isoproterenol
   Phenylbutazone, oxyphenylbutazone
   Bromide poisoning
   Chronic heavy-metal poisoning (lead, mercury)
   Thiocyanate
   Thiouracil
   Phenothiazines

V. Metabolic
   Malnutrition (protein deficiency ?)
   Rapid refeeding after malnutrition
   Obesity
   Diabetes mellitus, overt and latent
   Alcoholism (malnutrition ?)
   Gouty parotitis
   Uremic parotitis

VI. Miscellaneous
   Sarcoidosis (uveoparotid fever)
   Mikulicz's disease–Sjögren's syndrome–benign lymphoepithelial lesion
   Waldenström's macroglobulinemia
   Systemic lupus erythematosus
   Fatty atrophy
   Menopausal hypertrophy
   Excessive starch ingestion
   Cystic fibrosis
   Fibrous parotitis
   Pneumo-parotitis (glass blowers, trumpet players)
   "Anesthesia" mumps

VII. Conditions resembling parotitis
   Intraparotid, anterior cervical, lymphadenitis
   Lymphoma
   Dental abscess
   Severe otitis externa
   Caffey's disease (infantile cortical hyperostosis)
   Cervicofacial actinomycosis
   Masseter hypertrophy (bruxism, excessive gum-chewing)
   Branchial cleft cysts
   Prominent transverse process of atlas

POLIOMYELITIS *

By JOHN M. LEEDOM, M.D.
Los Angeles, California

SYNONYMS

Acute anterior poliomyelitis, infantile paralysis, Heine-Medin disease.

DEFINITION

Poliomyelitis is an acute infectious and communicable disease. Its major clinical manifestations — paresis and paralysis of striated muscles — result from destruction of, or injury to, the motor neurons of the spinal cord and medulla. Less frequently, there is involvement of neurons of the cerebral cortex, cerebellum, and autonomic nervous systems.

ETIOLOGIC AGENTS

Most cases of clinically evident poliomyelitis are caused by one of three immunologically distinct types of small (25 to 30 mμ) RNA viruses, termed respectively polioviruses types 1, 2, and 3; unless otherwise qualified, the term "poliomyelitis" as used in this article refers to disease caused by one of these three poliovirus types. However, it should be emphasized that acute anterior poliomyelitis is a clinical syndrome, and not all cases of clinical poliomyelitis are caused by polioviruses. Other viruses such as coxsackieviruses types A7, B3, and B4, and echoviruses types 2, 4, 6, 9, and 16 are rare causes of acute paralytic illnesses identical to those caused by polioviruses.

EPIDEMIOLOGIC CONSIDERATIONS

The polioviruses are indigenous to man. Nonhuman primates can be infected, and some strains of polioviruses can infect other laboratory animals. However, animal reservoirs play no role in the transmission of polioviruses to humans.

In temperate climates most cases of poliomyelitis cluster in the late summer and early fall, although sporadic cases may occur at any time. The median incubation period is 12 days with a range of 7 to 20 days.

Most human infections with polioviruses are asymptomatic or result in nonspecific febrile illnesses. The ratios of such inapparent and mild infections to those causing paralytic disease vary from outbreak to outbreak but generally range from 100:1 to 1000:1. Infected persons shed polioviruses in their pharyngeal secretions and feces, and because of their continued normal daily activities, persons with asymptomatic or mild infections are of special epidemiologic importance in the spread of polioviruses.

Polioviruses have been recovered from the pharynges of persons who subsequently remained well and from the pharynges of poliomyelitis patients during a period ranging from 5 days before to 14 days after onset of paralysis. Polioviruses have been isolated from the stools of patients as early as 19 days before the onset of paralysis, and fecal harborage of polioviruses for as long as 100 days has been reported.

Although oral-oral spread of polioviruses occurs, the fecal-oral route is probably the most important mode of virus transmission. Such fecal-oral spread occurs very readily among preschool children, because their personal sanitary habits, such as thorough handwashing after defecation, are often not yet well established. Furthermore, young children frequently place toys and other objects in their mouths and subsequently share them with playmates, thus facilitating the spread of viruses.

All three types of polioviruses spread readily within a nonimmunized population, particularly if sanitary standards are poor. Even in the United States, prior to the advent of effective inactivated and live attenuated poliovirus vaccines, serologic surveys often showed that 80 to 90 per cent of the older children and adults studied had neutralizing antibodies to all three poliovirus types. Despite such serologic evidence of widespread infection with all three poliovirus types, the three types clearly differed in their potential for causing paralytic disease. In most years, type 1 was the most frequent cause of paralytic illness in the United States and was responsible for 80 to 90 per cent of the cases. Type 3 was second in importance, causing 10 to 20 per cent of the annual total of cases, whereas the type 2 virus customarily accounted for only about 0.5 to 3.0 per cent of the cases of paralytic disease.

Subsequent to the widespread use of oral live attenuated poliovirus vaccine (Sabin) (OPV) in the United States, paralytic poliomyelitis has become a very rare disease, and poliovirus type 2 has been responsible for a much larger proportion of the annual totals of cases. For example, during the 8-year period 1969 through 1976, only 132 cases of paralytic poliomyelitis were reported to the United States Public Health Service, Center for Disease Control (CDC), Atlanta, Georgia. This repre-

* Supported in part by the Hastings Foundation Fund.

sented the lowest total of any 8-year period to date. Of these 132 cases, the CDC had data allowing serotypic association of specific poliovirus types in 113. Type 1 accounted for 54 cases (48 per cent), type 2 for 29 cases (26 per cent), and types 3 for 30 cases (27 per cent). In contrast, during the preceding 8-year period 1961 through 1968, of 1214 serotypically diagnosed cases, 827 (68 per cent) were associated with type 1, 60 (5 per cent) with type 2, and 327 (27 per cent) with type 3 polioviruses. Thus, during the most recent 8-year period, there was a marked decrease in the relative importance of types 1 and 3 polioviruses and a fivefold increase in the relative frequency of the association of type 2 polioviruses with paralytic disease. It is also of interest to note that, of the 132 cases of paralytic poliomyelitis reported to the CDC during the period 1969 through 1976, 10 patients (7 per cent) had received OPV within 4 to 30 days before onset of illness, and 34 more (26 per cent) had onsets of illnesses within 4 to 60 days after OPV had been fed to a contact, with illness occurring within 30 days of that contact. Within the 8-year period 1969 through 1976, 11 patients with paralytic poliomyelitis and immune deficiency states were reported. All 11 patients had histories of recent receipt of OPV or recent contact with a recipient. In addition, 15 (11 per cent) of the 132 patients were judged to be imported cases of poliomyelitis, with their illnesses acquired abroad.

In summary, paralytic poliomyelitis has become a rare disease in recent years. If a patient has the paralytic poliomyelitis syndrome, the physician should look for a history of recent ingestion of OPV, contact with an OPV recipient, or evidence of immune deficiency, or recent entry into the United States from an endemic area.

CLINICAL FEATURES

Important Predisposing Factors. Certain host factors are known to predispose nonimmune individuals to more severe and extensive paralytic disease, or to localization of paralysis in a specific area, upon infection with a virulent poliovirus strain.

Age is an important factor. In one study, the case fatality rates for adults over 25 years of age were two to five times greater than those among children under 7 years of age. Among nonfatal cases, the average extent of paralytic involvement increases with age, as does the frequency of severe bulbar and respiratory involvement. Clinical studies, confirmed by experiments using monkeys, show that stress, severe exercise, and undue fatigue all have adverse effects on persons incubating poliomyelitis or in the early clinical stages of the disease. Pregnancy has seemed to enhance susceptibility to paralytic poliomyelitis in many studies. Prior tonsillectomy and adenoidectomy also seem to predispose to the occurrence of paralytic poliomyelitis and to more serious disease. Finally, if poliomyelitis occurs within 1 month after an injection of any kind of antigen, there is increased likelihood that paralysis will occur in the injected extremity.

Presenting Complaints. The initial symptoms of poliomyelitis are usually quite nonspecific and are of value in alerting the physician to watch for later paralysis only in the face of an epidemic. In about 20 per cent of the patients with paralytic poliomyelitis, the illness has a biphasic course. That is, the nonspecific symptoms constitute a minor illness of 24 to 36 hours' duration, which is separated from the onset of paralysis by an interval of 1 to 4 days or occasionally longer. This biphasic course is often called "the dromedary phenomenon."

The primary minor illness usually has an acute onset with headache, fever, anorexia, sore throat, nausea, and occasional vomiting. The temperature is usually not very high, generally ranging from 99 to 101 F. The patient does not complain of a stiff neck or back.

Although the biphasic illness, in which the onset of the secondary illness follows an asymptomatic interval, is considered "classic" for acute paralytic poliomyelitis, it should be re-emphasized that about 80 per cent of the patients fail to follow this "classic" course. In those patients the primary illness is followed immediately by the onset of central nervous system (CNS) symptoms and paralysis, or CNS symptoms or paralysis or both occur without a recognized antecedent illness.

When the secondary or paralytic phase of the illness begins, there is usually a recrudescence or worsening of fever, often to markedly hyperpyrexic levels. Frontal headache is a common complaint, as is vomiting. Stiffness of the neck and back, often painful, usually precedes the development of paralysis.

If weakness has developed, the patient may complain of muscle pain and spasm involving areas other than the neck and back, although such pain and spasm are far from constant complaints, particularly on admission. Cutaneous hyperesthesia and hyperhidrosis are also frequent complaints.

Findings on Physical Examination. At the time of admission to the hospital, most patients are febrile, and some are dramatically hyperpyrexic. Most patients appear "toxic." They are usually flushed and often sweaty, restless, and apprehensive. Most patients are mentally alert. If obtundation occurs, it is usually later in the course of the illness and results from hypercapnia and hypoxia caused by ventilatory insufficiency or, more rarely, from encephalitic involvement.

Tachycardia is usual; hypertension may be present; and respiratory irregularity, most marked during sleep, may be noted. Vasomotor abnormalities, such as flushing, localized pallor, or generalized mottling of the skin, are often seen.

Nuchal rigidity is usually present. Kernig's and Brudzinski's signs are positive. The back is stiff, and there is often painful tightness, contraction, or spasm of the paraspinal muscles, the extensors of the thighs, and the hamstrings. It is well to remember that infants often lack these signs.

In addition, head drop (inability to raise the head when the shoulders are elevated) and the tripod sign (inability of the patient to sit erect with the legs and thighs extended without using both arms extended behind him as props to maintain the sitting position) are often present.

Characteristics of the Motor Involvement. In poliomyelitis the onset of paresis or paralysis or both is typically acute, asymmetrical, and quasi-segmental. Unless the patient's paralysis is very profound indeed, careful muscle function testing usually elicits appreciable differences in the strengths of adjacent involved muscles. There are no sensory changes. Very early (during the first few hours) after onset of weakness, there may be hyperreflexia of an affected muscle group, but hyporeflexia and areflexia quickly supervene. The paralysis is of the flaccid variety. Superficial reflexes (abdominal and cremasteric) are characteristically lost early in patients who develop weakness of the muscles of the abdominal wall or thighs and may be lost prior to the onset of clinically detectable muscle weakness.

During the early phase of the paralytic illness, involved muscle bellies are tender to deep pressure or upon stretching. Spontaneous painful muscle spasm in the muscles innervated by the affected neurons may also occur but is not an invariable complaint. Painful spasms may also develop in the antagonists of the weakened musculature.

The distribution of the muscle weakness and the occurrence of other clinical signs that localize the sites of CNS involvement have resulted in a widely accepted system of classification of paralytic poliomyelitis: *spinal, bulbar, bulbospinal,* and *encephalitic.* It should be emphasized that, although encephalitis with clinical signs limited to those of cerebral or cerebellar dysfunction can occur, encephalitic poliomyelitis usually occurs in conjunction with evidence of involvement of the medulla or spinal cord or both.

Complications. Ventilatory insufficiency is the immediate, life-threatening complication of spinal poliomyelitis. Significant arm and shoulder weakness should alert the clinician to the possibility of impending diaphragmatic and intercostal muscle weakness.

Ventilatory failure as a result of involvement of the medullary respiratory center has an ominous prognosis and is manifested by irregularities in the rate, depth, and rhythm of breathing (Biot type respiration). Another acute life-threatening manifestation of severe bulbar disease is pharyngeal paralysis, with difficulty in swallowing, which results in accumulation of secretions in the oropharynx, aspiration, and ventilatory obstruction. Lability of the pulse rate and blood pressure secondary to involvement of the medullary vasomotor centers may cause life-threatening circulatory insufficiency.

Encephalitic patients have one or more of the following: hyperpyrexia, cerebellar signs, delirium, stupor, or coma. As most of the signs of polioencephalitis can be produced by hypoxia or hypercapnia or both, in the absence of actual involvement of the cortical neurons, polioencephalitis should not be diagnosed unless the signs of supramedullary involvement fail to subside, despite correction of abnormal Po_2, Pco_2, and pH values. Seizures are so uncommon in patients with encephalitis caused by polioviruses that the occurrence of a seizure renders the diagnosis unlikely.

Acute urinary retention lasting from a few hours to many weeks is a frequent complication of paralytic poliomyelitis. Indeed, most patients who have weakness in the lower extremities develop urinary retention, at least transiently. For this reason urinary output should be carefully monitored, and if the patient fails to void after adequate hydration, diagnostic catheterization should be performed after 8 to 12 hours of observation. If retention is detected, and the patient continues to be unable to void, he should be recatheterized at 8-hour intervals on an "in and out" basis two more times before an indwelling catheter is inserted. The urinary retention frequently lasts less than 24 hours, and the problems incident upon the insertion of an indwelling catheter can be avoided by using the aforementioned procedure.

Other common complications secondary to the paralytic process, which may arise in the first few days to weeks, include atelectasis and pneumonia and thrombophlebitis with pulmonary embolism. Acute duodenal ulcers, often resulting in massive gastrointestinal hemorrhage, may occur and are especially common in patients with paralysis of the respiratory musculature who are managed with mechanical aids to ventilation.

Ordinarily, muscle paralysis may progress throughout the febrile course of the disease, which may last as long as 10 days but more frequently has a duration of 1 to 4 days. However, it should be emphasized that paralysis may progress in the absence of fever, especially in small children. Indeed, paralysis may occur without a recognized febrile illness in infants and young children.

LABORATORY FINDINGS

Routine Blood and Urine Studies. There are no characteristic abnormalities of the total peripheral white blood cell and differential counts. Urinalysis and blood chemistry determinations are within normal limits or show abnormalities of fluid and electrolyte balance, pH, PCO_2, or PO_2 secondary to ventilatory failure or dehydration, vomiting, and fever.

Cerebrospinal Fluid Findings. A lumbar puncture usually discloses a normal cerebrospinal fluid (CSF) pressure. Grossly, the CSF is clear to hazy. Upon microscopic examination, there is usually mild to moderate pleocytosis, characteristically lymphocytic, although particularly during the first few days after onset of CNS signs and symptoms, polymorphonuclear leukocytes may predominate. The total CSF cell count seldom ranges outside the limits of 10 to 500 per cu mm and is usually 100 to 200 cells per cu mm. The CSF glucose concentration is within normal limits. Initial CSF protein values usually fall within the range of 25 to 150 mg per dl(100 ml). Characteristically, modest CSF protein elevations are found during the first week after onset of CNS signs and symptoms. CSF protein levels tend to decrease toward the tenth day, but may increase again in a secondary stage (100 to 400 mg per dl) during the third and fourth weeks, and sometimes even during the second week. With this secondary rise in CSF protein, the CSF white blood cell count does not rise. Indeed, cells may be completely absent. Thus there is albuminocytologic dissociation during the latter stages of the acute disease.

Virus Laboratory Studies. Modern tissue culture techniques permit ready isolation and identification of polioviruses. They can be isolated from blood early in the course of illness but only rarely have been recovered from CSF specimens. Pharyngeal secretions and feces regularly yield polioviruses during a period that extends from several days prior to onset of the acute paralytic disease, throughout the acute illness, and, for feces, sometimes for many weeks thereafter.

Today, poliomyelitis is such a rare disease in the United States that each patient has epidemiologic significance. For that reason, virus isolation studies should be done in every case in which the diagnosis is suspected. Specimens for virus isolation from every patient should include CSF, pharyngeal secretions (throat swab), and feces (rectal swab). In fatal cases, CNS tissue should also be cultured.

The CSF specimen (1 to 5 ml.) should be stored at −20 to −70 C until it can be inoculated into tissue culture. A CSF specimen should be obtained, in spite of the fact that polioviruses are almost never isolated from CSF. Nonpolioenteroviruses, such as echovirus type 9, which may cause a clinical syndrome of acute anterior myelitis indistinguishable from that caused by polioviruses, can frequently be isolated from the CSF during the acute illness. Thus CSF is useful as a virus isolation specimen chiefly because the recovery of some other virus from the CSF may lead to the exclusion of polioviruses as etiologic in a given case of acute anterior myelitis.

Pharyngeal secretions should be collected on a cotton swab as soon as poliomyelitis is suspected. Fecal material should be collected on a similar swab. Both swabs should be placed in tightly closed tubes containing 10 to 15 ml of veal infusion broth or a similar medium. These specimens should be stored at −20 to −70 C until inoculation into tissue culture.

If the patient dies during the acute phase of the illness, it may be possible to recover a poliovirus from CNS tissue taken at necropsy. The tissue should be removed aseptically. Samples of cerebral cortex, medulla, and cervical, thoracic, and lumbar sections of the spinal cord should be studied. Each tissue sample should be stored in a separate sealed container at −20 to −70 C until it can be inoculated into tissue culture.

Primary rhesus monkey kidney tissue culture (RMKTC) constitutes the system of choice for the isolation of polioviruses from clinical specimens. Polioviruses in clinical specimens may produce detectable cytopathic effects in RMKTC as early as 24 hours after inoculation of the tubes, although longer incubation is frequently necessary.

Cytopathogenic agents, recovered in RMKTC, are identified as specific poliovirus types by neutralization with type-specific hyperimmune sera.

In addition to the virus isolation specimens discussed earlier, every patient suspected of having poliomyelitis should have an acute serum sample drawn and stored for serologic tests at the time the diagnosis is first suspected, and a convalescent serum should be obtained 2 to 3 weeks later. These sera are separated from the clots and stored frozen until tested. It is important that the serologic test be performed on the acute and convalescent samples simultaneously. Serologic confirmation of a poliovirus infection is obtained by demonstrating a four-fold or greater rise in neutralizing antibody titer against a prototype strain of one of the three poliovirus types. Fourfold or greater rises in type-specific complement-fixing antibodies also constitute serologic confirmation of infection.

PITFALLS IN DIAGNOSIS

Neurologic conditions that are sometimes confused with acute CNS symptoms caused by polioviruses include cerebrovascular accidents; syringomyelia; hematomyelia; myelitis resulting from infection with bacteria, acid-fast bacteria, or fungi; epidural abscess; neoplasms of the brain and spinal cord; acute anterior myelitis associated with nonpolioenteroviral infections; acute encephalitis with myelitis caused by arboviruses; radiculomyelitis, particularly the Guillain-Barré syndrome; and multiple sclerosis. Of the conditions listed, the last four are the most troublesome. As stated previously, non-polioenteroviruses can cause the clinical syndrome of acute paralytic poliomyelitis. They can be distinguished only by recourse to the virologic laboratory. Arboviruses such as the St. Louis encephalitis virus, the Western equine encephalitis virus, and the Eastern equine encephalitis virus may cause acute encephalomyelitis or acute myelitis indistinguishable from acute poliomyelitis. Sometimes such infections can be ruled out, or suspected, on epidemiologic grounds, or the development of neurologic abnormalities not seen in poliovirus infections will suggest that a poliovirus is not responsible for the illness. Nevertheless, final positive confirmation of arbovirus infections must be done by the virus laboratory. Patients with the Guillain-Barré syndrome characteristically have subjective or objective sensory abnormalities; the paralysis is typically ascending and symmetric; and the patient is afebrile. However, the Guillain-Barré syndrome with rapidly developing severe paralysis, particularly in a small child in whom sensory changes may be difficult to detect, can be confusing. The ultimate differentiation of such cases usually requires careful observation over a period of several days, with repeated physical examinations and lumbar punctures. Acute myelitis, or encephalomyelitis, as the first manifestation of multiple sclerosis, can also usually be suspected after careful observation over a period of several days. Rarely do the neurologic signs and symptoms remain confined to the anterior horn cells and/or the neurons of the cerebral cortex or cerebellum.

Perhaps even more important as pitfalls in the diagnosis of poliomyelitis are pseudoparalytic disorders. In these conditions, the physician incorrectly attributes failure to move an extremity or stiffness and limitation of motion of the neck and back to dysfunction of the motor nerves. Such diagnostic errors are most common in infants and young children who are too young to possess verbal facility. Some examples of disorders seen at the Communicable Disease Service of the Los Angeles County–University of Southern California Medical Center with referring diagnoses of poliomyelitis include congenital syphilis with osteitis; trauma, including fractures, dislocations, sprains, and hemarthrosis; rheumatic fever with arthritis; rheumatoid arthritis; pyarthrosis; and acute hematogenous osteomyelitis of extremities and spine.

COXSACKIE AND ECHO VIRAL INFECTIONS

by SIDNEY KIBRICK, M.D., Ph.D.
Boston, Massachusetts

The coxsackieviruses were discovered in 1948 during attempts to use newborn mice for isolation of polioviruses from feces of patients diagnosed clinically as having poliomyelitis. These agents were subsequently divided into two groups, A and B, on the basis of the pathology they induce in suckling mice. At present coxsackievirus A types 1 to 24 and coxsackievirus B types 1 to 6 are recognized.

The existence of echoviruses (Enteric Cytopathogenic Human Orphan) was revealed about 1951 when previously unrecognized viral agents were encountered during application of the tissue culture technique to the isolation of polioviruses from feces. Initially called orphan viruses because their relationship to specific illness was obscure, they were subsequently renamed echoviruses as more descriptive of their properties. At present echovirus types 1 to 34 are recognized.

Since the coxsackie-, echo- and polioviruses are all transient inhabitants of the human enteric tract and since they share many biophysical, epidemiologic and clinical properties, these three virus groups were classified together as enteroviruses in 1957.

The coxsackieviruses and echoviruses, initially differentiated from each other on the basis of pathogenicity for newborn mice and certain other properties, have been found to be more closely related than previously suspected, and their differences less marked. Accordingly, the decision was made that additional enteroviruses discovered since 1969 would no longer be designated as coxsackieviruses A, B, or echovirus types but would instead be assigned numbers beginning with enterovirus type 68 (allowing for 3 poliovirus types, 24 coxsackievirus A, 6 coxsackievirus B, and 34 echovirus types for a total of 67). At present, the last such virus to be assigned has been designated as enterovirus type 71.

Studies of these agents have revealed that they are widely distributed among man, that subclinical infections are common and that infection may be manifested clinically by a variety of overlapping and often nonspecific syndromes, not only among members of each group but also among the three groups. Since many of these syndromes may also be produced by other agents, a specific diagnosis often cannot be made in such illness except through viral laboratory studies. Certain of these syndromes, however, are sufficiently characteristic of infection with coxsackieviruses or echoviruses or both to permit a presumptive diagnosis as to cause. Others, less specific, may be strongly suspected on the basis of epidemiologic observations. General considerations helpful in recognizing these infections are outlined. The syndromes commonly associated with specific agents are then described.

GENERAL CONSIDERATIONS

1. In temperate climates, coxsackieviruses and echoviruses are most prevalent in the summer and fall.

2. The incubation period for infection with these agents averages from 2 days to 2 weeks with a mean of 3 to 5 days.

3. Infection is followed by long-lasting immunity but only to the infecting type of virus.

Since many of these viruses can produce similar clinical manifestations, a clinical syndrome due to these agents may occur more than once.

4. Epidemiologic support for a diagnosis of coxsackievirus or echovirus disease is provided by the presence of these agents or their manifestations among close associates of the patient or when these viruses are known to be prevalent in the community. It is common to have more than one member of a family affected, with different clinical features in each one.

ASEPTIC MENINGITIS

This is a mild, self-limited syndrome, clinically like other viral meningitides, which may result from infection with any of the enterovirus groups. It may be preceded by a several-day prodrome with malaise, anorexia, nausea, vomiting, and, especially in children, abdominal pain. Spinal fluid cell counts are usually below 500 per cu mm. Initially neutrophils predominate but later the cells are characteristically mononuclear. Spinal fluid protein is usually mildly elevated and glucose is normal. Occasionally the pleocytosis may persist for several weeks. The illness is generally over within a week but fatigue and irritability may persist for weeks to months.

There are no distinctive clinical signs whereby aseptic meningitis due to coxsackieviruses or echoviruses can be distinguished from that of other agents. These viruses, however, are among the commonest causes of this syndrome, especially in the summer. The findings of a biphasic fever and course and/or thoracic or abdominal muscle pain are suggestive of coxsackievirus group B infection. The presence in the patient, his family, or his close associates of other manifestations associated with these viruses further implicates these agents. Of special significance in this regard are pleurodynia, exanthematous disease, and pericarditis (vide infra).

PARALYSIS, ENCEPHALITIS

Illness clinically indistinguishable from paralytic or bulbar poliomyelitis, as well as encephalitis, ataxias, and other signs of cerebral dysfunction, may occasionally result from coxsackievirus A, B, or echovirus infection. Such disorders have generally but not always been self-limited and reversible. These illnesses, especially clinical paralytic or bulbar poliomyelitis, in patients adequately immunized against the polioviruses, should suggest a coxsackievirus or echovirus cause. Differentiation from poliomyelitis is based on virus isolation and serologic tests.

FEBRILE EXANTHEMATOUS DISEASE

Infection with a number of these agents is manifested by febrile exanthematous disease, occasionally misdiagnosed as rubella and occurring either alone or in conjunction with aseptic meningitis. The rashes are most commonly maculopapular; however, vesicular, petechial, and various mixed eruptions have also been observed. Their extent is variable. In general, enteroviral rashes are nonpruritic, do not desquamate, and heal without discoloration. They are most commonly seen in infants and young children. Although adenopathy may be present, it is not generally a prominent feature. Occasionally, the illness is associated with a papular or vesicular exanthem or with small ulcerative or typical herpanginal lesions (vide infra) in the oropharynx.

Several general patterns of exanthems have been noted with the enteroviruses, in addition to features specific for certain agents. With some of these viruses the rash is chiefly maculopapular, most concentrated on the face and trunk, and associated with fever. This central pattern has especially been noted with echovirus 9 and coxsackievirus A9. Exanthematous disease caused by echovirus type 9 usually appears first on the face and neck, spreads rapidly to the trunk, and may involve the extremities. It clears rapidly on the body, but on the face, especially the cheeks, it often becomes semiconfluent with a violaceous tint and clears more slowly (average of 5 days). Occasionally petechiae are present, the rash resembling that of meningococcemia. In some patients an enanthem of small yellow or gray-white lesions may be seen in the oropharynx.

A second pattern is a maculopapular rash with a predominantly central distribution, which tends to appear as the fever subsides and persists for 2 to 4 days. This feature is fairly characteristic but not pathognomonic of echovirus 16 (Boston exanthem). It has also been seen with several other enteroviruses, with some adenovirus infections, and in roseola.

In certain patients with maculopapular eruptions due to enteroviruses, some of the lesions may progress to form clear vesicles, which subsequently regress. Such rashes may be primarily central, as occasionally noted in coxsackievirus A9 infection or they may predominantly involve the extremities and oral cavity as seen in hand, foot, and mouth disease. This latter syndrome is generally associated with group A coxsackieviruses, especially A16. It is characterized by fever, an oral vesicular enanthem, usually involving the tongue and buccal mucosa, and a symmetrically distributed sparse maculopapular eruption that may progress to vesicles. Although the hands and feet are primarily affected, other parts of the body may be involved, especially the buttocks, in infants and young children.

HERPANGINA

This is a self-limited infection, usually seen in infants and children and caused chiefly by group A coxsackievirus. Onset is acute with fever (up to 4 days), sore throat and dysphagia and less frequently, abdominal pain and headache. The distinctive feature is the presence of small (1 to 2 mm) scattered oropharyngeal vesicles, each surrounded by an erythematous zone, most commonly in the posterior oropharynx. The lesions average about 5 to 10 during infection, progress to shallow ulcers, and are generally gone within a week.

ACUTE LYMPHONODULAR PHARYNGITIS

This illness, found only with coxsackievirus A10 to date, resembles herpangina in many respects but differs in that the lesions are discrete, solid, white to yellow papules surrounded by a zone of erythema. They occur on the uvula, palate, tonsillar pillars, and posterior pharynx, develop simultaneously, and resolve without ulceration after 6 to 10 days.

EPIDEMIC PLEURODYNIA (EPIDEMIC MYALGIA, BORNHOLM DISEASE)

This is an acute disease resulting chiefly from infection with group B coxsackievirus. Following a vague prodrome, there is sudden onset of fever, headache, and a sharp, stabbing pleuritic-like pain in the muscles of the chest or upper abdomen or both. The pain is intensified by respiration and movement and when substernal may simulate myocardial infarction. In children it may be localized to the abdomen, resembling acute appendicitis. The pain, however, is muscular rather than deep. Sore throat and myalgias are often also present. Physical examination may reveal only a mild pharyngitis. Chest films and laboratory findings are usually normal. The illness may subside within days or persist for several weeks. In about one third of the patients the course is multiphasic, with recurrences of the fever and symptoms.

About one quarter of the patients develop fibrinous pleuritis and an intermittent pleural friction rub. Some develop aseptic meningitis and occasionally, as a late complication, orchitis. Other infrequent complications include pericarditis and in adults, myocarditis.

Pericarditis and Myocarditis

Coxsackie B viruses and infrequently other enteroviruses may sometimes cause an acute benign pericarditis or myocarditis or both. Usual findings include fever, tachycardia, dyspnea, and precordial pain. A pericardial friction rub may be the only distinctive sign; in some patients congestive failure and myocarditis may also be present. Electrocardiography reveals changes compatible with pericarditis and occasionally with myocarditis, and radiography may show pericardial or pleural effusion or congestive failure. The acute pericardial illness varies in severity and lasts about 2 to 4 weeks with complete recovery usual. When myocarditis is present the prognosis is more grave.

Generalized Disease in the Newborn

Infection with group B coxsackievirus in the first month of life may result in severe, frequently fatal disease characterized by myocarditis and involvement of various other organs, especially central nervous system and liver. Onset is usually abrupt; prominent findings include lethargy, feeding difficulties, frequently fever, and signs of cardiac or respiratory distress. Serial electrocardiograms may be needed to detect transitory changes suggestive of myocarditis. Although signs referable to the central nervous system are present in only about 25 per cent of patients, pleocytosis is common, making examination of the spinal fluid helpful in diagnosis. The illness usually terminates rapidly with circulatory failure and death within days or with recovery over the next few weeks. Infection is generally acquired during a nursery outbreak or from an immediately preceding illness consistent with a coxsackie B infection in the mother, often a nonspecific febrile or respiratory illness.

Additional Syndromes

A type of coxsackievirus A (enterovirus 70) has been implicated in acute hemorrhagic conjunctivitis. This syndrome is associated with preauricular adenopathy, swollen eyelids, lacrimation, and occasionally subconjunctival hemorrhage. Patients are usually afebrile and they recover in 1 to 2 weeks.

Several types of group B coxsackievirus have been associated with glomerulonephritis and with the hemolytic uremic syndrome, an illness characterized by acute renal failure, hemolytic anemia, and thrombocytopenia, usually in infants.

A higher incidence of coxsackievirus B infection has been noted in mothers of infants with congenital heart disease.

Coxsackieviruses A and B and echoviruses have been implicated as causes of diarrheal disease especially in infants, acute upper respiratory disease, pneumonia, and nonspecific or minor febrile illnesses. In patients with such nonspecific disorders, an etiologic diagnosis cannot be made without supporting epidemiologic or laboratory data.

Laboratory Diagnosis

Peripheral blood tests and the erythrocyte sedimentation rate are generally of little value in diagnosis of enteroviral infection.

Coxsackieviruses and echoviruses are easily isolated from throat swabbings during the acute stage of illness and from feces for some time thereafter. If clinical and epidemiologic observations are suggestive of enteroviral infection, laboratory support for the diagnosis may be obtained by virus isolation and/or a significant increase in neutralizing antibodies to the suspected agent during the course of the illness. Virus isolations from extraparenteral sources are less significant than isolations from parenteral sources. The most rigid proof of cause is obtained, however, when the virus is isolated from the site of the pathologic process (e.g., from spinal fluid in aseptic meningitis).

COLORADO TICK FEVER

By RICHARD W. EMMONS, M.D.
Berkeley, California

Synonyms

Mountain fever, American mountain tick fever (historical).

Definition

Colorado tick fever (CTF) is an acute, febrile disease caused by a virus (CTF virus) that is transmitted by bite of the wood tick, *Dermacentor andersoni*. The natural cycle involves ticks, small rodents, and other mammals, and is limited to mountain or foothill areas of a dozen western and Pacific coast states and southwestern Canada. Several hundred cases occur annually from March through September, coinciding with adult tick activity.

PRESENTING SIGNS AND SYMPTOMS

The disease begins abruptly, 3 to 6 days after tick bite, and consists of high fever, severe headache, photophobia, retro-ocular pain, malaise, myalgias, and arthralgias. A history of exposure in endemic areas can be elicited but the patient may not be aware of a tick bite. The onset of Rocky Mountain spotted fever, which is transmitted by the same tick species in similar areas of western United States, is very similar.

COURSE

The disease is often biphasic, with a 2 to 3 day fever, a remission of signs and symptoms for 1 to 2 days, then a recurrence of fever and worse symptoms for 2 to 3 days. There may be only a single febrile period, or rarely 3 episodes. Anorexia, nausea and vomiting, cloudy sensorium, and disorientation may occur. Convalescence may be prolonged for many weeks, with weakness, weight loss, and lethargy. There is no specific treatment for the disease.

PHYSICAL FINDINGS

A mild, macular, or petechial rash on the trunk occurs briefly in a few patients, but it is not persistent, progressive, or involving the limbs, palms, and soles as in Rocky Mountain spotted fever. There may be conjunctival injection. The spleen is sometimes palpable, but otherwise the physical findings are unremarkable.

COMMON COMPLICATIONS

There are no common complications; however, myocarditis, meningitis, or a frank encephalitis has been seen, and a hemorrhagic diathesis is noted rarely. Renal failure and disseminated intravascular coagulation have also occurred. These complications are more frequent in children. Only two fatal cases have been recorded, although others may have been falsely attributed to Rocky Mountain spotted fever. Cases during early pregnancy might result in spontaneous abortion.

LABORATORY FINDINGS

Transient leukopenia is a hallmark of CTF. Depression of the leukocyte count to 3000 or 2000 cells per cu mm or lower occurs, most striking during the second febrile period. A "left shift" of granulocytes may occur, with metamyelocytes and even myelocytes in peripheral blood. There is usually a relative lymphocytosis during the recovery phase. Thrombocytopenia is also frequent, and probably accounts for the hemorrhagic tendency. There may be mild anemia, followed by reticulocytosis during recovery. The cerebrospinal fluid (CSF) may show lymphocytosis in patients with encephalitis.

The CTF virus has a tropism for bone marrow and infects all blood cells, depressing their production temporarily. The persistent viremia, which is so characteristic of CTF, is due to the presence of the virus within erythrocytes, where it is protected from antibodies. The erythrocytes are not lysed, but continue to circulate up to 3 to 4 months, long after clinical recovery of the patient. The blood can thus transmit infection by transfusion or laboratory accident, but the disease is not otherwise contagious.

The diagnosis is readily confirmed by isolation of the virus from peripheral blood and by serologic tests. Clotted blood samples can be sent without refrigeration to most state health department laboratories in the endemic areas. The virus is isolated by inoculating newborn mice with a suspension of the blood clot, and the acute- and convalescent-phase sera are tested for complement-fixing or neutralizing antibodies. Since antibody development is sometimes slow, the convalescent blood sample should be taken 3 to 6 weeks after the acute one. Fluorescent antibody staining methods are available in a few laboratories and can rapidly confirm the diagnosis by detecting the infected erythrocytes in peripheral blood smears, even during the first few days of illness. The virus can sometimes be isolated from the CSF in encephalitic cases.

PITFALLS IN DIAGNOSIS

The initial symptoms of Rocky Mountain spotted fever are similar, as just described, but this disease has a more severe course and the characteristic progressive rash involving the extremities. Tick-borne relapsing fever in western United States mountain regions follows the bites of infected soft (argasid) ticks, of which the patient is rarely aware. Several to many relapses of fever are characteristic, and the causative spirochete can be demonstrated in stained smears of peripheral blood taken during the fever. Tularemia rarely can occur following tick bite, but lymphadenopathy, a septic, nonremittant course, and tests for specific agglutinating antibodies are helpful clues. Various enteroviral and respiratory viral diseases are similar to CTF in some respects and may occur coincidentally with exposure to ticks. A patient may develop CTF following return to a nonendemic area where the disease is unfamiliar to health care personnel and laboratory tests are not available, so that a travel history is essential. About one fourth of the patients will not recall having a tick bite, but all will have been in a tick-infested environment.

VARICELLA

(Chickenpox)

By PIERCE GARDNER, M.D.,
Chicago, Illinois

and WILLIAM BERENBERG, M.D.
Boston, Massachusetts

DEFINITION

Varicella is a highly contagious disease of childhood, caused by a large DNA virus and characterized by (1) a well-defined incubation period, and (2) a vesicular rash that typically occurs in successive crops and is most marked on the trunk. In healthy children, the disease is usually mild with clinical symptoms limited to the skin; but in immunosuppressed children and adults, life-threatening illness caused by deep visceral involvement is not uncommon. After a primary infection, varicella virus generally persists in a latent form in dorsal root sensory ganglia. In response to various stresses the virus may reactivate to produce herpes zoster (shingles), a painful vesicular eruption in a dermatomal pattern most commonly seen in adults. Lifelong immunity to exogenous varicella infection usually follows the primary infection. Patients with either chickenpox or herpes zoster represent a source of infection to susceptible persons.

PRESENTING SIGNS AND SYMPTOMS

The classic presentation of varicella is that of a young child (highest incidence between 2 and 8 years of age) with a history of exposure to chickenpox 10 to 21 days previously (usually, 14 to 16 days), who has mild prodromal symptoms of malaise and low-grade fever, followed within 12 to 36 hours by a centripetal (maximally truncal) rash. Early recognition of varicella is of greatest importance in the hospital setting, where exposed immunosuppressed children with no previous history of varicella should be identified and treated with zoster immune globulin (ZIG)* or plasma in order to prevent or modify the clinical course of varicella. Since the benefit of passive immunization of exposed contacts is greatest during the period immediately after exposure, early recognition of the index case is important for optimal management. Recipients of zoster immune globulin or plasma who do develop modified varicella often have a prolonged incubation period (up to 42 days) and prolonged clinical course (with prolonged viral shedding).

PHYSICAL EXAMINATION AND COURSE

Typically, the rash begins with erythematous macules that rapidly progress to papules, which vesiculate to form the classic "dewdrop on a rose petal." Itching is a common and sometimes intense early symptom. In contrast to vaccinia and variola, the lesions are located in the superficial layers of epidermis and have thin, easily ruptured walls. The vesicular lesions are often elliptical, rarely exceeding 3 to 4 mm in diameter. Drying results in central depression (umbilication) of vesicles, followed by crusting. Characteristically, successive crops of vesicles appear for 3 or 4 days after the first rash, so that in a given area lesions may be seen in all stages of development from macules to vesicles to lesions that are becoming encrusted. Only rarely do new lesions appear after the seventh day of rash except in immunocompromised hosts. Lesions may involve any mucous membrane, most commonly the mouth, conjunctiva, or genital area, producing local irritation and pain. Local lesions may account for the occasional complaints of abdominal pain, dysuria, and cough. The evolution of the lesions from vesicles to crusting is variable but is usually complete within 7 to 10 days. Once crusted, the lesions are probably no longer contagious. Temporary depigmentation is common, but generalized scarring is rare in the absence of secondary bacterial infection. Systemic symptoms and fever are generally mild. The presence of high

---

*Available from Sidney Farber Institute, Boston, MA (617) 732–3121.

fever or significant toxicity should lead the physician to suspect one or more of the complications listed below.

Rarely, a hemorrhagic form of varicella has been noted, marked by high fever and hemorrhage into vesicles and other areas. This often fatal syndrome appears to be related to intravascular coagulation of clotting factors and platelets, and has been noted predominantly in children with impaired host defenses (i.e., leukemia).

COMPLICATIONS

Secondary Bacterial Infection. Skin lesions often become superinfected by staphylococci or streptococci. Impetigo and cellulitis are the most common infections and may in severe cases result in generalized sepsis or metastatic infections (especially septic arthritis). Poststreptococcal sequelae, including glomerulonephritis or rarely acute rheumatic fever, may occur.

Pneumonia. Chest infiltrates can be detected roentgenographically in as many as 16 per cent of patients with varicella. Respiratory symptoms are usually mild or absent. Clinically, significant pneumonia has been detected most frequently in adults and immunosuppressed patients. Symptoms of cough and tachypnea typically begin several days after the rash appears. In certain patients, severe hemorrhagic pneumonitis with marked impairment of respiratory function may cause life-threatening illness. This complication is important to recognize, as preliminary studies suggest that the antiviral agent adenine arabinoside (Ara A) may be of therapeutic benefit.

Varicella pneumonia also may be complicated by bacterial superinfections, most commonly with *Staphylococcus aureus*. The bilateral nodular densities characteristic of varicella pneumonia may subsequently calcify and appear indefinitely on chest x-rays.

Dissemination to Other Viscera. Involvement of the liver and other viscera is rare except in the immunosuppressed patient. Fever, right upper quadrant pain, toxicity, and elevated hepatocellular enzymes are the hallmarks of hepatic involvement by varicella. Widespread visceral dissemination is associated with high mortality. Neonates who contract varicella are also at increased risk of visceral involvement. The risk is greatest for infants developing the rash at age 5 to 11 days or born of mothers with onset of varicella within 4 days of delivery. Early recognition of disseminated varicella is important, because prompt therapy with Ara A may be beneficial.

Central Nervous System Complications. Varicella has now supplanted measles as the most commonly identified cause of fatal encephalitis in the pediatric age group. Encephalitis, which occurs approximately once per 1000 cases, usually represents a postinfectious encephalitis in which hypersensitivity mechanisms are thought to be important in the pathophysiology. Characteristically, the symptoms of headache, altered sensorium, meningeal irritation, and secondary fever begin 3 to 7 days after the appearance of the rash. Cerebrospinal fluid pleocytosis (predominantly lymphocytes) and protein elevation are common. Although many patients recover completely, death occurred in 15 per cent of patients as reported to the National Communicable Disease Center recently. Residual neurologic deficit is not uncommon.

Other neurologic complications of varicella include cerebellar ataxia, transverse myelitis, polyneuritis, and aseptic meningitis. Recovery from these complications is usually complete. Lumbar punctures performed on children with varicella often show mild pleocytosis (lymphocytes) in the absence of neurologic signs or symptoms.

Coagulation Complications. Thrombocytopenic purpura or disseminated intravascular coagulation with hemorrhage into vital organs may occur in unusual cases.

Rare Complications. Varicella infection of the cornea may threaten vision. Lesions in the larynx may produce edema with airway obstruction requiring tracheostomy. On occasion, varicella, as well as a number of other infectious agents, has been associated with Reye's syndrome (acute fatty degeneration of the liver together with "toxic" encephalopathy, often with hypoglycemia), or myocarditis.

LABORATORY FINDINGS

Laboratory tests are seldom necessary to secure the diagnosis of varicella. However, if doubt exists, the following tests are useful:

1. Examination of scrapings of the vesicle base (stained with Wright or Giemsa stain) usually will reveal multinucleated giant cells, often with inclusions. These cells may also be seen in herpes simplex but not in other diseases associated with vesicles.

2. Acute and convalescent sera taken 14 days apart may be expected to show an elevation of complement-fixing and neutralizing antibodies.

3. Demonstration of virus can be achieved by isolation in human tissue culture or by direct electron microscopy of scrapings from the base of a lesion.

Differential white blood cell count and urinalysis are seldom of diagnostic importance.

PITFALLS IN DIAGNOSIS

The characteristic epidemiology and clinical appearance usually serve to distinguish varicella from other diseases associated with vesicles. Early lesions may be confused with insect bites, dermatitis herpetiformis, eczema vaccinatum, eczema herpeticum, smallpox, or rickettsialpox. Later lesions may be confused with pemphigus or bullous impetigo. With the exception of infections caused by herpes simplex, none of these diseases is associated with multinucleated giant cells in scrapings of the vesicle base, and microscopic demonstration of these giant cells by Giemsa or Wright stained smears (see above) is a most useful rapid diagnostic test. Hemorrhagic chickenpox may mimic meningococcemia or hemorrhagic smallpox, but epidemiologic and other clinical features provide a basis for differentiation.

CHRONIC DIARRHEA

By J. RAINER POLEY, M.D.
Norfolk, Virginia

Numerous conditions cause chronic diarrhea in infants and children. Three major factors are responsible for the production of diarrhea: deranged enterosorption of water and electrolytes, disturbed intestinal motility, and decreased rectal holding capacity. Diarrhea is probably better defined by total fecal weight rather than fecal frequency. In diarrhea, more than 90 per cent of the total weight is water.

For the production of excess fecal water, a single pathophysiologic mechanism may be operative, or it may be the result of interactions between more than one such mechanism. A brief review of pathophysiologic mechanisms responsible for chronic diarrhea is presented in Table 1.

In the assessment of severity or chronicity or both of chronic diarrhea in children, the status of growth and development is important. Normal growth and weight gain are unlikely to be associated with a process of a severe nature.

It is rather difficult at times to arrive at a diagnosis in a relatively short time, and some situations are puzzling. A schematic approach to a stepwise diagnostic evaluation and helpful procedures is given in Table 2.

DISTURBANCES IN THE DIGESTION AND ABSORPTION OF CARBOHYDRATES

DISACCHARIDASE DEFICIENCIES

Hereditary Defects. *Isolated Lactase Deficiency.* This is probably quite rare in infants (there is usually an acquired and reversible lactase deficiency secondary to mucosal damage). By contrast, frequency is great (70 to 95 per cent) among adults of many populations, such as blacks, North and South American Indians, Eskimos, Asians, and Africans, but only about 6 to 20 per cent in populations of central and northern European origin. Manifestations such as diarrhea, abdominal pain, and increased intestinal gas after lactose ingestion may begin in childhood: after age 5 to 8 years in black and Indian children and after 12 to 15 years in whites.

The disorder is inherited. Some evidence suggests autosomal recessive; some favors autosomal dominant inheritance. There is loss of most of brushborder beta-galactosidase activity, with some activity of hetero-beta-galactosidase remaining.

Diagnosis: Hydrogen breath test; oral lactose tolerance test; assay of lactase activity on biopsied small intestinal mucosa: Sucrase:lactase ratio > 4; normal histology.

Sucrase-Isomaltase Deficiency. Probably caused by the presence of inactive enzymes, this heritable (autosomal recessive) disorder is less frequent than isolated lactase deficiency. However, manifestations may begin in early childhood. These include diarrhea, bloating, evidence of fermentation in stool (bubbles); there is association of diarrhea with sucrose intake. Growth and development usually are normal.

Diagnosis: Be aware of possibility! Sucrose in stool after ingestion; abnormal sucrose tolerance test; assay of sucrase activity on biopsied intestinal mucosa: sucrase:lactase ratio < 0.6; normal histology. Usually the activity of isomaltase is strongly decreased, and, less so, of maltase.

Complications: Nephrolithiasis in adults on liberal diet (enteric hyperoxaluria).

Bonus: No caries (on sucrose-restricted diet)!

Acquired Defects. Acquired defects are secondary disaccharidase deficiencies, because they result from small intestinal mucosal damage. Uusually two or more enzymes (lactase, sucrase, isomaltase, maltase, trehalase) are deficient. Defects are reversible with recovery of mucosal structure.

Table 1. *Pathophysiology of Chronic Diarrhea*

Etiology	Mechanism	Disorder
Villus atrophy, crypt cell hyperplasia	Impairment of intestinal transport of water and electrolytes (exsorption > insorption)	Gluten-sensitive enteropathy; cow's milk and soy protein hypersensitivity
Osmotic water retention	Increased amount of osmotically active particles; unabsorbed mono- and disaccharides; medium chain fatty acids; amino acids, di- and tripeptides; sulfates	Primary and secondary disaccharidase deficiencies; monosaccharide malabsorption Excess medium chain triglyceride in diet; combination of excess monosaccharide, medium chain fatty acids and amino acids in elemental diets; water with high sulfate content
Stimulus-secretion coupling		
Bacteria	Elaboration of enterotoxins with subsequent stimulation of synthesis of vasoactive substances, as vasoactive intestinal polypeptide (VIP) or prostaglandins; secretory stimulus via adenylate cyclase Direct invasive action of microorganisms; deconjugation of bile acids and synthesis of hydroxy fatty acids	Conditions characterized by intestinal bacterial overgrowth in the small intestine Local disease: diverticula, blind loop, pouches after side-to-side enteroanastomoses Systemic disease: chronic pancreatic and liver disease; diabetes mellitus; so-called contaminated bowel syndrome; immunodeficiency disease; ileocolonic anastomosis (absence of ileocecal valve); Hirschsprung's disease
Bile acids, fatty acids	Promotion of water and sodium secretion into colon, inhibition of colonic water and sodium absorption	Excess bile acid loss into large intestine: ileal resection or ileal disease, cystic fibrosis Long-chain fatty acids and hydroxy fatty acids in states characterized by steatorrhea
VIP, prostaglandins	Stimulation of secretory apparatus, mediated via adenylate cyclase	Neurogenic tumors; non-beta islet cell tumors of pancreas (gastrinoma); medullary carcinoma of thyroid
Unknown	Secretory stimulus: ?pathway, ?target organ, ?system	Acrodermatitis enteropathica; congenital chloride diarrhea; congenital rubella or cytomegalovirus diarrhea; food hypersensitivities

Symptoms: Those of hereditary defects plus those of the underlying disease (milk hypersensitivity, celiac disease, bacterial overgrowth, etc.). Usually failure to thrive, irritability, mood changes, poor sleep.

Diagnosis: Disaccharidase assays on biopsied small intestinal mucosa (abnormal histology, several enzymes depressed). Screen with breath hydrogen test, oral carbohydrate tolerance tests, or 1-hour D-xylose test if celiac disease is suspected. Screen stool for pH, reducing substances, and occult blood.

TRANSIENT MONOSACCHARIDE MALABSORPTION

Transient monosaccharide malabsorption may be a sequel of acute or chronic diarrhea (bacterial overgrowth in small intestine). If there is excess glucose in diarrheal stool, if stool pH is less than 5.5, or if definite symptoms appear after glucose ingestion, monosaccharide should be omitted from feedings for 1 week or longer, if necessary.

GLUCOSE-GALACTOSE MALABSORPTION

Rare; less than 30 patients on record. Watery diarrhea, which may be severe, occurs upon ingestion of these sugars. Symptoms begin in early childhood with failure to thrive. The disorder is due to defective active intestinal transport of glucose and galactose. Renal glucosuria may be present.

Diagnosis: Abnormal (flat glycemic response) oral glucose and galactose tolerance tests with diarrhea (do tests under intravenous fluid coverage). Normal tolerance for fructose. Normal intestinal histology.

STARCH INTOLERANCE

Although not proved, the existence of such a disorder is possible. Patients with hereditary sucrase-isomaltase deficiency may be intolerant to starch. Too much starchy food may cause loose stools in certain infants (? decreased activity of brush border glucoamylases).

Table 2. Diagnostic Steps and Tests in Chronic Diarrhea

Most important: Good history, particularly feeding history; onset, duration of diarrhea; organic qualities of symptom complex (nature of stools and subjective complaints, night stools); good physical examination.

Step I:	Feces	Serum	Oral Carbohydrate Tolerance Test	Miscellaneous	Remarks
	Weight Bacteriology pH (<5.5) Reducing substances ($>1/2$%)° Occult blood	Screening for lipid malabsorption: cholesterol, prothrombin time, vitamin E Screening for protein maldigestion or loss of protein: electrophoresis Electrolytes Acid-base balance Immunoglobulins Peripheral smear for RBC morphology Serum-iron Sedimentation rate (chronic inflammatory bowel disease)	Lactose Saccharose (Infants, 50 gm/m²; children, 1 gm/kg; blood glucose at 0, 30, 60, 120 min) Mean average rise of blood glucose, 42 ± 3 mg/dl after lactose (abnormal: <25 mg/dl); 58 ± 4 mg/dl sucrose (abnormal: <35 mg/dl) 1-hr D-xylose test (0.5 gm/kg, maximum 5 gm D-xylose P.O.); normal: rise of serum D-xylose: >20 mg/dl over baseline	Sweat chloride determination: values > 60 mEq/L diagnostic of cystic fibrosis. Do not perform sweat test when peripheral edema present (falsely low results)	Decrease of stool pH and presence of reducing substances not always reliable, but helpful when abnormal If abnormal, suspect disaccharidase deficiency or monosaccharide malabsorption, with or without mucosal damage

Step II:	Feces	Small intestinal biopsy	Radiology	Miscellaneous	Remarks
	Fat (normal absorption coefficient >95% in children, >90% in infants) Note: adequate fat intake! Electrolytes: when Cl-concentration $>$ sum of K + Na concentration: congenital chloridorrhea	Histology Disaccharidase activities Enterokinase activity; immune histology. Indication for biopsy: to rule out mucosal damage, diagnosis of primary vs. secondary disaccharide deficiencies (do smear-prep for Giardia, bacteria).	Bone age ± demineralization (significant failure to thrive) Upper GI series (see remarks) Small bowel Colon IVP	Endoscopy (rectum, colon) Breath analysis (if feasible): H₂-breath test; ¹³C-trioctanoin breath test; ¹³C-cholylglycine breath test (see remarks); electrophoresis of serum lipids; ⁵¹Cr-albumin turnover test (protein-losing enteropathy)	Upper GI series and small intestinal x-ray unrewarding in patients below 2 yrs old even in presence of mucosal damage H₂ breath test for lactose malabsorption ¹³C-cholylglycine breath test for bile acid malabsorption ¹³C-triolein breath test for lipid malabsorption (latter two tests may not yet be routinely performed—mass analysis of stable isotope required)

Step III:	Feces	Pancreas	Urine	Miscellaneous	Remarks
	Bile acids (normal: <100 mg/24 hr/m²) Hydroxy fatty acids (normal: almost none) Prostaglandins (elevated in chronic inflammatory bowel disease)	Secretin-pancreozymin test PABA test (see remarks) Enterokinase assay	Vanillylmandelic acid Homovanillic acid Oxalate (enteric hyperoxaluria)	Duodenal juice: special bacteriology Serum: VIP, prostaglandins Test ileal function: bile acid excretion test or postprandial rise of cholylglycine in serum (see remarks) TORCH screen (CMV rubella-CF) RAST test for presence of food hypersensitivity	Bile acid excretion test: after IV injection of 3ᴴ (or whenever possible, 2ᴴ cholic acid): check 24-hr stool excretion of isotope: >50% excreted, significant ileal disease Postprandial rise of serum cholylglycine reflects clearance of cholylglycine from ileum and spill-over into systemic circulation. No or poor rise: ileal disease likely (normal hepatic function required) PABA test; after feeding of L-benzoyl-L-tyrosyl-para-aminobenzoic acid tyrosyl-PABA peptide bond split exclusively by chymotrypsin. PABA absorbed, excreted, and measured in the urine (convenient screening for pancreatic function)

°With Clinitest tablet on stool supernatant. To detect sucrose, acidify first and warm for 1 minute, then add tablet. Sucrose is not a reducing sugar!

DISTURBANCES IN THE DIGESTION AND ABSORPTION OF FAT

The increase of fecal weight (fecal water) in conditions characterized by steatorrhea probably results from secretory activity of nonabsorbed long-chain fatty acids and of hydroxy fatty acids. The latter are synthesized by intestinal bacteria from unsaturated long-chain fatty acids and have fairly strong secretory properties. Best test for fat maldigestion and malabsorption is quantitative fecal fat. Screen: ^{13}C-trioctanoin breath test (see Table 2).

INTESTINAL DISEASE

Mucosal Damage (villous atrophy). Decreased penetration of long-chain fatty acids and monoglyceride through mucosa is observed in celiac disease, milk and soy hypersensitivity, and increased bacterial activity in small intestine. In general, stools of patients with steatorrhea are loose and foul smelling and float on water, but they can also look normal. An occasional patient may be constipated!

Diagnosis: 1-hour D-xylose test; stool fat determination; diagnosis of mucosal damage by intestinal biopsy.

Decreased Absorbing Surface. Steatorrhea with or without diarrhea may follow resection or disease, or both, of upper jejunum of distal ileum. Diarrhea or steatorrhea, or both, following disorders affecting the distal ileum are mediated through bile acid malabsorption (see below).

PANCREATIC DISEASE

Observation of oil droplets in stool is evidence of undigested triglyceride, i.e., indicative of lipase deficiency. This valuable information may be obtained by history.

Cystic Fibrosis. Clinical symptoms are malabsorption and failure to thrive. Most often there is also associated bronchopulmonary disease. Isolated involvement of the pulmonary or digestive tract is possible.

Diagnosis: Sweat chloride > 60 mEq per liter.

Exocrine Pancreatic Insufficiency. Various forms of the Shwachman syndrome are seen, with or without metaphyseal dysostosis. An occasional patient will have chronic pancreatitis, usually of the hereditary type. Diabetes mellitus may appear in later life in both.

Diagnosis: Clinical evidence of pancreatitis, cyclic neutropenia, or bone marrow dysfunction. Documentation of pancreatic insufficiency by either secretin-pancreozymin test or para-aminobenzoic acid (PABA) test (Table 2). X-ray of large joints for metaphyseal dysostosis. Bone marrow evaluation.

Isolated Lipase Deficiency. Rare; 12 patients have been reported. Presence of greasy-oily stools since infancy, but no failure to thrive. Lipase activity is markedly depressed or undetectable, and other pancreatic enzymes, bicarbonate, and electrolyte secretion are normal. Colipase is present.

Diagnosis: Pancreatic function tests (Table 2).

LIVER DISEASE

Chronic (mainly) cholestatic liver disease results in greatly decreased secretion of bile salts into the intestine. Bile salt concentration is not adequate for efficient micellar dispersion of lipolytic products (fatty acid and monoglyceride), which are absorbed poorly. Unabsorbed fatty acids, and hydroxy fatty acids synthesized by bacteria, stimulate intestinal secretion. Since bile salts seem necessary for intraluminal activation of enterokinase, protein digestion may be deficient as well.

METABOLIC DISEASE

Steatorrhea, diarrhea, and failure to thrive are features of abetalipoproteinemia or hypobetalipoproteinemia. Because of a defect in the synthesis of normal apolipoprotein C peptides (major component of β-LP class), chylomicrons cannot be formed. The absorbed fat remains in the intestinal villus as triglyceride. A small intestinal mucosal biopsy with an oil-red O stain is diagnostic. Blood smear may show spiny red blood cells (not pathognomonic). Low serum cholesterol; very low β-lipoproteins on electrophoresis of serum lipids.

DISTURBANCES IN THE DIGESTION AND ABSORPTION OF PROTEIN

INADEQUATE ACTIVATION OF PANCREATIC PROTEOLYTIC ENZYMES

Enterokinase Deficiency. Intermittent diarrhea, failure to thrive, and response to a casein hydrolysate formula are the principal features. Further, there may be signs of deficient protein metabolism such as hypoalbuminemia, anemia, and edema.

Diagnosis: Assay of enterokinase activity either in biopsied small intestinal mucosa or in fasting duodenal juice.

INADEQUATE PRODUCTION AND EXCRETION OF PANCREATIC PROTEOLYTIC ENZYMES

This is a feature of chronic and acute pancreatic disease. The contamination of the small bowel with bacteria in chronic pancreatic disease may be in part responsible for the diarrhea.

EXCESSIVE INTESTINAL PROTEIN LOSS

Numerous conditions such as inflammatory bowel disease are associated with intestinal protein loss. It can also occur on the basis of intestinal lymphangiectasis (diffuse or segmental) with or without combined malformation of peripheral lymphatics (lymphedema) and/or chylous ascites. Usually present are hypoalbuminemia, hypogammaglobulinemia, lymphopenia, and recurrent infections.

Diagnosis: Excessive intestinal (endogenous) protein loss as shown by ^{51}Cr-albumin turnover studies. Intestinal biopsy.

HYPERSENSITIVITY TO DIETARY PROTEIN

COW'S MILK PROTEIN

One tries to distinguish between "quick reactors" (milk hypersensitivity) and "slow reactors" (milk intolerance). Patients with milk hypersensitivity respond immediately or within 24 hours to milk challenge with severe reactions, including diarrhea (which may be bloody), with great intestinal water loss. Marked intestinal mucosal damage and secondary disaccharidase deficiencies may be seen, as is significant failure to thrive. The intestinal lesions are often indistinguishable from those seen in celiac disease but, in contrast to celiac disease, may show a patchy distribution. Villous atrophy is probably not observed in children beyond 1 year of age. Diarrhea after milk intake can persist for several years despite normal lactase activity.

Patients with milk intolerance are not as severely affected, although some intestinal mucosal damage and low-grade disaccharidase deficiencies may be present. Upon challenge, they usually respond with diarrhea within a few days but not as severely as infants with milk hypersensitivity. Signs of milk intolerance usually persist only for several months.

Cow's milk proteins most often implicated are α-lactalbumin, β-lactoglobulin, and occasionally casein. Patients sensitive to β-lactoglobulin will also have diarrhea after goat's milk (β-lactoglobulin!).

Methods of diagnosis are controversial, for many physicians are reluctant to perform three challenges as proposed by Goldman. This is particularly true in babies with milk hypersensitivity, who may respond with severe reactions. One to two well-documented challenges with expected response should be sufficient. A good immunologic test is needed but is not presently available. Serum milk antibodies are nonspecific. A decreased serum IgA is often observed, but its relationship to the pathogenesis is obscure. An occasional patient may develop celiac disease at a later age.

Options for formulas are shown in Table 3.

GLUTEN-SENSITIVE ENTEROPATHY

Definition: Celiac disease or gluten-sensitive enteropathy is a permanent hypersensitivity of the small intestinal mucosa to gluten, with variable clinical expression, in a genetically predisposed individual.

Gluten-sensitive enteropathy is more common in Europe, Canada, and Australia than in the United States. Symptoms may begin at any age, but diagnosis is most commonly made between 12 and 24 months. Symptoms include: irritability and mood changes, abdominal distension, and failure to thrive with loss of weight. There is stool pathology, with frequent bulky, foul-smelling, and floating stools. Anorexia is common. Vomiting may be a presenting symptom on occasions (flat abdomen!). Stools may be normal in some patients, and constipation has been observed. Unusual presentations should be kept in mind: sudden unmasking of disease after acute (enteric or extraenteric) illness; a poor maternal-child relationship that may detract from diagnosis; diarrhea that may be very watery; iron deficiency anemia refractory to oral therapy; hyperphagia; or a history of frequent formula switching, which does not cure the problem.

On physical examination, the following signs should also be watched for: long, straight silky eyelashes, smooth tongue, peripheral edema, and clubbing. An occasional patient may present with hypothyroid features.

Diagnosis: Demonstration of total villous atrophy on biopsied intestinal mucosa, clinical and histologic response to a strict gluten-free diet, and recurrence of intestinal damage following challenge with gluten. Because of great variability of clinical expression, mucosal damage after challenge with a regular diet may not become apparent until 3 to 5 years. More rapidly, gluten sensitivity may be established in vitro using organ cultures. In patients with established diagnosis, gluten restriction should be maintained for life. Adults with celiac disease

Table 3. *Useful Formulas in Chronic Diarrhea*

Formula	Protein	Fat°	Carbohydrate	Remarks
Nutramigen	Casein hydrolysate	LCT	Sucrose, starch	If patient is sucrase deficient, do not feed.
Portagen	Casein	MCT	Glucose	Patient with intolerance to casein will continue to have diarrhea. Start slowly with ¼ strength, and gradually increase; otherwise, osmotic effect of medium chain fatty acids may prolong diarrhea. MCT formulas may be tolerated full strength after several days.
Pregestimil	Casein hydrolysate	MTC	Glucose (starch)	Recommended in severe mucosal damage. Start slowly (see above).
Isomil (and others)	Soy protein	LCT	Sucrose	Note: most babies with milk intolerance tolerate soy protein.
CHO-Free	Soy protein	LCT	Traces	In about one third to two thirds of patients with milk hypersensitivity, soy protein is poorly tolerated and diarrhea continues; consider also digestibility of carbohydrate and lipid in formula (intestinal biopsy!)

°LCT = long chain triglyceride; MCT = medium chain triglyceride.

are more prone to malignancies in structures arising from the foregut. Further, there may be peripheral neuropathy, pulmonary complications (fibrosing alveolitis), and ulcerations in the large and small intestine. The latter carry an unfavorable prognosis.

The presence of gluten antibodies in serum or stool is nonspecific.

SOY AND RICE PROTEIN

Usually considered hypoallergenic, these proteins produce severe reactions (vomiting or diarrhea or both) in susceptible patients (rice: anaphylactoid; soy protein: anaphylactoid and severe mucosal damage with villous atrophy, which may be patchy, diarrhea and malnutrition).

Diagnosis: Rests with cautious challenge. Intestinal biopsy is indicated in patients suspected of having soy protein hypersensitivity (flat mucosa).

INFECTIOUS DIARRHEA

Enterotoxigenic *Escherichia coli,* some strains of Klebsiella, and Salmonella elaborate enterotoxins that stimulate the intestinal secretory apparatus. This stimulus-secretion coupling is probably mediated via activation of adenylate cyclase. Prostaglandins or vasoactive intestinal polypeptide (VIP) may be mediators.

ENTEROPATHOGENIC ESCHERICHIA COLI

Numerous strains are known and can be typed routinely. Occasionally outbreaks occur in nurseries, the infection often being traced to an asymptomatic carrier handling infants. Bacteria are pathogenic to prematures, newborns, and young infants.

ENTEROTOXIGENIC ESCHERICHIA COLI

These strains of *E. coli,* also responsible for traveler's diarrhea, cannot yet by typed in a routine laboratory, so clinical suspicion must suffice. A routine stool culture showing "pure culture" or 3+ growth of *E. coli* is suspicious.

KLEBSIELLA

Some strains of Klebsiella elaborate a toxin that, by stimulating active intestinal secretion, produces watery diarrhea.

SALMONELLA

Chronic reservoirs are human asymptomatic carriers, pets, and pet foods. Infection may mimic chronic ulcerative colitis. Osteomyelitis is a known complication.

SHIGELLA

Like certain strains of *E. coli* responsible for disease in man, Shigella is invasive of tissue, mainly colon. Diarrhea with macroscopic blood and mucus, as well as tenesmus, is frequent.

Complications: Bacteremia, central nervous system involvement, pneumonitis.

CHRONIC INFLAMMATORY BOWEL DISEASE

CHRONIC ULCERATIVE COLITIS (CUC)

Etiology and pathogenesis are still unknown, but local immunologic processes may be responsible for perpetuation of the disease.

CUC may start at any age, but it is rare in infants and children under 5 years of age. In infants, milk hypersensitivity may mimic CUC clinically, endoscopically, and radiologically.

Diagnosis: Made via proctosigmoidoscopy and radiology. The rectosigmoid is almost always involved, with diffuse superficial ulcerations in a red, granular, and friable mucosa. Crypt abscesses are present histologically. On barium enema diffuse superficial ulcerations are noted, impressing as fine serrations and fuzziness. "Thumb-printing" with submucosal hemorrhage may be seen.

Most common extracolonic manifestations are (1) arthralgias or acute toxic arthritis, usually involving large joints of lower extremities; and (2) liver involvement (pericholangitis, portal fibrosis, "chronic active hepatitis"), or dysfunction as manifested by elevations of serum glutamic oxaloacetic transaminase (SGOT) and serum glutamic pyruvic transaminase (SGPT), elevation of alkaline phosphatase, and increased bromsulphalein (BSP) retention.

CROHN'S DISEASE

The frequency of Crohn's disease is increasing. No cause is known; however, viruses produce disease in animal models, and a transmissible agent (? virus) seems to have been isolated from human tissue. However, no proof is available yet that Crohn's disease is caused by an infectious agent. Pathogenesis is not clarified, but local immunologic processes could determine site and depth of lesions. Bloody diarrhea is observed in only 40 to 50 per cent of patients; more common are progressive crampy abdominal pains, fever (sometimes of unknown origin), and loss of weight. Anal lesions such as fissures and fistulas may precede abdominal manifestations by months. Joint involvement (knees, ankles, wrists) is more frequent than in CUC. Recurrent aphthous lesions of oral mucosa should be watched for.

Diagnosis: Confirmed by endoscopy (proctosigmoidoscopy, colonoscopy, if available) and barium contrast studies. The rectosigmoid may be normal in 50 per cent, but hemorrhoids and telangiectasis lead one to suspect more proximal disease. Endoscopically, there is edema of the bowel wall; deep ulcers, which may be discrete or linear or cross-hatched, usually do not involve the entire circumference, as in CUC.

Radiologically, there may be continuous or discontinuous involvement (skip lesions), deep ulcers, or fistula (paracolonic or enteroenteric). Ileocolonic involvement is probably the most common presentation of Crohn's disease in children. Growth retardation is a serious complication of untreated disease and probably related to inadequate nutrition.

SUBSTANCES PROMOTING ACTIVE INTESTINAL SECRETION

The mechanism by which bile acids, fatty acids, prostaglandins, and vasoactive intestinal polypeptide induce intestinal secretion is not yet clearly defined. Stimulation of adenyl cyclase is a possibility, as is increased "leakiness" of junctional membranes and blocking of the Mg- and NA'-K'-dependent ATP-ase dependent sodium pump.

BILE ACID DIARRHEA

The secretory organ is the colon. Excess bile acids are lost into the colon after ileal resection or disease. Limited resections and loss of the ileocecal valve result in bile acid diarrhea, extensive reactions, usually in significant steatorrhea, and fatty acid diarrhea. Induction of colonic secretion is effected only by dihydroxy bile acids, i.e., chenic and deoxycholic acids, in concentrations above 3 mM. In ileal resection, lipid conservation is mainly a function of length of ileum resected; water conservation depends on length of colon remaining.

Diagnosis: Watery diarrhea after ileal resection, loss of excess bile acids in stool, and response of diarrhea to cholestyramine. Test for ileal function (see Table 2).

FATTY ACID DIARRHEA

Target organs are probably the small and large intestine. Fatty acid diarrhea (including hydroxy fatty acids) is related to steatorrhea and the presence of bacteria (see Table 1).

VASOACTIVE INTESTINAL POLYPEPTIDE AND PROSTAGLANDINS

The target organ is probably the small intestine. Profuse watery diarrhea occurs with hypokalemia. These substances may be produced in differentiated neurogenic tumors (ganglioneuroma and ganglioneuroblastoma), in non-β islet cell tumors of the pancreas, and probably also in medullary carcinoma of the thyroid.

The presence of profuse watery diarrhea (stool weight > 500 grams per day) with hypokalemia should initiate the search for a "diarrheagenic" tumor.

ENDOCRINE DISORDERS

DIABETES MELLITUS

Chronic or intermittent diarrhea is observed in children when difficulties exist in controlling diabetes. In adults, there may be associated autonomic neuropathy of the intestine, causing hypomotility, which is conducive to bacterial overgrowth. Whether the excess spilling of sugar into the intestine observed in children with poorly controlled diabetes is contributory to the diarrhea remains conjectural.

HYPERTHYROIDISM

Hyperthyroidism is observed occasionally, but other clinical symptoms of hyperthyroidism should not make diarrhea a diagnostic puzzle.

ADRENAL INSUFFICIENCY

This is an occasional occurrence. The mechanism has not been elucidated. However, it is known that glucocorticoids influence the absorption of water and sodium in the gut.

HYPOPARATHYROIDISM

The disturbance of intestinal motility with or without diarrhea that is occasionally observed may be due to hypocalcemia. Restoration of normocalcemia abolishes the diarrhea.

IMMUNODEFICIENCY DISEASES

Isolated IgA deficiency does not, by itself, cause diarrhea. It is probable that the complement system is also engaged in the pathogenesis of diarrhea, although its role is not yet understood.

Intractable diarrhea is common in severe combined immunodeficiency. It is not an early manifestation, but its appearance may be an ominous sign. Diarrhea is also a manifestation of the graft-versus-host reaction after bone marrow transplants. In a child with failure to thrive and chronic, refractory diarrhea that does not fit other categories, disorders of the immune systems should be sought: serum immunoglobulins, monilia skin test, granulocyte function test, T and B cell population studies, mixed lymphocyte cultures, and the like.

MISCELLANEOUS DISORDERS

HIRSCHSPRUNG'S DISEASE

In a child with intermittent symptoms of constipation, abdominal distension, and explosive diarrhea, the suspicion of aganglionic megacolon should arise. The enterocolitis of Hirschsprung's disease is probably related to increased bacterial activity above the aganglionic segment.

Chronic diarrhea starting shortly after birth, even in the absence of vomiting, may be a presenting symptom of segmental aganglionic colon.

ACRODERMATITIS ENTEROPATHICA

Diarrhea is quite common and may precede the appearance of the typical skin lesions. The diarrhea may be watery, and fecal water may contain excess sodium. Decreased urinary zinc excretion and decreased serum zinc are present.

CONGENITAL CHLORIDORRHEA

Diarrhea, hypokalemia, and alkalosis with excess wasting of fecal chloride are characteristic. Diarrhea and failure to thrive may have been present since early childhood. Occasionally, the diagnosis is not made until early adulthood. Etiology and pathogenesis are related to a disturbance of ileal ion transport, in which chloride is exchanged for bicarbonate. In the stools, the concentration of chloride is always in excess of that of sodium and potassium combined. This is the only type of chronic diarrhea with this unique pattern of fecal ion excretion.

DIARRHEA ASSOCIATED WITH CONGENITAL RUBELLA AND CYTOMEGALOVIRUS INFECTION

The pathogenesis has not been elucidated. Diarrhea usually develops early and is present in 10 to 20 per cent of patients. Small intestinal histology shows nonspecific changes, and disaccharidase activities may be depressed. If this is documented, the respective sugars are best eliminated from the feedings. An elemental diet such as glucose, medium chain triglycerides, protein hydrolysate formula (Pregestimil) may be helpful.

These viral agents should be suspected in an infant with chronic diarrhea and hepatospleno-megaly.

CHRONIC NONSPECIFIC DIARRHEA

The most common form of diarrhea in a "healthy" child and a problem for physicians caring for children is chronic nonspecific diarrhea (probably a better label than "irritable colon" of childhood, which seems an embarrassing diagnosis).

Onset of diarrhea is most common after the first year of life and may follow acute gastroenteritis. The diarrhea may be watery, with three to six bowel movements a day or occasionally more. The smell of the stools is very foul. There is excess flatulence and abdominal distension. These children are often irritable and do not sleep well. However, they have grown and developed normally. Boys are twice as often affected as girls. A family history of allergy is common, as is marked factitious whealing of the skin.

There is excessive bacterial overgrowth (anaerobes and aerobes) in the upper small intestine. Thus the designation of "contaminated bowel syndrome" has also been used.

Small intestinal biopsy shows nonspecific abnormalities and/or more or less visible edema of the lamina propria, patchy infiltration of mononuclear inflammatory cells. Disaccharidase activities are usually normal, but there is often intolerance to oral sucrose (diarrhea!).

Diarrhea caused by food allergy does exist. When suspected, it must be looked for; diagnosis is usually established on a challenge-trial-and-error basis. A radioallergosorbent (RAST) test may be helpful in trying to find offending foods, particularly in those patients with nasal, bronchial, or skin symptoms (urticaria), and elevated serum IgE.

RICKETTSIAL DISEASE *

By LTC DAVID R. HABURCHAK, M.D., *and* COL. WILLIAM L. MOORE, JR., M.D.

Fort Gordon, Georgia

The diagnosis of the rickettsioses in many ways tests the breadth of knowledge of the clinician. In particular, his skills at geography, zoology, world history, and immunology are challenged as significantly as his ability to elicit a detailed history of symptoms or demonstrate physical findings. Laboratory methods are constantly improving to aid in early diagnosis, but the clinician still must rely on his skills in epidemiology and physical diagnosis to institute appropriate and sometimes life-saving therapy before confirmation is available.

As a group, the rickettsioses should be considered in the differential diagnosis of any patient with fever and headache. Fever is classically sustained and the headache severe. A rash enhances the diagnosis considerably, but never occurs with Q fever. Rash may be difficult to detect in dark-skinned individuals or may never be present, even in fatal cases. Because all the rickettsioses are predominantly infectious vasculitides, the spectrum of organ systems involved may be extensive and confusing, but the triad of fever, rash, and headache is often all that is needed to start the process of assessment in the right direction.

ROCKY MOUNTAIN SPOTTED FEVER

SYNONYMS

Spotted fever, tick typhus, black measles, tick fever, fiebre manchada, São Paulo typhus, Tobia fever.

ETIOLOGIC AGENT

Rickettsia rickettsii.

EPIDEMIOLOGY

A true zoonosis, this disease is transmitted to man by hard-shelled ticks. It has been increasing in incidence in the past decade, possibly because of changes in outdoor recreation and suburban living. Although the disease is named for the originally studied endemic focus in the Bitterroot Mountain range on the Idaho–Montana border, recently more than 90 per cent of the reported cases have occurred in the United States east of the Mississippi River, especially in Virginia, the Carolinas, Maryland, and Georgia. Most are in children under 15 years of age. April through August is the peak season, but in Southern and mild regions the disease may be seen year round. Asymptomatic tick infestation and crushing of ticks during removal are the common modes of inoculation.

About 60 per cent of patients give a history of tick bite. A history of exposure to dogs or woodlands may also be helpful. Laboratory accidents have been responsible for more unusual occurrences of this disease and emphasize the extreme danger of working with this organism.

CLINICAL FEATURES

After an incubation period of 3 to 12 days, there is an abrupt onset of headache, rigor, and prostration. Fever rises over 2 days to approximately 104 F (40 C) and is sustained. Myalgias, arthralgias, and muscle tenderness are common. The rash, the most helpful diagnostic feature of the illness, usually is evident on the fourth day of fever, starting as 2 to 6 mm pink blanching macular lesions about the wrists, ankles, palms, and soles. It spreads centrally within 6 to 12 hours and often becomes petechial or frankly purpuric within days. Capillary fragility is frequently demonstrable. In severe cases frank necrosis of skin, digits, ears, and nose may occur.

Multiple organ system involvement is common. Headache is severe, persistent, predominantly frontal and is associated with malaise, restlessness, and insomnia progressing to frank encephalopathy in severe cases. Overt myocarditis, pneumonitis, hepatitis, and nephritis are unusual but can occur. Dehydration and ileus are common late manifestations in severe cases. Splenomegaly is said to occur in about one half of the patients. Without proper antibiotic therapy, the illness may last up to 3 weeks and terminate fatally in 20 per cent of patients, usually with disseminated intravascular coagulation and shock.

LABORATORY FINDINGS

Mild to moderate thrombocytopenia is common; if marked, disseminated intravascular coagulation should be suspected. Anemia and normal to low leukocyte counts are to be expect-

*The opinions or assertions contained herin are the private views of the authors and are not to be construed as official or reflecting the views of the Department of the Army or the Department of Defense.

ed. The occurrence of hyponatremia has recently been emphasized and is probably a manifestation of inappropriate antidiuretic hormone (ADH) secretion. Azotemia and hypoalbuminemia may reflect renal and liver involvement, respectively.

At present only serologic confirmation is available at most reference laboratories. A fourfold complement-fixation antibody rise to *R. rickettsii* is diagnostic and considerably more sensitive and specific than the Weil-Felix reaction. The latter may be positive in Proteus infections, leptospirosis, borreliosis, and severe liver disease.

Although the complement fixation test is the currently recommended method of serologic diagnosis, it may soon be replaced by more sensitive tests that are not affected by early treatment. These include microimmunofluorescence, microagglutination, and hemagglutination assays.

Most promising for early diagnosis is a newly developed indirect immunofluorescent test for identification of the organism in biopsy specimens of skin lesions. When widely available, this could allow rapid diagnostic confirmation and timely institution of antibiotic therapy.

PITFALLS IN DIAGNOSIS

The most common disease confused with spotted fever is measles. The absence of coryza, lacrimation, and Koplik spots should lead one away from the diagnosis of measles. Patients with meningococcemia and gonococcemia generally have rashes not in the distribution of the rash of spotted fever. Frank arthritis and meningitis do not occur in spotted fever. In murine typhus the rash begins centrally and spares palms and soles.

If the rash is absent, the diagnosis may be difficult unless actively considered. Prompt response to tetracycline or chloramphenicol is strong presumptive evidence of the diagnosis when such therapy is instituted upon epidemiologic and clinical evidence.

OLD WORLD TICK TYPHUSES

ETIOLOGIC AGENTS

Fièvre boutonneuse	*R. conorii*
North Asian tick typhus	*R. siberica*
Slovakian tick typhus	*R. slovaka*
Queensland tick typhus	*R. australis.*

EPIDEMIOLOGY

These similar diseases are all spread by hard-shelled ticks in a manner similar to Rocky Mountain spotted fever, which they resemble antigenically as well. Recent extensive outbreaks of disease due to *R. siberica* have occurred in Central and East Asia. Dutch, German, and Swiss tourists have contracted fièvre boutonneuse after camping in or visiting infected areas in the Mediterranean and Africa.

CLINICAL FEATURES

The clinical illness of each is similar and represents a milder version of Rocky Mountain spotted fever. At the time of the abrupt fever onset, a primary lesion of *tache noire* is frequently seen. This is a single black crusted ulcer ringed with erythema and associated with regional lymphadenopathy. A maculopapular rash similar in distribution to that of Rocky Mountain spotted fever usually appears about the fifth day. After 10 to 14 days the patient defervesces and the rash soon resolves. Fatalities are rare except in the elderly and infirm.

LABORATORY FEATURES

Diagnosis may be confirmed with specific complement-fixing antibody rise. All the tick typhuses, including Rocky Mountain spotted fever, can react to Proteus OX–19 and OX–2 in the Weil-Felix test.

Q FEVER

SYNONYMS

Query fever, Balkan grippe.

ETIOLOGIC AGENT

Coxiella burnetii.

EPIDEMIOLOGY

Q fever is seen worldwide, chiefly in areas with extensive cattle, sheep, and goat herds and associated industry. It is a zoonosis capable of transmission by fomites, infected dust, and ticks. Large outbreaks have occurred in the Mediterranean and in Northern California, but individuals especially at risk of endemic disease appear to be herdsmen, shepherds, veterinarians, and dairy and slaughterhouse workers.

CLINICAL FEATURES

An incubation period of 2 to 4 weeks precedes the abrupt onset of fever, chills, frontal headache, malaise, and myalgia so characteristic of all the rickettsioses. Chest pain may be a feature specifically suggestive of Q fever but has been described infrequently in recent outbreaks. Fever is usually remittent, 101 to 104 F (38.3 to 40 C) and persists 9 to 14 days. A mild dry cough may appear about the fifth day of illness. Physical examination commonly reveals tachypnea, relative bradycardia, hepatomegaly, and splenomegaly. Examination of the chest discloses few physical signs, whereas the chest roentgenogram may reveal surprising homogenous consolidation suggestive of pneumococcal pneumonia. Pneumonia is not universal in confirmed cases, however, and when present probably reflects the mode of transmission. Pneumonia has been demonstrated in 33 to 80 per cent of patients in various reports. Infrequent complications are pleurisy, pleural effusions, thrombophlebitis, endocarditis, granulomatous hepatitis, orchitis, and uveitis. Prolongation of illness occurs in 20 per cent of patients. No rash is seen in Q fever.

LABORATORY FINDINGS

A fourfold complement-fixation titer rise is diagnostic. The Weil-Felix test is negative. Hematologic and blood chemistry profiles are sufficiently variable to be of no diagnostic value.

PITFALLS IN DIAGNOSIS

Q fever should be considered in the differential diagnosis of atypical or viral pneumonia in patients with a livestock exposure. Because of the frequent absence of pneumonia in confirmed cases, Q fever should be considered in the differential diagnosis of febrile illness in anyone exposed to livestock or their excretions.

EPIDEMIC TYPHUS

ETIOLOGIC AGENT

Rickettsia prowazekii.

EPIDEMIOLOGY

Epidemic typhus has been the decisive enemy of armies and peoples destitute by war since the time of the Romans. In this century, louse-borne typhus devastated the Soviet Union after World War I and was extensive in Eastern Europe during World War II. Because of public health measures, especially the use of effective insecticides against the louse, the epidemic disease has been virtually eliminated from Europe, Asia, and South and North Africa. Most recent cases have been in Central Africa, mainly Rwanda, Burundi, and Ethiopia. There

also have been small foci of infection in Mexico, Bolivia, Ecuador, Peru, and Guatemala. The African outbreaks appear to be in part related to DDT-resistant lice. Although not reported in North America, the potential for epidemic typhus remains because of the population of East European émigrés who may develop Brill-Zinsser disease (discussed later) and the recently well-documented increase in louse infestation in all social strata.

CLINICAL FEATURES

Abrupt onset of headache, chills, and fever begins about 7 days after exposure. On day 5 of the illness, a blanching macular pink rash begins in the axillary folds. In 1 to 2 days it spreads to the trunk, then the extremities, ultimately becoming nonblanching, petechial, and possibly confluent. The palms, soles, and face are spared. The fever is sustained at 102 to 104 F (38.9 to 40 C) until therapy, recovery, or death.

Neurologic disturbances may be impressive and give the disease its name, typhus, from the Greek for "stupor." Cardiovascular collapse, cyanosis, and renal failure are late manifestations of the severe, widespread vasculitis that may occur in untreated patients. Thrombosis of small and medium blood vessels resulting in gangrene and death may occur in severe cases during the 9th and 18th day of illness. Secondary bacterial infection is a common cause for delayed death. Mortality is highest in older age groups.

LABORATORY FEATURES

Anemia and neutropenia are common. Leukocytosis usually is a manifestation of secondary bacterial infection. Hematuria, proteinuria, and azotemia are common. The electrocardiogram may have nonspecific ST–T wave changes and chest roentgenogram may demonstrate patchy pulmonary infiltrates. Cerebrospinal fluid (CSF) examination is usually normal except for mild elevation of opening pressure. Specific complement-fixation test and the relatively nonspecific Weil-Felix Proteus OX-19 provide retrospective serologic confirmation.

BRILL-ZINSSER DISEASE

SYNONYMS

Recrudescent typhus, sporadic typhus.

ETIOLOGIC AGENT

Rickettsia prowazekii.

EPIDEMIOLOGY

Brill-Zinsser disease represents a milder endogenous recrudescence in persons with previous epidemic typhus. Relapse usually occurs 10 to 20 years after the initial illness but may appear after as many as 40 years. The best documented cases have come from Yugoslavia, Czechoslovakia, and Romania. Diminished host resistance is speculated to play some role in the recrudescence because most patients are elderly, and other infections such as influenza, paratyphoid fever, leptospirosis, and shigellosis have been associated with Brill-Zinsser disease. A significant epidemiologic concern is that the patients with Brill-Zinsser disease may transmit the infective agent to lice and initiate epidemic typhus.

CLINICAL FEATURES

The illness is similar to typhus but is usually ameliorated by partial host immunity. Rash may be absent, the vasculitis less severe, and complications infrequent. Age-specific mortality is considerably lower than in epidemic disease.

LABORATORY FEATURES

An anamnestic rise in IgG complement-fixing antibodies to *R. prowazekii* as early as the fourth day of illness is diagnostic. In the primary attack, specific IgM CF antibodies are found no earlier than day eight. The Weil-Felix titers are lower in Brill-Zinsser disease than in typhus.

MURINE TYPHUS

SYNONYMS

Endemic typhus, urban typhus, rat typhus.

ETIOLOGIC AGENT

Rickettsia mooseri.

EPIDEMIOLOGY

A zoonosis of rats and other rodents transmitted by fleas, murine typhus affects man as an accidental host. The disease has been reported most heavily in Vietnam, Thailand, Malaysia, Mexico, and Guatemala. It is seen in United States coastal areas in the Southeast, and in Texas. It appears most commonly when rat populations fluctuate widely or come into close contact with humans. Granary workers appear to be at high risk, especially in summer and fall. Urban renewal and disruption of rat harborage may also play a role in dispersal of the reservoir. It has been estimated that up to 10 per cent of a large urban rat population may carry *R. mooseri* in their brains. One outbreak in Texas in 1968 was associated with cat fleas.

CLINICAL FEATURES

Murine typhus presents as a milder version of epidemic typhus. After an incubation period of 8 to 16 days, onset may be gradual with a prodrome of headache, chills, and myalgias. As the disease progresses, frontal headache intensifies and is accompanied by rigors and fever. Nausea, vomiting, and prostration are common. Children may be less symptomatic than adults.

Fever is usually sustained, reaching 104 F (40 C) and it lasts about 12 days. The macular rash begins in the axilla on the fifth day and soon spreads to the trunk and upper extremities. The pea-sized macules blanch within the first 24 hours, then become persistent and papular. Petechiae and purpura are extremely rare, however, and sparing of the palms and soles helps to differentiate the disease from Rocky Mountain spotted fever. The rash often persists for 4 to 8 days then fades before the patient becomes afebrile.

Nonproductive cough and abdominal pain with constipation are common complaints.

LABORATORY FEATURES

Most laboratory findings are unremarkable except for hypochloremia in severe cases. Specific diagnosis may be confirmed using complement-fixing antibody rise or a rise in Proteus OX–19 by the third week of illness.

SCRUB TYPHUS

SYNONYMS

Tsutsugamushi disease, mite-borne typhus.

ETIOLOGIC AGENT

Rickettsia tsutsugamushi.

EPIDEMIOLOGY

A mite-borne typhus, this disease is a zoonosis of small rodents in East Asia and the southwest Pacific. It has appeared most frequently in servicemen and in field and plantation workers in the area.

CLINICAL FEATURES

An incubation period of 10 to 12 days precedes an illness of insidious onset in two thirds of the patients. Characteristically there is a prodrome of headache, chilliness, and anorexia lasting about 5 days before the patient seeks medical attention. Fever up to 104 F (40 C) is common at the time of presentation and is typically unremittent. About one half of patients have a nonproductive cough.

The most consistent and typical finding is generalized lymphadenopathy, occurring in up to 85 per cent of patients by the seventh day of illness. An eschar is seen in about one half of patients, most commonly on the legs. A maculopapular eruption occurs on the trunk in about one third of patients between the third and eighth day and persists for about 4 days. In the absence of rash and eschar, the most common mistaken clinical diagnosis made has been infectious mononucleosis. Fever usually lasts 14 days in the untreated patient, and complications such as pneumonia, thrombophlebitis, and neurologic disturbances are unusual.

LABORATORY FEATURES

Mean leukocyte count is about 8,000 per cu mm with 70 per cent of patients developing lymphocytosis. Twenty per cent of patients have abnormal urinalysis, most commonly proteinuria. Blood chemistries, spinal fluid, and chest roentgenogram are usually normal or show mild, nonspecific changes. Serologic confirmation has been most consistently obtained by fluorescent-antibody testing. Proteus OXK antibody rise in either Weil-Felix or hemagglutination technique appears to be less sensitive and is somewhat strain specific.

RICKETTSIALPOX

ETIOLOGIC AGENT

Rickettsia akari.

EPIDEMIOLOGY

Like scrub typhus, rickettsialpox is a zoonosis of small rodents, transmitted by mites. Rickettsialpox is usually an urban disease, however, transmitted to man after depletion of the usual murine hosts for the mite. The initial cases were reported in New York City, but it has occurred in other American and European cities.

CLINICAL FEATURES

A nonpainful red papule 1 cm in diameter appears 7 to 10 days after the mite bite. Within a few days the papule vesiculates and has a zone of erythema. Regional lymphadenopathy develops. An abrupt onset of fever with temperature of 103 to 104 F (39.4 to 40 C), chills, headache, and photophobia occurs 3 to 7 days after onset of the lesion, either accompanied or followed by the exanthem. Rickettsialpox is unique among the rickettsioses because of the vesicular component of the maculopapular rash. It may even involve the oral cavity, but it spares the palms and soles. Constitutional symptoms are mild and the rash resolves without scarring within a week. It is somewhat easily mistaken for varicella. The latter is rare in adults and does not have a primary lesion. Smallpox and more exotic pox viruses have more severe constitutional signs, and the viral poxes, especially in the unvaccinated, become pustular.

LABORATORY FEATURES

The Weil-Felix test is negative. A complement-fixation test using *R. akari* antigen appears to be useful, but does cross react with *R. rickettsii*.

TRENCH FEVER

ETIOLOGIC AGENT

Rochalimea quinata.

EPIDEMIOLOGIC FEATURES

Man is believed to be the only reservoir of this louse-borne disease, which was widespread in armies of both world wars. Like typhus it is manifested during periods of social upheaval and general lousiness. Few data are available about current epidemiology, but within the past few decades it has been thought to exist in Eastern Europe, Central America, and North Africa. Like typhus it also appears capable of causing recrudescent disease in a previously infected individual up to 32 years later.

CLINICAL FEATURES

After an incubation period of 10 to 30 days there is often an abrupt onset of fever lasting 3 to 5 days with retro-orbital headache, myalgias, weakness, and prostration. The clinical course has been highly variable and prone to relapse. Splenomegaly and transient macular rash may appear in as many as 70 to 80 per cent of the patients. The more severe manifestations of systemic vasculitis are rare.

The differential diagnosis is that of other "camp" diseases, including influenza, typhus, and dengue. Specific laboratory diagnosis is not routinely available.

BACTERIAL PNEUMONIAS

By JAMES R. TILLOTSON, M.D.
Albany, New York

DEFINITION

Bacterial pneumonias are acute inflammatory reactions of the parenchyma of the lung caused by a variety of bacterial species. Persons with altered resistance are most often afflicted, but certain organisms may infect young, previously healthy persons.

DIAGNOSIS

Knowledge of the characteristic clinical features and the background in which a particular infection occurs may provide important clues to help differentiate the many causes of bacterial pneumonia, but for the most part diagnosis is contingent upon the proper interpretation of Gram stains and cultures of appropriately collected sputum specimens. Since the pharynx harbors many of the bacteria that can cause pneumonia, and pharyngeal secretions routinely contaminate sputum, microscopic examination of any sputum submitted for culture should be considered routine. Throat cultures correlate poorly with the lower respiratory flora in pneumonia and should not be relied upon for diagnosis. When sputum is not available, aspiration of secretions from the trachea by the transtracheal or nasotracheal route should be performed. In addition, several blood cultures should be collected before therapy is initiated, and culture of infected pleural fluid, if present, should be considered the most reliable aid to diagnosis.

PNEUMOCOCCAL PNEUMONIA

The pneumococcus remains the major cause of bacterial pneumonia, accounting for 60 to 80 per cent of the bacteriologically proven cases. The onset is often abrupt, occurring during or immediately after an acute upper respiratory infection, with a rigor or chest pain, or both, followed by fever, dyspnea, cough, and expectoration of yellow or rusty sputum. Conditions producing inadequate clearance of organisms from the lungs, such as congestive heart failure, chronic bronchitis, recent surgery, or altered states of consciousness, also predispose to pneumococcal pneumonia, often with a more insidious onset. Unless one of these conditions exists, however, the diagnosis of pneumococcal pneumonia should be questioned.

The physical signs in the chest and the roentgenographic picture may show a rapid progression from early congestion to consolidation, often confined to a single lobe, but today nonconsolidating pneumonias predominate. Prompt institution of effective antimicrobial therapy may abort the disease before the characteristic picture is fully developed but host factors are generally the major determinants of the clinical presentation. Leukocytosis is usually present; moderate but early leukopenia may occur in severely ill or debilitated patients. An extreme degree of leukocytosis or multiple chills usually denotes a purulent complication. Properly collected, stained smears of the sputum demonstrate encapsulated, grampositive, elongated cocci in pairs. Blood cultures may yield pneumococci in up to 30 per cent of patients.

Complications are more frequent in debilitated patients or with delay in therapy and include empyemas, lung abscesses, meningitis, endocarditis, pericarditis, septic arthritis, metastatic abscesses, peritonitis, postpneumonic sterile effusions, and delayed resolution.

STAPHYLOCOCCAL PNEUMONIA

Pneumonias due to coagulase-positive *Staphylococcus aureus* generally occur in specific settings, resulting in different clinical manifestations. Infants with bronchogenic staphylococcal pneumonia show a characteristic roentgenographic picture with pneumatoceles and pyopneumothorax. In older patients following an acute respiratory infection or in elderly debilitated patients, especially after treatment with antibiotics or tracheostomy, a descending infection occurs, characterized by tracheobronchitis and a perihilar infiltrate, lobar consolidation, or diffuse bronchopneumonia. Abscess formation is seen within a few days and empyemas are common, but bacteremia occurs in only 10 per cent of patients. A fulminating form of this disease may occur after measles or influenzal pneumonia with extreme dyspnea, cyanosis, cough, scant bloody sputum, high fever, and a rapid downhill course. In patients with persistent bacteremia an embolic type of staphylococcal pneumonia occurs, characterized by discrete, usually subpleural nodules that undergo early cavitation and abscess formation.

The sputum in staphylococcal pneumonia is usually blood streaked, and gross hemoptysis may occur. Gram-stained smears of the sputum demonstrate large gram-positive cocci, often in tetrads or grape-like clusters.

HEMOLYTIC STREPTOCOCCAL PNEUMONIA

Once a common cause of atypical pneumonia, this disease is rare today. Previously healthy children or young adults are most commonly infected, usually after a bout of pharyngitis or tonsillitis, or occasionally after influenza or measles. This infection produces thin, bloody or blood-streaked sputum, retrosternal soreness, patchy bilateral bronchopneumonia, and early large, serous or serosanguineous effusions; recovery is slow. Positive blood cultures are rare. Characteristic chains of cocci are seen on smears of sputum or pleural fluid. Residual abscesses, bronchiectasis, and fibrosis are common.

KLEBSIELLA PNEUMONIA

Klebsiella pneumonia (Friedländer's bacillus) causes pneumonia in patients with debilitating diseases, especially alcoholism and chronic bronchopulmonary disease, and is becoming more common as a nosocomial bacterial pneumonia. Preceding upper respiratory infections are unusual, but 2 to 3 weeks of bronchitis often precedes the pneumonia and most patients have significant periodontal disease. The sputum may be gelatinous, bloody, or purulent and demonstrates encapsulated gram-negative bacilli on stained smear. Early leukopenia, severe acidosis, and cyanosis or rubor are common in patients with severe disease, many of whom die within a few days. Bacteremia occurs in about 10 per cent of the patients.

The initial pulmonary lesion is patchy but may rapidly become confluent, producing a massive, dense consolidation with sharply defined and rapidly advancing borders. Necrosis with abscess formation occurs frequently in the first week. Survivors usually have parenchymal fibrosis or residual abscesses or both.

PNEUMONIA DUE TO HEMOPHILUS INFLUENZAE

In infants and children and in adults with immunologic deficiencies (including alcoholism and diabetes) this organism produces a confluent bronchopneumonia simulating the lobar pneumonia caused by the pneumococcus. Bacteremia, empyema, and anemia are common. On the other hand, patients with chronic lung disease more frequently manifest a diffuse bronchopneumonia with a miliary pattern that is rarely complicated by bacteremia or empyema. This type accounts for up to 15 per cent of all adults hospitalized for pneumonia. The sputum in both types is copious owing to the associated tracheobronchitis and may be green in color. On Gram-stained smears, many small pleomorphic gram-negative coccobacilli are seen. Arthralgia and myalgia are common in both types, while secondary localization of the bacteremia in bones, joints, or meninges may occur, especially in children.

PSEUDOMONAS PNEUMONIA

Persons with severe cardiac or pulmonary disease seem to be particularly predisposed to the bronchogenic pneumonia caused by *Pseudomonas aeruginosa*, especially following tracheal intubation or antibiotic therapy or both. Characteristics of this infection often include an initial normal total white blood cell count with an increased number of immature polymorphonuclear leukocytes, extreme toxicity with mental confusion and hallucinations, cyanosis, jaundice, a diffuse bilateral infiltrate with microabscesses, and small serosanguineous pleural effusions. Often initial clinical improvement occurs only to be followed by progressive hypotension, congestive heart failure, gastrointestinal bleeding, and death 7 to 10 days later. The sputum is yellow or yellowish-green and copious and contains many large, pleomorphic gram-negative bacilli. Bacteremia is common but often transient. The prognosis is grave even with the use of appropriate therapy.

PNEUMONIA DUE TO ESCHERICHIA COLI

The colon bacillus generally causes pneumonia following a bacteremia from a urinary or gastrointestinal source. These infections produce moderate leukocytosis and fever and lower lobe bronchopneumonias. Large empyemas develop 1 to 2 weeks after the onset if the pneumonia is unrecognized and not properly treated initially. Smears and cultures of the sputum and pleural fluid reveal relatively few gram-negative bacilli; blood and urine cultures are frequently positive. The mortality is high but death can usually be prevented by recognition and appropriate early therapy. These pneumonias are probably much more frequent than generally recognized, up to 25 per cent of *E. coli* bacteremias being associated with secondary pulmonary infection.

ANAEROBIC PLEUROPULMONARY INFECTIONS

Recent improvement in techniques of specimen collection and handling and of culturing has resulted in better definition of the role of anaerobic bacteria in lower respiratory tract infections. These infections, usually caused by more than one species in contrast to those caused by aerobic or facultative bacteria, may result from aspiration of infected upper respiratory secretions or by bacteremic spread to the lung, usually from the gastrointestinal or genital tract. Only the Gram-stained smear can effectively distinguish the infectious pneumonias due to anaerobic bacteria from the other types of aspiration (e.g., chemical). Empyemas are common and not infrequently the only or the predominant roentgenographic finding. The onset may be abrupt or insidious with localized or diffuse, consolidating or nonconsolidating, and necrotizing or nonnecrotizing pneumonias. A foul taste or smell to the sputum and the presence, in properly collected sputum or pleural fluid, of mixed flora consisting of small or large and pleomorphic gram-negative bacilli and tiny or pleomorphic gram-positive cocci is virtually pathognomonic of an anaerobic bacterial pneumonia. Microscopic examination of the sputum and pleural fluid is of particular importance since sputum is not, and usually should not be, cultured anaerobically.

LEGIONNAIRES' DISEASE

Following extensive speculation and investigation, the cause of Legionnaires' disease was eventually determined to be a previously unrecognized bacterium, named *Legionnella pneumophila*. The initial manifestations of this disease often simulate a viral or mycoplasmal infection but the distinctive clinical features should permit an appropriate diagnosis, or at least a strong clinical suspicion early. The onset is generally abrupt with high fever and systemic symptoms of myalgias and headache, but these may be preceded by upper respiratory symptoms. Lower respiratory manifestations occur several days later with cough, dyspnea, and parenchymal infiltrates, but sputum is scant and free of the usual acute inflammatory response or bacteria characteristic of most bacterial pneumonias. Abdominal pain, liver enzyme elevations, abnormal renal function studies, alterations in mental status, and markedly elevated erythrocyte sedimentation rates are common and should suggest the diagnosis of Legionnaires' disease. The organism requires special media for isolation, but early diagnosis can be made with fluorescent antibody studies of sputum, pleural fluid, or lung tissue obtained by biopsy, or confirmed by a diagnostic rise in antibody titers during the convalescent stage. Patients with chronic pulmonary disease or on immunosuppressive therapy are most susceptible and have the more severe cases.

OTHER BACTERIAL PNEUMONIAS

Pulmonary infections may develop in the course of systemic infections caused by a variety of bacteria including salmonella, pasteurella, brucella, vibrio, listeria, and meningococci, and many other genera may produce localized pulmonary infections. In fact, virtually every bacterium known to be pathogenic for man has been implicated in pneumonia.

Despite the reduced morbidity and mortality of certain types of pneumonia resulting from the availability and use of antibiotics, this means of therapy has been at least partially responsible for the introduction of many previously unrecognized causes of bacterial pneumonia. Some of these occur as secondary infections superimposed on a treated pneumococcal pneumonia or in patients receiving antibiotics for other diseases. Bacteria isolated from the sputum after antimicrobial therapy, however, should not be considered causative of a coexisting pulmonary parenchymal infiltrate unless there is a deterioration in the clinical course, a secondary fever rise, and appropriate findings on the smears and cultures of the sputum. The morbidity and mortality of pneumonia have shown little change in the past 30 years and will be significantly reduced only when appropriate diagnostic procedures are properly performed in all patients with bacterial pneumonia, and inappropriate use of antibiotics ceases.

INFECTIONS OF THE THROAT

By MICHAEL A. GERBER, M.D.,
and EDWARD L. KAPLAN, M.D.
Minneapolis, Minnesota

SYNONYMS

Tonsillitis, pharyngitis, tonsillopharyngitis, sore throat.

DEFINITION

This discussion covers acute infections involving the pharynx, tonsils, and soft palate. Numerous infectious agents have been implicated in acute pharyngitis. Bacteria including groups A, C, and G beta-hemolytic streptococci, *Corynebacterium diphtheriae, Neisseria gonorrhoeae,* and *Mycoplasma pneumoniae,* as well as viruses such as adenovirus, Epstein-Barr virus (infectious mononucleosis), herpes simplex, coxsackievirus group A, influenzae, and parainfluenzae have been etiologically associated with sore throat. However, an infectious agent cannot be identified in a large percentage of patients with pharyngeal infections; these are presumably also caused by viruses. From a practical standpoint, the primary diagnostic challenge to the clinician is differentiating streptococcal from nonstreptococcal pharyngitis because streptococcal pharyngitis requires antibiotic therapy to prevent nonsuppurative sequelae, whereas nonstreptococcal pharyngitis (except diphtheria) requires no specific therapy.

PRESENTING SIGNS AND SYMPTOMS

The cause of a throat infection cannot be determined clinically with any certainty.

There is a great deal of variability in the clinical presentation of streptococcal pharyngitis. Patients with this infection characteristically present with the acute onset of fever, sore throat, painful swallowing, and headache. On examination there is typically redness and edema of the pharynx, tonsillar pillars, and tonsils and a creamy exudate on the tonsils or pharynx, or both. Petechiae are often present on the soft palate. Enlarged, but more importantly, tender anterior cervical lymph nodes (adenitis) are palpable. A scarlatiniform rash may also be evident. Typical streptococcal pharyngitis is unusual in children less than 3 years of age.

These children usually present with an indolent course with fever, cough, coryza, with no exudate.

A community outbreak or direct contact with a person who has a diagnosed specific infection may suggest a particular infectious agent, proving very helpful to the clinician. While streptococcal pharyngitis occurs most commonly during the winter and early spring, coxsackievirus A infections characteristically occur in the late summer and fall. Nonstreptococcal pharyngitis may be clinically indistinguishable from streptococcal pharyngitis. There is also a clinical syndrome of chronic tonsillitis with large cryptic tonsils, which are often injected and occasionally have minute amounts of exudate. Frequently, cultures do not demonstrate beta-hemolytic streptococci, thus suggesting some other cause. Clinical observations would suggest that antibiotic therapy may not be related to resolution of this infection. Diphtheria is suggested by the presence of a tough gray-white pseudomembrane and a history of inadequate immunization. A history of oral sexual exposure suggests gonococcal pharyngitis, while generalized lymphadenopathy with hepatosplenomegaly suggests infectious mononucleosis. Viral pharyngitis is often accompanied by evidence of inflammation in other parts of the respiratory tract, such as hoarseness and cough as well as myalgia and lymphadenopathy. Both herpes simplex and coxsackievirus A infections usually produce small vesicles or superficial ulcers in the pharynx; the presence of similar mouth or lip lesions suggests herpes.

COURSE

The symptoms of streptococcal pharyngitis usually resolve within 2 or 3 days with or without treatment. Patients with nonstreptococcal pharyngitis tend to have a more protracted and less predictable course that is, with the exception of diphtheria, usually self-limited.

COMPLICATIONS

Streptococcal pharyngitis may be followed by suppurative complications, but only group A beta-hemolytic streptococcal pharyngitis may be followed by nonsuppurative complications. The suppurative complications usually occur during the acute phase of the illness and include acute sinusitis, cervical lymphadenitis, peritonsillar abscess, and otitis media. The nonsuppurative complications usually occur 2 to 3 weeks after the acute phase of the illness and include acute rheumatic fever and acute glomerulonephritis. Appropriate antimicrobial treatment initiated within approximately 1 week of the onset of the pharyngitis will prevent acute rheumatic fever, but acute glomerulonephritis may occur even with antibiotic therapy.

For the complications of diphtheria and infectious mononucleosis the reader is referred to the articles dealing with those infections. Gonococcal pharyngitis may be complicated by disseminated gonococcal disease. Complications of viral throat infections are usually limited to the lower respiratory tract and include laryngotracheobronchitis and pneumonitis.

LABORATORY FINDINGS

A throat culture is essential for making the diagnosis of streptococcal pharyngitis. Betahemolytic streptococci can be identified by colony morphology when grown on sheep-blood agar for 18 to 24 hours at 37 C; a subculture using a special bacitracin disc sensitivity test will usually differentiate group A from nongroup A streptococci (approximately 95 per cent of the time). Capillary precipitation and immunofluorescent and slide agglutination tests for grouping streptococcal isolates are also available. The diphtheria bacillus can be isolated on Loeffler medium, gonococcus on Thayer-Martin medium, and *Mycoplasma pneumoniae* on Mycoplasma isolation agar. Routine viral cultures, while available in many hospitals, are of little practical value in the management of acute pharyngitis, except perhaps for epidemiologic purposes.

Determination of streptococcal antibody titers (e.g., antistreptolysin-O [ASO], anti-DNase B, anti-hyaluronidase, streptozyme-measured-antibodies) is helpful when considering acute rheumatic fever and acute glomerulonephritis and in retrospectively differentiating streptococcal carriers from those with acute streptococcal infections but is of essentially no clinical value during the acute illness. Tests for heterophil antibodies are important in diagnosing infectious mononucleosis. The serologic diagnosis of mycoplasma or viral pharyngitis also requires acute and convalescent sera and is also of limited value at the time of the acute illness.

The total leukocyte count and differential have been felt to be helpful by some clinicians, but since leukocytosis also accompanies viral disease they are usually not helpful in differentiating streptococcal from nonstreptococcal infections. The presence of atypical lymphocytes, however, suggests infectious mononucleosis.

THERAPEUTIC TESTS

A trial of antibiotics as a diagnostic test for streptococcal pharyngitis or nonstreptococcal pharyngitis is of no value.

PITFALLS IN DIAGNOSIS

The major pitfall in the diagnosis of throat infections is attempting to diagnose streptococcal pharyngitis using clinical criteria alone without a properly obtained throat culture. There is currently no totally reliable way to distinguish those patients with acute streptococcal pharyngitis from streptococcal carriers with intercurrent viral pharyngitis except retrospectively by examination of acute and convalescent sera for streptococcal antibody titer rises.

Staphylococci, pneumococci, and other bacteria are frequently recovered from throat cultures; however, there is no convincing evidence that these organisms actually cause pharyngitis.

SEPTICEMIA [*]

By A. MARTIN LERNER, M.D.
Detroit, Michigan

Septicemia is an inexact term meaning the circulation of bacteria, fungi, parasites, viruses, or their byproducts (e.g., endotoxins or exotoxins) in the blood. The diagnosis of septicemia assumes that (1) multiplication of the pathogenic organism in infected tissues of the host has reached a sufficient concentration to overwhelm local and humoral defenses, permitting dissemination, and (2) the patient is, as a direct result of these events, sick. Malaise, chills, fever, hyperventilation, and prostration are common. Unless prompt and vigorous specific therapy is initiated, renal failure, peripheral vascular collapse, disseminated intravascular coagulation, and death may ensue.

[*]Aided by a grant from The Skillman Foundation and another from the Schering Corporation for the general support of infectious diseases research at Wayne State University School of Medicine.

Minute amounts of endotoxin from the outer cell membrane of gram-negative bacilli in the blood produce septicemia with its component clinical signs, fever, chills, and hypotension. Nanogram amounts of this lipopolysaccharide-protein macromolecular complex can be assayed by its characteristic gelling of the otherwise soluble lysate of the leukocytes (amebocytes) of the horseshoe crab (limulus lysate test). Endotoxin can also be measured with about a ten times less sensitive assay, the rabbit pyrogen test. Intravenous injection into the rabbit ear vein induces fever and falls in blood pressure. The sensitivity of the rabbit to these ill effects is remarkably like that of humans.

The molecular weight of most endotoxins is in the millions. These large substances, although soluble, are not cleared by the glomerulus and are dependent upon the mononuclear phagocytic (reticuloendothelial) system predominantly, the fixed macrophages of the liver, spleen, and lungs. Generally, the latter system is efficient in clearing endotoxin from the blood within 5 to 10 minutes. Prolonged circulation of endotoxin can occur when the amounts are massive (saturating the phagocytic capacity), or when corticosteroids are given concomitantly. These agents markedly inhibit mononuclear phagocytic function. Unrestricted endotoxemia leads to prolonged septicemia and activation of the alternate complement pathway and ultimate microvascular conversion of fibrinogen to fibrin. The prolonged circulation of other macromolecular components from gram-positive bacteria, fungi, parasites, or viruses probably evokes a similar mechanism, but limulus lysate tests are negative.

Effective therapy of septicemia requires accurate diagnosis dependent upon the earliest possible exact definition of the invading bacterium, fungus, virus, or parasite and an understanding of the subsequent pathologic physiology in the affected patient. Here a method is outlined that attempts to obtain a *presumptive bacteriologic diagnosis* before results of appropriate cultures are available. This method frequently allows the institution of directed rather than empiric antimicrobial therapy. It is axiomatic that the premature and indiscriminate use of antibiotics may render cultures negative and prohibit specific etiologic diagnosis often required for the recovery of the patient with septicemia.

HISTORY

Often the patient is unable to give a comprehensive synopsis of his illness, but he should be questioned briefly. If even this is not possible, a member of the family should be interrogated. If the condition of the patient permits, a brief but a complete history should be obtained. This must include a record of previous drug allergies or idiosyncrasies, because drug fevers may mimic sepsis.

Sometimes it will be learned that the prostrate person has a history of tuberculosis, frequent urinary infections, chronic bronchopulmonary disease, diverticulitis, or inflammatory bowel disease, or has been taking corticosteroids (raising the possibility of miliary tuberculosis), has been a hide or wool worker (suggests anthrax), is a butcher or has drunk unpasteurized milk (brucellosis, Q fever), has handled or eaten wild rabbit or squirrel (tularemia), is a farmer or gardener (sporotrichosis, aspergillosis, histoplasmosis), has traveled through an area of endemic coccidioidomycosis, has attempted to end an unwanted pregnancy (gas gangrene), or has had rheumatic heart disease (endocarditis). Moreover, the season may be an important factor in reaching an early diagnosis. In temperate climates enterovirus infections (including pleurodynia, myocarditis, and meningoencephalitis) are more common in the summer and early fall. During an epidemic of influenza A infections, staphylococcal or, if antibiotics have been used, gram-negative bacillary pneumonias might be expected.

Often septicemia occurs in an immunosuppressed patient already in the hospital with a malignancy or other chronic disease. The presence of a tracheostomy tube raises the possibility of a nosocomial antibiotic-resistant gram-negative bacillary pneumonia, and a urinary catheter suggests a similar gram-negative bacteremia. An indwelling intravenous catheter may herald bacteremia or fungemia from an unobtrusive area of phlebitis. In addition to the usual members of the family Enterobacteriaceae (Erwinieae, Escherichieae, Proteeae, Salmonelleae, Serratieae), Providencia, Acinetobacter, Aeromonas, Citrobacter, and Pseudomonas are increasingly common causes of nosocomial sepsis.

PHYSICAL EXAMINATION AND PHYSIOLOGIC EVALUATION OF THE PATIENT WITH SEPTICEMIA

This must be thorough and complete. Spinal or paraspinal tenderness may lead to a diagnosis of osteomyelitis or a paravertebral abscess and Pott's disease. Pneumonia may become evident. In patients on anti-cancer or immunosuppressive treatments, *Pneumocystis carinii, Legionella pneumophila* (Legionnaire's disease) and Cytomegalovirus pneumonias must be con-

Table 1. *Physiologic Evaluation of the Patient with Septicemia*

A. *Physical Signs*   *Observations*
1. Temperature — Record rectal temperature F every 2–4 hr
2. Pulse, blood pressure — Record every 2–4 hr
3. Respirations — Record every 2–4 hr
4. Urine — Record every hr (should exceed 30 ml/hr)

B. *Special Laboratory Tests*   *Normal Values*
1. Central venous pressure — 6–12 cm H_2O
2. Cardiac output — 3.0 liters/min/sq meter body surface area
3. Arterial blood
   pH — 7.35–7.45
   PO_2 — 80–104 mm Hg
   PCO_2 — 34–46 mm Hg
4. Coagulation platelet count — >100,000/mm^3
   Prothrombin time (one-stage) — 11–12.5 sec
   Fibrinogen, plasma — 200–400 mg per 100 ml

C. *Other Tests*
1. Hb, total WBC and differential counts, urinalysis, serum electrolytes, including Na, K, CO_2, Cl, BUN, creatinine
2. Serum albumin
3. X-rays (chest, upright abdomen)

sidered. Abdominal guarding or rebound tenderness may indicate an acute abdomen. Tenderness at the costovertebral area may indicate pyelonephritis or a perinephric abscess. Pelvic or rectal examination may indicate pelvic inflammatory disease or an appendiceal abscess. Localized collections of pus may be confirmed by ultrasound, gallium, or computerized body scans.

Much can be learned by carefully charting recordings of rectal temperature and pulse every 2 to 4 hours. In my experience, even carefully taken oral temperatures are inaccurate. It is my practice to connect the line of the daily peak in the rectal temperature curve of a septic patient, noting an ascending (worsening) or descending (improving) slope. Relative bradycardia may indicate typhoid fever or Pseudomonas exotoxemia. Peaks in the diurnal temperature curve during the day rather than in the evening, when they are expected, could indicate miliary tuberculosis or typhoid. Respiratory rates and urinary output must be carefully noted (Table 1).

LABORATORY AIDS

A number of simple and immediately available laboratory procedures are crucial if a *physiologic diagnosis* is to be transformed quickly into an accurate *presumptive bacteriologic diagnosis*. Blood cultures, complete blood counts, and urinalysis of a noncentrifuged and clean-voided specimen should be done on every septicemic patient. Leukocytoses generally accompany bacterial infections, but transient leukopenia is found during the peripheral vasoconstriction that accompanies rigor. During the sweat that immediately follows, a leukocytosis is again seen. A single bacterium seen at Gram stain per high power microscopic field of an uncentrifuged and clean-voided sample of urine indicates that there are more than 100,000 organisms per milliliter and an associated significant infection. Pyuria may be present without bacteriuria if there is renal tuberculosis, funguria, or ureteral obstruction. Bacteriuria may be present without pyuria if there is severe leukopenia or occasionally in enterococcal urinary infections.

The history or physical examination may necessitate lumbar puncture, thoracentesis, removal of an indwelling intravenous catheter, aspiration of the peritoneum or of an involved joint, or a cul-de-sac puncture. Of course, whenever possible, sputum should be obtained. Valid sputum is recognized by a ratio of 10:1 leukocytes to epithelial cells. If sputum is unobtainable, transtracheal aspirates, bronchoscopy (sometimes with transbronchial biopsy), or open lung biopsy may be needed. These vital materials must be obtained and promptly and intently studied before the initiation of antimicrobial therapy. As appropriate, Gram, Wright, crystal violet, silver, or acid-fast stains, bacterial or fungal cultures, cytologic studies, and chemical studies (protein, sugar, mucin content) must be done. Preferably they should be performed by the responsible physician or should be closely supervised by him. Practice by the physician leads to expertise. It is best that examination of stains for bacteria amid a polymorphonuclear exudate not be left solely to a technician who may not realize the gravity of the therapeutic decision that is to result. It should be noted that in the leukopenic patient under immunosuppression, polymorphonuclear exudates ordinarily accompanying infection may be absent.

If the patient's circulation or respiration is dubious or if bleeding ensues, cardiac output, central venous pressure, arterial blood gases, and coagulation should be assessed (Table 1). A decreasing cardiac output and forward cardiac failure usually precede an increase in central venous pressure. A PO_2 of less than 50 mm Hg and a PCO_2 of over 50 mm Hg indicate respiratory failure. Simultaneously decreased platelet count, prothrombin time, and concentration of fibrinogen may indicate diffuse intravascular coagulation.

Some procedures indicated by the initial physical examination are shown in Table 2. Here also are listed the pathologic microorganisms that may be responsible.

Erythrocyte sedimentation rates are generally elevated in bacterial infections. A normal value

Table 2. *Presumptive Microbiologic Diagnosis in Patient with Suspected Septicemia, as Determined by Physical Examination and Immediately Available Laboratory Aids*

Anatomic site	Pathologic process	Procedure°	Presumptive microbiologic finding
Blood	Bacteremia, fungemia, viremia, parasitemia; continuous or intermittent	Culture, every 5 to 60 minutes, three times	Bacteremia (aerobic, anaerobic) fungemia, viremia, parasitemia
Skin	Phlebitis at site of indwelling intravenous catheter	Culture, tip of catheter	Staphylococci, various gram-negative bacilli; several species of Candida
	Abrasions, excoriations	Needle aspiration (Gram and acid-fast stains; culture)	Group A, β-hemolytic streptococci; *Staphylococcus aureus, Clostridium tetani*
	Abscesses	Needle aspiration (Gram and acid-fast stains; culture)	*S. aureus,* species of Actinomyces
	Erysipelas	Needle aspiration (Gram and acid-fast stains; culture)	Group A, β-hemolytic streptococci ALSO: *Sporotrichum schenckii, Bacillus anthracis*
Lymph nodes		Needle aspiration (Gram and acid-fast stains; culture)	*M. tuberculosis,* staphylococci, streptococci, *Pasteurella tularensis*
Head	Pharyngitis	Throat swab (Gram stain, culture)	Group A, β-hemolytic streptococci, *S. aureus, Hemophilus influenzae*
	Otitis media		*Streptococcus pneumoniae,* β-hemolytic streptococci, *H. influenza, Mycoplasma pneumoniae*
	Meningitis	Lumbar puncture (Gram stain, cell count, cultures [routine, fungus, acid-fast bacilli])	*S. pneumoniae, N. meningitidis, E. coli, Listeria monocytogenes, Cryptococcus neoformans, M. tuberculosis,* Mucor, Leptospira
	Brain abscess	Lumbar puncture (Gram stain, cell count, cultures [routine, fungus, acid-fast bacilli])	Bacteroides species, anaerobic streptococci
	Encephalitis	Lumbar puncture, electro-encephalogram, brain scan, carotid angiogram	Herpes simplex virus, type 1 or type 2 (HSV–1 or HSV–2), Arboviruses, Enteroviruses, *M. pneumoniae*
	Subdural, epidural empyema	Lumbar puncture, electro-encephalogram, brain scan, carotid angiogram	*S. aureus*
Lung	Pneumonia ± (abscess, empyema, pericarditis)	Sputum, transtracheal aspirate, fiberoptic bronchoscopy with brushing, open lung biopsy, thoracentesis (Gram, Dieterle Silver impregnation for *Legionella pneumophila* and acid-fast stains; cultures [routine Mueller-Hinton agar with 1% hemoglobin and 2% Isovitalex, acid-fast fungi; specific gravity, protein on fluids])	*S. pneumoniae, Klebsiella pneumoniae, S. aureus,* Proteus species, *Pseudomonas aeruginosa, E. coli,* Bacteroides species, other gram-negative bacilli, *H. influenzae, M. pneumoniae, L. pneumophila*

Table continued on the following page

Table 2. *Presumptive Microbiologic Diagnosis in Patient with Suspected Septicemia, as Determined by Physical Examination and Immediately Available Laboratory Aids* (Continued)

Anatomic site	Pathologic process	Procedure°	Presumptive microbiologic finding
	Lung abscess	Sputum (Gram and acid-fast stains; cultures [routine, acid-fast fungi]) Acute and convalescent sera for complement-fixation titers (histoplasmosis, coccidioidomycosis, *M. pneumoniae*); fluorescent antibodies to *L. pneumophila* Skin tests: tuberculosis,[+] histoplasmosis, coccidioidomycosis	Anaerobic streptococci, fusiforms, various spirochetes, Actinomyces species, *Histoplasma capsulatum*, *C. neoformans* (Torula), *Coccidioides immitis*, *M. tuberculosis*, *Nocardia asteroides*, Aspergillus, psittacosis agents, *M. pneumoniae*
Heart	Endocarditis	Wright stain of ear-lobe puncture for histiocytes Examine sediment of urine for microscopic hematuria	Viridans group, streptococci, *S. aureus* or *albus*, enterococci; *P. aeruginosa*, various other bacteria occur less commonly
Abdomen	Peritonitis (pelvic, sub-hepatic, or subdia-phragmatic abscesses)	Aerobic and anaerobic culture and Gram stain of exudates from drains	*Bacteroides fragilis*, various gram-negative bacilli
	Enterocolitis	Gram stain of feces Examination of feces for amebae (trophozoites) and leukocytes	Various species of Salmonella, Shigella, Vibrio; *S. aureus*, enterotoxin-producing *E. coli*, other gram-negative bacilli, *Clostridium difficile*, plus all enterobacteria listed as possible causes of cholecystitis
	Cholecystitis	Serum, alkaline phosphatase, cholesterol, bilirubin, cholecystogram	*E. coli*, *Enterobacter aerogenes*, Proteus or Bacteroides, Salmonella, Pseudomonas, enterococci, Clostridia
	Pyelonephritis (peri-nephric abscess)	Examine noncentrifuged urine for pyuria and bacteriuria (Gram stain) Intravenous pyelogram Serum urea nitrogen	*E. coli*, *Enterobacter aerogenes*, Proteus, *P. aeruginosa*, enterococci, occasionally staphylococci
	Appendicitis (rupture, peritonitis or abscess)	Possible needle aspiration of abdomen for Gram stain, culture X-rays of abdomen (upright, flat-plate)	Same enteric organisms as listed under Cholecystitis
Genitourinary tract	Pelvic inflammatory disease, septic abortions, primary HSV–2 infection, etc.	Gram stain, culture of cervical exudate; similar treatment of material obtained by cul-de-sac, Tzanck smear, virus culture	*N. gonorrhoeae*, enteric organisms, listed under Cholecystitis, *Acinetobacter calcoaceticus*, Clostridia
Joints	Septic arthritis	Needle aspiration of joint for Gram stain, acid-fast stain, and appropriate culture; tuberculin skin test	*N. gonorrhoeae*, *S. pneumoniae*, *S. aureus*, *M. tuberculosis*
Bone	Osteomyelitis	Bone scans, x-rays of involved bone, tuberculin skin tests, Gram and acid-fast stains, appropriate cultures	*S. aureus*, *M. tuberculosis*, Brucella

°Blood cultures, complete blood counts, urinalysis, urine culture by the clean-voided method, and erythrocyte sedimentation rate should be obtained before the initiation of therapy in all patients.
[+]Intermediate strength PPD preferred.

may indicate a virus disease or trichinosis. Polymorphonuclear leukocytic exudates generally indicate active bacterial disease, whereas mononuclear cells may be present in mycoplasma or virus infections. On the other hand, in bacterial infections lymphocytes appear with healing or after the institution of antibiotic therapy. In a patient with asthma and pneumonia (or bronchitis), the reappearance of eosinophils in sputa heralds recovery. Infective organisms in sputa, cerebrospinal, or synovial fluids are usually present in pure culture (usually in large numbers). However, in tuberculous pericarditis, peritonitis, or pleural effusions, cultures for acid-fast bacilli are frequently negative, even when obtained before the initiation of anti-tuberculous therapy. In these latter instances, a predominantly lymphocytic exudate along with biopsies of affected tissues is helpful in suggesting *Mycobacterium tuberculosis*. In pneumococcal meningitis, gram-positive lancet-shaped encapsulated diplococci are predominantly extracellular and very numerous in relation to the numbers of white blood cells, whereas in meningococcal meningitis gram-negative diplococci are intracellular and much less numerous. A total cerebrospinal fluid cell count of several hundred with varying numbers of mononuclear and polymorphonuclear leukocytes may indicate a brain abscess or mycotic aneurysms(s). The latter, of course, suggests bacterial endocarditis. Examination of a blood smear may reveal malarial or filarial parasites (the latter only from blood specimens drawn at night). Similarly, an upright film of the abdomen may show free air under and fluid in the pleural space above a diaphragmatic leaf, indicating a subdiaphragmatic abscess. An intravenous pyelogram may reveal an acute hydronephrosis.

If the method is successfully applied, the diagnosis of septicemia is insufficient. A specific pathophysiologic and a presumptive microbiologic diagnosis are substituted, and specific therapy can be initiated.

RHEUMATIC FEVER

(Acute Rheumatic Fever, Acute Articular Rheumatism)

By LEO M. HENIKOFF, M.D.
Chicago, Illinois

Rheumatic fever is a disease process that is poorly understood and thus is imprecisely defined. Although it is generally agreed that this disease is part of or closely associated with the immune response to infection with group A beta-hemolytic streptococci, the mechanism remains unknown. The disease itself is characterized pathologically by inflammation of many tissues including skin, subcutaneous tissues, joints, the central nervous system, and the three layers of the heart. Although a characteristic pathologic lesion is produced in the myocardium (the Aschoff body), lesions with some similarities have been observed in nonrheumatic myocardial inflammation. There is no specific laboratory test for this disease, and thus diagnosis is made on the basis of a constellation of clinical and laboratory findings that indicate a high degree of probability of the presence of acute rheumatic fever.

In 1944, criteria for this purpose were proposed by Dr. T. Duckett Jones, and these criteria were subsequently modified in 1955 and again in 1965. The 1965 revision is presented in Table 1.

It is indicated that the diagnosis of rheumatic fever is likely if two major manifestations are present or if one major manifestation is present in conjunction with two minor manifestations. In each circumstance there must be supporting evidence of preceding streptococcal infection or the diagnosis of acute rheumatic fever is unlikely. A set of criteria such as this will function to exclude some actual cases of rheumatic fever that fail to meet the criteria and to include some instances of other disease processes mimicking rheumatic fever. The more specific and stringent the requirements, the fewer false positives will be diagnosed, but the greater number of true cases of rheumatic fever will fail to meet the criteria. The Jones Criteria, then, must be viewed as a diagnostic aid with deficiencies of both overdiagnosis and underdiagnosis and must be applied with judgment. Further comment will be made when differential diagnosis is discussed.

Children aged 5 to 15 years are most commonly affected, with the peak incidence at 9 years. Initial attacks may occur at any age, however, and have been recorded in the geriatric population. Peak incidence coincides with the school year. A good clinical history of the antecedent streptococcal infection is often lacking and cannot be obtained in over two thirds of patients.

PRESENTING SIGNS AND SYMPTOMS

Rheumatic fever presents with signs and symptoms of one or more of the five major criteria and most often is associated with fever. Fever is present in almost all patients with polyarthritis and in a high percentage of patients with other major manifestations except for chorea. Chorea is a late manifestation of rheumatic fever and usually is observed after the acute inflammation in non-nervous system tissues has subsided. For this reason fever is uncommon in those patients who present with chorea. Erythema marginatum and subcutaneous nodules are relatively uncommon findings in acute rheumatic fever and are apparently less frequent now than in previous years. Older reports documented their occurrence in 10 to 20 per cent of cases of acute rheumatic fever. More recent observations are in the 5 per cent or less range.

Table 1. *Jones Criteria (Revised)**

Major Manifestations	*Minor Manifestations*
Carditis	Fever
Polyarthritis	Arthralgia
Chorea	Previous rheumatic fever or
Erythema marginatum	rheumatic heart disease
Subcutaneous nodules	Elevated ESR or positive CRP
	Prolonged PR interval

Plus

Supporting evidence of preceding streptococcal infection: history of recent scarlet fever; positive throat culture for group A streptococcus; increased ASO titer or other streptococcal antibodies.

*Jones Criteria (revised) for guidance in the diagnosis of rheumatic fever. Circulation 32:664, 1965.

The vast majority of patients will present with carditis or arthritis or both. Chorea is unusual in that it is most frequently encountered in females, is uncommon after puberty, and is very rare after the teens. The incidence of chorea as part of acute rheumatic fever has decreased markedly over the years from early reports of approximately 50 per cent of cases to more recent estimates at under 10 per cent.

Carditis. Forty to 50 per cent of patients with acute rheumatic fever will show evidence of carditis during the acute attack. This percentage is higher in areas of the world other than the North American continent. Carditis may involve endocardium, myocardium, or pericardium alone or in any combination. Although the entire endocardium may be inflamed, inflammation of the mural endocardium does not produce specific signs or symptoms. Inflammation of the valvular structures, however, often produces valvular malfunction characterized by turbulent blood flow and auscultatory murmurs.

The most frequent murmur encountered in acute rheumatic fever is that of mitral valve insufficiency. This murmur may be caused by inadequate approximation of the mitral valve leaflets owing to endocardial inflammation in the absence of myocardial inflammation or myocardial dysfunction. In that circumstance a murmur of mitral insufficiency would be present with a normal cardiac size and probably a normal cardiac rate. Myocardial inflammation, rheumatic or otherwise, may lead to left ventricular dilatation and dilatation of the mitral annulus, which is a separate factor responsible for incomplete closure of the mitral leaflets. In that circumstance one would expect tachycardia to be present. Viral myocarditis can masquerade as rheumatic disease in this manner.

The murmur of aortic insufficiency may be produced by valve inflammation, but not by ventricular dilatation. This murmur in conjunction with mitral insufficiency serves to substantiate the diagnosis of acute rheumatic fever but is present in fewer than 25 per cent of cases. It is extremely rare to encounter aortic insufficiency as the only murmur of acute rheumatic fever. In that circumstance the diagnosis should be suspected and bacterial endocarditis should be carefully considered. A mid-diastolic apical rumble may occur, sometimes transiently, in the acute phase of rheumatic fever. This murmur is indicative of mitral valve irregularity resulting from inflammation and is enhanced by the augmented flow across the mitral valve in mitral insufficiency.

In those instances in which carditis is clinically apparent as part of the acute rheumatic episode, it is usually observed within the first 7 days from the time of diagnosis of the disease. Evidence of myocardial inflammation is (1) tachycardia out of proportion to fever, (2) cardiac dilatation, and (3) congestive heart failure in severe cases. The myocardial inflammation of rheumatic fever cannot be distinguished from that of viral myocarditis. Signs of pericardial involvement are relatively infrequent and include a friction rub, clinical evidence of pericardial effusion, electrocardiographic changes of pericarditis or pericardial effusion, x-ray changes of pericardial effusion, and in rare circumstances pain associated with pericarditis. The pericarditis of acute rheumatic fever is not distinctive. It is exceedingly uncommon to have pericarditis as the only cardiac manifestation of acute rheumatic fever.

Arrhythmias may be encountered during the acute phase of myocarditis but are uncommon in children. Prolongation of the P-R interval occurs in approximately 40 per cent of patients with acute rheumatic fever but is not selectively distributed in those patients showing signs of carditis. Therefore, prolongation of the P-R interval cannot be used as evidence for carditis and of itself is not a major criterion.

Arthritis. Most patients with acute rheumatic fever present with joint complaints. Approximately 75 per cent of patients with acute rheumatic fever will display objective evidence of arthritis. The larger joints are most commonly involved, a distinguishing pattern from rheumatoid arthritis, which commonly involves smaller joints. The temporomandibular joint and the upper cervical spine are almost never involved in acute rheumatic fever. Knees, ankles, wrists, and elbows are most often involved. The fingers and toes are usually spared. The pain is severe and responds quickly to therapeutic levels of salicylates. Both the severity of the pain and the immediacy of response are valuable diagnostically in differentiating this disorder from others. The arthritis is migratory, usually involving a particular joint from 1 to 4 days. The migratory nature of arthritis in acute rheumatic fever may be masked by even suboptimal doses of aspirin. Of those patients with objective evidence of arthritis, between 25 and 40 per cent will show evidence of carditis during the acute attack. The involved joint is characteristically exquisitely tender, hot, red, and swollen. Pain on motion is usually so severe that the patient is quite apprehensive about examination.

Chorea. Chorea consists of spontaneous uncontrolled spasmodic movements that interfere with voluntary motor control, most commonly evident in the arms and face. Concomitant muscular weakness is present. Emotional lability and speech abnormalities coexist. Chorea may occur as a late finding during the acute phase of rheumatic fever or may occur in an isolated fashion without other criteria being present. In the latter circumstance the laboratory assessments, which will be subsequently described, may all be normal. Chorea is much more frequently seen in females than in males and has an unexplained association with the subsequent development of rheumatic mitral stenosis.

Erythema Marginatum. Erythema marginatum is an evanescent rash that occurs in a small percentage of patients and is usually on the upper extremities or upper thorax; the face is rarely involved. A serpiginous raised erythematous border surrounds an apparently uninvolved center. Shape and color change rapidly, so that the total duration of rash may be only several hours. A single lesion that remains unchanged for a 24-hour period is unlikely to represent this entity. The rash is nonpruritic and is most often seen during the initial phases of the illness. A hot bath is said to enhance observation of this phenomenon but perhaps reflects merely its enhancement of observation of children in the unclothed state. Erythema marginatum may be seen in conditions other than acute rheumatic fever.

Subcutaneous Nodules. Subcutaneous nodules appear later than arthritis and carditis during the acute phase of rheumatic fever and statistically are associated with patients who exhibit findings of carditis. These nodules are nontender, movable lumps that are usually quite firm. They may be found over the extensor surfaces of hinged joints and on the scalp. They range in size from 1 to 10 mm in diameter and are histologically observed to be composed of fibrinoid necrosis surrounded by connective tissue cells and lymphocytes. They disappear over a period of weeks to months.

Minor Manifestations. Fever has been previously discussed. It is an indicator of the magnitude of the inflammatory process.

Arthralgia without objective evidence of arthritis may indeed represent mild arthritis, but since arthralgia may have multiple causes, its significance is far less than that of arthritis. Elevation of the erythrocyte sedimentation rate and the C-reactive protein are discussed under Laboratory Findings. A prolonged P-R interval is not evidence for carditis, but it is of statistical significance in the diagnosis of acute rheumatic fever. Careful attention must be paid to a previous diagnosis of acute rheumatic fever without sequelae. Records of the episode should be obtained and reviewed. The presence of existing rheumatic heart disease should be carefully documented, as congenital heart disease may mimic this condition.

Other clinical findings that are not designated as minor manifestations include abdominal pain (which is uncommon, but may be severe), rheumatic pneumonitis, and epistaxis.

COURSE

Acute symptoms persist for a variable period of time that may be as short as 1 week and as long as 6 months or more. Usually, however, the duration of the acute phase of this disease is from 6 to 12 weeks. Persistent inflammation, when present, is usually cardiac. Permanent sequelae are limited to the heart with the exception of the extremely rare occurrence of Jaccoud's rheumatic arthritis of the metacarpalphalangeal joints. Whether the latter results from acute rheumatic fever is a disputed question. Death during the acute phase of the disease is extremely uncommon owing to improved methods for management of myocardial inflammation and congestive heart failure. Individuals with evidence of valve involvement during the acute phase will usually continue to exhibit evidence of valve abnormality as chronic rheumatic heart disease. One fourth to one third of patients exhibiting mitral insufficiency in the acute phase will lose this murmur within 10 years in the absence of recurrent acute rheumatic fever. Aortic regurgitation disappears less frequently. Mitral stenosis and aortic stenosis are late complications of rheumatic heart disease, taking years to develop. Involvement of the tricuspid and pulmonic valves is uncommon.

LABORATORY FINDINGS

The erythrocyte sedimentation rate (ESR) is elevated in almost every patient with acute rheumatic fever with the exception of those who present with pure chorea. The elevation usually lasts from 1½ to 3 months and may be shortened with treatment. The magnitude of abnormality of the ESR does not correlate with the presence or the magnitude of cardiac involvement in acute rheumatic fever. It does correlate, however, with the degree of tissue inflammation in general.

The C-reactive protein (CRP) fluctuates more rapidly than the ESR and often returns to normal more quickly when therapy is instituted.

Various antibodies against streptococcal products may be elevated during the acute phase of rheumatic fever. Commonly used antibody tests include antistreptolysin-O (ASO), antihyaluronidase (AH), and anti-DNAase B. Infection with group A beta-hemolytic streptococcus is likely to produce a measurable abnormality in any one of these titers 80 per cent of the time. Therefore, if any one test is used it will be about 80 per cent accurate; if two tests are used the accuracy will be over 90 per cent; and if three tests are used over 95 per cent. When two or more tests are employed, an abnormality in any single test is considered positive for the series.

Often a mild anemia is present. Gamma globulins are frequently elevated, as are alpha-1, alpha-2, and beta globulins. Serum haptoglobin is often increased as well. The serum glutamic oxaloacetic transaminase (SGOT) is elevated in an inconsistent manner. None of these abnormalities is specific nor consistent enough to be of importance in diagnosis.

Heart reactive antibodies may be studied by special techniques. However, they are not specific for acute rheumatic fever and are elevated in only approximately one half of the patients.

X-ray abnormalities are those of cardiac enlargement, pericardial effusion, pulmonary edema, or rheumatic pneumonitis.

Electrocardiographic abnormalities include first degree atrioventricular block, and evidence of pericardial effusion by voltage criteria or pericarditis by ST segment elevation and T wave abnormalities.

A throat culture positive for group A beta-hemolytic streptococci must be interpreted with the knowledge that from 12 to 20 per cent of asymptomatic grade school children will have such positive cultures. Whether this fact documents the carrier state or indicates the frequency of mild infection is a question of considerable debate.

PITFALLS AND DIFFERENTIAL DIAGNOSIS

Carditis. The carditis associated with acute rheumatic fever may be difficult to differentiate from acute viral myocarditis when the other four major manifestations of rheumatic fever are absent. When there is evidence of myocarditis alone, without valvular murmurs, the diagnosis of rheumatic carditis is unlikely except in the very young child. When there is little or no cardiac dilatation and the development of a mitral insufficiency murmur is noted, the diagnosis of valvulitis and thus rheumatic disease is highly probable. When there is cardiac dilatation and mitral insufficiency, the distinction between viral myocarditis and acute rheumatic fever may be difficult and will depend more heavily upon the presence of minor criteria and documentation of a preceding streptococcal infection. Aortic insufficiency with mitral insufficiency excludes viral myocarditis and is almost pathognomonic for acute rheumatic fever. Isolated aortic insufficiency is extremely uncommon in acute rheumatic fever and should raise the question of bacterial endocarditis. Cardiac manifestations of systemic lupus erythematosus, rheumatoid arthritis, and sickle cell anemia should be of secondary importance to other manifestations of those diseases.

Differentiation from congenital cardiac defects that produce mitral insufficiency may sometimes be difficult. The chronic nature of these conditions may be helpful, but all too often they are first discovered at the time of a sore throat, and the diagnosis of acute rheumatic fever is entertained. Such congenital cardiac lesions would include ostium primum atrial septal defect with mitral insufficiency, other endocardial cushion defects, congenitally corrected transposition of the great vessels with Ebstein's anomaly of the posterior atrioventricular valve, anomalous left coronary artery, and endocardial fibroelastosis. The latter diagnosis is usually evident in infancy and thus not confused with rheumatic fever.

Arthritis. The arthritis of acute rheumatic fever is most often confused with that of rheumatoid arthritis. Rheumatoid arthritis often has an onset prior to age 4, while rheumatic fever is very rare at this age. The differences in specific joint involvement have been described previously, as has their differing response to salicylate therapy. Rheumatoid arthritis is a chronic disease and is associated with muscle wasting. Often the spleen and lymph nodes are enlarged, and a macular rash different from erythema marginatum is present.

Systemic lupus erythematosus may closely mimic rheumatic fever in its involvement of the heart and the joints. The characteristic rash and nephritis, if present, serve to differentiate this disease.

Septic arthritis is most commonly unifocal, but when caused by gonococcus may involve several joints. Aspiration of the joint fluid may be helpful in isolating an organism or in documenting the presence of over 100,000 cells per ml, which would suggest infection.

Sickle cell disease, if considered, is readily diagnosed by the hemoglobin electrophoresis. The anemia may cause cardiomegaly and murmurs of the high output state. These murmurs associated with joint involvement might lead the unsuspecting to conclude that two major criteria are present.

Other conditions that affect the joints include serum sickness (often identified by associated angioneurotic edema or urticaria), post-infectious arthritis (following rubella, rubella vaccination, or other viral infections), Henoch-Schönlein purpura (which is often characterized by petechiae), traumatic arthritis, leukemia, and the arthritis of bacterial endocarditis.

Chorea. Chorea may be confused with tics or habit patterns, abnormal movements in Wilson's disease, drug reactions (particularly prochlorperazine), and Huntington's chorea.

GONORRHEA

By NICHOLAS J. FIUMARA, M.D.

Boston, Massachusetts

Although no groups of people are immune to this disease, gonorrhea, like syphilis, appears more commonly in metropolitan centers. Young adults 20 to 24 years of age have a higher incidence, followed by teenagers of 15 to 19. To date, the youngest boy reported with sexually acquired gonorrhea was 6 years of age. Gonorrhea is a ubiquitous disease and an attack confers no immunity to subsequent reinfections, often caused by the same untreated partner.

The organism of gonorrhea can be found in the genital tract, oropharynx, and anal canal. Thus the disease almost always is contracted sexually except for conjunctivitis and, occasionally, vulvovaginitis in preadolescent girls. Anogenital exposure may result in proctitis, and fellatio (orogenital contact) may cause pharyngitis. Transmission of this disease via toilet seats, bath towels, drinking glasses, and so on is but a face-saving myth.

The causative organism is *Neisseria gonorrhoeae*, commonly called the gonococcus. It is a gram-negative diplococcus of the genus Neisseria, to which belong also *N. meningitidis*, the other important human pathogen, and about 30 other species found in human and animal mucosa.

CLINICAL PICTURE

Symptoms can occur as soon as 1 day or as late as 2 weeks following sexual contact, and the average incubation period for males is 3 to 5 days. In the female it is difficult if not impossible to know when symptoms first begin, because about 75 per cent of infected females are asymptomatic in contrast to about 10 per cent of the males. The diagnosis of acute gonorrhea in the male presents little or no problem to the practicing physician. There is a history of sexual exposure within the prior 2 weeks. The earliest symptoms are uncomfortable sensations along the course of the urethra, followed by frequency of urination. By this time, the gonococcus has penetrated the columnar epithelium of the anterior urethra and has gone into the submucosa. An inflammatory response is triggered, manifested by a mucoid urethral discharge with dysuria. This is followed, usually in a matter of hours, by a purulent, dirty yellow urethral discharge. Constitutional symptoms, if present, are mild. The laboratory confirmation of gonorrhea in the male is relatively easy. There are no gram-negative diplococci normally present in the male genitourinary tract.

Laboratory confirmation is afforded by discovery of the gram-negative intracellular diplococci in the smears. This is practically 100 per cent sensitive and specific in acute gonorrhea in the male. However, very early in the course of the disease and in old untreated cases, the organism may be seen extracellularly. If the patient has taken penicillin or a broad-spectrum antibiotic within several hours of the smear examination (and many patients do), the gonococci will appear swollen and stain very poorly, making a laboratory confirmation by smear almost impossible. A male patient who has been exposed to a female with gonorrhea may be asymptomatic, yet a urethral smear and culture will be positive. He represents the male carrier. The incidence of male carriers is low, and in our experience is about 10 per cent of infected males.

In the female, acute gonorrhea involves the urethra, Skene's gland, Bartholin glands and the cervix; the vagina is never affected after the age of puberty. Symptoms are therefore referable to the structures involved. However, about 75 per cent of women have no subjective symptoms of infection, which is not too surpirsing when one considers that the carrier state is also seen with other Neisseria such as *N. meningococci*.

It is much more difficult to make the diagnosis in the female. The smear of the cervix is unreliable both in sensitivity — too few organisms — and specificity: false-positive gram-negative diplococci such as *N. flavescens* and *N. sicca* often are present. Thus the physician must rely on a culture to confirm the diagnosis. Specimens of pus for cultures should be taken from the urethra and cervix, not from the vagina. No lubricant should be used on the speculum or gloves, since surgical jelly often will kill whatever gonococci may be in the specimen. There is no contraindication to taking a cervical specimen during menstruation. The culture medium of choice today is the Thayer-Martin VCN medium, consisting of chocolate agar to which have been added vancomycin, colistin, and nystatin. These antibiotics will suppress the growth of all other organisms, including the saprophytic Neisseria. Minor modifications of the Thayer-Martin VCN plate are available on the market, such as the Transgrow bottle and Jembec. However, the Thayer-Martin VCN medium still is the best and it has a sensitivity of about 70 per cent. Physicians are advised to treat prophylactically all females who are sexual contacts of a male patient with gonorrhea pending the results of the culture. If the culture is positive, the diagnosis of gonorrhea is confirmed, but if the culture is negative, the patient's record is closed out as noninfection.

In addition to these problems peculiar to the genitourinary tract of males and females, other complications occur. Proctitis, when it occurs in males, almost always is a result of homosexual contact, but in women it may be caused by anal aspiration of the vaginal discharges as in defecation or from genitorectal exposures. The latter mode of spread is being seen more frequently, particularly among married women.

Pelvic Inflammatory Disease (Salpingitis, Parametritis)

Acute pelvic inflammatory disease (PID) develops 1 to 2 months following infectious exposure and occurs in 9 to 20 per cent of untreated females. It is an ascending infection from the cervix to the tubes. The risk of PID is less in patients with tubal ligation and more in those patients who use an intrauterine device (IUD). The disease may be gonococcal or nongonococcal on the basis of a positive or negative cervical culture.

The diagnosis of PID may be made when the patient complains of low abdominal pain with tenderness and spasm, pain on moving the cervix (chandelier sign), and adnexal tenderness. There may be fever, increased white blood cell count, and sedimentation rate. The differential diagnosis is that of a surgical abdomen (e.g., acute appendicitis, ovarian cysts, ectopic pregnancy, endometriosis, diverticulitis). Therapy should be initiated immediately, without waiting for the results of the cultures.

Disseminated Gonococcal Infection (Gonococcemia)

Disseminated gonococcal infection (DGI) occurs in 1 to 3 per cent of recently infected patients whose infective exposure occurred within the past 2 months. It is a disease principally of the female, with onset in the premenstrual period. It is also seen in pregnancy. The onset is abrupt, with chills, fever, pain in the joints, particularly the weight-bearing joints, and tenosynovitis, particularly of the wrists and fingers. The arthritis is nonsuppurative at this time. An eruption then appears on the acral areas: the hands, the feet, the fingers, and the toes. There is first an inflammatory macule, in the middle of which a vesicle develops, which rapidly becomes pustular and then purpuric. One should look for the inflammatory macules on the dorsum of the fingers particularly. Seldom are meningitis and endocarditis seen, but they may occur.

The diagnosis of DGI is confirmed by a blood culture taken, preferably during the chill phase, by a scraping from a skin lesion for smear and culture and by cervical culture in the female and urethral culture in the male. Interestingly enough, a number of the male contacts of these patients are infected asymptomatically.

Gonorrheal arthritis of the monopolyarticular variety may occur in 1 to 3 per cent of untreated patients and may be accompanied by tenosynovitis, particularly at the wrists or dorsum of the hands. It formerly was a disease principally of the male, but today it is seen more often in the female. The arthritis may be of two types. The first is the acute, painful type, characterized by swollen, hot, red joints, which, when tapped, reveal fluid under pressure. The fluid is purulent and loaded with gram-negative intracellular diplococci; the culture usually is positive, and the patient usually has symptoms and signs of gonorrhea. The second type involves painful joints with little or no swelling, no increased heat and, on aspiration, the joint fluid is not under pressure. There are few, if any, cells, but the smear and culture of the joint fluid are negative for the gonococcus or other organisms. Clinically, the patient has no subjective symptoms of gonorrhea; however, a cervical discharge is present that is positive by smear and culture for the gonococcus.

Gonococcal Pharyngitis

Gonococcal pharyngitis is seen often today. It always is the result of penile-oral (fellatio) exposure, not the result of kissing or cunnilingus. The examining physician may see three different types of throat effects. The first is the strep-like throat with diffuse erythema and edema with or without small punctate pustules in the tonsillar area. Next is the so-called viral throat, with patchy erythema and edema and minute pustules of the tonsillar area and uvula. The third type is the normal-appearing throat — the gonococcal carrier. In each instance, the diagnosis is established by culture and sugar fermentation or a direct fluorescent antibody test on the culture. It is my practice to take routine throat cultures on all prostitutes and homosexuals and others as indicated. Fortunately, gonococcal pharyngitis responds to the same treatment as cervicitis and urethritis.

Gonococcal Proctitis

Gonococcal proctitis is a result of penile-rectal exposure or in the female the aspiration of a gonococcal vaginal discharge into the rectum at defecation or contamination of the rectum with vaginal discharge either from wiping the anal area or from tight-fitting underclothes. Clinically, three symptom patterns may occur. The first is seen in the patient who walks with a wide gait, complaining of pain and swelling of the anal area and tremendous pain on defecation. On examination, the anal area is red and swollen and a purulent discharge can be readily seen extruding from the rectum. In the second type, the patient complains of pain on defecation with pus and blood staining of the underclothes. The third category of patient has no complaints and is a carrier. The diagnosis is established by obtaining a positive culture from a rectal specimen.

PENICILLIN-RESISTANT GONOCOCCI

Today, physicians need to be aware that the occasional patient with gonorrhea whose condition does not respond to penicillin therapy may be harboring a penicillin-resistant strain of gonococcus. Since January of 1976, beta-lactamase-producing gonococci have been found, particularly if the exposure and subsequent disease was acquired in the Far East, although since 1976 these strains of gonococci have been identified in most parts of the world. These strains contain a plasmid (which contains DNA) that secretes the enzyme that inactivates penicillin. Clinically, the disease is the same.

CHANCROID

By M. BRITTAIN MOORE, JR., M.D.
Lakeland, Florida

SYNONYMS

Soft chancre, ulcus molle, Ducrey's disease (infection).

DEFINITION AND PRESENTING SIGNS AND SYMPTOMS

Chancroid, the most common of the minor venereal diseases, produces, after a short incubation period, painful, tender, multiple superficial ulcerations in the anogenital region, associated with inflammatory regional lymphadenopathy. It is caused by the gram-negative Streptobacillus *Hemophilus ducreyi*, a

fastidious organism only as regards its growth requirements on artificial media.

CLINICAL COURSE AND PHYSICAL FINDINGS

One to three days after exposure, an exquisitely tender, small, painful, ragged ulceration appears (following an evanescent papule or pustule), most commonly just proximal to the glans penis, at the site of first entry of the Ducrey bacillus. By autoinoculation, multiple lesions often develop on skin and mucous membrane in direct apposition to the primary lesion(s). The ulcerations grow rapidly with undermining and coalescence and may encircle the penis at the coronal sulcus. Tender regional lymphadenopathy occurs within a week and is bilateral in up to 50 per cent of cases. Unilocular fluctuation develops several days later. Despite the severity of the local inflammatory disease, constitutional symptoms (low-grade fever, malaise) are rare.

Immunity does not develop well and reinfection is common. Reported cases are 20 to 50 times as frequent in males as in females, but it has been shown that women may harbor the organism as part of their vaginal flora for prolonged periods without symptoms.

COMPLICATIONS

If the condition is untreated or with delayed treatment, horrible, foul-smelling, phagedenic ulcerations and chronically draining, suppurative regional lymphadenopathy develop. Phimosis or paraphimosis is common, and urethral fistuli may develop when intraurethral lesions are present.

LABORATORY AIDS

With great difficulty, *Hemophilus ducreyi* can be grown on blood agar at 37 C (98.6 F) from material taken from beneath the undermined edges of ulcers. Smears from ulcers or lymph node aspirates stained with Gram or Wright stain may be helpful *if* the short gram-negative Streptobacillus can be found. It usually cannot and these studies are time consuming and disappointing. A much more helpful direct immunofluorescent staining procedure has been developed and should be used where available.

Years ago an intradermal skin test (Igo-Reenstierna) was used. Generally, it did not become positive before the third week of infection, thus limiting its usefulness in the fast-moving venereology practice of today in which acute conditions are treated immediately. The material for this skin test presently is not available commercially.

There is no serologic test for chancroid.

PITFALLS IN DIAGNOSIS (DIFFERENTIAL DIAGNOSIS)

The differential diagnosis includes granuloma inguinale, lymphogranuloma venereum, syphilis, and anogenital herpes simplex infection.

Granuloma inguinale is excluded by absence of pain and regional lymphadenopathy, as well as its diagnostic findings on biopsy. Lymphogranuloma venereum is excluded by absence of genital lesions at the time of presentation and by the character of the suppurative lymphadenopathy (unilocular in chancroid, multilocular in lymphogranuloma venereum).

Primary syphilis with multiple chancres can be ruled out by negative darkfield examination of *painful, non-indurated,* "dirty" chancroid lesions associated with *tender* lymphadenopathy as contrasted with indurated, nontender syphilitic chancres accompanied by rubbery, discrete, nontender satellite bubos. The serologic tests for syphilis detecting reagin (e.g., Venereal Disease Research Laboratory [VDRL], and rapid plasma reagin [RPR]), are reactive in only about 50 per cent of those with primary syphilis on first examination but will become reactive soon (and always within 1 month after appearance of primary lesion) if no antitreponemal therapy is administered.

Chancroid is most often confused with secondarily infected anogenital herpes simplex infection in which prompt erosion of the grouped vesicles occurred before the patient or examining physician saw them, or with primary herpes *without* secondary infection. After syphilis is excluded, a therapeutic test with tetracycline is reasonable. Before syphilis is excluded, sulfonamide therapy can be given without interfering with the diagnosis of syphilis.

Failure to recognize syphilis with multiple chancres is the most serious pitfall in the diagnosis of chancroid, and there is little reason for this to happen. Overdiagnosis of herpes infection as chancroid is of little consequence.

Incision and drainage of an abscessed lymph node for material for culture and sensitivity determinations should not be done, for chronic draining sinus tracts may persist despite adequate treatment. Material should be aspirated only through a needle inserted through normal adjacent skin (preferably above the node).

Chancroid is almost never seen in a circumcised male and, for all practical purposes, rarely occurs in anyone with good hygiene. As our standard of living has improved, the incidence of chancroid has decreased and the relative frequency of its most common differential diagnostic problem, genital herpes simplex infection, has increased.

WHOOPING COUGH

By JAMES W. BASS, M.D.
Washington, D.C.

SYNONYMS

Pertussis, chin cough, tosferira (Spanish), Keuchhusten (German), coqueluche (French), and pertoss (Italian).

DEFINITION

Whooping cough is an infection of the respiratory passages characterized by prolonged and protracted episodes of cough, usually ending in an inspiratory whoop. Greater than 95 per cent of cases are caused by *Bordetella pertussis* and less than 5 per cent by *B. parapertussis,* with *B. bronchiseptica* an even rarer cause of the disease. Recent studies have also etiologically implicated certain adenoviruses alone or in concert with *B. pertussis* organisms. Whooping cough is highly contagious with attack rates from 80 to 100 per cent in susceptible household contacts. The disease confers a fairly high degree of lasting immunity. Immunization produces relative protection, most field trials showing 70 to 80 per cent reduction in attack rate in vaccinees. This lasts only 2 to 3 years with declining protection thereafter and little or no evidence of protection after 12 years. Although the incidence of the disease has declined dramatically over the past few decades, a small number of cases have still been reported annually throughout the United States. The case fatality rate is now less than 1 per cent in this country; however, this disease is still a serious threat to young infants under 6 months of age. Most deaths occur in the 2 to 3 month age group. Whooping cough is still a major cause of sickness and death in developing countries throughout the world where broad-scaled immunization against the disease has not been achieved.

PRESENTING SIGNS AND SYMPTOMS

After an incubation period of 10 days (range, 5 to 16) the disease presents as a simple cold with nasal stuffiness, clear mucosal discharge, and a cough. This is referred to as the "catarrhal" stage and usually lasts 6 to 7 days. It may on some occasions persist up to 2 weeks, whereas in others it may be so mild as to even go unrecognized.

COURSE

The cough of the catarrhal stage worsens, and the subsequent clinical course of the disease varies depending upon age. Violent paroxysms of cough occur, numbering from only several to numerous bouts daily. This "paroxysmal" stage of the disease lasts from 1 to 3 weeks, but usually averages about 2 weeks in duration. In infants under 6 months these severe paroxysms of cough are usually so exhausting as to leave the infant limp, cyanotic, and apneic; death may occur if resuscitation measures are not immediately instituted. The characteristic whoop is seldom heard in these small, weak infants. In older, stronger infants and preschool children, the cough is usually followed by the classic inspiratory whoop which most often leads to the diagnosis. Schoolage children and young adults may simply have severe paroxysmal coughing bouts without a whoop. The "convalescent" stage of whooping cough consists of a persistent occasional cough for an additional 3 to 4 weeks, the whole illness then lasting a total of several weeks. *Formes frustes* of whooping cough do occur, with the entire illness so modified as to resemble only a mild cold with an occasional cough.

PHYSICAL EXAMINATION

Pertussis organisms are not invasive beyond the ciliary border of the tracheobronchial mucosa, so that fever does not occur unless complications develop. Thick tenacious nasal and tracheobronchial secretions cause nasal obstruction and sometimes choking episodes if aspiration occurs. These, along with frequent bouts of severe paroxysmal cough, often produce numerous facial petechiae, primarily around the eyelids and cheeks and on the neck. Conjunctival and scleral hemorrhages may be extensive. Epistaxis is common. When the disease is severe, there may be puffy edema of the face, most pronounced in the periorbital tissues. Laceration of the frenulum of the tongue may develop as a consequence of repeated protrusions of the tongue against the lower incisors with cough paroxysms. Scattered coarse wet rales and rhonchi are commonly heard; fine moist rales are not heard unless pneumonia complicates the disease. Vomiting occurs frequently at the termination of severe cough paroxysms. In small infants, this may lead to dehydration and metabolic alkalosis with tetany. Weight loss and malnutrition may develop if the course is protracted.

COMPLICATIONS

High fever seldom occurs unless complications ensue. Atelectasis, bronchopneumonia, and otitis media are the most frequent complications. Convulsions may occur in small infants, with severe and persistent paroxysmal bouts of cough complicated by cyanosis and apnea. They may occur at any time during the course of illness but are more commonly seen in the earlier paroxysmal stage. A transient hemiplegia (Todd's paralysis) may follow these seizures when they are severe. Convulsions followed by lethargy progressing to coma are an ominous sign; should recovery occur, prominent neurologic residua are often seen.

LABORATORY FINDINGS

The white blood cell count with differential smear is a most helpful diagnostic aid. An absolute lymphocytosis is usually observed, with the total white cell count often above 20,000 cells per cu mm and the differential smear showing greater than 60 to 70 per cent small mature lymphocytes. Lymphocytic leukemoid reactions with counts varying from 50,000 to 125,000 per cu mm are most often seen in association with severe complications. In younger infants, particularly those under 6 months of age, the characteristic lymphocytosis of whooping cough is frequently absent. The erythrocyte sedimentation rate is normal or, more frequently, low. Should it become elevated, a secondary complication should be suspected. The chest x-ray may show hilar peribronchial infiltrates, producing the "shaggy heart" appearance characteristic of whooping cough. Lobar atelectasis, particularly involving the right upper lobe, as well as a patchy segmental atelectasis occurs commonly. Fluffy alveolar infiltrates diagnostic of secondary bacterial pneumonia develop in about 10 per cent of children with the disease.

Most large medical centers and state laboratories can now quickly confirm the presence of *B. pertussis* organisms by the use of fluorescent antibody staining. Smears are made from posterior nasopharyngeal swabs of patients suspected of having the disease, and these can be tested by skilled technicians in a few minutes. Fluorescent antibody staining is more sensitive than culture and often remains positive even after effective antibiotic administration has cleared the patient of viable organisms. Best results in the culturing of *B. pertussis* organisms are achieved utilizing calcium alginate nasopharyngeal swabs smeared directly onto fresh Bordet-Gengou medium containing 20 per cent sheep's blood. Characteristic, small pinpoint metallic-like colonies with a mercurial sheen are first noted after 72 hours or more incubation at 37 C. Swabs taken from the oropharynx and cough plate specimens yield less reliable results. The nasopharyngeal smear for fluorescent antibody (FA) studies and culture is usually positive within the first 1 to 2 weeks of illness. Organisms disappear thereafter, and these tests are seldom positive after 3 to 4 weeks.

PITFALLS IN DIAGNOSIS

The most common pitfall in the diagnosis of whooping cough is the frequent absence of the whoop in infants under 6 months of age and in the older child and adult, causing the clinician to fail to suspect the diagnosis. Another is the misconception that immunization confers protection against the disease. Vaccine protection is relevant and declines considerably with time, so that prior immunization does not preclude the diagnosis of whooping cough in a patient otherwise suspected of having the disease.

GRANULOMA INGUINALE

By THOMAS W. JOHNSON, M.D.

Nashville, Tennessee

SYNONYMS

Granuloma venereum, Donovanosis, ulcerating granuloma of the pudenda, granulomatosis, infective granuloma, sclerosing granuloma, granuloma contagiosa, chronic venereal sores.

DEFINITION

Granuloma inguinale is a chronic ulcerogranulomatous disease caused by the microbacillus *Donovania granulomatis*, also referred to as the Donovan body. Although the disease is worldwide in its distribution, it is more common in tropical and subtropical areas. The frequency of cases of this disease is low. Primary manifestations of the disease involve the genitalia in a majority of patients, and the disease is generally considered to be one of low contagiousness.

PRESENTING SIGNS AND SYMPTOMS

The incubation period of granuloma inguinale may vary from 8 days to 4 months with an average of 14 to 50 days. The majority of patients are in the age group from 20 to 45 years, although the disease has been reported in infants and children. The incidence is greater in males than in females.

The initial lesion is a solitary, plane, flat-topped papule or subcutaneous nodule of the skin or mucous membranes and occurs on the external genitalia in over 90 per cent of the patients. Extragenital lesions, when present, usually represent sites of autoinoculation from primary lesions of the genitalia and most commonly involve the lips, oral cavity, face, neck, upper trunk, posterior aspects of the hands, and the digits. Direct orogenital contact may also account for the presence of extragenital lesions. Pain is not a prominent symptom of the primary lesion, which breaks down within a few days of its initial occurrence to yield a shallow, well-demarcated ulcer with a rolled edge and a vivid, pink base of granulation tissue. Extension of the lesion may occur by contiguity through advancement of the border of granulation tissue or by autoinoculation in satellite or more distant locations with eventual coalescence of lesions. The lesions may undergo spontaneous arrest or continue to spread slowly, especially in warm, moist intertriginous areas. Eventually, untreated or inadequately treated lesions progress to marked atrophic, depigmented scarring. The intervention of secondary infection complicates the course of the lesions and increases the possibility of systemic complications and debility.

CLINICAL COURSE

With the exception of the primary lesion, which rapidly sloughs to form a shallow, well-demarcated ulcer, the course of granuloma inguinale is characterized by a slow, progressive spread of granulomatous tissue. Spontaneous arrest of the spread can occur, or the lesions may continue a destructive course for many years. Superinfection of the lesions may occur with fusospirochetal organisms with resultant acceleration and accentuation of the destructive process. Lymph node involvement, although not characteristic of granuloma inguinale, can occur with the formation of indurated swellings or fluctuant abscesses (pseudobuboes) that eventually rupture and add to the ulcerative process. Hematogenous dissemination of the organisms is rare.

PHYSICAL EXAMINATION

The initial lesion tends to occur on the external genitalia of the male and on the labia, clitoris, and fourchette in the female. Characteristically, the lesion is a solitary, plane papule or subcutaneous nodule that breaks down in a few days to form a shallow, well-demarcated ulcer with a pink, velvety base and rolled edges of granulation tissue. A serosanguineous exudate is present. Four clinical types of granulation tissue are seen: (1) Nodular — pink to beefy red, well-defined, exuberant granulation tissue. (2) Ulcerovegetative — the most frequently observed type. Extension occurs by contiguity or by the formation of satellite papules and nodules that eventually ulcerate and coalesce with the parent lesion. Serpiginous borders are characteristic, and the formation of deep scars may occur. (3) Hypertrophic — formation of large, granulomatous lesions. (4) Cicatricial — rapidly forming areas of fibrosis are interspersed among areas of ulcerations. Secondary keloid formation may occur as well as hypo-and depigmentation.

COMMON COMPLICATIONS

The most common complication of granuloma inguinale is superinfection with fusospirochetal organisms. A rapidly spreading, destructive ulceration covered by a foul-smelling exudate results. Interference of the lymphatic drainage from extensive genitoinguinal scarring may result in pseudoelephantiasis of the external genitalia, particularly in females. In males, penile destruction and deformities may occur. Cicatricial narrowing of the urethra, vagina, and anus may also occur. Squamous cell carcinomas of the penis, vulva, and cervix may develop, particularly in those instances in which the disease has a protracted course.

LABORATORY FINDINGS

Slide Preparations. It is essential that the clinical diagnosis of granuloma inguinale be confirmed by demonstration of the causative organisms, the Donovan bodies, in smear preparations. This is best done by obtaining a small specimen from the granulation tissue at the border of an ulcer, crushing the specimen between two clean glass slides, and then smearing the specimen on the slides by rubbing the slides together as they are separated. Smears can also be made from a punch biopsy by smearing the undersurface of the specimen on a slide prior to placing the specimen into a fixative solution. Slides should be air dried and then stained by Gram, Giemsa, Wright, or pinacyanole stain. Giemsa stain is preferred. Donovan bodies are rod-shaped microorganisms that can usually be demonstrated in the large mononuclear cells found in the granulation tissue. They occur individually or in clusters, have a bipolar appearance owing to the concentration of chromatin material found at both ends, and may contain a well-developed capsule. Morphologically and antigenically (based on capsular antigens) they closely resemble Klebsiella sp. By Gram stain, the organisms are gram-negative; by Giemsa stain, the organisms are red. Wright-stained organisms are bluish to deep purple surrounded by a pink capsule; with pinacyanole stain, they are blue-black with a pink capsule. Material aspirated from pseudobuboes can also be used for staining purposes.

Biopsy. Because of the possibility of squamous cell carcinoma occurring at the site of lesions of granuloma inguinale, a biopsy is recommended. As stated previously, the biopsy specimen is suitable for the preparation of a smear prior to essential fixation for histopathologic processing. The histopathology reveals an absence of the epidermis in the center of the lesion with acanthosis at the border of proportions sufficient for it to be called pseudocarcinomatous hyperplasia. A dense infiltrate is present in the dermis, composed predominantly of histiocytes and plasma cells. Scattered throughout this infiltrate are a small number of lymphoid cells. Donovan bodies are present within a variable number of histiocytes. Donovan bodies are best demonstrated by Giemsa or silver stain.

Culture. Culture is generally not a useful, practical means of isolating the organisms because of the need for special enriched medium under strict cultural conditions.

PITFALLS IN DIAGNOSIS

In spite of the apparent decreasing incidence of granuloma inguinale, the disease must be considered as a diagnostic possibility in the presence of chronic ulcerogranulomatous processes. This is particularly significant if the lesions involve the genital, genitoinguinal, or perineal areas. Syphilis, chancroids, and lymphogranuloma venereum, in particular, must be considered on a differential basis as well as tuberculosis (ulcerative type), streptococcal and phagedenic ulcers, and squamous cell carcinoma. Clinical impressions must be confirmed by laboratory identification of the causative organisms.

DIPHTHERIA

By EDWARD B. SHAW, M.D.

San Francisco, California

Diphtheria was recognized in antiquity and in 1826 was given the name of diphtherite by Bretonneau. For many years in the past it was known as the "curse of childhood."

ETIOLOGY

The specific cause, *Corynebacterium diphtheriae*, is a gram-positive slender rod that is best recognized with methylene blue, Albert stain, or others that reveal polychromatic bands or granules not apparent in the Gram stain. In smears from cultures, the organisms are arranged in somewhat geometric patterns, "Chinese letters." Pathogenicity is not revealed by morphology, for other corynebacteriae have identical appearance but do not produce the powerful toxin that is responsible for illness and death. Curiously, these nontoxigenic strains may be rendered toxin producers by the addition in the laboratory of a specific phage that is present in toxin producers, but apparently this does not happen spontaneously in nature.

The organism is lacking in invasive properties and is essentially a surface saprophyte; it is rarely found in deeper tissues or blood cultures except agonally. Exposure is probably effected by hand-to-mouth contact from another patient or a carrier. Initially the organism develops on a speck of necrotic tissue or desquamated epithelium. There it produces its toxin that destroys surrounding tissues and affords the opportunity for local extension and finally for the production of more toxin for local and systemic damage and the spreading pseudomembrane.

The organism may set up its effect in numerous locations but is most commonly in the tonsillopharyngeal area. In this typical localization the throat may at first be mildly reddened and then a few spots of yellowish exudate may appear. During the next 24 hours or so these affected areas spread, coalesce, and form a dense pseudomembrane that is tightly adherent to underlying structures. If it is forcibly removed, bleeding will follow. As this membranous process extends, it first covers the tonsils and the pillars, then extends to the posterior pharynx and to the soft palate and uvula, the anterior extension being quite characteristic of diphtheria. Along with this advancing inflammation the adjacent tissues become extremely edematous, sometimes, especially in adults, almost obscuring the membrane, At the same time the cervical glands are swollen, but especially the surrounding soft tissues may be greatly swollen to produce the classic "bull neck." When this tremendous swelling is mistaken for a peritonsillar or cervical abscess and incised, the result is almost invariably fatal because of increased access of toxin to the circulation. In late stages the child develops a fetid breath, but this is evidence that should not be awaited for diagnosis.

Initially the child often does not appear to be very ill and convulsions, common to many other serious infections, are infrequent. The temperature is often not very greatly elevated, the pulse is often increasingly rapid, out of proportion to the rise in temperature, but all of these symptoms are quite variable and never should be insisted upon for the diagnosis. With progression the serious nature of the illness becomes apparent with extreme prostration and evident toxemia. Curiously, even with advanced disease the child may complain very little of sore throat.

DIFFERENTIAL DIAGNOSIS

Most younger pediatricians, and for that matter many older faculty members, have never encountered a case of diphtheria. For this reason the clinical evidences of this disease should be strongly impressed in teaching. Today most diphtheritic patients are at first thought to have infectious mononucleosis or beta-streptococcal infection, but these conditions are characterized more by purulent exudate than by a pseudomembrane. Some of the virus infections of the oral cavity, such as those of herpesvirus or coxsackievirus, will sometimes be confused by the inexpert. Often in smears from the affected areas spirillae and fusiform bacilli may be present. These organisms were believed to be the cause of "Vincent's angina," but they usually have very little to do with oral infection and are common to any necrotic process in the mouth, including advanced diphtheria. I have seen diagnostic problems presented by secondary syphilis, leukemia and other blood disturbances, and during treatment of malignancy.

In children the inexorable course of the disease is crescendo for 4 or 5 days, at which point therapy becomes much less effective and the disease ends in death or slowly in recovery. Late complications may occur during recovery. Early treatment with antitoxin often leads to rapid regression. In adults the course may be somewhat more protracted and marked edema of the tonsils and palate may be more impressive than the extent of visible pseudomembrane; the profound edema may somewhat obscure the pseudomembrane.

With progression of the local disease the patient becomes increasingly ill; exudate and edema may cause respiratory obstruction. Death in the untreated case usually occurs on the fifth to the eighth day and is due to respiratory obstruction or to the mounting effects of the toxin on the heart and circulation, the adrenals, the kidneys, and the nervous system. Numerous complications may occur up to 6 or 8 weeks after recovery, whether or not treatment has seemed immediately to be effective.

OTHER FORMS

Tonsillopharyngeal diphtheria is the classic form of disease, and when the pseudomembranes occur elsewhere they are also tightly attached to underlying structures.

Nasal diphtheria was formerly common and characterized by obstruction of one or both nares, with a serous and sometimes bloody discharge, which could be mistakenly thought to be caused by a foreign body; sometimes a foreign body constitutes the initial insult, producing the lesion on which the organisms are implanted. These organisms are toxigenic but for some unexplained reason in this location there is little or no evidence of toxemia. This form of disease was previously important in transmission of virulent organisms such as in schoolroom epidemics.

Nasopharyngeal diphtheria, when the exudate occurs high in the nasopharynx and is not readily seen, may be difficult to diagnose and is sometimes manifested by extraordinary toxemia and high mortality.

Laryngeal diphtheria was previously called true croup or membranous croup. We then spoke of true croup and false croup; the former was diphtheria of the larynx and the latter was spasmodic croup that occurs in very young children, usually in the early hours of the eve-

ning. At this time there was little knowledge of epiglottitis caused by *H. influenzae* and all infections from *H. influenzae* were less frequently encountered than at present. When laryngeal disease occurs in older children and adults it is an extension of diphtheria of the tonsils and pharynx. I have seen it follow infection of the post-tonsillectomy slough that resembles the diphtheritic pseudomembrane, the disease being recognized only when it spread to the larynx. Although this form of infection usually complicates infection of the tonsils and pharynx, it can occur in children of 6 months to 2 years of age; primarily these patients may have no exudate in the tonsillar area.

Laryngeal localization begins with hoarseness and a brassy, croupy cough that advances in 2 or 3 days to increasing respiratory obstruction, loss of voice, and finally the unmistakable appearance of the child who is indifferent to everything except his agony in breathing. Because of the small diameter of the infant larynx, a very small amont of exudate and edema can be a disastrous impediment to respiration.

In early times it was customary to treat small children with any suspicion of this illness promptly with antitoxin to avoid the horrendous methods then in use to provide an airway. The O'Dwyer tube, designed to fit within the larynx, was available in different sizes for different ages. This tube was inserted blindly, which was very difficult to accomplish; sometimes the larynx was irreparably damaged by an inexpert operator. In addition, the child might cough up the tube at any time, leaving him with even more severe laryngeal obstruction. This form of treatment was succeeded by the almost universal use of tracheostomy, which provided an airway to the trachea below the level of the obstructed larynx.

Today this form of obstruction will usually be treated with an endotracheal tube. This does have a disadvantage: if the child coughs up some of the exudate that separates after treatment with antitoxin, this may block the tube and lead again to obstruction. This form of diphtheria demands early recognition and a maximum dose of antitoxin. With this treatment it is unnecessary for any form of artificial airway to be left in for more than a very few days.

OTHER LOCATIONS

1. Somewhat rarely, the diphtheritic pseudomembrane will occur in the conjunctivae.
2. The newborn is usually protected by transplacental globulin from the mother, although a few severe infections have occurred in the umbilical stump or the circumcision wound.
3. Wounds may be infected, especially in

cases in which there is a large area that is healing slowly; the cause may not easily be detected.

4. The vulva and vagina may be the site of infection.

5. Skin infection has been troublesome in tropical geographic areas, localizing in an area of scratch or abrasion and producing a more or less impetigo-like lesion that has a prolonged course and is sometimes followed by the late complications due to toxin.

LABORATORY FINDINGS

Routine laboratory studies are not especially helpful. There is usually moderate leukocytosis. The urinalysis may show some increase in protein, especially in advanced and more toxic cases. Toxic damage to the kidney occurs but postinfectious glomerular nephritis does not follow. As the disease progresses, the electrocardiogram will reveal myocardial changes indicating the severity of involvement of the heart muscle and conduction system.

Material for detection of *C. diphtheriae* should be collected by a swab inserted slightly underneath the margin of an area of membrane. Direct examination of the smear requires a great deal of skill and often leads to errors. Cultures are far more reliable but involve a delay of 12 to 24 hours before there is sufficient growth on special media to permit microscopic examination. Special culture media have been devised to indicate something of the nature of the organism that grows. Cultures cannot instantly establish that an organism isolated is a toxin producer, but in the presence of clinical symptomatology the morphology of the isolate should be accepted as corroborative. Management based purely on sound clinical judgment should not be derided.

The *Schick test* was originally devised to show that the patient had an adequate amount of antitoxin in his blood. This was first proposed when it was customary to give daily doses of antitoxin until there was definite clinical improvement—this is now thought unnecessary because a very large initial dose of antitoxin is employed. As originally devised, this test was supposed to show that the patient had been given adequate antitoxin to control his disease; at the present time it is indicative of the presence of antitoxin in the patient from whatever source. The Schick test consists of the intradermal injection of diluted diphtheria toxin in an amount of one fiftieth minimum lethal dose (MLD). The result of this cannot be determined in less than 48 hours and is more reliable after 96 hours, when an area of extreme inflammation and induration constitutes a positive reaction, indicating the *absence* of antitoxic immunity. This test is of value for detecting the success of immunization but is of no use for guidance during the treatment of the disease. This test has largely been abandoned, because the success of toxoid immunization is trusted, and most physicians prefer to give a booster dose of immunizing toxoid instead of testing resistance by means of the Schick test. It is unfortunate that this test is no longer available, for it not only indicates the presence of immunity but, more importantly, indicates the capacity of the patient to respond to an antigenic stimulus.

COMPLICATIONS

In the acute course of the disease the patient often shows evidence of seriously affected heart muscle; this may be the cause of death. Severe cardiac complications may also occur after the local process has subsided, with or without treatment. The cardiac symptoms may become very severe after 1 or 2 weeks, with softening of the first sound, loss of the diastolic pause, and a tic-tac rhythm to the heart sounds. The electrocardiogram may show bizarre evidences of disturbances of conduction that may be a late cause of death. (Years ago it was a custom to refer to the patient who temporarily recovered only to succumb to the late effects of the toxin as "recovered from the disease but died from the treatment!") Late in the convalescent course there may be severe neurologic damage with involvement of the vagus nerve that may also produce abnormalities of the heart action. In advanced toxic cases late cardiac damage may be very severe. In the ultimate course the degree of recovery in those who survive very severe cardiac damage may be amazingly complete.

The neurologic complications of diphtheria are numerous. Fairly early in the acute phase the patient may develop a nasal voice, regurgitation of fluids through the nose, and difficulty in swallowing. This is apt to be worse on the side on which there has been more membrane in the throat. The latency of neurologic damage may be extreme and may first appear only 4 to 6 weeks after the acute disease in the patient with pharyngeal palsy, evidence of extremity weakness, loss of tendon reflexes, foot drop, and paralysis of the diaphragm and intercostal muscles leading to respiratory failure. (It is of interest to remember that the tank respirator, later extensively employed in treating poliomyelitis, was initially designed for use for postdiphtheritic respiratory paralysis.)

Very late, after 6 weeks or more, ocular paralyses of various types may appear, principally loss of accommodation to near vision. All these forms of late neurologic damage may be minimal or extensive, particularly in those with a long, untreated course, such as the extensive skin lesions that were encountered in war time and went unrecognized for a long time. With extensive muscular weakness the spinal fluid may show a definite increase in protein so that such patients have often been diagnosed, perhaps even entirely correctly, as having the Guillain-Barré syndrome. Complete recovery is the rule in neurologic complications unless they are immediately fatal. Rarely are there such prolonged residua as loss of tendon reflexes, foot drop, or nasal voice, but there are some exceptions.

THE CARRIER STATE

Healthy carriers of the organism, who are themselves insusceptible, were formerly a source of infection to others, but this means of spreading diphtheria has become less important because of widespread immunization. In those who have had the disease the organism may remain in the nose and throat for many weeks. The antitoxin will arrest the progress of the disease but will not eliminate the organism. Antitoxin disappears from the patient's circulation after a very few weeks, but some patients have been known to have a second attack only a few weeks after the initial one, the antitoxin having disappeared and the organism remaining in the tonsils and pharynx. The disease is not always followed by immunity and some who have had the disease earlier may develop it again in later life. The organisms have usually disappeared after about 3 weeks but this may take a great deal longer.

Antibiotics are quite inappropriate for treatment of the disease, for which only antitoxin is effective, but generous doses of penicillin or erythromycin accelerate the disappearance of organisms and terminate the carrier state. Tonsillectomy was formerly recommended for prolonged carrier states but immediately after this operation the area was so sensitive that cultures sometimes were not adequately taken. Public health regulations require isolation until two successive cultures are negative for the organism, but often the inept physician will get his patient out of quarantine much more quickly than the one who takes cultures with more care.

Before the introduction of antitoxin into therapy, the death rate from diphtheria was 40 to 50 per cent. In the huge epidemics of the 1880's it may have been much greater than this. With the use of antitoxin early in this century the death rate dropped to about 10 per cent. With the introduction of immunization of children, the morbidity and mortality have steadily declined, although about 200 cases are reported annually in the United States, emphasizing the need for universal and complete immunization.

It is worthy of emphasis that the physician who is unaware of the criteria for the diagnosis of diphtheria and does not include this disease in his differential diagnosis of throat infections risks losing the only such patient he may ever encounter.

TETANUS

By WESLEY FURSTE, M.D.,
and GEORGE W. PAULSON, M.D.
Columbus, Ohio

SYNONYM

Lockjaw.

DEFINITION

Tetanus, a severe and dreaded infectious complication of wounds, is caused by the toxin-producing *Clostridium tetani*. This disease is characterized by tonic spasms of the voluntary muscles, by a tendency toward episodes of respiratory arrest, and over the entire world by a mortality rate of about 50 per cent. Although tetanus is uncommon in developed countries, the World Health Organization estimates that about 1,000,000 tetanus deaths, including about 900,000 from neonatal tetanus, occur per year throughout the world.

ETIOLOGIC AGENT

C. tetani is a ubiquitous, large, motile, anaerobic spore-forming, gram-positive bacillus without a capsule. It is an obligate anaerobe and can be cultivated on artificial media in the absence of atmospheric oxygen. Characteristic spherical terminal spores are produced, which are highly resistant; if protected from direct sunlight, they can survive for many years. Tetanus spores are often present in the intestinal contents of man and animals and have been found in soil and street dust in many parts of the world. Under suitable conditions of growth, *C. tetani* elaborates a powerful exotoxin. Following invasion by the specific microorganism and

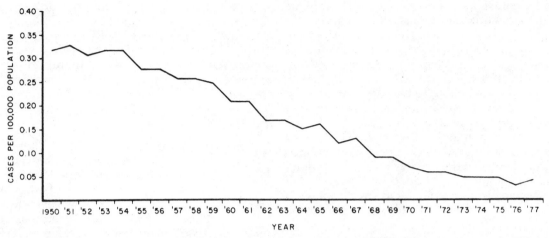

Figure 1. Reported cases of tetanus per 100,000 population by year. United States, 1950–1977. (From: MMWR Annual Summary 1977. Center for Disease Control, Atlanta.)

production of the specific neurotoxin, the central nervous system is altered with hyperexudation. Tetanus is thus a toxi-infection, being neither simply a toxic state nor solely an infection.

PATHOGENESIS

  C. tetani is carried into human tissues by contamination of a wound. A variety of lesions, both large and small, may offer a suitable haven for growth: lacerations, compound fractures, gunshot wounds, septic abortions, and lesions produced by nails, slivers, and human and animal bites. For example, tetanus with death resulted when a 49-year-old woman was bitten by a pet rooster. Cases have been due to the use of unsterile surgical supplies and unsterile biologic materials. Infections of the postpartum uterus and the umbilical stump (tetanus neonatorum) were once common but now can be rare with proper tetanus toxoid immunization of the mother and with aseptic obstetric techniques. Cultural habits can be important etiologic considerations; the practices of rubbing the umbilical cord with dirt or dung, piercing of earlobes, or, in the United States, "skin popping" of contaminated heroin, may be responsible for tetanus. *C. tetani* is so ubiquitous in the human environment that almost any contaminated wound may contain the organisms; hence tetanus may occur wherever man is living.

  The mere fact that *C. tetani* is present does not necessarily mean that the patient has tetanus or that he will develop it. In a wound, the organism will proliferate only in the presence of an oxidation-reduction potential far lower than that existing in normal living tissue. Once the organism begins to grow, it produces an exotoxin. This neurotoxin is known to block release of

inhibitory amino acids, such as glycine; although peripheral synapses can be affected, the major effect is to produce central disinhibition with increase in reflex excitability of all spinal efferents.

PRIOR HISTORY OF PATIENTS SUSPECTED OF HAVING TETANUS

  The amount of the very potent tetanus necessary to produce tetanus is so small that it will not incite an active antibody level high enough to prevent a second attack of tetanus. Consequently, tetanus is a nonimmunizing disease; hence a history of tetanus does not rule out the possibility of a second attack of tetanus.

  If a patient has had a traumatic wound during the previous days or few weeks, tetanus should be considered. In these days of numerous auto-

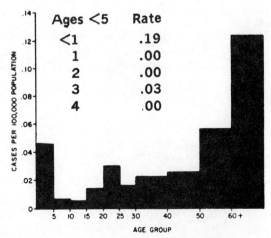

Figure 2. Reported cases of tetanus per 100,000 population by age group, United States, 1977. (From: MMWR Annual Summary 1977. Center for Disease Control, Atlanta.)

mobile collisions, burns, occasional airplane crashes, and other accidents, deep wounds are caused in which tetanus toxin can be produced. Tetanus has occurred as a complication of wounds of all sizes, including lacerations, compound fractures, burns, abrasions, and even hypodermic injections. Not uncommonly tetanus may develop in a neglected or forgotten trivial wound considered by the patient not important enough to require a visit to the physician and may even occur in persons in whom a wound of entry of the organism cannot be demonstrated. Since many patients with tetanus will not have an obvious wound and since tetanus is a toxic state, a diagnosis can be made in the absence of cultural proof.

The incidence of tetanus caused by contaminated catgut or surgical instruments has fortunately become very low. Rarely tetanus has occurred after operations on the intestinal tract, which has been a source of the etiologic *C. tetani.*

Definite proof that a wounded person has previously had adequate tetanus toxoid immunization is reassuring and — according to follow-up studies on World War II veterans — just about eliminates the possibility of tetanus if a booster dose of tetanus toxoid is given to a wounded patient. The efficiency and safety of tetanus toxoid as a prophylactic agent were proved by the World War II experiences of the United States Army. Twelve cases of tetanus occurred in a series of 2,734,819 hospital admissions for wounds and injuries for an incidence of 0.00044 per cent. Of these 12 patients, only 4 had been given adequate basic immunization plus emergency stimulating toxoid injections.

Unfortunately, not all civilians have adequate active tetanus immunization; hence, if wounded, they may develop tetanus. For example, data from the Center for Disease Control indicate that during the past 13 years only about three of four children in the 1 to 4 year age group have had three or more injections for diphtheria, tetanus, and pertussis (Fig. 3).

INCUBATION PERIOD

The incubation period may be as short as 1 day or as long as 54 days. Prognosis is generally better when the incubation period is longer. The longer incubation periods are particularly likely to occur when the patient has received partial protection from human or equine antitoxin or when secondary surgical revision or manipulation of wounds, especially war wounds, is performed. Rarely, when a scar of a wound has of necessity been surgically explored, tetanus has occurred many years after the time of the primary wound.

CLINICAL MANIFESTATIONS

The disease almost always appears in a general form (Fig. 4), but may occasionally appear as local tetanus. Uncommon in man, local tetanus may start in the muscles near the infection, probably because of the path of ascent of the neurotoxin, or in the facial muscles, particularly if the ear or jaw is the source. With local tetanus, usually sooner or later, general symptoms occur, but then the disease is likely to be milder and less often fatal than the general type usually seen.

In the familiar general form, the earliest indications of tetanus infection usually become evident from 1 to 2 weeks after injury. The severity

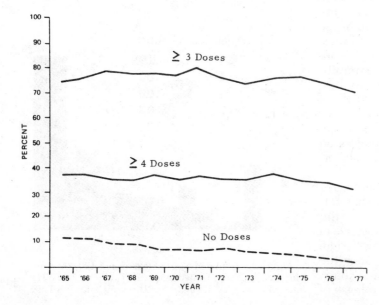

Figure 3. Diphtheria–tetanus–pertussis immunization status of 1- to 4-year-old children, United States, 1965–1977. (From United States Immunization Survey: 1977. Center for Disease Control, Atlanta.)

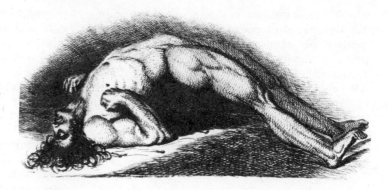

Figure 4. Opisthotonos as illustrated in London in 1865 in Sir Charles Bell's *Anatomy and Philosophy of Expression.* (Courtesy of the National Library of Medicine.)

of the clinical picture and the mortality rate are roughly inversely proportional to the duration of the incubation period.

Some patients have prodromal symptoms of restlessness and headaches. In others, the first symptoms are those stemming from the developing muscular rigidity, with vague discomfort in the jaws, neck, or lumbar region. At an early stage, spasm of the muscles of mastication causes trismus and difficulty with chewing, i.e., lockjaw. Sustained contraction of the facial muscles produces a distorted grin (risus sardonicus). Figure 4 demonstrates risus sardonicus and carpopedal spasm as well as opisthotonos. Spasm of the pharyngeal muscles makes swallowing difficult. Stiff neck and opisthotonos are also among the early signs. Progressively, other muscle groups become involved, with tightness of the chest and rigidity of the abdominal wall, the back, and the limbs. Generalized tonic convulsions are frequent and exhausting. Any sudden jar or sound, such as a hypodermic injection or the fall of a broom outside the patient's door, will excite such generalized convulsions. Generally speaking, touch or position change is more likely to trigger the convulsions than is stimulation by light or sound. In association with these convulsions, spasm of the laryngeal and respiratory muscles is present, sometimes with a resulting respiratory arrest and possibly fatal acute asphyxia. Respiratory complications are the most common cause of death; and, in neonatal tetanus in particular, the inability to swallow and aspiration can lead to a rapid demise.

The patient is mercilessly mentally clear throughout the course of the disease and he suffers great pain from the muscular spasms. The pulse rate is elevated and there is profuse perspiration. Vegetative disturbances including increased or decreased blood pressure and even respiratory irregularities can originate from the effects of the toxin on the medulla, but the major neurologic findings are hyperactive reflexes, clonus, and the stimulus-sensitive myo-

clonus or spasms. Sensory changes are absent. Fever may or may not be present.

If the patient survives, the intensity of the muscular contractions begins to diminish during about the second week. Even with adequate treatment, improvement may be slow; contractions can continue for over a week. Complete recovery may take several months.

Occasionally, mild cases occur in which there is only moderate muscle rigidity without tetanus seizures. The administration of tetanus antitoxin to a person who has not had tetanus toxoid prophylaxis before injury may forestall the development of severe tetanus and may result in development of only a mild tetanus or a local tetanus involving only the muscles around the site of injury.

Even when treatment is adequate, the mortality rate may be 50 per cent or higher. Older children and younger adults respond better than infants, younger children, and older adults. Most deaths occur within 10 days of the onset of the illness. Patients who live as long as a week and a half have good prospects of complete recovery.

LABORATORY DATA

The diagnosis of tetanus must be based on the clinical picture, for laboratory examinations are of little assistance. The demonstration of *C. tetani* in a wound does not prove the diagnosis of tetanus; the failure to demonstrate the organism in a wound does not eliminate the possibility of tetanus. The urine is normal unless secondary urinary tract infection occurs. Tetanus itself produces a slight elevation in the leukocyte count, but secondary infection may produce greater elevation. The cerebrospinal fluid is often under increased pressure, but it is otherwise not remarkable. There may be an increase in serum creatine phosphokinase (CPK) that roughly parallels the severity of the muscle tonus. Electromyograph studies, so useful in peripheral neuropathic conditions and Guillain-

Barré syndrome, are of little value in tetanus. Electroencephalograms may be useful in estimating the extent of cerebral involvement, especially in patients who have had hypoxia. The activity recorded on electroencephalograms is not specifically diagnostic of tetanus, but serial electroencephalograms at the proper time during the course of the disease may be of considerable importance in the long-range evaluation and care of the patient and in respect to liability problems.

COMMON COMPLICATIONS

Complications and death in early tetanus are almost solely due to respiratory difficulty and can often be avoided by adequate control of the muscle spasms. Pulmonary atelectasis may be followed by pneumonia, which is especially to be dreaded, for it seriously lessens the chances of recovery. Traumatic glossitis is seen frequently. Compression fractures of the vertebrae may result from the convulsive seizures. Decubitus ulcers are likely to occur in patients under heavy sedation. Constipation, fecal impaction, and urinary retention are often encountered. Cystitis and pyelonephritis may develop in patients requiring catheterization. One to three weeks after the administration of heterologous equine or bovine antitoxin, serum sickness may occur. If homologous human antitoxin (tetanus immune globulin [human]) is given, such sickness will not occur. Foot drop and muscle contractures may follow prolonged unconsciousness with the limbs in poor position. Asphyxia from respiratory or laryngeal muscle spasm or from aspiration of secretions, vomitus, or food may be the immediate case of death.

DIFFERENTIAL DIAGNOSIS

Other toxic states rarely mimic tetanus; strychnine poisoning is the classic example. Whereas spasms tend to persist in tetanus, the muscles are relaxed between seizures in strychnine poisoning, and this toxic state can clear rapidly. Rabies is indicated by the patient's inability to swallow as an early symptom, by drooling of saliva, and by spasms of the muscles of deglutition. Hypocalcemia, especially in the neonate, may produce rigidity but usually not the severe sensitivity of tetanus. Tetany when related to parathyroid dysfunction is rarely severe and may affect only the upper limbs. The laboratory will clarify these problems. The remarkably common acute dystonic reaction secondary to phenothiazines can be diagnosed by history as well as by the rapid response to treatment. Toxicity secondary to penicillin or haloperidol may produce a tetanus-like condition. Heterologous serum sickness can be confused with early tetanus.

In addition to such toxic problems, infectious states can produce some increased tone, particularly meningitis or encephalitis. In these conditions tremor or myoclonus can also occur, but they usually have more cerebral involvement than tetanus and can be diagnosed by cerebrospinal fluid examination.

Local infections of the jaws or tumors and infections of the oropharynx will rarely lead to diagnostic confusion. Growth of a primary or secondary tumor is rarely missed, although we have seen one patient with severe trismus due to pressure of a large craniopharyngioma on the trigeminal region.

The spasms of a localized group of voluntary muscles caused by soft tissue or bone injuries may simulate local tetanus.

Hysteria or malingering can be confusing in all branches of medicine. One unusual patient presented such a picture to remain near a ward nurse and be with her, particularly at night. In such cases, the electroencephalogram can be of value. Hyperventilation syndrome, with concomitant carpopedal spasm, is usually brief and readily identified. The rigidity of parkinsonism, Jakob's disease, or the "stiff man" syndrome will not be confused with tetanus because of the long course and distinctive clinical pattern in each of these entities.

Neonatal tetanus, though uncommon in developed countries, may be confused with many serious conditions of the neonate, such as meningitis, sepsis, hypocalcemic tetany, hypomagnesemia, metabolic alkalosis, and intracranial hemorrhage. Newborns of drug-addicted mothers may temporarily present a clinical picture suggesting tetanus.

While diagnostic efforts are under way, the response of the spasms to adequate therapy will help not only with diagnosis but with prognostication. This toxi-infection must first be suspected to be diagnosed and may appear when least suspected.

TYPHOID FEVER

By R. L. HUCKSTEP, C.M.G., M.D.,
F.R.C.S., F.R.A.C.S.
Sydney, Australia

INTRODUCTION

Typhoid fever in the 1980s is still epidemic in many of the developing countries of the world, and epidemics also occur in North America, Europe, and other economically rich countries, usually where a carrier has infected a static water supply, ice cream, or some other food. In March 1973, for instance, 65 confirmed cases were reported near Miami, Florida from contaminated well water.

Two large epidemics of typhoid fever occurred in the 1960s in Zermatt in Switzerland and in Aberdeen, and many other epidemics have been reported from Europe and North America since then. They have caused consternation, as the United States, Switzerland, and Britain have supposedly high standards of education and hygiene and pure water supplies. The World Health Organization figures for 1976 reported 384 cases from the United States, 7001 from Italy, 2092 from Spain, 1935 from Mexico, 8746 from Algeria, 3633 from Sri Lanka, 7469 from Chile, and many thousands of new cases from other parts of the world. When it is realized that only a fraction of all new cases of typhoid are diagnosed or reported, and that for each new case there are many asymptomatic carriers, it will be apparent that the problem is a huge one. It will remain so until a protective vaccine is developed that is considerably better than the present typhoid, paratyphoid A, and paratyphoid B (TAB) vaccine, which gives relatively incomplete protection.

Over 20 cases in the Aberdeen epidemic alone occurred among people who had had previous TAB vaccine inoculation. This indicates even more the importance of maintenance of high standards of hygiene as the first line of defense and reinforces the statement about the relative lack of value of TAB vaccine. The drug that is still the first choice in treatment (chloramphenicol) is potentially dangerous, while the disease has still an appreciative mortality, even when treated adequately and well. The asymptomatic carrier is difficult both to trace and to treat, and an epidemic such as the one in Aberdeen, with well over 400 confirmed cases, is bound to leave both known and unknown carriers in its wake.

The diagnostic criteria given in this chapter are based on a series of over 1300 typhoid cases that I treated in East Africa from 1954 to 1972. Nine hundred and seventy-five of these patients were documented, and much of the material in this article is the result of investigation of these cases, most of which has been already reported in the monograph entitled "Typhoid Fever and Other Salmonella Infections."

CLINICAL DIAGNOSIS (Fig. 1)

During an epidemic the problem of diagnosis is simplified. Many isolated cases of typhoid, however, still occur each year, as just mentioned, in the United States, Britain, and Europe, and these cases may be misdiagnosed, especially if mild or asymptomatic.

Typhoid fever and the paratyphoid fevers may present identical diagnostic problems, and the clinical and laboratory pictures are similar in most respects.

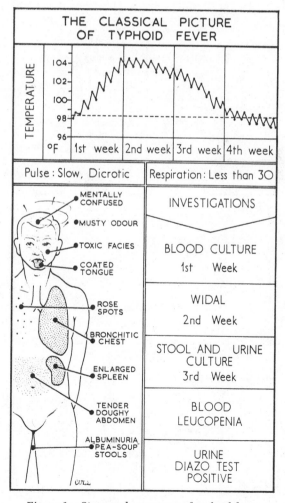

Figure 1. Signs and symptoms of typhoid fever.

The severity of an attack of typhoid depends not only on the dosage and virulence of the particular organism but also on the resistance of the patient and the stage of the disease at the time treatment is started. Epidemics undoubtedly vary, and those occurring in the developing countries of the world tend to be more severe, possibly because of the combination of a more virulent strain of organisms, larger doses of bacteria, late diagnosis and treatment, and low resistance of patients.

Symptoms (Fig. 2)

The symptoms of typhoid fever may be very variable and range from a completely asymptomatic patient, only diagnosed on routine stool culture, to an extremely virulent and rapid onset of a disease very much like a severe salmonella gastroenteritis.

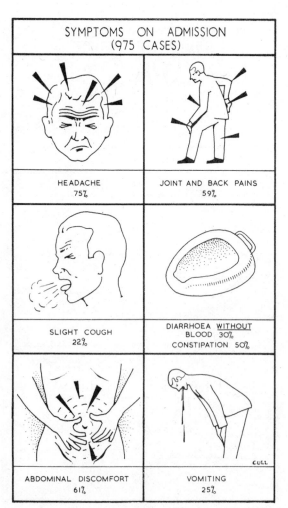

SYMPTOMS ON ADMISSION
(975 CASES)

HEADACHE 75%	JOINT AND BACK PAINS 59%
SLIGHT COUGH 22%	DIARRHOEA WITHOUT BLOOD 30% CONSTIPATION 50%
ABDOMINAL DISCOMFORT 61%	VOMITING 25%

Figure 2. Some of the varied symptoms of typhoid fever seen on admission.

A good clinical history is essential, and this may be difficult to obtain if the patient is mentally dull or confused. Delirium and mental confusion are particularly likely to occur in patients who are seen relatively late in this disease.

The incubation period is usually from 10 to 14 days, but it may vary from 7 to 21 days, and sometimes in even less than 7 days. In the Aberdeen outbreak the first two students to be affected became ill after an incubation period of only 5 days. In the case of the paratyphoid fevers the incubation period is shorter than in typhoid.

A history of exposure to a likely infected source is important, as in the case of a recent trip to a country with endemic typhoid such as Spain, Italy, or Mexico. Infected water, milk, and ice cream are still the most important worldwide sources of infection despite the epidemics in Britain caused by contaminated meat from South America.

The insidious onset helps to differentiate typhoid from influenza, gastroenteritis, acute bronchitis, malaria, and bacillary dysentery. In children the onset tends to be much more sudden, and the diagnosis is therefore more difficult. Massive infection in adults may also cause an acute onset similar to that seen in influenza or gastroenteritis.

General malaise, anorexia, and lassitude early in the disease are almost invariable symptoms, and they tend to be longer-lasting than in many other conditions. Headache is common, usually occurring within the first 2 days, and is generally dull and continuous rather than acute.

Vague abdominal discomfort is an early symptom and very common. Vomiting tends to be mild and not sustained. Constipation occurs more frequently than diarrhea, but if diarrhea does occur it is nearly always without blood, a useful point of differentiation from bacillary dysentery. Diarrhea plus vomiting is rare in typhoid but common in gastroenteritis.

Mild joint pains and backache are common, but the joints are *not* swollen except following the rare complication of typhoid arthritis, in which case the pain is not usually severe. A dry cough is common but tends to be slight unless a complication has supervened. Epistaxis sometimes occurs and varies from epidemic to epidemic.

General Signs (Fig. 3)

Superficially the typhoid patient has a dull, expressionless, lethargic face, which is typical of very few other diseases except typhus. The patient, however, can sometimes be roused into

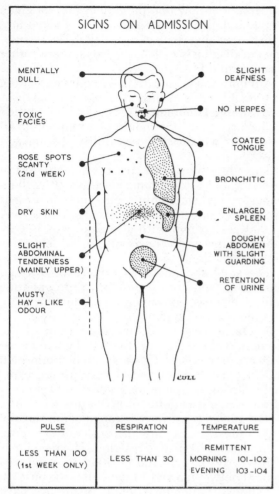

SIGNS ON ADMISSION

MENTALLY DULL

TOXIC FACIES

ROSE SPOTS SCANTY (2nd WEEK)

DRY SKIN

SLIGHT ABDOMINAL TENDERNESS (MAINLY UPPER)

MUSTY HAY – LIKE ODOUR

SLIGHT DEAFNESS

NO HERPES

COATED TONGUE

BRONCHITIC

ENLARGED SPLEEN

DOUGHY ABDOMEN WITH SLIGHT GUARDING

RETENTION OF URINE

PULSE	RESPIRATION	TEMPERATURE
LESS THAN 100 (1st WEEK ONLY)	LESS THAN 30	REMITTENT MORNING 101–102 EVENING 103–104

Figure 3. Admission signs. The so-called "toxic facies" is typical of few other diseases.

a state of mental alertness that is often belied by an inaccurate history. The mental state may vary within the wide limits of normal mentality through muttering delirium to frank mental confusion, but rarely violence.

The cheeks are usually flushed and the eyes bright during the first week of illness. In the second and third weeks the expression becomes dull, the pupils dilated, and the skin and lips dry.

Other signs on general examination, which may be of value, are a dry skin, a lack of marked coughing or sputum, the absence of a crop of vesicles due to herpes simplex, and the presence of a rather musty odor. The patient often shows a rather indefinite state on admission that can best be described as "toxic."

Slight deafness is common during the first week and may become more marked in later stages of the disease.

Rose spots usually occur between the seventh and tenth day of illness. Each spot lasts for 3 to 4 days and then disappears completely. The spots may continue to appear for another 1 to 2 weeks. The spots are rose-colored, slightly raised, and fade on pressure. They occur mainly on the abdomen and chest and occasionally on the back, upper arms, and thighs. The spots usually number less than 12 in typhoid but are more numerous in the paratyphoids. Their presence and number bear no relation to the severity of the attack. They *can* be seen on a black skin despite teaching to the contrary, and a drop of oil will make them easier to see.

SPECIFIC SIGNS

1. Pyrexia. Fever varies greatly in typhoid, and the classic temperature pattern may be present only in the untreated and uncomplicated cases. The classic chart in the untreated case shows a stepladder rise during the first week with an evening rise of about 2 F (1.1 C) and a morning fall of about 1F (0.55 C). Toward the end of the first week the temperature usually reaches about 104 F (40 C), and during the second week the evening temperature is about 103 to 104 F (39.4 and 40 C) with a morning temperature of about 101 to 102 F (38.3 to 38.8 C).

The pyrexia in the third week in an uncomplicated case begins to fall in much the same way as it rose, i.e., a fall of 2 F (1.1 C) in the morning with a rise of 1 F (0.55 C) in the evening. There are many other temperature patterns, and this may lead to difficulty, especially if the patient is seen late or a complication has set in. A sudden rise at an early stage of the disease may be due to a complication such as typhoid lobar pneumonia, and a sudden fall may be seen in the later stages of the disease or after a complication such as sudden intestinal hemorrhage or perforation. A low pyrexia may occur in mild cases or occasionally in older patients. In the paratyphoid fevers the pyrexia tends to be lower than in typhoid. A rise in pyrexia in convalescence may be due to a relapse or a complication.

The temperature after treatment with chloramphenicol usually shows a drop to normal in about 4 days, but there is a latent period during the first 2 days when very little alteration is noted.

Thus, it can be seen that the temperature pattern in typhoid may be deceptive. In the typical uncomplicated case, however, it can be a very useful clinical sign, especially when correlated with other diagnostic criteria.

2. Respiratory System. In the majority of cases the respiration rate is from 20 to 30 per minute. It is rare to find a rate of over 30 per minute in adults, which is a useful differential diagnostic sign from lobar pneumonia.

A bronchitic chest is a common finding, and 56 per cent of my patients presented with this. This finding may vary from a few rhonchi to a frank acute bronchitis. It may be of considerable diagnostic value, especially when correlated with the typical abdominal findings of typhoid fever, and together these constitute the two most valuable diagnostic signs.

3. Cardiovascular System. The pulse rate is classically described as a bradycardia. A better description, however, is that the pulse rate is relatively slow compared with the temperature during the first week of illness and it seldom exceeds 100 per minute. It also tends to be dicrotic. In children and in severe cases the pulse rate may be much more rapid, even during the first week of illness.

4. Gastrointestinal System. The tongue may be dry and coated on admission. In severe cases it may be covered by a brown fur on the dorsum with a marked diminution of saliva, especially during the second and third weeks in an untreated patient.

The abdominal signs of most value are a combination of slight upper abdominal tenderness in the liver and splenic regions, while a tender palpable spleen may be a valuable positive finding in countries where hypersplenism is uncommon. There is often slight guarding and generalized tumidity of the abdomen similar to the "doughiness" of tuberculous peritonitis, and moderate abdominal distention is common in the second and third weeks of illness.

5. Central Nervous System. There is often some mental dullness in typhoid, although this may not be present in mild cases of paratyphoid.

Meningism may be seen at an early stage of the disease, sometimes mimicking a true meningitis. There may be neck retraction, photophobia, and severe headache, which gradually regresses as the ordinary signs of typhoid develop. Meningism is particularly common in children.

6. Skeletal System. Joint, muscular, and back pains may be complained of by the patient on admission. Clinical examination, however, is usually negative.

7. Genitourinary System. Apart from retention of urine, which may occur in the early stages, there are no early signs attributable to the genitourinary system.

INVESTIGATIONS

1. Simple Ward Tests. The stool in typhoid should always be inspected. The "pea soup" stool of the classic papers on typhoid fever is less frequent now that purgatives are not given in typhoid, but it should always be looked for.

Blood in the stool early in the illness indicates a diagnosis of bacillary dysentery rather than typhoid fever.

Albuminuria is an extremely common finding in typhoid but is of little diagnostic value.

2. Simple Laboratory Tests. The blood slide for malarial parasites should be examined in all cases in which the possibility of malaria exists.

The white blood cell count is a useful test in typhoid, and a low count with a relative lymphocytosis is commonly seen. The converse is much truer, and a white blood cell count of over 10,000 per cu mm with a leukocytosis is very much against a diagnosis of enteric fever, except in children.

The stool specimens examined for ova and entameba may be useful in differentiating schistosomiasis and amebiasis from the more chronic forms of typhoid in endemic areas.

3. Diazo Test of Urine. The froth of the urine of typhoid patients turns red when mixed with diazo reagents. This test can be performed quickly in the ward and is very useful, especially during an epidemic. Eighty to 90 per cent of the typhoid patients in my series who were tested gave a positive reaction at some stage of their illness, while only 5.7 per cent of control patients gave a positive reaction. The reaction is particularly likely to be positive in a pyrexial patient between 5 and 14 days after the onset of the illness. Laboratory details of the test have been described elsewhere.

The diazo reaction is particularly useful when the blood has been sterilized by chloramphenicol or the Widal reaction invalidated by previous TAB vaccine inoculations. It has definite limitations but is a quick screening test in countries where typhoid is widespread and particularly where laboratory facilities are scarce.

4. Culture of the Typhoid Bacillus. Culture of the typhoid bacillus is the only sure method of making the diagnosis of typhoid fever.

A blood culture may be positive at any stage of the clinical illness, particularly during the first week. Chloramphenicol usually sterilizes the blood within 2 hours, and it is therefore important to take a blood sample before chloramphenicol is started.

Blood clot culture, however, has been shown to be positive more often than whole blood culture, and it may remain positive several days after the administration of chloramphenicol.

Stool culture is not positive as often as blood culture. It is, however, a valuable diagnostic test, and several stool specimens should always be cultured. Contrary to the usual teaching, it is often positive before the third week of illness and may be positive at any stage of the disease.

Urine culture is not positive as often as stool culture, and then only after the second week of illness. Culture of pus from abscesses and postmortem culture will occasionally yield a positive result when other results have been negative.

5. Agglutination Tests. The diagnostic value of the Widal reaction has been diminished by the widespread use of TAB vaccination. In an unimmunized patient it does not become positive until after 7 to 10 days of illness.

In an endemic area, or in patients who have had previous TAB vaccine inoculations, the H antibody level can be raised by many nonspecific illnesses and therefore yields little specific data. The O antigen agglutination is of much more value, and an O antigen agglutination of 1:200 in a patient with a rising titer and a pyrexia clinically resembling typhoid is very suggestive of typhoid but is not diagnostic. In patients in nonendemic areas who have not had previous TAB vaccine, the Widal reaction is of much greater value.

DIFFERENTIAL DIAGNOSIS

Typhoid fever may be confused with a large number of diseases. In the United States and Britain the diagnosis is particularly liable to be missed in isolated cases, while in the tropics many conditions may resemble typhoid fever.

1. Paratyphoids A, B, and C. The laboratory is usually required as the final authority. The paratyphoids tend to run a milder course with profuse rose spots. Geographic distribution sometimes simplifies the matter; the paratyphoids are rare in East Africa, but paratyphoid B is not uncommon in Britain.

2. Salmonella Infection and Gastroenteritis. Salmonellae, the dysentery group, and staphylococci may occasionally cause an invasive illness that resembles typhoid fever with bacteremia. Usually, however, the gastrointestinal symptoms are more acute than the general manifestations and the pyrexia much lower and of shorter duration.

3. Other Disease in Differential Diagnosis. There are many other conditions that may mimic typhoid fever. A careful history and examination, with the aid of the laboratory when necessary, will often resolve the difficulty.

Malaria may be mistaken for typhoid in countries where both are endemic, but a history of previous attack, the more rapid onset, the shivering and sweating, the high early pyrexia, the relative infrequency of abdominal symptoms and signs, and a positive blood slide all point to a diagnosis of malaria.

Influenza may also be confused with typhoid, but it is usually of much more rapid onset, with high temperature, severe sore throat, cough, and the absence of a palpable spleen and rose spots.

Bacillary dysentery seldom causes much difficulty in diagnosis. The onset is usually acute, with severe bloody diarrhea, although in mild cases the blood may be absent. Diarrhea with blood is rare in early typhoid. The signs and symptoms in dysentery are usually abdominal and remain so, the mental state and chest being clear.

Typhus and other rickettsial infections are important to consider in the differential diagnosis, as both typhus and typhoid can cause a febrile illness with delirium, chest signs, and abdominal discomfort. In typhus, however, the onset is acute and the temperature high at an early stage. Shivering attacks are common at the onset, and prostration is rapid. The rash is quite different (brownish red in color and much more profuse) and does not fade on pressure as does the rose spot in typhoid. There is a leukocytosis, and the Weil-Felix test becomes significantly positive at about the tenth day.

In economically poor countries pulmonary tuberculosis and atypical abdominal tuberculosis are probably the most difficult diseases to differentiate from typhoid fever. The pyrexia and vague symptoms and signs may be very similar, and an x-ray of the chest or laboratory confirmation of typhoid may be the only sure method of diagnosis.

Brucellosis may cause difficulty, but the onset tends to be more insidious, the patient is alert, and a painful joint is frequently present. Trypanosomiasis in endemic areas should also be considered in the differential diagnosis.

The other diseases that enter the diagnostic field are too numerous to mention individually. Suffice it to say that there are few conditions that cannot mimic, or be mimicked by, typhoid fever.

TYPHOID AS A COMPLICATION
(Fig. 4)

Typhoid itself may first present as a complication such as typhoid pneumonia, meningitis, orchitis, nephritis, or abscess. An acute abdominal emergency may prove to be a perforated ileum in an otherwise unsuspected case of typhoid fever.

COMPLICATIONS

There are many complications in typhoid fever, and it may sometimes be difficult to differentiate between a complication and the

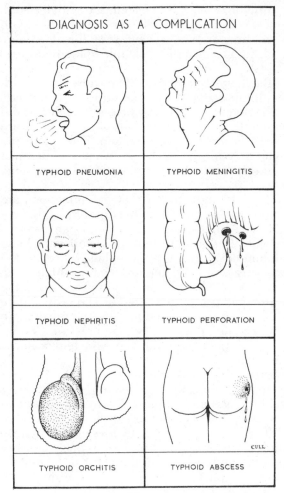

DIAGNOSIS AS A COMPLICATION

TYPHOID PNEUMONIA

TYPHOID MENINGITIS

TYPHOID NEPHRITIS

TYPHOID PERFORATION

TYPHOID ORCHITIS

TYPHOID ABSCESS

Figure 4. Typhoid fever as a complication.

natural course in so variable a disease. Complications are often associated with the gross toxemia and prostration of the disease and are especially common if nursing care is inadequate.

1. General Complications. The general complications include typhoid abscesses, boils, bed sores, otitis media, Zenker's degeneration of muscle, severe mental confusion, deafness, severe dehydration, and tonsillitis.

The importance of typhoid abscesses is that they are often missed, as they tend to be deep in the buttocks. They may, however, be superficial and present exactly like boils.

Zenker's degeneration of muscle is rare, but it may affect other muscles besides the classic site of rectus abdominis.

Mild deafness is common, but severe inner ear deafness is rare. Other complications are mainly due to intercurrent infection or difficulties of nursing in a debilitated patient.

2. Medical Complications. The medical complications include acute bronchitis and frank typhoid lobar pneumonia, toxic myocarditis, venous thromboses, hemolytic anemia, acute typhoid nephritis, typhoid meningitis, and peripheral neuritis.

Acute bronchitis is so common that it should be considered as a manifestation of the disease itself rather than as a complication. Typhoid lobar pneumonia presents with the typical symptoms and signs of lobar pneumonia except that "rusty" sputum is uncommon and the white blood cell count low; it responds well to chloramphenicol.

Myocarditis is extremely common, particularly in the very toxic patient. The cardiac muscle is affected, even in convalescence, and this is shown by a rapid deterioration of the cardiovascular system in a relapse or after administration of a general anesthetic.

Typhoid meningitis, which is rare, must not be confused with meningism, which is common. Mild hemolytic anemia is fairly common in the very toxic typhoid patient. A marked degree is rare, and the mortality rate is high.

Febrile albuminuria is common, but a true acute typhoid nephritis rare. Peripheral neuritis and "tender toes" should be treated with large doses of vitamin B complex, which should also be given in typhoid fever as a prophylactic measure.

3. Major Surgical Complications. The major surgical complications of typhoid fever may include parotitis, intestinal perforation and hemorrhage, acute cholecystitis, paralytic ileus, orchitis, pyelitis, cystitis, retention of urine, empyema, arthritis, and osteomyelitis.

Intestinal perforation may be associated with peritonitis. This is one of the most serious complications of typhoid and rarely occurs before the third week of illness. Diagnosis may be difficult, and many of the usual symptoms are masked by the general toxic state of the patient and by local adhesions around the leakage. In many cases, especially in the very sick, the first indication of perforation may be the presence of free fluid, either generalized or localized, with deterioration of the condition of the patient, absent bowel sounds, and vomiting. Sometimes the classic signs of perforation will occur, but deterioration in the general condition is always rapid.

Intestinal hemorrhage may be a very serious complication of typhoid fever; it usually occurs from 14 to 21 days after the onset of the illness and is often "silent." The patient may bleed small amounts from several areas, or there may be a massive silent hemorrhage, and the first evidence may be a shocked patient with very pale conjuctivae.

Typhoid cholecystitis, like cholecystitis due to other organisms, occurs more frequently in women than in men. Diagnosis may be difficult because of the upper abdominal tenderness that is often present in typhoid fever.

Paralytic ileus may be secondary to a perforation or primary to a severe toxemia. Intestinal obstruction may be due to a localized abscess or adhesions.

Typhoid orchitis usually occurs in convalescence, while acute pyelitis is more common than is generally recognized. Typhoid arthritis and osteomyelitis are uncommon, and a true typhoid spine is rare and a late complication. Infection of bones due to other salmonellae, however, such as *Salmonella typhimurium*, is common, especially in sickle cell anemia.

CONCOMITANT DISEASES

In tropical countries concomitant diseases such as bacillary dysentery, malaria, amebiasis, and worm infestations are common. They should always be borne in mind, as they may confuse the diagnosis.

TYPHOID FEVER IN CHILDREN

The incubation period in children tends to be shorter and the onset more acute than in adults, and in some cases the disease simulates a gastroenteritis due to other causes. The child often, but by no means invariably, has a less severe attack than the adult, with pyrexia settling earlier. Complications tend to be less common, but when they do occur they usually progress more rapidly. Dehydration and mineral loss may be particularly severe.

TYPHOID FEVER IN PRIMITIVE CONDITIONS

Despite the publicity given to outbreaks in the United States, Britain, and Europe, the problems associated with them are trivial compared with the rest of the world. Most cases occur in countries in which hygiene is poor, equipment and trained medical and nursing staff are extremely short, and transportation to hospital is sometimes nonexistent.

Diagnosis must be made mainly on clinical findings plus simple tests such as a low blood cell count and the diazo test for urine. Confirmation is obtained from a single specimen of clotted blood that can be used for both culture and the Widal reaction, while a culture of feces in glycerol will allow for delay in transport of the specimen. Finally, in doubtful cases, a therapeutic test with chloroquine for malaria, peni-

cillin for pneumonia, and sulfaguanidine for bacillary dysentery may be unscientific but is essentially practical.

THE CARRIER

The screening of all patients, suspects, and contacts is essential in countries in which adequate medical facilities exist. Three, and preferably 6, negative stool and urine cultures and a negative Vi antigen test of blood should be the minimum requirements before a proved case of typhoid is discharged from hospital.

THE PARATYPHOID FEVERS

The paratyphoid fevers A, B, and C resemble typhoid fever and usually, but not always, run a milder course. *Salmonella paratyphi*, however, requires a medium in which to multiply, and meat pies, synthetic cream, and milk are the usual vehicles for this. Paratyphoid fever resembles other nonspecific salmonella infections in this respect, and paratyphoid B may occasionally also have an onset similar to Salmonella gastroenteritis. Despite this, paratyphoid fever is primarily an invasive type of disease like typhoid fever.

Paratyphoid A, however, is less likely to cause complications than typhoid fever but is more likely to relapse. Paratyphoid B, which is common in Europe, is milder than typhoid but is more likely to result in carriers and to cause jaundice, thromboses, and suppurative lesions. Paratyphoid C differs clinically from typhoid fever and the other paratyphoids by causing more septicemic manifestations such as arthritis, cholecystitis, and abscesses, with little in the way of gastrointestinal lesions.

CONCLUSIONS

The enteric fevers, and particularly typhoid fever, are still very much a worldwide problem, and many hundreds of thousands, if not millions, of new cases occur each year throughout the world. It will be many years before the hygiene of the world is improved and the incidence of the disease drastically diminished.

In the future, it will be not only the practitioner in the hygienically backward country who will have to contend with the disease but his colleague in the so-called developed countries as well. As air travel increases, so will actual cases in visitors and vacationers returning from abroad and also epidemics caused by unknown carriers. Other sources of infection, such as preserved foods from abroad, will also undoubtedly continue to be a source of infection, as it will obviously be impossible to examine every can of meat or improve world standards of hygiene overnight. Sooner or later the practitioner will fall into the diagnostic trap that the sporadic unsuspected case presents, unless he constantly bears in mind the many guises of this "international" disease.

ACKNOWLEDGMENTS

I am indebted to Mr. Robert Duncan, Managing Director of Churchill Livingstone for permission to reproduce Figures 1–4 from my monograph, "Typhoid Fever and Other Salmonella Infections."

BACILLARY DYSENTERY

By ROBERT H. GILMAN, M.D.,
and FREDERICK KOSTER, M.D.
Baltimore, Maryland

SYNONYM

Shigellosis.

DEFINITION

Bacillary dysentery or shigellosis is an acute intestinal infection caused by organisms of the genus Shigella and is characterized by diarrhea, fever, abdominal cramps, and, when severe, tenesmus and bloody mucoid stools. Complications are rare in adults, but convulsions and dehydration are common in infants and children.

PATHOPHYSIOLOGY

After ingestion of as few as 100 organisms, shigellae proliferate in the lower small bowel and colon. Shigella produces a cytotoxic enterotoxin that may contribute to the symptoms of watery diarrhea. The ability of the organism to invade and proliferate in the epithelial cells of the colonic mucosa is responsible for the symptoms of dysentery. The disease is associated histologically with a polymorphonuclear leukocyte inflammatory response in the lamina propria, the formation of crypt abscesses, and, when severe, destruction of the epithelium and pseudomembrane formation.

CLINICAL PICTURE

Shigella organisms are responsible for a wide spectrum of clinical illness. Usually, fecal excretion of shigellae is associated with asymptomatic infection or moderate diarrhea without fever, although fulminant dysentery preceded by high fever, toxemia, and abdominal pain is not uncommon.

Although any Shigella species can produce severe dysentery, S. sonnei tends to be associated with milder disease than S. flexneri or S. dysenteriae species. Infection with Shiga bacillus, Shigella dysenteriae type 1, is associated with the most severe disease and can occur in pandemics. In Central America and Bangladesh, epidemics occurred with Shiga strains, resistant to multiple antibiotics, which produced severe disease characterized by hypoproteinemia, hyponatremia, and leukemoid reactions. In some cases the disease in patients with leukemoid reactions then progressed to microangiopathic hemolytic anemia with or without acute renal failure (hemolytic-uremic syndrome).

After an incubation period of 36 to 72 hours or occasionally up to 8 days, fever may initiate the illness, followed by abdominal cramps, malaise, and anorexia. After this brief prodrome, watery diarrhea ensues in almost all patients and can be severe enough to require oral or intravenous rehydration. Diarrhea may continue for several days as frequent loose motions accompanied by tenesmus and then may abate or be followed by frank dysentery consisting entirely of blood and mucous in the stools. Fever, tenesmus, abdominal pain, and vomiting may persist. Shigellosis in the majority of patients, excepting infants, is a mild self-limiting disease lasting 3 to 5 days. In children and in adults with more severe cases of dysentery and toxemia, appropriate antibiotics rapidly lyse fever, decrease stool frequency, and eliminate fecal excretion of the organism. Rare chronic asymptomatic carriers have also been described.

Infants and young children commonly present with high fever, toxemia, dehydration, and a history of a convulsion. Meningismus may be present, although the cerebrospinal fluid is completely normal. Rectal prolapse and hypoproteinemia are often sequelae of shigellosis in endemic areas. Although rare in mild cases, bacteremia occurs in approximately 5 per cent of severe cases but carries no special prognostic significance.

PHYSICAL EXAMINATION

There are no characteristic findings. Signs of dehydration and toxemia are often prominent.

Proctoscopic appearance of the rectal mucosa is a useful prognostic guide and correlates with the severity of clinical disease. In mild disease, mucosal edema, erythema, and copious mucus are seen. In more severe disease a thin white exudate is apparent, with scattered hemorrhages and ragged mucosa. In severe Shiga dysentery shallow mucosal ulceration and a heavy pseudomembrane are striking.

Development of abdominal distension and ileus are ominous signs occurring only in very severe cases. One per cent of young adults may have a monoarticular arthritis, usually in the knee, with a culture-negative effusion. In some series arthritis has been accompanied by conjunctivitis or urethritis.

LABORATORY STUDIES

Although the white blood cell count is variable, it is often mildly elevated with a shift to the left. In children, leukemoid reactions can be seen. Stool examination reveals an abundance of fecal leukocytes but not eosinophils. Fecal leukocytes may also be abundant in idiopathic ulcerative colitis and in dysentery caused by invasive E. coli, Vibrio parahemolyticus, Endamoeba histolytica, and rarely in rotavirus and nontyphoid salmonella. Fecal leukocytes are present but few in number in diarrhea owing to noninvasive agents such as enterotoxigenic E. coli and Vibrio cholera and in many cases of rotavirus diarrhea. Collar-button ulcers seen in barium enemas of ulcerative colitis are also seen in prolonged shigellosis.

A specific diagnosis of shigellosis can be made in most instances within 48 hours by routine stool culture. A combination of a selective media such as Salmonella-Shigella (S-S) or xylose-lysine-desoxycholate (XLD) agar and a differential (noninhibiting) medium such as MacConkey's agar should be used. Suspicious colonies should be subcultured to triple sugar iron agar; those giving typical Shigella reactions should be tested for agglutination with typing sera.

Serologic tests, using serotype-specific shigella lipopolysaccharide, are useful for epidemiologic studies only.

DIFFERENTIAL DIAGNOSIS

Idiopathic ulcerative colitis, and dysentery caused by invasive E. coli, Vibrio parahaemolyticus, Campylobacter fetus, Yersinia enterocolitica, amebic dysentery, and rarely heavy infestation with Trichuris trichura or Strongyloides stercoralis, may mimic shigella dysentery. Only shigella and invasive E. coli when inoculated into guinea pig or rabbit eye will produce keratoconjunctivitis (Sereny test). When watery diarrhea or loose stools alone are present, it is difficult to distinguish shigella from disease caused by enterotoxigenic E. coli, salmonella, giardia, parvovirus, and rotavirus agents. Stool culture and microscopic examination of stool for fecal leukocytes, hematophagous trophozoites of Entamoeba histolytica, and trophozoites or cysts of giardia will assist in differentiation.

TULAREMIA

By MORTON I. RAPOPORT, M.D.
Baltimore, Maryland

DEFINITION

Tularemia is an acute bacterial infection with remarkable similarity to plague. It is caused by the gram-negative coccobacillus *Francisella tularensis*. This disease is encountered worldwide and is epizootic and enzootic in numerous species of animals. In addition, a variety of acarina and insects, including ticks and deer flies, have been established as vectors in the transmission of the disease. The Center for Disease Control (CDC) has reported more than 138 cases per year for the last 3 years.

The clinical course of this disease is dependent on the route of infection. While tularemia can be divided into five basic clinical patterns, frequent overlap can hinder definitive categorization. Variant forms of the disease include ulceroglandular, oculoglandular, enteric or typhoidal, and pulmonary. Most human infections are of the ulceroglandular type, although primary and secondary pulmonary infections are frequently encountered.

The infection may be transmitted by arthropod vector or animal bite, by handling of infected animal tissues, or by exposure to infected aerosols. Diagnosis is frequently suspected by historic exposure; however, only serologic and cultural findings are confirmatory.

CLINICAL COURSE

The various forms of infection, while occasionally overlapping, are distinctly different and generally reflect the route of inoculation. The two major types of infection, pulmonary and ulceroglandular, are both associated with prominent lymphatic involvement.

Ulceroglandular Tularemia. Direct inoculation of the organism is associated with ulceroglandular infection. Patients with this illness become clinically ill within 1 week of contact. The classic lesion begins as a small erythematous papule that rapidly progresses to ulceration. Within 1 to 2 days regional lymph nodes are noted to enlarge and become painful. In many patients systemic influenza-like symptoms including chills and fever, headache, and toxicity become manifest. Occasionally, the inoculation site and the regional lymphatic involvement go unrecognized and constitutional and pulmonary symptoms predominate. These latter infections may be mistaken for primary pulmonary infections. In the more typical patients with ulceroglandular tularemia, the lymph nodes are the most prominent sites of involvement. Over a period of several weeks tender nodes become fluctuant and may progress to suppuration and frank drainage. Microscopic examination of the lymph nodes show large numbers of organisms in association with granulomatous lesions and abscesses remarkably similar to tuberculous infection.

A mortality rate of 3 to 7 per cent has been reported in ulceroglandular infection.

Pulmonary Tularemia. Primary pulmonary infection or pneumonia due to *Francisella tularensis* is almost invariably associated with inhalation of the organism, although the circumstance of exposure may vary widely. Hunters and trappers may be exposed to aerosols during the process of skinning and dressing game, farm workers can be exposed during threshing of grain that has been contaminated by rodent feces, and laboratory workers likewise can be exposed in the process of diagnostic or cultural handling of the organism. It should be noted that the organism is exceedingly infectious and inhaled counts of as few as 10 organisms may be associated with disease.

The incubation period varies between 2 and 4 days and tends to reflect the intensity of the aerosol. Illness is abrupt in onset with constitutional symptoms becoming most prominent. Initial symptoms including headache, chills, high fever, and malaise with nonproductive cough are recognized. With delayed diagnosis or therapy the illness proceeds to a more virulent form characterized by bloody sputum, prostration, and refractory hypoxemia. In as many as 50 per cent of patients, physical findings may be absent and therefore not reflective of the fulminance of the disease.

More reliable diagnostic findings include a radiologic picture that shows diffuse broncho-pneumonic or lobar infiltrate. In addition, pleural effusion and hilar or mediastinal adenopathy may be associated with parenchymal involvement.

Rarely, as just noted, secondary pulmonary involvement may be encountered in patients with advanced ulceroglandular disease. These patients may present with severe toxicity in association with advanced roentgenologic evidence of parenchymal and mediastinal disease.

Untreated or delayed treatment of pulmonary infection is associated with a mortality rate considerably higher than that encountered with ulceroglandular disease, possibly as high as 30 per cent.

Oculoglandular Tularemia. Considerably less common is the infection caused by direct inoculation of the organism into the mucous membranes of the eye. Diagnosis is frequently delayed because of the relatively nonspecific complaints and findings. Symptoms of severe pain, lacrimation, and photophobia may be encountered. Physical findings include formation of yellowish, white granulomatous lesions on the palpebral conjunctiva. In addition, conjunctival suffusion, chemosis, or conjunctival edema is also present. Characteristically, regional lymph nodes, particularly preauricular and cervical, may be enlarged and tender. Delayed recognition may result in corneal perforation or optic atrophy.

Typhoidal Tularemia. Much less common is the enteric or typhoidal form of tularemia associated with infection by the oral route. The organism has been isolated from mud and water, and water-borne infection has been documented.

Chills and high fever in association with nausea, vomiting, diarrhea, and severe abdominal pain may suggest a diagnosis of typhoid fever. Similarity to typhoid may extend to development of ulcerative lesions in the gastrointestinal tract as well. Complications including significant gastrointestinal hemorrhage and perforation may also be encountered. The mortality rate approximates that experienced with pulmonary tularemia.

LABORATORY DIAGNOSIS

Leukocyte counts and acute phase reactants are of little diagnostic value in that they may be normal or slightly increased. Using selected media isolation of the organism from ulcers, secretions, blood, and biopsy specimens serves to establish the diagnosis given. The organism is easily propagated on glucose cystine blood agar (GCBA). Extreme care in the handling of this organism is required because of its remarkable propensity for producing laboratory infection. Similarly, laboratory animal inoculation is discouraged, owing to the frequency of laboratory-acquired disease.

Surprisingly, serologic diagnosis may be extremely useful even in the early diagnostic process. Indeed, significant increases in agglutinating antibodies may be detected within the first 10 to 14 days of clinical illness.

As with most serologic studies, diagnosis is established most effectively using paired or sequential sera in an effort to document titer increases. In tularemia, the importance of sequential sera is also underscored by virtue of the characteristic persistence of antibodies for many years. Cross-reactivity of serum obtained from patients with brucellosis has also been reported, although comparative studies will reflect higher titers using the homologous antigen.

A diagnostic intradermal skin test using a purified killed suspension of *F. tularensis* as described by Foshay is highly specific. Positive reactions are encountered after one week of illness and reactivity persists for many years. The reaction is analogous to the tuberculin reaction in that inoculation intradermally is followed by an erythematous indurated papule within 48 hours in patients with positive reaction.

PITFALLS OF DIAGNOSIS

Ulceroglandular tularemia must be distinguished from the myriad conditions that are associated with cutaneous ulceration and draining lymphadenopathy. These include plague, cat-scratch fever, rat-bite fever, anthrax, lymphogranuloma venereum, sporotrichosis and other cutaneous fungal infections, including histoplasmosis and coccidioidomycosis. While historic and epidemiologic information may exclude most diagnostic possibilities, serologic and cultural data are particularly relevant to the array of conditions that mimic ulceroglandular tularemia.

Pulmonary tularemia must be distinguished from a variety of pulmonary infections not readily diagnosed by bacteriologic smears. These include primary fungal infections, mycoplasma infection, Legionnaires' disease, rickettsial infections (specifically, Q fever), and an acute viral infection, particularly influenza.

BRUCELLOSIS

By IAN M. SMITH, M.D.
Iowa City, Iowa

SYNONYMS

The disease is frequently called Bang's disease by farmers and veterinarians. Veterinarians sometimes refer to it as infectious abortion or epizootic abortion. Other names for the disease are undulant fever, Malta fever, and Mediterranean fever.

DEFINITION

Brucellosis is a septicemic disease with occasional localization in lung, bone, or soft tissue. It is caused by one of the four principal species of the genus Brucella, *B. abortus, B. melitensis, B. suis,* or *B. canis.* These organisms are primarily, but not exclusively, isolated from cattle, goats, hogs, or dogs, respectively. A number of biotypes that differ from one another in one chemical or biologic characteristic exist for each species. The disease occurs in domestic animals and rarely in wild animals. Man acquires the disease from infected animals directly or indirectly. A proper understanding of the disease in animals aids the physician in diagnosing the disease in man. Animals are infected in the sale barn or on pasture or in other contact by a variety of methods. They can be infected by drinking infected milk, licking aborted fetuses or placentas, licking the external genitalia of other animals, by intravaginal, intrauterine, conjunctival, or cutaneous routes, by artificial insemination, or rarely by flies, mosquitoes, and ticks. The organism grows to a titer of 10^4 in regional lymph nodes at the point of entry. After a week or two it circulates in the blood at a titer of 10^2 and settles in tissues with a high content of erythritol. These tissues are the placenta, seminal vesicles, or testicles, where it grows to a high titer of 10^7 organisms per gram of tissue. In the regional lymph nodes near the udder, organisms will be present at a titer of 10^3. Spread can occur from the aborted fetus, all fluids associated with this, or from milk infected by the paraudder lymph nodes. Infection is particularly prone to occur in veterinarians who extract a retained placenta without using the usual protective rubber gloves. Therefore, all human infection occurs by direct contact with animals or through the ingestion of unpasteurized contaminated dairy products. In this country brucellosis is primarily a disease of farmers, veterinarians, and packing house workers. Veterinarians can also infect themselves from accidental inoculation with the cattle protective strain 19 live vaccine.

Until recently *B. abortus* was uncommon because of the effective control program in cattle. Because of reduced expenditure in this area, there has been an upsurge in *B. abortus* disease. Most other cases are caused by *B. suis,* but foreign cheeses or goats may cause occasional cases of *B. melitensis* infection. Rarely, man is infected by *B. canis.* Approximately 10 per cent of stray dogs are infected with this strain and 2 per cent of home pets.

PRESENTING SIGNS AND SYMPTOMS

I find it convenient to classify brucellosis as; (1) asymptomatic brucellosis, (2) acute brucellosis, (3) relapsing brucellosis, (4) brucellosis localized in various organs, and (5) strain 19 vaccine disease.

About one half of packing house workers and about one third of veterinarians who have high titers or fourfold rises in titer to brucellosis are unaware of an acute infection.

Approximately 7 to 21 days after exposure to infected animals or animal products, the patient develops a generalized illness characterized by shaking chills and fever. Fever, sweats, weakness, chills, headache, depression, backache, and generalized aching occur in varying combinations. In addition, about one fifth of the patients have a monoarticular arthralgia affecting the knee, shoulder, ankle, or elbows, and about 50 per cent complain of weight loss averaging 15 pounds, with a range of 5 to 50 pounds depending on the length of undiagnosed illness.

Of patients with the disease who receive adequate treatment, approximately 5 per cent have relapse. This occurs particularly in veterinarians. In their second attack, they have more fever, more fatigue, more weakness and chills, and nocturnal sweating attacks are more frequent. It is possible that more severe disease is likely to relapse or that some degree of sensitivity to the toxins of the Brucella has developed. Rarely, veterinarians will develop an allergic response to Brucella with swelling of the hand and arm that have been in contact with the organism. This is accompanied by fever and chills, but blood cultures are negative.

Localized brucellosis has occurred in the lungs, kidneys, bones, and joints, and rarely in the central nervous system or cardiovascular system. Female patients predominate in this group, and the onset is often insidious. Fever occurs in 30 per cent (in contrast to 95 per cent in acute infections), weight loss in 12 per cent (versus 50 per cent), chills in 12 per cent (versus 65 per cent), and the titer against Brucella is often low. Diagnosis is by biopsy culture. In many ways this localized disease mimics tuberculosis.

Veterinarians have repeated accidents with strain 19 vaccine—in one study, 35 per cent on two occasions, 10 per cent on three, and 3 per cent on four. The number of veterinarians with strain 19 disease is more than 10 per cent of the total cases of brucellosis in veterinarians. The disease is generally milder with less fever, fatigue, weakness, chills, headache, and nocturnal sweats.

COURSE

My colleagues and I have made a study of untreated brucellosis in Iowa. With the *Brucella suis* cases a third last for up to 3 months, another third for 4 to 6 months, and the remainder are mostly resolved within 2 years, but cases of longer duration have been found. With *B. abortus*, the cases usually last 3 months or less, but about one quarter last for 4 to 6 months and a few longer than this. With *B. melitensis*, the distribution is approximately the same as that for *B. abortus*. In summary, two thirds of untreated cases last less than 6 months. Most acutely ill patients respond promptly within 4 to 7 days to adequate chemotherapy, which needs to be continued for 4 weeks. Approximately 5 per cent have relapse and need to be re-treated.

PHYSICAL EXAMINATION

In general, there is little to find on physical examination, but about one quarter of the patients have splenomegaly. Hepatomegaly with tenderness is occasionally found, and lymph nodes may be enlarged. Splenomegaly is found in 32 per cent of children and 19 per cent of adults, hepatomegaly in 11 per cent of children and 5 per cent of adults, lymphadenitis in 19 per cent of children and 3 per cent of adults. A rash has been described in 15 per cent of children and 7 per cent of adults. Appropriate physical findings may relate to localization in the vertebral column, in the long bones, or in the lung or kidney.

COMMON COMPLICATIONS

Localized brucellosis may follow the occurrence of acute brucellosis, but it can occur independently. In our experience, the organisms have localized in the bones or joints in 20 per cent of cases with local findings, caused endocarditis in 20 per cent, occurred in the lung or pleura in 15 per cent and in the genitourinary system (primarily the kidney) in 12 per cent, produced neurologic disease in 10 per cent and abscesses in 8 per cent, and affected miscellaneous organs such as the spleen, gallbladder, and lymph nodes in 15 per cent. Orchitis can occur in a small number of patients. When the disease localizes in the bony system, the lumbar or thoracic vertebrae are common areas for this to occur. *B. suis* is particularly likely to cause localized disease.

LABORATORY FINDINGS

The diagnosis of brucellosis should be suspected in farmers, veterinarians, and meatpackers with an occupational exposure to infected animals. It should also be expected in travelers who have eaten unpasteurized dairy products or in persons who have a conscientious objection to pasteurization. Brucellosis patients are likely to have leukopenia or a normal white blood cell picture.

BLOOD CULTURES

Three to 5 blood cultures should be kept for at least 3 to 4 weeks; to retain these cultures, most laboratories have to be specially notified that brucellosis is suspected. In early acute disease up to 75 per cent of the blood cultures will be positive, but 20 to 50 per cent is more usual. About 20 per cent of urine cultures are also positive, but they are almost never positive if the blood culture is negative. If there is no evidence of a heart murmur or emboli, we take 3 blood cultures 2 hours apart. If endocarditis is suspected, we take 5. Rarely, if the disease is still suspected after negative blood cultures, we will take a second group of 3 or 5 blood cultures. *Brucella abortus* requires a carbon dioxide atmosphere to grow adequately.

CULTURE OF TISSUES

The incorporation of erythritol (1 μM per ml) in Morris medium produces the earlier appearance of colonies of *Brucella abortus* and *B. melitensis* organisms. On Albimi agar erythritol accelerates the growth of *B. melitensis* but not *B. abortus*. *B. suis* growth is not accelerated on either medium. At concentrations higher than this, strain 19 vaccine organisms are inhibited. Below this level, there is neither inhibition nor stimulation of the growth of strain 19 Brucellae.

When tuberculosis is suspected, or in a routine screen of a patient who may have cancer,

Table 1. *Identification and Characteristics of Members of the Genus Brucellae That Infect Man*

	Number of Biotypes	Preferential Host	Growth in Presence of Dyes		H_2S PRODUCTION	CO_2 REQUIREMENT
			THIONINE 1:50,000°	BASIC FUCHSIN 1:25,000°		
B. abortus	9	cattle	−	+	‚++	+
B. melitensis	3	goats	+	+	+	−
B. suis	4	swine	+	−	+++	−
B. canis	1	dogs	+	−	++	−

°Varies with different batches of dye.

particularly in a patient with an occupational hazard, biopsy tissue should be cultured for Brucella. Again, the cultures have to be kept for 4 weeks. The tissues needing culture are lung, kidney, bone marrow, liver, or lymph nodes.

Once isolated, Brucellae strains are typed into their six species by: (1) their requirements for added carbon dioxide for growth, (2) growth in the presence of dyes, (3) production of hydrogen sulphide, (4) the urease test, (5) agglutination in specific sera. Further identification can be obtained through reference centers by (6) susceptibility to Brucella phage and (7) oxygen uptake in selected amino acid and carbohydrate substrates. The main reactions are summarized in Table 1.

The brucellin skin test can be negative when the serology and clinical findings are positive for brucellosis. The skin test will stimulate the production of antibody. The brucellin skin test has no place in the diagnosis of brucellosis and is no longer available commercially.

AGGLUTINATION TEST

A phenolyzed suspension of heat-killed smooth bacilli is used as the standard strain that is agglutinated by the antiserum to all three species commonly encountered. *B. canis* requires a special bacillary suspension, and titers against this organism must be requested separately. Titers over 1:80 are indicative of old or possibly active infection. A titer of 1:160 or higher is highly suggestive of recent disease on the tube agglutination test. A prozone phenomenon can occur; that is, a certain sera can react only when diluted several hundredfold. The cause of this is the presence of blocking antibodies. Dilution in sodium chloride or albumin or adding Coombs' reagent will overcome this problem.

In the past the use of brucellergen to desensi-

tize patients caused a cross-reaction. Rarely at the present time tularemia or tularemia vaccination, cholera or cholera vaccination, and *Vibrio fetus* or Yersinia infection can induce agglutinins against Brucella. A patient who has had brucellosis in the past may have a low titer serum such as 1:80 long after; fever due to an unrelated disease can be confusing in this case. We have noted a few patients, perhaps 1 to 2 per cent (who usually have localized disease), who have a positive culture for Brucella organisms and a negative agglutination reaction. The newly admitted patient usually has a titer of 1:1280 because this is a long incubation period disease. The titer usually falls to 1:320 in the first 6 months and 1:160 or 1:80 after a year.

Recently an enzyme-linked immunosorbent assay (ELISA) using phenol water extracted lipopolysaccharides as antigen was found to be tenfold to one hundredfold more sensitive than the commonly used tube agglutination assay. This has not yet entered general use. Radioimmunoassay (RIA) has been used as a primary type assay and avoids the difficulties with blocking or nonagglutinating antibody. This also has not been used in large diagnostic laboratories.

Counterimmunoelectrophoresis is another useful test presently under development.

The antihuman globulin (Coombs') agglutination, standard agglutination test, mercaptoethanol treated standard agglutination test, and complement fixation tests for brucellosis, when positive, usually react in a titer ratio of 16:8:2:1.

BIOCHEMICAL FINDINGS

If streptomycin is being used in treatment, it is mandatory to monitor the renal function at the beginning of therapy and at least weekly thereafter.

PULMONARY TUBERCULOSIS

By MAURICE SONES, M.D.

Philadelphia, Pennsylvania

DEFINITION

Pulmonary tuberculosis is a bacterial infection most commonly of the lungs caused by the *Mycobacterium tuberculosis*. When disseminated, lesions may also occur in the meninges, kidneys, bones as well as many other organs and tissues of the body.

PRESENTING SIGNS AND SYMPTOMS

Fatigue, anorexia, weight loss, and inanition may herald the onset of clinical pulmonary tuberculosis, followed by respiratory symptoms of cough, increased expectoration, hemoptysis, dyspnea, and chest pain. It is not unusual to find active tuberculosis in a routine chest x-ray in an asymptomatic patient. Pleural effusion is not infrequently an early manifestation of pulmonary involvement, which is preceded often by pleuritic pain, and friction rub may be noted on physical examination.

Patients with advanced disease may present with symptoms of marked weight loss, severe cough, copious expectoration, hemoptysis, and anorexia. These are hard-core cases, usually older male alcoholics who are notoriously noncompliant on any treatment schedule and are commonly seen in hospital emergency rooms often in acute respiratory failure.

PHYSICAL EXAMINATION

In early pulmonary tuberculosis, physical findings may be few or completely absent. Slight, persistent afternoon fever and occasional crepitant rales, especially after cough, may be the only manifestations noted. Sometimes in primary tuberculosis with compression of a bronchus by enlarged hilar nodes, an evanescent wheeze may be elicited. Symptoms more often associated with pneumonia or bronchitis are noted in acute forms of pulmonary tuberculosis, namely severe cough, chest pain, bloody expectoration, high fever, myalgias, chills and sweating and signs of consolidation, impaired percussion note, bronchial breathing, and coarse rales or rhonchi. In long-standing tuberculosis, one finds deviation of the trachea, dullness on percussion, coarse rales and rhonchi and signs associated with cavity formation,

egophony, whispered pectoriloquy, and, with large cavities, tympany. Because physical findings can be so variable, the value of the x-ray examination is increasingly most important.

X-RAY EXAMINATION OF THE CHEST

Standard posterior-anterior and lateral films of the chest will demonstrate most early lesions seen in pulmonary tuberculosis. Occasionally, an apical lordotic or oblique view or tomograms or both will be required to reveal lesions hidden by shadows created by ribs or clavicles or the heart (viz.: lateral tomograms). Nodules, cavities, cysts, and calcifications may best be visualized by tomography. Bronchograms will delineate bronchiectasis.

Primary tuberculosis is characterized most often in children by unilateral hilar adenopathy (uncommonly, bilateral), and x-rays will demonstrate the enlarged lymph nodes; if compression of a bronchus occurs, atelectasis will result with volume shrinkage and retraction of the lung to the side of involvement. When healing takes place, x-rays will often reveal the calcified primary complex with its Ghon lesion.

Reinfection tuberculosis, which, as noted, usually occurs in adults and is a manifestation of endogenous breakdown, will be seen on x-ray as lesions involving most often the apical and posterior segments of the upper lobes or the superior segments of the lower lobes. These lesions may be nodular or streaky in character and involve subsegments, segments, or an entire lobe. Atelectasis may also be seen in reinfection tuberculosis with retraction of the hilum and deviation of the trachea. If hematogenous spread has occurred x-rays will demonstrate miliary nodules throughout both lungs, uniform in size with symmetrical distribution. Pleural effusion, either unilateral or bilateral, may also occur.

It should be emphasized that pulmonary tuberculosis may result in almost any form of x-ray abnormality and should always be considered in differential diagnosis.

THE TUBERCULIN TEST

Purified protein derivative (PPD) is a protein fraction of tubercle bacilli that has replaced OT (old tuberculin) as the accepted skin testing material for tuberculosis. It was originally prepared in the laboratories of Florence Seibert at the Henry Phipps Institute in Philadelphia. Currently the preparation is stabilized by the addition of Tween 80 (antiabsorbent polysaccharide) in a testing dose of 5 tuberculin units (TU) — intermediate test. First strength PPD contains 1 TU and second strength, 250 TU. These test doses have been calibrated and approved by the United States Public Health Service. It is an intradermal skin test and should be read in 48 to 72 hours. Induration of 10 mm or more is a positive test and indicates tuberculosis, active or dormant; activity will be determined by clinical and x-ray manifestations. A reaction 5 to 9 mm in diameter is of doubtful significance and may suggest cross-reactivity with other (mycobacterial) diseases. Anything under 4 mm in diameter is a negative test.

A positive test results as a delayed hypersensitivity reaction caused by triggered release of lymphokines and dependent on an adequate number of sensitized T lymphocytes. The intermediate skin test may be negative in clinical tuberculosis if an inadequate number of sensitized T cells are present because of high fever, severe clinical illness, or large pleural effusions. In such cases one should test with PPD No. 2; if this test is negative, the disease present is not likely to be tuberculosis. However, sometimes dying patients with advanced tuberculosis are skin test negative to even PPD No. 2. Negative skin tests are observed in patients with active tuberculosis who may also have sarcoidosis, acute febrile illness, exanthems, and immunosuppressive diseases. Corticosteroid drugs or other immunosuppressive agents may also inhibit the tuberculin reaction.

SPUTUM EXAMINATION

The only absolute proof of the presence of tuberculosis is culture of the organism from the sputum or tissue involved. Cultures are made either on solid egg medium (Lowenstein-Jensen) or Middlebrook 7H-11 medium using 20 to 40 mm Hg pressure of carbon dioxide to speed growth. However, the sputum smear using the standard Ziehl-Neelsen stain or auromine-rhodamine stain for fluorescence microscopy will reveal the organisms, especially in patients who are expectorating sputum containing considerable numbers of bacilli. This will enable the physician to start treatment without waiting until positive identification is made by culture. Of course, one must be aware that saprophytic organisms will stain like tubercle bacilli; this is particularly evident in gastric aspirates (children swallowing sputum). But even in this case, with good clinical evidence, one may start treatment in a patient with a positive gastric smear.

Sputum specimens are best obtained in the morning after a good deep cough or after inhalation of heated, nebulized saline as an aerosol. Bronchial washings, brushing, and tracheal aspiration are also good sources of adequate material. Often multiple specimens will be required to demonstrate the organisms.

Characteristics of human *Mycobacterium tuberculosis* that are helpful for proper identification include rough strain, no pigment in the dark or after exposure to light, cord formation, and a positive niacin reaction. Guinea pig inoculation is no longer necessary.

OTHER LABORATORY STUDIES

Elevation of white blood cells is not common in the average case of pulmonary tuberculosis. However, leukocytosis may be seen in tuberculous pneumonia and may herald a complicating pyogenic infection. Miliary tuberculosis may be accompanied by leukocytosis, which is considered to be a leukemoid reaction. Increased erythrocyte sedimentation rate is usually seen as with any infection. Anemia may be present, which represents that noted in long-standing infection. Urinalysis is usually negative, but it should be noted that 10 per cent of patients with pulmonary tuberculosis excrete tubercle bacilli in the urine even without detectable urinary tract lesions.

Biopsy of mediastinal lymph nodes, lung tissue, pleura, liver, and bone marrow (by needle aspiration) may reveal caseating lesions with demonstrable acid-fast bacilli. These techniques enable one to start definitive therapy early.

Abnormal liver function may indicate liver involvement. Hypercalcemia has been demonstrated in pulmonary tuberculosis and is considered to be related to increased absorption of vitamin D as is also noted in sarcoidosis.

COMPLICATIONS

Cavitation and hemoptysis are common complications of pulmonary tuberculosis; cavitation indicates advanced disease. Since the numbers of tubercle bacilli are markedly increased, this complication usually requires triple drug therapy. Hemoptysis characterized by blood streaking occurs often, but frank hemorrhage is rare and is due to the formation sometimes of a mycotic aneurysm (Rasmussen's aneurysm). Emergency surgery may be necessary to control the bleeding.

The common manifestation of pulmonary tuberculosis is usually that of an indolent process that may take weeks to develop. However, an uncommon presentation would be an acute tuberculous pneumonia that may often be misdiagnosed and treated as a bacterial pneumonia, unless smears are ordered specifically for tubercle bacilli.

Pleural effusion often results from a silent focus in the lung. This focus invades the subpleural surface, then erodes into the pleural cavity, causing an immunologic reaction and pleural pain. Since the tuberculin test may be negative, pleural biopsy should be done. In positive cases a granuloma will be shown, which may be noncaseating with an absence of acid-fast bacilli. This complication occurs usually in young adults and the tuberculin test may be negative. Therefore PPD No. 2 should be applied and invariably will be positive. Antituberculosis treatment may be started under such circumstances even in the absence of the demonstration of tubercle bacilli.

Tuberculosis of the larynx, trachea, and bronchi may complicate pulmonary tuberculosis and is usually associated with advanced cavitary disease in the lungs. Rarely do these sites become involved as the primary focus of the disease. When this does occur, one must particularly exclude carcinoma and fungal diseases.

Miliary tuberculosis is the result of an overwhelming tuberculous infection that seeds all organs and tissues of the body. Small, discrete, symmetrical lesions are shown in the lungs by x-ray. Triple drug therapy is required to combat the disease. Sometimes endogenous foci in other organs will break down and cause meningitis, bone and skin involvement, and genitourinary, adrenal gland, peritoneal, and pericardial disease.

Differential Diagnosis

The most common diseases that may simulate pulmonary tuberculosis in order of frequency are sarcoidosis; bronchogenic carcinoma; bacterial, viral, and aspiration pneumonia; fungal infection; silicosis; and bronchiectasis. In endemic areas, fungal disease moves higher on the list.

Sarcoidosis usually presents with bilateral hilar adenopathy; is often asymptomatic in this stage. Rarely, unilateral hilar adenopathy will be seen. The tuberculin test is negative in all strengths in the majority of patients; however, the patient with primary tuberculosis will invariably have a positive PPD First or intermediate strength. On biopsy noncaseating granuloma will be observed in both conditions but tubercle bacilli will be absent in sarcoid granulomata. The parenchymal lesions of sarcoidosis may simulate tuberculosis. PPD testing and sputum studies will aid in differentiation.

Bronchogenic carcinoma is seen frequently in older males who are also the prime target for tuberculosis, especially when malnutrition and alcoholism are associated. Not infrequently carcinoma develops on an old tuberculous scar. Skin testing, sputum studies (mycobacteria and cytology), and tissue biopsies must all be used to arrive at a diagnosis.

The bacterial, aspiration, and viral pneumonias may be confused with pulmonary tuberculosis. If one thinks about this at the time of presentation, a simple sputum smear may show large numbers of tubercle bacilli. Fungal disease, histoplasmosis, blastomycosis, cryptococcosis, coccidioidomycosis, and aspergillosis are the common fungal diseases to be considered. Appropriate studies should be instituted, especially if the patient resides in an endemic area. Aspergillosis often complicates cavitary tuberculosis — "fungus ball."

Silicosis may present both clinically and radiographically like pulmonary tuberculosis. Because of lung destruction by silicosis, tuberculosis frequently complicates the disease. A patient with silicosis and a positive tuberculin test should be treated with prophylatic isoniazid (INH). This rule also applies to patients with bronchiectasis that has resulted from previous lung disease and bronchial damage, often seen in children.

If a situation arises in which tuberculosis is suspected but not proven in a patient who is seriously ill, antituberculous therapy would be justified while cultures and other tests are awaited. These drugs may then be discontinued if the diagnosis is other than tuberculosis.

HISTOPLASMOSIS

By RAJENDRA KAPILA, M.D.,
and DONALD B. LOURIA, M.D.

Newark, New Jersey

SYNONYM

Darling's disease.

DEFINITION

Histoplasmosis is an infectious disease caused by a dimorphic fungus that is acquired through the respiratory route, the primary focus of infection being in the lungs. Dissemination to reticuloendothelial tissues, including liver, bone marrow, and spleen, occurs either hematogenously or via lymphatics. The fungus exists in yeast phase at the body temperature of mammals and in mycelial form in nature, especially in certain types of soils fertilized by bat, chicken, and other bird droppings.

In the United States the Ohio and Mississippi Valleys are major endemic areas; the states with the highest prevalence are Kentucky, Tennessee, Arkansas, and Missouri. Histoplasmosis is also present in southern Canada, parts of Mexico, and in Puerto Rico. Although originally described in Panama, it has only been recently recognized that infections caused by *Histoplasma capsulatum* have a broad geographic distribution including Central and South America, the tropical western parts of Africa, and rarely Southeast Asia. In Africa the predominant histoplasma species is *H. duboisii*; the clinical disease caused by *H. duboisii* is very different from that caused by *H. capsulatum*, being characterized by cutaneous lesions, skeletal involvement, and lymphadenopathy.

It is estimated that in the United States about 30 million persons have been infected, with 500,000 new histoplasma infections and 800 deaths occurring each year.

The endemicity of *H. capsulatum* infection in a given area has been determined by intensive skin testing programs; in some areas of Middle Tennessee and Kentucky, 90 to 95 per cent of the people are positive reactors.

Epidemics have been associated with dry weather and dusty conditions affecting chicken coops, starling roosts, bat-infested caves, attics, lofts, and hollow trees, especially during bulldozing or "earth day" activities.

Chickens and starlings do not suffer from histoplasmosis, presumably because their body temperature is too high to support the replication of the fungus; in contrast, the bat is susceptible supposedly because of its lower body temperature.

Primary infection occurs when the spores of *H. capsulatum*, inhaled by a non-immune person, germinate in the alveoli or interstitial spaces. Transformation to the yeast form occurs rapidly and thereafter multiplication occurs within mononuclear cells in the lungs or, after the organisms have disseminated, in spleen, liver, lymph nodes, and bone marrow. Polymorphonuclear cells are capable of ingesting and killing *H. capsulatum*, but control appears to depend on the development of delayed immune mechanisms (the lymphocyte-macrophage system). The characteristic cellular response is the granuloma; sometimes granuloma formation is associated with caseation necrosis.

CLINICAL MANIFESTATIONS

The spectrum of illness is variable and depends both on inoculum size and the host reaction.

Infection with *H. capsulatum* can be primary or a reinfection. A mild exposure in either case produces an asymptomatic infection and this accounts for at least 95 per cent of the cases in an endemic area. With primary infections the incubation period is usually between 2 and 3 weeks, while symptoms starting within 10 days suggest reinfection.

The true incidence of symptomatic pulmonary histoplasmosis is unknown; many cases develop in epidemic situations in which a number of persons have encountered a heavy inhalation exposure at the same time. Symptoms of primary pulmonary histoplasmosis include malaise and headache, followed by fever, chills, nonproductive cough, aching, and substernal discomfort, often indistinguishable from virus influenza. Physical examination of the lungs may show a few moist rales; only infrequently is there evidence of consolidation. Occasionally skin lesions such as erythema nodosum and erythema multiforme accompany the pulmonary manifestations.

Roentgenograms show patchy pneumonic infiltrates with soft hazy edges in one or more areas. Occasionally nodular lesions, smaller in size, may be present. Hilar and mediastinal adenopathy may be seen and in some patients may be the predominant x-ray abnormality.

Complete recovery usually occurs over a 2 to 4 week period and the roentgenographic changes ordinarily resolve in 2 to 3 months, often with residual "buckshot" calcification. In some patients single or multiple primary nodules may increase and decrease in size over a period of months; these roentgenographic findings may or may not be accompanied by exacerbations and improvements in the clinical manifestations. In those recovering from acute histoplasmosis, splenic calcifications may occur, indicating that dissemination probably occurs frequently and as with acute pulmonary disease resolves without treatment. Rarely, in acute pulmonary infection, blood cultures are positive in the absence of any clinical evidence suggesting dissemination. Mortality is less than 0.5 per cent and is related to acute respiratory failure or to dissemination.

In the reinfection type of acute histoplasmosis the incubation period is shorter, the symptoms are milder, and roentgenographic findings often consist of miliary nodulation with no adenopathy or pleural involvement. In infants and young children and rarely in adults, the patient suffers from a cough that may be brassy in character and from variable amounts of fever lasting for 3 to 4 weeks. Roentgenographs show primarily hilar and mediastinal lymphadenopathy, sometimes with patchy parenchymal infiltrates. Most of the cases resolve spontaneously.

CHRONIC PULMONARY HISTOPLASMOSIS

This mimics chronic pulmonary tuberculosis in clinical features as well as roentgenographic changes and is more frequent in persons predisposed to chronic disabling pulmonary disease such as centrilobular and bullous emphysema. Clinical features include cough, sputum production, night sweats (less common than in tuberculosis), fever, and weight loss. The chest pain often is referred to deeper structures and this may suggest a neoplastic process. Hemoptysis occurs in more than one third of the patients. Roentgenographic findings include pneumonic lesions in the apicoposterior areas of the lung, a reticular pattern of interstitial pneumonitis that undergoes scarring, and rarely a wandering form of pneumonia in which new areas become involved as the disease appears to resolve in areas of previous involvement. In chronic pulmonary disease cavitation occurs frequently. Bullous lesions, persistent thick-walled cavities, and nodular fibrosis may lead to progressive pulmonary insufficiency over a period of years.

CLINICALLY APPARENT DISSEMINATED HISTOPLASMOSIS

This occurs infrequently in otherwise healthy adults, most of the cases being in children below the age of 6 months. Compromised patients with hematopoietic and lymphatic malignancies who are receiving corticosteroids or immunosuppressive drugs are more susceptible to the disseminated form of the disease.

The incidence is estimated to be 1 per 6000 cases of acute infection. In adults the incidence is highest in the sixth and seventh decades and male-to-female ratio is 4 to 1.

The clinical spectrum of disseminated disease is wide and can range from a mild chronic disease to a severe overwhelming process. Cough, malaise, irregular fever ranging from 38.3 to 40 C (101 to 104 F), anorexia, and weight loss are frequent findings. Hepatosplenomegaly is almost always present, the spleen and liver often extending at least 5 cm below the costal margin. Interstitial pneumonia and generalized peripheral lymphadenopathy may also be present. Other manifestations include diarrhea caused by gastrointestinal ulceration, papulonodular or ulcerative skin lesions, tongue or buccal mucosal ulcerations, and acute nephritis. Arthritis has been reported rarely. Adrenal involvement is seen in 70 to 80 per cent of the patients, with 5 to 10 per cent developing clinical evidence of adrenal insufficiency. In the milder forms of disseminated disease, the fever may be intermittent and low grade, with only mild fatiguability and gradual weight loss.

In those compromised by hematologic malignancy the most frequent finding is diffuse interstitial lung infiltrates; hepatosplenomegaly is reported less often.

SPECIAL FORMS OF PULMONARY HISTOPLASMOSIS

Histoplasmoma. This is the primary focus equivalent of the Ghon complex in primary tuberculosis. The lesion starts as a 2 to 4 mm mass with a 1 to 2 mm fibrous capsule. Rarely it may grow concentrically by 1 to 2 mm per year to reach a size of 3 to 4 cm in 10 to 20 years. This often mimics a neoplasm but can be distinguished from a tumor if it shows a central area of calcification with concentric rings of lamination around it.

Mediastinal Fibrosis (Collagenosis). This is seen in hypersensitive persons. Progressive fibrous reaction around a lymph node in the mediastinum in the right paratracheal area can cause a superior vena caval syndrome and often stenosis of the right main stem bronchus. In the subcarinal area this may involve the right or left main stem bronchi, while in the hilar area stenosis of the pulmonary artery and bronchial tree occurs.

Mediastinal Granuloma. This occurs when

large caseous lymph nodes break down and mat together, forming a single large mass 8 to 10 cm in size, usually in the right paratracheal area.

DIAGNOSIS

Microbiologic Diagnosis. In pulmonary disease the sputum should be cultured on Sabouraud's or blood agar; after incubation at 30 C or room temperature, colonies appear in 3 to 14 days. In disseminated disease intracellular organisms may be seen in the buffy coat or bone marrow. Indeed, marrow aspiration for smear and culture is the most effective technique for establishing the diagnosis in compromised hosts suffering from hematologic disorders. Mucosal and cutaneous lesions should be smeared and stained with Wright or Giemsa stain; biopsies can be stained with a variety of silver stains and cultured on Sabouraud's or other agars.

Serologic. Two types of antigens are used: (1) histoplasma mycelial antigen and (2) whole or ground yeast antigen. There are two techniques presently employed in most laboratories: complement fixation and immunodiffusion.

Complement Fixation. Either antigen can be used for this test. Antibody appears 2 to 3 weeks after the exposure. A titer of more than 1:16 or a fourfold rise in titer is presumed to indicate active infection; most patients with histoplasmosis have titers higher than 1:32. However, some with severe infection may have lower titers. After several months antibody titers usually decline to less than 1:2 to 1:16; persistently elevated titers of 1:32 or greater suggest progressive disease.

False elevations of antibody levels, especially against the histoplasma mycelial antigen, may be seen in 10 to 20 per cent of patients who develop a positive reaction to the histoplasma skin test. The intradermal test has limited utility in establishing a diagnosis of acute histoplasmosis and should be done only after serum for the histoplasma serologic tests has been drawn. On occasion even a negative skin test can induce a positive serologic reaction.

Immunodiffusion Tests. Histoplasmin antigen is ordinarily used. Two precipitin lines are important; these are called the H and M bands. The M band appears earlier in the course of the illness, may persist in the asymptomatic patient, and may be induced by the skin test, while the H band is usually associated with active infection and is not affected by the skin test. The H band may be absent early in the course of active infection and in some chronic infections, especially those localized to the lungs.

Other Serologic Techniques. Radioimmunoassay (RIA) and gas liquid chromatography (GLC) analyses look promising. The RIA test for antibody detection is said to be less influenced by cross-reactions with other fungal antigens and is said to provide better quantitation of low-titer sera. Sera from patients with histoplasmosis studied by GLC reportedly show increased amounts of mannose, galactose, and *N*-acetyl glucosamine. Neither RIA nor GLC has yet been adequately tested.

Other Laboratory Tests. Leukopenia or thrombocytopenia, or both, and anemia are found in at least 75 per cent of patients with disseminated disease. However, in chronic pulmonary disease anemia is not commonly present and the white blood cell count is normal.

Abnormal liver function tests, especially alkaline phosphatase elevations, often suggest disseminated disease; biopsy and culture of liver tissue can be very useful in establishing a diagnosis in these patients.

OTHER COMPLICATIONS AND UNUSUAL SYNDROMES

1. Subacute vegetative endocarditis
2. Pericarditis
3. Massive lymphadenopathy resembling lymphoma
4. Cerebral histoplasmoma (space-occupying lesion)
5. Meningitis (basilar) resembling tuberculosis
6. Ulceration of the gums, larynx, penis, or bladder — with or without regional lymphadenopathy
7. Uveitis
8. Gastrointestinal ulceration, perforation, hemorrhage, or obstruction
9. Bone or spinal cord involvement

COCCIDIOIDOMYCOSIS

By ROBERT D. LIBKE, M.D.

Fresno, California

SYNONYMS

Cocci, San Joaquin Valley fever, desert rheumatism, coccidioidal granuloma.

DEFINITION

Coccidioidomycosis is a disease caused by the fungus *Coccidioides immitis.* The organism, present in the soil in endemic areas, usually enters the body by inhalation of the arthrospore phase and causes an acute respiratory, flu-like illness. In most persons the infection is self-limiting and confined to the lungs, hilar nodes, and pleural space. A few patients, especially those with compromised host defenses, pregnant patients, those of certain ethnic background, and those receiving a large infecting dose may have dissemination to extrapulmonary sites with progressive disease and death.

PRESENTING SIGNS AND SYMPTOMS

Primary Disease. The majority (60 per cent) of patients with acute coccidioidomycosis have subclinical infection. The symptoms in the remainder vary widely from a brief flu-like illness to severe respiratory complaints with marked systemic toxicity. Nonproductive cough, chest pain, and fever are often accompanied by myalgia, headache, and anorexia. Early in the illness transient, erythematous skin rashes may be seen, especially in children. Erythema nodosum or erythema multiforme occurs later in about 20 per cent of patients and is most commonly seen in females. At this stage arthralgia and arthritis may also occur and if transient, do not necessarily indicate dissemination. Patients may have hemoptysis and, when this is associated with chest pain, have an illness easily confused with pulmonary embolism.

Disseminated Disease. When disease occurs, outside the lungs or the pleural space, almost any tissue may be involved, but most often the effect becomes apparent in lymph nodes, skin, meninges, bones, and joints. Localized manifestations depend on the area of involvement and may be preceded by prolonged fever and nonspecific complaints. Lymph node involvement results in enlargement and tenderness and is most frequently detected in the cervical area. Mediastinal adenopathy noted on chest x-ray is considered by most clinicians to represent dissemination, whereas hilar adenopathy is regarded as part of primary disease. Bone involvement is accompanied by local symptoms and occasionally by draining sinuses. Synovitis most often occurs in the knees and ankles but can involve any joint. Skin lesions have a variety of forms that usually begin as small pustules; these persist or enlarge to form chronic ulcers or granulomas. Meningitis may present as the only site of dissemination or, rarely, be part of widespread, rapidly progressive disease. Meningitis often presents with insidious onset of headache, mentation abnormalities, and minimal nuchal rigidity.

COURSE

Symptomatic primary coccidioidomycosis usually resolves in 1 to 3 weeks; however, malaise and fatigue may persist for longer periods. Persistence of symptoms, especially fever, for longer than 1 month is associated with an increased risk of dissemination. In patients with dissemination, the signs and symptoms are often chronic with exacerbations and remissions. Two thirds of untreated patients with extrapulmonary disease will eventually have progressive deterioration and death. Those with untreated meningitis have almost 100 per cent mortality within 2 years.

Although no more susceptible to primary disease, certain ethnic groups, especially Filipinos and blacks, are at increased risk for the development of extrapulmonary spread and death.

PHYSICAL EXAMINATION

The findings on physical examination are nonspecific and in primary disease consist of fever, rales, and occasionally signs of pleural effusion. The transient erythematous and maculopapular rashes sometimes seen in children may be found only during the first few days of illness. Erythema nodosum or erythema multiforme occurs somewhat later and tends to be more persistent. When noted in patients residing in, or travelers exposed to, the endemic areas, these later rashes are highly suggestive of coccidioidomycosis.

COMMON COMPLICATIONS

In a small number of patients, convalescence from the primary disease may be prolonged and does not necessarily imply poor outcome. Patients who have the illness longer than 4 weeks, however, should be evaluated for evidence of dissemination or intrathoracic complications.

Such complications associated with primary coccidioidomycosis include cavity formation, pleural effusion, empyema, pneumothorax, and chronic granuloma. Spread to the pericardium occurs by local extension and does not imply extrathoracic spread of the organism.

LABORATORY FINDINGS

Routine laboratory evaluation often shows leukocytosis and variable eosinophilia. Chest x-rays during the acute phase usually reveal localized densities with ipsilateral hilar adenopathy. Diffuse pulmonary changes can occur when a large number of spores have been inhaled. Variable pleural effusion may be present and may be the major roentgenographic abnormality.

Skin tests may be informative but in an endemic area are seldom diagnostic unless the patient is shown to have conversion from negative to positive with an illness. Coccidioidin, derived from the mycelial stage, and sherulin, derived from the spherule stage, should both be used in difficult cases to increase the likelihood of detecting delayed hypersensitivity to *C. immitis*. A negative skin test does not entirely exclude coccidioidomycosis, especially early in the illness or when disseminated disease is present.

Detection of antibody response is useful in the diagnosis of coccidioidal infections and, in many instances, is the only method of proving disease caused by *C. immitis*. IgM immunoglobulin antibodies are first to be detected and comprise most of the components detected in the precipitin test. The precipitin reaction usually becomes positive by the second week of illness and reverts to negative by 5 months in most patients with uncomplicated disease. The latex agglutination test is quite sensitive and, like the precipitin test, is used in the early stages of disease when IgM antibodies are predominant.

IgG immunoglobulins rise later and are detected by immunodiffusion and complement-fixation test. A positive titer of 1:4 is suggestive of coccidioidal infection. The height of the complement-fixation titer correlates with the severity of disease, and titers of 1:32 or greater are often associated with dissemination. Antibodies measured by immunodiffusion and countercurrent immunoelectrophoresis correlate with the complement-fixing antibodies.

The immunodiffusion test kit is commercially available and the test can be performed in most laboratories. These diffusion tests are particularly useful in patients with anticomplementary serum.

In patients with meningitis, the detection of complement-fixing antibodies in the cerebrospinal fluid (CSF) is frequently the only method of specific diagnosis since cultures are often negative. Occasionally, patients without meningitis may have low titers of antibody in the CSF if a parameningeal focus of infection is present.

A positive culture of *C. immitis* from sputum, CSF, draining lesions, or biopsy material is diagnostic of coccidioidomycosis. Microscopic examination of clinical material can be used to detect the distinctive spherules. Staining of sections with hematoxylin and eosin, para-aminosalicylic acid (PAS) and methenamine silver is useful and may be supplemented with fluorescent antibody techniques in difficult cases. The finding of organisms in tissues outside of the thoracic cavity, except in the rare case of primary cutaneous coccidioidomycosis, is indicative of disseminated disease.

PITFALLS IN DIAGNOSIS

The diagnosis of coccidioidomycosis must be considered in patients who develop illness after having been in an endemic area, even for brief periods. Failure to elicit a history of travel into such areas will lead to missed or late diagnosis when disease occurs in locales where the illness is seldom seen.

Serologic and skin tests may be negative early in the disease and should be repeated after 7 to 10 days if coccidioidomycosis is suspected. Cross reactions with histoplasma and blastomyces infections are seen.

Meningitis due to *C. immitis* may have findings similar to viral processes with sterile cultures and lymphocytic response in the CSF. A low CSF glucose often will distinguish coccidioidal from most viral meningites but will require consideration of mycobacterial or other fungal disease.

Coccidioidomycosis should be included in the differential diagnosis of infections in compromised hosts since late reactivation has occurred in such circumstances. Occasionally, patients responding poorly to appropriate therapy for proven tuberculosis have been found to be infected with *C. immitis* also.

BLASTOMYCOSIS

By BRANCH T. FIELDS, JR., M.D.

Little Rock, Arkansas

SYNONYMS

North American blastomycosis, Gilchrist's disease, the Chicago disease.

DEFINITION

Blastomycosis is a chronic disease of mixed suppurative and granulomatous pathology affecting principally the lungs, skin, bones, and genitourinary tract. It is caused by the dimorphic fungus *Blastomyces (Ajellomyces) dermatitidis*. Because the perfect or sexual stage of this fungus has been discovered, the correct name of this organism is *Ajellomyces dermatitidis*. However, *Blastomyces dermatitidis*, the accepted name of the imperfect or asexual stage of the microorganism, will probably also continue to be used. The perfect stage has only been observed in rigorous laboratory experiments. The imperfect stage, that which is cultured from patients with the disease, is itself dimorphic. It exists in a mycelial phase that grows at room temperature. The belief that mycelia live in soil is unproved; spores, called conidia, probably infect man via inhalation into the lung. What actually exists and is observed in human clinical exudates, however, is the yeast-like phase of the imperfect stage of the organism, which grows at 37 C in vitro and in vivo.

CLINICAL PRESENTATION

Active blastomycosis of dogs and humans confines itself mainly to the Mississippi, Ohio, and St. Lawrence River valleys, the Middle Atlantic and Southeastern United States, and a part of Southern Manitoba. However, there are many well-documented cases from certain parts of Africa and a few reports from Mexico and South America. The disease is not contagious from man to man nor from animal to man. The illness occurs much more frequently in males than in females. Although it affects all ages, higher incidences occur between ages 20 and 50. Although the disease is said to occur more commonly in persons with a soil-related occupation, convincing evidence for this is lacking; the dictum that a chronic lung infection in a bulldozer operator is likely to be blastomycosis appears unsubstantiated.

SYMPTOMS

Patients with active blastomycosis usually have systemic disease that has begun in the lung and has subsequently disseminated most commonly to skin but also commonly to bones and to the prostate gland. The illness usually begins gradually with malaise, fever, cough, and weight loss and progresses within a few weeks to a few years with more specific symptoms of the organ systems involved. Disease limited to one organ has been seen in one third to one half the patients in recent series. About half of these one-organ cases involve lung and the other half involve skin. Rarely seen today are skin-inoculation blastomycosis with regional lymphadenopathy and the benign primary pulmonary form, sometimes caused by laboratory accident.

Lung. Primary disease, as manifested by frank infiltrates on chest roentgenograph and often accompanied by sputum production, pleuritic pain, and occasionally hemoptysis, was present in 50 to 80 per cent of patients with blastomycosis and was the presenting manifestation in 33 to 45 per cent of patients in recent series.

The patient may have fever, chills, and night sweats, and appear toxic, or he may be afebrile and appear only chronically ill. Chest examination is often nonrevealing. The roentgenographic features are not specific and include perihilar adenopathy suggesting carcinoma, consolidation, cavities, cysts, and fibronodular or miliary infiltrates. The infiltrates may involve one or many lobes and may be bilateral. Pneumothorax occurs occasionally; solitary nodules are rare. Upper lobe infiltrates have often led to a mistaken diagnosis of tuberculosis.

Skin. Cutaneous lesions have occurred in up to 80 per cent of patients in recent reports, and they were the presenting manifestations in 25 to 40 per cent of patients. Multiple lesions occurred in 60 to 90 per cent of patients who had skin involvement. Lesions usually begin on exposed areas such as the nose, face, lower legs, hand, and wrist, and appear later on the trunk and other unexposed surfaces. It is unusual for the palms, soles, and scalp to be affected. The commonest lesions are subcutaneous nodules or papulopustules that ulcerate and evolve into the characteristic raised, wart-like granulomas with serpiginous, abruptly sloping borders. These lesions are usually so characteristic that the experienced clinician makes a presumptive diagnosis after inspection. However, frankly ulcerative skin lesions may occur. Involved areas expand peripherally and heal centrally with scarring. Mucous membrane lesions not adjacent to skin lesions are seen in 5 per cent of patients. Weeping sinus tracts occur over bone lesions. Skin lesions vary from 1 to 10 cm in diameter; pain and significant purulent discharge are uncommon manifestations.

Bone. Osteomyelitis occurs in 20 to 50 per cent and is a presenting manifestation in 10 to 20 per cent of patients with blastomycosis. Radiologically these osteolytic defects are indistinguishable from neoplastic, pyogenic, and tuberculous lesions. The pelvis, skull, ribs, and epiphyseal ends of long bones are common sites of involvement. In addition, lumbar and thoracic vertebrae are often affected with erosion anteriorly of vertebral bodies and destruction of discs. Occasionally, monoarticular infective arthritis occurs in the absence of a contiguous bone lesion.

Genitourinary System. Blastomycosis, unlike other deep mycoses, involves the prostate, epididymis, testis, or seminal vesicles in 10 to 33 per cent and presents with involvement of one of these organs in 4 to 8 per cent of patients. A persistently indurated prostate, pyuria without dysuria, and perineal discomfort usually lead to surgical biopsy and diagnosis. Swelling of the testis or epididymis may also occur.

COMMON COMPLICATIONS

Occasionally, pericarditis produces symptoms and signs mimicking congestive heart failure. Endocarditis has occurred, as has adrenal cortical insufficiency. Other unusual sites of involvement include meninges, brain, esophagus, appendix, tonsils, trachea, colon, rectum, anus, cornea, uveal tract, paranasal sinuses, diaphragm, and the pituitary gland.

LABORATORY FINDINGS

Mild normochromic anemia, hypoalbuminemia, and leukocytosis each occur in about 25 per cent of patients, and nonspecific hyperglobulinemia and elevated erythrocyte sedimentation rate are very common. The blastomycin skin test is usually negative in patients with active disease. Because of this, the antigen is no longer available. There is evidence suggesting that skin testing is consistently positive in rare epidemics of primary pulmonary blastomycosis; perhaps the few patients who subsequently develop disseminated blastomycosis then become anergic and can no longer react to the skin test antigen — after the pattern so well established in coccidioidomycosis. Serum complement-fixing antibodies against *B. dermatitidis* are detectable only in about 50 per cent of cases and cross-react with *Histoplasma capsulatum* antigens. Thus, while this fungal serol-

ogy test is not sufficient for even a presumptive diagnosis, a titer of 1:32 or higher should stimulate aggressive efforts to identify the microorganism.

COURSE

Untreated systemic blastomycosis progresses either rapidly or slowly to disability, it occasionally remits, and in various series it has caused death in 21 to 92 per cent of patients. Of the patients who die, 90 per cent do so within 3 years after diagnosis. It is said that cutaneous involvement alone carries a good prognosis for longevity, but that the skin lesions rarely clear without therapy. Multiple organ involvement worsens the prognosis.

DIAGNOSIS

Any combination of skin, lung, bone, or urinary tract disease in a patient from the appropriate geographic area strongly suggests blastomycosis, as does the appearance of the skin lesion itself. The presence of a gastrointestinal lesion suggests neoplasm, ameboma, tuberculosis, or histoplasmosis rather than blastomycosis.

Once suspected, a presumptive diagnosis sufficient for initiating antimicrobial therapy can be made by: (1) identification by a trained microscopist of yeast-like forms resembling *B. dermatitidis* in wet coverslip preparations of patient exudates, or (2) demonstration of the yeast-like forms in histologic sections of tissue. The diagnosis is confirmed by isolation of *Blastomyces dermatitidis* from exudates or lesions. Examination of pus from skin lesions, sputum, and urine should be performed; and in addition, biopsies of lung, bone, prostate, epididymis, or other lesions will be rewarding. The prostate should be massaged in almost all male patients. Skin biopsies should be done at the periphery of the involvement. Liver biopsy and bone marrow examination have only occasionally been helpful.

Direct coverslip mounts are made by collecting a drop of fluid onto a slide, placing a coverslip and examining at 500 times magnification (high-dry objective). The 10 to 16 micrometer yeast-like form is a single cell having usually one bud connected to the parent cell by a wide 4 to 5 micrometer neck. Cells without budding are also present but are not adequate for a diagnosis. There is no capsule. The large yeast-like form, 1.5 to 2 times the size of an erythrocyte, stands out in such contrast to cells and debris that neither staining nor 10 per cent potassium hydroxide (KOH) is usually necessary. However, the endospores of *Coccidioides immitis* may resemble *B. dermatitidis* cells until either budding or a *C. immitis* spherule is identified. *Histoplasma capsulatum* yeast-like cells cannot be seen in wet exudate preparations. Candida cells are 3 to 4 micrometers in size, they take the Gram stain intensely, and they usually have pseudohyphae, unlike *Blastomyces*. Unlike *B. dermatitidis, Cryptococcus neoformans* yeast-like forms usually have large capsules; *Paracoccidioides brasiliensis* cells generally have multiple buds attached to the parent cell by a narrow base, and they are rarely seen in the United States.

Histologically, a mixed reaction comprising granulomas, giant cells, and central polymorphonuclear leukocytes is seen. However, this is not specific for blastomycosis, since a mixed granulomatous and neutrophilic reaction is also seen in sporotrichosis and coccidioidomycosis. Skin lesions in blastomycosis show pseudoepitheliomatous hyperplasia, which is sometimes misdiagnosed as epidermoid carcinoma; crusts, tiny abscesses, necrosis, ulcer, and scar are also seen.

In tissue, the yeast-like forms are discernible with hematoxylin and eosin stain, but visualization is greatly enhanced by periodic acid–Schiff (PAS) or Gomori methenamine-silver stains. Mayer's mucicarmine stain usually illuminates *C. neoformans* brilliantly and *B. dermatitidis* faintly. The "double-contoured" appearance of the cell wall, a confusing term, refers to either the inner and outer limit of the cell wall or alternatively to the inner limit of the cell wall and the outer limit of the cytoplasm retracted away from the wall in fixed specimens. Bronchoscopic or gastric washings and cytologic examination of sputum can demonstrate the fungus.

Isolation and identification of *B. dermatitidis* requires an interested, trained technologist; training is available in many universities and at a course at the Center for Disease Control in Atlanta, Georgia. Alternatively, an organism may be isolated and sent to a reference laboratory for identification. Because of contaminants, mailed sputum specimens would seem to be unsatisfactory but have not been shown to be so.

Sabouraud's agar is adequate, and 0.5 to 1 ml of exudate should be inoculated onto each of several slants or plates. If cultures are incubated at 37 C, the granular yeast-like colony of *B. dermatitidis* will appear; but if incubated at room temperature, the yeast-like forms will convert to the mycelial phase as they grow, and the tightly entangled white to light brown mold will be seen. Cultivation of the mycelial phase at 23 to 30 C is more reliable than cultivation of the yeast-like phase. Although negative cultures should be held for a month, growth usually appears in 4 to 7 days. The laboratory diagnosis of *B. dermatitidis* is established by the presence of smooth, round, or pyriform spores (conidia) emanating from the hyphae, absence of the tuberculate macroconidia characteristic of the mycelial phase of *H. capsulatum*, and most importantly by demonstration of dimorphism — conversion of the mycelial to the yeast-like phase by incubating freshly inoculated subcultures at 37 C. Most other fungi are not dimorphic. *H. capsulatum* is dimorphic but has spiny conidia and tuberculate macroconidia (large round structures with multiple knobby projections). By electron microscopy *B. dermatitidis* is multinucleate, whereas *H. capsulatum* and *C. neoformans* are uninucleate.

PITFALLS IN DIAGNOSIS

The primary pitfall is failure to consider blastomycosis, particularly in an endemic area. Another is eliminating blastomycosis because of a negative fungal serology test. Still a third is the pitfall of allowing a positive blastomycosis complement-fixation test to be the only laboratory evidence for a diagnosis. As mentioned, the decision to treat should rest on visualizing or isolating and identifying the causative fungal organism. An exception to this is the critically ill patient with clinical evidence strongly suggestive of blastomycosis. In addition, seriously ill patients from the blastomycosis geographic area whose chest radiographs show a miliary pattern should be studied carefully for blastomycosis with multiple wet coverslip preparations of good-quality sputum specimens. In "miliary" blastomycosis, the prognosis is grave unless therapy is instituted quickly; coverslip preparations of sputum are usually positive.

The suspected diagnosis of blastomycosis can be elusive if lung by itself is affected and coverslip preparations of sputum fail to reveal the yeast-like forms. It may then take 1 to 2 months for multiple sputum cultures containing few yeasts to distinguish this illness from neoplasms, tuberculosis, histoplasmosis, coccidioidomycosis, actinomycosis, nocardiosis, anaerobic bacterial pneumonia, and other chronic infiltrative diseases.

ACTINOMYCOSIS

By KENNETH K. LEE, M.D.,
and ELLIOT GOLDSTEIN, M.D.

Davis, California

SYNONYMS

Lumpy jaw, leptothricosis, streptothricosis.

DEFINITION

Actinomycosis is an uncommon, chronic, noncontagious, granulomatous infection characterized by suppuration, abscess formation, and sinus tract drainage secondary to tissue invasion by endogenous bacteria of the genus Actinomyces. Although originally considered fungi, actinomyces are now classified as true bacteria on the basis of similarity of cell wall components and structure, nuclear composition, and antibiotic susceptibility patterns. Actinomyces are anaerobic or microaerophilic, non-acid fast, gram-positive microorganisms that form vegetative mycelia that fracture into bacillary, coccoid, and filamentous elements.

PATHOGENESIS

Most human infections are caused by *Actinomyces israelii*, *A. naeslundii*, *A. viscosus*, *A. odontolyticus*, *Bifidobacterium eriksonii*, and *Arachnia propionica* produce infections similar to those of *A. israelii* but do so less frequently. Actinomyces are part of the flora of the oropharynx and alimentary tract. Normally, the oxidation-reduction potential of intact mucosal tissues prevents actinomycotic proliferation; therefore, antecedent trauma to mucosal membranes and the presence of devitalized tissue are necessary for the initiation of infection. In a large series of patients, however, the majority had no record of antecedent operation, disease, or trauma. Even in such circumstances of antecedent trauma actinomyces may be insufficiently virulent to sustain infection, and "helper" bacteria such as *Bacterium actinomycetumcomitans*, fusiform bacteria, anaerobic streptococci, and gram-negative bacilli are invariably present in actinomycotic lesions.

Once established, spread occurs from the primary focus to contiguous tissues. Dense scarring, abscesses, and multiple draining sinuses are common sequelae. Exudates from these lesions often contain "sulfur granules," which, although not pathognomonic of actinomycosis, are highly presumptive of the diagnosis. Continued tissue destruction results in disfigurement and on occasion death. Septicemia and dissemination are rare complications that in most instances are consequences of underlying pulmonary infection.

CLINICAL MANIFESTATIONS

Actinomycosis occurs in all age groups, with slightly higher prevalences among males and without apparent predilection for those with immunologic deficiencies. The commonest sites for infection are cervicofacial, thoracic, and abdominal. Involvement of other sites such as brain, liver, kidney, female pelvic organs, or bone is rare. Actinomycosis of the hands is an infrequent complication of human bites. Patients with cervicofacial actinomycosis present with enlarging, painful, firm paramandibular swellings of several weeks' duration. A history of poor oral hygiene, dental surgery, or trauma is often obtained. If the infection progresses, multiple fistulas, the clinical hallmark of cervicofacial actinomycosis, develop in the overlying skin. Continued progression of infection results in periostitis followed by cyst formation, osteomyelitis, and bone destruction. Such infections may spread into contiguous areas of the cervical spine, orbit, cranial bones, meninges, middle ear, and tongue. In extremely severe cases, the lesions extend into the scapula, upper extremities, lungs, and pleura.

Primary pulmonary actinomycosis results from the inhalation or aspiration of infected oropharyngeal materials into pulmonary regions, permitting anaerobic growth. These slowly progressive pulmonary infections are associated with low-grade fever, cough, purulent sputum, and hemoptysis. Dyspnea, night sweats, anorexia, weight loss, and pleuritic pain indicate more extensive disease.

Chest roentgenograms show mass lesions, chronic alveolar infiltrates, fibrosis, or cavitary disease. Penetration of a pulmonary lesion through an interlobar fissure or involvement of the pleural space and chest wall with evidence of osteomyelitis is highly suggestive of actinomycosis, and in such cases empyema, chest wall osteomyelitis, and sinus tract formation are prominent features. Fistula formation into the trachea, esophagus, or abdomen as well as pericarditis and myocarditis can also occur.

Gastrointestinal infections tend to originate in ileocecal areas, frequently following an attack of appendicitis. Surgical and traumatic perforations of the intestinal wall are other antecedent causes for abdominal actinomycosis. The onset of illness is insidious, with abdominal discomfort and fever being the earliest symptoms. As the disease progresses, chills, night sweats, weight loss, vomiting, and jaundice become prominent manifestations, and an abdominal mass may be palpated. In the past, most infections were undiagnosed prior to exploratory laparotomy or the development of sinus tracts, at which time extension of the infection into the liver, kidneys, vertebrae, and perirectal regions was common. Routine roentgenographic examinations are of limited diagnostic value because of difficulties in delineating the ill-defined intraabdominal masses. Vertebral periostitis may be an early roentgenographic finding. Although unproven, the newer computerized tomographic, ultrasonic, and scintigraphic techniques using radioactive gallium (^{67}Ga) or technetium 99m should permit earlier diagnosis of actinomycotic lesions.

On occasion, the major site of infection is in the brain, spinal cord, urinary tract, uterus, and adnexal structures (often secondary to an infection from an intrauterine device), and bone. Except for brain infection, which results from septicemia, these less common infections are usually due to extension from a cervicofacial, thoracic, or abdominal focus. As a general rule, metastatic lesions are uncommon.

LABORATORY FINDINGS

Examination of the peripheral blood may show a slight to moderate normocytic, normochromic anemia, an increase in the erythrocyte sedimentation rate, and a leukocytosis, with an increase in "band" forms. Blood chemistries, bone marrow examinations, and urinalysis are not diagnostically helpful.

There are no skin or serologic tests of diagnostic value. Agglutinating and complement-fixing antibodies against actinomyces are demonstrable in the sera of patients, but these tests are of unproven reliability. Animal inoculation studies are of no practical value in isolating actinomycetes.

Microscopic examination using low-power objectives of pus or infected tissues may suggest the diagnosis by revealing white to yellowish so-called sulfur granules, 0.25 to 2.00 mm in diameter. When these granules, which represent growing microcolonies of actinomyces, are crushed, dense rosettes of radially arranged, club-shaped filaments are seen. Gram stain of the crushed material reveals a meshwork of delicately intertwined gram-positive filaments and interspersed bacillary and coccoid bodies. Actinomyces is not acid-fast; this property aids in differentiating the microorganism from Nocardia, which forms integumentary but not visceral sulfur granules and is acid-fast

when examined following acid decolorization. Sulfur granules are also found in infections caused by Streptomyces, Actinomadura, and *Staphylococcus actinophytosis* (botryomycosis).

These microorganisms are differentiated from actinomycetes by their aerobic growth and by their appearance on Gram stain — the mycelium of streptomyces do not fragment; staphylococci are gram-positive. Because of the usefulness of demonstrating sulfur granules, materials suspected of containing microorganisms should be strained through gauze dressings to increase the likelihood of discovery. However, sulfur granules are not always present, and even when present may be so small or few in number as to be nondetectable by laboratory means.

Except for the demonstration of sulfur granules and filamentous microorganisms, actinomycotic lesions have a nondistinctive pathologic appearance. Sections from these lesions demonstrate microabscesses, chronic granulation tissue, and extensive fibrosis.

Successful culture of actinomyces is the principal means of establishing the diagnosis. Specimens can be obtained from pus from a draining sinus, irrigation fluid from a sinus tract, material collected on gauze dressings, and biopsied tissues. They should be washed if granules are present and plated without delay on blood agar, brain heart infusion, and thioglycollate broth for anaerobic and aerobic incubation. Characteristic colonies appear in a few days; definitive identification requires 10 to 24 days.

PITFALLS IN DIAGNOSIS

Failure to consider actinomycosis or to perform anaerobic cultures, early use of antibiotics, and overgrowth by competing bacteria on culture plates are the principal pitfalls in the diagnosis of actinomycosis. Because of these errors, visible facial lesions often remain undiagnosed for prolonged periods. Once taken into consideration, cervicofacial actinomycosis is easily proved by microscopic examination and anaerobic culture. Thin needle aspiration of cervicofacial lesions has been described as useful in obtaining specimens for culture and histology. Other causes for persistent facial infection (tuberculosis, nocardiosis, blastomycosis, staphylococcal infection) usually do not produce sulfur granules and have distinctively different microbiologic characteristics.

Because of their hidden and relatively asymptomatic nature, the slowly progressive thoracic and abdominal infections are even harder to diagnose than are the cervicofacial ones. The time from clinical presentation to diagnosis is often measured in terms of months to years. Their diagnosis depends entirely on a high index of suspicion, roentgenographic, ultrasonic and scintigraphic testing, and the surgical procurement of tissue for anaerobic cultures. Pulmonary lesions detected by roentgenography are usually indistinguishable from those caused by mycobacteria, fungi, nocardia, pyogenic bacteria, and neoplasms. The same lack of etiologic specificity applies for actinomycotic lesions detected in abdominal roentgenograms. The newer scintigraphic, ultrasonic, and computerized tomographic techniques are likely to improve detection of abdominal lesions but not their etiologic identifications. As such, surgeons must be advised of the possibility of actinomycosis to ensure submission for anaerobic culture of appropriately procured pulmonary or abdominal materials. Lastly, it is worth emphasizing that actinomycetes are part of the normal oropharyngeal flora, and therefore culture of these microorganisms from expectorated sputa is not a reliable means of diagnosis.

SYPHILIS

By A. PAUL KELLY, M.D.,
and ALICE FAYE SINGLETON, M.D.
Los Angeles, California

SYNONYMS

Lues venerea, pox, morbus gallicus, "the French disease," "bad blood," "hair cut," "old Joe," and "sif."

DEFINITION

Syphilis is an infectious disease caused by the spirochete *Treponema pallidum*. It is usually transmitted from person to person by intimate contact, but it may be acquired prenatally and by blood transfusion. The disease is characterized by the florid primary and secondary types, which resolve and enter into a period of latency that may progress into a tertiary stage.

PRESENTING SIGNS AND SYMPTOMS AND COURSE

Since all stages of syphilis may mimic other medical problems it is often called the "great imitator"; as Sir William Osler said, "He who knows syphilis, knows medicine."

Syphilis in an adult passes through several stages: inoculation during sexual contact, an incubation period of approximately 3 weeks; a *primary* lesion and silent systemic dissemination for 1 to 2 months; a *secondary* stage of approximately 6 weeks; resolution; and a latent stage lasting from 1 year to a lifetime or progressing to a *tertiary* stage, which is manifested by central nervous system, cardiovascular, and granulomatous lesions. *Congenital syphilis*, on the other hand, results from the transmission of spirochetes from an infected mother to the fetus. It is divided into early and late stages and stigmata.

Primary Syphilis. The initial lesion of primary syphilis is the chancre, which usually develops at the site of treponemal inoculation after an incubation period of 9 to 90 (average 21) days. During this incubation period, spirochetes multiply at the inoculation site, in regional lymph nodes, and in various organs throughout the body. Constitutional symptoms, however, are absent in primary syphilis.

Since syphilis is usually transmitted by sexual contact, most chancres appear on the genitals. They begin as papules that ulcerate. The typical ulcer (chancre) has a smooth, well-defined, raised border with a hard and finer granular base. Sometimes, owing to secondary infection, the ulcer may be covered with a yellowish crust or have a necrotic base. Chancres are usually solitary but may be multiple. They vary in size from a few millimeters to 1 to 2 cm in diameter and, although most are annular, they may assume any morphologic appearance. Typically, they are painless, although extragenital and secondarily infected lesions are often painful.

The neighboring lymph nodes usually become enlarged, hard, nonsuppurative, and nontender ("satellite bubo") within a week after the chancre appears. The nodes have a rubbery consistency, are discrete, and are not adherent to the skin or underlying tissues; there is no overlying erythema or skin change. Initially, the adenopathy associated with genital chancres is unilateral but subsequently becomes bilateral. Approximately one third of the patients with primary syphilis have no adenopathy. In addition, lymphadenopathy is not usually detectable in patients with cervical or rectal chancres.

In males most chancres appear on the penis, especially on the prepuce, coronal sulcus, frenulum, or glans; in homosexual males, however, they are more common in the anorectal area. In infected females the most common sites are the labia majora, labia minora, and the fourchette. Fourchette chancres are often multiple and coalescent. Common, but often missed because they are not looked for, are chancres of the male urethra, which may be accompanied by mucoid discharge. In females, urethral and cervical lesions often go unnoticed.

Foreplay and various sexual practices may give rise to extragenital chancres, which can be found anywhere on the body, with the lips being the most common location. Other more common extragenital locations are the breasts, fingers, toes, tongue, tonsils, face, and eyelids. In males, chancres contracted by kissing are more common on the upper lip, whereas in females they usually appear on the lower lip.

Since the primary lesions of syphilis are often asymptomatic, they may go unrecognized and untreated. Without treatment they usually heal within 3 to 6 weeks, leaving a thin atrophic scar.

Syphilis secondary to blood transfusion or puncture wounds is often devoid of a chancre in the primary stage and usually presents with signs and symptoms of the secondary stage. This appearance of secondary lesions without a primary chancre is called "syphilis d'emblée."

Clinically, primary syphilis should be differentiated from the following diseases: chancroid, herpes simplex, granuloma inguinale, balanitis, lymphogranuloma venereum, carcinoma, trauma, and fixed drug eruption.

Secondary Syphilis. In untreated individuals the secondary stage of syphilis occurs 2 to 12 (average 3) weeks after the appearance of the chancre or within 6 months (average 2) after exposure. A resolving primary chancre may still be present when secondary lesions appear. Secondary syphilis is the most contagious stage of early syphilis, because there are usually many contagious lesions in contradistinction to a single lesion of primary syphilis.

Patients with early secondary syphilis often have influenza-like symptoms: fever, headache, sore throat, malaise, anorexia, and generalized arthralgia. Generalized painless lymphadenopathy, as well as spleen and liver enlargement, may also occur.

Skin lesions are usually the hallmark of secondary syphilis. They may be macular, papular, follicular, papulosquamous, or pustular. Any of these types may occur singly or, more commonly, in combination. Vesiculobullous lesions do not occur in adults but may be seen in congenital syphilis. Except for follicular skin lesions, eruptions are usually nonpruritic. Initially they are usually generalized and symmetrical, often becoming localized. Untreated lesions of secondary syphilis may last from weeks to months.

Macular lesions of secondary syphilis are copper colored in light-skinned persons and of a deep brown hue in persons with dark skin, in whom they often go unrecognized. These lesions tend to be discrete and oval, following the lines of cleavage, especially on the trunk. The face is usually spared.

Papular lesions are the most common and characteristic skin manifestation of secondary syphilis. They may arise in macular lesions or independently. Their color varies according to the skin color of the patient: reddish-brown (salmon) on light skin and brown to gray on dark skin. Papular lesions are usually diffuse and symmetrical, with the most characteristic location being on the palms and soles. Macular and papulosquamous lesions also appear on the palms and soles. Here, because of the induration of the lesions and the thickness of the epidermis, they often appear flat or slightly elevated. Discrete, hyperkeratotic, centrally pitted papules (syphilis cornée) may appear on the palms and soles. Occasionally, a large papule may be surrounded by smaller satellite papules, producing a configuration called corymbiform (corymbose) syphilis. Split eroded papules at the corners of the mouth are also diagnostic of syphilis.

Grouped papules may coalesce to form annular ("nickel and dime") lesions, which are most commonly seen on the mid face. Contrary to popular belief, they are seen in whites as well as in blacks. Lesions of condyloma lata are whitish moist papules and plaques that occur in moist intertriginous areas, especially the anogenital region. Lesions may vary from few to many in number. Clinically they are similar to lesions of condyloma acuminata. Papulosquamous lesions are common and must be differentiated from psoriasis, pityriasis rosea, and drug eruption.

Pustular lesions are usually the last to appear in secondary syphilis. They may resemble impetigo, acne, or chickenpox. A rare form, characterized by necrosis and ulceration with systemic symptoms, is called "lues maligna" or "malignant syphilis."

The skin lesions of secondary syphilis usually heal without scarring in 2 to 10 weeks, regardless of whether the patient is treated or not.

Mucous membrane lesions may occur alone or with any of the cutaneous lesions just discussed. They are usually 1 to 2 cm grayish-white erosions that may be surrounded by a dull erythematous margin (mucous patch). The lips, oral mucosa, tongue, pharynx, and larynx are most often involved. When the larynx is involved a sore throat or hoarseness, or both, may occur. Mucous membrane lesions are highly infectious and usually last for several weeks but may be present for only a few days.

Alopecia is a common manifestation of secondary syphilis. It may present either as a diffuse thinning of the scalp hair or as patchy hair loss, giving the characteristic "moth-eaten alopecia." The scalp lesion resembles alopecia areata, whereas, when the eyebrows are involved, the hair of the lateral portion is lost, resembling changes seen in leprosy and hypothyroidism. The hair loss is temporary and non-scarring regardless of whether or not the patient receives treatment.

Since secondary syphilis is a systemic disease, signs and symptoms often originate from organs other than the skin. These may appear in any time relationship to the skin lesions. Most patients disregard constitutional symptoms but, with thorough questioning, often admit to headache, sore throat, low-grade fever, malaise, arthralgias, and anorexia. Generalized lymphadenopathy usually precedes the skin lesions, with the cervical, epitrochlear, popliteal, and suboccipital nodes being characteristically involved. As in primary syphilis, the nodes are nontender, discrete, and rubbery in consistency. Concomitant spleen and (less commonly) liver enlargement may be present. Ophthalmic lesions may consist of iritis, uveitis (decreased vision, eye pain, photophobia, tearing) and corneal opacities. Nephropathy, probably secondary to immune complex deposition, may cause proteinuria and edema. Anorexia, nausea, vomiting, and epigastric pain secondary to ulcerations or strictures, or both, may be present. Syphilitic myositis characterized by aching muscles and progressive proximal muscle weakness, without muscle wasting, may occur. Severe aching pains of the long bones (osteocopic pain) are sometimes present; however, this is more common in congenital syphilis. Bone destruction, especially of the frontal bone, tibia, and clavicle, has been reported. Headaches may indicate acute syphilitic meningitis. Additional (although uncommon) central nervous system findings are transverse myelitis, nerve deafness, papilledema, and thromboses of the cerebral or spinal arteries. Other often neglected findings are transient electrocardiographic abnormalities, which clear with adequate treatment.

Latent Syphilis. Even without treatment the signs and symptoms of secondary syphilis clear in 2 to 8 weeks. Latent syphilis then supervenes. Latent syphilis is that stage in which, although there are no clinical signs and symptoms of the disease, serologic tests for syphilis are reactive. Latency is divided into two periods: early and late. There is disagreement as to the duration of early latency. Some experts use 2 years from the onset, while others use 4 years from the onset. Regardless, in early latency approximately one half of the patients may have one or more relapses of mucocutaneous secondary syphilis, especially during the first year of infection. Therefore, early latency, along with the primary and secondary stages, is considered to be part of infectious syphilis. As the time of latency increases, the infectiousness decreases. At the end of this stage approximately two-thirds of patients will enter the late latent phase, and the other third will enter the tertiary stage.

Late latent syphilis of more than 4 years' duration is not communicable, except in pregnant women who, if not treated, may transmit syphilis to the fetus. Also, if the spinal fluid examination is negative at 4 years, it will probably remain so for the lifetime of the patient, unless he or she is reinfected. Approximately one half of late latent patients do not develop tertiary syphilis and become seronegative.

Tertiary Syphilis. Tertiary syphilis may involve any organ system, but cutaneous, bone, cardiovascular, and central nervous system lesions predominate, developing 5 to 20 years after the primary stage, although a small percentage of cases occur earlier or later.

Gummatous lesions may develop in any organ system, but the skin, liver, and bone are the most common sites. They are usually benign, but lethal cases have been reported secondary to heart or brain involvement. Cutaneous gummas often begin as erythematous or flesh colored painless nodules that enlarge slowly and are often arranged in a polycyclic fashion. Sometimes these nodules ulcerate, forming noduloulcerative lesions. The nodular lesions heal without residua, but ulcerative lesions usually heal with atrophic scars and hyperpigmentation. Some lesions start as deep subcutaneous indurations with an overlying dusky-red appearance of the skin or mucous membrane. They rapidly break down and form punched-out ulcers with an arciform border.

These lesions tend to be quite destructive, often causing damage to the underlying bone and cartilage with resulting perforation of the hard palate or nasal septum. Serologic tests for syphilis are always positive in patients with active gummata, but spirochetes are not demonstrable in the lesions. This fact has led many syphilologists to postulate that gummas result from a hypersensitivity reaction rather than from direct tissue invasion by the spirochetes. Gummas are not infectious.

Neurosyphilis. Neurosyphilis develops in approximately 10 per cent of patients with untreated syphilis. It is more frequent in males than in females and is seen more frequently in whites than in blacks. Although invasion of the central nervous system occurs during early stages of syphilis, symptoms usually do not appear for at least 2 years after the initial infection. Neurosyphilis occurs in two forms: meningovascular and parenchymatous, but the classic clinical presentation of each type is usually not observed because routine antibiotic treatment of nontreponemal disease alters the pattern of disease.

In asymptomatic neurosyphilis there is no clinical evidence of disease, the patient having been identified because of positive routine serologic tests. Spinal fluid examination usually reveals an increased leukocyte count (5 or more per cu mm), a total protein count of over 40 mg per dl (100 ml), and a positive serologic test for syphilis (STS). In tabes dorsalis the spinal fluid examination is normal in approximately 20 per cent of the patients.

Meningovascular syphilis (syphilitic meningitis) may be acute or chronic. Acute involvement (within the first 2 years of infection) is manifested by symptoms of headache, fever, stiff neck, and a positive Kernig's sign. It is rare, occurs usually in males, and may clear with or without treatment.

The clinical manifestations of chronic meningovascular syphilis vary according to which blood vessels or areas of the central nervous system are involved. Vessel involvement may cause psychosis, dizziness, mental confusion, aphasia, and hemiplegia. Extraocular muscle and facial palsies result from chronic meningitis of the base of the brain. Vertex involvement results in headache, seizures, increased intracranial pressure, nausea, and vomiting. Optic neuritis or optic atrophy or both may result from syphilitic inflammation of the optic nerve. Other cerebral manifestations may include irregularity and inequality of the pupils with a normal reaction to accommodation but a sluggish reaction to light (Argyll Robertson pupil) and inequality of deep tendon reflexes.

Degeneration of the ganglion cells and axons may result in parenchymatous neurosyphilis. There may be frontal lobe involvement (general paresis) or involvement of the posterior columns and posterior roots of the spinal cord (tabes dorsalis). The midbrain and sympathetic nervous system may also be involved in tabes.

Initially, paresis is often associated with subtle nonspecific symptoms such as headache, insomnia, poor concentration, and behavioral changes before overt mental changes are noted; some patients, however, may have seizures that are diagnosed as epilepsy and other patients may have small strokes that are usually diagnosed as a cerebrovascular accident. The full-blown mental symptoms consist of varied psychoses such as mania, euphoria, dementia, depression, and schizophrenia. Neurologically, the symptoms may be varied, but slurring of speech and pupillary irregularities are common.

The classic symptoms of tabes dorsalis are ataxia, lightning pains, paresthesias, visceral crises, bladder disturbances, impotence, and diplopia. Ataxia is manifested by loss of position sense (high stepping-slapping gait), especially in the dark. Lightning pains occur most commonly in the legs. They start suddenly, are severe and intermittent, and may last for minutes or days. Abdominal pain with visceral crises may be so severe that patients undergo surgery. The classic Argyll Robertson pupil or optic atrophy or both may be present. Loss or impairment of pain sensation may lead to trophic joint changes (Charcot's joints), the knee being the most common joint affected. Loss of deep pain sensation may lead to chronic indolent ulcers on the soles or toes (mal perforant).

The signs and symptoms of paresis and tabes dorsalis may coexist in the same patient (taboparesis).

Cardiovascular Syphilis. Cardiovascular involvement may occur as early as 5 years after primary infection but is seldom detected before 10 years and may not be discovered for 30 years after primary involvement. There are no early electrocardiographic changes. Approximately 10 per cent of untreated syphilitics will develop cardiac disease, males being more frequently affected than females.

The basic lesion of cardiovascular syphilis is aortitis, which has been reported only in acquired syphilis. In aortitis the elastic tissue of the media and the intima is destroyed and replaced by rigid fibrous tissues, producing saccular aneurysms that may be filled with organized blood clots. The ostia may become narrowed, leading to myocardial ischemia and (rarely) death.

Involvement of the aortic valve rings and cusps may produce incompetence, resulting in regurgitation of the blood in the left ventricle. A diastolic murmur is produced that is best heard in Erb's area with the patient sitting and leaning forward in forced expiration. The pulse rises and falls quickly (Corrigan's, collapsing or water-hammer pulse).

Large aortic aneurysms may exert pressure and cause problems with the trachea, bronchi, lungs, vagal nerve, diaphragm, recurrent laryngeal nerve, and vertebrae.

Congenital Syphilis. *Treponema pallidum* will not pass through the placenta until after weeks 16 to 20, apparently because the Langhans' cell layer of the placenta, which completely atrophies by week 16, prevents its passage. As a result, congenital syphilis dates from after the fourth or fifth month of gestation. If a mother is adequately treated before this time, the product of gestation will have no evidence of syphilis.

Congenital syphilis is classified as early (up to 2 years, wherein the lesions are infectious); late (2 years and later, with primarily noninfectious lesions), and stigmata (permanent changes resulting from the disease in either stage).

Early Congenital Syphilis. The disease in the newborn is extremely variable in severity of onset. Local skin findings may erupt in an infant who appears to be quite well. Other infants may present with snuffles (coryza) and mucosal fissures or patches, rashes and periostitis and osteochondritis; a disseminated maculopapular rash, particularly prominent on the palmar and plantar surfaces, associated with mucous membrane lesions; or a classic picture of snuffles and rhagades, with hepatosplenomegaly and a generalized rash. Other clinical presentations include those of an isolated anemia, thrombocytopenia, leukocytosis, jaundice, lymphadenopathy, fever, and failure to thrive. What is most difficult for the practitioner is that an infant may be entirely well, with negative serology, only to subsequently develop the full-blown disease.

Vesiculobullous lesions ("syphilitic pemphigus") are the earliest skin manifestations of congenital syphilis, often being present at birth. This is the only time of life when syphilis will be associated with a vesicle or bulla. On physical examination, the infant often has grouped vesiculobullous lesions, symmetrically distributed, particularly on the palms and soles. These lesions may also be present at the anorectal junction, periorally and, on rare occasions, may be generalized. The rash may be scant or diffuse, with fluid contents that are serous or seropurulent. Darkfield examination reveals that the contents are loaded with *T. pallidum*, thus being highly infectious. The lesions usually progress to superficial crusted erosions. During this phase, the child may often appear to be gravely ill.

Superficial desquamation, particularly of the palms and soles, is a quite frequent finding. It may, indeed, be the only dermatologic manifestation of congenital syphilis.

Later in onset are macular, papular, maculopapular, and papulosquamous eruptions, which constitute the typical syphilide. The palms and soles may be so intensely involved that they appear to be diffusely inflamed. Cutaneous lesions also appear on the face, chin, buttocks, genitals, and diaper area (presenting as a persistent diaper rash). In moist intertriginous areas, these may progress to become condylomata lata. The eruption may be scant or diffuse

in quantity, and of a reddish color. Some experts attribute the development of rhagades to the secondary bacterial infection of the eruption around the mouth.

Other cutaneous manifestations include circinate lesions, raised plaques, café au lait–like patches, and shallow ulcers.

Mucous patches identical to those of acquired secondary syphilis develop, particularly on the palate, at the commissures of the mouth, and at various mucosal sites of the mouth, nose, anus, and genitals. They begin as maculopapular lesions, developing a central fissure with ulceration, becoming covered with a grayish membrane. The patient usually has accompanying systemic symptoms, including fever and malaise.

Mucous patches in the nose give rise to "snuffles," the signs and symptoms of which are coryza and rhinitis, which do not respond to decongestants and topical medications, and produce symptoms of obstruction. The amount of discharge may be profuse or slight, but the discharge is highly infectious, as demonstrated by a plethora of spirochetes on darkfield examination. It is serosanguineous, mucoid, purulent, or mucopurulent. Eventually, it excoriates the upper lip. By interfering with the development of the nasal bones, the infection in the nose gives rise to syphilitic facies, including the saddle nose (flat nasal bridge), small maxilla, and high-arched palate. The development of rhagades (linear circumoral scars) has also been attributed to this manifestation of syphilis.

Bony involvement has been given many names (Parrot's periostitis, osteomyelitis, periostitis, metaphysitis, osteochondritis). It consists of a panosteomyelitis, with most prominent effects on the growth plate of the metaphysis. Bone destruction and bone production are characteristic of this disease. The long bones and skull bones are involved most often, although involvement of the scapulae and ribs has been reported. Symptoms range from none (positive x-ray only) to pseudoparalysis, resulting from pain on motion. One may also find pyarthrosis, crepitation, and dislocation of joints. Pathologic fractures, usually in the metaphysis, have been reported in the diaphysis as well. Untreated bony lesions may resolve without residua or may progress into the bony lesions of late congenital syphilis.

Central nervous system involvement in early congenital syphilis may be the initial manifestation of a florid syphilitic infection. Although symptoms or signs (bulging fontanel, seizures, nuchal rigidity, increasing head circumference, etc.) may be present, it is asymptomatic in half of the patients. There are several forms that the central nervous system disease may take: acute meningovascular syphilis, which has severe sequelae including mental retardation and low-grade hydrocephalus; acute syphilitic meningitis with seizures; and meningoencephalitis.

Visceral involvement includes hepatosplenomegaly, lymphadenopathy, nephrotic syndrome, acute nephritis, and severe hepatitis, among others. Eye lesions include iritis and chorioretinitis. Edema may develop, resulting from hypoproteinemia, the major cause of which is thought to be malnutrition, rather than the renal loss of protein. Orchitis, pneumonia, fever, failure to thrive, gastrointestinal disturbances, hemorrhage, and restlessness have also been reported. Death attributed to pulmonary hemorrhage, bacterial infection, or severe hepatitis may occur.

Late Congenital Syphilis. Untreated early congenital syphilis is the origin of late congenital syphilis. Sixty per cent of cases of late congenital syphilis remain latent, however, being diagnosed only by a routine serologic test. Among the 40 per cent that become clinically evident, the spectrum of disease differs widely from that of acquired late syphilis, aside from the fact that cardiovascular syphilis rarely if ever occurs in congenital syphilitics. Except for rhagades and gummas, lesions of the skin are not present. Bone and joint lesions include Clutton's joints and gummatous periostitis. Clutton's joints (chronic syphilitic hydrarthrosis) are characterized by symmetrical painless swellings of knees more often than of elbows or other joints. These lesions present primarily in pubertal or adolescent males. Joint tap produces no *T. pallidum*, but 10,000 to 45,000 white blood cells, primarily lymphocytes, are found. X-ray reveals no bony changes. It is thought that Clutton's joints represent a hypersensitivity reaction to the *T. pallidum*. Treatment with penicillin is ineffectual. Joint tap is followed by a reaccumulation of fluid, until the disease burns itself out.

Gummatous periostitis may, as in the bony lesions of early congenital syphilis, be bone-producing or bone-destroying. Bone-producing lesions are found in the tibias (leading to the development of saber shins), phalanges, and skull. Lesions of the scapulae, clavicles, and shoulder girdle have been reported. Sternoclavicular swelling (Higouménakis' sign) has also been described. Bone-destroying lesions occur primarily in the palate, producing palatal perforation. They also occur in the bony ridge of the nose. In contrast to the lesions of early congenital syphilis, wherein the defects in the nose and face result from the *prevention of development* of bones, in late congenital syphilis they result

from actual *destruction* of bone. The age of onset is 4 to 20 years.

Visceral lesions include gummas of the liver and other organs.

Central nervous system lesions that are asymptomatic are present in one third of untreated patients lacking other clinical manifestations. A positive spinal tap is the only manifestation of disease in these patients. Symptomatic neurosyphilis occurs in one fourth of untreated congenital syphilitics over the age of 6 years. It consists of parenchymal disease (juvenile tabes dorsalis, juvenile paresis), meningovascular syphilis, and eighth nerve deafness. The last finding, limited to the auditory portion of the nerve, occurs in 25 to 38 per cent of late congenital syphilitics. It may occur in isolation, leading to rapidly progressive deafness. It is characterized by the sudden onset, at age 8 to 10 years, of bilateral, symmetrical, sensorineural deafness. No vestibular signs are present. This finding is often associated with interstitial keratitis or Hutchinson's incisors (an affliction of the permanent incisors, usually the upper central pair but involving other teeth at times), or both.

The most common lesion of late congenital syphilis is interstitial keratitis. Although it usually presents at the same age as does palatal perforation, it may present at any time. Like Clutton's joints, this lesion is thought to result from a hypersensitivity reaction to the *T. pallidum*. The patient presents with acute photophobia, pain, and lacrimation in one or both eyes. Even if the affliction begins unilaterally, however, it eventually — after weeks or years — involves the other eye. The condition leads to progressive corneal opacity and blindness. Treatment with penicillin alone will not be effective. Other ocular lesions include chorioretinitis, vascular occlusion, and optic atrophy. The combination of eighth nerve deafness, Hutchinson's incisors, and interstitial keratitis is called Hutchinson's triad.

Stigmata. By definition, the stigmata of congenital syphilis are the scars and defects that remain as permanent evidence of congenital syphilis. They usually result from the more severe lesions. Stigmata of early congenital syphilis include old chorioretinitis (resulting from active chorioretinitis); frontal bossing (from osteomyelitis of the skull); syphilitic facies (maxillary underdevelopment, high arched palate, saddle nose) resulting from the mucous patches in the nose; rhagades (either from snuffles that excoriate the skin around the mouth, aggravated by grimacing or smiling, or from secondary bacterial infection of moist lesions around the mouth); pupillary changes from iritis. Hutchinson's incisors and Moon's (mulberry) molars also arise from this stage and may be seen on x-ray prior to eruption.

The stigmata of late congenital syphilis include old chorioretinitis (also arising from active disease), frontoparietal bossing (from sclerotic osteoperiostitis), and saber shins (from the waxing and waning of sclerotic periostitis).

LABORATORY FINDINGS

The clinical diagnosis of syphilis should be confirmed by laboratory tests that demonstrate the presence of spirochetes in the lesions, classic histopathologic findings on biopsy and/or antibodies in the serum or spinal fluid. Syphilis antibodies are of two main types: those to the organism itself and those secondary to the interaction of the spirochete with the tissue (reagin).

Darkfield Examination. This is the direct visualization of spirochetes in the lesions of primary and secondary syphilis. Darkfield examination of late secondary or tertiary lesions is usually negative. To perform a successful darkfield examination: (1) Abrade the lesion with gauze so as to produce a serous exudate with little or no bleeding. (2) Squeeze the lesion between your gloved thumb and forefinger. (3) Wipe away the first few drops in order to get more spirochetes from the depth of the lesion. (4) Touch the exudate with a glass slide (from the vagina and cervix collect the serum with a capillary pipette). (5) Place a coverslip on the drop of serum and, in order to prevent drying and death of the spirochetes, seal the coverslip with petrolatum.

Oral and genital mucous membrane lesions often have other spirochetes that are confused with *T. pallidum.* Darkfield examination in these patients is best done by injecting 0.5 to 1 ml. of sterile saline solution into an enlarged regional lymph node, using the needle tip to macerate the tissue, aspirating the materials and examining it for spirochetes. If the patient has used topical antiseptics, or if the lesion is secondarily infected, the spirochete may be temporarily destroyed in the surface serum. In these cases, advise the patient to compress the lesions with saline solution 20 to 30 minutes 3 or 4 times a day and return in 24 hours for darkfield examination.

SEROLOGY

The humoral antibodies produced in syphilis are measured by treponemal and nontreponemal tests. The nontreponemal tests are further divided into flocculation (VDRL, Hinton, Kahn,

Kline) and complement-fixation (Wasserman, Kolmer) types.

Nontreponemal Tests. There are over 100 different nontreponemal tests for syphilis but the most commonly used flocculation tests are the Venereal Disease Research Laboratory test (VDRL) and a modification developed for rapid screening, the rapid plasma reagin (RPR) test. The Kolmer is the most commonly used complement-fixation test. The VDRL may be positive in 10 to 25 per cent of the patients having a chancre of 1 week's duration, increased to 50 per cent positivity by the end of the second week of the chancre and usually reaching 75 per cent positivity in primary syphilis. The reactivity increases to 100 per cent in secondary syphilis but decreases thereafter. A negative test in suspected patients should be repeated at least two times. False-positive tests may be secondary to acute viral infections, bacterial infections, other spirochetal diseases, malaria, leprosy, collagen vascular disease, recent vaccination, chronic intravenous narcotic use, pregnancy, and old age.

An advantage of the VDRL is its quantitativeness. Serum is diluted serially and the test repeated at each dilution until it is no longer reactive. The last dilution producing a positive result is the titer, e.g., a titer of 1:32 means that the serum was reactive at 1:32 (7-tube dilution) but negative (nonreactive) at 1:64. In active disease the titer usually increases on subsequent testing. If the patient is not treated in late syphilis, the titer remains the same; with treatment, however, it decreases. The VDRL becomes nonreactive with treatment within a year in almost 100 per cent of those with primary syphilis, and in 95 per cent of those treated in the secondary stage it becomes nonreactive within 18 months. Occasionally with nontreponemal tests, the excess production of antibody (especially in the secondary stage of syphilis) results in the prozone phenomenon. Undiluted serum will give a weakly reactive, atypical or, on rare occasions, nonreactive reading, whereas testing at higher dilutions will give reactive test results. Treponemal tests are nonspecific but are more expensive and more difficult to perform. They become positive earlier in primary syphilis and remain positive for indefinite periods of time after treatment. The highest percentage of positive tests is found in secondary syphilis.

One of the most specific tests is the *Treponema pallidum* immobilization test (TPI), which is a complement-fixation test using live treponema. Owing to the slow development of antibodies, the TPI test becomes reactive later in primary syphilis than do the nontreponemal tests. The test is difficult to perform and is only done at the Center for Disease Control (CDC) in Atlanta, Georgia, and a few research laboratories. This test should be used only if one suspects syphilis in a patient with any condition that may cause other tests to be falsely positive.

The most widely used treponemal test is the fluorescent treponemal antibody-absorption test (FTA-ABS). It is quite specific and sensitive, but intravenous narcotic addiction, hypergammaglobulinemia, systemic lupus erythematosus, pregnancy, and rheumatoid arthritis with a high titer rheumatoid factor may cause a false positive reaction. The FTA-ABS test becomes positive in primary syphilis at approximately the time that the chancre appears and remains positive longer in treated and in late untreated syphilis than any of the treponemal or nontreponemal tests.

Other Tests.   The most promising new test is the treponemal isohemagglutination test (TPHA). It seems to approach the specificity of the TPI test and is much easier to perform. It is more specific and more sensitive in all stages beyond primary syphilis than the nontreponemal tests. The TPHA becomes positive in primary syphilis later than the VDRL and FTA-ABS tests. At present, its place in the diagnosis of syphilis has not been established.

LABORATORY TESTS IN CONGENITAL SYPHILIS

If the mother is treated late in pregnancy, even if the baby is negative at birth — serologically and clinically — the physician should follow the baby's serology and clinical picture, since these may change. The most difficult diagnosis to make is on the infant whose VDRL titer is the same as the mother's. In this case, one should do the long bone x-rays as soon as possible, since these may be positive early; one should also send a blood specimen for quantitative IgM, which may indicate an intrauterine infection of some kind if the level is over 20 mg per dl. All newborns with suspected or definite congenital syphilis should have a spinal fluid examination. A FTA-ABS–IgM should also be done. If it is positive, it is helpful, although in 10 per cent of cases it may be positive because of anti-IgM produced by the infant in response to other antigens, including maternal IgG, which is passively transferred to the fetus. The major drawback to this test, however, is that it will fail to detect the condition in up to 35 per cent of patients having delayed-onset disease!

Any moist lesion may be examined under darkfield, although this examination may not distinguish between pathogenic and nonpathogenic spirochetes. Other useful tests include a complete blood count with a differential cell count, and cell morphology.

When in doubt, the best regimen is to treat the patient for neurosyphilis. Those physicians who prefer to wait for definitive evidence of the disease may follow the VDRL and clinical picture. If the antibody is passively transmitted to the fetus, the VDRL will decline promptly and become negative by 3 months of age. An increase in titer or the failure of the titer to decline is suggestive of active disease. It is essential to follow the titer until it becomes completely nonreactive, because occasionally there will be an initial decrease followed by progressive increases. In late congenital syphilis, it is common for the VDRL titers to vary from measurement to measurement.

Histopathology.   The fundamental pathologic changes in syphilis are swelling and proliferation of the endothelial cells and a perivascular infiltrate that is composed of lymphocytes and numerous plasma cells. In tertiary syphilis one finds these changes, in addition to a granulomatous infiltrate of epitheloid and giant cells. Caseation necrosis is often present in the center. Although plasma cells are the hallmark of syphilitic tissue, there are few to none in some biopsy specimens. Spirochetes are difficult to demonstrate except in condyloma lata. If present, they can be demonstrated with silver stains such as the Warthin-Starry or Levaditi's stain. They are more common in the epidermis than the dermis and will not be present if antibiotic therapy has been given prior to biopsy.

DIFFERENTIAL DIAGNOSIS

Primary Syphilis.   A genital chancre must be differentiated from chancroid, herpes simplex, granuloma inguinale, erosive balanitis, trauma, and carcinoma. Primary cervical chancres must be differentiated from carcinoma. Extragenital chancres, according to their sites, must be differentiated from various diseases: oral lesions due to tuberculosis, Behçet's disease, herpes simplex, and carcinoma; nipple lesions due to Paget's disease; tonsillar lesions secondary to infectious mononucleosis, agranulocytosis, and acute tonsillitis; finger chancres from paronychiae, sarcomas, carcinomas, felons, or herpetic whitlow; and anal or rectal lesions must be differentiated from cancer, thrombosed hemorrhoids, or Bowen's disease.

Secondary Syphilis.   This may mimic any cutaneous disease and any cutaneous disease may coexist with syphilis. Macular and papular lesions must be differentiated from pityriasis rosea, lichen planus, urticaria pigmentosa, drug eruption, leprosy, sarcoid, infectious mononucleosis, measles, and erythema multiforme. Papulosquamous lesions may resemble psoriasis, pityriasis rosea, seborrheic dermatitis, and tinea. Syphilitic alopecia resembles alopecia areata. Granuloma annulare, sarcoid, and tinea corporis must be differentiated from the annular lesions of secondary syphilis. Hemorrhoids, condyloma acuminata, Behçet's disease, and pemphigus vegetans may resemble condyloma lata. Cutaneous lesions of congenital syphilis must be differentiated from atopic eczema, from diseases causing hepatomegaly and splenomegaly, and from diseases causing lymphadenopathy.

Tertiary skin lesions may resemble any granulomatous disease, especially tuberculosis, leprosy, sarcoidosis, and deep mycoses.

Diagnostic Guidelines. Any patient treated for gonorrhea should have a serologic test for syphilis 6 to 12 weeks later. Darkfield examination of a chancre or an enlarged lymph node is indicated in any patient suspected of having primary syphilis. If the darkfield examination cannot be performed, then serum should be drawn for a nontreponemal test. If the test is negative, but suspicion remains high, a FTA-ABS should be performed.

Both treponemal and nontreponemal serologic tests are reactive in almost 100 per cent of patients with secondary syphilis. If, however, a false-positive reaction is suspected, a darkfield examination should be performed on all suspected lesions or on a lymph node aspirate.

In late syphilis nontreponemal tests may become negative, therefore the FTA-ABS or other treponemal tests must be ordered. These patients should all have spinal fluid examinations.

RELAPSING FEVER

By WILLIAM B. DEAL, M.D.

Gainesville, Florida

SYNONYMS

Tick fever, fowl nest fever, vagabond fever, bilious typhoid, febris recurrens, spirillum fever.

DEFINITION

Relapsing fever is a systemic illness caused by spirochetes of the genus *Borrelia*, resulting in acute febrile episodes with interim afebrile periods usually lasting at least a week.

EPIDEMIOLOGY

Two distinct epidemiologic types of relapsing fever occur: *louse-borne*, which is transmitted from man to man by the human body louse, and *tick-borne*, which is the only endemic form of relapsing fever in the United States.

The reservoir is small rodents in the western United States and the disease is transmitted to man by *Ornithodoros* ticks, so-called soft ticks. Because the soft tick feeds in the dark for short periods and the bites are not painful, the bite goes unnoticed.

In January, 1978, a case of endemic relapsing fever was reported from Ohio, thus possibly reflecting the spread of the host or reservoir or both.

CAUSATIVE AGENT

Borrelia recurrentis is a slender (10 to 20 microns by 0.3 micron), loosely coiled (5 to 7), motile, gram-negative spirochete. It has the capacity for antigenic change during the infection and thus relapses occur. *Borrelia* cannot be cultured but may be kept viable in suspension for extended periods.

PRESENTING SIGNS AND SYMPTOMS

Following an incubation period of 5 to 7 days, the patient develops fever, arthralgia, and myalgia. Because of the severity of symptoms, the patient is acutely ill. Hepatosplenomegaly may occur with associated icterus. Occasionally, respiratory and central nervous system involvement occurs. Respiratory involvement may include frank bronchopneumonia. With neurologic involvement, meningismus and cerebrospinal fluid pleocytosis can occur. Classically, patients are febrile for less than 1 week, then defervescence occurs to be followed by a relapse in about 7 days. Patients may have as many as five relapses. Tick-borne disease has a case fatality rate of about 5 per cent.

During the period of fever, spirochetemia is prominent. As relapses occur, the duration of fever becomes shorter and the number of circulating spirochetes diminishes.

DIAGNOSIS

If an exposure in an endemic area is elicited, the patient's blood should be examined by direct observation of unstained wet preparations by either lightfield or darkfield microscopy. The examination of thin and thick-stained blood films by light microscopy may also be productive. Thick blood smears stained with Wright or Giemsa stain will reveal the purple-stained spirochete. Since *Borrelia* is the only human blood-borne spirochetal disease-causing organism that stains with aniline dyes, diagnosis is thereby facilitated. Direct examination should be limited to the acute febrile period. At best, in only 70 per cent of patients can the microorganism be demonstrated, but the yield does increase when multiple smears are taken.

Differential diagnosis should include Colorado tick fever, Rocky Mountain spotted fever, Q fever, leptospirosis, and meningococcal disease.

There are no specific serologic tests.

The presence of spirochetes in peripheral blood and a history of exposure is diagnostic. White blood cell counts are not helpful because they may be normal, high, or low.

PITFALLS IN DIAGNOSIS

The failure to take a proper history and suspect the disease are the most common errors made in evaluating a patient with an acute relapsing febrile illness.

AMEBIASIS

By P. N. CHHUTTANI, M.D., D.T.M., F.A.Sc., F.A.M.S.

Chandigarh, India

Amebiasis — infection with *Entamoeba histolytica* — has a worldwide incidence of around 10 per cent of humanity, but this alarming estimate should be viewed with some reservation. The disease is not a major health problem in the developed world, but most developing nations, especially China, India, and the Philippines, are hotbeds of the disease, with high morbidity and a significant mortality in the hepatic form. Positive cytologic studies for the parasite are not reliable in evaluating the importance of the infection and its morbidity potential in a particular population. Positive seroepidemiologic surveys may prove more useful because they imply contact at some stage between tissues and *Entamoeba histolytica* or its products, thus suggesting its role as a pathogen. Identification of the protozoan and its cys-

tic forms is not difficult for a trained protozoologist. However, the question of its pathogenicity in a particular patient, especially when there are no symptoms, remains an unsolved problem.

It is well established that infection with *Entamoeba histolytica* is mostly transmitted through the fecal-oral route. The infection may be asymptomatic, may be associated with mild to severe colonic symptoms, or may produce a liver abscess that may prove fatal. Uncommonly, the protozoan may invade tissues other than the colon and the liver — namely, the lungs, pleura, brain, genitals, and the skin.

COLONIC AMEBIASIS

The symptomless cyst carrier and the patient with fulminant amebic dysentery are the two extremes in a wide range of signs and symptoms of the colonic form of the disease. A great variety of clinical presentations are seen between these two ends of the spectrum.

The symptomless carrier, discovered when routine stool examination of a healthy person or a patient suffering from a totally unrelated disease shows the presence of *Entamoeba histolytica* cysts, poses a problem. In temperate climates of the developed world, where invasive clinical amebiasis is unusual, the carriers generally are merely of academic interest. But in the tropics or wherever symptomatic disease is seen, the problem assumes considerable importance. My rule of thumb is to treat everyone shown to be infected. We see persons in this category frequently, because every member of the family of a patient suffering from clinical colonic amebiasis is screened. A sizable proportion of such persons have *Entamoeba histolytica* cysts in the stool while having no symptoms of the disease.

Dysentery as such (i.e., loose stools with blood and mucus) is not the rule in colonic amebiasis; neither is it the exception. The textbook tables for distinguishing amebic from bacillary dysentery are of limited use. Repeated microscopic examination of fresh stools is the most crucial aid in diagnosis. It is worth remembering that amebic and bacillary dysenteries can rarely occur simultaneously.

Vague colonic symptoms of discomfort in the abdomen, bowel irregularity, constipation, diarrhea, griping, tenesmus, and a malabsorption-like picture can occur in various combinations. Low-grade fever, loss of weight, pallor, and generalized nonspecific aches and pains are not uncommon. In the more acute forms of the disease passage of loose stools with blood and mucus in varying quantities, griping, and tenesmus are common. In severe forms of the disease the picture can closely resemble acute to fulminant bacillary dysentery. The patient may be seriously ill and toxic, and may exhibit electrolyte imbalance with its own clinical picture. Fulminant forms may be accompanied by severe hemorrhage, extreme prostration, and innumerable stools, and may be complicated by perforation with localized or generalized peritonitis and secondary bacterial infection.

The role of proctoscopy and sigmoidoscopy in the diagnosis of colonic amebiasis is established enough to warrant these procedures being routinely carried out in every patient with colonic disease. They are useful not only in detecting the classic amebic ulcers and obtaining direct smears for parasitologic diagnosis but also for the differential diagnosis of amebiasis from ulcerative colitis, bacillary dysentery, polyposis, and carcinoma. A biopsy should be taken routinely from any lesion even remotely suggestive of a neoplasm and this will also enable a positive diagnosis of ameboma or rarer isolated colonic tuberculosis. However, it must be stated that sigmoidoscopy and proctoscopy are frequently of no diagnostic help in parasitologically confirmed clinically active colonic amebiasis.

The usefulness of repeated fresh stool examinations for detecting *Entamoeba histolytica* cysts or trophozoites is well established. Ideally, the internist should be able to recognize vegetative and cystic forms of the parasite as well as the bacillary exudate of bacillary dysentery. In any case, the fresher the stool, the better the chance of an accurate identification of *Entamoeba histolytica*, especially its vegetative trophozoite forms. In case of delay in the transit of a specimen of stool to a reference laboratory, polyvinyl alcohol (PVA) can be used as a preservative. Use of amebicidals interferes with cytologic diagnosis of amebiasis, as do vigorous purgatives or even a barium study.

The role of serologic diagnosis in colonic amebiasis as an epidemiologic community study has been referred to earlier: its value in any individual case of colonic amebiasis is negligible, as most of the tests remain positive even when disease has been cured. However, in case of a possible ameboma (amebic granuloma) serologic positivity will help the physician in deciding about the indication of a full therapeutic trial with emetine or metronidazole or both. In tropical practice with limited facilities, differential diagnosis of any colonic mass must include the possibility of ameboma, the other two main possibilities being carcinoma and tuberculous granuloma (i.e., hypertrophic cecal tuberculosis).

HEPATIC AMEBIASIS

Invasion of the liver with *Entamoeba histolytica* is the commonest extraintestinal form of the disease. It is seen with a steady frequency wherever colonic amebiasis is endemic. The onset is usually insidious but, exceptionally, a rapid course can also be seen. The usual presenting symptoms are pain in right upper quadrant or fever or both. Uncommonly, the first indication of the disease may occur via pulmonary or pleural signs or symptoms. A tender hepatomegaly is a highly suggestive finding. The liver may, on account of location of the abscess, enlarge only upward, raising the right diaphragm. It may first be detected by the finding of a collapse consolidation of the right base of the lung, clinically or on radiologic examination. The abscess may spread to the pleura, providing a pleural reaction that may progress to an effusion. The abscess can burst into the pleural cavity, leading to empyema, or may rupture into the lung, forming a lung abscess.

The presence of jaundice, once thought to be so rare as to suggest an alternative diagnosis, is now known to be not infrequent, although when present it denotes a more serious form of the disease. Abscess in the left lobe of the liver can present difficulties in diagnosis, especially when it is deep-seated or is situated near the inferior surface. Left lobe liver abscess, for obvious anatomic reasons, has a proclivity to rupture into the pericardium and, indeed, its first discovery may arise when pericarditis with effusion has developed and an aspiration is done to determine its cause.

Pyrexia of uncertain origin is a common problem in the tropics, and one of the causes that have to be remembered is hepatic amebiasis. Although telltale bedside clues to this possibility are usually elicitable by a physician with a high index of suspicion, mistakes are common and it may be months before the diagnosis becomes obvious. However, with modern serologic methods as well as scanning facilities the confirmation of diagnosis has become simplified.

OTHER FORMS OF EXTRAINTESTINAL AMEBIASIS

Metastatic amebic abscess in the lungs but away from the bases is occasionally seen, and the diagnosis can be difficult if there is no overt liver involvement.

Similarly, an amebic brain abscess can also occur, although the diagnosis, as a rule, is not made in life.

Cutaneous amebic ulceration is not very rare.

Disaster awaits the unwary surgeon and his patient if the former should drain an appendicular mass in the causation of which *Entamoeba histolytica* has played an undetected role. Extensive ulceration of the abdominal wall can occur before someone thinks of making direct smears and looking for easily detected trophozoites of this protozoan. The other favorite site for cutaneous involvement is around the anus and genitals. Penile amebic ulceration, also well described, is often the result of homosexual contact.

LABORATORY DIAGNOSIS

Invasive colonic amebiasis is best diagnosed by detecting the cystic or trophozoite forms of the parasite in the stool. Repeated examination of fresh stools may be required, as the parasite is not excreted consistently in every stool. Mild aperients can help in the detection. Should mucus or blood be present, selection of the adjoining stool pays the best dividends.

Hepatic amebiasis is as a rule accompanied by a leukocytosis with mild shift of the neutrophils to the left. However, this may be absent. Hepatic functions are well maintained, although a rise of serum alkaline phosphatase is common. A marked rise of serum bilirubin is uncommon but when present its conjugation is not affected.

Radioisotope scanning of the liver is usually of material help not only in making a firm diagnosis but also in giving a lead to selection of a site for aspiration.

Radiologic studies are of little help in invasive colonic amebiasis but are quite useful in detection of hepatic amebiasis. Since the right upper quadrant of the liver is a common site, elevation of the right diaphragm, its slower movement, and involvement of the pleura or right pulmonary lung base are all expected confirmatory findings. In case of left lobe liver abscess, radiologic studies may show similar findings on the left side. The stomach may be pushed aside by the abscess in the left lobe. As previously mentioned, pericarditis with effusion may be present, apart from involvement of left pleura and left lower lobe.

Barium enema study is valuable in diagnosis of ameboma, which will need to be differentiated from carcinoma by tissue diagnosis. However, a therapeutic test with powerful amebicidals such as emetine or metronidazole or both can also resolve the difficulty successfully.

Direct smears examined fresh in isotonic saline solution are invaluable in diagnosis of cutaneous amebiasis because of the ease with which the pathogenic vegetative forms can be recognized.

Serologic diagnosis of amebiasis has made rapid strides. The main tests available are complement fixation, indirect hemagglutination, (HA) fluorescent antibody (FA) and immune diffusion. The FA test is more specific but less sensitive than the HA test. This is a rapidly developing field and more helpful tests are in the offing but those mentioned are good screening procedures. However, they do not replace the importance of demonstrating the parasite, especially in colonic forms of the disease. It is worth remembering that serologic tests remain positive long after the disease has been cured.

ROLE OF THE THERAPEUTIC TEST

A therapeutic test with a potent amebicidal is a standing temptation in clinical practice but this should be resisted to the extent of not allowing it to become a habit. However, judiciously employed, a therapeutic test can be very valuable and can save considerable morbidity and on occasions even prevent mortality. Metronidazole is effective in both intestinal and hepatic forms of the disease. Emetine is quite effective in hepatic and acute colonic forms but not so in chronic bowel amebiasis. Chloroquine is effective only in hepatic form of the disease, especially when combined with one of the former two drugs. Luckily, there is no contraindication to combining two of the three powerful amebicidals.

PITFALLS IN DIAGNOSIS

Any large series of autopsies in the tropics will show the pitfalls in diagnosis of amebiasis in its colonic and hepatic forms. Simultaneous presence of carcinoma of the colon or nonspecific ulcerative colitis is not very rare. Misdiagnosis of ameboma is the rule rather than the exception. In the tropics, most patients with an irritable colon syndrome have to suffer repeated courses of amebicidals because there is a great deal of overlap in their symptoms. This can be prevented by a thorough clinical history, detection of positive clues to the diagnosis of an anxiety state and, above all, by repeated search for the protozoa by a competent laboratory. The hepatic form of the disease is even more prone to pitfalls in diagnosis. Secondaries in the liver, even hepatoma and chronic liver disease, all have to be carefully excluded.

The greatest help to a correct diagnosis is a very high index of critical suspicion coupled with competent help to identify the parasite, and also the availability of supportive help by radiology, serology, and a radioisotope scan.

PARASITIC DISEASES OF THE INTESTINES

By CHARLES B. BEAL, M.D.

Palo Alto, California

INTESTINAL PROTOZOAN INFECTIONS

There are several protozoa that inhabit the human intestines and are associated with illness in some degree. Other species commonly found are considered nonpathogenic. These are *Entamoeba hartmanni* (previously known as small race *E. histolytica*), *Entamoeba coli, Entamoeba polecki, Endolimax nana, Iodamoeba bütschlii, Chilomastix mesnili,* and *Trichomonas intestinalis.* These are significant only in that their presence suggests probable exposure to the pathogenic protozoa. Not included in this section is amebiasis caused by *Entamoeba histolytica.* The diagnosis of amebiasis is discussed on page 213.

GIARDIASIS

SYNONYM

Infection with *Giardia intestinalis,* or *Giardia lamblia.*

DEFINITION

Etiologic agent is *Giardia intestinalis,* or *Giardia lamblia,* a flagellate living in the upper small bowel and biliary tract, although rarely observed in this location. Both trophozoites and cysts occur in the human, the cysts being quite resistant to the external environment and sometimes found in community water supplies and mountain streams. This parasite is one of the less frequent organisms associated with traveler's diarrhea. The disease is being recognized much more frequently now than in the past.

PRESENTING SIGNS AND SYMPTOMS

Probably at least three fourths of infected persons are asymptomatic. Symptomatic persons usually exhibit epigastric discomfort and distention, flatulence, intermittent nausea, lassitude, and foul-smelling, loose or watery stools.

COURSE

Asymptomatic infections may disappear spontaneously in a few days, or last several years. Symptoms usually begin from 6 to 18 days after exposure and resolve spontaneously after several weeks or be intermittently present for months or years. Or there may be rapid progression to an acute, debilitating diarrhea with 10 or more watery stools daily. A typical malabsorption syndrome may develop, and milk intolerance is common. In immunodeficient persons the disease may be particularly chronic and recur repeatedly after therapy.

PHYSICAL EXAMINATION FINDINGS

Findings usually are minimal, sometimes with a vaguely uncomfortable abdomen and hyperactive bowel sounds.

LABORATORY FINDINGS

Blood and urine is normal. The stool often is semiformed or liquid, and negative for blood. Microscopic examination of a direct smear of the stool in saline occasionally reveals the readily visible motile trophozoites. Usually, however, only cysts are present, and these may be best observed in a concentrated, iodine-stained specimen. Quite frequently the parasite cannot be found in the stool, and duodenal sampling by intubation and aspiration, or by the simpler string capsule method (Entero-Test, Hedeco, Mountain View, CA) must be done. Observe direct smear for motile trophozoites. The string capsule method is most effective when the string is left in place overnight. If both stool and duodenal specimens are negative, jejunal mucosal biopsy may reveal the trophozoites. The mucus clinging to the biopsy tube also should be examined by direct smear. In patients with steatorrhea the biopsy may show partial or severe villous atrophy, as well as the parasite. Small bowel x-rays may be consistent with an inflammatory process, usually limited to the duodenum and jejunum. In severe cases tests for fat, D-xylose, and vitamin B_{12} malabsorption may be positive.

THERAPEUTIC TESTS

When typical symptoms and a history of probable exposure are present, yet the parasite cannot be found, a trial of therapy sometimes is done using mepacrine or metronidazole. This action may compound the diagnostic dilemma, however, because one frequently observes the symptoms to subside after such therapy, only to recur a short time later. In such a case the tentative diagnosis of giardiasis probably was in error, although organisms resistant to the usually prescribed dosage level are known to exist.

COCCIDIOSIS

SYNONYM

Isosporiasis.

DEFINITION

Etiologic agents are the sporozoan small bowel epithelial parasites *Isospora belli* and *I. hominis.* They are relatively uncommon, generally, but increased prevalence rates have been reported from Rumania, Holland, Chile, the Philippines, and the Southwest Pacific. *I. hominis* probably is a sarcocyst.

PRESENTING SIGNS AND SYMPTOMS

There is usually acute onset with fever, headache, asthenia, and diarrhea. There may be considerable abdominal pain and colic.

COURSE

The disease usually is self-limiting, lasting from a few weeks to 6 months. But it may persist, flaring up intermittently for many years, and may be associated with malabsorption and steatorrhea.

PHYSICAL EXAMINATION FINDINGS

Generally there is a rather nonspecific abdominal tenderness. However, the pain and tenderness may be severe enough to lead to an exploratory laparotomy.

LABORATORY FINDINGS

Typical parasites may be found in the stool, duodenal contents, or small bowel biopsy. Other tests usually are normal.

BALANTIDIASIS

SYNONYM

Balantidial dysentery.

DEFINITION

Mucosal infection of the large bowel due to the ciliate *Balantidium coli.* This is primarily an infection of pigs, rats, and guinea pigs, affecting humans only accidentally, but may be transmitted from person to person.

PRESENTING SIGNS AND SYMPTOMS

Infected persons may be asymptomatic, have mild diarrhea with abdominal cramps, or have an actual bloody dysentery.

COURSE

The course generally is asymptomatic or mild and self-limiting but may be severe and prolonged. Rarely, it is fatal.

PHYSICAL EXAMINATION FINDINGS

There may be pain on palpation over the sigmoid colon. Proctosigmoidoscopic examination may reveal discrete, sometimes hemorrhagic mucosal ulcerations. Concurrent *Trichuris* infection may be found and probably favors tissue invasion by the protozoan.

DIENTAMOEBA DIARRHEA

DEFINITION

This is a large bowel infection in which the ameba *Dientamoeba fragilis* is present, but in which no pathologic effect on tissues has been demonstrated.

PRESENTING SIGNS AND SYMPTOMS

This condition is asymptomatic or with mild, sometimes recurrent diarrhea, with lower abdominal discomfort and flatulence.

LABORATORY FINDINGS

The characteristic amebic trophozoite is present in the stool. Cyst stage is unknown. The parasite begins to disintegrate soon after the stool is passed, so fresh specimens should be examined. A low-grade eosinophilia sometimes occurs.

INTESTINAL NEMATODE INFECTIONS

Of the many species of roundworms that have been found in the human gut, only a few are of worldwide importance. A few others are mentioned briefly because they are of considerable regional importance in various parts of the world.

ENTEROBIASIS

SYNONYMS

Pin worm or seat worm infection, oxyuriasis.

DEFINITION

Enterobiasis is infection of the lower small intestine and large bowel by the ubiquitous nematode *Enterobius vermicularis.*

PRESENTING SIGNS AND SYMPTOMS

Most infections are asymptomatic. There may be anal itching and sometimes pain, particularly at night. Restlessness during sleep may be observed. Pruritus ani may be intense.

COURSE

The infection usually is self-limiting, lasting a few weeks. Longer infections are known, and reinfection is quite common.

PHYSICAL EXAMINATION FINDINGS

Generally, there are no positive findings except that the gravid female worms may be observed at night, and occasionally during the day, on and around the anus.

COMMON COMPLICATIONS

In young girls the parasite may migrate to the vulvovaginal area with resultant itching. Rarely, the worms will migrate through the female genital tract and produce peritoneal granulomas, which usually are asymptomatic. Worms have been reported in pathologic specimens from various other parts of the body, but these are quite rare. Although pin worms sometimes are found in the appendix, it is doubtful that they are the cause of appendicitis.

LABORATORY FINDINGS

Generally, all standard tests are normal. Rarely, a slight eosinophilia exists, particularly if the worms are in ectopic locations. Diagnosis is made by observation of the adult worms or finding the eggs on the anus. For this purpose the Scotch tape slide technique is useful. The tape is placed over the end of a tongue depressor with the sticky side out. The gummed surface is pressed against several areas of the perianal region, and the tape is then attached to a microscope slide, sticky side down. The test should be taken in the morning before the patient bathes or defecates. The procedure can be done at home by a parent and should be carried out on 2 or 3 mornings, after which the slides are brought in to the physician or laboratory for examination. Diagnosis is made by observation of the typical embryonated eggs that are flattened on one side. If considerable detritus is on the tape, then it can be lifted and a drop of 0.1 per cent sodium hydroxide (NaOH) placed on the slide and the tape replaced. The NaOH clears the field.

ASCARIASIS

SYNONYMS

Large round worm infection; giant intestinal round worm.

DEFINITION

This condition is small bowel infection with *Ascaris lumbricoides,* a cylindrical worm with pointed ends and measuring up to 4 mm in diameter and 40 cm long. The common pig ascarid *A. suum,* nearly identical to *A. lumbricoides,* also occurs in man, but with much less frequency. The dog and cat ascarids, *Toxocara canis* and *T. cati,* infect man, usually infants and children, but do not reach maturity, the larvae migrating for a time in various organs, particularly the liver, producing the disease visceral larva migrans.

PRESENTING SIGNS AND SYMPTOMS

In heavy *A. lumbricoides* infections the developmental stage in which the larvae are passing through the lungs may cause a brief pneumonitis with cough, fever, shortness of breath, and occasionally asthma. More commonly, first symptoms, if there are any, are vague abdominal discomfort and distention. There may be colicky epigastric pain, nausea, and vomiting. During an attack, worms may be passed in vomitus or stool.

COURSE

Pulmonary symptoms generally subside within 2 weeks. The life span of the adult worm is about 1 year, but in endemic areas reinfection regularly occurs, so that people, particularly children, may be chronically infected.

PHYSICAL EXAMINATION FINDINGS

In most patients there are no positive findings. When observed, pulmonary signs are indistinguishable from pneumonitis or asthma of other cause. There may be upper and midabdominal discomfort, and in infants occasionally a large bolus of worms can be palpated in the abdomen.

COMMON COMPLICATIONS

Most complications occur in infants and small children. Small bowel and common bile duct obstruction both may be fatal if not recognized and properly treated. Migrating worms may enter any duct or body cavity connected to the gastrointestinal tract, as a nasal sinus, for example. A bolus of worms may initiate an intussusception. Worms actually may perforate the bowel.

LABORATORY FINDINGS

A moderate to high blood eosinophilia may be present during larval migration through the lungs. Otherwise, there generally are less than 8 per cent eosinophils. Typical fertile or nonfertile eggs usually are seen in abundance in a direct smear of the stool, using an iodine or thiomersal-iodine-formalin stain. Stool concentration techniques rarely are necessary.

OTHER TESTS

Worms may appear on x-ray films as linear tissue densities, and a bolus of worms as a tangled, thick cord. The worm may ingest barium, with a consequent "GI series" of the worm itself, revealing a linear opacity about 1 mm wide.

TRICHURIASIS

SYNONYMS

Trichocephaliasis, whipworm infection.

DEFINITION

The thin, nearly nonpathogenic *Trichuris trichiura*, with a whip-like shape, lives in the cecum and ascending colon, and in heavy infections in the entire large bowel. The tip of the narrowed anterior portion of the worm is buried in the intestinal mucosa.

PRESENTING SIGNS AND SYMPTOMS

Usually there are no signs, symptoms, or positive physical findings. Occasionally there are vague abdominal complaints or diarrhea, and in very heavy infections rectal prolapse may be seen, with worms attached to the mucosa.

COURSE

As the worms live several years and reinfection is common, people in endemic areas may harbor the parasite for much of their lives.

LABORATORY FINDINGS

Eosinophilia occurs rarely if at all. A slight iron deficiency anemia may be seen in patients with quite heavy infections. Typical barrel-shaped eggs with transparent polar plugs generally are found in abundance in direct smears of the stool. Concentration techniques may reveal very light infections, but these are of little or no significance.

HOOKWORM DISEASE

SYNONYMS

For *Ancylostoma duodenale* infections: uncinariasis, ancylostomiasis, old world hookworm infection. For *Necator americanus*: necatoriasis, new world hookworm infection, American hookworm infection.

DEFINITION

Hookworm disease involves upper small bowel infection with *Ancylostoma duodenale* or *Necator americanus*. Tissue destruction and blood loss from parasitic attachment to the mucosa and ingestion of blood are proportional to the numbers of the worms present. The dog hookworm A. *braziliensis* may accidentally invade humans, producing only a skin infection, cutaneous larva migrans.

PRESENTING SIGNS AND SYMPTOMS

Usually there are no symptoms and no positive physical findings. Repeated and heavy skin penetration (usually of the feet) may produce an itching, erythematous, papulovesicular rash, termed ground itch. Pulmonary migration of the parasite larvae rarely may cause a mild cough with dyspnea and eosinophilia.

COURSE

The worms have a life span of up to 5 years, and reinfection is common in endemic areas. Thus the disease may last many years.

COMMON COMPLICATIONS

In malnourished persons, particularly children, moderate and heavy infections may produce an iron deficiency anemia, which may be severe. Malabsorption also may occur in intense infections. A profound anemia may induce cardiac failure.

LABORATORY FINDINGS

Hemoglobin levels may be below 3 grams per cent, and red blood cell counts below 1,000,000 per cu mm. Eggs usually are found readily in the stool, and measure from 55 to 76 microns in length. Direct examination of the stool specimen may be aided by an iodine or thimerosal-iodine-formalin stain. Infections light enough to require stool concentration techniques for diagnosis are of no clinical significance.

PITFALLS IN DIAGNOSIS

In stool samples that are held a day or so before examination the egg may hatch into larvae that resemble *Strongyloides* larvae. There are a few slight anatomic differences that will distinguish them, however. Occasionally in very constipated persons eggs will hatch before the stool is passed. The eggs cannot be used to differentiate the two species of hookworm, and for clinical purposes this is not important. If differentiation is desired, the larvae may be used for that purpose. Hookworm disease and strongyloidiasis may coexist, and this is clinically important. Thus if larvae are found, they should be definitively identified.

STRONGYLOIDIASIS

SYNONYMS

Strongyloidosis, strongyloid threadworm infection.

DEFINITION

An invasion of the upper small bowel mucosa by the 2 mm long nematode *Strongyloides stercoralis*. This worm can reproduce and multiply in the human host. *S. fülleborni*, a simian parasite, also is found in man occasionally.

PRESENTING SIGNS AND SYMPTOMS

It is estimated that a third of the patients have no symptoms or physical findings. Epigastric pain, burning, and tenderness may occur, with occasional nausea, vomiting, and diarrhea. Symptoms are those of a duodenitis, and may mimic peptic ulcer disease. Epigastric pain with eosinophilia in persons who have lived in rural, warm, and moist environments is strongly suggestive of the disease.

COURSE

There is an early migratory phase through the lungs, sometimes associated with a pneumonitis, and even pleural effusion. However, this phase often passes unnoticed. The disease may last decades with few symptoms, or with episodic attacks of the symptoms as noted. Urticaria occurs intermittently in up to 20 per cent of the patients, and sometimes may be serpiginous-appearing, usually most prominent on the lower abdomen, buttocks, and thighs. A malabsorption syndrome or protein-losing enteropathy may occur in heavy infections.

COMMON COMPLICATIONS

If for any reason the patient's immune system becomes depressed, autoinfection may lead to a massive, frequently fatal hyperinfection syndrome with larvae being found in several organs, particularly the lungs. There often are abdominal pain, distention, wheezing, dyspnea, high fever, and shock with neurologic signs. A gram-negative septicemia often precedes death. In this condition there may be a moderate leukocytosis, but eosinophilia may be absent.

LABORATORY FINDINGS

An eosinophilia of 35 per cent or higher may be found, particularly in the more symptomatic patients. In chronic cases peripheral eosinophils usually are in the 6 to 10 per cent range. During the early migratory phase some filariform larvae may be found in the sputum. In the hyperinfection syndrome the slightly smaller rhabditiform larvae usually are present in abundance. Since the eggs of the mature worms usually hatch while still in the small bowel, larvae are found in the stool, but these generally are few in number. Thus, both a direct unstained smear (to search for the motile larvae) and zinc sulfate or other concentration method should be used for the stool examination. In suspected cases several specimens should be studied, and then only about 75 per cent of cases are diagnosed. Both Baermann and Harada-Mori have described relatively simple techniques for attracting the larvae from the stool so that they might be more easily observed. Probably the most reliable results are obtained by observing a direct smear of duodenal fluid for the motile larvae. A sample of fluid may be obtained by duodenal intubation and aspiration, or by the much simpler string capsule method (Entero-Test, Hedeco, Mountain View, CA). Mucosal biopsy may reveal the organism as well as the associated tissue pathology.

X-ray Findings

The duodenitis of the more severe cases produces mild dilatation and mucosal edema. Nodularity or ulceration may be noted. The radiographic abnormalities may involve the stomach and jejunum as well, but rarely beyond.

Pitfalls in Diagnosis

In duodenal sampling, both eggs and larvae may be seen. The eggs resemble hookworm eggs, which also may be present in the duodenum. However, *Strongyloides* eggs will be embryonated and the hookworm eggs will be at the four-nucleus stage.

In patients who have resided in endemic areas, particularly in rural locales, and who are to undergo immunosuppressive therapy, a search for the larvae should be made before institution of the therapy. Otherwise a fatal hyperinfection syndrome may result.

INTESTINAL NEMATODES PRIMARILY OF REGIONAL IMPORTANCE

In trichostrongyliasis, or pseudohookworm infection, caused by *Trichostrongylus orientalis* and related species, the eggs may be confused with hookworm eggs. However, they are slightly longer, measuring 73 to 95 microns. This disease is endemic, particularly in Korea, Japan, the Middle East, and the USSR. Symptoms and signs usually are minimal. However, abdominal pain and diarrhea may occur, accompanied by an eosinophilia.

Anisakiasis, known also as herring worm and eosinophilic phlegmon, occurs in people who frequently eat raw, unfrozen sea fish or squid infected with *Anisakis* larvae. The disease is seen particularly in Japan and to a lesser extent in northern Europe. The larvae inside the gastric or intestinal wall produce an eosinophilic granuloma, often of sufficient size and causing severe enough abdominal pain to require emergency surgery and resection of the lesion. A peripheral eosinophilia of 60 per cent is not uncommon. Diagnosis usually is confirmed only by pathologic examination of the specimen. Chronic cases also may occur.

Intestinal capillariasis was first recognized in 1966 in Central Luzon, the Philippines, during an intense epidemic of severe diarrhea with a mortality rate of about 35 per cent. The parasite, living primarily in the jejunum, was named *Capillaria philippinensis*. The disease also has been reported in Thailand. The disease often presents as would a severe strongyloidiasis. Death results from a protein-losing enteropathy. Typical eggs are in the stool.

Intestinal angiostrongyliasis, caused by *Angiostrongylus costaricensis*, is another recently recognized disease found primarily in Central America. The parasite is related to *A. cantonensis*, the cause of eosinophilic meningitis, but in this case lives mostly in the small arteries of the terminal small bowel and cecum. Symptoms generally are acute, suggesting appendicitis, but with a peripheral eosinophilia. Significant necrosis of tissue supplied by the parasitized arteries may occur. Subacute and recurrent attacks also have been reported.

INTESTINAL CESTODE INFECTIONS

At least 10 varieties of tapeworms have been found in the human intestine, but only 3 have worldwide significance. These are the beef tapeworm, *Taenia saginata*, the pork tapeworm, *T. solium*, and the fish tapeworm, *Diphyllobothrium latum*. All live in the small bowel and are acquired through eating inadequately cooked beef, pork, or fresh-water fish. In spite of tales to the contrary, most infections with these huge worms cause very few symptoms. There may be some abdominal discomfort, anorexia, and occasionally nausea. *T. saginata* is quite innocuous but inconvenient in that living segments of the worm may spontaneously wiggle their way through the anus. *T. solium*, on the other hand, is dangerous because the egg can hatch within the gastrointestinal tract, the larvae migrating throughout the body and forming small cysts or cysticerci. In the brain particularly these cysts act as space-occupying lesions and may be responsible for seizures, cerebrospinal fluid obstruction, and other disabilities. *D. latum* competes with the human host for vitamin B_{12} and may be responsible for a pernicious anemia–like syndrome.

Laboratory Findings

Generally the tapeworms produce no eosinophilia or other hematologic changes. Diagnosis of all the intestinal cestodes is made by finding the characteristic eggs or proglottids in the stool. In *D. latum* infections, tests for B_{12} deficiency are positive in less than half the cases. Gastric acidity is unaffected by the worm. *T. solium* cysticerci in the central nervous system are readily demonstrated by computerized axial tomography (CT) scanning.

INTESTINAL TREMATODE INFECTIONS

As many as 20 trematode species have been identified as inhabiting the intestinal lumen, peri-intestinal venules, or the bile ducts. The parasites are known as flatworms, or flukes. They have a life cycle involving asexual reproduction in the snail, the intermediate host, and sexual reproduction in the human definitive host.

SCHISTOSOMIASIS

SYNONYMS

Schistosoma mansoni: intestinal or Manson's bilharzia, Egyptian splenomegaly; *S. japonicum*: oriental schistosomiasis, Katayama disease, Yangtse River fever, urticarial fever.

DEFINITION

There are several schistosomes that affect man. The three major ones are *Schistosoma haematobium*, *S. mansoni*, and *S. japonicum*. Of these three, the latter two inhabit the intestinal and mesenteric venules. The eggs from each mated pair of worms penetrate the vessel walls, enter the intestinal mucosa, and are slowly extruded into the lumen. Some eggs are washed into the hepatic portal system and thence to the liver. Apparently through shunt mechanisms some eggs may be deposited in the lungs, brain, spinal cord, and elsewhere. Some worm pairs also may live in ectopic sites, producing eggs wherever they may be. The tissue response to each egg is a minute granuloma, and millions of eggs in an organ can produce profound pathologic changes.

The geographic distribution of these diseases is determined by the natural distribution of the various specific intermediate snail hosts.

PRESENTING SIGNS AND SYMPTOMS

Light infections may be virtually asymptomatic. Early heavy primary infections produce an acute febrile illness with cough, lymphadenopathy, hepatosplenomegaly, and eosinophilia. This phase usually is more severe with *S. japonicum* than with *S. mansoni*, and in addition there may be giant urticaria and central nervous system symptoms, probably of a toxic or edematous origin. Usually, however, patients seek medical help when the disease is in a more chronic phase, in which the symptoms are quite nonspecific, with some fatigue, diarrhea, and abdominal pain. In the advanced stage, characterized by hepatic cirrhosis, there are hepatomegaly and splenomegaly, with eventual development of esophageal varices.

COURSE

In general, *S. japonicum* produces a more virulent disease than *S. mansoni*. The rate of the progression of the disease in either case is proportional to the worm burden. Heavy infections may progress to fatal hepatic failure in less than a year. The worms themselves may live for several years, or even decades, so that there usually is slow progression of the disease, as eggs are being deposited continuously in the liver.

COMMON COMPLICATIONS

Bleeding eosphageal varices, when occurring, has about a 60 per cent mortality. Hepatic failure is much less common, as the liver retains quite normal function until late in the cirrhotic process. These patients also may develop pulmonary hypertension and cor pulmonale. Ectopically localized worms may produce a diffuse cerebral disease, focal epilepsy, or transverse myelitis.

LABORATORY FINDINGS

Typical eggs are present in the feces, although usually in small numbers. Thus, if a direct smear does not reveal the eggs, a stool concentration technique should be used. If three specimens are negative, rectal biopsy should be done. Three or four snips should be taken. The tissue may be placed between two glass slides and examined microscopically for the presence of the eggs. If they are found, it is useful to replace the upper glass slide with a coverslip, and observe the eggs under oil immersion, looking for the small undulating flame cell, indicating that the eggs are viable and presumably fairly recently deposited. Liver function tests usually are normal, or nearly so, and the hemogram normal or with an eosinophilia of 8 to 10 per cent. However, in the early acute stages, particularly in *S. japonicum*, the eosinophil count may reach 80 per cent.

Serologic tests are positive even when no eggs can be found, but this test is not completely reliable because of some cross-reactivity, particularly with schistosome dermatitis, caused by exposure to certain animal schistosomes. The test is quite useful, however, as a screening procedure for persons who have lived or traveled in endemic areas. For this purpose a 5 ml sample of serum may be sent to the Center for Disease Control, Parasitic Disease Division, Atlanta, Georgia 30333.

PITFALLS IN DIAGNOSIS

The initiation of the entire diagnostic process is dependent on a positive history of potential exposure, such as swimming in possibly infected water in endemic areas. For S. *mansoni* these areas are Egypt, the Sudan and the remainder of Africa south of the Sahara, the Arabian peninsula, Brazil, Surinam, Venezuela, and much of the Caribbean. For S. *japonicum* endemic areas exist in China, Taiwan, Japan, the Philippines, Cambodia, Laos, Thailand, and the Celebes.

The proper diagnosis of schistosomiasis involves an estimate of the worm burden, and whether or not they are still alive and producing eggs. These considerations help determine future management. A positive serologic test without finding the eggs, except in special circumstances, is inadequate to make the diagnosis of the disease. Further, in advanced cases in which eggs are identified, it is important to determine the viability of the eggs, since they persist in the tissue long after the adult worms have died.

TREMATODES OF THE INTESTINAL LUMEN AND BILIARY TRACT

Fasciolopsis buski and several similar species inhabit the small bowel of man. The symptoms generally are quite nonspecific, but sometimes mimic peptic ulcer disease. Most of these parasites are endemic in various parts of Asia, and occasionally in Europe and Africa. None are of worldwide distribution. Diagnosis is made by finding characteristic eggs in the stool.

Clonorchis (Opisthorchis) sinensis, O. felineus, and *O. viverrini* all are similar and live in the biliary passages. Clonorchiasis is quite prevalent in China, Hong Kong, Vietnam, Korea, and Taiwan. The other species are endemic mostly in Thailand and eastern Europe. Light and moderate infections are asymptomatic, whereas quite heavy worm burdens may present as a pyogenic cholangitis, single or multiple liver abscesses, biliary carcinoma, or, rarely, pancreatitis. Diagnosis is made by finding the typical but minute eggs in the stool or duodenal contents.

Fasciola hepatica, the sheep liver fluke, is an accidental parasite of man but is not rare in sheep and cattle-raising areas of the world that are damp. The fluke inhabits the biliary tract, but also may invade the liver parenchyma. Heavy infections may produce a multiplicity of gastrointestinal symptoms, plus fever and eosinophilia, sometimes greater than 50 per cent. Late effects include significant liver parenchymal necrosis and fibrosis, resulting in a tender, painful hepatosplenomegaly, jaundice, and ascites. Diagnosis is by finding characteristic eggs in stools or duodenal contents.

MALARIA*

By EDWARD J. COLWELL, M.D.,
and CRAIG J. CANFIELD, M.D., COL., M.C.
Washington, D.C.

DEFINITION

Malaria is an acute or chronic disease of vertebrates caused by parasitic protozoans of the genus Plasmodium, class Sporozoa. Human infections are generally attributable to any of four species of these parasites and, for precision and rational chemotherapy, the type of malaria infection should be distinguished according to the causative species as falciparum malaria, vivax malaria, malariae malaria, and ovale malaria. Although naturally acquired infections in man with subhuman primate plasmodia have been reported, they are very rarely encountered.

SYNONYMS

Before discovery of the causative organisms, "malarial fevers" were designated by such ecologic terms as swamp fever, marsh fever, paludism, miasmatic fever, estivo-autumnal fever, and jungle fever. After demonstration of the causative agents at the beginning of this century, infections were frequently characterized by a periodicity of recurrent paroxysms that presumably reflected synchronous development of parasites in the human host. Periodic paroxysms occurring every 72, 48, or 24 hours were called quartan, tertian, or quotidian fevers, respectively. Malaria parasites generally associated with these intermittent fevers were *P. malariae* (quartan), *P. vivax* (tertian), and *P. falciparum* (quotidian, subtertian). Although *P. malariae* infections are nearly always associated with quartan paroxysms, *P. vivax* and *P. falciparum* infections are frequently characterized by remittent or continuous fevers, especially in initial attacks, because of asynchrony of parasite maturation or mixed plasmodial infections.

LIFE CYCLE OF THE ORGANISM

Knowledge of the life cycle of the malaria parasite in man is essential in order to understand the pathogenesis and clinical manifestations and to institute appropriate antimalarial chemotherapy for termination of the acute attack, prevention of recurrences, and reduction of further transmission.

*This is contribution #1,157 of the Army Malaria Research Program.

The development of the parasite requires two hosts. Asexual development (schizogony) occurs in an intermediate vertebrate host, and sexual development (sporogony) takes place in a definitive mosquito host. Man usually contracts the disease through inoculation of sporozoites from an infected anopheline mosquito during a blood meal. Sporozoites are rapidly cleared from the circulation and are sequestered in the liver, where the pre-erythrocytic stage of schizogony is initiated. The parasites multiply within the hepatocytes and eventually are released into the circulation. The interval between initial exposure to sporozoites and detection of parasites in blood is called the prepatent period, and is variable for the human plasmodia. The prepatent period is about 8 to 12 days for *P. falciparum, P. ovale,* and *P. vivax* infections and about 24 days for *P. malariae* infection. However, the duration of the prepatent period may be considerably longer in vivax and malariae infections — many weeks and months, and even years in malariae infections.

The entry of parasites into the peripheral circulation initiates the erythrocytic stage of schizogony. Parasites released from the liver penetrate red blood cells and at this stage consist of a single nucleus with a thin ring of cytoplasm. They are called trophozoites or, in laboratory jargon, "ring forms." When the nucleus divides, the parasite is designated a schizont and, upon completion of a successive series of nuclear replications, the mature schizont ruptures the erythrocyte with release of many individual, uninuclear forms called merozoites. Merozoites penetrate other red blood cells, after which they are morphologically indistinguishable from trophozoites, and erythrocytic schizogony is repeated.

Concurrent with erythrocytic schizogony, the development of sexually differentiated forms (viz., gametocytes) takes place. Circulating male and female gametocytes can be ingested by a noninfected mosquito, thereby initiating the sporogonic or sexual stage.

PRESENTING SYMPTOMS AND COURSE

There are no symptoms associated with pre-erythrocytic schizogony. Early symptoms of malaria are attributed to rupture of parasitized erythrocytes with release of pyrogenic substances. Therefore the incubation period extends a few days beyond the prepatent period. Prodromal symptoms include malaise, myalgia, arthralgia, headache, backache, cough, and gastrointestinal irritability. Most of these symptoms are related to vascular congestion of involved organs in which definitive pathogenetic mechanisms are not completely elucidated.

Patients often present with a febrile paroxysm associated with intensification of the prodromal symptoms. The pyrexial attacks are usually characterized by three stages. The patient first experiences a shaking chill, followed soon by a febrile phase, with a temperature usually over 104 F (40 C) and frequently as high as 106 F (41.1 C). After defervescence to normal or below normal, a period of profuse diaphoresis ensues, and the patient becomes lethargic and somnolent. Although such chills and fever are classic for malaria, a history of exposure in a malarious area associated with a febrile illness should immediately alert the diagnostician.

The course of vivax, malariae, and ovale infections is usually uncomplicated, and spontaneous resolution of symptoms is not uncommon, particularly in residents of a malarious area. Certain developmental characteristics of the parasites interacting with defense mechanisms of the host contribute significantly to this reduction in disease severity. *Plasmodium vivax* and *P. ovale* parasites attack almost exclusively the young red blood cells and appear incapable of infecting mature erythrocytes. Conversely, *P. malariae* parasites have a predilection for infecting older erythrocytes. These developmental peculiarities tend to impose a limit on the magnitude of parasitemia, which usually ranges from 8000 to 15,000 per cu mm and rarely exceeds 50,000 per cu mm. This relatively benign course of parasitemia may afford sufficient time for development of a protective immune response by the host. Recent investigations have demonstrated that the latter may be mediated in part by circulating antibodies of the IgG and IgM classes that can inhibit merozoite penetration of red blood cells, thereby limiting amplification of erythrocytic schizogony.

Plasmodium falciparum, however, invades all erythrocytes, irrespective of age. Consequently, the course of falciparum malaria may be much more fulminant with an overwhelming parasitemia, particularly in a nonimmune patient in whom diagnosis and treatment are delayed.

PHYSICAL EXAMINATION

Corresponding to the stage of the malaria paroxysm, many patients, particularly Caucasians, are noted to be "cold and blue" or "hot and pink." During the initial chill, the skin is cold, dry, and dusky, and the patient may experience violent shaking. During the hyperthermic stage, the skin becomes hot, dry, and erythematous, and the face is usually flushed. With defervescence, the skin is wet with profuse diaphoresis.

Localized signs are often absent during the early phase of an uncomplicated infection. If treatment is delayed, tenderness may be elicited over the hepatic and splenic areas, and the spleen becomes enlarged and palpable. Scleral icterus and jaundice occasionally may be observed, depending on the degree of unconjugated hyperbilirubinemia associated with intravascular hemolysis. The conjunctivae are usually injected, probably a peripheral reflection of visceral congestion.

COMMON COMPLICATIONS

Several characteristic complications of *P. falciparum* and *P. malariae* infections have been recognized, especially in subjects in whom chemotherapy is delayed (Table 1). Complications of falciparum malaria are usually fulminant and portend a fatal outcome unless prompt treatment with antimalarial agents and supportive measures are instituted. Complications of *P. malariae* infections are more chronic and indolent and are generally associated with prolonged, low-density parasitemias or repeated infections. It is probable that a variety of interacting mechanisms contribute to the pathogenesis and severity of these complications.

Acute renal insufficiency is one of the more common complications of falciparum malaria. Predisposing factors in the development of this syndrome are reduced renal perfusion secondary to salt and water depletion, and hypoxemia associated with intravascular hemolysis. Profound hemolysis is often observed in patients with extremely high levels of parasitized erythrocytes and/or in those with erythrocytic glucose-6-phosphate dehydrogenase deficiency who have received oxidant drugs. Blackwater fever refers to the passage of hemoglobin or its breakdown products in the urine secondary to severe hemolysis. It may or may not be associated with renal insufficiency.

Cerebral malaria is another complication of *P. falciparum* infections, with neurologic deficits ranging from mild disturbances of mentation to decerebrate rigidity. Contributing factors in this grave complication are hypoxemia secondary to an overwhelming parasitemia and sludging of infected erythrocytes, leading to vascular occlusion and increased capillary permeability of cerebral blood vessels.

Severe pulmonary insufficiency complicating *P. falciparum* infections was recognized in American servicemen in Southeast Asia. This complication was originally confused with acute pulmonary edema in patients with renal failure and fluid overload. However, the lack of an elevated central venous pressure and the absence of cardiomegaly served to distinguish this syndrome from congestive heart failure. Pulmonary insufficiency in malaria patients is usually associated with high levels of parasitemia and either renal or cerebral complications. However, it may occur suddenly several days after initiation of therapy when the level of asexual parasitemia is considerably reduced. Other manifestations include rapid and labored respirations, tachycardia, cyanosis, and diffuse pulmonary infiltrates. Pathologic studies of lung tissue have shown capillary congestion, scattered hemorrhages, and hyaline membranes within the alveoli. There is a striking clinicopathologic similarity of "malaria pneumonitis" with the "shock lung" syndrome.

In addition to hemolytic anemia, another hematologic complication described in falciparum malaria is the syndrome of disseminated intravascular coagulation. Accelerated clotting can lead to a generalized consumption of coagulation factors, small vessel thrombosis, and excessive fibrinolysis. Because of hypofibrinogenemia, massive internal hemorrhage may occur.

The complications of *P. malariae* infections, namely tropical splenomegaly and the nephrotic syndrome, have been attributed to immunopathologic reactions. Malariae malaria is often associated with chronic, recurrent, low-density parasitemias that may be undetectable with conventional light microscopy. The chronic antigenemia provides repeated stimuli for specific immunoglobulin responses, and the circulating antigen-antibody complexes are subsequently trapped by the renal glomeruli. Cellular trapping of these soluble immune complexes then activates the complement cascade reactions, and the cytolytic effect disrupts the structural integrity of the glomerular basement membrane. Massive proteinuria ensues.

The pathogenesis of tropical splenomegaly is less well defined. Presumably, chronic antigenemia provides stimuli for continued lymphoid hyperplasia, particularly in tissues that sequester parasitized erythrocytes (e.g., the spleen). Splenomegaly can attain massive proportions, extending across the midline and down to the iliac crest. A functional hypersplenism with pancytopenic complications (viz., bacterial in-

Table 1. *Malarial Complications*

Complications with falciparum malaria
  Acute renal insufficiency (e.g., blackwater fever)
  Cerebral malaria
  Malaria pneumonitis
  Consumptive coagulopathy
  Malaria hepatitis (bilious malaria)
  Enteritis
Complications with malaria (quartan) malaria
  Nephrotic syndrome
Idiopathic tropical splenomegaly
Miscellaneous: Ruptured spleen

fections, severe anemia, bleeding diathesis) may be observed in these patients.

LABORATORY FINDINGS

Blood Smear. Definitive identification of the plasmodial species is mandatory for selection of appropriate chemotherapy and cognizance of impending complications. Species identification is accomplished by visualization of the parasites on stained blood films.

The preparation, staining, and examination of peripheral blood films requires training and experience without which parasites may be missed or confused with platelets and artifacts such as precipitated stain, dust, fungi, and other contaminants. It is recommended that the glass slides be thoroughly cleansed by soaking in dilute acid, washing in distilled water, and subsequent air drying in a dust-free atmosphere.

A thick film is prepared by depositing a drop of blood approximately 5 mm in diameter from an earlobe or finger puncture onto the end of the slide. A corner of another slide is used to spread the drop to 10 to 15 mm. A thin smear is made on the same or another slide with standard technique. Both films are dried, preferably in a desiccator in areas of high ambient humidity. Only the thin smear is fixed with absolute methanol for retention of red blood cell morphology. Both films are then stained with a Romanowsky polychrome stain such as Giemsa. Multiple slides should not be exposed simultaneously to a common staining solution because of the possibility of transference of parasites from infected blood smears to noninfected smears. In the early stages of the infection or in a partially immune subject with a low-density parasitemia, it may be necessary to obtain peripheral blood smears every 4 to 6 hours before the level of parasitemia exceeds the microscopic threshold (i.e., about 10 parasites per cu mm).

The thick film is examined for demonstration of malaria infection, and the thin film is inspected for speciation of the plasmodial parasites. Examination of the thick film is often sufficient for differentiation of single falciparum from single vivax, ovale, and malariae infections. In falciparum infections, only trophozoites are generally observed in peripheral blood. If a sufficient interval (7 to 9 days) has elapsed from the onset of patent parasitemia to time of laboratory diagnosis, the characteristic crescent-shaped falciparum gametocytes may be visualized. In the other three plasmodial infections, many developmental stages of asexual parasites may be demonstrable, although several repeated examinations at hourly intervals may be necessary.

Differentiation of *P. vivax, P. ovale,* and *P. malariae* infections is best accomplished by examination of the thin blood films; however, this is tedious because of the low density of parasitemia usually observed in these infections. Erythrocytes invaded by *P. vivax* and *P. ovale* are usually large and polychromatophilic and exhibit eosinophilic stippling (Schüffner's dots). The cytoplasm of vivax trophozoites is ameboid in character, whereas that of *P. ovale* is more compact and band shaped. The margin of ovale-infected erythrocytes is often crenated or fimbriated, and the red blood cell tends to be oval.

Erythrocytes infected with *P. malariae* are normal in size and do not exhibit Schüffner's dots. The mature schizont of *P. malariae* is quite characteristic and usually contains from 6 to 12 merozoites arranged concentrically around the pigment, giving rise to a "daisy head" or rosette appearance.

Complete Blood Count and Bone Marrow Examination. These parameters may be normal in the early stage of the infection. With disease progression a normocytic normochromic anemia and thrombocytopenia may become apparent. The total leukocyte count is often below normal. The eosinophil count is depressed during acute infections, but may become elevated during convalescence and should alert the diagnostician to search for other disorders such as helminthiasis. Examination of the bone marrow in subjects with adequate nutritional balance usually reveals only hyperplasia of erythrocytic precursors and malaria pigment (hemozoin). Parasitized erythrocytes may also be visualized. Hemozoin is distinguished from hemosiderin by its dusky, nonrefractile appearance and its nonreactivity with Prussian blue iron stains. In malaria patients with nutritional imbalance as iron, vitamin B_{12}, or folate deficiency, bone marrow elements may exhibit the characteristic morphologic abnormalities.

Serodiagnostic Tests. Recent investigations have indicated that malaria serology may be useful as both an epidemiologic and a diagnostic tool. Malaria antibodies appear in the plasma from 4 to 8 days after the onset of patent parasitemia, attain peak concentrations several weeks thereafter, and may persist for many months, and even years after termination of the infection, albeit at low titer.

Indirect hemagglutination and indirect fluorescent antibody techniques are available at some institutions for detection of malaria antibody. These tests are simple, rapid, inexpensive, and highly sensitive. Although these tests are valuable diagnostic adjuncts, particularly in patients with very low density parasitemias, their use is limited because of their unavailability at most hospital laboratories and their inability for definitive speciation. In acutely ill subjects, treatment should not be delayed pending outcome of a serologic test.

Malaria serodiagnostic tests must be interpreted in light of the history and physical examination. A high serotiter in a febrile patient after potential exposure to malaria is presumptive evidence for a malaria infection. Conversely, a negative titer in serum obtained 2 or more weeks after the onset of symptoms in an immunocompetent subject decreases the likelihood that the illness is due to malaria. A low titer could indicate the early period of rising malaria antibody levels, or it could reflect persistent antibody in a patient without an active malaria infection. Demonstration of a significant rise in serotiter in a subsequent specimen would be useful in distinguishing between these two alternatives.

Urine and Biochemical Findings. Abnormalities of these tests are nonspecific and of little aid in diagnosis. Transient abnormalities of liver function tests with mild choluria may be present. Urinalysis in uncomplicated infections usually reveals only mild albuminuria and cylindruria. In severe falciparum infections, protein casts, hemoglobinuria, hemosiderinuria, and a fixed isosthenuric urine may be demonstrable.

SPECIAL CONSIDERATIONS

Two special considerations related to accidental infusion of malaria-infected blood merit discussion; viz., transfusion-induced malaria and needle-induced malaria in parenteral drug abusers.

Malaria parasites can survive for weeks in bank blood, and an increasing number of accidental transfusion-induced malaria cases have been reported in recent years. According to recommendations of the American Association of Blood Banks, prospective donors are excluded if they have a history of malaria, and are deferred for 2 years if they have received malaria chemoprophylaxis while exposed in a malarious area. Conceivably, the availability of rapid, simplified, sensitive, and inexpensive serodiagnostic techniques for detecting malaria antibody should be valuable for donor screening.

Outbreaks of needle-induced malaria among drug addicts sharing injection equipment have been reported in recent years. During 1970 and 1971, an epidemic of 47 cases of vivax malaria occurred among heroin addicts in California. The index case was shown to be an asymptomatic Vietnam returnee who had a history of malaria while in Vietnam.

PITFALLS IN DIAGNOSIS

Demonstration of the parasite by thick and thin blood smear examinations in patients with the nephrotic and hypersplenic complications of *P. malariae* infections is often very difficult. Difficulties arise because of the low density of parasitemia and because of the prolonged intervals between tissue release of parasite broods. It may be necessary to examine blood films twice daily for several weeks before the parasite is demonstrable. The value of sensitive and specific serodiagnostic techniques is obvious in these situations.

TOXOPLASMOSIS

By B. H. KEAN, M.D.,
and ANNE C. KIMBALL, Ph.D.
New York, New York

Toxoplasmosis, caused by *Toxoplasma gondii*, is probably the most common infectious disease; it is estimated that 1 billion human beings harbor the parasite. About 1 per cent of adults become infected each year.

T. gondii is an intracellular protozoan parasite (subphylum Sporozoa, subclass Coccidia) with a sexual cycle in the small intestines of felines (cats being of dominant importance), and an asexual cycle that can occur in any warm-blooded animal, including man.

The disease is acquired by the ingestion of *T. gondii* cysts in muscles of infected animals (asexual cycle) or by the ingestion (or inhalation followed by ingestion) of oocysts from the feces of cats (sexual cycle). Raw or poorly cooked pork or mutton (lamb) have been incriminated more often than beef or poultry. Ground beef (hamburger) has been documented as a source of infection; however, it must be remembered that "pure" beef often contains pork. The oocyst from cat feces is the sturdiest form of *T. gondii* and with sufficient moisture can survive in soil for over a year. The oocyst's role as a source of infection for humans is probably especially important in less affluent countries where meat is a luxury and in which toxoplasmosis is frequently acquired by children who play in areas contaminated by cat feces. Contaminated environment (corrals, barns, barnyards, gardens, stables, milking stalls, feeding pens, etc.) may be more important in the affluent countries than has been appreciated previously.

PATHOGENESIS

Trophozoites (tachyzoites) derived from either the cyst or oocyst forms penetrate the intestinal wall and during the proliferative phase invade a wide variety of cells in many tissues. When an as yet undetermined level of immunity develops, most infected cells are cleared of the active stage of the parasite but cysts remain in muscle, brain, retina and, less frequently, in other tissues. Later, even decades later, these cysts can rupture, often producing no symptoms, but in the retina, retinochoroiditis may become evident. In immunosuppressed patients, cysts rupturing in the brain may cause encephalitis, often localized and simulating tumor. A few studies suggest that *T. gondii* is a cause of polymyositis and cyst rupture may precede this manifestation of toxoplasmosis.

TYPES OF TOXOPLASMOSIS

Asymptomatic. The majority of toxoplasmic infections are subclinical or cause such minor illness that the patient does not seek medical attention. About 30 per cent of 30-year-olds have toxoplasma antibodies; 50 per cent of 50-year-olds have been infected.

Acute Adult Lymphadenitis. This is the most frequently observed clinical type. The symptoms may vary from mild, transient lymphadenopathy to a febrile illness with myalgia and malaise lasting for weeks. Typically, the patient presents with a syndrome resembling infectious mononucleosis but with a negative test for heterophil antibodies.

The cervical nodes, *particularly the posterior chain,* usually are enlarged, rubbery, and nontender. Axillary and inguinal node enlargement is not uncommon, but hilar and mesenteric lymphadenopathy have been observed only rarely. Leukocytosis and lymphocytosis are usually present but the percentage of atypical lymphocytes is usually under 15. Leukopenia occurs occasionally, and there may be a slight increase in eosinophils. Splenomegaly may be absent or prominent and transient or may persist for several months. Hepatomegaly is rarely observed; liver function tests usually are normal. During the first few days of the symptomatic period a few patients (approximately 10 per cent) develop a transient, diffuse, nonpruritic maculopapular rash that may involve the trunk and the extremities. Myositis may be mild and transient or severe and persistent.

Histologic examination reveals a constellation of morphologic findings that helps to alert the pathologist to the presence of this disease. Epithelioid foci are the most notable features in toxoplasmic lymphadenitis; the clusters of histiocytes are found principally in the pulp of the lymph node but also within or adjacent to germinal centers or capsular areas. The foci consist of about 20 to 30 cells, often less, with pale vacuolated eosinophilic cytoplasm and oval-to-elongate vesicular nuclei with one or more small nucleoli. Typical Langerhans or foreign body giant cells and caseation are not seen. Reactive follicles with large germinal centers are quite common. There is necrosis in these centers and karyorrhectic debris is prominently engulfed by macrophages.

Another feature in the typical case of toxoplasmic lymphadenitis is distension of the subcapsular and trabecular sinusoids by large numbers of benign mononuclear cells. Some of these cells may represent reactive sinusoidal lining cells and others true macrophages, but they are usually admixed with scattered neutrophils and eosinophils. In the classic case, these cells spill into perinodal connective tissue. It must be pointed out that the distension of sinusoids and spillage into adjacent tissue may be a localized phenomenon. The parasitic cysts containing merozoites or free trophozoites are rarely observed.

Congenital Toxoplasmosis. Toxoplasmosis is transmitted to the fetus in 40 to 50 per cent of instances when the mother, previously uninfected, acquires the disease, usually without symptoms, during pregnancy.

Asymptomatic Congenital Toxoplasmosis. In the United States about one infant per 1000 births is infected with *T. gondii* and about 60 per cent of these are asymptomatic at birth. These subclinical infections have been identified only with serologic testing in prospective studies. The asymptomatic type is important because it includes those individuals who may develop toxoplasmic retinochoroiditis years later.

Generalized Congenital Toxoplasmosis. The severely infected infant may be aborted, stillborn, or born alive prematurely or at full term. Many organs may be involved and severely damaged by the necrosis resulting from cells ruptured by the proliferating *T. gondii.*

Fever is common, and a hemorrhagic rash may be seen. Generalized infection frequently will resemble erythroblastosis or severe infections with rubella or cytomegalovirus. Hydrocephaly or microcephaly present at birth or hydrocephaly developing after birth is common. Cerebral calcifications in the periventricular region may be demonstrable at birth or may develop a few weeks later. Healed or active retinochoroiditis is often present. The spinal and ventricular fluid may show pleocytosis and xanthochromia, and *T. gondii* may be isolated from these fluids. High-titered toxoplasma antibodies in both mother and infant will support the diagnosis if the infant maintains a high titer after birth.

When only the central nervous system is involved, clinical signs may not be recognized in infancy; but later, slow physical development, mental retardation, or seizures may be noted. Cerebral calcification may or may not be observed, but scars of healed retinochoroiditis can often be detected. The older the child when diagnosis is attempted, the less firm is the support from the serologic tests. The titers in both mother and infant will fall with the passage of time, but both will remain positive.

Acute Ocular Toxoplasmosis. Evidence accumulated in the last 3 decades indicates that toxoplasmosis is the most frequently diagnosed inflammatory disease of the posterior uveal tract. Onset is more frequent in the second and third decades of life and is predominantly a late sequel of congenitally transmitted infection. Recently, a few cases have been recognized following the acquired disease but it appears to be a rare sequel of this frequently acquired infection.

The onset is insidious, and the major complaint is hazy vision. The lesions usually are unilateral. Healed pigmented scars of prior retinochoroiditis may be seen. Active lesions are frequently contiguous with healed lesions. Recurrent bouts may occur with subsequent development of pain, glaucoma, and blindness; occasionally, enucleation may be required. Specific diagnosis is difficult because antibody titers usually are low, but the ophthalmologic examination usually is definitive.

TOXOPLASMOSIS IN THE IMMUNOSUPPRESSED

T. gondii infection can become recrudescent in immunosuppressed patients, particularly patients with lymphomas or leukemias, or in those involved in organ transplants. *T. gondii* cysts in the brain rupture and the organisms proliferate causing necrosis; the lesions may be single or localized in a few areas, or the infection may be generalized. Fever with symptoms suggesting

intracerebral lesions, the absence of any other demonstrable cause of infection, and positive toxoplasma antibody tests prompt a therapeutic trial that is often successful. Serologic titers may be low in a few of these patients.

ISOLATION OF T. GONDII SPECIMENS

Specimens of spinal fluid, ventricular fluid, buffy coat of heparinized blood, or triturated biopsy tissue (lymph node, bony marrow, muscle, brain) are inoculated intraperitoneally into 4 mice. Two mice are sacrificed 7 to 10 days later; peritoneal fluid is stained by the Giemsa method and examined for *T. gondii*. If no organisms are found, a blind passage of peritoneal cavity washings and triturated spleen is made to 4 additional mice. The remaining 2 mice inoculated with the specimen are sacrificed 6 weeks after inoculation, bled from the orbital plexus, and fresh brain is examined for *T. gondii* cysts. Antibody tests are performed on the mouse serum. If cysts are not found but high titered toxoplasma antibodies are found in the mouse serum, a passage of fresh brain to 4 mice is advisable. In our experience, the successful isolates are most often identified in the peritoneal fluid examination at 7 to 10 days. A failure to isolate is not reported until all the original and blind-passage mice are examined, which may be 8 to 12 weeks after primary inoculation.

The *skin test* for toxoplasmosis is no longer used clinically.

SEROLOGIC TESTS

Two tests*, the Sabin-Feldman Dye Test (DT) and the indirect fluorescent antibody test (IF), give similar results; both become positive early (10 to 30 days after acquisition) and achieve high titers (1: ≥1024) rapidly. Conversion from negative to positive is seldom "caught," but a rise in titer is seen when patients report early. With these tests the titers fall gradually but remain positive for decades and probably for life.

Three other tests detect antibodies that do not persist for decades. (1) The complement-fixation test using soluble (light) antigen becomes positive slightly later than the DT and IF, usually reaches a titer of 1:32 or higher, and

---

*The indirect hemagglutination test (IHA) also detects long-lasting antibody but it is not recommended for diagnosis because it becomes positive late, occasionally as late as 2 months after infection, and the titer rises very slowly; the height of the titer (1:≥2048) may not be achieved until 6 or 8 months after acquisition.

falls to negative in a few months or occasionally not until a few years later if the titer achieved was very high (1:≥512). (2) The gel diffusion test (GD) detects antibodies within a time span similar to the CF but is difficult to quantitate. (3) The indirect fluorescent test for toxoplasma IgM antibodies (TIgM) becomes positive as soon as the DT and IF tests do and usually becomes negative in a few weeks or months but will occasionally persist for a year.

The use of two tests is recommended for diagnosis — one for early and long-lasting antibody (DT or IF) as a screen test and one for the shorter-lasting antibody (CF, GD, or TIgM) on all specimens positive to the screen tests.

The new enzyme-linked immunosorbent assay technique (ELISA) has been applied to toxoplasmosis. When fully evaluated, it may prove useful for demonstrating both long- and short-lived antibodies by the use of heavy and light antigens, respectively.

INTERPRETATION OF ANTIBODY TEST RESULTS

Laboratory support for the diagnosis of clinically apparent infection is usually provided by demonstrating conversion, a rise in titer, or very high initial titers to one or both tests (long- and short-lived antibody). In adults with chorioretinitis, the antibody titers are seldom high.

The interpretation of high titered positive antibody tests on obstetric patients with no clinical symptoms of recently acquired toxoplasmosis is difficult but important. If the patient is past the period of possible abortion, advance preparations for thorough examination of the newborn, including ophthalmologic examination and serologic tests on cord blood, should be made so that therapy for symptomatic disease in the infant can be started promptly. If the newborn is asymptomatic, serologic tests at 2 months and 4 months of age are recommended. The antibody tests on cord blood will be almost identical to the mother's whether or not the fetus was infected. The titers will fall at the rate of about 50 per cent per month if there was no transmission of infection but will remain at the same level, rise, or fall slightly and then rise later (when the infant-produced antibodies appear) if the fetus was infected. Therapy for asymptomatic congenital disease is recommended.

Conversion from negative to positive or a significant rise (two-tube) in titer observed early in pregnancy should prompt the consideration of abortion. *T. gondii* is transmitted to the fetus somewhat less frequently in the early months of pregnancy but may be more dangerous in this period. When toxoplasma titers initially are moderate, tests should be repeated. Happily, most titers in pregnant women are low and do not rise so that no action but reassurance is required. Tests positive before conception mean that there is no risk to the fetus. Negative tests should prompt educating the patient to avoid cats (especially cleaning the litter box) and to eat meat that is well cooked.

TRICHINOSIS

By HERMAN ZAIMAN, M.D.

Valley City, North Dakota

SYNONYMS

Trichiniasis, trichinellosis, trichinelliasis.

DEFINITION

Trichinosis, a disease with protean manifestations, is initiated by ingesting meat containing infective larvae of *Trichinella spiralis*. Such larvae may be present naturally in many homeothermic carnivores. Hogs, however, are the main source of human infection with interesting small epidemics occurring when bear and arctic mammals are eaten. Epidemics have even been reported from as unlikely a delicacy as badger.

Once ingested, the larvae are freed from their capsules by host ferments. They attach to the mucosa, grow, then migrate into the gut lumen to find partners, mate, and produce embryos that are deposited in villous lacteals and venules. The embryos are subsequently distributed throughout the body by the circulatory system. The adult life span in the host gut is limited by: (1) parasite genetics, (2) trauma suffered by the parasites, (3) host resistance, (4) age, (5) health, and (6) acquired immunity.

The longer the adults persist, the greater the number of embryos produced. The literature is filled with the concept that 1500 larvae is the average number produced, but this is true only in specific standardized laboratory animals. It is probably higher in debilitated patients.

Larval production begins about the fifth day of infection. The larvae (embryos) are probably "strained" from the circulation within one to three "passes" and cause local damage wherever they are trapped. Those that do not reach striated muscles probably die. Those that do, invade the muscle cells. Subsequently, capsule (cyst) formation is initiated by the host. Such cysts become calcified in less than a year but the larvae within them may live on for years.

Continuation of the life cycle requires ingestion of the infected host muscle. Hence, human infections are essentially dead ends. In nature, the carcasses of infected, sick or dying animals are quickly eaten by predatory or scavenging carnivores. This spreads the infection. In the past, hogs were often infected by scraps of infected meat in garbage. Recently, when it became mandatory that garbage fed to hogs be cooked, a profound reduction in hog infections occurred. As a result, new human infections with *Trichinella* have become rare in the United States.

COURSE

Human infection with *Trichinella* varies from the asymptomatic to the fulminant fatal case. The severity of any specific infection depnds on the number of worms ingested and the genetic and environmental histories of both the parasite and the host. Thus, a susceptible patient ingesting large numbers of virulent parasites will suffer severely. Conversely, a resistant host who ingests small numbers of avirulent parasites will suffer little.

During the early stages of infection, the worm and pathology are limited to the gut. Thus, for the first week, enteric symptoms and malaise may predominate.

Subsequently, and in association with migration and tissue invasion, systemic, allergic, and localized phenomena are prominent. These include fever, edema, skin, muscle, cardiac, pulmonary, and neurologic signs and symptoms.

Convalescence may begin about the fourth week or the patient may die from one or a combination of factors.

PRESENTING SYMPTOMS AND PHYSICAL EXAMINATION FINDINGS

Because the parasites are distributed throughout the body, a wide variety of symptoms are possible. This creates multiple false initial diagnostic impressions. Involvement of more than one family member and a history of ingestion of a common source such as a family-slaughtered pig or a hunted bear are extremely helpful in suggesting the correct diagnosis.

Fever of 38 to 41 C (100 to 106 F) is common, remitting, and long lasting (10 to more than 40 days). Muscle stiffness, soreness, and cramps occur. The pain may be so severe that paralysis is mimicked. It may be impossible to chew food, turn the eyes, or talk. Respiration may be extremely painful. Edema of the eyelids, the periorbital space, or the entire face is common. Pulmonary signs and symptoms may result from passage of the larvae through the lungs or poor toilet secondary to muscle pain and decreased respiratory excursion. Bronchitis, pneumonia, and dyspnea are frequent.

Cardiac involvement occurs with considerable frequency and is associated with trauma to the myocardium by larvae traveling through or dying in the heart muscle. Tachycardia, bradycardia, and arrhythmias are frequent. Precordial pain with or without congestive failure may occur. Myocardial damage is by far the most frequent cause of death.

Ocular changes often follow invasion of the extraocular muscles. Chemosis, conjunctival hemorrhages, edema, exophthalmos, optic neuritis, and invasion of the retina are all possible. Nearly 75 per cent of all patients have periorbital edema. Neurologic changes were of grave prognostic value before the use of corticosteroids. Headaches, vertigo, tinnitus, deafness, aphasia, insomnia, convulsions, abnormal reflexes, polyneuritis, hemiplegia, and psychiatric changes occur.

LABORATORY FINDINGS

Peripheral Blood. A moderate leukocytosis is usually present. Almost always (90 to 95 per cent of all patients), this is associated with an eosinophilia, involving up to 90 per cent of all circulating white cells. The granules are often paler and smaller but occasionally larger than those in normal eosinophils. An absence of eosinophils or a precipitous decrease in eosinophils has grave prognostic significance.

Biochemical Findings. Electrophoretic patterns show decrease in albumin gamma globulin and an increase of alpha$_2$ globulin. Hypoproteinemia may occur. Enzymes of muscle origin usually increase so that lactic acid dehydrogenase, creatine phosphokinase, myokinase, glutamic-oxaloacetic and pyruvic acid transaminases may all be elevated.

Electrocardiogram. Prolongation of the P-R interval and alterations in QRS complex indicate myocardial damage. Elevation of the ST segment and inverted T waves suggests myocardial infarction. Electrocardiographic changes have been recorded in experimental animals prior to invasion of the myocardium by migrating larvae.

Urinalysis. Creatinine excretion is usually increased.

Immunologic Diagnosis. Intradermal test antigens are available commercially. The tests are easy to perform and are of the immediate type that are read within 15 minutes. Unfortunately, false-negative and false-positive results occur. Positive tests may indicate old, rather than current, infection.

Multiple serologic tests are also available. Of these, the complement-fixation, the direct precipitation, and the bentonite flocculation tests are most commonly available. These tests usually become positive in the second or third week of infection and positive results may persist for years. Changing titers must be demonstrated by repeated tests to prove that positive titers are related to the current clinical problems rather than old infections. Multiple false-negative and false-positive results occur.

Parasitologic Examination. The search for adult trichinae in feces is unpleasant, time-consuming, and very rarely rewarding. It is not recommended. Migrating larvae are infrequently demonstrated in the blood. Differentiation of larvae found in the cerebrospinal fluid from other migrating nematodes is extremely difficult.

The demonstration of larval trichinae in patients' muscle is the definitive diagnostic technique. While this can be done early in the course of the disease, chances for a positive biopsy increase with duration of infection as a result of increase in (1) larval population, (2) larval size, and (3) cyst formation. After the twentieth day of infection, a muscle biopsy near tendinous insertions is obtained by surgery. At least 0.5 gram of tissue is cut into very small pieces and compressed between glass slides. These are then immediately examined under the microscope. Encapsulated larvae are easily seen. Unencapsulated larvae may be confused with muscle fibers unless motion is observed. Many may migrate from the tissue and can be found in expressed fluid.

A portion of the biopsy specimen is reserved for histologic sectioning. This, however, is inferior to the press preparation, since smaller areas are examined in each microscopic field. Other portions of the biopsy may be digested with a 1 per cent pepsin, 0.5 per cent hydrochloric acid solution. Still other sections may be fed to mice that are sacrificed some 4 weeks later and examined by press preparation or pepsin digestion or both.

DISCUSSION

Trichinosis is a relatively rare disease in the United States at this time. In an era devoted to cost containment, the diagnosis will probably be best derived by muscle biopsy following discovery of eosinophilia in a patient who shows enteritis, facial edema, myositis, fever or other appropriate signs and symptoms, has an appropriate dietary history, or is part of a group involved in an epidemic. Unfortunately, the biochemical and immunologic tests available at this time are neither reliable nor definitive.

GAS GANGRENE AND SIMILAR ANAEROBIC SOFT TISSUE INFECTIONS

By WESLEY FURSTE, M.D.,
and HUGO CABRERA, Ph.D.
Columbus, Ohio

Many of the great men of medicine have been interested in gas gangrene as a complication of wounds because of its spectacular nature, fulminating course, profound toxemia, mutilating effects, and high mortality. During the past few decades, gas gangrene has become a general term that has been loosely applied to a number of conditions (Table 1).

SPECIFIC CONDITIONS

Gas Gangrene Resulting from Soft Tissue Trauma. Clostridial myositis of the spreading or diffuse type represents true gas gangrene resulting from trauma. It may be manifested clinically as the crepitant type, the noncrepitant or edematous type, the mixed type, or the profound toxemic type. Diffuse clostridial myositis is essentially an affection of the muscles, and, comparatively, at first, connective tissues may be little affected.

Three distinct zones in gas gangrene can be recognized:
1. A central or dead zone that consists of disintegrated muscle destroyed by trauma, organized clot, and a vast number of organisms.
2. A second or dying zone that contains devitalized muscle fibers covered by masses of bacteria and the products of infection. The anatomic arrangement of these muscle fibers remains undisturbed even though the fibers become separated by an exudate that is or is not packed with leukocytes, according to the

Table 1. *Gas Gangrene and Similar Anaerobic Soft Tissue Infections*

I. Deep infections with muscle involvement
   A. Gas gangrene
      1. Gas gangrene resulting from soft tissue trauma; clostridial myositis; clostridial myonecrosis
      2. Abdominal wall gas gangrene; postoperative clostridial sepsis of the abdominal wall; clostridial myonecrosis of the abdominal wall
      3. Uterine clostridial infections
      4. Gas gangrene of the heart
   B. Streptococcal myositis; anaerobic streptococcal myonecrosis; anaerobic streptococcal myositis
   C. Infected vascular gas gangrene; nonclostridial gas gangrene; nonclostridial myositis
II. Superficial infections
   A. Hemolytic streptococcal gangrene
   B. Acute infectious staphylococcal gangrene
   C. Anaerobic cellulitis; creptitant phlegmon; clostridial cellulitis
   D. Necrotizing fasciitis
   E. Synergistic necrotizing cellulitis
III. Simple clostridial contamination of wounds
IV. Infiltration or injection of gas into wounds
   A. Battle wounds
   B. Pranksters' jokes
   C. Self-inflicted wounds (malingering)
V. Gas in tissues after industrial accidents
   A. Magnesiogenous pneumagranuloma
VI. Gas in tissues after injections of chemicals
   A. Injection of drugs
   B. Accidental injection of a foreign agent
      1. Benzene

This table consists of diagnoses that have been reported in the literature or to the authors. Closely related diagnoses are grouped together.

type of infection. Local leukocytosis usually is associated with mixed infections.

3. A third or normal zone in which the muscle is normal except for some cellular infiltration.

The *incubation period* between the occurrence of the injury and the onset of gas gangrene varies from a few hours to a few days.

Pain is nearly always the earliest symptom. Although it may result in part from the effects of injury, it is caused principally by the rapid infiltration of the tissues by fluid and gas. In some instances, what is felt has been described at first as a sensation of heaviness or tension and later as a burning, but rarely as a throbbing pain.

The *temperature* varies considerably but frequently it is less than 101 F. (38.3 C). Although it is not a reliable index of the severity and extent of the infectious processes, it has prognostic value, for a low temperature with a rapid pulse suggests a grave outlook.

An alarming rapidity and a feebleness of the pulse, which are out of proportion to the temperature, follow soon after the onset of pain.

Such a condition often becomes increasingly apparent and may progress to an abrupt, progressive, and severe circulatory collapse. Initially, the blood pressure may be slightly elevated, but later becomes significantly low.

Hemograms usually reveal a marked reduction in the number of erythrocytes per cu mm and in hematocrit and hemoglobin levels. The total leukocyte count is seldom elevated above 12,000 to 15,000 per cu mm. *In general, no satisfactory laboratory tests exist for the early diagnosis of gas gangrene. For this reason, immediate surgical exploration of any wound suspected of harboring clostridial myositis is advisable.*

Microscopic examination of the watery discharge usually reveals numerous red blood cells, a few pus cells, and many large grampositive bacteria. In contrast to pyogenic infections, few pus cells are seen. When *Clostridium perfringens* is present in tissues, it does not have spores, but other toxigenic clostridia do often sporulate.

Three groups of clostridia are found in association with traumatic wounds. The first, including *C. perfringens (welchii), C. novyi (oedematiens),* and *C. septicum,* are toxigenic and proteolytic organisms capable of causing the clinical syndrome of gas gangrene. Of these, *C. perfringens* is the most frequent. It occurs in 56 to 80 per cent of cases, although in the majority of wounds containing clostridia more than one species of these bacteria are found. The second group, including *C. sporogenes, C. histolyticum, C. bifermentans,* and *C. fallax,* are nontoxigenic, but, because of their proteolytic enzymes, augment the infection by supplying additional nutrients for bacterial growth. The third group includes nontoxigenic and nonproteolytic strains, such as *C. butyricum* and *C. tertium,* that appear only as contaminants in these wounds. Rarely, other clostridia, such as *C. tetanomorphum, C. putrificum, C. aerofoetidus, C. capitovale,* and *C. sphenoides,* have been associated with gas gangrene.

Roentgenograms taken at intervals of 2 to 4 hours may aid in the diagnosis by differentiating gas in the soft tissues that has been produced by clostridial invasion from gas that has been produced by mechanical or chemical causes. When the visible gas increases in amount or when it presents a linear spread along the muscle and fascial planes, a diagnosis of gas gangrene can be made.

Abdominal Wall Gas Gangrene. Abdominal wall gas gangrene is associated with abdominal surgery or trauma. The provoking event is contamination of the wound with histotoxic clostridia in the intestinal flora. Thus, this complica-

Table 2. *Differential Diagnosis of Some Anaerobic Soft Tissue Infections*

Characteristic	Clostridial Cellulitis	Clostridial Myonecrosis	Anaerobic Streptococcal Myonecrosis	Necrotizing Fasciitis	Synergistic Necrotizing Cellulitis
Toxemia	±	++++	++	++	+++
Local pain	±	++++	Late	±	++
Local swelling	±	+++	+++	++	++
Gas	++ to ++++	++	++	±	±
Appearance of skin	Essentially normal	Tense, white, or gangrenous with bullae	Sometimes coppery	Brawny; pale red or gangrenous	Swollen, red, or gangrenous
Gross characteristic of exudate	Putrid, brown	Thin, serous; sometimes sweetish or putrid	Seropurulent, sour	Variable	Purulent, putrid
Gram stain of exudate	Abundant PMNs; gram-positive rods	Few PMNs; gram-positive rods	Many PMNs; gram-positive cocci	Many PMNs; variable, sometimes mixed organisms	Variable PMNs; Mixed organisms
Etiology	Clostridia	Clostridia	Anaerobic streptococci; ± aerobic streptococci, staphylococci	Aerobic and anaerobic staphylococci and streptococci; enteric bacilli: occasionally Bacteroides	Mixed: anaerobic streptococci, Bacteroides, and coliforms
Surgical therapy	*Judicious incision and debridement*	Extensive removal of *all* infected muscle	Removal of necrotic muscle	Widespread filleting incisions if no response to antibiotics	Widespread filleting incisions

Except for several minor changes, this table is reproduced with permission of M. Barza from his chapter in Current Therapy 1977 (H. Conn, Ed.), Philadelphia, W. B. Saunders Co.

Table 3. *Microorganisms That May Produce Gas in Human Tissues*

Gram Stain Result	Aerobes	Anaerobes
Gram-positive microorganisms		
Cocci	Staphylococcus aureus (Staphylococcus pyogenes) Group A Streptococcus (Streptococcus pyogenes: beta-hemolytic Streptococcus)	Peptostreptococcus (anaerobic Streptococcus)
Bacilli		Clostridium perfringens Clostridium novyi Clostridium septicum Clostridium histolyticum Clostridium sporogenes Clostridium tertium and other clostridia species that may be responsible for gas gangrene
Gram-negative microorganisms		
Bacilli	Escherichia coli Klebsiella pneumoniae Enterobacter species	Bacteroides fragilis

tion can follow operations for intestinal malignancies, volvulus, diverticulitis, biliary tract disease, and appendicitis with rupture, and can be a complication of intra-abdominal procedures during which the bowel has been opened. Tissue gas is a relatively late finding (often 3 to 5 days after the other signs evolve). When gas does make its appearance, it is widely disseminated; crepitance may be palpated from the symphysis pubis to the clavicle.

Large bowel cancer occasionally reveals itself by perforation and the subsequent development of abdominal wall gas gangrene. The clinical features in such instances are subtle and often difficult to diagnose in the early stages. The condition can begin 2 to 3 days after the precipitating episode with low-grade fever and insidious renal failure; hemolysis and jaundice are relatively common. Local findings at this stage are usually minimal. There may be some abdominal pain, but there is often no visible change in the abdominal wall until several days into the course.

Uterine Clostridial Infections. *C. perfringens* is present in the genital tract of about 5 per cent of women. Following abortion, or uncommonly after prolonged labor, this organism may invade the uterine wall, producing extensive necrosis, high fever, and circulatory collapse. Bacteremia, unusual in gas gangrene, is characteristic of this process. Severe intravascular hemolysis caused by the alpha-toxin (lecithinase) of *C. perfringens* results in hemoglobinemia, which can produce acute renal shutdown.

Gas Gangrene of the Heart. With widespread systemic clostridial infection, there may be invasion of the cardiac muscle. Cardiac lesions consist of foci of myonecrosis containing numerous organisms, myocardial gaseous cysts, and clumps of organisms within the lumina of cardiac, vascular, and lymphatic channels.

Streptococcal Myositis. In this condition there is a massive infection of muscle, together with discoloration, edema, serous exudate, gas formation, local pain, and generalized toxemia. Neglected cases may progress to a true gangrene of muscle. The chief points of differentiation between streptococcal myositis and clostridial myositis are: (1) streptococcal myositis' more pronounced and extensive cutaneous erythema; (2) its involvement of muscle which, although edematous and discolored, is still alive and reactive to stimuli at exploratory operation; (3) its different odor; and (4) the microscopic appearance of a muscle smear stained by Gram's method that reveals no gram-positive bacilli but vast numbers of gram-positive cocci among masses of pus cells. Although *Peptostreptococcus* (anaerobic *Streptococcus*) is the causative agent of streptococcal myositis, *Staphylococcus aureus* and Group A *Streptococcus* are sometimes present as well.

Infected Vascular Gas Gangrene. Although the infecting organisms show little proclivity to invade healthy tissue, infection may supervene in any site that has become devitalized through loss of its blood supply. This is especially common in elderly patients with atherosclerotic vascular disease. The infection can involve anaerobic as well as aerobic bacteria, such as *Bacteroides*, *Peptostreptococcus*, *Escherichia coli*, and *Klebsiella*.

Hemolytic Streptococcal Gangrene. Hemolytic streptococcal gangrene occasionally follows some relatively minor operative procedure or injury. The lesion is essentially an epifascial, spreading subcutaneous gangrene with thrombosis of the nutrient vessels and resultant slough of the overlying skin. It usually develops in the extremities, although the perineum, face, and other parts of the body may be involved. Hemolytic streptococcal gangrene is characterized by the onset of pain and marked swelling at the site of the wound, chills, elevation of the temperature from 101 to 104 F (38.3 to 40 C), rapid pulse, toxemia, prostration, and a rapidly spreading painful cellulitis that undergoes bullous formation and a peculiar patchy and extending necrosis. Group A *Streptococcus* is found in the subcutaneous gangrene and bullae, often in pure culture.

Acute Infectious Staphylococcal Gangrene. Acute infectious staphylococcal gangrene rarely simulates gas gangrene. After an injury or in cases of acute fulminating osteomyelitis, patients develop a rapidly spreading cellulitis with pain, swelling, brawny induration, patchy discoloration of the skin, and elevation of temperature to high levels. In acute infectious staphylococcal gangrene, *Staphylococcus aureus* is the sole organism to be demonstrated on aerobic and anaerobic cultures of the pus obtained by aspiration of or multiple incisions in the involved tissues.

Anaerobic Cellulitis. Anaerobic or clostridial cellulitis is a crepitant septic process of the epifascial, retroperitoneal, or other connective tissues that usually have been devitalized by trauma. Ordinarily, there is no extensive invasion of living muscle as is found in true gas gangrene. Anaerobic cellulitis is most commonly seen in extensive lacerations of soft tissues other than muscle, the anaerobic organisms (clostridia and other anaerobes) multiplying freely in necrotic debris; it may also occur in association with enteric fistulas and after abdominal and pelvic cavity operations. The incubation period of anaerobic cellulitis is usually 3 or 4 days, and the onset is more gradual than that of true gas gangrene. Systemic effects may be slight unless the wound is also very septic, and this relative mildness of the general reaction is helpful in distinguishing between it and true gas gangrene. Anaerobic or clostridial cellulitis, however, is not a condition to be regarded lightly. The spread of infection in the tissue spaces may be rapid and extensive and may necessitate radical surgical drainage even within a few hours.

Necrotizing Fasciitis. This infection is defined on the basis of its most striking target organ, the fascia, which, rather than serving to limit its spread, provides a natural tissue plane along which the process runs rampant. The disease occurs most commonly in patients who are diabetic, have severe atherosclerotic vascular disease, or who use illicit drugs parenterally. Although there is often no evident site of initial injury, the infection may appear in the extremities at sites of trauma or vascular compromise, in the perineal area at a focus of trivial injury, or in proximity to stay sutures or drainage tubes in the chest or abdomen. Its progress is often evident by the production of a rapidly advancing margin of woody induration and bronze discoloration of the skin.

Necrotizing fasciitis is somewhat of a misnomer in that there is extensive involvement of the skin and subcutaneous fat, with only secondary destruction of the deep enveloping fascia. Rarely are muscle compartments invaded. The process is not as rapidly progressive as is the case with gas gangrene or synergistic necrotizing cellulitis.

It is sometimes difficult to differentiate necrotizing fasciitis from synergistic necrotizing cellulitis. A variety of causative organisms have been recovered, including aerobic and anaerobic staphylococci and streptococci, enteric bacilli, and *Bacteroides* species.

Synergistic Necrotizing Cellulitis. This syndrome is closely related to necrotizing fasciitis and occurs in many of the same situations. The distinction is based chiefly upon the tissue layers of major impact.

In contrast to other infections caused at least in part by *Streptococci,* synergistic necrotizing cellulitis is more similar to gas gangrene, for there is widespread involvement of the deeper tissues. Necrosis of muscle and fascia is the rule, while gangrenous changes in skin and subcutaneous fat are the direct consequence of a more extensive infectious process beneath.

A common site of this infection is in the perineal area (perineal phlegmon or Fournier's gangrene), in which a rapidly progressive cellulitis spreads over the scrotum and base of the penis. This may advance within hours to involve the lower trunk, perineum, and upper thighs. Systemic toxicity may be severe. The causative agents are similar to those found in necrotizing fasciitis; aerobes appear to act in concert with anaerobic bacteria, in a manner that is incompletely understood, to produce this dangerous infection.

Simple Clostridial Contamination of Wounds. Many incisions and wounds harbor clostridia, often mixed with other bacteria, such as noninvasive saprophytes. The lesions appear clean or can contain a superficial exudate. There is no local pain, tissue necrosis, or systemic toxicity.

It has been established that *C. perfringens* is practically ubiquitous in the human environment. The dust collected from a battleship has been found to be contaminated by pathogenic strains of *C. perfringens.* The soil of countries that has been cultivated for centuries has always been heavily contaminated with clostridia. Samples of dirt from the major street intersections of Cincinnati contained viable spores of *C. perfringens* as well as of other clostridia. *C. perfringens* was likewise present in samples obtained during World War II from cultivated areas of the African desert.

Wool clothing is also an important source of clostridial contamination. The uniforms of wounded soldiers have often been found to harbor *C. perfringens* and other clostridia. Clothing made from wool harbors *C. perfringens* and other anaerobic gas-producing bacteria because of the sheep's association with soil and its contaminants. Less common sources of contamination have been (1) unsterile and imperfectly sterilized dressings and instruments, (2) the unprepared skin of the abdominal wall, and (3) the ice used for refrigeration anesthesia.

Battle Wounds with Gas Not Produced by Bacteria. Cases in which air has been sucked into tissues by *penetrating or perforating missiles* have in some instances been confused with true gas gangrene so that unnecessary and incorrect radical surgical intervention — such as amputation — has been effected. Clinical examination of these patients, who do not show the signs of severe toxemia, reveals palpable crepitation in the tissues. However, roentgenologic examinations usually show that collections of air lie along the course of the wound rather than in the planes of the tissue.

Pranksters' Jokes. Pranksters, not understanding the danger of their actions, may inject gas under pressure into the tissues. An example of such an action resulting in very serious consequences is the insertion of the tip of a gasoline station air hose (normally used for inflating tires) into the anorectal canal. With such an act, the prognosis is, of course, extremely guarded, for the large intestine can be ruptured and numerous aerobes and anaerobes can be blown into the peritoneal cavity to produce an overwhelming peritonitis.

Gas Infiltration in Tissues of Wounds Self-Inflicted by a Malingerer. One such individual, whose actions were described for the authors, deliberately lacerated his hand and, with an air hose, injected gas into the laceration in an effort to obtain an industrial compensation award.

Magnesiogenous Pneumagranuloma. Subcutaneous crepitant masses around lacerations have developed in the hands of patients who have been blowing an alloy containing 90 per cent finely powdered magnesium under pressure during the production of airplanes.

Injections of Drugs. Injections of drugs have rarely been followed by the development of gas infections. In many cases, it has been postulated that the contaminating, gas-producing organisms were injected simultaneously with such drugs as digitalis, epinephrine-in-oil, suramin, crude liver extract, amobarbital, insulin, and other drugs or combination of drugs.

Accidental Injection of Benzene. An unusual condition that may be confused with gas gangrene is caused by the accidental injection of benzene. A series of 15 patients developed crepitant necrosis of muscle a few hours after injection, into the pectoralis muscle, of material thought to be typhoid vaccine but that later proved to be benzene. No bacteria were found in the exudate.

Concluding Comments

If the responsible surgeon is in doubt about the possibility of the diagnosis of gas gangrene, he should seriously consider a longitudinal incision of the involved area to be certain that a potentially lethal gas gangrene is not present.

Many individuals — nurses, hospital administrators, public health officers, government officials, lawyers — can be involved in the care of patients with anerobic soft tissue infections. Therefore, it is strongly recommended that physicians and other medical scientists, who are held medically, morally, and legally accountable, *document in writing their observations and decisions in regard to the diagnosis of gas gangrene and similar anaerobic soft tissue infections.*

Section 3

DISEASES OF THE EAR

OTITIS MEDIA

By DAVID N. F. FAIRBANKS, M.D.
Washington, D. C.

DEFINITION

Otitis media is an inflammatory process of the middle ear, the anatomic area that includes the tympanic membrane, the ossicles, the mastoid and tympanic air spaces with their mucous membrane linings, and the eustachian tube. The term is inclusive of several differing pathologic entities, as noted in the following outline:

1. Acute otitis media: bacterial or viral infection of the middle ear
   a. Acute suppurative otitis media
   b. Acute coalescent mastoiditis
   c. Acute necrotizing otitis media
   d. Bullous myringitis
2. Serous-mucoid otitis media: retention of secretions in the middle ear
   a. Unresolved acute otitis media
   b. Allergic otitis media
   c. Baro-otitis
   d. Congenital-mechanical eustachian tube dysfunction
3. Chronic otitis media–tympanomastoiditis
   a. With perforation
   b. With cholesteatoma
   c. Tuberculous

SIGNS, SYMPTOMS AND PHYSICAL FINDINGS

Acute otitis media is characterized by pain and a stuffy or blocked sensation in the ear. In the first few hours of the disease the inflammation affects the mucosa of the middle ear space and the eustachian tube, yet the tympanic membrane is deceptively normal: The normal tympanic membrane is somewhat translucent and has the color, thickness, and tensile strength of waxed paper. Minute blood vessels can be seen coursing around the periphery of the membrane and down the long process ("handle") of the malleus bone where it is attached to the membrane. Acute otitis media is first detectable when these vessels become engorged, but the examiner may not detect this change as abnormal unless he compares the painful ear with the one on the opposite side.

Within 24 hours the entire tympanic membrane becomes erythematous and overvascularized, and in the ensuing days the membrane loses its concave appearance and bulges because of the accumulation of inflammatory secretions in the middle ear space. The light reflex on the membrane is often (but not always) lost when the membrane bulges. Pus in the middle ear adds a yellow hue to the reddened membrane.

If untreated, the inflammation will lead to such pressure and weakening of the membrane that spontaneous perforation occurs, releasing yellow secretions into the ear canal. The perforation is usually pinhole-sized and is not seen by the examiner if secretions obscure the view. The secretions are usually pulsatile, which reflects the state of vascular engorgement of the membranes.

In acute necrotizing otitis media the vascular supply of the tympanic membrane is infarcted and the central portions of the membrane become necrotic and virtually disappear, which results in a large horseshoe-shaped perforation. This is seen in children with high fever and concurrent infections such as scarlet fever or measles.

Bullous myringitis, on the other hand, does not lead to perforation or suppuration but rather to blister-like lesions on the surface of the membrane. They resemble the labial lesions of herpes simplex. Usually they contain only serous clear fluid, but they may become hemorrhagic and look like blood blisters. This type of infection is extraordinarily painful.

Acute coalescent mastoiditis is an extension of acute suppurative otitis media into the mastoid air spaces and bone. It follows the acute episode by about 10 to 14 days and is characterized by a recurrence of pain and ear discharge. Tenderness and swelling behind the ear and a bulging displacement of the ear forward and away from the head are ominous signs.

Serous-mucoid otitis media is a prevalent disease in children and it is occasionally seen in adults as a sequel to acute otitis media with incomplete recovery of eustachian tube function. Any event that compromises the function of the tube will lead to such a condition. Notable examples are allergies of the upper airways, infections of the adenoids and nasopharynx, and the cleft palate deformity. Barotitis, barotrauma, and tympanic squeeze are terms describing malfunction of the eustachian tube during rapid changes in air pressure such as those encountered in airplane travel and scuba diving, especially when the patient has a respiratory infection.

Most adults find the stuffy, blocked sensation in the ear caused by serous-mucoid otitis media distressing enough to seek medical attention. However, many children do not, and the disease is discovered on routine physical examinations or on school screening tests for hearing. Tuning fork tests show better hearing by bone than by air, but not always. Changes in the appearance of the tympanic membrane are subtle and easily overlooked. They include any of the following:

1. Air-fluid levels (bubbles) behind the membrane

2. Retraction of the membrane with rotation of the malleus handle posterior-superiorly

3. Discoloration of the membrane due to color in the fluid behind it, usually an amber or "old dishwater" color, but sometimes blue or black from hemorrhage

4. Increased vascularity and thickening of the membrane with loss of its translucency

5. Decreased mobility of the membrane to changes in air pressure.

The last named sign (5) is demonstrated by the application of alternating positive and negative air pressure against the drum, utilizing the pneumatic otoscope. Decreased mobility suggests fluid in the middle ear space. Absent mobility suggests a perforation.

Chronic otitis media is characterized by hearing loss from damage to the tympanic membrane and ossicles, and by recurring drainage from the ear. The tympanic membrane appears thickened with calcific white patches in some patients; in others there are thin atrophic areas, and perforations of various sizes and shapes are usually present. Contamination of the middle ear occurs through the perforation whenever the patient allows water to enter his ear, such as when swimming or showering, and this is followed by drainage of yellow-brown or gray pus through the perforation. During such an active infection the middle ear mucosa (visible through the perforation) is reddened and edematous. When no active infection is present there are no visible secretions, and through the "dry" perforation the middle ear mucosa is seen as a transparent glistening covering over the white bone.

A "perforation" in the superior part of the membrane may actually be a retraction pocket where skin from the tympanic membrane is inverted into the mastoid air cells. If it becomes large and deep, it will retain the keratin that epidermal cells shed, and an epidermal inclusion cyst will develop in the mastoid. This condition is known as cholesteatoma and is today's most common form of mastoiditis. On examination the perforation appears to be filled with cheesy seborrheic debris and, when infected, with foul-smelling discharge.

Tuberculous otitis begins with multiple small perforations that subsequently coalesce into a larger one, and painless drainage with hearing loss ensues.

COMMON COMPLICATIONS

All varieties of otitis media produce a conductive hearing loss. Mastoiditis is the notable complication of otitis media. From the mastoid the infection can extend into the labyrinth (labyrinthitis), intracranially (subdural empyema, brain abscess, meningitis), into the facial or abducens nerves (seventh or sixth nerve paralysis), or into the deep tissue planes of the neck (Bezold's abscess).

LABORATORY FINDINGS

Audiometry reveals the presence and severity of conductive hearing loss characteristic of otitis media. It is unnecessary in acute otitis unless the diagnosis is in question; in serous-mucoid otitis it aids considerably in confirming the diagnosis. Fluid in the middle ear creates mild losses from 5 to 40 decibels. Patients with small perforations due to chronic otitis media may exhibit no hearing loss; those with larger perforations show mild losses in the range of 20 to 40 decibels. A hearing loss of 40 to 60 decibels suggests destruction of the ossicular chain. Tympanometry (impedance audiometry) showing impaired mobility of the middle ear structures suggests serous-mucoid otitis. Exaggerated mobility suggests disruption of the ossicular chain, and failure to obtain an air-tight seal suggests a perforation.

Cultures taken from middle ear secretions in acute suppurative otitis media reveal the pneumococcus as the predominant pathogen: *Hemophilus influenzae* is common in younger patients; the streptococcus is an occasional pathogen, but the prevalence is increased if anaerobic culturing techniques are used. Bullous myringitis may be caused by any of the foregoing, or by the *Mycoplasma pneumoniae* organism. Nasopharyngeal cultures correlate with middle ear cultures in only 50 per cent of instances.

Chronic otitis media pathogens are those of external origin that commonly contaminate open wounds: *Pseudomonas aeruginosa, Bacteroides fragilis, Staphylococcus aureus,* and *Proteus.*

Mastoid x-rays are helpful only when mastoiditis is suspected, and such films are easily overinterpreted since even acute suppurative otitis media produces clouding of the mastoid air cells. However, when the bony partitions between such cells are eroded, the condition is termed coalescent mastoiditis, which is a surgical emergency. Chronic otitis media produces a sclerotic, constricted mastoid air system that has little clinical significance.

PITFALLS IN DIAGNOSIS

Otitis media is probably overdiagnosed as a cause of fever in children. Young children when screaming and restrained often demonstrate a flushed, erythematous appearance not only of the face but of the eardrum as well. The appearance is indistinguishable from that of early acute otitis media. The child should therefore be examined when he is quietly sitting in his mother's lap.

Otitis media must be distinguished from otitis externa, as discussed in the following article, since the disease processes and treatments are entirely different.

Earache does not necessarily signal ear infection. Indeed, the ear is the target of referred pain from almost any structure in the head and neck. Ear pain that is transitory, waxing and waning without treatment, is almost certainly a "referred" otalgia. Following is a list of anatomic sites that refer pain to the ear:

1. Temporomandibular joint: dysfunction due to malocclusion, teeth grinding, or faulty chewing patterns

2. Teeth: caries, abscess, or "cutting" teeth in children

3. Tonsils: inflammation or tumor, especially ear pain after tonsillectomy

4. Adenoids and nasopharynx: inflammation or tumor

5. Sinuses: inflammation or tumor

6. Salivary glands: inflammation or tumor

7. Base of tongue: inflammation or tumor

8. Larynx or hypopharynx: inflammation or tumor

Any patient with earache, normal-appearing tympanic membrane, and normal hearing deserves a thorough examination of these structures.

OTITIS EXTERNA

By DAVID N. F. FAIRBANKS, M.D.
Washington, D.C.

DEFINITION AND SYNONYMS

Otitis externa is an inflammatory process of the skin of the external ear canal. The term is inclusive of several differing pathologic entities as noted in the following outline:

1. Acute otitis externa ("swimmer's ear")
2. Otomycosis ("fungus ear," "jungle ear")
3. Seborrheic otitis externa
4. Allergic otitis externa

SIGNS, SYMPTOMS, AND PHYSICAL FINDINGS

Acute otitis externa is characterized by severe pain and tenderness in the ear, with scanty greenish-gray discharge that obstructs the ear canal and impairs hearing. It usually occurs the evening or day after the patient has been swimming or after some other event that allowed water into the ear canal, such as hair washing, showering, or washing the ear with water for removal of ear wax.

The characteristic physical finding is tenderness to pressure on the tragal cartilage. Similar pain is elicited when the ear is pulled. The skin of the ear canal is red and swollen, and usually is too tender to allow the examiner to insert the ear speculum. For this reason, and also because of purulent secretions mixed with ear wax, the tympanic membrane is often not seen.

Otomycosis, by contrast, creates only mild pain, but rather a sensation of itching and blockage of the ear with a fluid that sloshes back and forth. The ear canal contains a whitish secretion the texture of cottage cheese, with surface patches of black, which, on magnified inspection, prove to be fuzzy spores. There is little swelling of the ear canal skin or tenderness of the ear or tragus.

Seborrheic otitis externa is characterized by chronic itching of the ears and a reddened scaly ear canal skin with overproduction of scaly ear wax. It may be the only site of seborrheic dermatitis in the patient, but more often other sites are also affected, such as the scalp. Patients with this condition are prone to develop acute otitis externa easily when water is allowed into their ear canals.

Allergic otitis externa is a reaction to ear drops that have been used to soften ear wax or to treat infection. The history is suggestive. The patient exhibits pain, tenderness, reddening, swelling, and blistering of the ear canal and nearby skin. Another type of allergic reaction occurs against fungal infections of skin elsewhere on the body. It causes itching and scaliness similar to seborrheic otitis externa.

COMPLICATIONS

Necrotizing (malignant) otitis externa involving the ear and scalp and extending intracranially is a rare complication of acute otitis externa. It occurs in elderly, diabetic, or debilitated patients with compromised host defenses.

LABORATORY FINDINGS

Culture studies of secretions in acute otitis externa yield *Pseudomonas aeruginosa* in most instances. Occasionally *Staphylococcus aureus* or *Proteus* will be present. Otomycosis yields *Aspergillus niger*.

PITFALLS IN DIAGNOSIS

Otitis externa is frequently misdiagnosed as acute otitis media because of the pain and otorrhea. Tenderness of the tragus is the distinguishing diagnostic sign because pressure on the cartilage stretches the ear canal skin, creating pain in external canal infections but not in otitis media. Furthermore, the tympanic membrane, when visible, is seen as normal in most external ear infections. Postauricular swelling due to cellulitis and postauricular lymphadenopathy in advanced otitis externa may mimic some signs of acute coalescent mastoiditis, and the mastoid x-rays may even show haziness owing to inflamed overlying skin. However, otitis externa runs a rapid course with pain and swelling appearing in a few days. Mastoiditis, on the other hand, takes 10 to 14 days to develop after the initial onset of acute suppurative otitis media.

Folliculitis or furunculosis of the ear canal skin may mimic acute otitis externa, but the inflammatory lesion is more localized and generally does not extend deeply into the ear canal.

Herpes zoster can affect the ear canal. It also affects the seventh and eighth cranial nerves, creating facial paralysis, neural hearing loss, and vertigo. The ear canal, the ear, and nearby facial skin exhibit painful vesicular eruptions.

Section 4

NECK TUMORS

NECK TUMORS

By STANLEY W. COULTHARD, M.D.
Tucson, Arizona

INTRODUCTION

Neck tumors noted as a "lump in the neck" are common clinical problems. Even though much has been written about the ominous results of a delay in diagnosis and inappropriate timing of biopsy procedures, it is still mandatory to reinforce these facts. An organized and direct approach to the evaluation of a neck tumor is necessary to give the patient the most efficient and efficacious medical care. This means extracting from the history, physical examination, and diagnostic evaluation information that allows a reasonable working differential diagnosis and therapeutic approach. As a differential diagnosis is formulated, the cause of the tumor is classified as (1) neoplastic, (2) congenital, or (3) inflammatory.

This article deals with the approach a physician should use in evaluating a "lump in the neck." Particular emphasis is placed on the sequence of the evaluation, the completeness of the head and neck history and examination, and proper timing of biopsy procedures of the primary lesion or the metastatic mass in the neck.

NEOPLASMS

Neoplasms may occur as primary lesions in the neck or may be metastatic from a primary site elsewhere. An enlarged cervical lymph node is usually the site of a metastatic neoplasm to the neck. The neck has numerous lymph node groups that drain the head and neck region. Seventy to 80 per cent of all asymmetric cervical lymph node enlargements are malignant neoplasms that have arisen from a primary in the head and neck region. Squamous cell carcinoma is the most common histologic subtype that is metastatic to cervical lymph nodes. A squamous cell carcinoma usually arises from the mucous membrane surfaces of the upper aerodigestive system and spreads via the cervical lymph channels to lymph nodes.

Lymph node lesions caused by Hodgkin's disease, lymphosarcoma, and reticulum cell sarcoma are less frequent in the neck than are metastatic neoplasms.

Malignant salivary gland neoplasms metastasize to the carotid and submandibular lymph nodes of the neck. The neoplasms are frequently asymptomatic and noticed only by chance when the patient is washing or looking in a mirror. Lipomas, fibromas, neuromas, and carotid body tumors are frequent in the neck and must be included in the physician's differential diagnosis.

CONGENITAL LESIONS

Thyroglossal duct and branchial cleft cysts present as congenital neck tumors. They may be present for long periods of time before medical attention is sought. Each of these cysts can have superimposed infections that confuse the definitive diagnosis.

The thyroglossal duct cyst is typically in the midline of the neck, moves on swallowing, and is noted sometime before the midteen years. It is not uncommon that the cyst will become infected and require incision and drainage prior to definitive surgical removal.

Branchial cleft cysts are identified along the anterior border of the sternocleidomastoid muscle in its upper or middle portion. The cysts may become suddenly obvious during an upper respiratory infection. The cyst may be connected to the neck skin or pharynx by a sinus tract.

Dermoid cysts frequently present in the submandibular triangle or at the angle of the mandible. The cysts are asymptomatic and, once noted, usually do not change significantly in size. It is uncommon for the dermoid cyst to become acutely infected and require incision and drainage.

INFLAMMATORY PROCESSES

Inflammatory processes, including specific granulomas and bacterial infections, may pre-

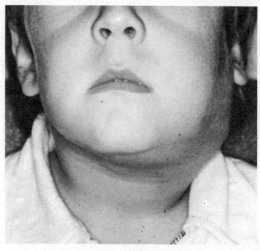

Figure 1. Eight-year-old male with nasal congestion, epistaxis, left ear serous otitis, and left neck tumor. A large nasopharyngeal lymphoepithelioma with left neck metastasis was found.

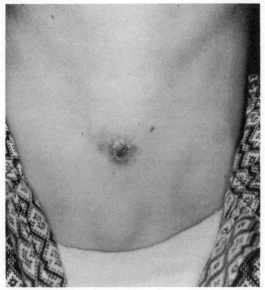

Figure 2. Sixteen-year-old male with a six-year history of a thyroglossal duct cyst. Previous attempts at removal were unsuccessful and the sore continued to drain periodically.

sent as a neck tumor. When these infections do present in the neck, the cervical lymph nodes are responsible for the neck swelling. The nodes enlarge in response to the inflammatory reaction and may progress to abscess formation. Unfortunately, many patients have neck tumors treated with antibiotics first, and only when there is worsening or no change in the neck mass are the history, physical, and laboratory evaluation completed.

HISTORY

The history is extremely important. A history directed toward the symptoms and signs of the neck tumor should be considered first. The patient should be asked for duration of signs and symptoms, pertinent changes in the neck mass, and associated problems.

Duration of the neck mass is one of the better indicators of its cause. Neoplasms in the neck are commonly present for weeks to months before the patient seeks medical attention. The reason for this delay is that neoplastic masses are asymptomatic and can easily be disregarded for long periods of time. The history in an inflammatory neck mass shows that the patient has had symptoms for only a short while and has sought medical attention relatively soon after the onset of symptoms. There will frequently be associated systemic indicators of infection such as fever, chills, and malaise. Congenital masses are usually present for several years. It is not uncommon that a congenital mass will be noticed at the time of birth or early childhood.

Symptoms of hoarseness, dysphagia, trismus, shortness of breath, and ear pain may be good indicators that the patient's neck mass is related to a primary problem in the mouth, pharynx, or larynx.

Other factors in the family, social, smoking, and drinking history are somewhat ancillary to making the actual diagnosis, but can direct the physician's suspicion and can help in his overall understanding of the patient and his disease. The relationship between smoking, drinking, and squamous cell carcinoma of the mucous membrane surfaces of the upper aerodigestive tract is well documented.

PHYSICAL EXAMINATION

Physical examination, like the history, must be specifically directed toward the local head and neck region but must also be general in terms of examining all body systems. The physical examination starts with a general inspection of the head and neck region. The astute observer can notice many important clues simply by observing the patient for a short while. In this sense, the physical examination starts as the physician begins his interview. This is particularly true of head and neck problems, which may often be easily observable and manifest as the patient speaks and moves. Neck tumors may cause noticeable asymmetry of the neck. The tumor should be examined from the standpoint of size, consistency, mobility, and specific location in the neck.

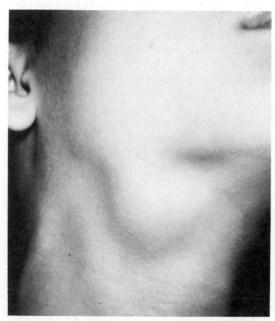

Figure 3. Fourteen-year-old female with a submandibular mass since birth. Excision revealed a dermoid cyst.

Palpation is the examiner's most important tool for determining these factors. The examining physician must position himself to comfortably palpate the entire neck with specific emphasis on comparing both sides of the neck. Bilateral neck palpation gives the examiner the opportunity to detect asymmetric contours in the neck. The palpating fingers should grasp the neck structures deeply and determine the location of the tumor in relationship to the sternocleidomastoid muscle, the laryngotracheal structures, and the jugular vein. It is particularly important to identify whether the mass is in the anterior or posterior triangle of the neck. The sternocleidomastoid muscle divides the neck into the anterior and posterior triangles. Further delineation of the neck mass location can be in relationship to specific jugular lymph node groups such as the digastric, carotid, and omohyoid lymph nodes. The submandibular and supraclavicular regions are also points of ready reference.

In a complete head and neck examination palpation of the tongue, floor of mouth, buccal mucosa, and nasopharynx is extremely important. Submucosal neoplasms in these areas can only be detected by careful palpation.

It is important to differentiate tumors that may be located in the parotid, submandibular, and thyroid glands. A mass that is in the tail of the parotid gland may be misdiagnosed as a jugular lymph node. Appreciation of the boundaries of the parotid gland and its relationship to the neck, mandible, and mastoid tip will make this differentiation easier. Masses in the submandibular gland will not roll over the edge of the mandible when palpated because of their fascial attachments. In contrast, large lymph nodes in the submandibular triangle will easily move over the mandible. Bimanual palpation also helps in determining submandibular mass locations. The thyroid gland is palpable low in the midline of the neck and moves on swallowing. Many examiners prefer standing behind the patient for this examination.

Once the tumor mass has been inspected and palpated, other physical examination techniques such as auscultation and transillumination can be used. Tumor masses causing interference in blood flow will create a bruit that can be heard with the stethoscope over the involved artery. Transillumination can be performed in a darkened room by placing a light source behind the mass and looking for dispersion of light on the skin surface. If this occurs, it is indicative of a fluid-filled cyst.

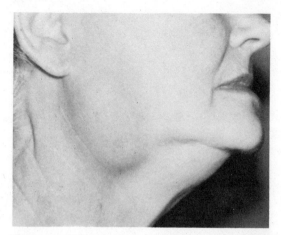

Figure 4. Fifty-nine-year-old female with a gradually enlarging tail of parotid tumor for 5 years. Superficial parotidectomy revealed a benign mixed cell tumor.

A complete head and neck examination must be performed in all patients with a neck tumor, as the majority of patients with neck tumors will have a cause of the tumor identified in this region.

The head and neck examination proceeds from the neck to the examination of the nose, mouth, pharynx, and larynx. The mucous membrane surfaces of these areas can be directly or indirectly examined if the proper techniques are utilized. These techniques involve the use of the headlight and examining mirror. Areas of nasopharynx and pyriform sinuses may require further investigation with direct endoscopy if a diagnosis is not made on the general physical examination. After the head and neck examination a general physical examination is performed to determine the possible relationship of the tumor to other body systems. The physical examination also allows a summary of the patient's general health.

LABORATORY AND RADIOGRAPHIC EVALUATION

After the history and physical examination, further diagnostic evaluation is pursued by using hematologic, biochemical, and radiographic techniques to investigate the neck tumor and the patient in general.

Patients with a neck tumor should have a chest x-ray and hemogram at the beginning of the evaluation. This allows for an early general inspection of the lung parenchyma and identifies any areas suspicious for metastatic or in-

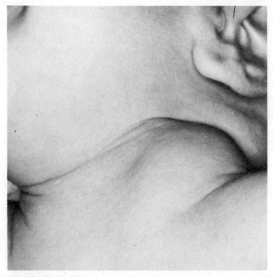

Figure 5. A newborn male with a soft, cystic neck mass. The mass transilluminated. Diagnosis was cystic hygroma.

fectious origins. This is particularly important in patients who may have tuberculosis that is manifested in the neck. An x-ray of the paranasal sinuses is frequently necessary, as this is one area of the head and neck region that evades a direct inspection. Special contrast studies of the digestive and genitourinary tracts are very helpful when the cause of a neck tumor is elusive.

Arteriography is used when it is thought that the neck tumor is intimately associated with the carotid system or when the tumor is felt to be extremely vascular.

When the diagnostic evaluation has progressed through the history, physical examination, and routine diagnostic laboratory studies with no definitive diagnosis apparent, a thyroid scan should be included in the work-up of the patient. This is particularly important if the neck mass is considered to be a thyroglossal duct cyst. In this instance, the mass may contain the patient's only thyroid tissue and removal would be detrimental to the patient.

ENDOSCOPY

When a neck tumor evaluation proceeds to the point of looking for an occult primary in the head and neck area, direct endoscopic techniques are used for closer inspection of the mucous membrane surfaces and biopsy of suspicious areas. Direct laryngoscopy, bronchoscopy, and esophagoscopy are the endoscopic techniques used for this inspection. During this investigation the base of tongue, nasopharynx, and pyriform sinus are particularly noted and biopsies obtained. These areas have been found to be sites of occult primaries.

SURGICAL EXPLORATION

When the evaluation has proceeded through an exhaustive search for a definitive cause of the neck tumor with no firm conclusions, a neck exploration for definitive treatment or biopsy is indicated. It is extremely important that this be done at the end of an exhaustive diagnostic study. The surgeon who proceeds with a neck exploration should be able to deal with any of the numerous problems that may be identified. He should be aware not only of the technical aspects of treating the tumor but also of the best therapeutic measures available. Incisions in the neck should be well planned to accommodate further extension of the surgery if necessary.

CONCLUSION

Evaluation of a neck tumor must involve close scrutiny of not only the neck but also the regional and systemic aspects of the patient. A cervical lymph node enlargement is considered metastatic carcinoma from a primary neoplasm of the head and neck region until proved otherwise. A complete head and neck examination is performed, using both direct and indirect endoscopic techniques with headlight and mirror. A neck mass is biopsied only after an exhaustive history, physical examination, and laboratory evaluation fail to reveal a diagnosis. Finally, if the physician initiates a neck exploration, he should be capable of coping with all the numerous possible neoplastic, inflammatory, and congenital problems he may encounter.

Section 5

DISEASES OF THE RESPIRATORY SYSTEM

DISORDERS OF THE PARANASAL SINUSES

By STEPHEN L. LISTON, M.D., F.R.A.C.S., F.R.C.S.

Minneapolis, Minnesota

INTRODUCTION

The paranasal sinuses are air-containing cavities within the facial bones. They are connected with the nasal cavity and are lined by respiratory epithelium. They are named for the bones in which they are located: the maxillary, ethmoid, frontal, and sphenoid sinuses. The major disease processes affecting the sinuses are infections, allergic disorders, and neoplasms.

PRESENTING SIGNS AND SYMPTOMS

Acute Sinus Infections. The commonest symptoms of an acute purulent infection within the paranasal sinuses are discomfort and pressure. This discomfort and pressure, which is felt in the face, between the eyes and across the forehead, follows viral upper respiratory infections that involve the nose and spread to the contiguous sinus mucosa. These symptoms usually resolve once the viral infection runs its course. However, in a number of patients, the openings of the sinuses to the nasal cavity become closed by edematous mucosa and a secondary bacterial invasion occurs. This results in the sinus' becoming a closed cavity containing pus. At this point the pain becomes worse and may take on a throbbing character. Coughing, straining, and bending over make this pain much more severe. Usually several of the paranasal sinuses are infected at the same time, producing a "pansinusitis." Unilateral radiologic opacification of a paranasal sinus that does not clear promptly with treatment should alert the physician to be suspicious of a noninflammatory cause.

Maxillary sinus pain is felt in the cheek and, as the roots of the upper posterior teeth project into the maxillary sinus, dental pain may occur. Ethmoid sinus pain is felt between the eyes. Photophobia may be noted. Frontal sinus pain produces headache and is felt in the forehead, particularly in the supraorbital region. This pain may not be noticeable when the patient wakes but becomes worse as the day progresses. Sphenoid sinus pain is referred to the vertex. Purulent sinus infections are associated with a low-grade fever.

Another route of infection of the maxillary sinus is secondary to infection of the roots of the upper posterior teeth owing to caries or via an oroantral fistula following an extraction of one of these teeth.

Chronic Sinus Infections. Chronic sinus infections follow inadequately treated acute infections. They may also occur in the presence of such underlying conditions as severe nasal allergy, nasal obstruction from a deviated nasal septum, a compromised state of immunity, bronchiectasis, or cystic fibrosis. The mucosa becomes so thickened and chronically infected that it does not return to normal even when drainage into the nose is re-established. In the maxillary sinus, the nasal ostium is not at the most dependent site and ciliary action is required to clear the normal secretion. When this ciliary action breaks down, pooling of secretions leads to chronicity. A constant mucopurulent discharge occurs that drains posteriorly. Patients complain of this postnasal discharge and of associated sore throats, eustachian tube obstruction, hoarseness, and cough. Chronic sinusitis is rarely very painful but may cause a dull headache.

When the nasal opening of the sinuses is obstructed, rapid changes in the air pressure associated with diving or flying may produce bleeding within the sinus and pain. The history usually makes the diagnosis of barotrauma obvious.

In children, a unilateral nasal discharge is usually secondary to an intranasal foreign body.

Allergies. Allergies are usually manifested by nasal obstruction, sneezing, and a watery rhinorrhea. Itch is another common symptom and it occurs in the eyes, nose, and palate. The allergy is usually an inhalant but ingested allergens may also produce these symptoms. Some patients may be aware of which particular allergens incite these symptoms: for example, dust, pollens, or animal danders. Other patients cannot be so specific. Allergies also cause edema of the nasal mucosa. This mucosal edema may become so severe as to produce nasal polyposis. Patients may have a family of allergies or asthma. A triad of aspirin sensitivity, asthma, and nasal polyps exists, and in such patients aspirin may cause severe asthma. Nasal polyps in children suggest a diagnosis of cystic fibrosis. Most patients complaining of "sinus" symptoms have allergic rhinosinusitis.

Neoplasms. Neoplasms of the sinuses are unfortunately relatively silent and do not cause symptoms until they break through the bony wall of the sinus. Most tumors occur in the maxillary sinus and may spread medially to produce nasal obstruction. Epistaxis may occur and a unilateral blood-stained nasal discharge is highly suspicious of a neoplasm. Spread inferiorly may produce dental pain or anesthesia, loosening of the teeth, or palatal swelling. Dentures that were previously satisfactory may no longer fit. Anterior spread may cause swelling of the cheek and pain or anesthesia over the distribution of the infraorbital nerve. Superior spread invades the orbit and can result in proptosis and ophthalmoplegia resulting in diplopia. Blockage of the nasolacrimal duct may produce epiphora. Posterior spread reaching the pterygomaxillary fossa may cause trismus or symptoms of trigeminal nerve pressure as it exits the base of the skull.

Ethmoid sinus neoplasms may involve the nose with nasal obstruction, epistaxis, or blood-stained discharge. Lateral spread will produce orbital problems, including proptosis, ophthalmoplegias, and epiphora. Spread to the anterior cranial fossa occurs but usually does not produce obvious symptoms.

Frontal sinus neoplasms are not common and benign osteomas are the commonest neoplasms of this sinus. The osteoma may block the nasal frontal duct and cause painful localized sinusitis and headache, or spread beyond the confines of the sinus to produce orbital displacements.

Sphenoid neoplasms are rare. They spread to involve the optic chasm and cause visual loss in the upper outer quadrant of the visual field, or the pituitary causing hypopituitarism. Lateral spread may involve several cranial nerves. Oculomotor nerve involvements produce a dilated pupil, ptosis, and a downward and outward displacement of the globe of the eye. Trochlear nerve involvement causes superior oblique paralysis while involvement of the abducens nerve causes paralysis of the lateral rectus muscle. The ophthalmic nerve may be affected, causing hypoesthesia of the cornea and forehead.

COURSE

Acute infections of the sinuses usually resolve once drainage to the nasal cavity is reestablished. Chronic sinusitis persists until it is adequately treated or until the underlying cause is removed.

Nasal allergies may be a constant problem, but remissions and exacerbations are more common. Nasal polyps tend to continue to recur following their removal, unless their specific cause is well controlled.

PHYSICAL EXAMINATION

Infections. Patients with a severe purulent pansinusitis appear febrile and ill. The nasal mucosa is congested and contains mucopus. The cheek and eyelids may be edematous. Tenderness can be elicited on percussion of the cheek. Digital pressure or percussion to the inner canthral area and floor of the frontal sinus will produce pain and tenderness. Percussion of the upper posterior teeth may also cause pain. Postnasal examination will show a mucopurulent postnasal drainage. Lesser degrees of symptoms and signs are common. In the case of chronic sinus infections the nose may be congested and contain mucopus and a postnasal drainage can be seen.

Some indication of which sinuses are involved may be gained from observing mucopus in the middle meatus (frontal maxillary and anterior and middle ethmoid sinuses) or the superior meatus (posterior ethmoid and sphenoid). Sinuses do not normally drain into the inferior meatus.

Allergies. The lining mucosa of the nose is usually found to be edematous with a bluish coloration. The turbinates are covered with polypoidal mucosa and nasal polyps may be visible. A clear nasal discharge may be present. One may distinguish between polyps and edematous mucosa covering the turbinate by palpation with a small applicator. Polyps will be mobile, while the bony skeleton will be palpable within a turbinate. It should be noted that "nasal allergy" cannot be diagnosed by examination of the nose alone as other conditions can mimic this appearance.

Neoplasms. When a neoplasm is confined within the sinus, physical examination may be normal. As the neoplasm starts to extend beyond the walls of the sinus, physical signs become manifested. Neoplasms of the maxillary and ethmoid sinuses may produce nasal obstruction from the tumor or associated polyposis; therefore, all polyps should be examined histologically. A unilateral mass or polyp should arouse suspicion, as should a unilateral blood-stained nasal discharge. There may be swelling of cheek and palate, loosening of the teeth or denture, or hypoesthesia of the area supplied by the infraorbital nerve. Epiphora or dacrocystitis may follow nasal-lacrimal duct obstruction. Extension to the orbit causes proptosis and ophthalmoplegias. Trismus may occur from posterior extension. Frontal sinus neoplasms (and mucoceles) tend to displace the globe of the eye laterally and down. Sphenoid neoplasms cause visual field defects; ophthalmoplegias from third, fourth, and sixth nerve involvement; and facial pain or hypoesthesia owing to ophthalmic and maxillary nerve involvement.

Endocrine abnormalities may result from hypopituitarism. Squamous carcinomas of the sinuses tend to spread locally and metastases to the cervical lymph nodes are not common.

COMPLICATIONS

Infections of the frontal sinus may erode the posterior bony table and reach the dura mater. Here, the infection may cause an epidural abscess, meningitis, or a localized arachnoiditis. This arachnoiditis may seal off the cerebrospinal space and allow the infection to spread to produce cerebritis or an abscess within the frontal lobe. This frontal lobe abscess may manifest itself as a personality change. Infection of the frontal bone secondary to frontal sinus infection produces a frontal osteomyelitis. This causes a pitting edema of the frontal region originally described by Percivall Pott and called Pott's puffy tumor. Infection may also spread inferiorly to involve the orbit.

Mucoceles occur as a complication of frontal (and more rarely, maxillary) sinus infections. The mucopus cannot drain via the frontonasal passage so an expanding cyst occurs. Frontal mucoceles usually erode the bone inferiorly and cause downward and lateral displacement of the globe of the eye. Frontal mucoceles can also erode posteriorly to form a pathway for infection of the dura mater. The mucocele itself may become infected, producing a pyomucocele.

Ethmoid sinus infections may erode the lamina papyracea of the ethmoid and thus spread laterally to involve the orbit. This is more common in children. Initially, a periorbital abscess is formed. The eyelids and conjunctivae are markedly swollen. The periorbital abscess may penetrate the periosteum to produce an orbital cellulitis or an intraorbital abscess. Another complication of ethmoid sinus infection is retrobulbar neuritis owing to spread of infection from the posterior ethmoid cells to the adjacent optic nerve.

Maxillary sinus infections are less likely to become complicated but may spread to involve the orbit. Maxillary osteomyelitis is usually secondary to a tooth infection in infants. A swollen inflamed cheek is more commonly due to a dental abscess than to sinusitis.

The complications of sphenoid sinusitis produce signs and symptoms similar to those already described for neoplasms in this area. Cavernous sinus thrombosis may follow infection of any of the paranasal sinuses because venous drainage is in this direction. Proptosis of the eye will occur with edema of the lids and ophthalmoplegias due to involvement of third, fourth, and sixth cranial nerves. The retinal veins are distended and papilledema is present.

Such patients are extremely ill, with high fever and signs of meningeal irritation.

RADIOGRAPHIC, LABORATORY, AND ENDOSCOPIC EVALUATION

Radiologic examination is basic to the diagnosis of paranasal sinus disorders. Sinusitis cannot be adequately diagnosed without x-ray. The standard radiologic views are Water's (upright), Caldwell, submental-vertex, and lateral view. An "upright" Water's view shows the maxillary sinus well, whereas the Caldwell is better for the frontal and ethmoid sinuses. The lateral view is needed for evaluation of frontal and sphenoid sinuses, and the submental-vertex view is confirmatory.

Pus within a sinus may produce an air-fluid level. Mucosal swelling produces clouding of the sinuses. Mucoceles have a characteristic ground-glass appearance, while osteomas are densely calcified. Bone destruction is the hallmark of neoplastic processes. Tomography (particularly hypocycloidal tomography) may demonstrate this bone destruction before it is evident on plain films. Computerized axial tomography will show the extent of a neoplasm and may demonstrate extension to involve the central nervous system, orbit, or pterygomaxillary space. Destruction of the pterygoid plate is indicative of posterior spread of neoplasms. Dental radiographs may be necessary when a sinus infection is secondary to dental infection or an oroantral fistula. A chest x-ray will demonstrate any associated bronchiectasis.

Any nasal discharge can be examined and cultured. Eosinophils in the nasal drainage suggest an allergy etiology. Allergy tests may then be obtained.

Pus from the maxillary sinus cavity can be obtained by inserting a trocar and cannula via the inferior nasal meatus or the canine fossa of the maxilla under the lip. These same routes can be used to introduce a sinoscope, an instrument that enables one to examine the interior of the sinus visually. Any pus obtained can be examined by Gram stain and culture. Fungal cultures may be useful in patients who are diabetic or taking corticosteroid or immunosuppressive drugs as these patients are prone to fungal infections. In children with sinusitis or nasal polyps a sweat chloride should be obtained to rule out the possibility of cystic fibrosis.

The central nervous system complications of sinusitis may require electroencephalography, brain scanning, computerized axial tomography, lumbar puncture, or blood culture to make a definitive diagnosis. Any abnormal tissue noted on examination should be biopsied and submitted for histologic examination.

PITFALLS IN DIAGNOSIS

The most serious pitfall in diagnosis is to ascribe all the symptoms and signs to an infectious process and hence delay the diagnosis of a neoplastic process. In this regard tissues involved in any sinus problem that is unilateral or refractory to treatment should be biopsied. A second pitfall is to tell patients who have headaches that they have "sinus." Unless they are acutely ill and have confirmatory x-rays, the diagnosis of "sinus headache" is unlikely to be correct.

CHRONIC BRONCHITIS

By BURGESS GORDON, M.D.
Narberth, Pennsylvania

This is a long-standing disease or condition of the bronchial tree characterized by inflammation, fibrosis and atrophy of mucous membrane with relationships to certain pulmonary, nasal, and systemic problems.

SYNONYMS

Winter cough, wheezing, hacking, cigarette cough.

CLINICAL OBSERVATIONS

In a speculative sense certain phenomena involving this condition tend to make its development inevitable, e.g., by harboring infection and, coincidentally, in favoring repetitious symptoms and physical signs. The outcome may be influenced by physical-physiologic states: malpositions of the abdominal viscera, notably in obesity, and a low, poorly functioning diaphragm. These add complexity to the bronchi and their function.

Systemic diseases may be a factor in chronic bronchitis: heart disease, especially with associated hypertension, and aneurysm of the aorta. These conditions unfavorably influence chronic bronchitis by direct impairment of the circula-

tion and/or indirectly by certain pressure phenomena, somewhat anatomic in type. Malformations of the thorax may interfere with proper "physical" respiration, as in chronic pleurisy with contracture of the chest. Coincidentally, faulty posture accentuates breathing difficulties.

Ventilationary studies reveal the presence and usually the degree of malfunction, notably with the use of "timed" volume estimations or inflow measurements. Thus the expiratory volume is usually low, while the vital capacity estimations may be normal or slightly decreased. The vital capacity tends to be low, as are the maximum voluntary ventilation and maximum expiratory flow rate.

The physician's powers of observation combined with pharmacologic and technical aids may throw important light on the etiology and physical signs, as well as contributing or aggravating influences during the course.

Patients with chronic bronchitis have a normal diffusing capacity with low arterial oxygen saturation; those with emphysema have a lower diffusing capacity with relatively normal oxygen saturation. A low diffusing capacity of the lung may result from a destruction of the alveolar wall, a reduction in the number of pulmonary capillaries, and increases in thickness of the alveolar capillary membrane.

In the presence of severe obstruction of the bronchioles, the area of diffusion of oxygen is decreased by nonventilation of the alveoli. This results in a low diffusing capacity of the lung.

SYMPTOMS AND SIGNS

Cough is a primary manifestation followed by expectoration — possibly more striking at night, while the patient is in the recumbent position as during sleep or resting. Intercurrent infection brings on attacks of coughing. Paroxysmal cough is common, especially during exercise; blood spitting with foul expectoration may occur in advanced cases.

The contour of the chest may be "normal," flat, rounded, or restricted. Movements are guarded during cough and discomfort. Thoracic movements tend to be more prominent than abdominal breathing. Breathing may be restricted unilaterally, as in chronic pleurisy.

At auscultation, breathing is characterized generally by prolonged expiration, and tends to be wheezy in type. Rales are heard over affected parts, especially in the hilar regions and bases; cough precipitates adventitious sounds, notably rales. With expiration, high-pitched, piping sounds may be heard throughout. Fever is uncommon during acute episodes.

DIAGNOSTIC STUDIES

Laboratory Studies. Cultures and microscopy are essential in the study of bronchial secretions, notably if obtained following cough or via bronchoscopy. Certain diseases should be excluded by laboratory study as well as history: asbestosis; byssinosis; bagassosis; and berylliosis. Hematology may suggest relations to systemic conditions, notably disturbances of the blood-making system.

Radiology. Graphic alterations of the lungs may be noted in standard flat plates or films, in fluoroscopy, and following the introduction of an opaque substance into the bronchi. Areas of increased or decreased density or both may be noted, with accentuations during forced inspiraton and expiration. Special methods are available through the specialties of radiology. These include studies to identify pulmonary edema, atelectasis, aspirated foreign body, tumor, or pneumonia.

Bronchoscopy. Inspection of the bronchial tree by bronchoscopy is essential in the study of suspected chronic bronchitis to determine cause and physiologic function of the bronchi and related lung areas. Alterations in the size, contour, position, and behavior of the bronchus are pertinent in critical study. Opaque substances are introduced for associated studies in radiology; materials for microscopic and bacteriological examinations are invaluable, as are tissue biopsies for special examination.

MANAGEMENT

Management of chronic bronchitis begins with a systematic study of the patient with use of selective measures for prevention and the control of manifestations. Realization should be paramount that chronic bronchitis is a many-sided condition, that broad as well as specific relationships may come into play and that the outcome depends on general care as well as definitive treatment. It is interesting to mention that the results of treatment tend to clarify the causes and mechanisms of the disease.

PULMONARY EMPHYSEMA

By JAMES KIERAN, M.D.
Berkeley, California

DEFINITION

The word emphysema is derived from the Greek, modified by the French, and can be loosely interpreted as "a blowing into" or "inflated." This term refers to the end stage of pulmonary emphysema, when there is marked overinflation of the lungs. It was probably Laennec who first used this word to describe the entity in its anatomic terms and it has been so described ever since.

The basic pathologic process is a destruction of the alveolar septa, which are the walls that separate the alveolar spaces one from another. When such a septum is destroyed, two formerly small alveoli effectively become one larger alveolus. As the process continues and more septa are lost, air spaces become larger and larger. In the process, the anatomic elements that traverse the alveolar septa, primarily elastic tissue and blood vessels, likewise disappear.

The exact mechanism by which this anatomic septal destruction occurs is as yet unclear. However, it appears that the normal chemical balance between the proteolytic enzymes (known as proteases, which destroy lung tissue) and the protease inhibitors (which prevent such destruction) is upset in favor of the proteases. As a result, there is more degradation of protein than there is reparation. This is particularly true of the protease *elastase*, which degrades elastin, the primary elastic fiber in the lung.

Furthermore, it is known that there are several specific clinical situations in which this equilibrium between the proteases and the protease inhibitors is upset in favor of the proteases. The first of these is genetic. It occurs when there is a deficiency of the protease inhibitor alpha-1-antitrypsin. Other causes that can upset the equilibrium are bronchial infection and certain air pollutants. The most important cause of enhanced activity of the proteases, however, is the inhalation of cigarette smoke. Once again, the exact mechanisms of its action are not entirely clear. It appears to act by mobilizing macrophages and causing them not only to increase in number but also, and at the same time, to increase their proteolytic activity.

The process of destruction, and therefore the anatomic entity known as chronic pulmonary emphysema, occurs slowly and over a long period of time. There is evidence that it may start in some people as early as the late teens, and certainly during the 20s. But, because the destructive process is quite slow, and because man has approximately twice as much lung tissue as he really needs to carry on his daily activity (and therefore can lose a large amount of lung tissue before becoming clinically aware of the fact), the clinical manifestations of emphysema do not occur until much later in life, usually in the mid 40s and early 50s.

The clinical diagnosis of pulmonary emphysema, therefore, pedagogically should be divided into two stages. The first stage is *early*, or asymptomatic, or subclinical emphysema. The second stage is *late*, symptomatic, or clinical pulmonary emphysema.

PRESENTING SIGNS AND SYMPTOMS

There are two specific characteristics of patients with pulmonary emphysema. First, almost all are cigarette smokers. Second, most are male, although the gap between the numbers of males and females with this disease is slowly narrowing, probably owing to the increased number of women who are now smoking cigarettes.

The diagnosis of early pulmonary emphysema is extremely difficult to make. Unfortunately, the primary symptom, shortness of breath on exertion, occurs only quite late in the disease. And, since the age group in which this illness is centered is 45 years or older, this symptom is frequently interpreted, both by the patient and, occasionally, by the physician, as a sign either that he is growing older or that he is in poor physical condition, or both. In addition, the patient may already have made some adjustment either consciously or unconsciously, to his obviously decreasing ability to exercise. He may have begun to take the elevator instead of walking up the stairs, or use a cart instead of walking the golf course, and so forth. Therefore, the presenting symptom in a patient with early pulmonary emphysema is usually no symptom at all. If specifically asked, he will usually respond that he is *not* short of breath on exertion.

If, as is usually the case, he also has chronic bronchitis, he may describe cough and sputum. But, providing that his problem is merely early pulmonary emphysema, if he has any cough at all it will be minor, and it will produce, if anything, only small amounts of whitish, viscid mucus, occasionally containing bubbles of air. This mucus may be somewhat difficult to raise. However, if the physician investigates further in response to the negative answer to the question about shortness of breath on exertion and asks about changes in exercise habits, e.g., "Are you still hiking in the mountains?" or "Do you still play tennis?" or "Do you still walk up the three flights of stairs at your office?" in many cases the patient will answer in the affirmative.

In late pulmonary emphysema, the situation is entirely different. The patient is obviously clinically ill. He is thin and complains of shortness of breath on slight exertion or on bending. He may also have a history of bronchitis with cough and sputum. He may or may not wheeze, either on exertion or when his bronchial tubes contain a large amount of mucus. In the latter case, the wheeze will be relieved by coughing up the mucus. If his disease is not too far advanced, his symptoms of shortness of breath will be relieved by resting, especially lying down. He will have no difficulty sleeping flat. However, in the final stages of the disease, orthopnea supervenes and he will be more comfortable sitting up.

Course

Pulmonary emphysema advances at a quite slow but otherwise unpredictable rate. It probably has been present for many years, perhaps as many as 20, before the patient becomes aware of any symptoms. Once the symptoms occur, they progress at a variable rate. But, as time goes on, the patient usually notes that his shortness of breath occurs with less and less exertion, until he is finally completely bedridden.

Blood gas values are usually maintained well into the final stages of the disease, usually by the mechanism of hyperventilation.

Thus these patients are known as "pink puffers." However, eventually the equilibrium can no longer be maintained. The oxygen value is the first to fall, with carbon dioxide elevation occurring usually only in the terminal phases. At that time the patient is completely bedridden and requires oxygen therapy in order to have enough strength to turn over in bed. The end is frequently sudden, probably secondary to a cardiac arrhythmia owing to hypoxemia, or right ventricular failure. Or it may occur over the course of a few days from what would otherwise be a relatively minor pulmonary infection.

Physical Examination Findings

In early pulmonary emphysema no significant positive findings are seen on physical examination. Careful evaluation of thorax and lungs reveals them to be within normal limits. As the disease progresses, however, the loss of elastic recoil in the lungs will lead to obstruction of expiratory air flow. The earliest physical sign is noted to be prolongation of the pulmonary expiratory note. This is best determined with the stethoscope. If the patient with early pulmonary emphysema is asked to inhale to maximum inspiratory capacity and hold his breath for a second, and then to breathe out as rapidly and as completely as he can, it may be noted that the expiratory phase is prolonged, usually beyond 4 seconds.

In late pulmonary emphysema, the picture is entirely different: the patient exhibits all the textbook signs of classic pulmonary emphysema. He is thin. He may be hyperventilating at rest. Inspection of the neck will reveal the accessory muscles of respiration to be sharply outlined and in use. The clavicles are prominent; the supraclavicular fossae are deep and may increase in depth with inspiration. Likewise, the trachea may descend during inspiration. However, the neck veins will usually be flat.

Inspection of the thorax reveals the rib cage to be thin and the ribs sharply outlined. The intracostal muscles are usually visible as they contract. The inferior portion of the thorax may be drawn inward during inspiration. There may be such dorsal kyphosis and anterior bowing of the sternum that the anteroposterior diameter of the chest is increased. Thoracic excursions are usually rapid and shallow. On auscultation, the breath sounds are noted to be faint, or absent. When they are heard, there is prolongation of the expiratory note, which can easily be accentuated by asking the patient to exhale rapidly. Rales and rhonchi are usually absent.

Heart sounds are frequently distant and difficult to hear, and the apex beat is usually impalpable. Cardiac pulsations may be seen and felt in the epigastrium. The heart sounds are usually heard best within this location. The percussion note reveals hyperresonance throughout both lung fields. It may also reveal that the diaphragms are low and move only slightly, if at all.

Common Complications

Complications of pulmonary emphysema are relatively uncommon. Unless emphysema is accompanied by chronic bronchitis, as it so frequently is, pulmonary infection occurs relatively uncommonly, and then usually only in late stages of the disease. Pneumothorax may occur occasionally. It may be quite difficult to diagnose clinically because of the hyperresonance and decreased-to-absent breath sounds already caused by the underlying emphysema.

In the terminal phases of emphysema, as a result of the marked decrease in the number of pulmonary capillaries and the resultant loss of the vascular bed, pulmonary hypertension and right ventricular failure may occur.

LABORATORY FINDINGS

The earliest positive findings in pulmonary emphysema, usually occurring before the appearance of the symptom of exertional shortness of breath, are in the pulmonary function tests. Simple spirometric studies are usually sufficient to uncover the defect in expiratory flow. The most useful spirometric studies are measurements of the vital capacity (VC) and the forced expiratory volume in one second (FEV_1). In emphysema, the FEV_1 is reduced, while the VC is normal or only slightly reduced. The value of the FEV_1 will be unchanged after the use of a potent bronchodilator. This is in marked contrast to the result of such testing in asthma, and occasionally in bronchitis.

Many other spirometric measurements evaluating various sections of the spirometric curve can be made directly from the curve itself.

In addition to providing the earliest means of diagnosing emphysema, these tests can be performed on relatively simple and accurate equipment, easily available not only in all laboratories but also in a doctor's office.

There are numerous other reasons why an FEV_1 can be reduced. The results depend on the effort and cooperation of the person being tested. There may be a lack of understanding of the instructions on the part of the patient, malingering, or other entities such as bronchitis or asthma may be present. Therefore, if these extrapulmonary causes are ruled out, as soon as the FEV_1 is noted to be reduced, the patient should be referred to the pulmonary function laboratory for more sophisticated testing, not only to confirm the diagnosis but also to provide a base line for following the course of the disease and evaluating response to therapy as well as estimating prognosis.

In the pulmonary function laboratory, the tests to be done should include lung volumes, diffusing capacity, and arterial blood gases. The lung volumes should include repeat and confirmatory measurements of expiratory flow, such as the FEV_1, as well as total lung volume (TLC) and residual volume (RV), and the ratio of the two (RV/TLC). All of these are increased in pulmonary emphysema, the residual volume increasing more than the total lung capacity, and their ratio therefore increasing from the normal range of 25 to 30 per cent to the abnormal range of 45 to 50 per cent, and even beyond.

Diffusing capacity may be normal in early, asymptomatic emphysema, but as the disease increases and the vascular bed decreases in size, the diffusing capacity becomes abnormal at rest and fails to increase during exercise. This abnormality in the diffusing capacity progresses with the course of the degenerative process. At this later stage, this is a useful diagnostic test to differentiate emphysema from bronchitis and asthma. In these two entities, the diffusing capacity remains normal.

Arterial blood gases are usually well maintained and will be normal in early pulmonary emphysema, and, indeed, until the late phases of the illness. At that time, the arterial blood oxygen is usually the first to become abnormal. It will slowly decrease in value. Elevation in arterial carbon dioxide and decrease in arterial pH occur only extremely late, or in response to some complication such as a pulmonary infection or pneumothorax.

In addition to these simple pulmonary function tests, the chest x-ray may be helpful. In early pulmonary emphysema, it is usually normal. On the typical x-ray, findings of pulmonary emphysema are noted only late in the course of the disease. Positive x-ray findings in late pulmonary emphysema include hyperaeration of the lung fields, decreased-to-absent markings in the periphery, and low, flat diaphragms. On the lateral film, dorsal kyphosis and an increased anteroposterior diameter of the chest may be seen, with retrosternal and retrocardiac hyperaeration. If the x-rays are taken in expiration, as well as in inspiration, it will be noted that the diaphragms move poorly if at all, and there may be air trapping.

OTHER LABORATORY TESTS

In early pulmonary emphysema the other laboratory tests are normal. Blood counts, sputum analyses, and chemistry panels are all within normal limits. But as the disease progresses, changes may be noted. In late pulmonary emphysema, red cell volume and hematocrit may increase in response to developing hypoxemia and the white blood cell count may rise in response to infection. Sputum studies are normal unless there is pulmonary infection or unless there is accompanying bronchitis or asthma.

In early pulmonary emphysema the electrocardiogram is normal. In late pulmonary emphysema, arrhythmias are frequently seen, both atrial and ventricular. The signs of right ventricular hypertrophy, imperfect as they are, such as tall, symmetrically peaked P waves and rightward shift of the P wave axis, begin to appear.

MORE ELABORATE STUDIES

The specific pulmonary function test that indicates pulmonary emphysema is the measurement of lung compliance, or the volume change per unit of pressure change in the lung. The compliance is increased in emphysema as a result of the loss of elastic recoil. Although this test has come to be recognized as specific for late pulmonary emphysema, it is complicated and requires sophisticated equipment and usually the placement of an intraesophageal balloon. It is usually done only in academic institutions interested in pulmonary research.

Measurement of airway resistance has yet to be proved as a specific aid in diagnosing emphysema. Results are conflicting, and the test requires a body plethysmograph.

In late pulmonary emphysema, the inspired air is distributed unevenly into the lungs. This lack of uniformity of distribution of ventilation can be measured by a nitrogen washout method that can record such abnormal distribution.

Because of the inexorable progressive course of pulmonary emphysema, more sophisticated studies aimed at finding the disease earlier do not appear to be warranted at this time, especially since most of these tests have not yet been fully evaluated and their prognostic significance is unknown. Facilities for these tests are usually found only in academic institutions. Such tests are measurements of such factors as closing volumes and frequency dependency of compliance.

THERAPEUTIC TESTS

Therapeutic tests are not very helpful in emphysema. Antibiotics, bronchodilators, and steroids have all been used in this category, in the absence of specific reasons so to do. However, improvement in the patient's condition secondary to the use of these modalities usually means that another entity, such as asthma or bronchitis, is present along with the emphysema.

PITFALLS IN DIAGNOSIS

The main pitfall in the diagnosis of pulmonary emphysema is not suspecting that this disease may be present. This is true not only in patients who are asymptomatic but also in those whose exertional shortness of breath is minimal, and in whom the physical examination and the chest x-ray are normal.

All patients who complain of mild shortness of breath on exertion for which there is no other immediate obvious explanation deserve a spirometric evaluation. This test should also be done on all cigarette smokers 45 years of age and older, symptomatic or asymptomatic, unless the diagnosis of emphysema has already been made. In this way the diagnosis of early pulmonary emphysema can be made. Armed with this information, the physician can help his patient chart an intelligent course of action to cope with the problem.

BRONCHIECTASIS

By RICHARD A. MARCUCCI, M.D., *and* JOHN W. JENNE, M.D.
Hines, Illinois

INTRODUCTION

Bronchiectasis, although basically an anatomic, morphologic change in the bronchi, has recently been associated with several biochemical and immunologic diseases. It may be diffuse or localized within the tracheobronchial tree. The ectatic bronchi may result in prominent x-ray changes and are found to be of several different shapes. Bronchiectasis is accompanied by the symptom of chronic disabling cough, with large quantities of grossly purulent sputum produced. This disease may result as the consequence of pneumonia and is a common cause of repeated episodes of pneumonia in affected areas of lung. It still remains the single most frequent cause of hemoptysis. Epidemiologically, since the advent of the antibiotics and immunization its frequency appears to be diminishing.

CLASSIFICATION

There have been several different classification schemes developed for the morphologic pathology of bronchiectasis. The three basic ectatic changes described in a commonly used scheme are (1) *cylindrical*, (2) *saccular*, and (3) *varicose*. It is extremely important to recognize that temporary cylindrical bronchial changes may accompany and follow severe pneumonias. Those changes may persist for at least 6 weeks before resolving completely. Obviously this is of great clinical significance when considering surgical resection of localized disease.

Cylindrical bronchiectasis is characterized by the absence of distal tapering of the bronchial segment. Cylindrical ectatic areas are of nearly uniform diameter, and generally are larger in caliber than similar generation bronchi. Although this change is reversible in a fair percentage of patients with resolving pneumonias, it may persist and occasionally can be found in patients without a history of prior pneumonia.

Saccular bronchiectasis is seen as balloon-like outcroppings of the bronchial wall and mucosa. These saccular lesions are seen at the terminal ends of visible bronchi, and although they are not blind-ending pouches, the exits from these bronchi may be difficult to trace.

Varicose ectatic lesions are produced by alternating constriction and dilatation of the bronchi. This pathologic change can produce prominent plain x-ray abnormalities.

ETIOLOGY

The vast majority of bronchiectatic abnormalities have, in the past, been directly attributable to childhood infectious diseases. Most commonly implicated were childhood measles, bronchiolitis, and whooping cough (pertussis), although many other viral and bacterial bronchopulmonary infections have also been implicated.

The pathogenesis of this bronchiectasis is thought to follow the pattern of, first, infection, then, obstruction by mucus plugging, and consequent inflammatory thickening and destruction of the bronchial wall. Bronchial obstruction, if severe and persistent, results in distal bronchiectasis. Bronchiolitis may be followed by parenchymal scarring, with retraction of the bronchial wall by this mechanism as well.

Such a cause need not be restricted to childhood. Similar changes also occur in adults, although with diminished frequency. Indeed, such changes have been reported in adult tuberculosis, and occasionally after pneumococcal pneumonia. It has been postulated that this smaller incidence may result from the larger caliber of adult bronchi, and the fact that they are less likely to become obstructed. In any case, since the development of antimicrobial and antituberculous chemotherapy and immunotherapy (specifically, reduction and control of certain childhood diseases by vaccination), this cause of bronchiectasis has been observed less frequently.

Mucoviscidosis, a disorder characterized by the recessive autosomal inheritance of diffuse exocrine gland dysfunction, may also produce bronchial ectatic lesions. Destruction and fibrosis are most commonly observed in the pancreas, but lung changes are also quite frequent. The pathogenesis is thought to be related to an increased viscosity of glandular secretions and diminished tracheobronchial clearance. There

may also be significant mucus plugging with bronchial damage distal to these obstructions, secondary to infection. Since the disease affects clearance from all areas of the lung, it is observed in both upper and lower lobes. In contrast, bronchiectasis of other causes is more frequently found in dependent areas of the lung.

Since the pulmonary pathology of cystic fibrosis occurs more diffusely and is associated with some degree of pulmonary fibrosis, more lung destruction and irreversible pulmonary artery hypertension is observed here. Because the disease is genetically determined and hence present from birth, the associated pulmonary changes observed here usually become clinically apparent early. Modern medical management has, however, prolonged the life of these patients, and many are surviving to middle age. We may soon see increasing numbers of these patients in our adult medical practices.

Another recently described development is the occurrence of pulmonary abnormalities associated with minimal extrapulmonary pathology. These individuals are identified later in life (viz., late adolescence or early adult life) by a positive test for increased sodium chloride content in sweat. It is important to identify this group of patients so that intensive medical management can be instituted, and, hopefully, can slow progression of the pulmonary disease.

Bronchiectasis as caused by the two previously described mechanisms results in hyperstimulation of the immunologic system. Immune system insufficiency is another cause for the development of bronchiectasis. Here, the patient's immune defenses are inadequate to prevent frequent sinopulmonary infections with pyogenic organisms. These frequent and in general more severe infections result in repeated inflammatory injury to the lower respiratory tract. The resultant effect is persistent ectatic change of the tracheobronchial tree.

Many of the congenital and acquired immunodeficiencies are associated with bronchiectasis. It has been observed with the hypogammaglobulinemia and decreased secretory globulins that accompany congenital lymphocyte deficiency, that is, Bruton's type of congenital hypogammaglobulinemia. Combined T and B lymphocyte defects may also be associated with bronchiectasis, if the affected patients survive long enough. These are usually the acquired combined defects, since most patients with congenital combined defects die in infancy. Acquired hypogammaglobulinemia and isolated IgA deficiency, both seen primarily in adults, are probably the most common immune defects associated with bronchiectasis.

The prognosis of these syndromes is usually quite grave, but intensive medical management, with treatment of acute infections, prophylactic suppression of bacterial populations in the tracheobronchial tree, and globulin administration, may decrease morbidity and mortality.

There are several congenital developmental abnormalities that may result in bronchiectasis. Localized bronchiectasis is usually the rule here, although Kartagener's syndrome (sinusitis, situs inversus, and bronchiectasis) and a syndrome of abnormal lymphatic and bronchial development may exhibit diffuse changes. These are all rare conditions, but simple congenital cystic bronchiectasis is most frequently observed. Other congenital abnormalities are bronchial cysts and pulmonary sequestration. These do not differ from congenital cystic bronchiectasis developmentally. The former, however, is associated with bronchial noncanalization, whereas the latter is found associated with systemic vascular supply to the ectatic segment.

Congenital abnormalities may be differentiated pathologically from acquired by the absence of inflammatory cell infiltration of the bronchial wall, and intact muscular, elastin, and cartilaginous layers of the bronchi. This is somewhat misleading, however, since subsequent infection may obscure purely developmental changes.

Bronchiectasis may also result from bronchial obstruction by aspirated foreign bodies, or by exposure to toxic and allergenic substances, when they elicit an intense bronchial inflammatory reaction. Most commonly reported is the concentric bronchiectasis seen as a complication of allergic pulmonary aspergillosis.

Finally, there has recently been observed a syndrome consisting of immobile cilia, associated in males with totally immobile but apparently normal spermatozoa. Mucociliary transport in the tracheobronchial tree has been observed to be quite slow in these syndromes. This leads to poor elimination of aspirated bacteria, repeated tracheobronchial infections, and the development of bronchiectasis. Further investigation of these conditions by electron microscopy has revealed abnormal ultrastructure of the cilia and sperm tails in affected individuals. The abnormalities consist of absent spoke, nexin link, and dynein arm connections in the microtubular ultrastructure of the functionally abnormal cells. It is felt that these connectors, especially the dynein arms, are contractile elements that normally are responsible for sperm locomotion and ciliary action. This type of abnormality has been observed occasionally in a familial distribution; however, its true frequency is not known.

CLINICAL SIGNS AND SYMPTOMS

Bronchiectasis may occasionally be completely asymptomatic. Much more frequently the clinical presentation is that of frequent, recurrent bronchopulmonary infections, and expectoration of rather large quantities of purulent sputum. The sputum produced is classically described as revealing three distinct layers: an upper layer consisting primarily of mucus, saliva in the middle, and pus; inflammatory cells; and mucus plugs settling to the bottom layer. Three-layered sputum is not, however, pathognomonic for bronchiectasis and may be observed in other inflammatory pulmonary conditions.

Historically, affected patients can give evidence of repeated bronchopulmonary infections and pneumonias since childhood. They usually have a chronic cough with paroxysms often precipitated by a change in position. Occasionally, the first of such infections may have been preceded by a childhood disease such as measles or pertussis. Since widespread vaccination programs have decreased these childhood disorders, many more patients give a history of or are found to suffer from underlying immunologic deficiencies or mucoviscidosis.

Recurrent pneumonias in the same pulmonary lobe or segment should alert the physician to a possible localized structural abnormality such as bronchiectasis. Repeated pneumonias in different lobes or bronchial segments may be a consequence of diffuse tracheobronchial bronchiectasis or can reflect an underlying immune deficiency.

Hemoptysis, in the form of massive hemorrhage or more frequently blood-tinged sputum, is a common symptom of bronchiectasis. Bronchiectasis is, in fact, the single most common cause of hemoptysis. This symptom is usually observed in combination with other symptoms but may occur in an otherwise completely asymptomatic patient.

PHYSICAL FINDINGS

Physical findings vary with the severity of involvement. Examination in localized bronchiectasis will reveal only crepitant rales and rhonchi when the examiner auscultates over affected lobes or segments. More diffuse disease will obviously be accompanied by more diffuse auscultatory findings and may be associated with cyanosis, respiratory insufficiency, and clubbing.

CHEST X-RAY ABNORMALITIES

Chest roentgenograms are normal in approximately 7 per cent of patients with bronchiectasis. The remainder exhibit several different radiologic abnormalities, including atelectasis, honeycombing, patches of irregular fibrosis, and increased lung markings such as tubular shadows and "gloved-finger" shadows.

Tubular shadows and double-lined parallel or tapered shadows are normally seen close to the hilum, and are a radiographic reflection of air-filled large bronchi. If these shadows are observed distal to the hilum, bronchiectasis should be considered, since this disease is the commonest cause of tubular shadows in the distal lung. Pathologically thickened, inflamed walls of smaller bronchi cause the projection of these shadows. Other commonly seen lung markings are "gloved-finger" shadows. These represent bronchiectatic segments with retained mucus or pus and are seen as homogenous band-like densities in the distal lung. Both are not pathogenic for bronchiectasis and may also be seen in chronic bronchitis or bronchial asthma. Occasionally the multiple cysts of cystic bronchiectasis, sometimes with fluid levels, are seen on careful inspection.

DIAGNOSTIC TESTS

Bronchography provides a morphologic diagnosis of bronchiectasis and helps to localize its extent and distribution. Many roentgenographic techniques and contrast media have been employed in bronchographic studies. The most commonly used technique is transglottic injection of radiopaque material through a soft rubber urethral catheter placed transnasally into the main bronchi. Contrast material (12 to 15 ml) is injected under fluoroscopic control, with the patient positioned so that the segment of interest is most dependent. The patient is instructed to breathe deeply and one third of the contrast material is injected during expiration. The patient is then instructed to cough and breathe deeply for 5 minutes, so the required segment is visualized.

Another approach that has been employed successfully is the bronchoscopic injection of contrast material, usually propyliodone (Dionosil), warmed to 37 C, into the lobe or subsegment to be studied. This procedure is carried out under direct bronchoscopic visualization and usually gives excellent results in the segment under study. Often spillover from reflex coughing may cause visualization of other segments of the same lung but obviously multiple injections are required to visualize large areas of the tracheobronchial tree. Demonstrating diffuse disease with this technique is somewhat impractical, but it is an easy method to establish the presence of bronchiectasis.

Respiratory insufficiency is the major contraindication for bronchographic examinations of the lung. No patient should be studied if clinical respiratory insufficiency is present. Vigorous medical management may improve a patient's condition sufficiently for bronchography to be indicated, but in irreversible respiratory failure limited therapeutic options temper the decision to test further.

Complications following bronchography include worsening of respiratory function secondary to impairment of ventilation and diffusion; atelectasis, particularly in children; foreign body reaction; and allergic reactions to the contrast materials.

OTHER LABORATORY TESTS

Routine laboratory tests are, in general, nonspecific and quite variable. During an infectious exacerbation, the white blood cell count may be elevated with a left shift. Chronic uncontrolled infection in bronchiectasis may also result in a normochromic, normocytic anemia as seen in other chronic disorders. Gammaglobulin levels may be diffusely elevated secondary to chronic inflammatory stimulation or may be quite low when associated with immunodeficiency disease. Secondary amyloidosis may occur in advanced, longstanding cases.

As mentioned previously, sodium chloride content in sweat, if increased, is diagnostic for mucoviscidosis, and therefore may indicate the specific causes of bronchiectasis in these patients.

Microbiologic examinations of the sputum are helpful if pathogens such as a Pneumococcus, *Hemophilus influenzae*, Staphylococcus and Pseudomonas are identified in pure culture. The patient can then be treated for exacerbations with antibiotics directed against the isolated organism. More frequently, however, multiple organisms are recovered on culture.

Several other laboratory tests may occasionally be helpful for diagnosis of bronchiectasis. Perfusion lung scans often show crowding of vascular structures in an affected segment. This adds confirmatory evidence to the diagnosis but usually is an impractical and nonspecific aid.

In the rare instance when mucociliary clearance dysfunction is suspected, a sperm count and check of sperm motility will be helpful. The total sperm count is normal in this disease but the sperm are immobile. Further electron microscopic studies must be done for definitive diagnosis in these syndromes.

PULMONARY FUNCTION TESTS

Pulmonary function test abnormalities in this disease are a function of the degree of involvement. When disease is localized to a segment or several subsegments, no abnormalities may be observed. However, when lung involvement is more diffuse, pulmonary function tests usually reveal evidence of obstructive pulmonary disease. In these patients diminished forced vital capacity, expiratory flow rates and maximum voluntary ventilation will be observed. There are also significant ventilation-perfusion ($\dot{V}/\dot{Q}$) abnormalities seen at this stage of the disease. These $\dot{V}/\dot{Q}$ abnormalities are the result of perfusion of alveoli that are underventilated because of mucus plugging or atelectasis. Patients who have patchy fibrosis may have normally ventilated areas that are underperfused owing to fibrotic obliteration of the capillary bed. This will increase the ventilation-perfusion abnormality. Many patients are also found to have significant arteriovenous shunting. These shunts, which may approach 10 to 15 per cent, are a result of arteriovenous communication in areas of severe pulmonary destruction.

It should be quite apparent at this point that bronchiectasis is a disease with multiple causes, presenting as a broad spectrum of clinical illness. It is extremely important to consider all these factors when establishing the diagnosis of bronchiectasis.

PNEUMOCONIOSIS

By JOHN W. G. HANNON, M.D.

Washington, Pennsylvania

DEFINITION

The term "pneumoconiosis," coined by Zenker, was used to describe abnormal lung conditions caused by the inhalation of dusts associated with metal mining. The scope of the context has been increased by the purists to encompass all dusts that can be inhaled and retained in the lungs, whether they be harmful or not. Therefore each living person has inhaled and retained in his lungs many types of dust during his lifetime, and in the majority of instances has suffered no ill effects. The dusts found in the lungs at autopsy may be of academic interest only. However, we do encounter dusts that, when inhaled and retained in the lungs in sufficient quantities, can and do produce changes that are of clinical importance. It is these abnormalities that concern us most.

A practical working definition of pneumoconiosis is as follows: Pneumoconiosis is a condition of the lungs caused by the inhalation of and retention in the pulmonary tissues of dusts, which can be demonstrated by x-ray films of the chest or functional impairment or both. The broad use of the all-inclusive term "pneumoconiosis" has led to a subgrouping of various biologic states such as silicosis, asbestosis, anthracosis, bagassosis, byssinosis, siderosis, and stannosis. Subgroups resulting from mixed exposures have been established, such as anthracosilicosis, asbestosilicosis, and siderosilicosis.

CAUSATIVE AGENTS

No dusts are "good" if they are inhaled and retained in sufficient quantities. Basically, dust particles may be classified as follows: (1) Organic dusts of animal, vegetable, and synthetic origin. Dusts in this category do not produce fibrosis but can produce asthma and local respiratory irritation. In some instances the inhaled material may be accompanied by infective agents and produce a severe type of pneumonitis accompanied by extreme malaise, fever, and abnormal shadows on the chest x-ray film. Examples of these types of reaction are byssinosis (cotton, flax, soft hemp), bagassosis (dried and aged sugar cane fibers), and farmer's lung. (2) Inorganic dusts. These can produce fibrosis (asbestosis, silicosis). (3) Those causing x-ray changes because of their high molecular density (siderosis, barytosis, stannosis), or by their physical presence in displacing normal air-bearing pulmonary tissue (clay, coal, and other inert dusts).

DIAGNOSIS

As most of the pneumoconioses of clinical importance are legal diseases and are so defined by federal, state, and provincial statutes, one must proceed with caution and scientific effort in establishing a diagnosis. Perhaps the most valuable asset of the chest physician is a thorough knowledge of the working environment in the industrial establishments of his community. The diagnostic tools most commonly used can vary as much as the suspected type of lung condition; however, the following must be ascertained:

1. Occupational history of adequate exposure to the suspected dust.

2. Abnormal chest x-ray findings that are compatible with the suspected condition.

3. Symptomatology characteristic of the condition.

4. History, physical examination, chest x-ray study, or other laboratory tests that reveal physical conditions that could masquerade, subjectively or objectively, as the suspected condition.

5. Studies that may be of value in the diagnosis: biopsies of lung, pleura, and scalene node; studies of blood, sputum, and urine; skin tests; electrocardiogram; and lung function studies. Because of the legal aspect one must be prepared to classify the condition as minimal and only of academic importance or as an advanced state and of clinical importance and subject to compensation rulings.

Occupational History

The industrial occupation history should be as complete as possible and should start with a notation of the birth date, listing subsequent activities in chronological order. A record of full-time industrial jobs should be made, indicating the name of company, the kind of job held, the duration of employment, and the potential health hazards if any. Of equal importance is a history of hobbies. Amateur ceramic workers can show silicosis. Experimentation with electric units that produce high concentrations of ozone may cause physiologic damage to the lungs. The present-day trend to sniff various chemicals presents a potential danger to the lungs. Sniffing scouring powders has been known to produce a severe type of silicosis.

Evaluation of the exposures is of great importance. A workman may be exposed to a certain substance, but the concentration may be so low as to be of academic importance only; however, the concentration may be high enough to present a hazard. All exposures are not necessarily productive of demonstrable lung pathology.

Chest X-Ray Examination

The x-ray examination of the chest should be made with proper techniques, so that a film of good quality and density is produced. Light films may accentuate the normal lung markings to such an extent as to cause errors in interpretation. A dark overexposed film may mask some or most of the abnormalities. Previous periodic x-ray films may be of great aid. It is a bit embarrassing to make a diagnosis of silicosis based on nodular shadows on a single chest film and find that the chest film of 10 months before was negative, and after further study to find that the patient had a fungal or a nonindustrial pulmonary disease. The 14 by 17 film is prefera-

ble. The abnormalities present should be compatible with the occupational history. Mixed exposures can create disturbing situations. A proper appraisal of the working environment is a "must" — there are no substitutes. Dust counts are usually available and are helpful.

Symptomatology

The usual symptoms of those pneumoconioses that cause impairment of lung function are these, in order of importance: dyspnea, tightness in the chest, fatigue, and a lessened capacity for work or exercise. Cough may be present in some patients, but it is not always productive.

Special Studies. Incineration of microscopic sections of lung tissues to burn out the organic material is useful in identifying silica particles and asbestos fibers. Further treatment in warm-concentration hydrochloric acid will leach out the soluble salts and leave the refractory material as a residue.

Incinerating the sputum and finding concentrations of silica in the residue is proof of exposure but not an index to the degree of pathology or impairment of function that may be present.

Blood and urine studies for the presence of silica are not always reliable, as the silica may represent material that has been absorbed from the gastrointestinal tract.

Biopsy. Scalene node biopsy may be of great aid in the diagnosis. Pleural biopsy may be used in selective cases. Lung biopsy is of great help. The needle biopsy is not satisfactory, as it fails to supply sufficient tissue for a complete study. The wedge biopsy supplies adequate tissue for a complete histologic examination and a chemical analysis.

The electrocardiographic and lung function studies may furnish valuable information in the differential diagnosis.

Estimation of Pulmonary Dysfunction

Once a diagnosis of a pneumoconiosis is firmly established, it then becomes imperative to determine the amount of pulmonary dysfunction that may be present. Office procedures in evaluating pulmonary impairment must be simple and accurate.

The pulmonary ventilation tests that are most commonly used are the FEV_1 (1 second forced expiratory ventilation), the vital capacity (VC), and the maximum voluntary ventilation (MVV). The values obtained from these tests are dependent upon the effort and cooperation of the

Applicant's Name			Date
			Social Security No.
Height cm.	Weight Kg.		Date of Birth
Age BSA	Temp.		Telephone Number

Ventilation Studies:

	Observed	Predicted	Per cent of Predicted
FEV$_1$			
Vital Capacity			
MVV			

	FEV$_1$	VC	MVV
Effort			
Dyspnea After			
Cough			
Wheezing			
Dizziness			
Cooperation			

Remarks:

Figure 1. Form for recording pulmonary ventilation test values and effort and cooperation and any signs of respiratory embarrassment due to abnormalities in ventilation.

person being tested. A poor or fair effort gives a value that can be well below the predicted values that are based upon age, height, weight, and body surface area (BSA).

The degree of effort and cooperation is graded as excellent, good, fair, and poor. If the poor amount of effort is made there should be dyspnea immediately after the test, possibly a cough, wheezing, or dizziness, and these findings are graded in degrees of 1+ through 4+. It is important that the person's effort and cooperation be obtained at all times. The findings of the ventilation tests should be compatible with the observations made during the examination (clinical and laboratory), and during any physical activity during these periods.

We have found the form shown (Fig. 1) to be very helpful in recording the data obtained prior to and after the ventilation tests.

ASBESTOSIS

DEFINITION

Asbestosis is a diffuse pulmonary disease in which fibrosis is the dominant reaction to prolonged retention in the lungs of asbestos fibers.

ASBESTOS

The name derives from the Greek word meaning "unquenchable." Of the 30 or more asbestoid minerals, only six are of economic importance. They are amosite, anthophyllite, actinolite, chrysotile, crocidolite, and tremolite.

Their chemical constituents include silicon, magnesium, iron, fluorine, nickel, cobalt, aluminum, sodium, and chromium in various molecular states, and hydrated to different degrees. Their chief chemical properties are resistance to moisture, to corrosion, and to the action of acids. Their principal physical properties are the flexibility and high tensile strength of the fibers, the protective action against heat and cold, and the ease of separation into filaments of fibers. Because of their unusual chemical and physical properties, these minerals now have some 3000 industrial applications.

PATHOGENESIS

Two theories, chemical and physical, have been proposed by various groups of investigators. Those who favor the chemical theory believe that some unknown fibrogenic agent is released by the leaching action of the body fluids on the fibers. This is supported by the long delay between exposure and the development of fibrosis. These investigators make use of the C × T (concentration times time) factor. Exposure to high concentrations of asbestos dust produces fibrosis in a much shorter time than does exposure to low concentrations of the same dust.

The physical or mechanical irritation concept is supported by the observation that fibrosis occurs first and is more severe in those portions of the lungs where respiratory movements are the greatest.

There is no evidence that asbestos fibers are toxic or have allergenic properties.

PULMONARY LESIONS

The principal pulmonary lesions are interstitial, focal, mucosal, and bronchiolar fibrosis, with distortion, distention, and stenosis of the finer bronchial segments. The lesions may occur throughout both lungs, but the highest concentration is at the bases and subpleurally. In advanced disease, perivascular fibrosis can contribute to the development of cor pulmonale. The finding of "asbestos bodies" in the lungs or the sputum does not necessarily mean that the patient has asbestosis. Many fibers of exogenous and endogenous origin can simulate asbestos bodies. Because of this, it is impossible to definitely identify an asbestos body with the ordinary microscope, and x-ray diffraction studies must be used. Asbestoid fibrosis may be concentrated around previous scar tissue in the lung. Pleural plaques have been described by some authors, but there is nothing characteristic of these types of lesions, as in most cases it has been impossible to demonstrate asbestos fibers or lesions of asbestosis. The plaques are small and do not cause disability.

SEQUELAE AND COMPLICATIONS

Acute and chronic right-sided heart disease and progressive cardiorespiratory failure are the most common terminal sequelae. An association between asbestosis and tuberculosis has never been proved by statistical or epidemiologic studies. Bronchitis and pneumonia are relatively infrequent.

Reports from some geographical locations have favored a relationship between asbestosis and pulmonary new growths and also pleural mesothelioma, whereas those from other areas do not indicate such a connection. Statistically, amosite and crocidolite exposures appear to be significant. Many investigators are studying the problem, and some are of the opinion that substances adsorbed to the fibers during processing may be the causative factors. Others believe that the presence of different chemicals in the various types of fibers may play a significant part. It appears that cigarette smokers are more susceptible to neoplasia, and crocidolite (blue asbestos) causes the greater number of mesotheliomas. About 15 per cent of patients with mesothelioma relate no exposure to asbestos, and other causes may be found. There is no relationship between length and severity of exposure and the development of neoplasia.

ROENTGENOLOGY

The early radiologic pattern of asbestosis is characterized by a ground-glass appearance on the x-ray film, and sometimes by a fine stippling. Later the cardiac silhouette may be blurred by linear fibrotic lesions, resulting in the "shaggy" or "porcupine" heart. With progression the lesions become larger and sometimes assume massive proportions. The lesions develop in direct proportion to the severity of exposure and may require from 12 to 20 years to develop.

SYMPTOMS AND SIGNS

The onset of symptoms is insidious, as in most slowly developing pneumoconioses. The principal symptom is dyspnea, which may be out of proportion to the extent of x-ray changes. A dry, irritating cough may be present. Tightness of the chest and wheezing are not common features. Cyanosis may be present. Chest expansion is usually decreased. The breath sounds are usually within normal limits, but forced ventilation, as in panting, can elicit moist rales throughout the bases of the lungs. Complications can cause alterations in the breath sounds.

PULMONARY FUNCTION STUDIES

There is usually no evidence of obstructive lung disease. The findings are those of restrictive lung disease with little impairment in the vital capacity, forced expiratory flow, and maximum ventilatory capacity. The principal disabling factors are interference with the gaseous diffusion across the alveolar capillary membrane and reduced pulmonary elasticity. Anoxemia may be the only abnormal finding. The severity of disease, the patient's age, and the presence of infection or other factors may influence the pulmonary function.

DIFFERENTIAL DIAGNOSIS

Before proceeding with the differential diagnosis, one should have just cause to strongly suspect that the patient has asbestosis. Diagnosis can be approached through the following steps: (1) Exposure. Is there an accurate history of adequate exposure to asbestos dust? A careful work history must be taken and exposure must be proved. (2) Chest x-ray study. Are the abnormalities on the x-ray film compatible with a diagnosis of asbestosis? Access to several periodic radiographs of the chest should be obtained when possible. The abnormalities on the chest films of asbestos workers appear only after long exposure. It is indeed very embarrassing to make a diagnosis of advanced asbestosis and then find that the x-ray film of 6 months before was negative and that one is dealing with a nonoccupational diffuse interstitial fibrosis. (3) The symptoms of asbestosis are not unlike those of other pulmonary diseases, and can be simulated by heart disease, anemia, and a host of other diseases. (4) A physical examination should be made with a complete evaluation of organic and functional disturbances. Asbestosis can be simulated by a diffuse interstitial fibrotic disease of the lungs. Diffuse inflammatory or infectious lung diseases caused by chemicals and biologic agents should also be considered. Special tests such as lung biopsy should be considered at certain times. The finding of asbestos bodies in the sputum indicates an exposure only, not necessarily asbestosis. As there are some 80 fibers that when retained in the lungs can give the gross appearance of an asbestos body, one must proceed with great caution in establishing a relationship between the unidentified body and the lung fibrosis. It has been suggested that the term "ferruginous bodies" be used to classify this type of reaction to inhaled fibers of all types.

BAGASSOSIS

Bagassosis results from the inhalation of dusts produced in the handling of dried sugar cane fiber.

Symptoms and Signs

The symptoms and signs usually do not develop after short exposure, but may appear after a few weeks' exposure if the concentrations of the dust are sufficiently high.

Dyspnea is the outstanding symptom, but cough, weakness, and fever usually are present. The fever may vary from 99 to 103 F (37 to 39.5 C).

The physical signs may include cyanosis, labored breathing, and coarse rales throughout both lung fields.

Roentgenology

The chest film may show miliary shadows, or lesions up to 1 cm. in diameter. There may also be patchy areas of a larger size that enlarge to massive shadows. There are no residuals on the x-ray film after complete recovery.

Pulmonary function studies show ventilatory impairment, airway obstructions, and a decrease in diffusion.

Diagnosis

The essential factors in diagnosis are a history of exposure plus the presence of compatible signs, symptoms, and x-ray findings. Without a definitive history, the abnormalities seen on the x-ray film are not unlike those found in pneumonitis resulting from inhalation of nitrous or cadmium oxides.

BERYLLIUM-ASSOCIATED DISEASE

Definition

Inhalation and retention of certain compounds of beryllium can produce two specific pulmonary conditions, one of which, acute beryllium pneumonitis, is caused by inhaling the soluble compounds of beryllium such as the acid salts. Berylliosis is a chronic pulmonary disease caused by inhaling and retaining the relatively insoluble compounds of beryllium such as the oxide and the beryllium phosphors.

ACUTE BERYLLIUM PNEUMONITIS

The onset is usually characterized by pain in the pharynx, larynx, or trachea, and may last for several hours up to 36 hours; a tentative diagnosis of tracheolaryngitis may be made. As the process develops, there is bronchial and bronchiolar involvement with a progressive nonproductive cough and dyspnea of a severe type. This is followed by malaise, physical weakness, and rapid weight loss. The respiratory rate is increased, the pulmonary excursions are decreased, and auscultation of the chest reveals sibilant rales, particularly at the bases. Later the breath sounds resemble those found in pulmonary edema and can be heard at some distance from the patient. There is little alteration in temperature except in the presence of a secondary infection.

Laboratory Findings

Acute beryllium pneumonitis lesions are found in the alveolar regions of the lung; edema and cellular debris may fill the affected alveolar spaces of the involved area. Laboratory studies are usually negative except for a transient hypergammaglobulinemia. X-ray studies are usually negative until about the seventh day when diffuse mottling appears throughout both lung fields, which may progress for several days and disappear in 2 to 4 weeks. There are no x-ray residuals after recovery.

Lung function studies show an impairment of diffusion in addition to a decrease in ventilatory capacity. The diagnosis is based upon a history of exposure to the soluble compounds of beryllium and x-ray findings plus the characteristic symptoms. The finding of beryllium in the urine and tissues is of value for confirmation of exposure only.

BERYLLIOSIS

The principal etiologic agent is usually either beryllium oxide or one of the beryllium phosphors. Some patients may be asymptomatic, but they are in the minority. The onset is insidious with a long latent period between first exposure and the development of symptoms or signs. Cough is usually the first symptom. The cough is mild and is usually associated with fatigue. Later there is a progressive dyspnea, which may be present even at rest. Weight loss, chest pain, and physical weakness may occur. Cyanosis has been noted in about 40 per cent of patients and clubbing of the fingers in about 30 per cent.

ROENTGENOLOGY

The chest film may show progressive abnormalities ranging from a ground-glass appearance to a diffuse stippling throughout both lung fields. As further progression occurs the lesions appear nodular and may coalesce.

LUNG FUNCTION STUDIES

The principal finding is low arterial oxygen tension and incomplete saturation of arterial blood at rest. The ventilatory capacity usually shows no deviation from the normal unless emphysema is present.

DIAGNOSIS

A history of known exposure to beryllium, a chest x-ray film showing a stippling, punctate, or nodular pattern, plus a clinical picture of pulmonary insufficiency and weight loss should suggest beryllium. The differential diagnosis should include Boeck's sarcoid, farmer's lung, Hammond-Rich syndrome, and the many pneumoconioses. Lung biopsy is of great diagnostic value provided that a wedge biopsy is obtained; this provides adequate tissue for a complete histologic and chemical analysis. The Kveim test may help in the differentiation between sarcoid and berylliosis. Study of the sputum is helpful in determining the presence of fungi or other organic or inorganic substances that may contribute to symptoms, signs, or the abnormal x-ray pattern. Calciuria and phosphaturia are often associated with chronic beryllium disease. The patch test is of some value in the differential diagnosis.

BYSSINOSIS (BROWN LUNG)

Byssinosis is caused by the inhalation of dusts produced in the handling of cotton and flax. The condition is confined to persons employed in opening, blow, and card rooms, but lately there is increasing evidence that persons employed in the winding room may also be affected but to a lesser degree.

Although, statistically, airborne cotton and flax fibers have been shown to be the causative agents, fungi, molds, and other contaminants have received attention.

Exposure to dusts of soft hemp (*Cannabis sativa*) is reported by some investigators to cause byssinosis, whereas others maintain that the characteristic symptoms of "Monday feeling" are absent and have called the condition cannabosis. Hemp is used in the manufacture of rope, and both soft and hard hemp fibers are used, but as yet there is no evidence that inhalation of the hard fibers causes pulmonary symptoms. Exposure to soft fibers may cause slight dyspnea and a decrease in pulmonary ventilation.

SYMPTOMS

The principal symptoms are tightness of the chest, dyspnea, or both. The symptoms are first noticed when the person returns to work after the weekend ("Monday feeling") or after a vacation period. The symptoms come on from 1 to 6 hours after the start of the work shift and are usually absent the next day. However, after many years of exposure the symptoms may become more severe, occur on more days in the week, and be associated with a cough and wheezing. The classification of byssinosis is usually made on the basis of symptoms as follows: grade I, occasional chest tightness on Mondays; grade II, chest tightness, dyspnea, or both every Monday; grade III, chest tightness, dyspnea, or both on Mondays and other days of the week.

LABORATORY AND X-RAY FINDINGS

X-ray studies show no characteristic demonstrable lesions.

Lung function studies show impaired ventilation, with a decrease in forced expiratory volume and maximum voluntary ventilation rates.

DIAGNOSIS

The diagnosis is based on the following findings: (1) History of adequate exposure to cotton dust. (2) History of long-standing and progressive "Monday feeling." (3) History of constant and progressive effort dyspnea. (4) Radiologic evidence excluding other chest diseases.

COAL MINER'S LUNG (BLACK LUNG)

There is no uniformity of opinion regarding a specific definition of the pneumoconiosis that occurs in coal workers. The mining of coal produces dusts that can vary from relatively pure carbonaceous material on the one hand to relatively pure silica on the other, with a mixture of coal and silica between these.

Because of the many fluctuations that can occur in the dusts found in the industrial atmosphere, pathologic changes in the lungs assume many and bizarre patterns. The quality and the quantity of the dust produced can differ from mine to mine in the same general area, from job to job in the same mine, and even from man to man on the same job. These variations can be accounted for by the following factors:

1. Production methods. The production method has a definite influence on the amount of dust produced. Mechanical mining produces more dust and smaller particle sizes than hand methods.

2. Dust control. The high incidence of coal miner's pneumoconiosis in Welsh pits is best explained by the introduction of mechanization without adequate dust suppression. The patchiness of cases in the United Kingdom is best explained by differences in dust concentrations.

3. Geology. Mines having thin coal seams require considerable roof drilling, which causes dustiness with high silica content. A fault in the coal seam caused by siliceous rock also requires drilling of this rock, with production of high concentrations of silica dust. The geology can vary greatly from mine to mine in the same general area. Anthracite coal mining produces a more serious hazard than does bituminous coal mining owing to the large amount of rock drilling that is necessary in order to remove the coal.

4. Type of work. The specific job of the miner has a definite bearing on his exposure. Men engaged in rock drilling are exposed to high concentrations of silica dust and a small amount of coal dust. Coal-face workers are exposed to relatively pure concentrations of coal dust and show characteristic lung changes. Coal trimmers who load ships at the dock are also exposed to coal dust and show the same lesions as coal-face workers.

The tendency of some coal miners to move from mine to mine, with associated changes in jobs, production methods, dust control, and geology, is of etiologic significance. These complicating environmental factors can contribute to an involved pathologic pattern in the pneumoconioses associated with coal mining.

FORMS OF COAL MINER'S LUNG

The industrial pulmonary conditions found in coal mining may be grouped into the following classifications: coal dust — anthracosis; mixed dusts — anthracosilicosis; silica dust — silicosis.

Any of these forms may be modified by infection or overwhelming concentrations of the particular dust to produce progressive massive fibrosis.

Anthracosis. A condition of the lungs caused by pulmonary retention of coal dust and subsequent pigmenting of the pulmonary tissues.

Anthracosilicosis. A condition referred to by the British as mixed pneumoconiosis and by others as a modified silicosis. There are some who would discard the term "anthracosilicosis," whereas others believe that the term adequately and accurately describes a condition that occurs among coal miners. It is contracted through exposure to a mixed dust or by moving from one job to another, with a change in exposure from relatively pure coal to relatively pure silica or vice versa. Anthracosilicosis produces a clinical picture similar to silicosis.

Silicosis. Classic silicosis can be found in coal miners, and its clinical course does not differ from that found in other industries. There are progressive stages in silicosis, and in the advanced stages it may cause dyspnea, cough, tightness in the chest, fatigue, and a lessened capacity for work.

Progressive Massive Fibrosis. A disorder sometimes occurring in the lungs of coal workers. There are massive lesions that may involve one or both upper lobes.

PULMONARY LESIONS

Anthracosis. The causative factor is the retention of coal dust that has been phagocytized and carried by the lymph channels and mixes with the lymphatic fluid. Here the concentrations may build up after repeated exposures until a coal macule is formed and is of sufficient size to be identified on the x-ray film. Fibrosis is not present, and the macule produces a shadow on the x-ray film by displacing normal oxygenated pulmonary tissue. Anthracosis does not usually produce disability.

Anthracosilicosis. The picture is similar to

silicosis. The pathologic lesions are not discrete, like those found in silicosis, and the areas are diamond-shaped rather than round. Coalescence may occur as a result of continuous exposure, and cavitation caused by avascular necrosis can occur without evidence of a tubercular infection. The x-ray presents diffuse, irregularly shaped lesions scattered throughout both lung fields. Impairment of lung function can occur and follows the pattern of that found in silicosis.

Silicosis. The silicosis found in coal workers may present a typical picture, pathology, x-ray findings, and lung function not deviating from the usual pattern.

Progressive Massive Fibrosis. The etiology of massive fibrosis in coal miner's lung has not been established. Some believe that tuberculosis is an essential factor. Another view is that primary exposure to coal dust and subsequent exposure to high concentrations of silica are the causative factors. Personal observations on workmen who had 8 to 12 years of exposure in coal mines and who later worked in the silica brick industry showed that massive pulmonary lesions developed acutely without demonstrable evidence of tuberculosis. Massive lesions can result from (1) overwhelming concentration of dust and (2) patchy areas of atelectasis with secondary nontuberculous infection, causing localized pneumonitis, abscess formation, or both.

Progressive massive fibrosis can cause severe vascular changes. Endarteritis and thrombotic obliteration are not uncommon. A thrombus can propagate from an area of massive fibrosis along the branches of the pulmonary artery to the hilus of the lung. Massive arterial obstruction is a major cause of hypertrophy of the right ventricle of the heart. Dilatation often accompanies the hypertrophy. Disturbances in the pulmonary circulation as well as massive fibrosis in the lung bring about severe disability. Cor pulmonale can be present as a direct result of advanced emphysema or massive fibrosis. Advanced emphysema, which usually accompanies these massive lesions, is capable of producing total disability and may lead to dilatation of the right side of the heart.

The x-ray film shows massive shadows, particularly in the upper lobes. Pulmonary function studies show evidence of increased residual air, and progressive anoxemia on exercise.

COMPLICATIONS

Focal Emphysema. In this disturbance there is a coal macule plus emphysematous changes in the adjacent tissues. On pathologic study, the macule of dust is observed surrounding the respiratory bronchioles of the third and fourth orders. There is destruction of the elastic framework around the respiratory bronchioles, and marked dilatation of the respiratory bronchioles. The dilated respiratory bronchioles represent the areas of focal emphysema that are best demonstrated in large lung sections, i.e., a sagittal section (400 to 500 mμ in thickness) of the whole lung. The incidence and severity are in direct proportion to the concentration of coal dust and the length of exposure. The disorder occurs only in coal miners who have well-developed areas of dust retention around the respiratory bronchioles. The x-ray film shows only the coal macules as in anthracosis. Disability is uncommon except in the aged.

Tuberculosis. Tuberculosis may be a complication. Clinical evidence of active tuberculosis with pulmonary changes caused by "coal dusts" is sufficient evidence of disability.

Chronic Bronchitis. Earlier studies indicated that chronic bronchitis was a complication of exposure to coal dusts, but later studies revealed that the incidence of chronic bronchitis was as high in the unexposed groups as in the coal miners. Further studies indicated a higher incidence of bronchitis among some of the wives of miners. Chronic bronchitis is a bacterial disease until proved otherwise.

DIAGNOSIS

The diagnosis is based upon (1) industrial history of adequate exposure, (2) x-ray changes that are compatible with the history of exposure, and (3) physical examination to rule out those conditions that might mimic coal miner's pneumoconiosis. Lung biopsy should rarely be performed, but is extremely valuable in a controversial situation.

DIATOMACEOUS EARTH PNEUMOCONIOSIS

Diatomaceous earth pneumoconiosis is a disease of the lungs caused by the prolonged inhalation of diatoms. Diatoms are algae that were deposited on the floors of freshwater inland lakes as well as in sea waters. There is some evidence that the diatoms found in extinct inland lakes cause less fibrosis than the diatoms from sea water.

SYMPTOMS AND SIGNS

Workers exposed to the natural diatomaceous dusts usually do not present symptoms, but those exposed to the flux of calcined powders may have exertional dyspnea that is progressive. Tightness in the chest is also common, and in the advanced stage there may be cough and wheezing. Clubbed fingers have been found in some cases.

ROENTGENOLOGY

The abnormalities vary in degree of severity. The first change observed is increased linear markings. Later there is a particular pattern. As the condition progresses, there is mottling of the lung and finally in some cases massive fibrosis with involvement of both upper lobes, without superimposed infection. There may be evidence of bullous emphysema, a spontaneous pneumothorax, or both.

LUNG FUNCTION

Lung function studies have no diagnostic value because of the obstruction as well as the difficulties in diffusion resulting from the thickened alveolar walls.

DIAGNOSIS

With a history of adequate exposure over a sufficient number of years the diagnosis is not difficult. Serial x-ray studies and those taken at the time of the most recent examination are of great value in establishing a diagnosis. The symptomatology is not unique in the advanced stage. Incinerating the sputum and finding concentrations of the specific dust establishes the history of exposure but does not give an index to the degree of pathology or the extent of pulmonary dysfunction. Lung biopsy may be indicated as a last resort.

SIDEROSIS

Siderosis is a condition of the lungs caused by inhaled and retained iron, and by iron oxide fumes and dusts. It can occur in iron ore miners, welders, metal grinders, and polishers. Pure siderosis is considered a benign pneumoconiosis.

ROENTGENOLOGY

The typical shadow is usually 1 mm or smaller in its greatest diameter, and the gross appearance is of fine stippling throughout both lung fields.

LUNG FUNCTION

There are no abnormalities in the respiratory pattern in pure siderosis.

DIAGNOSIS

Diagnosis is usually not difficult. The history of exposure is of great value. The absence of symptoms is to be expected. Siderosis must be differentiated from silicosis (which produces a larger nodular shadow on the x-ray film). Iron deposits in the lungs secondary to congestive heart failure or repeated transfusions can present some diagnostic difficulties, but these can be resolved by an accurate history. Exposure to tin oxides (stannosis) and barium salts (barytosis) produces a similar picture because of the high molecular density of these elements, but such exposure can be ruled out by history. Metastatic calcification of the lungs must be eliminated in the differential diagnosis. Lung biopsy usually is not employed, but it can be of great value. Exposure to both iron and silica dust may produce siderosilicosis that gives a clinical picture of modified silicosis.

SILICOSIS (MINER'S PHTHISIS, POTTER'S ROT)

DEFINITION

Silicosis is a disease of the lungs caused by the prolonged inhalation and retention of silicon dioxide and characterized by diffuse fibrotic changes in the lungs that can be demonstrated by suitable x-ray films and in pathologic specimens. Silicosis occurs in many stages of severity; in the severe forms it is capable of producing shortness of breath, cough, tightness in the chest, fatigue, and a lessened capacity for work.

The severity and rate of development depend chiefly on the amount of silica in the atmospheric dust, the fineness of the particles, the concentration of the dust, and the duration of the exposure. The presence of admixed dusts may accelerate, retard, or inhibit the usual fibrosis-producing action of silica. The presence of a tuberculosis reaction can also modify the progression and severity of the condition.

ENVIRONMENTAL ASPECTS

Silica dust exposure is present in many industries, but mining, ceramics, and foundry industries employ the greatest number of exposed workers. The types of silica encountered in these industries are as follows: (1) crystalline — quartzite, quartz, rock crystal; (2) cryptocrystalline — chert; (3) amorphous — opal, diatomaceous earth; (4) conversion products (silica, silicates, and heat) — crystobalite, tridymite, silica fume.

All of these are termed "free silica" and are capable of producing pulmonary fibrosis. Crystobalite and tridymite cause more fibrosis than quartzite. Basic clays that contain no free silica and are considered inert may become fibrogenic when subjected to prolonged or repeated exposure to temperatures in the range of 1600 to 2000 F. The clays can be converted to a product containing 40 to 50 per cent crystobalite. In assessing a silica exposure one must not think in terms of the qualities of the raw material, but must give due recognition to the way it is processed and what conversion products may be expected.

SYMPTOMS AND SIGNS

Not all subjects with demonstrable changes on the x-ray film have a pulmonary impairment of sufficient magnitude to produce symptoms. The nodule, which is the diagnostic lesion, has little or no bearing on the symptoms. The onset of symptoms is insidious and the first one is usually dyspnea. Tightness in the chest with bronchiolar spasm occurs later, and respiratory wheezing on exertion is not uncommon in the far advanced cases. Clubbing of the fingers is seldom seen, as is cyanosis, except in those patients with massive lesions and right heart strain.

LYMPHATIC SILICOSIS

This is the common type of silicosis. The principal diagnostic lesion, the nodule, is formed in the lymphatic aggregates of the lung. The phagocytes engulf the silica dust and are caught in the lymphatic aggregates in the peribronchial areas as they exit from the alveoli by way of the lymph channels. Some of the cells may gain access to the lymphatic plexuses and be deposited in the hilar lymph glands. Long exposure causes an increase in the number of nodular lesions, and there may be coalescence of nodules that may be patchy or massive and usually are seen in the upper lung fields. In massive lesions the width of the pleura may be increased to 1 inch. With these lesions cor pulmonale, with right heart dilatation, hypertrophy, or both, can be caused by blockage of the pulmonary blood vessels or by retraction of fibrotic tissue. Emphysema, although not of significance in the classic type of silicosis, can be of serious consequence when associated with massive lesions. Tuberculosis, which was once a common and serious complication, is not as frequent today thanks to control measures in the general population.

ROENTGENOLOGY

The chest film varies with the degree of pathology. The earliest findings are increased linear markings extending out from the hilar regions of the lung and particularly the right hilar region. As exposure continues and retention of silica dust is increased, the linear markings assume a cross-hatch pattern with beading. With further progression the nodules appear and with sufficient exposure coalescence and, in some patients, massive shadows are seen.

LUNG FUNCTION ASPECTS

Many workmen with classic silicosis have no apparent physiologic impairment. Others have only restrictive lung impairment. They are comfortable at rest but dyspneic on exercise. The pulmonary compliance is decreased. Another group may have obstructive lung disease caused by bronchiolar spasm, which is the chief cause of respiratory symptoms in silicotics. The maximum voluntary ventilation is markedly decreased. Those with massive lesions present a picture of advanced emphysema with increased residual air and low oxygen saturations.

DIAGNOSIS

The diagnosis is based on the history of adequate exposure, x-ray findings, and symptoms if present. Microincineration of the sputum and a large number of silica particles in the residue are proof of exposure only. Lung biopsy may be valuable if indicated. As silicosis is the most common occupational disease of the chest, it presents many problems in differential diagnosis. Conditions that may mimic silicosis are discussed under Pitfalls in Diagnosis.

SUBEROSIS

DEFINITION

Suberosis is a disease of the lungs caused by the inhalation of cork dusts and associated fungi and bacteria in factories processing cork bark.

PATHOGENESIS

Cork dust is highly irritating and causes burning sensations of the skin. The particles produced in forming operations are of respirable size. Circulating precipitins against penicillin frequentans were found in 38 per cent of workers.

SYMPTOMS

The symptomatology varies with the severity of the exposure. Some workers developed asthma-like reactions during the first days of exposure and hence were not suitable for this type of work. However, in most workmen the disease develops insidiously, and they fall into two groups: (1) workmen with bronchial asthmatic reactions who showed obstructive ventilatory defects; (2) workmen with disease affecting the peripheral gas exchange tissues. This type can also appear acutely.

Those with insidious onset complained of cough, severe and progressive dyspnea, malaise, and loss of weight. Patients with acute onset had, in addition, febrile episodes. The acute attacks usually resolved 24 to 48 hours after removal from exposure, but reappeared on re-exposure.

X-RAY FINDINGS

Diffuse fine miliary mottling is seen. Some patients with chronic disease show irreversible lesions thought to be due to irreversible fibrosis. Restriction and gas exchange defects are found in this latter group.

DIAGNOSIS

1. The workmen who strip the bark from the cork oak are not affected.
2. The disease affects only those who work in the cork factories and are exposed to cork dust and fungi.
3. The use of precipitin tests must be employed in making a specific diagnosis, as the x-ray findings and subjective symptoms can be found in many pulmonary diseases.
4. Lung biopsy can be used as a last resort in making the diagnosis.

TALCOSIS

Talcosis is caused by the inhalation of a variety of dusts that are commonly called talc. The chemical and physical properties of the dust or its mixtures vary to such an extent that the biologic action can range from a foreign body response to a severe fibrogenic reaction.

Talc — $H_2Mg_3(SiO_3)_4$ — is a natural anhydrous magnesium silicate used in the manufacture of paint, ceramics, rubber, roofing paper, toilet preparations, and insecticides. There are three basic types of talc used in industry: tremolite talc, pure talc (alpine talc), and talc with admixtures of other substances such as pure silica, chromates, and many other substances.

DIAGNOSIS

The diagnosis is based on the history of exposure, the clinical features, and the x-ray film. Lung biopsy may be needed to make a specific diagnosis. The tremolite type of talc, because of its biologic properties, is the only type that produces the clinical picture of asbestosis.

PITFALLS IN DIAGNOSIS

MIXED PNEUMOCONIOSES

One of the great problems that confronts the clinician is to evaluate the patient who has been exposed to several different dusts that produce anatomic and physiologic changes in the lungs. In compensation hearings it is the last employer who is usually liable, but he is not necessarily responsible for the lung changes and impairment of pulmonary function that may result from multiple exposures. Study of this type of patient involves the following aspects:

1. A careful industrial history, listing the different exposures as to duration, severity, possible conversion of inert raw materials by heat to fibrogenic or toxic materials, and the amount of effort expended in each job. In heavy work there is a greater demand for oxygen, and hence the body utilizes an increased amount of air that may be polluted by dusts in the working atmosphere.
2. History of hobbies and possible exposures.
3. Does the abnormality on the x-ray film show any characteristic type of lesion that, when correlated with the history, seems to be significant? Are serial films available?
4. Does a specific alteration in the lung function studies suggest a certain type of exposure?
5. Lung biopsy of the wedge type may be indicated to allow for a histologic and chemical analysis.
6. Autopsy studies sometimes cause problems in evaluation of the abnormal lung changes. The complexity of the picture produced by mixed dusts deserves a meticulous study.

IMITATORS

Although any of the pneumoconioses may be mimicked by nonindustrial diseases, exposure to silica presents the greatest problems because it is most common.

Silicosis has been known for many centuries, is worldwide in distribution, and occurs in many types of industry. Despite its prevalence it is frequently misdiagnosed, causing adverse economic, sociologic, familial, and public relations results.

Workmen have been told by laymen and physicians whose knowledge of occupational diseases of the chest is limited that their subjective symptoms or the objective findings are due to silicosis. The diagnosis may be accurate, but the condition may be one that simulates silicosis through the subjective symptoms or the objective findings on the chest x-ray film.

A serious problem exists when the workman, because of a faulty diagnosis, is told he has silicosis in a late stage. In all probability he is told that he must quit his job, thus impairing his economic security. His family feels that their security and plans for the future are shattered. The workman is sometimes shunned by his neighbors, and his employer receives adverse publicity from the community and the employee's union.

The symptoms of disabling silicosis are shortness of breath, cough, tightness in the chest, and fatigue. Any and all of these symptoms can be found in many nonindustrial diseases of the lungs, heart, chest wall, and blood, as well as in systemic diseases and chronic infections.

Dyspnea, the most common symptom of silicosis, is also found in the following chronic disorders: asthma, chronic bronchitis, bronchiectasis, lung tumors, laryngeal tumors, tuberculosis, bronchiolitis, emphysema, heart disease, diseases of the blood, kidney disease, liver disease, systemic disease, chronic infection, and metabolic diseases.

Cough is a common symptom of disorders of the respiratory tract, but these disorders can be nonindustrial as well as industrial in origin. The cough of respiratory origin is usually accompanied by production of sputum. The more productive cough occurs in bronchiectasis. Cough can also be extrarespiratory in origin. This is a dry ("useless") cough that is purposeless and avails nothing. Tumors or local irritations of the ear, nose, throat, pleura, or diaphragm can cause this type of cough.

Tightness in the chest is usually associated with bronchiolar spasm, which is a common symptom of asthma, chronic bronchitis, bronchiolitis, bronchiectasis, emphysema, organic obstructions of the airways, coronary heart disease, and far advanced fibrosis of nonindustrial origin. Tightness of the chest usually is triggered by primary or secondary lung exercise.

Fatigue is a symptom that is usually more common in the older age groups but can occur in all age groups when caused by anemia, debilitating disease, emphysema, or infection. In fact any condition that causes dyspnea can cause fatigue.

A diagnosis of silicosis cannot be made with any degree of accuracy if based on subjective symptoms alone.

These imitators of silicosis that present as objective findings on the chest x-ray film can be eliminated by differential studies.

Silicosis has been defined as a condition of the lungs characterized by diffuse fibrotic lesions that are fairly equally distributed throughout both lung fields. Government bodies have specified that the typical fibrotic nodule of silicosis is the criterion on which a diagnosis is based. However, when one realizes that this medicolegal definition places the roentgenologic differential diagnosis among some hundred pulmonary diseases showing miliary nodules — either primary lung disease or a pulmonary manifestation of systemic disease — then one must proceed with great caution in interpreting mottled shadows of the lung as being due to inhalation of silicon dioxide. Conditions that must be considered in the differential diagnosis of silicosis are as follows:

1. The proliferative pneumoconioses such as asbestosis.

2. The inert pneumoconioses. (a) Dusts of high molecular density such as iron oxide, tin oxide, and barium salts, which can cast shadows on the x-ray film by reason of their high molecular density and without producing fibrosis. (b) Retention deposits of large amounts of inert dusts which cast a shadow on the x-ray film by virtue of their physical presence (coal, clays).

3. Coal miner's pneumoconiosis, which produces a bizarre lung picture.

4. Chemical pneumonitis. The inhalation of certain chemicals such as cadmium oxide and the oxides of nitrogen and beryllium compounds can result in the appearance of shadows on the x-ray film that are not dissimilar to the fibrotic change of silicosis.

5. Bacteria. Conditions such as histoplasmosis, tuberculosis, wood fungal infections, and other infections cast shadows on the x-ray film similar to the lesions of silicosis.

6. Allergy of the pulmonary type, which can simulate silicosis.

7. Diseases of the blood. Pulmonary hemosiderosis, polycythemia, hemorrhagic disease, leukemia, and myeloma frequently simulate silicosis on the chest film.

8. Malignancy, primary or metastatic.

9. Diseases of the skin and mucous membranes that frequently have associated pulmonary lesions, such as scleroderma and Boeck's sarcoid.

10. Metabolic diseases. Histiocytosis, amyloidosis, and metastatic calcification of the lungs can frequently simulate silicosis.

11. Shadows cast by substances outside the pleural cavity, such as hair, skin tumors, clothing, and the like.

HYPERSENSITIVITY PNEUMONITIS

By J. O. HARRIS, M.D.,
Gainesville, Florida

DEFINITION

Hypersensitivity pneumonitis (extrinsic allergic alveolitis) is an immunologically mediated lung disease usually caused by inhalation of organic dusts. The initial pathologic changes are located primarily at the alveolar level and consist of a predominantly mononuclear inflammatory reaction with infiltration of the pulmonary interstitium by lymphocytes, plasma cells, and histiocytes. Along with these interstitial changes there are increased numbers of lymphocytes and macrophages in alveolar spaces. Bronchiolitis also may be present in many patients. The acute changes give way to granulomatous lesions with multinucleated giant cells and thickened alveolar septa. Usually these pathologic changes resolve with return to normal lung architecture, but chronic interstitial fibrosis may result if exposure to the causative antigens is repeated or continuous. Extensive histologic information is not available regarding hypersensitivity pneumonitis caused by different antigens (Table 1), but the available information suggests that similar abnormalities are induced by many of them. Therefore, a specific etiologic diagnosis cannot be made by histologic examination of the lung.

The pathologic changes in the lung are most consistent with a cell-mediated immune reaction, and there is substantial clinical and experimental evidence to support the explanation of a cell-mediated mechanism in the pathogenesis of the disease. Available clinical and experimental evidence also suggests that an immune-complex, complement-fixing reaction (humoral) may be involved. It has not yet been resolved whether either cell-mediated or humoral immune reactions or both are responsible for the lung lesions. Additionally, mycotoxins have been suggested as a third mechanism by which lung damage could occur after inhalation of dusts containing fungi.

CLINICAL FEATURES

Patients with hypersensitivity pneumonitis may have acute, subacute, or chronic symptoms. The determinants for the type of symptoms a patient has are the intensity and duration of exposure, frequency of exposure, and the immunologic reactivity of the individual.

The principal symptoms of acute hypersensitivity pneumonia are fever, chills, and dyspnea occurring 4 to 8 hours after exposure to the antigen. In addition, the patient may complain of malaise, headache, and anorexia and after repeated exposure may have weight loss. Physical examination typically reveals the patient to be tachypneic and febrile (38.3 to 40 C). Fine-to-medium inspiratory crackles can be heard over the posterior chest with greatest intensity at the bases. Wheezing is not a usual finding, but some atopic patients have bronchoconstriction soon after exposure to the antigen. In severe cases, peripheral cyanosis may be present. A peripheral blood leukocytosis of 12,000 to 20,000 is usually present, and acute phase reactants may be elevated. Arterial blood gases reveal hypoxemia with hypocapnia. The x-ray film of the chest sometimes appears normal, but usually some type of parenchymal infiltrate is visible.

The most suggestive x-ray pattern is diffuse, finely nodular densities that tend to spare the extreme periphery of the lung. Associated with this nodularity there is often a soft patchy interstitial infiltrate confined to the same areas of lung. Pulmonary function studies show a restrictive ventilatory abnormality, with decreased vital capacity, lung volumes, and diffusing capacity.

When exposure to the offending antigen is interrupted for a period of time, the acute form of hypersensitivity pneumonitis usually resolves completely. In a matter of hours to a few days, the temperature elevation subsides, but the dyspnea, rales, abnormal x-ray of the chest, and cough take longer to improve, usually resolving in 2 to 3 weeks. A few persons, particularly those who have had repeated exposure, are left with permanent respiratory disability after exposure to the antigen is terminated and the acute symptoms subside.

Occasionally, hypersensitivity pneumonitis

Table 1. *Causes of Hypersensitivity Pneumonitis*

Probable Antigen	Source	Exposure
Thermophilic actinomycetes		
Micropolyspora faeni	Moldy hay	Farming
Thermoactinomyces vulgaris	Moldy compost	Mushroom workers
T. vulgaris	Moldy bagasse (pressed sugar cane)	Bagasse processing
T. sacchari		
T. vulgaris	Contaminated humidifiers, air conditioners, and heating units	Humidifier lung
T. candidus		
Fungi		
Aspergillus sp.	Moldy grain (corn, oats, barley)	Farming, animal husbandry, malt workers
Cryptostroma corticale	Maple logs	Saw mill
Penicillium caseii	Cheese mold	Cheese workers
Alternaria sp.	Contaminated wood pulp	Wood pulp workers
Penicillium	Moldy cork	Cork workers
Graphium sp.	Contaminated sawdust	Saw mill
Pullularia sp.		
Mucor stolonifer	Moldy paprika pods	Paprika workers
Avian proteins		
Pigeon serum	Droppings, dust, feathers	Pigeon breeding, chicken and turkey raising, pet birds
Chicken proteins		
Turkey proteins		
Parakeet proteins		
Other		
Sitophilus granarius	Wheat weevils	Milling grain
Bacillus subtilis	Washing detergents	Detergent use or manufacture
Sodium cromolyn	Drugs	Drug use
Nitrofurantoin		
Hydrochlorothiazide		
Toluene diisocyanate		Polyurethane production

presents as a hyperacute illness with the patient rapidly proceeding to respiratory failure; however, the prognosis is good if supportive measures are adequate to carry the patient through the crisis.

Intermediate between the patients with acute and chronic symptoms are those who continuously have cough, malaise, dyspnea, and weight loss. These symptoms may fluctuate, but acute exacerbations with fever and chills are infrequent and less dramatic than in the acute form of disease.

The chronic form of hypersensitivity pneumonitis begins insidiously with slowly progressive dyspnea on exertion and mildly productive cough. Acute episodes with fever and chills do not occur, and weight loss is frequent. The patient does not associate the symptoms with exposure to dust as easily as in the acute form; therefore, the diagnosis is not as readily suspected. The chest x-ray is seldom normal and is likely to show more linear densities associated with the nodular lesions. In advanced cases there may be "honeycombing" of the lung. Histologic examination usually reveals a degree of fibrosis; consequently, withdrawal from exposure to the antigen is less likely to result in complete resolution of symptoms and normali-

zation of pulmonary function. Chronic hypersensitivity pneumonitis may progress to severe respiratory insufficiency with cor pulmonale.

LABORATORY FINDINGS

Precipitating antibodies to the offending antigen can be shown to be in the serum of most patients with hypersensitivity pneumonitis by agar-gel double diffusion. However, this finding is not specific because many asymptomatic persons exposed to the antigen will also have these antibodies. Both symptomatic and asymptomatic persons may respond to intradermal injection of the specific antigen with an immediate wheal and flare followed by an area of erythema and edematous induration 4 to 8 hours later. This cutaneous reaction, thought to be an Arthus reaction, subsides over the next 24 hours.

Typical delayed hypersensitivity reactions with induration at 24 to 48 hours do not occur. However, both peripheral blood and bronchoalveolar lymphocytes from patients with hypersensitivity lung disease have been shown to produce macrophage migration inhibition factor when exposed in vitro to the offending antigen. This indicates that cell-mediated immune mechanisms are stimulated by these antigens. Unfortunately, some persons who are exposed to the antigen but do not develop symptoms also have sensitized peripheral blood lymphocytes, which renders this type of test nondefinitive. At this time we do not know whether examination of bronchoalveolar lymphocytes can distinguish symptomatic from asymptomatic individuals exposed to antigen.

The inhalation provocative challenge is the most definitive test for hypersensitivity pneumonitis because it distinguishes between symptomatic and asymptomatic persons who have been exposed and have circulating precipitating antibodies and T-lymphocytes sensitized to the specific antigen. For this test, subjects inhale an aerosol of antigenic extract and patients with clinical illness develop fever, chills, rales, and leukocytosis 4 to 8 hours after challenge. Associated with these findings is a decrease in vital capacity and diffusing capacity. This test is not likely to become widely used because of the nonavailability of different antigen preparations and because the test induces illness in the susceptible subjects that entails some risk for them.

The histologic appearance of a lung biopsy specimen during the early stages of disease is suggestive of hypersensitivity pneumonitis, although the specific antigen is not evident. However, once extensive fibrosis is part of the pathologic picture, it is more difficult to distinguish this disease from other causes of chronic pulmonary fibrosis.

DIAGNOSIS

Because no simple definitive test is readily available for hypersensitivity pneumonitis, the diagnosis usually must be established by the following criteria:

1. Clinical, radiologic, and physiologic features compatible with the diagnosis.

2. Documentation of exposure to a possible antigen. The patient may readily recognize such exposure, but if not, the success of documenting exposure depends on the questions that the physician puts to the patient. It is important to establish a clear picture of the patient's work, home, and recreational environments. Specific inquiries should be made concerning the hobbies of the patient and his family, prescription and nonprescription medications, exposure to birds, and the type of heating and cooling systems at home and at work.

3. Demonstration of serum precipitating antibody to the suspected antigen. Commercial kits are available for the most common causative antigens; therefore, this supportive laboratory test should be available to most physicians.

4. Clinical improvement in response to avoidance of the antigen.

5. Histologic features of lung biopsy specimen. One would hope that this criterion would not be necessary, since it is no more specific than the clinical criteria listed and is expensive and of greater risk to the patient.

PULMONARY EMBOLISM AND INFARCTION

By KENNETH M. MOSER, M.D.
San Diego, California

DEFINITION

Venous thrombi may originate in any of the systemic veins and, less commonly, in the right cardiac chambers. When such thrombi detach, are carried to the pulmonary vasculature and lodge in the pulmonary arterial vessels, pulmonary embolism has occurred. Occasionally, embolism leads to pulmonary infarction, that is, hemorrhage, collapse and, rarely, actual death of the lung tissue distal to the embolic destruction.

PATHOGENESIS

Since pulmonary embolism is but a complication of venous thrombosis, the pathogenesis of embolism is the pathogenesis of venous thrombosis. The basic factors involved in the genesis of venous thrombosis are stasis, injury to the vascular intima, and thrombogenic alterations in the coagulation system. These alterations are poorly understood and there are no specific coagulation measurements that reliably predict thrombotic tendency (aside from the rare heritable condition of antithrombin III deficiency). However, stasis or intimal injury or both occur in a number of well-recognized clinical contexts, in which the incidence of venous thrombosis and pulmonary embolism is high. Such situations include the postoperative period, pregnancy and the postpartum state, traumatic injuries (particularly to the pelvis and lower extremities), burns, congestive heart failure, and any cause of prolonged immobility. Obesity and cancer are other known risk factors. A number of studies have disclosed a substantial incidence of venous thrombosis and pulmonary embolism in all of these "high-risk" situations.

NATURAL HISTORY

In approaching the diagnosis of pulmonary embolism, it is important to recognize its natural history. Embolism is a dynamic disorder. After an embolus lodges in the vasculature, it undergoes changes over hours to days. Most frequently, resolution of the embolus occurs due to fibrinolysis. This is a relatively rapid process, which, in man, can result in total dissolution of the embolus over a period of several days. With even minimal dissolution, an embolus may move distally, obstructing a smaller segment of the pulmonary vasculature.

If fibrinolytic resolution proceeds slowly, emboli resolve by the process of organization — fibroblastic ingrowth followed by endothelialization. This "scar" leaves a permanent, though usually quite small, residual in the vessel wall. Rarely, fibrinolysis and organization lead to little resolution, and extensive, chronic obstruction persists.

Additionally, recurrence of emboli may develop from the original thrombotic source; or, in some instances, the embolus itself may grow further in situ by accretion of platelets and fibrinogen.

Thus, the status of the patient with pulmonary embolism may change rather rapidly in terms of symptoms, signs, and the findings on certain laboratory tests.

Another consideration of diagnostic importance is the factors that condition the severity of the cardiopulmonary consequences of embolism. One major one is the *extent* of obstruction per se; i.e., the more vascular bed is occluded, the more severe the impairment of cardiac and pulmonary function. Another is the release of vasoactive and bronchoactive amines (e.g., serotonin) from the platelets that are known to coat emboli. Such a sequence occurs in dogs and may occur in man. Finally, the pre-existing cardiopulmonary status of the patient conditions the consequences. Patients with reduced function may have serious responses to relatively small emboli; otherwise healthy individuals may tolerate rather extensive embolism with minimal symptoms.

Pulmonary infarction is an uncommon consequence of embolism. In individuals without prior cardiopulmonary disease, it occurs in well under 10 per cent; in those with, in as high as 40 per cent. This fact is important diagnostically because the clinical and laboratory findings of *infarction* are absent in the majority of patients with *embolism*.

DIAGNOSIS

Conceptually, there are two major categories of approach to the diagnosis of embolism: (1) by detection of the consequences of embolism, and (2) by direct visualization of the emboli.

Consequences. Among the potential consequences are symptoms and physical findings, i.e., the clinical diagnosis of embolism. Unfortunately, the clinical diagnosis is notoriously unreliable. Signs and symptoms of embolism are nonspecific; they are shared with many other cardiopulmonary diseases. Therefore, they suggest — but cannot make — the diagnosis. The most common symptom of embolism is *dyspnea of sudden onset*. In general, the more extensive the occlusion, the more severe the dyspnea. A sense of "impending doom" is commonly reported. Substernal chest discomfort, mimicking that which occurs with coronary occlusion, may be reported, usually with extensive obstruction; syncope may occur. Pleuritic chest pain and hemoptysis are less frequent symptoms because they are manifestations of infarction, which follows embolism in a minority of patients.

Among physical findings, *tachycardia* is the most common. Cardiac examination is frequently otherwise normal; only with embolism of sufficient magnitude to cause significant pulmonary hypertension are such findings as a palpable right ventricular "tap" along the left sternal border, a right ventricular S_3, fixed splitting of the second sound, and accentuation of the pulmonary closure sound detected.

The lung fields are usually clear to examination. With infarction, a pleural rub and the physical findings of consolidation and pleural effusion may be present. Clinical evidence of peripheral venous thrombosis is absent in more than 50 per cent of patients with embolism. Fever, usually not exceeding 101.5 F (40.5 C), occurs in a minority of patients, particularly in those with infarction.

Thus, symptoms and signs are often quite modest, particularly when small emboli occur in patients with no pre-existing cardiopulmonary disease. In all patients, the findings are nonspecific. Therefore, definitive diagnosis of embolism depends upon laboratory tests.

The majority of such tests, again, mirror the consequences of embolism and so are variable and nondefinitive. Leukocytosis often occurs but does not assist in diagnosis, although it rarely exceeds 20,000 per cu mm. There are no definitive "blood tests" that confirm or rule out embolism. Serum glutamic oxaloacetic transaminase (SGOT), lactic dehydrogenase (LDH), fibrin degradation products, and other tests proposed have such a high incidence of false positives and false negatives that they are useless. The most frequent electrocardiogram shows only tachycardia; occasionally, with extensive obstruction, evidence of acute right atrial and ventricular overload is seen ("S_1, Q_3 pattern," peaked P waves, nonspecific ST-T changes, R axis shift). The chest roentgenogram is notoriously unreliable. Without infarction, one looks for disparities in the size of major pulmonary arteries that *should* be of similar size, or regional hypoperfusion — both are subtle and nondiagnostic findings. With infarction, pulmonary infiltrate(s) or pleural effusion(s) or both may be seen. Despite prior suggestions, there are no shapes or locations of infiltrate that are definitive for infarction, except that all do abut a pleural surface.

Similar nonspecificity characterizes the values of arterial blood gases seen in embolism. It is certainly true that some degree of hypoxemia is common in embolism, and that the more extensive the occlusion, the more frequent and severe the hypoxemia (low PaO_2). However, it is equally true that (1) a normal PaO_2 (>80 mm Hg) is seen in a substantial proportion of patients with embolism, and (2) hypoxemia is common in many nonembolic disorders that mimic embolism. Therefore, whereas measurement of the PaO_2 is useful in patient management, it is not a valuable diagnostic tool.

The only laboratory tests that rely on embolic consequences that are at all reliable are the perfusion and ventilation lung scans. A perfusion lung scan should be performed in all patients suspected of embolism. The reason for this is that a normal, six-view (posterior, anterior, both laterals, both posterior obliques) well-performed perfusion (Q) scan excludes the diagnosis of embolism. While a negative Q scan in embolism is a theoretical possiblity, no angiographically proved embolus with a negative scan (performed immediately before or after) has been reported.

But what if the scan is "positive," that is, shows one or more "defects" indicative of reduced or absent pulmonary blood flow? It is true that many disorders other than embolism can cause such abnormalities in the distribution of pulmonary blood flow. In my view, the discovery of perfusion defects in a patient with a negative chest x-ray who has no history or physical findings of cardiopulmonary disease is compelling evidence of pulmonary embolism. Depending upon the clinical context, a positive Q scan may suffice as an indicator of embolic

disease. However, if these criteria are not satisfied or if the potential risks of heparin therapy are high, additional confirmation is useful.

Often this can be obtained with a radionuclide ventilation (V) scan using a radioactive gas (most commonly xenon-127 or xenon-133). The use of the $\dot{V}/\dot{Q}$ scan is based on the physiologic fact that vascular obstruction (including embolism) produces a zone of the lung in which *perfusion* is absent but *ventilation* remains normal. Thus embolism results in $\dot{V}/\dot{Q}$ "mismatch" (normal V, absent Q), whereas parenchymal pulmonary diseases (e.g., emphysema) result in $\dot{V}/\dot{Q}$ "match" (abnormal V and abnormal Q). However, the *technique* of V scanning is crucial to proper interpretation. First, with proper doses of radionuclides, a V scan can and should be performed immediately after an abnormal Q scan is obtained. The prior Q scan does not interfere with interpretation of the V scan. Second, a "single breath" V scan is not satisfactory. The most useful component of the V study is the *washout* phase. Therefore, the study should be performed by having the patient rebreathe xenon-133 to equilibrium (washin), then washout. Patients with embolism washin and washout normally. Patients with parenchymal disease washin and, particularly, washout slowly. The V study should be done in that view (e.g., posterior) in which the Q defect(s) is best seen.

Should a Q (and $\dot{V}/\dot{Q}$) scan be done in someone with an infiltrate on chest x-ray? Yes, because emboli often (more than 30 per cent) are multiple, and characteristic $\dot{V}/\dot{Q}$ "mismatch" may be seen in other, noninfiltrated zones of the lung.

How reliable is the finding of $\dot{V}/\dot{Q}$ "mismatch" in the diagnosis of embolism? In my judgment, the finding is highly reliable. Normal washout in an area of perfusion deficit indicates that vascular occlusion is present. One need go further diagnostically only when the V/Q results are equivocal or certain therapeutic procedures (such as embolectomy and inferior vena caval ligation) are being contemplated.

Procedures That Visualize Emboli. At present, short of thoracotomy, only one procedure is available by which an embolus can be directly visualized: pulmonary angiography. However, the limitations of this procedure must be weighed against its benefits. First, it is an invasive procedure that is not without some risk. Second, both risk and yield are conditioned by the experience of those performing the angiogram. When angiograms are performed infrequently, the risk is increased, the quality of the study reduced, and the interpretation rendered uncertain. Even pulmonary angiograms of high quality are not "easy" to interpret. Those of poor quality may be impossible to evaluate.

Third, there are only two diagnostic findings by angiogram: the "filling defect," in which the thrombus creates a negative image within the stream of opaque medium, and the "cut off," in which there is abrupt cessation of the dye stream. Other findings such as absence of capillary filling are nonspecific and nondiagnostic.

One advantage of performing angiography is that the hemodynamic status of the patient also can be determined; that is, pulmonary arterial pressure, cardiac output, and so forth can be measured.

Thus, our indications for angiography are (1) the presence of an experienced angiographic team, and (2) the need for a high degree of diagnostic certitude either because of the equivocal nature of other studies (or lack of access to them) or the contemplation of high risk or high morbidity medical or surgical therapy.

OTHER DIAGNOSTIC CONSIDERATIONS

New techniques are being introduced that may allow visualization of emboli. The two most promising are direct labeling of emboli with gamma-emitting radionuclides (e.g., ^{111}indium-labeled platelets) and fiberoptic angioscopy (transvenous insertion of a fiberoptic device directly into the pulmonary arterial system). The true potential of these techniques awaits elucidation.

Another approach suggested by some is to study the lower extremities for deep venous thrombosis (in lieu of angiography). Whether this is done by contrast venography or impedance phlebography, the thesis is the same: If there are no venous thrombi present, the diagnosis of embolism is highly unlikely. Unfortunately, this attractive thesis is flawed. In my experience, some 20 per cent of patients with emboli do not have evidence of venous thrombosis in the legs. How can this be, if more than 95 per cent of all emboli arise from leg thrombi? Our presumption is that, in these patients, the entire thrombus detached as an embolus. (In a small additional percentage, the emboli arose from the right cardiac chambers.)

Furthermore, venous thrombi can occur in patients whose cardiopulmonary symptoms are not due to emboli. Thus, although establishing the presence or absence of venous thrombosis certainly is useful in planning the management of patients with embolism, it does not allow exclusion (or inclusion) of the diagnosis of embolism.

Finally, it should be noted that the extent of diagnostic "work-up" in a given patient that needs to be completed before therapy is instituted depends heavily on the potential risk of that therapy in the specific patient. Unless that risk is high (e.g., bleeding due to heparin), therapy usually is initiated before such procedures as scans and angiograms are obtained.

ATELECTASIS

By DAVID C. BUDSON, M.D.,
Vallejo, California

and PHILIP A. BROMBERG, M.D., F.A.C.P.
Chapel Hill, North Carolina

DEFINITION

Translated literally from its Greek source, atelectasis means "imperfect stretching." The term was originally applied to a lung or a portion of lung that did not fill with air at birth but was later used to denote collapse of a previously expanded portion of lung. Atelectasis has been defined by a number of authors as any state associated with a loss of lung volume. This definition unfortunately includes the loss of volume owing to pulmonary fibrosis, for which a category of "cicatrization" or "contraction" atelectasis has even been designated. However, the loss of volume secondary to fibrosis is due to replacement of alveoli with fibrous tissue rather than to the collapse of intact alveoli, and in reality, few clinicians or physiologists think of fibrosis in the lungs as a form of atelectasis. It would seem therefore that a better definition of atelectasis would be "the collapse of anatomically intact alveoli associated with a loss of lung volume."

CLASSIFICATION

The most rational classification of atelectasis is based on an understanding of the mechanisms that are responsible for maintaining lung volume and the ways in which these may be altered. On the basis of a discussion of these mechanisms, we will describe three general types of atelectasis: relaxation atelectasis, atelectasis related to altered surfactant, and resorption atelectasis.

Lung Elastic Recoil and Relaxation Atelectasis. The force with which the lungs tend to collapse at a given volume (retractive pressure or elastic recoil) arises from elastic forces in lung tissue as well as surface-related forces at the alveolar-air interface. At functional residual capacity (FRC), the elastic recoil of the lung is balanced by the passive expansile tendency of the chest wall, resulting in a subatmospheric intrapleural pressure. (At lung volumes higher than FRC, active chest wall muscle contraction is required to balance the increased lung elastic recoil.) Alteration of the resting position of the chest wall or interference with the coupling of the chest wall to the visceral pleural surface, which may occur with thoracoplasty, pneumothorax, or pleural effusion, may allow retraction of the underlying lung. A similar mechanism is responsible for retraction of lung tissue adjacent to a space-occupying lesion in the lung parenchyma (e.g., solid masses, cysts, bullae, or lobar emphysema in infants). This form of atelectasis is referred to as *passive* or *relaxation atelectasis*. Other synonyms include *mantle atelectasis* and *compressive atelectasis*, but the latter term is not entirely accurate since the lung in this situation collapses owing to its own passive recoil rather than to active compression.

Surface Forces and Atelectasis. Surface forces also contribute to the tendency of the lung to retract, and high surface tensions at the alveolar-air interface render alveoli unstable, particularly at low lung volumes and low distending pressures. Alveoli are lined by a phospholipid-containing surface active film, or surfactant, that promotes alveolar stability by its inherent property of lowering surface tension as alveolar surface area decreases. If surfactant activity is reduced by impaired synthesis, destruction, or increased removal, alveoli become unstable and collapse. This form of atelectasis has been variously termed *adhesive, congestive,* and *nonobstructive atelectasis*. It is likely to be spotty or focal but is often diffuse in distribution. Deficiency of lung surfactant due to decreased synthesis is well established in the neonatal respiratory distress syndrome, in which diffuse atelectasis is a prominent feature.

Normal lung expansion is thought to be necessary for continual renewal of surfactant, and conditions associated with decreased transpulmonary pressure (e.g., recumbency, obesity, ascites, and diaphragmatic weakness) may predispose to atelectasis. The resulting alveolar collapse in such cases may be inapparent radiographically, so-called *microatelectasis* or *miliary atelectasis*, or it may result in linear radiographic densities, so-called *discoid* or *plate-like atelectasis*. Altered surfactant has also been implicated in atelectasis associated with pulmonary thromboembolism and a variety of other lung insults.

Airway Obstruction and Resorption Atelectasis. The maintenance of noncollapsed alveolar units depends on the patency of the airways supplying these units. If these airways are blocked, and if there are no other pathways by which air may enter these units, then the remaining air distal to the obstruction is gradually absorbed until collapse occurs. This is usually termed *resorption* or *obstruction atelectasis*.

Airway obstruction may result from intraluminal causes such as a neoplasm, foreign body, blood clot, or mucus plug, or from extrinsic compression by a neoplasm, enlarged lymph nodes, an aortic aneurysm, or an enlarged left atrium. In addition, airway narrowing from bronchoconstriction, secretions, or intramural edema may act in concert with any partial intrinsic or extrinsic obstruction to cause complete obstruction. Although collapse of a lobe or segment may be due to obstruction of its supplying main airway, it may also occur as a result of obstruction of multiple small airways, with the more proximal larger airways remaining widely patent.

Atelectasis is not an inevitable result of bronchial obstruction. Even an obstruction that appears bronchoscopically to be "complete" may allow enough air to pass to avoid atelectasis, although total obstruction may then result from minor additional changes in the airway. An obstructing tumor or foreign body may at times behave as a check-valve, permitting air to enter the obstructed region during inspiration but preventing its egress, leading to the paradoxical situation of hyperinflation of the obstructed region, characteristic of foreign body aspiration in children.

The development of obstructive atelectasis may also be modified by pneumonic consolidation or the accumulation of fluid in the air spaces distal to an obstruction. Infection is a common complication of obstructing neoplasms or foreign bodies, and consolidation developing distal to an obstruction may at least partly counteract the collapse that would usually result from air resorption. In acute obstructive atelectasis, there is often some degree of exudation of fluid in the alveolar spaces that again limits the volume loss. This exudation is a result of the increasingly negative pleural pressure that occurs with collapse and that is transmitted to the interstitial space, pulling fluid from the vascular bed. This accumulation of fluid distal to an obstruction has been referred to as the "drowned lung." If the obstruction persists, excess fluid is gradually absorbed, resulting in further volume loss.

The composition of the inspired gas mixture is important in the development of collapse following bronchial obstruction. Nitrogen is poorly soluble in blood and is slowly absorbed from a closed space. Replacement of nitrogen (which comprises 78 per cent of room air) by high concentrations of oxygen or by highly soluble anesthetic gases (both of which are relatively rapidly absorbed) hastens the collapse that may occur following bronchial obstruction. Also, lung units that are very poorly ventilated but not totally devoid of air may be converted to completely collapsed units if their gas composition is changed to one that may be absorbed at a rate faster than can be replaced by inspired ventilation.

Finally, the development of atelectasis following bronchial obstruction may be modified by the presence of collateral ventilation, i.e., ventilation of alveoli by pathways other than direct airway connections. Diminished collateral ventilation to the right middle lobe compared to other lobes is thought to be an important factor in the development of chronic or recurrent atelectasis of this lobe, so-called *middle lobe syndrome.*

CLINICAL FEATURES

The clinical features of atelectasis depend on the volume of lung involved, the acuteness or chronicity of the collapse, the mechanism by which the collapse occurs, and the underlying disease or conditions that predispose the patient to developing atelectasis.

Symptoms and Physical Signs. In all cases, the history and physical examination should be directed toward revealing the underlying disease or conditions responsible for the atelectasis. It is important to seek clues for foreign body aspiration, bronchial neoplasms, conditions associated with bronchial plugging (e.g., asthma, cystic fibrosis, or pneumonia), conditions associated with decreased diaphragmatic mobility (e.g., neuromuscular diseases, sedation, obesity, and the postoperative period), and conditions associated with nitrogen washout (e.g., administration of anesthetic gases of high concentrations of oxygen).

In general, dyspnea, tachypnea, and tachycardia are more prominent with collapse that occurs acutely and involves larger volumes of lung than with collapse that evolves gradually, is chronic, or involves only small losses of volumes. In the former circumstance, there is usually an increase in tidal volume and respiratory frequency, leading to increased total minute ventilation and hypocarbia. This ventilatory response results from a vagal reflex induced by the effects of lung deflation on pulmonary stretch receptors, irritant receptors, or both. Stimulation of arterial chemoreceptors may also contribute to the increased ventilation when atelectasis results in significant arterial hypoxemia.

Fever and cough may be present owing to either the underlying condition or to the development of secondary infection. Unproductive cough may also be a result of stimulation of irritant receptors by deflation. Chest pain, usually of a pleuritic nature, is often a prominent feature of pneumonia, pneumothorax or pleural effusions, but may also occur with acute obstructive atelectasis secondary to mucus plugging.

The chest examination in resorption atelectasis reveals signs of absent air entry (dullness to percussion, decreased breath sounds, decreased fremitus, and inspiratory lag). If the collapse is extensive enough, there may be tracheal or cardiac deviation toward the atelectatic side, and hemidiaphragmatic elevation and rib space approximation on the atelectatic side, all a result of more negative local pleural pressures. With relaxation atelectasis due to a space-occupying process, there are also decreased breath sounds over the affected region. The percussion note, however, depends on the nature of the space-occupying process — whether it is air or fluid. The mediastinum shifts away from the atelectatic side owing to local pleural pressure becoming less negative. With a large pneumothorax or pleural effusion, the rib spaces may also be widened owing to expansion of the thoracic cage; i.e., part of the volume of fluid in the pleural space is taken up in the expansion (relaxation) of the chest wall. If there is enough mediastinal shift, as in the case of a "tension" pneumothorax, the volume of the contralateral lung may also be seriously compromised.

Arterial Blood Gases. Arterial blood gases reflect the effects of atelectasis on total ventilation and on the distribution of ventilation and perfusion. As previously indicated, decreased arterial P_{CO_2} and a corresponding rise in pH may occur in acute collapse because of an increase in total ventilation. However, respiratory acidosis is more likely in a patient with severe underlying lung disease. Hypercapnia and acidosis are also frequent accompaniments of the neonatal respiratory distress syndrome. This is due to the immature infant's inability to increase total ventilation enough to eliminate the high P_{CO_2} that is present at birth as well as to the presence of multiple alveolar units that maintain ventilation but are poorly perfused (increased dead space).

A widened alveolar-arterial oxygen tension difference is frequently an important feature of atelectasis. Overt hypoxemia usually results from the persistence of pulmonary arterial blood flow to lung units that are completely unventilated, resulting in increased venous admixture of the blood entering the systemic circulation (a right-to-left shunt). Hypoxemia resulting from this mechanism is characterized by its unresponsiveness to the administration of increased concentrations of oxygen, in contrast to hypoxemia resulting from less extreme ventilation-perfusion inequality or from overall alveolar hypoventilation, in which increased inspired oxygen concentrations cause a substantial increase in arterial PO_2.

A number of factors may affect the pulmonary arterial blood flow to atelectatic lung, thereby determining the degree of intrapulmonary shunting and hypoxemia that occurs. Two very important factors are the state of lung inflation and the alveolar oxygen tension. Pulmonary vascular resistance is increased at low lung volumes (particularly below residual volume), owing to passively decreased caliber of the conducting vessels. Alveolar hypoxia is known to cause active local pulmonary arterial vasoconstriction. Both of these mechanisms may act to decrease pulmonary blood flow to atelectatic lung (which is both deflated and hypoxic), thereby limiting the extent of right-to-left shunting and arterial hypoxemia. However, following acute obstructive atelectasis as well as collapse from pneumothorax, there is commonly a prompt fall in arterial PO_2. Usually the degree of hypoxemia is not as great with pneumothorax as with resorption atelectasis, and in the former the PO_2 usually reverts toward normal within hours, whereas in the latter situation significant hypoxemia is more likely to persist.

Several factors may contribute to these differences. With resorption atelectasis, the increased negative pleural pressure on the side of the collapse causes the contralateral lung to hyperinflate. If there is enough overinflation of that lung, its capillaries are compressed, thus increasing pulmonary vascular resistance, and limiting the amount of pulmonary blood flow that can be diverted away from the collapsed lung. In addition, some recent experimental work has indicated that the local hypoxic pulmonary vasoconstrictor response may be attenuated by the presence of systemic hypoxemia operating via arterial chemoreceptors. Such an effect might create a self-perpetuating mechanism for hypoxemia. Another consideration is that if infection develops distal to a bronchial obstruction, pneumonic consolidation might maintain pulmonary blood flow to that region.

Also of importance in determining the degree of hypoxemia caused by intrapulmonary shunting are the effects of posture, exercise, and mixed venous oxygen saturation. The distribution of pulmonary blood flow is greatly affected by hydrostatic pressure differences, with the most dependent lung regions receiving the greatest proportion of pulmonary arterial blood. The blood flow to an atelectatic region may therefore increase when that region is placed in a dependent position. Blood flow to an atelectatic lung may also increase with exercise. Finally, in the presence of intrapulmonary shunt of blood through an atelectatic area, the oxygen saturation of the mixed venous blood will affect the degree of desaturation in the systemic arterial blood. For the same degree of shunt, as a fraction of total cardiac output, there will be greater arterial oxygen desaturation if the mixed venous oxygen saturation is low. Conditions that are associated with low mixed venous oxygen saturations, such as anemia, low cardiac output, or increased O_2 consumption, may therefore magnify the degree of arterial hypoxemia resulting from atelectasis.

Hypoxemia is a major feature of the extensive atelectasis characteristic of the neonatal respiratory distress syndrome. The right-to-left shunt in this condition is often quite large (up to two thirds of the cardiac output), and is attributable mainly to perfusion of nonventilated alveoli, although shunts through the foramen ovale or patent ductus arteriosus are also contributory. Surface atelectasis of a more limited nature, such as diffuse microatelectasis or more focal plate-like atelectasis, is characterized by an increased alveolar-arterial oxygen gradient owing to perfusion of nonventilated alveolar units. Atelectasis of this sort may produce no clinical findings other than hypoxemia.

Re-expansion and Complications. Elimination of a bronchial obstruction or removal of a space-occupying process, such as pneumothorax, large pleural effusion, or large emphysematous bulla, often results in re-expansion of a collapsed lung or lobe with relief of symptoms and of hypoxemia. Similarly, one or two full lung inflations can reverse the microatelectasis seen in conditions associated with decreased diaphragmatic movement. Several factors, however, may interfere with expansion of the collapsed region, even when the initiating cause of the collapse is reversed. In a completely airless lung or lobe such as that resulting from resorption atelectasis, considerable pleural negative pressures are required to overcome the surface forces of apposed alveoli and bring about their reopening. The critical opening pressure required to expand alveoli in lungs that are atelectatic owing to nonresorptive mechanisms is not as great, because some gas may remain trapped in bubbles within the terminal air spaces; i.e., the lung or lobe is not as completely airless as in resorption atelectasis. The large opening pressure required to expand lungs or lobes following removal of an offending obstruction may not be attainable by patients with respiratory muscle weakness, and in this circumstance atelectasis may persist despite removal of the obstruction that initiated the atelectasis. It is also possible that surfactant may be altered with long-standing atelectasis, especially if there is complicating infection or if local pulmonary blood flow is markedly decreased, and this may hinder the ability of the lung to re-expand.

Following obstructive atelectasis, infection and inflammation frequently develop because of impairment of mucociliary clearance and the cough mechanism in the bronchial tree distal to an obstruction. Bronchiectasis, with chronic suppuration and scarring, is a complication of long-standing atelectasis, and may prevent complete re-expansion of the involved portion of lung, leading to chronic respiratory impairment if the volume loss is great enough. In relaxation atelectasis, however, bronchial clearance mechanisms are more likely to be maintained, and secondary infection is not as great a problem as in obstructive atelectasis. However, long-standing pleural effusions or pneumothoraces may result in pleural changes limiting re-expansion of the collapsed lung.

A well-recognized complication of collapse owing to pneumothorax or pleural effusion is the development of unilateral pulmonary edema following the rapid re-expansion of the underlying collapsed lung. The setting in which this may occur is that of a large pneumothorax or hydrothorax that is rapidly removed after having been present for at least several days. The pulmonary edema is usually limited to the side of the re-expanded lung. The development of edema may be preceded by a sensation of chest tightness and coughing during the thoracentesis, following which symptoms of respiratory distress may develop. Typically, such edema resolves spontaneously within a few days. The pathogenesis of re-expansion pulmonary edema is not well understood, but it is clearly noncardiogenic and may be at least partly related to a sudden marked increase in negative intrapleural pressure. This pressure is transmitted to the lung and may alter Starling forces in a way that leads to the transudation of fluid from the microvascular bed.

Radiologic Features

The definitive diagnosis of atelectasis is made with the posteroanterior and lateral chest roentgenograms. The importance of the lateral projection cannot be overemphasized. In the case of right middle lobe collapse or lingular collapse, it is the lateral view that most clearly demonstrates the triangular densities cast by these collapsed lobes, the findings on the frontal projection being more subtle. The lateral projection is also extremely useful in differentiating complete pulmonary collapse from massive consolidation or massive pleural effusion. In the case of total lung collapse, the contralateral lung becomes hyperinflated and the anterior mediastinum is displaced to the affected side, rotating laterally and posteriorly. This gives the appearance on the lateral projection of increased depth and radiolucency of the retrosternal airspace as well as a general increase in density posteriorly. In the case of massive consolidation or effusion, the x-rays passing through the chest in the lateral projection are absorbed uniformly, and no such differences in radiolucency or density are observed.

Resorption (Obstructive) Atelectasis. The basic radiologic principles governing lobar and segmental atelectasis secondary to bronchial obstruction are similar, the differences between them owing only to the volume of lung that is collapsed. Generally, collapse results in a triangular density with its apex directed toward the hilum and its base situated on the pleura. Description of distinctive roentgenographic patterns cast by each individual lobe or segment are beyond the scope of this article but may be found in several excellent references (Felson: *Chest Roentgenology*, W. B. Saunders, 1973; Fraser and Paré: *Diagnosis of Diseases of the Chest*, Vol. I, W. B. Saunders, 1977). The basic radiologic signs common to lobar and segmental collapse will be discussed briefly.

Since atelectasis involves the loss of lung volume, the direct sign of lobar collapse is displacement of interlobar fissures. With lesser degrees of volume loss in segmental collapse, displacement of fissures is usually minimal. Indirect signs of atelectasis include increased radiodensity of the collapsed zone, crowding of bronchovascular markings, and signs that occur because of compensation for the volume loss. These signs include hemidiaphragm elevation, mediastinal and hilar displacement, compensatory overinflation of nonobstructed lung, and approximation of ribs.

Hemidiaphragmatic displacement is a more prominent feature of lower rather than upper lobe atelectasis, and mediastinal shift is generally a more helpful sign in upper lobe collapse, in which tracheal position may be assessed. (The degree of mediastinal shift is always greatest in the region of the major pulmonary collapse.) Compensatory overinflation of the noncollapsed portion of the involved lung is a helpful sign, but since it takes time to develop, it is not helpful immediately following collapse. In contrast, mediastinal and diaphragmatic displacement tends to be greatest acutely and becomes less prominent as atelectasis becomes chronic. Hilar displacement occurs more predictably in upper lobe than in lower lobe collapse and is more marked the longer the atelectasis has been present. Rib approximation may be noted in situations of chronic volume loss but is generally not a reliable compensatory sign in atelectasis.

Two conditions that may sometimes be confused radiologically with lobar collapse are consolidation and encapsulated pleural fluid. In consolidation without collapse, there is no displacement of the interlobar fissures. Encapsulated pleural fluid can be more difficult to distinguish but may be suspected from the presence of pleural thickening elsewhere in the thorax, the absence of air bronchograms, the visualization of a lobar septum that is separate from the density, and its rounded contours.

The presence or absence of an air bronchogram may be a useful clue in atelectasis. If enough bronchial obstruction occurs to cause air resorption from the parenchyma, it must also cause all air to be absorbed from the bronchial tree. In the situation in which pneumonitis develops distal to such an obstruction and the degree of consolidation prevents significant volume loss, the absence of an air bronchogram may help in identifying the primary process as an obstructing lesion with a secondary infection rather than a simple bacterial pneumonia.

Relaxation (Passive) Atelectasis. A discussion of the radiographic features of pneumothorax and pleural effusion will not be attempted here except to indicate several important features of the collapse associated with these conditions. In the case of a large pneumothorax or pleural effusion, many of the compensatory signs of obstructive atelectasis are reversed. Hence, if there is any shift of mediastinal and hilar structures, it is to the side away from the atelectasis. Similarly, in the case of pneumothorax, the chest springs outward as the underlying lung collapses so that the distance between ribs is widened rather than narrowed. The collapse resulting from pneumothorax produces no increase in radiodensity until approximately 90 per cent of the lung is collapsed. This is due to the presence of air in the pleural space anterior and posterior to the collapsed lung, as well as to the concomitant decrease in pulmonary blood flow that occurs with pneumothorax. In contrast to the absence of an air bronchogram with resorption atelectasis, an air bronchogram is usually present with relaxation atelectasis. This may provide a useful clue in lung collapse secondary to pneumothorax, in which case the absence of an air bronchogram may be indicative of an otherwise unsuspected endobronchial obstruction.

Surface Atelectasis. As indicated before, this form of atelectasis commonly exists without any radiographic manifestations, the diagnosis of "microatelectasis" being inferred from the presence of mild or moderate hypoxemia in the appropriate clinical setting. Plate-like atelectasis, which has similar pathophysiologic significance, is manifested radiographically by single or multiple linear densities ('Fleischner's lines"), 1 to 3 mm in thickness and up to several centimeters in length, always extending to a pleural surface. They are usually located in the lung bases, unilaterally or bilaterally, and are horizontal or slightly oblique in orientation. These areas of atelectasis are usually transient, often appearing or disappearing within a few hours. Despite this, they are important to recognize because of the pathophysiologic significance they have in terms of ventilation-perfusion abnormalities.

The radiographic appearance of the extensive atelectasis seen in the neonatal respiratory distress syndrome (hyaline membrane disease) is that of a diffuse mottling and granularity with prominent air bronchograms.

OTHER ROENTGENOGRAPHIC STUDIES

Oblique projections may permit better visualization of a collapsed segment, depending on which segment is involved. Regular lung tomography and computerized axial tomography may help define segmental collapse that is not as apparent on ordinary chest roentgenograms. These techniques may also be valuable in identifying enlarged lymph nodes or tumors that have caused a lobe or segment to collapse. Bronchography may be useful when chronic collapse occurs with a patent lobar or segmental bronchus, in which case peripheral plugging of multiple small airways may be demonstrated.

FIBEROPTIC BRONCHOSCOPY

Fiberoptic bronchoscopy, which allows direct visualization of the tracheal bronchial tree to the level of subsegmental bronchi, is an invaluable aid in identifying various causes of obstructive atelectasis. Endobronchial obstructions such as tumors, foreign bodies, blood clots, or mucus plugs may be identified, or extrinsic bronchial compression may be noted.

Material may be aspirated for cultures and cytologic examination, and brushings and biopsies of lesions may also be obtained. In the case of obstructive atelectasis due to mucus plugging or foreign bodies, fiberoptic bronchoscopy may be therapeutic as well as diagnostic.

OTHER LABORATORY TESTS

Pulmonary function tests such as spirometry, lung volumes, and carbon monoxide diffusing capacity are not helpful in the diagnosis of atelectasis per se, but may be quite useful in the diagnosis of such underlying pulmonary diseases as asthma or chronic bronchitis, and in the evaluation of pulmonary functional impairment resulting from chronic atelectasis.

Other laboratory tests such as urinalysis, complete blood count, eosinophil count, blood chemistries, and sputum examination are essential in evaluating the underlying conditions and should be selected on the basis of the clinical setting.

PULMONARY HYPERTENSION

By CLIFFORD ZWILLICH, M.D., *and* JOHN T. REEVES, M.D.

Denver, Colorado

DEFINITION

Pulmonary hypertension exists when the mean pulmonary arterial pressure exceeds 20 mm Hg. This increase in pressure results from obstruction of flow within pulmonary precapillary, capillary, or postcapillary vessels, or from increased pressures within the left heart. Therefore pulmonary hypertension is a syndrome of many possible causes. The exact cause of pulmonary hypertension should be sought in each patient with this abnormality, because it is often reversible. Mean pulmonary arterial pressures of more than 50 mm Hg constitute severe pulmonary hypertension. Table 1 lists the more *common causes* of pulmonary hypertension.

SYMPTOMS AND SIGNS

Unfortunately, symptoms of hypertension per se usually occur late in the natural history of the

Table 1. *Causes of Pulmonary Hypertension*

  I. Left ventricular failure
   A. Atherosclerotic heart disease
   B. Hypertensive cardiovascular disease
   C. Aortic valvular disease
   D. Cardiomyopathy
   E. Mitral insufficiency
 II. Left atrial disease
   A. Mitral stenosis
   B. Left atrial tumor or thrombosis
   C. Cor triatriatum
III. Pulmonary venous obstruction
   A. Mediastinal fibrosis
   B. Pulmonary venous thrombosis
 IV. Pulmonary parenchymal disease
   A. Chronic obstructive lung disease
   B. Severe pulmonary fibrosis
     1. Sarcoidosis and other granulomatous lung diseases (many types)
     2. Diffuse interstitial fibrosis (many types)
   C. Acute severe pulmonary injury
     1. Adult respiratory distress syndrome
     2. Severe diffuse pneumonitis
  V. Pulmonary artery disease
   A. Primary pulmonary hypertension
   B. Recurrent or massive pulmonary emboli
   C. In situ thrombosis or vasculitis
   D. Pulmonary arterial stenosis
   E. Increased pulmonary blood flow: Congenital heart disease with left-to-right shunt (atrial and ventricular septal defects, patent ductus)
 VI. Hypoxia and/or hypercapnia
   A. Some patients with chronic obstructive lung disease
   B. High altitude exposure
   C. Primary hypoventilation
     1. Obesity-hypoventilation syndrome
     2. Primary alveolar hypoventilation

syndrome, because pulmonary, like systemic, hypertension tends to be asymptomatic. If the pulmonary hypertension is due to left heart disease, the most common symptoms are exertional dyspnea and fatigue. Frequent also are cough and either anginal or pleuritic chest pain. Syncope or hemoptysis may direct the physician to consider diseases affecting the pulmonary circulation. Eventually the patient may present with right-sided congestive heart failure.

PHYSICAL EXAMINATION

The classic findings of pulmonary hypertension are as follows: (1) Elevated jugular venous pressure with prominent "a" waves. The "a" waves reflect the forceful atrial contraction necessary to fill the hypertrophied or failing right ventricle. (2) A sustained systolic thrust (lift) along the left sternal border, reflecting right ventricular hypertrophy. (3) Accentuation of the pulmonary valve closure sound. With extremely high pressure or in patients with thin chest walls, the pulmonary valve closure may be palpated. The pulmonary hypertension itself may cause either no murmurs or a short, soft, systolic ejection murmur over the pulmonary area (second left interspace). If pulmonary hypertension develops in patients with ventricular septal defect (Eisenmenger's syndrome) or a patent ductus arteriosus, there may be no murmur because there is little or no pressure gradient across the defect. Nevertheless, murmurs suggesting rheumatic or congenital heart disease as the cause of the pulmonary hypertension should be sought. An ejection click may be heard in pulmonary hypertension from the sudden tensing of the pulmonary valve or pulmonary artery. If the pulmonary valve ring becomes dilated, a diastolic murmur of pulmonic insufficiency may be heard. If the cardiac output is low, the peripheral arterial pulses may be of small volume. Cool extremities may also be noted, along with cyanosis resulting from peripheral capillary stasis. More commonly, cyanosis indicates systemic hypoxemia caused by one or more of the following: (1) pulmonary parenchymal disease, as in chronic bronchitis and emphysema; (2) severe mismatching of ventilation with perfusion, as in pulmonary embolism; (3) right-to-left shunting, as in Eisenmenger's syndrome or through a patent foramen ovale in primary pulmonary hypertension; or (4) alveolar hypoventilation, as in the pickwickian syndrome. If there is incipient or overt right heart failure, there may be a third or fourth heart sound heard best at the left sternal border during inspiration, a murmur of tricuspid insufficiency, or peripheral edema.

CHEST X-RAY

In severe pulmonary hypertension the frontal chest x-ray shows a prominent main pulmonary artery often with rather abrupt decrease in caliber of secondary branches (Fig. 1A). Because the two ventricles are superimposed in the frontal view, it is not a satisfactory view for distinguishing right from left ventricular hypertrophy. However, the lateral view (Fig. 1B) may show encroachment of a hypertrophied and dilated right ventricle on the retrosternal anterior clear space. In addition, the x-ray combined with fluoroscopy will often be helpful in identifying many of the causes of pulmonary hypertension.

The most common cause of pulmonary hypertension, left heart failure, is accompanied by a large left ventricle, enlarged pulmonary veins, and Kerley B lines at the periphery of the lung bases. Rheumatic mitral valve disease may be revealed by calcification of the mitral valve and enlarged left atrium. The presence of restrictive or obstructive pulmonary parenchymal disease may be indicated, respectively, by interstitial infiltrates or by overexpanded radiolucent lungs with flattened diaphragms.

ELECTROCARDIOGRAM

The electrocardiogram (Fig. 2) is more helpful than the chest x-ray in separating right from left ventricular hypertrophy. Right axis deviation, right ventricular hypertrophy, and right atrial enlargement provide strong evidence favoring pulmonary hypertension (unless there is right ventricular outflow obstruction). One criterion for right ventricular hypertrophy is either (1) a frontal QRS mean axis of $+110°$ or more, or (2) an R or R^1 wave in V_1 of 5 mm or more with an R/S ratio in V_1 of 1.0 or more. Electrocardiogram evidences of left ventricular hypertrophy may obscure the evidence for right hypertrophy.

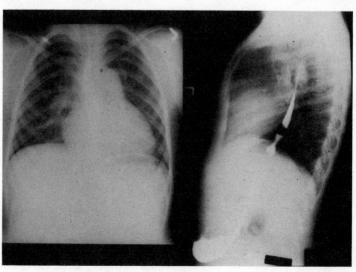

Figure 1. *A,* The posteroanterior view of the chest shows an enlarged heart and pulmonary arteries. The lung fields are normal in this patient with primary pulmonary hypertension. *B,* The lateral view shows that the retrosternal anterior clear space is filled by the dilated right ventricle.

A   B

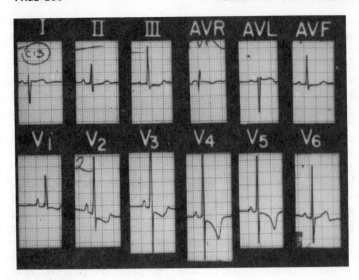

Figure 2. This electrocardiogram demonstrates the findings of pulmonary hypertension. The QRS axis is right shifted ($+120°$), and tall p waves are present in leads V_{1-2}. The very tall R wave in V_{1-2} plus the deep S wave in V_6 is additional evidence of right ventricular hypertrophy.

ARTERIAL BLOOD GASES

In patients with primary pulmonary hypertension or left heart failure the arterial oxygen tension may be normal. Carbon dioxide elevation with hypoxia points toward either chronic obstructive pulmonary disease or primary alveolar hypoventilation. Acute massive pulmonary embolism is almost always associated with lowering of the arterial oxygen tension (PO_2). In congenital heart disease with pulmonary hypertension, a reduced arterial PO_2 not fully corrected (>500 mm Hg) by 100 per cent O_2 inhalation suggests the presence of a right-to-left shunt.

PULMONARY FUNCTION TESTS

Pulmonary function tests are of importance in establishing the presence or absence of pulmonary parenchymal disease. Simple spirometric measurement of vital capacity and 1-second forced expired volume (FEV_1) provides an index of the severity of lung disease and indicates whether the disease is obstructive or restrictive. Values less than 50 per cent of predicted indicate pulmonary disease sufficiently severe to account for or contribute to pulmonary hypertension. More sophisticated tests of total lung volumes, pulmonary compliance, airway resistance, and carbon monoxide diffusion will better document the nature of the pulmonary abnormality.

ECHOCARDIOGRAPHY

Echocardiography is useful in establishing whether or not mitral valve stenosis or left atrial myxoma is present. Either may present initially as severe pulmonary hypertension without cardiac murmurs. The echogram can also demonstrate an enlarged left atrium, an insufficient mitral valve, or a dilated left ventricle, thus providing evidence for left heart dysfunction as a cause of pulmonary hypertension.

CARDIAC CATHETERIZATION

Cardiac catheterization is undertaken for two reasons: (1) to quantitate the severity of suspected pulmonary hypertension, and (2) to determine the cause of the pulmonary hypertension. In general, diagnostic catheterization in pulmonary hypertension should be restricted to those patients in whom surgery is contemplated for correction of rheumatic or congenital heart disease, to those in whom the cause of the suspected pulmonary hypertension is not known, and to those with suspected but otherwise unproved pulmonary embolism. Restrictions are indicated because of catheter trauma to the right ventricle, increased vasoreactivity from contrast media during angiography, or release of small emboli during the procedure, which may trigger sudden or delayed death in patients with long-standing pulmonary hypertension.

In patients in whom the cause of pulmonary hypertension is not known, measurement of the pulmonary arterial wedge pressure, which measures left atrial pressure, differentiates pulmonary hypertension of precapillary origin from that caused by left heart disease. The normal mean pressure gradient from pulmonary artery to wedge (left atrial pressure) is less than 8 mm Hg, and the normal wedge pressure is 12 mm Hg or less. Higher pressure differences indicate precapillary obstruction and high wedge pressures reflect left heart pressure elevation as the cause of pulmonary hypertension.

One reservation is that small pulmonary vein obstruction cannot be detected by measurement of wedge pressure. Fortunately, such instances are rare.

In patients with congenital heart disease and pulmonary hypertension, the measurement of pulmonary flow is essential. This procedure is to determine to what extent the pulmonary hypertension is due to increased lung blood flow. Although pulmonary arterial pressure may approach systemic levels, the blood flow may be sufficiently increased that calculated resistance is but moderately increased. Patients with calculated pulmonary vascular resistances less than two thirds systemic resistance may be candidates for surgical closure of a congenital cardiac defect even though pulmonary hypertension is severe. Also part of the diagnostic procedure is to determine, insofar as possible, the reversibility of the pulmonary hypertension by the use of pulmonary vasodilators (inhaled 100 per cent oxygen, intravenous tolazoline or isoproterenol) or by muscular exercise. These maneuvers not only may establish the cause of the pulmonary hypertension but may also have therapeutic implications.

PRIMARY PULMONARY HYPERTENSION VS. RECURRENT PULMONARY MICROEMBOLISM

These two diseases are fortunately uncommon causes of pulmonary hypertension. Primary pulmonary hypertension is a disease of unknown cause that may occur at any age but largely appears in women less than 45 years old. Apparently it begins as hypertrophy of the small pulmonary arteries progressing to vascular sclerosis and obliteration of small vessels. Most patients die within 3 years of diagnosis. It has been frequently described in association with collagen vascular diseases such as systemic lupus erythematosus, periarteritis nodosa, progressive systemic sclerosis, and occasionally rheumatoid arthritis, leading to the suggestion that it results from altered immune mechanisms.

Recurrent pulmonary microembolism usually develops in persons older than 45 years and may be associated with hypercoagulable states such as with cancer. Rarely, patients with cirrhosis of the liver develop pulmonary hypertension from recurrent emboli. The disease has been reported in younger persons with emboli originating from hepatic veins, children with hydrocephalus having surgical drainage of cerebrospinal fluid to the right atrium, and young women taking oral contraceptives. The clinical, radiographic, electrocardiographic, and hemo-

dynamic findings in these patients do not distinguish them from patients with primary pulmonary hypertension. At present, differentiation can be made only by a skilled pathologist during microscopic examination of lung tissue.

LUNG ABSCESS

By MURRAY N. ANDERSEN, M.D.
Buffalo, New York

DEFINITION

A lung abscess is an area of tissue necrosis in the lung that has progressed to formation of a cavity filled with pus. Although lung abscesses may develop in tuberculosis, mycoses, and other diseases, the term is commonly applied to pyogenic suppurative pneumonitis caused by various aerobic and anaerobic bacteria. Although commonly occurring after aspiration, particularly in patients who are unconscious from alcoholism or other causes, lung abscesses also develop as a complication of certain types of pneumonia, particularly staphylococcal and streptococcal. Abscess formation may also develop as a secondary event after pulmonary infarction or as a complication of pre-existing pulmonary cysts.

SIGNS AND SYMPTOMS

The onset of symptoms is typically that of a pulmonary infection, which usually precedes the development of frank abscess. Initial symptoms are usually cough, fever, pleuritic chest pain, and frequently hemoptysis. When the infection has progressed to abscess formation, the patient typically has copious and particularly foul-smelling sputum, the latter characteristic being typical of infection with anaerobic organisms. The associated hemoptysis is usually in the form of blood-streaked sputum, but on occasion it may be massive and even fatal.

A history of alcoholism with preceding episodes of unconsciousness is frequent.

In some patients the abscess ruptures into the pleural space, presenting as an empyema. In this event the existence of the abscess may not be apparent until the empyema is drained, at which time the presence of a bronchopleural fistula confirms the presence of a pre-existing abscess.

Physical signs are not specific for lung abscess and are those associated with consolidation of the underlying lung or intrapleural fluid. Clubbing of the fingers is seen on rare occasions.

DIAGNOSIS

In the early stages of developing pulmonary abscess it may be impossible to differentiate abscess from pneumonia with consolidation. It is only when partial evacuation of the necrotic content occurs and cavitation is visible on the x-ray that the true diagnosis is apparent. The principal diagnostic tool is the radiograph of the chest showing cavitation with surrounding pulmonary infiltrate as a result of adjacent pneumonitis. On many occasions carcinoma of the lung will present with cavitation and surrounding inflammation quite similar in appearance to an abscess; however, the presence of a thick, irregular wall will usually suggest that the lesion is necrosis within a tumor rather than an abscess.

The location of the lesion is not helpful in differentiating abscess from other conditions, for although it occurs somewhat more commonly in the upper lobes than in lower or middle lobes, this is also true of other lesions such as tuberculosis, pulmonary cysts, and carcinoma, and each also occurs in the lower lobes in a substantial number of cases.

Bacteriologic studies are an essential part of the treatment in determining appropriate antibiotics; however, the bacteria found in the sputum are not of diagnostic importance in distinguishing between abscess and pneumonitis, and a variety of organisms may be found in either condition.

General laboratory findings are not useful diagnostically, as they do not provide a differentiation between lung abscess and other types of intrathoracic infection.

The initial chest x-ray commonly shows consolidation typical of pneumonia, which may be localized or diffuse. As central necrosis and subsequent evacuation develop, an area of radiolucency appears, confirming the diagnosis of abscess formation. Typically, initial evacuation is incomplete so that the cavity presents with an air-fluid level, with greater or lesser proportions of the cavity filled with pus. When complete drainage has been accomplished with evacuation of all pus and disappearance of the fluid level, the patient commonly improves clinically, much as with any other abscess that has drained.

As the surrounding inflammatory process sub-

sides with treatment, the adjacent pulmonary infiltration may disappear, leaving a relatively thin-walled and empty cavity that will decrease in size at a variable rate. Even though closure may be slow, the majority of cavities will eventually disappear completely, leaving only a residual scar.

Bronchoscopy is generally carried out in patients with suspected lung abscess to rule out the presence of a proximally obstructing tumor and also to aid in evacuation of the contents of the abscess with aspiration of pure sputum samples for culture. The dramatic evacuation of the abscess that frequently follows bronchoscopy is most likely due to associated severe coughing on the part of the patient rather than to direct aspiration of the abscess content, as the cavity cannot ordinarily be entered.

Bronchography is not of any specific diagnostic value, because the location is evident, and communication with the bronchial tree can be assumed when an air space is present.

PITFALLS IN DIAGNOSIS

The principal conditions that may present in a similar way to lung abscess are carcinoma of the lung, tuberculosis, fungal diseases, infection of pre-existing pulmonary cysts, and pulmonary infarction with necrosis.

Carcinoma of the lung may usually be distinguished by the presence of an irregular thick wall of the cavity, usually with lesser degrees of surrounding pneumonitis. The age of the patient, smoking history, and clinical course are often suggestive. Failure of resolution of the surrounding pneumonitis with complete evacuation after therapy is also suggestive of malignancy with central necrosis.

Tuberculosis can usually be distinguished fairly early in the course of events by a positive skin test and positive sputum for acid-fast bacilli. The x-ray appearance also frequently suggests chronicity and long-standing fibrosis when cavitation is present. Cavitation in the lower and middle lobes in patients with tuberculosis is also much less common than in the upper lobes.

An infected pulmonary cyst is, in effect, a lung abscess, and the primary importance of making a distinction lies in its prognostic significance. If infection has developed in a preexisting cyst, the cyst will not disappear as the infection resolves, and surgical removal will be necessary to prevent recurrence. An infected cyst is usually thin walled and with little surrounding inflammation, presenting as a rather benign-appearing cavity partially filled with fluid.

Fungal infection with cavitation is usually

suggested by exposure in an endemic area, the radiologic appearance, the absence of foul-smelling sputum, and positive skin, serologic, and sputum tests. The most common fungal infections that produce cavitation and may be misdiagnosed as pyogenic lung abscess are pulmonary histoplasmosis and coccidioidomycosis. Cavitation is unusual in blastomycosis and actinomycosis but occurs on rare occasions.

Pulmonary infarction usually presents with an acute onset of chest pain and a typical radiologic appearance. Lung scans will frequently show multiplicity of pulmonary defects even when only one lesion is visible on the x-ray, and this finding is of particular diagnostic importance. When central necrosis in an area of infarction develops, it is, in effect, a pulmonary abscess even though the cause and management are then different.

LUNG CANCER

By MARTIN H. COHEN, M.D.
Washington, D.C.

SYNONYMS

Bronchogenic carcinoma, bronchial carcinoma, carcinoma of the lung.

DEFINITION

Bronchogenic carcinoma is the most common form of cancer in the United States. Approximately 100,000 new cases were diagnosed in 1979. This cancer is, in large part, a result of chronic exposure to environmental and occupational carcinogens, with cigarette smoke being of primary importance. Occupational lung carcinogens include asbestos, radiation exposure, chloromethyl ether, other organic carbon-containing products originating from coal or petroleum, arsenic, nickel, chromium, and hematite. For those exposed to most occupational carcinogens, concomitant cigarette smoking markedly increases lung cancer risk. While previously lung cancer was mainly a disease of males over 40 years of age, the incidence of lung cancer in women is markedly increasing. Epidemiologically, this relates to a dramatic increase in cigarette consumption by females beginning in the late 1930s. While lung cancer risk has decreased somewhat with the introduction of low-tar, filtered cigarettes, the risk for a

smoker remains considerably higher than for the nonsmoker. For ex-smokers the risk of lung cancer decreases in proportion to the number of years of abstinence.

Lung carcinomas usually arise in segmental or subsegmental bronchi, at sites of bronchial bifurcations. These areas are susceptible to injury because of turbulent airflow and decreased mucus flow rates. Normally the tracheobronchial tree, down to terminal bronchioles, is lined with pseudostratified, ciliated, or mucin-containing columnar epithelial cells. Interspersed between these cells are basal (reserve) cells, some of which contain neurosecretory granules. Repetitive lung injury leads to loss of ciliated columnar cells and to mucous cell hyperplasia. Basal cells are stimulated to proliferate. Mucous cell hyperplasia progresses to epidermoid metaplasia by conversion of columnar mucous cells to cuboidal or flattened cells with associated keratin production. With progressive injury the basal portion of the metaplastic epithelium becomes disorganized, while the superficial mucosa retains an organized pattern. This is the stage of "atypical metaplasia" or "dysplasia." Eventually the entire mucosal thickness is replaced by proliferating disorganized neoplastic cells (carcinoma in situ). When the basal membrane is penetrated, the carcinoma is invasive.

This mechanism of carcinogenesis particularly pertains to epidermoid carcinoma. Pulmonary adenocarcinoma may occasionally arise in this fashion, or the cell of origin may be derived from submucosal bronchial mucous glands or from bronchiolar Clara cells. Small cell anaplastic carcinoma probably derives from granular basal cells (Kulchitsky cells). These cells may also give rise to bronchial carcinoids. Large cell anaplastic carcinoma is a wastebasket category for tumors showing no maturation or differentiation by light microscopy. Electron microscopy is sometimes useful in classifying these tumors as either poorly differentiated epidermoid or adenocarcinomas.

In addition to epidermoid carcinoma, small cell anaplastic carcinoma, adenocarcinoma, and large cell anaplastic carcinoma—which make up over 90 per cent of primary pulmonary malignancies — the World Health Organization lists nine other diagnostic categories: combined epidermoid and adenocarcinoma, carcinoids, bronchial gland tumors, papillary tumors of surface epithelium, "mixed" tumors and carcinosarcomas, sarcomas, unclassified tumors, mesotheliomas, and melanomas. These nine categories will not be discussed further.

Epidermoid and adenocarcinoma are subdivided by degree of differentiation into well-differentiated, moderately differentiated, and poorly differentiated varieties. Degree of differentiation may be of prognostic importance for survival. Small cell anaplastic carcinoma has been divided into lymphocyte-like (oat cell) and intermediate type, including fusiform and polygonal cells. At present there is no basis for this subclassification as the clinical behavior and response to therapy of the various small cell histologies is identical. For well-differentiated and moderately well-differentiated carcinomas and for small cell anaplastic carcinoma, there is good agreement between cytologic diagnosis and histologic diagnosis. For poorly differentiated tumors histology provides more accurate classification.

The biologic behavior of the major histologic subtypes of lung cancer varies considerably. Epidermoid lung cancer is characterized by an apparent slow volume doubling time and by a tendency to grow locally to large size. The duration of symptoms prior to diagnosis tends to be long. Early metastases are relatively uncommon in patients with well-differentiated and moderately well-differentiated tumors. Epidermoid carcinoma is the cell type most likely to show cavitation on chest x-ray.

Small cell anaplastic carcinoma differs from epidermoid carcinoma in that the course of disease appears to be compressed into a shorter time frame, consistent with the more rapid doubling time of this tumor. Symptom duration before diagnosis is short. Evidence of tumor dissemination to regional lymph nodes or to systemic sites is often noted at the time of presentation. At many institutions patients with small cell anaplastic carcinoma are not considered as candidates for curative surgery.

Adenocarcinoma of the lung is characterized by peripheral location of the primary tumor on chest x-ray and by the frequent lack of symptoms at the time of tumor discovery. The metastatic potential of adenocarcinoma is intermediate between epidermoid carcinoma and small cell anaplastic carcinoma.

Large cell anaplastic carcinoma, like adenocarcinoma, is generally located peripherally on chest x-ray. These tumors grow locally to larger size than do adenocarcinomas. The metastatic potential of this cell type is similar to adenocarcinoma and to poorly differentiated epidermoid carcinoma.

SIGNS, SYMPTOMS, AND FINDINGS

Signs and symptoms in lung cancer relate to primary tumor growth, to regional extension into the mediastinum, and to systemic metastatic spread. Primary tumor symptoms vary depending on whether the tumor is centrally or peripherally located on chest x-ray. Epidermoid carcinoma and small cell anaplastic carcinoma are most often centrally located. Bronchoscopic examination in patients with these types generally reveals exophytic mucosal tumor masses in proximal bronchi. These masses produce greater or lesser degrees of bronchial obstruction. Symptoms associated with this type of tumor growth include cough, dyspnea related to loss of lung volume, vague chest pain owing to involvement of peribronchial and perivascular nerves, hemoptysis, wheezing, and pneumonic symptoms secondary to infection behind a bronchial obstruction. Physical examination findings in these patients are dependent upon the degree of bronchial obstruction and on whether there is associated pulmonary infection.

By contrast, primary tumor symptoms of peripherally located adenocarcinomas and large cell anaplastic carcinomas include pleuritic chest pain, dyspnea on a restrictive basis (pleural effusion or severe pain), and a less prominent cough except in the bronchioloalveolar variant of adenocarcinoma. Bronchoscopy in these patients rarely demonstrates large mucosal tumor masses, so that hemoptysis and obstructive symptoms are uncommon. Physical examination of the chest is either normal or reveals findings consistent with pleural involvement, including a pleural friction rub or signs of a pleural effusion.

Less common symptom complexes related to intrapulmonary tumor growth include acute febrile and toxic illnesses resulting from lung abscesses in necrotic tumor cavities (epidermoid and large cell anaplastic carcinoma) and the superior sulcus or Pancoast's syndrome. The latter is most frequently associated with epidermoid carcinoma. Pancoast tumors growing in the lung apex expand to involve the first thoracic and eighth cervical nerves, resulting in characteristic pain in the shoulder and ulnar-innervated portion of the arm. Further growth results in erosion of the first and second ribs. Paravertebral extension with sympathetic nerve involvement produces Horner's syndrome (ptosis, miosis, enophthalmos, anhidrosis).

Mediastinal spread of lung cancer, either by direct extension or via the lymphatics, leads to characteristic regional disease symptoms. These symptoms are extremely important, since their presence indicates that the patient is not a candidate for surgery. Regional symptoms arise from nerve entrapment, from vascular obstruction, or from direct extension to involve the pericardium or esophagus. The most common manifestation of nerve entrapment is hoarseness secondary to involvement of the recurrent laryngeal nerve. Laryngoscopy reveals paralysis of the vocal cord in abduction. Left-sided tumors most often cause this symptom because of the long intrathoracic course of the left recurrent laryngeal nerve. The phrenic nerve may also be involved by either left- or right-sided tumors. This produces diaphragmatic paralysis with decreased, absent, or paradoxic diaphragmatic excursion during respiration.

The major vascular syndrome in lung cancer is the superior vena cava syndrome. Obstruction of the vena cava, generally by right-sided lung tumors, produces venous suffusion and edema of the face, neck, and arms along with dilated tortuous collateral vessels over the upper chest and back. Presence of superior vena caval obstruction may constitute a medical emergency requiring early treatment with radiation therapy or chemotherapy if the tumor is a small cell carcinoma.

Pericardial tumor involvement may also constitute a medical emergency with death resulting from cardiac tamponade or from an acute arrhythmia. Physical findings are those of pericarditis in general, including paradoxic pulse, decreased heart sounds, increased cardiac dullness, pericardial friction rub, Kussmaul's sign and Ewart's sign.

The frequency of tumor metastatic symptoms varies by the type of lung cancer. Small cell anaplastic carcinoma and epidermoid carcinoma are at opposite ends of the spectrum of metastatic potential. Nearly every organ or tissue in the body is a potential site for lung cancer metastases so that the number and variety of metastatic symptoms is vast. One metastatic syndrome, namely epidural spinal cord compression, is singled out for mention because it represents a medical and surgical emergency. The presenting symptom is usually back pain. Neurologic examination reveals evidence of sensory or motor impairment with or without abnormalities in bowel or bladder sphincters. Bone x-rays and nuclear scans often demonstrate vertebral tumor involvement. After myelography to localize the obstruction, treatment consists of decompressive laminectomy or radiation therapy or both, depending on the radiosensitivity of the tumor and the rapidity of development of the neurologic deficit.

Paraneoplastic (extrapulmonary, nonendocrine) manifestations may also be seen in lung cancer patients. These include coagulation disorders, either hemorrhagic or thrombotic; osseous abnormalities; neurologic deficits; myopathies; and cutaneous findings. The paraneoplastic osseous lesion associated with lung cancer is hypertrophic pulmonary osteoarthropathy, a clinical syndrome consisting of clubbing of the digits and periostitis of long bones. Symptoms include pain over affected bones with or without an associated polyarthritis. This syndrome is most common in adenocarcinoma patients.

In patients presenting with neurologic abnormalities the differential diagnosis is between a paraneoplastic syndrome versus a metastasis to the nervous system. Helpful clinically in pointing to a paraneoplastic symptom is a symmetrical neurologic deficit that involves several levels of the nervous system simultaneously (e.g., cerebellar findings with a myopathy or with a myasthenia-like picture).

Acanthosis nigricans is the most common cutaneous manifestation of lung cancer. This skin finding is nonspecific, however, in that it may be associated with nonmalignant disease.

Symptoms may also result from the production of hormones or hormone-like substances by lung cancers. Hypercalcemia with its associated clinical symptoms is usually seen in patients with epidermoid lung cancer. Hyponatremia secondary to inappropriate secretion of antidiuretic hormone is noted in patients with small cell anaplastic carcinoma. Occasionally either Cushing's syndrome or carcinoid syndrome is also seen in patients with small cell cancer. Gynecomastia, probably relating to ectopic hormone secretion, is associated with all lung cancer types.

COURSE

Prognosis in lung cancer is determined by histologic type of tumor and by the stage of disease at presentation. In many institutions, the diagnosis of small cell anaplastic carcinoma is a contraindication for surgery. Appropriate therapy consists of combination chemotherapy alone or with radiation therapy. Such treatment is capable of producing disease-free survival of long duration, and possibly cure, in approximately 10 per cent of treated patients.

For non–small cell carcinoma (epidermoid, adenocarcinoma, and large cell anaplastic carcinoma) disease stage determines prognosis. Staging is usually recorded in the tumor-node-metastases (TNM) system. Factors of importance with regard to the primary tumor include the diameter of the lesion, the most proximal extent of tumor on bronchoscopy, whether such sequelae of bronchial obstruction as atelectasis or pneumonitis are present, and whether there is direct tumor extension into adjacent structures such as the pleura or pericardium.

For regional nodal involvement the first lymph node barrier consists of ipsilateral hilar (bronchopulmonary) lymph nodes. Mediastinal (tracheobronchial) nodes and more distant lymph nodes are involved subsequently. For distant metastases only presence or absence is important. Patients with operable lesions generally have primary tumors (T) that do not invade adjacent structures and that by bronchoscopy are greater than 2 cm from the carina. If atelectasis or pneumonitis is present, it involves less than the entire lung. Pleural effusions are absent. Patients whose lesions are operable may have involved ipsilateral hilar lymph nodes (N). With rare exceptions involvement of mediastinal lymph nodes is a contraindication to surgery. The presence of distant metastases (M) is also a contraindication to surgery. If physiologically feasible, all patients with favorable stage epidermoid carcinoma, adenocarcinoma, and large cell anaplastic carcinoma should have a thoracotomy with an attempt at curative resection. The surgeon should sacrifice as little normal lung tissue as possible consistent with complete tumor resection. Thus, when feasible, lobectomy is preferred to pneumonectomy and, on occasion, wedge resections of peripheral lesions may be done. The reason for operations of lesser extent than pneumonectomy is a decreased operative mortality (3 to 5 per cent for lobectomy versus 12 to 15 per cent for pneumonectomy) with equivalent 5-year survival in appropriately staged patients. Further, since patients with resected lung cancer have a high risk of developing a second primary lung cancer, additional lung tissue may have to be resected in the future.

For patients with favorable primary tumors, with no lymph node involvement or only ipsilateral hilar nodes involved, and with no systemic metastases, the 5-year survival after curative surgery exceeds 50 per cent. For all patients with resectable tumors 5-year survival is approximately 25 per cent. The major cause of surgical failure is the presence of undetected metastatic disease.

Unfortunately only 30 to 40 per cent of patients with newly diagnosed lung cancer are candidates for potentially curative tumor resection. The remaining patients are classified as inoperable either because regional or systemic tumor extension is evident during initial staging or because inoperable lesions are detected at thoracotomy. For these patients the median survival is approximately 1 year and only a rare patient survives 5 years. Radiation therapy and chemotherapy are useful in these patients for relieving tumor-related symptoms and for prolonging survival in responding patients.

Since surgery is the only curative treatment modality for non–small cell lung cancer, these lesions must be detected while they are confined to the lung. Pilot projects utilizing quarterly sputum cytology examination plus chest x-ray examination indicate that lung cancer detection may occur prior to the development of symptoms and prior to the appearance of a lesion on the chest x-ray. Tumor localization in such patients is accomplished by fiberoptic bronchoscopy or tantalum bronchography. Preliminary data on resectability rate and 5-year survival in this patient group look promising.

COMPLICATIONS

Complications of lung cancer may be disease- or treatment-related. A partial list of life-threatening complications related to local and regional tumor growth includes hemoptysis, cardiac tamponade, respiratory failure, tracheoesophageal fistula and esophageal obstruction. Since lung cancer metastasizes widely to nearly all organs and tissues of the body, the range of possible complications from metastatic disease is vast.

Complications may also result from paraneoplastic phenomena. Included here would be hemorrhagic and thrombotic side effects secondary to disseminated intravascular coagulation, migratory thrombophlebitis, or nonbacterial thrombotic endocarditis. A variety of neurologic manifestations — including encephalitis, neuropathies, myopathies, and myasthenia-like syndromes — may also be observed. As with other cancers, anorexia, weight loss, and cachexia may be prominent.

Complications may result from endocrine syndromes associated with lung cancer. Hypercalcemia in those patients with epidermoid carcinoma and hyponatremia in patients with small cell anaplastic cancer may pose significant management problems. Occasionally, clinical features of Cushing's syndrome or carcinoid syndrome may be seen.

Treatment-related complications of radiation therapy are acute or chronic. Acute complications include esophagitis with pain on swallowing and cutaneous toxicity with inflammation of the skin in the radiation field. These side effects are generally self-limiting. Chronic radiation complications include radiation pneumonitis and pulmonary fibrosis in nearly all patients treated intensively with radiation therapy. Uncommon complications include the possibility of developing radiation myelitis, carditis, and pericarditis.

Chemotherapy complications are primarily related to the gastrointestinal tract, hair follicles, and bone marrow and include nausea, vomiting, diarrhea, anorexia, mucositis, alopecia, and anemia, leukopenia and thrombocytopenia. Depending on the drugs employed, cardiac toxicity and renal toxicity may pose clinical problems.

LABORATORY STUDIES

Most lung cancer patients present with an abnormal chest x-ray. The first question when an abnormality on chest x-ray is detected is whether the lesion is benign or malignant. If older films are available, a determination of whether the lesion has changed in size can be made. It should be stressed, however, that a lesion may remain the same size for 2 to 3 years and still be malignant. Tomography to look for calcification of the lesion may be useful. If one sees laminated calcium deposition resembling the bull's eye of a target or if one notes a "popcorn" appearance with conglomerated calcium within the lesion, one can assume that the lesion is benign. The detection of a single central calcium deposit or several punctate foci of calcification does not rule out malignancy.

Laboratory studies can be divided into those used primarily for tumor diagnosis and those used for tumor staging. To establish a diagnosis of lung cancer requires that sufficient tissue be obtained and properly processed, so that a pathologist can unequivocally diagnose lung cancer and establish the histologic cell type. For well-differentiated and for moderately well-differentiated epidermoid carcinoma and adenocarcinoma and for small cell anaplastic carcinoma exfoliative cytology may be sufficient, since there is a greater than 90 per cent concordance between cytologic and histologic diagnosis. For poorly differentiated tumors generous tissue specimens are necessary.

Cytologic specimens may best be obtained by bronchoscopy. At presentation over 85 per cent of patients with epidermoid and small cell cancer have malignant cells demonstrable in bronchial washings. For patients with adenocarcinoma and large cell anaplastic carcinoma the yield of positive cytologies is lower. Since these tumors are generally located in the peripheral lung fields, diagnostic tissue may be obtained by needle biopsy if the patient's lesion is clearly inoperable or by thoracotomy if it appears to be resectable.

Sputum collection for cytologic diagnosis is also feasible. Three to five daily sputum specimens are optimal for cancer detection. Thus, in individuals eventually found to have a positive cytology, the detection rate rose from 45 per cent with a single sputum to 86 per cent for 3 sputums to 95 per cent when 5 sputums were collected.

As previously mentioned, sputum cytology examination may be one method of early cancer detection. The basis for this approach is the observation that many lung cancer patients shed cells that demonstrate increasing degrees of cytologic atypia for long periods of time before the detection of frank malignancy. For these early diagnostic techniques to be available to the general public, however, automated methods for sputum cytology reading will have to be developed.

Other surgical procedures useful for establishing a diagnosis of lung cancer include biopsy of any obvious tumor masses found on physical examination, or mediastinoscopy or mediastinotomy for individuals with abnormal mediastinal lymph nodes on chest x-ray. Exploratory thoracotomy should generally not be a diagnostic procedure except in patients with small peripheral lung lesions classified as potentially operable.

Lung cancer staging, for all histologic categories except small cell anaplastic carcinoma, is concerned with determining whether or not the patient is a candidate for surgery. The principal questions are whether the patient has mediastinal lymph node involvement and whether he has systemic metastases. For evaluation of mediastinal nodes roentgenographic, angiographic and/or surgical procedures may be used. Roentgenographic methods, which are the least useful clinically, include anteroposterior, lateral, and oblique pulmonary tomograms. Angiographic procedures include azygous venography or pulmonary angiography or both. These latter procedures are currently underutilized even though they can be performed in a relatively short time, do not require general anesthesia, and are associated with minimal morbidity.

Surgical staging procedures include mediastinoscopy for lesions of the right lung and left lower lobe and mediastinotomy for lesions of the left hilar region and left upper lobe. These procedures are more likely to be positive with centrally located tumors than with peripheral tumors. Mediastinoscopy has replaced blind scalene lymph node biopsy as a procedure to determine patient operability.

The principal difficulty with preoperative staging is in the detection of metastatic disease. Common sites of distant metastases are liver, bone, adrenals, abdominal lymph nodes, and brain. The routine use of radionuclide bone, liver, and brain scans is probably not justified in individuals in whom no clinical or laboratory evidence points to metastases in the specific organ to be scanned, owing to lack of sensitivity of these scans.

Since lung cancer may metastasize widely, staging by specific organ sites appears impractical. Use of radionuclides with affinity for tumor tissue may aid metastatic staging. Gallium-67 citrate is a radionuclide currently in clinical use for this purpose. The possibility of using radio-labeled antibodies to tumor-associated antigens or to fetal proteins produced by lung cancer cells is also being evaluated. Promising preliminary results have been obtained using an antibody to carcinoembryonic antigen.

For small cell anaplastic carcinoma, staging is primarily concerned with the determination of sites of tumor involvement so that response to therapy can be accurately determined. Bone marrow aspiration and biopsy are important, since this test will be positive in about 20 per cent of patients at presentation. Bronchoscopic examination is positive in over 90 per cent of patients. Liver biopsy, either percutaneously or by laparoscopy, is incorporated into many research protocols. Routine scans of bone, liver, and brain may have a place in small cell cancer because of the high frequency of metastases to these sites.

Laboratory tests also aid in following the course of a patient's disease and in assessing response to therapy. The marker most common-ly followed is carcinoembryonic antigen (CEA). CEA is elevated in about 70 per cent of lung cancer patients. Its greatest utility, when initially elevated, is in determining the completeness of surgical resection. CEA levels may also rise prior to clinical detection of tumor recurrence. CEA is not a useful marker for early diagnostic studies.

PITFALLS IN DIAGNOSIS

Too often physicians see patients in whom a chest x-ray abnormality or a new respiratory symptom or sign has been noted in the past but who have not been thoroughly evaluated as to the cause of the abnormality. Other patients may have been given long trials of antibiotic treatment to rule out pulmonary infection. This watch and wait attitude must be condemned if lung cancer is to be diagnosed at a time when it is surgically resectable. Until environmental and occupational carcinogen exposure can be eliminated, early diagnosis provides the best prospect for improving the survival of lung cancer patients.

DISORDERS OF THE PLEURA

By PETER A. EMERSON, M.D.
London, England

DRY PLEURISY

This term is applied to fibrinous pleurisy with fibrinous exudate only. There is pain on inspiration, sneezing, and rib cage movements and characteristically a pleural rub is heard.

Dry pleurisy is most commonly due to disease in the underlying lung. Any of the conditions causing pleurisy with effusion may present initially as dry pleurisy before the fluid accumulates. When a patient has a persistent dry pleurisy but an apparently normal chest radiograph, several conditions should be particularly considered. Tuberculosis can cause a low-grade dry pleurisy that can persist for months. The tuberculin test will be positive. Rheumatoid disease can be accompanied by dry pleurisy. Sometimes it is the presenting feature of systemic lupus erythematosus. Trauma can cause simple bruising of the parietal pleura with pain and a pleural rub that may persist long after the pain has subsided. A shallow pneumothorax may cause pleural friction as the lung re-expands; this presents as an apparent dry pleurisy. Dry pleurisy may be associated with pleural plaques owing to asbestos exposure in addition to being an initial presentation of a pleural mesothelioma. Radiation and certain cytotoxic drugs such as methotrexate can cause dry pleurisy. Although often diagnosed, viral infections rarely cause dry pleurisy unless there is pneumonia. An exception is epidemic myalgia, but even in this condition a pleural rub is unusual and an effusion rare.

EPIDEMIC MYALGIA (BORNHOLM DISEASE)

As its name suggests, this is primarily an infection of intercostal muscle caused by the Coxsackievirus Group B. Pain is severe, as is indicated by one of its eponyms, "the devil's grip"; it is aggravated by all movements of the chest and associated with intercostal tenderness. Pain in the shoulder from involvement of the diaphragm is common. Fever is not always present and the erythrocyte sedimentation rate (ESR) is normal or only slightly raised. Charac-

teristically, the pain and any fever may subside and recur several times before finally settling.

The diagnosis may be made by virus isolation from throat washings or stools during the acute phase but usually is made by the demonstration, in paired sera, of a rising titer of complement-fixing and neutralizing antibiotics to one of the Group B Coxsackie viruses.

PLEURAL EFFUSIONS

The cause may be obvious from pre-existing disease or from an easily demonstrated underlying lung lesion, but we are concerned with the presenting problem of fluid in the pleural space without obvious evidence of an underlying lung lesion. Fluid may be in the general pleural space or located between lobes, above the diaphragm, or against the chest wall or mediastinum.

Radiographic Appearances. Fluid causes a dense homogenous opacity. A moderate-sized effusion in the general pleural space appears as a triangular shadow based on the diaphragm with the apex curving up and out into the axilla. If one thinks of the lung as a balloon being pushed down into the chest half full of water, the reason for the increased radiographic density going up into the axilla is obvious. The upper level of the fluid is in fact always horizontal but is only seen as a horizontal fluid level if there is air as well as fluid in the pleural space (hydropneumothorax).

If radiographs are taken first upright and then in the lateral decubitus position, the fluid, unless encysted, can be observed to collect in the most dependent part of the pleural space and thus can be differentiated from consolidation and other conditions.

Ultrasound. With either B-mode or the M-mode ultrasound used for echocardiography, the site and depth of an effusion can be precisely defined. This is particularly useful before aspiration and in the elucidation of effusions caused by subdiaphragmatic infection.

Computerized Tomography (CT) Scan. This method is of particular value in assessing abnormalities of the pleura, particularly in deciding whether an effusion in a patient with parenchymal lung changes is a simple asbestosis effusion (pleura clear after aspiration) or is due to mesothelioma.

Diagnostic Pneumoperitoneum. The use of ultrasound now elucidates the problem of infrapulmonary collections of fluid and subdiaphragmatic infections, so pneumoperitoneum is no longer necessary. It can still be useful in demonstrating the small diaphragmatic defects referred to later. The air passes through into the pleura.

Examining the Fluid. The chest radiograph does not indicate whether the fluid is serous fluid, pus, chyle, or blood. This can only be determined by aspirating a small sample of fluid from any significant collection of fluid in the pleural space.

SEROUS EFFUSIONS

Cytologic examination of the fluid is of prime importance. Polymorphs favor an inflammatory cause other than tuberculosis when the predominant cells are lymphocytes. However, polymorphs are often replaced by lymphocytes in any serous effusion of some weeks' duration.

Eosinophilia in the pleural fluid most commonly occurs when there has been some minor extravasation of blood into the pleural space, for instance in pulmonary infarction. Pleural eosinophilia may also accompany peripheral blood eosinophilia as in polyarteritis nodosa and allergic lung disease. Bacteriologic examination by direct smear and culture for tuberculosis and other organisms is essential.

Chemical studies on pleural fluid are not practically helpful except in the diagnosis of effusion complicating acute pancreatitis, when the pleural fluid amylase concentration may be much in excess of that in the serum. The pleural fluid glucose is low in infections and effusions owing to rheumatoid disease. If infection can be excluded, a very low pleural fluid glucose (< 20 mg per 100 ml) is virtually diagnostic of rheumatoid effusion.

Pleural Biopsy

Needle biopsy of the pleura using an Abrams or Cope needle (taking several specimens) should be done at the time of initial diagnostic aspiration in all patients with undiagnosed pleurisy with effusion. Adequate biopsies are obtained in about 85 per cent. True positive results may be expected in about 65 per cent of patients whose effusions are due to tuberculosis and in about 50 per cent of those due to malignancy. A report of nonspecific inflammation does not exclude the more specific diagnoses. In these patients and those in whom a satisfactory biopsy is not obtained, the choice lies between thoracoscopy and pleural biopsy, limited thoracotomy and pleural biopsy, and full thoracotomy. The choice must depend on the circumstances and skills available. Provided that sufficient fluid can be aspirated and replaced with air, thoracoscopy and pleural biopsy will be the method of choice. When this is not possible, one or another form of thoracotomy is necessary.

The conditions listed in Table 1 must be considered when diagnostic aspiration yields straw-colored serous fluid.

PURULENT EFFUSIONS (EMPYEMA)

The following are causes of pus in the pleural space: lung infections such as lung abscess, pneumonia, tuberculosis, and fungal infections; subphrenic abscess; bronchopleural fistula, especially after lung resection; penetrating chest wounds with rupture of the esophagus. Sometimes there is no clinical evidence of a lung infection and the empyema appears to be the primary event — this is more likely to occur in diabetic patients or patients who are immunologically compromised.

Usually the diagnosis is made when an obvious collection of fluid in the pleural space is aspirated and pus is present. Severe and persistent pain suggests the presence of pus as opposed to serous fluid. Sometimes, however, the diagnosis is difficult and delayed. The underlying or preceding cause may not be apparent and the patient has some or all of the following indications: chronic ill health with persistent or intermittent low fever; peripheral blood polymorphonucleocytosis, anemia and raised ESR; finger clubbing; and unusual chest radiographic appearances that are difficult to interpret because they represent pockets of pus encysted along the chest wall or mediastinum or between lobes.

The key to the diagnosis is to keep in mind all the alternatives and to do chest aspiration, preferably after localizing any packets by ultrasound.

CHYLOTHORAX

Chylothorax is an unusual condition that is classically due to rupture of the thoracic duct. The duct may be ruptured by a nonpenetrating injury causing stretching of the thoracic duct over the vertebral bodies, such as landing from a jump, vomiting, and even coughing.

Usually a latent interval occurs after the injury. The duct ruptures and chyle starts to collect under the mediastinal pleura; the subpleural collection of chyle may resemble a tumor. Then, a week or month later the pleura gives way and the chyle escapes into the pleural space. The patient becomes short of breath and develops the physical and radiologic signs of chylothorax.

The thoracic duct is more likely to rupture if

Table 1.   Causes and Characteristics of Serous Fluid in the Pleural Space

Malignant disease, e.g., mesothelioma, metastatic carcinoma from lung, breast, ovary, also reticuloses and myeloma	Effusions often blood-stained and contain neoplastic cells; pleural needle biopsy positive in about 50 per cent of patients; thoracoscopy and biopsy useful.
Tuberculosis, e.g., post-primary tuberculosis in young adults or complicating established disease, usually in older persons	Straw-colored lymphocytic fluid; tubercle bacilli rarely seen on direct smear but grow on culture in about 60 per cent of patients; needle pleural biopsy diagnostic in about 65 per cent; tuberculin test positive.
Postpneumonic effusions	Serous fluid with polymorphs initially; untreated may proceed to empyema; causative organisms may be isolated.
Effusions secondary to subdiaphragmatic abscess or liver infection—whether amebic or simple abscess	Serous fluid with polymorphs; usually sterile unless an empyema develops; ultrasound diagnostic.
Asbestos effusions: benign pleural effusions; may be recurrent and occur unrelated to mesothelioma; usually evidence of parenchymal lung change due to asbestosis	Serous effusion: Cytology pleomorphic but no neoplastic cells and pleural biopsy nonspecific; history of asbestosis raises specter of mesothelioma; CT scan after aspiration clear.
Effusions due to acute pancreatitis	Serous fluid with amylase activity in the pleural fluid (500 to 2000 units), higher than in the blood; at autopsy pleura shows fat necrosis.
Pulmonary infarction	Straw-colored or blood-stained fluid; sometimes has a raised eosinophil content.
Acute rheumatic fever	Pleurisy with or without effusion in 10 per cent of cases.
Rheumatoid disease	Serous effusion; pleural fluid glucose much lower than the serum glucose; RA factor positive as in blood.
Systemic lupus erythematosus	A common manifestation; cytology pleomorphic; LE cells seen but more usual to identify ANF and DNA antibodies in blood.
Polyarteritis nodosa	Serous effusion with high eosinophil content.
Radiation pleurisy	Serous effusion usually several weeks after therapy; cytology pleomorphic; no malignant cells.
Adverse drug reactions, e.g., intramuscular methotrexate, oral practolol	Drug history is the clue. There may be others!
Massive onset of effusion (usually right sided) complicating ascites owing to malignant peritoneal involvement, ovarian fibroma (Meigs' syndrome), liver cirrhosis	Due to a small rupture of the tendinous part of the diaphragm; therefore ascitic and pleural fluids have the same characteristics; aspiration of pleural fluid relieves the ascites; communication can be demonstrated by pneumoperitoneum or other methods.
Transudates caused by cardiac failure or hypoproteinemia due to nephrotic syndrome, liver cirrhosis, protein-losing enteropathy	Cause usually clinically obvious; clear straw-colored fluid with few cells, low protein, low lactic dehydrogenase activity.

it is blocked centrally by, for instance, a mediastinal tumor; at other times it may actually be eroded by tumor. Other rare causes of obstruction are filariasis and tuberculosis.

Chylous Reflux. Apart from rupture of the thoracic duct in its mediastinal course, chylothorax may also occur when there is reflux of chyle and distended tributory lymphatics have ruptured, sometimes causing multiple small fistulas that weep chyle. This condition of chylous reflux is not necessarily associated with malignant disease. There may be a developmental blockage of the thoracic duct system.

Diagnosis of Chylothorax. The diagnosis may be suspected from the chest radiograph because the fat content of the collection of chyle makes it less radiopaque than other effusions. Confirmation depends on the aspiration of the chyle.

HEMOTHORAX AND HEMORRHAGIC EFFUSIONS

It is not always easy to distinguish between a blood-stained effusion and a true hemothorax. An originally serous effusion may be complicated by bleeding, especially if the patient is treated with anticoagulants; when primary bleeding occurs into the pleural space there is always a reactive outpouring of serous fluid that then dilutes the blood. For this reason, it is useful to measure the hemoglobin concentration of the fluid. Even in frank hemothorax, it will seldom be above 50 per cent and as time passes, the concentration falls further. Hemorrhagic effusions may be expected to have a concentration of under 10 per cent.

Causes of Hemothorax. The majority of cases of hemothorax and hemopneumothorax follow penetrating or nonpenetrating injuries to the chest. Spontaneous hemopneumothorax occurs when spontaneous pneumothorax is complicated by bleeding from a ruptured adhesion. In the majority of patients who present with blood, but no air, in the pleural space, there has recently been a hemopneumothorax from which the air but not the blood has been reabsorbed. Other causes of hemothorax are bleeding from pleural metastases and such rarities as endometriosis of the pleura.

Causes of Hemorrhagic Effusions. These are pleural metastases, pulmonary infarction, and tuberculous effusions (rarely).

PLEURAL FIBROSIS AND CALCIFICATION

Pleural Plaques. Local plaques on the parietal pleura are normally discovered on routine chest radiographs of persons who have been exposed to asbestos dust, either industrially or in the environment. A holly leaf pattern of calcification may develop and plaques are mainly seen on the chest radiograph when they are tangential to the x-ray beam on the lateral chest wall or along the diaphragm. There is almost certainly a relationship between the presence of such plaques and the eventual development of mesothelioma.

More Extensive Pleural Thickening. More extensive fibrosis of the visceral pleura occurs when the parenchyma of the lung is more extensively involved by asbestosis. It also occurs following incompletely resolved pleuropulmonary infections, after hemothorax and thoracotomy, as a result of radiation fibrosis, and as an adverse drug reaction to practolol. A particular apical form of fibrosis occurs in ankylosing spondylitis.

PNEUMOTHORAX

Table 2 shows the various causes of pneumothorax. The onset is usually signaled by the sudden onset of pain in the chest laterally and usually in the shoulder, accompanied by progressive shortness of breath. The pleural leak may seal itself spontaneously (closed pneumothorax); it may remain freely open so that the pleural space freely communicates with the atmosphere (open pneumothorax); or it may act as a one-way valve allowing air into the pleural space when the patient raises his intra-alveolar pressure by coughing or forced expiration. In this case air is never allowed out, so that the intrapleural pressure gets progressively greater (tension pneumothorax). This results in collapse of first the ipsilateral lung; then the mediastinum is displaced and even the contralateral lung collapses.

The clinical and radiologic signs of pneumothorax are as would be expected and are usually obvious. Difficulties arise, however, when the pneumothorax is a quite shallow one. The classical physical signs will be absent but if the pneumothorax is on the left there may be a "pleural click"; this is heard, not just with the stethoscope, but often by the patient and sometimes by other people in the room. It is due to a curious amplification of the heart sounds by the acoustic conditions of the shallow left pneumothorax. It is sometimes mistaken for the mediastinal crunch (Homan's sign) of pneumomediastinum.

When a pneumothorax is suspected but not seen on the routine chest radiograph taken in inspiration, it is essential to take a film in full expiration.

Table 2. *Examples of Occurrence and Causes of Pneumothorax*

1. In otherwise healthy young adults (usually males 5:1)	Lungs are usually normal apart from localized apical scars with associated bullae.
2. In patients with chronic lung disease with airflow obstruction	Older patients with chronic bronchitis and emphysema; asthmatics.
3. After certain invasive diagnostic and therapeutic procedures	Lung, pleural, liver biopsies; anesthetic blocks; operations on cervical fascia; acupuncture.
4. After trauma	Penetrating and nonpenetrating chest injuries.
5. Complicating neonatal respiratory distress syndrome	As a complication of IPPV, especially if PEEP used.
6. Complicating localized lung disorders	PTB; lung abscess; hydatid disease; metastases from bone sarcoma.
7. As a common complication of rare disease (∴ rare)	Tuberous sclerosis; lymphangioleiomyomatosis; eosinophilic granuloma; connective tissue disorders.
8. Decompression	In divers and air travelers.

PRIMARY PLEURAL TUMORS

Fibroma of the pleura is uncommon, and there is seldom an effusion unless the tumor becomes malignant. Clubbing is almost invariable and hypertrophic pulmonary osteoarthropathy may occur.

Diffuse malignant mesothelioma is becoming more common, and there are now about 300 cases reported each year in the United Kingdom. It is now recognized that the development of a mesothelioma of the pleura or peritoneum is often etiologically related to inhalation of asbestos up to 40 years previously. Contact with asbestos may have amounted only to living near or walking through the factory or merely cleaning workers' clothing — very much less than is required for the development of pulmonary asbestosis or even pleural plaques. It is also common in certain villages in Turkey where the size of the rock strata crystals are the same as those of asbestos, with obvious implications.

The name of one of the villages translated into English is "Pain in the Chest."

The course is more benign than for other pleural malignancies and the patient may survive for several years. Pain and shortness of breath result from the pleural involvement but episodes of pulmonary infarction may occur and give rise to additional contralateral chest pain.

The effusion is usually blood-stained and rapidly recurs after aspiration. Malignant mesothelial cells may be recognized on microscopy of the fluid.

The tumor does not metastasize to distant organs until late, but it is locally invasive, involving the chest wall, extruding through needle tracts or incisions or growing into the mediastinum or through the diaphragm. The tumor may also break through to the skin over areas where x-ray therapy has been given. For these reasons any interference does more harm than good and should be resisted. Patients who are left alone live longest.

Section 6

DISEASES OF THE CARDIOVASCULAR SYSTEM

CONGESTIVE HEART FAILURE

By NANETTE K. WENGER, M.D.,
Atlanta, Georgia

DEFINITION

Congestive heart failure is not a specific etiologic diagnosis but rather must be considered as a manifestation of numerous cardiovascular disease states. Thus the delineation of congestive heart failure requires identification of the underlying disease and precipitating factor or factors. It is defined as an inability of the heart to pump enough blood to supply the requirements of the body.

PATHOGENESIS

Congestive heart failure results from overloading of the compensatory mechanisms of the heart by an excessive pressure load (as with aortic stenosis), an excessive volume load (as with anemia, mitral regurgitation, patent ductus arteriosus), the loss of functional myocardial tissue (as with cardiomyopathy or myocardial infarction), or restriction to cardiac filling (as occurs with mitral stenosis, constrictive pericarditis, etc.). Dysrhythmias, characterized by an excessively slow or rapid rate, may also impair cardiac output.

The several compensatory cardiac mechanisms — dilatation, hypertrophy, increased sympathetic activity (with resultant tachycardia, increased myocardial contractility, sodium and water retention, etc.), and increased arteriovenous oxygen extraction — all function initially to sustain the previously described cardiac stresses. When these fail, congestive heart failure supervenes.

PRESENTING SYMPTOMS

The presenting symptoms of congestive heart failure vary considerably with the underlying cardiovascular disease, but they, as well as the physical findings and laboratory abnormalities, tend predominantly to reflect dysfunction of organ systems other than the heart. The majority of symptoms relate to excessive sodium and water retention and resultant pulmonary and systemic vascular congestion.

Dyspnea, an unpleasant awareness of breathing, difficulty in breathing, or breathlessness, reflects pulmonary venous congestion and hypertension. It initially occurs only with severe exertion (effort dyspnea), but as the severity of the heart failure progresses, may occur at rest. In describing dyspnea, the amount of effort required to precipitate it should be delineated.

Orthopnea, shortness of breath on recumbency that diminishes in the upright position, is due to the augmented systemic venous return on assuming the recumbent position; pulmonary vascular congestion increases and the vital capacity decreases. The severity of orthopnea is described by the elevation of the head required to relieve the symptom (e.g., one pillow, two pillows).

Paroxysmal nocturnal dyspnea, an almost specific finding for left ventricular failure, is characterized by the patient awakening from sleep with a feeling of suffocation, typically at the same hour of the evening, often 1 to 2 hours after falling asleep. Cough, anxiety, and at times wheezing are present, and the patient will sit up or run to the window seeking fresh air. The episode typically lasts 15 to 20 minutes. The genesis of the pulmonary congestion is a combination of the increased venous return associated with recumbency and resorption of edema fluid from previously dependent areas.

Acute pulmonary edema, a medical emergency, is caused by sudden transudation of fluid into the alveolar spaces as a result of acute elevation of the pulmonary capillary pressure. The patient sits upright, complaining of "smothering," gasping for breath, with pink frothy sputum coming from the nose and mouth. Pulmonary capillary rupture is the genesis of the pink tinge to the sputum.

Edema, a detectable increase of fluid in the interstitial spaces evident as soft tissue swelling, reflects the body's excessive content of sodium and water. The edema is initially dependent, beginning in the ankles, but progresses to involve the legs and genitals; initially the edema accumulates increasingly during the day but subsides overnight; severe, long-standing edema typically persists after a night of sleep. Although edema is typically encountered with right ventricular failure, it may also occur with isolated left ventricular failure, with the decreased cardiac output and diminished renal blood flow causing the sodium and water retention. In the bedbound patient, it may be seen in the presacral area.

Ascites, an accumulation of intraperitoneal fluid, is detected by the patient as an increase in abdominal girth. It may be associated with a complaint of right upper quadrant pain, reflecting hepatic congestion.

Additional symptoms of a decreased cardiac output include progressively severe fatigue and weakness as evidence of diminished muscle blood flow, as well as dizziness, somnolence, and confusion as evidence of diminished cerebral perfusion. Sweating and low-grade fever are seen owing to cutaneous vasoconstriction and poor heat loss. Anorexia, at times constipation, and nausea and vomiting may relate both to the diminished cardiac output and to visceral congestion; abdominal discomfort, particularly in the right upper quadrant, reflects distention of the hepatic capsule. Patients may also complain of nocturia (as tissue fluid is mobilized and renal perfusion increases in the recumbent position), in association with oliguria during the daylight hours when the patient is upright.

PHYSICAL EXAMINATION

As with the presenting symptoms, physical findings relate to pulmonary vascular congestion; to cardiac dilatation, hypertrophy, or restriction to diastolic filling; to fluid accumulation in the interstitial spaces and in the pleural, pericardial, and peritoneal cavities; and particularly to the elevation of the systemic venous pressure.

There is an increase in body weight over baseline level, typically associated with dependent edema, reflecting right ventricular failure; presacral edema is encountered in the patient at bed rest. When the edema is chronic, brawny induration, particularly of the feet and ankles, may be encountered. However, with long-standing, severe heart failure, cardiac cachexia with tissue wasting may be evident. Cool or cold extremities are evidence of peripheral vasoconstriction. Peripheral cyanosis reflects increased tissue extraction of oxygen.

Respirations are shallow and often rapid. Especially in older patients with cerebrovascular disease, severe congestive heart failure may be associated with Cheyne-Stokes respiration, alternating periods of hyperpnea, and apnea.

The blood pressure is variable; the patient with severe congestive heart failure, as typically encountered in the setting of myocardial infarction, often presents with hypotension. However, many patients with moderate to severe untreated congestive heart failure may have mild diastolic hypertension, reflecting compensatory sympathetic vasoconstriction; in this instance, blood pressure may return to normal with treatment of the congestive heart failure.

The heart rate may also vary considerably, as may the cardiac rhythm, typically dependent on the underlying disease. However, pulsus alternans, a regular alternation of strong and weak beats best felt at the femoral pulse, is a sign of severe left ventricular dysfunction.

Examination of the jugular veins for pressure and pulse contour is an important component of the evaluation of the patient with congestive heart failure. Elevation of the jugular venous column reflects elevation of systemic venous pressure. With the patient sitting at 30 to 60 degrees a jugular venous column over 3 cm above the sternal angle denotes an elevated systemic venous pressure. Additionally, the hand veins will remain distended when the hand is held above the level of the right atrium. As regards the jugular venous pulse contour, a large regurgitant systolic wave may reflect tricuspid regurgitation. Firm 30 to 60 second right upper quadrant pressure may force blood from a congested liver into the jugular venous system, raising the level of the jugular venous column, the hepatojugular reflux.

Palpation of the precordium typically shows an enlarged, diffuse, and sustained left ventricular impulse, reflecting left ventricular dilatation and hypertrophy. When right ventricular dilatation and hypertrophy are part of the underlying disease, a left parasternal or subxiphoid impulse or both may be prominent. On auscultation S_3 and S_4 sounds, reflected as a gallop rhythm when the heart rate is rapid, may be present; the S_3 is evidence of a noncompliant ventricle with an increased residual diastolic volume or a large volume load with rapid early diastolic filling; an S_4 is frequently encountered in the absence of heart failure when there is abnormal ventricular compliance. Murmurs of mitral or tricuspid regurgitation or both, reflecting valve ring dilatation and/or valve apparatus and papillary muscle dysfunction, are common with severe failure; they typically decrease or disappear as cardiac compensation improves.

Examination of the lungs shows moist rales owing to pulmonary congestion. Initially they are bibasilar, but as the severity of the congestive heart failure increases, they are audible higher in the lung fields. These rales persist after a cough or after deep breathing and may be associated with wheezing owing to bronchospasm or fluid or both, within the bronchi. In the patient with pulmonary edema, bubbling moist rales are present throughout the lung fields, associated with rhonchi and wheezes; supraclavicular and intercostal retraction are common. The patient with pulmonary edema has profound dyspnea, tachypnea, agitation, cyanosis, sweating, and flaring of alae nasae, and there is typically copious pink frothy sputum coming from the mouth and nose. With severe chronic congestive heart failure, the accumulation of pleural fluid may be reflected as dullness to percussion at the lung bases, associated with a decrease in tactile fremitus and decreased or absent breath sounds. Pleural effusion tends to occur bilaterally; when unilateral, it is almost invariably right-sided.

Ascites, the accumulation of peritoneal fluid, is due to a combination of hepatocellular dysfunction from liver congestion and sodium and water retention. This accumulation of peritoneal fluid is detected by a distended abdomen of increased girth, with a fluid wave and shifting dullness to examination. Hepatosplenomegaly may be detected.

LABORATORY TESTS

The *electrocardiogram* is of no value either to detect or to quantify the degree of congestive heart failure. Its main use is in providing a clue to the underlying cardiovascular disease.

X-ray examination of the chest is the most important laboratory test in the patient with congestive heart failure, reflecting variable degrees of cardiovascular dilatation and hypertrophy, dependent on the underlying disease. When left ventricular failure occurs, the radiographic changes reflect pulmonary venous hypertension. Initially, there is a redistribution of venous blood from the lower to the upper lobes of the lungs, with resultant prominence of the superior pulmonary veins. As the severity of the failure increases, interstitial pulmonary edema develops with evidence of fluid in the subsegmental fissures (Kerley lines) and in the perivascular and peribronchial spaces. Finally, with pulmonary edema, the lung fields are hazy and blurred, and there is blurring of the mediastinal margins with soft patchy perihilar (butterfly appearance) infiltrates. The pleural effusions may be unilateral or bilateral and occur late in the course of biventricular failure.

Blood tests typically reflect end organ dysfunction. Renal dysfunction may be evidenced by azotemia (typically with a normal creatinine level) and proteinuria, liver dysfunction by elevation of the liver enzymes serum glutamic oxaloacetic transaminase (SGOT) and lactic dehydrogenase (LDH) and at times by hyperbilirubinemia and prolongation of the prothrombin time. Hyperglycemia may be encountered as a reflection of increased sympathetic activity.

Examination of the pleural fluid should be consistent with a transudate; that is, it should have a low protein content, specific gravity, and osmolarity. The fluid should not clot on standing, should not be bloody, and should contain fewer than 1000 cells per ml.

Arterial blood gases may be valuable in distinguishing between heart failure and chronic obstructive pulmonary disease. The patient with chronic obstructive pulmonary disease typically has a depressed PO_2, an elevated PCO_2, and a decreased pH as evidence of respiratory acidosis; occasionally, an elevated bicarbonate may reflect metabolic compensation of this problem. The patient with left ventricular failure has a depressed PO_2, a normal or depressed PCO_2, and respiratory alkalosis evidenced by an elevated pH.

Determination of the venous pressure and circulation time is not commonly done. Elevation of the venous pressure may be documented by physical examination of the neck veins; however, a rapid circulation time in the presence of congestive heart failure is highly suggestive of a high-output etiology.

Echocardiography may help quantitate cardiac chamber dimensions, wall thickness, and ventricular function. As noninvasive tests, serial studies are possible and help define the response to therapy.

Pulmonary function tests help identify lung disease and differentiate its symptoms from those of congestive heart failure. ·

Cardiac catheterization, angiocardiography, and/or *radionuclide imaging* may be of value in elucidating the underlying cardiovascular problem.

In the patient with latent heart failure, provocative tests may be important. Exercise, such as sit-ups or isometric challenge with hand grip, may produce S_3 and S_4 sounds, an apical presystolic impulse, and/or the murmur of mitral regurgitation. Indeed, even more formal *multilevel exercise stress testing* may help differentiate the anxious patient from one with underlying cardiovascular disease. Exercise testing may help quantify cardiovascular dysfunction. It may identify cardiovascular dysfunction not evident at rest, which is provoked by varying degrees of activity, and may help, by serial functional assessment, to define the response to therapeutic interventions.

COURSE AND COMPLICATIONS

The course of congestive heart failure depends primarily on the type and severity of the underlying cardiovascular disease.

Typically, the patient responds well to management whose basic components include a decrease of activity, sodium restriction and diuretic agents to decrease sodium and water retention and thus systemic and pulmonary vascular congestion, digitalis to enhance myocardial contractility, and vasodilator therapy to enhance myocardial performance.

The major complications are those of thromboembolism, related particularly to relatively prolonged immobilization, and circulatory stasis. Pulmonary embolism with major pulmonary vascular obstruction may present as an acute cardiovascular emergency with dyspnea, pain, syncope, hypotension, and hypoxemia. Small recurrent emboli may be virtually symptomless, other than increasing the severity of the congestive heart failure.

Congestive heart failure may be precipitated or aggravated by a number of remediable factors: infection, dysrhythmia, anemia, undue physical activity, emotional stress, excessive sodium intake. Control of these may significantly improve cardiac compensation.

PITFALLS IN DIAGNOSIS

Many other diseases may also produce the symptoms commonly associated with congestive heart failure. Dyspnea may reflect respiratory disease, anemia, fever, obesity, or anxiety; similarly, orthopnea is common in the patient with lung disease. Edema may relate to renal disease, to hepatic disease, to malnutrition, and particularly to local venous or lymphatic disease. Fatigue may be seen with anxiety and depression or with severe lung disease, anemia, and many other systemic illnesses.

Congestive heart failure in the infant or young child may present a diagnostic challenge, because the presenting signs and symptoms differ from those in the adult. The infant and young child frequently present with cough, breathlessness, and difficulty in feeding. Other signs are tachypnea, sweating particularly at night, suprasternal and intercostal retraction, hepatomegaly and periorbital edema. Extremity edema is a relatively rare and late finding.

Similarly, the pregnant patient may have many findings that simulate congestive heart failure, which are related to the anemia, the hyperpnea, and the edema secondary to venous obstruction of the legs. The common complaints of fatigability, the observed hyperventilation, and the common third heart sounds and flow murmurs may cause further confusion.

CONGENITAL HEART DISEASE IN INFANTS AND CHILDREN

By WILLIAM B. BLANCHARD, M.D.,
and BENJAMIN E. VICTORICA, M.D.

Gainesville, Florida

Congenital diseases of the heart are one of the leading causes of death from birth defects in the first year of life. Consequently, any physician who provides care to infants and children should have a working knowledge of the pathophysiology of these anomalies and a sound approach to their diagnosis. In this decade alone significant advances in noninvasive technology have made the clinical evaluation of children with congenital heart disease more precise. While many of the more technically sophisticated methods may not be logistically available to the primary practitioner, the greatest accuracy in providing correct diagnosis still depends upon proper detailed physical examination and history supported by the conventional chest x-ray and 12-lead electrocardiogram (ECG). Additionally, the advent of M-mode echocardiography has provided useful insight into the basic anatomy and hemodynamic consequences of many of these lesions. In this chapter we emphasize the clinical presentation of the most commonly encountered congenital defects of the heart and outline their evaluation with these basic diagnostic tools.

The most common congenital heart defects encountered in the pediatric age range are shown in Figure 1. Acyanotic defects predominate, with left-to-right shunt lesions accounting for approximately 50 per cent of all congenital cardiac anomalies.

Usually, congenital cardiac defects occur as isolated anomalies but may on occasion be part of a chromosomal aberration or specific syndrome. Table 1 lists the most commonly encountered syndromes and genetic disorders with their associated cardiac defects.

DIAGNOSTIC CLUES AND TOOLS

CHEST X-RAY

Any child suspected of having a congenital cardiac anomaly should have a routine posteroanterior (PA) and lateral chest x-ray. Generally the approach to the chest x-ray should emphasize three stages of analysis: (1) evaluation of the bones, soft tissues, and other extracardiac structures; (2) evaluation of position of the aortic arch, great vessel relationship, cardiac size and contour; and (3) interpretation of the hemodynamic consequences of the underlying cardiac anomaly, particularly the status of the pulmonary vascularity.

Examination of the bony thorax will often provide evidence of previous surgical thoracotomy by showing narrowing of an anterior or posterior intercostal space, rib irregularities, or the presence of sternal wires. Many cardiac defects are associated with thoracic skeletal anomalies (hemivertebrae, kyphoscoliosis), particularly in tetralogy of Fallot.

The presence of a right aortic arch is important because of its higher association with cyanotic defects, as in 25 per cent of patients with tetralogy of Fallot.

The contribution of the different cardiac structures to the normal contour of the heart is

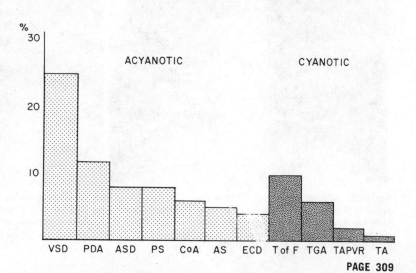

Figure 1. Overall incidence of the most common congenital heart defects. Key: VSD = ventricular septal defect; PDA = patent ductus arteriosus; ASD = atrial septal defect; PS = pulmonic valve stenosis; CoA = coarctation of the aorta; AS = aortic valve stenosis; ECD = endocardial cushion defect; ToF = tetralogy of Fallot; TGA = CTGV = complete transposition of the great arteries (vessels); TAPVR = total anomalous pulmonary venous return; TA = tricuspid valve atresia.

Table 1. *Common Syndromes and Genetic Disorders and Their Associated Cardiac Defects*

Syndrome	Characteristic Features	Associated Cardiac Defect
Down's syndrome (Trisomy 21)	Mental retardation, hypotonia, typical facies	ECD
Turner's syndrome (X0)	Short stature, ovarian dysgenesis, congenital lymphedema, broad chest with widely spaced nipples, webbing of the neck	CoA
Noonan's syndrome	Turner-like syndrome with normal chromosomes; mental retardation, short stature, hypertelorism, pectum excavatum, cryptorchidism	PS, ASD
Holt-Oram syndrome	Upper limb defects with hypoplasia and proximal placement of the thumb	ASD, atrial arrhythmias, VSD
Marfan's syndrome	Tall stature, arachnodactyly, subluxation of the lens, kyphoscoliosis	Dilatation of the aorta, AI, MVP with MI
Congenital rubella	Mental and growth deficiency, cataracts, nerve deafness, hepatosplenomegaly, thrombocytopenia	PDA, coarctation of pulmonary arteries
Fetal alcohol	Mental and growth deficiency, microcephaly, maxillary hypoplasia, altered palmar crease patterns	VSD, ASD, TOF

Key: See Legend, Figure 1. AI, aortic valve insufficiency; MI, mitral valve insufficiency; MVP, mitral valve prolapse.

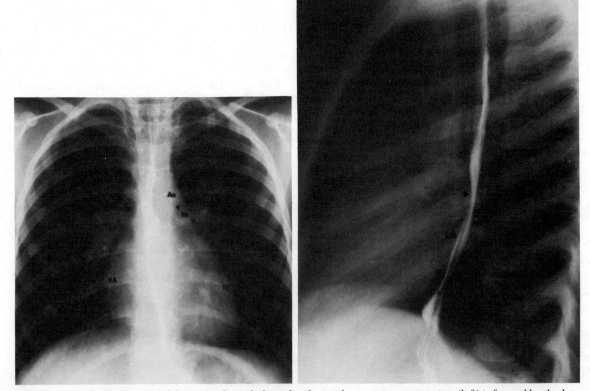

Figure 2.   Normal chest x-ray with barium. The right heart border on the posteroanterior view (left) is formed by the lower aspect of the superior vena cava (SVC) and the lateral wall of the right atrium (RA). The left heart border is made up by the aortic knob and the first portion of the descending aorta (Ao), the main pulmonary artery (PA), and the lateral wall of the left ventricle (LV). Note on the lateral view (right) the mild indentation produced by the posterior wall of the left atrium (LA) into the inferior portion of the barium-filled esophagus.

shown in Figure 2. The addition of barium swallow to the lateral view helps in determining the size of the left atrium. Recognition of the abnormal contour will assist the practitioner in determining the site of the underlying cardiac defect. Gross cardiomegaly rarely occurs with lesions that mainly cause ventricular hypertrophy (obstructive lesions).

Cardiomegaly is more often the result of volume overload such as in large left-to-right shunts or valve insufficiency lesions, or it may be due to congestive heart failure. Left atrial dilatation with posterior displacement of the barium-filled esophagus in the lateral view in the presence of volume overload of the left atrium (increased pulmonary venous return or mitral regurgitation) indicates an intact interatrial septum.

Right heart enlargement is characterized by either a dilated right atrium, an upturned cardiac apex, or a prominent pulmonary artery. In contrast, signs of left heart enlargement include a dilated left atrium, a down-turned apex with a straight left heart border, and a concavity in the area of the pulmonary artery.

Perhaps the most valuable radiographic clue in determining the functional or hemodynamic consequences of a cardiac defect is the assessment of the pulmonary vascularity. *Shunt vascularity* (large dilated arterial vessels throughout the lung fields) indicates the presence of an intra- or extracardiac left-to-right shunt. The associated finding of left atrial enlargement helps localize the level of the shunt to distal to the atrioventricular valves and implies an intact interatrial septum. In contrast, increased markings of the *pulmonary venous obstructive* type (redistribution of flow in the upper lobes with dilated pulmonary veins and ill-defined pulmonary arterial vessels in the lower lobes) implies the presence of anatomic or hemodynamic obstruction of flow within the left heart. *Decreased pulmonary vascularity* indicates obstruction to pulmonary blood flow with an associated right-to-left shunt.

ELECTROCARDIOGRAM

A similar systematic approach to the standard 12-lead electrocardiogram (ECG) may be equally helpful in localizing a specific cardiac defect. The initial step should involve a general scanning of the tracing to detect any technical error (for example, reversed arm leads) or a recording artifact.

The next phase should center on the analysis of the basic rhythm and rate. Most congenital heart defects will manifest normal sinus rhythm or sinus tachycardia as a consequence of con-

gestive heart failure. The presence of paroxysmal atrial tachycardia may be associated with Wolff-Parkinson-White syndrome characterized by a short P-R interval and initial slowing of the QRS complex (delta wave). Complete heart block may occur as an isolated congenital defect, be associated with a more complex congenital heart lesion, or be a complication of open heart surgery.

Determination of the mean frontal QRS axis by quadrant, utilizing leads I and aVF, is adequate for clinical purposes (Fig. 3). Defects that are associated with left axis deviation (0 to −90 degrees) include endocardial cushion defects, tricuspid valve atresia, and certain types of Wolff-Parkinson-White syndrome or those that develop following intracardiac surgery (left anterior hemiblock). Right axis deviation (+90 to +180 degrees) may be seen in lesions characterized by right ventricular hypertrophy as in tetralogy of Fallot, complete transposition

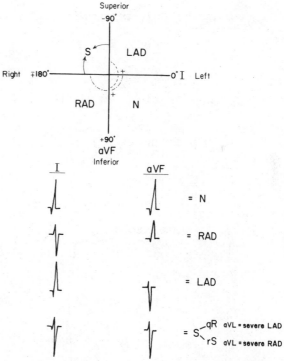

Figure 3. Plotting of the mean QRS axis by quadrant using the R/S ratio in leads I and aVF: A positive QRS complex (dominant R) in lead I places the axis leftward to the vertical line while a dominant R wave in aVF places the axis inferior to the horizontal line. A negative QRS complex (dominant S) in lead I or aVF would respectively indicate a rightward or superior axis. Thus, the presence of positive complexes in I and aVF results in a normal axis (N); the combination of negative complexes in I and positive in aVF results in right axis deviation (RAD), while the combination of positive complexes in I and negative in aVF results in left axis deviation (LAD). When the QRS complexes are negative both in I and aVF, the axis plots in the rightward and superior quadrant (S). In this case the QRS pattern in aVL (qR or rS) differentiates between severe LAD and RAD.

of the great vessels, pulmonic valve stenosis, or secondary to lung disease as in cor pulmonale. In the presence of a specific dysmorphic syndrome, the existence of an abnormal QRS axis deviation does not usually reflect the underlying hemodynamic situation (e.g., severe right axis deviation in mild pulmonic valve stenosis with Noonan's syndrome).

The next step should include evaluation of specific chamber enlargement. Configuration of the P wave helps in determining atrial enlargement. Right precordial leads (V_3R–V_1) directly reflect right ventricular hypertrophy, while left precordial leads (V_6–V_7) reflect left ventricular hypertrophy. Commonly encountered electrocardiographic patterns of atrial and ventricular hypertrophy are shown in Figure 4. These patterns may assist the clinician in a functional assessment of the hemodynamic effects of the specific cardiac defect. *Right ventricular volume overload* is primarily seen in atrial level left-to-right shunts (e.g., atrial septal defect),

while *right ventricular pressure overload* occurs in right ventricular obstructive lesions (e.g., pulmonic valve stenosis). *Left ventricular volume overload* may be the result of a hemodynamically large left-to-right shunt as in patent ductus arteriosus. *Left ventricular pressure overload* occurs secondary to an obstructive lesion of the left ventricle such as in aortic valve stenosis.

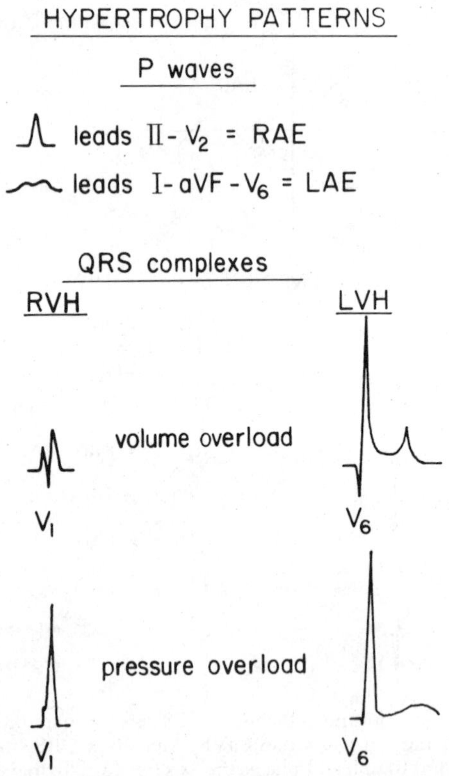

ECHOCARDIOGRAM

The advent of M-mode echocardiography (Echo) in the last decade has provided clinicians with much valuable information about cardiac anatomy and function. Using this portable, noninvasive technique, one can gain much information such as (1) determining the presence and relative size of the cardiac chambers and vessels, (2) ascertaining the presence of the four cardiac valves, and (3) establishing the normal anatomic continuity of the different intracardiac structures (Fig. 5). Here useful conclusions may be drawn regarding the hemodynamic effects of a suspected cardiac lesion. An example is dilatation of the right ventricular cavity secondary to volume overload of the right heart as seen in large atrial septal defects. Lack of normal continuity between the interventricular septum and the aorta (overriding aorta) in a cyanotic patient would suggest the diagnosis of tetralogy of Fallot.

HYPERTROPHY PATTERNS

P waves

leads II - V_2 = RAE

leads I - aVF - V_6 = LAE

QRS complexes

RVH   LVH

volume overload

V_1 V_6

pressure overload

V_1 V_6

Figure 4. P waves configuration: tall, peaked P waves indicate right atrial enlargement (RAE) while broad and notched P waves indicate left atrial enlargement (LAE). QRS complexes: (1) low voltage rsR' pattern in the right precordial leads (V_3R-V_1) indicate right ventricular hypertrophy of the volume overload type while tall R waves (greater than 15 mm) indicate right ventricular pressure overload; (2) deep q and tall R and T waves in the left precordial leads (V_6-V_7) indicate left ventricular hypertrophy of the volume overload type while small q with tall R waves and relatively small T waves indicate left ventricular pressure overload.

COMMON DIAGNOSTIC SITUATIONS

Three common diagnostic situations may confront the primary care physician in dealing with congenital heart disease. They include the evaluation of:

    1. Cyanotic newborn babies.

    2. Acyanotic infants with congestive heart failure.

    3. Children with a heart murmur.

We will discuss the systematic analysis of the different congenital cardiac defects as they present in these three patient groups in order to facilitate timely and accurate diagnosis. The scope of this chapter does not allow discussion of every complex heart defect. However, the lesions discussed account for more than 90 per cent of all congenital diseases of the heart.

CYANOTIC NEWBORN BABY

General Principles. Cyanosis is not always by itself diagnostic of a congenital cardiac defect. A normal newborn may exhibit *acrocyanosis* with mild transient bluing of the lips, hands,

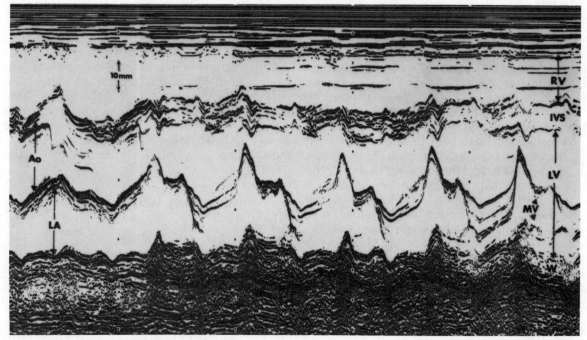

Figure 5. Normal echocardiogram showing normal continuity between the anterior wall of the aorta (Ao) and the interventricular septum (IVS). The left atrium (LA)–root of Aorta (Ao) dimensions and the IVS–left ventricular posterior wall (W) thickness are approximately the same. Both leaflets of the mitral valve (MV) are seen within the cavity of the left ventricle (LV). RV = right ventricular cavity.

and feet secondary to vasomotor instability. Cyanosis is usually encountered in newborns with lung disease such as respiratory distress syndrome or persistent fetal circulation. The presence of severe tachypnea, substernal or intercostal retractions, and grunting or nasal flaring or both should suggest a respiratory cause of cyanosis. Systemic desaturation may also occur with central nervous system insults, as in intracranial hemorrhage or with bacterial septicemia or various hemoglobinopathies. In general, cyanosis owing to congenital heart disease is not associated with signs of respiratory

distress other than mild tachypnea despite the presence of significant hypoxemia and metabolic acidosis. Cyanosis of cardiac cause may occur because of *inadequate mixing* between the systemic and pulmonary circulations (as in complete transposition of the great vessels), *decreased pulmonary blood flow* (as in pulmonary valve atresia), or *admixture of both circulations* (as in total anomalous pulmonary venous return).

Hyperoxia Test. Often it may be difficult to differentiate clinically between cyanosis of respiratory or cardiac origin. In these instances,

Figure 6. Hyperoxia test: values of arterial PO_2 (mm Hg) while breathing room air and 100 per cent oxygen: Group I, normal patients; Group II, patients with severe hypoxemia; Group III, patients with mild to moderate hypoxemia.

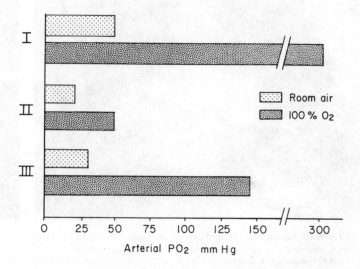

placing the baby in a pure oxygen environment can be of significant diagnostic value. In most lung diseases, despite significant alveolar-capillary block and intrapulmonary shunting, the arterial PO$_2$ on 100 per cent oxygen may reach levels greater than 150 mm Hg. In normal babies or in those with mild cases of respiratory distress, the arterial PO$_2$ is expected to exceed 300 mm Hg (Fig. 6–I).

In lesions characterized by inadequate mixing or decreased pulmonary blood flow, cyanosis will be severe and the arterial PO$_2$ during the hyperoxia test will usually not exceed 50 mm Hg (Fig. 6–II). This group of patients should be carefully monitored during the hyperoxia test, since oxygen-induced closure of a patent ductus arteriosus may result in rapid clinical deterioration.

In admixture lesions, despite common mixing of the systemic and pulmonary circulations,

Table 2. *Cyanotic Newborn Baby*

I. Severe cyanosis (arterial PO$_2$ on 100% O$_2$ = 30–50 mm Hg)
  A. Normal or shunt vascularity on x-ray
    1. Complete transposition of the great vessels
  B. Decreased pulmonary vascularity on x-ray
    1. Tetralogy of Fallot
    2. Pulmonary valve atresia with intact ventricular septum
    3. Tricuspid valve atresia
    4. Ebstein's anomaly of the tricuspid valve

II. Moderate cyanosis (arterial PO$_2$ on 100% O$_2$ = 50–150 mm Hg)
    1. Total anomalous pulmonary venous return
    2. Complex admixture lesions

cyanosis is usually mild, owing to the presence of excessive pulmonary blood flow. However, during the hyperoxia test the arterial PO$_2$ will usually not exceed 150 mm Hg (Fig. 6–III).

Utilizing a combination of the degree of cyanosis, the results of the hyperoxia test, and the radiographic assessment of pulmonary blood flow, we will discuss the diagnostic approach to the cyanotic newborn baby as outlined in Table 2. In this discussion we will present the six most common cyanotic cardiac defects of the newborn period.

I. NEWBORN BABY WITH SEVERE CYANOSIS

A. NORMAL OR SHUNT VASCULARITY ON X-RAY

1. Complete Transposition of the Great Vessels (CTGV)

Clinical Features. Babies with complete transposition of the great vessels (CTGV) frequently are males of greater than average birth weight and have no other associated congenital anomalies. Those with inadequate mixing are dusky and have a slate-gray color or may be deeply cyanotic. With significant systemic desaturation, a metabolic acidosis progressively develops. Cardiac auscultation is not helpful because of the lack of significant murmurs. The second heart sound is usually single, owing to the distant posterior position of the pulmonic valve. Signs of mild congestive heart failure may be present in those patients with intact ventricular septum and no pulmonic stenosis.

Chest X-Ray. In the immediate newborn

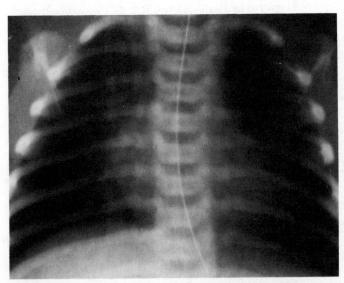
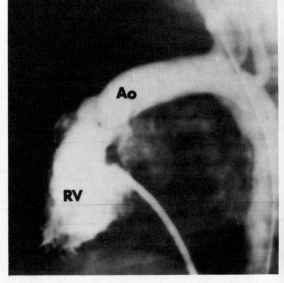

Figure 7. Chest x-ray (left) of a newborn baby with complete transposition of the great vessels. There is mild cardiomegaly and pulmonary vasculature is normal or slightly prominent and of the shunt type. Lateral view of the angiocardiogram (right) showing the anterior aorta (Ao) originating from the right ventricle (RV). There is a very small patent ductus arteriosus (arrow) with faint opacification of the posterior pulmonary artery.

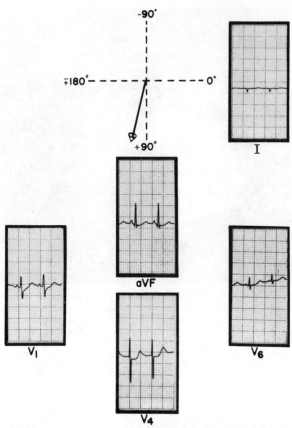

Figure 8. Electrocardiogram of a 36-hour-old baby with complete transposition of the great vessels. Normal tracing except for minimal ST segment depression in V_1.

period the chest x-ray (Fig. 7) may appear deceptively normal. Essential in the diagnosis is that the pulmonary vascularity is normal or even increased in the presence of severe cyanosis. Heart size may be normal or increased and the cardiac contour often demonstrates an oval, or egg, shape with a narrow superior mediastinum and an absent pulmonary artery segment. There is usually a decrease in thymic proportion owing to the effects of hypoxia and stress.

Electrocardiogram. The ECG in the first few days of life is frequently normal for a newborn baby (Fig. 8). Within days, however, signs of right atrial enlargement and abnormal degrees of right ventricular hypertrophy may appear, manifested by a pure R wave or a qR pattern in the right precordial leads (V_3R through V_1). Signs of left ventricular hypertrophy rarely exist, even in the presence of significant pulmonic stenosis with increased left ventricular pressure.

Echocardiogram. Various subtle echocardiographic abnormalities have been described in CTGV. For the most part they involve recording the anterior great vessel more rightward (as opposed to the normal leftward position of the pulmonary artery). Additionally the posterior pulmonic valve opens before and closes after

the anterior aortic valve, a sequence that is the reverse of that encountered in normal hearts. Generally these criteria are difficult to confirm and may not be of great practical value.

Cardiac Catheterization and Angiocardiography. Oxygen saturation in the venae cavae, right atrium, right ventricle, and transposed aorta is significantly decreased and directly related to the magnitude of mixing between the parallel systemic and pulmonary circulations. In contrast, the left atrium, left ventricle, and transposed pulmonary artery contain fully saturated blood. Angiography shows the classic anteriorly positioned, transposed aorta in the lateral plane (Fig. 7).

B. DECREASED PULMONARY VASCULARITY ON X-RAY

1. Tetralogy of Fallot (TOF)

Clinical Features. These babies are severely cyanotic from birth and may become intensely worse with crying. Generally they are small for gestational age and have a high incidence of associated bony anomalies. Signs of congestive heart failure are virtually never present unless associated with severe anemia. The presence of a palpable thrill or systolic murmur at the lower left sternal border implies patency of the right ventricular outflow tract.

At times of crying or straining with bowel movements or during a cyanotic spell, there is a dynamic narrowing of the right ventricular infundibulum and the intensity of the murmur may decrease or disappear completely. With atresia of the right ventricular outflow tract, there are no palpable thrills or ejection murmurs. On auscultation only a faint systolic or continuous murmur may be audible secondary to flow through a patent ductus arteriosus or dilated bronchial collateral vessels. There frequently is an ejection click audible at the cardiac apex and upper left sternal border, which is aortic in origin. The second heart sound is single.

Chest X-Ray. The heart is characteristically normal or small in size. The apex of the heart is upturned; coupled with the absent pulmonary artery segment, this produces the typical "boot-shaped" appearance of the cardiac contour (Fig. 9). The lung fields are markedly hypovascular. A right-sided aortic arch is present in 25 per cent of the patients. Skeletal anomalies are frequently present.

Electrocardiogram (Fig. 10). The mean QRS frontal axis is usually rightward and there may be signs of right atrial enlargement. The precordial pattern, even in newborn babies, shows evidence of right ventricular hypertrophy pressure overload with either pure R waves, rR'

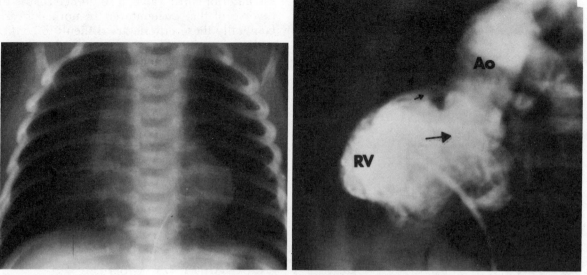

Figure 9.   Chest x-ray of a newborn baby with severe tetralogy of Fallot (left). Note the normal heart size with an upturned apex and the superior vena cava laterally displaced by a large ascending aorta. The pulmonary vascularity is decreased with very small peripheral vessels. Angiocardiogram (right): Lateral view of the right ventriculogram (RV) showing a small infundibulum (small arrow) leading into a hypoplastic pulmonary artery. The majority of the contrast material crosses the ventricular septal defect (large arrow) with opacification of the large overriding aorta (Ao).

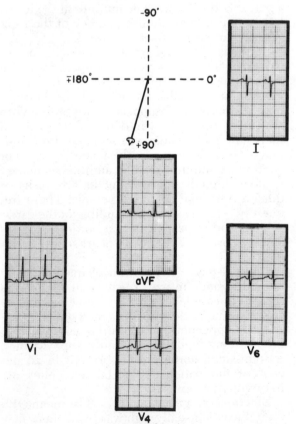

Figure 10.   Electrocardiogram of a 1-week-old baby with tetralogy of Fallot. 100 per cent R waves in V_1 suggest right ventricular hypertrophy.

complexes, or a qR pattern in the right precordial leads.

Echocardiogram.   M-mode echocardiography may provide confirmatory evidence of the anatomic diagnosis. The dimension of the aortic root is typically increased and the left atrial dimension is small owing to decreased pulmonary venous return. On a sweep from the aortic root to the body of the ventricles (Fig. 11), there is absence of the normal continuity between the anterior wall of the aorta and the interventricular septum (overriding of the aorta). The pulmonic valve is often difficult or impossible to record, particularly in patients with severe obstruction to the right ventricular outflow tract.

Cardiac Catheterization and Angiocardiography.   Oxygen saturation in the right heart and aorta is significantly decreased. Right ventricular peak systolic pressure is increased at systemic levels. Right ventriculogram typically shows a normal-sized but thick-walled right ventricular cavity and evidence of a right-to-left shunt through a high interventricular septal defect (Fig. 9). Anterior displacement of the crista supraventricularis creates varying degrees of outflow tract obstruction ranging from mild narrowing to complete atresia.

2. Pulmonary Valve Atresia With Intact Ventricular Septum (PA)

Clinical Features.   These infants are severe-

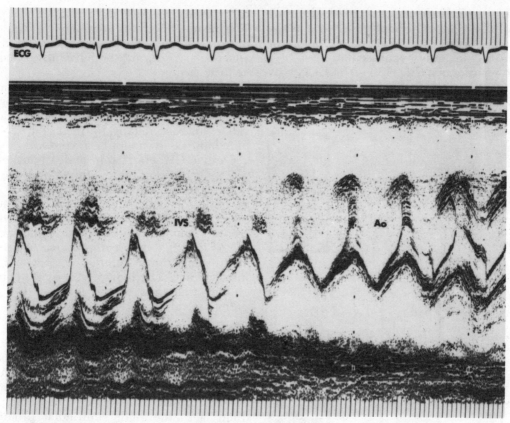

Figure 11.   Echocardiogram in tetralogy of Fallot. The root of the aorta (Ao) overrides the plane of the interventricular spetum (IVS) with obvious lack of anatomic continuity between the anterior Ao wall and the IVS.

ly cyanotic and hyperpneic and, with progressive hypoxia, metabolic acidosis ensues. Signs of congestive heart failure are frequently present. The auscultation may reveal no murmurs in patients with a competent tricuspid valve or there may be a smooth, high-frequency holosystolic murmur at the lower left sternal border in patients with significant tricuspid valve incompetence. The second heart sound is single and there are no diastolic murmurs. These babies are prone to sudden clinical deterioration.

Chest X-Ray.   The   cardiac   silhouette   is

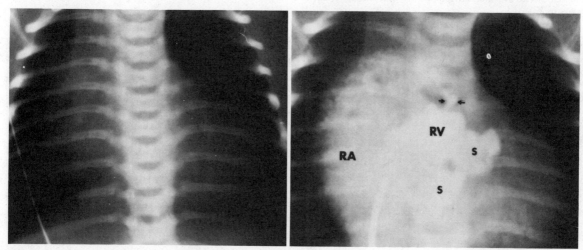

Figure 12.   Chest x-ray of a newborn baby with pulmonary valve atresia and an intact ventricular septum (left). Note the marked cardiomegaly with a large right atrium and almost complete lack of pulmonary vascularity. Frontal view of the angiocardiogram (right) showing the hypoplastic right ventricle (RV) with a very small infundibulum (arrows) ending at the atretic pulmonic valve. Note retrograde filling of myocardial sinusoids (S) and the presence of tricuspid valve insufficiency with faint opacification of a dilated right atrium (RA).

characteristically enlarged with marked prominence of the right heart border due to massive dilatation of the right atrium (Fig. 12). The lung fields are significantly hypovascular.

Electrocardiogram (Fig. 13). The ECG typically shows marked right atrial enlargement. The mean QRS axis is normal or rightward. The precordial leads show dominance of the left ventricular forces and a relative absence of right ventricular forces.

Echocardiogram. The echocardiogram in the majority of patients shows a diminutive right ventricular cavity. The small tricuspid valve can occasionally be recorded, while the pulmonic valve cannot be recorded.

Cardiac Catheterization and Angiocardiography. Oxygen saturation throughout the right and left heart is significantly decreased owing to obligatory mixing of venous and arterial blood at the left atrial level and markedly decreased pulmonary blood flow. Angiocardiography (Fig. 12) shows a diminutive right ventricle, usually with significant tricuspid valve insufficiency. The hypoplastic right ventricular outflow tract fills to the level of the atretic pulmonic valve.

3. Tricuspid Valve Atresia (TA)

Clinical Features. Newborn babies with tricuspid valve atresia (TA) usually have significant decreases in pulmonary blood flow and are deeply cyanotic. They are typically poor feeders and may have marked dyspnea. The precordium lacks the right ventricular prominence encountered in the normal newborn. Auscultation usually reveals a single first heart sound, a harsh systolic murmur of a ventricular septal defect, and a single second heart sound. Prominent third and fourth heart sounds or an apical diastolic mitral flow murmur may be present.

Chest X-Ray. The heart size is frequently normal (Fig. 14) with prominence of the right heart border secondary to dilatation of the right atrium. The pulmonary artery segment is absent and the lungs are characteristically hypovascular.

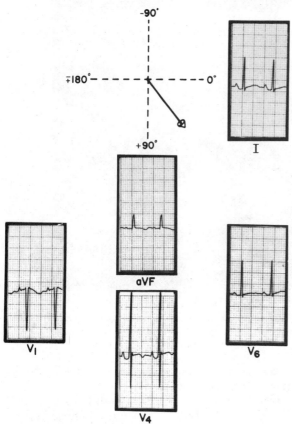

Figure 13. Electrocardiogram of an 8-week-old baby with pulmonary valve atresia and an intact ventricular septum. Note the presence of a leftward but inferior mean QRS axis associated with absence of right ventricular forces (small r waves in V_1).

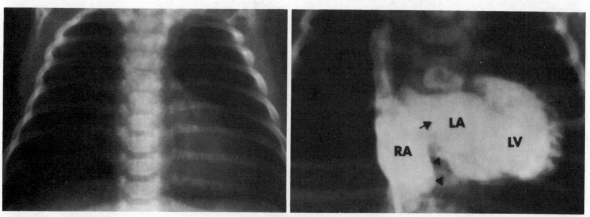

Figure 14. Chest x-ray of a newborn baby with tricuspid valve atresia (left). The heart is of normal size but has a left ventricular configuration. The pulmonary vascularity is obviously decreased. Angiocardiogram (right): Frontal view of a right atriogram (RA) showing the intact floor of the right atrium (arrowheads) with all the contrast material crossing an atrial septal defect (arrow) with dense opacification of the left atrium (LA) and ventricle (LV).

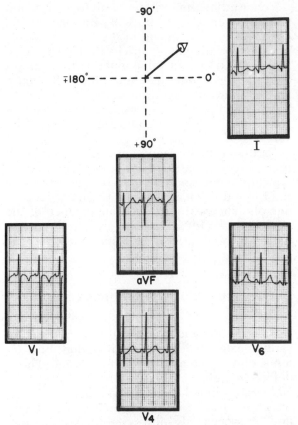

Figure 15. Electrocardiogram of a newborn baby with tricuspid valve atresia. There is left axis deviation of the mean QRS axis and left ventricular hypertrophy pattern in the precordial leads (deep S waves in V_1 and dominant R waves in V_6).

Electrocardiogram. The ECG shows marked right atrial enlargement. The mean frontal QRS axis is shifted leftward and superiorly between 0 and −90 degrees (Fig. 15). Typical of the anatomically small right ventricular cavity, the precordial leads show decreased right ventricular forces.

Echocardiogram. The tricuspid valve cannot be recorded. The right ventricular dimensions are decreased or absent, while the left ventricle is often dilated with volume overload.

Cardiac Catheterization and Angiocardiography. Because of common mixing at the left atrial level, oxygen saturations are decreased and equal in the left atrium, left ventricle, and aorta. Right atrial injection (Fig. 14) typically shows absence of the right ventricle, producing a "window" type effect by the floor of the right atrium. The diminutive right ventricle fills through a small ventricular septal defect.

4. Ebstein's Anomaly of the Tricuspid Valve

Clinical Features. Clinically, these babies may be difficult to distinguish from those with pulmonary atresia with an intact ventricular septum. Sometimes they may present with supraventricular tachycardia. Despite the usual presence of massive tricuspid valve insufficiency, these babies may have no murmurs or have a short, high frequency systolic murmur maximal at the lower left sternal border. The second heart sound may be single or widely

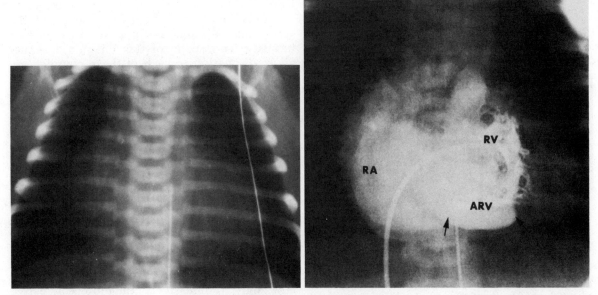

Figure 16. Chest x-ray of a newborn baby with Ebstein's anomaly of the tricuspid valve (left). Note the marked cardiomegaly with a prominent right atrium and decreased pulmonary vascularity. Angiocardiogram (right): Right ventriculogram in the frontal view clearly shows the functioning right ventricle (RV), the atrialized portion of the right ventricle (ARV), and the right atrium (RA).

split. Characteristically, prominent third and fourth heart sounds are present and associated with a mid-diastolic tricuspid flow murmur.

Chest X-Ray. Heart enlargement may vary from mild to massive, with prominent right atrial dilatation (Fig. 16). The pulmonary vascularity is typically decreased.

Electrocardiogram (Fig. 17). There is marked right atrial enlargement and occasionally the P wave may be taller than the QRS complex. Generally, two different ECG patterns are observed: those with right bundle branch block and those with a pattern of Wolff-Parkinson-White syndrome. The right bundle branch block pattern displays rightward deviation of the mean QRS axis and rsR' complexes in leads V_3R–V_1 with a broad, low-voltage R' wave. Those with Wolff-Parkinson-White syndrome have a short P-R interval and initial slowing of the QRS complexes (delta wave) best seen in the left precordial leads. The Wolff-Parkinson-White pattern in Ebstein's anomaly is always type B, displaying posterior QRS forces with dominant S waves in leads V_3R–V_1.

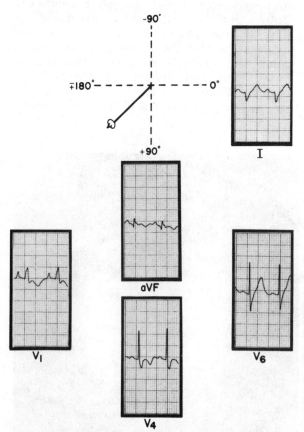

Figure 17. Electrocardiogram in Ebstein's anomaly of the tricuspid valve showing first degree A-V block (P-R interval 0.16 second, right atrial enlargement (peaked P waves in V_1) and right ventricular conduction delay (low-voltage broad R waves in V_1).

Echocardiogram. Signs of right ventricular volume overload are present. Because of the downward displacement of the tricuspid apparatus into the right ventricle it is possible to record the tricuspid valve much farther toward the left precordium than in normal individuals. On simultaneous recording of the atrioventricular valves, the tricuspid valve closure may be considerably delayed compared to mitral closure.

Cardiac Catheterization and Angiocardiography. Oxygen saturation in the left heart is typically decreased owing to the presence of a right-to-left shunt at the atrial level. Angiocardiography shows the trilobed appearance of the right heart with a smooth atrialized portion between the dilated right atrium and the distal functioning right ventricle (Fig. 16).

II. NEWBORN BABY WITH MODERATE CYANOSIS

General Principles. Moderate cyanosis of cardiac cause in the newborn period most often is due to a complex admixture lesion. These defects are characterized by mixing of arterial and venous blood at some level that, combined with the usual increase in pulmonary blood flow, produces only mild systemic desaturation. The hyperoxia test in these instances usually reveals an arterial PO_2 in the 50 to 150 mm Hg range (Fig. 6–III); a few admixture lesions with excessive pulmonary blood flow may rarely reach 200 mm Hg. Congestive heart failure may often be present. Representative examples of admixture lesions include common atrium (cor triloculare), single ventricle (double inlet left ventricle), common ventricle (absence of the ventricular septum), and persistent truncus arteriosus. The scope of this chapter does not allow discussion of each of these complex anomalies. However, we will discuss the commonest defect in this group and the most surgically amenable of all these lesions — total anomalous pulmonary venous return.

1. Total Anomalous Pulmonary Venous Return (TAPVR)

Clinical Features. Because of mixing of arterialized and venous blood and generous pulmonary blood flow, oxygen saturation may be as high as 90 per cent and clinical desaturation may be difficult to appreciate. The hyperoxia test will show an arterial PO_2 generally in the 50 to 150 mm Hg range. Patients with the unobstructed variety and increased pulmonary blood flow may progressively develop congestive heart failure. There is volume overload of the right heart, and thus the auscultatory findings are similar to that of an atrial septal defect: a soft

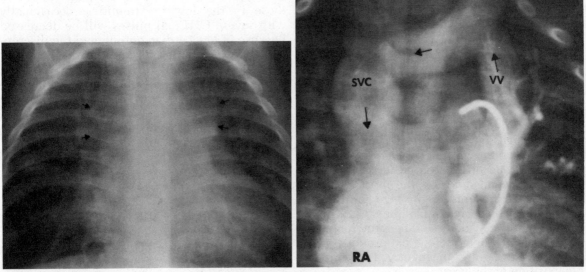

Figure 18. Chest x-ray of a baby with total anomalous pulmonary venous return, supradiaphragmatic (left). There is prominent shunt vascularity. The large heart plus the wide superior mediastinum, due to dilated left vertical vein and right superior vena cava (arrows), form the characteristic "snowman" configuration. Angiocardiogram (right): Frontal view showing the levophase of a pulmonary arteriogram. The arrows indicate the direction of blood flow via a left vertical vein (VV) toward the superior vena cava (SVC) and right atrium (RA).

pulmonic flow murmur heard best at the second left intercostal space, with a widely split second heart sound and a mid diastolic murmur at the lower left sternal border of tricuspid flow. Newborn babies with the less common infra-diaphragmatic form and obstruction to pulmonary venous return become symptomatic within the first few days of life and the clinical features may resemble severe hyaline membrane disease.

Chest X-Ray. Patients with the most common supradiaphragmatic form show cardiomegaly and widening of the superior mediastinum, producing a characteristic figure of eight or "snowman" appearance of the cardiac silhouette (Fig. 18). The pulmonary vascularity is significantly increased of the shunt type and there is no left atrial enlargement.

Electrocardiogram. The ECG invariably shows evidence of right atrial enlargement and severe right ventricular hypertrophy (Fig. 19).

Echocardiogram. In the usual unobstructed variety, signs of right ventricular volume overload are seen with increased internal dimension of the right ventricle and paradoxical motion of the interventricular septum. The left atrial dimension is often small.

Cardiac Catheterization and Angiocardiography. Depending upon the site of entry of pulmonary venous return, saturation in either the vena cava or coronary sinus will be higher than normal. Typical of admixture lesions, oxygen saturations distal to the right atrium and

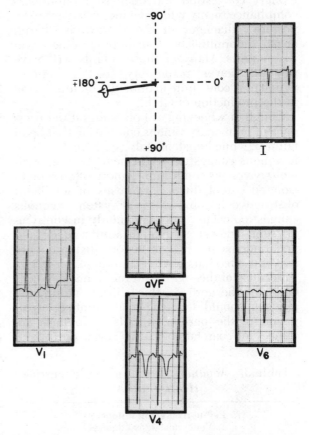

Figure 19. Electrocardiogram of a newborn baby with total anomalous pulmonary venous return. There is right atrial enlargement (peaked P waves in aVF) and severe right ventricular hypertrophy (qR pattern in V_1).

throughout the left heart are equal. Injection in the main pulmonary artery will show the anomalous pathway of pulmonary venous return (Fig. 18).

ACYANOTIC INFANT WITH CONGESTIVE HEART FAILURE

General Principles. Acyanotic lesions that produce congestive heart failure in infancy can be classified into two functional types: left-to-right shunts and obstructive lesions (Table 3). Ventricular septal defect is the most common anomaly that presents in this age group, followed closely by coarctation of the aorta with or without associated defects. The principal *cyanotic* congenital heart defect that produces congestive heart failure in infancy is complete transposition of the great vessels.

Detailed physical examination plays a significant role in the evaluation of the infant with congestive heart failure (CHF). These infants are thin, tachypneic, and diaphoretic; feeding is difficult. Additionally, they have persistent tachycardia, even during sleep. Because of pulmonary congestion and decreased pulmonary compliance, many will have increased anterior-posterior diameter of the thorax, or "barrel chest" deformities, with scalloping of the lower rib margins. Many of these infants will have frequent lower respiratory tract infections, which may contribute to or be the inciting event in the production of CHF.

Cough or wheezing or both suggest the presence of pulmonary venous congestion (left heart failure), while hepatomegaly is a sign of systemic venous congestion (right heart failure). Pulmonary venous congestion is more often seen in isolated patent ductus arteriosus or left heart obstructive lesions, whereas systemic venous congestion occurs more commonly in ventricular septal defect. Unlike in adults, facial and pedal edema and jugular venous distention are late and rare signs of CHF in infants.

Because of the significant incidence of coarctation of the aorta in this clinical group, the clinician should devote special attention to palpation of the peripheral pulses. In most instances of coarctation of the aorta, peripheral

Table 3. *Acyanotic Infant with Congestive Heart Failure*

A. Left-to-right shunt lesions
   1. Ventricular septal defect
   2. Patent ductus arteriosus
   3. Endocardial cushion defect
B. Obstructive lesions
   1. Coarctation of the aorta

----

pulses in the arms will be much stronger than those in the lower extremities; occasionally with severe CHF, all pulses will be decreased because of low cardiac output, and the discrepancy between the upper and lower extremities will not be clinically obvious. However, blood pressure recordings in all extremities, particularly by Doppler technique, will confirm the diagnosis. The presence of bounding pulses in all extremities indicates an aortic "run-off" lesion, as in patent ductus arteriosus.

A. LEFT-TO-RIGHT SHUNT LESIONS

1. Ventricular Septal Defect (VSD)

Clinical Features. The infant with a large ventricular septal defect (VSD) exhibits poor growth and has little subcutaneous fat and decreased muscle mass. The infants are tachypneic at rest and have the previously described barrel chest deformities and prominent precordium. Signs of congestive heart failure may be present, including persistent tachycardia, diaphoresis, and hepatomegaly. The precordium is hyperactive. There is a palpable thrill associated with a harsh, pansystolic murmur at the lower left sternal border. The second heart sound varies according to the presence of any associated pulmonary hypertension. In the group with large left-to-right shunts, pulmonary artery pressure is usually increased, producing narrow splitting of the second heart sound and increased intensity of the pulmonic component. Third and fourth heart sounds are often audible at the apex. Owing to increased pulmonary venous return, a mid diastolic mitral flow murmur (relative mitral stenosis) is also audible in this region.

Chest X-Ray. The heart is uniformly enlarged and the pulmonary vascularity is increased of the shunt variety (Fig. 20). The left atrium is enlarged in the lateral barium swallow projection.

Electrocardiogram. There is usually left atrial enlargement. In patients with congestive heart failure, signs of right atrial enlargement may also be present. The precordial complexes often show isolated criteria for both left and right ventricular hypertrophy and additionally show large (greater than 50 mm) equiphasic QRS complexes in the mid precordial leads (Fig. 21).

Echocardiogram. The left atrium is dilated and the left ventricle is characterized by a volume overload pattern with increased internal dimension and hyperkinetic motion of the interventricular septum and posterior wall. In rare instances, a VSD may be suspected by demonstrating interruption of the ventricular septal

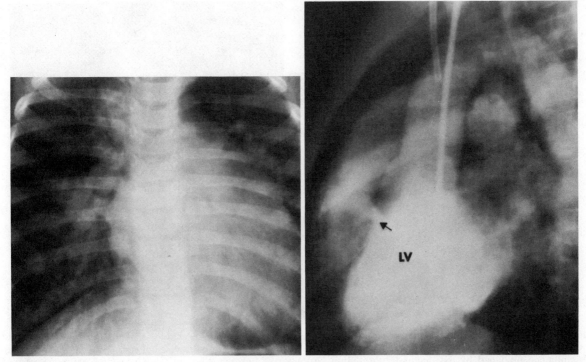

Figure 20. Chest x-ray of an infant with a large ventricular septal defect (left). Note the cardiomegaly and the prominent shunt vascularity. Angiocardiogram (right): Lateral view of the left ventriculogram (LV) showing the jet of contrast material crossing an infracristal defect (arrow) into the right ventricle.

echoes on a sweep into the aortic root. This generally is an unreliable sign and may occasionally be artifactually simulated.

Cardiac Catheterization and Angiocardiogra- phy. The left-to-right shunt is detected by increased oxygen saturation in the right ventricle. Pressure in the right ventricle and main pulmonary artery will depend on the magnitude of the

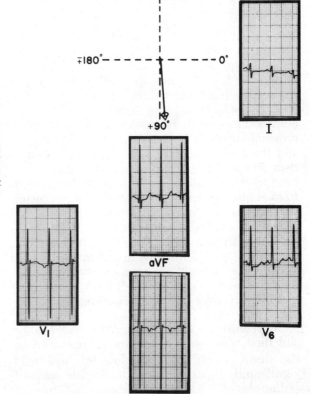

Figure 21. Electrocardiogram of a 9-month-old infant with a large ventricular septal defect. Large QRS complexes over the midprecordium (V_4) with increased posterior QRS forces (deep S waves in V_1) indicate biventricular hypertrophy (left greater than right).

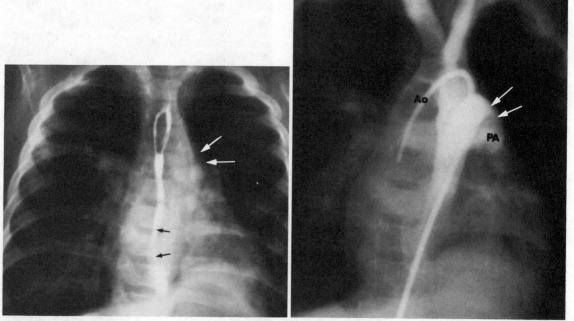

Figure 22. Chest x-ray of an infant with a patent ductus arteriosus (left). There is shunt vascularity (in addition to a right upper lobe infiltrate) and left atrial enlargement causing deviation of the barium-filled esophagus (arrows). Note the extra prominence produced by the ductus infundibulum (arrowheads) between the aortic knob and the pulmonary trunk. Angiocardiogram (right): Aortogram (Ao) showing the patent ductus arteriosus (arrowheads) with opacification of the pulmonary artery (PA).

shunt or the pulmonary vascular resistance or both. In the presence of CHF, the hemodynamic situation is usually one of a high flow, high pressure VSD. Left ventricular angiography will show the site of the septal defect with subsequent opacification of the right ventricle (Fig. 20).

2. Patent Ductus Arteriosus (PDA)

Clinical Features. PDA is often seen in females and premature babies. Some present within the first few months of life with signs of congestive left heart failure that may be manifested by wheezing or frank signs of pulmonary edema. The peripheral pulses are bounding, an unusual situation for a patient in heart failure, and the blood pressure shows a wide (greater than 40 mm Hg) pulse pressure owing to aortic run-off. The typical continuous murmur of a PDA is often heard in the second left intercostal space or left supraclavicular area and may be accompanied by a palpable thrill. Often the second heart sound is obscured by the crunchy, machinery-like continuous murmur. Third and fourth heart sounds are prominent and a pronounced mid diastolic mitral flow murmur at the apex (relative mitral stenosis) may be present.

Chest X-Ray. There is usually cardiomegaly and the pulmonary vascularity is increased of the shunt variety (Fig. 22). The left atrium is significantly enlarged and radiographic signs of pulmonary edema may be present.

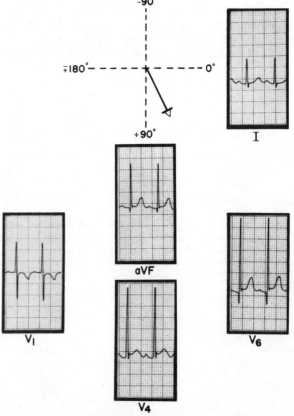

Figure 23. Electrocardiogram of a female infant with a large patent ductus arteriosus. Note the presence of left atrial enlargement (broad P waves in leads I and V_6) and a left ventricular volume overload pattern (deep q waves, tall R waves in V_6 with "coving" of the ST segment).

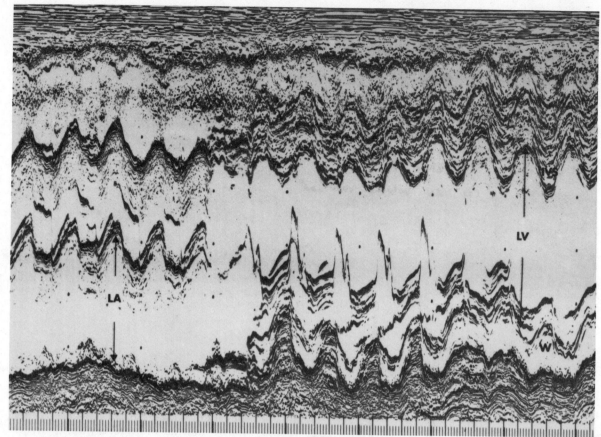

Figure 24.   Echocardiogram of an infant with a large patent ductus arteriosus. There is left atrial enlargement (LA) and left ventricular volume overload: dilated left ventricular cavity (LV) with increased systolic excursion of the interventricular septum (IVS) and left ventricular posterior wall (W).

Electrocardiogram.   Electrocardiographically, the tracing may be identical to that of a large ventricular septal defect, showing left atrial enlargement and biventricular hypertrophy, left greater than right. Characteristically, the left ventricular hypertrophy is of the volume overload type (Fig. 23).

Echocardiogram.   The left atrium typically is dilated with a ratio of the left atrium to aortic root dimensions greater than 1.0. Signs of left ventricular volume overload are usually present (Fig. 24).

Cardiac Catheterization.   The venous catheter can often be manipulated from the pulmonary artery, across the PDA, and into the descending aorta. There are significant increases in oxygen saturation in the pulmonary artery. Pulmonary artery pressure may be moderately elevated in patients with large left-to-right shunts. Left atrial and left ventricular end diastolic pressures are often markedly elevated. The aortogram (Fig. 22) shows a left-to-right shunt through the PDA with subsequent filling of the pulmonary arteries.

3. Endocardial Cushion Defects (ECD)
Clinical Features.   This defect occurs most commonly in babies with Down's syndrome. As with most patients with high flow, high pressure left-to-right shunts, infants with complete atrioventricular (A-V) canal have marked growth failure, frequent respiratory infections, and signs of congestive heart failure. The precordium is quite active and a variety of systolic murmurs may be heard, including the harsh, pansystolic murmur of a ventricular septal defect at the lower left sternal border or an A-V valve insufficiency murmur toward the cardiac apex. The second heart sound is frequently narrowly split with increased intensity of the pulmonic component. Gallop rhythms are common and mid diastolic A-V valve flow murmurs are often present.

Chest X-ray.   Areas of pneumonia or atelectasis or both are often seen (Fig. 25). The heart is typically enlarged with significant dilatation of the right atrium. The pulmonary vascularity is markedly increased both of the shunt variety and pulmonary venous congestion type, but without signs of left atrial enlargement.

Electrocardiogram.   The ECG is the most helpful diagnostic aid in this entity. Typically, the mean frontal QRS axis in complete A-V canal is deviated superiorly between −60 and

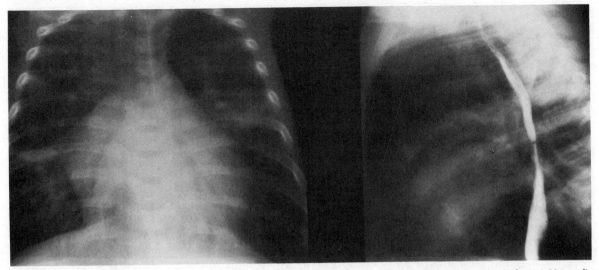

Figure 25. Chest x-ray of an infant with Down's syndrome and an endocardial cushion defect (complete A-V canal). Anteroposterior view (left) showing moderate cardiomegaly, shunt vascularity and multiple pulmonary infiltrates. Despite increased pulmonary blood flow, the lateral view (right) shows no left atrial enlargement.

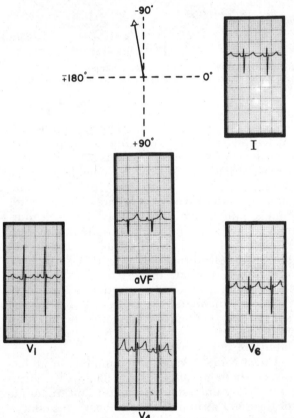

Figure 26. Electrocardiogram of a 4-month-old infant with Down's syndrome and endocardial cushion defect (complete AV canal). Note the superior mean QRS axis (severe left axis deviation) characteristic of this condition. The precordial leads indicate right ventricular hypertrophy (positive T waves in V_1 and deep S waves in V_6).

−120 degrees (Fig. 26). This axis deviation is thought to result from abnormal orientation of the conducting fascicles. The precordial pattern usually shows biatrial enlargement and biventricular hypertrophy, right greater than left.

Echocardiogram. Isolated ostium primum atrial septal defect will manifest signs of right ventricular volume overload. In complete A-V canal, however, there is often evidence of biventricular hypertrophy and volume overload of both ventricles. The leaflets of the common A-V valve may be seen crossing the plane of the interventricular septum in diastole (Fig. 27).

Cardiac Catheterization and Angiocardiography. There are increases in oxygen saturation at both the atrial and ventricular levels. Often the atrial level communication is the most significant because of A-V valve incompetence resulting in a functionally direct left ventricle to right atrial shunt. Pulmonary artery and right ventricular pressures are elevated often at systemic levels. Left ventricular angiography typically shows the elongated "goose neck" deformity of the left ventricular outflow tract (Fig. 28) and varying degrees of A-V valve insufficiency.

B. OBSTRUCTIVE LESIONS

1. Coarctation of the Aorta (CoA)

Older children with isolated coarctation of the aorta (CoA) are often asymptomatic; the condition is generally detected only because of the murmur of an associated bicuspid aortic valve

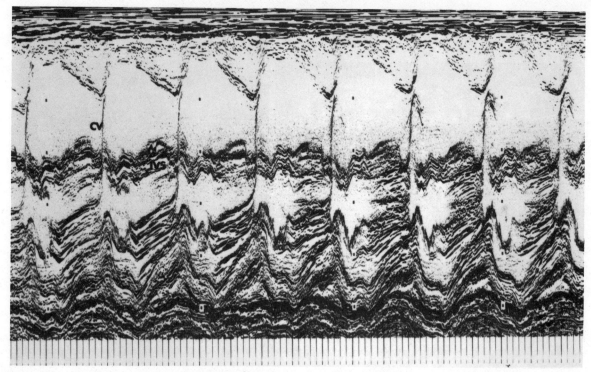

Figure 27.   Echocardiogram of a 5-month-old infant with an endocardial cushion defect of the complete atrioventricular canal type. The large common A-V valve (CV) appears to cross the plane of the interventricular septum (IVS) as it opens in diastole.

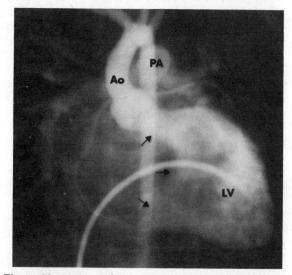

Figure 28.   Angiocardiogram in endocardial cushion defect. Frontal view of the left ventriculogram (LV). Note the characteristic "gooseneck" deformity of the left ventricular outflow tract (arrows) produced by the abnormal insertion and opening of the common atrioventricular valve. The large ventricular septal component causes simultaneous opacification of the aorta (Ao) and pulmonary artery (PA).

or because of systemic hypertension. The latter is not invariably present if the patient has had time to develop significant systemic collateral vessels via the internal mammary and intercos-

tal arteries. CoA is extremely rare in the presence of a right aortic arch.

Clinical Features.   The infant with severe CoA usually presents between 1 and 3 months of age in congestive heart failure. Pulses in the lower extremities are usually faint or absent compared to the brisk pulses palpable in the arms. With severe heart failure and low cardiac output, however, all pulses may be uniformly decreased and the diagnosis cannot be made unless blood pressures are obtained. The precordium is prominent and there is a palpable left ventricular-apical lift. A soft systolic murmur may be audible in the back at the interscapular region or there may be a systolic ejection click or murmur or both of a bicuspid aortic valve at the cardiac base. A loud fourth heart sound is an important finding and suggests marked decrease in compliance of the left ventricle.

Chest X-Ray.   The overall cardiac silhouette is enlarged with a left ventricular contour (Fig. 29). In severe left ventricular failure, the left atrium is often dilated and there is evidence of pulmonary venous obstruction. In the older, asymptomatic patient, it is often possible to visualize the site of coarctation in the first portion of the descending aorta. Additionally, one may see notching of the undersurface of the fourth and lower ribs posteriorly secondary to marked dilatation of the collateral intercostal vessels.

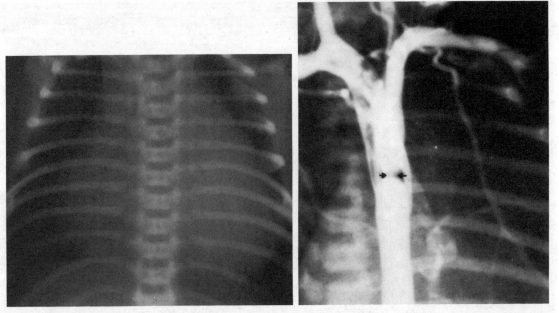

Figure 29. Chest x-ray of a one-month-old infant with coarctation of the aorta in congestive heart failure (left). There is marked cardiomegaly and pulmonary venous congestion (prominent but ill-defined vascularity, particularly in the upper lobes). Aortogram (right) showing a severe coarctation of the aorta (arrows) just distal to the origin of the left subclavian artery.

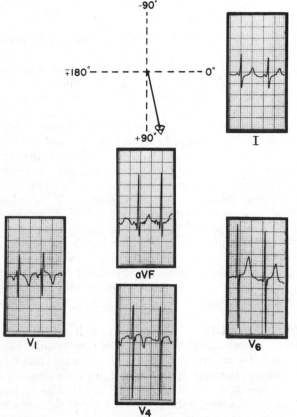

Figure 30. Electrocardiogram of a 1-month-old infant with coarctation of the aorta in congestive heart failure. There is left atrial enlargement (notched P waves in V_6) and biventricular hypertrophy (greater than 20 mm R and S waves in V_6).

Electrocardiogram (Fig. 30). The ECG manifests signs of left atrial enlargement and biventricular hypertrophy, left greater than right. The older child may show a mild right ventricular conduction delay pattern with an rSr′ complex in leads V_3R through V_1, in addition to signs of left ventricular hypertrophy.

Echocardiogram. The echocardiographic signs of coarctation of the aorta are secondary to pressure overload of the left ventricle. There is usually symmetric hypertrophy of both the interventricular septum and left ventricular posterior wall. In those patients with a bicuspid aortic valve, one may see multiple eccentric diastolic closure echos of the abnormal aortic valve.

Cardiac Catheterization. In severe CoA the pulmonary wedge or left atrial pressures or both are elevated and there may be systemic arterial hypertension. The pressure difference across the coarctation depends on the severity of the stenosis, the degree of collateralization, and the presence or absence of systemic hypertension. Aortogram often shows a bicuspid aortic valve and a discrete coarctation distal to the left subclavian artery (Fig. 29).

CHILD WITH A HEART MURMUR

General Principles. In this section we present a few common, contrasting diagnostic problems that may confront the primary care physician in evaluating an older child with a heart murmur. As physical growth is frequently normal in this group and all are acyanotic, special emphasis will be placed on *location* and *quality* of the respective cardiac murmurs.

At this juncture several points need to be made about a more detailed cardiac examination. The patient should be fully undressed in order to allow adequate inspection and eliminate any extraneous noise from clothing or bed sheeting during auscultation. On palpation of the precordium the examiner may gain information about the patient's heart rate and any irregular cardiac rhythms. Increased parasternal lift would suggest the presence of right heart pathology, whereas an increased apical lift indicates left heart involvement. Palpable thrills at the lower left sternal border most commonly accompany a ventricular septal defect, whereas a thrill at the base of the heart and suprasternal notch suggests great vessel pathology. An apical thrill may be encountered in mitral valve incompetence.

The auscultatory portion of the examination should best begin with the patient in the supine position. Four specific areas should be examined: (1) the cardiac apex, (2) mid precordium and lower left sternal border, (3) upper left sternal border, and (4) upper right sternal border. High-frequency sounds or murmurs are best heard with the stethoscope diaphragm, whereas low frequency sounds (third and fourth heart sound and diastolic flow murmurs) are best heard with light pressure of the stethoscope bell. The examiner should determine: (1) timing and intensity of the first heart sound; (2) presence of any ejection click; (3) tonal quality, intensity, and duration of any systolic murmur; (4) splitting of the second heart sound and intensity of the pulmonic component; (5) quality and timing of any diastolic murmur; and (6) presence of any third or fourth heart sounds.

Using the auscultatory points just emphasized, we will discuss several diagnostic situations that commonly confront the clinician on the basis of location and quality of any murmurs heard (Table 4).

Table 4.   *Child with a Heart Murmur*

I. Murmur at the cardiac base
   A. Flow quality murmur
      1. Functional pulmonary flow murmur
      2. Atrial septal defect
   B. Ejection quality murmur
      1. Pulmonic valve stenosis
      2. Aortic valve stenosis
II. Murmur at the midsternal border
      1. Functional vibratory murmur
      2. Small ventricular septal defect
III. Murmur at the cardiac apex
      1. Mitral valve prolapse
      2. Rheumatic mitral valve insufficiency

I. Murmur at the Cardiac Base

A. *FLOW QUALITY MURMUR*

The flow quality murmur is often heard at the upper left sternal border (cardiac base) and is a low-to-medium frequency systolic murmur that is often unimpressive in intensity. We will emphasize the distinction between the functional or innocent pulmonary flow murmur and its pathologic cousin encountered in atrial septal defect.

1. Functional Pulmonary Flow Murmur

This type of murmur is the most common innocent murmur encountered in the pediatric age group and is believed to originate from vibrations of the pulmonary trunk during right ventricular systole.

The murmur is of maximal intensity at the upper left sternal border. It begins shortly after the first heart sound and ends well before the second heart sound. The characteristic features are that it is soft, medium in frequency and of low intensity. This murmur is loudest in the supine position and may be intensified by exercise, fever, or anemia. There are no ejection clicks. The second heart sound is normally split and varies with respiration. Because these murmurs do not reflect any hemodynamic abnormality, the chest x-ray and electrocardiogram are normal.

2. Atrial Septal Defect (ASD)

Clinical Features.   This defect is well tolerated in infancy and growth is not affected. The majority are females and are asymptomatic or show mild decrease in exercise tolerance. A palpable parasternal lift is present secondary to right ventricular dilatation. A medium frequency, low intensity pulmonic flow quality murmur is heard at the upper left sternal border. This murmur may have all the characteristics of the functional pulmonary flow murmur discussed. The main diagnostic clue is that the second heart sound is widely split and does not vary with respiration. The other pathognomonic sign is a short, mid diastolic tricuspid flow murmur at the lower left sternal border (relative tricuspid valve stenosis). An apical murmur of mitral insufficiency may be present owing to an associated cleft or prolapse of the mitral valve.

Chest X-Ray.   The heart is of normal size or may be mildly enlarged and the pulmonary artery prominent (Fig. 31). The pulmonary vascularity is increased of the shunt variety. On the lateral view there is no left atrial enlargement.

Electrocardiogram.   In ostium secundum ASD, there is often right axis deviation. There may be signs of right atrial enlargement and a prolonged P-R interval. The precordial complexes show evidence of right ventricular hy-

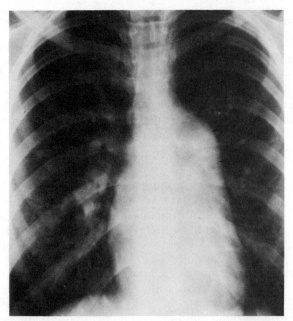

Figure 31. Chest x-ray of a 15-year-old female with an atrial septal defect. Note the prominent pulmonary artery (arrows) and the shunt vascularity.

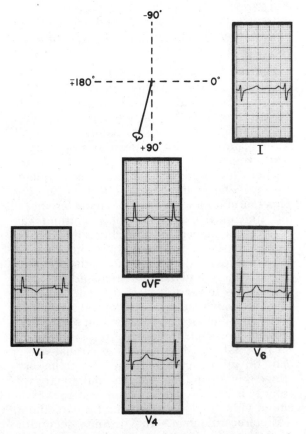

Figure 32. Electrocardiogram of a 15-year-old female with an ostium secundum atrial septal defect. Note the right axis deviation and right ventricular volume overload pattern (low voltage slow R wave in V₁).

pertrophy of the volume overload type (Fig. 32). Similar precordial patterns are seen in both ostium primum and sinus venosus atrial septal defects. However, the ostium primum ASD manifests a frontal QRS axis that is deviated leftward and superiorly (0 to −90 degrees). The sinus venosus ASD is frequently associated with an ectopic atrial pacemaker, identified electrocardiographically by a left and superior P axis and frequently a short P-R interval.

Echocardiogram. The common echocardiographic findings in ASD are those of right ventricular volume overload (Fig. 33). In ostium primum ASD, since it is part of the spectrum of endocardial cushion defect, the anterior leaflet of the mitral valve may appear in closer apposition to the interventricular septum in diastole than normal.

Cardiac Catheterization and Angiocardiography. The catheter can easily be manipulated across the defect into the left atrium and pulmonary veins. There is an increase in oxygen saturation at the right atrial level. There may be a small associated right-to-left shunt owing to streaming of blood from the inferior vena cava toward the ostium secundum ASD or from the superior vena cava toward the sinus venosus defect. Right heart pressures may be normal or mildly elevated. The anatomic type of defect can be defined by selective angiocardiography.

B. EJECTION QUALITY MURMUR

The ejection murmur at the cardiac base is of harsher tonal quality, occupies all of systole, and is of greater intensity than the flow quality murmur. It is crescendo-decrescendo in configuration and may obscure the heart sounds. The two most common pathologic entities producing ejection murmurs at the cardiac base are pulmonic valve stenosis and aortic valve stenosis.

1. Pulmonic Valve Stenosis (PS)
Clinical Features. Growth and development are usually not affected even in severe pulmonic valve stenosis (PS). Characteristically, children with this defect are chubby and have a round face with hypertelorism. Patients with mild or moderate PS are asymptomatic, whereas those with severe stenosis may have decreased exercise tolerance. A suprasternal notch thrill is usually present, while a precordial thrill may be present only in moderately severe cases. A systolic ejection click is heard at the upper left sternal border that may vary in intensity with respiration, being louder during expiration. This is followed by a harsh crescendo-decrescendo systolic ejection mur-

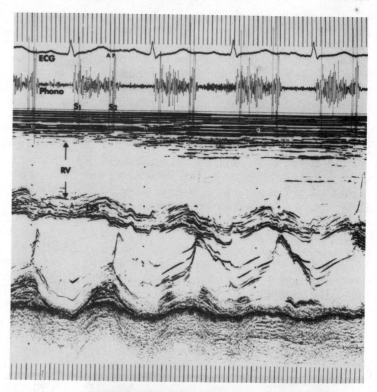

Figure 33. Simultaneous phono and echo-cardiogram of a 14-year-old female with an atrial septal defect. Note the constant splitting of the second heart sound (S₂) and the presence of right ventricular volume overload: dilated right ventricle (RV) and paradoxical anterior systolic movement of the interventricular septum (IVS).

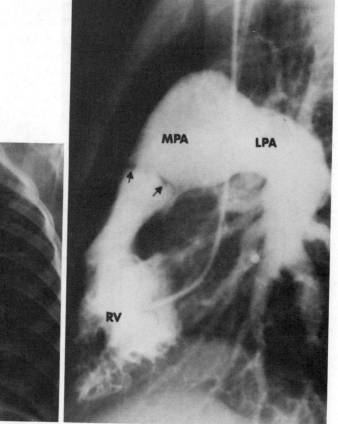

Figure 34. Chest x-ray of an 8-year-old female with pulmonic valve stenosis (left). Note the prominence of the main pulmonary artery (large arrows) and of its axial continuation, the left pulmonary artery (small arrows). Angiocardiogram (right): The lateral view of the right ventriculogram (RV) clearly shows a thickened and domed pulmonary valve (arrows) and poststenotic dilatation of the main (MPA) and left pulmonary artery (LPA).

mur that ends before the second heart sound in mild stenosis or may extend through aortic closure to the pulmonic component in severe stenosis. The second heart sound is typically widely split because of prolonged emptying time of the right ventricle secondary to the obstruction. The pulmonic component is diminished in intensity. Occasionally there is a short diastolic murmur of pulmonic valve insufficiency.

Chest X-Ray. The most characteristic radiographic finding is poststenotic dilatation of the main and left pulmonary arteries (Fig. 34). Heart size and pulmonary vascularity are normal.

Electrocardiogram. In mild PS, the ECG may show minimal signs of right ventricular hypertrophy, often manifested only by a positive or upright T wave in the right precordial leads. In moderate or severe PS, the ECG shows progressive degrees of right ventricular pressure overload, varying from pure R waves with normally inverted T waves in patients with near systemic right ventricular pressure (Fig. 35) to a qR pattern with ST segment depression in patients with suprasystemic right ventricular pressure. Signs of right atrial enlargement may also be present.

Echocardiogram. The echocardiogram is the least useful tool in evaluating isolated PS. In mild PS, the pulmonic valve echo may be normal. In moderate to severe stenosis, owing to decreased right ventricular compliance and secondary forceful right atrial contraction, there is exaggeration of the normal posterior or presystolic motion of the pulmonic valve leaflet ("a" dip). Thickening of the anterior wall of the right ventricle may be present.

Cardiac Catheterization and Angiocardiography. Right ventricular peak systolic pressures are elevated in direct proportion to the severity of the stenosis. With severe obstruction, pressure in the right ventricle may be greater than systemic pressure. Right atrial and right ventricular end diastolic pressures are also elevated secondary to decreased compliance of the right ventricle. Angiocardiography will disclose the thickened pulmonic valve leaflets with doming of the valve in systole (Fig. 34).

2. Aortic Valve Stenosis (AS)

Clinical Features. A bicuspid, nonstenotic aortic valve may statistically be the most common congenital heart defect. Patients are usually males and are asymptomatic and have normal radiographic and electrocardiographic findings. It is associated with coarctation of the aorta in 75 per cent of patients.

Patients with moderate aortic valve stenosis are usually asymptomatic throughout the pediatric age range and are often robust and athletic individuals. Symptoms of chest pain or syncope or both, if present, are ominous signs of severe stenosis. There is a palpable apical lift and usually a suprasternal notch thrill. A precordial thrill at the upper right sternal border usually indicates a moderate-to-severe stenosis. A prominent ejection click is heard both at the cardiac apex and upper right sternal border and does not vary in intensity with respiration, an important point in differentiating this click from that heard in pulmonic valve stenosis. The systolic murmur is harsh and crescendo-decrescendo in quality, beginning after the ejection click and ending at the second heart sound. The second heart sound may be normal in mild or moderate stenosis. In severe stenosis there is prolonged emptying of the left ventricle, with delayed closure of the aortic valve resulting in a narrowly split or single second heart sound. A high-frequency, early diastolic murmur of aortic valve insufficiency is sometimes present.

Chest X-Ray. The most characteristic radiographic sign of aortic valve stenosis is post-

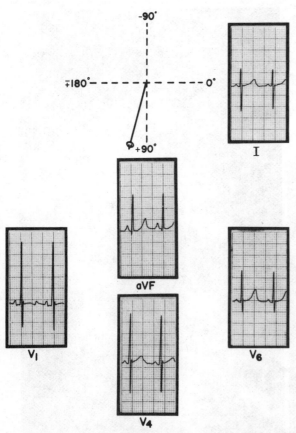

Figure 35. Electrocardiogram of a 3-year-old child with moderately severe pulmonic valve stenosis. Note the right axis deviation and right ventricular hypertrophy of the pressure overload type (tall R waves and biphasic T waves in V_1).

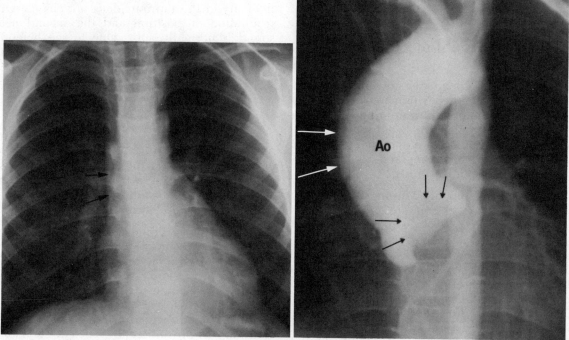

Figure 36. Chest x-ray of a boy with aortic valve stenosis (left). Note the laterally displaced superior vena cava (arrows) by the poststenotic dilated ascending aorta. The heart has a left ventricular configuration. Aortogram (Ao) in aortic valve stenosis (right) showing the domed valve in systole (arrowheads) and the poststenotic dilatation of the ascending aorta (arrows).

stenotic dilatation of the ascending aorta, which may produce rightward displacement of the superior vena cava. The heart size is usually normal or may have an abnormal left ventricular configuration in the frontal view characterized by a concavity in the area of the pulmonary artery and downward displacement of the apex (Fig. 36). Pulmonary vascularity may be normal or show pulmonary venous congestion.

Electrocardiogram. Those with a bicuspid aortic valve or mild stenosis may have a normal ECG or show left ventricular hypertrophy (Fig. 37). The ECG may not reflect the degree of hemodynamic obstruction but those with severe AS will manifest signs of left ventricular pressure overload with ST-T segment changes of ischemia or strain or both.

Echocardiogram. There is frequently symmetric hypertrophy of the left ventricle and increased diameter of the aortic root. The diastolic closure lines of the aortic valve may appear multiple and dense or eccentrically placed. The degree of aortic cusp separation in systole is not a reliable indicator of the severity of the stenosis with single crystal echocardiography.

Cardiac Catheterization and Angiocardiography. Left ventricular peak systolic pressure is elevated in proportion to the severity of the stenosis. In severe cases the left atrial and left ventricular end diastolic pressures are increased owing to decreased left ventricular compliance. Angiocardiography often demon-

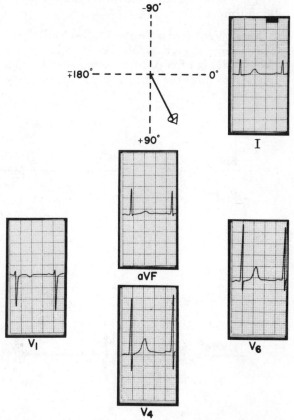

Figure 37. Electrocardiogram of a 10-year-old girl with moderate aortic valve stenosis. The tracing is suggestive of a left ventricular pressure overload pattern (small q and tall R waves in V_6).

strates thick leaflets that dome during systole (Fig. 36).

II. Murmur at the Midsternal Border

The two most commonly encountered murmurs in this anatomic position are the functional, innocent vibratory murmur and the murmur of a small ventricular septal defect (VSD). As both of these situations are of no hemodynamic significance, the chest x-ray and electrocardiogram are within normal limits.

1. Functional Vibratory Murmur

This is another very common innocent cardiac murmur. It is rarely heard in infancy but occurs frequently after the age of 3 years.

The vibratory murmur is best heard at the mid to lower left sternal border or mid precordium. It is loudest in the supine position, and may diminish when the patient is sitting up. Characteristically, the murmur has a musical, harmonic frequency and has been likened to a "twanging string." It begins after the first heart sound and ends well before the second heart sound (Fig. 38). The second heart sound is normally split and moves with respiration. There are no associated ejection clicks or diastolic murmurs.

2. Small Ventricular Septal Defect (VSD)

The murmur of a small ventricular septal defect (VSD) is of very high frequency, begins immediately after the first heart sound, and may occupy only the first portion of systole. The intensity of the murmur does not change with respiration or position and the second heart sound is normally split. Due to the hemodynamic insignificance of the left-to-right shunt, there are no mitral flow murmurs.

III. Murmur at the Cardiac Apex

Generally, any high-frequency murmur that originates at the cardiac apex should be considered pathologic regardless of the intensity. We will emphasize the two most commonly encountered apical systolic murmurs in children and their clinical features.

1. Mitral Valve Prolapse (MVP)

Clinical Features. Children with mitral valve prolapse (MVP) are asymptomatic or may complain of vague chest pain and shortness of breath. Auscultation typically reveals an apical mid systolic click that may occur as an isolated finding or be followed by a late systolic murmur of mitral valve insufficiency. The click and murmur vary with position and are often absent with the patient supine and intensified in the sitting, standing, or squatting position.

Chest X-Ray. Cardiac size and pulmonary vascularity are usually normal. Skeletal anomalies are frequent including kyphoscoliosis or straight back syndrome (Fig. 39).

Electrocardiogram. Characteristically there is flattening or inversion of the T waves in standard leads II, III, and aVF, although this

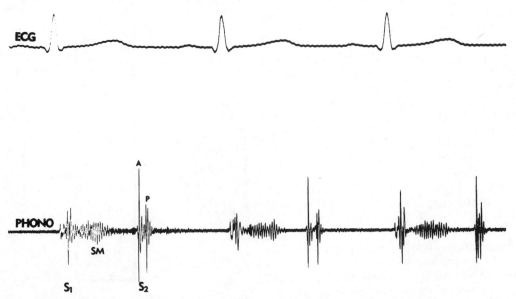

Figure 38. Phonocardiogram showing the characteristic "picket fence" pattern produced by the harmonic vibratory type functional murmur. Note the variable splitting of the second heart sound. Key: S_1 = first heart sound; SM = systolic murmur; S_2 = second heart sound (A = aortic, P = pulmonary components).

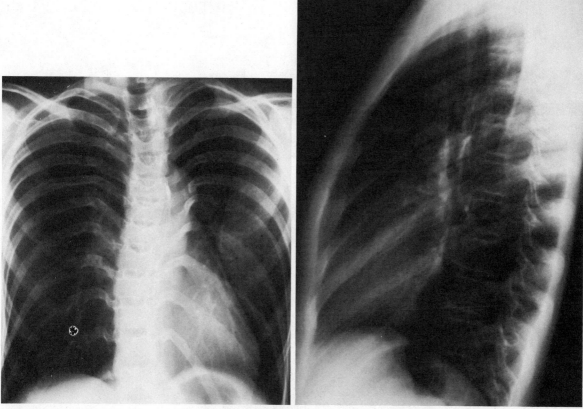

Figure 39. Chest x-ray of an adolescent with mitral valve prolapse and scoliosis (left). Lateral view of another patient (right) showing a narrow anteroposterior diameter and a straight back.

Figure 40. Electrocardiogram of a 13-year-old girl with mitral valve prolapse and insufficiency showing left atrial enlargement (broad P waves in V_6) and the characteristic ST-T changes (flat T waves and prolonged QT interval).

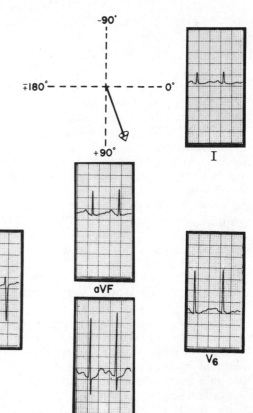

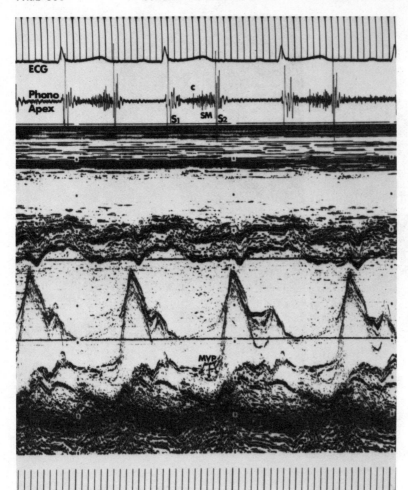

Figure 41. Simultaneous phono and echocardiogram of a 10-year-old female with mitral valve prolapse. Note the mid systolic click (c) and the late systolic murmur (SM) timing with the posterior prolapse of the mitral valve leaflet (MVP).

finding is not a constant feature (Fig. 40). Those patients with significant mitral insufficiency may show signs of left atrial enlargement. Supraventricular or ventricular dysrhythmias may occur in the young adult population.

Echocardiogram. The echocardiographic findings of MVP are pathognomonic. There are various degrees of prolapse of the posterior mitral leaflet, the most common occurring in late systole with its onset coinciding in timing with a mid systolic click (Fig. 41). In some instances the prolapse may be pansystolic, with posterior "hammocking" of the mitral leaflet throughout all of systole.

2. Rheumatic Mitral Valve Insufficiency (MI)

Clinical Features. Patients with mild mitral insufficiency (MI) are asymptomatic. Those with severe MI often are dyspneic and complain of easy fatigability or orthopnea. These patients manifest an active precordium with a hyperdynamic apical impulse, often with a palpable thrill. The murmur of MI is very high

frequency, begins with the first heart sound, and extends all through systole to the second heart sound (holosystolic or pansystolic). There are no ejection clicks. The second heart sound is usually normal with mild MI or, in severe cases with pulmonary hypertension, may have increased intensity of pulmonic valve closure. Third and fourth heart sounds are present. A mid diastolic mitral flow murmur is often heard. Not uncommonly there is an associated murmur of aortic valve insufficiency.

Chest X-Ray. Heart size and pulmonary vascularity may be normal in mild cases. With significant MI or rheumatic carditis, cardiomegaly is usually present. Pathognomonically there is prominence of the left atrial appendage (Fig. 42). The body of the left atrium itself is also dilated with posterior displacement of the barium-filled esophagus. The pulmonary vascularity is increased of the pulmonary venous obstructive type with redistribution of flow to the upper lobes.

Electrocardiogram. Patients with mild MI may have a normal ECG. Patients with moder-

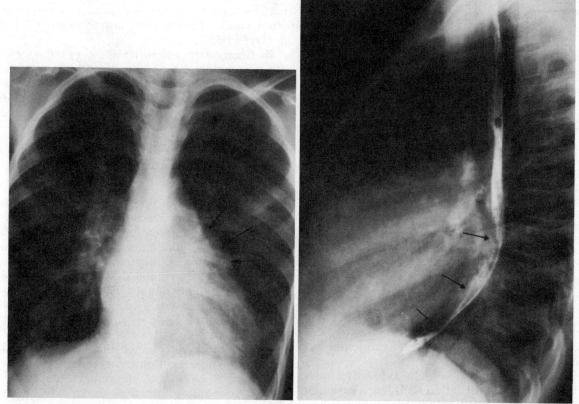

Figure 42.   Chest x-rays of an 8-year-old girl with severe rheumatic mitral valve insufficiency. Posteroanterior view (left) showing the characteristic dilatation of the left atrial appendage (arrowheads) seen in patients with rheumatic heart disease. The pulmonary vascularity shows venous congestion with redistribution of blood flow to the dilated upper lobe veins. The lateral view (right) shows the indentation on the barium-filled esophagus (arrows) by the dilated left atrium.

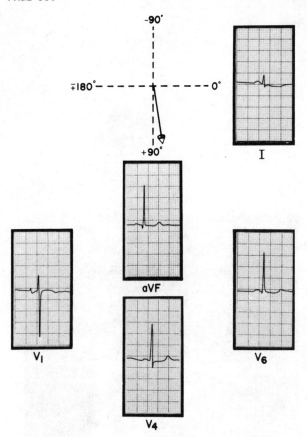

Figure 43. Electrocardiogram of a 13-year-old female with chronic rheumatic heart disease and severe mitral valve insufficiency. There is marked left atrial enlargement (broad and notched P waves in leads I and V_6). Despite the presence of a left ventricular volume overload lesion, the left precordial leads characteristically show small q waves and relatively flat T waves.

ate to severe insufficiency will show signs of left atrial enlargement and left ventricular hypertrophy (Fig. 43).

Echocardiogram. The echo typically shows signs of left atrial dilatation with left ventricular volume overload. Patients with associated aortic valve insufficiency will have abnormal diastolic vibrations of the anterior mitral leaflet.

VALVULAR HEART DISEASE

By ROBERT S. FRASER, M.D.
Edmonton, Alberta, Canada

The incidence of rheumatic fever has fallen over the past 30 years and this has increased the relative importance of some formerly unrecognized or infrequently occurring valvular abnor-

malities. Nevertheless, rheumatic and congenital heart disease remain important causes of heart murmurs. Many can be correctly identified with noninvasive investigation, in which auscultation retains pride of place.

MITRAL STENOSIS

ETIOLOGY

A. *Congenital mitral stenosis* is a rare condition generally associated with maldevelopment of the left side of the heart. Parachute mitral valve, characterized by one papillary muscle, may be recognized beyond infancy, when most other cases of congenital mitral stenosis have declared themselves.

B. *Rheumatic valvulitis* is accepted as the most common precedent of mitral stenosis, which is characterized by loss of mobility of the leaflets, fusion of the commissures and chordae tendineae, and finally, calcification of the valve leaflets.

CLINICAL AND HEMODYNAMIC FEATURES

Obstruction of the blood flow through a narrowed mitral orifice leads to restriction of cardiac output and an increase in pressure in the left atrium and the pulmonary venous system. The initial symptoms of fatigue, decreased exercise tolerance, and exertional dyspnea reflect these changes in hemodynamics. Elevation of pulmonary vascular resistance may lead to an increase in right ventricular pressure, fluid retention, and signs of congestive failure. Orthopnea results from pulmonary congestion, and cough is a common symptom. Pulmonary edema may be precipitated by effort, emotion, sexual intercourse, respiratory infection, pregnancy, or the onset of atrial fibrillation.

Hemoptysis may be sudden and profuse owing to rupture of an endobronchial vein. It usually stops spontaneously. It is rare in the presence of high pulmonary vascular resistance and is an earlier rather than a later symptom in the natural course of the disease. Blood-stained sputum may be seen with respiratory infections, pulmonary edema, or pulmonary infarction.

The course from the initial involvement of the mitral valve appears to be abbreviated in direct relation to the number of recurrences of streptococcal infection. Significant obstruction may occur in as soon as 5 years but is generally delayed for 20 years after the initial attack.

The clinical findings are those indicative of obstruction of the mitral orifice and those secondary to an increase in left atrial pressure and its consequences. The apical impulse is brief

Table 1. *Clinical Diagnosis of Valvular Heart Disease*

	Mitral Stenosis	*Mitral Regurgitation*	*Aortic Stenosis*	*Aortic Regurgitation*
Arterial pulse	Small volume	Normal or slightly collapsing	Anacrotic small bisferious when stenosis and regurgitation combined; "jerky" pulse in IHSS	Collapsing
Venous pulse	Increased pulmonary pressure reflected in prominent "a" wave; atrial fibrillation; → loss of "a" wave	Same as for MS	Normal, unless in failure	Normal, unless in failure
Palpation	Apical first sound palpable; diastolic apical thrill may be present; RV overactive with elevated pulmonary pressure	May be systolic apical thrill	Sustained forceful apical thrust	Diastolic thrill may mean retroversion of aortic cusp, perforation, luetic disease
Heart sounds and murmurs	Diastolic, rumbling crescendo; localized apical murmur; first sound increased; second sound may be loud with elevated pulmonary pressure; splitting inconstant; opening snap heard widely indicative of mobile cusp	Pansystolic apical murmur transmitted to axilla; abnormal wide splitting of second sound; third heart sound at apex	Systolic ejection murmur apex to 2nd R space; transmission to left carotid; paradoxical splitting of second sounds (also in LBBB) with significant stenosis; systolic ejection click with mild stenosis	Diastolic decrescendo, left sternal border; diastolic murmur max. in 3rd right space suggests disease of aortic root; Austin Flint murmur at apex vs. mitral stenosis; third sound common

and tapping, and both the first sound and a diastolic thrill may be felt.

In the presence of sinus rhythm, the diastolic murmur is rumbling and crescendo in character, leading to an accentuated first sound. The left atrial pressure (and the severity of obstruction) is reflected roughly in the length of the murmur and by the shortening of the interval between the apical second sound and the opening snap. The latter is best heard in the apicosternal region but is well transmitted to the base, where it can be mistaken for an accentuated pulmonary second sound.

Elevation of the pulmonary vascular resistance leads to accentuation of the pulmonary component of the second sound, which may become palpable, together with a left parasternal heave of a hypertrophied right ventricle. Pulmonary hypertension gives rise to a prominent jugular "a" wave in the presence of sinus rhythm.

LABORATORY STUDIES

A. The *electrocardiogram* may be normal. The presence of broad notched P waves in lead 2 and a biphasic P wave in lead V_1, with a wide negative component, is indicative of overload of the left atrium. Evidence for right ventricular hypertrophy may be recognized when pulmonary hypertension is present. The waves of atrial fibrillation in patients with mitral stenosis are generally rather coarse.

B. *Radiologic findings* consist of left atrial enlargement, as identified by the prominence of the left atrial appendage along the left cardiac border, a "double shadow" in the posteroanterior view, and displacement of the barium-filled esophagus in the lateral and oblique views of the heart. The presence of lymphatic congestion is recognized in the horizontal linear markings (Kerley lines) near the costophrenic angles. Chronic edema is further shown by bilateral prominence of the hila.

Redistribution of venous blood flow with prominence of the upper lobe vasculature is indicative of pulmonary venous hypertension. Further changes may include enlargement of the right heart (right ventricle and right atrium).

C. *Echocardiography* can provide valuable information concerning the severity of mitral stenosis by measurement of the movement of the cusps. The size of the left atrium can also be calculated.

D. *Cardiac catheterization* and *angiocardi-*

ography are useful in assessing the amount of associated regurgitation. Calculation of pulmonary vascular resistance may be desirable in a small number of patients and in some instances pressure measurements may be useful in sequential appraisals of the patient's progress.

DIFFERENTIAL DIAGNOSIS

A. *Myxoma* of the left atrium is seldom confused with mitral stenosis if the complaints and physical findings are carefully evaluated. Intermittent syncope, particularly positional, emboli in the absence of atrial fibrillation, positional variation of the diastolic apical murmur, and infrequent occurrence or uncharacteristic quality of an opening snap suggest this diagnosis in a patient whose left atrium is normal in size and who may have a fever, elevated sedimentation rate, and arthralgia. The frequent use of echocardiograms in assessing mitral stenosis should further reduce the possibility of confusion through recognition of a tumor in the left atrium.

B. An *Austin Flint murmur* of aortic regurgitation may simulate a mitral diastolic murmur. An Austin Flint murmur may be suspected if there is no opening snap and no other reason for the absence of an opening snap is found (e.g., a heavily calcified mitral valve). Further evidence for the aortic origin of the murmur is the presence of an apical third heart sound, a reduction in intensity of the murmur after peripheral vascular resistance is reduced with amyl nitrite, and echocardiographic evidence for fluttering of the anteroseptal mitral leaflet with delay in opening of the valve.

C. *Atrial septal defect* (ostium secundum) can be mistaken for mitral stenosis when the widely split second sounds in the pulmonary area provide the illusion of an opening snap. However, there is no characteristic opening snap of the apex, and although a diastolic "flow" murmur may be heard internal to the apex, it has no crescendo quality. There will also be no radiologic evidence for an enlarged left atrium.

COMPLICATIONS

A. *Atrial fibrillation* may not occur for 20 to 30 years after the initial recognition of mitral valvulitis. The rapid ventricular rate, shortened diastolic filling time, and resultant increase in pulmonary venous pressure may precipitate pulmonary edema.

B. *Systemic emboli* occur in up to 15 per cent of patients and the majority end in the cerebral circulation. The occurrence is not related to the severity of mitral stenosis. Paroxysmal atrial fibrillation may contribute to thrombus formation and lead to emboli in those patients who later present in sinus rhythm.

C. *Hemoptysis* is rarely sufficient to be life-threatening.

D. *Infective endocarditis* is a rare complication of pure mitral stenosis but the incidence increases with the association of even trivial mitral regurgitation.

E. *Severe pulmonary vascular obstruction* with pulmonary artery pressure nearing systemic levels is uncommon, but when present may lead to persistent right ventricular failure, effort dyspnea, exertional angina and syncope.

MITRAL REGURGITATION

ETIOLOGY

Regurgitation through the mitral valve may result from a wider variety of causes than those that may lead to stenosis. Effective functioning of the valvular apparatus depends on the integrity of the valve leaflets, the annulus, the infravalvular apparatus (chordae and papillary muscles), and the left ventricular myocardium. The more important causes of dysfunction of any of these are classified as nonrheumatic and rheumatic.

Nonrheumatic Mitral Regurgitation

A. *Congenital clefts* of the mitral leaflets may be either isolated or associated with maldevelopment of the atrioventricular junction (ostium primum defect or atrioventricular canal). *Congenitally long or short chordae* may interfere with the mutual buttressing effect of the leaflets, permitting regurgitation. *A single papillary muscle and parachute mitral valve* may be incompetent in systole.

B. *Infective endocarditis,* arising on a valve damaged by rheumatic valvulitis, on a prolapsing or "floppy" valve, or on a cleft mitral valve, may produce or exacerbate mitral regurgitation.

C. *Mitral valve prolapse* generally involves the posterior cusp and in its milder forms may not produce regurgitation. Floppy valves, associated with Marfan's syndrome, polychondritis, and Ehlers-Danlos syndrome, are included in this category.

D. *Rupture of chordae* can occur with an apparently normal mitral valve but may also be associated with mucoid degeneration of mitral cusps or infective endocarditis, and can produce sudden severe mitral regurgitation.

E. *Blunt injury* to the chest may disrupt the papillary muscles and chordae or damage the valve cusps.

F. *Infarction of papillary muscles* may interfere with the normal support of the edge of the cusps by the chordae and produce regurgitation after inferior or posterior myocardial infarction. Regurgitation may also occur during episodes of angina, presumably from ischemia of the papillary muscles.

G. *Dilatation of the left ventricular cavity* may distort normal relations and produce mitral regurgitation.

Rheumatic Mitral Regurgitation

About one half of patients with rheumatic mitral disease with regurgitant lesions have no obstruction; the other half have mixed stenosis and regurgitation. There is usually a history of acute rheumatic fever and early recognition of the holosystolic apical murmur.

CLINICAL AND HEMODYNAMIC FEATURES

The clinical presentations of chronic and acute mitral regurgitation are different, probably because of the difference in compliance in the left atrium. When enlarged and distensible, the left atrium protects the pulmonary vascular bed from systolic surges of blood under high pressure. Pulmonary edema is a frequent presenting sign in patients suffering acute disruptions caused by ruptured chordae, perforated cusps, or infarcted papillary muscle.

Fatigue, exertional dyspnea, and palpitation are the major symptoms of chronic regurgitation. Patients with mitral prolapse are frequently asymptomatic if regurgitation is minimal. They may complain of atypical pains in the left chest, generally unrelated to activity. Atrial and ventricular arrhythmias are not unusual.

Examination of the patient with mitral regurgitation discloses a hyperdynamic apical impulse, extending beyond the diameter of a 50-cent piece. There may be a left parasternal rocking impulse, even in the absence of pulmonary hypertension. This has been attributed to the transmitted systolic expansion of a large left atrium. The first sound at the apex is usually normal except when the anterior cusp is rigid or destroyed. Merging of the first sound with a loud holosystolic murmur may give an illusion of softness to it. The holosystolic murmur of rheumatic mitral regurgitation tends to continue with constant intensity to the second sound, whereas the nonrheumatic regurgitant murmur is early, mid, or late systolic, and more diamond-shaped in character.

Widely split second sounds over the base and a sharp third heart sound over the apex are signs of moderate to severe regurgitation. An opening snap occurs in 10 per cent of those with mitral regurgitation (with a large anterior and a small mural cusp) and is not necessarily indicative of mitral stenosis.

Prolapse of the posterior cusp permits a systolic jet to transmit the murmur to the base of the heart and superficial examination may lead to an incorrect diagnosis of aortic stenosis. Prolapse of a mitral cusp characteristically produces a single systolic click or a series of clicks, which are followed by a mid or late systolic murmur. Both the click and the murmur appear earlier in systole when the patient stands and are delayed in appearance with an increase in afterload such as that induced by isometric hand-grip.

LABORATORY FINDINGS

A. The *electrocardiogram* shows voltage criteria and ST segment changes of left ventricular hypertrophy (LVH) in less than one half the patients. The P wave may be lengthened and biphasic in lead V_1. Atrial fibrillation is present in most patients 15 to 20 years after their initial illness.

B. *Radiologic findings* consist of enlargement of the left ventricle and moderate-to-aneurysmal dilatation of the left atrium. In acute mitral regurgitation the atrium is frequently normal in size.

C. The *echocardiogram* is useful in identifying a prolapsing mitral cusp. It does not identify mitral regurgitation directly but may show irregular, bizarre diastolic motion of a cusp, evidence suggestive of ruptured chordae. The size of the left atrium and left ventricle can be estimated.

D. *Cardiac catheterization* and ventriculography can be useful in estimating the amount of regurgitant flow and identifying prolapsing cusps as well as recording changes in pulmonary vascular resistance.

DIFFERENTIAL DIAGNOSIS

A. The *murmur of aortic stenosis* may be transmitted to the apex and conversely that of a prolapsing mural cusp may be best heard over the base. The changes in the murmurs induced by standing and the use of amyl nitrite are useful in distinguishing these. (The aortic murmur is intensified and the mitral reduced.)

B. *Rupture of the ventricular septum* may produce a murmur that can be heard well at the apex as well as the left sternal border. Catheterization may be necessary to distinguish between this on the one hand and ruptured chordae or infarction of a papillary muscle on the other in a patient with a myocardial infarction.

C. *Tricuspid regurgitation* can be distinguished from mitral regurgitation by the behavior of the jugular veins and the inspiratory increase in length and intensity of the tricuspid murmur.

COMPLICATIONS

A. *Atrial fibrillation* may be intermittent initially, to be succeeded 15 years or so after the initial damage by a persistent arrhythmia.

B. *Infective endocarditis* seems to have a predilection for cases of mild mitral regurgitation. It has also been reported in patients with prolapsing mitral cusps. The hazard is unrelated to the severity of the regurgitation.

C. *Emboli* may arise from left atrial thrombi.

AORTIC STENOSIS

ETIOLOGY

A. *Congenital* valvular aortic stenosis is the most common congenital lesion involving the outflow tract of the left ventricle. The aortic valve is thickened and rigid; the commissures, which are incompletely developed, may be two or three in number. A congenital bicuspid valve generally becomes thickened and calcified by the fifth decade. Other but uncommon congenital forms of obstruction are *supravalvular* and *discrete subvalvular stenosis.* The left ventricular outflow tract can also be obstructed by hypertrophy of the septum and left ventricular wall *(idiopathic hypertrophic subaortic stenosis).*

B. *Rheumatic* aortic stenosis results from fusion of aortic cusps at the commissures and secondary calcification of thickened, rigid, and distorted leaflets.

CLINICAL AND HEMODYNAMIC FEATURES

This lesion, which is twice as common in men as in women, may not become manifest until a combination of restricted cardiac output and coronary artery disease results in angina, dyspnea, and syncope with or without effort, in the sixth decade. More severe degrees of obstruction caused by congenital aortic stenosis may produce symptoms in infancy or childhood.

Physical signs consist of a small sustained arterial pulse, a low pulse pressure, a basal systolic thrill, and a mid systolic murmur. An aortic ejection click indicates continuing mobility of the aortic cusps, more often noted in the patient with congenital aortic stenosis. The effect of amyl nitrite may be useful to distinguish between an apical systolic murmur arising from the aortic valve and the murmur of mitral origin. A faint early diastolic murmur is often heard along the left sternal border and is indicative of minimal aortic regurgitation.

LABORATORY FINDINGS

A. *The electrocardiogram* generally shows voltage criteria for left ventricular hypertrophy but is not specific and is not sufficiently sensitive to identify those at risk. It is particularly unreliable in the elderly patient with tight stenosis.

B. *X-rays* or *cardiac fluoroscopy* frequently shows a calcified aortic valve. There may be poststenotic prominence of the ascending aorta with evidence of hyperactivity noted at fluoroscopy. The left ventricle may be prominent as a result of hypertrophy.

C. *Echocardiography* helps to identify a bicuspid aortic valve and sometimes the level of obstruction in the other less frequent abnormalities of the left ventricular outflow tract and aorta.

D. *Cardiac catheterization* permits measurement of the gradient across the stenotic aortic valve and calculation of the valve orifice.

COMPLICATIONS

A. *Syncope* may result from atrioventricular block (generally caused by periannular calcium extending into the septum), from restricted cardiac output insufficient for a given level of exercise, from ineffective cerebral flow secondary to postexercise vasodilatation, and from arrhythmias. Death may result from any one of these mechanisms.

B. *Emboli* originating from a calcified valve may enter the cerebral or coronary circulation and cause infarction.

C. *Infective endocarditis* accounts for less than 20 per cent of deaths.

D. *Atrial fibrillation* is much less common in aortic stenosis than in patients with mitral disease, but its onset may lead to abrupt decompensation.

AORTIC REGURGITATION

In contrast to aortic stenosis, aortic regurgitation may be attributed to several causes and may be either chronic or acute in onset.

ETIOLOGY

A. *Rheumatic valvulitis* is a major cause of aortic regurgitation (80 per cent) and affects males twice as often as females.

B. *Syphilitic aortic regurgitation* results from aortitis of the ascending aorta that weakens and dilates the valve ring. It is frequently accompanied by angina because of coronary ostial involvement by the inflammatory changes. The disease is now uncommon.

C. *Congenital bicuspid aortic valves* may exhibit minor degrees of incompetence. *High ventricular septal defects* may interfere with the normal support of the aortic valve and lead to aortic regurgitation in addition to a left-to-right shunt.

D. *Blunt trauma* to the chest may produce tears in the aortic valve cusps, leading to acute regurgitation and left ventricular failure.

E. *Infective endocarditis* on either normal or minimally diseased valves may lead to perforation of a valve cusp.

F. *Aortic valve involvement* may occur in association with Marfan's syndrome, spondylitis, or Reiter's syndrome.

G. *Dissecting aortic aneurysm* may cause acute aortic regurgitation. Rupture of a *sinus of Valsalva aneurysm* into the left ventricle may simulate aortic regurgitation but may also disrupt an aortic cusp, leading to regurgitation.

CLINICAL AND HEMODYNAMIC FEATURES

Aortic insufficiency is often well tolerated for many years. Heart failure or death can be predicted within 2 years in 50 per cent of patients who exhibit (1) moderate or marked left ventricular hypertrophy clinically or radiologically, (2) electrocardiographic evidence for left ventricular hypertrophy, and (3) a systolic blood pressure greater than 140 and a diastolic less than 40 mm Hg.

The increase in stroke volume and reduction in peripheral vascular resistance results in the peripheral signs of aortic insufficiency (collapsing pulse, increased pulse pressure, and capillary pulsation). Breathlessness, orthopnea, and palpitations signal the beginning of decompensation. A few patients experience tachycardia and attacks of substernal pain at rest, often at night, which are relieved by nitroglycerin. The heaving apex is displaced down and to the left. The length of the diastolic decrescendo murmur heard along the left sternal border is not a reliable measure of the severity of the lesion. There is frequently a mid systolic murmur indicative of increased forward flow through the slightly stiffened valve leaflets. At the apex an Austin Flint murmur (discussed before) may be difficult to distinguish from the murmur of mitral stenosis. A diastolic thrill along the sternal border may be indicative of perforation of an aortic cusp, prolapse of the cusp into the left ventricular outflow tract, or syphilitic aortitis.

Decompensation may lead to a reduction in the length and intensity of the diastolic decrescendo murmur and some increase in the diastolic pressure, thereby obscuring the severity of the lesion.

LABORATORY STUDIES

A. The *electrocardiogram* may show a pattern of left ventricular hypertrophy with diastolic overloading.

B. *X-rays* demonstrate enlargement of the left ventricle and minimal if any enlargement of the left atrium until frank decompensation occurs.

C. The *echocardiogram* may be useful in identifying vegetations on the aortic leaflet or suggesting the presence of a bicuspid aortic valve.

D. *Cardiac catheterization* and angiocardiography may be required to exclude complicating lesions.

DIFFERENTIAL DIAGNOSIS

A. *Patent ductus arteriosus* can be recognized by the continuous nature of the murmur and the radiologic evidence for plethoric lung fields, often with some left atrial enlargement.

B. *Rupture of a sinus of Valsalva aneurysm* in either ventricle can best be recognized by aortography, which is indicated in patients with an acute onset of aortic regurgitation.

C. The *diastolic decrescendo murmur* of pulmonary hypertension may be suspected when other evidence points to pulmonary pressures at systemic levels. Such a murmur may intensify on inspiration.

COMPLICATIONS

Bacterial endocarditis constitutes a significant risk and is more frequently encountered than is the case with stenotic lesions.

PULMONIC VALVULAR DISEASE

ETIOLOGY

For practical purposes, only congenital pulmonic valvular stenosis need be considered.

Rare occurrences of carcinoid disease or acute infective endocarditis of the pulmonic valve (usually related to narcotic addiction) are listed only for completeness. Pulmonic regurgitation occasionally results from severe pulmonary hypertension, or as a rare congenital lesion.

CLINICAL AND HEMODYNAMIC FEATURES

Isolated pulmonic valvular stenosis is an uncommon congenital lesion that may present in infancy as a result of severe obstruction or may remain asymptomatic, characterized only by a systolic ejection murmur throughout adult life. The lesions of those with right ventricular pressures less than 55 mm Hg do not appear to progress to more severe degrees of obstruction.

Findings include a left parasternal lift indicative of right ventricular hypertrophy when significant obstruction exists, a systolic thrill over the outflow tract of the right ventricle, and a systolic ejection murmur with radiation through to the back at the left of the spine. Significant obstruction may be recognized by a prominent jugular "a" wave and a delayed pulmonic second sound. A systolic ejection click is variably present.

LABORATORY STUDIES

A. The *electrocardiogram* may show evidence for right ventricular hypertrophy.

B. *Radiologic findings* consist of prominence of the main pulmonary artery segment and right heart (right ventricle and right atrium).

C. *Cardiac catheterization* provides a measurement of the gradient across the stenotic valve.

DIFFERENTIAL DIAGNOSIS

A. *Aortic stenosis* with a basal systolic ejection murmur can sometimes be difficult to distinguish from pulmonic stenosis. The presence of a thrill, a delayed pulmonary second sound, and radiation of the murmur through to the back tend to favor pulmonic origin. Both murmurs may be transmitted to the carotids. An ejection click, if present, will diminish or disappear on inspiration only with pulmonic stenosis.

B. *Idiopathic dilatation* of the pulmonary artery can often be differentiated from pulmonary stenosis only by catheterization of the right heart.

C. *Atrial septal defects* are accompanied by a systolic ejection murmur but *fixed* splitting of the aortic and pulmonary second sounds. There is seldom an ejection click. The chest x-ray generally shows pulmonary plethora.

COMPLICATIONS

Infective endocarditis is most infrequent.

TRICUSPID VALVE DISEASE

ETIOLOGY

A. *Congenital tricuspid stenosis,* tricuspid atresia, and Ebstein's anomaly of the tricuspid valve are rare conditions. The first two usually lead to investigation in infancy.

B. *Trauma* is an infrequent but recognized cause of damage to the tricuspid valve, leading to regurgitation.

C. *Rheumatic tricuspid valvulitis* is relatively uncommon and practically never occurs as the only form of valvulitis in rheumatic disease. Tricuspid regurgitation may occur secondary to right ventricular enlargement and in most cases results from rheumatic aortic or mitral disease.

CLINICAL AND HEMODYNAMIC FINDINGS

Both regurgitation and stenosis result in a picture of right-sided failure and a noteworthy ability of the patient to tolerate lying flat. The symptoms and signs may mimic those of cirrhosis, with ascites rather than dependent edema being a prominent feature.

The diastolic murmur of tricuspid stenosis tends to be shorter than that of mitral stenosis and lacks a crescendo quality. An opening snap may be present. Both this murmur and the systolic murmur of tricuspid insufficiency increase in a characteristic fashion with inspiration except when the pressure in the right atrium is significantly increased. The neck veins show characteristic giant "a" waves with tricuspid stenosis and a prominent "y" descent with tricuspid regurgitation.

LABORATORY STUDIES

A. The *electrocardiogram* may reveal right ventricular and right atrial hypertrophy.

B. *X-rays* of the chest show a prominent right ventricular border. In the presence of tricuspid stenosis the lung fields may appear unusually normal for a patient with this degree of fluid retention. Other abnormalities are those of the associated valvular lesions.

C. *Cardiac catheterization* will permit measurement of the gradient across the stenotic tricuspid valve or may demonstrate the typical pressure tracing of tricuspid regurgitation.

Table 2. *Clinical Diagnosis of Valvular Heart Disease*

	Tricuspid Stenosis	Tricuspid Regurgitation	Pulmonary Stenosis	Pulmonary Regurgitation
Arterial pulse	Normal to small volume	Normal to small	Normal to small	Normal to small
Venous pulse	Large jugular "a" waves; prolonged "y" descent: inspiratory filling sometimes present in jugular	Prominent "cv" wave, rippling in character	Prominent "a" wave reflects RVH	Prominent "a" wave reflects pulmonary hypertension and RVH
Palpation	Mid-diastolic thrill, low left sternal border	Systolic thrill over lower sternum, some-times R parasternal interspaces	Systolic thrill over outflow RV	L parasternal systolic heave with severe insufficiency
Heart sounds and murmurs	Diastolic murmur over low left sternal border; increase with inspir-ation; opening snap may be heard	Sometimes paradoxical splitting of second sounds due to early pulmonary closure	Wide splitting of second sounds with moderate-severe stenosis but normal variation	Congenital pulmonary regurgitation may cause wide split second sounds; diastolic de-crescendo murmur, left sternal border

DIFFERENTIAL DIAGNOSIS

Tricuspid disease is generally missed be-cause it is not thought of. Other forms of central venous obstruction and hepatic cirrhosis may present similar clinical features and must be considered.

COMPLICATIONS

Tricuspid regurgitation may very occasion-ally produce a protein-losing enteropathy and an immunologic deficiency.

ISCHEMIC HEART DISEASE

By LOFTY L. BASTA, M.D.,
and JOHN F. COYLE, II, M.D.

Tulsa, Oklahoma

PATHOPHYSIOLOGY OF MYOCARDIAL ISCHEMIA

Myocardial ischemia results from failure of myocardial oxygen supply to match myocardial oxygen demands.

Oxygen delivery to the myocardium is affect-ed by coronary artery patency, coronary perfu-sion pressure, an autoregulation mechanism adjusting coronary arteriolar resistance to myo-cardial metabolic needs, oxygen content of the coronary artery blood, and the ability of myocar-dial cells to extract and utilize available oxygen. Given patent coronary arteries, coronary flow is controlled by myocardial metabolic demands, with tissue hypoxia and accumulation of adeno-sine leading to decreased coronary arteriolar re-sistance.

INTERPLAY BETWEEN DEMAND AND SUPPLY

Myocardial ischemia results from a discrep-ancy between myocardial oxygen demand and supply. Increased demand alone, without com-promised supply, rarely if ever causes myocar-dial ischemia. This is because of the built-in autoregulation of coronary flow. Table 1 lists causes of reduced oxygen supply. In most in-stances of transient myocardial ischemia, there is a transient increase in demand without a matched increase in supply.

Patients with stable angina usually experi-

Table 1. *Causes of Reduced Myocardial Oxygen Supply*

Coronary artery disease
Coronary artery spasm
Small vessel coronary disease
Aortic stenosis
Aortic insufficiency
Hypotension
Elevated left ventricular end-diastolic pressure
Hypoxia
Anemia and polycythemia
Abnormal oxygen dissociation curve of red cells or myo-
  globin
Cytotoxic agents

Table 2. *Factors Influencing Myocardial Oxygen Demand*

1. Myocardial muscle mass
2. Heart rate
3. Cardiac work/beat is dependent upon:
     Wall tension
       (Systolic BP × Ventricular Radius)

Less important
- Stroke volume
- Ejection phase
- Velocity of contraction
- Blood viscosity
- Electric depolarization

HR × Systolic BP × 10^{-2} (double product) correlates well with myocardial oxygen demand

endocardial layers caused by elevated left ventricular diastolic pressure.

In tachyarrhythmias, there is increased oxygen demand from increased heart rate and decreased supply caused by shortened diastolic period, and transient myocardial ischemia may occur with or without coronary occlusive disease.

Myocardial ischemia may result from decreased oxygen supply without an increase in demand. This is seen with acute coronary artery occlusion (thrombosis, embolism, or dissection), and in patients with spontaneous coronary artery spasm. In spasm, manifestations of cardiac ischemia occur without antecedent change in heart rate or blood pressure.

ence the manifestations of myocardial ischemia at a given double product (HR × Systolic BP $\times 10^{-2}$), which tends to be constant in a given patient, regardless of the rate or type of exercise causing angina.

In coronary atherosclerosis, clinical symptoms are present only at high work load with arterial stenosis of less than 50 per cent, and are often present on exertion with greater than 70 per cent stenosis. Pain that occurs at rest is almost always accompanied by total or near total coronary occlusion.

Patients with aortic stenosis often experience angina without significant coronary artery disease. Excessive oxygen demand is caused by increased muscle mass and left ventricular systolic pressure, causing increased LV wall tension (especially pronounced in patients with dilated left ventricles), and to a lesser extent by prolonged ejection phase (Table 2). Coronary supply is relatively compromised by the specific flow characteristics leading to reversal of systolic coronary flow (Venturi effect) and decreased effective coronary perfusion to the sub-

MANIFESTATIONS OF CARDIAC ISCHEMIA

Transient myocardial ischemia leads to metabolic, mechanical, electrical, and subjective changes expressed clinically and detectable by special tests (Table 3).

Recent reports indicate that pain is not an early manifestation of cardiac ischemia. Hemodynamic monitoring often shows impaired ventricular performance before the patient experiences angina. Similarly, ambulatory electrocardiography may show "transient ischemic changes" preceding chest pain or in the absence of chest pain.

Transient impairment of myocardial contractility is further expressed in complaints of shortness of breath, fatigue, or exertional hypotension.

During myocardial ischemia, disordered repolarization in ischemic tissue may be manifest in ST changes and can predispose to arrhythmias and conduction abnormalities.

Although chest pain is the hallmark of myo-

Table 3. *Manifestations of Myocardial Ischemia*

ISCHEMIA

METABOLIC ABNORMALITIES
(TISSUE HYPOXIA, ADENOSINE ACCUMULATION, LACTIC ACID PRODUCTION, ETC.)

Impaired Contractility	*Electric Abnormality*	*Pain*
Impaired segmental wall motion	ST changes	Exertional angina
Depressed LV ejection fraction	(depressed in subendocardial)	Angina at rest
Elevated LV end-diastolic pressure	(elevated in transmural)	Myocardial infarction
	Abnormality in impulse formation	
	Conduction abnormalities	
Shortness of breath	Ectopic activity	
Fatigue	Re-entrant arrhythmias	
Pump failure	Ventricular fibrillation	
Papillary muscle dysfunction		

cardial ischemia, the intensity, duration, and radiation of pain may be influenced by factors other than the ischemic process. This is discussed subsequently.

ANGINA PECTORIS

Chest Pain. It has become customary to classify angina chest pain into *typical* and *atypical* types, depending on whether the pain conforms to Heberden's original description of angina pectoris.

It should be emphasized that, short of coronary arteriography, careful history taking is the most important tool in the assessment of coronary artery disease. Significant coronary artery occlusion is expected in over 95 per cent of patients with a history of "typical angina pectoris." In contrast, over 85 per cent of patients with chest pain that is "unlike angina pectoris" will show no significant occlusive disease in coronary arteriograms. Some sex variation is present and women have a higher "false-positive" history rate.

The important features that characterize most episodes of ischemic chest pain are: (1) they occur in response to precipitating factors such as exercise, emotion, or exposure to cold, or following a heavy meal or, in severe cases, at rest; (2) they have a limited duration, usually of a few minutes; and (3) they are relieved by cessation of activity and by nitroglycerin. Belching is commonly encountered with angina pectoris and is often associated with pain relief. This phenomenon should not lead to the misdiagnosis of an upper gastrointestinal cause of pain. Ischemic chest pain is characteristically diffuse and ill defined and, when it spreads to the arms, is usually perceived as pressure or weakness rather than as numbness or tingling; the latter suggests somatic (root or nerve) pain rather than visceral pain.

Certain categories of ischemic chest pain are particularly likely to be misinterpreted or overlooked and therefore warrant special description. Among these are prodromal pains that occur before acute myocardial infarction, rest angina, Prinzmetal's angina, nocturnal angina, and linked angina. Over half the patients sustaining an acute myocardial infarction experience prodromal symptoms in the few days or weeks before the infarction; of these symptoms, chest pain is the most common prodrome. Pain often recurs without definite provocation and sometimes lasts longer than a few minutes. However, pain usually has the typical features of ischemic cardiac pain in that it tends to be perceived as diffuse, ill-defined chest oppression.

Unstable angina pectoris is a state of new or changing pattern of chest pain. Almost 20 per cent of patients admitted to the coronary care unit with the diagnosis of unstable angina pectoris do not subsequently show significant proximal coronary artery stenosis in the coronary angiograms. Detailed history in those with normal coronaries often provides clues suggesting a functional nature of the pain, such as (1) precipitation by certain emotional situations; (2) lack of consistency in quality, location, or radiation at different times; or (3) somatic, rather than visceral, characteristics. Monitoring of the patient during pain episodes can be of great help in distinguishing ischemic from nonischemic chest pain; patients with angina exhibit changes in pulse rate (usually an increase), blood pressure (usually an increase), and often in the electrocardiogram (usually depression of the ST segment) during ischemic episodes. Patients in whom pulmonary wedge pressure is monitored by a Swan-Ganz catheter often exhibit an increase in pulmonary wedge pressure during episodes of angina pectoris. Chest pain during which these parameters remain unchanged is therefore unlikely to be true angina pectoris.

Prinzmetal's angina refers to episodes of chest pain during which there is ST segment elevation rather than the usual depression. Many patients with extensive coronary artery disease and a long history of exertional angina pectoris may conform to these criteria. In its typical form, however, Prinzmetal's angina is usually encountered in relatively young women, is not associated with limitation in exercise tolerance, tends to recur at certain times of the day without significant provocation, tends to last longer than is usual for classic angina, is accompanied by a decrease in pulse rate and in blood pressure, and is quite frequently complicated by arrhythmias during attacks. Patients with this syndrome often have periods of days or weeks without chest pain. Prinzmetal's angina is believed to be due to coronary artery spasm with or without occlusive coronary artery disease — which, when present, is usually limited to one vessel.

Patients whose exercise capacity is limited because of disease in the lower extremities involving bone, joint, or the nervous system and particularly those with severe intermittent claudication of the legs may experience angina pectoris only with arm exercise, at meals, or on lying down and may therefore be mislabeled as having "atypical" rather than "advanced" angina pectoris.

Nocturnal angina is usually found in patients also having exertional pain. Otherwise, nocturnal angina often reflects left ventricular failure or may be due to "a cold bed"; the cold hours of winter nights may be associated with an increase in blood pressure and in pulse rate sufficient to increase myocardial oxygen consumption beyond the capacity of the compromised blood supply in patients with occlusive coronary artery disease.

Occasionally, "atypical" chest pain represents *linked angina pectoris*. This signifies the coexistence of myocardial ischemia and another disease capable of producing pain that radiates to the area of ischemic cardiac pain so that the two pains may enhance each other and link together. Peptic ulcer, hiatal hernia, gallbladder disease, cervical spondylosis, and rheumatoid arthritis are examples of diseases producing pain that can link with angina. In such circumstances, angina pectoris pain may start in the adjacent painful area or may show a predilection to radiate toward it. Furthermore, exacerbation of the associated disease may make angina pectoris episodes more frequent, more prolonged, and less responsive to treatment. For example, in addition to exercise-induced pain, a patient with hiatal hernia and angina pectoris may experience similar pain after a meal, on lying down, or on stooping. The pain often starts in the epigastric region but exhibits the other characteristics of angina pectoris. Improvement of the symptoms of hiatal hernia often leads to amelioration of angina pectoris, which may then recur more typically with exercise. In patients with "linked angina," the symptoms are often misinterpreted as being due "exclusively" to the noncardiac disorder; the coexistence of ischemic heart disease may thereby be overlooked.

Patients with significant left ventricular outflow obstruction, such as aortic valve stenosis, often present with "classic" angina pectoris. In contrast, patients with severe aortic incompetence tend to experience angina pectoris only after they have exhibited features of left ventricular failure. Furthermore, in aortic incompetence, angina pectoris attacks may represent autonomic dysfunction. They tend to recur at rest or during the night, are usually prolonged, are often associated with vasomotor phenomena such as excessive sweating, throbbing, and flushing, and are likely to be relieved with mild exercise.

Physical Findings. In the vast majority of angina pectoris patients, the physical examination shows no abnormality. Clues to risk of coronary disease may be detected, including xanthelasma, premature arcus senilis, tuberous xanthoma, and hypertension.

Cardiac examination may reveal a cause of ischemia, such as aortic valve disease, idiopath-

ic hypertrophic subaortic stenosis (IHSS), or luetic aortic aneurysm. Left ventricular enlargement due to associated hypertension or prior myocardial infarction may be seen. A palpable presystolic atrial "kick" over the apical impulse may be detected, with or without an audible fourth heart sound, caused by decreased left ventricular compliance.

Clinical assessment should also include evaluation of the vascular system. Conditions that can contribute to mycardial ischemia should be sought, such as pulmonary disease, anemia, polycythemia, as well as abdominal and musculoskeletal abnormalities.

Exercise Tolerance Test. Patients with stable angina tend to experience chest pain at a remarkably constant double product (HR × systolic BP × 10^{-2}) regardless of the precipitating mechanism. The exercise tolerance test provides diagnostic confirmation, functional quantitation of the severity of the disease, and prognostic information. Correlation with coronary arteriography has shown that exercise tolerance test is normal in 60 per cent of patients with single-vessel disease, 30 per cent of patients with two-vessel disease, and in only 10 per cent of patients with "significant" three-vessel disease. It has to be emphasized that exercise testing provides "functional evaluation," whereas coronary arteriography provides "anatomic evaluation" and is subject to observer variation concerning the significance of disease.

The value of exercise ST segment changes in the assessment of coronary disease has stimulated a considerable amount of research.

Generally, flat or downsloping ST segments of 1 mm or more 0.08 second after the J point are considered significant. More significance is given to ST depression of 2 mm or more (or rarely ST elevation), particularly if it appears early during the exercise protocol, persists during recovery period, and is associated with 20 per cent or more increase of R amplitude in the lead showing most ST depression (usually V_5).

An abrupt drop of blood pressure or the appearance of arrhythmias during chest pain or during ST changes is a further indicator of ischemia.

Since repolarization is influenced by a variety of conditions, exercise-induced ST segment depression can be encountered without significant coronary disease. Female sex, digitalis, tranquilizers, hyperventilation, mitral valve prolapse, intraventricular conduction abnormalities and electrolyte abnormalities are often associated with "false-positive" ST depression. Among asymptomatic middle-aged men, 50 per cent stenosis of one or more coronary arteries is expected in 30 to 60 per cent of those showing exercise-induced ST depression. Therefore, the value of exercise-induced ST changes in the routine screening of asymptomatic individuals is subject to controversy.

Radioisotope Studies. *"Cold Spot" Imaging.* In *cold spot imaging*, radioisotopes are taken up by normally perfused myocardium, with ischemic regions showing little or no radioisotope activity. Many radiopharmaceutical drugs are available for this purpose but thallium 201 is generally preferred because it forms high concentrations in the myocardium and has favorable emission characteristics. Thallium 201, a potassium analog, is taken up by cells in which the sodium-potassium pump is active.

In the diagnosis of transient myocardial ischemia, thallium 201 is usually injected intravenously near peak exercise, the patient is instructed to continue exercise for 1 minute, and an image is taken within a few minutes and repeated in 2 to 4 hours. Comparison of the images taken at peak exercise and at rest helps to delineate the ischemic zones and provides a semiquantitative assessment of ischemia. Although the sensitivity and specificity of exercise screening for myocardial ischemia approaches 90 per cent with combined exercise and thallium study, technical difficulties still exist regarding detection of small ischemic zones, and comparable ischemia in two adjacent segments. There is also difficulty with diffuse hypoperfusion related to left main coronary artery disease and with inferior wall ischemia, since it is often difficult to separate myocardial from liver radioactivity. The test is also fairly expensive.

Detection of Mechanical Dysfunction. Since impaired myocardial contractility is an early manifestation of myocardial ischemia, assessment of left ventricular performance and segmental wall motion at rest and peak exercise could be of utmost value in the detection and quantitation of myocardial ischemia. Several methods (apex-cardiography, systolic time intervals, radar kymography, echocardiography, and contrast left ventriculography) have been utilized, but all have major limitations. Biplane single-pass radioisotope ventriculography using the patient's own tagged red cells or radioactive albumin holds great promise as a sensitive and reliable noninvasive test. By contrast to normally perfused myocardium, which shows more vigorous contractility in response to exercise, ischemic myocardium shows impaired contractility that is often reversed with successful revascularization surgery.

Coronary Arteriography. The coronary arteriogram provides definitive information about the extent and severity of coronary disease and the feasibility of aortocoronary bypass surgery. Combined with left ventriculography, it provides a reliable prognostic indicator.

In most laboratories, coronary arteriography carries a relatively low morbidity (less than 1 per cent) and mortality (0.1 per cent). It is indicated for the evaluation of unstable angina, stable angina not controlled satisfactorily with medical treatment, ischemic heart disease in a relatively young individual, and atypical chest pain. Also, it is often required as part of the evaluation of middle-aged or older patients with valvular heart disease.

When coronary artery spasm is suspected from the clinical history, provocative diagnostic measures may be utilized, preferably during cardiac catheterization. The most popular method used is an intravenous injection of ergonovine in sequential doses of 0.05, 0.1, and 0.25 mg. In a typical case, the patient will experience chest pain associated with marked ST elevation. Repeat coronary arteriogram during the pain should show spasm in the artery supplying the ventricular wall corresponding to the ST elevation. Nitroglycerin administered sublingually, intravenously or in the involved coronary artery should cause immediate relief of the spasm.

MYOCARDIAL INFARCTION

With the death of myocardial cells, a constellation of diagnostic features usually appears. Of chief importance are symptoms and electrocardiographic and enzyme abnormalities.

Symptoms. Prodromal symptoms occur in about 60 per cent of patients suffering acute myocardial infarction. The prodromal stage is usually characterized by ischemic pain of the type described under Angina Pectoris. However, the prodrome of acute myocardial infarction is distinguishable from chronic stable angina pectoris by the *recurrence* of symptoms plus occurrence in a *crescendo pattern.* Prodromal symptoms are more common in patients with anterior myocardial infarction and nontransmural infarcts. Psychologic stress may be involved in production of the prodrome. Another interesting prodromal characteristic is the occurrence of nocturnal angina in about 10 per cent of patients experiencing myocardial infarction. Again, patients with anterior and subendocardial infarction have this symptom far more commonly than do those with inferior myocardial infarction (MI), probably owing to more severe left ventricular dysfunction caused by left coronary artery disease.

Herrick described classic symptoms of acute

myocardial infarction in 1912. The most common presenting complaint is severe chest pain that is precordial, crushing, or squeezing, with radiation to the arms (in about 25 per cent), jaws, back, or epigastric area. The pain may be associated with sweats, nausea, vomiting, and shortness of breath. This chest discomfort typically lasts more than 20 minutes. The duration of pain is significant, as 20 minutes of myocardial ischemia probably results in some loss of myocardial cells in all instances. Although the classic presentation of acute myocardial infarction is frequently encountered, many patients have myocardial infarction without chest pain. Symptoms of this "atypical" group may include respiratory difficulty with dyspnea and nonproductive cough, extreme fatigue, abdominal or epigastric distress, and syncope. Mortality in these patients is high, in part owing to delayed recognition of myocardial infarction. Frequency of "painless" or "silent" myocardial infarction is probably about 20 per cent.

Physical Examination. Typically, the patient is anxious, restless, and uncomfortable. His face is pale; he may have cold sweats. Heart rate is usually normal, although tachycardia is sometimes encountered. Severe bradycardia may be found in patients with high vagal tone, sinus node ischemia, or a variety of conduction abnormalities. Blood pressure is usually normal or elevated, but the patient in severe distress may show hypotension and other signs of shock. Auscultation of the lungs may occasionally reveal rales, indicating left ventricular dysfunction. Wheezing or "cardiac asthma" is sometimes encountered. The jugular venous pressure is frequently normal but may be elevated, especially with right ventricular infarction. Carotid pulse contour sometimes shows small volume. The precordium is usually quiet during the early stages of infarction, although an atrial filling wave may be palpable. The heart sounds are frequently distant or muffled with abnormal resonance of the first heart sound. The second heart sound may be normal, but wide or paradoxical splitting of the second heart sound may be encountered in instances of bundle branch block or severe ventricular dysfunction. The presence of a third heart sound suggests left ventricular failure. The fourth heart sound, suggestive of decreased left ventricular compliance, is commonly heard at the apex. An apical systolic murmur with radiation to the left axilla, or occasionally to the left lower sternal border, suggests mitral regurgitation secondary to papillary muscle dysfunction. This murmur will occur during the hospital course in more than 50 per cent of patients with acute myocardial infarction. A pericardial friction rub will be found in a large number of patients. Unless the patient has pre-existing congestive heart failure, ankle edema, hepatic distention, and presacral edema are uncommon on presentation.

Electrocardiography. A normal electrocardiogram does not exclude the diagnosis of acute myocardial infarction. The electrocardiographic changes of acute myocardial infarction are highly variable and depend on the location, magnitude, and duration of ischemia. The initial electrocardiogram (ECG) may be normal, show ST segment depression, ST segment elevation, or tall, peaked T waves. Serial ECGs over several days are often required to adequately assess the possibility of infarction. It must be remembered that all of the ECG changes of infarction may eventually disappear. New Q waves of 0.04 second duration usually indicate infarction. Only 25 per cent of the thickness of the ventricular wall need undergo necrosis in order to produce a Q wave. Standard classification of location of infarction by ECG abnormalities includes new changes in leads II, III, and aVF representing the inferior wall; changes in leads I, aVL, and V_{4-6} representing the lateral wall; and changes in I, aVL, and V_{1-4} indicating anteroseptal infarction. Two special cases deserve mention: true posterior infarction that may be electrocardiographically silent except for ST-T changes in lead V_1, and "normalization" of previously inverted T waves, rendering a previously abnormal ECG "normal." Some areas of the heart are electrocardiographically silent and an infarction in those regions may not produce typical ECG changes. These include the subendocardium, the posterior wall of the left ventricle, the cardiac apex, the papillary muscles, the interventricular septum, the right ventricle, and the atrium. In patients with left bundle branch block or ventricular pacemakers, ECG changes of myocardial infarction may be obscured.

Enzyme Determinations. The use of quantitative measurements of cardiac cell enzyme activity to provide an indicator of myocardial damage has been a major advance in the diagnosis of acute myocardial infarction. The most commonly used determinations are creatine phosphokinase, glutamic oxaloacetic transaminase, lactic dehydrogenase, and myoglobin.

Creatine phosphokinase (CPK). CPK activity levels usually rise above normal 6 to 12 hours after myocardial damage, reach peak levels at 24 hours, and fall to the normal range by 3 to 4 days after onset of symptoms. CPK exists in three enzymic forms, termed BB (brain), MB (myocardium), and MM (muscle). For all practical purposes CPK–MB is released only by myocardium. The CPK–MB isoenzyme may be present in serum for as few as 24 hours following onset of symptoms, and early sampling after onset of symptoms is essential. Samples may need to be collected every 8 hours for 24 hours following admission in order to demonstrate CPK–MB peak. Use of CPK isoenzyme determinations is extremely useful, as this test has sensitivity for myocardial infarction of 96 per cent and specificity of 99 per cent.

Glutamic Oxaloacetic Transaminase (SGOT). Activity of this enzyme rises above normal 8 to 12 hours after onset of symptoms, peaks at approximately 18 to 36 hours, and usually falls to the normal range by day 3 or 4. A characteristic rise in SGOT occurs in more than 95 per cent of patients with clinically proved myocardial infarction. Unfortunately, this enzyme is found in numerous tissues and elevation of SGOT is a relatively nonspecific finding.

Lactic Dehydrogenase (LDH). LDH is released from necrotic myocardial cells and exceeds normal values at 24 to 48 hours after onset of symptoms, peaks at approximately 3 to 6 days, and returns to normal by day 8 to 14. Although LDH is also widely distributed in the body, use of LDH isoenzyme determination allows accurate diagnosis of acute myocardial infarction. LDH_1 is found in high concentration in myocardial cells, red cells, and renal cells. An LDH_1:LDH_2 ratio greater than 0.76 carries a sensitivity and specificity of over 95 per cent for acute myocardial infarction. Intravascular hemolysis and renal infarction can also produce this abnormality of isoenzyme ratio. The great benefit of LDH isoenzyme assay is in its use in patients who present more than 24 hours after onset of symptoms, since, by the time of initial evaluation, CPK may have returned to the normal range. Owing to the prolonged elevation of LDH, accurate diagnosis of acute myocardial infarction can often be made in spite of late presentation.

Myoglobin. Although it is not an enzyme, assay for myoglobin falls into the same general category as the tests just listed. Use of radioimmunoassay for detection of myoglobin in serum for diagnosis of acute myocardial infarction has recently received attention. Although this technique appears to offer a relatively sensitive and specific estimation of the presence of myocardial damage, it does not show any clear-cut advantages over other tests, especially CPK–MB determination.

Radionuclides. The use of radionuclides in the assessment of myocardial infarction is primarily limited to two agents, thallium 201 and technetium 99m pyrophosphate. With thallium 201, a scintigraphic "hole" or "cold spot" occurs seconds after occlusion of a coronary artery. Thallium 201 scans appear to be most sensitive within 6 hours of the onset of chest pain, with a sensitivity of 100 per cent, falling to 94 per cent by 6 to 24 hours after onset of chest pain, and 74 per cent when performed after 24 hours. These changes in sensitivity may be due to formation of collateral blood supply. With its specificity of 95 per cent, a negative thallium 201 scan makes acute MI very unlikely. Technetium 99m pyrophosphate acts as a bone-seeking radionuclide and accumulates in areas of calcium hydroxyapatite deposition. Calcium hydroxyapatite deposits form in the mitochondria of cardiac tissue that has undergone necrosis. The "infarct-avid" imaging becomes useful between 12 and 24 hours following infarction and remains positive for up to 1 week following infarction. Optimal images are obtained 1 to 3 days postinfarction, and the scan has usually returned to normal after 2 weeks. Owing to higher blood flow (30 to 40 per cent of normal) in the periphery of lesions, infarct-avid agents such as technetium 99m pyrophosphate are taken up more in the periphery than in the center of infarction where blood flow is even lower. Technetium pyrophosphate scans are diagnostic in about 80 per cent of patients with acute transmural, anterior, or inferior infarctions, but in only 70 per cent of patients with subendocardial infarctions. Unfortunately, a faintly positive technetium pyrophosphate scan can be obtained in disorders other than acute myocardial infarction, including unstable angina, pericarditis, and ventricular aneurysm.

Diagnosis of infarction using radionuclide scanning has been highly successful in patients with anterior and lateral infarctions, but inferior and posterior infarcts and nontransmural infarcts have been more difficult to detect. It has been suggested that thallium 201 scanning is perhaps more accurate than technetium 99m pyrophosphate scanning in detecting and localizing acute myocardial infarction in patients without prior infarction. However, the exact role of radionuclide scanning remains undetermined.

Estimation of Myocardial Infarction Size. Estimation of myocardial infarction size has two important uses. First, it makes possible evaluation of therapeutic interventions designed to reduce the amount of myocardial damage occurring with acute infarction. Second, important prognostic information can be obtained from determination of infarct size. Numerous techniques have been used to estimate infarct size, but no widely accepted solution to the problem of infarct sizing has been found. It must be recalled that myocardial infarction in humans is frequently not the result of a single abrupt event. Rather, it is often the final stage of a chronic process that may have already led to fibrosis, hypertrophy, collateral formation, and other pathologic abnormalities. Furthermore, the area of infarct is not always a homogeneous mass but may be a "marbled" region in which zones of viable tissue lie adjacent to and intermingled with areas of infarction.

Among the techniques used to measure infarct size, several have been prominent:

1. ST segment change, usually determined by integration of multiple ST segments recorded by the use of an ECG grid over the precordium.
2. Summation of CPK isoenzyme activity found in serial blood samples.
3. Angiographic evaluation of the extent of left ventricular wall abnormality.
4. Radionuclide scan with determination of area of abnormality.
5. Two-dimensional echocardiography.

Although each has its advocates, none of these methods is perfect. It is useful to remember that pathologic correlation of the extent of myocardial infarction as related to the 12 lead electrocardiogram shows electrocardiographic changes to underestimate seriously the extent of myocardial infarction. It is of interest that peak levels of serum creatine kinase (CPK) correlate well with cumulative CPK release. This roughly reflects the extent of myocardial infarction. Total mortality within a year after infarction has been reported to increase twofold to threefold when peak creatine kinase level exceeds eight times the upper limit of normal, or when peak transaminase level exceeds five times the upper limit of normal. Infarct sizing with thallium 201 scanning is generally accepted to provide a rough index of myocardial damage, allowing classification of infarct size as "small, medium, or large."

Hemodynamic Monitoring. Numerous recent studies have demonstrated that stratification of mortality risk in patients with acute myocardial infarction can be carried out by analysis of hemodynamic variables. Bedside measurement of hemodynamic parameters has been made possible by the development of the balloon-tipped flow-directed catheter. With this device, right atrial, right ventricular, pulmonary artery, and pulmonary artery wedge pressures can be measured. Cardiac output determinations, using the thermodilution technique, can be quickly and easily carried out. Measurement of oxygen content in mixed venous samples from the pulmonary artery gives a good indication of whole body perfusion. Serial sampling from the various chambers will reflect the presence of left-to-right shunting, which can be caused by ventricular septal defect.

Indications for placement of a balloon-tipped catheter into the pulmonary artery in patients with acute myocardial infarction include hypotension, cardiogenic shock, pulmonary edema, suspected ventricular septal rupture, severe mitral regurgitation, or persistent tachycardia, possibly related to hypovolemia. The procedure carries very little risk and is of special usefulness in the differential diagnosis of shock states in association with acute myocardial infarction. The primary differential diagnostic consideration is severe left ventricular dysfunction versus hypovolemia. The interrelation of left ventricular filling pressure (as measured by the pulmonary artery end-diastolic pressure) and the left ventricular stroke work index, derived from stroke volume and blood pressure, has great prognostic power.

Patients with pulmonary artery end-diastolic pressure greater than 15 mm Hg have a poor prognosis, with mortality risk of over 25 per cent. When this is combined with markedly depressed left ventricular stroke work index, the mortality risk increases substantially. If direct hemodynamic measurements are not available, a rough estimation of left atrial pressure may be based on evaluation of upright PA chest film. Under normal conditions, the size and number of vessels seen in the lower lung is greater than in the upper lung zones, owing to the effect of gravity. Equality of upper and lower vessel sizes indicates mild elevation of left atrial pressure. When upper zone vessels are larger than lower zone vessels, left atrial pressure is 15 to 25 mm Hg. If interstitial edema is present, pressure is 25 to 35 mm Hg.

Two caveats are in order. First, changes in chest x-ray may persist for hours or even days after resolution of the hemodynamic abnormalities that produced the changes. Second, in longstanding pulmonary venous hypertension, interstitial fibrosis may occur, producing "permanent Kerley-B lines" that do not reflect left atrial pressure.

Complications of Myocardial Infarction. *Arrhythmias.* Diagnosis of cardiac arrhythmias is dealt with extensively in other articles. Sinus bradycardia, often reflecting increased vagal tone, or narcotic effect, is frequently seen early in the hospital course. Sinus tachycardia may indicate continuing pain, anxiety, dehydration, pericarditis, or left ventricular failure. Atrial fibrillation probably occurs in 10 per cent of patients with acute myocardial infarction, usually within the first few days. Atrial flutter occurs in about 5 per cent. Junctional rhythms occur frequently (40 per cent) and may indicate ischemia, digitalis toxicity, congestive heart failure, hypokalemia, or hypoxemia. Premature ventricular contractions (PVCs) are seen in virtually all patients, and frequency greater than 5 per minute suggests important ventricular irritability owing to ischemia, hypokalemia, or congestive heart failure. Unfortunately, absence of frequent or high-grade ventricular arrhythmias in the early stages of acute myocardial infarction (first 4 days) does not exclude appearance in the late phase (day 12 to 21) Persistent ischemia, left ventricular segmental dyssynergy, or both predispose to late hospital PVCs and sudden death.

Conduction Abnormalities. First degree atrioventricular (A-V) block (prolonged P-R interval) occurs frequently owing to high vagal tone, A-V nodal ischemia, or drug effects. The significance of A-V block varies with respect to anatomic location of infarction. Second degree and third degree A-V block in inferior infarction is usually due to A-V nodal ischemia. Occurrence of such block in anterior infarction may indicate interventricular septum necrosis and carries a more ominous prognosis. New right bundle branch block in the setting of inferior MI seems to carry less hazard than in anterior wall infarction. However, new left bundle branch block and other bifascicular blocks, regardless of the site of infarction, are potential harbingers of complete heart block with emergence of slow, unreliable pacemakers.

Congestive Heart Failure and Cardiogenic Shock. As outlined above, these conditions are usually due to left ventricular dysfunction. Evaluation of left ventricular function may be carried out in a variety of ways, including determination of ejection fraction by gaited frame nuclear imaging or by echocardiography. Cardiogenic shock is usually defined as systolic blood pressure less than 90, with urine output less than 30 ml per hour, signs of hypoperfusion of the brain, including confusion, and peripheral hyperperfusion with cold clammy skin. Hypovolemia must always be excluded in the evaluation of "cardiogenic shock."

Papillary Muscle Dysfunction or Rupture. Papillary muscle dysfunction with murmur of mitral regurgitation occurs in more than half of the patients with acute myocardial infarction at some time in the hospital course. Rupture of the papillary muscle is associated with severe, acute mitral regurgitation, florid left ventricular failure, and a 50 to 80 per cent mortality. Rupture most commonly occurs on day 2 or 3 of the course and may be associated with subendocardial or transmural infarction.

Anterolateral papillary muscle rupture is less common (1:4) than posteromedial rupture. A new murmur occurs more frequently in partial than complete papillary muscle rupture. Diagnosis of papillary muscle rupture is aided by echocardiography, which will show abnormal motion of the mitral leaflets. Swan-Ganz catheterization will usually show large V waves in the pulmonary artery wedge trace.

Rupture of the Interventricular Septum. Septal rupture is an uncommon complication of acute myocardial infarction. It often occurs between day 2 and 3 of infarction and is always associated with transmural infarction involving the interventricular septum. Septal rupture produces a holosystolic murmur along the left sternal border and may mimic the murmur of severe mitral regurgitation. One fourth of the patients die on the first day and over half die during the first 2 weeks. Free wall rupture may occur concomitantly. In approximately one third of the patients with ventricular septal rupture, there is A-V block, in distinction to papillary muscle rupture, in which A-V block almost never occurs. Diagnosis of interventricular septal rupture is confirmed by passage of a balloon-tipped catheter with serial blood oxygen saturation measurements from the right atrium, right ventricle, and pulmonary artery; left-to-right shunting is indicated by a step up of greater than 1 volume per cent between the right atrium and the right ventricle. Echocardiography has been used by some in diagnosis of this abnormality, but its exact role remains undetermined.

Pericarditis. Pericarditis occurs in between 10 and 50 per cent of the patients with acute myocardial infarction and usually implies epicardial or transmural infarction. Pericarditis may occur in anterior or inferior infarctions. Physical examination reveals a typical three-component rub resembling "the squeaking of a leather saddle," usually at the PMI or the lower left sternal border. Pleuritic chest pain, fever, and sinus tachycardia may also be present. Echocardiography often reveals pericardial effusion. ECG shows ST segment elevations and P-R depression.

Myocardial Rupture. This dread complication is 8 to 10 times more common than rupture of the interventricular septum or papillary muscles. It probably occurs in 10 per cent of myocardial infarction fatalities. Myocardial rupture usually occurs in the first week of myocardial infarction but may be found in the first few hours. Patients may die suddenly without premonitory symptoms or they may have prodromal chest discomfort for a few hours. ECG abnormalities include bizarre, M-shaped QRS configuration in the precordial leads. Also, monophasic RS with an upright T wave has been described. The frequency of these findings is unknown.

Psychiatric Complications of Acute MI. Segregation by sex occurs in the psychiatric complications of myocardial infarction: men are susceptible to denial and depression, while women are more likely to become overly dependent. Some of the marked personality changes observed in the context of acute myocardial infarction are probably related to its unique ability to cause sudden death.

Aneurysm. Ventricular aneurysm is usually a left ventricular finding, typically involving the anterior and apical areas. Signs of left ventricular aneurysm include refractory congestive heart failure, arrhythmias, and systemic arterial embolism. Physical examination reveals a large, paradoxically bulging apical impulse. Chest x-ray may show left ventricular deformity and, eventually, calcification. ECG usually reveals ST segment elevation persisting more than 6 weeks postmyocardial infarction, with T wave inversions and significant Q waves. Two-dimensional echocardiography is frequently of benefit in demonstrating the location and size of the aneurysm, but definitive diagnosis requires left ventricular angiography.

Ischemic Cardiomyopathy. It is debatable whether diffuse coronary atherosclerosis could lead to diffuse myocardial scarring and congestive heart failure without history of angina pectoris or myocardial infarction.

Hypoxia is known to increase myocardial vulnerability to cardiotropic viruses and myocardial toxins such as alcohol.

As in other forms of congestive cardiomyopathy, the patients present with cardiac enlargement associated with features of congestive heart failure and propensity for arrhythmias and thromboembolism.

HYPERTENSION

By ARAM V. CHOBANIAN, M.D.

Boston, Massachusetts

DEFINITION

Blood pressure levels in any population represent a continuum and follow a relatively normal distribution. Any definition of abnormality must take into consideration the pressure level above which a harmful effect can be expected. Since age is a factor influencing blood pressure, it also needs to be considered. Epidemiologic studies have demonstrated a progressive increase in risk from cardiovascular complications at levels above 130 mm Hg systolic and 85 mm diastolic pressure. For practical purposes, adult blood pressures of less than 140/90 can be considered as relatively normal, between 140/90 and 160/90 as borderline elevated and more than or equal to 160/95 as hypertensive. In children, these numbers would need to be revised downward.

The distribution of blood pressure and the relative prevalence of hypertension in the United States is illustrated in Figure 1. The values represent the data obtained in more than 150,000 individuals who were screened as part of a hypertension detection and follow-up program. Approximately 25 per cent of adults have diastolic blood pressure more than or equal to 90 mm Hg. The prevalence rates in blacks is almost twice that in whites.

MEASUREMENT OF BLOOD PRESSURE

The measurements should be made with the arm at the level of the heart. When using the indirect method, the cuff should be wide enough to allow adequate transmission of pressure to the center of the arm and long enough to permit firm application to the arm. A 13 by 27 cm cuff is adequate for most adults, although larger cuffs may be essential for obese individuals and smaller ones for children. Either the fourth phase (muffling) or fifth phase (disappearance) Korotkoff sounds can be used, the latter now being recommended. On initial examination of a hypertensive patient, blood pressure should be evaluated in both arms and in the lower extremities to rule out obstructive vascular disease. Upright as well as recumbent or sitting pressures should be obtained to determine the presence of orthostatic hypotension, particularly if hypertensive medications are being administered. In general, casual blood pressures in the sitting and standing position are adequate for follow-up purposes. Three successive blood pressure readings should be taken and the last two averaged. In patients with mild hypertension or with marked lability of blood pressure, frequent recordings may be required to assess adequately the need for therapy. Home blood pressure measurements are of particular value in this group as well as in patients with severe disease the management of which may be difficult.

DIAGNOSTIC EVALUATION

The extent of the diagnostic work-up will vary from patient to patient. The overall cost

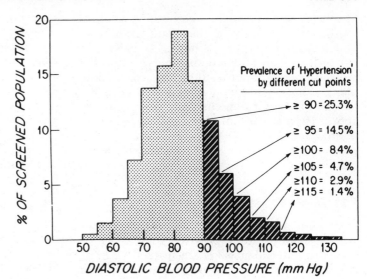

Figure 1. Frequency distribution of diastolic blood pressure in 158,906 persons, 20 to 69 years of age, studied as part of a hypertension detection and follow-up program. (From Circulation Research *40:*I–106–109, 1977.)

and the possible risk to the patient need to be considered in making the decision on how far to proceed. In general, the younger the patient and the more severe the hypertension, the more extensive should be the evaluation. In patients with mild and easily controlled hypertension, a minimum of studies are needed, whereas in patients with accelerated or malignant hypertension, every possible measure may be warranted to uncover a curable secondary cause of hypertension or to obtain data that would be helpful in selecting the most effective antihypertensive drugs.

All hypertensive subjects should have a thorough history to rule out obvious reversible secondary causes such as use of oral contraceptive drugs and sympathomimetic agents, and to assess the cardiovascular and renal background, diet, family history, and so forth. A careful physical examination is needed to evaluate such essential items as the degree of retinopathy, cardiac and neurologic status, peripheral pulses, and vascular bruits. Routine laboratory studies in everyone should include measurement of serum creatinine or blood urea nitrogen, blood sugar, serum electrolytes, calcium, thyroxine, uric acid, cholesterol, and triglycerides. An electrocardiographic tracing also is mandatory. Urine culture would be useful on at least one occasion, as well as assays of urinary metanephrine or vanillylmandelic acid (VMA) excretion.

Intravenous pyelography is a relatively expensive procedure (generally costing in excess of $100) and is required in less than half of hypertensive patients. These would include very young individuals who have a higher percentage of renal causes of hypertension; patients with genitourinary symptoms, abdominal bruits, known renal disease or impaired renal function; or subjects with severe or refractory hypertension.

Measurement of plasma renin activity (PRA) is of value in some individuals, particularly those with spontaneous hypokalemia in whom the differentiation between primary and secondary forms of mineralocorticoid excess is important. PRA assays also help in decisions regarding antihypertensive therapy in severely hypertensive patients. Renin-suppressing drugs have been found to be extremely useful in patients with high PRA, while diuretics and salt depletion particularly benefit low PRA subjects. Renin assays also are of value in the evaluation of patients for renovascular disease or other potentially curable angiotensin-dependent states.

Random measurements of PRA generally do not have much merit unless some standardized approach is utilized. One system widely employed involves administration of the diuretic furosemide (80 mg orally) and removal of blood 3 hours later for PRA assay. A PRA of less than 2.5 nanograms per ml per hour in the stimulated state is considered abnormally low and greater than 12 to 15 nanograms per ml per hour as abnormally elevated. The PRA can also be related to 24-hour urinary sodium excretion and to a nomogram developed from values obtained in a large group of normal subjects. Both methods have disadvantages associated with them and are not practical for use in the total hypertensive population.

Several specialized studies are available for the work-up of hypertension and these are discussed later. They involve measurement of specific hormones, angiography, and selective venous catheterizations. They generally are expensive and often can involve some risk to the patient. They therefore need to be restricted to specific subgroups such as those in whom (1) routine screening studies have suggested a secondary form of hypertension, (2) a major need exists to identify a remediable cause, or (3) data are required to assist in their medical management. Those patients with known secondary forms of hypertension currently represent only about 10 per cent of the total hypertensive population, and selectivity needs to be employed in the utilization of these diagnostic procedures.

ETIOLOGIC CLASSIFICATION

Systolic Hypertension. Systolic hypertension without diastolic pressure increase is observed in clinical states characterized by either decreased distensibility or obstruction of the aorta or by increased stroke output of the left ventricle (Table 1).

It occurs most commonly in aged individuals as a result of calcification of major arteries and degeneration of aortic elastin with reduced arterial compliance. Systolic hypertension by itself is an important risk factor in the development of ischemic heart disease, heart failure, or strokes. It may be difficult to treat, particularly when present in elderly patients who may require potent antihypertensive drugs but who cannot tolerate marked blood pressure reductions because of coexisting cerebrovascular or coronary disease.

Coarctation and other obstructive disease of the aorta lead to reduced blood pressure in the lower extremities and decrease in amplitude and delay in appearance of pulses. Pressures in the upper part of the body and the left ventricle will be markedly increased, and a prominent collateral circulation above the level of obstruction may be apparent. Notching of ribs may result from dilatation of intercostal arteries. The markedly increased pressures may lead to left ventricular failure, cerebrovascular accidents, or dissecting aneurysms of the aorta. If diastolic hypertension becomes prominent with coarctation, involvement of the renal circulation and

Table 1. *Etiologic Classification of Systolic Hypertension*

Decreased aortic distensibility
    Arteriosclerosis
    Coarctation
Increased stroke output of left ventricle
    Hyperthyroidism
    Arteriovenous fistula
    Anemia
    Paget's disease
    Complete heart block
    Aortic insufficiency
    Left-to-right shunts

---

superimposed renovascular hypertension should be suspected.

Combined Diastolic and Systolic Hypertension. *Idiopathic or essential hypertension* accounts for approximately 90 per cent of the population with diastolic hypertension. This group undoubtedly is not a homogeneous one but probably reflects multiple potential causes that have not been defined as yet (Table 2).

Renal disease appears to be the most important of the secondary causes. The renal abnormality may involve either the parenchyma of the kidney, its collecting system, or its circulation. Chronic pyelonephritis is probably the most common parenchymal cause, but the mechanism for the hypertension is uncertain and is probably unrelated in most instances to abnormalities in the renin-angiotensin system. The severity of the hypertension may not reflect that of the pyelonephritis. Chronic glomerular or interstitial nephritis of any type may produce hypertension, particularly when renal function is impaired significantly. Renal tumors or space-occupying lesions such as renal cysts also may induce hypertension. Juxtaglomerular cell tumors and some Wilms' tumors may produce renin-like material and severe hypertension, hyperreninemia, and hypokalemia. Hydronephrosis is another cause often associated with excess renin secretion.

Renovascular hypertension may be present in approximately 1 to 2 per cent of the hypertensive population. The diagnosis can be made on clinical grounds alone, although certain clinical features may raise the index of suspicion. These include the presence of an abdominal bruit, accelerated hypertension, abrupt increase in severity of hypertension, or the onset of hypertension before age 20 or after age 50. Screening procedures such as intravenous pyelography or radioisotope renography may be useful but have the drawback of a relative high rate (approximately 20 per cent) of false-negative results. Ultimately, the decision to proceed with more intensive work-up depends on the clinical severity of the hypertension and the ability to lower blood pressure medically.

Renal angiography and renal vein assays are both required to confirm the diagnosis of renovascular hypertension. The arterial abnormality is usually one of 2 types — renal artery atherosclerosis or fibrous stenosis. The former is much more common in older persons, particularly males, and usually involves the proximal portion of the renal artery. Fibrous stenosis occurs primarily in females and affects the mid and distal portion of the renal artery with an unusual intimal or medial fibrosis that leads to aneurysmal dilatation of the vessel. Both types of arterial disease may be bilateral in nature in a significant fraction of patients. Since renovascular

Table 2. *Etiologic Classification of Combined Diastolic and Systolic Hypertension*

Idiopathic or essential hypertension
Renal hypertension
  Parenchymal
    Pyelonephritis
    Glomerulonephritis
    Interstitial nephritis
    Diabetic nephropathy
    Connective tissue diseases
    Renal tumors (juxtaglomerular cell tumor, hyper-
      nephroma, Wilms' tumor)
    Renal cysts and polycystic kidneys
    Developmental abnormalities (Ask-Upmark)
    Other (amyloidosis, gouty nephritis, hematomas)
  Obstructive–hydronephrosis
  Renovascular
    Renal artery atherosclerosis
    Fibrous stenosis of renal arteries
    Thrombotic or embolic occlusion
    Other diseases (tumors, inflammation, pseudoxanthoma
      elasticum)
  Renoprival
    Renal failure
    Anephric state
Adrenal hypertension
  Mineralocorticoid
    Primary aldosteronism
    Idiopathic aldosteronism
    DOC hypertension
    18-hydroxy-DOC hypertension
    Hydroxylation deficiency syndromes
  Pheochromocytoma
  Cushing's disease
  Adrenogenital syndrome
Other endocrine
  Myxedema
  Hyperparathyroidism
  Acromegaly
Coarctation of the aorta
Toxemia of pregnancy
Neurogenic hypertension
  Increased intracranial pressure (brain tumors,
    hematomas)
  Neuroblastomas
  Neuropathies (polyneuritis, porphyria, lead poisoning,
    tabes)
  Spinal cord transection
  Encephalitis
  Bulbar poliomyelitis
  Diencephalic syndrome
  Acute porphyria
  Lead poisoning
Drug-induced
  Oral contraceptives, estrogens
  Monoamine oxidase inhibitors with tyramine
  Sympathomimetics (amphetamines, cold remedies, etc.)
Other
Hypercalcemia
  Carcinoid syndrome
  Licorice excess

significance. Elevated levels of renin activity in renal venous blood from an ischemic kidney should exceed that from a normal contralateral kidney by at least 50 per cent. However, with branch arterial lesions or focal disease of other types, lesser ratios may be present, and selective catheterization of the veins from individual segments of the kidney may be required to delineate the local site of hyperreninemia. Several other causes of hypertension associated with unilateral renin excess can be present (Table 3). A particular problem in this regard is the fact that 10 to 20 per cent of patients with essential hypertension will have a 50 per cent or greater differential in renal vein renin activity between the two sides. Drugs that stimulate renin release, such as diuretics, vasodilators, and inhibitors of angiotensin converting enzyme activity, typically increase the difference in renal vein renin activity between the two sides and may enhance the sensitivity of the procedure. However, beta-adrenergic blockers and other hypertensive drugs as methyldopa and clonidine, which reduce sympathetic activity and renin secretion, may narrow the differential and should be avoided.

Saralasin (Investigational), a peripheral competitive antagonist of angiotensin II, may have value in determining whether the hypertension is angiotensin-dependent. A positive response is present if the blood pressure is reduced by more than 7 to 10 mm Hg with acute infusions of saralasin. Approximately 90 to 95 per cent of patients with renovascular hypertension respond to saralasin, and in 85 to 90 per cent of patients, the blood pressure decrease correlates with the surgical result. Its diagnostic value, however, is limited by the fact that the state of sodium balance will affect the antihypertensive response. If salt depletion is present, a blood pressure reduction can be induced even when the hypertension originally was not angiotensin-mediated. In addition, increases in blood pressure may occur with saralasin in patients with low renin hypertension because of its agonist properties in inducing contraction of vascular smooth muscle. Finally, in occasion-

Table 3. *Hypertension with Unilateral Increase in Renal Vein Renin Activity*

Renovascular
Renal tumors
  Juxtaglomerular cell
  Wilms'
  Hypernephromas and cysts
Unilateral hydronephrosis
Unilateral chronic pyelonephritis
Renal trauma (scars, compression)
Unilateral renal malformations
Essential hypertension

lesions are relatively common in normotensive as well as hypertensive patients, a cause-and-effect relationship is not established unless functional evidence also can be provided.

Selective renal vein renin measurements continue to be the most useful test of functional al patients with severe hyperreninemia, a marked rise in blood pressure may develop upon cessation of saralasin because of the marked stimulation of renin activity occurring during angiotensin II blockade.

Surgical treatment of renovascular hypertension depends to a great extent on the severity of the disease and the ease and success of controlling the blood pressure medically. Even with complete diagnostic assessment, revascularization procedures or nephrectomy may produce a cure or substantial improvement in hypertension in only 70 to 80 per cent of patients, and the risks of renovascular surgery are not insignificant. It goes without saying that if a patient is not considered to be a candidate for surgery, invasive studies such as angiography or venous catheterizations are unwarranted.

Mineralocorticoid hypertension may be secondary to several endocrine abnormalities. The most common is primary hyperaldosteronism, which is caused by an aldosterone-secreting adenoma of the adrenal cortex. The most characteristic feature of the disorder is potassium depletion and hypokalemia, which is present even without diuretic therapy. Marked hypokalemia (serum potassium < 3.0 mEq per liter) on diuretics also may be suggestive of the diagnosis. The typical clinical symptoms and signs of muscle weakness, polyuria, tetany, metabolic alkalosis, cardiac arrhythmias, and carbohydrate intolerance are related to the potassium wasting. PRA is suppressed in primary aldosteronism and other forms of mineralocorticoid hypertension, and its measurement is extremely valuable for differentiating between primary and secondary causes of aldosterone excess. Renin activity typically is reduced in the former instance but increased in the latter case.

Several other causes of low PRA in hypertensive patients may be present (Table 4). Of particular importance is the fact that approximately 20 per cent of patients with essential hypertension fall into this group, although no unusual mineralocorticoid has as yet been uncovered in them. Some of the low PRA patients have diminished peripheral sympathetic activity that would serve to impair renal renin secretion. Black subjects have a much higher prevalence of low PRA. In addition, the PRA appears to decrease with age, presumably as a result of reduction in renal responsiveness, and many hypertensive patients in the low renin group may thereby be demonstrating this age-related phenomenon.

Plasma or urinary aldosterone measurements or both are required to confirm the diagnosis of primary aldosteronism. In addition, localization

Table 4. *Hypertension and Low Plasma Renin Activity*

Essential hypertension (20 per cent patients)
Black race
Decrease renal tissue or renin responsiveness
  Aging
  Chronic renal disease (volume expanded)
  Diabetes
Adrenergic blocking drugs (beta blockers, clonidine, methyldopa, etc.)
Mineralocorticoid excess syndromes
  Primary aldosteronism
  Idiopathic aldosteronism
  Deoxycorticosterone excess
  18-Hydroxydeoxycorticosterone excess
  17-α-Hydroxylase deficiency
  11-β-Hydroxylase deficiency
  Cushing's syndrome
  Congenital adrenal hyperplasia
  Acromegaly
  Licorice excess

of the tumor is important by assay of adrenal venous aldosterone activity to determine whether a unilateral excess of secretion is present. The latter procedure is useful in distinguishing between primary and "idiopathic" aldosteronism, in which bilateral hyperplasia of the adrenal cortex is present. The latter appears to account for approximately 15 to 20 per cent of patients with the syndrome of primary aldosteronism who, in contrast to patients with solitary adenomas, respond relatively poorly to adrenal surgery. Computerized axial tomography (CT) scans of the adrenal areas and scintillation scanning using radiolabeled iodocholesterol also are valuable tools for localization of adrenal tumors. Surgery is not always necessary, even in patients with solitary adenomas, since the blood pressure may respond quite well to spironolactone or other diuretics. However, if medical therapy is selected, careful attention should be given to potassium balance.

Several other quite rare causes of mineralocorticoid hypertension may be present (Table 4).

18-Hydroxydeoxycorticosterone (18-OH-DOC) is characterized by hypertension, low plasma renin activity, and low aldosterone secretion in association with increased secretion of 18-OH-DOC. Hypokalemia is a variable finding in this syndrome.

17-α-Hydroxylase deficiency hypertension results from a genetic defect of 17 α-hydroxylase activity in the adrenal, which may produce hypertension, hypokalemia, and reduced plasma renin concentration. Aldosterone secretion is low, but increased production of deoxycorticosterone (DOC) occurs. Because of the defect in 17 α-hydroxylation, there also is a reduction in the synthesis of the sex hormone precursors 17 α-hydroxypregnenolone and hydroxyprogesterone, and gonadal insufficiency occurs. Treatment with dexamethasone corrects the hypertension and hypokalemia.

11 β-Hydroxylase deficiency hypertension results from a defect in adrenal 11 β-hydroxylase activity that interfers with the conversion of 11 β-desoxycortisol to cortisol and of DOC to corticosterone. The increased levels of DOC appear to be responsible for the hypertension.

Deoxycorticosterone (DOC) hypertension may occur in rare instances with tumors or with other disorders of adrenal cortical metabolism (see later discussion).

Some patients with *Cushing's syndrome* or *acromegaly* also may have aldosterone excess, and the hypertension may be on the basis of mineralocorticoid excess.

Licorice (50 to 100 grams per day) may produce a reversible form of hypertension that is associated with hypokalemia. The effects appear related to the presence in licorice of glycyrrhizinic acid, which produces a mineralocorticoid effect.

Pheochromocytoma is an uncommon cause of hypertension (less than 0.5 per cent of cases) that is characterized by a tumor of chromaffin tissue that secretes excess amounts of catecholamines. The tumors originate typically from the adrenal gland but in 5 to 10 per cent of patients occur at other sites, such as the organ of Zuckerkandl, sympathetic nerve ganglia, bladder, or thorax. Pheochromocytomas may involve both adrenal glands in 5 to 10 per cent of patients and may be malignant in a similar percentage.

The most common symptoms and signs are headaches, excessive sweating, paroxysmal hypertension, orthostatic hypotension and tachycardia, fever, carbohydrate intolerance, and unusual blood pressure increases occurring during induction of anesthesia or childbirth. Sustained hypertension may occur in approximately one half of patients. Pheochromocytomas may be familial in nature and may be associated with medullary thyroid carcinomas, parathyroid adenomas, neuromas, and adrenal cortical hyperplasis, the so-called multiple endocrine adenomatosis type II. The inheritance appears to be autosomal dominant, and the disorder may involve a generalized dysplasia of neural crest cells. Multiple and recurrent pheochromocytomas at various sites are common in this syndrome. Neurocutaneous disorders, cerebellar hemangioblastomas, polycystic disease, coarctation of the aorta, and Turner's syndrome also may occur with increased frequency in patients with pheochromocytoma.

The diagnosis of pheochromocytoma is made by biochemical means. Assay of urinary metabolites of norepinephrine, particularly urinary metanephrines and vanillylmandelic acid, should uncover almost all patients. Measurement of plasma catecholamines also may be of value. False-negative results are rare, but several causes of false increases in urinary catecholamines are present. These include methyldopa therapy, amphetamines and sympathomimetic agents found in nosedrops or proprietary cold remedies, tetracycline, bananas, coffee, and vanilla-containing products. In addition, certain anxious persons may exhibit marked increases in plasma or urinary catecholamines and may be mistaken for patients with pheochromocytoma.

It generally is important to localize the site of a pheochromocytoma preoperatively to minimize the possibility of a negative surgical exploration. This can best be achieved with either CT scans of the abdomen or angiography, although the latter can be hazardous. Regional venous catheterization with assay of venous blood for catecholamines is also quite useful for localization, particularly if the other studies have proven to be unrewarding. In addition, since the conversion of norepinephrine to epinephrine occurs only in the adrenal medulla or in tissues of adrenal origin, urinary assays for norepinephrine and epinephrine derivatives may be of value. A nonadrenal site for the tumor may be expected if norepinephrine derivatives represent more than 90 per cent of the total.

Toxemia of pregnancy is characterized by hypertension, albuminuria, and edema developing during the latter half of pregnancy. Blood pressure normally does not change appreciably with pregnancy in normotensive persons or

Table 5. *Hypertension and Elevated Plasma Renin Activity*

Essential hypertension (10 per cent patients)
Therapy
   Diuretics, salt depletion
   Estrogens
Reduced renal perfusion
   Renovascular disease
   Accelerated hypertension
   Heart failure
Renal tumors
   Juxtaglomerular cell
   Wilms'
   Hypernephroma and cysts
Other renal disease
   Chronic renal failure
   Hydronephrosis
   Acute glomerulonephritis
Increased adrenergic activity
   Pheochromocytoma
   Hyperthyroidism

patients with idiopathic hypertension. The levels tend to decrease during the first trimester, return to normal during the second, and remain unchanged or slightly increased in the final. The factors leading to the development of toxemia and hypertension are unknown. The increases in renin and aldosterone activity normally observed with pregnancy may actually be inhibited with the development of toxemia or its more severe manifestations, preeclampsia or eclampsia.

Oral contraceptive drugs represent the most important reversible cause of hypertension. While the incidence rates have varied markedly in different studies, hypertension appears to develop in approximately 5 per cent of subjects treated with the "pill" for prolonged periods. The hypertension may take weeks or months either to develop or to recede following discontinuation of the drug. The mechanism has not been clearly delineated but appears to involve abnormalities in the renin-angiotensin-aldosterone system. Increases in plasma renin activity and aldosterone secretion have been noted with therapy, the former occurring presumably as a result of increased renin substrate. Both estrogens and progestagens are capable of producing the hypertension, although the estrogens clearly are more important. Many patients who develop hypertension may have a positive family history of the disease, suggesting that a genetic predisposition to hypertension may influence the response to the drugs. Oral contraceptive drugs also should be avoided by women with a prior history of toxemia during pregnancy and by obese subjects. Postmenopausal patients receiving estrogen therapy also may be susceptible to its hypertensinogenic action.

COURSE AND COMPLICATIONS

Epidemiologic studies have shown that hypertension is the most important risk factor for most of the major cardiovascular complications occurring in Western society. Striking correlations have been observed between the levels of both systolic and diastolic blood pressure and ischemic heart disease, sudden deaths, strokes, peripheral vascular disease, and congestive heart failure. Several of the clinical manifestations can be attributed to the blood pressure elevation itself; these are congestive heart failure, cardiomegaly, cerebral hemorrhage, malignant hypertension, hypertensive crisis, renal failure, and dissecting aortic aneurysms. More than 75 per cent of patients with these disorders

have an underlying background of hypertension. On the other hand, complications such as myocardial and cerebral infarction and peripheral vascular insufficiency are related to the influence of hypertension in accelerating atherosclerosis. Incidence of hypertension in these disease states appears to be at least 50 per cent.

A number of factors influence the risk for cardiovascular disease in the hypertensive patient. Hyperlipoproteinemia and cigarette smoking are the most important in this regard. Cardiomegaly and left ventricular hypertrophy also increase risk appreciably. The combination of hypertension and diabetes mellitus may have a devastating effect on the circulatory system, particularly since many such patients also have hyperlipoproteinemia and are obese.

The overall mortality rate in hypertensives has been estimated to average twice that of normotensive persons. The life expectancy of adults at each age group decreases with increasing levels of blood pressure. In nonmalignant hypertension, the major causes of death are acute myocardial infarction, hypertensive heart disease, and strokes, while in accelerated or malignant hypertension, renal failure predominates. Malignant hypertension can develop in any hypertensive patient with marked pressure elevation, regardless of the underlying cause. Widespread damage to small arteries and arterioles develops, with resulting necrosis, edema, and acute inflammatory reaction in the vessel wall. All organs can be involved, even though the major clinical effects occur as a result of impairment of renal function. While the survival rate is negligible in untreated patients with malignant hypertension, excellent results are achieved with therapy, particularly if renal function is reasonably unimpaired.

Antihypertensive therapy has a markedly beneficial effect on the hypertensive complications. The incidence of thrombotic strokes is also reduced appreciably by lowering the blood pressure, but it is not entirely clear as yet whether other disorders related to advanced atherosclerosis, such as myocardial infarction and peripheral vascular insufficiency, are affected. It is also unclear whether antihypertensive therapy has a favorable effect in elderly patients with systolic hypertension, and there is a major need for prospective studies to examine this question. The presence of other risk factors multiplies the risk for the atherosclerotic complications of hypertension, and control of such abnormalities will probably prove to be important for the prevention of these complications.

CARDIAC ARRHYTHMIAS

By GALEN S. WAGNER, M.D.,
Durham, North Carolina

BARRY W. RAMO, M.D.,
Albuquerque, New Mexico

and ROBERT A. WAUGH, M.D.,
Durham, North Carolina

The normal cardiac rhythm is initiated by a series of electrical impulses or depolarizations. Each impulse is formed spontaneously within the sinus node. The impulse is then conducted sequentially through the atria, atrioventricular (A-V) node, His bundle branch system, and ventricles. If the electrical wave front advances homogeneously, no second entry (reentry) is possible, owing to the refractory state of the recently depolarized cells. Therefore, each succeeding impulse must be newly formed by a recurrent spontaneous depolarization in the sinus node. Both the rate of sinus impulse formation and the speed of impulse conduction, particularly through the A-V node, are dependent upon the balance of sympathetic and parasympathetic activity. A cardiac arrhythmia is defined here as any alteration of this impulse formation or conduction. Such an alteration might be evident as either a bradyarrhythmia or tachyarrhythmia or might be detectable only by analysis of the electrocardiogram; for example, a delay in impulse conduction caused by a block in one of the bundle branches.

This presentation has been designed to provide simplicity and order to the subject of cardiac arrhythmias. This approach should provide a foundation both for therapeutic decisions regarding current problems and for the addition of new concepts as they result from electrophysiologic research.

DEFINITIONS

It is important initially to define certain key terms. *A-V association* occurs when the atria and ventricles are activated sequentially by a common electrical impulse. *A-V dissociation* occurs when atria and ventricles are activated independently. The *P-R interval* is measured from the beginning of a P wave to the beginning of the resultant QRS complex. The *R-R interval* extends between the onsets of two consecutive QRS complexes. A *premature impulse* is one that occurs before the time of the next expected impulse and an *escape impulse* is one that occurs later than the time of the next expected impulse.

Supraventricular describes impulses that arise proximal to the branching of the His bundle. These impulses will result in QRS complexes identical to those occurring with normal sinus rhythm unless there is a rate-related bundle branch block. Bundle branch block, either fixed or rate-related, is an example of *aberrant conduction*, in which the QRS complex is most altered in its terminal aspects. However, aberrancy also occurs due to preexcitation of the ventricles via an anomalous A-V pathway, and this produces marked slowing of the initial part of the QRS complex (as is seen in the Wolff-Parkinson-White syndrome). A *ventricular* impulse originates distal to the branching of the His bundle, resulting in a QRS different in appearance from supraventricular and $\geqslant 0.12$ second in duration.

Paroxysmal and *nonparoxysmal* refer to the mode of onset and termination of an arrhythmia. A sudden onset and termination indicates that the arrhythmia is paroxysmal, and a gradual onset and termination implies that it is nonparoxysmal.

Reentry refers to a situation in which the electrical impulse is able to continually find receptive tissue. The impulse will then continue to reenter as long as the conduction velocity is sufficiently slow and the refractory period sufficiently brief. A reentry tachyarrhythmia starts and stops abruptly and is therefore termed paroxysmal. Reentry may occur in any part of the heart.

It is termed *macro* if the circuit involves major aspects of either atria or ventricles, and *micro* if it occurs within the A-V node or other relatively circumscribed areas. When reentry is macro in the atria, no discrete P wave will be seen and when it is macro in the ventricles, no discrete QRS or T will occur. Instead, the baseline will continually undulate: regularly as in flutter or irregularly as in fibrillation. Only the large muscle masses of atria and ventricles generate sufficient electrical activity to be apparent on the surface electrocardiogram. Thus, when there is micro reentry, the continuing activity is not apparent on the ECG. Only the resultant spread of activity through atria and ventricles is apparent. Cells other than those in the sinus node are capable of spontaneous depolarization and may serve as cardiac pacemakers. Either escape or premature pacemaker activity may occur in cells scattered around the atrial endocardium or cells organized into the bundle of His or bundle branches. Both intrinsic rate and reliability of pacemaker activity are greatest in the sinus node and decrease progres-

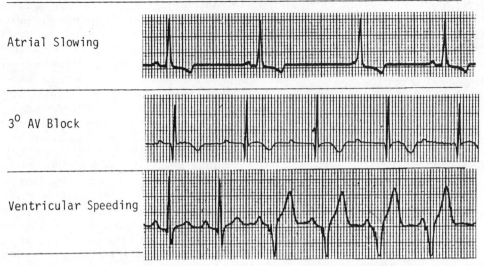

Figure 1. The three causes for A-V dissociation are shown: atrial slowing (<60/min), complete (3°) A-V block, and ventricular speeding (>60/min). In the upper and lower examples, the dissociation is intermittent and sinus capture of the ventricles affirms the competence of A-V conduction.

sively in more distal areas. Pacemakers tend to change rate gradually, and thus pacemaker tachyarrhythmias are nonparoxysmal.

DIAGNOSTIC LIMITATIONS

Usually, it is possible to reach a specific diagnostic conclusion regarding a cardiac arrhythmia by careful observation of a single lead recording. At times, observations of multiple leads is required. On other occasions a recording of a single lead during an intervention is helpful. Sometimes, however, no single diagnosis can be established and one must conclude that two or more possibilities exist. It is important to note these limitations of arrhythmia diagnosis; they are indicated in the subsequent text.

DIAGNOSTIC GROUPS

For this discussion, the cardiac arrhythmias are presented in four major groups: (1) A-V dissociation, (2) intraventricular conduction delays, (3) bradyarrhythmias, and (4) tachyarrhythmias.

1. A-V DISSOCIATION

The term is descriptive only and thus analogous to a symptom rather than a disease. This condition requires the electrocardiogram for its identification and is defined when there is a variation in the P-R interval with a concurrent regularity of the R-R interval. A varying P-R interval, accompanied by a varying R-R interval, suggests A-V association with variable A-V block. Often, lengthy electrocardiogram (ECG) strips are required to document the P-R variation, since independent atrial and ventricular rhythms may at times be "isorhythmic" (occur at similar rates).

There are three mechanisms that produce A-V dissociation. Dissociation occurs when the atrial rate is sufficiently slow to permit an escape pacemaker in the His bundle or bundle branches to emerge and capture the ventricles (Fig. 1) (see Bradyarrhythmias). A-V dissociation is also caused by independent acceleration of ventricular activity (see Tachyarrhythmias) that may result from either abnormal pacemaker activity or reentry originating below the A-V node. In both of these situations, the dissociation persists as long as the ventricular rate exceeds the atrial rate. If, during A-V dissociation, the atrial rate is less than 60 per minute and the ventricular rate is more than 60 per minute, either or both mechanisms might be responsible.

The third cause for A-V dissociation is complete or third degree A-V block (see Bradyarrhythmias). In this situation, appropriately timed atrial impulses are incapable of activating the ventricles because of impaired conduction either in the A-V node or His bundle branch system. Complete heart block should be diagnosed only when a P wave occurs at a time when it would have been expected to conduct; that is, following the T wave and >0.2 second before a QRS complex.

Often, it is apparent that more than one of the possible factors are present concurrently and that their individual roles in producing the dissociation cannot be determined. One may be able only to conclude, for example, that the A-V dissociation is due to both ventricular speeding and a "high degree" A-V block. In this situation, some of the atrial impulses might have been conducted to the ventricles if there were no interference caused by the accelerated ventricular rate. The term "A-V dissociation" should always be followed by an indication of its cause: atrial slowing, ventricular speeding, A-V block, or a combination of these.

Both digitalis and ischemia are common causes for A-V dissociation. They may produce any of the mechanisms of dissociation by slowing atrial activity, delaying A-V conduction, and accelerating independent lower pacemaker activity.

2. INTRAVENTRICULAR CONDUCTION DELAYS

A delay in the transmission of electrical impulses occurs either in the bundle branches or in the ventricular myocardium. These delays may result in alterations of the QRS morphology with or without an increase in the total QRS duration. One depends entirely upon the electrocardiogram for diagnosis of the delay, although complete left bundle branch block is suggested by paradoxical splitting of the second heart sound and complete right bundle branch block by an extremely wide physiologic splitting of the second heart sound. It is important to understand the limitations of the electrocardiogram in indicating the precise diagnosis. An identical alteration of the QRS complex may result from altered conduction in the bundle branches or in the myocardium. Thus, left bundle branch block could be simulated by left ventricular hypertrophy and right bundle branch block by right ventricular hypertrophy. One may be able only to diagnose that the QRS has been altered in a specific manner and that there are several possible causes.

Bundle Branch Delay. The common A-V bundle, or His bundle, branches into the right and left bundles that differ greatly from each other anatomically. The right bundle branch is single and subdivides only toward the distal aspect of the right side of the interventricular septum. However, the left bundle may not even exit from the common bundle as a single branch. Near the point of exit from the His bundle, the fibers of the left bundle diverge in three directions. A part of the left bundle enters the interventricular septum and produces the earliest activation of ventricular muscle. A second group of fibers extends posteriorly toward the posterior papillary muscle of the mitral valve as the left posterior fascicle. The remain-

ing fibers extend anteriorly toward the anterior papillary muscle of the mitral valve as the left anterior fascicle. A delay in any part of the bundle branch system will cause an area of myocardium that is normally activated early during the QRS complex to be activated at some later point. If the delay is minimal, the QRS will be altered but not prolonged; however, progressively longer delays can both alter the morphology and increase the duration of the QRS.

Identification of the specific part of the bundle branch system responsible for intraventricular conduction delay can be accomplished by noting the direction of the terminal forces of the QRS complex. Since the right ventricle lies primarily anteriorly and the left ventricle posteriorly, an electrocardiographic lead with anterior-posterior orientation (V_1) is most capable of differentiating between right and left bundle branch block. If the late forces are directed toward V_1, then delayed activation of the anterior or right ventricle is suggested and right bundle branch block is diagnosed. If, however, the late forces are directed away from V_1, the delayed activation of the posterior or left ventricle is suggested and left bundle branch block is diagnosed.

Observation of leads that provide left-right and superior-inferior orientation (1, 2) is necessary for diagnosis of partial left bundle branch involvement, either in the presence or absence of concurrent right bundle branch block. In the posteriorly positioned left ventricle, the anterior aspect lies leftward and superiorly and the posterior aspect lies rightward and inferiorly in the chest. Therefore, delay in the left anterior fascicle results in late forces directed leftward and superiorly (extreme left axis deviation) and delay in the left posterior fascicle produces late forces directed rightward and inferiorly (extreme right axis deviation).

Conduction delays within the bundle branches can result from acute anterior septal myocardial infarction. Less often, involvement of the posterior aspect of the bundle branches, including the right bundle and the posterior fascicle of the left bundle, can be produced by inferior infarction. Unlike the conduction delays in the A-V node that occur in the setting of inferior infarction and are discussed later, the bundle branch blocks either persist or recur intermittently after the acute phase of the infarct and, if bilateral, may result in complete heart block.

The most common cause of bundle branch disease is the development of idiopathic fibrosis within the proximal aspects. This process may begin relatively early in life, producing first partial and then total bundle branch block. Subsequently, there may be bilateral involve-

Table 1. *Characteristics of A-V Block in Varying Locations*

						Etiology			
	Degree	Type	QRS	Site of Escape	Vagus	Dig	IMI	AMI	Fibrosis
AV node	1–2–3	I	WNL	His	Y	Y	Y	N	Y
HIS	1–2–3	II	WNL	Bundles	N	N	N	N	Y
Bundles	1–2–3	II	≥.12	Distal bundle	N	N	N	Y	Y

IMI = Inferior myocardial infarction.
AMI = Anterior myocardial infarction.

ment and, when the process involves all aspects of both bundles (occurring at an average age of 70 years), complete heart block will result.

Global involvement of the bundle branches from any cause may therefore result in a clinically significant consequence such as heart failure, presyncopal episodes, Stokes-Adams syncope, or sudden death. Complete block of the bundle branches is particularly dangerous, as will be noted later (Table 1), both because it may occur paroxysmally without preexisting first or second decree A-V block, and because there is minimal reliability of escape pacemakers within the distal parts of the bundle branches.

Myocardial Delay. All of the manifestations of delay within the bundle branches can be simulated by conduction delay within the ventricular myocardium. There are five principal causes of myocardial delay: (1) acute myocardial infarction, (2) ventricular hypertrophy, (3) preexcitation, (4) electrolyte imbalance, and (5) pharmacologic agents.

Acute myocardial infarction that spares the bundle branches can still produce abnormalities in the terminal as well as in the initial aspect of the QRS complexes. In the left ventricular free wall, the distal aspects of the left anterior fascicle insert near the base of the anterior papillary muscle and those of the left posterior fascicle near the base of the posterior papillary muscle. The electrical activation then spreads from endocardium to epicardium. In these areas, coronary blood flow occurs in an epicardial-to-endocardial direction. Therefore, the endocardial areas are in greater danger of acute infarction. Involvement of these areas may infarct the myocardium into which a fascicle of the left bundle inserts. Then, if more superficial layers of myocardium are spared, these will be activated circuitously and therefore later during the QRS complex. Thus involvement of the anterolateral aspect could cause lateral "peri-infarction" block and simulate left anterior fascicular block. Involvement more posteriorly could cause inferior "peri-infarction" block with simulation of left posterior fascicular block. These bundle branch and myocardial origins for an intraventricular conduction delay may cause identical QRS alterations. When delay is within the fascicle of the bundle branch system, however, the initial Q wave tends to be minimal and the terminal R wave maximal both in amplitude and duration. Alternatively in peri-infarction delay, the initial Q wave is of greater and the terminal R wave of lesser prominence (Table 2).

Severe left or right ventricular hypertrophy may simulate complete left or right bundle branch block, respectively. Less severe left or right ventricular hypertrophy may simulate left anterior or left posterior fascicular block, respectively. Thus extreme left axis deviation can be caused by left ventricular hypertrophy and extreme right axis deviation by right ventricular hypertrophy. The resultant QRS morphologies

Table 2. *Differentiation of IVCD Due to Bundle Branch Block and Peri-infarction Block*

	Most Prominent QRS Abnormality				
ECG Lead	Initial Q wave duration	Terminal R wave duration	Terminal R wave amplitude	Terminal S wave duration	Terminal S wave amplitude
V₁	—	Right bundle branch block	Right ventricular hypertrophy	Left bundle branch block	Left ventricular hypertrophy
aVL	Lateral peri-infarct block	Left anterior fascicular block	Left ventricular hypertrophy	—	
aVL	Inferior peri-infarct block	Left posterior fascicular block or Right ventricular hypertrophy		—	

may be identical or may vary, in that the involvement of the bundle branch system has maximal effect on the QRS duration while hypertrophy primarily affects QRS amplitude. Thus, in the presence of a terminal R′ in lead V_1, the greater the amplitude of the R′, the more likely the cause is right ventricular hypertrophy; the longer the duration of the R′ the more likely the cause is right bundle branch block. Conversely, when there is prominence of the terminal S wave in lead V_1, the greater the amplitude the more likely the cause is left ventricular hypertrophy, and the longer the duration the more likely the cause is left bundle branch block. Similarly in the frontal plane, when there is prominence of the terminal R wave in lead avl, the greater the amplitude the more likely the problem is left ventricular hypertrophy and the longer the duration the most likely it is left anterior fascicular block. No such differentiation regarding the appearance of the prominent terminal R wave in lead avl has been found helpful in distinguishing right ventricular hypertrophy from left posterior fascicular block (Table 2).

Intraventricular activation is also changed when there is antegrade conduction over a congenitally abnormal muscular connection (Kent bundle) between atria and ventricles. The QRS alterations that occur with bundle branch block, myocardial infarction, and ventricular hypertrophy are due to delayed activation of a part of the ventricular myocardium, but an anomalous atrioventricular pathway causes "pre" or early activation. Therefore, the P-R interval is shortened, a slurred Q or R wave occurs, and the total time from onset of the P wave to end of the QRS is not prolonged.

Intraventricular conduction delays, wherein the QRS duration is prolonged without prominent changes in morphology, are commonly produced by both hyperkalemia and various pharmacologic agents such as the quinidine group of antiarrhythmic drugs (quinidine, procainamide, and disopyramide). Unlike the delays in the bundle branch system that can result in any degree of A-V block, these intramyocardial conduction delays can only result in alterations in the morphology of the QRS complex. Thus, although the conditions may be arrhythmogenic, they are not in themselves arrhythmias. They are included here only because of their place in the differential diagnosis of alterations in QRS morphology.

3. BRADYARRHYTHMIAS

A. Sinus Bradycardia. Slowing of the sinus node (sinus bradycardia) may occur physiologically and nonparoxysmally owing to predominance of parasympathetic autonomic activity. However, sinus bradycardia may occur paroxysmally as a result of either a sudden increase in parasympathetic activity or an intrinsic problem within the sinus node. Such an intrinsic problem could be a defect in either the formation of the impulse or in its transmission from the node to the surrounding atrial myocardium. Paroxysmal sinus slowing can cause presyncope, Stokes-Adams syncope, or sudden death. The clinical effect of any paroxysmal bradyarrhythmia is dependent upon the escape capabilities of more distal areas. It should be noted that the appearance of an escape pacemaker is a physiologic phenomenon and therefore the arrhythmia should not be named solely on the basis of the electrocardiographic appearance. For example, the problem is sinus bradycardia regardless of whether the heart rate of 40 has normally appearing P waves for each QRS complex or abnormal or no P waves. These latter appearances are not the result of atrial, nodal, or junctional bradycardia but rather sinus bradycardia with atrial, junctional, or ventricular escape.

A paroxysmal sinus slowing becomes clinically important only when there is an inadequate escape rate by a lower pacemaker. When the problem is within the sinus node, escape rates are usually adequate and no clinical consequences occur. However, when the sinus slowing results from a sudden increase in parasympathetic activity, there may be concomitant suppression of both escape pacemakers and conduction through the A-V node. Thus, in most patients with symptomatic paroxysmal sinus bradyarrhythmias, the cause is extrinsic to the sinus node, i.e., enhanced parasympathetic activity.

Diagnostic Subgroups. When a sudden slowing of atrial rate is noted on the electrocardiogram, one must differentiate between the simulation of pacemaker malfunction that may be induced by a blocked premature atrial impulse and true malfunction caused by either failure of impulse formation (sinus arrest) or failure of impulse conduction to the surrounding myocardium (sinus exit block). A blocked premature atrial impulse may not be easily recognized on a single ECG lead but should be suspected any time an apparent sinus pause is noted. The preceding T waves should be closely inspected for any variation from the normal that would suggest a superimposed premature P wave. This alteration may be apparent on all, some, or none of the electrocardiographic leads. If no P waves are detected, a true sinus pause may be erroneously diagnosed because such premature atrial activity can be proven only by intraatrial or esophageal recording. In the presence of a premature atrial impulse, A-V block may be a physiologic disturbance. Indeed, it is those impulses occurring most prematurely that are likely both to be hidden within the T wave and to arrive at the A-V conduction system during its refractory period.

Physiologic A-V block becomes even more likely if there is some preexisting delay in A-V conduction (first degree A-V block). A premature atrial impulse will usually prematurely activate (reset) the sinus node. Therefore, the delay between the premature P wave and the subsequent sinus-originated P wave should be at least equal to the previous sinus node cycle length. At times, however, this interval will be prolonged because the premature impulse will result in transient suppression of the sinus rate.

When, in the presence of a sudden slowing of the atrial rate, a blocked premature atrial impulse is not present, a true sinus pause should be diagnosed. The differential diagnosis between sinus arrest and sinus exit block is only possible in that rare circumstance when there is minimal preexistent sinus arrhythmia (beat-to-beat variation in the P-P interval owing to physiologic alterations of sympathetic and parasympathetic balance) and when the P-P interval surrounding the pause is a precise multiple of the basic sinus cycle length. In all other instances of a paroxysmal sinus slowing not caused by blocked premature atrial impulse, one should diagnose a sinus pause and note that this could be produced either by true arrest of pacemaker capabilities or by block of impulses from reaching the atrial myocardium. This diagnostic limitation does not present a clinical problem because the therapeutic considerations are identical.

B. A-V Block. *Degree versus Type.* Blocked transmission of impulses between the atrial and ventricular myocardium may be characterized either by severity or location. The degree of the block describes the severity: first degree, P-R >0.20 sec with all impulses conducted; second degree, only some of the impulses conducted; and third degree (complete), none of the impulses conducted. Block may be located (Fig. 2) in the A-V node, the His bundle, or the bundle branches. Electrocardiographic clues concerning location of the block may be obtained from observation of both the P-R interval of conducted beats and of the QRS interval of either conducted or escape beats. It is important to note that typing of block (Figs. 2 and 3) is possible only in the presence of either first or second degree block, because typing requires observation of conducted beats: a nonconducted beat is not required. Thus, types 1 and 2 are not merely subsets of second degree A-V block. These types are frequently called "Mobitz" types in recognition of the physician who was responsible for their original electrocardiographic description.

It is important to note the electrophysiologic phenomenon that makes the typing of A-V block useful for diagnosing its specific location. Figure 4 illustrates the contrasting recovery characteristics in schematic form in the A-V node and in a representative part of the His-bundle branch system. Each activation is followed by a refractory period. This period may be absolute and permit no reactivation or it may be relative, permitting reactivation that propagates with a slower conduction velocity. Each activation of the A-V node is

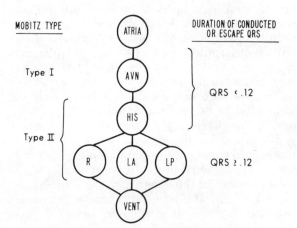

ECG CLUES TO SPECIFIC
LOCATION OF AV BLOCK

Figure 2. There are three possible sites for A-V block: A-V node (AVN), His bundle, and bundle branches (R, LA, LP), because an electrical impulse must traverse all to progress from atria to ventricles. Clues to this differential diagnosis from the surface ECG are Mobitz type and QRS duration.

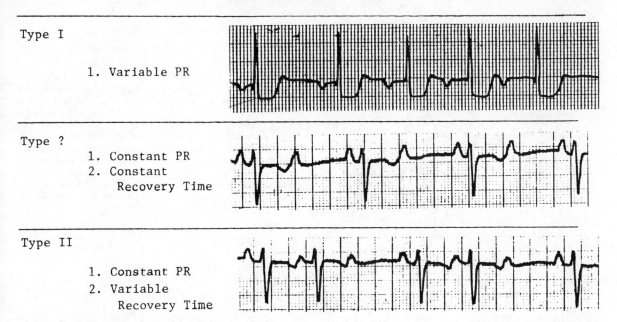

Type I

    1. Variable PR

Type ?

    1. Constant PR
    2. Constant
       Recovery Time

Type II

    1. Constant PR
    2. Variable
       Recovery Time

Figure 3. There are three types of A-V block: I, II, and indeterminant. Type I is diagnosed when any variation in the P-R interval is observed; however, type II is diagnosed only when a constant PR interval is observed in the setting of a variable recovery time for the A-V conduction system. The recovery time is measured from the beginning of the QRS complex of a conducted impulse until the onset of the P wave of the next conducted impulse.

followed by a relatively brief period of absolute refractoriness and then a long period of relative refractoriness. In contrast, each activation of the His-bundle branch system is followed by a long absolute refractory period with essentially no relative refractory period present.

In Figure 5, the results of progressively more premature stimulation of both the A-V node and the His-bundle branch system are illustrated. Activation of the A-V node during the relative refractory period results in a reactivation with slower rate of rise of the action potential and thus slower conduction velocity. The more pre-mature the activation the slower the resultant conduction. It is only when the impulse is so premature that it enters the A-V node during the absolute refractory period that no conduction will result. By contrast, premature activation in the His-bundle branch system either falls after the absolute refractory period and thus results in normal speed of conduction or falls into the absolute refractory period resulting in no conduction.

The A-V node is a structure capable of widely varying conduction times. The speed of conduction is determined both by the timing of entry of

Figure 4. The electrophysiologic basis for the capability of typing A-V block is the variation in refractory properties of the A-V node (long relative refractory period depicted above by slow return from depolarized to repolarized state of A-V nodal cell) and the His-bundle branch system (absent relative refractory period depicted above by sudden return from depolarized to repolarized state of right bundle branch cell).

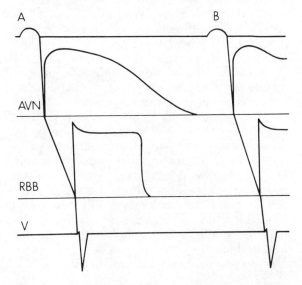

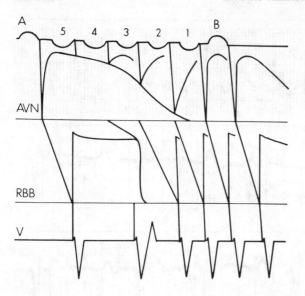

Figure 5. The results of presentation of sequentially earlier premature atrial impulses (1–5) into the two electrophysiologically different aspects of the A-V conduction system: progressively longer conduction times through the A-V node during its relative refractory period (impulses 2–4) then failure to conduct for impulse 5 that encounters the absolute refractory period, versus "all or nothing" conduction through the right bundle branch. Impulses 1, 2, and 3 would result in the appearance on ECG of normal-appearing QRS complexes, impulse 4 would be aberrantly conducted, and impulse 5 would produce the pause characteristic of a blocked premature atrial impulse.

the impulse into the A-V node and by the underlying sympathetic and parasympathetic balance. Parasympathetic excess will prolong the relative refractory period of the A-V node and sympathetic excess will decrease it. By contrast, conduction through the His-bundle branch system either occurs at a constant conduction time or fails to occur at all. "Type I" then refers to block in an area that is capable of variable conduction time, and "type II" refers to block occurring in tissue that is capable of only a constant conduction time.

As is shown in Figure 3, the diagnosis of type I block is quite simple: there is variability of the P-R interval. The mere presence of P-R variation indicates type I block, and it is not necessary to search for the classical example of type I block, Wenckebach. The diagnosis of type II block is more difficult, requiring that the P-R interval remain constant despite variability in the time between sequentially conducted impulses (recovery time). When the constant P-R occurs in the setting of a constant recovery time (e.g., 2:1 A-V block), typing of block is impossible. This is true because the A-V node's capability of conducting at varying velocities does not dictate an inability to conduct at a constant velocity when conditions are stable. If there is a constant interval between presentation of impulses to the A-V node and if the sympathetic parasympathetic balance remains stable, the resultant conduction time remains constant. Only when the P-R interval remains constant in the presence of conditions that would cause the A-V node to conduct variably can type II block be diagnosed and the conclusion reached that the problem is located within the His-bundle branch system.

A second clue to the location of the A-V block

is also noted in Figure 2. If the duration of the QRS complex of either conducted or escape beats is less than 0.12 second, the site of block must be proximal to the branching of the His bundle; i.e., A-V node or His. A QRS duration more than or equal to 0.12 second is not as helpful. It may mean that the block is resulting from complete involvement of the bundle branches or that there is block both in the A-V node or His and in some aspect of the bundle branches. For example, a patient with preexisting left bundle branch block who receives excessive amounts of digitalis might be expected to have a delay in A-V nodal conduction and thus demonstrate type I block with a QRS duration of greater than or equal to 0.12 second.

Characteristics of A-V block in the varying locations are shown in Table 1. Any degree of block is possible in any location. However, block within the His bundle is quite rare. Thus, most A-V block is either in the A-V node or in the bundle branches. The causes and consequences for block in these two locations are quite different. Complete block in the A-V node usually occurs gradually, with progression through first and second degrees of block. Also, the emergence of an effective escape pacemaker is quite likely since the entire His-bundle branch system lies distal to the site of block. However, as was just noted regarding the sinus node, A-V nodal block may occur precipitously as a result of a sudden increase in parasympathetic activity. This may produce symptoms of presyncope, Stokes-Adams syncope, or even sudden death, because the high level of parasympathetic activity can suppress both A-V nodal conduction and the emergence of escape pacemakers. In contrast, complete heart block occurring in the His bundle and bundle branches almost always occurs suddenly without progress through first and second degrees of block. Also, the emergence of an effective escape pacemaker is much less likely because the mass of ventricular muscle is not capable of the spontaneous diastolic depolarization necessary for pacemaking. The causes of block are noted both in Table 1 and in the preceding discussion of intraventricular conduction disturbances.

4. Tachyarrhythmias

A. Premature Impulses. Single premature impulses are nonsustained tachyarrhythmias and are therefore considered in this section. They may be either supraventricular or ventricular in origin. Supraventricular premature impulses originate in the atria, A-V node, or His bundle proximal to the branching and usually are conducted normally to the ventricles, resulting in a narrow QRS complex. Those from the atria, however, may be blocked in the A-V node as noted in the discussion on bradyarrhythmias. Since this is particularly likely when the impulses are most premature, the P wave may be concealed within the T wave of the normal impulse and thus be difficult to recognize on the ECG. A supraventricular premature impulse that is conducted through the A-V node may encounter refractoriness in one of the bundle branches (rate-related bundle branch block). The impulse will then be conducted abnormally, producing an alteration and widening of the QRS complex. This is an example of aberrant conduction and may simulate a premature ventricular impulse. Rate-related bundle branch block usually involves the right bundle branch in people without cardiac disease because of the somewhat longer refractory period of this fascicle. However, the premature supraventricular impulse could fail to propagate normally through either the right or the left bundle branch. Thus an important diagnostic differential occurs when a premature QRS complex of ≥0.12 second is present: premature supraventricular impulse with aberrancy or premature ventricular impulse.

Supraventricular versus Ventricular. When single premature impulses occur, the only differential diagnosis of clinical significance is supraventricular versus ventricular. Further attempts to subdivide supraventricular prematures into groups such as atrial, nodal, junctional, and so forth is not useful for clinical management. It is only when a premature QRS of ≥0.12 second occurs that an effort should be made to diagnose the site of origin. This differential diagnosis requires observation of the appearance and timing of the atrial activation and is attended by varying degrees of difficulty.

When a premature QRS is different in morphology and ≥0.12 second in duration, it is important to determine whether it is preceded by a premature P wave. This may be difficult from observation of only a single ECG lead because of concealment of the P wave in the preceding T wave. However, observation of a distortion in a T wave of any ECG lead confirms a supraventricular origin for the premature QRS complex. If no such distortion of the T wave is present, the premature impulse could be supraventricular (A-V node or His bundle) or ventricular in origin. The differential diagnosis is quite difficult and requires intracardiac recording to determine whether His bundle activation precedes the premature QRS. There is rarely a clinical indication for proceeding with this differential diagnosis, and one should consider a premature abnormal QRS not preceded by a premature P wave to be ventricular in origin. Measurement of the "pause" between the premature impulse and the subsequent normal impulse to determine if it is fully "compensatory" has not proven to be useful in the differential diagnosis. A supraventricular premature may fail to have retrograde propagation to the sinus node and thus result in a "full compensatory" pause. Alternatively, a premature impulse arising in the ventricles may propagate retrograde to the sinus node, causing a pause that is "less than compensatory."

The differential diagnosis of the supraventricular versus ventricular origin of a premature QRS complex is more difficult if atrial flutter-fibrillation rather than sinus rhythm is present. Several parameters may be helpful, including the appearance of the QRS complex, the coupling interval, and the atrial and ventricular rates.

Even if the premature QRS has an abnormal appearance, a duration of less than 0.12 second is indicative of aberrancy of conduction of a supraventricular impulse. A QRS complex that arises from the ventricles (distal to the branching of the His bundle) will almost always result in a QRS of at least 0.12 second in duration. It is also unusual for aberrancy owing to rate-related bundle branch block to result in a QRS duration of >0.14 second and thus, in the absence of ventricular preexcitation, QRS complexes of this duration are most likely ventricular in origin. Therefore, it is only when the QRS complexes are 0.12 to 0.14 second in duration that the differential diagnosis is difficult.

Observation of the QRS morphology may also be helpful. One should search for examples of

Table 3. *Spectrum of Atrial Flutter-Fibrillation*

Atrial rate	200	220	300	360	400	500+
Ventricular rate	200	180	150	120	100	70
Regularity	Regular	Regularly irregular	Regular	Regular	Irregularly irregular	Irregularly irregular
Name	Flutter		Flutter-fibrillation			Fibrillation
Stability	Little					Very
May use digitalis to ↑ AVB	No		Difficult			Effective
Converts with DC shock	Low energy					Higher energy
Converts with pacing	Easily					Impossible

premature wide QRS complexes during sinus rhythm when the differential diagnosis is less difficult for comparison with those occurring during atrial flutter-fibrillation. Also, an rSR[1] configuration in lead V_1 is highly suggestive of aberrant conduction.

Insight into this differential may be obtained from observation of either the atrial or ventricular rate. As is noted in Table 3, atrial flutter-fibrillation is a spectrum extending from slow flutter at a rate of approximately 200 per minute to fine fibrillation where no atrial rate can be determined. Whereas at the flutter end of the spectrum there may be regularity of A-V nodal conduction producing ratios of A-V block of 2:1, 3:1, and so forth, no such regularity is possible at the fibrillation end of the spectrum. Therefore, a constant interval between a QRS of normal duration and a premature wide QRS in the presence of atrial flutter might be due either to aberrancy of conduction or a premature ventricular impulse. This constant coupling, however, would be diagnostic of primary ventricular activity in the presence of atrial fibrillation. Likewise, if there were regular intervals between a series of wide QRS complexes in the presence of atrial fibrillation, ventricular impulses or ventricular tachycardia could be diagnosed. Therefore, there is diagnostic advantage at the fibrillation end of the spectrum that is not present at the flutter end. Also, measurement of the ventricular rate may be helpful. The less A-V nodal delay, the faster the ventricular rate and the more likely that impulses will fail to propagate through all the aspects of the bundle branches. Therefore, aberrancy of conduction is suggested when the ventricular rate is rapid and is less likely when more A-V block is present.

The differential diagnosis between primary ventricular prematures and aberrant conduction is most important in the patient who has been receiving digitalis. The presence of primary ventricular premature impulses might indicate digitalis excess, while insufficient A-V block might indicate inadequacy of digitalization. Here the observation of the ventricular rate is most useful. If excess digitalis were responsible for causing the ventricular premature impulses, the effect of the drug at the A-V node might be expected to produce a relatively slow ventricular rate. Therefore, when the patient on digitalis therapy presents with atrial flutter-fibrillation and a rapid ventricular rate, premature wide QRS complexes are most likely due to aberrancy of conduction. Exceptions do occur, however, particularly when intrinsic sympathetic tone is extremely high as with thyrotoxicosis, acute myocardial infarction, pulmonary edema, or pulmonary emboli. Carotid sinus massage may be additionally helpful when a slowing of the ventricular rate by the induction of A-V block results in disappearance of the premature wide QRS complexes. If they persist despite vagally induced slowing of the ventricular rate, the presence of primary ventricular prematures is more likely.

Many other guidelines have been suggested to help in this difficult differential diagnosis. It is often suggested that the sequence of long cycle-short cycle preceding the premature QRS in question has diagnostic significance favoring aberrancy (Ashman-Hull phenomenon). However, this sequence also favors the emergence of a premature ventricular impulse (the rule of bigemini). Often, when premature wide QRS complexes are seen in the setting of atrial flutter-fibrillation, differentiation between aberrancy and ventricular prematurity is impossible. This is particularly true when (1) the atrial rate is at the flutter end of the spectrum, (2) the atrial rate is at the fibrillation end of the spectrum but neither fixed coupling nor fixed interectopic intervals is present, or (3) the ventricular rate is rapid and the patient is either not on digitalis or on digitalis but has an illness that is characterized by high sympathetic tone.

B. Sustained Tachyarrhythmias. By definition, all sustained tachyarrhythmias begin with a premature supraventricular or ventricular impulse. However, in the presence of sustained tachyarrhythmias, it is mandatory that the differential diagnosis be refined beyond a simple supraventricular versus ventricular consideration. Further diagnostic decisions are both clinically possible and important. Tachyarrhythmias have been given many names based on their electrocardiographic appearance. It is important to know which separate tachyarrhythmia entities exist and, more importantly, to know which occur at an incidence sufficient to be of clinical significance. It is also important to have a system for classification that is based both upon the site of origin and the mechanism for sustaining the tachyarrhythmia. For single premature impulses, it was sufficient to divide sites of origin into supraventricular and ventricular. For sustained tachyarrhythmias, it is important that supraventricular be divided into sinus node, atria, and A-V junction (A-V node, His bundle, and anomalous A-V pathway). Ventricular should be divided into bundle branch and myocardium. The mechanisms are accelerated pacemaker activity and reentry or circus movement. Each of these mechanisms occurs at only some of the possible sites. Therefore, although there are 12 possible tachyarrhythmic entities, in fact there are only 8 that are clinically important (Table 4).

Accelerated Pacemakers. Since the only cells with pacemaking capabilities are the cells that lie in the sinus node, the cells scattered around the subendocardial areas of the atria, and the Purkinje cells of the His bundle and bundle branches, accelerated pacemaker tachyarrhythmias can originate only from these four areas. The sinus node provides a model for a pacemaker-induced tachyarrhythmia. The pacemaker has a certain intrinsic rate of discharging. Sinus tachycardia occurs "nonparoxysmally" as defined earlier, and also disappears nonparoxysmally. There is a maximal rate depending upon the limits of automatic frequency of the pacemaker cell. Usually, the other cardiac sites with pacing capabilities are activated by the spread of the impulse from the more rapidly discharging sinus node. These sites serve an important escape function if the sinus node fails, as noted in the discussion on bradyarrhythmias. Their pacemaking rate can also be accelerated, and thereby cause a tachyarrhythmia. Fortunately, pacemaker-induced tachyarrhythmias other than sinus tachycardia are not common and constitute a quite small percentage of the clinically important tachycardias.

Reentry. It is important that a model for reentrant tachycardias that is as easy to understand as sinus tachycardia be identified as a "touchstone." The congenital anomaly of a persistent muscle bridge between atria and ventricles leading to ventricular preexcitation and the Wolff-Parkinson-White syndrome provides such a model. In the absence of this anomaly, there is

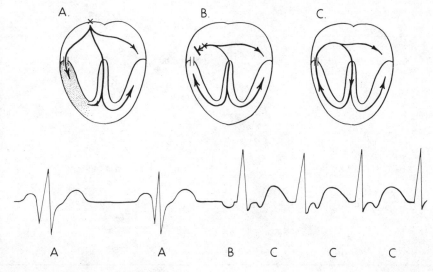

Figure 6. In the presence of an abnormal A-V connection, such as the right atrial to right ventricular muscle bridge above, there may be either antegrade conduction (A) resulting in aberrant conduction to the ventricles or antegrade block as depicted in B when a premature atrial impulse arrives at the muscle bridge before it has completed its refractory period. The result may be initiation of a reentrant tachycardia (C) if the impulse is able to continually encounter receptive tissue.

only one pathway for electrical conduction between atria and ventricles — the A-V node. In all other areas of the A-V ring, there are no tissues capable of electrical conduction. When a muscle bridge exists between atria, it provides an alternate route for atrioventricular conduction. As can be seen in Figure 6, this may result in premature activation of the ventricular muscle at the distal end of the connection. The QRS complex has a slurred upstroke or delta wave followed by a more rapid terminal aspect produced by the normally conducted impulse activating the areas of myocardium farthest from the site of the anomalous pathway. For this fusion to occur, both the A-V node and the anomalous pathway must be receptive to antegrade conduction of the electrical impulse. If either pathway is refractory (e.g., not yet fully repolarized following the previous activation), the ventricles might be activated via only one route. Then, if the anomalous pathway had lost its refractoriness by the time the impulse arrived at its ventricular end, it might be activated in a retrograde direction. Thus, "unidirectional block" would have occurred and, if the impulse traversing the anomalous pathway then encounters atrial myocardium that is no longer refractory, reentry will occur. This reentry will continue as long as receptive tissue is encountered. It may result in a single premature impulse or, when a circuit is established, may produce a sustained tachycardia. In the case of the Wolff-Parkinson-White syndrome, this circuit typically includes A-V node, His bundle, bundle branches, ventricular myocardium, anomalous pathway, and atrial muscle. The appearance on ECG is similar to that of a tachycardia produced by recycling within the A-V node (Tables 4, 5, and Fig. 8). These arrhythmias have been previously termed PAT (paroxysmal atrial tachycardia) but, since they are the result of reentry either within the A-V node or involving an abnormal A-V pathway, the name *paroxysmal A-V junctional tachycardia* is more appropriate.

During a reentry tachycardia, all cells with pacemaker capability would be activated as the wave front spreads through that area, and thus their pacemaking capabilities would not be required for sustaining the tachycardia. Whereas the rate of a pacemaker tachycardia is dependent upon the frequency of spontaneous activation, the rate of reentrant tachycardia is dependent upon the speed of conduction of the impulse, the length of the refractory period of the various tissues, and the length of the circuit. The rates of both may change gradually, but only a reentrant tachycardia will appear and disappear suddenly or paroxysmally.

One important reason for distinguishing between these two mechanisms of tachycardia is their very different response to electrical shock (Fig. 7). The shock is capable of depolarizing or activating all the various regions of the heart. Following the electrical shock, the rhythm will be reinitiated by the area with the most rapid pacemaking capabilities. If the tachycardia was caused by a rapidly discharging pacemaker, this will recur after electrical shock although the rate may be transiently altered by autonomic imbalance induced by the current. A reentrant tachyarrhythmia is entirely dependent upon continually encountering receptive areas. If all areas of the heart are rendered refractory by an electrical shock, the reentrant tachycardia must

Table 4.   *Sites and Mechanisms of Tachyarrhythmias*

	Mechanism	
	---	---
Site	*Pacemaker*	*Reentry*
Supraventricular		
Sinus node	Sinus tach	—
Atria	Nonparoxysmal atrial tach with block	Atrial flut-fib
AV node	—	Paroxysmal A-V junctional tach
His bundle	Nonparoxysmal His tach	—
Ventricular		
Bundle branches	Nonparoxysmal vent tach	Paroxysmal vent tach
Ventricles	—	Vent flut-fib

Table 5. *Supraventricular Tachycardias*

	Rate	Mechanism	Vagal Response of the Tach	Etiology	A:V Ratios
Sinus tach	100 200	Pacer	Gradual slowing	Sympa- thetic	1:1
Nonparoxysmal atrial tach with block	100 200	Pacer	Gradual slowing	Digitalis	>1:1
Paroxysmal A-V junctional tach	150 250	Micro reentry	Sudden breaking	Congenital	1:1
Atrial flut-fib	200 500+	Macro reentry	Gradual speeding	↑ Atrial size ↑ Sympa- thetic tone	>1:1
Nonparoxysmal His tach	60 120	Pacer	None	Dig/Isch	Dissoc/ retrograde

stop. Asystole will follow and will then be terminated by the most rapidly discharging pacemaker. Reentry may then subsequently recur but only after an impulse has been initiated by an area with pacemaking capabilities. Thus, the characteristic of termination by an electrical shock is unique to a tachyarrhythmia with reentrant mechanism.

Macro versus Micro Reentry. The terms macro and micro reentry are defined in the introductory section of this chapter. The reentry that occurs in the Wolff-Parkinson-White syndrome is an example of macro reentry. The other varieties are noted in Table 4 and Figure 8. When macro reentry occurs within the atrial muscle, the result is atrial flutter-fibrillation; when macro reentry involves the ventricular muscle, ventricular flutter-fibrillation is produced. The most common site for micro reentry is the A-V node, wherein the tachycardia is sustained by recycling of the impulse within the A-V node. Since such A-V nodal recycling is not apparent on the surface electrocardiogram, the resultant P and QRS waves are the only data available for analysis. There is a tendency to name the tachyarrhythmia depending upon the sequence of the P and QRS; if the P wave precedes the QRS, it has been termed *paroxysmal atrial tachycardia;* if the P wave is concealed or follows the QRS, it has been termed *paroxysmal nodal* or *junctional tachycardia.* The sequence of P and QRS, however, is irrelevant. The electrocardiographic appearance of this arrhythmia is identical to the macro reentry that was previously described for the Wolff-Parkinson-White syndrome. An all-inclusive term for this supraventricular arrhythmia is *A-V junctional tachycardia.* The other common site of micro reentry is the ventricles. This may either be localized to the bundle branches or to some abnormal area of the ventricular myocardium. Because the area itself is not of sufficient size for its activation to be apparent on the surface electrocardiogram, only the resultant QRS complexes and their T waves will be seen.

Supraventricular Tachycardias. Clinical

Figure 7. There is an important difference in the response to DC shock of the two mechanistically different types of tachycardia. Since the rhythm after the shock will always be determined by the most rapidly discharging pacemaker, DC shock will not terminate an accelerated pacemaker tachycardia. However, current sufficient to simultaneously bring the areas necessary for the propagation of a recycling impulse into a state of refractoriness will terminate a reentrant tachycardia.

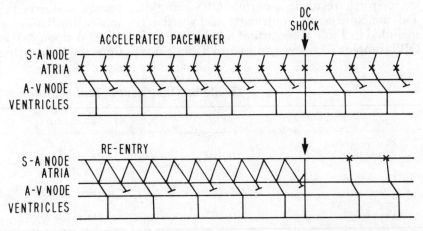

x *represents pacemaker discharge*

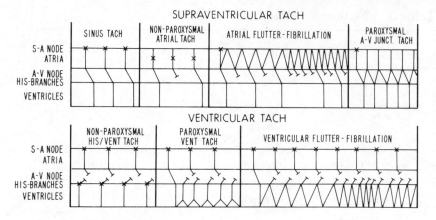

Figure 8. The seven tachyarrhythmias are depicted schematically, indicating the two important diagnostic aspects: site and mechanism. X is site of pacemaker activity, (〰〰) is a continually recycling impulse (reentry), and (∨) is block of the impulse. Paroxysmal AV junctional tachyarrhythmia may be alternatively produced by reentry involving an anomalous A-V pathway (Fig. 6).

characteristics of the supraventricular tachycardias are noted on Table 5 and a schematic diagram of their mechanisms is shown in Figure 8. It should be noted that pacemaker-induced tachycardias have a relatively lower maximal rate than reentry tachycardias. Also, the maximal rate of the sinus node and atrial pacemaker cells is higher than that of Purkinje cells located in the His bundle and bundle branches. Any generalized increase in sympathetic activity usually results in maximal acceleration of the sinus pacemaker and thus sinus tachycardia. A pacemaker tachycardia other than sinus typically occurs only if (1) the sinus node is inadequate, (2) there is a local problem such as ischemia in the area of other pacemaker cells with pacemaking capabilities, or (3) digitalis toxicity is present. Although digitalis has a readily apparent parasympathetic effect on the A-V node, it has a sympathetic effect upon areas with pacemaking capabilities. It may result in either nonparoxysmal atrial or His-bundle branch tachycardia. When the atrial pacemaker is accelerated, there will be attendant A-V block because of the parasympathetic effect at the A-V node. When the His or bundle branch site is accelerated, A-V dissociation will occur. The nonparoxysmal His tachycardia is included in Table 5 as a supraventricular tachycardia because it may result in a narrow QRS complex, and nonparoxysmal ventricular tachycardia is included in Table 6 because it results in a wide QRS complex. However, in Figure 8, nonparoxysmal His and ventricular tachycardias are combined into a single tachyarrhythmic entity, since both the cause and the methods of management of these accelerated pacemakers are identical. The only differences are that Purkinje cells proximal to the site of bundle branching have a somewhat more rapid intrinsic pacing rate and result in a narrow QRS complex, while those distal to the site of branching have a somewhat slower intrinsic pacing rate and result in a widened QRS complex. Therefore, the term *nonparoxysmal His-ventricular tachycardia* is used to describe accelerated pacemaker activity in the His or bundle branches, regardless of the QRS appearance.

Vagal Response. The response to vagal stimulation noted in Table 5 refers to the change in the tachyarrhythmic problem itself. It is important to note that a parasympathetic intervention may influence the tachyarrhythmia either directly or indirectly through its effect on the A-V node. In the instances of sinus tachycardia and paroxysmal A-V junctional tachycardia, the clinician is most concerned with the vagal effect directly upon the tachycardia wherein gradual slowing occurs with sinus tachycardia and sudden breaking occurs with paroxysmal A-V junctional tachycardia. In the presence of either nonparoxysmal atrial tachycardia with block or atrial flutter-fibrillation (with block), the primary vagal effect is upon A-V nodal conduction rather than upon the tachyarrhythmia itself. The vagally me-

Table 6. *Ventricular Tachycardias*

	Rate	Mechanism	Etiology
Nonparoxysmal vent tach	60–120	Pacer	Dig/Ischemia
Paroxysmal vent tach	150–220	Micro reentry	–
Vent flut-fib	200–500+	Macro reentry	–

diated induction of A-V block is important because it removes QRS complexes from the electrocardiogram, allowing one to accurately diagnose the tachyarrhythmia by observation of the uncovered atrial activity. The differential diagnosis between nonparoxysmal atrial tachycardia and atrial flutter-fibrillation is quite important, because the former is frequently caused by digitalis toxicity while the latter is almost never caused by digitalis. Indeed, with atrial flutter-fibrillation, it is important that sufficient digitalis be maintained to optimize the ventricular rate. This differential, however, may be quite difficult because, as noted in Table 5, the upper limit of the rate spectrum for nonparoxysmal atrial tachycardia is 200 per minute, which is the same as the lower limit of the rate spectrum for atrial flutter (200 ± 20 beats per minute). Therefore, when the atrial rate is 200 ± 20 beats per minute, the rate alone does not distinguish between these two entities.

Another important aid in diagnosis is observation of the morphology of the atrial activity. Since atrial flutter-fibrillation is a macro reentry within the atria, there is never a time when all the atrial muscle is activated or another time when it is all recovering. Instead, part of the atria is activated while another part is recovering. This results in a continually undulating baseline rather than in discrete P waves separated by a flat baseline. Since the nonparoxysmal atrial tachycardia is due to an accelerated pacemaker within the atria, discrete P waves separated by a flat baseline are seen. One may be misled in this differential diagnosis if only the right precordial leads of the electrocardiogram are observed.

Discrete positive waves separated by a flat baseline may appear in leads V_1 and V_2 while simultaneous recording of frontal plane leads 2, 3, or aVF will reveal a typical "saw-toothed" pattern of undulating baseline. This occurs in atrial flutter because a portion of the route of the circus movement is perpendicular to the transverse plane or the body, so that during this time there is neither net anterior nor posterior predominance of electrical forces, resulting in a flat baseline on the electrocardiogram. Such a flat baseline between P waves may be due either to no electrical activity or to electrical activity that has equal distribution toward and away from the monitoring lead. The absence of electrical activity explains the flat baseline in right precordial leads in the presence of nonparoxysmal atrial tachycardia, while the "cancellation effect" applies to atrial flutter: the differential diagnosis requires observation of inferiorly oriented frontal plane leads. It is important to emphasize this point because the right precordial leads are optimal for identifying atrial activity but they are not capable of this particular differentiation.

"*PAT*". Note (Tables 4, 5 and Fig. 8) the totally different sites and mechanisms for the two tachyarrhythmic entities: nonparoxysmal atrial tachycardia with block and paroxysmal A-V junctional tachycardia. These are usually referred to as *PAT with block* and *PAT*, respectively. The term PAT (paroxysmal atrial tachycardia) is a misnomer for both of these different tachyarrhythmia entities. Nonparoxysmal atrial tachycardia with block is usually produced by digitalis toxicity and is due to acceleration of pacemaker activity within the atria. It may, in fact, be either acceleration of the sinus node or of the pacemaker cells scattered around the atrial endocardium. Careful observations during the onset of digitalis toxicity have shown the atrial rate to gradually accelerate to a maximal rate of about 200 per minute and then to gradually decrease as the toxicity spontaneously abates or is reversed by administration of potassium. Therefore, this PAT is truly an AT (atrial tachycardia) but is nonparoxysmal rather than paroxysmal. The other tachyarrhythmic problem known as PAT is due to reentry within the A-V junction. Therefore, this PAT is truly a PT (paroxysmal tachycardia) but is A-V junctional rather than atrial in origin.

Atrial Flutter-Fibrillation. In Tables 4 and 5 and Figure 8, atrial flutter-fibrillation is combined as one tachyarrhythmic entity because it is due to a single mechanism — macro reentry within the atria. There is a spectrum, as is noted in Table 4 and Figures 8, 9, and 10, within this arrhythmia. At the one end is atrial flutter with a relatively slow and quite regular atrial rate. At the opposite extreme is atrial fibrillation, which is very rapid and irregular. In the middle of the spectrum the appearance may resemble more closely either that of flutter or fibrillation. The differential diagnosis between flutter and fibrillation is not important, since it is a single tachyarrhythmic entity. Some patients are able to move spontaneously to different rates within the spectrum. Others will remain at a particular rate even in the presence of interventions that are capable of altering atrial conduction velocity and refractoriness and therefore could potentially alter the rate and regularity of atrial flutter-fibrillation. Other patients will not change their rates spontaneously but will move toward the flutter end of the spectrum when quinidine-like drugs are administered and will move toward the fibrillation end owing to either use of digitalis or vagal stimulation (Fig. 10).

It was noted previously that, in the presence of atrial flutter-fibrillation, the most obvious vagal effect is the production of further A-V block. When one observes the atrial activity during vagal stimulation, it may be seen to move toward the fibrillation end of the spectrum. This occurs

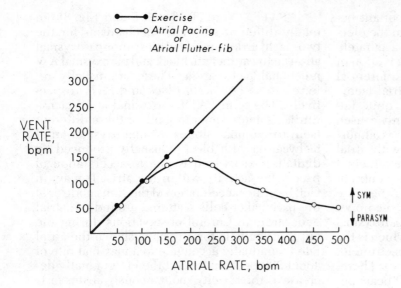

Figure 9. The effects of increasing the atrial rate by exercise versus pacing or the tachyarrhythmia, atrial flutter-fibrillation are contrasted. The high sympathetic tone during exercise causes both an acceleration of the atrial rate and a shortening of the A-V nodal refractory period causing a 1:1 A-V ratio. During atrial acceleration due to either pacing or atrial flutter-fibrillation, however, the A-V nodal refractoriness remains at the baseline level, impairing impulse conduction. The nonconducted beats cause further A-V nodal refractoriness and thus the greater their number the slower the resultant ventricular rate.

because the acetylcholine has an opposite effect upon conduction velocity and refractoriness within the atria, versus the A-V node. Note that acetylcholine shares this paradoxical effect with digitalis (Fig. 10). This speeding of the atrial rate during vagal stimulation provides convincing evidence that the mechanism of atrial flutter-fibrillation is reentry and not acceleration of a pacemaker. Even though a reentrant tachycardia occurs paroxysmally, changes in rate are quite possible. This may occur over a wide spectrum as in atrial flutter-fibrillation or, as will be noted later, ventricular flutter-fibrillation, or over a more narrow range in the presence of micro reentry either within the A-V node or ventricles.

Table 3 and Figures 8 and 10 illustrate that there is an inverse relationship between the atrial rate within the atrial flutter-fibrillation spectrum and the resultant ventricular rate. This relationship occurs because the ventricular rate depends on the amount of A-V block. The nonconducted atrial impulses do not stop at their point of entry into the A-V node. They penetrate the node to variable degrees, rendering it refractory to the following impulse. Therefore, the very occurrence of multiple atrial impulses is a cause for A-V nodal block. Digitalis may induce A-V nodal block both by parasympathetic effect on the A-V node and by its ability to accelerate the atrial rate from flutter toward fibrillation. This relationship between atrial and ventricular rates is further illustrated in Figure 9.

During exercise, there is a 1:1 relationship between atria and ventricles because the same sympathetic stimulation that is producing the sinus tachycardia is speeding the conduction velocity and shortening the refractory period of

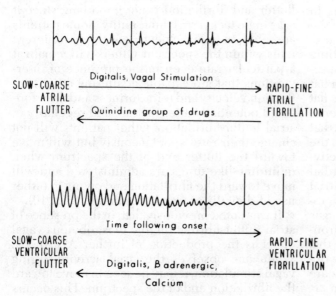

Figure 10. The comparison between the atrial and ventricular flutter-fibrillation spectra is depicted. Both occur when the electrical impulse continues to encounter receptive tissue, and this may proceed along an orderly (flutter) or disorderly (fibrillation) pathway. Flutter and fibrillation are not two different tachyarrhythmic entities, but there are important differences between the extremes of both the atrial and ventricular flutter-fibrillation spectra.

the A-V node, facilitating 1:1 atrioventricular relationship with a persistently normal P-R interval. When the atrial rate is accelerated by either artificial atrial pacing or the presence of atrial flutter-fibrillation, no such sympathetic effect is present. Rather, the A-V node remains at its baseline level of conduction velocity and refractoriness. Therefore, as is shown in Figure 5, the atrial impulses reach the A-V node during its refractory period. Some occur during the relative aspect and are conducted slowly toward the ventricles, while others occur earlier during the absolute refractory period and are not conducted at all. The most slowly conducted may fail to reach the His bundle, but their penetration may produce further refractoriness within the node. As is shown in Figure 9, as the atrial rate is increased further, there may be resultant slowing of the ventricular rate.

Progressively more rapid atrial pacing in normal individuals would result in an initial increase in ventricular rate with prolongation of the P-R interval. At an atrial rate of approximately 150 per minute, however, second degree A-V block typically occurs, and further increase of the atrial rate results in further decreases of the ventricular rate. As shown in Table 3, the regularity of the ventricular rate varies depending on the atrial rate. At the flutter end of the flutter-fibrillation spectrum, the ventricular rate may be regular with 1:1 conduction. Such a situation, with a ventricular rate of about 200 per minute, is poorly tolerated clinically and may be avoided by the use of digitalis. Use of a quinidine-like drug in the absence of digitalis might cause this 1:1 atrioventricular relationship because, as shown in Figure 10, the quinidine group of drugs slows the atrial rate from fibrillation toward flutter.

As shown in Table 3, at more rapid atrial rates the ventricular rate may be regularly irregular. A 6:2 atrioventricular ratio is commonly seen in atrial flutter. As the atrial rate increases further, the ventricular rate may become regular with 2:1 or even 3:1 or 4:1 block. At the fibrillation end of the atrial flutter-fibrillation spectrum, no regularity of the ventricular rate is possible, and it is typically irregularly irregular. This expectation of irregular irregularity is an important diagnostic clue to the origin of early wide QRS complexes in the presence of atrial flutter-fibrillation, as is noted in the previous section on single premature impulses.

There are other differences shown in Table 3 between the characteristics at the flutter end versus the fibrillation end of the spectrum. Flutter tends to be more transient while fibrillation is more stable. Relatively small amounts of digitalis may increase the A-V block at the fibrillation end of the spectrum. Digitalis is much less effective in achieving an optimal ventricular rate in the presence of atrial flutter. Digitalis produces an additive effect to the amount of block that is intrinsically present, but toxic amounts of the drug are necessary to produce any A-V block when none initially exists, as in sinus tachycardia. A quite small amount of digitalis may effectively enhance the A-V block caused by the multiple atrial impulses of atrial fibrillation. Atrial flutter is somewhere between these two extremes and thus an intermediate therapeutic effect will be noted. If, in the patient with atrial flutter, administration of digitalis results in speeding of the atrial rate toward the fibrillation end of the spectrum, one may expect to achieve optimal slowing of the ventricular rate. If, despite the use of digitalis, the atrial rate remains at the flutter end of the spectrum, it is difficult to achieve a similarly low ventricular rate without inducing digitalis toxicity.

At the flutter end of the spectrum where the impulses circuit the atria along a constant pathway, the tachyarrhythmia may be interrupted either with low-energy DC shock or with atrial pacing. At the fibrillation end of the spectrum, however, higher energy is required for cardioversion and atrial pacing is ineffective. This difference in response to electrical intervention at the ends of the flutter-fibrillation spectrum is further noted in the discussion of ventricular flutter-fibrillation.

Ventricular Tachycardias. The ventricular tachycardias are classified in Table 4, characterized in Table 6, and illustrated in Figure 8. There are only three, and one of these — nonparoxysmal ventricular tachycardia — has already been discussed as a part of the nonparoxysmal His-ventricular tachycardia problem. Since the upper limit of pacing rate for the Purkinje cells of the bundle branches is relatively low (approximately 120 per minute), there is rarely either a clinically significant hemodynamic problem or a difficult differential diagnosis versus reentrant ventricular tachycardias.

There are two distinctly different reentrant ventricular tachycardias: paroxysmal ventricular tachycardia caused by micro reentry and ventricular flutter-fibrillation owing to macro reentry. Differences in the sites and electrocardiographic appearances of these tachyarrhythmias have been discussed earlier. The ventricular flutter-fibrillation spectrum has many characteristics that are similar to those of the atrial flutter-fibrillation spectrum. The electrocardiographic appearances are similar: a continually undulating baseline. The contrast between the two ends of the spectrum is illustrated schematically in Figure 8 and electrocardiographically in Figure 10.

If the normal A-V node is the only electrical

connection between atria and ventricles, atrial flutter-fibrillation will not result directly in ventricular flutter-fibrillation. If, however, there is a preexcitation pathway as in the Wolff-Parkinson-White syndrome, all or most of the atrial impulses can reach the ventricles, resulting directly in ventricular flutter-fibrillation. When the A-V node is the only electrical pathway between atria and ventricles, digitalis will enhance A-V block. However, since digitalis has an opposite effect upon conduction velocity and recovery time within muscle, it may, in the presence of an anomalous pathway, produce a paradoxical increase in the ventricular rate.

When ventricular flutter-fibrillation is initiated by a premature ventricular impulse, its appearance is that of "coarse ventricular fibrillation," or ventricular flutter. The resultant lowered cardiac output is insufficient to maintain the stability of this rhythm within the myocardium. If the heart is perfused by another source (as during cardiopulmonary bypass), this "ventricular flutter" typically persists. In the usual clinical situation, its appearance quickly changes to the irregular irregularity of ventricular fibrillation. As mentioned for atrial flutter-fibrillation, response to electrical current is very different at the two ends of the spectrum. A thump to the chest or a 1 watts-second current may break ventricular flutter, whereas even the maximal output of a defibrillator may be insufficient to break "fine" ventricular fibrillation. For this reason, efforts are made to "coarsen" the ventricular fibrillation, as noted in Figure 10, by use of either beta-adrenergic stimulating agents or calcium. If sufficient electrical current is delivered to activate all of the heart simultaneously, any reentrant tachycardia will break.

Toward the fibrillation end of both atrial and ventricular flutter-fibrillation, however, the delivery of sufficient current may not be possible. When a "failure to convert" occurs, one should make the very important distinction between no conversion versus conversion with subsequent return of the reentrant tachyarrhythmia. This can be best accomplished if equipment is used that permits continual observation of the electrocardiogram during the cardioversion procedure. Even during continuous recording, the electrocardiographic signal may be transiently lost because of the capacitance charging following the shock.

With some equipment, the recording device may be protected from receiving this capacitance discharge by persistent compression of the "defibrillation button." The patient will, of course, receive only one shock, but the resultant stable electrocardiographic baseline will permit diagnosis of the immediate post-shock rhythm. Only if failure to convert has occurred should additional current be used, an alternate paddle site chosen, a "coarsening" agent administered, or a different defibrillator employed. If a break in the reentrant tachycardia has occurred but reentry has been reinitiated, the therapeutic efforts should be made toward prevention of recurrence following subsequent DC shocks.

There is also the important decision of whether synchronization of the DC shock should be assured by timing the discharge to the patient's QRS complex. This decision requires attention to the differential diagnosis of whether discrete QRS complexes are present. Discrete QRS complexes will occur in all the reentrant tachyarrhythmias other than ventricular flutter-fibrillation. Here, even at the flutter end of the spectrum, no discrete QRS complexes or T waves are present. Therefore, synchronization would not be possible. In all other instances, synchronization is indicated because an electrical discharge during the T wave could cause initiation of the ventricular flutter-fibrillation spectrum.

CONCLUSION

This article is based on an organized approach that has been designed to expand understanding of the cardiac rhythm and arrhythmias. In this system only four general classifications of cardiac arrhythmias are used: A-V dissociation, intraventricular conduction delays, bradyarrhythmias, and tachyarrhythmias. There are three different reasons for AV dissociation, two different sites for intraventricular conduction delay, two sites and mechanisms for producing bradyarrhythmias, and seven different tachyarrhythmic entities. It is a system that avoids use of classical nomenclature, uses electrophysiologically proven principles only when they contribute to clinical understanding, and relies heavily upon tables and figures to provide illustrations that may be quickly recalled to guide clinical management when a precise diagnosis of the cardiac rhythm is required.

PERICARDITIS

By EDWARD JOHN PERRINS, B.Sc., M.B.,
M.R.C.P.,
and RICHARD SUTTON, M.B., M.R.C.P.,
F.A.C.C.
London, England

DEFINITIONS

The heart is invested by two layers of pericardium, visceral and parietal, that are separated by a potential space. Although not essential to life, the intact pericardium is thought to exert considerable influence on cardiac physiology, particularly on the diastolic properties of the ventricles. Pericardial disease may therefore cause profound hemodynamic upset. Pericardial disease is either congenital or inflammatory (pericarditis). Pericarditis may be acute or chronic, and associated with effusion, tamponade or constriction. Pericarditis is usually part of a more generalized disease process.

CONGENITAL PERICARDIAL DISEASE

PERICARDIAL CYSTS

Pericardial cysts are not uncommon. They are usually recognized as a mass on routine chest x-ray. They rarely produce symptoms unless extremely large, when they may compress neighboring structures. The cysts are usually coelomic and not actually in communication with the pericardial lumen. In over 80 per cent of patients, they are situated anteriorly and at the right pericardiophrenic angle. Differential diagnosis includes foramen of Morgagni diaphragmatic hernia, large right pericardial fat pad, or tumors of the heart, pericardium, and mediastinum.

CONGENITAL DEFICIENCY OF THE PERICARDIUM

This is a rare cardiac anomaly. The defect is usually on the left side and may be partial or complete. Pectus excavatum may be an associated finding. On chest x-ray, there is a shift of the heart to the left, a prominent pulmonary artery segment, and flattening of the left ventricular segment. Herniation or even strangulation of cardiac structures has been described in incomplete defects.

PERICARDITIS

Pericarditis may be acute or chronic and may be accompanied by effusion or progress to constriction or tamponade. The causes are legion and are summarized in Table 1.

SYMPTOMS

Pain is the cardinal symptom of acute pericarditis and is invariably present in the idiopathic group. The pain may be severe; it is precordial and is usually aggravated by inspiration or coughing. Inflammation of the adjoining diaphragmatic pleura may cause radiation to the supraclavicular region and shoulder tip. The pain is classically eased by sitting up. A sensation of dyspnea may be experienced owing to the pain, but genuine dyspnea does not occur without hemodynamic embarrassment, which is the result of effusion.

Other symptoms are those of the associated disorder, but the idiopathic variety is often heralded by fever, joint pains, headache, and general malaise.

SIGNS

A pericardial friction rub is the pathognomonic sign of pericarditis, although it is not always

Table 1. *Etiology of Pericarditis*

1. Acute idiopathic (probably viral)
2. Specific infections
   Bacteria (TB, gonococcal)
   Rickettsiae (Q fever)
   Fungal (Histoplasmosis, nocardiosis)
   Protozoal (amebiasis)
   Viral
   Bacterial endocarditis
3. Disease of adjoining structures
   Myocardial Infarction and Postinfarction
      (Dressler's syndrome)
   Dissecting aortic aneurysm
   Pleurisy
4. Primary *or* metastatic neoplasm
5. Connective tissue disease
      (rheumatoid, SLE, scleroderma)
6. Iatrogenic–Thoracotomy
   Cardiac catheter
   Pacemaker lead
   Radiotherapy
   Drugs: Hydralazine, procainamide,
      anticoagulants, penicillin
7. Trauma
8. Miscellaneous
   Sarcoid
   Myxedema
   Amyloid
   Uremia
   The commonest cause is undoubtedly the acute
   idiopathic variety, which is almost certainly due to
   a viral infection.

present. The rub may be localized and heard with the patient in one particular posture, for example, sitting up. The rub is a short, high-pitched, scratchy sound, best heard with the diaphragm of the stethoscope and typically has three components corresponding to atrial systole, ventricular systole, and ventricular diastole. The rub is intensified by increasing the force with which the diaphragm is applied to the chest and varies in intensity with respiration. When only two components are present, a to and fro sound is heard. If the rub is heard only in diastole or in systole (the latter circumstance is extremely rare), then it should be viewed with suspicion. However, frequent observations will reveal the evanescent quality of a true rub. Other signs are those of the underlying condition or accompanying effusion (see later discussion).

LABORATORY FINDINGS

There is no diagnostic investigation for pericarditis. The erythrocyte sedimentation rate may be raised. The white cell count may be normal or show a relative lymphocytosis in the idiopathic variety. The electrocardiogram is helpful. Typically, there is ST segment elevation, convex upward, in all leads except aVR, without pathologic Q waves or reciprocal ST-T changes. The ST elevation usually persists for only a few days. The T wave change, however, may be permanent and extensive; this finding may indicate a poorer prognosis. Chest x-ray is normal, unless an effusion or associated cardiac disorder is present. Echocardiography and cardiac blood pool scanning are similarly unhelpful in the absence of effusion. Negative serial cardiac enzymes and technetium pyrophosphate scan may, however, be helpful in excluding myocardial infarction.

DIFFERENTIAL DIAGNOSIS

The principal differential diagnoses are myocardial infarction, pulmonary embolism, dissecting aortic aneurysm, and pleurisy. Chest pain together with a pericardial or pleuropericardial rub may be present in any of these conditions.

The presence of cardiac failure makes pericarditis unlikely, unless there is clear evidence of effusion. If clinical suspicion is high, then specific investigations such as isotopic lung or cardiac scanning may be helpful.

COURSE

Acute idiopathic pericarditis is generally a self-limiting disease, running a benign course. However, it may be recurrent and progression to constriction does rarely occur. The course of other varieties of pericarditis depends entirely upon the underlying disorder. It should be emphasized that pericarditis may be completely silent clinically, and become apparent only when effusion or constriction has occurred.

CHRONIC CONSTRICTIVE PERICARDITIS

Constrictive pericarditis is the result of fibrosis, calcification, and adherence between the visceral and parietal layers of pericardium. An effusion may also be present. Constrictive pericarditis is a rare disorder and may result from any of the causes of acute pericarditis, although frequently there is no antecedent history. Tuberculosis has been blamed for up to 40 per cent of cases, but this view is now being challenged, despite the decreasing incidence of this disorder.

SYMPTOMS

The clinical picture is dominated by the hemodynamic embarrassment caused by restriction of ventricular and atrial filling. Pain is unusual. The picture is one of chronic congestive failure, with fatigue, dyspnea, ascites, and edema as principal complaints. There is a tendency for the ascites to develop before peripheral edema, and the patient may present as hepatic cirrhosis, the cause of which will be missed without careful cardiac observation. Orthopnea and paroxysmal nocturnal dyspnea are uncommon in pericarditis, in contrast to other causes of congestive failure.

SIGNS

Examination of the venous and arterial pulses is of the utmost importance. The venous pulse is always elevated and shows a rapid Y descent. When in sinus rhythm a rapid X descent may sometimes be observed as well. Kussmaul's sign (elevation in venous pulse on inspiration) may also be noted. The venous pulse may be so elevated as to be overlooked. The arterial pulse is usually of low amplitude and may exhibit pulsus paradoxus. The apex beat may be impalpable or occasionally exhibit systolic retraction. Atrial fibrillation is present in approximately one third of patients. Auscultation reveals soft heart sounds, a physiologic second sound, and a high frequency early diastolic third heart sound (pericardial knock) may be heard. A friction rub is generally absent. There may be ascites, hepatosplenomegaly, and stigmata of chronic liver disease. There may be signs of an underlying disorder.

LABORATORY FINDINGS

The chest x-ray may be very helpful. Pericardial calcification is present in approximately one half of the patients. The calcification tends to encircle the heart in contrast to posttraumatic and postrheumatic calcification, which tends to occur in isolated plaques. The lung fields are usually clear because the major effect of the constriction tends to weigh on the right heart, and the heart size may be normal.

The electrocardiogram shows low-voltage QRS complexes and nonspecific T wave change. The presence of other electrocardiographic abnormalities such as hypertrophy or bundle branch block would suggest another diagnosis, such as cardiomyopathy.

Echocardiography is of great value, but mainly in excluding occult left heart disease. Occasionally, the pericardial thickening may be visualized directly. The presence of reduced left ventricular function does not, however, exclude the diagnosis, as occasionally the pericardial calcification invades the myocardium, causing reduced function. A pericardial effusion may also be detected by echo.

Cardiac catheterization is of importance. Characteristically, all the cardiac pressures are elevated, with the pulmonary wedge, pulmonary artery, right ventricle and right atrial pressures all very close to one another. There is an M-shaped pattern to the right atrial tracing and and early diastolic dip in the right ventricular trace. Wood has described a characteristic response of the pulmonary wedge and right atrial pressures during deep inspiration. When the two pressures are recorded simultaneously, the left atrial (wedge) pressure paradoxically rises faster than the right atrial pressure.

DIFFERENTIAL DIAGNOSIS

This is chiefly from cor pulmonale, tricuspid valve disease, cardiomyopathy, or occult left-sided heart disease. The lack of signs of elevated pulmonary venous pressure, despite gross congestive cardiac failure, is strongly suggestive of constrictive pericarditis. Restrictive cardiomyopathy may be extremely difficult to distinguish from constriction, as the catheter findings may be quite similar. Occasionally, surgical exploration or myocardial biopsy is required.

COURSE

The clinical course is rapid and relentless, with severe congestive failure. However, surgical resection of the pericardium usually produces dramatic and sustained improvement.

PERICARDIAL EFFUSION

Pericardial effusion may occur in association with any of the causes of acute or chronic pericarditis just described, or it may occur without evidence of pericardial disease. When small, an effusion is generally symptomless. Larger effusions produce cardiac enlargement on chest x-ray and produce cardiac constriction or compression (tamponade).

SYMPTOMS

The symptoms of effusion depend on both the size and rate of accumulation of pericardial fluid. If there is no underlying cardiac disorder, then very large effusions may be symptomless. If there is preexisting cardiac or pericardial disease, tamponade may rapidly ensue. Effusions causing constriction produce the symptoms of congestive failure.

Cardiac tamponade occurs when the intrapericardial pressure rises to a point at which ventricular filling is severely impeded. This produces a fall of stroke volume, which initially is compensated for by tachycardia. Further elevation of outer pericardial pressure then causes reduced cardiac output with hypertension or syncope.

The important causes of tamponade are:
1. Trauma
2. Malignant disease with effusion
3. Tuberculous pericarditis
4. Rupture of heart or great vessels
5. Uremic pericarditis in patients on hemodialysis
6. Iatrogenic causes: needle aspiration of effusion, cardiac catheter, pacemaker leads, and so forth.

SIGNS

The classic picture of cardiac tamponade is one of rapidly rising venous pressure with falling systemic arterial pressure, tachycardia, and a "quiet heart" on auscultation. The arterial pulse classically displays pulsus paradoxus, i.e., a respiratory fall of peak systolic pressure greater than 10 mm Hg. This sign is not specific, however, and can occur also in constrictive pericarditis or more commonly in severe respiratory distress — for example, an acute asthmatic attack. It is important to realize that, in the presence of severe myocardial disease or aortic regurgitation, pulsus paradoxus may be absent, despite severe tamponade.

LABORATORY INVESTIGATIONS

Echocardiography is undoubtedly the most sensitive method available for the detection of an effusion. The demonstration of an echo-free space between the mobile posterior left ventricular wall and immobile posterior pericardium is diagnostic. Quite small effusions may be detected in this way. Septal motion may also be abnormal, but this is a more nonspecific sign. In large effusions, the whole heart can be seen to be moving within the fluid-filled sac, a finding particularly dramatic on two-dimensional echocardiography. There is sometimes an associated electrical alternans on the ECG.

The M-mode echo can give only an approximate guide to the size of the effusion, generally speaking, but the recent advance of two-dimensionsal scanning has increased the accuracy and allows loculated effusions to be visualized. Recently in cardiac tamponade, echocardiography has demonstrated marked respiratory variations of ventricular dimension associated with pulsus paradoxus.

The chest x-ray will show cardiac enlargement that is globular in shape and serial films are useful in documenting changes in size of the effusion. The lung fields are generally clear.

The electrocardiogram shows nonspecific changes, similar to constrictive pericarditis.

Other routine investigations are not helpful, but, particularly in cases in which the cause of the effusion is in doubt, aspiration of pericardial fluid is of importance. The fluid should be cultured, examined cytologically for malignant cells, and rheumatoid factor and antinuclear factor estimations carried out on it. Aspiration may be safely performed by the subxiphoid approach, with careful ECG monitoring of the exploring needle, the appearance of ST elevation signifying that the needle is touching epicardium.

COURSE

This again depends upon the underlying disorder. Small effusions may persist for years without symptoms; those due to malignant disease, uremia, or infection are generally rapidly progressive to fatal tamponade, unless pericardial aspiration is undertaken. In recurrent tamponade, surgical creation of a pericardial window or anterior pericardectomy is indicated.

PITFALLS AND POINTERS IN DIAGNOSIS

1. Pericardial disease in generally part of a systemic disorder.

2. A clinical picture of cirrhosis with distended neck veins may be constrictive pericarditis.
3. A clinical picture of cardiomegaly, clear lung fields, and heart failure usually indicates a pericardial effusion.
4. A clinical picture of pericardial effusion with congested lung fields is usually caused by primary myocardial or valvular heart disease.

CARDIOMYOPATHIES

By AMJAD I. SHEIKH, M.D., and RAYMOND J. PIETRAS, M.D.

Chicago, Illinois

SYNONYMS

Some synonyms for cardiomyopathy are idiopathic cardiomyopathy, primary myocardial disease, myocardiopathy, myocardiosis, and idiopathic cardiac hypertrophy. The subgroup of patients with idiopathic cardiac hypertrophy includes patients with asymmetric septal hypertrophy, hypertrophic obstructive cardiomyopathy, and idiopathic subaortic stenosis.

DEFINITION AND CLASSIFICATION

Those disorders that primarily affect the myocardial cell in initiating cardiac dysfunction are referred to as cardiomyopathies. This broad term encompasses a heterogeneous group of disorders in which cardiac involvement may be evident or be inconspicuous during the course of an illness. Cardiomyopathy can also be considered a possibility after exclusion of hypertensive cardiovascular disease, ischemic myocardial disease, rheumatic heart disease, and congenital heart disease. A detailed discussion of specific causes of the cardiomyopathies is beyond the scope of this presentation, but a partial etiologic classification is outlined in Table 1. This classification is meant to stimulate the physician to consider etiology, early recognition, and prevention of these disorders. Idiopathic cardiomyopathy is the most common form of this disorder; however, early recognition of known causes of cardiac muscle pathology, the so-called secondary cardiomyopathies,

Table 1. *Etiologic Classification of Cardiomyopathies*

I. Idiopathic
  A. Postinfectious (infectious agent not identified)
  B. Peripartal
  C. Idiopathic (unknown antecedent event)
II. Secondary
  A. Inflammatory (myocarditis)
    1. Known agents
      Viral: Coxsackievirus B, echoviruses, cytomegalovirus, *Chlamydia psittaci* (psittacosis)
      Rickettsial: mycoplasma, typhus
      Parasitic: *Trichinella spiralis, Trypanosoma cruzi* (Chagas' disease)
      Bacterial: *Corynebacterium diphtheriae*, streptococci
      Spirochetal: *Treponema pallidum* (syphilis), *Leptospira*
      Borrelia (relapsing fever)
      Mycotic: Blastomyces, *Actinomyces israelii*, Aspergillus
    2. Unknown Agents
      Allergic: drug reaction, serum sickness.
      Collagen disease: rheumatoid arthritis, lupus erythematosus, dermatomyositis, scleroderma
  B. Toxic
    1. Alcohol
    2. Heavy metals: antimony, cobalt (beer drinker's heart), arsenic, anesthetics
    3. Drugs: emetine, phenothiazines, tricyclics, ergot alkaloids, doxorubicin, daunomycin
  C. Familial
    1. Idiopathic familial cardiomyopathy
    2. Hypertrophic obstructive cardiomyopathy
    3. Neuromuscular disorders: Friedreich's ataxia, myotonic muscular dystrophy, pseudohypertrophic muscular dystrophy, Duchenne type muscular dystrophy, fascioscapulohumeral muscular dystrophy, limb girdle type of muscular dystrophy
  D. Endocrine
    1. Thyrotoxicosis
    2. Myxedema
    3. Pheochromocytoma
    4. Acromegaly
  E. Infiltrative
    1. Amyloidosis
    2. Sarcoidosis
    3. Neoplastic (primary and metastatic tumors)
    4. Hemochromatosis
    5. Glycogen storage diseases
    6. Lipid storage disease
    7. Mucopolysaccharide storage disease
  F. Nutritional
    1. Kwashiorkor
    2. Beriberi

is only possible if they are kept in mind during management of early heart disease of an obscure nature. This is the crucial stage at which withdrawal of a noxious agent may revert the pathologic process or early treatment may arrest progression of the disease.

Depending on the nature of the pathophysiologic process, varied hemodynamic disturbances are found on physical examination and cardiovascular investigation of these patients.

Classification of these clinical patterns into three types — congestive, hypertrophic, and restrictive — has been useful. The fact that the pathophysiologic patterns overlap should not obscure their clinical value.

Congestive cardiomyopathy implies that myocardial involvement is clinically manifested as congestive heart failure. This is the most prevalent type of cardiomyopathy and is due to many causes of acquired myocardial disease. Common examples are postinfectious cardiomyopathy, alcoholic cardiomyopathy, and acute myocarditis. The main features are marked dilatation of ventricles with generalized hypokinesis, mild ventricular hypertrophy, and biventricular failure.

Hypertrophic cardiomyopathy is present when the width of the left ventricular wall is increased. Outflow tract obstruction may occur with asymmetric septal to free wall hypertrophy. Hypertrophic cardiomyopathy involves mainly the left ventricle with reduced ventricular cavity size and restricted filling owing to increased ventricular stiffness; despite good pump function, stroke volume is reduced.

In restrictive cardiomyopathy, ventricular filling is reduced by a rigid, unyielding myocardium that produces clinical and laboratory features resembling constrictive pericarditis. Amyloidosis and sarcoidosis and infiltrative heart diseases are examples of this type of cardiomyopathy. Obliterative cardiomyopathy hemodynamically resembles restrictive cardiomyopathy and has been regarded as a subgroup of the latter. In this variety of cardiomyopathy, the intense endomyocardial fibrosis and overlying thrombus gradually obliterate the ventricular cavity.

SIGNS AND SYMPTOMS

The clinical manifestations of cardiomyopathy are diverse, since they depend on the extent, site, and nature of the myocardial disorder and consequent disturbances of hemodynamics. Although the majority of patients have symptoms in the late stages of the disease, a considerable number may be entirely asymptomatic at the onset. They are usually referred for evaluation of ventricular premature beats, cardiac enlargement, and an abnormal electrocardiogram or heart murmur; these abnormalities are usually discovered on routine examination.

Left-sided congestive heart failure is by far the most common presentation. Initially, fatigue owing to decreased cardiac output is followed by dyspnea, paroxysmal nocturnal dyspnea, and orthopnea; right heart failure with edema and ascites complete the sequence of events. Palpitations and variable degrees of dizziness to overt syncope have been observed secondary to cardiac arrhythmias in about one third of the patients. In obstructive hypertrophic cardiomyopathy, syncope occurs frequently after exertion and is related to a sudden decrease in venous return, which produces increased outflow tract obstruction and a reduced cardiac output.

Chest pain, sometimes resembling angina, and symptoms owing to systemic and pulmonary emboli are also common. Unfortunately, some patients die suddenly without any preceding symptoms referable to the cardiovascular system.

History

A detailed history is very important in the search for a specific cause. The diagnosis of cardiomyopathy is based on both positive findings and on the exclusion of common forms of heart disease. A history of recent respiratory infection or febrile illness should be sought to exclude a viral cause. A scrupulous history of alcohol ingestion or exposure to toxins and drugs that produce cardiac damage cannot be overemphasized. Of all the cardiomyopathies, the hypertrophic are most likely to give a positive family history of heart disease.

Specific clinical settings can be helpful in diagnosis. Cardiomyopathy is likely when a woman without a previous history of heart disease develops congestive heart failure in the third trimester of pregnancy or after delivery without evidence of toxemia, pulmonary emboli, rheumatic heart disease, or hypertension. An increased incidence of congestive cardiomyopathy is known to be associated with certain inherited neuromuscular disorders. On the other hand, patients with known risk factors — diabetes mellitus, arterial hypertension, and heavy cigarette smoking — are more likely to have arteriosclerotic heart disease than cardiomyopathy.

Physical Examination

Sinus tachycardia is the most frequent manifestation of cardiomyopathy. In the presence of acute infection, tachycardia out of proportion to the degree of fever has been regarded as an important clue to myocardial involvement. Cardiac enlargement is next in frequency to tachycardia and may be detected by palpation of a precordial impulse displaced laterally and inferiorly. However, early in the course or when restrictive fibrosis prevents dilatation of the heart, cardiomegaly may not be impressive. The precordial impulse may be sustained, nonsustained, or double; palpable gallops and pulmonary sounds may be found.

In the presence of tachycardia the first sound may be distant and muffled, and the heart tones may be indistinguishable and produce a rhythm of embryocardia. The diminished intensity of first sound in the presence of tachycardia should suggest cardiomyopathy, since most other conditions associated with tachycardia increase its intensity. The second heart sound may be accentuated and closely split with increasing degrees of pulmonary hypertension. This, in the absence of significant left ventricular failure, suggests pulmonary embolism. With right bundle branch block or right ventricular failure, the second sound may be widely split, and with left bundle branch block or left ventricular failure or both, paradoxical splitting can be auscultated.

A gallop rhythm is the hallmark of cardiomyopathy. In the early stages when loss of ventricular compliance is the main abnormality, an atrial gallop may be heard at the left ventricular apex or in the suprasternal notch. This is particularly common in hypertrophic cardiomyopathy in which there is marked stiffness of the ventricle. Later, when ventricular volumes increase, a diastolic gallop may become audible and is accentuated by overt failure. With rapid heart rates the presence of both atrial and diastolic gallops may produce a summation gallop or may simulate a rumbling diastolic murmur suggestive of mitral stenosis.

Patients with idiopathic hypertrophic subaortic stenosis have unique physical signs. The pulse rises rapidly and suggests aortic incompetence, but a search for a diastolic murmur is unrewarding. Instead, there is a systolic murmur loudest along the left lower sternal border and cardiac apex radiating to the base without transmission to the carotids. The murmur varies in intensity with various maneuvers that help distinguish this condition from aortic valvular stenosis and mitral regurgitation. Maneuvers that decrease the venous return to the heart — the Valsalva maneuver, sudden standing, and amyl nitrate inhalation — reduce the size of the ventricular cavity and increase the outflow tract obstruction and the intensity of the murmur. On the other hand, maneuvers that increase venous return, such as sudden squatting and leg raising in the supine position, increase the size of the ventricular cavity and reduce the outflow tract obstruction and the intensity of the murmur. Augmentation of contraction by postextrasystolic beats and isoproterenol administration will increase the outflow tract obstruction and enhance the murmur; an increase in peripheral resistance by isometric exercise and angiotensin administration reduces the outflow tract obstruction and diminishes the intensity of murmur.

A murmur of mitral regurgitation may be present owing to either malalignment of the papillary muscles as in hypertrophic cardiomyopathy or, more commonly, papillary muscle dysfunction or dilatation of mitral annulus or both owing to cardiomegaly as in congestive cardiomyopathy. The murmur of tricuspid regurgitation is less often heard, and it occurs late in the course of biventricular failure. At this time elevated jugular venous pressure with systolic pulsations can be observed. The liver enlarges and frequently pulsates, and signs of fluid retention manifested by peripheral edema, ascites, and pleural effusion are found. As the patient is treated, evidence of congestive failure disappears along with the atrioventricular valvular insufficiency; however, the gallop sounds usually persist unless the underlying cardiomyopathy regresses.

COURSE

The clinical course of cardiomyopathy varies depending on the cause. The majority of patients with viral myocarditis recover without residual abnormalities. If myocardial dysfunction persists long after the acute infection is over, the prognosis is poor. Abstinence from alcohol before marked cardiac dilatation occurs results in marked improvement with a return to good cardiac function, although a decrease in left ventricular compliance persists. A heart damaged by other causes is generally more sensitive to alcohol ingestion, which may precipitate congestive heart failure or malignant arrhythmias or both. Thiamine deficiency, beriberi, usually responds dramatically to replacement therapy. Cardiac function usually returns to normal after withdrawal of the toxins and drugs presumed to cause the cardiomyopathy. Nonetheless, permanent damage does occur if exposure is prolonged and significant irreversible damage has already been produced.

Peripartal cardiomyopathy has a variable course, depending on the duration of the disease. If the heart size returns to normal after 6 months, as happens in almost one third of patients, cardiac function returns to normal. Another third, although improved, have residual changes that prohibit subsequent pregnancy. The remaining third ultimately succumb to intractable congestive heart failure. Most infiltrative and metabolic cardiomyopathies and those associated with neuromuscular disorders are apparently unaffected by treatment and have a relentless downhill course.

The prognosis in hypertrophic cardiomyopathy seems to depend in part on the degree of outflow tract obstruction. Although complete beta-blocking doses of propranolol alleviate symptoms in most patients irrespective of the severity of subvalvular obstruction, no significant difference in mortality has been shown with this therapy. Patients with idiopathic hypertrophic subaortic stenosis do not tolerate atrial fibrillation, and onset of this arrhythmia may precipitate congestive heart failure. Diminution or loss of the outflow tract mumur in a patient with obstructive hypertrophic cardiomyopathy occurs with congestive heart failure; presumably, left ventricular dilatation and reduced myocardial contractility decrease the gradient across the left ventricular outflow tract and the intensity of the systolic murmur.

COMPLICATIONS

The most common complications of the cardiomyopathies are emboli, arrhythmias, and pulmonary hypertension.

Both pulmonary and arterial emboli have been common features of congestive cardiomyopathy. Arterial emboli to the brain, kidneys, and extremities originate from mural thrombi in the dilated left ventricle and left atrium. Factors that favor embolization are cardiac enlargement, congestive heart failure, and atrial fibrillation. Patients have been hospitalized and presumed to have had a cerebral vascular accident; in them, the diagnosis of cardiomyopathy was initially overlooked. With right heart failure, pulmonary embolism is common with thrombi originating in peripheral veins of the lower extremities.

Serious tachyarrhythmias and bradyarrhythmias are not common until late in the course of most cardiomyopathies; notable exceptions are myocarditis of viral and diphtheritic etiology, obstructive hypertrophic cardiomyopathy, and cardiomyopathy associated with neuromuscular disorders. Cardiomyopathy due to amyloid and sarcoid infiltration may involve the conduction system and lead to bradyarrhythmia. Ventricular preexcitation or the Wolff-Parkinson-White syndrome has been observed in 25 per cent of patients with idiopathic hypertrophic subaortic stenosis and may underlie recurrent tachyarrhythmias. Some patients with cardiomyopathy manifest an increased sensitivity to digitalis; this produces serious arrhythmias or conduction disturbances. Severe pulmonary hypertension may eventually develop in some patients with cardiomyopathy, and an erroneous diagnosis of primary pulmonary hypertension may be entertained. This complication is due to long-standing left ventricular failure or repeated subclinical pulmonary emboli or both.

LABORATORY FINDINGS

Electrocardiogram. The electrocardiogram is almost always abnormal. The most common finding is nonspecific ST-T changes. Left ventricular and left atrial enlargement is usual in both congestive and hypertrophic cardiomyopathy, although more marked in the latter. Right ventricular enlargement occurs late in the clinical course and follows recurrent pulmonary emboli. It almost always is accompanied by left ventricular enlargement.

In idiopathic hypertrophic subaortic stenosis, pathologic Q waves in leads II, III, aVF and the left precordium are a frequent finding produced by marked hypertrophy of the interventricular septum. Many patients with these are diagnosed incorrectly as having previous myocardial infarction. Q waves may also be seen in other varieties of cardiomyopathy owing to loss of cardiac muscle by fibrosis or infiltration. One fourth of patients with idiopathic hypertrophic subaortic stenosis have at least two of the three components of Wolff-Parkinson-White syndrome, viz., a short P-R interval, a delta wave, and QRS prolongation.

Atrial fibrillation is the most common arrhythmia observed with congestive cardiomyopathy, but atrial flutter, junctional rhythm, supraventricular tachycardia, and ventricular tachycardia have all been noted. Left bundle branch block is present in about 10 per cent of patients. Right bundle branch block is in general unusual, but more common than left bundle branch block in alcoholic cardiomyopathy.

Chest X-ray. About one half of patients with idiopathic hypertrophic subaortic stenosis demonstrate cardiac enlargement on x-ray examination; however, the size of the heart does not correlate with the degree of obstruction or disability. Aortic dilatation and aortic valve calcification are conspicuously absent. In congestive cardiomyopathy, the findings on x-ray films depend on the stage of disease. Cardiomegaly is usual, even in earlier stages, and redistribution of pulmonary blood flow with equalization in the upper and lower lung fields is seen. The main pulmonary arteries are enlarged and pulmonary infarction may be seen. Dilatation of all four chambers of the heart and pericardial effusion account for gross enlargement of cardiac silhouette in the later stages.

Echocardiography. Echocardiography is the most useful noninvasive technique for the diagnosis and characterization of idiopathic hypertrophic subaortic stenosis. The two principal echocardiographic findings are asymmetric septal hypertrophy, that is, an increase in the width of interventricular septum relative to the posterior free wall to more than 1.3 to 1, and abnormal systolic motion of anterior mitral valve leaflet. Less commonly found is the midsystolic closure of the aortic valve corresponding to the period of maximal obstruction of the left ventricular outflow tract.

The echocardiographic findings in congestive cardiomyopathies are ventricular dilatation, poor movement of a thin posterior left ventricular wall, and paradoxical motion of thin septum. These findings contrast with the infiltrative cardiomyopathies, in which the size of the left ventricular cavity is normal to small, and the septum and posterior wall are thickened. Reduced wall motion in restrictive cardiomyopathy helps to distinguish this entity from constrictive pericarditis, in which wall motion is normal. Lack of thickening of valve cusps and their normal mobility assists in the exclusion of valvular heart disease.

Blood. The underlying systemic disease in primary myocardial disorders may be reflected through changes in the immune systems. Complement level, rheumatoid factor, acute and convalescent viral and parasitic sera, and other serologic tests may all aid in diagnosis. Measurement of creatine phosphokinase (CPK), lactic dehydrogenase (LDH), and serum glutamic oxaloacetic transaminase (SGOT), particularly the cardiac fraction, may help identify myocardial involvement in systemic disease. Although a rise in cardiac enzyme is observed during active myocardial damage in neuromuscular disease, the cardiac fraction may not be distinguished from enzymes produced by skeletal muscle damage.

Radionuclide Studies. Gated radionuclide cardiac blood pool scanning is a noninvasive technique that can be used to assess cardiac chamber size, regional wall motion, and ejection fraction. It is helpful in following the course of disease and evaluating therapeutic interventions. In patients with idiopathic hypertrophic subaortic stenosis, a disproportionate upper septal thickening, cavity obliteration, and a filling defect in the region of the left ventricular outflow tract can be demonstrated, and this technique may prove to be a useful diagnostic adjunct to echocardiography in the noninvasive evaluation. Thallium 201 myocardial perfusion scans performed at the height of exercise are useful in detecting ischemic myocardial lesions, which are most often associated with significant coronary artery disease, a major differential in the diagnosis of cardiomyopathies.

Cardiac Catheterization. Coronary arteriography is the only absolute way to exclude the diagnosis of suspected coronary artery disease in a patient who is considered to have a cardiomyopathy. The hemodynamics in congestive cardiomyopathy are those of failure of the heart as a pump and lack any specific diagnostic value. The hemodynamic findings in idiopathic hypertrophic subaortic stenosis, however, are specific. The arterial pulse pressure rises rapidly and falls in mid systole followed by a second elevation, producing a spike and dome pattern. On withdrawal of the cardiac catheter from the left ventricle, the muscular obstruction can be localized to the subvalvular region. The gradient across the subaortic obstruction can be accentuated or diminished by various maneuvers and vasoactive substances. The Valsalva maneuver and amyl nitrate and isoproterenol administration increase the gradient, while methoxamine and phenylephrine reduce or abolish the gradient. On angiocardiography, the normal pear-shaped contour of the left ventricle is replaced by a diffusely enlarged and generally hypokinetic ventricle in congestive cardiomyopathy, whereas in idiopathic hypertrophic subaortic stenosis there is marked thickening of the ventricular wall with a small irregular cavity, frequently with complete obliteration during systole.

Myocardial Biopsy. Except for patients with suspected allograft rejection, amyloid, sarcoid, or hemachromatosis, endomyocardial biopsy with a cardiac biotome has proved to be of only limited value. In general, the yield has been poor and risk of complications significant. Rarely, open myocardial biopsy may be performed if a definitive diagnosis is necessary to treat a patient.

Pitfalls in Diagnosis. The correct diagnosis of cardiomyopathy depends largely on the clinician's awareness of the various disorders and their characteristic findings. Nonetheless, a cardiomyopathy is easily confused with other forms of heart disease. Clearly, cardiomyopathy is a diagnosis of exclusion, and in any given case, hypertensive heart disease, coronary artery disease, and rheumatic heart disease must always be excluded.

In men over the age of 40 years, diagnosing cardiomyopathy as coronary artery disease has been the most common error. Some patients with cardiomyopathy have angina-like chest discomfort, but it is usually atypical and almost always accompanies significant congestive heart failure. The electrocardiogram may mimic old infarction without clinical evidence of prior myocardial infarction. The occurrence of typical angina in the absence of congestive heart failure or findings of obstructive cardiomyopathy and in the presence of risk factors for coronary atherosclerosis strongly favors the diagnosis of coronary artery disease. On clinical evaluation the correct diagnosis can be reached in 90 per cent of patients, but a definite diagnosis requires coronary arteriography and should be performed, since its results may lead one to significantly alter management.

In idiopathic hypertrophic subaortic stenosis, the clinical presentation of a patient with angina, syncope, and congestive heart failure may be confused with aortic stenosis. The variation of intensity of the systolic murmur with various maneuvers in idiopathic hypertrophic subaortic stenosis versus the delayed pulse, soft aortic sound, calcified aortic valve, and poststenotic dilatation of the aorta in aortic stenosis are characteristic findings allowing a clinical distinction that can be confirmed by echocardiography.

In severe congestive heart failure, a markedly enlarged heart associated with pulsus paradoxus can be confused with cardiac tamponade. Echocardiography can be used to identify pericardial effusion and make the correct diagnosis. Normal myocardial contractility demonstrated by echocardiography, nuclear studies, and angiocardiography in constrictive pericarditis helps to distinguish this from restrictive cardiomyopathy, in which myocardial contractility is diminished. However, pericarditis may progress to constriction and have considerable myocardial involvement that makes distinction very difficult. Surgical exploration may be necessary to make the diagnosis.

INFECTIVE ENDOCARDITIS

By O. M. KORZENIOWSKI, M.D.,
and M. A. SANDE, M.D.
Charlottesville, Virginia

SYNONYMS

Subacute bacterial endocarditis, acute bacterial endocarditis, infectious endocarditis.

DEFINITION

Infective endocarditis is an infection involving the endocardium. This usually occurs on the cardiac valves but occasionally involves a septal defect, a mural thrombus, or the aortic endothelium distal to a coarctation. The disease was historically classified as acute or subacute on the basis of the infecting organism and the usual progress of untreated disease.

The acute form of endocarditis killed the patient in days or weeks and was usually caused by coagulase-positive staphylococci, *Streptococcus pneumoniae, Neisseria gonorrhoeae,* or group A beta-hemolytic streptococci. The cardiac valves were often reported normal before infection but once endocarditis occurred, rapid and severe value destruction was frequent. Subacute bacterial endocarditis typically occurred on a deformed heart valve or congenital cardiac lesion, slowly produced additional valvular damage, and was caused by a streptococcus (most commonly either a viridans streptococcus or an enterococcus). It usually led to death in 6 weeks to 3 months.

The relationships between course, type of infecting organism and underlying heart disease have changed in the last 3 decades. A number of factors may have contributed to this change. First, there has been a decreasing incidence of rheumatic heart disease (37 to 76 per cent of patients with endocarditis) and an increasing prevalence and identification of degenerative heart disease (30 per cent of patients with endocarditis), while patients with congenital, rheumatic, and arteriosclerotic heart disease now survive longer (over 50 per cent of patients with endocarditis are now > 35 years of age).

The widespread use of antimicrobial agents has not only changed the mortality of this disease but also probably affected the causative organism. Advances in medical sciences leading to cardiac surgery, intravenous hyperalimentation and indwelling intravenous catheters, and a popularization of parenteral drug use ("mainlining") by substantial segments of the young populations have introduced new forms of the disease with a markedly altered clinical course. Patients now less frequently give a history of prolonged illness when first seen, many have infected prosthetic valves, and the infecting organisms now include unusual bacteria (gram-negative bacilli, diphtheroids) and microorganisms other than bacteria (e.g., fungi such as Candida).

Presenting Signs and Symptoms

Infective endocarditis accounts for 0.15 to 5.4 patients per 1000 hospital admissions in the United States. There is consistently a preponderance of male over female patients (1.7:1). Fifty-four per cent of patients are between the ages of 31 and 60.

The presenting complaints are typically nonspecific. Daily fever occurring primarily at night is the most common presenting symptom. Fever may not be present in the elderly, in patients who have received prior antibiotic therapy, and in patients with renal failure, severe congestive heart failure, and with terminal illnesses owing to other causes.

An organic heart murmur is present in the majority of patients with endocarditis but may be absent in 10 to 20 per cent. It is most common in those who have had a longer course of infection. Patients with an acute onset of disease may not as yet have developed sufficient valvular destruction to produce hemodynamic changes. Thus, the development of a new or changing murmur (10 to 15 per cent of cases), especially a regurgitant murmur, is particularly ominous as it implies functional valvular disturbance by large vegetations or valve rupture.

Approximately one half of patients also complain of chills, weakness, and dyspnea. Dyspnea may be due to pulmonary emboli in addicts or to congestive heart failure resulting from insufficient aortic or mitral valves. Night sweats, anorexia, weight loss, malaise, and cough occur in one fourth of all patients with endocarditis. Cough and hemoptysis are frequently (75 per cent) the presenting complaints in drug addicts with pulmonary emboli from infected tricuspid valves. Cerebral emboli resulting in a stroke have been reported to occur in up to 20 per cent of patients and are most common in patients with prosthetic valve endocarditis. Other potential central nervous system presentations include delirium or coma caused by ruptured mycotic aneurysms, meningitis, cerebritis (especially in staphylococcal endocarditis), or intracranial abscesses.

Course

Untreated infective endocarditis is almost uniformly fatal. In the preantibiotic era, survival was about 1 per cent, with uncontrolled infection accounting for 64 per cent of the deaths. At the present time, survival in patients with natural valve infections is influenced by age, duration of infection before diagnosis, antibiotic selection, and the nature of the infecting organism. Institution of appropriate antibiotic therapy results in a feeling of well-being and a reduction in the fever after several days to a week of treatment, depending on the organism. Blood cultures become sterile in 2 to 5 days. However, although the clinical response is rapid, it takes a much longer time to sterilize the infected vegetations. Thus, in order to achieve a bacteriologic cure and prevent relapse, treatment of infective endocarditis usually requires

2 to 6 weeks. Organisms such as streptococci of the viridans group that are highly susceptible to antibiotics are eradicated in 2 to 4 weeks of treatment. The bacteriologic cure rate approaches 100 per cent. Enterococci, *Staphylococcus aureus, Staphylococcus epidermidis* and gram-negative bacilli generally require 4 to 6 weeks of treatment for cure. Prosthetic valve or fungal endocarditis, in general, has an extremely low cure rate with medical therapy alone and usually requires surgical intervention with replacement of the infected valve.

Despite the fact that the bacterial infection can be cured, mortality from bacterial endocarditis still ranges from 30 to 35 per cent and has remained unchanged from the early antibiotic era. Congestive heart failure (47 to 55 per cent of patients) or emboli to vital organs (cerebral emboli 30 to 35 per cent) are the major causes of death. Death may also result from rupture of a mycotic aneurysm or renal failure.

PHYSICAL EXAMINATION FINDINGS

Fever is present in more than 90 per cent of patients with endocarditis. It is usually low grade 38.3 to 38.8 C (101–102 F) and remittent with nightly spikes. Temperature elevations in excess of 39.4 C (103 F) *rarely* occur and suggest acute staphylococcal disease. The administration of antipyretic agents or subtherapeutic antibiotics may alter the curve and produce an intermittent fever pattern.

Cutaneous Signs. Petechiae, found in 20 to 40 per cent of endocarditis patients, are found on the conjunctivae, palate, buccal mucosa, and extremities. These red, nonblanching lesions, which become brown and barely visible within several days, are caused by extravasation of blood from superficial capillaries injured by the vasculitis, which may be associated with endocarditis. Splinter hemorrhages are linear, dark-red streaks beneath the finger or toe nails. Both petechiae and splinter hemorrhages may result from local trauma (e.g., poorly-fitting dentures). Osler's nodes are probably manifestations of an acute vasculitic process and are firm, raised, painful intracutaneous lesions found on the pads of fingers and toes. They range from 2 to 15 mm in diameter and have a reddish-purple cast with frequently a white center or they may be invisible. Janeway's lesions are macular, hemorrhagic, nontender areas found on the palms and soles. They are probably embolic and occasionally organisms have been cultured from them. Clubbed fingers may be present in patients with long-standing endocarditis.

Eye Findings. Roth's spots, oval, pale, retinal lesions surrounded by an area of hemorrhage, are usually located near the optic disc. They are seen in less than 5 per cent of patients with endocarditis and may also occur in patients with hematologic and collagen vascular diseases. Retinal artery emboli are uncommon. Panophthalmitis may occasionally be seen in pneumococcal or staphylococcal endocarditis.

Cardiac Findings. A changing heart murmur has been regarded as a characteristic and major diagnostic feature of endocarditis but occurs in only 5 to 10 per cent of patients. Changing murmurs are most frequently associated with a fulminant endocarditis such as that produced by staphylococcus. Organic heart murmurs (aortic and mitral) are commonly (80 to 90 per cent) present in patients with endocarditis and reflect the high incidence of underlying cardiac valve lesions in patients who acquire the disease. Murmurs are more likely to be absent in intravenous drug users. When present (one third of patients) or if it develops during the course of the disease, the murmur is commonly that of tricuspid regurgitation and may be accompanied by distended neck veins and hepatomegaly. Insufficiency murmurs of paraprosthetic leaks in patients with prosthetic valves are common manifestations of valve dehiscence resulting from infection.

Pulmonary Findings. Pulmonary emboli with infarction are common in patients with endocarditis involving the right side of the heart, while congestive heart failure is particularly common in patients with aortic valve endocarditis.

Abdominal Findings. Enlargement of the spleen has been noted in 25 to 60 per cent of patients with endocarditis and is most common in patients with disease of long duration. Left upper quadrant pain with a splenic friction rub or a left pleural effusion are associated with embolic infarction of the spleen. Flank tenderness may be caused by renal infarction. Abscesses may occur in any organ.

Central Nervous System Findings. Hemiplegia, cortisensory losses, aphasia, or ataxia may be present in patients with major cerebral artery emboli. Mental confusion, meningismus, or coma may result from ruptured mycotic aneurysms, toxic encephalopathy, cerebritis, or meningitis.

COMMON COMPLICATIONS

Complications of endocarditis may be cardiac or extracardiac. Congestive heart failure (CHF) is the most common cause of morbidity and mortality. It usually results from valve destruction by infection, rupture of supporting structures such as chordae tendineae or papillary muscles, or by valve obstruction by large vegetations. The development of CHF, especially in patients with aortic insufficiency, requires prompt surgical intervention. Recognition of myocardial infarction, which may be produced by embolic occlusion, thrombosis, or mycotic aneurysm, is more frequent now. Involvement of the myocardium or valve ring by microabscesses may result in arrhythmias or heart block. Pericarditis is rare except in staphylococcal or pneumococcal infections.

Extracardiac complications of endocarditis include peripheral emboli, which may be noninfectious or suppurative. Large emboli are most common with fungal endocarditis. Emboli from lesions on the left side of the heart distribute themselves randomly throughout the systemic circulation and may involve the brain, kidney, spleen, skin, and limb arterial supply. In lesions involving the right side of the heart, pulmonary emboli are dominant.

Rupture of a cerebral mycotic aneurysm or a cerebral abscess is usually a catastrophic terminal event.

Diffuse vasculitis resulting from circulating immune complexes may involve the central nervous system, myocardium, renal glomerulus, and skin.

Metastatic abscess may lead to meningitis, brain abscess formation, osteomyelitis, septic arthritis or abscess involving the liver, spleen, and kidney.

Besides complications related to the infection itself, complications produced by prolonged antibiotic administration are also encountered. Long-term administration of high doses of penicillin for endocarditis results in colonization by penicillin-resistant bacteria and fungi, which may then produce superinfections. Seizure activity may be induced by the high doses of penicillin used in the treatment of streptococcal endocarditis, especially in patients with diminished renal function in whom toxic penicillin serum concentrations can accumulate. Rashes, fever, and hemolytic anemia may be induced by the penicillins and cephalosporins. Neutropenia is commonly observed in patients receiving long-term penicillin and cephalosporin derivatives. Renal toxicity is common and includes interstitial nephritis caused by penicillin derivatives and azotemia caused by aminoglycosides alone or in combination with vancomycin and cephalosporins. The frequency of ototoxicity varies with the type of aminoglycoside administered.

LABORATORY FINDINGS

The single most important finding in patients with endocarditis is persistent bacteremia or fungemia. In patients with endocarditis, if any blood cultures are positive, nearly all the blood cultures drawn will be positive. The incidence of blood-culture negative endocarditis is probably less than 10 per cent in all patients. Negative blood cultures result usually because the patient has had previous antibiotic treatment or because the infecting organism displays fastidious culture requirements such as an anaerobic environment, prolonged incubation (diphtheroids), or supplementation of standard blood culture media. In fungal endocarditis other than that caused by Candida (i.e., Aspergillus or Histoplasma), blood cultures are rarely positive. Diagnosis of fungal endocarditis should be attempted by staining and culturing emboli surgically removed from peripheral vessels. Intraleukocytic bacteria may occasionally be seen on Giemsa-stained leukocyte monolayers prepared from leukocyte concentrates of venous blood.

Hematologic manifestations of infective endocarditis usually include a normocytic, normochronic anemia of chronic disease that responds to therapy for the underlying disease. Rarely, acute hemolytic anemia may be present. Impact hemolytic anemia is associated with malfunctioning prosthetic heart valves in patients with endocarditis. Thrombocytopenia may result from entrapment of platelets in enlarged spleens of some patients with endocarditis or rarely as a result of disseminated intravascular coagulation. The usual white blood cell count in patients with a subacute form of infective endocarditis is within normal range, although the differential may show a shift to the left. The exceptions are patients with a staphylococcal, pneumococcal, or gonococcal endocarditis who generally present with a leukocytosis of 15,000 to 25,000 per cu mm. The sedimentation rate is usually elevated and resolves with therapy. Histiocytic cells have been seen in the first drop of blood obtained from the ear lobe in 25 per cent of patients with endocarditis.

Urinary abnormalities are frequently seen and include hematuria, proteinuria, red blood cell casts, or white blood cell casts. The most common findings are proteinuria with microscopic hematuria (30 to 60 per cent of patients). The blood urea nitrogen (BUN) or serum creatinine may also be elevated. Such abnormalities can result from either sterile or septic emboli and/or glomerulonephritis. Occasionally, significant bacteriuria ($> 10^5$ organisms per ml) may be present in patients with enterococcal or staphylococcal endocarditis.

Although the cerebrospinal fluid (CSF) is typically sterile, the CSF findings of patients with staphylococcal endocarditis commonly include pleocytosis, increased protein concentrations, and normal sugar levels. Acute purulent meningitis with positive cultures occurs occasionally with pneumococcal endocarditis.

Serologic studies are helpful but not absolutely diagnostic in infective endocarditis. A positive rheumatoid factor is present in 50 per cent of patients with endocarditis of at least 6 weeks' duration. A reduction in titer may be helpful in monitoring response to treatment. Serum complement may be low, especially in those patients with acute glomerulonephritis associated with endocarditis. Circulating cryoglobulins have been reported. Circulating immune complexes can be detected in the serum by means of the Raji cell assay in many patients with bacterial endocarditis, especially those with manifestations of vasculitis. Detection of specific antibodies to teichoic acids present in the walls of staphylococci (coagulase positive) may be particularly useful in the diagnosis of *S. aureus* endocarditis, especially in those patients with negative blood cultures resulting from previous antibiotic treatment. A reduction in the serum titer of teichoic acid antibody occurs with successful treatment and relapse is associated with a rapid reappearance or rise.

Echocardiography, especially two-dimensional echocardiography, has been successfully used in the detection of vegetations on aortic, mitral, and tricuspid valves of patients with bacterial, fungal, and culture negative endocarditis. Vegetations of ≥ 2 mm can be detected. Echocardiography can also be helpful in ascertaining significant valvular insufficiency before the development of frank congestive heart failure. It may be useful in monitoring resolution of valvular vegetations with successful therapy.

Recently, experimental studies have indicated the potential future usefulness of scintigraphic detection of radiolabeled platelets deposited on valvular vegetations.

Therapeutic Tests

It is important to determine the exact antibiotic sensitivities of organisms causing endocarditis. Quantitative results may be obtained with broth dilution sensitivity tests and are an aid in the selection of the most effective antibiotic for eradication of each organism. For example, demonstration of a high degree of sensitivity to penicillin (inhibitory concentration of < 0.1 microgram per ml) by staphylococci or streptococci of the viridans group allows their successful treatment with penicillin without fear of the development of resistance.

Tests for synergism of antibiotic combinations are helpful in choosing optimal antibiotic treatment in endocarditis caused by unusual organisms. Assays for synergism of penicillin with streptomycin or gentamicin should also be performed in enterococcal endocarditis because of the appearance of resistance of 10 to 40 per cent of all recent enterococcal isolates to the penicillin-streptomycin combination.

Adequacy of therapy can be monitored by means of serum bactericidal levels. Clinical experience suggests that patients whose serum at the antibiotic peak (1 hour after administration of antibiotic) kills the causative organism in at least a 1:8 dilution are probably receiving adequate antibiotic therapy. Weekly serum assays for antibiotic concentration are important to monitor the maintenance of a therapeutic level and to monitor the potential development of toxicity in patients receiving aminoglycosides.

Pitfalls in Diagnosis

Failure to diagnose endocarditis most commonly is due to failure to consider the diagnosis. If blood cultures are obtained before the administration of antibiotics to febrile patients with a poorly defined focus of infection, endocarditis will rarely be missed. Furthermore, the diagnosis of endocarditis *must be considered* in febrile patients with underlying congenital, rheumatic, or degenerative valvular disease and in young patients with unexplained cerebrovascular accidents or in febrile users of parenteral drugs, even in the absence of a heart murmur.

The high incidence of valvular involvement in patients with pyogenic infections caused by staphylococci, gonococci, or pneumococci demands careful observation of patients presenting with bacteremia caused by these organisms. Any signs of endocarditis are indications for both an increased dose of antibiotics and a longer duration of treatment. Similarly, pyogenic bacteremias (especially *S. aureus*) occurring in patients with central intravenous catheters or arteriovenous shunts may result in the seeding of cardiac valves or other intravascular sites. The commonly accepted short-course antibiotic treatment (10 to 14 days) for such bacteremias may be inadequate for eradicating these foci of infection. Endocarditis should also be considered in all febrile patients with prosthetic valves and in those who demonstrate increased intravascular hemolysis or valvular dysfunction due to obstruction or paraprosthetic leaks.

ANEURYSMS OF THE AORTA

By R. CLEMENT DARLING, M.D.,
DAVID C. BREWSTER, M.D.,
and JOHN W. HALLETT, Jr., M.D.

Boston, Massachusetts

Aneurysms of the aorta remain one of the most life-threatening forms of cardiovascular disease. Surgical advances over the past 25 years now allow successful treatment with low morbidity and low mortality in elective cases in most instances. This is often the primary result of early recognition and diagnosis before the development of complications.

CLASSIFICATION AND DEFINITION

An aneurysm may be defined as a permanent, usually localized dilatation of an artery. *True* aneurysms involve all three layers of the arterial wall and generally result from a degenerative process involving the elastic and muscular components of the medial layer. Most true aneurysms are acquired as a result of arteriosclerosis, although other degenerative diseases such as syphilis, cystic medial necrosis, or infection may be involved. *False,* or pseudoaneurysms, in contrast, have an outer wall composed only of adventitia or perivascular tissues. They are usually the result of an aortic dissection, trauma, or disruption of an arterial anastomosis. *Dissecting* aortic aneurysms, frequently associated with cystic medial necrosis or hypertension, result from an intimal tear in the thoracic aorta with extravasation of blood into the medial layer. An intramural hematoma forms and arterial pressure causes antegrade or retrograde propagation for varying distances.

Aneurysms may also be classified by anatomic location. *Thoracic* aortic aneurysms are limited to the chest cavity and account for approximately 25 per cent of aortic aneurysms. They may involve the ascending thoracic aorta, aortic arch, or descending thoracic aorta. If the aneurysmal process extends below the diaphragm a *thoracoabdominal* aneurysm results, usually involving the origin of the celiac axis, superior mesenteric or renal arteries. *Abdominal* aortic aneurysms comprise nearly 75 per cent of all aneurysms of the aorta and are located in an infrarenal location in about 95 per cent of cases.

CLINICAL PRESENTATION

In this country most aortic aneurysms are now discovered while asymptomatic. The patient may notice a pulsatile mass himself, or the doctor may palpate an aneurysm during a routine physical examination. More widespread use of chest x-rays and various abdominal radiologic procedures has also led to a more frequent diagnosis of aortic aneurysms that are detected by the characteristic calcification in the aortic wall.

The most common symptom of a thoracic aneurysm is deep, diffuse, aching chest or upper back pain. Large thoracic aneurysms can also compress mediastinal structures such as the recurrent laryngeal nerve, tracheobronchial tree, lung, esophagus, or vena cava, and cause possible hoarseness, cough, hemoptysis, dysphagia or a superior vena cava syndrome.

Dissecting aortic aneurysms tend to have an acute onset, marked by a sudden episode of severe pain in the anterior chest or infrascapular region, which may progress downward into the lumbar region. The dissection may compromise the origin of the major aortic branches, producing possible manifestations of cerebrovascular insufficiency, acute arterial insufficiency of an upper or lower extremity, or possible intra-abdominal or renal ischemia if these vessels are involved. If retrograde dissection occurs, acute aortic valvular insufficiency may result or acute myocardial infarction may occur if coronary artery origins are compromised.

Asymptomatic abdominal aortic aneurysms are usually detected by the presence of a pulsatile epigastric mass or on incidental abdominal x-rays. With expansion, pressure on vertebral bodies and paravertebral sensory nerves may produce characteristic low back pain, unrelated to activity and usually located in the mid and lower lumbar region. The abdominal pain that may occur may mimic that of renal colic or diverticulitis. Ruptured aneurysms present with a characteristic triad of severe back or abdominal pain, hypotension, and a tender pulsatile abdominal mass.

NATURAL HISTORY

Aneurysms of the aorta generally form and progressively expand over a period of years. The natural history of aneurysms of the aorta terminates in rupture unless the death of the patient occurs from other causes. The rate of expansion, however, is often unpredictable, with some aneurysms remaining stable in size for long periods of time, while others undergo sudden enlargement and rupture.

Many aortic aneurysms may remain asymptomatic for long periods. Symptoms, when present, are usually due to expansion and compression of adjacent structures. Occasionally, peripheral arterial emboli may result from atheromatous debris shed from the lining of such aneurysms. Rarely, an aortic aneurysm may thrombose, particularly when associated with arteriosclerotic occlusive disease distal to the aneurysm.

Rupture of the aneurysm, whether in the abdomen or the chest, is a common complication and may be the first sign of the disease process. Rupture occurs most commonly in the retroperitoneum, where temporary tamponade of hemorrhage may occur. Rupture anteriorly of an abdominal aneurysm into the free peritoneal cavity is less common and more often fatal. Less commonly, rupture may occur into the adjacent duodenum or inferior vena cava, resulting in an aortoenteric fistula and gastrointestinal bleeding or an aortocaval arteriovenous fistula, both of which produce unusual findings associated with abdominal aortic aneurysms.

Most authorities agree that the likelihood of rupture is determined primarily by aneurysmal size, particularly in the abdomen. A large aneurysm over 7 cm is clearly at greater risk of rupture than a smaller aneurysm. In our experience, however, little difference in the rate of rupture exists for aneurysms between 4 and 7 cm in size; therefore, there is no "critical" size for an aneurysm for which the risk of rupture can be considered negligible. Once the aneurysm, particularly in the abdomen, increases above 10 cm in size, the vast majority of patients, regardless of their associated medical history, die from rupture of the aneurysm.

DIAGNOSIS

Diagnosis of aneurysms of the thoracic aorta depends mainly on radiologic tests, since physical examination is often unrevealing. Chest x-rays, often with oblique views, and chest fluoroscopy usually demonstrate the presence of a thoracic aneurysm, usually by revealing a mass contiguous with part of the aortic shadow. With fluoroscopy this may be seen to pulsate in some instances. Displacement of the trachea or esophagus may be evident. Direct contrast aortography delineates the problem more accurately and should eliminate possible diagnostic errors based on the less invasive radiologic tests. Ultrasonography of the thoracic aorta has generally been unsuccessful because the surrounding lung transmits sounds poorly. The place of computerized axial tomography (CT scan) in the diagnostic work-up of aortic aneurysmal disease is not yet well defined.

Dissecting aortic aneurysms may be diagnosed frequently by characteristic history and physical examination, including a difference in arm pressures, a murmur of aortic regurgitation, or abnormalities of carotid and other peripheral pulses. A chest x-ray will often reveal a widened mediastinum and perhaps obliteration of the aortic knob or a double density aortic contour. Again, definitive diagnosis is made by contrast aortography, which should reveal a double aortic channel and perhaps the actual site of origin of an intimal tear.

Abdominal aortic aneurysms may be diagnosed by a variety of techniques. An experienced examiner may make an accurate diagnosis in most instances by findings of a pulsatile and laterally expansile abdominal mass. In approximately 10 per cent of patients, the aneurysm may not be palpated reliably owing to obesity, or other abdominal masses may be present with transmitted pulsations. In addition, a tortuous aorta in a thin patient may give a mistaken impression of an abdominal aortic aneurysm. This is often associated with a lumbar lordosis in the middle-aged woman. Physical examination is often variable and somewhat unreliable in accurate estimation of true aneurysmal size.

A lateral lumbosacral spine x-ray taken using bone technique remains perhaps the most reliable, easily obtained, and relatively inexpensive diagnostic test. Characteristic curvilinear calcification sufficient to allow diagnosis and accurate measurement of aneurysm size is present in about 75 per cent of patients.

Aortic ultrasound examination is a safe, noninvasive method that is now widely available. This is an accurate diagnostic test that is applicable to all patients, unless the aorta is obscured by intestinal gas at the time of examination. Advances in ultrasonography, particularly in the use of the gray-scale devices, now allows rather accurate measurement of aortic size if such an examination is obtained by experienced personnel. Such an examination should be obtained if the lateral lumbar spine film is nondiagnostic but need not be necessarily used in all patients because of its greater expense.

Aortography has little place in the diagnosis of an abdominal aortic aneurysm. The opacified lumen of the aneurysm may be near normal because of the frequent presence of intramural thrombus. Aortography alone is notoriously inaccurate in determining aneurysm size. We believe, as do other authorities, that the use of aortography before operation for abdominal aortic aneurysms is particularly helpful. The presence of accessory renal arteries, mesenteric and celiac artery occlusive disease, and associated aneurysms of the iliac, femoral or popliteal region can be ruled out. The procedure, however, is useful basically for providing anatomic information rather than for diagnosis.

PITFALLS IN DIAGNOSIS

Thoracic aneurysms, usually presenting as radiologic abnormalities, may be confused with other mass lesions of the lungs or mediastinum. The differential diagnosis can usually be made with certainty by angiography.

Acute dissecting thoracic aortic aneurysms may be difficult to differentiate by clinical and historical means from acute myocardial infarction or pulmonary emboli. The finding of pulse abnormalities or aortic insufficiency may help differentiate between the three common causes of spontaneous severe chest pain. Only a skilled angiographer can establish the diagnosis of a dissecting aortic aneurysm. Suspicion of the diagnosis in any patient with acute chest or upper back pain, particularly if he is hypertensive, is of paramount importance.

Other abdominal masses with transmitted pulsations, such as gastrointestinal or pancreatic malignancies, retroperitoneal lymphoma or abscess, pseudocyst or lymphadenopathy, may cause confusion with diagnosis of abdominal aortic aneurysm based only on physical examination. Properly performed lateral lumbosacral spine x-rays or ultrasound examination or both should eliminate such errors and indicate the direction for further evaluation.

CHRONIC ARTERIAL OCCLUSIVE DISEASE OF THE LOWER EXTREMITY

By HENRY HAIMOVICI, M.D.
New York, New York

Atherosclerosis is the most common cause of chronic arterial disease of the lower extremities, in contrast to thromboangiitis obliterans (Buerger's disease), which is by far a much rarer entity.

THROMBOANGIITIS OBLITERANS (TAO)

Until about 1950 this entity was diagnosed fairly often. Thereafter its incidence decreased dramatically. Based on recent data, an eightfold decline in its rate over the past 25 years has been estimated. The reason for this decline is rather obscure. The age at clinical onset of the disease is known to be between 20 and 35 years. Ninety per cent of cases occur in men and only 10 per cent in women.

TAO involves the lower extremities more commonly and usually more severely than it does the upper. It begins in medium-sized or small arteries. The lesions are distinctly segmental and follow an episodal course. Larger arteries (popliteal, femoral, or brachial) may also be affected if the disease is severe and progressive. In the major arteries (aorta, iliac) the distinctive lesions of TAO have never been reported.

Migrating thrombophlebitis, in contrast to atherosclerosis, is often the presenting feature in many patients and is considered to be a specific component of TAO. The course of TAO is characterized by periods of remission and relapse directly attributable to cigarette smoking. Relationship between recurrence of the disease and its progression with resumption of tobacco smoking is quite striking. Arteriography may reveal features considered specific of TAO, of which the most significant is the smooth outline of the arterial tree, in contrast to intimal irregularities so characteristic of atheromatous lesions. While these arteriographic signs may be important in the differential diagnosis, they are not pathognomonic. Noninvasive methods for evaluating the hemodynamics in TAO are important and are described later (see Atherosclerosis).

The vascular lesions of TAO are those of an inflammatory process. Their histopathology has been, and still is, the subject of much controversy. This may be partially due to the relatively wide spectrum of lesions, ranging from the acute stage to the healed thrombus. Absence of both intimal atheromatous plaques and medial calcification is an important negative finding necessary to rule out atherosclerosis. A definitive diagnosis may sometimes require a biopsy of an occluded vessel or examination of specimens obtained at amputation or at autopsy.

In brief, TAO is a rare entity but distinct from arteriosclerosis (ASO). It begins at an earlier age than does ASO. Thrombophlebitis may precede the appearance of calf claudication and the upper extremities are often involved. Ulcerations and gangrenous changes of toes and fingers are due to involvement of the small arteries and are the source of severe to excruciating pain. Complete abstinence from tobacco smoking and local management of lesions may limit tissue loss. Lumbar or thoracic sympathectomy or reconstructive surgery may be indicated in selected patients. Otherwise, staged amputations are the alternative.

ATHEROSCLEROSIS

The pathogenesis of atherosclerosis, despite recent progress, is not entirely elucidated. In its simplest definition, atherosclerosis, a degenerative process, is characterized by lipid deposition in the tissue layer that lines the arteries and by focal fibromuscular proliferation.

STRUCTURAL FEATURES

The atherosclerotic process may be divided into three major stages. (1) The *asymptomatic* stage is represented early by fatty streaks and later by fibrous plaques. The *fatty streaks* appear soon after birth. Lipids are found in the intima, some of it being in macrophages, as foam cells or intimal smooth muscle cells. *Fibrous* plaques appear later on, increasing slowly between the second and fourth decades. (2) The *potentially symptomatic* stage is characterized by lesions in which secondary changes such as calcification, hemorrhage, and ulceration occur. (3) In the *symptomatic* stage, due to complicated lesions, the changes just described result in marked occlusion of the vessel. The chronologic relationship between these three stages is still uncertain. However, a great deal of evidence indicates that this process begins in childhood and does not become apparent until middle or late age. At an advanced stage, the endothelial lining is disrupted, leading to a thrombotic occlusion at the site of the atheromatous plaque.

ATHEROGENIC MECHANISMS

The most important of the atherogenic risk factors are metabolic, chemical, physical, biological, and mechanical. Of these, the origin of lipids and their role in atherogenesis have received the greatest attention from biologists and clinicians alike. It is well known that arterial lesions cannot generally be produced experimentally without an increased intake of cholesterol and fat. Recent biochemical studies of blood lipoproteins in humans are of considerable interest. There are four main types of lipoproteins, which are classified according to their size and density: (1) chylomicrons, (2) very low density lipoproteins (VLDL), (3) low-density lipoproteins (LDL), and (4) high density lipoproteins (HDL). Of these four main types it is currently accepted that LDL may play the

most important role in atherogenesis. It is generally accepted that most lipids enter the arterial wall in a lipoprotein vehicle by crossing the endothelial barrier. The major components of the lipid composition of the atheromatous lesions derive from the circulating cholesterol and other lipids, particularly in the form of LDL. Clinically, the determination of HDL seems to be an important index of the risk factors concerned with cholesterol. An increased HDL is indicative of a negative risk factor for coronary atherosclerosis as well as for peripheral. This lipoprotein fraction has been found to be consistently higher in animal species resistant to atherosclerosis. The reason for the protective effect of HDL in humans is not known.

Other factors important in atherogenesis are arterial hypertension and diabetes mellitus, the latter representing a most serious prognostic feature.

DISTRIBUTION OF ATHEROSCLEROTIC LESIONS

The atherosclerotic process usually involves somatic and visceral arteries in various degrees. Knowledge of the relative incidence of distribution of arterial lesions is largely lacking. Most studies have focused attention either on the peripheral arterial tree or individual visceral arteries. In general, it is recognized that the pathologic features of atherosclerosis are quite variable from individual to individual and from one arterial segment to another. As a result, the patterns emerging from the innumerable combination of lesions are varied and complex. However, in terms of location and extent of the atherosclerotic process, in the lower extremity it is possible to identify a certain number of regional patterns that lend themselves into an overall classification of three major groups: (1) aortoiliac, (2) femoropopliteal, and (3) tibioperoneal-pedal.

1. Aortoiliac Arteriosclerotic Occlusive Disease. The atherosclerotic process of the aortoiliac segment may begin at the bifurcation or most frequently in one or both common iliac arteries. The development of these lesions is slow, insidious, and progressive. From a clinical pathologic standpoint it may be emphasized that this syndrome ("Leriche's syndrome") may go through two distinct phases — stenotic and occlusive. The reported incidence of these two phases varies with published statistical studies. The degree of stenosis and occlusion of the infrarenal abdominal aorta and that of the iliac arteries is also variable. The variability of these anatomical features is translated into a great number of patterns that in turn determine the clinical manifestations, prognosis, and management. The degree of ischemia is further complicated by the often associated atherosclerotic stenosis or occlusion of the femoral-popliteal or tibioperoneal vessels.

Collateral circulation in aortoiliac occlusive disease varies according to whether the lesions are confined to this segment or are combined with lesions below the inguinal ligament.

The intermittent claudication in this group is characterized by pain affecting primarily the thigh or back musculature. In combined lesions the dominant pain is mostly in the calf and much less above. Some degree of atrophy of the lower extremities is present, which may be symmetrical or asymmetrical depending on the degree of arterial involvement. Femoral pulses may be diminished in stenotic arterial lesions but are absent in complete and extensive occlusions. Audible bruits may be heard over the distal iliac or femoral vessels.

Evaluation of these lesions, in addition to the physical examination, is achieved by the noninvasive Doppler methods as mentioned later. If surgery is contemplated, translumbar or transfemoral aortography and arteriography are essential.

Indications for arterial reconstruction depend on the severity of the intermittent claudication or the nonhealing of ulcers or gangrenous changes of the toes. Although aortoiliac occlusive disease confined to this segment may go on for years before serious ischemic manifestations occur, in the combined patterns with distal occlusive disease the process is progressive and usually requires reconstruction, mostly of the proximal arterial tree, for adequate revascularization of the lower extremities.

2. Femoral-Popliteal Arteriosclerotic Occlusive Disease. The occlusive process of the femoral-popliteal segment is the commonest lesion of the lower extremity, especially in patients over 60. It has been estimated that, of the 73,000 reconstructions of major arteries performed in the United States every year, more than 20,000 (over 27 per cent of the total) involved the femoral-popliteal segment. These statistical data reflect both the high incidence of these lesions and the widespread use of surgical procedures for their reconstruction.

The extent and location of the lesions in the femoral-popliteal segment are extremely variable. Initial lesions are characterized by mild to severe stenosis. One of the most common locations is at the junction between Hunter's canal and the initial segment of the popliteal. Another frequent location is in the distal popliteal or below the origin of the anterior tibial. A complete occlusion of the superficial femoral artery may occur from Hunter's canal up to the bifurcation of the common femoral. The incidence of isolated lesions of the femoral-popliteal segment is much smaller than that of those combined with the proximal or distal arterial tree.

Clinical manifestations consist of intermittent claudication of variable degrees, rest pain without or with ulcers or gangrene of the toes or foot when the occlusive process is quite widespread and when it affects also the distal vessels (see later discussion).

3. Tibioperoneal Occlusive Disease. Occlusion of leg arteries alone occurs in over 25 per cent of the patients. Combined occlusions of leg arteries with other arterial segments occurs in all the other arterial locations. Comparison of the incidence of various patterns in nondiabetic and diabetic groups shows that the atherosclerotic process is more discrete in the nondiabetic and more diffuse in the diabetic group. Involvement of a single artery of the leg is noted more often in nondiabetic than in diabetic patients. Conversely, occlusion of two or all three leg arteries occurs in about two-thirds of the diabetic and only in about one third of the nondiabetic patients. This is of considerable importance when considering revascularization of the leg and foot in the presence of limb-threatening, severe ischemia.

Collateral pathways compensating for the different patterns of occlusion are provided by preexisting major branches of the femoral, popliteal, and leg arteries. Their efficiency depends on the extent of the occlusive process of the major branches as well as of the involvement of the profunda femoris, which is the major collateral of the thigh and leg. The alternate collateral pathways for the salvage of the foot are provided by the dorsalis pedis and plantar arteries through the pedal anastomotic networks. The main arterial arch of the foot is completed in a dorsoplantar direction. The existence of these dorsal and plantar arterial arches providing the metatarsal arteries will determine whether any proximal reconstruction of the arterial tree would be successful enough to salvage the foot and prevent the need for amputations.

CLINICAL MANIFESTATIONS

The clinical manifestations of chronic arterial insufficiency, as just stated, vary with the location and extent of the vascular lesions. They are divided into three major groups of increasing severity: (1) intermittent claudication, (2) rest pain, and (3) ischemic ulcers and gangrene.

Intermittent claudication, indicating inadequate blood supply to contracting leg and foot muscles, varies in intensity according to the degree of arterial involvement. Mild to moderate intermittent claudication is generally not considered an indication for reconstructive surgery. By contrast, marked intermittent claudication, greatly restricting the patient's walking ability often to the point of disability, is a major indication. This is especially true if this symptom is a serious handicap in the lifestyle of a younger person. However, an older inactive person whose livelihood is not threatened by this type of claudication is not to be considered a candidate for reconstruction, especially if systemic manifestations of arteriosclerosis are present.

The degree of intermittent claudication is largely related to the extent and progression of the arterial disease. In the course of the evolution of the arteriosclerotic process, a superimposed acute segmental occlusion may occur, with a corresponding sudden aggravation of the claudication. In such instances, arterial reconstruction may assume a more urgent indication than in the chronic stage.

Rest pain is a well-known clinical indication of advanced arterial insufficiency, and is due to a fall in the blood flow when the limb is in the supine position. Clinically, rest pain involves the toes and the adjacent metatarsal area and occurs mostly at night. The patient awakes and hangs the involved limb over the side of the bed to relieve his pain. If further dependency of the limb is necessary to improve the capillary flow, the patient walks about the room before he can return to sleep. In a further advanced stage, rest pain may become continuous and be present not only during the night but also during waking hours. Associated signs of end-stage ischemia often present are a cold, anesthetic or a cold, edematous, and discolored foot.

Ischemic ulcerative and gangrenous lesions, to be amenable to reconstructive arterial surgery, should be localized either in the toes or the heel or a combination thereof. In these patients, use of antibiotics and avoidance of any trauma will usually limit the lesions to a small area. However, spreading gangrene may occur if local infection is not controlled, especially in diabetic patients, if a venous thrombosis is superimposed and if cardiac failure is present.

In attempting to establish any therapy, it is important to take into account: (1) the type of onset, (2) the age of the patient, (3) the pattern of occlusive arterial disease, and (4) the presence of diabetes.

The mode of onset may be insidious: sudden without prior claudication or sudden with prior claudication and a combination of associated trauma, venous occlusion, arterial embolism, and vasospastic conditions. As to age, the majority of patients fall within the sixth, seventh, and eighth decades and over 80 per cent are males. It is noteworthy that the relative age incidence in nondiabetic and diabetic patients varies inversely with the advance in decades. In a study of vascular lesions in these two groups of patients by me and my colleagues, there were slightly more than 50 per cent under the age of 60 in the nondiabetic group, whereas only 33 per cent were found in the diabetic group. Conversely, after 60 the incidence in the diabetic group was 67 per cent and 48.6 per cent in the nondiabetic.

Diabetic foot lesions deserve a special mention. They are frequently associated with, and sometimes dominated by, two other important clinical manifestations: diabetic neuropathy and local infection. The association, in varying degrees, lends to the lesions a truly characteristic clinical picture, often referred to as the "diabetic foot." Because of their quasi specificity, these lesions justify a separate description. The clinical manifestations may be classified under the following four headings: (1) arteriosclerosis obliterans, (2) peripheral neuropathy, (3) infection, and (4) combined lesions. In treating a diabetic, one has to take into account the possibility of the three major factors in order not to overlook any of them.

CLINICAL EVALUATION OF ARTERIAL INSUFFICIENCY

Prior to undertaking noninvasive instrumental or arteriographic assessment of the arterial insufficiency, its clinical evaluation is the most important part of the physical examination. The *color* of the leg, especially of the foot and toes, in the supine and dependent, as well as elevated, positions, may provide a clue as to the severity of the arterial ischemia at the capillary level. The *temperature* of the skin, examined under basal conditions, may provide an indication of the degree and the location of the arterial impairment, especially if there is a difference between the two sides. Unilateral foot coolness or coldness carries a significant sign of ischemia. It is interesting to note that in an occlusion of the distal superficial femoral or proximal popliteal, *the knee* on the affected side is much warmer than on the contralateral side. This finding, which I call "hyperemic knee sign," indicates an increased collateral circulation around the knee provided by the genicular system and branches of the profunda femoris. The difference between the two knee temperatures may range from 2 to 5 F.

Systematic *palpation* of all the pulses from

the abdominal aorta down to the pedal ones should provide a first indication about the degree and location of the arterial occlusion. *Auscultation* along the arteries from the abdominal aorta down to the popliteal may indicate the presence of marked stenosis when a systolic bruit is audible. *Oscillometry,* when other noninvasive methods for evaluation are not available, will provide semiquantitative information concerning the amplitude of the pulsations and should be carried out at several levels of the extremity on both sides. Today, the *Doppler ultrasonic* blood velocity determination is commonly used and is an important means for comparative flow assessment and for localizing the lesions. A permanent record of these blood velocities and blood wave determinations should be kept for future reference. Usually these noninvasive methods are carried out by experienced technicians in especially equipped vascular laboratories. Thus, the interpretation of the graphic flow patterns, analysis of segmental pressure measurements, and interpretation of postexercise ankle blood pressure obtained with this method may aid greatly in the evaluation of the arterial insufficiency and help in deciding the type of treatment to be applied.

CLINICAL ASSESSMENT OF GENERAL CONDITION

A routine systematic evaluation of all the vital organs is essential, especially if they are considered for arterial surgery: electrocardiogram (ECG); cerebral symptomatology; the renal function, especially in diabetic patients; a chest film; blood pressure determinations over a period of several days; and a complete lipid profile.

ARTERIOGRAPHIC EVALUATION

If surgery is contemplated, a comprehensive assessment of the arterial lesions of the lower extremity is mandatory and should include the entire arterial tree from the terminal abdominal aorta to the pedal vessels. This method is essential to provide information not only about the lesions of the femoral and popliteal arteries but also about the state of the aorta and iliac arteries (inflow tract) as well as about the tibial and pedal vessels (outflow tract). This can be achieved by serial aortoarteriography, performed under general anesthesia and consisting of a percutaneous puncture of both common femoral arteries and using Teflon catheters. Bilateral arteriography should be carried out routinely since in the majority of instances the arteriosclerotic process involves both lower extremities. Interpretation of arteriographic findings is usually not difficult, especially in centers in which angioradiology is a specialized section of the x-ray department. Patients with symptomatic arterial insufficiency rarely display arterial lesions of a monosegmental type and the lesions are most often multiple and complex.

The complete occlusion of a segment is easily interpretable, but intimal lesions encroaching upon the lumen are often difficult to assess in terms of their hemodynamic significance. The degree of stenosis assigned to an atheromatous lesion radiologically visible may be often misleading. Operative findings are usually more severe than the arteriographic outline would indicate. The nature of the lesions may range from a soft atheromatous to a hard fibrous or calcified plaque. The extent of the latter is rarely detectable from the angiographic image. Because of possibility of misinterpretation of these observations, it is essential to obtain an adequate opacification of the angiographic outline of the entire vascular tree.

Diagnosis of the nature and degree of chronic arterial insufficiency of the lower extremity can be achieved by clinical, noninvasive, and arteriographic evaluations. Classification of the lower extremity arterial insufficiency is I, intermittent claudication ranging from mild to severe; II, rest pain; and III, ulcers or gangrene.

Conservative management is indicated in most cases, except in those patients in whom conservative measures fail to relieve rest pain or heal minor ulcers or limited gangrene of toes. Reconstructive surgery is then indicated.

PERIPHERAL VENOUS DISEASE

By JOHN J. CRANLEY, M.D.
Cincinnati, Ohio

Almost all peripheral venous disease states fall into one of two major categories, those in which there is some form of intravenous thrombosis and those in which there is venous insufficiency owing to incompetent valves with or without mainstream obstruction.

THROMBOPHLEBITIS

Thrombophlebitis is the accepted term for intravenous thrombosis of whatever cause,

Table 1. *A Clinical Classification of the Etiologic Factors of Thrombophlebitis Based on the Classic Triad of Virchow*

I. An endothelial lesion
  1. Sclerosing solution for varicose veins
  2. Any irritating intravenous solution
  3. Mechanical trauma
    a. Needle puncture
    b. Strain (axillary vein thrombosis)
    c. Wounds of violence
    d. Prolonged compression
  4. Ischemia
  5. Sepsis
II. Hypercoagulability of the blood
  1. Tumor, malignancies
    a. Blood dyscrasias (polycythemia vera, leukemia)
  2. Heart disease
  3. Thromboangiitis obliterans
  4. Contraceptive pills
  5. Gram-negative septicemia
  6. Postpartum, postoperative
  7. Vasculitides
III. Decreased blood flow (stasis)
  A. Cardiac failure
  B. Interference with venous return
    1. Postoperative
    2. Prolonged sitting
    3. Immobilization
      a. Fractures
      b. Prolonged bed rest
      c. Compression of veins
        (1) Swelling (subfascial)
        (2) Casts (swelling)
        (3) Tumor (pelvic, mediastinal)
        (4) Gravid uterus
      d. Varicose veins
IV. Idiopathic factors

whether the thrombus is loosely attached to the vein wall or involved in the inflammatory reaction in the vein wall and therefore firmly attached. A loosely attached thrombus may embolize, but if it does not, it becomes firmly attached, may propagate, and in turn form a soft portion that may be loosely attached. Both firm and loose clots may exist in different portions of the same vein at the same time. Therefore, it seems best not to define different types of deep venous thrombosis on the basis of adherence (or lack of it) to the vein wall.

ETIOLOGY

The classic triad of Virchow (an endothelial lesion, hypercoagulability of the blood, decrease in the velocity of blood flow) is the basis of Table 1. A fourth category, idiopathic, is added to cover thrombophlebitis of unknown cause. It should be noted that some overlapping necessarily occurs. For example, trauma may cause thrombophlebitis by injuring the intima, by disturbing the coagulability of the blood, or by venous stasis due to compression.

DIAGNOSIS

A practical clinical classification is as follows:

Superficial
Superficial and deep
Deep
  Soleal sinus thrombi
  Tibial vein thrombi
  Popliteal and femoral vein thrombosis
  Femoral and iliac vein thrombosis

Phlegmasia cerulea dolens
  Benign
  Malignant
Upper extremity thrombophlebitis
  Ulnar-radial
  Brachial
  Axillary-subclavian

SUPERFICIAL THROMBOPHLEBITIS

The presence of pain, tenderness, erythema, and a palpable cord in the known course of the vein establishes the diagnosis of superficial thrombophlebitis. The erythema may vary from mild to intense. When intense, the redness may suggest acute cellulitis or lymphangitis. This is the sole problem of differential diagnosis. In superficial thrombophlebitis, the patient's temperature is normal, the white blood count rarely exceeds 10,000, and there is no shift to the left. In acute cellulitis, there is no palpable cord and the tenderness is more apt to be confined to the area of the lymph nodes.

Spontaneous resolution can be expected almost invariably in chemical thrombophlebitis of the upper extremities. In thrombophlebitis of the saphenous vein and its tributaries, spontaneous resolution occurs in the vast majority of the patients. When spontaneous resolution does not occur, the thrombosis may progress either slowly or rapidly toward the saphenofemoral junction. If this occurs, treatment consists of anticoagulant therapy or excision of the phlebitic veins with ligation of the saphenous vein at the saphenofemoral junction. If the thrombus extends into the common femoral vein, a soft clot may also be formed and a pulmonary embolus occur. In the absence of involvement of the common femoral vein, we have been unable to document a single example of pulmonary embolism following superficial thrombophlebitis.

DEEP THROMBOPHLEBITIS

The most important advance in this field over the past decade has been the recognition that the clinical diagnosis of deep venous thrombosis is fallible, with an error of approximately 50 per cent. Not only may there be a complete absence of signs and symptoms in a patient with advancing deep venous thrombosis, but also the classic symptoms and signs may occur in the absence of deep venous thrombosis.

Indeed, the diagnosis of deep venous thrombosis is so frequently in error that my colleagues and I believe we have the absolute responsibility of establishing the diagnosis in every patient. A summary of the diagnostic problems follows, adhering to the outline presented, after which a more detailed analysis of the methods of objective diagnosis is discussed.

Soleal Sinus Thrombi. The muscle of the calf may be painful, feel tight on palpation, and there may be pain on passive dorsiflexion of the foot (Homans' sign), or there may be no symptoms whatever. The diagnosis may be established by venography. The radioactive fibrinogen uptake test offers the only other practical means of diagnosing this type of deep venous thrombosis.

Tibial Vein Thrombi. Clinically, such thrombosis may be totally "silent" or there may be calf swelling, calf tenderness, pain in the calf on dorsiflexion of the foot, and superficial vein distention when the limb is in neutral position. Objectively, venography is the most accurate in diagnosing tibial vein thrombi; other methods include radioactive fibrinogen, phleborheography, and the Doppler velocity detection technique.

Popliteal and Superficial Femoral Vein Thrombosis. This type is less likely to be "silent." There may be swelling, superficial vein distention, tenderness, and tightness of the calf. Venography, radioactive fibrinogen, phleborheography, Doppler velocity detection, assessing maximal venous outflow by the impedance technique, and the mercury-in-rubber type strain gauge are methods of diagnosing this form of venous thrombosis.

Femoral and Iliac Vein Thrombosis. In the presence of acute swelling, and particularly in the absence of prolonged sitting, this type of venous thrombosis can be diagnosed clinically most of the time. In rare instances, we have seen patients without swelling in proven femoroiliac venous thrombosis, but these patients have been at bed rest. Usually there will be significant swelling of the entire extremity in the majority of such recumbent patients, and also in those who have been sitting or ambulant. Distention of the superficial veins in the neutral position, pain (particularly in the calf muscles but also in the thigh muscles), and tenderness in the calf muscles and over the femoral triangle are the usual symptoms. Diagnosis is confirmed by venography and also by phleborheography, the Doppler technique, and the methods of recording maximal venous outflow. Clots in the upper thigh and pelvis are not detected well by the use of radioactive fibrinogen.

Phlegmasia Cerulea Dolens. *Benign.* When the venous outflow of the limb is blocked sufficiently to cause stagnation of the venous blood in the limb, the color of the skin becomes violaceous and the diagnosis of phlegmasia cerulea dolens can be made. Clinically, it is established with a high degree of accuracy. One sees a patient with a massively swollen limb that is bluish in color. Further examination reveals superficial vein distention, tenderness in the muscles of the leg and thigh, and usually, tenderness over the femoral triangle. The diagnosis can be confirmed by venography, phleborheography, the Doppler technique, and the methods of measuring venous outflow. That the thrombosis is due to purely physical blockage of the venous outflow can be demonstrated by the prompt subsiding of swelling and the return to normal color of the skin following thrombectomy of the major veins of the thigh and pelvis.

Malignant Type. This is a special type that is rarely encountered and is diagnosable on inspection at a glance. In many instances, it is identical to what has been called "venous gangrene." We have preferred not to use this term in the hope (unrealized to date) that some such limbs might be treatable, particularly by enzymatic action.

The thrombotic process starts in the toes in almost all instances and spreads proximally slowly, although we have seen it start on the dorsum and then spread in both directions. The color of the skin is deeply violaceous with a sharp line of demarcation between the involved and the normal skin proximal to it. Once seen, this cannot be forgotten. We recall no instance in which the diagnosis has not been made correctly on first sight of the patient's extremity. On at least two occasions, we have had the opportunity of seeing a patient with a very faint violaceous discoloration of the toes on the first day and the fullblown picture on the next day.

The diagnosis can be confirmed at amputation, autopsy, or by venography, or by any of the plethysmographic techniques, or by the Doppler method. We have seen only one patient (of 20) who survived, with above-the-knee amputation. All others have been either terminally ill or nearly so, most with a malignancy of some type, including hematologic disorders, but some with cachexia from other causes. Heparin appears to have no effect whatever on the thrombotic process. Pathologically, every single vein in the limb is thrombosed, including the major veins, muscular veins, and in one instance at least, the veins of the nerves were observed to be thrombosed.

VENOUS THROMBOSIS OF THE UPPER EXTREMITY

The incidence of "silent" thrombosis of the veins of the upper extremity is unknown. We believe that most cases are undiagnosed. If a patient has swelling of the upper extremity, particularly with venous distention, one is led to suspect the diagnosis of venous thrombosis. Pain is less than that in lower extremity venous thrombosis. Diagnosis is made by venography, and occasionally, by the Doppler technique. In our experience, phleborheography has not been accurate in the upper extremity, and we have had no experience in the use of the other diagnostic techniques.

OBJECTIVE METHODS OF DIAGNOSING DEEP VENOUS THROMBOSIS

Venography. In our experience with over 700 venograms, we have at times employed all published techniques. The most satisfactory in our hands has proved to be as follows: A British Columbia Medical (BCM) table is used that incorporates 5 separate 14 by 51-inch plates. Each exposure enables one to evaluate the entire contrast length. The dorsal vein in the foot is cannulated by a 19-gauge thin-walled butterfly needle with the tip directed toward the toes in a retrograde fashion. A smaller needle may be used if necessary. The saphenous vein and its major tributaries are avoided. A cut-down has rarely been necessary. If the foot is edematous, local compression is applied until the vein becomes visible. If the veins are too small, warm towels are used. A tourniquet is placed tightly around the thigh just above the knee. At this point, the intravenous solution of 250 ml of isotonic saline solution containing 2500 units of heparin is allowed to drip in rapidly until it slows down precipitously, indi-

cating that the limb veins are filled with blood and fluid. A second tourniquet is then placed just above the ankle and injection of approximately 100 ml of Renografin-60 (diatrizoate meglumine) is begun.

The first film is taken with the foot in external rotation after 25 ml of contrast medium has been injected. The lower tourniquet is removed, a second 25 ml of dye is injected, and the second film is taken. Now the final 50 ml of contrast medium is injected and the upper tourniquet is removed and two films are taken. During the second picture, the pretrained patient performs the Valsalva maneuver. This causes a rapid rise in venous pressure and produces reflux of blood down some of the tributaries both large and small. Finally, the limb is elevated and a film taken, to show the iliac veins and the vena cava. Following examination, the legs are wrapped snugly from toes to knee with a 4 by 6-inch elastic tensor bandage. In the absence of existing acute thrombophlebitis, active ambulation is encouraged immediately. If the patient is hospitalized, the limbs are elevated during the night.

Phleborheography. Phleborheography is a name selected to describe a plethysmographic method of diagnosing deep venous thrombosis developed in the vascular laboratory of Good Samaritan Hospital, Cincinnati, Ohio. Phleborheography is based on three principles. The first is that acute thrombosis in the main venous stream diminishes or obliterates the respiratory waves normally visible in the dependent extremity, analogous to the elimination of the sound of respiratory waves detected by Doppler examination that are present in the normal, and absent in the clotted, vein. Second, compression of the limb by squeezing or use of blood pressure cuffs momentarily increases the flow of blood proximally in the limb. Any obstruction to this flow of blood will cause minute swelling of the extremity, which is detected by the pneumatic cuff attached to a volume recorder. The third principle takes advantage of the fact that compression of the limb, in addition to propelling blood proximally, siphons blood from the foot in a normal extremity and this too is decreased or absent in the limb with deep venous thrombosis.

The phleborheograph detects mainstream occlusive clots, particularly when acute. It does not detect clots outside the mainstream — in the saphenous vein, the soleal sinuses, the profunda femoris, and the hypogastric vein. This has not proved to be a drawback to date. Clots in the saphenous vein are easily detected clinically. If clots in the soleal veins propagate, to the tibial or particularly to the popliteal, they

Table 2. Results: Acute Deep Venous Thrombosis of the Lower Extremities

	Phlebographic-Phleborheographic Correlations in 649 Extremities	
A. False negatives		20/240 (8.3%)
Equivocal	2/240 (0.8%)	
Error in interpretation	5/240 (2.1%)	
Test error	13/240 (5.4%)	
B. Infrapopliteal false negatives	12/57 (21%)	
C. False positives		20/409 (4.8%)
Equivocal	3/409 (0.7%)	
Technical error	5/409 (1.2%)	
Error in interpretation	3/409 (0.7%)	
Test error	9/409 (2.2%)	

(Four cases of venous compression secondary to tumor were not counted as test errors.)

will be detected. Clots in the deep femoral vein that do not propagate to the common femoral are probably rare. We have not documented their occurrence. We have encountered three patients with clots in the hypogastric vein that embolized, but probably because of their small size, did not prove fatal.

Accuracy. For acute occlusive clots in the popliteal, femoral, and iliac veins, phleborheography has been 100 per cent accurate in our experience. We have encountered seven extremities with occlusive disease of the femoral vein not detected by phleborheography, but in each instance it was evident both clinically and by the venogram that the occlusion was of chronic nature with very large collateral circulation. For clots in the named veins below the knee — the anterior tibial, posterior tibial, and the peroneal — there has been a false negative rate of 25 per cent. When our errors due to the learning experience, technical problems, or to interpretation are excluded, our overall accuracy rate is 5 per cent false negatives and 2 per cent false positives (Table 2). In a survey recently conducted among laboratories using the phleborheograph, the gross error rate was found to be 9 per cent of extremities in which the diagnosis was confirmed by venography. About half (4.5 per cent) of these errors were inherent in the method and the rest were artifacts or interpretive errors.

Clinically, three situations arise in which phleborheography has been of inestimable value: (1) The patient with massive swelling of the extremity, in which the phleborheogram is negative. In this instance, one can be certain that the swelling is not due to deep venous thrombosis. Usually, the edema is due to the gravitational effect of prolonged sitting. (2) If the tracing is positive for any reason, the patient should be hospitalized and treated with anticoagulant therapy. (3) If the patient has pain in the lower calf and the phleborheogram is negative, he is not admitted and not given heparin; rather, the phleborheogram is repeated in 2 or 3 days. If positive then, the patient is hospitalized and treated with anticoagulant agents. If not positive on repeat testing, if it seems clinically warranted, the patient may be followed further.

The phleborheographic technique differs from all others as regards method, and therefore must be learned. Most physicians can learn to interpret tracings in from 3 to 5 days. The technique is technician-sensitive. It takes about 2 weeks to train a technician to carry out the test properly.

Doppler Ultrasound Velocity Detection. The Doppler velocity detector may be used to identify deep venous thrombosis with a high degree of accuracy if the physician makes a determined effort to learn the method. It is possible to become expert in its use for diagnosing venous disease, although few of our associates have found time to do so. The overall accuracy in published reports varies from 83 to 92 per cent.

Impedance Plethysmography. Impedance plethysmography involves the principle of recording the maximal venous outflow. This principle is also employed in other plethysmographic techniques, such as the use of the mercury-in-rubber strain gauge and the pulse volume recorder. Reports of the accuracy of the impedance technique from Wheeler, its originator, and from Hirsh and Bergan, who use it in combination with the Doppler velocity detector, are excellent for thrombi in the popliteal and femoral veins. Most authors have not found it useful for thrombi in veins below the knee. We do not have experience with this technique or with the mercury-in-rubber strain gauge method. We have a modest experience with the pulse volume recorder, but our results have shown an accuracy rate of scarcely better than 50 per cent.

Radioactive Fibrinogen. This method has become popular in Europe, but it is not widely used in the United States. The prime reason is that the cost in our country is many times that of using it in Canada or Europe. In Cincinnati, the average cost of using this technique is $250 for screening a patient for 7 days. Since many hospital patients need screening for at least 14 days, the amount should be doubled. The incidence of clinically significant deep venous thrombosis is not high enough to justify this cost.

Other problems existing with the radioactive technique are its insensitivity to clots in the common femoral or pelvic veins, where large, potentially lethal clots are formed; the high incidence of false-positives due to hemorrhage in the tissues, serous effusion, or to other unexplained causes; its contraindication in a limb upon which an operation has been performed; its failure to detect old organized clot; its invasiveness and the less than ideal equipment for detecting radioactivity in a limb. A very slight movement of the probe may convert a positive to a negative tracing, and vice versa. The greatest advantage of this method lies in detecting acute fresh clots in the soleal and tibial veins.

Radionuclide Venography. In this technique, technetium[99] MTc is injected into a vein in the foot below an ankle or lower-leg tourniquet and it is then visualized by means of a gamma camera as it flows proximally in the deep veins. It is useful for clots in the large vessels (femoral, iliac, vena cava) but not for those in the smaller calf and leg veins.

CHRONIC VENOUS INSUFFICIENCY OF THE LOWER EXTREMITY

This term describes symptoms and signs due to malfunctioning of the peripheral venous heart. The condition may be divided into groups in which the incompetency is of the superficial system alone (varicose veins), the deep veins alone, or in some combination of superficial and deep veins. The symptoms and signs, whether they be of the superficial or deep venous systems, are similar. The patient complains of discomfort in the limb that is related to the duration of time he has been standing. The symptoms are described as a feeling of tired-

ness, heaviness, fullness, and dull, aching pain that is absent when the patient is recumbent and early in the morning, and that becomes progressively more severe as the day progresses, particularly if the patient is standing still (e.g., while ironing or at a work bench). Symptoms are relieved by elevation of the extremities. During sleep the patient may experience muscular cramps, particularly if varicose veins are present, but this is not specific.

VARICOSE VEINS

Varicose veins are diagnosed by inspection, although there may be a difference of opinion between what the patient calls "varicose veins" and the physician's definition. Frequently patients consider any visible vein to be "varicose." Some of these are small intracutaneous veins, often called "spider veins," which are visible venules of a millimeter or less in diameter. The second type is subcutaneous veins that are entirely normal but visible, of uniform size, without bulging, and usually smaller than the visible veins on the dorsum of the hand. True varicosities are usually at least 5 to 10 mm in diameter or larger, are tortuous, and if the limb is elevated and the vein compressed while the patient is standing, it can usually be seen that the blood flows in a retrograde fashion (Trendelenburg test). Most patients with varicose veins have no abnormal discoloration of the skin or daily swelling of the ankles. However, we believe that in approximately 25 per cent of limbs seen with ulceration owing to chronic venous insufficiency the condition is caused by incompetent superficial veins and in 75 per cent by a combination of superficial and deep veins. Since the clinical picture is similar, it is described in the following section.

CHRONIC VENOUS INSUFFICIENCY DUE TO INCOMPETENT SUPERFICIAL AND DEEP VEINS (POSTPHLEBITIC SYNDROME)

The clinical picture can best be visualized by the natural history of the untreated disease. The patient reports a history of having had deep thrombophlebitis for which he was hospitalized and treated with anticoagulant therapy. After a few months most of the swelling had disappeared, except the daily swelling of the ankles, which has been present from that time on. This is a cardinal event. The syndrome does not occur in the absence of daily swelling and can be prevented entirely if the swelling is controlled. This swelling is believed to represent transudation of fluid from the circulating blood volume into the tissues as a result of the higher than normal ambulatory venous pressure. In time, the capillaries dilate to the point that the formed elements of the blood, such as the red cells, the white cells, and proteins, escape into the tissues, where they are then trapped. The brownish discoloration is due to hemosiderin of the red cells. The loss of hair and scaliness of skin, followed by induration of the subcutaneous tissue and by weeping, eczema, and ulceration, are believed to be due 'to malnutrition of the skin and subcutaneous tissue in some way caused by this extravasation of formed elements in the blood, as well as the elevation of the pressure itself.

Ulceration. Ulceration due to venous insufficiency is most common on the medial aspect of the legs and above the ankles but may occur on the lateral aspect as well. The typical venous ulcer is irregular in shape, surrounded by deeply pigmented skin. This deep brownish pigmentation is rarely absent in an ulcer caused by venous insufficiency. The ulcer may be grossly infected and even contain necrotic portions; however, it rarely penetrates the deep fascia. These features distinguish it from ulceration owing to arterial disease, which is, initially at least, surrounded by skin that appears normal. The ulcer is sharply punched out. The tissues are actually necrotic in appearance. Arterial ulcers usually penetrate the deep fascia.

OBJECTIVE METHODS OF DIAGNOSIS

Venography. In chronic venous insufficiency the venogram shows large, dilated veins. Incompetent perforating veins may be detected, and evidence of thrombosis in the major trunks may be disclosed. In descending venography, dye is injected into the common femoral vein of the patient, who is in the erect or semierect position. Under the fluoroscope one sees "dancing" of the dye due to the pulsation of the adjacent artery. Overcoming this pulsation, the column of dye slowly progresses proximally in the normal extremity. This presents a dramatic contrast to what happens in the extremity in which the femoral valve is incompetent. In this case, the dye can be seen dropping precipitously down the extremity through the superficial femoral vein and either continuing on through the leg or coming to rest whenever a competent valve is encountered. Incompetency of the common femoral, superficial femoral, and popliteal veins is easily detected. This method has been popularized by Kistner.

Phleborheography. The phleborheograph can be used to detect some but not all instances of deep venous insufficiency. If the tracing shows obstruction of the main channels plus large respiratory waves, one can be quite certain that there is chronic deep venous insufficiency. A second method of diagnosing old thrombosis is by the shortened refilling time of the foot after compression of the calf.

Doppler Ultrasound Velocity Detection. An incompetent vein can usually be detected by the Doppler method. Its most valuable place in our experience is in listening to the common femoral vein to detect incompetency and thus select patients for descending venography. If one listens to the venous sound over the femoral triangle and the patient performs the Valsalva maneuver, one can readily hear the rush of blood through the incompetent valve and the absence of such a sound in the patient with competent valves. Similarly, incompetence may be detected at the knee, although it is more difficult to discern through the confluence of veins and there is uncertainty as to exactly which vein is being heard. In the lower leg, incompetent valves can be discovered by placing the probe over a superficial vein and compressing the calf. In our experience, a problem has been that there is such an abundance of incompetent veins in chronic deep venous insufficiency that it is well nigh impossible by this method to detect any one isolated incompetent communicating vein.

Recently, Bergan and associates have used a photocell at the ankle to record refilling time of the foot after calf compression, which they correlate with venous pressure measured directly through a vein on the dorsum of the foot. Their preliminary results are excellent.

Section 7

DISORDERS OF THE BLOOD AND BLOOD-FORMING ORGANS

ANEMIA DUE TO INADEQUATE ERYTHROCYTE PRODUCTION

By WILLIAM E. BARRY, M.D.

Philadelphia, Pennsylvania

SYNONYMS

Hypoproliferative anemia, aregenerative anemia.

DEFINITION

Anemia due to inadequate erythrocyte production occurs when a quantitative deficiency of erythroid precursors exists in bone marrow of sufficient magnitude that normal concentrations of erythrocytes or hemoglobin cannot be maintained in peripheral blood. It also occurs when there is an inadequate marrow response to physiologic or pathologic demands for increases in marrow erythroid production. Thus, the erythropoietic "balance sheet" requires *quantitative* and *functional* integrity of the erythroid marrow.

A classification of the anemias due to inadequate erythrocyte production is shown in Table 1. Although the principal mechanism of anemia in these disorders is *inadequate production*, it should be pointed out that in some instances other mechanisms, such as a hemolytic component or diminished iron supply to the marrow, represent contributing factors.

ABSOLUTE DECREASE IN MARROW ERYTHROID PRECURSORS

APLASTIC ANEMIA

Aplastic anemia, a time-honored term despite its lack of precision, is characterized by destruction of marrow precursors of erythrocytes, granulocytes, and platelets, resulting in pancytopenia.

ETIOLOGY

Recognizable causes occur in only about 50 per cent of patients with aplastic anemia. In such patients, drugs, certain infections, and immunologic mechanisms have been implicated. Although numerous drugs have been incriminated in isolated case reports, chloramphenicol, phenylbutazone, and gold salts are

Table 1. *Anemia Due to Inadequate Erythrocyte Production—Classification*

I. Absolute decrease in marrow erythroid precursors
  A. Aplastic anemia
  B. Pure red cell aplasia
  C. Aplastic crisis in hemolytic disorders
  D. Marrow infiltrative diseases

II. Decreased erythropoietin response
  A. Anemia of renal failure
  B. Anemia of chronic disease
  C. Endocrine disorders
  D. Anemia of protein malnutrition

especially suspect. Viral hepatitis has been reported in association with aplastic anemia in children and adults. Immunologic mechanisms have been suspected owing to reports of successful treatment with immunosuppressive drugs.

A congenital type of aplastic anemia, *Fanconi's anemia*, occurs in children in association with other structural anomalies.

SIGNS AND SYMPTOMS

Typically, patients with aplastic anemia present with generalized bleeding phenomena (purpura, epistaxis, bleeding gums, hematuria, melena). Fatigue and skin pallor is usually present. Secondary bacterial infections of skin, respiratory tract, or urinary tract are seen less commonly in early stages, depending on the degree of granulocytopenia. Enlargement of spleen, lymph nodes, or liver is notably absent. In the absence of complicating infection, fever is usually not present.

COURSE

Historically, about 50 per cent of patients with aplastic anemia die in less than 2 years, usually because of bleeding or infection. Some patients have spontaneous complete or incomplete recovery after months or years, or continue to have mild cytopenia without clinical disease. If numerous transfusions of red blood cells have been required, residual iron overload, especially in the liver, can occur, representing a potential hazard if coincidental transfusion-related viral hepatitis also occurs. Therapeutic trials of bone marrow transplantation or immunosuppressive drugs pose additional problems too complex to discuss here.

LABORATORY FINDINGS

The peripheral blood shows pancytopenia, accompanied by a low reticulocyte count. The anemia is normocytic, normochromic in type. Polychromasia and nucleated red cells are absent. Bone marrow aspiration, done with ease, shows considerable fat with markedly diminished or absent cellularity, except for stromal elements and lymphocytes. Increased lymphocytes or plasma cells or both are sometimes seen. Whether they represent residual, unaffected cells or signify a possible immunologic etiology has not been clearly established. Rarely, small foci of apparently normal marrow cells are seen, but if adequate material is obtained, particularly by trephine biopsy, the overall histologic pattern of reduced cellularity is readily apparent.

The serum iron level is invariably high, often greater than 200 micrograms per dl (100 ml), with a normal or reduced total iron-binding capacity. Elevated fetal hemoglobin is sometimes seen.

Ferrokinetic studies with ^{59}Fe demonstrate a low *plasma iron turnover*, with extremely low red cell incorporation. Organ counting with scintillation detectors shows increased uptake of the isotope in liver.

PITFALLS IN DIAGNOSIS

In patients in whom the degree of marrow depletion of precursor cells is not complete, or if marrow aspiration discloses equivocal hypocellularity, aplastic anemia can be confused with a "preleukemic" state, which may be manifested by varying degrees of peripheral blood cytopenia and a nondiagnostic bone marrow. The "preleukemic" syndromes more commonly have normal or increased cellularity but in those cases in which the cellularity is decreased, mimicking aplastic anemia, qualitative abnormalities in the immature granulocytes are frequently seen. These include "nuclear-cytoplasmic asynchrony" in which there is a discrepancy between the maturity of the nucleus and that of the cytoplasmic contents. For example, the nucleus may have prominent nucleoli but the cytoplasm may contain sufficient granules, suggesting a fully matured segmented cell. Alternatively, cells with segmented, mature nuclei may have sparse granules ("granule-poor polys"). In addition, the "preleukemic" states may have "ringed sideroblasts." These qualitative abnormalities are not found in typical aplastic anemia. Occasionally, it may be impossible to distinguish true aplastic anemia from early, atypical acute leukemia except by long-term observation.

Paroxysmal nocturnal hemoglobinuria is often characterized by pancytopenia and a hypoplastic marrow. If the other features of this syndrome, viz., chronic intravascular hemolysis with episodic hemoglobinuria, are not prominent or are overlooked, it may be indistinguishable from typical aplastic anemia. Therefore, in all patients with apparent aplastic anemia, a Ham's test or sugar water test is advisable.

PURE RED CELL APLASIA

Two different categories of this disorder have been observed. One, occurring in infancy and childhood, is characterized by reduced or absent red cell precursors in marrow (Blackfan-Diamond syndrome). In adults, an anemia characterized by lack of red cell precursors in marrow, with preservation of granulocyte and megakaryocytes, has been associated frequently with thymoma. Some cases have been associated with drugs and rarely with carcinoma. Others have been reported with no discernible cause. In recent years, attention has been directed to immunologic mechanisms owing to the finding of antibodies to erythroblast nuclei or erythropoietin, as well as reports of cases responding to corticosteroids, immunosuppressive drugs, or anti-thymocyte globulin.

The symptoms and signs relate to the anemia, which is often severe. Occasionally, myasthenia gravis occurs when a thymoma develops. The clinical course is often chronic. In most patients, the need for repeated red cell transfusions leads to iron overload with adverse effects on liver and myocardium.

The peripheral blood shows a normocytic, normochromic anemia with decreased reticulocyte count. The white cell count and platelet count are normal. Bone marrow shows virtual absence of erythroid precursors, with normal granulocytes and megakaryocytes. A slight increase in small lymphocytes and plasma cells may be observed. The serum iron level is high, with increased saturation of the total iron-binding capacity.

PITFALLS IN DIAGNOSIS

Transient erythroblastic hypoplasia occurs in chronic hemolytic anemias in association with infection. If bone marrow aspiration is delayed, the lack of red cell precursors may be missed, or the recovery phase of erythroblastic proliferation may be confused with the megaloblastic erythropoiesis of folate depletion that occurs occasionally in the same hemolytic states.

Pure red cell aplasia is rarely the forerunner of acute leukemia, especially the monocytic variety.

MARROW INFILTRATIVE DISEASES

Infiltration of bone marrow by malignant cells or granulomatous diseases usually results in significant depression of normal marrow elements, including red cell precursors (*mye-lophthisic anemia*). Presenting signs and symptoms vary, depending, in part, on the degree and type of marrow inadequacy. Fatigue and weakness are common owing to the anemia but also to the type and severity of the underlying disease. Bleeding phenomena may occur from thrombocytopenia. Physical findings, in addition to pallor, may include hepatosplenomegaly if extramedullary hematopoiesis occurs.

The peripheral blood characteristically shows a normocytic, normochromic anemia with variation in size and shape of the red blood cells. Tear-shaped red blood cells are usually seen. Nucleated red blood cells commonly occur. The reticulocyte count is variable and may be inappropriately high. The white cell count may be low, normal, or high. Immature granulocytes, including a few myeloblasts, are often seen. These so-called *leukoerythroblastic* blood findings strongly suggest marrow infiltrative disease, but bone marrow examination is needed to distinguish marrow infiltrative disease from typical *myelofibrosis*.

Bone marrow may be difficult to aspirate, as in myelofibrosis. Bone marrow biopsy is necessary to identify the character of the marrow infiltration.

PITFALLS IN DIAGNOSIS

Marrow infiltrative disease is occasionally spotty in distribution and marrow aspirate or biopsy can reveal only normal marrow elements. The presence of a "leukoerythroblastic" blood picture should prompt one to obtain repeated marrow specimens until the mechanism can be identified.

In agnogenic myeloid metaplasia, the bone marrow may not reveal collagen fibrosis but rather a cellular marrow. In such cases, however, the marrow elements are markedly hyperplastic and there is virtually no fat, in contrast to the normal cellularity in uninvolved sites, when marrow infiltrative disease is "spotty."

DECREASED ERYTHROPOIETIN RESPONSE

ANEMIA OF RENAL FAILURE

The severity of anemia in chronic renal disease is roughly correlated with the degree of renal failure. The mechanism of the anemia is inadequate availability of erythropoietin. Other factors, such as folate or iron deficiency, may compound the anemia. In some forms of renal failure, microangiopathic hemolytic anemia may occur. Disturbance of aerobic glycolysis may also shorten red blood cell survival.

The presenting signs, symptoms, and physical findings are nonspecific. If the anemia is severe (less than 7 to 8 grams of hemoglobin per dl) the symptoms may be largely related to the effects of anemia (e.g., fatigue, pallor, dyspnea, tachycardia, etc). Purpura or other bleeding manifestations may occur from a qualitative platelet defect, but the platelets are quantitatively normal.

LABORATORY FINDINGS

The anemia is normocytic and normochromic unless it is complicated by iron or folate deficiency. The bone marrow is usually normally cellular but occasionally may show erythroid hypoplasia when renal failure is severe.

The serum iron level is variable, depending on iron supply. A bone marrow iron stain is helpful to distinguish those patients with iron deficiency, who may profit by supplemental oral or parenteral iron. Ferrokinetic studies may show normal plasma iron turnover and red blood cell incorporation, consistent with the interpretation that this represents an inadequate response in the face of anemia. More severely affected individuals demonstrate an expected decrease in red blood cell production.

PITFALLS IN DIAGNOSIS

Since the level of hemoglobin in renal disease is only roughly correlated with the degree of azotemia, it is sometimes difficult to decide when a given level of hemoglobin is related entirely to renal failure, or if there is some superimposed complicating feature. Significant (less than 10 grams hemoglobin per dl) anemia rarely is found when the blood urea nitrogen level is less than 40 mg per dl or the creatinine less than 2.0 mg per dl. Severe anemia is usually present if the creatinine clearance is less than 20 ml per minute.

ANEMIA OF CHRONIC DISEASE

The anemia of chronic disease is the most common anemia seen in hospitalized patients, and ranks second only to iron deficiency anemia in unselected patients with anemia. It is a useful category that includes anemia due to *infection, malignancy,* and *rheumatoid arthritis.* The mechanism of anemia appears to be identical in all these disorders. That the anemia of chronic disease is not confined to these readily identified causes is shown by observations that "anemia of chronic disease" can occur in patients in whom an identifiable "chronic disease" cannot be found.

PATHOGENESIS

The anemia is characterized by three features: (1) marrow erythroid inadequacy, (2) decreased iron delivery from the reticuloendothelial system to marrow via transferrin, and (3) slight shortening of red blood cell survival. The marrow erythroid inadequacy appears to be primarily related to diminished erythropoietin secretion, possibly aggravated by decreased iron supply to marrow. Whatever the contribution of decreased iron supply is to marrow erythroid production, it is a most useful diagnostic marker. The reason for the decreased iron supply to marrow is a "block" in release of iron from the reticuloendothelial system, resulting in a characteristically low serum iron level. The reason for the associated decrease in total iron-binding capacity (that is, in transferrin level) is not understood fully, but the combination of a low serum iron *and* a low total iron-binding capacity (TIBC) is invariably found in anemia of chronic disease.

The slight shortening of red blood cell survival is insufficient by itself to account for the anemia, but it underscores the importance of inadequate erythroid marrow compensation. The anemia of chronic disease is usually asymptomatic. The underlying disease dominates the clinical picture.

LABORATORY FINDINGS

The level of hemoglobin is usually between 10 and 12 grams per dl, and rarely below 9 grams per dl. The red cell indices show a normocytic, normochromic picture. Occasionally, there is a slight degree of hypochromia. The reticulocyte count is invariably normal or low. Changes in the white blood cell counts, if they occur, reflect variations in the underlying disease. The platelet count is normal.

Both the serum iron and the TIBC are reduced. Transferrin saturation (serum iron ÷ TIBC × 100) is usually between 5 and 15 per cent. The bone marrow is normally cellular. Bone marrow iron stain characteristically shows decreased or absent sideroblasts and normal or increased tissue iron stores. Ferrokinetic studies show normal plasma iron turnover and slightly increased red blood cell incorporation. In the face of anemia, the plasma iron turnover values are inappropriately low and reflect marrow inadequacy.

PITFALLS IN DIAGNOSIS

Anemia of chronic disease is rarely complicated by absolute iron deficiency. In the presence of chronic disease, the characteristic increase in TIBC that occurs in iron deficiency is masked by the depressed TIBC in chronic disease. The level of serum iron may be identical in both disorders. Lack of stainable marrow iron serves to identify the uncommon coexistence of iron deficiency in a patient with a low serum iron and TIBC characteristic of anemia of chronic disease. Iron therapy is totally useless in the anemia of chronic disease. Furthermore, even if the two disorders coexist, viz., anemia of chronic disease and iron deficiency, the presence of the former usually inhibits any response to iron in the latter.

ENDOCRINE DISORDERS

Endocrine deficiency states involving the thyroid, pituitary, adrenal, and gonads result in a decrease in red cell mass. In adrenal insufficiency, however, the hemoglobin level is usually normal, owing to a greater decrease in plasma volume compared with the decrease in red cell mass.

In most of these deficiency states, the anemia is "adaptive" in nature, that is, it reflects a decrease in oxygen requirements owing to disordered cellular metabolism.

The presenting signs, symptoms, and physical findings are related to the particular endocrine disorder, and the anemia usually is asymptomatic.

LABORATORY FINDINGS

In general, the anemia is normocytic and normochromic. Coexistent B_{12}, folate, or iron deficiency may cause red cell changes consistent with these deficiencies. This has been noted particularly in hypothyroidism.

Ferrokinetic studies demonstrate reduced plasma iron turnover and erythron iron turnover, confirming the fact that the anemia is due to reduced red cell production.

PITFALLS IN DIAGNOSIS

The slow, insidious development of hypothyroidism often is not appreciated by the physician caring for a patient over long periods of time, although it may be immediately apparent to a new observer. The presence of anemia is frequently helpful in stimulating a reappraisal of possible mechanisms. In a patient with mild, normocytic (or macrocytic), normochromic anemia with normal or low reticulocyte count, hypothyroidism must be considered. Once considered, confirmation is not difficult by standard clinical and laboratory observations of thyroid function.

PROTEIN MALNUTRITION

Anemia due to protein deficiency in man occurs only in severe disorders such as kwashiorkor, rarely found in the United States. The coexistence of deficiencies of iron and folate and the possible contribution of erythropoietin lack and infection make it difficult to be certain of the role of protein in the development of anemia. Indeed, there is much evidence that the protein requirements for hemoglobin synthesis are met at the expense of other body tissues. Consequently, mild degrees of protein deficiency are not accompanied by anemia. It is only when severe degrees of protein-calorie starvation occur that anemia owing to protein deficiency should be suspected.

PERNICIOUS ANEMIA AND OTHER MEGALOBLASTIC ANEMIAS

By JOHN LINDENBAUM, M.D.
New York, New York

The pathophysiology, diagnosis, and therapy of the megaloblastic anemias have been the subject of intense interest for more than a century, and perhaps more is known about them than almost any other medical condition. Nonetheless, they remain a diagnostic challenge. The recent availability of automated Coulter Counter cell sizing in thousands of hospitals has led to the renewed recognition of the many causes of macrocytic anemia other than deficiencies of vitamin B_{12} and folate, and has also provided increasing opportunities for the early diagnosis of megaloblastic anemias, since mean corpuscular volume (MCV) elevations regularly can be detected before the development of anemia.

Megaloblastic anemias can be defined as anemias due primarily to bone marrow failure, with the typical findings in the peripheral blood of erythrocytes that are macrocytic and oval in shape as well as neutrophils with hypersegmented nuclei, and in the bone marrow of nuclear-cytoplasmic dissociation in erythroid precursors, and giant bands and metamyelo-

cytes. When all these findings are present, the condition is almost invariably the result of deficiency of vitamin B_{12}, folic acid, or both vitamins.

SYNONYMS

In the past, the term "pernicious anemia" has been used rather broadly to refer to any megaloblastic anemia or to B_{12} deficiency from any cause. More precisely, *pernicious anemia* should be defined as a B_{12} deficiency state resulting from lack of gastric intrinsic factor (IF). "Macrocytic anemias" should not be used interchangeably with "megaloblastic anemia," since there are many causes of anemia associated with macrocytosis that are not accompanied by a megaloblastic marrow or evidence of B_{12} or folate deficiency.

PRESENTING SIGNS AND SYMPTOMS

In many patients the presenting symptoms are nonspecific, since they are those occurring in any chronic anemia: fatigue, weakness, dyspnea, edema, palpitations, or angina pectoris. Anorexia is frequent, as is the resulting weight loss, which can be substantial and be misinterpreted as a sign of an underlying malignancy. Soreness of the tongue and mouth (and, occasionally, recurrent buccal ulcerations) is somewhat more specific for folate or B_{12} lack, although they sometimes occur with depletion of other nutrients, as in iron deficiency anemia. Tongue complaints are curiously intermittent, tending to remit and recur spontaneously. Diarrhea is a frequent symptom, occurring in about a quarter of patients with B_{12} or folate deficiency, even in the absence of an underlying malabsorption syndrome. Constipation is even more common in patients with depleted B_{12}. Difficulty in swallowing, of unknown cause, which rapidly clears after vitamin therapy, is an occasional chief complaint in B_{12} deficiency. Purpura due to thrombocytopenia is unusual.

Relatively more specific for vitamin B_{12} lack are certain neurologic complaints. These include paresthesias, ataxia, difficulty walking down stairs, impaired fine movements of the fingers, and partial loss of memory. In some patients dementia may be prominent. Rare neurologic manifestations include loss of visual acuity due to optic atrophy and orthostatic hypotension. Advanced central nervous system involvement may progress to paraplegia, impotence, and loss of sphincter control. Neurologic signs and symptoms occur in only one fourth to one half patients with B_{12} deficiency seen at the present time. Some patients with striking neurologic deficits may have little or no anemia, although almost all such patients will have an elevated MCV and hypersegmented neutrophils on blood smear.

Contrary to previous dogma, pernicious anemia is frequently seen in virtually all ethnic groups, and is common in blacks, Jews, and peoples from the Caribbean. It is predominantly a disease of the elderly, but 10 per cent of patients first present below the age of 40.

Other signs and symptoms not directly related to the presence of B_{12} or folate lack may be a reflection of the underlying disorder causing the deficiency state, as in some patients with sprue or regional enteritis. On the other hand, in some patients, megaloblastic anemia is the only clinical sign of an otherwise completely asymptomatic gastrointestinal condition, such as multiple jejunal diverticula or tropical sprue.

PHYSICAL EXAMINATION FINDINGS

Physical findings, which may be present depending on the severity of anemia, include pallor, a lemon-yellow tint to the skin, signs of congestive heart failure, and retinal hemorrhages. Minimal icterus is common. About a quarter of patients will have either a smooth, atrophic tongue with loss of papillae or an inflamed tongue that is beefy and red. Increased pigmentation, most common over the fingers and toes and reversible after vitamin therapy, is equally common but will not be elicited as a complaint without specific questioning. The spleen is occasionally palpable. Low-grade fever is seen in many patients.

Any of these physical findings may occur with either folate or B_{12} deficiency. In contrast, certain neurologic signs are not a feature of folate lack but are characteristic of B_{12} depletion (although, as stated earlier, many B_{12}-deficient patients lack neurologic signs and symptoms). These include (1) impairment of position and vibration sense, usually symmetrical, more marked distally, and tending to involve the lower extremities earlier and more severely than the upper; (2) in more severe cases, ataxia and a positive Romberg sign are typical and ankle jerks are commonly absent; (3) in advanced cases, in addition to these findings, spasticity, hyperreflexia, positive Babinski signs, ankle clonus, paraplegia, loss of sphincter function, and impairment of sensation extending to the trunk may be encountered.

Other B_{12}-depleted patients will present with a nonspecific peripheral neuropathy, with impairment of touch, pain, and temperature sensation, often in a glove or stocking distribution. Also, some diminution of memory can frequent-

ly be demonstrated in B_{12}-deficient patients. Varying degrees of irritability, mood disturbance, mental confusion, and dementia are not rare, especially in elderly patients. Frank psychosis is much less common.

COURSE

Since the introduction of liver therapy, fatal cases of pernicious anemia have become extremely rare. Irreversible neurologic damage continues to be encountered, however, in patients in whom the diagnosis of B_{12} deficiency has not been made for many years, or in whom prolonged folic acid therapy (which often improves the hematologic picture without reversing the neurologic disorder) has been mistakenly given. In general, when neurologic symptoms have been present for less than 6 months before therapy, they will be completely reversible; if they have been present for more than 3 years, complete return of neurologic function will not occur, although almost all patients show some improvement.

The tendency for B_{12} deficiency states such as those owing to pernicious anemia, tropical sprue, regional enteritis, or ileal resection to recur after cessation of maintenance B_{12} therapy must be emphasized. In such patients anemia, glossitis, or neuropathy recurs 1 to 12 years after stopping vitamin injections. Marrow failure progresses insidiously, and an elevated MCV without anemia or a mild, initially nonprogressive anemia may persist for months or years before becoming more severe or giving rise to symptoms.

COMMON COMPLICATIONS

Iron deficiency anemia occurs at some time in about 10 per cent of patients with pernicious anemia. Myxedema, thyrotoxicosis, and less commonly, vitiligo, hypoparathyroidism, and myasthenia gravis all are seen in increased frequency in association with pernicious anemia. Carcinoma of the stomach, previously more common, now develops in 1 to 2 per cent of patients with pernicious anemia.

PERIPHERAL BLOOD FINDINGS

Unlike iron deficiency anemia, which is often normochromic and normocytic when mild in degree, B_{12} and folate deficiency are manifested by morphologic abnormalities in the peripheral blood even before the development of anemia. The erythrocyte MCV is usually in the range of 100 to 140. The mean corpuscular hemoglobin (MCH) is also elevated and the mean corpuscular hemoglobin concentration (MCHC) is normal. *Macroovalocytes* are a characteristic finding on blood smears. With moderate or severe anemia, striking *anisocytosis* and *poikilocytosis*, often with red cell fragmentation, may dominate the picture, and if the macroovalocytes are overlooked, a primary hemolytic state may be suspected. Nucleated red blood cells, which may show megaloblastic morphology, and Howell-Jolly bodies are common. The percentage of reticulocytes is low or normal in the face of anemia, indicating a bone marrow failure state.

Hypersegmentation of neutrophils (most reliably defined as the presence of one or more granulocytes with six or more lobes) is another early finding that typically appears before anemia develops. It is detectable in 98 per cent of anemic patients. Those who are profoundly neutropenic or who have a marked shift to the left in the white blood cell differential owing to an associated inflammatory condition may not show hypersegmentation. Hypersegmentation is not specific for megaloblastic anemias, since it may be seen in iron deficiency anemia, renal failure, and chronic myeloproliferative disorders, and as a congenital anomaly.

Macrocytosis on blood smear and MCV elevations commonly occur in other conditions. These include liver disease, chronic alcoholism in the absence of folate deficiency, marked reticulocytosis, hypothyroidism, idiopathic acquired sideroblastic anemias, acute myelocytic leukemia, and myelofibrosis. It also occurs in patients having marrow replacement by hematologic or solid tumors, and during therapy with a host of antimetabolite drugs. In liver disease, chronic alcoholism, reticulocytosis, and hypothyroidism, the macrocytes are typically round. In the other conditions just listed oval macrocytes may be encountered. Neutrophil hypersegmentation, however, is not associated with any of these disorders, with the exception of treatment with some of the antileukemic agents such as methotrexate or cytosine arabinoside.

When anemia is moderately severe (hematocrit below 30 per cent), *thrombocytopenia* is quite common. *Neutropenia* is somewhat less frequent. Profoundly anemic patients frequently exhibit a *pancytopenia*, and B_{12} and folate deficiency must be considered among the common causes in the differential diagnosis of pancytopenia. Isolated neutropenia or thrombocytopenia, in the absence of anemia, is not encountered.

BONE MARROW

In patients with all of the classic findings in the peripheral blood (viz., high MCV, macro-

ovalocytes, *and* hypersegmented neutrophils), a bone marrow examination may be unnecessary if serum folate and B_{12} levels are readily available. If any question as to diagnosis exists, and especially in the alcoholic patient, in whom anemia is often multifactorial, a bone marrow aspiration is advisable to demonstrate the typical findings of a megaloblastic anemia. These include erythroid hyperplasia, nuclear-cytoplasmic dissociation in red cell precursors (that is, failure of the nuclear chromatin to aggregate to a degree appropriate to the stage of differentiation of the cytoplasm), and giant metamyelocyte and band cells, often with ribbon-like nuclei. Megakaryocytes may be increased or decreased in number and do not show clear-cut diagnostic morphologic features. Erythroid hypoplasia is an uncommon finding.

Megaloblastic marrow red cell precursors morphologically indistinguishable from those seen in B_{12} and folate lack may be present in a number of other conditions, including refractory macrocytic anemias, preleukemic states, acute myelocytic leukemia, and erythroleukemia. In these disorders, hypersegmented neutrophils in the peripheral blood and giant bands and metamyelocytes in the bone marrow are usually not seen. The absence of these associated granulocytic abnormalities essentially rules out B_{12} or folate deficiency as a cause of megaloblastic erythropoiesis.

OTHER LABORATORY FINDINGS

Owing to the destruction of red cell precursors in the bone marrow (so-called "ineffective erythropoiesis"), other laboratory findings common in B_{12} and folate deficiencies may mislead the physician toward a diagnosis of hemolytic anemia. Most patients show a mild elevation of the unconjugated bilirubin (typically 1.5 to 3 mg per dl [100 ml]) and plasma haptoglobin is usually low or absent. Serum lactic dehydrogenase (LDH) levels are elevated (often astronomically) in 90 per cent of patients, owing to increases in the LDH_1 and LDH_2 isozymes. Serum iron is typically elevated or normal.

In B_{12} deficiency, cerebrospinal fluid protein concentrations are moderately increased in half of the patients.

SERUM VITAMIN LEVELS

Once a patient has been shown to have a megaloblastic anemia, the next step is to determine whether it is due to B_{12} or folate deficiency, or both. Serum vitamin levels usually allow for precise diagnosis. Serum B_{12} concentrations are invariably low in untreated B_{12} deficiency, with the proviso that when certain commercially available radioassay kits are used, some deficient patients will have values of 200 to 400 picograms per ml, which is in the lower end of the normal range. (This is an avoidable technical problem that hopefully will be corrected in the near future.) Antibiotic therapy may cause a falsely low B_{12} or folate level if measured by microbial assay methods. In addition, 10 per cent of patients with pure folate deficiency will have a low serum B_{12} concentration, so that measurement of both vitamin levels is essential in diagnosis.

Serum folate as assayed by microbiologic or radioisotopic methods is typically low (less than 4 nanograms per ml and usually less than 2 nanograms per ml) in megaloblastic anemia due to folic acid lack. Unfortunately, serum folate levels often become subnormal after a few weeks of decreased dietary intake or alcohol ingestion, before body stores have been depleted. Thus, a low serum folate in the absence of morphologic evidence of tissue deficiency (viz., macroovalocytes, hypersegmentation, megaloblastic marrow) should not be interpreted as evidence of significant folate deficiency. Red cell folate concentrations are a more reliable indicator of depletion of body stores but are low in some patients owing to B_{12} deficiency. In pure B_{12} lack, serum folate concentrations are usually normal or elevated. Low levels are seen in 10 per cent of patients, usually with marked anorexia. In patients with malabsorption syndromes, such as tropical sprue, combined deficiency of both vitamins may be encountered.

Patients with megaloblastic marrows in whom serum levels of both vitamins are clearly normal will usually be found to have one of the "nondeficiency" causes of megaloblastic states just mentioned, such as refractory anemia or acute leukemia.

WORK-UP OF THE B_{12}-DEFICIENT PATIENT

The possible causes of B_{12} deficiency are listed in Table 1. Virtually all patients who are encountered clinically will have a disorder of the assimilation of dietary cobalamin. In 75 per cent, this is due to lack of gastric IF secondary to chronic inflammatory disease of the stomach (pernicious anemia). One half to two thirds of these patients will have serum antibodies to IF, which can be easily demonstrated by a simple in vitro test. In the patient with B_{12} deficiency who has serum antibodies to IF, the diagnosis of pernicious anemia due to chronic atrophic gastritis can be considered established, and no further diagnostic work-up is necessary. (Anti-

Table 1.   *Causes of Vitamin B_{12} Deficiency*

A. Poor intake
    1. Strict vegetarianism
    2. Infants of B_{12}-deficient mothers
B. Lack of intrinsic factor
    1. Pernicious anemia
        a. Adult type (chronic atrophic gastritis)°
        b. Congenital
    2. Total or partial gastrectomy°
    3. Congenitally abnormal intrinsic factor
    4. Diffuse gastric damage
        a. Infiltrative disease
        b. Corrosive ingestion
C. Jejunal bacterial overgrowth ("blind loop syndrome")
    1. Multiple jejunal diverticula°
    2. Following gastrointestinal surgery°
    3. Intestinal obstruction due to strictures
D. Fish tapeworm (*D. latum*) infestation
E. Ileal dysfunction
    1. Regional enteritis°
    2. Ileal resection°
    3. Tropical sprue°
    4. Ileal tuberculosis
    5. Radiation ileitis
    6. Lymphoma of ileum
    7. Congenital selective B_{12} malabsorption
F. Congenital deficiency of transcobalamin II

°Relatively common causes.

bodies directed against parietal cells are even more common in pernicious anemia, but there are too many false positives for the test to be diagnostically useful.)

If antibodies to IF are absent or the determination is not available, serial Schilling testing is the next diagnostic maneuver. In most hospitals, the Schilling test is performed first without added IF (so-called part I). If low, it is then repeated with IF (part II). With the exception of the very rare individual (in Western countries) with a pure dietary B_{12} deficiency, all patients who have developed B_{12} lack will have a low Schilling test without added IF (Table 2). Furthermore, if the test is low with IF, it will invariably be low without IF. Therefore, we believe that it makes more sense to do part II of the test first. Only if and when part II is normal is it meaningful to do the test without IF (part I). The expected results of serial Schilling tests in the clinically common causes of B_{12} deficiency are shown in Table 2. The Schilling test is usually performed by the 24-hour urinary excretion method, but some workers have found measurement of plasma radioactivity 8 to 12 hours after an oral dose of ^{57}Co-B_{12} equally reliable.

Since B_{12} deficiency itself may cause a megaloblastic gut, in 50 to 75 per cent of patients this may be associated with a transient impairment

Table 2.   *The Schilling Test in Patients with Vitamin B_{12} Deficiency*

Cause of B_{12} Deficiency	Without IF (Part I)	With IF (Part II)
Lack of intrinsic factor (IF)	Low	Normal
Bacterial overgrowth	Low	Low
Ileal dysfunction	Low	Low

of ileal function. Therefore, the Schilling test with IF may be low before B_{12} treatment or during the first 1 to 8 weeks of vitamin replacement. Since this ileal dysfunction is corrected after 1 week of treatment in most patients, we routinely defer Schilling testing until that time.

In IF antibody-negative patients in whom results of part II are persistently low, x-rays of the upper gastrointestinal tract, including small bowel "follow-through," are indicated and will usually demonstrate the cause of bacterial overgrowth or ileal dysfunction. In patients with tropical sprue or gluten-sensitive enteropathy, however, intestinal x-rays may be normal. Xylose testing (performed a week after initiating B_{12} therapy) and jejunal biopsy are helpful in the diagnosis of the sprue syndromes. In patients with one of the causes of jejunal bacterial overgrowth listed in Table 1, the Schilling test, without IF, may be repeated after 3 to 5 days of therapy with tetracycline or ampicillin and should be normal at that time.

The patient with a low part II Schilling test and normal x-rays and xylose absorption will usually be found to have pernicious anemia with a Schilling test (part II) that will return to normal within 2 months. However, in 5 to 10 per cent of patients with pernicious anemia, the test remains slightly low despite years of therapy. In such individuals (or in IF antibody-negative patients in whom Schilling testing is impossible because of renal disease or inability to collect a 24-hour urine), gastric analysis for acid secretion before and after pentagastrin (or betazole) injection will be helpful. Gastric pH should remain above 6 if the diagnosis of pernicious anemia due to chronic atrophic gastritis is to be entertained. Routine gastric analysis is no longer necessary in the average patient with this disease, since the diagnosis is established by more specific tests (serum antibody to IF or serial Schilling tests).

WORK-UP OF THE
FOLATE-DEFICIENT PATIENT

The possible causes of megaloblastic anemia due to folic acid deficiency are listed in Table 3. In most patients in whom folate lack has been

established the cause can be determined by history alone (alcoholism, poor diet, pregnancy, anticonvulsant drug therapy), and no further diagnostic tests are necessary or indicated. In patients in whom these factors cannot be identified by history, a small intestinal disorder should be suspected even if diarrhea is absent, and a xylose test, fecal fat analysis, and small intestinal x-ray (and possibly a jejunal biopsy) are indicated.

THERAPEUTIC TESTS

Therapeutic trials to differentiate folate from B_{12} lack are time-consuming, sometimes misleading, and usually unnecessary, unless serum folate and B_{12} concentrations are not available. If such trials are performed, small doses of the vitamins (1 to 2 micrograms of parenteral B_{12} or 100 micrograms of parenteral folic acid daily) should be used to avoid nonspecific responses. Reticulocyte elevations should occur within 7 to 10 days. The first trial is best undertaken with folic acid rather than B_{12}, because "spontaneous" reticulocytosis may occur during the first week in the hospital in folate-deficient patients owing to withdrawal of alcohol and resumption of folate intake.

Table 3.   *Causes of Folate Deficiency*

A. Poor intake
    1. Inadequate diet*
    2. Parenteral alimentation
B. Alcohol ingestion combined with poor intake*
C. Small intestinal disease
    1. Gluten-sensitive enteropathy*
    2. Tropical sprue*
    3. Regional enteritis
    4. Massive jejunal resection
    5. Intestinal lymphoma
    6. Congenital folate malabsorption
D. Increased requirements
    1. Pregnancy*
    2. Hemolytic anemia
    3. Infancy
E. Drug therapy
    1. Anticonvulsants
    2. Sulfasalazine
    3. ? Oral contraceptives
F. Inborn errors of folate metabolism
G. Combinations of the above*

   *Relatively common causes.

PITFALLS IN DIAGNOSIS

Some important pitfalls in diagnosis have already been mentioned, including the many possible causes of macrocytosis and macroovalocytosis, other conditions associated with neutrophil hypersegmentation, and various caveats in the interpretation of serum B_{12} and folate levels. In addition, certain other problems in diagnosis may occur.

1. A small percentage of patients with megaloblastic anemia due to B_{12} or folate deficiency will have a normal red cell MCV. Most commonly, a dimorphic blood smear containing both macroovalocytes and hypochromic microcytes will be observed. These patients will usually have another disorder in addition to B_{12} or folate lack, such as iron deficiency, thalassemia minor (present in 3 to 5 per cent of American blacks), alcohol-related sideroblastic anemia, or the anemia of chronic disease. In some iron-deficient patients who are also lacking in B_{12} or folate, the serum iron may be misleadingly normal. In addition, megaloblastic changes in erythroid precursors may be unimpressive or even absent in the iron-deficient state, although giant bands and metamyelocytes and hypersegmented neutrophils will be seen.

2. It is now recognized that many well-nourished chronic alcoholics will have a mildly elevated MCV (usually in the 100 to 110 range) without anemia. On blood smear, round rather than oval macrocytes are present and no hypersegmented neutrophils are found. In such patients the macrocytosis is not usually due to folate deficiency and does not respond to folic acid therapy, but will disappear only after several months of abstinence.

3. Alcoholics with all the typical features of folate deficiency anemia may also have prominent neurologic signs that are unrelated (e.g., due to thiamine deficiency). These patients may be mistakenly thought to be B_{12} deficient unless serum vitamin levels are obtained.

4. In addition to the problems in the interpretation of the Schilling test just discussed, it should be remembered that renal insufficiency (including that associated with minimal elevations of serum creatinine) and incomplete 24-hour urine collection are common artifactual causes of abnormal Schilling tests. Recently some batches of "intrinsic factor" commercially available in the United States and Canada have been shown to be inactive in promoting B_{12} absorption in the Schilling test in patients with pernicious anemia. Hopefully this problem will be corrected in the near future. Patients with pancreatic disease often have abnormal Schilling tests, but this is of little clinical significance since B_{12} deficiency does not develop as a result of pancreatic disease.

5. Some patients with apparent megaloblastic anemia caused by documented vitamin deficiency may fail to respond to B_{12} or folic acid therapy with an elevation of the reticulocyte count or hematocrit. Most commonly this is because of the presence of a second cause of anemia, such as iron deficiency or the anemia of chronic disease, or a coexistent infection. In such cases, repeat bone marrow examination after vitamin treatment will show disappearance of the megaloblastic changes. If such morphologic changes persist after 2 weeks of therapy with pharmacologic doses of B_{12} and folate, they are not due to deficiency of these vitamins, and other diagnoses such as refractory anemia, erythroleukemia, or a preleukemic state should be entertained.

IRON DEFICIENCY ANEMIA

By ARTHUR HAUT, M.D.
Little Rock, Arkansas

SYNONYMS

Iron lack anemia; anemia of chronic blood loss; incorrectly, hypochromic-microcytic anemia. The latter is incorrect as a synonym because iron deficiency is but one and not the only cause of hypochromic-microcytic anemia. That misconception is widely held.

DEFINITION

Anemia in which lack of iron per se is the limiting factor in erythropoiesis is correctly termed *iron deficiency anemia*. It is differentiated from *latent iron deficiency*, in which iron stores are exhausted but anemia is not present; *iron depletion*, in which iron stores in the bone marrow and elsewhere are less than normal, irrespective of the presence of anemia of any cause; and *iron-deficient erythropoiesis*, a general term referring to less than optimal delivery of iron to the erythron. The latter circumstance can result not only from lack of iron per se but also from chronic inflammatory diseases in which body iron stores are adequate but the mechanism for release of iron from the reticuloendothelial system is defective.

CLASSIFICATION

Iron deficiency anemia may be the leading cause of anemia, world wide. It is among the most common causes of anemia in the United States. It results from conditions in which either the supply of iron or its absorption from the intestine is subnormal, or else the loss of iron from the body is excessive. The only exceptions are idiopathic pulmonary hemosiderosis, in which the body iron is sequestered in the pulmonary macrophages, and the very rare congenital atransferrinemia, in which iron cannot be transported to erythroblasts, rather than actually being deficient in the body taken as a whole. In aspects other than retention of iron in the lung and marrow, respectively, these conditions are like other examples of iron deficiency anemia.

The diagnosis of iron deficiency anemia is best considered in three aspects: (1) grounds for suspecting its presence, (2) definitive tests for establishing the diagnosis, and (3) the diagnosis of the condition underlying the development of the iron-deficient state. Symptoms and signs provide the clues that lead to suspicion of iron deficiency anemia. When they are found, the physician should order the tests listed in Table 1. When positive, the test results establish the diagnosis of iron deficiency anemia. Nevertheless, iron deficiency anemia must be considered to be only one symptomatic manifestation of an underlying disease. Correct diagnosis of the underlying disease is the means for preventing recurrence of the iron deficiency anemia and may prevent serious and perhaps fatal consequences that could arise if the underlying disease, such as carcinoma of the colon, were to be undiagnosed.

PRESENTING SYMPTOMS AND SIGNS

In the healthy adult, body iron losses average about 1 mg per day, somewhat more in the menstruating female; iron absorption is of the same order from a diet that provides about 15 mg per day. In infancy, childhood, and pregnancy, wherein growth requires a greater supply of iron than that needed to offset normal losses, diet and dietary supplements play a greater role in the development of iron deficiency anemia than in other circumstances. In most patients,

Table 1. *Results of Differentiating Tests in Iron Deficiency and Simulating Anemias*

No.	Test°	Units	Common Test Results			
			NORMAL	IRON DEFICIENCY	THALASSEMIA HETEROZYGOTE	CHRONIC DISEASE
1	Hemoglobin concentration	gram/dl	♀ > 12 ♂ > 14	4–11	10.5–12.5	7.0–12.0
2	MCV	cu micra	83–96	70–80	65–77	77–90
3	MCHC	gram/dl rbc	32–36	25–32	29–33	28–34
4	Plasma iron	micrograms/dl	65–175	2–40	40–140	25–125
5	TIBC	micrograms/dl	250–400	275–425	225–425	150–375
6	Transferrin saturation	%	20–50	2–15	20–50	12–60
7	Serum ferritin	micrograms/dl	♀ > 35 ♂ > 69	1–10 1–10	♀ > 35 ♂ > 69	40–100 70–100
8	Marrow iron, (Prussian blue stain)	(Visual)	Normal	0–trace	Normal	Normal or increased
9	Marrow sideroblasts	%	30–50	0–8	> 10	6–30
10	Hb A_2	%	2.4–3.0	1.8–2.8	3.0–5.5	2.4–3.0
11	FEP	micrograms/dl	30–90	200–500	30–90	90–200

Abbreviations: Hb, hemoglobin; MCV, mean corpuscular volume; MCHC, mean corpuscular hemoglobin concentration; TIBC, total serum iron binding capacity; FEP, free erythrocyte protoporphyrin

°The first six tests usually suffice to identify iron deficiency anemia; less often, 7, or 8, and 9 are required. Test 10 differentiates beta-thalassemia heterozygotes from iron deficiency anemia. Tests 7 and 11 are used in population surveys for iron deficiency anemia. The combination of 2 and 10 surveys for beta-thalassemia.

excessive loss of iron, which generally occurs as pathologic blood loss, causes the development of iron deficiency anemia. For convenience of recall, the symptoms of iron deficiency anemia may be grouped as (1) symptoms common to cases of any cause and also according to the basis of the iron-deficient state, (2) excessive loss of iron, (3) deficient supply of iron or deficient absorption of iron.

Symptoms Common to All Patients. Weakness, fatigue, lassitude, pallid complexion, intolerance of cold, exertional dyspnea, and tachycardia are commonly found but are nonspecific. They are most prominent when anemia is severe or of more recent or more rapid development. Patients may also complain of dysphagia, angular stomatitis, or thin, brittle fingernails with spoon-like deformity (koilonychia).

Blood Loss–Related Symptoms. These may be of diverse causes (Table 2). Since iron deficiency anemia is most often the result of pathologic blood loss, the following symptoms are most important and most frequent: menorrhagia and intermenstrual vaginal blood loss, hematemesis, hematochezia, melena, hematuria, hemoglobinuria, chronic hemoptysis, and a history of therapeutic phlebotomies, polycythemia, multiple diagnostic venesections, or recurrent donations of blood for transfusions. Pregnancy causes an average net loss of about 700 mg of iron (about 2.5 mg per day) and lactation causes an additional loss of 0.5 to 1.0 mg per day. When those physiologic events occur and the diet is not supplemented with iron, excessive iron loss results. Therefore, those events may be considered as symptomatic evidence and signs suggesting the presence of iron deficiency anemia in the anemic woman.

Menorrhagia is notoriously difficult to recognize in many instances, even by women considered to be medically sophisticated. Any of the following should be considered to be evidence of menorrhagia: menstruation for more than 7 days; the passage of clots, especially after the first day, or of more than about 1 cm in size; the use of "double" pads or pads and tampons at the same time, or "super" pads or tampons for three or more days; or, possibly, the use of more than four pads or tampons in a day.

Occult blood loss is not recognizable as such by history, but it should be suspected if there are symptoms consistent with peptic ulcer, gastritis, or hiatal hernia. Daily ingestion of aspirin or alcohol is often associated with gastritis and occult blood loss, and therefore suggests iron deficiency anemia. Persistent or recurrent diarrhea, progressive constipation, or other major change in bowel habits may also be accompa-

Table 2. *Predecessors of Iron Deficiency Anemia: Conditions That Most Often Explain Pathologic Blood Loss*

Genital tract
  Dysfunctional uterine bleeding
  Submucosal uterine fibroids
  Grand multiparity

Gastrointestinal tract
  Hiatal hernia
  Gastritis due to aspirin or alcohol
  Gastric ulcer
    Benign and malignant
  Duodenal ulcer, peptic
  Leiomyoma of intestine
  Meckel's diverticulum
  Hookworm infestation
  Regional enteritis
  Celiac syndrome
  Carcinoma of colon and rectum
  Polyps of colon and rectum
  Diverticulosis coli
  Ulcerative colitis
  Bleeding hemorrhoids
  Hereditary hemorrhagic telangiectasia

Urinary tract
  Carcinoma of kidney
  Carcinoma of urinary bladder
  Hemoglobinuria and hemosiderinuria
    Due to traumatic hemolysis because of prosthetic heart valve
    Due to paroxysmal nocturnal hemoglobinuria

Respiratory tract
  Pulmonary hemosiderosis
  Goodpasture's syndrome

Phlebotomy
  Therapeutic
  Diagnostic
  Surreptitious

nied by occult blood loss. The stool should be tested for blood to evaluate those suspicions.

Diet-Related Symptoms. The average American diet is said to contain about 6 mg of iron per 1000 calories. Economic constraints, cultural and sociologic factors, food fadism that is especially significant for teenaged and obese females, and dependence upon unsupplemented milk diets in infancy are factors that can lead to diets deficient in iron. Inadequate food intake and iron intake due to those factors, anorexia, or pica, are important considerations in iron deficiency anemia. (Pica is the habitual ingestion of non-food substances.) It, particularly, should suggest iron deficiency anemia. Pica includes pagophagia (eating ice), geophagia (eating clay and other earths), and amylophagia (eating laundry starch). The last two may be culturally motivated but all seem to be associated with iron deficiency anemia. Certain clays retard the absorption of food iron.

Malabsorption-Related Symptoms. Steatorrhea, dumping syndrome, a history of gastric or intestinal resection, and geophagia are historical points that may be clues to the diagnosis of iron deficiency anemia.

PHYSICAL SIGNS

Pallor is most common. The sclerae are notably white and remarkably clear. Occasionally, atrophy of the lingual papillae may be seen. If koilonychia is found, iron deficiency anemia is strongly suggested. The spleen is rarely enlarged; when it is, it extends not more than 1 or 2 cm below the left costal margin. The discovery of hemorrhoids or a polyp or mass on rectal examination or sigmoidoscopy, or of uterine myomata on pelvic examination, are important clues. The telltale lesions of hereditary hemorrhagic telangectasia may be found on the vermilion border of the lips, or on the tongue, nasal septum, or finger tips, indicating the presence of that rare familial disorder that gives rise to iron deficiency anemia. However important these symptoms and physical signs may be as a guide, none of them are definitive evidence that iron deficiency anemia is present. This conclusion must come from certain laboratory tests (see later discussion).

COMMON COMPLICATIONS

The major complications are either cardiovascular or the consequence of failure to diagnose and treat the disease that caused the iron deficiency anemia. Examples of the former relate to the severity of the anemia and include angina pectoris, tachyarrhythmias, and congestive heart failure. Examples of the latter are metastatic carcinoma of the stomach, colon, or kidney, or acute hemorrhage or perforation from a duodenal ulcer. Esophageal web, retinal hemorrhages, and increased intracranial pressure are rare complications of iron deficiency anemia.

LABORATORY FINDINGS

Whereas symptoms and signs lead to the suspicion of iron deficiency anemia, the diagnosis is made only with certain laboratory tests (Table 1). Anemia must be present; that is, the hemoglobin concentration is less than 14.0 grams per dl (100 ml) in the adult male and less than 12.0 grams per dl in the adult female. In children, the lower limit of normal hemoglobin concentration is related to age. After infancy, less than 10 grams per dl is always abnormal,

whereas higher values may be subnormal at other ages of childhood.

Classically, this finding signifies iron deficiency anemia: a hypochromic-microcytic anemia as indicated by microscopic examination of the blood film showing small, pale red blood cells and subnormal red cell indices (low mean corpuscular volume [MCV] and low mean corpuscular hemoglobin concentration [MCHC]), with hypoferremia, an increased total serum iron-binding capacity, and the serum transferrin saturation being less than 16 per cent (Table 1). If the symptoms and signs discussed are present, and especially if there is objective evidence of pathologic blood loss, further laboratory tests are not needed. When the data are equivocal or conflicting, the serum ferritin may be measured.

Bone marrow examination is usually not needed. It is uncomfortable for the patient and less well accepted and more expensive than blood studies. For these reasons, it is reserved for cases not resolved by the tests listed before it. If the marrow is examined, aspiration is usually sufficient rather than routinely doing a biopsy as well. If iron is found in any more than trace amounts, the diagnosis of iron deficiency anemia may be excluded. Marrow examination is most helpful in the latter context. However, if satisfactory marrow particles are not obtained on aspiration, bone marrow biopsy may be needed.

In iron deficiency anemia the marrow is hypercellular and has erythroid hyperplasia, poor hemoglobinization of the normoblasts, and a low myeloid-to-erythroid ratio. Most importantly, iron stores are absent when aspirates or biopsies are studied by the Prussian blue reaction or when wet mounts of unstained, fresh marrow aspirates are examined. Sideroblasts are normoblasts that contain fine ferritin granules demonstrable by the Prussian blue reaction. Sideroblasts are rarely found in iron deficiency anemia (average 2.5 per cent of all normoblasts), whereas in most other kinds of anemia sideroblasts are at least four times as common. The red cells of sideroblastic anemia resemble those of iron deficiency anemia morphologically, but finding of large numbers of sideroblasts in the marrow and of ringed sideroblasts readily distinguishes this condition from iron deficiency anemia. Hemoglobin electrophoresis and the hemoglobin A_2 fraction are normal in iron deficiency anemia.

Except for the absence of iron in the bone marrow, not all of these classical findings may occur in every case. Furthermore, even the absence of iron in the bone marrow does not establish that an anemia is due to iron deficiency. That is because iron depletion itself is not rare, and it may coexist with an anemia of another cause. No single test should be considered the sine qua non of the diagnosis of iron deficiency anemia. Rather, the concurrence of findings assures the correctness of the diagnosis. When the anemia is of slight degree, or of recent onset, either the MCV and the MCHC, or both, may be normal. In that circumstance, when symptoms or signs suggest iron deficiency anemia, it is best that many of the tests be done. The tests most useful for the diagnosis of iron deficiency anemia, and the common results in that condition and in differentiating it from anemias that mimic it, are given in Table 1. Other tests are useful less often. The absorption of an orally administered tracer dose of radioactive cobalt is increased in iron deficiency anemia, and that is revealed by the increased excretion of the isotope in the urine. The plasma transferrin clearance (t ½) is abnormally short on ferrokinetic study with radioactive iron. Values of 10 to 20 minutes are commonly found, whereas the normal range is 60 to 120 minutes. The urinary excretion of an iron-chelate complex after the parenteral administration of deferoxamine or diethylenetriaminepentacetic acid (DTPA) is less than normal in patients with iron deficiency anemia, whereas in those with anemia of other causes it is normal or greater. These tests are of limited usefulness because of the time involved and the inconvenience to the patient. The chelation test is further limited by some overlap between results in some normals and in patients with iron deficiency anemia.

OTHER BIOCHEMICAL FINDINGS

The free erythrocyte protoporphyrin (FEP) is increased in iron deficiency anemia, often to about 200 to 500 micrograms per dl, and generally it is greater than 100 micrograms per dl. However, in other conditions, including the anemia of chronic disease, malignancy, and lead poisoning, the FEP is also elevated. The highest values occur in lead poisoning. The normal minor hemoglobin component of adults, designated hemoglobin A_2, is normal or somewhat reduced in iron deficiency anemia. Best determined by column chromatography, it differentiates beta thalassemia from iron deficiency anemia, because in the former the A_2 fraction is increased. When both conditions coexist, the increase in A_2 may not be appreciated until the iron deficiency is treated. In that circumstance the persistence of microcytosis provides the clue.

URINALYSIS

Routine urine analysis is normal, unless there is hematuria or hemoglobinuria as a sign of the condition that caused the iron deficiency anemia. Hemosiderinuria, detected by the Prussian blue reaction on the urine sediment, is found when iron deficiency is the result of paroxysmal nocturnal hemoglobinuria (Marchiafava-Micheli syndrome) or traumatic hemolysis owing to a prosthetic heart valve, or, rarely, owing to an abnormal natural valve.

THERAPEUTIC TESTS

The ultimate proof of the diagnosis of iron deficiency anemia lies in the therapeutic test, that is, the complete recovery of the patient and the restoration of the abnormal laboratory tests that were interpreted as due to iron deficiency to normal soon after the administration of therapeutic amounts of iron. When 0.3 gram of ferrous sulfate is taken by mouth once to three times daily, the reticulocyte count should rise from about 1 per cent to a peak of from 5 to 15 per cent, commonly 5 to 8 per cent, within 5 to 8 days. The hemoglobin concentration in the blood should be restored to normal values in 4 to 8 weeks, regardless of the degree of anemia at the outset, if iron deficiency is the *sole cause* of the anemia. However, a therapeutic test is not advised as the means to make the diagnosis. That is because improvement coincident with the administration of iron does not prove a cause-and-effect relationship. For example, improvement in a transient hemolytic anemia, such as that associated with administration of a drug to a patient with glucose-6-phosphate dehydrogenase deficiency, would have occurred whether or not iron was being given. The false inference of iron deficiency anemia would then lead to unwarranted search for pathologic blood loss, and the failure to protect the patient from the subsequent administration of the offending drug.

Particularly, one should never administer a combination "hematinic" preparation containing, in addition to iron, folic acid and vitamin B_{12}, as a therapeutic test for iron deficiency anemia. The inclusion of the other compounds deprives the physician of the opportunity of confirming the diagnosis by the response to a single agent or discovering that failure of the patient to respond has upset the diagnosis. A misdiagnosis or an incomplete diagnosis can prove to be unnecessarily expensive and detrimental to the patient, and eventually for the physician as well.

PITFALLS IN THE DIAGNOSIS

Whereas the presence of a hypochromic-microcytic anemia or of hypoferremia is generally an indicator of iron deficiency anemia, either or both of these may be found less often in other conditions. The administration of iron is not beneficial in other types of anemia and is sometimes harmful. Thalassemia heterozygotes are the patients who are probably most frequently misdiagnosed as having iron deficiency anemia. However, in these patients hypochromia on the blood film appears greater than that suggested by the MCHC, because the leptocytes of thalassemia are thinner than normal red cells and thus appear very pale. The MCV in thalassemia is generally quite low, 65 to 75 cu micra, even though in the heterozygote the anemia may be slight (hemoglobin concentration 10 to 12 grams per dl). Thalassemia rather than iron deficiency anemia should be suspected in a hypochromic microcytic anemia if splenomegaly is found, target cells are seen on the blood film, or the anemia is familial. The tests listed (Table 1) should permit differentiation. Anemia of chronic disease, sideroblastic anemia, or lead poisoning should be suspected if the preliminary tests are equivocal or conflicting. The bone marrow iron or serum ferritin should differentiate them, since in conditions other than iron deficiency anemia, normal or even greater than normal marrow iron stores may be seen owing to the diversion of iron from circulating hemoglobin to the marrow reserve pool.

The most common pitfall is to consider the diagnosis of iron deficiency anemia to be complete before the mechanism for the development of iron deficiency has been discovered. Unless there is incontrovertible proof of grossly inadequate iron intake or malabsorption, one must look for the source of pathologic blood loss. However, even in children with iron-deficient diets and adults after gastrectomy, pathologic blood loss has often been shown to be a contributing factor.

THE SIDEROBLASTIC ANEMIAS

By EDWARD R. EICHNER, M.D.

Oklahoma City, Oklahoma

SYNONYMS

Refractory sideroblastic anemia, iron-loading anemia, pyridoxine-responsive anemia, sideroachrestic anemia, refractory normoblastic anemia, chronic refractory anemia with sideroblastic bone marrow.

DEFINITION AND CLASSIFICATION

The sideroblastic anemias comprise a diverse group of disorders that has the following features in common: (1) hypochromic red blood cells, (2) elevated serum iron and elevated saturation of total iron-binding capacity, (3) ineffective erythropoiesis, and (4) bone marrow findings of erythroid hyperplasia and numerous pathognomonic ringed sideroblasts, i.e., erythroblasts with a ring of Prussian blue–positive iron granules around the nucleus. The hypochromic red cells reflect the block in formation of heme; the hyperferremia reflects the ineffective erythropoiesis, which can be documented by ferrokinetic studies that show an increased plasma iron turnover and erythroid iron turnover but a subnormal adult red cell incorporation of iron; and the ringed sideroblasts reflect the deposition, because of the block in heme formation, of nonheme iron in the mitochondria.

Ringed sideroblasts, which are pathologic, must be differentiated from normal marrow sideroblasts. In normal persons, 20 to 80 per cent of the nucleated erythroid cells are sideroblasts, which contain one to six minute granules of nonheme, ferritin iron. These Prussian blue–positive granules, containing iron beyond that needed for normal heme formation, do not form a ring around the nucleus because they are too few and because they are in the cytoplasm, not in the mitochondria.

Inasmuch as the sideroblastic anemias are heterogeneous, several different classifications have been put forward. Some investigators have divided sideroblastic anemias into (1) primary, either hereditary or acquired; (2) secondary; and (3) pyridoxine-responsive forms. Since most of the hereditary forms are variably pyridoxine-responsive and most of the acquired forms do not show much response to pyridoxine, the classification shown in Table 1 groups sideroblastic anemias into hereditary and acquired forms, and the acquired forms are grouped according to presumed common pathophysiology.

The hereditary sideroblastic anemias are a heterogeneous group with variable response to pyridoxine. In the majority, a sex-linked inheritance is evident, but some kindreds seem to have an autosomal recessive pattern. In the classic sex-linked, pyridoxine-responsive type, affected males are usually diagnosed in youth, but occasionally not until adulthood. The female carriers (heterozygotes) usually have little or no anemia but have some hypochromic red cells and occasionally a high serum iron. Female heterozygotes tend to have a dimorphic smear, and isolation in such heterozygotes of two red cell populations differing in red cell

Table 1.   *Sideroblastic Anemias — Classification*

I. Hereditary (variably pyridoxine-responsive)
   A. Sex-linked
   B. Autosomal recessive

II. Acquired
   A. Idiopathic refractory
   B. Drugs or toxins (reversible)
      1. Alcohol, lead, chloramphenicol
      2. Isoniazid (INH), pyrazinamide, cycloserine
      3. Azathioprine
   C. Associated with acute myelocytic leukemia, preleukemia, di Guglielmo's syndrome, multiple myeloma, aplastic anemia, myelofibrosis, or other hematologic malignancy
   D. Complicating other diseases
      1. Plausible link: severe malabsorption, certain hemolytic anemias, erythropoietic porphyria, porphyria cutanea tarda
      2. Possibly coincidental: rheumatoid arthritis, polyarteritis, systemic lupus erythematosus, thyroid disease, carcinoma

antigens and in porphyrin content supports the concept of two clones of red cells. Presumably, affected males inherit the X chromosome that codes for a defective delta-aminolevulinic acid synthetase, the rate-controlling mitochondrial enzyme of heme synthesis. Large pharmacologic doses of pyridoxine, the coenzyme for delta-aminolevulinic acid synthetase, normalize the hemoglobin but do not completely correct the peripheral smear or bone marrow, in about 20 per cent of cases, presumably by mass action by saturating the defective apoenzyme with coenzyme. Other patients get some improvement with pyridoxine therapy, but a few show no response. The patients who respond are not nutritionally deficient in pyridoxine; they do not respond to physiologic doses.

The acquired sideroblastic anemias are far more common than the hereditary. Of these, the most common is idiopathic refractory sideroblastic anemia, which usually occurs in older adults of both sexes and also gives evidence of being a clonal disease, perhaps from a stem cell mutation. The dimorphic smear suggests two clones of red cells, and the population of smaller, hypochromic cells has elevated protoporphyrin content, decreased iron incorporation, and decreased survival as compared to the population of normal red cells.

Drugs or toxins can cause reversible sideroblastic anemia. Alcohol is probably the most common cause of reversible ring sideroblastic anemia. Up to 30 per cent of skid row alcoholics hospitalized because of complications of alcoholism have folate-deficient megaloblastic anemia with numerous ring sideroblasts, but sideroblastic anemia is uncommon in alcoholics

still functioning in the community. Ring sideroblastic changes, along with megaloblastic changes, have been induced in volunteers ingesting alcohol under controlled conditions.

The mechanism by which alcohol induces ring sideroblasts is still debated. Initially, it was thought that red cell levels of pyridoxal phosphate were subnormal because alcohol-inhibited pyridoxine kinase or because acetaldehyde, a metabolite of alcohol, enhanced degradation of pyridoxal phosphate. Recent work suggests that erythrocyte pyridoxine kinase activity is normal in alcoholics and that there is no major intracellular deficiency of pyridoxal phosphate. In vitro, alcohol inhibits the heme synthetic pathway at several loci, mainly at delta-aminolevulinic acid synthetase. Also, it seems likely that prerequisites for the formation of ring sideroblasts may be (1) structural damage to mitochrondria induced by alcohol and (2) rapid cycling of iron induced by the ineffective erythropoiesis of the concomitant folate deficiency.

Lead causes ring sideroblasts by inhibiting the heme synthetic pathway at several loci, primarily at amino-levulinic acid dehydrase but also at delta-aminolevulinic acid synthetase and at heme synthetase. Chloramphenicol causes ring sideroblasts primarily by inhibiting mitochondrial protein synthesis and causing ultrastructural damage to mitochondria. Azathioprine has caused anemia with macrocytosis and ring sideroblasts in renal transplant patients and when used for immunosuppresive therapy for autoimmune hemolytic anemia.

The three antituberculosis drugs listed in Table 1 have all caused ring sideroblastic anemia. The main offender has been isoniazid (INH), which combines with pyridoxal to form a hydrazone that inhibits pyridoxal kinase. The number of reported cases of sideroblastic anemia in patients receiving INH is small in relation to the widespread use of this drug. Thus, perhaps certain individuals are genetically or nutritionally predisposed to developing ring sideroblastic anemia from INH. In this light, it has recently been shown that the mean erythrocyte pyridoxine kinase activity in American blacks is approximately 50 per cent lower than in American whites. There have been a few reports of ring sideroblastic anemia from pyrazinamide (mechanism unknown) and from cycloserine, which inactivates pyridoxal by binding with it and which also directly inhibits pyridoxine kinase.

Acquired sideroblastic anemia occurs in association with a wide variety of serious and malignant diseases of bone marrow. This association, along with the aforementioned evidence for clonality of the anemia, suggests that some sideroblastic anemias arise as a mutation of a multipotent marrow stem cell. This concept is further strengthened by the demonstration of chromosomal abnormalities, such as an extra C chromosome, in some cases of sideroblastic anemia, and by certain "leukemia-like" abnormalities when stem cells from sideroblastic marrows are grown in vitro in culture. The transformation of sideroblastic anemia into leukemia will be dealt with later in the discussion.

Ring sideroblastic anemia has complicated diverse diseases. In some instances, a causative association seems plausible. One example is a patient with severe malabsorption from adult celiac disease treated with folic acid and massive doses of iron, but not with pyridoxine. Other examples are patients with mechanical hemolytic anemia treated with massive parenteral doses of iron and a few patients with certain types of porphyria, such as erythropoietic porphyria, in which heme synthetase is deficient, and porphyria cutanea tarda, in which red cell uroporphyrinogen decarboxylase is deficient. In other instances, the relationship may be coincidental. Sporadic cases of sideroblastic anemia associated with rheumatoid arthritis, polyarteritis, systemic lupus erythematosus, thyroid disease, carcinoma, lymphoma, and infectious mononucleosis have been reported, but the mechanisms responsible for the sideroblastic anemia and the relationship, if any, to the associated diseases remain uncertain.

PRESENTING SIGNS AND SYMPTOMS

The mode of presentation of the sideroblastic anemia is influenced by the age of the patient and by the type and duration of sideroblastic anemia involved. The sex-linked type occurs mainly in boys and young men who present with pallor but few or no symptoms; the anemia is usually mild-to-moderate in degree. In up to 50 per cent of these patients, tissue iron-loading occurs slowly, presumably from lifelong increased absorption of dietary iron and from chronic hyperferremia from the ineffective erythropoiesis; in time, some patients develop the clinical picture of hemochromatosis. Female heterozygotes usually have little or no anemia, and therefore no symptoms.

The older patients (most are over 50) with idiopathic refractory sideroblastic anemia usually have moderately severe anemia and present with fatigue, but some present with angina, congestive heart failure, or cerebral dysfunction. Nonspecific symptoms of the anemia include easy fatigability, weakness, general lassitude, dyspnea on exertion, headache, and nausea. The symptoms may develop insidiously and be present for years before the patient sees a doctor. Splenomegaly, usually mild but occasionally considerable, occurs in about half of these patients, and hepatomegaly also occurs, although the degree of tissue iron-loading is usually mild.

In the sideroblastic anemias from drugs or toxins, the clinical picture is dominated by the effects of the drug or toxin. The typical patient with alcoholic ring sideroblasts is a derelict who has concomitant folate deficiency, malnutrition, and liver disease. In adults with lead poisoning the cardinal features are abdominal cramps, constipation, or peripheral neuropathy, along with a lead line on the gums; symptoms of anemia play only a minor role. With antituberculosis drugs the anemia develops insidiously during many months on the drug; the patient can present with severe anemia and symptoms therefrom.

When the sideroblastic anemia is associated with another disease, the features of the other disease usually predominate. An exception is the ring sideroblastic anemia that serves as a harbinger of late leukemia in multiple myeloma. A recent study showed that 4 of 75 patients with myeloma developed sideroblastic anemia, and, within 6 months, all 4 developed acute myelomonoblastic leukemia. Late leukemia now occurs in about 2 per cent of patients with myeloma. It is probably related to the mutagenic effects of melphalan therapy, although it may be an unmasking of a hitherto unrecognized aspect of the natural history of myeloma because of the prolonged survival induced by the chemotherapy. So far, the late leukemia that occurs in Hodgkin's disease patients, especially those treated with both chemotherapy and irradiation, and in patients with ovarian cancer has not been reported to be preceded by a clear-cut sideroblastic anemia, although this may be found if sought. There is at least one report of sideroblastic anemia as an early feature of di Guglielmo's erythroleukemia that developed in a patient with Hodgkin's disease.

PHYSICAL EXAMINATION FINDINGS

Physical findings vary with the type of sideroblastic anemia, the age of the patient, and the severity and duration of the anemia. There may be no findings, or only pallor. There may be tachypnea, hyperpnea, venous distension, hemic murmurs, gallops, rales, edema, and other signs of congestive heart failure. Hepatosplenomegaly is variable. Eventual hemochromatosis, especially in the hereditary forms, can cause hyperpigmentation of the skin, some jaundice, and even testicular atrophy.

LABORATORY FINDINGS

Peripheral Blood. In the hereditary, sex-linked variety, usually the entire red cell population is hypochromic and microcytic, with marked variation in size and shape, so that it closely resembles comparably severe cases of iron deficiency or thalassemia. Female heterozygotes have a dimorphic population, one normal and one hypochromic, microcytic. Patients with idiopathic refractory sideroblastic anemia also have a dimorphic smear, suggesting the emergence of an abnormal clone. One population of red cells is normal-to-macrocytic (presumably macrocytic because of elevated levels of erythropoietin), while the abnormal population (clone) is distinctly hypochromic microcytic. Although there is great variability, the abnormal clone usually predominates. Depending upon the severity of anemia, nucleated red cells may be seen. Basophilic stippling (especially in the hypochromic cells) is common, and one usually sees a few siderocytes. Leukocytes and platelets are usually normal, although some patients with idiopathic refractory sideroblastic anemia have moderate-to-marked thrombocytosis. Hypersegmentation of the polymorphonuclear leukocytes is not seen in these patients. Because of the ineffective erythropoiesis, reticulocytes, which appear as polychromatic cells on Wright stain, are not as frequent as marrow erythroid activity would predict.

In alcoholics, while there are a few hypochromic microcytes, there is not really a dimorphic population, as the macrocytosis of concomitant folate deficiency usually predominates and is associated with hypersegmentation of the polymorphonuclear leukocytes. Likewise, in the sideroblastic anemia from antituberculosis drugs the smear is generally hypochromic and microcytic, not dimorphic.

In the cases of sideroblastic anemia associated with acute myelomonoblastic leukemia, a few myeloblasts or monoblasts may be seen in the smear, along with other young myeloid forms, and thrombocytopenia. During the preleukemic phase, one may see abnormal neutrophils with stunted granule formation and hyposegmentation, the pseudo–Pelger-Hüet anomaly.

The degree of anemia is variable. Older patients with the idiopathic form usually have hemoglobin concentrations from 7 to 10 grams per dl (100 ml), whereas young boys with the sex-linked form range from almost normal to as low as 5 grams per dl, and patients taking antituberculosis drugs can present with a level as low as 4 grams per dl. The mean corpuscular volume is usually subnormal in the sex-linked form (and in that caused by antituberculosis drugs), and usually high-normal to macrocytic (sometimes low-normal) in the idiopathic refractory form. Since the latter disorder comprises a bimodal size population, one small and one normal-to-large, the resultant mean corpuscular volume obviously must vary with the relative size of each clone. Alcoholics with ring sideroblasts usually have macrocytic indices because of folate deficiency.

Bone Marrow. The bone marrow is hypercellular with marked erythroid hyperplasia. Except in alcoholics, the erythroid series, although often "macronormoblastic," probably because of a high level of erythropoietin drive, is not megaloblastic. In the preleukemic or leukemic forms of acquired ring sideroblastic anemia, the red cell series may be megaloblastoid or may show the multinuclearity (2, 4, or even 8 nuclei in 1 erythroblast) characteristic of erythroleukemia. Granulocytic precursors are normal in numbers and maturation except in preleukemic or leukemic patients, who show increased numbers of myeloblasts or promyelocytes and in patients with folate deficiency, who show giant myelocytes and metamyelocytes. Megakaryocytes are usually normal, although an occasional patient with idiopathic refractory sideroblastic anemia may have marked thrombocytosis and marked proliferation of megakaryocytes.

The pathognomonic hallmark is the ringed sideroblast best seen on Prussian blue–stained films of aspirated marrow. Characteristically, a dense ring of 10 to 20 coarse blue granules, mainly iron-laden mitochondria, is seen around the nucleus of 40 to 80 per cent or more of the erythroblasts. By electron microscopy, these cells contain massive amounts of non-heme iron as ferruginous micelles within the interstices of the inner cristae of the mitochondria, often producing distortions of the inner membrane of the mitochondria. Iron deposits in the reticuloendothelial cells are often massively increased. In thalassemia major, in certain hemolytic anemias, and in pernicious anemia and some cases of folate deficiency, the erythroblasts, because of high serum iron levels, have increased numbers of small ferritin granules distributed randomly in the cytoplasm; these are not in mitochondria, and these abnormal sideroblasts, which have no pathophysiologic significance, should not be mistaken for ring sideroblasts.

ADDITIONAL LABORATORY FINDINGS

All sideroblastic anemias characteristically have high-normal or elevated serum iron levels and an increased per cent saturation of the total iron-binding capacity. In some patients with excessive body iron, the serum iron is very high and transferrin is completely saturated. Serum ferritin levels increase in proportion to the progressive expansion of the body iron load.

The erythrocyte protoporphyrin concentration is subnormal (or normal) in the sex-linked, pyridoxine-responsive type, reflecting deficient formation of the precursor, delta-aminolevulinic acid. In most of the other types, erythrocyte protoporphyrin level is increased, ranging from 40 to as high as 500 micrograms per dl, suggesting an accompanying functional deficiency of heme synthetase, either primary, or secondary to mitochondrial iron-loading. In lead poisoning and erythropoietic porphyria, and in the clone of hypochromic, microcytic cells in preleukemic acquired sideroblastic anemia, the protoporphyrin level may be strikingly elevated (over 1500 micrograms per dl) compared to the normal range of 10 to 35 micrograms per dl.

Hemoglobin electrophoresis and hemoglobin F and A_2 levels are normal. In up to two thirds of patients with idiopathic refractory sideroblastic anemia, serum and red cell folate levels are low or subnormal, and leukocyte alkaline phosphatase values are low. Radioactive chromium (^{51}Cr)–labeled red cell survival is usually only slightly shortened, although the survival of the abnormal clone is markedly shortened. Ferrokinetic studies reveal the aforementioned pattern of ineffective erythropoiesis, resulting from destruction of developing red cells within the marrow. Bilirubinemia is usually mild. Tests of hepatic and renal function are normal unless affected by associated disease. Patients with alcoholic ring sideroblasts have subnormal serum levels of pyridoxal phosphate, along with laboratory evidence of folate deficiency, but their red cell content of pyridoxal phosphate may be normal or near-normal.

BIOCHEMICAL FINDINGS

These have been adequately covered in the preceding discussion. The exact pathogenesis of most types of sideroblastic anemia remains unproved, but there are increasing reports of a primary defect in the formation of delta-aminolevulinic acid, presumably because of an abnormality in delta-aminolevulinic acid synthetase, the rate-limiting enzyme of heme synthesis, in both the hereditary and idiopathic refractory forms of sideroblastic anemia. Although the response to pyridoxine in idiopathic refractory sideroblastic anemia is usually disappointing, a few reports have appeared of partial response to the active form of the coenzyme, pyridoxal phosphate. These reports, however, need to be confirmed more widely before pyridoxal phosphate is advocated as a possible therapy.

THERAPEUTIC TESTS

There is no reliable therapeutic test for ring sideroblastic anemia. The diagnosis is made by demonstrating the ring sideroblasts by marrow iron stain.

Perhaps 20 per cent of patients with hereditary sideroblastic anemia will correct their anemia with pharmacologic (50 to 200 mg per day) doses of pyridoxine. Their marrow and peripheral blood will still show subtle abnormalities. If the pyridoxine is discontinued, a full relapse will occur within 2 months. The remaining 80 per cent of patients with hereditary sideroblastic anemia show little or no response to pyridoxine.

Most American investigators agree that most patients with idiopathic acquired sideroblastic anemia show little response to either folic acid or pyridoxine, alone or together, although, as mentioned in the preceding discussion, some report partial response to pyridoxal phosphate. Some British investigators report partial responses to folic acid or pyridoxine or both in apparently similar patients.

Alcoholics respond promptly to withdrawal of alcohol and institution of a nutritious diet. Patients with sideroblastic anemia from antituberculous drugs improve when the drugs are halted or when pyridoxine is given along with the drugs.

COURSE AND COMPLICATIONS

There are two subsets of patients with hereditary sideroblastic anemia. The smaller group are the boys who are severely anemic in their first decade and who require frequent transfusions. They follow a course much like that of thalassemia major, with death in childhood. The larger group have a milder anemia, usually first diagnosed in adolescence or early adulthood. They require few or no transfusions and follow a chronic course, often progressively complicated by signs of tissue iron overload and, finally, the clinical picture of hemochromatosis. The present and future use of chelating agents by continuous subcutaneous infusion may greatly improve the long-term outlook of such patients by preventing or ameliorating iron overload. Splenectomy is contraindicated in hereditary sideroblastic anemia; it does not improve the anemia, and it may be followed by marked thrombocytosis with lethal thromboembolism.

Adults with idiopathic refractory sideroblastic anemia can also be divided into two groups. Those with mild, stable anemia not requiring transfusion usually follow a mild, nonprogressive course lasting from 5 to more than 15 years, with most deaths from causes unrelated to the sideroblastic anemia. The prognosis is worse in the other group, those requiring transfusions. These patients tend to die earlier of complications of the anemia; some have a transformation into acute myelomonoblastic leukemia.

While there is no way to predict with certainty whether an individual patient will develop leukemia, there are recent reports that patients with thrombocytosis (from 500,000 per cu mm to 2 million per cu mm) are less likely to develop leukemia than those with normal or low platelet counts, and that patients with acquired hemoglobin H (beta chain tetramers, also seen in erythroleukemia) are more likely to develop acute leukemia than those lacking this "preleukemic marker" on routine hemoglobin electrophoresis. The estimates of the rate of transformation of idiopathic refractory sideroblastic anemia into acute leukemia range from a low of 7.5 per cent to a high of 50 per cent, and the growing consensus is that the "true" incidence is around 20 per cent. Leukemic transformation does not occur in hereditary sideroblastic anemia.

PITFALLS IN DIAGNOSIS

The major pitfall in the diagnosis of ring sideroblastic anemia is the failure to think of it and thus the failure to look carefully at an iron stain of an aspirated bone marrow film. The most common misdiagnosis is probably iron deficiency anemia. Oral iron therapy of sideroblastic anemia is, of course, contraindicated, because it may augment the tissue iron overload and will not improve the anemia. Sometimes the dimorphic smear is initially confused with iron plus folate or vitamin B_{12} deficiency. The serum iron values should easily separate iron deficiency anemia, with a subnormal serum iron level and a per cent saturation of total iron-binding capacity usually under 15 per cent, from sideroblastic anemia, with a high-normal or elevated serum iron level and a per cent saturation usually well over 70 per cent. Serum ferritin, subnormal in iron deficiency and elevated in ring sideroblastic anemia, should also help in the differential diagnosis. The definitive test is the bone marrow iron stain, which shows absent iron stores and markedly decreased to absent sideroblasts in iron deficiency, but the pathognomonic ring sideroblasts and increased iron stores in sideroblastic anemia.

Thalassemia major or intermedia presents more difficulty in differential diagnosis, because this autosomal recessive anemia shares the hypochromic red cells, the elevated serum iron, the increased marrow iron stores, the tissue iron overload, and even an increase in marrow sideroblasts, although there are few or no actual ring sideroblasts. Other helpful differentiating tests are the frequent Mediterranean ancestry of patients, the equal sex incidence, and the elevation in hemoglobin A_2 or F in thalassemia.

Hypoplastic or aplastic anemia, despite the associated high serum iron level, should not be confused with sideroblastic anemia. The red cells in a hypoplastic anemia should look fairly normal, not hypochromic, and the bone marrow will be hypoplastic, not hypercellular with erythroid hyperplasia, as with ring sideroblastic anemia. Marrows in hypoplastic or aplastic anemias do not show ring sideroblasts. There are a few instances in which sideroblastic anemia followed recovery from aplastic anemia.

Primary sideroblastic anemia may be temporarily masked by blood loss. If an elderly patient with idiopathic refractory sideroblastic anemia has major gastrointestinal bleeding, for example, marrow iron may be depleted, serum iron may fall, and ring sideroblasts may disappear. The underlying sideroblastic anemia may nevertheless be suspected because of the dimorphic peripheral smear and a few residual siderocytes that can be confirmed by doing a Prussian blue stain on the peripheral smear. When iron is repleted in such a patient, the ring sideroblastic anemia will again become fully manifest.

THALASSEMIA

By FRANCES McNIELL GILL, M.D.
Philadelphia, Pennsylvania

The thalassemic disorders result from decreased production of one or more of the globin chains of hemoglobin. Each hemoglobin molecule is composed of four polypeptide chains. The composition of the hemoglobins normally present is hemoglobin A (Hb A) $\alpha_2 \beta_2$; hemoglobin A_2 (Hb A_2) $\alpha_2 \delta_2$; and hemoglobin F (Hb F) $\alpha_2 \gamma_2$. Production of each globin chain is under specific gene control. Presence of a thalassemia allele results in decreased production of all the hemoglobin types containing that globin chain. The common forms are beta and alpha thalassemia. Other thalassemic disorders and thalassemia-like states are mentioned briefly.

BETA THALASSEMIA

There are two beta thalassemia alleles. The beta⁰ thalassemia allele is associated with absent beta chain production and the beta⁺ thalassemia allele with decreased levels of beta chain production. The beta thalassemia alleles are widely distributed but are most common in people from the Mediterranean area, Southeast Asia, India, and parts of northern and western Africa. However, the gene occurs sporadically in all populations and cases of beta thalassemia trait have been described in people of many ethnic origins, including Northern European peoples.

BETA THALASSEMIA TRAIT

Synonyms. Beta thalassemia minor, heterozygous beta thalassemia, beta thalassemia trait of the high Hb A_2 variety.

Definition. Beta thalassemia trait is the heterozygous condition characterized by decreased beta chain production and mild hematologic abnormalities.

Clinical Course and Findings. Patients with beta thalassemia trait are usually asymptomatic, although fatigue is a common complaint. Physical findings are mild pallor in some patients and minimal splenic enlargement in a few. During pregnancy anemia may be accentuated and may in a few women be severe enough to require the transfusion of red blood cells.

There are no common complications unless iron therapy, particularly with intramuscular preparations, has been given long enough to cause excessive iron storage in the body.

Laboratory Findings. Mild anemia is present, generally at the level of 9 to 11 grams per dl(100 ml) in children and women and 12 to 14 grams per dl in men and postpubertal boys. The red cell count is mildly elevated in many patients. The mean cell volume (MCV) is reduced usually to 55 to 70 cu micra and the mean cell hemoglobin (MCH) is decreased to about 20 to 23 picograms, while the mean cell hemoglobin content (MCHC) is normal or almost so. Mild reticulocytosis of 2 to 4 per cent is commonly present. Examination of the peripheral blood smear reveals small red cells with poor hemoglobin content and some variation in red cell size and shape. The degree of anisocytosis and poikilocytosis varies from minimal changes in some patients to moderate abnormalities in others.

Several families with beta thalassemia trait of unusual severity have been described. The clinical course is more severe with symptomatic anemia, gallstone formation, leg ulcers, and need for splenectomy in some patients. The anemia has been moderate with marked reticulocytosis and red cell changes on peripheral smear that are more similar to beta thalassemia major than to beta thalassemia trait. Elevations of Hb A_2 and F, however, are similar to those found in beta thalassemia trait.

Other Laboratory Studies. The free erythrocyte protoporphyrin level (FEP) is normal, in contrast to the elevation present in iron deficiency or lead poisoning.

Hemoglobin electrophoresis on starch gel or cellulose acetate at pH 8.6 shows a normal pattern of Hb A and A_2. The hemoglobin A_2 level is elevated, usually in the range of 3.5 to 8 per cent, the mean being 5 per cent. In approximately half of the patients the Hb F level is also elevated, usually comprising 1 to 6 per cent of the total hemoglobin content.

There has been recent interest in population screening for beta thalassemia trait. The most efficient plan for screening is use of an electronic cell counter to identify people with an MCV below 79 cu micra followed by measurement of their Hb A_2 level. Several other diagnostic aids have been suggested, including several discriminant functions using the red cell parameters measured on the electronic counter and the degree of variation in red cell size distribution. However, the most reliable diagnostic plan for an individual is a blood count with red cell indices, an FEP measurement to eliminate the presence of iron deficiency, and quantification of the Hb A_2 level.

Biochemical Findings. Measurement of globin chain synthesis by reticulocytes shows that beta chain production is about one half that of alpha chain (β/α synthetic ratio of 0.5). In normal persons this ratio is 1. Although this technique is valuable for specific problems, including prenatal diagnosis of beta thalassemia major, it is too expensive for routine use in diagnosis.

Pitfalls in Diagnosis. The red cell morphology may suggest iron deficiency anemia, but in thalassemia trait the degree of microcytosis and hypochromia is more marked than would be expected for the hemoglobin level. In iron deficiency, changes of this degree usually occur at hemoglobin levels below 10 grams per dl. In addition, the red cell count is usually normal or slightly elevated in beta thalassemia trait. Iron deficiency can result in decreased levels of Hb

A_2, and the diagnosis may be missed if iron deficiency is not treated and the measurement repeated.

A few patients with beta thalassemia trait have normal red cell indices. Measurement of the Hb A_2 and F levels will identify most of these patients, although these are also normal in the silent carriers who must be identified by globin synthesis studies.

Hemoglobin electrophoretic techniques and the methods for quantifying hemoglobin A_2 and F levels must be carefully standardized. Densitometric scanning of the Hb A_2 band on cellulose acetate strips is not a reliable measurement of the A_2 level.

The physician must be aware that beta thalassemia trait can occur in any ethnic group and should consider the diagnosis in any one with a hypochromic anemia that does not respond to iron therapy.

Beta Thalassemia Major

Synonyms. Homozygous beta thalassemia, Cooley's anemia, Mediterranean anemia.

Definition. Beta thalassemia major is the homozygous state in which beta chain production is severely decreased or absent and significant anemia occurs. Anemia develops and clinical symptoms occur as gamma chain production decreases and beta chain production fails to rise to normal levels.

Clinical Findings and Course. The symptoms usually begin by 5 to 6 months of age and include poor appetite, irritability, diarrhea, and failure to gain weight normally. Physical findings are pallor, tachycardia and other cardiac findings secondary to the anemia, and in almost all infants significant splenomegaly with hepatomegaly of a lesser degree. The hemoglobin level falls gradually to about 2 to 4 grams per dl. Patients usually require regular transfusions by 1 year of age although some are not diagnosed until the second year. Patients who do not receive transfusions on a regular basis die by 4 to 5 years of age of infection or of congestive heart failure from the chronic anemia. Bone changes owing to expansion of the active bone marrow include frontal bossing, zygomatic arch and maxillary enlargement with protrusion of the front upper incisors, producing a "chipmunk facies." Bronzing of the skin is prominent. Extramedullary hematopoiesis may be marked and cause massive lymph node enlargement in the mediastinum and abdomen; compression of the spinal cord may occur.

The child who receives regular transfusions of red cells designed to keep his hemoglobin level above about 9 grams per dl usually grows and develops normally for the first 6 to 8 years. Poor growth and delayed sexual maturation are evident in the second decade. Early institution of this transfusion program may minimize the degree of splenomegaly and prevent some or all of the marked bone changes, but some children develop some of the stigmata despite adequate transfusion therapy.

Complications. The complications of hemolytic anemia include gallstone formation, fractures due to cortical thinning, and in a few patients folic acid deficiency. The bone changes and extramedullary hematopoiesis have been described earlier. Leg ulcers are infrequent. Hypersplenism is a common complication even in children receiving regular transfusions. Epistaxis occurs frequently in some patients and may be worsened if thrombocytopenia is present.

The most serious complications, however, result from excessive iron accumulation in vital organs and include pericarditis, arrhythmias, and congestive heart failure, liver fibrosis and eventual cirrhosis, diabetes mellitus, and, less commonly, hypoparathyroidism. Most patients die in the late second or early third decade, usually from the cardiac problems secondary to excessive iron accumulation from the multiple red cell transfusions.

Children receiving regular transfusions do not seem to have an increased risk of infection. After splenectomy, however, the incidence of overwhelming infection is quite high, although this risk seems to have been significantly reduced recently in patients receiving regular prophylaxis with penicillin.

Beta thalassemia major in the black patient is a milder disease. Anemia is moderate, and transfusions are not usually required until the third decade. Successful pregnancies have occurred in some women. Splenectomy may be of particular benefit to these patients. Once regular transfusions are begun, excessive iron accumulation with the problems mentioned earlier occurs.

Laboratory Findings. The anemia is moderate or severe depending on the age of the patient. The MCV and MCH are decreased; the reticulocyte count is usually 5 to 15 per cent; nucleated red blood cells are present. Leukocytosis and mild thrombocytosis are common unless there is concurrent hypersplenism. Examination of the peripheral smear shows marked variation in the size of the red cells, from some large cells to many extremely small cells that are almost devoid of hemoglobin content. Hypochromia is marked, as is the variation in red cell shape. Polychromasia, target cells, ovalocytes, and basophilic stippling are present. The hypochromia and marked anisocytosis and poikilocytosis are the most pronounced abnormalities.

Examination of a bone marrow aspirate shows marked erythroid hyperplasia with predominance of the early red cells. Late red cells may have torn cytoplasm. If a bone marrow sample is incubated with methyl violet, large inclusion bodies composed of precipitated alpha chain are seen in many of the red cells. These may also be demonstrated in the peripheral blood of patients who have been splenectomized and of some newborn infants with thalassemia major in the first day or so of life.

Other Laboratory Tests. Serum chemistry abnormalities include mild elevation of the indirect bilirubin level, increased LDH level, and decreased levels of cholesterol and uric acid.

Hemoglobin electrophoresis on starch gel or cellulose acetate shows greater than 10 per cent Hb F, usually from 35 to 90 per cent. The Hb A_2 level may be decreased, normal, or slightly increased. If the patient is homozygous for beta^0 thalassemia, no Hb A is present. Globin synthesis studies will confirm the absence of beta chain production. If the patient has one or two beta$^+$ thalassemia alleles, some Hb A will be seen. The hemoglobin F is heterogeneously distributed on a Betke-Kleihauer preparation.

Pitfalls in Diagnosis. There is usually no difficulty in making this diagnosis once it is considered. During the early stages thalassemia major can be confused with moderate or marked iron deficiency anemia. However, in thalassemia there is usually marked splenomegaly by this stage, and nucleated red cells are present in the peripheral blood. Measurement of the FEP level and hemoglobin electrophoresis will establish the correct diagnosis. Beta thalassemia major has been diagnosed in fetuses using globin synthesis studies of fetal blood. It may be possible in the future to diagnose some cases by analysis of DNA structure in fibroblasts obtained by amniocentesis but it seems unlikely at this time that all cases can be diagnosed by this technique. Diagnosis of the newborn infant requires globin synthesis studies unless methyl violet inclusion bodies can be demonstrated in the red cells.

BETA THALASSEMIA OF INTERMEDIATE SEVERITY

Synonym. Thalassemia intermedia.

Definition. A thalassemic disorder that is intermediate in clinical severity between beta thalassemia trait and beta thalassemia major. It may be caused by one of several different genetic disorders.

Clinical Findings and Course. The patient may have symptoms, particularly fatigue and decreased exercise tolerance, from the moderate anemia. Splenomegaly is usually present and may be marked. Other complications of thalassemia major may be present, such as bone changes, leg ulcers, and gallstones. The patient does not require regular red cell transfusions, although these may be necessary during infections or pregnancy. If hypersplenism develops, splenectomy will usually postpone or prevent the need for transfusions. Iron overload and tissue damage do not become major problems if regular transfusion therapy is not required.

Laboratory Studies. The anemia is generally in the range of 6 to 10 grams per dl. The red cell changes are usually more marked than those in beta thalassemia minor. The indirect bilirubin and LDH levels may be elevated. The findings on hemoglobin electrophoresis depend on the nature of the underlying genetic disorder. As mentioned before, beta thalassemia major in blacks is milder, and some white patients with homozygous beta thalassemia also have this milder form. The findings in beta thalassemia trait of unusual severity have been mentioned. Patients with some of the more unusual forms of thalassemia, such as homozygous delta-beta ($\delta\beta$) or $\delta\beta$-β thalassemia, and Hb Lepore-β thalassemia, may have a milder course or may be clinically identical to patients with beta thalassemia major. Interactions of the beta thalassemia allele with the silent carrier allele, an alpha thalassemia gene, or with a structurally abnormal hemoglobin such as Hb E or the unstable Hb Saki, have resulted in an intermedia picture. The exact nature of the hemoglobin disorder can usually be delineated by careful electrophoretic studies and other techniques such as globin synthesis studies. However, evaluation of family members, and particularly the parents, remains a very important part of diagnosis.

OTHER DISORDERS

In delta-beta thalassemia there is absence of delta and beta chain production from the affected allele. The heterozygous state is similar to beta thalassemia minor in lack of clinical symptoms and blood picture. Hemoglobin electrophoresis, however, shows a normal or slightly decreased level of Hb A_2 and a moderate increase in Hb F level, usually to 5 to 15 per cent. The patient with homozygous $\delta\beta$ thalassemia or one doubly heterozygous for $\delta\beta$-β thalassemia is clinically similar to the patient with beta thalassemia major, although some patients have a milder clinical course. Hemoglobin electrophoresis shows only Hb F or F and A if a β^+ allele is present. The distribution of Hb F is heterogeneous.

Hemoglobin Lepore is a structurally abnormal hemoglobin with two normal alpha chains but a pair of abnormal chains that have the initial sequence of delta chain and the terminal sequence of beta chain. The abnormal hemoglobin is produced in decreased amounts. The clinical picture of Hb Lepore trait is like that of beta thalassemia trait, and the severity of Hb Lepore-β thalassemia or homozygous Lepore is usually comparable to that in beta thalassemia major. In Lepore trait, the Hb A_2 level is normal or slightly decreased, and there is 5 to 15 per cent of the abnormal hemoglobin that migrates as S on cellulose acetate or starch gel but does not sickle. In homozygous Lepore, about 20 per cent of the hemoglobin is Lepore and the rest is Hb F. There is no hemoglobin A. The Hb F is heterogeneously distributed.

In hereditary persistence of fetal hemoglobin (HPFH), hemoglobin F is produced at elevated levels throughout life. There are several varieties of HPFH, and the exact findings depend on the form present. There are no clinical symptoms and no significant hematologic abnormalities. Some microcytosis may be evident on peripheral smear. In the form described in American blacks, people with heterozygous HPFH have 15 to 30 per cent Hb F. Blacks with homozygous HPFH have been described who have 100 per cent Hb F without clinical effects except for a slight increase in red cell count. In the Greek variety heterozygotes have 5 to 15 per cent Hb F. The Hb F is distributed homogeneously in the red cells, in contrast to the heterogeneous distribution seen in other thalassemias.

Pitfalls in Diagnosis. Homozygous $\delta\beta$ thalassemia or doubly heterozygous $\delta\beta$-β^0 thalassemia may be confused with homozygous beta^0 thalassemia, since the clinical findings are generally the same and there is no Hb A on electrophoresis. Study of the parents and other family members is of particular importance in establishing the precise diagnosis. Since hemoglobin Lepore migrates close to the position of Hb S, interpretation of the electrophoretic pattern may be confusing initially. However, Hb Lepore does not sickle, microcytosis and hypochromia are present with Lepore, and the percentage of Hb Lepore is less than that of S in sickle cell trait.

ALPHA THALASSEMIA

The genetic basis of the alpha thalassemia states is not completely known, but recent studies of the structure of the DNA of globin genes have yielded new insight. In most populations there are two loci with four genes for alpha chain production. However, some populations studied had some people with only two or three genes for alpha chain. Alpha thalassemia in almost all cases results from gene deletion, the severity of the disorder increasing as the number of genes deleted increases. In the fatal form, hydrops fetalis, all four alpha genes are deleted and there is no alpha chain produced. Hemoglobin H disease, the other symptomatic form of alpha thalassemia, results in most cases from deletion of three alpha genes. However, in a few studied cases it results from a combination of gene deletion and abnormal gene function. In addition, some cases in people of oriental descent result from the interaction of alpha thalassemia with the abnormal hemoglobin Constant Spring. Hb Constant Spring contains an elongated alpha chain with 31 extra amino acid residues at the C-terminal end. It is produced in decreased amounts and acts as an alpha thalassemia gene.

Alpha thalassemia is common in Southeast Asia, the Mediterranean and Middle East areas, and in Africa. Alpha thalassemia trait is estimated to occur in 3 to 7 per cent of American blacks based on studies of Hb Bart's in cord blood screening surveys. The imbalance created by the decreased alpha chain synthesis leads to formation of tetramers of gamma chain, γ_4 (Hb Bart's). If significant imbalance persists beyond the newborn period, tetramers of beta chain are found (Hb H).

THE SILENT CARRIER

There are no clinical symptoms or hematologic abnormalities associated with this state except for some mild microcytosis evident on examination of the peripheral smear. Electrophoresis of blood in the newborn period shows 1 to 2 per cent Hb Bart's. This disappears by 6 months of age and hemoglobin electrophoresis thereafter is normal.

ALPHA THALASSEMIA TRAIT

Definition. There is a mild decrease in alpha chain production usually caused by deletion of two of the four alpha genes.

Clinical Findings and Course. No symptoms or physical findings are associated with this state. Mild anemia is present, generally in the range of 10 to 12 grams per dl in children and women and 12 to 14 grams per dl in men. The MCV and MCH are decreased, and the MCHC is normal. The reticulocyte count is normal. Examination of the peripheral smear reveals microcytic, hypochromic red cells with some target forms present. The values for MCV, MCH, and in some infants hemoglobin level are lower in infants with alpha thalassemia trait than in normal babies. However, because of the overlap in ranges of normal with those in alpha thalassemia trait, these differences cannot be used to make the diagnosis in an individual baby.

Other Laboratory Studies. In the newborn period Hb Bart's is present at levels of 5 to 10 per cent. After 6 months of age the electrophoresis is completely normal. Diagnosis may be made by studies of globin chain synthesis. The α/β ratio in Italian and Oriental patients has been about 0.77 and in American blacks about 0.85, as compared to the normal ratio of about 1. In a person heterozygous for one of the structurally abnormal hemoglobins such as S, C, or E, the percentage of the abnormal hemoglobin is decreased in the presence of alpha thalassemia trait. For example, the person with Hb AS and alpha thalassemia trait will have about 30 per cent Hb S instead of the usual 40 per cent.

Pitfalls in Diagnosis. Alpha thalassemia trait may be confused with iron deficiency anemia or beta thalassemia trait. Iron deficiency and lead poisoning also decrease the percentage of abnormal hemoglobin in people heterozygous for Hb S, C, or E. However, the FEP level is normal in alpha thalassemia and increased in iron deficiency or lead poisoning. Demonstration of other family members with microcytic, hypochromic anemia not due to other causes strengthens the diagnosis of alpha thalassemia trait.

HEMOGLOBIN H DISEASE

Definition. Hb H disease is a microcytic, hypochromic hemolytic anemia caused by a marked decrease in alpha chain production. The tetramers of beta chain, Hb H, are unstable and cause hemolysis.

Clinical Course and Findings. The patient usually has symptoms referable to a mild or moderate anemia. The severity of the disease varies greatly. Most patients have pallor and splenomegaly. Other findings may include scleral icterus and bone changes similar to those seen in beta thalassemia major. Hemolysis may increase, and thus anemia worsen, during infections or during treatment with oxidant drugs. The hemoglobin is usually in the range of 8 to 10 grams per dl. The MCV and MCH values are decreased, and reticulocytosis of about 2 to 8 per cent is present. Examination of the peripheral smear reveals hypochromia, microcytosis, and variation in red cell size and shape. Target cells and basophilic stippling are present. Bone marrow examination shows erythroid hyperplasia. Methyl violet inclusion bodies of beta chain may be demonstrated in bone marrow cells and in circulating red cells in patients after splenectomy.

Other Laboratory Studies. There may be mild elevations of the indirect bilirubin level and LDH. Incubation of red cells with brilliant cresyl blue (BCB) for 1 hour or more causes precipitation of the unstable Hb H. Examination of a slide made from this preparation shows dust-like particles in many red cells. Other tests for unstable hemoglobin, such as isopropanol screening or heat stability studies, will also be positive. Hemoglobin electrophoresis of fresh blood on starch gel or cellulose acetate will show the fast-moving band of Hb H. The cellulose acetate strip should be examined within 15 minutes of electrophoresis to be sure the unstable Hb H has not denatured. In those patients with Hb Constant Spring, this hemoglobin—which migrates more slowly than Hb A_2—is present in trace amounts. In the newborn period Hb Bart's comprises 20 to 25 per cent of the total hemoglobin. Globin synthesis studies have shown α/β ratios of about 0.35 to 0.60 in Italian and Oriental patients and 0.40 to 0.70 in American blacks.

Pitfalls in Diagnosis. A hemolytic anemia that is microcytic and hypochromic suggests the presence of Hb H disease. Similar morphology may occur in hemolysis due to cardiac valve disease if iron deficiency is present. Other unstable hemoglobins give positive results with BCB but usually require longer than 1 hour for precipitation. Hemoglobin H may be missed unless electrophoresis is done carefully.

HYDROPS FETALIS

Definition. In hydrops fetalis there is complete absence of alpha chain synthesis, and no Hb A or F can be formed. Hemoglobin Bart's and Hb H are present, but their oxygen affinity is so high that this condition is not compatible with extrauterine life. This form of alpha thalassemia has not been described in blacks.

Synonym. Homozygous alpha thalassemia.

Clinical Findings and Course. The fetus with homozygous alpha thalassemia develops severe anemia and congestive heart failure in utero, producing the hydropic state. In about two thirds of pregnancies, the mother develops preeclampsia. Delivery is usually premature, and the infant either is stillborn or lives only a few minutes. The infant is hydropic with edema and massive anasarca. Massive hepatic enlargement and splenomegaly to a lesser degree are present. The anemia is marked, with usual hemoglobin of 4 to 6 grams per dl. The MCV and MCH are very low for a newborn unless masked by the numerous circulating nucleated red cells. Reticulocytosis is pronounced. Examination of the peripheral smear shows extreme microcytosis and hypochromia, marked anisocytosis and poikilocytosis, polychromasia, target cells, basophilic stippling, and many nucleated red cells. Bone marrow examination shows marked erythroid hyperplasia. Methyl violet and BCB preparations are positive.

Other Laboratory Studies. There is usually elevation of the indirect fraction of bilirubin and decreased levels of albumin. Hemoglobin electrophoresis on starch gel or cellulose acetate shows about 80 per cent Hb Bart's, some Hb H, and a minor component of the embryonic hemoglobin Portland, which is composed of two ζ chains and two γ chains. This migrates slightly faster than Hb A at ph 8.6. There is no A present, unless fetal blood has been contaminated with maternal blood. Examination of the parents shows the presence of alpha thalassemia trait in both or alpha thalassemia trait in one and Hb H disease in the other.

Biochemical Studies. Globin chain synthesis studies show complete absence of alpha chain production. The gene deletion may be demonstrated by RNA or DNA hybridization studies or analysis of globin gene structure. These techniques have been employed using fibroblasts from amniotic fluid to diagnose this condition in utero.

Pitfalls in Diagnosis. This condition may be incorrectly attributed to an unusual blood group incompatibility unless the physician delivering the infant is aware of the existence of homozygous alpha thalassemia. The racial origin of the parents and the microscopic, hypochromic red cells should suggest this disease. A hemoglobin electrophoresis of cord or cardiac blood should be obtained on all infants with hydrops who do not have clearly documented blood group incompatibility. Correct diagnosis of this disorder is important so that genetic counseling and prenatal diagnosis in future pregnancies can be offered to the parents.

HEMOGLOBIN-OPATHIES

By RICHARD T. O'BRIEN, M.D.
Salt Lake City, Utah

The hemoglobinopathies comprise a group of well-defined inherited disorders. Although more than 200 human hemoglobin variants have been described, only a handful are of clinical importance. They are the result of single amino acid substitutions in the alpha or beta chains of adult hemoglobin that produce either hemoly-

sis, owing to changes in solubility or stability of the hemoglobin, or alterations in hemoglobin-oxygen affinity. This article deals with the diagnosis of the more common and clinically significant hemoglobinopathies.

The diagnosis of a hemoglobinopathy is generally suggested by the clinical presentation and routine hematologic data, including the examination of a well-made peripheral blood smear. The diagnosis is confirmed by demonstration of the abnormal hemoglobin in the red blood cells of the patient and his family. Although there are a variety of useful laboratory tests, quantitation of the abnormal hemoglobin by electrophoresis or column chromatography remains the definitive diagnostic tool.

HEMOGLOBIN S

Hemoglobin S (Hb S) results from the substitution of a valine for a glutamic acid in the sixth position of the beta chain. When deoxygenated, red cells containing hemoglobin S undergo a characteristic change in shape — sickle cells. The concentration of Hb S in the red cells is the most important variable influencing their ability to sickle. The homozygote for the Hb S gene (sickle cell anemia) has red blood cells that contain 85 to 95 per cent Hb S; the heterozygote (sickle cell trait), 35 to 45 per cent Hb S. The sickle cell gene is particularly common among blacks from equatorial Africa but is also found to a lesser extent among Mediterranean populations and in the Middle East and India. Approximately 8 per cent of American blacks carry the gene for hemoglobin S (heterozygotes) and sickle cell anemia is estimated to occur in 1 in 500 American blacks at birth.

SICKLE CELL ANEMIA
(HEMOGLOBIN SS DISEASE)

CLINICAL MANIFESTATIONS

General. The diagnosis of sickle cell anemia is usually made during the first few years of life. Although the clinical manifestations of the disease are legion, they are all the result of in vivo sickling of the red blood cells. These disorted cells are removed prematurely from the circulation, resulting in a partially compensated hemolytic anemia. Hyperbilirubinemia is common and gallstones occur with increased frequency. The medullary and extramedullary compensatory response to the chronic anemia includes marrow erythroid hyperplasia, which contributes to striking bone changes, and hepatosplenomegaly. The chronic anemia is associated with growth retardation and cardiomegaly. Cardiac dysfunction with murmurs of mitral or aortic insufficiency and congestive heart failure may occur later in life. Leg ulcers may also result.

Although the chronic anemia and its effects may be reasonably well tolerated at rest, particularly during childhood, the clinical course of the disease is punctuated by acute episodes traditionally referred to as "crises." These acute episodes may be either vaso-occlusive or hematologic in nature. In addition, infection represents another acute episode that is a frequent and serious complication of the disease.

Vaso-occlusive Crises. Vaso-occlusive crises are the hallmark of sickle cell anemia and exact a progressive toll of multiple organ dysfunction. Sickled erythrocytes obstruct small blood vessels, leading to a variety of acute or chronic effects. The clinical consequences of vaso-occlusion depend on the location, extent, and duration of the obstruction. Any organ may be involved. Vaso-occlusive episodes are generally not associated with changes in the hematologic values in the peripheral blood.

Acute vaso-occlusive episodes involving musculoskeletal or intra-abdominal structures are the most frequent and are typically associated with pain. In infants, obstruction of vessels to the small bones of the hands and feet produces painful, symmetrical swelling referred to as the hand-foot syndrome. The acute onset of abdominal pain may result from splenic infarction or the obstruction of blood flow to other abdominal organs. Repeated splenic infarcts reduce the spleen to a fibrous nub (autosplenectomy) so that splenomegaly is generally no longer evident after 5 to 6 years of age. These painful, vaso-occlusive crises are quite variable in their duration and frequency but may occur 2 to 10 times per year and yield symptoms for 1 to 10 days. Vaso-occlusive episodes may lead to strokes, retinopathy, priapism, nephrosis, hepatic necrosis, pulmonary infarction, or involvement of any other organ system. Although many of these vaso-occlusive crises occur spontaneously, others seem to be precipitated by infection, exposure to cold temperatures, or events that contribute to dehydration, acidosis, or hypoxia. General anesthesia imposes a definite threat and pregnancy is associated with an increased maternal risk and marked fetal wastage.

The sickling phenomenon may impede blood flow and induce shunting within an organ without producing infarction. In the kidney this results in hyposthenuria and in the spleen reticuloendothelial dysfunction. This effect on splenic blood flow is particularly important since it induces "functional asplenia," the major factor responsible for the inordinately high mortality from infection in sickle cell anemia during the first 5 years of life.

Hematologic Crises. In any chronic hemolytic anemia, factors that either contribute to hemolysis or suppress the bone compensatory effort may greatly aggravate the degree of anemia. A variety of viral infections may induce a transient suppression of red cell production. In patients with a hemolytic anemia such as sickle cell disease, a viral infection may induce marrow erythroid hypoplasia and reticulocytopenia. With the already shortened red cell survival, the hemoglobin level falls rapidly. This is called an aplastic crisis and is characterized by a falling hemoglobin concentration and reticulocytopenia. Although the hemoglobin may fall to such low levels that a blood transfusion is necessary, the process is self-limiting. Marrow recovery is followed by a brisk reticulocytosis and a return of hemoglobin concentrations to baseline values. If the patient is first seen during the recovery phase of an aplastic crisis, it might be interpreted as indicating a hyperhemolytic episode.

Children with sickle cell anemia whose spleens have not yet succumbed to multiple infarcts, or patients with sickle beta thalassemia or SC hemoglobin in whom splenomegaly persists into later life, are at risk for development of splenic sequestration crises. During splenic sequestration, for unknown reasons, the spleen suddenly pools vast quantities of blood and may present a life-threatening situation owing to hypovolemia. During a sequestration crisis the spleen enlarges, the hemoglobin falls rapidly but the reticulocyte count remains high. The sequestered blood may be quickly remobilized from the spleen and hematologic equilibrium restored by the transfusion of whole blood. Other factors that may increase hemolysis, such as infection or drugs, can also aggravate the anemia in sickle cell disease, causing so-called hyperhemolytic crises.

Infection. Infection represents the greatest life-threatening risk for the young child with sickle cell anemia. It accounts for most of the 20 to 30 per cent mortality from the disease that occurs during the first 5 years of life. The epidemiology of those infections is identical to that seen in asplenic individuals — overwhelming sepsis and/or meningitis usually owing to the pneumococcus or *Hemophilus influenzae*. The major factor contributing to that infectious risk is the development of functional asplenia (a deficit in splenic reticuloendothelial function despite palpably enlarged spleen) in young children with sickle cell anemia. Its development is directly related to the progressive replacement of fetal hemoglobin by sickle hemoglobin during the first year of life.

Patients with sickle cell anemia also have an increased risk of local infection in areas damaged by previous infarction, such as lung and bone. In addition, neutrophil functional abnormalities have been demonstrated.

Laboratory Findings. The anemia of sickle cell disease is moderately severe, with hemoglobin concentrations ranging from 5.5 to 9.5 grams per dl (100 ml) (average 7.5 grams per dl). The hemoglobin level is maintained fairly constant by expansion of the erythroid marrow and a reticulocytosis (5 to 30 per cent). The morphologic hallmark of the disease is the presence of sickled erythrocytes on a peripheral smear. The red cells are normochromic and normocytic; polychromasia, target cells, and occasional nucleated red blood cells may be seen. Elevations of the white blood cell count may also be found even in the absence of infection.

The sickle cell preparation with sodium metabisulfite and solubility tests using a reducing agent in a phosphate buffer are positive when hemoglobin S is present. As screening tests for sickle hemoglobin these tests have largely been replaced by hemoglobin electrophoresis on cellulose acetate, which can be performed inexpensively in minutes from a capillary blood specimen.

A definitive diagnosis of major sickle hemoglobinopathies requires demonstration and quantitation of the abnormal hemoglobin(s), either by microcolumn chromatography or hemoglobin electrophoresis. In sickle cell anemia no hemoglobin A is present. Eighty-five to 95 per cent of the hemoglobin is S. Hemoglobin F is moderately elevated. Hemoglobin A$_2$ is normal. In any major sickle hemoglobinopathy, electrophoresis at both pH 8.4 and 6.2 and careful family studies should be performed to differentiate between homozygous sickle cell anemia and other major sickle hemoglobinopathies such as sickle beta thalassemia or SC or SD disease. This is important because these other sickle states have a generally better prognosis.

Although clinical manifestations of sickle cell anemia are not evident during the first few months of life because of the protective effect of fetal hemoglobin, the disease can be readily diagnosed at birth. Cord blood screening programs for sickle cell diseases among high-risk populations are becoming increasingly common. Identification of the disease at birth is of dubious value unless it is accompanied by education of the family and provision of appropriate medical care.

SICKLE CELL TRAIT (HEMOGLOBIN AS)

Sickle cell trait, resulting from heterozygosity from the hemoglobin S gene, is associated with red blood cells containing 35 to 45 per cent hemoglobin S but no hematologic abnormalities. Under usual physiologic conditions sickle cell trait imposes few, if any, significant clinical consequences. Hyposthenuria and hematuria occur with increased frequency; under hypoxic circumstances, such as flight at high altitude in unpressurized aircraft, vaso-occlusive episodes such as splenic infarction can occur. There have been reports of unexpected deaths in persons with sickle cell trait and evidence of massive sickling discovered at autopsy. It is uncertain, however, whether sickling was the cause or result of death. There are no age-related differences in the prevalence of sickle cell trait, indicating that the condition does not affect life expectancy.

The major implication of sickle cell trait is genetic. Each offspring of two parents with sickle cell trait has a one-in-four risk of having sickle cell anemia. Screening programs for sickle cell trait have generally been aimed at identifying affected persons for the purpose of genetic counseling. Hemoglobin electrophoresis using capillary blood specimens has largely replaced the sickle preparation and solubility tests for this purpose.

OTHER SICKLE CELL DISORDERS

The inheritance of hemoglobin S plus another abnormal hemoglobin or thalassemia gene (double heterozygotes) yields a variety of well-defined clinical syndromes of varying severity. Hemoglobin SC disease and sickle beta thalassemia are those most frequently encountered. The clinical manifestations are similar to but less severe than in sickle cell anemia. Vaso-occlusive crises occur less often and overwhelming pneumococcal infections are unusual, probably because functional asplenia does not develop regularly. Aseptic necrosis of the femoral head and sickle retinopathy seem to occur more frequently in Hb SC disease.

Patients with Hb SC disease have red cells with approximately equal amounts of the two hemoglobins present. Hb A is absent. There is a moderate hemolytic anemia and the red cell morphology shows polychromasia, target cells, and infrequent sickled cells.

Sickle beta thalassemia may be more difficult to differentiate in the laboratory from sickle cell anemia because in a significant number of patients no Hg A is present. Sickle beta thalassemia is associated with microcytosis and family studies should reveal one parent to have sickle cell trait and the other thalassemia trait. The proportion of Hb A varies from 0 to 40 per cent. Hemoglobins F and A$_2$ are increased.

HEMOGLOBIN C

Hemoglobin C results from the substitution of a lysine for a glutamic acid in the sixth position of the beta chain. It is found almost exclusively among peoples of West African descent and 2.5 per cent of American blacks are heterozygous for Hb C.

HEMOGLOBIN C DISEASE (HEMOGLOBIN CC)

Homozygosity for hemoglobin C causes a mild to moderate chronic hemolytic anemia with hemoglobin concentrations between 9 and 12 grams per dl (100 ml) and an elevated reticulocyte count. Target cells are quite common on a peripheral blood smear. In addition, polychromasia, microspherocytes, and conch shell-appearing cells are seen. Splenomegaly is usually present but the patients are generally asymptomatic with an otherwise unremarkable physical examination. Life expectancy is probably normal.

Hg C is a slow migrating hemoglobin on electrophoresis at both acid and alkaline pH. In CC disease it accounts for more than 90 per cent of the total hemoglobin. Hb F is normal. Hb A_2 cannot be quantitated by usual techniques.

HEMOGLOBIN C TRAIT (HEMOGLOBIN AC)

Heterozygotes for hemoglobin C have red cells that contain 35 to 45 per cent hemoglobin C. Although target cells are seen in peripheral blood smears, there are no anemia, reticulocytosis, or other hematologic abnormalities and the individuals are well.

HEMOGLOBINS E, F, D, and G

Hemoglobin E is another beta chain variant. It is the most common abnormal hemoglobin found in Southeast Asia. Homozygotes have a mild, chronic hemolytic anemia with target cells and microcytosis. Heterozygotes are not anemic but mild microcytosis and a few target cells may be found. Hemoglobin E can be demonstrated by its characteristic electrophoretic mobilities at acid and alkaline pH.

Hemoglobin F (fetal hemoglobin), the major hemoglobin of intrauterine life, accounts for less than 2 per cent of total hemoglobin after the first year of life. It is moderately elevated in many major hemoglobinopathies and accounts for most of the hemoglobin present in beta thalassemia major patients who have not had transfusions. It is a hemoglobin with increased oxygen affinity. Hereditary persistence of fetal hemoglobin (HPFH) is a genetic mutation found with low frequency among blacks, Greeks, and Italians in whom the synthesis of hemoglobin F continues beyond infancy. It is a benign condition. Heterozygotes have 10 to 35 per cent Hb F. Homozygotes are rare, with virtually all their hemoglobin being Hb F. Quantitation of Hb F takes advantage of its relative resistance to denaturation by alkali — the alkali denaturation test. Hb F can also be differentiated inside red blood cells on a glass slide by the Kleihauer-Betke test. With the exception of HPFH, almost all conditions with increased Hb F have an irregular distribution of that hemoglobin among the red cells.

The terms hemoglobin D and hemoglobin G both refer to a variety of hemoglobin variants involving either the alpha or beta chains but having in common identical electrophoretic mobilities. These are all quite uncommon and produce few, if any, clinical problems.

UNSTABLE HEMOGLOBINS

The unstable hemoglobins comprise a group of about 50 uncommon hemoglobin variants. The amino acid substitutions or deletions occur at a critical location in either the alpha or beta chain, which results in molecular instability. Globin precipitation and Heinz body formation leads to hemolysis. These so-called congenital Heinz body anemias have an autosomal dominant pattern of inheritance.

The clinical and hematologic manifestations vary from mild anemia to severe hemolysis. Hemoglobin-oxygen affinity may also be altered. The red cell morphologic changes are nonspecific. Heinz bodies are not seen on regular Wright-stained smears but can be found after incubation with brilliant cresyl blue or crystal violet. The abnormal hemoglobin may not be demonstrable with electrophoresis, but when found it is usually present in relatively small amounts (5 to 20 per cent). Precipitation of unstable hemoglobins may occur with heating or in an isopropanol buffer solution. Following splenectomy an unstable hemoglobin may be more easily recognized.

HEMOGLOBINS WITH ALTERED OXYGEN AFFINITY

An increasing number of hemoglobin variants have been recognized to be associated with alterations in hemoglobin-oxygen affinity. They have an autosomal dominant pattern of inheritance. Most of these have been associated with increased oxygen affinity or a shift in the whole blood oxygen dissociation curve to the left (decrease in P_{50}). Erythrocytosis with increased red blood cell volume and hemoglobin concentration may result. The PaO_2 is normal and there are no other hematologic abnormalities. These benign, familial conditions must be differentiated from polycythemia vera or, more commonly, from cardiovascular or pulmonary diseases causing hypoxia.

A handful of abnormal hemoglobins with decreased oxygen affinity have been recognized, resulting in a right shift in the oxygen dissociation curve (increased P_{50}). The hemoglobin may be lower than normal without any symptoms of anemia, and cyanosis may be evident.

Finally, there are a group of hemoglobin variants that may also be a cause for familial cyanosis. These are collectively referred to as hemoglobin M disorders because the amino acid substitution results in the heme iron in the ferric form, or methemoglobin. Hemoglobin M can be detected spectrophotometrically or electrophoretically. It should be differentiated from other causes for methemoglobin formation such as congenital methemoglobin reductase deficiency.

ANEMIAS DUE TO ERYTHROCYTE ENZYME DEFICIENCIES

By WALTER E. DAVIS, M.D.
Durham, North Carolina

INTRODUCTION

Anemias that are due to erythrocyte enzyme deficiencies make up a large heterogeneous class of hereditary anemias whose only consistent similarity is that they are hemolytic anemias characterized by shortened red cell survival. With the exception of glucose 6-phosphate dehydrogenase (G6PD) deficiency, which is a common abnormality in certain southern European populations and black populations, these disorders are uncommon and are more often encountered in the pediatric age group than in adulthood. Definite diagnosis in all these anemias is made by demonstrating a decreased

activity of one or more red cell enzymes. The techniques used for red cell enzyme assays are rather sophisticated biochemical measurements not available in most hematology laboratories, and in fact are often unavailable in large commercial or university-based laboratories. For the individual practitioner the diagnosis of anemia secondary to a specific red cell enzyme deficiency is often one of exclusion and consultation for specialized biochemical assay.

The general outline of evaluation leading to diagnosis of these anemias consists of (1) demonstrating the presence of a hemolytic anemia, (2) exclusion of several more common hemolytic anemias, and (3) assay of red cell enzyme levels.

The presence of hemolysis requires the demonstration of a shortened red cell life span as measured by chromium-51 tagging of red cells or carbon monoxide excretion studies. In clinical practice the combination of several nonspecific abnormalities is often sufficiently suggestive of a hemolytic process to obviate the need for definitive red cell survival studies. Hemolytic anemias are characterized by a stable or falling hemoglobin with persistent reticulocytosis in the absence of bleeding, and an active bone marrow with red cell hyperplasia. The frequent presence of unconjugated hyperbilirubinemia and the variable presence of the following abnormalities — elevated serum lactic dehydrogenase levels, decreased or absent serum levels of haptoglobin, and elevated serum values for methemalbumin — are very strongly suggestive of a hemolytic anemia. Once it is determined that anemia is hemolytic in nature, one must exclude common causes of hemolysis such as Coombs-positive immune hemolytic anemia, schistocytic hemolytic anemia, hereditary spherocytosis, and hemoglobinopathy. After these more prevalent diseases are excluded by commonly available diagnostic studies, erythrocyte enzyme defects represent the vast majority of remaining cases.

For purposes of discussion it is most convenient to divide the anemias resulting from erythrocyte enzyme deficiency into two groups: diseases associated with intermittent hemolysis such as the African or North American variant of G6PD deficiency, and those associated with a chronic persistent anemia such as pyruvate kinase deficiency.

GLUCOSE 6-PHOSPHATE DEHYDROGENASE DEFICIENCY

This hemolytic anemia is due to inheritance of a variant red cell G6PD enzyme molecule that diminishes the red cell's ability to withstand oxidant stress by compromising hexose monophosphate shunt activity. The gene determining G6PD structure and function is carried on the X chromosome; consequently the defect is fully expressed in affected males and has a lesser manifestation in heterozygous females. Studies to date of G6PD deficiency have revealed that only rarely is there a complete absence of immunologically detectable enzyme, and that expression is due to functional variation rather than complete absence of enzyme protein.

The incidence of G6PD deficiency is not equally distributed in the population. The highest incidence has been described among Kurdish and Oriental Jews in whom it has been used as a population marker, but the disorder is commonly seen in Caucasian populations surrounding the Mediterranean and in black populations that originated in Central Africa. Various studies document the presence of this disorder in 13 per cent of black American males, and it is estimated that 20 per cent of black American females are heterozygous for G6PD deficiency.

G6PD variants in populations of Mediterranean origin may cause a chronic lifelong hemolytic anemia of varying severity, but the remainder of this discussion will be limited to the variant found in American blacks that makes up the vast majority of cases in the United States. In this racial group clinical manifestations consist of the episodic occurrence of acute hemolysis with spontaneous recovery. The usual patient with G6PD deficiency seen in the United States will experience episodes of acute hemolysis early in the course of an infectious disease or during the administration of an oxidant drug. Between episodes of hemolysis, this patient will have no signs or symptoms referable to the disease. This diagnosis should be considered when an acute hemolytic episode, characterized by weakness, jaundice, hemoglobinuria, and the general laboratory findings of hemolytic anemia, is induced by an acute bacterial or viral infection, an acute metabolic abnormality such as diabetic ketoacidosis, or the administration of one of the several oxidant drugs listed in Table 1.

Examination of the blood film and Heinz body preparations during acute hemolytic episodes caused by G6PD deficiency reveals reticulocytosis and the presence of typical Heinz body inclusions in a variable percentage of the red cells. Clinical jaundice, unconjugated hyperbilirubinemia, hypohaptoglobinemia, elevated lactic dehydrogenase (LDH) levels, and rarely, hemoglobinemia and hemoglobinuria may be noted. None of these findings is specific for this disorder, and definitive diagnosis of

Table 1. *Drugs Associated With Acute Hemolytic Episodes in G6PD Deficiency*

Antibiotics
  Primaquine
  Quinacrine
  Sulfonamides
  Sulfones
  Nitrofurantoin
  Chloramphenicol

Antipyretics and analgesics
  Acetanilid
  Aspirin
  Phenacetin

Miscellaneous
  Probenecid
  Vitamin K (water-soluble)
  Isoniazid
  PAS (para-aminosalicylic acid)
  BAL (British anti-lewisite, dimercaprol)

G6PD deficiency requires demonstration of abnormally low values of G6PD activity by biochemical measurement in patient erythrocytes. Two types of procedures are employed in the measurement of G6PD enzyme activity in red cells. The first type is a screening test, employing reduction of specific dyes, oxidation of an ascorbate-cyanide solution with resultant color changes, or differential fluorescence of dinucleotide cofactors. The second type consists of quantitative enzymatic measurement of G6PD activity in red cell hemolysates. This latter procedure is perhaps preferable in complicated situations, but generally exceeds the capability of most clinical laboratories. The characteristic clinical and laboratory manifestations appearing in a black patient with a history of exposure to drugs known to cause acute hemolysis and a positive screening test for G6PD deficiency are adequate to confirm the diagnosis in most situations.

The major pitfall in the laboratory diagnosis of G6PD deficiency arises from the occasional inability to demonstrate lowered G6PD levels during acute hemolytic events. G6PD is an erythrocyte age-dependent enzyme, and in the common variant of G6PD deficiency seen in the United States young red blood cells recently released from the bone marrow have a measurable level of G6PD. Thus in the face of a very brisk reticulocytosis, screening tests are often insufficiently sensitive to distinguish the G6PD levels in these young cells from normal. This generally is not a problem in male hemizygotes, for markedly reduced enzyme activity is present even with marked reticulocytosis. In female heterozygotes, however, enzyme levels determined on whole blood may fall within the normal range when the reticulocyte count is high. In this situation a definitive diagnosis, based on either the typical clinical situation and screening tests or definitive enzyme assay, may require delay until recovery of normal hemoglobin values and hence decrease in the reticulocytosis induced by acute hemolysis.

CHRONIC HEMOLYTIC ANEMIAS DUE TO OTHER ERYTHROCYTE ENZYME DEFECTS

Anemias associated with non-G6PD enzyme deficiencies are characterized by chronic, usually low-grade, hemolytic anemia that may vary in intensity with time, but which is detectable with careful study at any point in the course of the disease. This is in contrast to G6PD deficiency, in which hemoglobin values are intermittently normal. Many types of enzyme deficiencies, as outlined in Table 2, have been associated with this type of hereditary chronic hemolytic anemia. Pyruvate kinase deficiency is the most frequent representative of this group.

The clinical manifestations of these chronic hemolytic anemias include anemia, which may be mild or severe, jaundice, splenomegaly, intermittent hemoglobinuria, and a high incidence of gallstones. Hemolysis may be aggravated by intercurrent infection or other acute illnesses. Aplastic or aregenerative crises are rare occurrences thought to be related to acquired deficiency of folic acid or transient depression of erythropoiesis by acute illness. Diagnosis of the more severe varieties of these anemias is usually made during childhood, but milder forms may remain undetected until adulthood. Impairment of general development and growth through childhood and adolescence may occur in proportion to the severity of the anemia. Nonspecific abnormalities accompanying these anemias include reticulocytosis, the associated macrocytosis, and rarely spiculated cells (most common with pyruvate kinase deficiency), erythroid hyperplasia in the bone mar-

Table 2. *RBC Enzyme Deficiency Associated With Chronic Familial Hemolytic Anemia*

Some G6PD variants
Pyruvate kinase
Hexokinase
Glucose phosphate isomerase
Phosphofructokinase
Triosephosphate isomerase
Phosphoglycerokinase
Diphosphoglyceromutase
Glutathione synthetase

row, unconjugated hyperbilirubinemia, decreased serum haptoglobin levels, and variable elevation of serum LDH levels.

In all these hemolytic anemias, autohemolysis after 48 hours of sterile incubation is increased and variable correction of autohemolysis follows incubation with added glucose or adenosine triphosphate (ATP). Thus diagnosis depends upon the demonstration of a hemolytic anemia, absence of the more common causes, and the presence of increased autohemolysis. Demonstration of decreased specific enzyme levels in red cell hemolysates conclusively establishes the nature of the enzymatic defects.

HEREDITARY SPHEROCYTOSIS

By HUSSAIN I. SABA, M.D., Ph.D., *and* ROBERT C. HARTMANN, M.D.

Tampa, Florida

SYNONYMS

Hereditary hemolytic anemia, familial acholuric jaundice, congenital hemolytic anemia, chronic familial jaundice. With the greater specificity and clarity provided by the term hereditary spherocytosis, the synonyms are now largely of historical interest.

DEFINITION

Put briefly, hereditary spherocytosis (HS) is an autosomal dominant, chronic hemolytic anemia caused by an unknown erythrocyte membrane defect that in its full expression manifests anemia, jaundice, and splenomegaly clinically, spherocytic red blood cells (RBC) on blood smear and in vitro increased osmotic fragility and autohemolysis of such cells. Invariably, splenectomy leads to clinical cure such that in any seeming splenectomy failure, the diagnosis must be seriously questioned or thrown out. HS is the first described and most common heritable hemolytic disorder in Northern Europeans with an incidence of about 1 in 5000. It probably occurs in all ethnic groups including blacks, among whom it was formerly thought to be rare.

Inheritance. As expected from autosomal dominant inheritance, the sibling ratio is about

0.5. However, in about 10 to 20 per cent of HS patients, both parents are said to show no demonstrable abnormalities. The degree to which this is due to new mutations or to formes frustes is not known, but one exhaustive family study showed 50 per cent of patients with diagnosed cases of HS to have a mild, compensated hemolytic process and 15 per cent to "appear healthy." Thus, a negative family history by hearsay is inconclusive. Thorough personal historical interview, physical examination, and laboratory studies are necessary. In other families the clinical penetrance of HS may be more striking. Nonetheless, the highly varied clinical picture must be kept in mind in the ensuing discussion, which largely revolves around classic or full-blown clinical manifestations. Homozygous HS has not been clearly established, but in one family all 13 children were affected and 9 also manifested physical or mental retardation.

Erythrocyte Defect. The precise cause of the intrinsic membrane defect in HS RBC remains elusive but is manifested by (1) decreased membrane surface area relative to volume, (2) resultant rigidity and lack of deformability, (3) enhanced fragmentation during incubation in vitro, (4) a blistered and wrinkled surface on scanning electron microscopy, and (5) inability to find any consistent or significant primary abnormality in RBC lipids, hemoglobin, or enzymes. More recent studies suggest a genetic defect in RBC membrane microfilament protein (spectrin) to account for the rigidity and decreased survival of HS RBC, but more work is necessary to establish the significance of this intriguing observation. The increased Na^+ leak (influx) accompanied by compensatory increased glycolysis and cation pumping is an accepted feature of the membrane defect but is thought not to be importantly involved in hemolysis.

Regardless of the basic defect of the HS RBC, their shortened survival appears to result from splenic trapping, presumably associated with increased cell rigidity and enhanced by exposure to the deleterious splenic environment of low pH, low glucose concentration, and low O_2 tension. Each passage through the splenic pulp may result in loss of membrane lipid and protein with decrease in surface-to-volume ratio and further increase in rigidity; this becomes a vicious cycle until the cell disintegrates within the spleen and the fragments are then removed by macrophages.

PRESENTING SIGNS AND SYMPTOMS AND PHYSICAL EXAMINATION

The presenting features relate principally to anemia, jaundice, hemolytic crisis, splenomega-

ly, and the development of gallstones. The greater the severity of HS, the more striking are these features and generally the earlier the detection in life. Thus, severe HS may be manifest in the neonate or in infancy and presumably very mild HS only in old age. Nonetheless, in most cases anemia is first detected in childhood or adolescence. Frequently, jaundice is minimal but can increase in severity with fatigue, exposure to cold, emotional stress, and pregnancy. Even the clinically jaundiced patient with HS is commonly described as "more yellow than sick." However, once significant clinical jaundice sets in, it usually does not clear completely until after splenectomy. Cholelithiasis, hemolytic crisis, and aplastic crisis may also be presenting manifestations and will be discussed under Common Complications.

The spleen is clinically enlarged in about 80 per cent of patients, in the adult usually weighing 800 to 1500 grams. The liver in uncomplicated HS is not significantly enlarged and at the most felt 1 or several cm below the right costal margin.

HS is probably a more common cause of neonatal jaundice than generally appreciated. When diligently sought, a history of neonatal jaundice can be obtained from almost one half of the adults with HS. An unusually early or exaggerated form of "physiologic jaundice" of the newborn suggests the possibility. The differential diagnostic problem is compounded by the ordinary "physiologic jaundice" as well as by feto-maternal ABO incompatibility and sepsis, both of which can be accompanied by jaundice and spherocytosis. Some patients with neonatal HS have received exchange transfusions, and kernicterus has been reported in a few. In others, neonatal manifestation of HS has been a prelude to a severe course, forcing the issue of splenectomy in infancy. On the other hand, the degree of hemolysis in neonatal HS does not necessarily have predictive value as to the future of the disease. The various stressful circumstances of the neonatal period may bring out exaggerated hemolysis at that time, only to have the disorder settle down into a milder course later.

There are some complications of HS formerly considered prominent but now only rarely noted clinically, probably a phenomenon secondary to better detection of the disorder in its milder forms. These include chronic ankle ulcers, tower skull, and other roentgen findings that are similar to those of sickle cell anemia and thalassemia, albeit usually milder, and that may clear only after splenectomy. Extramedullary erythropoiesis may occasionally lead to paravertebral masses (heterotopia) visible on chest x-ray in children.

More than 20 different congenital abnormalities have been described in isolated cases of HS (e.g., of eyes, nose, palate, and digits), but the frequency may be no greater than in the population at large. Formerly, retardation of growth and development was prominently mentioned in HS. Nowadays, the threat of future potential retardation is not considered in itself an important factor in the decision for splenectomy in childhood.

COURSE

HS may be manifested or detected at any time from birth to old age. Patients most frequently come to medical attention for evaluation of anemia or unexplained jaundice (often attributed to hepatitis), during evaluation of cholelithiasis, or as part of a family study for HS. Mild HS itself is quite compatible with a normal life expectancy. However, the threat of severe and even fatal aplastic crisis and cholelithiasis remains. To obviate this, splenectomy is favored usually *after* the age of 7 if HS is well documented and the spleen is palpable, even if anemia and jaundice are mild. Surgery is usually less upsetting to school and employment records if performed during childhood. Once the spleen is removed (and the gallbladder, if cholelithiasis is present), the patient should have a normal life expectancy free of the complications of HS.

COMMON COMPLICATIONS

Cholelithiasis. This complication is seen in 43 to 85 per cent of HS patients over the age of 10 but has been detected in children as young as age 3. Multiple pigmented stones, predominantly calcium bilirubinate and hence radiopaque, are usually present. Once cholelithiasis is detected in HS, splenectomy and cholecystectomy are indicated. Preoperative work-up should include cholecystogram (and, if necessary, ultrasound visualization of the gallbladder) so that at the time of splenectomy, the patient's condition permitting, cholecystectomy can also be carried out. Preoperative diagnostic gallbladder studies are thus important to guide the surgical planning as well as in the occasional patient to detect "gallstone sand" at times difficult to ascertain solely by palpation of the gallbladder at operation. A particularly serious problem is the blockage of the entire extrahepatic biliary drainage system with thick, tenacious tar-like bile precipitate difficult to remove at surgery and sometimes causing death. All of this serves to emphasize the potentially serious nature of cholelithiasis in HS. Thus, a patient may have a lifelong relatively mild course with HS only to die in older age of the complications of serious cholelithiasis.

Hemolytic Crisis. From time to time the jaundice may deepen and the anemia increase, often accompanied by abdominal pain, vomiting, tachycardia, and fever. This so-called "crise de déglobulization" is described less than the aplastic crisis in recent years. This hemolytic crisis may develop in association with infection thought possibly to occur with secondary splenic hyperplasia.

Folate Deficiency. "Relative" folate deficiency (owing to increased demands of folate for the accelerated erythropoiesis) in patients with chronic hemolytic disease can be exaggerated, especially by dietary deficiency, intestinal malabsorption, drugs that interfere with folate absorption (e.g., oral contraceptives and certain anticonvulsants), pregnancy, liver disease, or alcoholism. Decrease in reticulocytosis, increased anemia, marrow megaloblastosis, and lastly, response to folate provide the diagnostic features.

Propensity to Infection. Whether there is truly an increased incidence of infections in children with severe HS is a moot question. However, infections can exacerbate the anemia, either by aplastic crisis or by splenic sequestration. Furthermore, it is clear that splenectomy during the first years of life carries a high risk of infection, particularly virulent and overwhelming pneumococcal sepsis and meningitis.

LABORATORY FINDINGS

In common with other hemolytic disorders HS manifests anemia, reticulocytosis, polychromatophilia, occasionally circulating nucleated red cells, marrow erythroid hyperplasia, normal to increased marrow iron, increased unconjugated bilirubin, and absent serum haptoglobin. Hemoglobin concentrations of 9 to 12 grams per dl (100 ml) are commonly seen but during a crisis may fall to 3 to 4 grams per dl. Persistent hemoglobin values less than 8 grams per dl are rare. Reticulocytosis is commonly at 5 to 20 per cent but may be as high as 90 per cent or during aplastic crisis as low as 2 per cent.

Slightly to moderately increased unconjugated serum bilirubin and increased fecal and, less often, urinary urobilinogen reflect the increased erythrocyte destruction and hemoglobin catabolism. Even in the occasional striking increase in serum bilirubin owing to hemolytic crisis, values greater than 6 to 8 mg per dl are suspect for other causes being involved as well, e.g., biliary obstruction or liver disease. The same is true if the conjugated bilirubin increases to greater than 25 to 30 per cent of the total bilirubin. Despite the increase in serum bilirubin, bile pigments and bile salts are absent from the urine in uncomplicated HS, hence the historical designation "acholuric jaundice." Although the RBC destruction is extravascular and hemoglobinemia and hemoglobinuria are not observed, unbound plasma haptoglobin is reduced or absent.

Examination of the peripheral blood smear usually provides the first specific clue, viz., the presence of a population of small, *densely* staining RBC lacking the normal central pallor. In moderate to severe cases, these microspherocytes are usually present in large proportion and readily detected. If only a few microspherocytes are present, they may often be more readily noted on scanning with the high, dry objective than with the use of oil immersion. The presence of varying proportions of these small spherocytes on the one hand and large reticulocytes and other young RBC on the other hand (as in any overt hemolytic anemia) leads to variable expression of RBC indices. Thus, the MCV may be low, normal, or high. The MCH is usually normal. However, as a consequence of the loss of membrane relative to cell volume, the MCHC is usually increased (commonly to 37 to 39 per cent) in the presence of a high proportion of microspherocytes, a finding shared by few other disorders. Thus, anisocytosis may be marked, but poikilocytosis is not usually striking even though a few fragmented forms may be seen. The polychromatophilia reflects the presence of reticulocytes. The presence of spherocytes in other disorders is discussed under Pitfalls in Diagnosis.

DIAGNOSTIC LABORATORY TESTS

The diagnosis of HS requires that it be kept in mind as a possibility and that other causes of chronic hemolysis be excluded. With proper testing the direct Coombs' test is negative as is also the indirect Coombs' test (unless there has been previous sensitization). The presence of microspherocytes on the peripheral blood smear is obviously the starting point in diagnosis.

Osmotic Fragility. HS RBC hemolyze more readily than normal RBC upon exposure to hypotonic solutions of buffered NaCl (increased osmotic fragility). The saline concentration at which hemolysis begins usually ranges from 0.51 to 0.72 gram per dl but may be as high as 0.85 gram per dl with hemolysis often complete at hypotonic NaCl concentrations at which hemolysis of normal cells just begins. The plotted osmotic fragility curve of HS cells is typically similar in shape to that obtained with normal cells but shifted to higher NaCl concentrations. However, there may be "tails" of the curve, owing at the high end of NaCl concentrations to very fragile HS RBC and at the low end owing to very immature and resistant cells.

"Incubated" Osmotic Fragility. In suspected mild cases exhibiting few spherocytes on blood smear or if the standard test on fresh blood is negative, it is essential to test the osmotic fragility of RBC *incubated* under sterile conditions at 37 C for 24 hours (heparinized or defibrinated blood). It is important to run a control on incubated normal blood since incubation per se increases osmotic fragility. However, that of HS RBC increases even more strikingly. The use of the "incubated" osmotic fragility test in family studies may be particularly helpful. Patients with only the incubated test positive apparently respond just as well to splenectomy. In neonatal manifestation of HS, incubation of the blood may be required to demonstrate the increased osmotic fragility.

The increase in osmotic fragility in HS does not correlate well with the degree of anemia but does with the degree of spherocytosis. Not unexpectedly, the osmotic fragility may be only minimally abnormal during an aplastic crisis. Testing has been simplified by the availability of a commercial kit.

Autohemolysis. Although not mandatory for diagnosis, the increased spontaneous hemolysis (10 to 50 per cent) of HS blood after incubation under sterile conditions at 37 C for 48 hours is a useful test, especially if in addition it is corrected to normal or near normal (<4 per cent) by the prior addition of glucose. These findings are characteristic of HS but not completely specific. Autohemolysis may also be increased in autoimmune hemolytic anemias and in hereditary hemolytic anemias owing to enzymatic defects. In the former, the addition of glucose is not usually protective, and in the latter, the response to glucose is variable.

DIAGNOSTIC CLINICAL INVESTIGATIONS

Erythrocyte Survival and Organ Sequestration. Determination of RBC survival with labeled erythrocytes is rarely required but may be of value to demonstrate the presence of intrinsic RBC abnormality in selected cases by employing cross-transfusion studies. Enhanced accumulation of radioactivity occurs in the spleen because of its selective trapping of HS RBC.

Family Studies. Strong confirmatory evidence for HS can be provided by the demonstration of clinical and laboratory findings similar to those of the patient in a familial pattern consonant with an autosomal dominant mode of inheritance. As mentioned previously, because of clinical mildness of HS in some family members, a negative family history may be reliable only if personal historical interview and examination and detailed laboratory testing are carried out.

Response to Splenectomy. Response to splenectomy with disappearance of anemia, hyperbilirubinemia, and reticulocytosis soon after the operation constitutes a gratifying diagnostic-therapeutic test. Spherocytosis and increased osmotic fragility persist with even more pronounced increments in osmotic fragility of incubated RBC owing to the more prolonged survival in the circulation of cells having potential for such changes upon incubation. It is not an uncommon event for the patient to deny easy fatigability before splenectomy only to note a most gratifying and unexpected increased sense of well-being and strength after splenectomy. After splenectomy the leukocyte count may be elevated (at times 20,000 to 30,000 per cu mm) for variable and even prolonged periods. This should be ascertained and the patient informed so that in the event of another illness, especially with abdominal pain, the leukocytosis is properly interpreted. Some elevation of the platelet count may also persist for years.

PITFALLS IN DIAGNOSIS

HS may occasionally be confused with a case of acquired autoimmune hemolytic anemia that is atypical because the conventional Coombs' test is negative. Spherocytosis and increased osmotic fragility may be seen in other hereditary or acquired hemolytic disorders. Therefore, appropriate studies to exclude the presence of abnormal hemoglobins, RBC enzymatic defects, RBC antibodies and toxins, and other diseases should be obtained. The spherocytosis and increased osmotic fragility are usually more striking or persistent or both in full-blown clinical HS than in the other disorders.

Furthermore, increased autohemolysis in other disorders is not usually corrected by the prior addition of glucose. In contrast to other disorders in which spherocytes are seen, the MCHC in HS is usually greater than 35 per cent. Finally, in extremely difficult cases, splenectomy, unless contraindicated on other grounds, may assist in resolving the issue.

HEREDITARY ELLIPTOCYTOSIS (OVALOCYTOSIS)

by HUSSAIN I. SABA, M.D., Ph.D.,
and ROBERT C. HARTMANN, M.D.
Tampa, Florida

DEFINITION

Hereditary elliptocytosis (HE) (or ovalocytosis), when accompanied by overt clinical hemolysis, is similar to hereditary spherocytosis in its clinical manifestations, associated complications, laboratory findings, and clinical cure with splenectomy. Thus, in the *hemolytic* group of HE there is clear-cut anemia, jaundice, and splenomegaly. However, the overtly *hemolytic* group probably comprises only a small proportion of cases of HE (10 to 15 per cent), and the large essentially *asymptomatic* group is difficult to define with precision.

The only practical diagnostic feature in the asymptomatic group may be the presence of a morphologic anomaly (viz., elliptocytosis) on the blood smear. "Ovoid" red blood cells (RBC) can be seen in a spectrum of shapes from "mildly oval" in up to 15 per cent of RBC in normal blood smears to more exaggerated oval forms in a variety of blood disorders (e.g., macro-ovalocytes in megaloblastic anemias) and finally a mixture of oval and rod-shaped forms comprising 25 to 90 per cent of RBC, which is diagnostic for HE. Thus, discrimination must be made as to type and percentage of oval cells.

Although hereditary elliptocytosis is said to be less common than hereditary spherocytosis, significantly increased numbers of elliptical cells have been reported in as many as 4 in 10,000 persons, an incidence similar to that of hereditary spherocytosis. There is no sex predilection, and HE is widespread throughout the world.

Inheritance. As with hereditary spherocytosis, the disorder is autosomal dominant. Linkage of the gene for HE with the Rh blood type has been demonstrated in families with mild or *asymptomatic* HE but not in those with the overtly *hemolytic* form. Although only 10 to 15 per cent have overt hemolysis, data are conflicting regarding the uniformity of hemolytic manifestations within families, in part perhaps because clear-cut differentiation between compensated hemolytic disease and complete freedom from hemolysis has not always been made. Nonetheless, in one family 57 per cent of the members showed signs of hemolysis at one time or another. Thus, the disease within a given family can have a relatively homogeneous expression. During the course of the disease the differentiation between asymptomatic and hemolytic groups may prove to be too arbitrary. It is likely that under certain stresses some of the asymptomatic group may show overt clinical hemolysis.

Erythrocyte Defect. Elliptocytes are characterized by an axial ratio (width-to-length) less than 0.78 (normal about 1.0). Nucleated RBC precursors and reticulocytes are round, not ovoid. Membrane cholesterol appears to be concentrated or polarized to the sites of greatest convexity, and on electron microscopy the hemoglobin appears similarly aggregated in a bipolar arrangement. The RBC glycolytic enzymes are normal as is the hemoglobin type, except in a few sporadic, probably coincidental cases. Upon in vitro incubation HE RBC show an abnormally rapid decline in adenosine triphosphate (ATP) and 2,3 diphosphoglycerate (2,3 DPG) with increased Na^+ efflux. However, neither the degree of these biochemical abnormalities nor the percentage of elliptocytes correlates with the degree of hemolysis in the HE patient. The hereditary elliptocyte appears to share many features with the hereditary spherocyte: abnormal cell shape, selective destruction in the spleen, and probably a somewhat similar membrane permeability defect. However, intracellular biochemical factors that differentiate the hemolytic variety of HE from the asymptomatic variety remain unknown.

SYMPTOMS, SIGNS, AND PHYSICAL EXAMINATION

The clinical picture is similar to that of hereditary spherocytosis but even more variable in its expression, consonant with the extremely large proportion of asymptomatic individuals. Thus, commonly mild elliptocytosis may be an incidental finding in an asymptomatic, nonanemic subject. In symptomatic patients neonatal jaundice, intermittent icterus, anemia, splenomegaly, and aplastic crisis may occur, the last especially in the course of intercurrent disease. There is also, as in hereditary spherocytosis, an increased incidence of cholelithiasis, especially early in life, which may be the lead to medical attention and diagnosis. Occasionally, skeletal deformities are seen as in hereditary spherocytosis.

COMMON COMPLICATIONS

These are identical to those of hereditary spherocytosis. As in hereditary spherocytosis, it is the complications that are particularly to be feared.

LABORATORY FINDINGS

There may be no laboratory findings except for the presence of elliptical cells on the blood smear. Upon closer scrutiny, a large proportion of supposedly *asymptomatic* patients may show laboratory manifestations of mild, largely compensated hemolysis with hemoglobin concentration of 12 grams per dl (100 ml) or more, reticulocytosis up to 4 per cent, and ^{51}Cr-labeled RBC survival normal or only slightly reduced.

Ten to 15 per cent of patients (hemolytic group) have a more severe hemolysis with hemoglobin concentrations of 9 to 10 grams per dl, reticulocytosis up to 20 per cent, and decreased red cell T½ survival, reported as low as 5 days. Some spherocytes and fragmented cells may also be seen on peripheral blood smears. Other laboratory findings of hemolysis with reference to increased hemoglobin catabolism, marrow erythroid hyperplasia, and reduced or absent unbound haptoglobin are present and as cited in the article on Hereditary Spherocytosis. Although the anemia has been described as normochromic and normocytic, the mean corpuscular volume (MCV) and mean corpuscular hemoglobin (MCH) can be low (50 to 76 cu micra and 18 to 28 picograms, respectively). Usually the mean corpuscular hemoglobin concentration (MCHC) is normal.

There is mixed opinion regarding the results of the osmotic fragility and autohemolysis tests in HE, perhaps arising from failure to separate consistently the results in the overtly hemolytic groups from those in the asymptomatic group. A major opinion is that the osmotic fragility tests (on both fresh and incubated cells) and the autohemolysis test are negative when there is no evidence of overt hemolysis, but that all three are positive when active hemolysis is present. Another opinion is that the osmotic fragility test on fresh RBC is normal but that on *incubated* cells, as well as the autohemolysis test, is positive. The abnormal autohemolysis test is supposedly corrected by the prior addition of glucose. In any event, it seems obvious that more work is necessary to clarify the situation.

DIAGNOSTIC LABORATORY AND CLINICAL FINDINGS

Since there are no other pathogenetic findings, the diagnosis revolves around the finding of a significant proportion of appropriate types of oval cells, that is, 25 to 90 per cent of ovalocytes, including rod-shaped forms. To eliminate artifactual effects one should see the oval forms diffusely throughout the smear and not in small collections with the axes all pointing in one direction. Unlike sickle cells, the elliptocytes do not change their shape in sealed fresh preparations. Average dimensions are 8.1 microns long and 5.3 microns wide, but the former may be as large as 12.2 microns and the latter as small as 1.6 microns. The disorder must be differentiated from other causes of mild-to-moderate elliptocytosis, such as thalassemia, sickle cell anemia, iron deficiency, myelofibrosis, macro-ovalocytosis (e.g., as in megaloblastic anemias), and certain red cell enzymopathies. The number of elliptical forms in a newborn with HE gradually increases until the child is 3 to 4 months of age. Hemolysis and hyperbilirubinemia requiring exchange transfusions have been observed in the newborn, at which time the morphologic picture more closely resembles pyknocytosis rather than elliptocytosis.

Further diagnostic help may be obtained from demonstration of findings in family members in a manner consonant with autosomal dominant mode of inheritance. Response to splenectomy with persistence of the morphologic abnormality in those with the classic disease serves to confirm the diagnosis.

PITFALLS IN DIAGNOSIS

Little confusion exists regarding the patient with a high percentage of elliptocytes on peripheral blood smear, frank hemolysis, splenomegaly, and response to splenectomy. As discussed earlier, the disorder must be differentiated from other causes of mild to moderate elliptocytosis. Appropriate tests should be obtained to exclude RBC enzymopathies, hemoglobin abnormalities, thalassemia, iron deficiency, myelofibrosis, and megaloblastic anemias not only as the primary diagnosis but even as a distinct and separate feature sometimes complicating a case of HE.

PAROXYSMAL NOCTURNAL HEMOGLOBINURIA

By ROBERT C. HARTMANN, M.D.
and HUSSAIN I. SABA, M.D., Ph.D.
Tampa, Florida

SYNONYMS

Strübing-Marchiafava-Micheli syndrome, chronic hemolytic anemia with perpetual hemosiderinuria.

DEFINITION

Paroxysmal nocturnal hemoglobinuria (PNH), the "great hematologic impostor," has attracted the attention of hematologists far out of proportion to its uncommon occurrence. For many reasons PNH has been considered a rather exotic "clue disorder." For example, it is the only *acquired* hemolytic anemia strictly caused by an intrinsic defect in the red blood cell (RBC). Furthermore, it is the prototype of *intravascular* hemolysis versus the more common type of hemolysis confined to the reticuloendothelial system. Thus, it readily permits the study of the long-term damaging effects of *intravascular* hemolysis on organ function that probably occurs largely from a remarkable chronic thrombotic state. Whatever its basic membrane defect, the crux of the disorder is that the *PNH erythrocyte possesses an exquisite sensitivity to the hemolytic action of complement* in the absence of detectable red blood cell (RBC) antibody. This phenomenon is the fundamental basis for the diagnostic tests and the initiating cause for most of the clinical picture.

Incidence. PNH is clearly not as extremely rare as formerly thought (i.e., two per 10^6). Some 85 cases have been seen at the Royal Postgraduate Medical School in London. Similarly large series have been reported from Asia. The increasing recognition may be due to: (1) greater awareness and availability of sensitive diagnostic tests, (2) increasing incidence of aplastic anemia, and (3) more prolonged survival in aplastic anemia allowing time for some patients to progress to PNH. In one half of the patients the onset is between the ages of 20 and 50 years. Not rarely it is seen between 10 and 20 years of age, but its onset is exceptional below age 10 and after age 70. The sex ratio is approximately equal. Family studies including those on identical twins have been negative.

Erythrocyte Defect. The membrane defect leading to the exquisite sensitivity to complement hemolysis remains unknown. Deficiency of RBC membrane acetylcholinesterase (AChE) activity is the most consistent biochemical anomaly detected. It may be extremely severe (e.g., 0 to 20 per cent of normal), and some deficient activity is present in all but those with the mildest hemolysis. However, the function of this enzyme in normal red blood cells (RBC) remains unknown. Furthermore, it is clear from extended studies that the deficiency of AChE activity is not the direct cause of the hemolysis, although the AChE deficiency serves as an excellent marker for that proportion of RBC susceptible to complement hemolysis. There is evidence that two (or more?) populations of RBC circulate in the PNH patient: (1) one complement-sensitive and lacking AChE activity, and (2) the other with normal or near normal complement-sensitivity and AChE activity. These findings taken in conjunction with the observed interrelationships between PNH and spontaneous or drug-induced aplastic anemia, acute leukemia, and myelofibrosis have led to the clonal theory of PNH. Accordingly, PNH is thought to arise from a clone of precursor cells in the setting of marrow damage.

Electron microscopy has revealed a patchy and pitted RBC surface and abnormal electron-dense material. Attempts to implicate abnormal membrane lipid composition or sensitivity to peroxidation have not met with consistent results. Recently the search has been directed more toward a membrane structural protein defect. Despite extensive research activity, to date no meaningful explanation for the exquisite sensitivity to complement has been forthcoming.

Granulocytes are often reduced in number; their phagocytic activity for certain organisms may be reduced; they are more susceptible to complement lysis and have reduced alkaline phosphatase activity. Platelets are often reduced in number but usually have a normal life span. They are more sensitive to antibody-induced, complement-dependent lysis. Therefore, PNH should be considered a disorder of hematopoiesis rather than just of erythropoiesis.

CLINICAL FEATURES:
PRESENTATION, SYMPTOMS, AND SIGNS

The symptoms and signs of PNH are so highly varied that it is impossible to present any typical clinical picture. It is in the main determined by varying combinations, degrees and changing patterns of hemolysis, bone marrow hypoplasia, thrombosis, and infection. At one end of the spectrum exist cases of severe anemia and hemolysis and complicating thromboses and infections; at the other end are quiescent, or "burned-out," cases with little or no anemia or gross hemoglobinuria. These variations exist both between patients and in the same patient at different times. Even in seemingly mild cases, sudden, disastrous complications can occur that require expeditious diagnosis and emergency treatment.

Delay in Diagnosis. PNH has seldom been diagnosed at the start of the patient's illness. Five to 10 years' delay in diagnosis is by no means rare. It is when features other than severe hemolysis dominate the picture that delay in diagnosis is prolonged.

Hemolysis. Twenty-five to 50 per cent of PNH patients have gross hemoglobinuria at the onset of the disorder, and eventually 80 to 90 per cent develop this manifestation. Typically it is nocturnal with progressive clearing during the day. It may occur in repetitive nocturnal cycles lasting 1 to 14 days (commonly 3 to 5 days). Such attacks occur with extreme variability, ranging from multiple times in a single month to but a few isolated episodes during the entire course of the disease. When carefully studied, it is discovered that the onset is after some 6 to 8 hours of sleep, and hence first noticed in the morning urine. Reversal of day-night sleep patterns proves that the hemoglobinuria is related to sleep. Many elegant studies (including diurnal patterns of pH, cortisol, complement and Mg^{++}) have failed to explain the nocturnal (or sleep) association.

There are, however, many exceptions. With severe episodes, notably those with recognized inciting factors, gross hemoglobinuria may be constant day and night. Inciting factors include infections, exposure to cold, drug and serum reactions, whole blood transfusions, surgery, iron therapy, severe exercise, and possibly certain foods. The common denominators probably include activation of complement and induction of systemic acidosis.

The chronic intravascular hemolysis is manifested by increased plasma hemoglobin, methemalbuminemia, hemoglobinuria, and hemosiderinuria. Clinical jaundice and unconjugated hyperbilirubinemia probably result from the catabolism of methemalbumin. *Perpetual hemosiderin* is the common denominator for all PNH patients.

Other presentations include those of an ill-defined chronic hemolytic process without gross hemoglobinuria. Such may remain un-diagnosed for years until an episode of gross hemoglobinuria provides the clue.

"Aplastic Anemia–PNH" Syndrome. As many as one fourth of PNH patients carry an initial diagnosis of aplastic anemia. When the "aplastic anemia" picture dominates the course, the acid and sucrose hemolysis tests may give relatively weak results and appear largely of secondary interest. Such cases behave clinically more like aplastic anemia.

Physical Findings. As in any hemolytic anemia, pallor and jaundice occur to varying degrees. Clinically detectable splenomegaly is not constant but may occur during episodes of gross hemoglobinuria. However, liver-spleen scans rather consistently reveal some degree of splenic enlargement. The liver may or may not be palpably enlarged. When the clinical picture is dominated by an "aplastic anemia" phase, the physical findings are frequently those associated with hemorrhage and infection.

COMPLICATIONS

The separation of complications from usual clinical manifestations is rather arbitrary since complications so frequently characterize much of the clinical course.

Infections. Formerly, infections were considered the principal cause of death in PNH, but this is no longer true with the advent of better management of infections in general. Neutropenia and impaired phagocytosis have been cited as factors leading to a propensity to infection. The major consideration is that infection is likely to set off severe hemolysis with gross hemoglobinuria.

Iron Deficiency. Because of the heavy urinary loss of iron in the form of hemoglobin and hemosiderin, iron deficiency develops sooner or later in most cases of PNH. The body distribution of iron is unusual with heavy renal siderosis, but other tissues are usually deficient in iron. Hypochromia may be difficult to appreciate because of macrocytosis owing to a young RBC population. Depression of serum iron may be masked by the ongoing hemolysis and the use of transfusions. Bone marrow examination is usually necessary to detect the iron deficiency. No extensive experience with serum ferritin determinations has been documented. In most PNH patients treatment with oral or parenteral iron precipitates gross hemoglobinuria sooner or later. Indeed, such has been cited as unmasking the diagnosis. Specific replacement treatment of the iron deficiency is thus not only hazardous but probably not highly essential, since iron stores are used at high priority for erythropoiesis.

Transfusion Reactions. Eventually, repeated transfusions of *whole blood* usually provoke episodes of gross hemoglobinuria that may provide the initial tip toward diagnosis. When studied, such patients usually have leukoagglutinins, but these are clearly not the cause of all hemolytic transfusion reactions in PNH.

Drug and Serum Reactions. Whether the alleged increased incidence of reactions is unique to PNH or simply what might be expected in a group of chronically ill patients with greater than usual exposure to such agents has not been clarified. In any event, such reactions are apt to induce serious episodes of gross hemoglobinuria, and great care should be exercised with the use of such agents.

Hemorrhage. Despite the relatively high frequency of thrombocytopenia in PNH, thrombosis rather than hemorrhage occurs. Spontaneous hemorrhage is probably more common in those with a predominantly "aplastic anemia" picture.

Association with Other Blood Dyscrasias. The intimate association of PNH with aplastic anemia has already been discussed. In a small number of cases there has been an association with myelosclerosis with myeloid metaplasia. In some the clinical picture of myeloid metaplasia predominated, with the presence of ancillary laboratory features of PNH. In several the presenting picture of myeloid metaplasia was subsequently supplanted by rather typical PNH.

There are now about a dozen cases of PNH reported to have terminated in leukemia, usually the acute nonlymphoid type. One patient went the route of successive development of chloramphenicol-induced aplastic anemia, PNH, and acute leukemia. Chromosomal studies have been widely quoted as normal in PNH, and this appears true for cultured lymphocytes from peripheral blood. However, when the *marrow* has been studied, a significant proportion have had varied but significant chromosomal abnormalities, suggesting the possibility of slow evolution of a preleukemic state.

Thrombotic Diathesis. Nowadays thrombosis is probably the most common cause of death in PNH. Major, large vein thrombosis has long been recognized, particularly peripheral vein thrombosis, pulmonary infarction, and cerebral and portal vein thrombosis. Only recently has the concept been extended to an undercurrent of chronic, smoldering low-grade thrombosis occurring in small veins and in the microcirculation and leading in some instances to eventual organ damage. The latter probably results in headaches, leg cramps, peculiar skin lesions, abdominal pain, gastrointestinal ulceration, progressive renal damage, and bone changes. Thrombosis is usually venous, but a few cases

have been arterial. Autopsy studies reveal that virtually all venous sites have been involved.

The osseous and renal changes in particular simulate those of sickle cell anemia, albeit milder. It had been considered remarkable that renal damage did not occur in PNH despite the severe renal siderosis. There is no solid evidence that renal siderosis per se is significantly harmful. However, when carefully studied, many patients demonstrate varying degrees of microscopic hematuria and proteinuria distinct from gross hemoglobinuria, fixed hyposthenuria, abnormal tubular function, declining creatinine clearance, and eventually hypertension. Radiologically, there are enlarged kidneys, cortical infarcts, and thinning and papillary necrosis, and in some patients eventual kidney shrinkage, all confirmed by autopsy.

Abdominal Pain. Abdominal pain in PNH can present a particularly difficult diagnostic problem between peptic ulceration; cholelithiasis; and mesenteric, portal, or hepatic venous thrombosis. There is an increased incidence of peptic ulceration in PNH. Cholelithiasis owing to pigmented gallstones occurs. Abdominal pain in PNH should be considered secondary to intra-abdominal thrombosis unless proved otherwise. Repeated attacks of mesenteric venous thrombosis are common in some patients and difficult to define and treat but in most instances clear eventually without sequelae.

Hepatic Venous Thrombosis. Probably the most dread, highly fatal complication of PNH is progressive, diffuse hepatic venous thrombosis (HVT) involving not only major venous branches but secondary and tertiary radicles as well. The clinical-laboratory picture has only recently been crystallized. Diagnosis is suggested by a clinical complex of abdominal pain, low-grade fever, (further) increase in liver size, occasionally liver tenderness, and when the condition is advanced, ascites. Certain laboratory results support the diagnosis of HVT: (1) further elevation of serum lactic dehydrogenase (LDH) and serum glutamic oxaloacetic transaminase (SGOT) (above baseline elevations due to chronic hemolysis alone); (2) elevated serum glutamic pyruvic transaminase (SGPT); (3) increased *conjugated* bilirubin (above 25 per cent of total even when the total is normal); and (4) an elevated titer of fibrin split products. Abnormal liver scans provide the most useful and least invasive procedure for the diagnosis of HVT and show hepatic and splenic enlargement, unequal distribution of colloid in the various lobes of the liver, and rapid changes in pattern and extrahepatic uptake. These changes also occur in advanced cirrhosis and must therefore be interpreted in the proper setting.

The rapidly progressing and highly fatal nature of HVT in PNH makes prompt diagnosis and institution of therapy mandatory. Given the typical clinical and biochemical findings plus an abnormal liver scan, heparin should be started immediately. If then deemed necessary, appropriate angiographic studies (e.g., hepatic venogram) can be carried out later. However, with increasing awareness of the clinical, laboratory, and liver scan patterns, angiographic studies, although of interest, should rarely if ever be necessary for the diagnosis. Liver biopsies are to be condemned since they rarely show a diagnostic lesion because of the spotty involvement even with *open* liver biopsies, which additionally carry a heavy risk in the face of the severe liver damage. Even needle biopsies carry the disadvantage of delaying the prompt institution of heparin therapy. Exploratory laparotomy for unexplained abdominal pain in PNH in ignorance of the possibility of hepatic venous or other thrombosis is clearly unwarranted. Although there have been but one or two well-documented cases with survival and complete return of liver function, earlier diagnosis and treatment may bring better success.

Pathogenesis of Thrombosis. There have been a legion of studies attempting to interrelate blood coagulation, platelets, and the complement system with respect to thrombosis in PNH. The results have been inconclusive if not conflicting, and to make a long story short, no cohesive, confirmed mechanism has yet been established.

COURSE

From the foregoing it is apparent that the course of PNH is so highly varied as to defy any simple categorization. Prognosis varies from several years to many decades, with a very few "burned-out" or seemingly spontaneously cured cases. Yet disastrous and even fatal complications can strike at any time. The frequent delays in diagnosis can play havoc with the patient's physical, mental, and financial well-being. Prognosis probably depends ultimately on the size of the patient's complement-sensitive RBC population, the degree of marrow aplasia, and the occurrence of serious thrombotic episodes.

LABORATORY FINDINGS

Although the degree of anemia varies widely, in most cases the hematocrit is less than 30 per cent. There are no distinct erythrocyte abnormalities on blood smears. The RBC indices and blood smear morphology reflect a mixture of macrocytes and polychromatophilia (paralleling the elevated reticulocyte count) and hypochromia owing to iron deficiency. The reticulocyte count ranges widely (e.g., 1 to 40 per cent) but commonly is 5 to 20 per cent.

The leukocyte count is low either regularly or at some time during the disorder in about 50 per cent of patients. It may be less than 1500 per cu mm and is principally associated with neutropenia. The leukocyte alkaline phosphatase activity is low or even zero but in the "aplastic group" may be normal. Platelet counts are less than 150,000 per cu mm in about two thirds of patients and less than 40,000 per cu mm in one fourth. Although pancytopenia has been cited as characteristic of PNH it is by no means constant from patient to patient nor within the same patient from time to time, and any combination of cytopenias can be seen. Marrow cellularity ranges from extreme hypoplasia to marked erythroid hyperplasia. Marrow iron is usually markedly reduced or absent.

The urine shows periodic gross hemoglobinuria and in many but not all cases, occult hemoglobinuria in the intervening chronic, steady state. In any event, some degree of perpetual hemosiderinuria is a sine qua non for the diagnosis. In active PNH the urine hemosiderin test gives a remarkably strong reaction with marked bluish-black discoloration of the Prussian blue reagents as well as the renal tubular cells in the urinary sediment — a finding strongly suggestive of PNH. Microscopic hematuria and fixed hyposthenuria are hallmarks of chronic renal damage owing to thrombosis. Urinary concentration tests should, however, be carried out with great care in view of the marked thrombotic tendency.

Serum chemistries typically reveal elevated unconjugated bilirubin, LDH, and SGOT activities, as seen with hemolysis. The additional changes owing to HVT have been discussed earlier in this article. One problem with serum chemistries in PNH is that clotted blood readily hemolyzes in vitro, giving inaccurate values. It is suggested that *heparinized plasma* be used for the usual serum chemistry determinations.

The following tests are normal in uncomplicated PNH: Coombs' test, osmotic fragility test on fresh RBC, serum antibodies and immunoglobulins, hemoglobin electrophoresis, and glycolytic as well as membrane enzymes (except for acetylcholinesterase). A few patients have had elevated hemoglobin F.

DIAGNOSTIC LABORATORY TESTS

The specific tests for PNH depend upon the demonstration of complement-sensitive erythrocytes in the absence of RBC antibody.

1. The Sucrose Hemolysis or "Sugar Water" Test. This test depends upon the activation of complement by low ionic strength media. One volume of blood anticoagulated with citrate or oxalate (but not with ethylenediamine tetraacetic acid [EDTA] or heparin) is mixed with 9 volumes of freshly prepared sugar water (1 volume of dry sugar diluted to 10 volumes with *distilled water*, not saline). The mixture is incubated at 37 C or room temperature for 30 minutes, centrifuged, and the supernatant inspected for evidence of gross hemolysis. The screening test is made more specific by utilizing saline-washed patient cells and fresh ABO compatible serum suspended in sucrose solution and similarly tested.

2. The Acid Hemolysis Test of Ham. This test depends upon the activation of complement by acidification of serum. One part of a 50 per cent suspension of saline-washed patient RBC is added to 9 parts of normal serum after its pH has been reduced by the addition of a small volume of dilute HCl (e.g., 0.2 N HCl). Hemolysis is evaluated after 30 minutes, incubation at 37 C.

The sucrose and acid hemolysis tests are the two most useful ones. The sucrose hemolysis test has the advantage of simplicity, not requiring special reagents and temperature and pH control, and is more sensitive. The acid hemolysis test is somewhat more specific. In the sucrose hemolysis test values of < 5 per cent hemolysis may occasionally be obtained with non-PNH cells; 5 to 10 per cent hemolysis is considered borderline; and > 10 per cent hemolysis definitely positive. Similar considerations hold for the acid hemolysis test. In both tests appropriate controls (which should yield no hemolysis) include the use of complement-inactivated heated serum (56 C for 30 minutes) and testing the patient's (acidified) serum against normal red cells.

Other diagnostic tests include the thrombin test of Crosby, the "heat test" of Hegglin-Maier, the inulin lysis screening test, and the antibody-induced lysis test. None of these possess the combination of specificity and simplicity of the sucrose and acid hemolysis tests, but several may be useful in research.

PITFALLS IN DIAGNOSIS

A high index of suspicion is paramount. Since PNH is the "great hematologic impostor," its diagnosis must always be considered in any patient with the following signs: unexplained hemolytic process, hemoglobinuria (especially cola beverage–colored urine on arising with clearing during the day), unexplained hemoglobinuric transfusion reactions, any combination of blood cytopenias, unexplained iron deficiency, precipitation of gross hemoglobinuria with iron therapy, recurrent bouts of abdominal pain, venous thrombosis, and, for that matter, any unexplained anemia. Patients with the condition may be referred by the urologist or nephrologist, particularly when pallor, weakness, and dark urine initially suggest glomerulonephritis or when gross "hematuria" actually turns out to be hemoglobinuria. A strongly positive test for hemosiderinuria is compelling evidence for PNH.

The diagnosis is made by the use of tests for the detection of complement-sensitive erythrocytes. Although these tests are simple in design and concept, false results may be obtained if they are not carefully performed with appropriate controls or if the serum used lacks adequate complement for any reason. An increase in acid hemolysis with 60 per cent of normal sera, but not in sucrose hemolysis, occurs in the rare disorder hereditary dyserythropoietic anemia.

ACQUIRED HEMOLYTIC ANEMIA

By EDWARD C. LYNCH, M.D.,
and CLARENCE P. ALFREY, M.D.

Houston, Texas

DEFINITION

Hemolytic anemia results from the premature breakdown of erythrocytes. Normally, erythrocytes survive approximately 120 days. When hemolysis is present, the life span of the red cells is shortened. A normal bone marrow responds to shortened red cell life span with a compensatory effort characterized by erythroid hyperplasia. When the degree of shortening of red cell life span exceeds the ability of the marrow to compensate, *hemolytic anemia* develops. A *compensated hemolytic state* exists when hemolysis is present, but no anemia is found because increased erythropoiesis fully compensates for the accelerated rate of destruction of erythrocytes.

The various hemolytic anemias are classified as either hereditary or acquired. In the evaluation of a patient with a hemolytic anemia of uncertain causation, one must consider both groups of hemolytic anemias. The hereditary hemolytic anemias are due to defects intrinsic to the red cells (intracorpuscular defects), whereas all the common acquired hemolytic anemias, with the exception of paroxysmal nocturnal hemoglobinuria, result from abnormalities extrinsic to the red cells (extracorpuscular defects).

CLASSIFICATION

A wide variety of disease states may result in an acquired hemolytic anemia. In the diagnostic approach to the patient with a hemolytic anemia, the physician should endeavor to establish the mechanism of the hemolytic anemia and then undertake further diagnostic steps to identify, if possible, an underlying disease process responsible for the hemolysis (Table 1).

A second useful classification relates to whether the hemolysis occurs predominantly intravascularly or extravascularly (organs of the reticuloendothelial system). Disorders in which the hemolysis is predominantly intravascular are (1) hemolytic transfusion reactions, (2) paroxysmal nocturnal hemoglobinuria, (3)

Table 1. *Acquired Hemolytic Anemia—Classification*

I. Immunohemolytic anemia
  A. Isoimmune type
    1. Hemolytic transfusion reactions
    2. Erythroblastosis fetalis
  B. Autoimmune, warm antibody type
    1. Idiopathic
    2. Secondary
      a. Lymphoproliferative disorders (chronic lymphocytic leukemia, lymphocytic lymphoma), Hodgkin's disease, histiocytic lymphoma
      b. Other neoplastic diseases (ovarian teratoma, carcinomas)
      c. Collagen disorders, particularly systemic lupus erythematosus
      d. Viral infections
      e. Sarcoid
      f. Drug-associated immune reactions
        (1) Hapten type (example: penicillin)
        (2) Innocent bystander type (examples: stibophen, quinidine)
        (3) Alpha-methyldopa
  C. Autoimmune, cold antibody type
    1. Primary cold agglutinin disease
    2. Secondary cold agglutinin–induced hemolysis
      a. *Mycoplasma pneumoniae*
      b. Infectious mononucleosis
      c. Lymphoproliferative disorders
    3. Paroxysmal cold hemoglobinuria
      a. Idiopathic
      b. Secondary
        (1) Syphilis
        (2) Viral infections

Table 1. *Acquired Hemolytic Anemia—Classification* (Continued)

II. Erythrocyte fragmentation syndrome
  A. Cardiac disorders
    1. Valvular prostheses
    2. Teflon patch repair of ostium primum defects
    3. Valvular heart disease
  B. Microangiopathic hemolytic anemia
    1. Thrombotic thrombocytopenic purpura
    2. Hemolytic-uremic syndrome
    3. Malignant hypertension
    4. Eclampsia and preeclampsia
    5. Disseminated carcinoma
    6. Microangiopathy due to immune mechanism (examples: systemic lupus erythematosus, micropolyarteritis nodosa, acute glomerulonephritis, and renal allograft rejection)
    7. Hemangiomas
    8. Disseminated intravascular coagulation
III. March hemoglobinuria
IV. Hypersplenism
  A. Portal hypertension
    1. Hepatic disease, particularly cirrhosis
    2. Portal vein occlusion
  B. Infiltrative diseases of the spleen
    1. Leukemia
    2. Lymphoma
    3. Myeloid metaplasia
    4. Reticuloendothelial disorders (example: Gaucher's disease)
  C. Collagen disorders
  D. Chronic infections
    1. Granulomatous infections
    2. Subacute bacterial endocarditis (SBE)
V. Paroxysmal nocturnal hemoglobinuria
VI. Metabolic disorders
  A. Uremia
  B. Spur cell anemia of liver disease
  C. Hypophosphatemia
VII. Environmental agents
  A. Microorganisms (malaria, bartonellosis, *Clostridium welchii* infection)
  B. Chemicals (arsine, lead, copper, water)
  C. Physical agents (thermal injury)

---

paroxysmal cold hemoglobinuria, (4) march hemoglobinuria, (5) erythrocyte fragmentation syndrome, (6) falciparum malaria, (7) *Clostridium welchii* sepsis, (8) intravenous administration of water or hypotonic solutions, and (9) thermal injury.

In some patients with warm antibody immune hemolytic anemia or cold agglutinin disease, particularly if the hemolysis is severe in degree, substantial intravascular hemolysis may occur.

PRESENTING SIGNS AND SYMPTOMS

Generally the presenting symptoms are those commonly seen in anemic patients: weakness, lassitude, malaise, dyspnea, and diminished exercise tolerance. When hemolysis develops over a short period of time, the symptoms are acute in onset. In contrast, when hemolysis causes only a slow decline in the hemoglobin level, symptoms may be minor until the hemoglobin value has decreased to 6 to 8 grams per dl (100 ml). In an anemic patient, the description of the passage of red or reddish-brown urine should raise the question of intravascular hemolysis.

A history of Raynaud's phenomenon is sometimes elicited in patients with cold agglutinin-induced hemolysis. Abdominal pain is a frequent symptom in patients with paroxysmal nocturnal hemoglobinuria and occasionally is experienced by persons with warm antibody autoimmune hemolytic anemia. Acquired hemolytic anemias commonly are associated with systemic disease processes and sometimes result from administration of certain drugs or exposure to environmental agents. Therefore, the physician in obtaining the history must thoroughly question the patient with the various causations of acquired hemolytic anemia in mind.

Physical Findings

Pallor is observed if the anemia is of sufficient severity. When the rate of hemolysis exceeds the capacity of the liver to take up and conjugate bilirubin, icterus may be detected. However, in a patient with normal hepatic and biliary tract function, jaundice will not be observed unless the hemolysis is rather severe in degree. Splenomegaly is ordinarily substantial in patients with hemolytic anemias resulting from hypersplenism and is found in patients with malaria. Mildly to moderately enlarged spleens may be palpated in 50 to 70 per cent of patients with autoimmune hemolytic anemias of the warm antibody type. Splenomegaly is sometimes detected in patients with hemolytic anemia associated with erythrocyte fragmentation. In most of the other acquired hemolytic anemias splenomegaly is uncommon. In patients who have hemolytic anemia associated with red cell fragmentation, cardiac murmurs are important diagnostically. Hemolysis in patients with prosthetic valves is commonly related to regurgitant flow resulting from a paravalvular leak, manifested clinically by the murmurs of valvular insufficiency.

Laboratory Findings

Demonstrating Hemolysis: Clinical Picture. Hemolysis should be suspected in the following clinical circumstances:

1. An anemic patient with acholuric jaundice (i.e., jaundice with no bilirubin in the urine).

2. Reticulocytosis in an anemic patient with no evidence of either blood loss or an erythropoietic response to a specific therapeutic agent (such as iron, vitamin B_{12}, or folic acid).

3. Development of an anemia (in the absence of blood loss) at a rate exceeding that which can be accounted for by total arrest of erythropoiesis. A decline in the blood hemoglobin concentration at a rate in excess of 1.0 gram per dl per week implies hemolysis, blood loss, or hemodilution. If the latter two causes can be excluded, the presence of hemolytic anemia is established.

4. The occurrence of hemoglobinuria.

Laboratory Confirmation of Hemolysis. Laboratory observations that may be useful in confirming the presence of hemolysis are as follows:

1. *An elevated value of the indirect-reacting serum bilirubin* with little or no elevation of the direct-reacting serum bilirubin. However, in patients with hemolytic anemia who have normal hepatic function, the indirect-reacting serum bilirubin will not be elevated unless the hemolysis is substantial in degree. Additionally, the indirect-reacting serum bilirubin may be elevated with a normal value of the direct-reacting serum bilirubin in patients with megaloblastic anemias (wherein breakdown of the megaloblasts in the marrow is the principal source of the elevated level of pigment), in persons with certain disorders of hepatic function such as Gilbert's disease and the Crigler-Najjar syndrome, and in association with extravasation of blood into tissues or body cavities. Thus the finding of an elevated value of the indirect-reacting serum bilirubin with a normal level of the direct-reacting serum bilirubin suggests hemolysis, but alternative explanations must be considered if other findings do not support the diagnosis of hemolytic anemia.

2. *Increased fecal and urinary excretion of urobilinogen.* The daily excretion of urobilinogen corresponds to the rate of production of bilirubin and therefore to the rate of degradation of hemoglobin. Fecal urobilinogen measurements, although usually valid as an indicator of excessive erythrocyte destruction, are infrequently conducted clinically because of the disagreeable task of carefully collecting timed stool samples for several days and analyzing them. Values for fecal urobilinogen are falsely low in patients receiving broad-spectrum antibiotics. The measurement of urinary urobilinogen is a less reliable assessment of hemolysis than determination of fecal urobilinogen.

3. *Elevated levels of free plasma hemoglobin and methemalbumin* are seen in patients with intravascular hemolysis but not in those with predominantly extravascular hemolysis.

4. *Hemoglobinuria and hemosiderinuria* are found in patients with intravascular hemolysis. The hemosiderin is formed in the renal tubular cells using iron from plasma hemoglobin filtered by the kidney. Hemosiderin is identified by staining the urinary sediment with Prussian blue. Ferritin also is excreted in the urine of these patients.

5. *Decreased or absent serum haptoglobins.* Haptoglobins are alpha-2-globulins that bind free hemoglobin. The hemoglobin-haptoglobin complex is rapidly removed from the blood by the reticuloendothelial system. The level of circulating haptoglobins declines in hemolytic anemias because the haptoglobins are consumed in the process of binding hemoglobin.

6. *Elevated values of serum glutamic-oxaloacetic transaminase (SGOT) and lactic dehydrogenase (LDH)* are often found in patients with intravascular hemolysis, because erythrocytes contain substantial amounts of these enzymes. However, tests for these enzymes have little specificity for hemolytic anemia, because values are elevated in many other disorders. The degree of elevation of the serum LDH closely parallels the severity of hemolysis in disorders in which hemolysis is intravascular.

7. *Increased carbon monoxide excretion in expired air and elevated carboxyhemoglobin level.* The alpha-bridge carbon of the protoporphyrin ring is the sole endogenous source of carbon monoxide. Thus increased hemoglobin degradation resulting from hemolysis causes increased carbon monoxide excretion. These tests are not valid in smokers. Carbon monoxide excretion is increased in some patients with ineffective erythropoiesis as well as in those with hemolytic anemias. The determination of carbon monoxide excretion, although a sensitive and prompt indicator of excessive red cell destruction, is not performed in most hospitals because of the requirement for special equipment.

8. *Shortened survival of ^{51}Cr-erythrocytes.* The half-disappearance time of autologous or compatible normal erythrocytes labeled with radiochromium and given intravenously to normal persons is 26 to 31 days. This half-disappearance time reflects a normal rate of destruction of the erythrocytes and a regular rate of elution of the isotope from the erythrocytes. When the erythrocytes of a patient with hemolytic anemia are labeled with ^{51}Cr and then returned to the patient, the half-disappearance time of the isotope from the blood is shortened. The study requires sampling of the patient's blood for 2 weeks to determine serially residual radioactivity. Results may not be valid if a "steady state" of the anemia does not exist throughout the 2 weeks. Splenic sequestration of erythrocytes may be assessed by determining, by external isotopic counting, the ratio of radioactivity detected over the spleen to that detected over the liver on the day at which half the radioactivity has disappeared from the blood. Ratios greater than 2:1 indicate significant splenic trapping of erythrocytes. In persons with autoimmune hemolytic anemia resulting from warm antibodies, ratios above 2.3:1.0 are an indication of a potentially favorable response to splenectomy.

PERIPHERAL BLOOD

Blood Counts. Leukopenia and thrombocytopenia may accompany the anemia in patients with paroxysmal nocturnal hemoglobinuria. Thrombocytopenia is commonly severe in degree in persons with microangiopathic hemolytic anemia; in contrast, patients with red cell fragmentation related to cardiac prostheses usually have normal platelet counts. The rare occurrence of thrombocytopenia with autoimmune hemolytic anemia (warm antibody type) has been termed Evans' syndrome. Patients with systemic lupus erythematosus may be pancytopenic, with both the anemia and the thrombocytopenia resulting from immune destruction of erythrocytes and platelets. Patients with hypersplenism caused by portal hypertension commonly have pancytopenia.

Red Cell Indices. In patients with acquired hemolytic anemias, the erythrocytes are usually normochromic and normocytic. However, because reticulocytes are larger than mature erythrocytes, the mean corpuscular volume (MCV) may be mildly to moderately elevated in patients wtih high reticulocyte counts. A second cause of an elevated MCV in a patient with chronic hemolysis is complicating folic acid deficiency; such patients do not have elevated reticulocyte counts. When intravascular hemolysis is chronic, the amount of iron lost in the urine (hemoglobinuria, ferritinuria, and hemosiderinuria) may be sufficient to cause iron deficiency with hypochromic microcytic red cell indices.

Erythrocyte Morphology. Examination of a peripheral blood film can be very helpful in directing the physician to a specific mechanism of a hemolytic anemia. An increased number of *polychromatophilic erythrocytes* correlates well with an elevated reticulocyte count. When the predominant morphologic abnormality is *spherocytosis*, the principal diagnostic considerations are hereditary spherocytosis and autoimmune hemolytic anemia. Observation of numerous *schistocytes, helmet cells, spherocytes, and other poikilocytes* is characteristic of the erythrocyte fragmentation syndrome. *Elliptocytes* are seen in large numbers in hereditary elliptocytosis and in smaller numbers in hypersplenism, myelofibrosis, thalassemia minor, and iron deficiency. *Acanthocytes* occur in substantial numbers in the spur cell anemia of patients with hepatic cirrhosis and in persons with abetalipoproteinemia. Lesser numbers of acanthocytes are seen in a wide variety of conditions, including disorders with erythrocyte fragmentation, uremia, and postsplenectomy. *Erythrophagocytosis*, that is, phagocytosis of red cells by monocytes, is occasionally observed in the blood of patients with autoimmune hemolytic anemia. In malaria, one may find *intraerythrocytic parasites* by examination of the peripheral blood film. When hemolysis is very severe, *normoblasts* may be identified in the blood. Excessive *aggregation of erythrocytes* on the slide suggests an antibody-induced mechanism for hemolysis.

Bone Marrow

Morphologic examination of the bone marrow is ordinarily not necessary in patients with acquired hemolytic anemias. Their elevated reticulocyte counts adequately reflect the erythroid hyperplasia of the marrow. When the reticulocyte count is not elevated in a patient with an established hemolytic anemia, megaloblastosis resulting from folic acid deficiency, rarely an "aplastic crisis," or an infiltrative disorder may be disclosed by examination of the bone marrow. In patients with leukopenia and/or thrombocytopenia, as well as hemolytic anemia, marrow aspirate should be obtained to assess the status of granulopoiesis and/or thrombopoiesis.

Determining the Mechanism of Hemolysis

By the use of various laboratory tests, one may often define the mechanism of hemolysis in patients with acquired hemolytic anemias. Several tests have a high degree of specificity in establishing a particular mechanism of hemolysis.

Direct Coombs' Test (Direct Antiglobulin Test). In patients with warm antibody autoimmune hemolytic anemia, erythrocytes are coated with immunoglobulin (IgG) or complement or both. Antibody-damaged erythrocytes are removed by macrophages of the reticuloendothelial system, particularly in the spleen. The antibody shows maximum reactivity with erythrocytes at temperatures around 37 C. The direct Coombs' test detects antibody or complement or both on the erythrocytes of patients with warm antibody hemolytic anemia.

The Coombs' reagent is a serum raised in rabbits previously sensitized by injection of human globulin. Therefore, the Coombs' reagent is an antiglobulin that reacts in vitro with human globulin (IgG or complement or both) on the membranes of red cells to cause agglutination of the cells (i.e., a positive direct Coombs' test). In order to identify whether IgG or complement or both are present on the red cells, further antisera have been developed (as reagents) that react specifically with IgG or complement when mixed with erythrocytes in vitro. The direct Coombs' reaction may be positive, but not indicative of autoimmune hemolytic anemia, in patients receiving cephalosporin drugs; the positive reaction is due to nonspecific absorption of globulins by red cells. Another cause of a positive direct Coombs' reaction in the absence of autoimmune hemolytic anemia is the occasional weakly positive reaction in patients with reticulocytosis of any cause resulting from binding of transferrin (a globulin) to the membranes of reticulocytes. Previously transfused patients may have a positive direct Coombs' test caused by minor blood group incompatibility of the transfused red cells.

Indirect Coombs' Test. The indirect Coombs' reaction will be positive if a person has free antibodies to erythrocytes in the serum. In this test, a patient's serum and compatible donor erythrocytes are mixed and incubated. Coombs' reagent is added. If antibodies to the erythrocytes are present in the patient's serum, agglutination occurs. The indirect Coombs' test is positive in many but not all cases of warm antibody hemolytic anemia. The severity of hemolysis is not necessarily related to the titer of antibody in the serum. By studying the reactivity of the serum antibody with a panel of erythrocytes obtained from multiple donors possessing many different red cell antigens, one can often ascertain whether the antibody is directed at a specific known red cell antigen (such as an Rh blood group antigen) or is "nonspecific." A patient who has a positive indirect Coombs' reaction but a negative direct Coombs' test does not have an autoimmune hemolytic anemia. The positive indirect Coombs' reaction in this circumstance has resulted from prior sensitization to a red cell antigen through transfusions or pregnancy.

Cold Agglutinin Test. In patients with hemolytic anemia resulting from cold agglutinins, hemolysis results from the action of agglutinating antibodies of immunoglobulin M (IgM) class. These antibodies show maximum reactivity between 0 and 20 C. The antibodies are generally directed at the "I" or "i" antigens of red cells. In blood containing cold agglutinins, agglutination occurs with cooling of the blood; antiglobulin reagent is not required. It is helpful clinically to determine the titer of the cold agglutinins in the serum and the thermal range of the agglutinating property of the antibodies. In patients with cold agglutinins, hemolysis is more likely to occur if the antibodies are present in high titer (1:500 or greater) and have a wide thermal range of reactivity with some activity against erythrocytes above 30 C. The direct Coombs' reaction is commonly positive in persons with cold agglutinin disease even though the erythrocytes are not cooled prior to testing.

Donath-Landsteiner Test. Paroxysmal cold hemoglobinuria is a rare hemolytic disorder in which an IgG antibody with specificity for the Pp blood group system is responsible for the hemolysis. Demonstration of the antibody is accomplished by the Donath-Landsteiner test, in which the antibody binds to erythrocytes in vitro in the cold followed by lysis of red cells by complement when the blood is warmed to body temperature.

Tests for Paroxysmal Nocturnal Hemoglobinuria (PNH). 1. Sucrose hemolysis test. PNH erythrocytes are susceptible to complement-related hemolysis when incubated in an isotonic solution of sucrose, whereas normal red cells are not likely to hemolyze.

2. Acid hemolysis test (Ham's test). PNH erythrocytes, compared to normal red cells, show higher levels of hemolysis when incubated in acidified (pH 6.5) serum containing complement.

3. Leukocyte alkaline phosphatase. The levels of this enzyme are very low in mature granulocytes of patients with PNH and those with chronic myelogenous leukemia.

4. Red cell acetylcholine esterase. The content of this enzyme in PNH erythrocytes is markedly reduced.

COURSE

The course of the illness in a patient with an acquired hemolytic anemia is quite variable because of the diverse mechanisms of hemolysis that result in acquired hemolytic anemias. Additionally, the availability of defined beneficial therapeutic programs in some of these anemias may alter the course of the illness significantly.

Hemolysis is usually self-limited in disorders such as cold agglutinin hemolysis related to *Mycoplasma pneumoniae* or infectious mononucleosis, march hemoglobinuria, and drug-related immune hemolysis. In patients with

PNH or with idiopathic warm antibody hemolytic anemia, hemolysis may be episodic or continuous. In persons with a hemolytic anemia secondary to an underlying disease process (examples: systemic lupus erythematosus, lymphoma), control of the underlying disease often ameliorates the hemolysis. Resolution of the hemolytic anemia caused by hypersplenism follows splenectomy. Improvement in the hemolytic anemia is observed frequently after splenectomy performed in patients with autoimmune hemolytic anemia, warm antibody type. Surgical correction of a malfunctioning valvular prosthesis commonly causes disappearance of a hemolytic anemia resulting from the prosthesis.

COMPLICATIONS

The decreased level of hemoglobin in the blood may result in myocardial hypoxia precipitating angina pectoris, cardiac arrhythmias, or congestive heart failure. Because of the increased formation of bilirubin by reason of increased hemoglobin catabolism, biliary tract stones are increased in incidence in patients with chronic hemolytic anemias. Folic acid requirements are greater in patients with hemolytic anemias than in normal persons because of utilization of folic acid in erythropoiesis. Thus with chronic hemolysis, folic acid deficiency may occur, manifested clinically by a decline in the reticulocyte count, macrocytic erythrocytes, hypersegmented neutrophils, and megaloblastic changes in the bone marrow. In patients with intravascular hemolysis, iron deficiency may appear owing to excessive loss of iron in the urine in the forms of hemoglobin, ferritin, and hemosiderin. Iron deficiency particularly may contribute to the severity of the anemia in patients with paroxysmal nocturnal hemoglobinuria (PNH) and those with hemolysis related to artificial valves. Rarely, "aplastic crisis" may appear during the course of an acquired hemolytic anemia. Sometimes an infection is the precipitating event in the aplastic crisis. Marrow aplasia is more common as a complicating event in PNH than in the other acquired hemolytic anemias. Additionally, in some patients presenting with aplastic anemia (but not hemolytic anemia) as an initial primary diagnosis, laboratory tests reveal the characteristic red cell abnormalities of PNH.

Venous thrombosis and pulmonary embolization are distinctly increased in incidence in patients with PNH and are somewhat more likely than expected in patients with other acquired hemolytic anemias such as the autoimmune group. The thromboses are apparently initiated by thromboplastic substances released from erythrocytes during hemolysis. Hemosiderosis may result from the chronic use of transfusional therapy. When a hemolytic transfusion reaction occurs, renal failure may develop.

Therapeutic Tests

Because rational therapy of an acquired hemolytic anemia is highly dependent upon understanding the mechanism of hemolysis and discovery in some cases of an underlying disease process, the diagnostic effort must be directed at defining carefully through laboratory tests the pathogenesis of the anemia. Most of the therapeutic modalities used in patients with acquired hemolytic anemias are potent and capable of producing complications if used inadvisably. Therapeutic tests using drugs such as corticosteroids are rarely or never helpful in establishing the specific diagnosis in the patient and should not be undertaken.

Pitfalls in Diagnosis

Major potential pitfalls in the diagnosis of an acquired hemolytic anemia are as follows:

1. Inadequate definition by laboratory means of the mechanism of hemolysis.

2. Lack of perseverence in seeking an underlying disorder (such as systemic lupus erythematosus, lymphoma, carcinoma, or prior drug therapy) to which the hemolytic anemia is secondary.

3. Failure to appreciate that certain congenital hemolytic anemias may not be recognized until adult life. Many patients with milder anemias caused by hemoglobinopathies, hereditary spherocytosis, or hereditary elliptocytosis are not diagnosed until careful evaluation of an anemia found by routine blood counts in adolescence or adulthood. Additionally, black patients with the hereditary disorder erythrocyte glucose-6-phosphate dehydrogenase deficiency experience hemolytic anemia principally after exposure to oxidant drugs. Therefore they may never be anemic until an encounter with such a drug in adult life.

4. Excessive dependence on the reticulocyte count as an indicator of hemolytic anemia. Although reticulocytosis is generally found in persons with hemolytic anemias, it is simply an indication of accelerated erythropoiesis and not specifically of hemolysis. Thus reticulocyte counts are elevated in persons with recent blood loss and those with deficiency anemias recently treated with a therapeutic agent specific for the deficiency, e.g., iron, vitamin B_{12}, or folic acid. In certain anemias related to leukemia, lymphoma, or myelofibrosis, hemolysis may be present, but the reticulocyte count may not be elevated because of infiltrative disease of the bone marrow.

5. Inappropriate reliance on the indirect-reacting serum bilirubin value. Although the value of the indirect-reacting serum bilirubin may be elevated in persons with moderate to severe hemolysis, values may be normal in patients with milder degrees of hemolysis. There are, in addition to hemolytic anemia, a number of other causes of an elevated indirect-reacting serum bilirubin such as ineffective erythropoiesis, pulmonary infarction, resolving hematomas, and Gilbert's disease.

6. Premature conclusions based upon examination of the peripheral blood film. For instance, whereas spherocytes are characteristically seen in hereditary spherocytosis, they are commonly observed in patients with autoimmune hemolytic anemia and accompany schistocytes and helmet cells in the disorders with erythrocyte fragmentation. Similarly, fragmented red cells are the morphologic hallmark of the red cell fragmentation disorders but are also observed, usually in smaller numbers, in thalassemia, iron deficiency anemia, sickle cell anemia, and myelophthisic disorders.

POLYCYTHEMIA VERA

By JOHN E. KURNICK, M.D.
Irvine, California

Synonyms

Erythremia, primary polycythemia, polycythemia rubra vera, Osler-Vaquez disease. The term polycythemia is used here to connote increases in all the cellular elements of the blood, as opposed to erythrocytosis that involves only increases in red cells.

Definition

Polycythemia vera (PV) is an acquired hematopoietic disorder characterized by excessive numbers of red blood cells, white blood cells, and platelets in the peripheral blood. Although its cause is obscure, the pathophysiology underlying these increases in all three circulating blood elements is bone marrow hyperplasia of erythroblasts, granulocytic precursors of all types, and megakaryocytes. This proliferation of all the cellular elements of the bone marrow, or panmyelosis, manifests itself early in the disease by obliteration of the fat spaces in the marrow of the axial skeleton and the appearance of cells in the normally entirely fatty marrow of the long bones. Small nests of erythroblasts, granulocytes, and megakaryocytes also appear in the enlarged spleen and liver.

As the disease progresses there is increasing myelofibrosis of the central marrow, while the cellular elements move progressively toward the peripheral skeleton, and the myeloid metaplasia in the spleen and liver may result in massive organomegaly. At this point the erythrocytosis disappears and anemia ensues, in what is termed the "spent" or "burned out" phase of polycythemia. The early panmyelosis and the ultimate myelofibrosis serve to differentiate PV from the various forms of secondary erythrocytosis, none of which reflects a primary bone marrow disorder and none of which is characterized by myeloid metaplasia.

CLINICAL AND LABORATORY FEATURES

Osler in 1903 provided an extremely accurate description of a syndrome characterized by polycythemia, splenomegaly, and cyanosis. Although acrocyanosis is commonly seen owing to sluggish peripheral circulation occasioned by the greatly increased whole blood viscosity, central cyanosis is not present in the classic case because of the usual requirement of normal arterial oxygen saturation for making the diagnosis. The Polycythemia Vera Study Group° has recently established a set of diagnostic criteria that are outlined in Table 1. Although imperfect for a number of reasons, they represent an excellent attempt to define the disease in terms of its clinical and laboratory parameters. Thus nearly every patient fulfilling the Polycythemia Vera Study Group's criteria will have PV. A small number of patients with PV will be missed by strict application of these criteria. Examples are patients with lowered blood volumes due to gastrointestinal bleeding, a frequent complication of PV, and patients with coexistent lung disease and hypoxemia.

Classically, the patient with PV presents as a ruddy-complexioned person with splenomegaly, slight hepatomegaly, and acrocyanosis. Splenomegaly is in fact present in at least 75 per cent and hepatomegaly in 25 to 50 per cent, while ruddy facies and acrocyanosis become more prominent as the hematocrit rises above 65 per cent. The patient may be asymptomatic, although complaints related to his increased vascular volume (headache, increased bleeding), elevated whole blood viscosity (impaired

mentation, peripheral circulatory failure, symptoms of heart failure), and thrombocytosis (thromboembolic events, paradoxical bleeding diathesis) are quite common. Pruritus, especially after a hot bath or shower, may be a prominent symptom and is probably related to histamine release from the increased basophils. Less common symptoms are related to complications such as gouty arthropathy or peptic ulcer disease, the latter also secondary to increased histamine levels. Quite significantly, there are no symptoms or physical findings to suggest a pulmonary, cardiac, or renal cause for the erythrocytosis.

Routine laboratory studies show the hematocrit to be well above the upper limit of normal, usually over 60 per cent and often over 70 per cent. Red blood cell morphology is most often characterized by microcytosis and hypochromia as erythrocyte production outstrips the available iron supply, but reticulocytes are seldom markedly elevated, and nucleated red blood cells are uncommon. The white blood cell count is modestly elevated, usually between 10,000 and 20,000 per cu mm, and there is a slight but definite increase in absolute numbers of eosinophils and basophils. Mild to moderate thrombocytosis is the rule, with platelet counts between 400,000 and 1,000,000 per cu mm. Occasionally one sees extreme thrombocytosis with platelet values as high as 3,000,000 per cu mm. Chest radiogram, electrocardiogram, and urinalysis reveal no specific findings, although quantitative 24-hour urinary uric acid will be increased.

More intensive laboratory investigation demonstrates elevated total body red cell volume by the ^{51}Cr technique (above 32 ml per kg in women and 36 ml per kg in men) in over 90 per

Table 1. *Polycythemia Vera Study Group Diagnostic Criteria*°

A1	Increased red cell volume (males $\geq$ 36 ml/kg; females $\geq$ 32 ml/kg)
A2	Arterial oxygen saturation $\geq$ 92%
A3	Splenomegaly
B1	Platelet count $\geq$ 400,000 cu mm
B2	White cell count $\geq$ 12,000 cu mm in the absence of infection
B3	Leukocyte alkaline phosphatase > 100 in the absence of infection
B4	Serum vitamin B_{12} > 900 pg/ml or unsaturated B_{12} binding capacity > 2200 pg/ml

---

°A cooperative group of hematologists from many centers in the United States and abroad under the chair of Dr. Louis Wasserman, funded by an NCI grant.

°The diagnosis of polycythemia vera requires all three parameters from category A *or* A1 and A2 plus any two parameters from category B.

cent of cases, with a median value close to 50 ml per kg and occasional values well above 60 ml per kg. Plasma volume by radio-iodinated serum albumin is normal or only slightly decreased, resulting in an elevated total blood volume. Arterial blood gases are characteristically normal. Leukocyte alkaline phosphatase score will be greater than 100 in 70 per cent of patients. Serum vitamin B_{12} level and unsaturated B_{12} binding capacity are frequently elevated above 900 picograms per ml and 2200 picograms per ml, respectively. Serum uric acid is often mildly elevated owing to increased marrow nucleic acid turnover, and slightly abnormal bilirubin levels may be present when the red cell mass is extremely high. Although rarely ordered, blood histamine levels will usually be above 0.1 microgram per ml. Erythropoietin is not detectable in the serum or urine in PV unless the patient is phlebotomized to a normal or low hemoglobin level. However, erythropoietin determinations are still a research tool with essentially no place in the initial evaluation of polycythemia.

When properly performed, the bone marrow examination provides extremely valuable diagnostic information in this bone marrow disorder. However, since the ratio of granulocytes to erythroblasts is not altered and cell morphology is normal, differential counts on smears of aspirated marrow particles are not helpful. Thus a histologic section of marrow core biopsy or of clotted marrow particles is necessary. On such preparations the normal marrow is seen to consist of cellular areas and fat spaces in approximately equal proportions. The cellular areas in the PV marrow nearly always comprise 80 to 100 per cent of the total marrow space with fat often absent and rarely comprising more than 20 per cent.

The increased marrow cellularity is characterized by hyperplasia of both granuloid and erythroid series, so their ratio remains normal, but megakaryocytes are increased, as are eosinophils. Iron stores are absent in over 90 per cent of patients. The hypercellularity with absent iron stores in PV is in direct contrast to the marrow of untreated secondary erythrocytosis, which is usually normocellular and often contains iron. Only with repeated phlebotomy does the marrow in secondary erythrocytosis approach the hypercellularity seen in PV, and then the hyperplasia is confined to the erythroid series.

COURSE AND COMPLICATIONS

PV runs a chronic course over about 5 to 15 years if serious complications can be avoided. During this course the active marrow extends peripherally and splenic and hepatic hematopoiesis become more prominent as the axial marrow becomes progressively fibrotic. Erythrocytosis lessens and the patient eventually becomes anemic, although the white cell and platelet counts may remain elevated. In this "spent" or "burned-out" phase, the disease is essentially indistinguishable from agnogenic myeloid metaplasia. Whether the natural history of the disease includes termination in acute granulocytic leukemia remains controversial. There is little doubt that ionizing radiation and radiomimetic therapy have contributed to an incidence of acute leukemia in the range of 20 per cent in PV patients treated with these agents.

Thrombotic and hemorrhagic complications are common and constitute the major causes of morbidity and mortality during the early stages of the disease. Venous thrombosis is abetted by sluggish flow of the abnormally viscous blood, while thrombocytosis contributes to the arterial thrombotic propensity. PV is a prominent cause of hepatic vein thrombosis. Thrombocytosis also creates a paradoxical bleeding tendency that makes surgical morbidity and mortality prohibitive in uncontrolled PV. With the elevated histamine levels contributing to a greatly increased incidence of peptic ulcer and the hemorrhagic tendency engendered by the thrombocytosis, gastrointestinal blood loss is quite common. Thus 10 per cent of PV patients will not have elevated red blood cell volumes at presentation, and a smaller proportion will actually be anemic. Gouty arthropathy and urate nephropathy complicated approximately 10 per cent of the cases before the advent of allopurinol therapy. Massive splenic enlargement later in the disease can result in splenic infarction and hypersplenism, which may necessitate splenectomy.

DIFFERENTIAL DIAGNOSIS AND DIAGNOSTIC PITFALLS

PV must be distinguished from (1) other primary bone marrow disorders such as chronic granulocytic leukemia (CGL), agnogenic myeloid metaplasia, and idiopathic hemorrhagic thrombocytosis, in all of which erythrocytosis is uncommon; and (2) other causes of erythrocytosis wherein there is no underlying bone marrow pathology (Table 2).

Distinction of PV from other hematopoietic disorders rarely presents a problem unless the PV patient is anemic with thrombocytosis and hemorrhage, or the CGL patient has an elevated hematocrit. In the first instance, the differential diagnosis may be impossible until after the hemorrhage has been controlled. In the unusual

Table 2. *Classification of Erythrocytosis*

I. Polycythemia vera
II. Secondary erythrocytosis
  A. Appropriate erythropoietin production
    (decreased tissue O_2 delivery)
    1. Lung disease
    2. Alveolar hypoventilation
      (pickwickian syndrome)
    3. Cyanotic heart disease
    4. Hemoglobinopathies with decreased
      O_2 release ("stingy" hemoglobins)
    5. Decreased 2,3-DPG
    6. High altitude
  B. Autonomous erythropoietin production
    1. Renal cysts
    2. Tumors, including hypernephroma, hepatoma,
      pheochromocytoma, cystic cerebellar hemangi-
      oblastoma, prostatic carcinoma, and
      uterine leiomyoma
III. Relative erythrocytosis (red cell volume normal)
    1. Hemoconcentration
    2. "Stress" erythrocytosis

the distinction may become impossible except by history.

In distinguishing PV from the other major causes of erythrocytosis (Table 3), it is essential first to obtain a measurement of total body red blood cell volume in order to rule out relative erythrocytosis, wherein red cell volume is normal and erythrocytosis is secondary to a decreased plasma volume. An elevated red cell volume does not differentiate true secondary erythrocytosis from PV. Arterial blood gases will indicate the large proportion of patients whose erythrocytosis is secondary to severe chronic lung disease. Here one should avoid the diagnostic pitfall of overly strict application of the Polycythemia Vera Study Group's criterion of arterial oxygen saturation over 92 per cent, since 10 per cent of PV patients will have mildly decreased saturations. The possibility of renal or hemoglobinopathic cause should be borne in mind when the cause of an increased red cell mass remains obscure. Finally, if the evaluation of erythrocytosis includes careful history and physical examination, radiochromium measurement of total red cell volume, arterial blood gases, leukocyte alkaline phosphatase determination, and bone marrow biopsy in cases in which arterial oxygen saturation is normal, the correct diagnosis will be ascertained in the vast majority of cases.

CGL patient with erythrocytosis, the presence of the Philadelphia chromosome and the low leukocyte alkaline phosphatase score serve to distinguish this condition from PV. In the polycythemic phase there is relatively little problem distinguishing PV from agnogenic myeloid metaplasia. As the PV progresses to myelofibrosis,

Table 3. *Differential Diagnosis of Erythrocytosis*

	PV	Secondary Erythrocytosis	Relative Erythrocytosis
Total blood volume	↑	↑	N
Red cell volume	↑	↑	N
Plasma volume	N	N	↓
White cell count	Usually ↑	N	N
Platelet count	Usually ↑	N	N
Bone marrow	Marked panhyperplasia	Mild erythroid hyperplasia	N
Arterial oxygen	Usually N	Usually ↓	
Leukocyte alkaline phosphate	Often ↑	N	N
Serum B_{12}	Often ↑	N	N
Splenomegaly	75%	N	N
Hepatomegaly	25–50%	N	N

N = normal or not present.

ACUTE TRANSFUSION REACTION

By DOUGLAS W. HUESTIS, M.D.

Tucson, Arizona

DEFINITION

An acute transfusion reaction may be defined as any untoward reaction occurring during or within a short time after transfusion of a blood component or components. There are many kinds of such reactions, and even more signs and symptoms that are reported as such but turn out on investigation to be unrelated to transfusion. Despite this, it is good practice to insist that any suspected reaction be reported to the blood bank and that it be appropriately investigated and interpreted.

The extent of investigation need only be sufficient to identify a reaction that could have serious clinical sequelae (e.g., immune hemolysis) and to classify a reaction so that preventive measures can be taken in future transfusions. Although traditional thinking has been that all reactions should be extensively investigated to rule out any remote possibility of hemolysis, such an approach is expensive, time-consuming, and largely productive of negative results. The investigative procedure outlined in this article entails a simple screening approach, supplemented when clinically indicated by more extensive serologic testing.

In the discussion of transfusion reaction, the customary emphasis is on the immune hemolytic transfusion reaction (HTR), since it is the most serious. But in fact HTR is uncommon compared with other transfusion reactions and is not necessarily the most serious. I am therefore focusing this article on the more frequent "minor" reactions, since they are the ones that often interfere with the completion of transfusions, causing wastage of blood, expenditure of time and effort in the laboratory, and erosion of patients' confidence in transfusion.

FREQUENCY

Table 1 shows a breakdown of 300 reported transfusion reactions at the University of Arizona Hospital in the transfusion of slightly less than 30,000 blood components. Reactions were thus reported for about 1 in 100 blood components transfused. With respect to patients transfused, reactions are generally reported in about 6 to 7 per cent.

In this series, there were three hemolytic

Table 1. *300 Reported Transfusion Reactions*

Type	Number	Percentage
Febrile nonhemolytic	184	61
Allergic	78	26
Miscellaneous other	18	6
Unrelated to transfusion	20	7
Total	300	100

episodes (listed under miscellaneous), none of which was caused by serologic incompatibility. (One was a transfusion of blood mistakenly given with water instead of saline; two were related to mechanical trauma in extracorporeal circulation.) Thus, 87 per cent of these reported reactions were either febrile or allergic. Since most of these occur during transfusion and result in the transfusion's being stopped, they cause appreciable blood wastage and interference with clinically needed transfusions.

The following outline and discussion of transfusion reactions is limited to those that occur during or immediately after transfusion, including delayed HTR, but does not include such late manifestations as disease transmission (e.g., hepatitis, malaria, syphilis) or iron overload.

INVESTIGATION OF TRANSFUSION REACTIONS

Since the occurrence of any untoward reaction during transfusion requires that the transfusion be stopped, thereby interfering with the patient's immediate treatment and potentially affecting his further therapy, such reactions must be promptly reported to the blood bank and must be investigated by a physician without delay.

Most serious and potentially dangerous transfusion reactions are caused by clerical misidentification, as in a patient receiving blood intended for someone else. For this reason, on report

Table 2. *Types of Transfusion Reactions and Mishaps*

1. Febrile nonhemolytic
2. Allergic and anaphylactic
3. Circulatory overload
4. Bleeding tendency
5. Contaminated blood, septicemia
6. HTR: immediate, delayed
7. Nonimmune hemolytic
8. Hypothermic: cold blood
9. Air embolism
10. Citrate toxicity
11. Potassium toxicity

Table 3. *Basic Transfusion Reaction Investigation*

1. Check blood bank and transfusion records to make sure patient received the blood intended for him.
2. Obtain post-transfusion clotted blood sample and do:
   a. Visual examination for hemoglobin, comparing with pretransfusion sample.
   b. Direct antiglobulin test.
   c. ABO and Rh typing.
3. Report results and interpretation to patient's physician.

of a reaction, the first thing to do is to make sure the patient got the right blood. The next is to draw a fresh clotted blood sample for the blood bank. This sample is examined visually for hemoglobin and compared with the pretransfusion serum. Any pink tinge indicates hemolysis to the extent of at least 20 mg per dl (100 ml); an actual red color, at least 30 mg per dl. Quantitative serum or plasma hemoglobin measurement is seldom indicated. On the same post-transfusion blood sample a direct antiglobulin test and repeat ABO and Rh blood type should be done. If there has been no blood mix-up, if there is no visible plasma hemoglobin, if direct antiglobulin reaction is negative, if the red cell typing conforms to that of the pretransfusion sample, and if no other reason is found to suspect red cell incompatibility, no further testing should be necessary. This procedure is simple and comparatively inexpensive (Table 3). The results and interpretation should be reported to the patient's physician.

If results of any of the investigative procedures suggest that incompatible blood may have been transfused (e.g., discrepancy in transfusion records, presence of hemoglobin, positive direct antiglobulin test, or inconsistent ABO or Rh typing), then a more detailed investigation must be carried out. The extent and nature of this will depend on the specific findings. If the wrong blood was given, it is essential to contact the patient's physician without delay, so that appropriate treatment may be started while further investigation proceeds. The presence of hemoglobin indicates red cell destruction but does not necessarily mean that the hemolysis was caused by red cell incompatibility (see later discussion). A positive direct antiglobulin reaction, if the same test was negative on the pre-transfusion sample, may have several meanings. The donor red blood cells may have been coated by an antibody in the recipient's plasma, or vice versa. It may even (rarely) indicate that there was a positive direct antiglobulin reaction on the donor red cells. In some cases, examination of the urine for hemoglobin may be worthwhile, particularly if an immediate post-transfusion blood sample was not obtained or if

hemolysis is suspected but no plasma hemoglobin is apparent. Similarly, a serum haptoglobin should be markedly decreased or absent if significant in vivo hemolysis has occurred. These latter two indications, and serum bilirubin at 5 to 7 hours, if positive, would tend to indicate that observed hemolysis in the post-transfusion blood reflected in vivo rather than factitious hemolysis. More extensive testing could include more detailed immunohematologic investigation and evaluation of renal function but are beyond the scope of this review.

FEBRILE NONHEMOLYTIC REACTION

Fever and chills during or shortly after transfusion arouse suspicion of hemolysis. This can usually be ruled out by the routine procedures given in Table 3. Until these investigations are completed, the transfusion should not be restarted.

These reactions are more common in women, especially multiparous ones, and in multitransfused patients. They are predominantly caused by antibodies directed against donor leukocytes or platelets, although serum protein antigens may also be involved.

Many patients experience chills without fever during transfusion if they are inadequately covered or in a cold or drafty location. Such "reactions" result in blood wastage and unnecessary investigative procedures. They can be prevented by ensuring that patients are warm and comfortably covered.

ALLERGIC REACTION

Urticaria (hives) is one of the most common reactions, usually in a patient with an allergic history. It may occur at any time during or shortly after transfusion. The blood should be discontinued and not restarted. Even with therapy, it is unwise to continue giving antigenic material to a patient who is reacting to it. Rarely, more severe allergic reactions may be seen, even anaphylactic ones. In such cases, investigation may be directed to the patient's immunoglobulins, since anaphylactoid reactions sometimes occur in IgA-deficient people who have been immunized to the IgA protein in normal donor blood.

CIRCULATORY OVERLOAD

This can result from overtransfusion or from use of whole blood, the latter particularly in the very young and the elderly. The signs and symptoms are those of congestive heart failure, and general measures to treat this may be needed.

BLEEDING TENDENCY

After one- or two-volume replacements with older stored blood, the patient's platelets and other clotting factors may be in effect washed out. This can cause bleeding, although it usually does not. Bleeding is more likely to occur in patients who have had prolonged periods on extracorporeal circulation. In addition, as pointed out earlier, disseminated intravascular coagulation may accompany an actual hemolytic transfusion reaction.

CONTAMINATED BLOOD

No matter how carefully blood is collected, bacteria may be introduced and some can survive and even grow under refrigeration, particularly strains of *Escherichia coli* and Pseudomonas. Fortunately, this is rare. Transfusion of contaminated blood results in septicemic shock with peripheral vasodilatation and hyperpyrexia, often fatal, probably the most severe form of transfusion reaction encountered. In such cases, the blood usually has an abnormal color and appearance, which is why it is important to examine the blood before any transfusion.

IMMUNE HEMOLYTIC TRANSFUSION REACTION

In the presence of sufficient circulating antibody, especially of the complement-binding type, incompatible red cells are attacked, complement is activated, and the cells are lysed. Free hemoglobin thus appears in the plasma. In addition, red cell thromboplastic substances may bring about disseminated intravascular coagulation, and the toxic byproducts of complement activation may cause shock and renal tubular damage or necrosis.

This kind of reaction is usually caused by ABO incompatibility, which should be preventable by proper blood selection and cross-matching. The reaction therefore results in most cases from some clerical mishap, such as improper sample identification or release of blood to the wrong patient. Poor laboratory technique is less commonly involved, but sensitive and rigorously controlled blood grouping and cross-matching techniques are essential.

Transfusion of plasma containing antibody directed against the patient's red cells, as in the use of group O whole blood for an A or B recipient, may cause hemolysis of the recipi-

---

Table 4. *Investigation* of Suspected Hemolytic Transfusion Reactions*

  A. Immunohematology: nature of incompatibility
    1. Major blood type: ABO, Rh. Compare pre- and post-transfusion blood and blood in container.
    2. "Minor" incompatibility: antibody in donor plasma. Check minor cross-match.
    3. Irregular blood group antibody
      a. Repeat antibody screening test and major cross-match on patient's serum, pre- and
         post-transfusion.
      b. Direct antiglobulin test, pre- and post-transfusion.
      c. Antibody identification. Use of appropriate panel of reagent red blood cells.
      d. Antibody titration. Comparison of pre- and post-transfusion serum.
    4. Known clinical characteristics of blood group antibody suspected.
  B. Evidence of hemolysis
    1. Direct measurement of plasma or serum hemoglobin.
    2. Urine hemoglobin.
    3. Serum bilirubin.
    4. Serum haptoglobin.
    5. Urine hemosiderin.
  C. Transfusion details
    1. Quantity of blood transfused.
    2. Concurrent intravenous fluids or medications, especially those in contact with blood.
    3. Age and storage conditions of transfused blood.
    4. Duration of transfusion.
  D. Condition of patient
    1. General status: shock, anemia, sepsis, etc.
    2. Renal function
      a. Serum urea, creatinine, etc.
      b. Clearance of hemoglobin.
      c. Urine flow rate.
    3. Other causes of hemolysis
      a. Paroxysmal hemoglobinuria: nocturnal, cold.
      b. Glucose-6-phosphate dehydrogenase deficiency.
      c. Other hemolytic anemias.

---

*The nature and extent of investigation should be determined by the blood bank physician in consultation with the patient's physician.

ent's own cells but does not often cause an overt reaction. This may also follow the use of non-group-specific platelet concentrates or cryoprecipitated antihemophilic factor. Rarely, hemolysis and even a clinical reaction may be caused by transfusion of donor blood containing an antibody, followed by another unit with the corresponding antigen.

Depending at least partly on the amount and nature of the antibody, clinical reactions to incompatible blood vary greatly as to type and severity. There may be no signs and symptoms (unusual), or only chills and elevation of temperature. More often, if the patient is conscious, there may be rapid onset of fever, shaking chills, burning pain along the course of the vein being infused, flushing, and pain or oppressive feeling in the chest or lower back. These manifestations often occur within a few minutes of starting the incompatible transfusion, and stopping the blood at that stage will prevent serious sequelae. This is one reason for requiring careful observation during the first 15 minutes or so of starting a transfusion. In the patient under anesthesia, symptoms are masked, and shock, abnormal bleeding or oozing, and hemoglobinuria may be the only signs. It is important to remember that some hemoglobinemia and even hemoglobinuria may be seen in patients undergoing cardiopulmonary bypass.

Any reaction characterized by fever or in which there is a reasonable suspicion of red cell incompatibility must be investigated at once, as just outlined. Further transfusions should be withheld except in an emergency until the reason for the reaction has been established. If any appreciable amount of incompatible blood has been given, particularly a full unit, the patient's serum or plasma will usually be dark red.

The moment a hemolytic reaction is suspected, and while investigation is proceeding, the transfusion must be stopped and a slow saline drip maintained pending further intravenous therapy. The blood container is disconnected and returned without delay to the laboratory.

Treatment is directed primarily to maintenance of blood pressure and promotion of diuresis and is not covered in this article.

DELAYED HEMOLYTIC REACTION

Occasionally a patient experiences an episode of hemolysis within the week or so after transfusion of apparently compatible blood. This may or may not be accompanied by an overt clinical reaction. On investigation, an irregular antibody is found that was not present in the original blood sample used for crossmatching. This type of reaction is caused by secondary antibody response, triggered by an antigen in the transfused blood to which primary immunization had taken place on some previous transfusion or pregnancy. The culprit is usually an antigen of the Rh–Hr system (other than Rh_o) or of the Kidd (Jk) system. Kidd antibodies are often difficult to detect and may cause severe reactions.

NONIMMUNE HEMOLYSIS

As a rule, only isotonic saline solution should be used to start transfusions or to pass through the same tubing with blood. Other solutions may be given directly intravenously, but many of them exert adverse effects on stored blood. Any solutions containing dextrose cause swelling of red cells and shortened post-transfusion survival. In addition, dextrose in water causes clumping of red cells; these may even block the needle. Hypotonic solutions, such as quarter-strength saline, are directly hemolytic. The same applies to distilled water, whether mistakenly used as an intravenous solution or during surgery on the urinary bladder (for irrigation).

Red cells that are deficient in glucose-6-phosphate dehydrogenase (G6PD) are subject to hemolysis when exposed to certain trigger drugs. This could happen to the patient's own cells or to transfused red cells, depending on which were defective, and could be mistaken for a hemolytic transfusion reaction. This is a rare complication, but both types have been reported.

In any case of observed post-transfusion hemolysis in which no incompatibility can be identified, investigation may need to be directed to the possibility of some form of osmotic, pharmacologic, or mechanical blood trauma, or to defective red cells.

COLD BLOOD REACTION

Very rapid infusion of large amounts of ice-cold blood can chill the heart and cause cardiac arrhythmia and even arrest. This is prevented by the use of some form of heat exchanger in any situation in which rapid infusion is likely to be needed, such as major surgery or exchange transfusion. It is entirely unnecessary to warm blood that is to be given at ordinary rates. Even if the patient has cold autoagglutinins, it is easier and better to warm the patient rather than the blood.

AIR EMBOLISM

This can occur when transfusions are given under direct air pressure through rigid containers. The resultant foaming of blood can severely reduce the cardiac pumping efficiency. The replacement of glass bottles by plastic bags as blood containers has almost eliminated this hazard, although it can still occur on changing infusion sets or erroneously venting a bag.

CITRATE AND POTASSIUM REACTIONS

These hazards, even in massive transfusions, are overrated. Both may affect cardiac function but seldom do. Excess potassium is of concern in patients with chronic renal disease, citrate in those with chronic liver disease. Citrate is, of course, automatically reduced when red blood cells are used rather than whole blood. This is not necessarily the case with potassium, since it leaks from the red cells during storage. However, while the *concentration* of potassium may be several times normal in older stored blood or red blood cells, the actual *amount* of it transfused to a recipient is usually insignificant. Appropriate measurements and calculations may be necessary if hyperkalemia is thought to have been caused by transfusion.

NEUTROPENIA AND AGRANULOCYTOSIS

By LEONARD H. BRUBAKER, M.D.
Augusta, Georgia

SYNONYMS

Granulocytopenia, agranulocytic angina.

While population studies indicate considerable variation in absolute neutrophil counts (total white blood cell count times fraction of neutrophils in the differential count), neutropenia is customarily defined as a neutrophil count less than 1500 per cu mm. Lower values than this, however, have been observed in asymptomatic and apparently healthy black Americans (especially males), black Africans, and Yemenite Jews.

Agranulocytosis usually refers to the sudden onset of severe neutropenia. Patients taking anticancer or immunosuppressive drugs who develop neutropenia as an expected drug side effect are not considered to have agranulocytosis. The term refers to an idiosyncratic response to a nonmyelosuppressive drug or chemical.

Neutrophil counts below 1000 per cu mm are associated with an increased risk of bacterial infections if the neutropenia is caused by lack of marrow production. If the neutrophil count goes below 500, the risk of fatal infection is much more serious. However, if neutropenia is due to abnormalities of pooling or increased destruction, such a risk is not necessarily present. For the most part, neutropenia is a secondary manifestation of a number of different diseases rather than a primary process.

PATHOPHYSIOLOGIC CAUSES OF NEUTROPENIA

The pathophysiologic causes of neutropenia can be divided into the following categories:
1. Decreased marrow production
2. Ineffective marrow production
3. Decreased survival in circulation
4. Abnormal pooling within the circulation.

Mixed pathophysiologies are sometimes found. Careful examination of the bone marrow provides considerable insight into the pathophysiologic mechanism of neutropenia, if one bears in mind certain pitfalls of random marrow sampling. For example, the cellularity of the marrow may vary from site to site. In older patients the posterior iliac crest may be markedly hypocellular or even aplastic, whereas the sternal marrow will show the normal cellularity of approximately 30 to 50 per cent cells and the rest fat. Previous radiation of a given bone marrow site may cause this area to be hypocellular while the rest of the marrow may be hypercellular.

There are also pitfalls associated with ineffective marrow production. This condition may be properly deduced when the marrow shows megaloblastic changes in the neutrophilic precursors. However, some causes of ineffective marrow production do not produce morphologic changes. In these situations the marrow is full of neutrophil precursors in contrast to the circulating blood neutropenia. Such myeloid hyperplasia can be confused with the appearance of the marrow when the pathophysiologic problem is decreased peripheral blood survival rather than ineffective production. One subtle difference between these two is that in ineffective production the marrow usually has a large number of mature polymorphonuclear neutrophils (polys), whereas in decreased peripheral survival the number of myelocytes, metamyelocytes, and band forms may be normal but there may be a sharp decrease in the number of mature polys.

A common cause of abnormal pooling is splenomegaly, regardless of its cause of origin. Splenic pooling or sequestration alone can produce neutropenia in some patients whose spleens are palpable at the umbilical level or below. The degree of splenic pooling is roughly proportional to the spleen size, the same as it is for platelets. Acute neutropenia due to abnormal pooling of neutrophils within the lungs can be produced in clinical situations in which there is a sudden activation of serum complement. Complement-mediated neutrophil pooling occurs during (1) hemodialysis and nylon-wool leukopheresis procedures as a trivial problem, (2) acute antigen-antibody reactions, (3) endotoxemia, (4) massive bacterial infections, and (5) shock. In situations 2 through 5 the complement activation may be massive, and the neutrophil pooling and breakdown in the lung may help cause pulmonary edema and other injury.

COMMON CAUSES OF NEUTROPENIA

Neutropenia from Drug Damage. Most anticancer or immunosuppressive drugs regularly produce neutropenia from transient depression of committed, actively cycling marrow stem cells. Some drugs in certain individuals may produce unexpectedly prolonged neutropenia. Busulfan, for example, can produce marrow aplasia lasting many months or years. Patients treated sequentially both by radiation of marrow-containing bones and by cytotoxic drugs also may have prolonged neutropenia owing to marrow aplasia. Several drugs, chemicals, and other agents may also produce marrow aplasia as an occasional, unpredictable side effect. Examples of these are chloramphenicol, phenylbutazone, benzene, and hepatitis virus. These reactions may lead to pancytopenia or to isolated neutropenia owing to selected suppression of marrow neutrophil precursors (agranulocytosis).

Another form of agranulocytosis due to drugs appears to be related to an immunologic reaction, exemplified by aminopyrine. Following a period of sensitization, the patient has abrupt onset of chills, fever, and collapse caused by the peripheral destruction of circulating neutrophils. These patients can recover quickly when the drug is withdrawn. They evince identical symptoms and develop neutropenia abruptly upon reexposure to the drug. Immunologic mechanisms may also be responsible for destruction of marrow neutrophil precursors. The drugs most commonly associated with agranulocytosis include phenothiazines, sulfonamides, antithyroid drugs, anticonvulsants, and some rarely used analgesics. There is a long list of other drugs reported to be rare causes of agranulocytosis. Every patient who develops neutropenia abruptly should be considered to have a drug- or chemically induced neutropenia, and all nonvital drugs should be discontinued.

Other Forms of Neutropenia Due to Decreased Marrow Production. *(1) Marrow stem cell defects.* A number of congenital syndromes have been described in which neutropenia is produced by lack of marrow neutrophil precursors. If this situation is present at birth the infant usually rapidly dies of infection. Sometimes this type of defect is characterized by a cyclic neutropenia, a condition in which fever, ulcerations of the mouth, skin, anus, or genitals, and extreme neutropenia recur for about 4 to 5 days out of each approximately 21 day cycle. At other times this situation is accompanied by a wide variety of other congenital defects, such as dysglobulinemia or agammaglobulinemia. *(2) Replacement of bone marrow.* Invasion of the bone marrow by tumors from the lung, breast, or other sites may produce neutropenia, pancytopenia, or some other combinations of cytopenias. The tumor involvement is often nonuniform, one iliac crest being involved and not the other, or the spine being involved and not the iliac crest. A positive bone scan will sometimes indicate the areas of involvement, but often the bone marrow is completely replaced by tumor while the bone scan in the area is negative. Plasma cell myeloma particularly causes that result. Agnogenic myeloid metaplasia may produce neutropenia but the opposite is usually true, since the enlarged spleen in this disease may produce greatly increased numbers of abnormal neutrophils.

Neutropenia Caused by Ineffective Marrow Production. Patients with megaloblastic anemia due to vitamin B_{12} or folic acid deficiency frequently are both thrombocytopenic and neutropenic. The morphologic changes in the marrow are readily apparent, including giant myelocytes, metamyelocytes, and bands and hypersegmented neutrophils in the marrow and circulating blood. The megaloblastic changes in the neutrophils may persist for many days following the B_{12}- or folate-induced reversion of the red cell changes to normal. Recognition of the persistence of giant bands and hypersegmented neutrophils within the marrow can lead to a diagnosis of pernicious anemia even when the red cell abnormalities have been eliminated by factors in hospital diet or blood transfusions.

Ineffective Marrow Neutrophil Production without Prominent Morphologic Changes. A diverse and vaguely defined group of patients with neutropenia, either isolated or in conjunction with other cytopenias, are considered to have "preleukemia." Several authors prefer the term "myelodysplasia," since only a minority of such patients, including those with refractory megaloblastic and sideroblastic anemias, will develop leukemia. The marrows of these patients are hypercellular and splenomegaly is rarely present. The percentage of blast forms on the marrow smear is slightly to moderately increased. Sometimes subtle morphologic abnormalities are present.

A small percentage of patients with rheumatoid arthritis develop splenomegaly and neutropenia (Felty's syndrome). The predominant pathophysiology of neutropenia in some of these patients is ineffective marrow production as shown by physiologic studies by several investigators and the well-known failure of some patients to respond to splenectomy. Lack of a better understanding of the pathophysiology of Felty's syndrome and of the ability to predict which patients are likely to respond to splenectomy has led to a great deal of controversy. Patients with systemic lupus erythematosus (SLE) may develop neutropenia by the same mechanism. Usually, these patients do not have splenomegaly. A practical differentiating feature between these conditions is the fact that patients with Felty's syndrome develop an isolated neutropenia, whereas patients with SLE usually develop panleukopenia. Rarely, however, patients with SLE develop isolated neutropenia with splenomegaly as a form of hypersplenism (see later discussion).

Neutropenia Due to Shortened Neutrophil Survival. Unequivocal antineutrophil antibodies in association with shortened neutrophil survival in neutropenia have only recently been demonstrated. The passive transfer of maternal antineutrophil antibodies may cause temporary neonatal neutropenia. Acquired antineutrophil antibodies can occur at any age. Several reliable tests for antineutrophil antibodies have now been described. Although these tests are much too difficult for routine laboratories, the patient's serum can be sent to one of several investigators for these studies. It should be noted here that leukoagglutinins do not correlate well with antineutrophil antibodies, since these leukoagglutinins are found in multiparas and multi-transfused patients and do not produce neutropenia or other illness.

Occasionally patients with slight or moderate splenomegaly from other causes have severe neutropenia. Several investigators have been able to demonstrate shortened neutrophil survival in these patients.

Neutropenia Due to Abnormal Neutrophil Pooling. Most patients with splenomegaly have sequestration of one or more cellular components of blood in the spleen. However, in the myeloproliferative disorders, extramedullary and medullary hematopoiesis may be balanced against the sequestration owing to splenic enlargement per se. Isotope dilution methods have been used to measure abnormal pooling,

but these are no longer available or are unproved. The magnitude of pooling is proportional to spleen size. Splenomegaly and neutrophil pooling are major parts of the pathophysiology of Felty's syndrome as well as congestive splenomegaly in association with cirrhosis or other causes. The lung can also be a site of abnormal pooling in patients who have massive complement activation. Examples have been listed previously.

Neutropenia Due to Mixed Pathophysiology. Here Felty's syndrome is a good example. These patients have been found to have varying degrees of all four of the major pathophysiologic mechanisms. Theoretically, patients who have marrow production problems with Felty's syndrome would not benefit from splenectomy. It would be logical that patients with the largest spleens, those filling a large proportion of the left abdomen, would be most likely to benefit from splenectomy, whereas patients whose spleens are barely palpable might be the ones who should not undergo splenectomy. Unfortunately, this is only a rough guide and there are many exceptions. Some investigators believe that the rationale for splenectomy in Felty's syndrome is to remove an antibody-producing organ. Patients with Felty's syndrome should be referred to research centers for special marrow and peripheral blood tests in order for practical solutions to this problem to be developed.

Patients with other causes of splenomegaly frequently have both shortened neutrophil survival and abnormal pooling. Many of these patients can go for long periods without problems from bacterial infections despite extremely low neutrophil counts.

CLINICAL SYNDROMES INCLUDING NEUTROPENIA

Benign Idiopathic Neutropenia. This is probably a mixture of several disorders that apparently include a variety of pathophysiologic causes. Some patients have a non–sex-linked dominant familial pattern, whereas others have acquired isolated neutropenia. The spleen is usually normal size. Despite profound neutropenia, there is little risk of infection. Pathophysiologic studies have shown some patients to have shortened neutrophil survival while others have bone marrow production defects.

Neutropenia in the Alcoholic. Evidently, this is also a mixture of pathophysiologic abnormalities. Alcohol-related neutropenia, in most cases, is caused by decreased or ineffective marrow neutrophil production. Patients with cirrhosis may in addition have a shortened neutrophil survival and pooling within an enlarged spleen. Since alcohol reduces neutrophil stickiness, a combination of neutropenia and depressed neutrophil function may help account for the frequent severe infections in alcoholics. Folate deficiency and other aspects of malnutrition may also play a role in the neutropenia and infection problem in alcoholics.

Lazy Leukocyte Syndrome. This rare congenital syndrome illustrates that neutropenia can be produced by abnormal neutrophil function. The neutrophils of patients with the syndrome respond poorly to chemotactic factors. The bone marrow appears normally cellular and is without morphologic abnormalities. The neutropenia is caused by the apparent difficulty of marrow neutrophils getting into circulation owing to their lack of response to chemotactic and other factors associated with marrow neutrophil release. Thus, this disorder appears to be a type of ineffective neutrophil production.

Pancreatic Insufficiency with Neutropenia. This is a congenital disorder with exocrine pancreatic insufficiency, neutropenia, dwarfism, and occasionally metaphyseal dysostoses. These patients have frequent infections and may die in infancy or childhood. The bone marrow is hyperplastic. Some patients have had a serum factor that is cytotoxic for neutrophils. This disorder may be differentiated from fibrocystic disease by the lack of chronic pulmonary disease.

Neutropenia with Hyperglobulinemia. This is a congenital disorder of which approximately half the cases are familial. The bone marrow demonstrates abundant early neutrophil forms with little maturation beyond the myelocyte stage. Since these children have two defects in their host resistance to infection, bacterial infections are frequent and severe. At times during bacterial infections, neutrophilia may be noted rather than neutropenia. The pathophysiology of this disorder is obscure.

PRESENTING SIGNS AND SYMPTOMS

Patients with agranulocytosis commonly present with a sore throat, chills, fever, weakness, and shortness of breath. Dyspnea and hypoxia without signs of congestive heart failure usually mean that pneumonia is present even if the chest roentgenogram is negative. The patient may have painful areas in the skin and mouth that may or may not be ulcerated. In contrast, many patients with chronic neutropenia have no symptoms and are discovered accidentally by routine blood counts.

COURSE

Acute agranulocytosis due to drug or chemical toxicity generally has a good prognosis and a short period of disability if the patient's infections can be controlled with antibiotics and the offending drug or chemical removed so that recovery can occur. The benign clinical course of most patients who are treated with anticancer marrow suppressive drugs demonstrates that transient neutropenia, even if severe, may not be associated with infections. Severe neutropenia (neutrophil count below 500 per cu mm), if present for several days, creates an increasing risk of infection. If infection occurs, the patient can die in shock in as short a time as 1 or 2 hours. The patients may recover uneventfully if antibiotics are given promptly and the neutrophil count returns to a normal level.

The course and outcome of chronic neutropenia due to other causes is dependent upon the nature of the associated disease and the pathophysiologic mechanism for the neutropenia.

PHYSICAL FINDINGS

The most specific physical findings concern the evidence of bacterial infections without signs of pus formation. As examples, skin infections may appear to be cellulitis, pneumonia may occur without early radiographic infiltrates, and urinary infections may not be associated with pyuria. Patients may develop multiple areas of cellulitis over the skin from which organisms may be cultured even though no pus is present. Patients who have *Pseudomonas aeruginosa* infections may develop a cellulitis with a central necrotic area (ecthyma gangrenosum). Such findings are characteristic of *Pseudomonas* infections in the setting of neutropenia, but rarely may be seen with *Staphylococcus* infections. Buccal and throat ulcerations are very common.

Other physical findings depend on the underlying associated disorder. For example, patients with physical evidence of rheumatoid arthritis who have splenomegaly probably will also have neutropenia (Felty's syndrome). Patients with enlarged spleens, as previously mentioned, have a strong tendency to pool neutrophils within the spleen and develop neutropenia if they do not have a myeloproliferative disease. The cause of splenomegaly may be elucidated by finding evidence of cirrhosis such as spider angiomas, palmar erythema, gynecomastia, testicular atrophy, and parotid enlargement, suggesting cirrhosis with alcoholism. The physician should be particularly sensitive to evidence of decreased vibration and joint position sense, a smooth tongue, and other signs suggestive of pernicious anemia. A skin rash may be found in some patients with hypersensitivity reactions to drugs. Free hemoglobin in the urine may suggest the presence of paroxysmal nocturnal hemoglobinuria, a rare condition that occasionally is associated with neutropenia.

LABORATORY STUDIES

Peripheral Blood. A number of clues regarding the underlying disorder may be found in the peripheral blood film. Hypersegmented polys and oval macrocytes may suggest that ineffective marrow production (megaloblastosis) is present. Patients who have shortened neutrophil survival with no marrow production problems are likely to have increased numbers of bands in proportion to the number of polys. Metamyelocytes may also be found occasionally in this setting, but the presence of large numbers of metamyelocytes, myelocytes, and more immature forms — especially with nucleated or teardrop red cells — suggests that the patient has myelofibrosis or tumor in the marrow. Many patients with neutropenia have an increased number of monocytes; this condition does not seem to be associated with an increased risk of infection. The presence of increased numbers of monocytes may also indicate that the bone marrow is beginning to recover from prior suppression. Patients with cyclic neutropenia may have an increased number of monocytes during the extremely neutropenic phase. These effects are probably due to the fact the it takes less time to mature from a promyelocyte to a monocyte than from a promyelocyte to a poly. The presence of neutropenia, other cytopenias, and a few circulating blast forms may indicate that the patient has acute leukemia.

Bone Marrow. As mentioned previously, a careful examination of the bone marrow is the most important means of detecting the pathophysiologic and occasionally the etiologic cause of the neutropenia. Lack of marrow neutrophil production may be immediately obvious. The so-called "maturation-arrest" picture can be misleading, however. Some patients' cells do not mature beyond the promyelocyte or early myelocyte stage, and these would appear to be examples of a true maturation arrest. However, neutropenic patients will be frequently found to have abundant neutrophil precursors except for the mature polys. These patients usually have shortened neutrophil survival or abnormal pooling in circulation or both, and the deficiency of polys reflects the premature extraction of these cells from the marrow in conjunction with their peripheral disappearance. On the other hand, the contrast between peripheral neutropenia and abundant polys in the marrow suggests a marrow releasing defect (ineffective marrow production).

Bone marrow biopsy from the iliac crest, the greater trochanter of the femur, or the posterior spine of a vertebra is most important for evaluation of the overall and neutrophilic cellularity. Tumor infiltrations of the marrow are most readily diagnosed by this technique. Large marrow biopsies may disclose variations in cellularity from place to place within the bone marrow and help avoid sampling error.

Other Diagnostic Procedures. Measurement of neutrophil survival with diisopropylfluorophosphate 32 (DF^{32P})-labeled neutrophils has been done in research centers in the past. This drug is no longer available in the United States. Radioactive chromium (^{51}Cr) has been proposed as a substitute, but this chemical labels monocytes and lymphocytes to a greater degree than neutrophils, making its effectiveness in neutropenic patients questionable. A procedure has been described (the "coil test") in which a neutropenic patient is phlebotomized of approximately 400 ml of blood with heparin anticoagulation. The blood is then placed in a hemodialysis coil for 15 minutes, which activates some of the complement in this blood. The activated blood is then returned to the patient. The procedure produces a 5-minute neutropenia followed by an overshoot neutrophilia. The magnitude of neutrophilia is a measure of marrow neutrophil reserves, while the rate of fall-off from the peak neutrophil count to the original baseline value is a measure of the neutrophil survival. The disadvantages of the procedure include the inability to measure neutrophil survival if the bone marrow does not put out enough cells to cause the overshoot neutrophilia and the lack of availability of the test except in a few centers. However, this test can be valuable in discovering the pathophysiologic cause of chronic neutropenia, especially in patients with Felty's syndrome and other patients who present the problem of distinguishing between ineffective neutrophil production and shortened neutrophil life span (previously mentioned as one of the major problems in interpretation of the bone marrow).

References have been made in several published articles to attempts to correlate levels of serum lysozyme and vitamin B_{12}-binding proteins with the neutrophil pathophysiology in neutropenic patients. The experience of most workers is that these tests are not helpful.

Fortunately, many patients have a transient neutropenia and do not require a pathophysiologic work-up. In other patients a careful examination of bone marrow gives sufficient evidence of the underlying pathophysiologic abnormality so that no further special tests are needed. Patients in whom more specialized tests are needed are those with Felty's syndrome, chronic idiopathic neutropenia, and patients with splenomegaly who are taking bone marrow suppressive drugs, a relatively common circumstance in patients with renal transplants or lymphomas involving the spleen and marrow.

Antineutrophil antibodies can be determined by several techniques. Frozen serum may be sent to investigators at several locations within the United States for this type of test.

Intravenous injection of small amounts of epinephrine with serial counts of the circulating white cells has been proposed as a procedure for measuring the marginated neutrophil pool. However, this test has not been adequately correlated with the isotope dilution method of determining the marginated neutrophil pool, and some investigators do not consider it reliable. It is rarely used because of this lack of substantiation.

Other tests that may be useful in the diagnosis of the underlying disorder associated with the neutropenia include serum B_{12}, folate, protein electrophoresis, rheumatoid factor, hepatitis-associated antigens, liver-spleen scans, and tests for neutrophil function. A list of diagnostic tests needed for neutropenic patients depends upon the suspected underlying disorders.

THE LEUKEMIAS

By LEWIS R. WEINTRAUB, M.D.
Boston, Massachusetts

INTRODUCTION

Leukemias in man have been classified in reference to their suspected cell of origin and whether the clinical course to death is acute or chronic. These guidelines are still in general use, but recent advancements have raised many questions as to the origin of some of the leukemic cells. In addition, advances in treatment have made survival in "acute lymphocytic leukemia" exceed that of many of the chronic forms of leukemia.

It is presently accepted that a pluripotential stem cell exists in the bone marrow. This cell divides slowly; with each division it gives rise to a daughter cell that remains as a stem cell and a second cell that under the appropriate stimulus will differentiate into the myeloid, erythroid, or megakaryocytic cell line. DNA-directed production of specific messenger RNA results in the synthesis of specific enzymes or structural proteins necessary for a specified function in the cell. Once this occurs, the cell can be recognized as "differentiated"; subsequent to this, maturation ensues. During the phase of maturation, several cell divisions may take place. Eventually the ability to divide is lost but the cell continues to mature to its functional state. The mature granulocyte, erythrocyte, or platelet is then delivered from the bone marrow to the peripheral blood to carry out its ultimate function. It is a disorder of the stem cell with subsequent abnormalities in differentiation and maturation that gives rise to the leukemic disorders.

MYELOGENOUS LEUKEMIAS

ACUTE MYELOGENOUS LEUKEMIA

Acute myelogenous leukemia is primarily a disease of adults. Its incidence rapidly increases in patients over the age of 50 and reaches a peak incidence of 14 per 100,000 in the eighth decade of life. Initial symptoms are variable but directly related to the decreased production of one or more of the three mature cellular elements in the peripheral blood: fatigue; decreased red cell and hemoglobin mass; and easy bruising, thrombocytopenia, and fever owing to infections due to neutropenia. Examination may reveal pallor and skin and mucous membrane hemorrhages. Peripheral adenopathy is relatively uncommon in acute myelogenous leukemia and its variants. Mild to moderate hepatosplenomegaly is common but massive splenomegaly as seen in the chronic leukemias or myelofibrosis with myeloid metaplasia is relatively rare.

The peripheral white blood cell count may be low, normal, or increased but in all instances the differential count is abnormal. In those patients in whom the white cell count is normal or increased, the predominant cell is a primitive myeloblast. In contrast, when the white count is low, one may see a marked reduction in or absence of mature neutrophils, a relative increase in lymphocytes, and only a small percentage of myeloblasts or in some cases no myeloblasts. Normochromic normocytic anemia and thrombocytopenia of varying degrees are present at the time of presentation. The bone marrow examination reveals a "hypercellular" marrow with the myeloblast as the predominant cell. The cell is large, with a large regular nucleus that has primitive fine reticular pattern with distinct nucleoli. In some instances Auer rod inclusions are noted in the cytoplasm. Histochemical stains may be of value in distinguishing the myeloblast from other primitive cells that may be seen in the bone marrow (Table 1). Megakaryocytes and erythroid precursors are markedly diminished.

Acute leukemia was initially believed to be a disease of rapid uncontrolled proliferation of the primitive myeloblast with replacement of the marrow cavity and suppression of normal hematopoiesis. More recent studies have demonstrated that the increased number of "blast" cells in the marrow of patients with acute leukemia is due to the "accumulation" of slowly dividing cells that fail to mature. The hypercellularity of the marrow is really a stagnation phenomenon. Radiation, viruses, and certain drugs have been incriminated as causes of acute leukemia in man. Each of these agents has the capability of disrupting DNA metabolism or the transcription of messenger RNA, thus inducing an abnormality in cell differentiation and maturation. If the etiologic agent affects the pluripotential stem cell, then one could explain the anemia and thrombocytopenia seen in patients with acute leukemia as a complete failure of the stem cell to differentiate into recognizable erythroblasts and megakaryoblasts.

VARIANTS OF ACUTE MYELOGENOUS LEUKEMIA

Acute Monocytic Leukemia. The monocyte is believed to be derived from the same pluripotential stem cell as the neutrophil. The monoblast is slightly larger than the myeloblast and the nucleus of the monoblast is convoluted. Auer rods are not seen in the cytoplasm. In addition to these features, histochemical stains help to differentiate the myeloblast from the monoblast (Table 1). The clinical features of acute monoblastic leukemia may be identical to those of acute myelogenous leukemia. In addition, there is a higher association of extramedullary infiltration of the leukemic cells in patients with acute monoblastic leukemia. The gingivae and skin are most frequently involved. Serum and urine muramidase (a lysosomal enzyme) are moderately elevated in contrast with normal or only slightly elevated levels in acute myelogenous leukemia.

Acute Myelomonocytic Leukemia. This is a disease variant in which the morphology and clinical features rest in between the classic descriptions of acute myelogenous and monocytic leukemia.

Acute Promyelocytic Leukemia. In this variant of acute leukemia the predominant cell in the bone and the peripheral blood is the promyelocyte. This cell represents the first step in maturation beyond the myeloblast. In contrast with the normal promyelocyte, the cells in this disorder may have increased numbers and larger nonspecific granules in the cytoplasm. There is also a high frequency of Auer rods. In addition to the clinical features of acute myelogenous leukemia, there is an increased incidence of a severe hemorrhagic disorder out of proportion to the degree of thrombocytopenia. This is explained on the basis of an associated disseminated intravascular coagulation syndrome and consumption coagulopathy. The prothrombin time and partial thromboplastin time are prolonged, with a reduction in the concentration of fibrinogen and an increase in fibrin degradation products and fibrin monomers. The leukemic cells are thought to be a source of a thromboplastin responsible for this syndrome.

Erythroleukemia. In erythroleukemia the predominant cell in the bone marrow is a primitive erythroblast that may have severe megaloblastic nuclear changes despite normal serum B_{12} and folate levels. One also sees an increase in primitive myeloblasts. The clinical presentation may be identical to acute myelogenous leukemia. Decreased numbers of all three forms of mature cells are noted in the peripheral blood. There may be a significant number of nucleated red blood cells, poikilocytosis of the mature red cells, and myeloblasts in the peripheral blood.

Table 1. *Histochemical Evaluation of Acute Leukemias*

Leukemia	Myeloperoxidase Sudan Black	Nonspecific Esterase	PAS
Acute myelogenous	++++	+	±
Acute promyelocytic	++++	+	−
Acute monocytic	±	++++ (Inhibition by NaF)	±
Acute myelomonocytic	+++	++	±
Acute lymphocytic	0	0	+++

Preleukemia Disorders. Several refractory hematologic abnormalities exist that eventually become transformed into the classic picture of acute myelogenous leukemia. In retrospect it becomes apparent that there are certain laboratory features suggesting that the initial presenting abnormality may be a "preleukemic disorder." The following are examples of this condition.

Unexplained Neutropenia. This may be associated with a mild monocytosis and the appearance of pseudo-Pelger-Huët cells (bi- and monolobed neutrophils) in the peripheral blood. Bone marrow examination may reveal a mild degree of hypocellularity with occasional small clusters of atypical myeloblasts with large nucleoli.

Unexplained Thrombocytopenia. In addition to being reduced in number, the platelets may be morphologically abnormal, large, and agranular. The platelets are qualitatively abnormal; this results in spontaneous clinical bleeding at platelet levels greater than 30,000 per cu mm. The bone marrow may show a slight decrease in megakaryocytes, many of which are abnormal with monolobed nuclei.

Refractory Macrocytic Anemia Associated with Normal Serum B$_{12}$ and Folate Levels. The bone marrow may reveal "erythroid megaloblastoid maturation" and ringed sideroblasts may be present. All of the conditions described may eventually undergo transformation into acute myeloblastic leukemia.

Chronic Myelogenous Leukemia

Chronic myelogenous (granulocytic) leukemia is a disease of adults with its peak incidence occurring in the fourth to fifth decade of life. Symptoms of fatigue related to anemia or left upper quadrant discomfort related to an enlarged spleen may be the patient's presenting complaint. In contrast to acute myelogenous leukemia infections, fever and bleeding are not common presenting problems, since the patients have adequate mature neutrophils and platelets at the initial manifestations of the disease. On physical examination, splenomegaly is a frequent finding and lymphadenopathy is not noted.

The characteristic laboratory finding is an elevated white cell count with all stages of myeloid development being present. The relative distribution of the cells is similar to that seen in a normal bone marrow, with less than 5 per cent of the cells being myeloblasts. Mild to moderate anemia is present with normal red cell morphology. Nucleated red cells are less commonly seen than they are in myelofibrosis with myeloid metaplasia. The platelet count in the early stages of the disease may be normal or increased. The leukocyte alkaline phosphatase score (a histochemical determination in peripheral blood neutrophils) is below normal or absent. In contrast, this is elevated in leukocytosis associated with infection, in a leukemoid reaction to tumor in the marrow, in polycythemia vera, or in myelofibrosis with myeloid metaplasia. The bone marrow findings reveal marked granulocytic and at times megakaryocytic hyperplasia. Maturation of the granulocytic line is normal. In contrast to acute leukemia, this disorder appears to represent a true hyperproliferative state owing to an increase in the rate of differentiation of the pluripotential stem cell into myeloid and at times megakaryocytic lines of development. One of the characteristic features of chronic myelogenous leukemia is the presence of an abnormal bone marrow chromosomal karyotype. The Ph^1 chromosome represents a translocation of a major part of the long arm of chromosome 22 to the chromosome 9. This abnormality is seen in karyotypes obtained from erythroid and megakaryocytic cells, supporting the concept of the stem cell origin of this disorder.

In the terminal stage of this form of leukemia, the bone marrow and peripheral blood findings become similar to those of acute leukemia, with the accumulation of primitive blasts associated with severe anemia and thrombocytopenia. The cells may have the appearance of "myeloblasts" or at times "lymphoblasts." These primitive cells have been shown to contain the primitive enzyme deoxyribonucleotidyl transferase in 20 per cent of the cases tested. It remains to be proved if these cells are truly lymphoblasts or if the cell we are calling a "lymphoblast" really represents the primitive stem cell.

LYMPHATIC LEUKEMIAS

Acute Lymphocytic Leukemia

Acute lymphocytic leukemia is primarily a disease of childhood. The peak incidence is in patients between the ages of 2 to 10. The disease occurs infrequently in young adults and rarely in the elderly patient. The symptoms of fatigue, weight loss, fever, and easy bruising are relatively acute in onset and are related to anemia, neutropenia, and thrombocytopenia, as in acute myelogenous leukemia. In addition, bone pain or tenderness or both are common symptoms. These symptoms are relatively uncommon in acute myelogenous leukemia. The bone pain may precede by weeks or rarely months any significant changes in the peripheral blood. Pallor, ecchymosis, peripheral adenopathy, and hepatosplenomegaly are common features on physical examination. Approximately 10 to 15 per cent of children with acute lymphocytic leukemia will have radiographic evidence of an anterior mediastinal mass at the time of presentation.

Examination of the peripheral blood reveals a significant leukocytosis in the majority of patients. Approximately one third of the patients may have a normal or reduced total white count. In all cases the differential is abnormal, with a significant neutropenia and the presence of the abnormal lymphoblasts. Anemia and thrombocytopenia of varying degrees are also present. The bone marrow is hypercellular and the predominant cell is the lymphoblast. The lymphoblast is smaller than the myeloblast. Cytoplasm is scant and agranular. The chromatin pattern is not as fine as the myeloblast and nucleoli are less frequent and distinct as compared with the myeloblasts. Histochemical stains may be of value in identifying the cell (Table 1).

Although we call the primitive cell a lymphoblast, there is still a question as to the origin of this cell. Utilizing surface immunologic markers, approximately 20 to 25 per cent of the patients with "acute lymphocytic" leukemia have the characteristic of a "T" lymphocyte (Table 2). It is of note that practically all patients with the mediastinal mass fall into this category. About 2 to 5 per cent have the characteristics of a "B" lymphocyte. Cells of the remaining 75 per cent of patients have *no* immunologic surface characteristics of either type of lymphocyte and are called null cells. Whether these are truly in the lymphoid series remains to be elucidated. Almost all of the patients with acute lymphoblastic leukemia will have the primitive enzyme deoxyribonucleotidyl transferase in the cells.

CHRONIC LYMPHOCYTIC LEUKEMIA

Chronic lymphocytic leukemia is a disease that primarily occurs in the older patient. Approximately 90 per cent of patients with this disorder are over the age of 50, and 60 per cent over 60 at the time of initial diagnosis. The disease may have a prolonged smouldering course with an initial asymptomatic phase. Not infrequently the diagnosis is made at the time of routine examination when an elevated white count is noted with a predominance of normal-appearing lymphocytes. As the disease progresses, diffuse lymphadenopathy and splenomegaly occur. Patients then develop anemia and thrombocytopenia with the appropriate associated symptoms. The anemia and thrombocytopenia are primarily due to impaired marrow

Table 2. *Characteristics of B and T Lymphocytes*

	B Cells	T Cells
Surface membrane immunoglobulins	+	0
Complement receptors	+	0
Sheep cell rosette formation at 4 C	0	+
Transformation to phytohemagglutinin stimulation	0	+

production, but the production of isolated autoantibodies against the patient's red cells or platelets by the abnormal lymphocytes may occur with the resultant shortened survival of both of these elements.

The typical peripheral blood findings reveal an elevated white blood cell count with 80 to 95 per cent normal-appearing lymphocytes. A small population of the lymphocytes may be larger with prominent nucleoli. These cells tend to be fragile and give rise to "smudge cells" on the peripheral blood smear. In the normal person approximately 70 per cent of the peripheral lymphocytes are T cells and 30 per cent B cells. Chronic lymphocytic leukemia is a B cell malignancy that results in a reversal of this ratio. This finding can be demonstrated by performing surface immunologic studies on the patient's lymphocytes (Table 2). Anemia and thrombocytopenia of varying degrees may be noted. In some instances the direct Coombs' test may be positive, indicating antibodies on the surface of the red cells, and platelet antibodies may be detected in the plasma. Not infrequently there is a significant hypogammaglobulinemia with reduction in all classes of immunoglobulins. As the disease progresses, the incidence and severity of hypogammaglobulinemia increases and plays a major role in the occurrence of frequent infections in these patients. The bone marrow examination shows a hypercellular marrow and the predominant cell is the small "normal-appearing" lymphocyte. Erythroid, myeloid, and megakaryocytic precursors are diminished.

Prolymphocytic Leukemia. This is a variant of chronic lymphocytic leukemia. The predominant cell is the larger lymphocyte with a prominent nucleolus. The white count is usually greater than the 100,000 to 150,000 per cu mm range and is associated with significant anemia and thrombocytopenia. Not infrequently the white count will be in the range of 300,000 to 500,000 per cu mm and produce clinical symptoms and signs of organ failure owing to leukostasis and poor perfusion. The patients have a rather rapid progressive downhill clinical course. This clinical syndrome may arise de novo or less frequently as a transformation of the more typical form of chronic lymphocytic leukemia. The cells in the peripheral blood are characterized by rather high concentrations of monoclonal immunoglobulins on their surface, as detected by immunofluorescence techniques.

Leukemic Reticuloendotheliosis (Hairy Cell Leukemia). A relatively uncommon disorder, this is initially characterized by splenomegaly, anemia, thrombocytopenia, and leukopenia. The differential white cell count reveals a predominance of mononuclear cells slightly larger than normal lymphocytes. The nuclear chromatin is finer than that of the lymphocyte; cytoplasm is more abundant, with fine hairlike projections on the surface. Although this cell was initially thought to be a reticuloendothelial cell, the application of surface immunologic techniques now reveal the B cell lymphocyte origin of this disorder. A unique feature of this lymphocyte is the presence of the acid phosphatase enzyme in the cytoplasm that is resistant to inhibition by tartaric acid. In contrast, the acid phosphatase in a normal lymphocyte is inhibited by tartaric acid. Bone marrow biopsies reveal an infiltration of the abnormal cells just described in a network of fine reticulin. Erythropoiesis, myelopoiesis, and megakaryopoiesis are diminished.

AGNOGENIC MYELOID METAPLASIA

By MURRAY N. SILVERSTEIN, M.D.
Rochester, Minnesota

SYNONYMS

Myelofibrosis, myelosclerosis, osteosclerosis, and myeloproliferative syndrome.

DEFINITION

Agnogenic myeloid metaplasia (AMM) is a myeloproliferative disease characterized by (1) striking splenomegaly, (2) leukoerythroblastic blood reaction, (3) significant teardrop poikilocytes on peripheral smear, and (4) bone marrow biopsy characterized by some evidence of fibrosis. The disorder has a close interrelationship with other chronic myeloproliferative diseases. Approximately 12 to 14 per cent of patients with polycythemia vera will evolve into a state indistinguishable from AMM. Chronic granulocytic leukemia in 8 per cent of patients will go through a myelofibrotic phase before the onset of blast transformation. In a recent series of 50 patients with primary thrombocythemia treated by me and my colleagues, 3 patients subsequently developed AMM. The condition of about 8 to 10 per cent of AMM patients will evolve into a syndrome indistinguishable from acute nonlymphocytic leukemia.

PRESENTING SIGNS AND SYMPTOMS

When first seen, approximately 70 per cent of patients are symptomatic and 30 per cent are asymptomatic. The disease in asymptomatic patients is usually picked up because of abnormalities on peripheral blood smear or the presence of splenomegaly. Of symptomatic patients, approximately 60 per cent have symptoms referable to the presence of normochromic anemia: dyspnea, weakness, fatigue, tachycardia, or frank congestive heart failure. Approximately 23 per cent of patients have symptoms related to pressure from the enlarged, uncomfortable spleen. Additional pressure symptoms related to splenomegaly may be reflected in flatulence, nausea, or early satiety owing to the enlarged spleen compressing various parts of the gastrointestinal tract. From 14 to 18 per cent of patients with AMM have symptoms related to bleeding. Bleeding in turn may be secondary to thrombocytopenia in about 33 per cent of patients or secondary to platelet function abnormalities that occur in at least 75 per cent of patients with this disease, or bleeding may be related to the onset of disseminated intravascular coagulation.

COURSE

Of the asymptomatic patients with myelofibrosis, approximately 80 per cent remain stable over a 5-year period. The other 20 per cent of patients develop symptoms referable to anemia, pressure from the enlarged spleen, or bleeding. In an overall cohort of patients with AMM, 5-year survivorship is approximately 57 per cent.

PHYSICAL EXAMINATION FINDINGS

On physical examination the striking abnormality is the enlarged spleen; splenomegaly occurs and progresses in every patient with the syndrome. More than 50 per cent of patients have hepatomegaly. Pallor may be seen in 60 per cent of patients, secondary to anemia. Ecchymoses seen in upwards of 40 per cent of patients are due to either thrombocytopenia or platelet function abnormalities.

COMMON COMPLICATIONS

Common complications of AMM are the development of normocytic, normochromic anemia leading in turn to predominantly cardiovascular or pulmonary symptoms. Twenty-three per cent of patients develop a large painful spleen that produces pressure represented as pain in the left upper quadrant or generalized abdominal discomfort. Patients with enlarged spleen in addition have various gastrointestinal manifestations depending on the location of pressure from it. Fourteen to 18 per cent of patients develop bleeding complications secondary to thrombocytopenia, platelet function abnormalities, or disseminated intravascular coagulation fibrinolysis.

About 6 to 8 per cent of patients with AMM develop portal hypertension or ascites. Portal hypertension most frequently is due to the marked increase in blood flow from the spleen to liver. In many instances this increased flow may be 10 to 15 times the normal hepatic blood flow. Ascites in AMM may be secondary to portal hypertension or due to metastatic implants of AMM in the peritoneum. In patients with portal hypertension, ruptured varices with catastrophic hemorrhage may be seen in more than 4 per cent of patients with AMM.

Eight to 10 per cent of patients with AMM develop acute nonlymphocytic leukemia, which has a rather virulent course and short survivorship. In reviewing the causes of death in myelofibrosis at our institution, I noted a very high incidence of degenerative vascular disease in more than 50 per cent of patients. This in turn leads to a high yield of patients with myocardial infarction or cerebrovascular accidents. Infection accounts for about one eighth of the deaths and leukemia approximately 10 per cent of the deaths.

LABORATORY FINDINGS

Approximately 95 per cent of patients develop normocytic, normochromic anemia. It is important in the work-up of an anemic patient with AMM to initially test total blood volume. As with other giant spleen syndromes, marked plasma dilution may occur on the basis of outstanding splenomegaly and thus lead to a dilutional picture in which the red cell mass is entirely normal. Obviously these patients are not anemic but simply have a dilutional problem similar to what is seen in patients with other giant spleen syndromes or pregnancy. The range of values for normocytic, normochromic anemia may vary from 5 to 10 grams per dl (100 ml) of hemoglobin. About 10 to 15 per cent of patients with AMM develop an overt hemolytic anemia that is often quite severe, leading to hemoglobin determinations between 3 and 6 grams per dl. These patients have almost routinely been Coombs' negative. At least 50 per cent of patients with normocytic, normochromic anemia of milder degree have been shown to have shortened red cell survival times.

Approximately 6 per cent of patients with AMM have iron deficiency anemia secondary to bleeding from the gastrointestinal tract. Leukopenia is seen in 12 to 14 per cent of patients with AMM and all patients with the syndrome have myeloid immaturity and the presence of normoblasts in the differential count. Approximately 33 per cent of patients develop thrombocytopenia with platelet counts below the level of 100,000 per cu mm. In addition to these abnormalities, hyperuricacidemia may be noted in upwards of 60 per cent of patients with AMM when first seen. A review of liver function studies by me and my colleagues revealed that approximately 30 per cent of patients have abnormal Bromsulphalein (BSP) retention and more than 17 per cent have elevations of serum glutamic oxaloacetic transaminase (SGOT) or alkaline phosphatase. The leukocyte alkaline phosphatase score is elevated, that is, above 100, in half the patients with AMM. It is normal in 25 per cent of patients and in 25 per cent of patients it is low.

PERIPHERAL BLOOD

A review of the peripheral blood smear shows leukoerythroblastic blood reaction in all patients and significant teardrop poikilocytosis. Giant platelets and occasionally megakaryocytic fragments may be seen in smears of patients with myelofibrosis. In about 12 per cent of patients there may be intense thrombocythemia. Platelet counts may be as much as 1,000,000 per cu mm and large platelet drifts may be seen on a peripheral smear.

BONE MARROW

The bone marrow of patients with AMM may be actually hyperplastic with areas of fibrosis. This picture may extend to the development of intense fibrosis with replacement of the marrow by dense fibrous tissue. All that remains in the interstices of this dense fibrous tissue is megakaryocytes.

OTHER LABORATORY TESTS

In relation to other laboratory tests, serum protein electrophoresis is normal in the vast majority of patients with AMM. On serum protein electrophoresis the most unusual abnormality is decreased serum albumin. This was seen in our series of patients in 12 of 70 consecutive protein electrophoreses conducted. Of importance is the fact that about 6 per cent of patients with AMM may have a homogeneous migrating spike in the serum. Whether this is merely due to a monoclonal gammopathy typical of the advanced age of some of these patients or whether this is related to the syndrome of myelofibrosis is still undecided.

Special coagulation studies in patients with myelofibrosis reveal the prothrombin time to be increased in three of every four patients tested. The major increase in the prothrombin time relates to the decrease in Factor V. Platelet function abnormalities are frequent, especially a lack of aggregation response to collagen and epinephrine, which is seen in almost every patient with AMM. Inapparent disseminated intravascular coagulation may occur in more than 12 to 15 per cent of patients with AMM. This is characterized by a syndrome with no actual clinical bleeding but on laboratory study low levels of Factors V and VIII and thrombocytopenia and increased fibrin split products. Studies in the normocytic, normochromic anemia of AMM reveal that with chromium and iron tagging, approximately 95 per cent of patients have ineffective erythropoiesis. This in turn is characterized by increased plasma iron turnover rates and low iron incorporation 8 days after the tag study has begun. Only about 6 per cent of patients have iron deficiency anemia and the occurrence of folate or B_{12} deficiency in patients with AMM in the United States has been extremely rare. Bone x-ray abnormalities are seen in approximately 45 per cent of patients. On x-ray the bones appear quite dense in general. Occasionally, scattered focal blastic areas may be seen in AMM and have been confused with metastatic carcinoma.

BIOCHEMICAL FINDINGS

In regard to biochemical findings, besides the values mentioned in the preceding discussion on leukocyte alkaline phosphatase (LAP) and hyperuricacidemia and those in the discussion of liver function and special coagulation studies, values for sodium, potassium, calcium, and phosphorus are usually normal. Interestingly, at least 40 to 50 per cent of patients with AMM have low levels of cholesterol and triglycerides. No reasonable explanation has been found yet for these findings.

URINALYSIS

Except for those patients who develop hyperuricacidemia and the renal complications of this event, the urine is unremarkable.

PITFALLS IN DIAGNOSIS

AMM may be confused with chronic granulocytic leukemia because of the huge spleen syndrome that accompanies both conditions. Differential diagnosis is quite easy because in AMM the white count is usually below 50,000, and there is orderly myeloid immaturity associated with the normoblast response. In chronic granulocytic leukemia, counts are usually in excess of 100,000 and a myelocyte bulge is seen in the differential count. Marrow findings in both diseases are quite diagnostic. In myelofibrosis the marrow tends to be quite hypocellular with a dense fibrotic reaction, whereas in chronic granulocytic leukemia the marrow is extremely hypercellular with very marked granulocytic hyperplasia. It is well to remember that more than 12 to 15 per cent of patients with polycythemia vera may develop a syndrome indistinguishable from myelofibrosis. Postpolycythemic myeloid metaplasia is a much more lethal syndrome than myelofibrosis, which arises de novo. Additionally, as pointed out earlier, primary thrombocythemia and chronic granulocytic leukemia may also become transformed marrow-wise into myelofibrosis. The clinical picture of patients developing myelofibrosis following primary thrombocythemia mimics quite well the syndrome of AMM. In patients with chronic granulocytic leukemia transforming to myelofibrosis, the myelofibrosis tends to be an extremely ominous sign, as blast transformation occurs rapidly after its occurrence in patients with chronic granulocytic leukemia.

Occasionally, metastatic carcinoma to the marrow may produce a syndrome indistinguishable from AMM. Differential diagnosis depends on a previous history of carcinoma and the presence of carcinoma cells in the marrow.

LEUKOCYTOSIS AND LEUKEMOID REACTIONS

By NANCY B. McWILLIAMS, M.D.,
and E. C. RUSSELL, M.D.

Richmond, Virginia

DEFINITION

Leukocytosis may be defined as an increase in the total number of white blood cells above normal levels for age (e.g., a total white blood cell count of 18,000 per cu mm constitutes leukocytosis in the adult but is within normal limits in the first week of life). The term "leukemoid reaction" has been used to describe a hematologic response that resembles leukemia because of exaggerated leukocytosis, usually in excess of 35,000 per cu mm and usually in the presence of immature cell forms. Clearly, a differential count and a careful evaluation of red cells and platelets are critical determinants in differentiating leukemoid reactions from leukemia. In most instances simple hematologic tools and clinical manifestations yield a ready answer. Rarely, diagnosis is elusive and close observation is necessary before the cause of the leukemoid reaction is apparent.

Leukocytosis and leukemoid reactions are best classified according to the predominant cell type. Neutrophilic leukocytosis of moderate (neutrophilia) or extreme (neutrophilic leukemoid reaction) degree is most common. Total leukocyte counts above 10,000 per cu mm with a predominance of neutrophilic leukocytes are a hallmark of many bacterial infections, especially those caused by gram-positive cocci. Usually the leukocyte count is between 15,000 and 25,000 per cu mm, but counts of 30,000 to 50,000 per cu mm not infrequently accompany severe infection.

Leukocytosis may accompany certain viral and fungal infections (such as varicella and actinomycosis, respectively), parasitic infestations such as liver flukes, and tuberculosis. Inflammatory reactions that occur in collagen vascular disease, burns, hypersensitivity states, and following surgery frequently produce moderate leukocytosis. Other causes include eclampsia, diabetic ketoacidosis, and heavy metal poisoning. Hemorrhage or acute hemolysis may precipitate a neutrophilic response and neutrophilic leukocytosis is common in certain chronic hemolytic states (e.g., sickle cell anemia). Corticosteroids induce a leukocytosis and a transient elevation of neutrophils follows the injection of epinephrine. In addition to severe infections, extreme neutrophilic leukemoid reactions may be produced by metastatic carcinoma, Hodgkin's disease, and myelofibrosis.

Eosinophilic leukemoid reactions may at times be striking, with total white counts as high as 100,000 per cu mm and 50 to 90 per cent eosinophils. Parasitic infestations, said to occur in a third of the world's population, are the commonest cause. In children, visceral larva migrans is the main offender, but exaggerated eosinophilia may also be produced by infestation with trichinella, ascaris, strongyloides, and hookworm. As the name suggests, the idiopathic hypereosinophilic syndrome or pulmonary infiltration with eosinophilia (PIE syndrome) may be associated with an eosinophilic leukemoid reaction. Other less common causes include Hodgkin's disease, periarteritis nodosa, and drug hypersensitivity.

Lymphocytic leukemoid reactions or lymphocytic leukocytosis may be produced by a number of infections including pertussis, infectious mononucleosis, infectious hepatitis, infectious lymphocytosis, and other viral disease. Drug hypersensitivity, thyrotoxicosis, and some chronic infections (e.g., tuberculosis and brucellosis) are less common causes.

Monocytic leukemoid reactions are rare but relative monocytosis may be encountered in granulomatous diseases, some infections such as subacute bacterial endocarditis, tuberculosis, and some carcinomas.

PRESENTING SIGNS AND SYMPTOMS

The clinical manifestations of leukocytosis are related to the condition producing it. Frequently, the history alone will suggest a diagnosis if one is attentive to details such as duration of illness, associated constitutional symptoms, drug exposure, pet exposure, and history of travel to areas where parasitic infection is endemic.

PHYSICAL EXAMINATION

As with the signs and symptoms, the physical findings are related to the underlying disorder. The patient may be acutely ill with a readily evident source of infection or obvious malignancy, or the physical examination may be within normal limits.

COURSE AND COMPLICATIONS

The course of leukocytosis or leukemoid reactions relates to their cause. Complications relate to the underlying disorder as a rule but may be iatrogenically induced if an incorrect diagnosis is made and improper therapy administered.

LABORATORY FINDINGS

A high white blood cell count is the sine qua non of leukocytosis. A careful differential must be done with attention to immature forms, presence or absence of toxic granulation, and/or Döhle's inclusion bodies. It is critical to obtain a complete hemogram including red cell indices, platelets, and reticulocyte count. Red cell and platelet morphology must be assessed and nucleated red blood cells searched for as clues to leukoerythroblastic reactions.

When severe bacterial infection is suspected, a Gram stain of the buffy coat may reveal organisms and aid in proper antibiotic selection. The leukocyte alkaline phosphatase score and the presence of the Philadelphia chromosome will confirm a diagnosis of chronic myelocytic leukemia (CML) in cases in which leukocytosis is extreme and there is a marked shift to the left.

If more than 12 per cent of the mononuclear cells are atypical lymphocytes, infectious mononucleosis, infectious hepatitis, or another virus is likely to be responsible and appropriate serologic tests should be ordered.

In exaggerated eosinophilic responses, stool examination for ova and parasites is of obvious importance, but negative results do not rule out parasitic infestation. Serologic tests, skin tests, biopsy, or even surgery may sometimes be necessary to secure a diagnosis.

Bone marrow examination is essential when leukemia is suggested by the blood film or cannot be ruled out, when a myelophthisic or granulomatous condition is suspected, or when special cultures for mycobacteria or fungi will aid in the diagnosis.

PITFALLS IN DIAGNOSIS

Leukocytosis and leukemoid reactions are not synonymous with leukemia and the physician should make every effort to secure the correct diagnosis. When the cause is elusive, careful follow-up with serial hemograms and other appropriate studies is essential.

INFECTIOUS MONONUCLEOSIS

By ROBERT J. HOAGLAND, M.D.
Warrenton, Virginia

DEFINITION

Infectious mononucleosis (IM) is an acute disease of the reticuloendothelial system, lymph nodes, and spleen; its cause is believed to be the Epstein-Barr virus (which has been demonstrated in lymphocytes of patients). Its hallmarks are relative and absolute lymphocytosis, many atypical lymphocytes, and production of many antibodies, among them the characteristic agglutinins for sheep erythrocytes.

PRESENTING SYMPTOMS

Sore throat, most frequently the presenting complaint, is preceded by 3 to 7 days of malaise. Rarely, sore throat is not complained of until the second week or not at all. Jaundice (infrequently the presenting complaint) is present in almost 10 per cent of patients, occurs in the second week, and ordinarily appears after the initial visit. Many jaundiced patients also have sore throat. About 10 per cent of patients seek medical attention only because of malaise and feverishness.

The subjective symptoms of IM are so few that any symptoms other than sore throat, mild myalgia, malaise, chills or fever, and headache should suggest a different diagnosis, a complication of IM or a concurrent illness.

PHYSICAL EXAMINATION

Some degree of bilateral posterior cervical or supraclavicular lymph node enlargement is a requirement for diagnosis. Anterior cervical lymph node enlargement, always present, is a feature of *any* type of acute pharyngitis. Other nodes also are enlarged. Enlargement may be minimal and may not become evident until the second week. Nodes are not tender (or, at most, are mildly so), and overlying skin is not inflamed; nodes are discrete and firm but not hard. Narrowing of the ocular aperture is often produced by slight edema of palpebral and orbital portions of the upper eyelids. Hyperplasia and inflammation of pharyngeal lymphatic tissue of variable degree are almost always apparent, and in about one third of the patients exudative tonsillitis is seen. Pinpoint to pinhead-sized red midpalatal lesions occur during the second and third weeks. They are not specific but are of great diagnostic value. After 7 to 10 days splenic enlargement may be evident. Jaundice is almost always mild (but one patient has been seen with a total bilirubin level of 31.5 mg per dl [100 ml]). A rash is so infrequent that it should suggest a concomitant disorder (especially reaction to ampicillin) or a different diagnosis. It must be emphasized that physical signs appear sequentially.

COURSE

Unless treated with corticosteroids, fewer than 10 per cent of patients are febrile fewer than 7 days and half are febrile 7 to 14 days; none are febrile for longer than 1 month. If sore throat is not abolished (by giving corticosteroids), it is likely to last 7 to 10 days. Weight loss is common. Fatigability persists after fever; its duration is directly proportional to amount of weight loss and duration of fever, and it is greater in women and asthenic males than in other patients. Well-motivated patients are able to resume *sedentary* activities a day or so after cessation of fever. In uncomplicated cases, normal stamina usually returns within 3 to 6 weeks after fever ends.

COMMON COMPLICATIONS

Splenic rupture occurs in 0.2 to 0.4 per cent of patients. Clues are left-sided abdominal pain, tenderness, and muscle spasm occurring 10 to 20 days after onset of mononucleosis. When shock is present, the diagnosis should be obvious.

Electrocardiographic changes, usually flat or inverted T waves, occurred in 6 per cent of the patients I have treated. Increased P-R and Q-T intervals and atrioventricular nodal rhythm were less frequent than merely T wave changes. I have never encountered pericarditis, but it has been reported. Functionally significant heart disease does not ensue.

Hemolytic anemia occurs in at least 3 per cent of patients, but as many as 25 per cent may have minimal hemolysis — not enough to produce anemia.

Thrombocytopenic purpura occurs in 0.2 per cent of patients, but regularly performed platelet counts reveal subnormal levels in 25 to 50 per cent.

Neurologic complications occurred in 8 of my first 500 patients (5 had mononeuritis or plexitis; 1 had meningitis; 1, meningismus; and 1, transverse myelitis). Only after seeing more than 500 patients did I encounter a patient with Guillain-Barré syndrome.

I believe that early use of corticosteroids has reduced the incidence of complications as reflected in the stated figures. Beta-hemolytic streptococcal pharyngeal involvement occurs in about 30 per cent of patients.

LABORATORY FINDINGS

Hematology. Absolute and relative lymphocytoses are characteristic and requisite for diagnosis. During the first week of illness the leukocyte count and distribution may be normal; infrequently there is moderate leukopenia, but never neutrophilia (unless it is due to a concurrent illness). In the second week the total leukocyte count and total and relative lymphocyte counts rise; they are essentially unchanged in the third week, then they decline. Total white blood cell counts at their zenith usually exceed 10,000; the highest count in my series was 31,000 per cu mm. Most patients achieve relative lymphocytosis of 70 per cent or higher; the highest in my series was 93 per cent. Relative lymphocytosis of at least 50 per cent is a requirement for diagnosis; over 90 per cent of my patients showed lymphocytosis of 60 per cent or higher. Lymphocytosis persists for at least 2 weeks unless a corticosteroid has been given or a bacterial infection supervenes. If intercurrent bacterial infection is present, there may be a transient neutrophil increase. (Usually there is still some increase in total number of lymphocytes.) Atypical lymphocytes are characteristic but not pathognomonic. During the second week such cells usually make up over 25 per cent of lymphocytes. The kinds of atypical lymphocytes change during the course of illness, and more than one kind is usually present in a blood smear. Bone marrow examination is not helpful.

Serology. The heterophil antibody reaction is a requirement for diagnosis but by itself is not diagnostic. It can usually be demonstrated between the eighth and twenty-first days of illness. Characteristically, there is agglutination of sheep erythrocytes after the patient's serum has been exposed to guinea pig kidney suspension but not after exposure to beef erythrocytes. Any titer after absorption with guinea pig kidney serves to confirm the diagnosis (if there is no titer after absorption with beef erythrocytes).

Antibodies are usually detectable for at least a month after onset of IM; they are rarely present after the eighth week but may recur during the course of an unrelated illness months or even years later.

Rapid slide tests — one using blood from the finger tip (the Monosticon test) —are suitable for confirmation of clinical diagnosis; however, the original Davidson differential test is advisable in research work and in doubtful cases.

BIOCHEMICAL FINDINGS

The performance of additional laboratory tests is needless. Liver function tests, in untreated patients, yield abnormal results in the second or third week. About one third of patients have serum bilirubin of over 1 mg per 100 ml, but alkaline phosphatase levels are often discordantly elevated.

THERAPEUTIC TEST

If a patient suspected of having IM does not regain a normal temperature 48 hours after initiation of corticosteroid therapy, he has either a complication or a different disease: of course, this is not an effect specific for IM.

PITFALLS IN DIAGNOSIS

1. Making a diagnosis despite negative results of serology 3 to 4 weeks after onset of illness (although rarely patients are incapable of making characteristic antibodies in amounts adequate to produce positive test results).

2. Disregarding the requirement of absolute lymphocytosis (i.e., at least 4500 cells per cu mm).

3. Accepting relative lymphocytosis of 50 per cent as sufficient.

4. Diagnosing "hepatitis" in a young person with jaundice and fever. If he has a sore throat also, he almost certainly has IM.

5. Believing the threadbare fallacy that IM is a "protean" disease, thus missing either complications or the correct diagnosis.

6. Failing to reexamine for lymph node enlargement for 14 days after onset of illness.

7. Forgetting that diagnostic physical signs, hematology, and serology may not appear until 12 to 18 days after onset of illness.

8. Basing diagnosis on serology alone.

MALIGNANT LYMPHOMAS

By JANE E. HENNEY, M.D.,
and VINCENT T. DeVITA, JR., M.D.
Bethesda, Maryland

DEFINITION

The lymphomas are a group of malignant diseases, usually arising in the lymph nodes or in the lymphoid tissues of parenchymal organs such as the gut, lung, or skin, with a characteristic histologic appearance. If untreated, they have a variable but progressive course leading to death.

Malignant lymphomas are generally classified in two groups: Hodgkin's disease in one and the lymphocytic and histiocytic lymphomas of Rappaport in the other. Each of these groups has been further divided into subcategories. The most common currently used classification of Hodgkin's disease that is readily reproducible and has prognostic relevance was described by Lukes and Butler (Table 1). The other lymphomas are generally described by the Rappaport classification (Table 2), which has two main subcategories based on lymph node architecture: diffuse and nodular. Lesions with the nodular pattern tend to follow a more indolent course while those with the diffuse pattern, with the exception of those with well-differentiated forms, have a rapid clinical evolution. The nodular and diffuse subtypes are further defined by describing the morphologic features of the cells, such as lymphocytic, histiocytic, and mixtures of the two cell types, the mixed lymphomas.

Classifications based on ultrastructural studies and immunologic techniques delineating T and B cells have recently been proposed by Lukes and Collins and others.

The term "histiocytic lymphoma" used by Rappaport to designate large histiocytic appearing cells is now known to be a misnomer but is still used by convention. About 80 per cent of all histiocytic and lymphocytic lymphomas are now known to arise from a proliferation of monoclonal B cells, including the lesions in all those patients with nodular forms of the disease. True T cell lymphomas are uncommon and are usually seen in children and adolescents with mediastinal adenopathy and a leukemic blood picture with large convoluted lymphoblasts in the peripheral blood. The only true form of a malignant histiocytic disease is histiocytic medullary reticulosis, although current evidence indicates that the cell of origin in Hodgkin's disease is a histiocyte.

Burkitt's lymphoma is a diffuse lymphoma of the follicular B cells that is primarily observed in African children. In the endemic regions of East Africa and New Guinea, evidence of infection with a herpes-like Epstein-Barr virus has been observed. The child in Africa most commonly presents with extra lymphatic tumor arising from the bone, often the mandible. The American child, on the other hand, presents with disease involving abdominal or pelvic sites, particularly the gastrointestinal tract, and infrequently the jaw is involved. Sites of secondary involvement for the African varieties include frequent spread to the abdominal viscera, ovaries, breast, and meninges and infrequent spread to the bone marrow. Both varieties of disease eventually involve the bone marrow and cerebrospinal fluid in over one third of the patients.

Angioimmunoblastic lymphadenopathy is not considered a histologically malignant disease but rather an extreme form of hypersensitivity reaction. This lymphoma-like systemic disorder most frequently occurs in adults and the clinical features often mimic those observed in the patient with advanced Hodgkin's disease or the other lymphomas. Generalized lymphadenopathy, hepatomegaly, splenomegaly, fever, sweats, and weight loss are often presenting features of this disease. In half of the patients, a generalized pruritic rash may precede the severe constitutional symptoms. In a small

Table 1. *Lukes-Butler Histopathologic Classification of Hodgkin's Disease*

Lymphocytic predominant

Nodular sclerosis

Mixed cellularity

Lymphocyte-depleted

Table 2. *Rappaport Classification of Lymphocytic and Histiocytic Lymphomas*

Type
 Nodular
  Lymphocytic: poorly differentiated lymphoma (NPDL)
  Mixed: (lymphocytic and histiocytic) lymphoma (NML)
  Histiocytic (NH)
 Diffuse
  Lymphocytic
   Well-differentiated lymphoma (DWDL)
   Poorly differentiated lymphoma (DPDL)
  Mixed: (lymphocytic and histiocytic) lymphoma (DML)
  Histiocytic (DHL)

number of patients a history of drug ingestion can be elicited.

Nearly all patients evidence anemia and in 25 per cent it is due to a Coombs' test–positive hemolytic anemia. Leukocytosis and eosinophilia may also be a part of the peripheral blood picture. The majority of patients have a polyclonal hypergammaglobulinemia as well.

When the enlarged lymph nodes are biopsied, alterations can be observed of nodal architecture or complete effacement with a pleomorphic cellular proliferation in which immunoblasts, lymphocytes, and plasma cells predominate. Vascular proliferation and prominent eosinophilic interstitial material are also often seen.

The remainder of the clinical course can vary greatly. Approximately 25 per cent of patients have a long survival, up to 4 years, with or without corticosteroid therapy and never require intensive chemotherapy. Another 25 per cent have a similar survival time but only when intensive chemotherapy is administered. The remaining patients have a rapid downhill course terminating in death regardless of the management approach. Among the terminal events, overwhelming infections, renal failure, and hepatic failure all have been reported.

PRESENTING SIGNS AND SYMPTOMS

Hodgkin's Disease. The young patient with Hodgkin's disease usually comes to the physician with adenopathy. This enlargement of lymph nodes can be either asymptomatic, discrete, or painless, or be associated with symptoms of fever, night sweats, weight loss, and sometimes pruritus. Fever, night sweats, and weight loss are referred to as "B" symptoms and have been demonstrated to be correlated with more advanced disease and a poor prognosis. Pruritus often accompanies fever but does not have significance when observed as an isolated finding. The disease in young people is often detected by finding mediastinal adenopathy on a routine chest x-ray or a film taken because of a persistent, dry, nonproductive cough. This presentation is most common if the Hodgkin's disease is of the nodular sclerosing variety.

In older patients with Hodgkin's disease the tumor commonly is associated with fever, night sweats, or both, followed by increasing malaise and weight loss. In some cases the enlarging lymph nodes are located exclusively in the abdomen. Those patients not having readily apparent lymph node enlargement usually are assigned by the physician a differential diagnosis of fever of undetermined origin. If the diagnosis establishes Hodgkin's disease, the lymphocyte-depleted variety is most frequent.

If fever has been among the presenting symptoms in the patient with Hodgkin's disease in either age group, it is usually remittent in nature.

A cyclical fever pattern known as Pel-Ebstein fever has also been observed in the patient with Hodgkin's disease. This temperature pattern is characterized by several days or weeks of fever alternating with afebrile periods. Pain coincident with the consumption of alcohol is uncommon, but when it does occur appears to correlate with heavy eosinophilic infiltration at the sites involved by tumor. Thus this may serve to direct attention to an involved site to biopsy and confirm the diagnosis of Hodgkin's disease. Infrequently, superior vena cava syndrome is the first symptom in a patient with Hodgkin's disease.

Lymphocytic and Histiocytic Lymphomas. Patients with the common nodular poorly differentiated lymphocytic lymphoma (NPDL) present with a more uniform clinical picture than those with the other types. The disease afflicts adults usually over the age of 40. Its occurrence in children is rare and such a diagnosis should suggest reactive hyperplasia to the physician. The patient with NPDL is commonly asymptomatic at the outset. Painless adenopathy in the cervical, axillary, and inguinal-femoral regions is the common presenting physical finding. Because the lymphocytic lymphoma commonly involves the gastrointestinal tract, large abdominal masses of retroperitoneal or mesenteric lymph nodes that cause acute gastrointestinal problems, including obstruction, hemorrhage, and intussusception, can occur. The symptoms of fever, night sweats, and/or weight loss are less common in patients with lymphocytic and histiocytic lymphomas, and their presence or absence is less related to prognosis.

The lymphadenopathy of the nodular lymphomas may have been present for a long period of time; often, a previous lymph node biopsy may have been interpreted as "atypical" or "hyperplastic." Subsequent review of the initial biopsy and comparison with a second biopsy often reveals that a lymphoma was present from the start. In many patients only one or several enlarged lymph nodes is obvious. Yet when more extensive examination with lymphangiography or other tests is conducted, widespread lymphadenopathy, often symmetrical, is easily revealed. The spleen of the patient with NPDL is often enlarged but generally asymptomatic at the onset of the disease. Involvement of the lymphoid tissue in Waldeyer's ring and epitrochlear lymph tissue is a more common clinical problem in patients with NPDL than in Hodgkin's disease. Paravertebral lymphoid masses may result in chylous pleural effusions or ascites or both. It is extremely rare for the central nervous system to become involved, although peripheral nerve compression and epidural tumor masses may develop. Some patients present with a clinical picture of lymphosarcoma cell leukemia, with white blood cell counts as high as 100,000 per cu mm, with evidence of nodular lymphoma in lymph nodes.

In contrast to patients with NPDL, those with the diffuse lymphomas, formerly called reticulum cell sarcoma, and diffuse lymphocytic lymphomas often present with localized lymph node enlargement or local extralymphatic manifestation. However, the natural history is more aggressive than in NPDL, with rapid growth of tumor masses. In approximately one fourth of the cases diagnosed, the disease is localized to only one side. The lymph nodes most frequently involved are predominantly located in the neck. Involvement of the gastrointestinal tract, bone, thyroid, testes, brain, and the lymph node tissue of Waldeyer's ring also occurs frequently. The bone marrow is involved initially in less than 10 per cent of the patients and is not commonly involved even late in the course of the disease. Patients with diffuse well-differentiated lymphoma have a natural history that mimics chronic lymphocytic leukemia, except that their disease begins by causing lymph node swelling before involvement of the blood or bone marrow. These patients often present with widespread asymptomatic modestly enlarged lymph nodes.

COURSE

Hodgkin's Disease. The asymptomatic adenopathy of a patient with Hodgkin's disease may wax and wane in size for extended periods of time before diagnosis. Previous chest x-rays occasionally reveal that evidence of mediastinal widening has been present for several years before the diagnosis. If left untreated, slow progression of the disease occurs, commonly by extension to contiguous lymph node areas. Once the hilar lymph nodes have been invaded, the tumor mass usually progresses to involve the pulmonary parenchyma. At some point in the progression of the disease, blood vessel invasion may occur. Involvement of the spleen, an organ that has no afferent lymphatics, occurs frequently in Hodgkin's disease. It suggests that vascular invasion may be a common occurrence, even in patients with apparently localized disease. Later, with further progression of the disease and clear evidence of vascular invasion, the bone marrow, liver, and other viscera are often invaded by tumor. Symptoms, if they

had not appeared initially, appear as the volume of tumor increases. Finally, cachexia, complicating infection, and widespread involvement of visceral organs by tumor usually overcome the host and cause death.

Lymphocytic and Histiocytic Lymphomas. The clinical course of nodular lymphoma is variable. In some, the course is indolent and lymphadenopathy may have been present for years before the diagnosis and may be well tolerated by the patient for 5 years or more after the diagnosis is established. The disease is malignant, however, and although there may be spontaneous regression of lymphadenopathy, clinical progression invariably occurs. In some patients the course of the disease progresses rapidly from the time of diagnosis. These patients may experience difficulties within months of the diagnosis.

When the disease becomes much more aggressive, lymph nodes enlarge rapidly, often in localized sites. Fever, night sweats, and weight loss can occur. If repeat biopsy is performed at the time of progression, the histologic appearance may be observed to have changed from nodular to that of a diffuse lymphoma. There are many similarities between nodular poorly differentiated lymphoma and the less frequently occurring nodular mixed lymphoma. The latter does differ, however, in overall prognosis, resembling that of those patients with diffuse large cell (histiocytic) lymphoma.

The diffuse lymphomas consist of a number of different types with a variable clinical evolution. The most indolent type is diffuse well-differentiated lymphocytic lymphoma. The clinical course and outcome is nearly the same as that of chronic lymphocytic leukemia. The diffuse poorly differentiated lymphocytic lymphomas and diffuse mixed-cell lymphomas present much like the nodular lymphomas but evolve much more rapidly.

"Histiocytic" lymphoma is highly invasive, and involvement of peripheral nerves, epidural tumors, compression of the vena cava or airways, and destruction of osseous tissue often occur during the course of the disease. The skin, liver, kidneys, lung, and even the brain may be involved. Occasionally, bone marrow invasion results with the appearance of large, undifferentiated cells in the peripheral blood.

HISTOPATHOLOGY

Hodgkin's Disease. The diagnosis and classification of Hodgkin's disease can be made only by biopsy and histopathologic examination of tissue under a light microscope. The Sternberg-Reed cell is the characteristic malignant cell of Hodgkin's disease. If such cells are

Table 3. *Staging Classification
for Lymphomas**

Stage	Definition
I	Involvement of a single lymph node region (I) or of a single extralymphatic organ or site (I_E).
II	Involvement of two or more lymph node regions on the same side of the diaphragm (II) or localized involvement of an extralymphatic organ or site and of one or more lymph node regions on the same side of the diaphragm (II_E).
III	Involvement of lymph node regions on both sides of the diaphragm (III), which may also be accompanied by involvement of the spleen (III_S) or by localized involvement of an extralymphatic organ site (III_E) or both (III_{SE}).
IV	Diffuse or disseminated involvement of one or more extralymphatic organs or tissues, with or without associated lymph node involvement.

The presence of fever, night sweats and/or unexplained loss of 10 per cent or more of body weight in the 6 months preceding admission are denoted by the suffix letter B. The letter A indicates the absence of these symptoms.

Biopsy-documented involvement of Stage IV sites is also denoted by letter suffixes: marrow = M+; lung = L+; liver = H+; pleura = P+; bone = O+; skin and subcutaneous tissue = D+.

*Adopted at the workshop on the staging of Hodgkin's Disease held at Ann Arbor, Michigan, April, 1971.

absent the diagnosis of Hodgkin's disease should rarely be made. However, the presence of a Sternberg-Reed cell by itself is not diagnostic, since cells simulating Sternberg-Reed cells have been found in patients with mononucleosis and breast cancer. However, if a patient's condition has been previously diagnosed as Hodgkin's disease, the presence of the mononuclear variety of the Sternberg-Reed cell is sufficient to diagnose Hodgkin's disease involving the liver or bone marrow.

Lymphocytic and Histiocytic Lymphomas. The diagnosis of the lymphocytic and histiocytic lymphoma is also made by histopathologic examination of biopsy material usually obtained from lymph nodes. The diagnosis and classification of tissue obtained from other extranodal sites may be more difficult.

PHYSICAL EXAMINATION AND STAGING

Hodgkin's Disease. Accurate staging is vital for planning long-term management (Table 3). The primary physician must take a detailed history, do a thorough physical examination, and look for any evidence of "B" symptoms. Fever, weight loss of 10 per cent or greater, and

soaking night sweats usually mean serious disease. The physician should be cautious to elicit a history of sweats that have taken place before the patient learned of his diagnosis, for soaking night sweats can occur in anxious patients.

The physician should carefully examine every lymph node area of the body. The presence or absence of nodal enlargement should be noted. If enlarged, the size, shape, and consistency of each node should be accurately recorded. The largest lymph nodes in a group should be selected for biopsy. Nodes in areas other than the primary site should be biopsied at the same time, especially if confirmation of spread of disease changes the stage of a patient. An examination of the oropharynx and nasopharynx by indirect laryngoscopy is essential to uncovering Waldeyer ring involvement by lymphoma.

The size of the liver and spleen should be recorded. In Hodgkin's disease, palpable splenomegaly is significant because if this is present, spleen involvement by the disease is likely and thus more generalized disease exists. The technical procedures required for staging patients with Hodgkin's disease under various circumstances are shown in Table 4.

Radiologic examination should include a routine chest film. If positive, whole chest tomography should be performed to identify the extent of mediastinal or hilar adenopathy or evidence of contiguous invasion of the lung from the hilar nodes. Lower extremity lymphangiogram is of paramount importance and should be required unless medically contraindicated. Occasionally, the lymphangiogram will not fill high retroperitoneal lymph nodes. Techniques that can be of use in supplementing lymphangiography are computerized axial tomography and ultrasound. The lymphangiogram is also of benefit in determining the status of bones in the majority of patients. If a patient is symptomatic with bone pain, separate skeletal survey and a technetium-99m pyrophosphate bone scan should be performed. The latter is the more sensitive test for identifying bone lesions.

Laparotomy should not be considered routine in the staging work-up. Since general treatment strategy may markedly influence the decision to perform a staging laparotomy, the type of treatment to be used by either the radiotherapist or medical oncologist should be considered before a decision is made to operate.

In the United States, the mortality from staging laparotomy in Hodgkin's disease is 1.5 per cent, with a complication rate of approximately 12 per cent. In institutions in which laparotomies are done infrequently, mortality rates up to 6.6 per cent and morbidity rates of more than 25 per cent have been reported. Thus, for some

Table 4. *Staging Work-up of Hodgkin's Disease*

1. Adequate surgical biopsy, reviewed by an experienced hematopathologist
2. A detailed history recording the absence or presence of and duration of fever, unexplained sweating and its severity, unexplained pruritus, and unexplained weight loss
3. A careful and detailed physical examination; special attention to all node-bearing areas, including Waldeyer's ring, and determination of size of liver and spleen
4. Laboratory procedures
   A. Complete blood count, including an erythrocytic sedimentation rate
   B. Serum alkaline phosphatase
   C. Evaluation of renal function
   D. Evaluation of liver function
   E. Bone marrow biopsy if A or B is elevated or there is evidence of bone disease by scan or x-ray
5. Radiologic studies
   A. Chest roentgenogram (posteroanterior and lateral) Whole-chest tomography if any abnormality is noted or suspected on the routine chest x-ray
   B. Intravenous pyelogram
   C. Bilateral lower extremity lymphogram Inferior cavography, ultrasonograph, or CT scanning to supplement equivocal lymphographic findings in the high retroperitoneal area
   D. Views of skeletal system to include thoracic and lumbar vertebrae, pelvis, proximal extremities, and any areas of bone tenderness
6. Exploratory laparotomy and splenectomy — only if identification of abdominal disease will change the proposed management plan

stages of Hodgkin's disease, the operative mortality may exceed the expected death rate at 5 years from the disease!

When performed, the laparotomy should always be complete. The procedure should include at least two needle biopsies of each lobe of the liver, a wedge biopsy of the liver edge, biopsies of suspicious areas, splenectomy, and biopsy of selected lymph nodes in the retroperitoneal area, marked on the lymphangiogram before the operation. Nodes in the porta hepatis should also be biopsied. A postoperative film should confirm that the proper lymph nodes were removed. Lastly, female patients in the reproductive years should have the ovaries moved laterally or centrally to avoid the majority of the radiation ports.

Laparoscopy has now been shown to be a useful alternative approach to laparotomy in staging abdominal disease. Liver involvement can be detected with equal facility using either approach.

Lymphocytic and Histiocytic Lymphomas. The staging classification developed for Hodgkin's disease is also used in the other lymphomas; the sequence of staging procedures differs, however, because extralymphatic presentations occur more frequently in non-Hodgkin's lymphomas than in Hodgkin's disease.

The histologic patterns of lymphocytic and histiocytic lymphomas correlate with specific disease patterns, response to therapy, and prognosis. Thus the patterns are a valuable aid in determining the staging procedures needed to select the appropriate treatment strategy for a particular patient. Further, since many physicians approach the treatment of Stage III and Stage IV disease in a similar manner, this distinction may be far less relevant in lymphocytic and histiocytic lymphomas than in Hodgkin's disease. Surgical staging clearly should not be considered a routine procedure in patients with lymphocytic and histiocytic lymphomas, since extensive disease can often be identified by simpler diagnostic technique. The major task of staging is to determine if the patient has limited nodal or extranodal "E" disease, which may be radiocurable (Stage I or II), or disseminated disease, which always requires systemic therapy (Stage III or IV). For patients who, after clinical staging, still appear to have localized disease and are considered eligible for curative radiotherapy, extensive surgical staging evaluation may then be justified. In those whose age or general medical problems limit therapy to local palliation with radiotherapy or systemic treatment with a single drug, few invasive staging procedures are indicated.

LABORATORY FINDINGS

Routine blood counts, erythrocyte sedimentation rate, urinalysis, liver function studies, and renal function studies are all necessary parts of the medical work-up of a patient with lymphoma, but by themselves they do not provide information on the extent of disease or specific organ involvement.

Patients with Hodgkin's disease who do not have symptoms and have disease localized above the diaphragm, with a negative lymphangiogram, do not need the bone marrow examination, since they rarely have bone marrow involvement. All other lymphoma patients should routinely have a bone marrow examination. Bone marrow involvement occurs most frequently with diffuse well-differentiated lymphocytic lymphoma and poorly differentiated lymphocytic lymphoma (nodular or diffuse) (50 to 60 per cent) but less frequently with diffuse histiocytic lymphomas (10 per cent). In Hodgkin's disease, initial bone marrow involvement is uncommon, occurring most often in patients with symptoms and in patients with the lymphocyte-depleted subtype.

If a bone marrow examination is to be done, a bone marrow biopsy rather than aspiration is required. Marrow aspiration does not yield results comparable to those obtained by biopsy. This is likely due to the fibrosis and granuloma formation in the marrow of patients with Hodgkin's disease. On smear or section, the myeloid-to-erythroid ratio may be increased and marrow eosinophilia is common; neither finding, however, is diagnostic of marrow involvement. Involvement of the marrow by tumor is demonstrated by finding either classic Sternberg-Reed cells or their mononuclear variant distributed focally or diffusely throughout the bone marrow. Marrow involvement marring the normal marrow architecture is often associated with reticular fibrosis. In a previously diagnosed patient with Hodgkin's disease, intense marrow fibrosis, even in the absence of the characteristic Sternberg-Reed cells, constitutes strong evidence of tumor in the bone marrow. Effective treatment by chemotherapy that results in a remission can lead to total resolution of this type of fibrosis.

Anemia, neutropenia, and thrombocytopenia can occur in either Hodgkin's disease or the other lymphomas and can be the consequence of bone marrow involvement. These conditions may also be caused by a variety of other conditions for which a systematic search must be conducted. Among these conditions are hypersplenism, immunologic mechanisms, blood loss secondary to gastrointestinal infiltration and ulceration, or complications of therapy. Patients with Hodgkin's disease frequently demonstrate a moderate normochromic, normocytic anemia associated with low serum iron and low iron-binding capacity but normal or increased iron stores in the bone marrow. This anemia has been shown to be due to both increased destruction and decreased production of red blood cells. In general terms, the anemia correlates with the extent and duration of the disease.

A Coombs' positive hemolytic anemia occurs in less than 1 per cent of patients with advanced diffuse or nodular lymphomas and Hodgkin's disease. It is seen with greater frequency in both the diffuse well-differentiated and the diffuse poorly differentiated types of lymphocytic lymphoma. Coombs' negative hemolytic anemia may also be present. Chronic illness resulting in a poor nutritional status and consequent folate deficiency may also contribute to the picture of anemia. Finally, radiotherapy or chemotherapy or both can result in diminished or ineffective erythropoiesis.

A moderate to marked leukemoid reaction is often observed in Hodgkin's disease. This is most common to those patients who are symptomatic. The leukemoid reaction disappears with successful treatment of the underlying Hodgkin's disease and does not indicate involvement of the marrow by tumor.

The leukemic phase of lymphoma is seen most frequently in the lymphocytic lymphomas, usually late in the disease. This type of leukemic invasion of the peripheral blood is rare in other lymphomas such as diffuse histiocytic lymphomas or Hodgkin's disease. In well-differentiated lymphocytic lymphomas, the leukemic cells are usually identical to those seen in chronic lymphocytic leukemia; in the leukemic phase of poorly differentiated lymphocytic lymphoma, they are larger and less mature and often have cleft nuclei, the so-called "buttock" cells. Leukopenia in an untreated patient suggests bone marrow infiltration or hypersplenism. In the patient undergoing therapy, leukopenia is usually due to the therapy. Thrombocytosis occurs occasionally in Hodgkin's disease and even less frequently in the other lymphomas. Frequently following staging splenectomy, the platelet count rises briefly. More often, thrombocytopenia occurs because of bone marrow replacement by lymphoma, hypersplenism, or therapy. Patients with Hodgkin's disease who have pruritus are often found to have a mild elevation of the peripheral eosinophil count.

In about 80 per cent of patients with Hodgkin's disease the erythrocyte sedimentation rate (ESR) is elevated, but less frequently so in lymphocytic and histiocytic lymphomas. The ESR may serve as a useful test to follow disease activity. However, its usefulness is limited by its sensitivity, for it may return to normal when residual disease is obviously still present. It can be a useful test to monitor patients who are in remission to determine the first evidence of recurrence. Caution must be used, however, for extensive radiation therapy may cause the ESR to be elevated for as long as 1 year after treatment without evidence of recurrent tumor. Numerous more complicated and usually more expensive laboratory tests such as C-reactive protein, fibrinogen, serum copper level, and haptoglobin and alpha$_2$ glycoproteins that indicate disease activity have not been shown to be superior to the ESR.

Jaundice may be caused by obstruction of the biliary duct by portal lymph nodes or by infiltration of liver secondary to hematogenous spread. The liver is most frequently involved at diagnosis in the three types of diffuse lymphocytic lymphomas (poorly differentiated, well-differentiated, and mixed-cell) and less often in histiocytic lymphoma. Splenomegaly or retroperitoneal lymphadenopathy or both can usually be demonstrated. Liver function abnormalities are poor indicators of Hodgkin's involvement of the liver but serve as a useful tool to rule out the presence of other complications or illnesses. In Hodgkin's disease, liver involvement is most commonly seen in patients with mixed cellularity of lymphocytic depletion type who have splenomegaly and symptoms. The differential diagnosis of jaundice must include hemolytic anemia and drug toxicity. Pathologic examination of the liver, spleen, lymph nodes, or bone marrow may show noncaseating granulomas. This sarcoid-like reaction is of no significance and does not indicate involvement of the liver by tumor.

Renal function tests may be abnormal secondary to renal obstruction, hyperuricemia, hypercalcemia nephropathy, or occasionally membranous glomerulopathy owing to immune complex deposition. Rarely, a nephrotic syndrome may result. Generally, other routine blood chemistry tests such as electrolytes, glucose, and blood lipids are normal.

Serum protein abnormalities occur most often in patients with Hodgkin's disease, and less often in the other lymphomas. A polyclonal hypergammaglobulinemia involving alpha$_1$, alpha$_2$, and beta fractions is the most frequent occurrence. This type of elevation is seen in 40 per cent of Hodgkin's disease patients; less frequently in the other lymphomas. Paraproteinemia may occur in lymphocytic lymphomas, especially in diffuse well-differentiated lymphocytic lymphoma, and has occasionally been observed in Hodgkin's disease. Hypogammaglobulinemia may precede the onset of either diffuse well-differentiated or diffuse poorly differentiated lymphocytic lymphoma, and occurs eventually in 60 per cent of these patients. This is seen less frequently in advanced Hodgkin's disease. Immunoglobulin levels are usually not decreased in patients with lymphoma. The presence of anergy, or decreased in vitro lymphocyte phytohemagglutinin response, has now been shown to have no influence on prognosis within a given clinical stage when modern therapy is used. Thus routine testing for these findings is unnecessary. This surprising observation indicates that effective antitumor treatment can eradicate disease in patients already immunosuppressed by their disease even when the drugs themselves are immunosuppressive. However, cellular immune function appears to be less affected in lymphocytic and histiocytic lymphoma patients than in Hodgkin's disease.

Radiologic findings such as the demonstration of a mediastinal mass may be the first clue to the diagnosis in an otherwise asymptomatic patient. Nodular infiltrates and pleural effusion secondary to tumor or lymphatic obstruction also occur. If extension of the tumor has led to the pericardium, an effusion and cardiomegaly may be noted on the chest x-ray. Gastrointestinal radiographs may demonstrate any number of abnormalities, including mass lesions, malabsorption pattern, splenomegaly, hepatomegaly, or obliteration of the psoas shadow, especially in patients with lymphocytic or histiocytic lymphoma.

PITFALLS IN DIAGNOSIS

The lymphadenopathy of Hodgkin's disease must be distinguished from adenopathy from other causes. Cervical or axillary adenopathy in young people commonly occurs as a result of infectious diseases with fever. However, headache and pharyngitis that occur in infectious disease usually do not occur in Hodgkin's disease. To be considered in the differential diagnosis are a number of diseases, including infectious mononucleosis, viral disease syndromes, or infection by *Toxoplasma gondii*. Local and lymphatic spread of head and neck cancers should also be included in the differential of older age populations. A good rule of thumb in all patients is that any lymph node 1 cm or larger in diameter that does not show signs of regression after 6 weeks of observation should be biopsied.

A patient presenting with mediastinal and hilar adenopathy may have sarcoidosis or primary tuberculosis. The former is distinguished from Hodgkin's disease in that it is nearly always pan-hilar. Tuberculosis, on the other hand, is unilateral like Hodgkin's disease but almost always has evidence of a resolving pulmonary infection and usually does not cause mediastinal lymph node enlargement. In older patients, one must also include primary tumors of the lung and mediastinum, specifically oat cell and epidermoid carcinomas, in the differential. Reactive mediastinitis and hilar adenopathy owing to histoplasmosis must be considered in patients who live or have travelled in regions where histoplasmosis is endemic. Further, histoplasma mediastinitis can involve the esophagus and should be considered if a history of difficulty in swallowing is obtained and subsequently confirmed by an abnormal esophagram. Occasionally, a biopsy may be necessary to confirm this diagnosis. Hodgkin's disease presenting as "fever of undetermined origin" may remain undiagnosed despite extensive investigations until an exploratory laparotomy is undertaken. Infrequently, patients present with autoimmune hemolytic anemia or idiopathic thrombocytopenia purpura and are found to have Hodgkin's disease only when splenectomy becomes necessary. It is of interest that in some of these cases Hodgkin's disease in the removed spleen has been the only focus of involvement with tumor.

COMPLICATIONS OF HODGKIN'S DISEASE AND LYMPHOCYTIC AND HISTIOCYTIC LYMPHOMA

The complications of lymphoma are many and may be due to progressive enlargement of lymph nodes, involvement of parenchymal organs, and hematologic, metabolic, or immunologic abnormalities.

Progressive lymph node enlargement causes compression or obstruction of surrounding structures such as vascular structures (superior vena cava syndrome), airway, esophagus, the urinary tract, or the gastrointestinal tract. Serious complications may ensue, depending on the site affected.

Direct infiltration of the lymphoma from involved mediastinal lymph nodes into the parenchyma of the lung, pleura, pericardium, and heart may occur. Infiltration from retroperitoneal lymph nodes through lymphatic channels leads to involvement of the gastrointestinal tract and may result in ulceration, perforation, hemorrhage, intussusception, or malabsorption.

Cord compression is the most serious acute neurologic complication caused by growing tumor masses and is usually observed in patients with progressive tumor whose primary treatment has failed. It can be caused by vertebral body involvement with collapse, which is easily seen on x-ray or bone scan, or by invasion of the epidural space from retroperitoneal lymph nodes with compression of the cord or compression of the vascular supply to the cord. Selective electromyelography is a useful way to detect regional denervation, but a myelogram is usually needed to confirm the diagnosis.

Central nervous system involvement may also occur by direct extension of tumor from the mediastinum or retroperitoneum to the spinal canal. Symptoms of cord compression produced in this way occur more often in Hodgkin's disease than with the other lymphomas. This is observed most frequently in those patients who have diffuse histiocytic lymphoma. Cranial nerves and brain may be affected by the lymphomas. Occasionally, lymphomatous meningitis may occur, and lymphoma cells, high protein, and low glucose appear in the spinal fluid. If a patient with diffuse histiocytic lymphoma has bone marrow involvement, a spinal tap is always indicated, since subsequent meningeal involvement occurs with such high frequency that prophylactic intrathecal therapy is recommended.

Bizarre neurologic manifestations occur rarely without demonstrable direct involvement by lymphoma. Progressive multifocal leukoencephalopathy, subacute cerebellar degeneration, myelopathy, and neuropathy have also been described. Occasionally, polymyositis may occur. The differential diagnosis of these central and peripheral nervous system complications includes bacterial and viral meningitis, herpes zoster, and drug toxicity, particularly when drugs such as the vinca alkaloids are used.

The lung may also be involved by direct extension either from mediastinal-hilar lymph nodes or by hematogenous spread. In the lymphocyte-predominant type of Hodgkin's disease and in nodular poorly differentiated lymphocytic lymphoma the lungs are rarely involved; in contrast, the nodular sclerosis type of Hodgkin's disease frequently involves the lungs. Pleural involvement by lymphoma with malignant effusion may occur with or without lymphoma of the lung. Pneumonia is a frequent complication of treatment and constitutes the major differential diagnosis of lymphoma. Bleomycin, methotrexate, and other drugs used to treat these diseases may cause pulmonary manifestations and their toxicity must be considered in the differential diagnosis of lung disease in patients undergoing treatment.

Skin involvement occurs as part of hematogenous dissemination of the lymphoma. A number of nonspecific skin lesions occur in lymphoma, including excoriations secondary to pruritus, urticaria, erythema multiforme, erythema nodosum, exfoliative dermatitis, and dermatomyositis.

Metabolic abnormalities may occur as a consequence of the lymphoma or therapy. Hyperuricemia is seen most often in patients who have a large volume of tumor. Effective therapy results in a rapid reduction of the tissue mass and may exacerbate the hyperuricemia, leading to a decrease in renal function and infrequently to gouty arthritis. Hydration and administration of allopurinol can prevent these complications. Hypercalcemia occurs in less than 10 per cent of patients, most frequently in diffuse histiocytic lymphoma and Hodgkin's disease of the lymphocyte-depleted and mixed cellularity types. The hypercalcemia is usually related to destruction of bone by the tumor but may be due to the release of parathyroid-like substance. Hypercalcemia also requires prompt and appropriate therapy.

Infections are common in patients with Hodgkin's disease. Those who have progressive tumor usually die of complications of bone marrow failure, bacterial septicemia, or disseminated fungal infections. Diffuse pulmonary infiltrates may appear in patients who are in remission between cycles of chemotherapy, radiotherapy, or both; infection with the protozoan *Pneumocystis carinii* should be suspected. Patients with Hodgkin's disease are also prone to develop cryptococcosis, either in the form of meningitis or as a primary pulmonary infiltrate with or without meningitis. Herpes zoster occurs in 10 per cent of treated Hodgkin's patients and in 20 per cent of treated patients who have had a splenectomy. Most patients who develop herpes zoster have a few scattered papules outside the involved dermatome; this minimal evidence of spread does not generally warrant systemic treatment.

SUMMARY

Malignant lymphomas can be diagnosed only after biopsy of involved tissue and histopathologic classification. A detailed history, physical examination, supportive laboratory, radiographic, and further biopsy information are useful in documenting the extent of the disease. Following these procedures, the physician is prepared to make appropriate management decisions that can result in long-term disease-free survival for the majority of patients afflicted with these highly treatable tumors.

MYCOSIS FUNGOIDES

By HARLEY A. HAYNES, M.D.
Boston, Massachusetts

Mycosis fungoides was first given its name by the French physician Alibert in 1835. He selected the name mycosis fungoides because of the mushroom-like appearance of the tumors and not to indicate any fungal disease. This name has been retained because of historical precedent.

DEFINITION

Mycosis fungoides is an uncommon neoplastic disease of the lymphoreticular system first manifested in the skin. The disease appears to be a disorder caused by dysplastic or neoplastic thymus-derived lymphocytes. Whereas lesions may remain confined to the skin for years, involvement of lymph nodes and internal organs usually occurs when the disease advances. The clinical course, although quite variable, is characteristically chronic and slowly progressive. Although it is disputed as to whether mycosis fungoides should appropriately be considered a hyperplasia, a dysplasia, or a neoplasia, the lesions in advanced stages are characteristic of malignant lymphoma and it seems appropriate to regard the entire process as a T cell lymphoproliferative disease.

SIGNS AND SYMPTOMS

In the undiagnosed early case the lesions may have the gross appearance of psoriasis, eczema, neurodermatitis, parapsoriasis en plaque, or poikiloderma. An atypical response to therapy or the histopathologic finding of atypical dermal infiltrate brings the diagnosis of mycosis fungoides under consideration. It is common for some lesions to clear spontaneously at the time others are appearing. Exposure to small doses of sunlight, ultraviolet or x-rays may cause lesions to disappear temporarily. Although early stages of lesions may persist, with spontaneous exacerbations and regressions for many months or years, progression eventually occurs in most patients. Lesions become more infiltrated and elevated plaques appear, followed by nodules or tumors. All types of lesions from early to late may be present simultaneously. Although pruritus tends to be a major manifestation of the disease even in early phases, the patient otherwise feels well until the disease is in an advanced stage.

It is characteristic for the skin lesions in mycosis fungoides to be randomly distributed over the cutaneous surface without any rhyme or reason, although in the early phases the areas of skin exposed to sunlight may be relatively less severely affected. The plaques that are formed on the skin tend to have a somewhat violaceous color rather than a bright pink color, although this is variable. The violaceous color is more pronounced as the degree of infiltration of the cutaneous lesions increases.

As the plaques become progressively more indurated, they clearly do not resemble banal dermatoses. It is not unusual for the lesions to clear centrally, forming annular or arcuate patterns. Areas of regression are commonly seen, leaving behind transient hyperpigmentation or hypopigmentation, generally without scarring. As the infiltration in the dermis increases, the cutaneous lesions become more elevated and firmer to palpation. The overlying epidermis, generally considerably scaly in the less infiltrated lesions, may remain scaly in the more indurated ones or may become smooth and taut. Alopecia may occur in lesions of considerable infiltration. Regrowth of hair may occur following regression of these plaques.

With increasing degrees of cellular infiltration, the lesions become sufficiently elevated to be termed tumors. Tumors may arise from a preexisting plaque or may arise from clinically normal skin. The number of lesions at any stage may be few, or there may be hundreds. The skin surface may at times be entirely involved. Ulceration may occur in plaques or tumors, and is often remarkably asymptomatic. In some patients a generalized erythroderma is the initial manifestation without occurrence of any of the individual plaques and tumors as just described. In other patients an erythrodermic stage supervenes after its initial presentation as plaques. When the erythrodermic picture is present and a peripheral blood leukocytosis showing a considerable proportion of atypical T lymphocytes is present, the condition is commonly referred to as Sézary's syndrome. While there has been question as to whether Sézary's syndrome represented a totally different disease entity from mycosis fungoides, it seems appropriate to consider Sézary's syndrome a variant of mycosis fungoides with a leukemic component.

OTHER PHYSICAL FINDINGS

In early stages of disease there are no characteristic physical findings other than the skin lesions. As the disease progresses, lymphadenopathy commonly occurs. Such lymph nodes are usually firm and nontender. The palpable lymph nodes may be few in number, or they may be many and generalized in distribution. Splenomegaly and hepatomegaly are uncommon except in the Sézary variant. Involvement of mucous membranes, particularly of the mouth and genitalia, occurs on occasion, as do laryngeal and gastrointestinal lesions. Shallow ulceration is the usual manifestation in those areas, although tumors that may hemorrhage can occur. Fever is common in patients with the tumor stage of disease. In patients who have a generalized erythroderma, inability to control the temperature may occur so that wide swings from high fever to hypothermia are seen. Peripheral edema is also usually found in patients who have generalized erythroderma, and even in patients who have significant numbers of plaques or tumors on the legs.

COURSE AND PROGNOSIS

If only minimally infiltrated lesions are present, the course is unpredictable and may be extremely chronic. There may be little change over many years; there may be spontaneous regressions and relapses, or the disease may progress directly into the infiltrated plaque and tumor stage. A protracted period may occur, when clinical and histologic diagnosis of mycosis fungoides cannot be made with certainty, although this diagnosis may be suggested by the clinician and by the pathologist.

Once the histologic diagnosis of mycosis fungoides is confirmed, the median survival for all patients, according to the literature, is 5 years. Patients under 50 years of age have a median survival twice as long as patients over 60 years of age. The presence of skin tumors, ulceration of skin lesions, or palpable lymphadenopathy, regardless of the histology of the lymph node, produces a median survival of less than 30 months. Patients having more of these unfavorable prognostic signs have a significantly poorer prognosis. Once lymphomatous involvement of viscera is diagnosed, survival is generally less than one year. At the present time it is not clear that therapy can prolong survival, although it clearly can drastically improve the quality of life. Some data indicate prolonged disease-free survival if electron beam therapy is used very early in the course of the disease.

COMMON COMPLICATIONS

Approximately one-third of the patients die from lymphomatous involvement of internal organs. The most common cause of death in the remaining two-thirds is infection, which is a major problem once there are many ulcerated cutaneous lesions. The cause of death sometimes is difficult to pinpoint, and may be termed generalized debilitation.

LABORATORY STUDIES

The diagnosis is usually made by skin biopsy. There are no specific findings on blood chemistry or on urinalysis. The primary histopathology of the lesions involves a dermal infiltrate that is usually located high in the dermis, abutting on and often invading the epidermis. The infiltrate is polymorphic, containing lymphocytes, histiocytes, eosinophils, polymorphonuclear leukocytes, and plasma cells. The relevant cell type is the T lymphocyte that, in this disorder, is often referred to as the mycosis cell, or the Lutzner cell. This cell has an enlarged nucleus with a very irregular contour that may be perceived on ordinary tissue sections but is much easier to see when 1 micron sections embedded in epon are stained and then viewed under the light microscope. A quite valuable histopathologic finding when present is the Pautrier's abscess.

This is a space within the epidermis containing the atypical T lymphocytes. A great deal of caution must be used in distinguishing this condition from benign eczematous dermatitis, in which activated but benign T lymphocytes may be infiltrating the upper dermis and into the epidermis in a somewhat similar manner.

Lymph node biopsy should always be done when there are palpable lymph nodes in a patient with the question of, or the diagnosis of, mycosis fungoides. Occasionally in patients whose skin biopsy is not quite diagnostic specific diagnoses may be obtained from histopathology of the lymph node. The commonest histopathologic change in the palpable lymph nodes is called dermatopathic lymphadenopathy. If these nodes are further examined on 1 micron sections, however, it is common to find multiple atypical T cells highly suggestive of the diagnosis of mycosis fungoides. At times lymphangiography is desirable to ascertain the presence of enlarged lymph nodes in the periaortic and iliac areas to determine the extent of disease or to locate abnormal nodes for biopsy purposes.

The peripheral blood should be carefully examined by a smear to look for circulating atypical T lymphocytes; these generally are seen as lymphocytes with a clefted or folded appearance to the nucleus. The morphology of the cells in the circulating blood can be better appreciated if a buffy coat pellet is fixed in epon and sectioned at 1 micron thickness. Small numbers of circulating atypical T cells may be found in patients with plaque or tumor stage mycosis fungoides, and these cells are an integral part of the Sézary syndrome.

Bone marrow biopsy is a reasonable procedure to be performed in these patients but usually is not revealing. An occasional patient has infiltration of the marrow by mycosis fungoides, but generally the marrow is reasonably free of disease even in late-stage patients, although those with circulating cells may have these cells present on marrow examination as well as in the peripheral blood.

Chest x-ray and liver-spleen scan are reasonable and noninvasive tests in the work-up of these patients, and may demonstrate infiltrates not clinically apparent. At the present time, routine laparotomy for staging purposes does not seem to be desirable.

THERAPEUTIC TESTS

While there are no specific therapeutic tests for mycosis fungoides, this diagnosis should come into consideration when a patient who is thought to have eczema or psoriasis fails to respond to therapy in the expected fashion. At this point a skin biopsy is the most reasonable diagnostic test. One must recall that potent topical steroids, or treatment with ultraviolet light, might be effective in mycosis fungoides in early stages in temporarily clearing the cutaneous lesions.

PITFALLS IN DIAGNOSIS

It is a quite difficult clinical problem to diagnose mycosis fungoides in its very early stages as the clinical and histopathologic appearance may resemble a subacute or chronic eczematous dermatitis. The finding of large numbers of atypical T cells in the infiltrate is strongly indicative of the diagnosis of mycosis fungoides. At the other end of the spectrum in very late disease, when the patient has tumor-stage disease, the histopathology may not be classic for mycosis fungoides in that the tumor infiltrates may be deeper seated in the dermis and may not involve to a large extent the overlying epidermis. Differentiation from histiocytic lymphoma, and from T-cell leukemia with leukemia cutis, must be pursued on the basis of cellular morphology, cytochemistry, and bone marrow examination.

MULTIPLE MYELOMA

By CHARLES I. JAROWSKI, M.D., *and* MORTON COLEMAN, M.D.
New York, New York

SYNONYMS

Plasma cell myeloma, myelomatosis, Kahler's disease.

DEFINITION

Multiple myeloma may be defined as a neoplastic proliferation of a single clone of plasma cells. The clinical manifestations of the disease result from the tumor cell burden in the marrow and from the effects of the monoclonal immunoglobulins secreted by the malignant plasma cells. It is the monoclonal immunoglobulins that produce the characteristic homogeneous peak when the serum or urine of these patients is studied electrophoretically.

The incidence of multiple myeloma has increased in recent years, perhaps secondary to the widespread use of improved diagnostic techniques. It now represents almost 1 per cent of all malignancy and nearly 10 per cent of all hematologic malignant disorders. More than 6000 persons each year in the United States will succumb to multiple myeloma and its complications. The peak incidence is in the sixth and seventh decades, although there have been reports of patients developing multiple myeloma before age 30. It appears to be more common in males than females. Although it occurs in all races and has been reported throughout the world, in the United States the incidence is higher in blacks than in whites.

PRESENTING SYMPTOMS AND SIGNS

One approach to the symptoms and signs of multiple myeloma is to divide the clinical manifestations into those secondary to the tumor cell mass and those related to the effects of the monoclonal myeloma protein.

From the Tumor Cell Mass. As the population of malignant plasma cells progressively infiltrates the marrow, the tumor cell burden results in the skeletal damage and hematopoietic compromise so typical of multiple myeloma.

At the time of initial clinical evaluation, nearly 60 per cent of patients will have some degree of bone pain. The most commonly involved bones are those with active marrows, such as the sternum, ribs, spine, clavicles, skull, pelvis, and proximal extremities. Back pain is the most common symptom. Some patients may develop chest deformity secondary to destruction of the sternum. Vertebral body collapse in other patients may result in a shortening of stature. Skeletal radiographs most frequently reveal osteoporosis and scattered lytic lesions. The classic radiographic findings of multiple small lytic lesions in the skull should suggest the diagnosis. Many patients are now found to have only a generalized osteoporosis, probably because of earlier diagnosis. Nearly one third of patients will develop hypercalcemia, in part secondary to bone resorption and immobilization. Stupor accompanied by polyuria and polydipsia should immediately suggest an elevated serum calcium.

Bone marrow compromise is manifested primarily by anemia and less frequently by leukopenia and thrombocytopenia. Sixty per cent of patients will have a normochromic, normocytic anemia and will complain of varying degrees of weakness, fatigue, and dyspnea on exertion. Leukopenia and thrombocytopenia occur in only one fifth of patients.

The tumor cell mass also results in hyperuricemia and hyperuricosuria, which are found in approximately 60 per cent of patients at diagnosis. The elevated uric acid levels contribute to the renal insufficiency that so often complicates the course of multiple myeloma. Uric acid stones and clinical gout, however, are rare developments.

From the Monoclonal Protein. Clinical manifestations related to the effects of the monoclonal myeloma protein consist in large part of the symptoms and signs of renal insufficiency. Less frequent complications are secondary to the development of amyloidosis, hyperviscosity syndromes, coagulopathy, and cryoglobulinemia.

Finally, these patients have an increased susceptibility to infection since normal immunoglobulin production is embarrassed. Pneumonia caused by encapsulated organisms is common. Recurrent pneumococcal pneumonia in an elderly patient should suggest the diagnosis of multiple myeloma.

COURSE

The course of multiple myeloma is one of progressive deterioration, ultimately resulting in death secondary to infection, renal insufficiency, cardiopulmonary failure, or an accelerated aggressive phase of the disease. Chemotherapeutic regimens can result in significant improvement in about half to two thirds of patients. Despite this, the overall median survival is less than 3 years. Poor prognostic features include evidence of a high tumor cell burden at presentation, specifically, an IgG monoclonal spike greater than 5.0 grams per dl (100 ml); an IgA monoclonal spike greater than 3.0 grams per dl; severe renal insufficiency; hypercalcemia; and advanced bone disease, i.e., lytic lesions.

COMMON COMPLICATIONS

Renal Insufficiency. Renal insufficiency occurs in nearly 65 per cent of patients with multiple myeloma. It probably results from the toxic effects of light chains on the renal tubules. Hypercalcemia, hyperuricemia, amyloidosis, and even plasma cell infiltration may contribute to the renal dysfunction in some patients. Diagnostic procedures that may result in dehydration (such as intravenous pyelography, computerized body scans with contrast, etc.) may cause the sudden onset of renal failure. These procedures may be undertaken if appropriate measures to preclude dehydration are employed. Some patients may show evidence of an acquired adult Fanconi syndrome, secondary to light chain damage to the renal tubule. A clinical picture of glucosuria, aminoaciduria, and even renal tubular acidosis may then be found.

Hypercalcemia. This occurs in up to one third of patients at some time during the course of their illness. It is due to bony resorption but may be aggravated by immobilization. Appropriate treatment (saline diuresis, prednisone, chemotherapy), including efforts to mobilize the patient, is essential to prevent deterioration of renal function secondary to hypercalcemic nephropathy.

Immunologic Abnormalities. Patients with multiple myeloma have depressed levels of normal immunoglobulins. These persons have also been shown to have decreased T cell responses to mitogens in vitro. These immunological abnormalities result in an increased susceptibility to infection. Patients with multiple myeloma have a six-times greater incidence of infection with encapsulated organisms, including *Streptococcus pneumoniae*, *Staphylococcus aureus*, and gram-negative rods. Three per cent of patients will develop disseminated herpes zoster during the course of their illness. This altered immunologic status may also play a role in the increased incidence of acute myelogenous leukemia and nonreticular neoplasms in patients with multiple myeloma.

Neurologic Complications. The most common neurologic complications occurring during the course of multiple myeloma are nerve root and spinal cord compression. Spinal cord compression secondary either to epidural myeloma tissue or collapsed vertebrae is uncommon but often results in paraparesis or even paraplegia. Peripheral neuropathy may also occur. This is unusually a complication of amyloidosis, as is the "carpal tunnel" syndrome, in which the median nerve may be compressed.

Amyloidosis. Amyloidosis may complicate the course of multiple myeloma. It results from deposition of the variable region of the light chains in various tissues. It most often results in macroglossia, salivary gland enlargement, purpura, malabsorption, congestive heart failure, and peripheral neuropathy.

Hyperviscosity Syndrome. This is not frequently seen in multiple myeloma except in the rare instances in which a monoclonal protein may exhibit high intrinsic viscosity or in which large quantities of protein are produced. When the syndrome is present, the patient may complain of vision impairment or develop central nervous system symptoms, including "coma paraproteinemicus."

Coagulopathy. In a small number of patients the paraprotein may interfere with fibrin monomer polymerization, or may couple with Factors II, V, VII, or VIII, thus blocking their action. In rare cases there may even be a paraprotein that coats the platelets, thus interfering with subsequent aggregation.

Cryoglobulinemia. This is a rare manifestation of multiple myeloma, usually seen only with paraproteins of IgG-subclass 3. It is much more frequently seen with IgM monoclonal proteins, as in Waldenström's macroglobulinemia. The clinical manifestations of the cryoglobulinemia include Raynaud's phenomenon, cold urticaria, and acral necrosis induced by cold exposure.

LABORATORY FINDINGS

Anemia is present in two thirds of patients at presentation and will develop in virtually all patients during the course of their illness. The anemia is usually normochromic and normocytic. In a small number of patients it may be macrocytic. This has been related to excess consumption of folic acid by the myeloma cell mass. Leukopenia and thrombocytopenia secondary to marrow replacement are not as common and occur in about one fifth of patients during the course of the disease. Other hematologic manifestations have included a mild lymphocytosis, neutropenia, and a rare unexplained eosinophilia. Circulating plasma cells are rarely seen. The monoclonal immunoglobulin is responsible for the characteristic elevated erythrocyte sedimentation rate and the rouleau formation seen on the peripheral smear.

Bone marrow aspiration and biopsy reveal increased numbers of plasma cells, often seen in focal collections. Although it is not possible to morphologically distinguish a plasma cell seen in the normal marrow from the malignant plasma cell occurring in patients with myeloma, certain features will strongly suggest myeloma. Plasma cells that are large or bizarre in shape or binucleated or trinucleated suggest multiple myeloma. Many plasma cells occurring in clumps or sheets also imply multiple myeloma. Myeloma is strongly suggested if the total percentage of plasma cells on marrow examination is more than 20. Several varieties of abnormal plasma cells can occasionally be seen. These include flaming plasma cells, thesaurocytes, morular cells, and Mott cells. Identification of these abnormal variants has no prognostic value.

Biochemical abnormalities include hypercalcemia (30 per cent of patients), hyperuricemia (60 per cent of patients), and some degree of azotemia (55 per cent of patients). Despite the presence of often extensive bony resorption and destruction, the serum alkaline phosphatase is usually within normal limits. Investigators in recent reports have commented on the presence of a lowered anion gap $(Na^+ + K^+) - (Cl^- + CO_2)$ in IgG multiple myeloma. This is thought to be due to the presence of cationic IgG paraproteins that cause a retention of excess chloride anions, thus lowering the anion gap. Rare hepatic dysfunction can be seen. Also the rare adult Fanconi syndrome has been reported with serum abnormalities, including hypophosphatemia and hypokalemia.

The skeletal survey most commonly reveals osteoporosis and scattered lytic lesions. Some patients will have only a generalized osteoporosis. The bone scan is often normal even in the face of extensive lytic lesions. This is best explained by the fact that multiple myeloma is almost entirely a lytic process and increased uptake of the radionuclide bone scan is dependent on increased osteoblastic activity. The usual normal serum alkaline phosphatase also reflects this fact.

Nearly all patients with multiple myeloma will demonstrate a monoclonal paraprotein in either the serum or urine. Cellulose acetate electrophoresis will demonstrate a monoclonal serum peak in the gamma to alpha-2 region. Immunoelectrophoresis of the serum will reveal an IgG peak in 50 per cent of patients, an IgA peak in 25 per cent of patients, and an IgD peak in only 1 per cent of patients. IgE serum peaks are not seen secondary to the rapid metabolism of this class of immunoglobulin. Immunoelectrophoresis of osmodialized urine will show kappa or lambda light chain monoclonal peaks in about 40 per cent of patients. One half of these patients will have a concomitant serum peak. Thus, 20 per cent of patients will have light chain disease (that is, no serum monoclonal peak with one type of light chain in the urine as the only paraprotein abnormality of their disease). Less than 2 per cent of patients will be nonsecretors with no demonstrable serum or urine paraprotein.

Diagnosis

The diagnostic criteria for plasma cell myeloma are shown in Table 1.

In order to establish the diagnosis of multiple myeloma, both bone marrow and immunoelectrophoretic criteria should be fulfilled. The bone marrow must demonstrate a percentage of plasma cells that is greater than 20 on a count of 1000 cells or sheet-like replacement of areas of the marrow by plasma cells. Immunoelectrophoretic abnormalities include a monoclonal serum spike of greater than 4.0 grams per dl

Table 1. *Diagnostic Criteria for Plasma Cell Myeloma*

I. Myeloma cells in excess of 20 per cent on a count of 1000 cells or sheet-like replacement by myeloma cells.

PLUS

II. Abnormality of immunoglobulin production
  A. Any of the following
    1. Monoclonal spike greater than 4 grams per dl
    2. Rising monoclonal spike followed annually
    3. Bence Jones protein in excess of 0.5 gram per 24 hours.

OR

  B. Any of the following
    1. Monoclonal spike less than 4 grams per dl with reciprocal depression of normal immunoglobulins
    2. (Pan) hypogammaglobulinemia.

AND

  C. Any of the following
    1. Osteolytic lesions when other causes have been excluded
    2. Absence of other diseases characterized by marrow plasmacytosis: collagen disease, chronic infection, metastatic carcinoma, rheumatoid arthritis, viral exanthem; the presence of amyloid does not necessarily exclude the diagnosis of myeloma.

(100 ml), or a rising monoclonal spike in the serum when followed semiannually, or Bence Jones proteins (light chains) in the urine amounting to greater than 0.5 gram secreted over a 24-hour period. If the criteria of these immunoelectrophoretic abnormalities are not met, a monoclonal spike of any size with reciprocal depression of the other immunoglobulin classes or hypogammaglobulinemia is acceptable evidence, provided that osteolytic lesions are present and other diseases characterized by reactive marrow plasmacytosis have been excluded. These other diseases include collagenvascular disease, chronic infection, and rheumatoid arthritis. There must, however, be an abnormality in serum immunoglobulins represented either by a monoclonal spike or hypogammaglobulinemia of one or more immunoglobulin groups.

Pitfalls in Diagnosis

Polyclonal Hypergammaglobulinemia. Polyclonal hypergammaglobulinemia may be confused with myeloma but is easily distinguished from monoclonal disease on protein electrophoresis. In contrast to a homogeneous monoclonal spike, polyclonal hypergammaglobulinemia is not considered an immunoglobulin abnormality. Polyclonal hypergammaglobuline-mia virtually excludes myeloma, since this type of immunoglobulin production represents a normal, adequate immune response. It usually reflects a reactive plasmacytosis in the bone marrow that may potentially be confused with myeloma if protein studies are not performed.

Monoclonal Hypergammaglobulinemia. While an abnormality in the immunoglobulin production pattern must be present for the diagnosis to be myeloma, an immunoglobu-lin abnormality alone does not automat-ically establish the diagnosis. Monoclonal hypergammaglobulinemia not due to myeloma has been described in various conditions, in-cluding aging, cholecystitis, solid neoplasms, and many chronic diseases. Recent studies, however, suggest that 10 per cent of patients with "benign" monoclonal gammopathy will develop overt multiple myeloma within 3 to 5 years of diagnosis. Benign monoclonal gammop-athy is rarely associated with a monoclonal spike greater than 4 grams per dl. Also, mon-oclonal gammopathy rarely will show a rise in concentration of the monoclonal paraprotein when followed over a series of years. Although reciprocal depression of normal immunoglobu-lins may occur in benign monoclonal gammop-athy, it is considerably more frequent in mye-loma. The mechanism for this reciprocal depression is not totally established but may represent multiple factors, including substrate utilization, replacement of normal marrow cells by myeloma, feedback ("chalone") inhibition, or higher catabolic rates of some immunoglobu-lins when the total immunoglobulin concentra-tion is elevated.

Hypogammaglobulinemia. Similar mechan-isms may produce hypogammaglobulinemia when no monoclonal component is present. Hypogammaglobulinemia is also seen in a number of other congenital and acquired dis-orders, especially the lymphoproliferative dis-eases, chronic lymphocytic leukemia, and lym-phoma; it is not solely a characteristic of myeloma.

Waldenström's Macroglobulinemia. The bone marrow in this disease is characteristically replaced by plasmacytoid lymphocytes rather than plasma cells. Sometimes it is difficult to distinguish the two cell types. In such in-stances, the diagnosis is based on the immuno-protein elaborated. In Waldenström's the mon-oclonal protein is always a macroglobulin (IgM), whereas myeloma is associated with the other immunoglobulin classes (IgG, IgA, IgD, and IgE). Osteolytic lesions are extremely rare in this disease and may suggest another neo-plasm. Bence Jones protein is seen less com-monly than in myeloma. An elevated serum viscosity is frequently present.

Heavy Chain Diseases. These are character-ized by the presence of a monoclonal protein consisting of a portion of the immunoglobulin heavy chain. Three types have been reported thus far. Gamma heavy chain disease is distin-guished by the presence of proteins related to Fc fragments of heavy chains of gamma speci-ficity in the serum and urine. The patient usual-ly presents with tonsillar enlargement and hepatosplenomegaly.

Alpha heavy chain disease usually presents as abdominal lymphoma.

Mu heavy chain disease clinically is similar to chronic lymphocytic leukemia.

Primary Amyloidosis. Patients with amyloi-dosis may have a monoclonal protein present in the serum and Bence Jones protein in the urine without concomitant myeloma. However, amy-loidosis is a known complication of multiple myeloma, and the distribution of amyloid is of the type seen in primary amyloidosis. There can be an increase in plasma cells in the bone marrow, but it rarely exceeds 20 per cent, characteristic of myeloma.

DISEASES OF THE SPLEEN

By RICHARD A. COOPER, M.D.

Philadelphia, Pennsylvania

INTRODUCTION

The spleen is an interesting organ that has a variety of roles to play in the physiology and pathology of human disease. It is a component of both the lymphatic and reticuloendothelial systems and in utero is even involved in hema-topoiesis. Anatomically, the spleen is made up of a capsule with trabeculae enclosing the white and red pulp. The white pulp represents the lymphatic portion of the organ and is composed of lymphocytes, plasma cells, and lymphoid follicles. A narrow marginal zone separates the white and red pulp and appears to represent a termination point for many small arterioles. The major bulk of the spleen is made up of the red pulp. This structure has replaced the capillary bed usually found in other organs and is com-posed of interconnecting vascular channels

Table 1. *Causes of Splenomegaly*

I. Inflammatory splenomegaly
   A. Acute infections, including endocarditis, infectious mononucleosis, and splenic abscess
   B. Chronic infection, including tuberculosis, histoplasmosis, toxoplasmosis, syphilis, brucellosis, and tropical parasitic disorders
   C. Collagen vascular disease, including systemic lupus erythematosus and rheumatoid arthritis
   D. Granulomatous disorders, including sarcoid and berylliosis

II. Congestive splenomegaly
   A. Cirrhosis of liver
   B. External compression or thrombosis of portal or splenic veins
   C. Chronic cardiac failure (rare)

III. Hyperplastic splenomegaly
   A. Congenital hemolytic anemia, including thalassemia, hemoglobinopathies, and abnormalities or red cell shape (spherocytosis) and metabolism
   B. Acquired anemia — most commonly immune hemolytic anemia (Coombs'-positive or cold agglutinins)

IV. Neoplastic splenomegaly
   A. Lymphoproliferative disease, including chronic lymphocytic leukemia and lymphoma
   B. Myeloproliferative disease, especially chronic myelocytic leukemia, myeloid metaplasia, and polycythemia rubra vera
   C. Acute leukemia
   D. Malignant tumors, primary (hemangioma, fibrosarcoma, leiomyosarcoma) or metastatic to the spleen

V. Infiltrative splenomegaly
   A. Amyloidosis
   B. Lipid storage disorders, including Gaucher's, Niemann-Pick, and Hand-Schüller-Christian diseases
   C. Letterer-Siwe disease
   D. Gargoylism
   E. Diabetes

VI. Miscellaneous
   A. Cysts — dermoid, echinococcal, multicystic disease, and false cysts (hemorrhagic or serous)
   B. Hematomas secondary to trauma

called cords and sinuses. The cords are narrow passageways rich in fixed and mobile macrophages. The sinuses are relatively large channels that carry the blood elements to the venous side of the splenic circulation. Blood cells entering the cords gain entrance to the sinuses through small openings between sinus lining cells, a process requiring considerable cell deformability. The red pulp with its sluggish circulation, intimate macrophage contact, and requirement for cell deformability provides the mechanism for filtration, sequestration, and ingestion of various particles, including bacteria and damaged or abnormal blood cells.

Diseases involving the spleen are generally recognized by the presence of splenic enlargement. This can be due to an enhanced normal splenic activity, proliferation of normal splenic elements, or abnormal cell proliferation or infiltration, as outlined in Table 1.

An enlarged spleen is usually detected by physical examination. Splenomegaly can be confirmed by x-rays of the abdomen, radioactive spleen scans, or echogram. Although the causes of splenomegaly are many, one can often narrow the choices down to a few on the basis of a good history, physical examination, and evaluation of the peripheral blood smear. These are the cornerstone of any diagnostic work-up for splenomegaly and will be emphasized in the discussion of the various diagnostic categories.

INFLAMMATORY SPLENOMEGALY

These disorders depend upon the response of the spleen to systemic infections and other inflammatory processes. Thus fever, night sweats, malaise, cough, or pharyngitis may suggest a systemic infection. Hyperplasia of the lymphoid system in response to infection is quite common in adolescents and children, so the age of the patient may be very helpful. A history of Raynaud's phenomenon, arthralgias, arthritis, or skin rash might implicate a collagen vascular disease.

On physical examination, fever, lymphadenopathy, skin rash, pneumonia, or other pulmonary process may suggest an inflammatory process. The laboratory evaluation should include a search for atypical lymphocytosis and serologic tests for infectious mononucleosis, hilar adenopathy and anergy of sarcoidosis; serologic tests for collagen disease; and appropriate cultures, skin tests, and serology for potential infectious agents.

CONGESTIVE SPLENOMEGALY

The most common cause of splenomegaly in patients over the age of 30 is portal hypertension resulting from chronic liver disease. These patients usually have a history of alcoholism, jaundice, or hepatitis. The presence of hepatomegaly, jaundice, spider angiomas, palmar erythema, or, in the male, gynecomastia, testicular atrophy, and pubic and axillary hair loss supports this diagnosis. The laboratory evaluation should include liver-spleen scan, liver function tests, serologic tests for the hepatitis B antigen, antimitochondrial and anti-smooth muscle antibodies, and possibly a liver biopsy. Thromboses of the portal or splenic vein are uncommon disorders usually accompanied by left upper quadrant pain caused by acute splenic congestion and require angiography to confirm the diagnosis.

HYPERPLASTIC SPLENOMEGALY

In these disorders, the spleen has undergone "work hypertrophy" owing to its role in the destruction of abnormal red cells. The inherited problems are usually associated with a history of long-standing anemia in the patient or family and often intermittent jaundice or pigment gallstones. The most important method of identifying this group of patients resides in the red cell morphology characteristic for each of these disorders. Laboratory identification may require hemoglobin electrophoresis, quantitation of A_2 and fetal hemoglobin, osmotic fragility, or autohemolysis tests. The most common cause for acquired splenic red cell destruction is immune hemolysis characterized by spherocytosis and identified by the Coombs' tests.

NEOPLASTIC SPLENOMEGALY

Certain manifestations may suggest neoplastic disease as the cause of splenomegaly. These may include weight loss, fever, night sweats, weakness, or pruritus. The lymphoproliferative processes often have associated lymphadenopathy and hepatomegaly. The myeloproliferative diseases often present with a history of spontaneous bleeding or episodes of thrombosis and frequently have massive enlargement of the spleen. The peripheral blood smear and bone marrow (aspirate and biopsy) are the crucial tests for documenting the diagnostic features of these hematologic malignancies.

The rare primary tumors of the spleen usually present as splenomegaly with or without pain, along with a space-occupying lesion on spleen scan. Angiography and splenectomy are required to document the disorder.

INFILTRATIVE SPLENOMEGALY

Deposition of amyloid in the skin, intestines, or kidney can lead to purpura, gastrointestinal bleeding, or the nephrotic syndrome. Rectal or skin biopsy can often document the diagnosis. The rare genetic disorders have characteristic clinical syndromes, and diagnostic cells or material may be found by bone marrow aspirate and biopsy or liver biopsy.

MISCELLANEOUS

A history of trauma to the left upper quadrant may suggest a splenic hematoma. Splenic cysts are often asymptomatic. A spleen scan or angiography or both may be necessary to confirm the diagnosis. In addition, splenic infarcts may produce acute abdominal pain. These usually occur in patients with substantial degrees of splenomegaly and are most common in the group of patients with neoplastic splenomegaly. Splenic rupture should be suspected in patients with a history of trauma and unexplained hemorrhagic shock.

HYPERSPLENISM

This term unfortunately has a variety of definitions and embraces a varying number of pathologic disorders. The three traditional criteria for this syndrome are splenomegaly, reduction of one or more blood elements, and a bone marrow with adequate or increased blood cell precursors. Thus any of the diseases listed in Table 1 may be associated with this syndrome of splenic sequestration and destruction of blood elements, including the diverse group of hemolytic anemias listed under hyperplastic splenomegaly. However, in this latter case, the spleen is carrying out its normal function of removing defective or abnormal cells. The pathophysiology and clinical characteristics of hypersplenism can be more clearly defined if these causes of hyperplastic splenomegaly are excluded to narrow the definition. Thus a fourth criterion is that the blood elements undergoing sequestration or destruction or both are not intrinsically defective.

Pathologic enlargement of the spleen results in aberrant sinusoidal circulation with prolonged cell transit time and sequestration. The red cells undergo metabolic deprivation and other ill-defined changes resulting in premature red cell destruction. Thrombocytopenia results from an increase in the splenic pool of platelets, and leukopenia probably results from a combination of pooling and shortened white cell survival. The peripheral blood morphology is usually unimpressive, with polychromatophilic macrocytes reflecting the degree of reticulocytosis. Mild spherocytosis may or may not be present. The reduction in white cells and platelets is not usually accompanied by any morphologic changes. The patients often have mild to moderate reticulocytosis, shortened red cell survival, and sequestration over the spleen. Radioisotope labeling of platelets reveals an increased platelet pool and normal survival.

It is distinctly unusual for hypersplenism, by itself, to produce cytopenias severe enough to result in a transfusion requirement, serious or spontaneous infection, or bleeding. However, it may contribute to the severity of these problems and, if hypersplenism is documented, improvement after splenectomy can be anticipated.

HISTIOCYTOSIS X

By DIANE M. KOMP, M.D.
New Haven, Connecticut

SYNONYMS

Reticuloendotheliosis, nonlipid reticuloendotheliosis, histiocytic reticuloendotheliosis, eosinophilic granuloma, Hand-Schüller-Christian syndrome, Letterer-Siwe disease.

DEFINITION

Histiocytosis X is characterized by the presence of granulomatous lesions, predominantly histiocytes, in a variety of organs. Patients whose biopsies show histiocytes without distinct cell membranes creating a syncytial pattern often have many eosinophils as well as fibrosis, focal necrosis, and multinucleated giant cells. These patients, whose condition is classified by Newton as "benign," often have a good prognosis. When histiocytes are mostly individual with folded, invaginated nuclear membranes and dark, basophilic, clumped, chromatic eosinophils, then multinucleated giant cells, necrosis, and fibrosis are rarely seen. These patients, whose condition is classified histologically as "malignant," frequently have a clinically more severe course characterized by organ dysfunction. Skin biopsy alone is inadequate to distinguish "benign" from "malignant" on these histologic grounds. Electron microscopy should demonstrate Langerhans granules.

It is no longer held valid that eosinophilic granuloma, Hand-Schüller-Christian syndrome, and Letterer-Siwe disease are distinct entities. Most authorities believe that they are different clinical expressions of the same process.

The cause is unknown. In cases in which bacteria, fungi, or viruses have been isolated, it is unclear whether these organisms were the cause of disorder or secondary invaders in a compromised host. Similarly, when cellular or humoral immune deficiencies have been noted, it has been unclear whether the deficiency was a primary one with a reactive histiocytosis or secondary to the histiocytosis. Immune "reconstitution" has been described after successful treatment with chemotherapy and remission of histiocytosis. The similarity of the clinical picture in infants to the graft-versus-host reaction is remarkable. The process cannot be considered neoplastic in the usual sense of the word.

GENETICS

The majority of cases that are clearly inheritable come under the category of "hemophagocytic lymphohistiocytosis." The histologic picture in these infants is reminiscent of histiocytic medullary reticulosis in adults. Hypofibrinogenemia and disseminated intravascular coagulation may be prominent. Phagocytic histiocytes may be identified in the bone marrow or spinal fluid. Attempts to demonstrate chimerism in these infants have been unsuccessful to date.

A second familial syndrome described is histiocytosis associated with eosinophilia and immune deficiency. These cases are not limited to males. Other cases of "familial Letterer-Siwe" have not been adequately studied to rule out eosinophilia and immune deficiency, although several children have survived for more than 5 years to die later of opportunistic infections.

CLINICAL MANIFESTATIONS

The symptoms and signs vary markedly, depending on the organs involved and the extent of involvement. The tissues most commonly involved are skin, bone, lymph nodes, lung, liver, spleen, bone marrow, and brain. The kidneys, salivary glands, thymus, thyroid, and intestinal tract are less frequent sites of involvement. Growth impairment is common even in the absence of growth hormone deficiency or skeletal defects. Diabetes insipidus may not be present at the time of initial diagnosis and is rarely associated with bony involvement of the sella turcica. Once it is clinically apparent — that is, with polyuria, polydipsia — it cannot be reversed by radiotherapy and chemotherapy.

Histiocytic accumulations can severely impair function of vital organs, leading to jaundice, hypoproteinemia, pulmonary fibrosis, seizures, optic atrophy, increased intracranial pressure, hypersplenism, and intractable diarrhea. Not life-threatening but significant problems can be caused by chronic otitis media, tooth loss, pathologic fractures, and hearing impairment.

Solitary bone lesions usually present as localized pain or swelling. The majority of patients with this presentation do not have further evidence of disease later in their course. Some, however, will later develop other bone lesions or soft tissue involvement or both. More often, patients with generalized bone plus soft tissue involvement will have evidence of more than bone involvement at initial diagnosis. The majority of patients with bone plus soft tissue involvement have a lengthy chronic course with signs of new disease involvement over a period of years despite chemotherapy and radiotherapy.

Disease confined to soft tissues is usually seen in infants under 2 years of age and may run a rapidly lethal course. Fever and multiple organ involvement are common.

RADIOGRAPHIC FINDINGS

The bone lesions of histiocytosis X are characteristically punched out with well-defined borders. As there is rarely surrounding sclerosis, radioactive scans of bone usually do not demonstrate lesions that are clearly osteolytic on skeletal survey. Multiple lesions are more common than single bone lesions. The bones most commonly involved are calvarium, jaw, vertebrae, pelvis, scapula, and long bones. Distal bony lesions are unusual.

Compression fractures of the vertebrae may not be detected until vertebra plana is established. Large lytic lesions may lead to pathologic fracture. When there is extensive gingival and alveolar bone involvement, the teeth may appear to be "floating in air." Although some patients with diabetes insipidus and exophthalmos also have destruction of adjacent bony structures, these lesions are basically "soft tissue" lesions.

Although isolated pulmonary disease is common in adults, it is rare or nonexistent in children. Pulmonary lesions are common in newly diagnosed patients with generalized disease but may develop 5 or more years after diagnosis. There may be disseminated nodular lesions or cystic "honeycomb" lesions. The radiographic pattern does not help distinguish histiocytosis of the lung from opportunistic infections that frequently complicate the course of these patients. The healing phase of lung involvement may be complicated by fibrosis and pneumothorax.

Both thymic enlargement and thymic aplasia may be noted in children with histiocytosis. Mediastinal node involvement is rare.

Involvement of the small intestine and stomach may lead to an abnormal mucosal pattern. Gastrointestinal complaints and involvement are unusual outside the infant age group.

OTHER LABORATORY FINDINGS

There is no specific test for this disorder. Abnormal laboratory findings reflect the pattern of organ involvement. Hypoproteinemia or hyperbilirubinemia or both may occur in the presence of severe liver involvement and abnormal pulmonary function studies in patients with severe pulmonary involvement. Water deprivation testing may demonstrate partial diabetes insipidus prior to clinically apparent diabetes insipidus. Growth hormone deficiency may be demonstrated in some patients.

The anemia and thrombocytopenia frequently seen in infants with histiocytosis are rarely associated with a myelophthisic bone marrow process. It is more commonly associated with massive splenomegaly. Normal-appearing histiocytes may be present in slightly increased numbers in the bone marrow of children with other organ involvement. Their significance is unclear. Although a hemolytic anemia may be present, iron deficiency anemia and the "dilutional anemia of massive splenomegaly" may also be present.

Cytocentrifugation of the spinal fluid is useful to demonstrate brain involvement. The presence of histiocytes and eosinophils may be documented by this technique even when cell counts and spinal fluid chemistries are normal.

The erythrocyte sedimentation rate may be elevated. Serum lipids and lactic dehydrogenase (LDH) are usually normal. Coagulation studies may be abnormal in familial erythrophagocytic lymphohistiocytosis and in severe liver involvement.

DIAGNOSIS

When the diagnosis of histiocytosis X is suspected on clinical grounds, appropriate tissue such as skin, bone, node, or gingiva should be biopsied. As with all tumors of childhood, material should be preserved in glutaraldehyde for electron microscopy if possible. When adequate material is available, bacterial, fungal, and viral cultures should be obtained. When lung is involved, biopsy is often required to rule out coexistent opportunistic infections such as *Pneumocystis carinii*, aspergillosis, histoplasmosis, and mycobacteriosis. Skin biopsy is not suitable for distinction of "benign" from "malignant" histology; the latter is suggested by severe organ dysfunction at diagnosis. This distinction on the basis of organ dysfunction may be useful when biopsy of tissue other than skin is not clinically feasible. Electron microscopy is necessary for the demonstration of Langerhans granules. Slide touch preparations of the skin may reveal large numbers of histiocytes suggesting the diagnosis.

SEQUELAE AND COMPLICATIONS

Children with bone plus soft tissue involvement have a high incidence of serious disabilities associated with long-term active disease. These include orthopedic difficulties, neurologic deficits, intellectual impairment, growth failure, chronic lung disease, and chronic liver disease. It is unclear whether intracranial neurologic problems such as focal demyelination, optic atrophy, cerebellar degeneration, hydrocephalus, and spasticity are consequences of histiocytosis or its therapy. Malignancies such as brain tumors, thyroid carcinoma, and osteogenic sarcoma have been seen in irradiated patients. These complications are more frequent when the length of active disease exceeds 5 years. Continuing but intermittent active disease has been documented far in excess of 20 years in some patients.

Patients with splenomegaly and cytopenias are exquisitely sensitive to chemotherapy and have difficulties with infections and bleeding. Middle ear infections can be chronic in the children with mastoid involvement.

Complications of chemotherapy are related to the specific drug. The most active agents have significant toxicity: corticosteroids, antimetabolites, alkylating agents, and vinca alkaloids.

DIFFERENTIAL DIAGNOSIS

The skin rash in infants can be confused with seborrhea (cradle cap) or eczema. The skin lesions are often scaly and hemorrhagic, located predominantly on the trunk. Erythema nodosum–type rashes may be seen in older patients.

Although lung findings may be mistakenly diagnosed as a primary infectious process, histiocytosis of the lung can often be complicated by an opportunistic infection.

The gingival lesions are not pathognomonic and frequently appear as punched-out lesions. Premature eruption of the teeth is commonly overlooked.

The lymphadenopathy can be massive, suggesting leukemia and lymphoma when not accompanied by a skin rash. Occasionally the multinucleated giant cells have been mistaken for Sternberg-Reed cells.

The bone lesions are quite typical on x-ray, although metastatic solid tumors may be considered in the differential diagnosis. The latter, however, are usually detectable by radioactive bone scan. Osteomyelitis may be suspected, especially when lung disease coexists.

Children with congenital infections caused by rubella or cytomegalovirus may have a reactive histiocytosis. It is unclear whether these truly represent histiocytosis X. Similarly, in children in whom immune deficiency is demonstrated, it is unclear which came first, the histiocytosis or the immune deficiency. The lipoid reticuloses and mast cell disease are ruled out by appropriate biopsies.

COURSE AND PROGNOSIS

Patients with disease limited to bone have an excellent prognosis without much risk of disability. Although children with bone plus soft tissue involvement usually survive (84 per cent), they may have significant disabilities if their disease is active for more than 5 years. Sixty-nine per cent of children who survive for at least 5 years will have one or more significant disabilities. Children whose disease is restricted to soft tissues do not run high risk of disability if they survive. Their major problem is survival.

Prognosis is affected by age at diagnosis, number of organs involved, and organ dysfunction. In addition, familial cases are usually fatal. It can no longer be said that "Letterer-Siwe" disease is uniformly fatal. Although the overall prognosis may be grave, responses to therapy warrant cautious optimism.

HEMOPHILIA AND OTHER HEREDITARY DEFECTS OF COAGULATION

By PHILIP M. BLATT, M.D.,
KENNETH D. ZEITLER, M.D.,
and HAROLD R. ROBERTS, M.D.
Chapel Hill, North Carolina

Hemophilia, as a congenital bleeding disorder, has been known since antiquity, and its familial nature has been recognized since early in the nineteenth century. As individual procoagulant proteins have become identified, and with better understanding of the role of platelets in hemostasis, hereditary coagulation defects have been shown to be a diverse group of disorders. Identification of and distinction between the various coagulation disorders is important, because each requires somewhat different therapy.

GENERAL APPROACH TO PATIENTS WITH SUSPECTED COAGULATION DEFECTS

Much information can be obtained from careful history and physical examination, although precise diagnosis requires specialized coagulation studies. The onset, extent, and duration of all bleeding episodes should be documented. The extent and duration of bleeding associated with sports participation, minor trauma and surgery, dental work, and menstruation should be ascertained. Association of bleeding with aspirin ingestion should be sought, and the patient should be queried about epistaxis, joint swelling and pain, skin and soft tissue hematomas, hematuria, and gastrointestinal bleeding.

A complete, careful family history is essential, with construction of a pedigree in as much detail as possible, giving attention to known bleeding episodes in all relatives. Hemophilia A (classic hemophilia) and hemophilia B are common and are the only X-linked recessive bleeding disorders; the family history is of great value in distinguishing them from autosomally inherited disorders. A negative family history does not exclude a hereditary bleeding disorder, as affected relatives may be unknown to the patient, the patient may be the only relative in whom a recessive trait has been expressed, or the patient may be a new mutant.

In the physical examination special attention should be given to the skin and mucous membranes to detect bruises, petechiae, and telangiectasia. Joints should be examined for symmetry, swelling, limitation of motion, and the characteristic hyperextensibility of Ehlers-Danlos syndrome.

Blood counts, including platelet count, should be performed, and the blood smear should be examined to detect blood loss anemia, diseases such as aplastic anemia and leukemia that may cause bleeding, and abnormal platelet morphology that may be present in certain congenital platelet disorders. The stool should be checked for occult blood and the urine for hematuria. Useful screening tests in all patients suspected of bleeding abnormalities include bleeding time, prothrombin time, partial thromboplastin time, and thrombin clotting time. More specific assays for blood clotting factors are discussed later.

BLOOD CLOTTING FACTORS AND RELATED DEFICIENCY STATES

Table 1 shows the known coagulation factors, the diseases that result from their deficiency or impaired function, and their inheritance pattern. The common abnormal screening tests are included.

THE HEMOPHILIAS

Originally, the term hemophilia referred to a bleeding disorder characterized by X-linked inheritance and severe bleeding manifestations, including hemarthrosis. By 1950, it was realized that two kinds of sex-linked hemophilia existed, which were indistinguishable on clinical grounds but were clearly differentiated by laboratory tests. These have been termed hemophilia A (classic hemophilia) and hemophilia B (Christmas disease).

Another hereditary coagulopathy that is separable from hemophilia A is von Willebrand's disease. This disease is typified by autosomal dominant inheritance, a prolonged bleeding time, abnormally decreased platelet retention on glass beads, and abnormal aggregation of platelets with the antibiotic ristocetin. These patients are, however, also typically deficient in antihemophilic factor as measured by clotting assays. These observations have suggested that antihemophilic factor is composed of at least two functional components. One component is synthesized under the direction of gene(s) on the X chromosome and is responsible for the procoagulant properties of Factor VIII. The other component is synthesized under the direction of autosomal genes and is responsible for "von Willebrand factor activity" as defined by the bleeding time, platelet adhesion, ristocetin-induced platelet aggregation, and delayed rise of Factor VIII clotting activity after infusion of normal or hemophilic plasma into a patient with von Willebrand's disease.

Studies of the molecular structure of Factor VIII support these observations in that it can be dissociated into two components, one of high molecular weight and the other of low molecular weight. The high molecular weight component possesses antigenic material precipitated by heterologous antisera (Factor VIII antigen, VIII:Ag) and corrects the defective ristocetin-induced platelet aggregation of von Willebrand's disease (von Willebrand factor, VIII:vWF), but does not support the clotting of hemophilic plasma. The low molecular weight component contains the procoagulant activity (Factor VIII coagulant, VIII:C), but is deficient in precipitating antigens and in the ability to support ristocetin-induced platelet aggregation. Whether the antihemophilic factor is one or more molecules and if so whether the bonds are covalent or noncovalent are questions that have not been settled. It has been shown that the high molecular weight component is synthesized by vascular endothelial cells, while the site of synthesis of the low molecular weight component is conjectural.

HEMOPHILIA A

Hemophilia A results from a physiological deficiency of Factor VIII clotting activity. Gen-

Table 1. *Coagulation Factors*

Factor	Synonyms	Deficiency State	Inheritance Pattern	Abnormal Tests
I	Fibrinogen	Afibrinogenemia	Autosomal recessive	BT, PT, PTT, TCT
		Dysfibrinogenemia	Autosomal dominant	PT, PTT, TCT
II	Prothrombin	Hypoprothrombinemia	Autosomal recessive	PT, PTT
		Dysprothrombinemia	? Autosomal recessive	PT, PTT
III	Tissue thromboplastin	None		
IV	Calcium	None		
V	Accelerator globulin (proaccelerin)	Factor V deficiency‡	Autosomal recessive	PT, PTT, BT (prolonged in 1/3)
VII	Proconvertin	Factor VII deficiency†	Autosomal recessive	PT
VIII	Antihemophilic factor	Classic hemophilia† (hemophilia A)	X-linked recessive	PTT
		von Willebrand's disease	Autosomal dominant	BT, PTT
IX	Plasma thromboplastin component	Hemophilia B† (Christmas disease)	X-linked recessive	PTT
X	Stuart factor	Factor X deficiency†	Autosomal recessive	PT, PTT
XI	Plasma thromboplastin antecedent	Factor XI deficiency†	Autosomal recessive	PTT
XII°	Hageman factor	Factor XII deficiency†	Autosomal recessive	PTT
Fletcher°	—	Fletcher factor deficiency	Autosomal recessive	PTT
Fitzgerald°	—	Fitzgerald factor deficiency	Autosomal recessive	PTT
Passavoy	—	Passavoy factor deficiency	Autosomal recessive	PTT
XIII	Fibrin stabilizing factor	Factor XIII deficiency†	Autosomal recessive	Clot solubility increased in 5 M urea

Key: BT = bleeding time; PT = prothrombin time; PTT = partial thromboplastin time; TCT = thrombin clotting time.
°No clinical symptoms.
†Genetic heterogeneity identified with some patients showing "true" deficiency of factor synthesis while other patients have abnormal molecules incapable of supporting procoagulant activity yet present in antigenically normal quantity.
‡Genetic heterogeneity suggested by variable levels of Factor V activity.

erally, only males will be bleeders, although rarely a female carrier will have a mild to moderate bleeding diathesis. Sons of affected males will be normal, and all the daughters will be carriers. Thus the disorder will appear to "skip generations," as only some of the male offspring of female carriers will be bleeders. As stated previously, the absence of a characteristic family history does not exclude hemophilia.

Hemophilia occurs in all degrees of severity corresponding to the level of Factor VIII clotting activity in the affected persons. Severely affected patients have less than 1 per cent Factor VIII activity and intermittently have spontaneous hemorrhages, especially into large joints and muscles. In patients with severe hemophilia A, symptoms may begin at birth with bleeding from the umbilical cord, although this does not occur frequently. Easy bruising may be noted in the child and, when he begins to walk, hemarthroses and muscle hematomas begin to be a problem. Bleeding can occur anywhere and mimic other diseases. For example, bleeding into the wall of the intestine may cause obstructive symptoms, whereas hemorrhage into the right psoas muscle may mimic appendicitis. Hematuria is a common problem. Bleeding into the central nervous system, either spontaneously or after trauma, results in a life-threatening situation and remains a major cause of death in hemophilia A. Affected patients also have a marked tendency to bleed after minimal trauma. The advent of Factor VIII concentrates has revolutionized the treatment of severe hemophilia A.

Moderately affected patients have approximately 1 to 5 per cent Factor VIII clotting activity. Spontaneous hemorrhage occurs much less frequently, but hemorrhage usually occurs after trauma of even minor degree. Mildly affected patients have greater than 5 to 7 per cent Factor VIII activity and generally bleed only after significant injury.

Although often termed "Factor VIII deficiency," hemophilia A may not be the result of the absence of the Factor VIII molecule, as most patients with this disorder have normal to increased amounts of circulating Factor VIII antigen (with decreased clotting activity) when tested using heterologous rabbit antibody. Thus hemophilia may result from an abnormal molecule that retains antigenic activity but relatively minimal coagulant activity.

Approximately one third of female carriers will have a subnormal level of Factor VIII clotting activity, whereas the remainder will have normal levels. Thus, one third of carriers (that is, those with low levels of Factor VIII) are susceptible to identification with reasonable certainty. Recently, a more discriminant test for the carrier state in hemophilia A carriers with normal Factor VIII levels has been developed, on the basis of the observation that the ratio of Factor VIII-related antigen to Factor VIII clotting activity is increased in the carrier state. The level of Factor VIII-related antigen is determined using a heterologous precipitating antibody to Factor VIII and the technique of immunoelectrophoresis. Early results suggest that 80 to 90 per cent of all carriers can be detected by this technique.

The proper diagnosis of hemophilia A is easy to make in patients with severe hemophilia A. These patients generally present with (1) a sex-linked disease; (2) "spontaneous" hemorrhage, leading to crippling hemarthropathy; (3) a prolonged partial thromboplastin time; (4) a low Factor VIII activity level; and (5) a normal bleeding time (see Laboratory Tests).

It is more difficult to diagnose *mild* hemophilia A because it must be distinguished from von Willebrand's disease, another congenital bleeding disorder characterized by low Factor VIII activity levels. In mild hemophilia A there is a decreased level of coagulant Factor VIII

(i.e., the Factor VIII level measured routinely in a coagulation laboratory using a one-stage method; see Laboratory Tests). The Factor VIII antigen, however, is normal or high when tested by immunoelectrophoresis using a heterologous precipitating antibody to Factor VIII. It is also important to recall that the bleeding time and the ristocetin-induced platelet aggregation test (which are abnormal in von Willebrand's disease) are normal in hemophilia A (both severe and mild). A further comparison of these two conditions is made in the discussion on von Willebrand's disease and is shown in Table 2, but it is important to emphasize that a low level of Factor VIII activity and a normal bleeding time do not confirm a diagnosis of mild hemophilia A. Some patients with hemophilia have a true deficiency of the clotting piece of the Factor VIII molecule, and others have an abnormality in this portion of the protein.

Factor VIII Inhibitors. Factor VIII inhibitors arise in 15 per cent of patients with severe classic hemophilia (rarely in patients with mild to moderate hemophilia) and in patients with a number of other conditions, including older people with no other associated illness, postpartum females, patients with allergic reactions to drugs, collagen vascular disease (especially systemic lupus erythematosus and rheumatoid arthritis), exfoliative skin disease, inflammatory bowel disease and patients with paraproteins.

It has been clearly established that anti-Factor VIII inhibitors are antibodies that are time, temperature, and pH dependent. In a patient with classic hemophilia and a high titer inhibitor, inhibitory activity can be detected by mixing the patient's plasma and normal plasma and performing a partial thromboplastin time (PTT) on the mixture. Instead of correcting the hemophilic defect as normal plasma does, the inhibitor in the patient's plasma will result in a prolonged PTT — usually at least 30 seconds longer than the control. Since this inhibitor is time and temperature dependent, the *immediate mix* may not detect this inhibitor, especially if the inhibitor is present in low titer. In this situation incubation of the mixture of normal plasma and the hemophilic plasma for 1 to 2 hours at 37 C, followed by a PTT, will most often demonstrate the inhibitor. It is essential that the control mixture also be similarly incubated. The inhibitor to Factor VIII can be specifically assayed in units. The various assays are based on the ability of the inhibitor to neutralize Factor VIII, and the units vary according to the method used. All patients with severe classic hemophilia should be screened before surgery for the presence of a specific inhibitor. The diagnosis of the inhibitor state is important in planning therapy.

Table 2. *Laboratory Differences Between Hemophilia A and von Willebrand's Disease*

	Hemophilia A	von Willebrand's Disease
Inheritance	Sex linked	Autosomal dominant
Factor VIII (procoagulant)	Low	Low to nearly normal (variable)
Bleeding time	Normal	Normal to prolonged (variable)
Ristocetin aggregation	Normal	Normal or low
Factor VIII-related antigen	Normal to high	Low to normal
De novo synthesis of Factor VIII after plasma or cryoprecipitate infusion	No	Yes
Platelet adhesiveness to glass beads	Normal	Decreased

VON WILLEBRAND'S DISEASE (vWD)

In 1926 Professor Erik von Willebrand described a bleeding disorder inherited as an autosomal dominant characteristic with variable penetrance and expressivity. Bleeding in this condition is variable but generally of the muco-cutaneous type (epistaxis, increased bruising, menorrhagia, or gastrointestinal hemorrhage). Bleeding during and after surgical procedures of varying types, including dental extractions, is quite common, whereas hemarthroses are rare.

Originally, the most consistent laboratory finding was a prolonged bleeding time. Later it was found that many patients with vWD also have a deficiency of Factor VIII clotting activity. The level of Factor VIII activity may vary from undetectable to normal levels. Although the Factor VIII activity levels in male patients with hemophilia A are reasonably constant throughout life, the Factor VIII activity levels in a given patient with vWD frequently fluctuate.

Because of the prolonged bleeding time and the fact that platelet adhesiveness is often decreased in vWD, a platelet defect was first suspected as the cause of the bleeding disorder. Actually, the defect appears to be due to a quantitative or qualitative "deficiency" in the Factor VIII molecule, which possesses not only coagulant and antigenic activity but also an activity required for the aggregation of platelets under certain circumstances. That part of the Factor VIII molecule related to platelet function has been termed the von Willebrand factor (vWF). The Factor VIII molecule therefore has at least two roles in hemostasis, one related to platelet function and the other to the coagulation sequence leading to fibrin formation. Patients with hemophilia A have normal platelet function and therefore normal bleeding times, because their circulating Factor VIII, although poorly functional from a coagulant point of view, is normal with respect to its role in platelet function.

The diagnosis of von Willebrand's disease is based on the family history, prolonged bleeding time, and decreased Factor VIII activity. Recently, platelet aggregation in the presence of the antibiotic ristocetin has been developed into an assay designed to detect the putative von Willebrand plasma factor. Ristocetin is an antibiotic that causes the spontaneous aggregation of normal platelets but fails to aggregate the platelets of patients with von Willebrand's disease when it is added to their platelet-rich plasma. Addition of von Willebrand factor to plasma from patients with von Willebrand's disease restores ristocetin-induced platelet aggregation to normal. Also helpful is the determination of the amount of Factor VIII-related antigen by the Laurell technique. In von Willebrand's disease the Factor VIII-related antigen is usually decreased, whereas in hemophilia A it is normal or increased.

A unique aspect of vWD involves the response to infusion of plasma or cryoprecipitate. Approximately 3 to 48 hours after this infusion, the Factor VIII activity level in the affected patient will begin to rise. This phenomenon has been termed "de novo synthesis of Factor VIII." Thus if Factor VIII has a normal plasma half-life of 8 to 12 hours, levels of Factor VIII activity in the transfused von Willebrand subject may continue to rise or may remain above expected values for many hours. This occurrence is unique to vWD, and serial (every 6 hours) Factor VIII activity levels should be tested in a patient with mild to moderate Factor VIII deficiency who requires treatment and in whom the diagnosis is uncertain.

The laboratory findings in von Willebrand's

disease are extremely variable, making the diagnosis more difficult than it might seem from the number of tests available. This variability takes two forms. There are now entire families thought to have vWD in whom one or more of the aforementioned tests are persistently normal, and yet in whom the bulk of clinical and laboratory evidence supports this diagnosis. Secondly, with a given patient, there can generally be marked variation from day to day or month to month in any or all of these tests. It is especially important to recognize that pregnancy and use of birth control pills can normalize many of the tests usually abnormal in vWD. Nevertheless, the diagnosis of von Willebrand's disease usually rests on five findings: (1) a long bleeding time, (2) a low Factor VIII activity level, (3) a decreased Factor VIII-related antigen, (4) a decrease in ristocetin-induced platelet aggregation, and (5) a delayed rise in Factor VIII activity after infusion of cryoprecipitate (Table 2). Variants of von Willebrand's disease have been reported. In some patients the von Willebrand piece of the molecule is undetectable; in others it is abnormal. Carbohydrate abnormalities have been reported.

Hemophilia B

Hemophilia B (Christmas disease) is the result of a deficiency of Factor IX. The bleeding manifestations vary from severe to mild and are virtually identical to those of Factor VIII deficiency. Like the latter, Factor IX deficiency results in a prolonged PTT and is inherited as an X-linked disorder. It can be distinguished in the laboratory from Factor VIII deficiency by specific Factor IX assay using a known Factor IX-deficient substrate. Several variants of Factor IX deficiency exist. One is known as hemophilia B$_m$, a variant of hemophilia B that has a prolonged ox-brain prothrombin time, but otherwise is similar to severe hemophilia B.

FACTOR XII DEFICIENCY

A deficiency of Factor XII (Hageman Factor) causes no bleeding symptoms. Affected patients have no abnormal bleeding even at surgery, and in almost all cases no replacement therapy is necessary. The unactivated partial thromboplastin time, however, may be greater than 200 seconds. The importance of recognizing this deficiency therefore lies in distinguishing it from other causes of a prolonged partial thromboplastin time, e.g., Factor VIII, IX, and XI deficiencies, which do produce bleeding syndromes and require therapy.

FACTOR XI DEFICIENCY

Factor XI deficiency was first recognized in 1953. It is inherited as an autosomal, incompletely recessive trait. Both homozygotes and heterozygotes may have increased bleeding, although the former have more severe symptoms. The incidence of this deficiency is highest in Sephardic Jewish people.

Bleeding in Factor XI deficiency is usually mild. Most commonly seen are bruising, epistaxis, and menorrhagia. Hemarthrosis is rare. Bleeding, which may be delayed, commonly follows dental extractions and surgery.

Factor XI deficiency can be suspected on the basis of a prolonged partial thromboplastin time, mild bleeding, and autosomal inheritance. It can further be distinguished from Factors VIII and IX deficiencies by mixing experiments. Fresh serum contains Factors XII, XI, IX, and X, whereas barium sulfate–adsorbed plasma contains Factors XII, XI, VIII, and V. Testing the ability of each of these reagents to correct the prolonged partial thromboplastin time of a patient's plasma yields considerable information about the patient's deficiency (Table 3). Distinguishing Factor XII from Factor XI deficiency, if the bleeding history is questionable, is best done by specific assay techniques based on the use of known deficient plasma as substrate in a one-stage assay.

FACTOR X DEFICIENCY

Deficiency of Factor X is a rare disorder, discovered in 1957 by Hougie, Barrow, and Graham, that is inherited as a highly penetrant autosomal recessive trait and has a heterozygous frequency of about one in 500 persons. The most common bleeding manifestations are epistaxis, hematomata, menorrhagia, and postpartum hemorrhage. Hemarthrosis may occur but rarely results in crippling arthropathy. Factor X deficiency classically results in a prolongation of both the prothrombin time and the partial thromboplastin time with a normal thrombin clotting time. The pattern is also seen in Factor V or II deficiency, and thus, to distinguish deficiencies of these factors, specific assays are required.

Variants of Factor X deficiency have been reported in which Factor X antigenic activity, as measured by its ability to neutralize heterologous antibody, is normal, while its clotting activity is deficient (Factor X Friuli). On the other hand, variants have also been noted with proportionately diminished clotting and antigenic activities (Stuart Factor). These findings

Table 3. *Use of Prothrombin Time (PT) to Identify Deficient Factor**

Deficient Factor	PT	PT + Serum†	PT + Adsorbed‡ Plasma
VII	Abnormal	Normal	Abnormal
X	Abnormal	Normal	Abnormal
V	Abnormal	Abnormal	Normal
II	Abnormal	Abnormal	Abnormal
I	Abnormal	Abnormal	Normal

*Normal PT is 12 to 14 seconds. Abnormal is greater than 14 seconds.
†See Table 4.
‡See Table 4.

suggest that some patients have normal numbers of functionally "abnormal" Factor X molecules, while other patients appear to have "true" deficiency of factor synthesis. The former patients are said to be positive for cross-reacting material (CRM⁺), while the latter lack cross-reacting material in proportion to their degree of clotting activity deficiency (CRM⁻). These findings imply genetic heterogeneity among patients otherwise typically Factor X-deficient and may lead to the identification of a variety of structural abnormalities of the Factor X molecule, as has by analogy been observed in the hemoglobinopathies.

FACTOR VII DEFICIENCY

Factor VII deficiency is inherited as an autosomal recessive trait with a homozygous frequency of about 2 per million individuals. Bleeding manifestations are most commonly epistaxis and menorrhagia, or gingival (especially after dental extraction) and subcutaneous. Other bleeding sites including hemarthrosis may occur but are unusual. The severity of postsurgical bleeding has varied considerably, and may not correlate with the level of Factor VII clotting activity. Factor VII deficiency is the only deficiency that results in an isolated prolongation of the prothrombin time and the diagnosis is confirmed by specific Factor VII assays.

Genetic variants of Factor VII have been reported (e.g., Factor VII Padua, Factor VII Verona). These variants display discrepancies of antigenic and clotting activity — that is, clotting activity reduced either in proportion to antigenic activity ("true" deficiency, CRM⁻) or in excess of antigenic activity (abnormal molecule, CRM⁺). This suggests genetic heterogeneity in the Factor VII deficiency state as noted for deficiencies of the other procoagulants.

FACTOR V DEFICIENCY

Factor V deficiency is a rare disorder transmitted as an autosomal recessive trait in which only the homozygotes have bleeding manifestations. Bleeding severity varies greatly and is often mild, consisting of epistaxis, easy bruising, menorrhagia, and postsurgical bleeding. In severely affected patients, gastrointestinal and central nervous system bleeding may occur. The carriers, however, are relatively easy to identify, as they have approximately one half the normal plasma level of Factor V. Carrier identification by specific factor assay is indeed generally possible in all the coagulation disorders characterized by autosomal recessive inheritance. Factor V deficiency results in both a prolonged prothrombin time and partial thromboplastin time. The bleeding time is prolonged in approximately one third of the patients. A specific assay of Factor V is required for accurate diagnosis.

PROTHROMBIN DEFICIENCY

Deficiency of Factor II is rare and inherited as an autosomal recessive trait. Bleeding manifestations generally correlate with the level of functional prothrombin, being insignificant with levels around 50 per cent and potentially life-threatening with levels less than 2 per cent. Severely affected patients may show postpartum hemorrhage, menorrhagia, and hemorrhage after surgery, circumcision, or trauma. Hemarthrosis is unusual. The prothrombin time and partial thromboplastin time are often slightly prolonged in this disorder; therefore, a specific prothrombin assay is required to make the diagnosis.

Genetic variation has been noted among patients with prothrombin deficiency as some patients have simply deficient factor synthesis, while others synthesize molecular variants (dysprothrombins). A number of such dys-prothrombins have now been investigated (e.g., prothrombins Cardeza, Molise, Metz, San Juan I and II, Brussels, Quick, Barcelona, and Padua) and specific molecular defects have been sug-gested.

FACTOR I DEFICIENCY

AFIBRINOGENEMIA

This disorder is inherited in an autosomal recessive fashion. Excessive hemorrhage is present from birth. Bleeding from the umbilical stump and after circumcision may be severe. Bruising, hematomas, epistaxis, and hemor-rhage after tooth extraction and surgery are common. Wound healing is often defective. For unclear reasons, despite the complete incoagu-lability of their blood, patients with this dis-order may go for long periods without spontane-ous hemorrhage, and in general have less disability than patients with severe hemophilia A or B. The blood is incoagulable, and the prothrombin time, partial thromboplastin time, and thrombin clotting time are grossly abnor-mal. Fibrinogen appears to be absent by both chemical and immunologic methods. The bleeding time is prolonged in about 50 per cent of patients.

Another group of patients have hypofibrin-ogenemia with levels ranging from 20 to 100 mg per dl (100 ml) (normal is 200 to 400 mg per dl). Bleeding manifestations are mild or absent, and the disorder often goes unrecognized.

DYSFIBRINOGENEMIA

Since 1963 more than 50 abnormal fibrin-ogens have been described. Ménaché first coined the term dysfibrinogenemia after discov-ering an abnormal fibrinogen called fibrinogen Paris I. Subsequent abnormal fibrinogens have also been named for the cities in which they were discovered. The inheritance pattern is usually autosomal dominant. The majority of the patients having this disorder are asymp-tomatic. Some have a mild hemorrhagic diathe-sis. An increased incidence of wound dehis-cence has been reported. A minority of patients have had thromboembolic disease. Most affect-ed patients will have a prolonged thrombin clotting time. The abnormality will not always be recognized, however, in the usual quantita-tive fibrinogen assays, because in many cases the abnormal fibrinogen is measured along with the normal fibrinogen present. In some cases, however, the fibrinogen level appears de-creased by clotting techniques as well as by immunologic techniques. Fibrinogen immuno-electrophoresis may identify the abnormal fi-brinogen, which will appear as a spur on the precipitating line of the normal fibrinogen, but this is not a reliable test. Most dysfibrinogen-emias have defective fibrin polymerization. Other dysfibrinogenemias are associated with hypercatabolism of the fibrinogen molecule. Rare abnormal fibrinogens (fibrinogen Oslo) have a short thrombin clotting time and are associated with thrombosis.

FACTOR XIII DEFICIENCY

Factor XIII deficiency, which was first de-scribed in 1960, is an exceptionally rare dis-order. Factor XIII is responsible for transform-ing a freshly formed, unstable, urea-soluble fibrin clot into a stable, cross-linked fibrin poly-mer. In its absence, the initial fibrin clot later fragments, allowing delayed bleeding. Clinical manifestations of deficiency include an almost universal history of umbilical bleeding at birth, easy bruisability and hematoma formation, and poor wound healing and delayed bleeding after surgery and dental extractions. Prothrombin time, partial thromboplastin time, and thrombin clotting time are *normal* in Factor XIII defi-ciency. Factor XIII deficiency can be detected by a simple screening test based on the solubili-ty of the clot in 5 M urea. In an affected patient, the clot will dissolve in 5 M urea solution within minutes to an hour or so. Normal clots formed in the presence of Factor XIII will be stable in 5 M urea for days. A specific assay based on the principle of Factor XIII catalyzing the incorporation of monodansylcadaverine into casein has been described by Lorand and colleagues.

OTHER FACTOR DEFICIENCIES

Recently several new clotting factor deficien-cies have been described. They are named for the patients in whom they were first discovered. All result in prolonged partial thromboplastin times. Fletcher and Fitzgerald factor deficien-cies are inherited as autosomal recessive traits and, like Factor XII deficiency, do not result in clinical bleeding. Deficiency of Passavoy factor is inherited in an autosomal dominant fashion. Affected persons have bleeding symptoms simi-lar to those of mild hemophilia. Specific assays using substrate plasma known to be deficient in the respective factor are required for the diag-nosis.

COMBINED FACTOR DEFICIENCIES

Aside from the statistically conceivable simultaneous inheritance of two rare recessive genes, specific combined congenital factor deficiencies resulting from a "common gene abnormality" have been strongly suggested by family studies. The most important combined deficiency to consider is that of Factors V and VIII. In this instance, of which approximately 30 cases have been reported, the deficiency of both factors is generally mild (each about 15 per cent of normal), and there have been notable associated congenital abnormalities (e.g., syndactylism, retardation). Therefore, it is important to assay for both factors in situations in which there is ostensibly mild deficiency of either factor, particularly if there are associated congenital malformations, as therapy should be tailored to the combined deficiency.

The heritable association of combined deficiency of Factors VII and X has been noted in conjunction with familial carotid body tumors and should be considered in the appropriate setting. An associated congenital deficiency of Factors VII and VIII has been reported but not widely verified. Two unrelated patients have been reported with the intriguing condition of combined congenital deficiency of all the vitamin K-dependent factors (II, VII, IX, and X).

ANTITHROMBIN III DEFICIENCY

Antithrombin III (ATIII) is a plasma protein that slowly inactivates thrombin and other clotting factors with active site serines. It appears that heparin's anticoagulant activity is mainly mediated by antithrombin III. Deficiency of ATIII is inherited as an autosomal dominant trait. The homozygous state is thought to be incompatible with life. Affected heterozygotes have a high incidence of phlebitis and thromboembolic disease, which usually appear in the second and third decades of life. Death from pulmonary embolism is common. A number of assays for antithrombin III are available, based on clotting, immunologic, or colorimetric techniques.

LABORATORY TESTS

BLEEDING TIME

The bleeding time is a measure of the time for bleeding to cease after a standardized cut has been made. Normal values vary according to the method used. The bleeding time is a measure of the adequacy of platelet function. If platelets are qualitatively normal, the bleeding time is usually normal at platelet counts greater than 50,000 per cu mm and often at counts below this number. The bleeding time is usually, but not always, prolonged in patients with qualitative platelet abnormalities. It may also be prolonged in the presence of circulating inhibitors of platelet function such as drugs (especially aspirin), metabolic byproducts that accumulate in renal and liver disease, and breakdown products of fibrin and fibrinogen that are released in great quantity during disseminated intravascular coagulation. We use the Ivy bleeding time routinely, whereas others use the template bleeding time.

WHOLE BLOOD (LEE-WHITE) CLOTTING TIME

This test determines the length of time required for a clot to form in freshly drawn blood contained in a glass tube. Because it is extremely variable, it is of little aid in the diagnosis of coagulation disorders. The Lee-White time is normal in hemophiliacs who have more than 2 per cent of the deficient factor.

PROTHROMBIN TIME

The one-stage prothrombin time, developed by Quick, measures the integrity of the extrinsic pathway. Citrated plasma is used and a lipoprotein extract of lung or brain tissue, commercially available, serves as a source of thromboplastin. After recalcification, the time for clot formation is noted. Prolongation of the prothrombin time indicates a deficiency in one or more of the factors of the extrinsic or common pathway. It can also be prolonged by specific antibodies to these factors or by any of the inhibitors mentioned in the discussion under Thrombin Clotting Time. Correction of the prolongation by addition of barium sulfate–adsorbed plasma or aged serum may aid in the identification of the deficiency (Table 3).

PARTIAL THROMBOPLASTIN TIME

Several procoagulant deficiencies can be detected by the partial thromboplastin time. As in the prothrombin time, fresh or frozen citrated plasma is used. After addition of a phospholipid extract (partial thromboplastin) and calcium, the clotting time is noted. Prolongation of the PTT indicates a deficiency in one or more of the factors of the intrinsic or common pathway. It can also be prolonged by specific antibodies to these factors or by any of the inhibitors mentioned under Thrombin Clotting Time. Substi-

Table 4. *Use of the Partial Thromboplastin Time (PTT)*
*to Identify Deficient Clotting Factor**

Deficient Factor	PTT	PTT + Serum†	PTT + Adsorbed‡ Plasma
XII	Abnormal	Normal	Normal
XI	Abnormal	Normal	Normal
VIII	Abnormal	Abnormal	Normal
IX	Abnormal	Normal	Abnormal

*Normal PTT is 45 to 65 seconds; abnormal is over 65 seconds.

†Serum should be aged to deplete thrombin and should be citrated (1 part 3.2 per cent citrate to 5 parts serum). Serum contains Factors VII, IX, and X and is devoid of I, II, V, and VIII.

‡BaSO$_4$-adsorbed oxalated plasma or Al(OH)$_3$-adsorbed citrated plasma removes Factors II, VII, IX, and X.

tution experiments with adsorbed plasma and aged serum again may point to the reason for a prolongation (Table 4).

THROMBIN CLOTTING TIME

The thrombin clotting time is performed simply by adding thrombin to citrated plasma. It will be prolonged when the fibrinogen level is very low (less than 50 mg per dl). It is prolonged by inhibitors of thrombin, such as heparin, or by substances that interfere with fibrin polymerization, such as fibrin degradation products and paraproteins found in multiple myeloma. It is also usually prolonged in the dysfibrinogenemias.

SPECIFIC FACTOR ASSAYS

Despite the aid in diagnosis of procoagulant deficiencies that is available from simple mixing experiments based on the prothrombin time and partial thromboplastin time (Tables 3 and 4)

and the clues to diagnosis that can be gained by looking at the results of the PT, PTT, and TCT (Table 5), all deficiencies need to be confirmed by specific assay. In our laboratory the assays for Factors XII, XI, IX, and VIII are based on the kaolin-activated partial thromboplastin time. Dilutions of the test plasma are mixed with a known deficient substrate plasma, and the resulting activated partial thromboplastin time is plotted versus dilution on semilog paper. A straight line and an average value for the factor level can be obtained after comparison with a standard curve. A similar type of assay based on the prothrombin time, rather than the partial thromboplastin time, is done for Factors VII, V, and X. The specific assay for prothrombin is based on the two-stage method. Fibrinogen is measured by the spectrophotometric quantitation of clottable protein. Factor XIII is measured qualitatively by clot solubility in 5 M urea. Radioimmunoassays and assays using chromogenic substrates are currently research tools for several factors, and will probably be clinically available in the near future.

Table 5. *Use of Prothrombin Time (PT), Partial Thromboplastin Time (PTT),*
*and Thrombin Clotting Time (TCT) to Identify Deficient Clotting Factor**

Deficient Factor	PT	PTT	TCT
I	Abnormal	Abnormal	Abnormal
II	Abnormal	Abnormal	Normal
V	Abnormal	Abnormal	Normal
VII	Abnormal	Normal	Normal
VIII	Normal	Abnormal	Normal
IX	Normal	Abnormal	Normal
X	Abnormal	Abnormal	Normal
XI	Normal	Abnormal	Normal
XII	Normal	Abnormal	Normal

*Normal PTT is 45 to 65 seconds; abnormal is over 65. Normal PT is 12 to 14 seconds; abnormal is over 14. Normal TCT is within 3 seconds of the control.

BONE MARROW ASPIRATION

A bone marrow aspiration is of little diagnostic aid in bleeding disorders except in the differential diagnosis of thrombocytopenia. It may usually be done without serious consequences in thrombocytopenic patients but should not be done without adequate factor replacement in patients with severe procoagulant deficiency.

PITFALLS IN DIAGNOSIS

In the use of the prothrombin time and partial thromboplastin time to evaluate a person with a bleeding history, *it is important to remember that these tests may be normal when there is greater than 20 per cent level of a given factor.* Thus with these tests it is possible to miss a case of mild hemophilia or mild von Willebrand's disease. Therefore, if the bleeding history or family history is suggestive, it is necessary to perform specific factor assays to rule out a deficiency.

PURPURA DUE TO CAPILLARY AND PLATELET DISORDERS

By MARIO G. BALDINI, M.D., *and* YASUO IKEDA, M.D.

Pawtucket, Rhode Island

INTRODUCTION

Purpura, i.e., spontaneous bleeding into the skin and mucous membranes, is the consequence of abnormalities in normal hemostasis, the physiologic process by which hemorrhage from a severed blood vessel is arrested. Four systems participate in this process: the *blood platelets*, the *capillaries*, the *blood coagulation mechanism*, and the *fibrinolytic system*.

Purpura may occur in the form of small, localized hemorrhages of pinpoint size, the petechiae; more expanded, superficial extravasations of blood, the ecchymoses; or deeper and larger tissue hemorrhages, the hematomas. A defect in the platelets or the capillaries or both is, as a rule, manifested mainly by petechiae

and small ecchymoses. Large ecchymoses and hematomas are usually a sign of a breakdown in the blood coagulation mechanism or of activation of the fibrinolytic system.

A pathogenetic classification of purpura is conveniently made on the basis of the four systems concerned with normal hemostasis, and four types of purpura are recognized: *vascular purpura, thrombocytopenic purpura, purpura of coagulation disorders,* and *fibrinolytic purpura.* The most common varieties are thrombocytopenic and vascular purpura.

VASCULAR PURPURA

A wide variety of disorders of small blood vessels are known to cause abnormal bleeding. As a rule, no quantitative or qualitative abnormalities in platelets or in blood clotting, and no increase in fibrinolysis, can be demonstrated in these patients. There is no single laboratory test that is diagnostic of vascular purpura. The bleeding time and the tourniquet test are found variably positive in this condition.

HEREDITARY HEMORRHAGIC TELANGIECTASIA

SYNONYM

Rendu-Osler-Weber syndrome.

DEFINITION

This is an hereditary disorder of blood vessels characterized by multiple, dilated, tortuous venules and capillaries throughout the body, but particularly in the skin and mucous membranes. These altered blood vessels become easily injured, giving rise to profuse bleeding. The basic defect is in the development of the vessel wall and mesenchymal tissue of the skin and mucous membranes. The walls of the dilated venules and capillaries are thinned out with no muscular and elastic layers. They cannot retract and, in case of injury, bleeding is always abundant. There is no defect in the blood coagulation system or in the platelets of these patients.

CLINICAL FEATURES

The condition is inherited as an autosomal dominant trait with a high degree of penetrance. The homozygous state may be lethal. Both sexes are equally affected. The patient's symptoms are related to recurrent hemorrhage and chronic anemia. The lesions are usually small (from pinpoint size to about 3 mm), flat, bright red or purple, and sharply demarcated from the surrounding normal skin or mucosa. Blanching with pressure is the rule. They are found most commonly on the lips, tongue, buccal mucosa, nasal mucous membrane, conjunctivae, face including the ears, and also the palmar and plantar surfaces. Visceral lesions are common in the stomach, respiratory tract, genitourinary tract, and liver, and hemorrhage in internal organs occasionally occurs.

The telangiectatic lesions appear usually in childhood and increase in number as age advances. Bleeding does not usually manifest itself until adult life. It may occur from any sites where the telangiectatic lesions are present and more often from lesions in the mucous membranes than from those in the skin. Recurrent epistaxes are the most common symptom. Hemorrhage from the mouth, gastrointestinal tract, or respiratory tract occurs less frequently. Iron deficiency anemia from chronic blood loss is the most common complication. Pulmonary arteriovenous fistulas have been found in patients with hereditary hemorrhagic telangiectasia and have caused recurrent hemoptysis and pulmonary infections, clubbing of the fingers, and hypoxemia. Arteriovenous fistulas of the retina and cerebral blood vessels and aneurysms of the splenic and hepatic arteries or aorta have been reported.

LABORATORY FINDINGS

Laboratory findings depend upon the severity of the hemorrhagic manifestations. Findings of acute posthemorrhagic anemia or of iron deficiency anemia are common. The degree of anemia is variable, depending upon the severity of the disease and the frequency of bleeding manifestations. Normal bleeding time and platelet count are the rule. Coagulation tests are normal. Occasionally, the tourniquet test may be positive, but this has no diagnostic meaning.

DIFFERENTIAL DIAGNOSIS

When the characteristic vascular lesions in the skin and mucous membranes are associated with recurrent hemorrhage and are familial in character, the diagnosis of hereditary hemorrhagic telangiectasia is not difficult. Diagnostic difficulties may arise when the vascular lesions are more discrete and are hidden in the nasopharynx or in the internal organs.

ANAPHYLACTOID PURPURA

SYNONYMS

Schönlein-Henoch purpura, allergic vascular purpura.

DEFINITION

Anaphylactoid purpura, also called Schönlein-Henoch purpura, is a nonthrombocytopenic disorder characterized by an erythematous and hemorrhagic vascular rash with acute joint symptoms. The purpuric rash is usually more intense about joints and buttocks and in most cases is only one manifestation of an acute, generalized syndrome, chiefly of children, including localized subcutaneous edema, fever, arthralgia with painful periarticular swelling, cramping abdominal pain at times with bleeding from the gastrointestinal tract, renal symptoms with hematuria, and hyaline and granular casts. Although the purpuric skin lesions are an invariable feature, the other manifestations can each occur in about half to two thirds of the affected patients, and less frequently in adults. In addition, inflammatory involvement of pleura and pericardium is noted in rare patients. An aseptic vasculitis of capillaries and arterioles with a marked perivascular inflammatory reaction represents the basic pathologic lesion. The histologic and clinical features have characteristics of a hypersensitivity phenomenon. An allergen from bacteria, foods, or drugs is often suspected to be the inciting agent. In most patients no causative factor can be identified.

CLINICAL MANIFESTATIONS

The Schönlein-Henoch syndrome is primarily a disease of small children, with a peak incidence between the third and seventh years of age. In most reports, the ratio of the disease in males to females is 3:2. In adults the disease is rare, and male sex predominance has not been observed. The disease is typically acute with a sudden onset and a self-limited course, although a more chronic variety is usually seen in adults.

In most patients with anaphylactoid purpura, the course of events suggesting a hypersensitivity phenomenon is quite impressive. There is often a history of a preceding infection, usually an upper respiratory infection, or of drug intake (antibiotics, antihistaminics, quinine, or others). After a lag period of 1 to 3 weeks, i.e., a period of "allergic build-up," the symptoms (purpuric, articular, abdominal, renal) appear in various combinations and variations. Headache, malaise, anorexia, moderate fever, skin rash, joint pain, and/or abdominal pain are often the presenting symptoms. Diagnosis of the disease is particularly challenging in about 20 per cent of patients when abdominal pain or joint pain or both precede the characteristic skin lesions or when these are very limited in number and may be overlooked. The purpuric rash, together with all the other symptoms, usually disappears in the course of several days to a few weeks. In most cases recovery is rapid and complete. In a few patients, however, albuminuria and hematuria may persist after all the other symptoms have disappeared, and a form of chronic glomerulonephritis may become established and persist for months or years. Rarely in other patients (usually adults), the purpura recurs and renal symptoms, in the course of months to years, may become indistinguishable from those seen in polyarteritis nodosa. The suggestion has often been made that anaphylactoid purpura and polyarteritis nodosa constitute the same condition, with the difference that in polyarteritis nodosa the arteries are involved but in anaphylactoid purpura the capillaries are more severely involved, depending on the pathogenetic variations operating in the individual patient.

The relationship between anaphylactoid purpura and other "autoimmune" disorders has repeatedly been emphasized. This concept points to the need for accurate and prolonged observation of these patients relative to the possible development of systemic lupus erythematosus or polyarteritis nodosa. True overlaps and combinations are, however, rare. Duration of the illness, number of recurrences, and frequency of complications do not appear to be affected by any form of treatment, which is usually directed to the relief of symptoms.

COMPLICATIONS

Gastrointestinal complications are commonly seen in patients who have a stormy clinical course. Massive gastrointestinal hemorrhage, intestinal obstruction caused by intussusception, and intestinal perforation have occasionally been seen, and at times surgical intervention has been required.

Abnormal urinary findings are commonly seen in 22 to 60 per cent of patients and represent a transient complication in most cases. In about 10 per cent of them, however, subacute or chronic glomerulonephritis develops, leading to chronic renal failure. Focal involvement of glomeruli is seen with features of allergic vasculitis. Diffuse glomerular lesions with crescent formation are observed in the most severe, usually fatal cases.

Localized edema, usually around the joints, is a common symptom, but it can become particularly prominent in some patients. In rare patients, edema of the central nervous system with convulsions is seen. Edema of the glottis with signs of acute respiratory obstruction has also been described.

Pleural pain, at times with pleural effusion and also pericardial effusion, has occasionally been reported.

LABORATORY FINDINGS

The diagnosis of anaphylactoid purpura is not made in the laboratory, because no specific laboratory findings exist for this disease. There is no autoantibody against the vascular endothelium and no antigen-antibody complexes can be demonstrated in the serum of the patients. The vasculitis is typical in its microscopic findings, but it is not characteristic or diagnostic of the disease. However, a few clinical findings are of help in supporting the diagnosis. Microscopic hematuria, the presence of granular and red cell casts, and albuminuria, as well as a positive test for occult blood in the stools, are very commonly found in this type of purpura. Peripheral blood counts show a normal platelet level together with a moderate degree of polymorphonuclear leukocytosis and eosinophilia. Furthermore, anemia is not found unless a large gastrointestinal hemorrhage has occurred. The bleeding time is regularly normal, and there is no abnormality in the coagulation mechanism. The erythrocyte sedimentation rate is increased only in the acute phase of illness. In the early stages, throat cultures are often positive for beta-hemolytic streptococci and for *Staphylococcus aureus*. The old belief, however, that allergy toward beta-hemolytic streptococci plays the fundamental role in the pathogenesis of the disease has been discredited. Studies of the antistreptolysin "O" titer (ASO) and isolation of group A, beta-hemolytic streptococci have so far failed to provide evidence that this organism is a fundamental causative factor in this disease. The antistreptolysin "O" titer is elevated in only about one third of patients, and the incidence does not differ statistically from that of a normal control population. The diagnosis of anaphylactoid purpura is, conclusively, based on a typical association of clinical signs and symptoms, and is supported by only a few laboratory findings.

DIAGNOSIS

The diagnosis of anaphylactoid purpura is first suspected on the basis of the typical rash and of the association of other known signs and symptoms. A normal platelet count and normal platelet aggregation with ADP, collagen, and epinephrine are important to confirm the diagnosis. The absence of an overt infection is also of importance, as a number of infections may be associated with purpuric skin lesions not caused by thrombocytopenia or disseminated intravascular coagulation. Drug purpura must also be ruled out in the process of differential diagnosis. A nonthrombocytopenic, vascular purpura related to the intake of a drug has, from time to time, been reported, and a wide variety of drugs have been incriminated. The effect of these drugs is supposed to be on an allergic basis, although a complete demonstration of this mechanism has been lacking in most patients. Penicillin, sulfonamides, barbiturates, iodides, chlorothiazide, salicylates, or chemicals such as mercury and bismuth have at times been associated with this type of purpura. Their effect has, however, not been seen to cause important hemorrhage unless thrombocytopenia develops. Some of these drugs have, in fact, been described as being capable of causing also thrombocytopenic purpura on an allergic basis in some susceptible patients. In the adult, one must also rule out other vasculitides such as cutaneous periarteritis nodosa, erythema multiforme, or those secondary to systemic lupus erythematosus and Sjögren's syndrome.

AUTOSENSITIVITY TO ERYTHROCYTES OR DNA (PSYCHOGENIC PURPURA, GARDNER-DIAMOND PURPURA)

Autoerythrocyte sensitization is a rare disorder characterized by spontaneous, large, and painful ecchymoses. All the reported cases have been described in women of middle age. In the majority of cases, a history of physical or surgical trauma preceding the onset of the disease is obtained. The spontaneous appearance of purpura is usually preceded by local itching, burning, and pain. The purpuric lesions, which are characteristically surrounded by erythema and edema, may appear at the site of trauma or elsewhere. They are commonly associated with headache, nausea, vomiting, diarrhea, syncopal attacks, or chest pain, which have often been considered of psychosomatic nature in these patients. The disease may persist for years, undergoing periods of remission and exacerbation. Exacerbation was found to correlate with periods of emotional stress. Psychiatric studies have revealed that patients tend to have a uniform personality pattern with tendency toward hysteria, anxiety, and, at times, masochism. Furthermore, hypnotic suggestion was shown to induce new skin lesions in four patients. Physical examination and hematologic laboratory findings are of no help for the diagnosis. Blood platelets are normal in number and function. Blood coagulation tests also give normal results. In some patients, the intradermal injection of autologous erythrocytes, red cell stroma, or even phosphatidylserine derived from the red cell membrane can produce the characteristic skin lesions, whereas the injection of DNA or autologous leukocytes has given largely negative results.

Rarely, autosensitivity to deoxyribonucleic acid (DNA) has also been described. It consists of a painful, erythematous, and indurated wheal, usually on arms or legs. It is not preceded by trauma. Itching of the skin in the area of the lesion is the very first symptom. The lesion expands in a few days to become a large ecchymosis. The lesion can be reproduced by the intradermal injection of a minute amount of DNA or of lysed autologous leukocytes. The nature of the lesion is not as yet completely clear, although autosensitization seems to be the preferable hypothesis at present.

PURPURA SIMPLEX

The persistent bruising tendency that some healthy young women have, either spontaneous or after minor trauma, is often challenging to the physician. It is usually called purpura simplex when it meets the following diagnostic criteria: (1) it is of mild to moderate severity; (2) it is not associated with other hemorrhagic manifestations such as epistaxis, menorrhagia, or postoperative bleeding; (3) it frequently has a familial incidence; (4) it usually disappears with advancing age. All hemorrhagic tests give negative results in these patients, although the tourniquet test has at times been found to be positive.

The diagnosis of purpura simplex has become less frequent in recent years now that physicians have become aware that a large number of common medications (aspirin and other antiinflammatory drugs) can interfere with platelet aggregation and cause a mild to moderate form of purpura which is not vascular in type.

SENILE PURPURA

Senile purpura is characterized by distinct and well-demarcated red to purple ecchymotic lesions seen in areas of the skin regularly exposed to sunlight (the face, neck, dorsum of the hands and forearms, and the legs). They usually appear spontaneously or in response to trivial trauma. The basic defect is in the degeneration of dermal collagen, which, together with subcutaneous fat, serves as the normally supporting structure of the capillary bed. These purpuric manifestations often leave a residual brownish pigmentation of the skin. A similar purpura is observed in severe cachexia. No qualitative or quantitative platelet defects are found in these conditions.

STEROID PURPURA

Purpura is seen in Cushing's disease or in patients on prolonged ACTH or corticosteroid therapy. This type of purpura is similar to senile purpura in character. It is thought to be related to an alteration in dermal vascular support. The purpura will often disappear with discontinuation of the corticosteroids.

PURPURA OF INFECTIONS

Purpura may be seen during the course of a variety of infections by means of vascular damage. Although thrombocytopenia or disseminated intravascular coagulation or both are responsible for the occurrence of hemorrhage in many patients, direct endothelial injury by the infectious agent (rickettsiae, some viruses) or vascular damage resulting from bacterial products or toxins may cause purpura. In bacterial endocarditis bacterial emboli in the microvasculature can cause purpura with a necrotic center. The same type of purpura is also seen in meningococcemia and other types of septicemia. In cases of bacteremia or viremia, thrombocytopenic purpura may also occur because of the sweeping-up effect that bacteria or viruses exert on the platelets in the circulation. Infections of severe degree may produce purpura and major hemorrhage by causing disseminated intravascular coagulation.

SCURVY

SYNONYMS

Ascorbic acid deficiency, vitamin C deficiency.

DEFINITION

Purpura in scurvy is principally vascular in nature. Deficiency of this vitamin causes a scarcity of perivascular supporting tissue of small blood vessels. Collagen becomes deficient, and there is a lack of intercellular cement substance. Increased permeability and fragility of small blood vessels is the major cause for petechiae and ecchymoses. Many studies have been published on the biochemistry of this disorder, but the nature of it remains obscure to a large extent.

CLINICAL MANIFESTATIONS

The clinical manifestations of hemorrhage in scurvy are well known. They include perifollicular petechiae and small ecchymoses, mostly in arms and legs. The medial surface of the thighs and buttocks is often covered with petechiae. Swollen bleeding gums develop, sooner or later, in every patient with the exception of the edentulous ones (the very old and the very young). After repeated hemorrhages, the hair follicles become hyperkeratotic and hair becomes short, brittle, tortuous, and "corkscrew"-like. Painful subperiosteal hemorrhages are characteristic of scurvy in infancy and are due to extravasation of blood from epiphyseal vessels. Hemorrhages at costochondral junctions are also common. Epistaxes, hematuria, and gastrointestinal hemorrhage are frequently seen.

In the United States and other countries with a high nutritional standard, scurvy is rare. It is common in areas of the world with a high incidence of malnutrition. Infants as well as old people are more liable than other age groups to vitamin C deficiency, because their diets are often inadequate and poor. When scurvy is prolonged and severe, infections become very common and represent the most frequent cause of death in this disease.

All manifestations of scurvy disappear in a very few days with the administration of vitamin C. This prompt response to this vitamin can be of diagnostic significance in some difficult cases. The diagnosis is, however, made with relative ease before treatment in the majority of patients. The typical perifollicular hemorrhages, the keratotic plugging of the hair follicles, the swollen and bleeding gums, the painful subperiosteal hemorrhages, and the history of inadequate food supplements or abnormal diet, together with the ascorbic acid level of peripheral white cells and platelets, usually provide enough documentation for a secure diagnosis. An increased capillary fragility is the most common and typical finding and can be demonstrated by the tourniquet test. The bleeding time and other hemorrhagic tests, on the other hand, are normal in this disorder in most patients.

HERITABLE DISORDERS OF CONNECTIVE TISSUE

Vascular purpura is also seen in Ehlers-Danlos syndrome. The lack of supportive structures for small and large blood vessels and the hyperextensible skin seen in these patients make it possible for small trauma to produce large ecchymoses. Extensive bleeding from small wounds is common. A bleeding tendency has also been observed in other types of mesenchymal dysplasia as in osteogenesis imperfecta, Marfan's syndrome, and pseudoxanthoma elasticum. The defect in these conditions is related to abnormalities in the structure of connective tissue in the vessel wall and in the perivascular supporting tissue.

In these disorders abnormalities in platelet Factor 3 activity and collagen-induced aggregation have also been described, and these may also contribute to the bleeding tendency seen in these disorders. The hemorrhagic symptoms are many and varied in these patients.

KAPOSI'S HEMORRHAGIC SARCOMA

This rare disease results from a neoplastic proliferation of vascular elements most commonly observed in the lower extremities with dark nodules and prominent superficial blood vessels, hemorrhage, edema, and brownish discoloration of the skin. The disease progresses slowly to invade visceral organs with severe and, at times, fatal complications in only about 20 per cent of patients. Diagnosis is suspected from the characteristic clinical features and confirmed by histologic examination.

PURPURA OF PLATELET DISORDERS

Whenever the number of blood platelets in the circulating blood is drastically reduced or their function is severely impaired, spontaneous bleeding is common. The majority of bleeding disorders are known to be associated with quantitative or qualitative platelet defects. In these conditions, the bleeding time is regularly prolonged, the tourniquet test is positive, the conversion of prothrombin to thrombin is defective, and clot retraction is incomplete or absent. These abnormalities are the direct consequence of a defect in the platelets, as it is known that if the patient is supplied with an adequate number of normal, fresh platelets, these findings will revert to normal and hemorrhage will temporarily be arrested.

Bleeding disorders associated with a low platelet count are frequently encountered in practice; these are the thrombocytopenic purpuras. Also frequently seen are hemorrhagic disorders caused by a qualitative rather than a quantitative platelet defect, i.e., the thrombocytopathic purpuras. Furthermore, bleeding manifestations may also be seen in patients with a platelet count that is too high. When the circulating platelets are greatly increased, hemorrhage, in addition to thromboses, may occur. The mechanism of this "paradoxic" hemorrhage in the hemorrhagic thrombocythemias and other thrombocytoses is poorly understood, but it is known that the bleeding manifestations

disappear when the platelet count is returned to normal after treatment.

THE THROMBOCYTOPENIAS

Thrombocytopenic purpura is the most common of all hemorrhagic disorders. Recent studies by radioisotopic techniques for measuring platelet survival have demonstrated that thrombocytopenias are mainly due to (1) deficient platelet production, (2) increased platelet destruction, or (3) abnormal platelet distribution. A decreased platelet production is, in most patients, associated with decreased numbers of megakaryocytes in the bone marrow (amegakaryocytic thrombocytopenia), although rarely, some patients may present a normal to increased number of megakaryocytes, which are, however, incapable of normal platelet production (ineffective thrombocytopoiesis). Thrombocytopenias caused by increased platelet destruction (thrombocytolytic thrombocytopenias) are typically associated with increased numbers of megakaryocytes in the bone marrow and a reduced platelet lifespan in the circulation. A third model of platelet kinetics is based on an abnormal platelet distribution as the principal cause of the thrombocytopenia. This occurs in "hypersplenism," in which large numbers of platelets become concentrated in the enlarged spleen, but they survive a normal or nearly normal lifespan. Megakaryocytes in the bone marrow are regularly increased in number in this condition.

Amegakaryocytic thrombocytopenias are commonly seen in patients with bone marrow failure caused by chemical agents or irradiation, in patients with aplastic anemia, or in those with very advanced myelophthisic states. Megakaryocytic thrombocytopenias with a shortened platelet lifespan are typically caused by an immunologic (mostly autoimmune) platelet destruction. Thrombocytopenia caused by ineffective thrombocytopoiesis is a relatively rare event, occurring usually in preleukemic states, in some patients with megaloblastic anemia, or in paroxysmal nocturnal hemoglobinuria (PNH).

A practical classification of the thrombocytopenic purpuras is given in Table 1.

Of the various tests available for the study of thrombocytopenic disorders, the bone marrow aspiration is without doubt the most useful diagnostic procedure. There is great difference in significance between a bone marrow depleted of megakaryocytes and a bone marrow with normal or increased numbers of these cells. The former situation implies a defect in platelet

Table 1.   *Classification of Thrombocytopenic Purpuras*

A. Amegakaryocytic
   1. Bone marrow hypoplasia (drug-induced, idiopathic, congenital, selective, or total)
   2. Myelophthisic bone marrow (leukemia, metastatic malignancy)
B. Megakaryocytic, thrombocytolytic
   1. Immunologic thrombocytopenic purpura (ITP) (idiopathic and secondary)
   2. Drug sensitization (quinidine, digitoxin, etc.)
   3. Neonatal, isoimmune thrombocytopenia
   4. Microangiopathic thrombocytopenias (thrombo-hemolytic thrombocytopenic purpura, disseminated intravascular coagulation, hemangioma, etc.)
   5. Septicemia, viremia
C. Megakaryocytic, nonthrombocytolytic
   1. Ineffective thrombocytopoiesis (preleukemia, PNH vitamin B_{12} or folic acid deficiency)
   2. "Hypersplenism" (pooling of platelets in the enlarged spleen)

production as seen in hypoplastic anemia or in cases of marrow replacement by leukemic or other malignant tissue; the latter situation indicates that a platelet-destructive mechanism has developed in the patient's circulation, usually an autoantibody as in idiopathic thrombocytopenic purpura, in systemic lupus erythematosus, or in drug sensitization. In some varieties of neonatal thrombocytopenia an antibody transferred through the placenta is the pathogenetic mechanism. In microangiopathic thrombocytopenic purpura, platelets are destroyed by contact with an altered vascular bed.

Although exceedingly important for the precise definition of a thrombocytopenic disorder, the bone marrow examination is only a part of the diagnostic approach to a bleeding patient with a low platelet count. Other investigations should be done, because the first step in the therapy of thrombocytopenic purpura is to clarify as definitively as possible the mechanisms whereby the platelet count is reduced. Detailed history, physical examination, and complete blood count, besides bone marrow examination, will usually indicate (1) any evidence of other diseases to which thrombocytopenia is secondary and (2) whether the thrombocytopenia is megakaryocytic or amegakaryocytic. A precise diagnosis has prognostic as well as therapeutic implications.

IMMUNOLOGIC THROMBOCYTOPENIC PURPURA

SYNONYMS

Idiopathic thrombocytopenic purpura (ITP), Werlhof's disease.

DEFINITION AND PATHOGENESIS

Immunologic thrombocytopenic purpura is a syndrome comprising diverse entities linked together by the following characteristics: petechiae and ecchymoses in variable numbers, a low platelet count in the peripheral blood, normal to increased numbers of megakaryocytes in the bone marrow, a shortened platelet lifespan, and an immunologic pathogenesis.

Originally, all forms of ITP seemed to be idiopathic, but in recent years secondary forms have been recognized, such as those following a viral infection, drug hypersensitivity (quinine, quinidine, penicillin or others), a lymphoproliferative disorder, systemic lupus erythematosus, autoimmune hemolytic anemia, repeated blood transfusions, or other conditions. The common link in all forms of ITP is the direct or indirect demonstration that an immunologic mechanism is the cause of increased platelet destruction and therefore of the thrombocytopenia. It is logical therefore that the ITP is presently understood to signify immunologic thrombocytopenic purpura rather than idiopathic thrombocytopenic purpura, as it was originally.

ITP is a typical autoimmune disorder, i.e., a disorder in which abnormal antibodies against the patient's own platelets arise in the circulation, causing the thrombocytopenia. The constant finding of a short platelet survival in all ITP patients is an important confirmation of this hypothesis. Other major points of evidence for the autoimmune nature of ITP are as follows:

1. Plasma from patients with ITP can cause thrombocytopenia when transfused to normal persons.

2. The thrombocytopenic factor in the plasma can be adsorbed onto platelets.

3. This factor is a 7S gamma globulin.

4. It is species-specific.

5. It is active against autologous as well as isologous platelets.

6. It can be transferred through the placenta, and often the babies of mothers with either relapsed or "cured" ITP are born with thrombocytopenic purpura lasting no more than 1 to 2 weeks.

7. Acute ITP caused by hypersensitivity to drugs (quinidine, quinine, Sedormid, or others) has clinical and hematologic characteristics very similar to those of the idiopathic form, yet an antibody can here be clearly demonstrated; this antibody is drug dependent for its action, and can be evidenced by practically all the techniques available for platelet antibodies.

8. Autoimmune hemolytic anemia and systemic lupus erythematosus are, at times, associated with ITP. These are disorders in which

autoantibodies against various blood cell constituents can be clearly demonstrated; their association with ITP is in favor of the autoimmune nature of this condition.

9. The clinical picture of ITP with thrombocytopenic purpura and plentiful megakaryocytes in the bone marrow is, at times, observed in the course of chronic lymphocytic leukemia and other lymphoproliferative disorders; it is well known that autoimmune diseases are observed with increased frequency in these conditions.

10. Corticosteroids given in adequate amounts can raise the platelet count and reduce the rate of platelet destruction in about 60 per cent of patients with ITP; although this is not necessarily indicative of the autoimmune nature of ITP, it is nevertheless in favor of this hypothesis.

All the evidence for the immunologic nature of the idiopathic form of ITP is indeed convincing, but it is all indirect. There is as yet no simple and reliable in vitro test by which the antiplatelet autoantibody can be detected and quantified and its structure and characteristics studied, although presently progress is rapidly being made in this area.

How, then, can one ascertain that the thrombocytopenic purpura in a patient is due to increased platelet destruction and has an immunologic pathogenesis? The diagnosis of ITP is regularly made by exclusion. One will first have to rule out all forms of "megakaryocytic" thrombocytopenia (i.e., thrombocytopenias with normal or increased numbers of megakaryocytes in the bone marrow) that are not sustained by an immunologic mechanism. These may present with either a normal or a reduced platelet lifespan. In the former, megakaryocytes are abundant in the bone marrow but do not produce platelets efficiently (ineffective thrombocytopoiesis); in the latter, the increased platelet destruction is not caused by an immunologic mechanism. The forms of ineffective thrombocytopoiesis are rare, and these can be rapidly excluded in making the diagnosis of ITP. They include the thrombocytopenia seen in vitamin B_{12} or folic acid deficiency, the one associated with paroxysmal nocturnal hemoglobinuria (PNH), and that seen in some cases of acute leukemia or preleukemia. The nonimmunologic, megakaryocytic thrombocytopenias associated with an abnormal platelet lifespan are also well defined and can be ruled out in most patients with ITP. They include those seen in septicemia, cavernous hemangioma, microangiopathic hemolytic anemia, thrombohemolytic thrombocytopenic purpura, disseminated intravascular coagulation, "hypersplenism," and some intracorpuscular platelet disorders,

typically the Wiskott-Aldrich syndrome. In some acute phases of bacteremia or viremia the platelets may be swept up from the circulation because of adhesion to the bacteria, activation by virus, and subsequent aggregation. The other disorders all involve an altered microvasculature together with various degrees of intravascular fibrin formation, both causing a rapid platelet destruction. These disorders are not ITP. In all these disorders the thrombocytopenia occurs during the acute phase of the disease rather than a few weeks after recovery, as in ITP. Until recently, it was believed that no drug could produce thrombocytolytic thrombocytopenia on a nonimmunologic basis. Ristocetin, however, may be an exception, as it apparently has a direct toxic effect on platelets and causes shortening of their lifespan.

"Hypersplenism" may be associated with a low platelet count in the circulation and increased megakaryocytes in the bone marrow independent of the pathologic process causing the splenic enlargement. In this syndrome, thrombocytopenia is often associated with anemia or leukopenia and is caused by pooling of the platelets in the enlarged spleen, together with a mild to moderate rate of platelet destruction. No antibody is at play in "hypersplenic" thrombocytopenia.

A severe intracorpuscular platelet defect (as in the Wiskott-Aldrich syndrome) may also cause increased platelet destruction with thrombocytopenia in the peripheral blood and increased numbers of megakaryocytes in the bone marrow. These disorders are very rare, are seen in early childhood, are hereditary in character, and are usually associated with other signs and symptoms which enable us to easily distinguish them from ITP.

The diagnosis of ITP is usually made in two successive steps: (1) Bone marrow examination first shows that the thrombocytopenia is associated with normal or increased megakaryocytes in the bone marrow (megakaryocytic thrombocytopenia). This is in itself an indirect demonstration that the thrombocytopenia is caused by increased platelet destruction, and this assumption is valid in most cases. (2) Nonimmune thrombocytopenias with increased platelet destruction or abnormal platelet distribution are then ruled out, and ineffective thrombocytopoiesis is excluded.

CLINICAL MANIFESTATIONS

Acute ITP. Acute ITP is predominantly a disease of childhood, 85 per cent of the patients being under 8 years of age. About two thirds of the patients give a clear history of an antecedent infection, usually viral, occurring a week or two before the onset of purpura. In adults, the acute manifestations are more commonly associated with hypersensitivity to a drug. Acute ITP, either truly idiopathic or following a viral infection or the intake of drugs, has characteristic hallmarks: (1) a sudden onset of purpura with blood blisters on mucous membranes, (2) a very marked thrombocytopenia with normal or increased numbers of megakaryocytes in the bone marrow, (3) a very short platelet survival time, (4) a self-limited course of 1 week to a few months, and (5) no palpable spleen.

A variety of infections can be associated with acute ITP. It is usually an upper respiratory infection or an exanthematous disorder of childhood or other nonspecific viral infections. Rubella, rubeola, and varicella are most common. Most patients become cured within a period of a week to 3 months. In a few patients the disease may last up to 6 months or longer. However, in about 10 per cent of the patients it will progress to the chronic, self-perpetuating form. It should be mentioned that acute ITP occurs with more severe manifestations in adults than in children. In adults, it is often associated with gastrointestinal bleeding, hematuria, epistaxis and extensive purpura, and a fatal outcome resulting from a central nervous system hemorrhage seen in the severe cases.

Acute ITP should not be confused with the severe thrombocytopenia that is occasionally observed during the acute phase of a viral infection, that is, during the viremic period.

Chronic ITP. Chronic ITP greatly predominates in young adults. Females are affected more frequently than males, with a ratio of approximately 3:1. The following are the main characteristics: (1) an insidious onset, with a prolonged history of easy bruising and prolonged menses; (2) relatively mild bleeding manifestations; (3) a moderately low platelet count, usually ranging from 30,000 to 80,000 per cu mm; (4) moderate to severe shortening of the platelet lifespan; and (5) no significant anemia or leukopenia, and, in the idiopathic variety, no splenomegaly. Chronic ITP is a self-perpetuating disorder that may last many years with remissions and relapses. During remission, the platelet count does not usually return to normal, but remains at one third to one half the normal value. After a number of years, the disease may become milder and then disappear. In rare patients, the disease may progress slowly to a more complex variety of autoimmune disorders with arthritis, vasculitis, kidney involvement, and, occasionally, the full picture of systemic lupus erythematosus.

Chronic ITP is usually not severe enough to threaten life in most patients. The severity of the bleeding manifestations is usually related to the degree of the thrombocytopenia. Infections and vaccinations are known to exacerbate the course of the chronic disease. Age of the patient is important in evaluating the prognosis, because in the older age group episodes of intracranial hemorrhage are most common.

Intermittent ITP. Rare cases with three to five attacks of acute ITP have been described. These have usually occurred for no apparent reason or have followed a cold or other upper respiratory infection, and have lasted a few weeks to 6 months in most of these patients. During the periods of remission the platelet count has been completely normal. Several of these patients have progressed, with time, to the development of systemic lupus erythematosus.

LABORATORY FINDINGS

Thrombocytopenia is always severe in acute ITP, with platelet counts below 20,000 per cu mm in most patients. In chronic ITP, thrombocytopenia is moderate to severe, usually ranging from 40,000 to 80,000 per cu mm. Prolongation of the bleeding time is well correlated with severity of the thrombocytopenia and with the degree of purpura and other bleeding manifestations. Anemia and leukopenia are not typical of the idiopathic form, although some anemia may be found as a consequence of blood loss. Significant anemia and leukopenia usually indicate that the disorder is not idiopathic. Moderate eosinophilia is commonly seen in acute ITP and not in the chronic variety.

Bone marrow changes in ITP are limited to the megakaryocytes except for the normoblastic erythroid hyperplasia, which may be seen as the result of blood loss. Megakaryocytes are increased in number in most patients, with a relative increase of immature forms. Signs of cytoplasmic and nuclear degeneration, vacuolization, lack of granular development, and deficient platelet budding around the cytoplasmic ridge may be found.

ITP does not usually present the common findings of other autoimmune diseases, such as hypergammaglobulinemia and a low complement level. Serum acid phosphatase may be elevated because of increased platelet turnover, but this occasional finding has little diagnostic value.

The platelet lifespan is shortened in all patients with ITP, and the shortest survival curves are obtained in the acute cases.

Although there is striking and convincing evidence that ITP is an autoimmune disorder, this evidence is all indirect, because there is as yet no easily reproducible and reliable laboratory test by which the antiplatelet autoantibody can be detected and measured in the patient's serum.

DRUG-INDUCED THROMBOCYTOPENIC PURPURA (PURPURA OF DRUG HYPERSENSITIVITY)

Immunologic thrombocytopenic purpura may occur after the intake of a drug to which the patient has become sensitized. In these patients, the drug in the presence of the patient's serum causes lysis of the platelets after fixation of complement. Without complement, only agglutination occurs. This type of thrombocytolytic thrombocytopenia is, at times, very severe, and patients may succumb because of massive hemorrhage. Petechiae and ecchymoses are here often associated with gastrointestinal bleeding, epistaxis, gum bleeding, and, at times, cerebral hemorrhage. Thrombocytopenia is usually very severe, although it is typically temporary, lasting only 3 to 4 days after the patient has discontinued the offending drug. It is now clear that this type of thrombocytopenia is caused by the effect of an antigen-antibody complex adsorbed onto the platelets and that the antibody in the serum is essentially directed against the drug. In vitro tests for demonstration of the antiplatelet factor in drug-induced purpura are simple, reliable, and reproducible. Various tests are used for the diagnosis. These are based on platelet agglutination or lysis, inhibition of clot retraction, complement fixation, or liberation of platelet Factor 3 activity. The diagnosis in these patients is also made, retrospectively, from the duration of the thrombocytopenia after the drug or, preferably, after all drugs have been discontinued. Prolonged delays of more than 1 week in the rise of the platelet count is a dependable indication that drug hypersensitivity is not the cause of the thrombocytopenia.

A number of drugs capable of causing thrombocytopenic purpura on a hypersensitivity basis have been studied. These include quinidine, quinine, digitoxin, chlorothiazide derivatives, chlorpropamide, and phenylbutazone, as well as antibiotics and antihistamines. Quinidine has been implicated most frequently.

THROMBOHEMOLYTIC THROMBOCYTOPENIC PURPURA

Synonyms

Thrombotic thrombocytopenic purpura (TTP), thrombohemolytic purpura, Moschcowitz's disease.

Definition

Thrombohemolytic thrombocytopenic purpura (TTP) is an acquired hemorrhagic syndrome, usually acute in nature, characterized by a pentad of (1) hemolytic anemia with fragmented erythrocytes; (2) thrombocytopenic purpura, usually severe; (3) fluctuating and transient neurologic abnormalities; (4) renal failure; and (5) fever. These clinical manifestations are caused by widespread hyaline microthrombi within arterioles and capillaries, and by hyaline material beneath the endothelium of patent blood vessels with little or no inflammatory reaction. Electron microscopic studies have demonstrated that the hyaline thrombi are principally made of fibrin and platelet aggregates.

The cause of TTP is presently unknown, and a multiplicity of hypotheses have been suggested to explain the origin and mechanism of the vascular abnormality supposed to represent the primary lesion originating the TTP syndrome. It is possible that multiple causative factors (infections, autoimmune phenomena, others) may lead to numerous focal injuries of the small blood vessel endothelium, which, in turn, may cause activation and aggregation of platelets and consequent deposition of fibrin. Microangiopathic fragmentation of red cells with severe hemolysis and destruction of platelets with thrombocytopenia would, then, be the final result of the microvascular alterations. The recent experience that whole plasma infusion has been highly effective in the management of patients with TTP seems to imply the deficiency of a factor in the patient's plasma. It has also been observed that when platelets are suspended in plasma from patients in the active state of the disease, aggregation occurs. Presently the association of plasma infusion and antiaggregating agents seems to be the most effective therapeutic approach available.

Clinical Features

The majority of patients described in the literature have been between 10 and 40 years of age, with a peak incidence in the 30's. Females are more frequently affected than males, with a ratio of 3:2. The disease is most frequently acute in onset, and its course has usually been fatal within a few days or weeks. However, in recent years, a chronic variety has been recognized with symptoms persisting for months or, sometimes, years. Hemolytic anemia or thrombocytopenic purpura or changing neurologic abnormalities are the presenting symptoms. The latter include paresthesias, seizures, aphasia, alterations in the state of consciousness, and transient, focal neurologic abnormalities. Typically, all neurologic symptoms in TTP may fluctuate in severity and are subject to rapid change. Renal insufficiency is present in practically all patients, with oliguria, anuria, and hyperazotemia. Fever, usually severe, is often the first symptom to appear in the acute variety of the disease. The liver and spleen are slightly enlarged in most patients. Abdominal pain, at times acute, has been described in a small percentage of patients and is presumably due to microinfarcts in various abdominal organs.

LABORATORY FINDINGS

Anemia is usually severe and jaundice with increased indirect serum bilirubin is often a prominent finding. The blood smear typically shows variable numbers of distorted and fragmented red cells. Reticulocytes are increased and the bone marrow shows erythroid hyperplasia. Thrombocytopenia is another prominent finding in the peripheral blood and is associated with normal to increased numbers of megakaryocytes in the bone marrow. A neutrophil leukocytosis in the peripheral blood is regularly seen. The Coombs' test is typically negative, and no direct or indirect evidence of abnormal antibodies in the serum is ever obtained. Surprisingly, there is no evidence of disseminated intravascular coagulation. Prothrombin time, partial thromboplastin time, fibrinogen level, and plasma fibrinolytic activity are usually normal.

Proteinuria, microscopic or gross hematuria, and abnormal casts are invariably present. Blood urea nitrogen and serum creatinine are typically elevated. The electroencephalogram may or may not indicate abnormalities of any sort. Usually, however, diffuse cortical changes are seen.

The diagnosis is usually confirmed by demonstrating in a biopsy specimen of skin, muscle, lymph node, bone marrow, or surgically removed spleen the typical microthrombi of hyaline material, giving a positive periodic acid–Schiff reaction and located in the lumina of arterioles and capillaries. In a number of patients with very acute disease, these anatomic changes are seen only after death at autopsy, most commonly in the vessels of the brain, heart, pancreas, kidneys, and adrenals. The diagnosis of TTP is, on many occasions, a clinical one, made only on the basis of symptoms and laboratory findings.

DIFFERENTIAL DIAGNOSIS

The first differential diagnosis that one must take into account is that of disseminated intravascular coagulation (DIC). Not only may there also be some hemolysis in these patients, but the microthrombi seen in patients with DIC may, at times, be difficult to differentiate from the hyaline thrombi of TTP. In these patients, one must rely on the laboratory findings not indicating DIC, and on the typical syndrome of hemolytic anemia, thrombocytopenic purpura, neurologic abnormalities, renal failure, and fever. Fragmented red cells in the peripheral blood are an essential finding for the diagnosis of TTP. Their presence helps in ruling out the Evans' syndrome with hemolytic anemia and thrombocytopenic purpura and, also, paroxysmal nocturnal hemoglobinuria. The hemolytic-uremic syndrome of Gasser is a variant of TTP. It is milder, with a shorter course, and is limited to children, with complete recovery in most cases. In these and other cases bordering with TTP, one must keep in mind that microangiopathic hemolytic anemia and thrombocytopenia may occur in a variety of small blood vessel changes, of various nature and localization, and that one cannot make the diagnosis of TTP on the evidence of microangiopathic hemolysis and thrombocytopenia alone. The complete pentad mentioned earlier must be present.

QUALITATIVE PLATELET DEFECTS

More rare are the hemorrhagic disorders caused by qualitative rather than quantitative platelet defects, i.e., the thrombocytopathic purpuras. Bleeding manifestations are usually less severe in thrombocytopathic than in thrombocytopenic purpuras. A simplified scheme of platelet function in hemostasis would summarize this complex phenomenon in four major steps: *adhesion* of the platelets to the altered vessel wall, *release* of nucleotides from the platelet storage granules and uncovering of platelet Factor 3 that has coagulant activity, platelet *aggregation* with formation of the early hemostatic plug, and platelet *contraction* with retraction of thrombosthenin filaments and stabilization of the early hemostatic plug. The qualitative platelet disorders, however, cannot all be classified along this scheme of platelet function, as most of them have overlapping functional defects.

Diagnostically, qualitative platelet disorders have a few common features: the bleeding time is prolonged, whereas the platelet count is normal and clotting tests are negative with the exception of clot retraction, which is impaired. Special tests of platelet function regularly indicate mechanism and degree of the intracorpuscular platelet defect. These tests include the measurement of platelet adhesion, platelet aggregation, platelet Factor 3 availability, and clot retraction.

Qualitative platelet disorders can be classified as follows:

1. *Congenital:* Thrombasthenia; thrombocytopathies (storage pool diseases, Bernard-Soulier syndrome, Fonio's syndrome, others); platelet defects associated with heritable disorders of connective tissue (Ehlers-Danlos syndrome, pseudoxanthoma elasticum, osteogenesis imperfecta) and other congenital disorders (Wiskott-Aldrich syndrome, May-Hegglin anomaly); von Willebrand's disease.

2. *Acquired:* Drug-induced platelet dysfunctions; uremia; myeloproliferative disorders; multiple myeloma and macroglobulinemia; fibrinolysis.

CONGENITAL QUALITATIVE PLATELET DEFECTS

THROMBASTHENIA

SYNONYM

Glanzmann's disease.

DEFINITION

Thrombasthenia is a rare congenital bleeding disorder transmitted as an autosomal recessive trait. The bleeding time is prolonged and the platelets fail to aggregate during coagulation or after addition of adenosine diphosphate (ADP). The basic defect seems to reside in the platelet membrane, which is unresponsive to ADP either added in vitro in any amounts or when released by the platelets themselves after the addition of epinephrine, collagen, or thrombin.

CLINICAL FEATURES

Spontaneous bleeding manifestations are usually moderate, but at times they necessitate blood transfusions. They begin early in life. Epistaxis, menorrhagia, gum bleeding, and easy bruisability are common. Serious or fatal hemorrhage has at times occurred after surgery or after severe trauma. There is great variability in clinical manifestations from patient to patient. The bleeding tendency usually becomes less marked as the patient grows older. The disease has a worldwide distribution. Being caused by an intrinsic platelet disorder, hemorrhage in these patients can temporarily be arrested by the transfusion of freshly prepared platelets from normal donors.

LABORATORY TESTS

These are a markedly prolonged bleeding time with a normal platelet count; absent platelet aggregation by ADP, collagen, epinephrine, or thrombin but normal aggregation with ristocetin and bovine Factor VIII; reduced platelet retention in glass bead columns; and decreased or absent clot retraction.

THROMBOCYTOPATHIES

It is uncertain whether this name points to one or several diseases with similar connotations. The Bernard-Soulier syndrome with giant platelets, the Fonio syndrome with agranular platelets, cases of storage pool disease, and other types of impaired collagen-induced aggregation have all, at times, been grouped under the generic name of thrombocytopathy. In most of these patients there is a decreased platelet Factor 3 activity. It is uncertain, however, whether this is a truly fundamental defect of the platelets or only an apparent defect owing to the inability of the platelets to undergo a complete release reaction and to aggregate properly in the kaolin test or after exposure to other inducers of the release reaction.

STORAGE POOL DISEASE

Synonyms. Thrombopathia, Portsmouth syndrome.

Definition. The storage pool of ADP and serotonin may be congenitally diminished in relatively rare patients or may be quantitatively normal, but the release mechanism may be defective. These two categories of patients typically have a life-long history of easy bruising and prolonged bleeding times. When epinephrine is added to a suspension of platelets from these patients, only a primary wave of aggregation occurs, whereas the secondary, complete aggregation is missing. Other inducers of the release reaction (collagen, ADP in small doses) also produce a defective aggregation. Although these defects appear congenital, the hereditary pattern is not known. It is furthermore believed that several types of platelet disorders are manifested by these two abnormalities, either a quantitative defect of the storage pool of nucleotides or a defect in ADP and serotonin release. The only possibility to separate these two defects in the individual patient is to determine the content of the storage pool of ADP and serotonin directly. In some patients with defect in the release reaction, an exaggerated sensitivity to aspirin (in vivo or in vitro) is noted, because aspirin is a typical inhibitor of the release reaction. Aspirin taken before a surgical operation usually causes dramatic bleeding in these patients.

BERNARD-SOULIER SYNDROME

Synonyms. Giant platelet syndrome, granulopenic thrombopathy.

Definition. The Bernard-Soulier syndrome is a relatively rare hemorrhagic disorder characterized by giant platelets and a prolonged bleeding time. Clot retraction is normal as well as platelet aggregation with ADP, collagen, and epinephrine. The platelets do not aggregate in response to ristocetin and to bovine fibrinogen similarly to what happens in von Willebrand's disease. However, the Factor VIII antigen level in the patient's plasma is normal, and normal plasma cannot correct the platelet defect. An impaired adhesion of platelets to subendothelium has been found. A defect in the platelet surface membrane is suggested by the findings of an abnormal platelet electrophoretic mobility and sialic acid content.

Clinical Manifestations. The clinical picture is characterized by moderate to severe bleeding manifestations, including purpura, epistaxis, and menorrhagia as the most frequent signs. The disease manifests itself in both sexes, and transmission appears to be autosomal recessive in most cases. The platelet count is normal to slightly decreased, and the bleeding time is prolonged although clot retraction is normal. The platelets are large and, in some cases, are devoid of granules. The giant-platelet syndrome is different from the May-Hegglin anomaly, in which there are giant platelets but mild to moderate thrombocytopenia is also present and patients usually have no hemorrhagic manifestations.

WISKOTT-ALDRICH SYNDROME

The Wiskott-Aldrich syndrome is a rare disorder of male children characterized by eczema, thrombocytopenia, and repeated infections. The disease is transmitted as an X-linked recessive character. In recent years it has been realized that the disease is not always fatal in early infancy or childhood, although 69 per cent of the reported patients have died at the average age of 3 years and 2 months. Two major aspects of the disease have been more clearly defined in the past few years: (1) the immunodeficiency aspect, and (2) the mechanism of the thrombocytopenia. The complex immunologic defect involves both cellular and humoral immune responses. Antibody responses to carbohydrates and some protein antigens are almost completely absent, and natural antibodies to blood group antigens are diminished. A low level of IgM is regularly found in the serum. Delayed hypersensitivity responses as assayed by skin tests are usually absent despite the presence of normal or only slightly reduced numbers of lymphocytes in the peripheral blood. Lymphocyte blastogenesis is impaired. Such broad defect has suggested a disorder of antigen processing or recognition, that is, a disorder in the afferent limit of immunity.

Studies to elucidate the mechanism of the thrombocytopenia have been done only recently. It was shown that platelets in this disorder have severe morphologic, biochemical, and functional defects, including a shortened lifespan. Megakaryocytes are normal or increased in the bone marrow. Although normal platelets survive a normal length of time in the patients' circulation, the patients' own platelets have a limited lifespan, indicating an "intracorpuscular" platelet defect. The platelets are smaller than normal in size; α-granules, glycogen granules, and mitochondria are reduced in number. Platelet adhesiveness to glass and to collagen fibers is defective; platelet aggregation with ADP, collagen, or epinephrine is reduced or absent; particle phagocytosis by platelets is severely impaired; and platelet aerobic glycolysis fails to respond with an outburst under stimulation.

Causes of death in these patients have been mainly infections and hemorrhage. About 60 per cent of the patients have died with bacterial or viral infections of various types. Among the bleeding manifestations, cerebral hemorrhage has been the most common cause of death. A high incidence of lymphoreticular malignancies occurs in these children when they survive long enough.

VON WILLEBRAND'S DISEASE

SYNONYMS

Vascular hemophilia, angiohemophilia, pseudohemophilia, von Willebrand–Jurgens thrombopathy.

DEFINITION

Von Willebrand's disease (vWD) is a hemorrhagic disorder, inherited as an autosomal dominant character, in which there are (1) a prolonged bleeding time in the presence of a normal platelet count; (2) a decreased level of Factor VIII activity; (3) reduced platelet adhesiveness while platelet-platelet interaction, that is, platelet aggregation, is normal; (4) decreased platelet retention in glass bead columns; (5)

absence of aggregation with the antibiotic ristocetin; (6) normal plasma or cryoprecipitate normalize platelet function in vitro and arrest hemorrhage in vivo.

In conclusion, the prolonged bleeding time in vWD results from impaired adhesion of platelets to the injured vessel wall. While platelets are intrinsically normal in this disease, a plasma factor necessary for their adhesion is lacking. This factor (the von Willebrand factor) is part of the Factor VIII system. Three components have now been recognized as part of this system: (1) a clot-promoting activity, (2) Factor VIII antigen (detected by the use of heterologous antisera), and (3) von Willebrand factor that, as the rest of the Factor VIII system, is synthesized by endothelial cells and is essential for normal platelet adhesiveness, that is, for a normal bleeding time, normal ristocetin induced aggregation, normal glass bead retention of platelets, and normal adhesion of platelets to blood vessel endothelium.

In classic vWD, all three of these activities are reduced, but there are variants of the disease in which there are low levels of von Willebrand factor, but normal or near normal levels of Factor VIII clotting activity and Factor VIII antigen. If all variants are considered, vWD is probably the most common hereditary hemorrhagic disorder. Furthermore, in addition to the congenital forms of vWD, rare acquired cases have been reported that apparently result from formation of an autoantibody.

CLINICAL FEATURES

The most common and characteristic forms of hemorrhage occur in the skin and mucosae. They appear early in childhood and tend to decrease at the time of puberty and adolescence. They include ecchymoses; bleeding from the gums, usually after brushing the teeth; bleeding after tooth extraction; epistaxes; and menorrhagia. The last of these may be troublesome for years and then subside with no set pattern. Gastrointestinal hemorrhage is rare. Petechiae are also uncommon. Joint bleeding is very rare. The length of the bleeding time is no secure indication of how much a patient will bleed from a major trauma or an operation. The postoperative bleeding in these patients is unpredictable and may be very severe.

When replacement therapy is indicated, cryoprecipitates are the treatment of choice. The infusion of cryoprecipitates is followed by an increase in all three components of the Factor VIII system. However, Factor VIII-related antigen has a shorter life span in the circulation than Factor VIII procoagulant activity. Von

Willebrand factor (i.e., ristocetin cofactor) has the most rapid disappearance rate with an average half-life of approximately 18 hours requiring the frequent administration of cryoprecipitate in the bleeding patient with vWD.

LABORATORY FINDINGS

Typically the bleeding time is prolonged, the platelet count is normal and Factor VIII level is reduced. The latter is usually higher than in hemophilia A and ranges from 5 to 15 per cent in most typical cases. Ristocetin-induced platelet aggregation, measuring von Willebrand factor, is abnormal, whereas platelet aggregation with ADP, epinephrine, and collagen is normal. Platelet retention in a glass bead column is reduced.

DIAGNOSIS

In severely affected patients, von Willebrand's disease is easily recognized from the dual finding of a prolonged bleeding time and a decreased Factor VIII value in the plasma. The positive family history is one additional important feature, particularly in making the diagnosis in incomplete forms of the disease as, for example, (1) a prolonged bleeding time but normal Factor VIII level, or (2) a normal bleeding time but decreased Factor VIII level. In the former, thrombasthenia and thrombocytopathia must be ruled out by appropriate platelet aggregation studies. In the latter, mild hemophilia A is the most probable diagnosis to be first screened out. Besides the platelet retention test in a glass bead column and the ristocetin aggregation test, both positive in von Willebrand's disease, the Factor VIII response and the response of the ristocetin test to plasma transfusion provides a reliable diagnostic clue.

ACQUIRED QUALITATIVE PLATELET DEFECTS

Acquired platelet dysfunctions have been described in a variety of disorders in which abnormal bleeding is, at times, a major complication. Prolonged bleeding time and abnormal platelet aggregation are the important hallmarks of these hemorrhagic conditions, whereas the platelet count is typically normal.

DRUG-INDUCED PLATELET DYSFUNCTIONS

A number of pharmacologic agents are now known to inhibit platelet function in hemostasis. They indirectly cause abnormal bleeding owing to platelet dysfunction. At times bleeding may be serious, particularly in persons who simultaneously have other mild or severe hemostatic defects.

Aspirin in commonly used dosage will inhibit platelet function and cause prolongation of the bleeding time. Its use has been implicated as a rather frequent cause of abnormal bleeding, although the percentage of aspirin users encountering overt hemorrhagic tendency is very small. Aspirin inhibits the platelet release reaction and prevents the aggregation that normally follows. As a result, platelet aggregation induced by collagen or epinephrine is abnormal. The primary phase of ADP-induced aggregation is not inhibited by aspirin, but secondary platelet aggregation is abolished. The mechanism by which aspirin inhibits ADP release has been extensively studied. Recently, inhibition of platelet prostaglandin biosynthesis has been proposed as the mechanism by which the release reaction is inhibited. After a single oral dose of aspirin, platelet abnormalities can be detected as long as 4 to 7 days, because the effect of aspirin is irreversible. There is a basic difference in laboratory results between patients on aspirin and those suffering from a "storage pool" defect. In the latter, both first and second waves of epinephrine-induced aggregation are impaired, while in the former only secondary aggregation is suppressed.

A number of nonsteroidal anti-inflammatory drugs (phenylbutazone, indomethacin, sulfinpyrazone, and others) also inhibit the platelet release reaction and thus platelet aggregation. However, their effect on platelets is of variable duration. A safe alternative is acetaminophen (Tylenol). Other drugs causing platelet dysfunction include antihistamines, tranquilizers, antidepressants, alpha-adrenergic blocking agents, local anesthetics, and others. The vasodilator dipyridamole is used deliberately to produce the same effect and prevent thromboembolism.

Dextran and other related plasma expanders also cause prolongation of the bleeding time by interfering with platelet function. Dextran decreases platelet Factor 3 activity and platelet adhesion by coating the platelets and altering their surface charge. Antidepressants (chlorpromazine, reserpine, imipramine), adrenergic blocking agents (phentolamine), ethanol, and antihistamines are also known to affect the platelet hemostatic function. Decreased platelet adhesiveness has been found with the administration of clofibrate (Atromid-S), local anesthetics, glyceryl guaiacolate, and dipyridamole.

UREMIA

Hemorrhage is frequent and, at times, fatal in chronic uremic patients, even in those whose platelet count is normal. Gastrointestinal bleeding is most common, but epistaxes, ecchymoses, and bleeding from the gums are also encountered. More than one aspect of platelet function has been shown to be responsible for the prolonged bleeding time and the occurrence of hemorrhage in uremia. Platelet adhesiveness, platelet aggregation, and platelet Factor 3 availability have all been shown to be defective by various groups of investigators. These platelet defects are "extracorpuscular" in nature, because all these abnormalities as well as the bleeding tendency can be corrected by hemodialysis or peritoneal dialysis. Furthermore, the platelet defect can be reproduced in vitro by incubating normal platelets with uremic plasma or metabolites of urea. There is good evidence that more than one plasma factor is inhibiting platelet function in uremia. Guanidinosuccinic acid, phenol, and hydroxyphenylacetic acid have all been implicated in this effect.

MYELOPROLIFERATIVE DISORDERS

Patients with myeloproliferative disorders (hemorrhagic thrombocythemia, polycythemia vera, myelofibrosis with myeloid metaplasia, and chronic myelogenous leukemia) frequently have a moderately prolonged bleeding time and may present bleeding manifestations or bleed overtly at surgery or after trauma. Patients with severe thrombocythemia with markedly increased platelet counts (over 1,000,000 per cu mm) tend to bleed the most. The severity of hemorrhage appears to be related to the magnitude of the platelet counts. Several qualitative platelet defects have been demonstrated in myeloproliferative disorders. These include bizarre platelet morphology, abnormal platelet adhesiveness and aggregation, and decreased platelet Factor 3 activity.

MULTIPLE MYELOMA AND MACROGLOBULINEMIA

The nature of bleeding diathesis in multiple myeloma and in macroglobulinemia is often a complex one. It seems clear, however, that increased blood viscosity and qualitative platelet defects may play the principal role. Decreased platelet Factor 3 activity and abnormal platelet aggregations have been thought to be caused by the coating of the platelet surface with macromolecules. Abnormal globulins, however, may also block the interaction of plasma clotting factors.

FIBRINOGEN DEGRADATION PRODUCTS

Proteolytic cleavage of fibrin or fibrinogen by plasmin results in the formation of fibrinogen degradation products (FDP). FDP may be found increased in the circulation in various disorders such as disseminated intravasacular coagulation, excessive fibrinolysis, and massive pulmonary embolism. Some of these degradation products, particularly those produced early in the proteolytic process, have been shown to inhibit platelet aggregation and adhesion by competing with fibrinogen on the platelet membrane. Impairment of platelet function by FDP therefore may cause prolongation of the bleeding time and may play an important role in the occurrence of abnormal bleeding in these conditions.

HEMORRHAGIC DISEASES DUE TO DISSEMINATED INTRAVASCULAR COAGULATION, ACCELERATED FIBRINOLYSIS, AND CIRCULATING ANTICOAGULANTS

By ROBERT W. COLMAN, M.D.
Philadelphia, Pennsylvania

DISSEMINATED INTRAVASCULAR COAGULATION

SYNONYMS

The term consumption coagulopathy describes the utilization of certain coagulation components by the action of thrombin but ignores changes that result from in vivo clearance of activated clotting enzymes. Defibrination syndrome is too narrow, describing only changes in fibrinogen. Disseminated intravascular coagulation (DIC), with its focus on the underlying pathophysiologic event, accelerated coagulation, is the preferred and widely accepted designation.

DEFINITION

Disseminated intravascular coagulation is an acquired bleeding and thrombotic disorder occurring in a wide variety of acute and chronic disease states, characterized by accelerated systemic coagulation, and almost always accompanied by secondary fibrinolysis. The manifestations are thought to be the result of the activation of circulating procoagulants leading to consumption and clearance of certain factors and diffuse deposition of thrombi, which in turn may become lysed. A decrease in Factors I, II, V, and VIII and platelets frequently occurs. The fibrinolysis results in circulating fibrinogen split products that are potent circulating anticoagulants.

PRESENTING SIGNS AND SYMPTOMS

DIC can be suspected on clinical grounds with a high degree of accuracy. The mode of presentation is frequently an acute bleeding or purpuric diathesis associated with sepsis, hypotension, or chemotherapy of neoplasias. Less common is a thrombotic presentation. Rarely, abnormal coagulation tests alone herald the onset of DIC. Examination of the skin is of great diagnostic value in patients with DIC. Patients may show petechiae, purpura, palpable purpura, hemorrhagic bullae, acral cyanosis, gangrene, and wound hematomas.

The duration of bleeding, acral cyanosis, or thrombosis from the onset of DIC until it is clinically recognized varies from minutes to weeks.

In most cases the time from onset to diagnosis is less than 2 days. The recognition that an acquired hemorrhagic diathesis exists is often delayed in three common situations. First, the critically ill patient often has multiple catheter insertions, venipuncture sites, and surgical wounds. Oozing of blood can occur at these sites but the presence of a bleeding diathesis goes unrecognized because the hemorrhage is attributed to the wounds and catheters alone. Similarly, thrombosis of vessels is often attributed solely to the mechanical effects of catheters. Second, when the patient suffers a major hemorrhage from a local site such as a gastrointestinal tract ulcer, other sites of concomitant bleeding such as purpura or hematomas may be overlooked. A third situation that may mislead is the occurrence of acral cyanosis, which may be attributed to hypotension or sepsis alone. This combination should be recognized as a clue to the diagnosis of DIC.

DIC is always a manifestation of an underlying disease or condition. Recognition of the underlying condition may lead to the removal of the cause, the most effective treatment of DIC. The common causes are summarized in Table 1.

COURSE

The evolution of disseminated intravascular coagulation depends to a great degree on the severity and course of the underlying conditions. Thus, in some patients it may be acute but self-limiting, particularly as seen with obstetric conditions. In other patients it may present as an acute fulminant bleeding diathesis, as observed in meningococcemia. DIC may also have a chronic course, such as in disseminated malignancies. The course of DIC may be modified by treatment of the underlying disease,

Table 1. *Etiologic Classification of Disseminated Intravascular Coagulation*

A. Obstetric
    Abruptio placentae
    Septic abortion
    Retention of dead fetus
    Amniotic fluid embolism
    Saline-induced abortion
B. Surgery and Trauma
    Extensive surgery (especially thoracic and
      neurosurgery)
    Burns
    Prostatic surgery
    Liver and renal transplantation
    Mismatched transfusions
    Extracorporeal circulation
    Heat stroke
    Hypothermia
    Prolonged shock or acidosis
C. Neoplastic
    Carcinoma of the prostate
    Acute promyelocytic leukemia
    Other disseminated malignancies
    Chemotherapy
D. Infectious
    Endotoxemia (particularly meningococcemia)
    Viral diseases
    Rickettsial infections
    Malaria
E. Miscellaneous
    Snakebite
    Kasabach-Merritt syndrome
    Thromboembolism
    Purpura fulminans
    Thrombotic thrombocytopenic purpura
    Hemolytic uremic syndrome

which may effectively reverse the coagulation abnormalities and clinical bleeding. Unfortunately, many of the underlying diseases described in Table 1 carry a grave prognosis in themselves and over half of patients with DIC die in the hospital. The patients who survive have less bleeding and their coagulation profile is less abnormal at the time of diagnosis.

PHYSICAL EXAMINATION FINDINGS

The signs reflect the underlying disease. In addition, manifestations of diffuse bleeding, especially purpura and hematomas, or skin necrosis may alert the physician to the concomitant development of disseminated intravascular coagulation.

COMMON COMPLICATIONS

Besides the complications arising from the underlying disease, problems arising from DIC relate to (1) hemorrhage, (2) thrombosis, or (3) effects of treatment. Excessive bleeding, in addition to the local effects, frequently results in shock, which may, in turn, exacerbate the coagulation abnormalities. Thrombi in the glomerular capillaries give rise to renal cortical necrosis; in the adrenals, to the clinical picture of Waterhouse-Friderichsen syndrome; and in the skin, to hemorrhagic necrosis, as seen in purpura fulminans. In the absence of heparin, administration of epsilon-aminocaproic acid, a fibrinolytic inhibitor, may prevent the secondary protective fibrinolysis and thus predispose to disseminated thrombosis.

LABORATORY DIAGNOSIS

A major difficulty in the care of patients with DIC had been a lack of accepted criteria for the diagnosis of DIC and its response to therapy. Three screening tests (prothrombin time, platelet count, and fibrinogen level) and two confirmatory tests (fibrinogen degradation products [FDP] and thrombin time) are of particular usefulness (Table 2). In the presence of clinical liver disease, abnormalities in all tests accurately permit the diagnosis of DIC. When possible, serial coagulation tests, prothrombin time, platelet counts, and fibrinogen levels should be performed in patients suspected of having a disease that acutely precipitates DIC. When the coagulation tests reach levels that are diagnostic — that is, the prothrombin time is greater than 15 seconds, platelet count is less than 150,000 per microliter, or fibrinogen is less than 160 mg per dl (100 ml) — approximately 80 per cent of the patients develop bleeding or throm-

Table 2. *Laboratory Diagnosis of DIC*

	Test Criteria°	Mean Value in DIC	Per Cent Abnormal
Screening			
Prothrombin time	>15 sec	18	90
Platelet count	<150,000 μl	52,000	93
Fibrinogen	<160 mg %	137	71
Confirmatory			
Fibrinogen degradation products	>1/8	1:84	92
Thrombin time	>5 sec above control	35 sec	59

°Criteria are set two standard deviations from normal mean values. For diagnosis one needs three screening tests abnormal or two screening tests and one confirmatory test abnormal. For patients with significant liver disease, more stringent criteria are needed: Prothrombin time, >25 sec; platelets, <50,000, and fibrinogen, <125, FDP >1/64.

bosis. In addition, usually when the coagulation tests begin to change in the direction predicted by the diagnosis of DIC, the prothrombin time will often become prolonged by more than 5 seconds, platelet count falls by as much as 200,000 per microliter, and the fibrinogen falls by an average of 150 mg per dl. These changes constitute dynamic evidence of the presence of DIC.

When only two of these three tests were abnormal, causes other than DIC were often found. For example, plasma or whole blood transfusions given during surgery might result in an elevation of the prothrombin time and a decrease of the platelet count, since blood kept in a bank for more than several days is deficient in platelets and Factor V. Thus, to establish the diagnosis of DIC when only two screening tests are positive, at least one confirmatory test must be positive. The most useful assay is FDP, since a positive titer was found in almost all of the patients. The thrombin time is positive in patients with more severe DIC but can be prolonged also when the fibrinogen level is less than 75 mg per 100 ml.

The diagnosis of DIC in the bleeding patient with liver disease poses special problems. In uncomplicated cirrhosis, tests measuring the state of the fibrinolytic system may be abnormal even though there is no clinically significant hemostatic abnormality. Patients with cirrhosis who are not bleeding appear to be in a state of compensated subclinical DIC. The half-life of fibrinogen is decreased by about one third and this abnormality is corrected by heparin. Since the usual criteria for clinically significant DIC appear not to be applicable, additional criteria have been applied. In these, values must be more than two standard deviations from the mean of uncomplicated cirrhosis to be considered diagnostic, thus the prothrombin time must be greater than 25 seconds, a platelet count less than 50,000 per microliter, or a fibrin-

ogen of less than 160 mg per dl, and the FDP titer greater than 1:64. We have found that these additional criteria permit the identification of most cases of clinically significant DIC in the presence of cirrhosis.

PERIPHERAL BLOOD

Examination of the peripheral blood smears may reveal the existence of thrombocytopenia or suggest a disease such as promyelocytic leukemia thought to be associated with DIC. In addition, in a minority of patients, severe abnormalities in red blood cell morphology such as are seen with microangiopathic hemolytic anemia may support the diagnosis of DIC, since fibrin deposits themselves have been shown to fragment red cells. The absence of schistocytes or helmet cells does not make the diagnosis less likely.

BONE MARROW

The bone marrow morphology is not specific for this disorder. Since platelets and to some extent red cells are rapidly destroyed, compensatory hyperplasia of their precursors may be found in the bone marrow. Certain underlying diseases such as leukemia or metastatic carcinoma may be revealed for the first time. If the cause of DIC is well established, a bone marrow examination may not be necessary.

THERAPEUTIC TRIALS

Although heparin therapy is indicated in selected cases of DIC, response to heparin may be coincidental with the resolution of the underlying disease. As a consequence a therapeutic trial of heparin is not indicated.

ACCELERATED FIBRINOLYSIS

SYNONYM

Pathologic fibrinolysis.

DEFINITION

Pathologic fibrinolysis is an acquired hemorrhagic disorder characterized by excessive systemic activation of the components of the fibrinolytic system. Most of the recognized cases of pathologic fibrinolysis are associated with DIC. Isolated pathologic fibrinolysis appears to be rare, except during the administration of urokinase or streptokinase. The bleeding diathesis is a consequence of consumption of clotting Factors II, V, VIII, and fibrinogen and of the anticoagulant effects of fibrinogen-split products (FSP). Concentrations of other coagulation factors are decreased, owing to hepatic clearance of activated clotting proteins. Nevertheless, the coagulation defect is isolated fibrinolysis such as occurs in fibrinolytic therapy and may be less severe than that in DIC, since the platelets as well as Factors II, IX, and X are unaffected. Localized fibrinolysis occurs in prostatic surgery and acute renal allograft rejection usually without systemic changes.

CLINICAL MANIFESTATIONS

The symptoms, signs, and complications are identical to those of DIC. If pathologic fibrinolysis is severe, the thrombotic complications of the latter are less frequent.

LABORATORY FINDINGS

There is so much overlap between the effects of consumption coagulopathy and those of pathologic isolated fibrinolysis that the laboratory distinction is difficult. Unlike in DIC or in therapeutic fibrinolysis (urokinase or streptokinase), the platelet count is normal.

THERAPEUTIC TEST

Epsilon-aminocaproic acid (Amicar), an inhibitor of the fibrinolytic system, has been recommended as a therapeutic test. Its use should be discouraged, since permanent thrombi and vascular occlusion may result from interference with fibrinolysis in the usual case due to coexisting DIC.

CIRCULATING ANTICOAGULANTS

SYNONYMS

Acquired anticoagulants, circulating inhibitors.

DEFINITION

These conditions are acquired disorders caused by circulating antibodies directed against coagulation proteins. The manifestations result from inhibition of the normal sequence of events leading to the formation of a fibrin clot. The conditions most commonly observed are the development of an inhibitor in Factor VIII or the appearance of a circulating antibody (lupus anticoagulant) directed against "prothrombinase," the enzymatic complex that converts prothrombin to thrombin. Instances of inhibitors of other specific clotting factors have been reported but are rare. The inhibitors of Factor VIII can be observed under four different circumstances: (1) in patients with congenital Factor VIII deficiency following multiple tranfusions; (2) in young women up to 2 years postpartum; (3) in elderly, previously healthy individuals; and (4) in patients with systemic lupus erythematosus.

PRESENTING SIGNS AND SYMPTOMS

The signs and symptoms of an acquired Factor VIII inhibitor relate to the occurrence of spontaneous bleeding, including hemarthroses, in a patient without previous hemorrhagic manifestations and may take any form, including hematomas and mucous membrane bleeding. In the case of the lupus anticoagulant, the patient is asymptomatic and generally a laboratory analysis is needed.

COURSE

The anticoagulants seen in patients with lupus erythematosus correlate with the severity of the disease and usually disappear if remission is obtained. Whereas the antiprothrombinase inhibitor usually does not represent a major hemostatic impairment, the Factor VIII antibodies may give rise to a severe clinical problem. In the hemophiliac with an acquired antibody to Factor VIII, resistance to Factor VIII infusions is evident. The inhibitor titer frequently increases with transfusion therapy; conversely, if transfusions are withheld, the titer usually decreases. In postpartum or elderly patients with Factor VIII antibodies, the anticoagulant may disappear within a few months to several years.

LABORATORY DIAGNOSIS

Factor VIII antibodies result in a prolonged PTT but a normal PT, whereas antiprothrombinase may affect both these tests, the PTT more than the PT. If an inhibitor is suspected, a simple mixing experiment will serve to confirm it: equal volumes of patient's plasma and normal plasma will result in correction of the abnormal test in the case of a clotting factor deficiency. In contrast, the test will remain abnormal if an inhibitor is present. This test is more sensitive for Factor VIII antibodies if the PTT is performed after the mixtures are incubated at 37 C (98.6 F) for 1 hour. In order to define the specific inhibitor, individual clotting factor assays are recommended. In this way an inhibitor specific for Factor VIII may be identified and its exact titer quantified. For the hemophilic patient who also develops an inhibitor, assays to assess the corrective effect of normal plasma or Factor VIII concentrates in vitro are performed. On the basis of these tests, the amount of Factor VIII needed to overcome the inhibition can be estimated. The antiprothrombinase can be confirmed by studies using dilutions of tissue thromboplastin in the prothrombin time, which makes the test more sensitive to this type of inhibitor.

OTHER LABORATORY TESTS

Tests to substantiate or rule out the diagnosis of lupus or related disorders are important, since their treatment of these disorders will influence the circulating inhibitor.

THERAPEUTIC TESTS

The differential diagnosis between a clotting factor deficiency and an inhibitor may be substantiated by infusing plasma or clotting factor concentrates. When an adequate dose fails to correct the abnormality, the presence of an inhibitor is confirmed if the patient is not actively bleeding and the preparation is proved to be active when assayed in vitro.

PITFALLS IN DIAGNOSIS OF ACQUIRED BLEEDING DISORDERS

1. Laboratory coagulation abnormalities may be produced artificially by poor venipuncture technique, high hematocrit (resulting in high citrate and low calcium concentration) and prolonged storage before assay.

2. Inadequate investigation may mislead — for example, congenital hypofibrinogenemia may present as DIC.

3. Heparin therapy temporarily aggravates coagulation abnormalities, although it may reverse the deficit eventually.

4. Liver disease makes the diagnosis of DIC difficult.

Section 8

DISEASES OF THE DIGESTIVE SYSTEM

NON-NEOPLASTIC LESIONS OF THE ORAL MUCOSA

By JERRY E. BOUQUOT, D.D.S., M.S.D.
Morgantown, West Virginia

INTRODUCTION

The oral mucosa is as adept in its reflection of systemic disease as it is varied in its production of local disease that may or may not eventually extend beyond the mouth. While a few systemic diseases with potential presenting signs on oral mucosa are discussed in this article, emphasis has been placed on the presentation of mucosal lesions somewhat unique to or commonly seen within the oral cavity. Much, and occasionally all, of diagnosis of such entities is based upon close visual and tactile inspection with special consideration of the intraoral site and the age of the patient; for the final diagnosis of oral complaints, relatively few sophisticated laboratory aids are required.

Lesions of the oral mucosa typically fall into one of the following broad categories: white plaques or macules, red or pigmented lesions, soft tissue masses, ulcers, and vesicles or bullae. It has long been established that the diagnosis of such lesions is much more dependent on an understanding of their potential clinical presentations than on a knowledge of their various causes. The entities following, therefore, have been listed and discussed in groups according to their most common presenting features in an attempt to aid the clinician in arriving at a rapid definitive or differential diagnosis. For disease entities not listed or for oral malignancies, the reader is referred to the article on Premalignant and Malignant Lesions of the Mouth or to readily available textbooks in oral pathology or oral diagnosis.

WHITE LESIONS (SLOUGHING)

CANDIDIASIS

SYNONYMS

Moniliasis, thrush, acute pseudomembranous candidiasis, candidosis, superficial monilial stomatitis.

DEFINITION

Candidiasis is an acute or chronic superficial infection of oral or other mucous membranes by the dimorphic yeast-like fungus *Candida albicans. Candida albicans* can be cultivated from most healthy individuals, and only under conditions of altered host resistance is its virulence enhanced enough to produce local, regional, or systemic manifestations of disease.

PRESENTING SIGNS AND SYMPTOMS

Candidiasis is found most frequently in patients at either extremity of the age spectrum, presenting usually as curd-like, white plaques that can be scraped off to leave a raw, painful, bleeding surface. Mild cases demonstrate fine, whitish papule-like deposits on an erythematous base, while severe cases showing invasion of deeper tissues are characterized by a more tenacious pseudomembrane or ulceration or both. Neonatal oral candidiasis, derived from a maternal vaginitis, usually becomes evident on the fifth to sixth postpartum day. Adult infections are typically promoted by dry mouth, aging, poor denture hygiene, antibiotic therapy, diabetes mellitus, pregnancy, cunnilingus, and lowered body resistance owing to such conditions as malabsorption, primary immune deficiencies, systemic malignancy, corticosteroid therapy, uremia, and various chronic nonfungal infections. An inherited syndrome of candidiasis, Addison's disease, and hypoparathyroidism has been described. The presence of candidal conjunctivitis and paronychial involvement of the nails of the hands is not necessarily indicative of systemic involvement, as direct spread of the fungus may be facilitated by hand-to-mouth and subsequent hand-to-eye contact.

CLINICAL COURSE AND COMPLICATIONS

In most otherwise healthy persons, oral candidiasis is a self-limiting disease that may produce intermittent or continuous burning sensations, tenderness, and/or pain for years if left untreated. The medication of choice is topical nystatin. The curd-like pseudomembranes may not always be prominent but can be replaced by a symptomatic erythema or a nonsloughing white plaque. Oral candidiasis in a debilitated patient tends to become deep-seated and to spread to the gastrointestinal and respiratory tracts, necessitating systemic therapy with amphotericin B.

LABORATORY AIDS

The most sensitive diagnostic procedure for oral candidiasis is the microscopic identification of pseudohyphae and spores via smears stained by a 10 per cent solution of potassium hydroxide; such a smear will seldom be positive in normal individuals. The organism is cultured on Sabouraud's agar, but a positive culture must be viewed with suspicion as this microorganism can be cultured from a large percentage of healthy mouths. Tissue sections from biopsy may show pseudohyphae or spores when processed with a fungal stain such as MacManus periodic acid–Schiff, (PAS), but such sections more often than not will be completely and frustratingly negative. An effective, albeit slow, diagnostic technique is a 4 to 8 week course of nystatin vaginal tablets (100,000 units dissolved in mouth 4 times daily) or oral suspension (less effective) for those patients with strictly oral manifestations and no underlying systemic process.

MATERIA ALBA

SYNONYMS

Plaque, food debris.

DEFINITION AND APPEARANCE

Materia alba is surprisingly often mistaken for the previously mentioned oral candidiasis because it presents as single or multiple curd-like white plaques on oral membranes. In reality, it is simply a mixture of food debris and bacteria, and is understandably most frequent in persons with poor oral hygiene. Unlike candidiasis, materia alba leaves a nontender, nonerythematous mucosal base after being removed by a tongue blade or with gauze.

ASPIRIN BURN

SYNONYMS

Chemical burn, contact burn.

PRESENTING SIGNS AND SYMPTOMS

The most frequent chemical burn in the mouth is caused by direct application of an aspirin tablet to an aching tooth. Other cases may result, however, from the dentist or physician inadvertently applying caustic medications to the mucosa. The clinical appearance of such lesions depends on the severity of tissue damage. Mild cases will produce a tender erythema, whereas more severe burns undergo necrosis and coagulate the surface of the tissue to produce a diffuse white plaque that can be scraped off to leave a painful, bleeding, erythematous surface.

CLINICAL COURSE AND COMPLICATIONS

Unless treated with a protective paste (Orabase), warm salt water rinses, and a bland diet, these lesions may provide 3 to 4 weeks of oral pain before healing (usually without scarring) and occasionally become secondarily infected. With palliative therapy most cases resolve within 7 to 12 days. Esophageal strictures may result if enough caustic was swallowed, but this is seldom the case except with small children who swallow household cleaners.

SECONDARY SYPHILIS

SYNONYM

Mucous patch.

PRESENTING SIGNS AND SYMPTOMS

Mucous patches are smooth-surfaced white plaques with a glistening, opalescent character; they may or may not scrape off easily and are usually painless. These lesions are single or few in number, usually seen on the tongue, lips, or soft palate 6 to 10 weeks after initial infection. Hoarseness, dysphagia, fever, swollen tonsils, and maculopapulary skin rash are other easily identifiable features that may be present. All moist lesions of secondary syphilis are extremely contagious.

CLINICAL COURSE AND COMPLICATIONS

Intraoral lesions of secondary syphilis persist for 1 to 3 weeks, after which they resolve without scar formation.

LABORATORY AIDS

A smear examined with darkfield microscopy will demonstrate motile spirochetes. The reader is referred to the syphilis article in this book for suggested approaches to the laboratory diagnosis of this disease.

WHITE LESIONS (NONSLOUGHING)

LEUKOPLAKIA

SYNONYMS

Benign hyperkeratosis, oral callus, linea alba, white patch, keratosis.

DEFINITION

While "leukoplakia" may, in fact, show microscopic dysplasia and be considered a premalignant entity, many physicians and dentists now use the term in a strictly clinical sense to refer to a keratotic white patch that cannot be scraped off and cannot be given another, more specific name. Many leukoplakias are nothing more than calluses formed in response to chronic trauma from the teeth or dental appliances. They typically appear as well-defined, painless, smooth-surfaced, nonindurated white plaques of variable thickness adjacent to a source of chronic mechanical irritation. They are usually quite small, even though they may have been present for several years. *Linea alba* is a thin keratotic line located bilaterally on the cheek mucosae and following the bite plane of the teeth.

CLINICAL COURSE AND COMPLICATIONS

The callus or nonpremalignant forms of leukoplakia are clinically indistinguishable from the premalignant forms, but the callus types will disappear upon removal of the causative ragged tooth or overextended denture. Any leukoplakia that has not disappeared within 4 to 6 weeks of the removal of a mechanical irritant should be considered premalignant and followed accordingly. The reader is referred to the article on oral premalignant and malignant lesions for further discussion of those aspects of leukoplakia.

NICOTINE PALATINUS

SYNONYMS

Nicotine stomatitis, smoker's palate, nicotinic palatal leukokeratosis.

PRESENTING SIGNS AND SYMPTOMS

Heavy tobacco smokers, especially pipe and cigar smokers, will usually develop a slight but diffuse grayish white appearance to the hard palate. With time, this appearance often alters to that of a thick, fissural, painless, white patch of the entire hard palate. Small red depressions with elevated white keratotic halos are an almost constant feature of the more severe cases of this nicotine palatinus, representing the inflamed ductal orifices of the numerous mucous glands of the palate. If a patient is a denture wearer, the lesions will be confined to mucosa not covered by the denture base. Patients are predominantly middle-aged and elderly males and may present with keratotic white plaques elsewhere in the mouth or throat.

CLINICAL COURSE AND COMPLICATIONS

With cessation of the smoking habit, nicotine palatinus will diminish rapidly and many lesions will completely disappear within 4 to 8 weeks. While this entity is, in fact, a form of smoker's leukoplakia and was for that reason once thought to be premalignant, it must be strongly emphasized that this is no longer considered to be the case; that is, nicotine palatinus is *not* considered now to be a precursor to oral malignancy. This is an anatomic-site diagnosis and prognosis: smoker's keratoses elsewhere in a patient's mouth *are* considered premalignant.

LABORATORY AIDS

Smears are useless relative to this entity. Biopsy will demonstrate nonspecific hyperkeratosis with minimal dysplasia, but nicotine palatinus is so characteristic clinically that microscopic evaluation is usually not necessary.

TOBACCO POUCH

SYNONYMS

Snuff pouch, snuff keratosis, snuff dipper's lesion.

PRESENTING SIGNS AND SYMPTOMS

Chronic tobacco or snuff chewers will often develop a well-circumscribed white or grayish white, opalescent fissured plaque of the vestibular mucosa of the area in which they habitually place their tobacco or snuff. This lesion often has a soft velvety feel, and further palpation of tobacco chewers will usually reveal a distinct "pouch" caused by the chronic stretching of the cheek muscles in the area. No erythema, ulceration, or pain is associated with this lesion, and it usually takes at least 5 to 10 years to become manifest.

CLINICAL COURSE AND COMPLICATIONS

Tobacco pouches may gradually show a thick, white leathery surface, but most remain unchanged for decades. While it is rare for a malignancy to develop from such lesions, when this does occur the cancer produced is most likely to be a verrucous carcinoma. This is a unique form of low-grade epithelioma that may locally enlarge for years without metastasis.

LABORATORY AIDS

Biopsy will show hyperkeratosis or intracellular edema, or both, of superficial epithelial layers; however, the characteristic clinical appearance combined with a history of tobacco or snuff chewing usually precludes the necessity of microscopic evaluation. Biopsy is definitely indicated for any ulceration or tumefaction, as these may show early malignancy.

LEUKOEDEMA

PRESENTING SIGNS AND SYMPTOMS

This condition most often presents as a filmy opalescence or a whitish gray wrinkling of the entire cheek mucosa bilaterally. It shows a racial predilection for blacks, is not associated with smoking or chronic irritation, and is usually manifest during young adulthood; there is no ulceration, erythema, or pain associated with it.

CLINICAL COURSE AND COMPLICATIONS

Once manifest, this "variation of normal anatomy" remains constant throughout life. There is no malignant potential.

LABORATORY AIDS

Smears are of no value. Biopsy will show characteristic hyperkeratosis or intracellular edema, or both, of superficial epithelial layers, but microscopic evaluation is usually not necessary because of the characteristic clinical appearance.

WHITE SPONGE NEVUS

SYNONYMS

Cannon's disease, congenital leukokeratosis, familial white folded dysplasia of mucous membranes, oral epithelial nevus.

PRESENTING SIGNS AND SYMPTOMS

This inherited disorder results from defective tonofibrils and typically presents as white or opalescent grayish white corrugated plaques of the buccal, gingival, oral floor or lingual mucosae. The lesions may be congenital or appear as late as puberty and may occasionally be found on mucosa of the esophagus, vulvae, vagina, anus, rectum, and nose.

CLINICAL COURSE AND COMPLICATIONS

The condition persists unchanged throughout life. There is no malignant potential.

LABORATORY AIDS

Buccal smears show paranuclear and perinuclear condensation of cytoplasm. Biopsy demonstrates marked spongiosis of the epithelium and is rather characteristic.

DIFFERENTIAL DIAGNOSIS

Many of the following entities are not discussed in this article, but all involve oral lesions similar to white sponge nevus and should therefore be ruled out before a final diagnosis is made: hereditary benign intraepithelial dyskeratosis (Witkop's disease), leukoedema, pachyonychia congenita, dyskeratosis congenita, Darier's disease, and chronic cheek bite.

CHRONIC CHEEK BITE

SYNONYMS

Cheek and lip biting, marsicatio buccarum, chronic lip bite.

PRESENTING SIGNS AND SYMPTOMS

Nervous individuals will occasionally develop a habit of sucking and "chewing" on their cheeks or lips, resulting in a macerated hyperkeratosis that is a white, often corrugated plaque with erythematous patches representing erosions or areas where the patient has peeled off the keratin layer of the epithelium. This condition is especially present in college and graduate students but may be seen at any age. The lesion is often bilateral on the cheeks and occasionally small hematomas may be seen.

CLINICAL COURSE AND COMPLICATIONS

This lesion will become more severe during times of increased stress and will otherwise persist as long as the habit persists. It has absolutely no tendency to develop into cancer. The lesion will disappear if the patient abandons the habit.

LABORATORY AIDS

Smears are not helpful, and biopsy will show nonspecific spongiosis and hyperkeratosis; therefore, neither technique is recommended.

LICHEN PLANUS

SYNONYM

Lichen ruber planus.

DEFINITION

Lichen planus is a rather common skin disorder of unknown cause. Up to 40 per cent of lichen planus patients, however, manifest oral mucosa lesions and many patients present with *only* oral lesions.

PRESENTING SIGNS AND SYMPTOMS

A variety of keratotic white patterns may occur on the oral mucosa of patients with lichen planus: reticular, annular and/or plaque-like lesions are most often seen on the buccal mucosa. Occasional patients will also demonstrate erythematous areas of erosion, ulceration, atrophy, or blister formation. The typical patient is a middle-aged woman who is "nervous," and while the cheeks are the most likely site, any oral membrane may be affected. A metallic taste or a burning sensation may accompany the oral lesions; the ulcers and bullae, when present, are painful. Skin lesions, when present, are small bluish-silver, flat-topped plaques or nodules that tend to coalesce or scale or both. Fine grayish lines (Wickham's striae) may be present on the surface of skin lesions, and pruritus may be prominent. The genital mucosa may also be affected.

CLINICAL COURSE AND COMPLICATIONS

Oral lesions may follow or precede skin lesions of lichen planus or may be the only lesions ever to develop. Once present, the lesions may last for months or years. The erosive or bullous forms, especially, tend to last a lifetime. If the disease does disappear in time, the patient should be informed that recurrences are common. Squamous cell carcinoma has occasionally developed in a preexisting lichen planus lesion, especially of the erosive or bullous type.

LABORATORY AIDS

The clinical manifestations of this disease are often so specific that no further testing need be performed. If such is not the case, however, biopsy of the oral keratotic areas will provide a definitive microscopic diagnosis demonstrating a band-like lymphocytic infiltrate of the lamina propria, hydropic degeneration of the basal cell layer, and hyperkeratosis.

LUPUS ERYTHEMATOSUS

DEFINITION

Lupus erythematosus, a so-called "collagen disease" of unknown etiology, is a multisystem disease that may be system-wide or may affect only a few tissues. Rather characteristic oral lesions may be the first presenting signs, but the reader is referred elsewhere in the book for a detailed discussion of extraoral aspects of this disease (page 1123).

PRESENTING SIGNS AND SYMPTOMS

Systemic and discoid lupus erythematosus present oral manifestations that are quite similar, although oral involvement is much more common with the systemic type. Oral lesions may present as erythematous papules, plaques, or ulcerations covered by a nonspecific white membrane, but more typically they present as rounded, well-circumscribed, slightly elevated white plaques (with a reticular or radial appearance) on an erythematous base. Centrally located areas of atrophy or ulceration are occasionally seen. Such oral lesions are usually painless and found most frequently on the lips, buccal mucosa, and palate. Palatal petechiae and gingival hemorrhage may be later signs of lupus erythematosus in the mouth. Patients treated with chloroquine or hydroxychloroquine may show a diffuse, brownish-black pigmentation of palatal mucosa.

CLINICAL COURSE AND COMPLICATIONS

White oral lesions may last for years; ulcerative and atrophic oral lesions heal in weeks or months with a tendency toward scar formation. There may be an increased tendency for patients with discoid lupus erythematosus to develop squamous cell carcinoma within lip scars.

LABORATORY AIDS

Biopsy of an intraoral white lesion of lupus erythematosus may be definitively diagnostic of the disease, but this is often not the case, especially with the systemic variant. Characteristic microscopic findings would include liquifactive degeneration of basal cells, atrophy, and mild hyperparakeratosis of the epithelium, and a marked cellular infiltrate of lymphocytes and plasma cells beneath the epithelium, in addition to vasculitis and a fibrinoid degeneration of perivascular and subpapillary connective tissue. The fibrinoid degeneration and a thickened basement membrane stain positively with the PAS stain. Deposits of immunoglobulins and complement and the basement membrane zone in oral lesions have been demonstrated as areas of granular fluorescence. IgM and complement are most frequently found, IgG less frequently, and IgA rarely.

FORDYCE GRANULES

SYNONYM

Fordyce's disease.

PRESENTING SIGNS AND SYMPTOMS

The heterotopic, usually nonfunctioning, sebaceous glands are seen in about 80 per cent of the population as numerous, small, yellowish white papules or superficial granules of the buccal mucosa, labial mucosa, and retromolar pad area. They are typically bilateral and asymptomatic and occasionally present a cauliflower appearance from coalescence of many glands (called sebaceous adenomas by some authorities). Rarely, patients will complain of altered taste, presumably secondary to sebum extrusion.

CLINICAL COURSE AND COMPLICATIONS

Fordyce granules increase in number until puberty or shortly thereafter, with no change after body growth stops. Because clusters of these glands may appear as nodular white plaques, they are occasionally mistaken by the patient or physician as carcinoma, but they are, in fact, completely benign and have no tendency to undergo malignant transformation.

LABORATORY AIDS

Most cases are so characteristic clinically that no further testing is necessary; however, biopsy showing normal sebaceous glands with or without ductal attachment to the overlying mucosal epithelium will provide a definitive diagnosis.

HAIRY TONGUE

SYNONYMS

White hairy tongue, black hairy tongue, yellow hairy tongue.

DEFINITION

Hairy tongue is a harmless elongation of the filiform papillae of the tongue to such lengths that they resemble hair. The condition is thought to be provoked by irritation from poor oral hygiene, antibiotic therapy, habitual use of oxidizing agents in oral preparations, and systemic disease debilitation. Chromogenic bacteria, food debris, tobacco, coffee, radiotherapy, and various coloring agents in medications and candies alter the normally white hairy tongue to a yellow, brown, or black appearance.

PRESENTING SIGNS AND SYMPTOMS

Numerous long, thin, white or discolored hairlike papillae are found on the dorsum of the tongue, especially toward the posterior aspect. Pain is not usually a feature, unless secondary infection by Candida albicans occurs, but the hairs may be long enough to produce a gagging problem. Alteration of taste may be present.

CLINICAL COURSE AND COMPLICATIONS

The condition is self-limiting and eliminated by treating the underlying systemic problem, eliminating the causative medicaments, and/or brushing the tongue daily.

LABORATORY AIDS

This entity is usually so characteristic clinically that further testing is unnecessary; however, biopsy or scrapings will reveal hyperkeratinized elongated papillae and bacterial aggregates.

GEOGRAPHIC TONGUE

SYNONYMS

Benign migratory glossitis, glossitis areata migrans, wandering rash.

PRESENTING SIGNS AND SYMPTOMS

This rather common disorder is of unknown cause and typically presents on the dorsum and lateral surfaces of the tongue as irregularly shaped red patches and white patterns resembling a map. The erythematous patches represent areas of desquamated filiform papillae and are usually surrounded by a small white rim of sloughed keratocytes and necrotic debris. The pattern of the lesions continuously changes and the "map" noticed initially may be completely altered within a week's time. The condition is unusual in children, and usually asymptomatic unless secondarily involved with Candida albicans or a limited bacterial infection. Similar changing lesions have recently been reported on vestibular mucosae.

CLINICAL COURSE AND COMPLICATIONS

The changing patterns of geographic tongue may persist for years with no detrimental effect. Spontaneous remissions and recurrences may be observed. While the tongue involved in such a disorder can look quite unusual, there is no tendency for malignant transformation.

LABORATORY AIDS

None.

BROWN-BLACK PIGMENTED LESIONS

PHYSIOLOGIC PIGMENTATION

SYNONYM

Racial pigmentation, Negroid pigmentation, melanoplakia.

PRESENTING SIGNS

Dark-complexioned people, especially blacks, frequently have single or multiple non-blanching brown macules of various configurations and sizes on the oral mucosa. Such pigmented macules are most frequently found on the gingivae, but buccal and palatal and labial mucosae are sites of lesser predilection.

CLINICAL COURSE AND COMPLICATIONS

The lesions are present from childhood and should not be changing size in an adult; there is no malignant transformation potential.

LABORATORY AIDS

Biopsy will show melanin pigment within the basal cell layer of the epithelium, but this technique is usually not required because the clinical appearance is so often diagnostic.

ORAL MELANOTIC MACULE

SYNONYM

Ephelis, freckle, lentigo, oral melanosis.

PRESENTING SIGNS AND SYMPTOMS

Single, nonblanching, brown macules on the oral mucosa of whites are an extremely rare phenomenon that can affect any site and are made manifest in middle-aged and older persons. They are usually painless, less than a centimeter in greatest diameter, well circumscribed, of the same consistency as normal mucosa, and of fairly recent onset.

CLINICAL COURSE AND COMPLICATIONS

Oral melanotic macules seem to reach their full maturity rapidly and then remain unchanged indefinitely. The major dilemma for the clinician lies in the fact that developing malignant melanomas are clinically similar or even indistinguishable from this benign macule. Excisional biopsy, therefore, of all doubtful lesions is strongly recommended.

LABORATORY AIDS

Biopsy will show melanin pigment within the basal cell layer of the epithelium as well as within histiocytes of the lamina propria.

AMALGAM TATTOO

SYNONYM

Amalgam pigmentation.

PRESENTING SIGNS AND SYMPTOMS

Abrasion of oral membranes during tooth preparation will allow dental amalgam particles to be entrapped within the soft tissues producing a smooth, irregularly outlined brown-black, nonblanching macule. Patients are often completely unaware of the initiating traumatic episode. The majority of amalgam tattoos will demonstrate radiopaque particles on radiographs. Graphite, dirt, or asphalt may produce a similar lesion if traumatically introduced into oral soft tissues.

CLINICAL COURSE AND COMPLICATIONS

The pigmented area remains unchanged after its initial appearance; the particles will not work their way to the surface, as with many other entrapped foreign bodies. The major problem is the occasional inability to differentiate between this entity and early malignant melanoma.

LABORATORY AIDS

Radiographs may detect the metal particles producing this lesion, otherwise a biopsy is required to microscopically reveal them. These particles are birefringent and seldom show evidence of a surrounding inflammatory reaction. The particles are usually not found within histiocytes, but are rather seen to be deposited along reticulum fibers.

PEUTZ-JEGHERS SYNDROME

SYNONYMS

Familial polyposis, intestinal polyposis II, periorofacial lentigines and visceral polyposis.

DEFINITION

Peutz-Jeghers syndrome is an inherited disorder with two main features: (1) mucocutaneous melanotic pigmentation and (2) benign intestinal polyposis.

PRESENTING SIGNS AND SYMPTOMS

All patients with this syndrome present with numerous small brown-black or blue-gray pigmented macules of the lips and 90 per cent have buccal mucosa macules, but any oral membrane may be involved. About half of the patients will have similar pigmented macules on the skin around the facial orifices. The pigmentation usually appears in infancy, which is usually a decade or more before the hamartomatous polyps appear in the intestines. Rarely, the pigment is present without polyps.

CLINICAL COURSE AND COMPLICATIONS

The skin pigmentation tends to fade somewhat after puberty, but this is not true for the intraoral macules. The oral lesions do not develop into malignancy. Intussusception, colicky pain, and melena may result from the intestinal polyps; a few cases of malignant transformation of these benign polyps have been reported.

LABORATORY AIDS

Biopsy of the skin or oral macules will show melanin pigmentation of the basal cell layer, but this technique is usually not necessary because the clinical appearance is so characteristic. Examination of the gastrointestinal tract by proctoscopic and roentgenographic means is recommended.

DIFFERENTIAL DIAGNOSIS

The following disorders may also present with multiple pigmented macules of the oral mucosa and should be ruled out before a final diagnosis is made: Addison's disease, Albright syndrome, drug ingestion (chloroquine), argyria, secondary syphilis, malignant melanoma, multiple melanotic macules (freckles), physiologic pigmentation.

RED MUCOSAL LESIONS

MEDIAN RHOMBOID GLOSSITIS

SYNONYM

Cherry patch tongue.

PRESENTING SIGNS AND SYMPTOMS

This anomaly typically presents as a painless, smooth or nodular red area (0.5 to 2.5 cm) in the posterior midline of the tongue. The red appearance is caused by the loss or lack of normal lingual papillae in the area. As this entity is seldom reported in children, current speculation implicates *Candida albicans* as a causative agent. The condition results in inflammatory or degenerative changes. Rarely, the surface may be white and keratinized or may be painful.

CLINICAL COURSE AND COMPLICATIONS

These lesions generally persist for years or a lifetime after diagnosis. Treatment with nystatin will reduce any tenderness but will not diminish the erythematous patch appreciably.

LABORATORY AIDS

While usually unnecessary, a biopsy of the area will provide an accurate diagnosis.

LINGUAL VARICOSITIES

SYNONYMS

Caviar tongue, phlebectasia linguae.

PRESENTING SIGNS AND SYMPTOMS

Oral varicosities, or distended veins, are a very common occurrence in older persons and typically present as superficial, painless, bluish blebs or tortuous vessels on the ventral surface of the tongue. These lesions blanch to palpation, are usually bilateral, are occasionally seen on the lip mucosa, and occasionally are grouped so densely as to mimic a hematoma or hemangioma. Phleboliths may be palpated or radiographically visualized.

CLINICAL COURSE AND COMPLICATIONS

Lingual varicosities slowly increase with age, but the rate is such that problems rarely develop, even in persons with numerous phleboliths.

LABORATORY AIDS

None are needed.

PAPILLARY HYPERPLASIA OF THE PALATE

SYNONYM

Palatal papillomatosis, inflammatory papillary hyperplasia.

DEFINITION

This is an inflammatory tissue response to chronic infection, probably by *Candida albicans,* beneath a full or partial denture.

PRESENTING SIGNS AND SYMPTOMS

Papillary hyperplasia is invariably confined to the palate and conforms to the patient's denture-bearing areas. Typical lesions consist of multiple red, edematous nodules, each of which is about 1 to 2 mm in diameter. The nodules often crowd together so as to appear clinically alarming. Tenderness or hemorrhage or both are occasional features, as are occasional white keratosis or fibrosis or both of long-standing lesions. About 10 per cent of denture wearers have papillary hyperplasia of the palate, especially those who do not remove their dentures at night. Occasionally, a case will be seen in a patient who does not wear dentures.

CLINICAL COURSE AND COMPLICATIONS

The condition persists indefinitely and tissue may become more fibrous, but a dramatic return to normal is often seen in those patients who are willing to forego wearing their dentures for 4 to 8 weeks. While this lesion can appear clinically aggressive, it has no tendency toward malignant transformation, a concept that is contrary to the implications in the older literature.

LABORATORY AIDS

While this entity is usually so clinically distinctive as to preclude further testing, a biopsy will show a characteristic microscopic appearance of multiple inflammatory, edematous polyps with pseudoepitheliomatous change.

ANGULAR CHEILITIS

SYNONYMS

Angular cheilosis, perlèche.

DEFINITION

This entity consists of erosions and fissures of the labial commissures secondary to *Candida albicans* infection, poor denture construction, vitamin B complex deficiency, and other factors.

PRESENTING SIGNS AND SYMPTOMS

As people age, they will tend to develop a skin fold at the corners of the mouth (commissure area), which is constantly moistened by saliva. The area eventually may become eroded, cracked, or macerated. Tenderness and a burning sensation are common complaints.

CLINICAL COURSE AND COMPLICATIONS

This is generally a chronic or recurrent condition that will not improve unless the initiating factor is removed.

LABORATORY AIDS

Smears for *Candida albicans* identification are used.

DENTURE SORE MOUTH

SYNONYMS

Denture-related candidiasis, denture stomatitis, chronic atrophic oral candidiasis.

DEFINITION

Denture sore mouth is an inflammatory atrophy of palatal mucosa secondary to trauma and candida overgrowth beneath a poorly fitting denture, especially one left in overnight during sleep.

PRESENTING SIGNS AND SYMPTOMS

The mucosa beneath the upper denture is fiery red and slightly edematous with possible petechiae or a burning sensation or both. The patient will have had the denture for some time and may also show evidence of other infection by *Candida albicans* (e.g., papillary hyperplasia of the palate, smooth and red tongue, angular cheilitis, and generalized burning sensation of all oral membranes). Rarely, the white curd-like manifestation of candida will be present.

CLINICAL COURSE AND COMPLICATIONS

Without treatment with nystatin, tissue conditioners, and improved denture hygiene, this inflammatory process will remain indefinitely.

LABORATORY AIDS

Smears for *Candida albicans* identification may be tried but are less successful than with acute pseudomembranous candidiasis.

XEROSTOMIA

SYNONYMS

Dry mouth.

DEFINITION

Xerostomia is not a disease but a nonspecific clinical condition of decreased salivation leading to minimal washing and lubrication effect for the oral tissues. A wide variety of underlying systemic conditions may produce xerostomia, including numerous drugs, sialadenitis, Sjögren's syndrome. Mikulicz's disease. Heerfordt's syndrome, hereditary ectodermal dysplasia, head and neck radiotherapy, diabetes mellitus, anemias, vitamin A deficiency, and simple aging.

PRESENTING SIGNS AND SYMPTOMS

Xerostomia patients often complain of soreness, burning, and pain of the oral membranes, which appear very atrophic and erythematous. The tongue often demonstrates a marked loss of papillae in addition to erythema and burning. Increased susceptibility to caries, intolerance to dentures, and speech or mastication difficulties are common features. Secondary infection by *Candida albicans* may produce angular cheilitis and more intense pain.

CLINICAL COURSE AND COMPLICATIONS

Unless the underlying causative factors are corrected, xerostomia will remain a problem indefinitely and the patient is forced to use artificial saliva.

INFECTIOUS MONONUCLEOSIS

SYNONYMS

Glandular fever, kissing disease.

DEFINITION

Infectious mononucleosis is a febrile condition affecting the lymphoreticuloendothelial system and the blood, and is probably caused by the Epstein-Barr and other viruses. The reader is referred to the article on the disease in this book for discussion of extraoral involvement.

PRESENTING SIGNS AND SYMPTOMS

Oral lesions of infectious mononucleosis may be the first indication of the disease. They include palatal petechiae, sore throat, tender and hemorrhagic gingivae, tonsillitis, ulceration of oral and pharyngeal membranes and/or generalized oral tenderness and redness. Cervical nodes are usually enlarged and tender.

CLINICAL COURSE AND COMPLICATIONS

Oral and pharyngeal involvement usually resolves within 5 to 14 days of onset.

DIFFERENTIAL DIAGNOSIS OF PALATAL PETECHIAE

Since palatal petechiae are an early and very characteristic sign of this disease process, the clinician should be aware of the fact that several other conditions will produce a similar phenomenon (e.g., measles, hemophilia, leukemia, severe cough, purpuras, fellatio trauma, hereditary hemorrhagic telangiectasia, and Fabry's disease).

ORAL ULCERS

TRAUMATIC ULCER

SYNONYMS

Denture sore spots.

PRESENTING SIGNS AND SYMPTOMS

This very common oral ulcerative lesion may be induced by mechanical, chemical, or thermal trauma and presents as a quite painful ulcer or crater with a clear or usually white pseudomembrane base and a red inflammatory halo of the surrounding mucosa. The size of the ulcer varies according to the severity of the trauma and there may be multiple lesions present at one time. Denture sore spots appear 1 to 7 days after placement of a new prosthesis and may be nothing more than a painful area of erythema. Ulcers on the vermilion border of the lips usually have a crusted surface because of the absence of saliva. Cervical lymphadenitis is common.

CLINICAL COURSE AND COMPLICATIONS

Most traumatic ulcers heal uneventfully within 7 to 10 days, but ulcers in areas that are continually receiving trauma may take 3 to 5 weeks or more to heal. Oral ulcers of longer duration should be biopsied, especially if nonpainful.

LABORATORY AIDS

There are none; biopsy will show only nonspecific inflammation and ulceration.

APHTHOUS ULCERS

SYNONYMS

Canker sores, aphthous stomatitis, recurrent aphthous stomatitis, minor aphthous ulceration.

DEFINITION

This is a common, self-limiting but recurring ulcerative condition of oral mucosa of unknown cause, but a host of theoretical causative factors, including trauma, psychologic stress, bacteria, autoimmunity, endocrine dysfunction, and allergy, have been postulated.

PRESENTING SIGNS AND SYMPTOMS

Patients are often aware of a burning sensation in the affected mucosa during the prodromal stage; the mucosa becomes focally erythematous, then necrotic. Lesions are usually single or few in number and tend to recur with or without identifiable irritating factors. The typical lesion is a round to oval, very painful ulceration between 3 to 10 mm in diameter with a grayish white fibrinous base and a red inflammatory halo around the periphery. These lesions are especially prominent on the lip, cheek, and tongue mucosae and occasionally reach 2 to 2.5 cm in diameter.

CLINICAL COURSE AND COMPLICATIONS

The ulcers heal without scarring in 10 to 14 days; recurrences may continue indefinitely at 1 to 12 episodes annually. Severe involvement may produce lymphadenitis, fever and/or malaise and the pain may make eating quite difficult.

LABORATORY AIDS

Culturing scrapings from an aphthous ulcer will prove nonproductive because of contamination by large numbers of bacteria normal to the oral environment. Biopsy will show only nonspecific ulceration.

MAJOR APHTHOUS STOMATITIS

SYNONYMS

Sutton's disease, periadenitis mucosa necrotica recurrens. Mikulicz's aphthae, recurrent scarring aphthae.

PRESENTING SIGNS AND SYMPTOMS

The individual oral ulcers in this nonhereditary condition of unknown cause are similar to routine aphthous ulcers except that they may be larger, deeper, and more numerous, and they tend to heal with scar formation. Remissions are short, and it is not unusual for a new ulceration to appear before a previous one has healed. Onset of these painful ulcers can take place at any age but is more common around puberty. Occasional involvement of laryngeal or genital mucosae has been noted.

CLINICAL COURSE AND COMPLICATIONS

The ulcers heal with scarring in 1 to 4 weeks, but continual recurrences are the rule and secondary infection of the ulcerations is a potential problem.

LABORATORY AIDS

A leukocyte and differential count will rule out agranulocytosis and neutropenia; biopsy is very nonspecific and not recommended.

SYPHILITIC CHANCRE AND GUMMA

SYNONYM

Lues, primary and tertiary syphilis.

PRESENTING SIGNS AND SYMPTOMS

The oral chancre of primary syphilis develops at the inoculation site 12 to 40 days after sexual contact. The lesion is a painless, round to oval clean-based indurated ulcer that usually begins as a nodule; if located on the lip, the lesion often has a crusted surface. Painless swelling of regional lymph nodes is common, and occasionally multiple chancres are seen. The oral chancre is an extremely contagious lesion.

The tertiary lesions of oral syphilis involvement consist of indurated and keratotic syphilitic glossitis or painless gummatous infiltration or both of the palate and tongue and occasional other oral sites. The gummas undergo necrosis to form sharply outlined punched-out ulcers that may have a granular appearance to their bases; they are usually single lesions and are not considered contagious.

CLINICAL COURSE AND COMPLICATIONS

Oral chancres heal without scarring within 2 to 4 weeks. Oral gummas heal with occasional scarring after several months; palatal gummas may perforate the bony palate before healing occurs. Syphilitic glossitis is considered to carry a malignant transformation rate of 25 to 30 per cent.

LABORATORY AIDS

The reader is referred to the article on syphilis elsewhere in the text. Biopsy should be performed on oral gummas in order to rule out squamous cell carcinoma, tuberculosis, histoplasmosis, blastomycosis, lethal midline granuloma, Wegener's granulomatosis, sarcoidosis, necrotizing sialometaplasia, and other chronic ulcerative-nodular disease entities.

BEHÇET'S SYNDROME

SYNONYMS

Behçet's disease, cutaneomucouveal syndrome, recurrent genito-oral aphthosis and uveitis with hypopyon.

DEFINITION

Behçet's syndrome is composed of the triad of aphthous stomatitis, genital ulcerations, and recurrent uveitis with hypopyon; its cause is unknown. Not all components of the syndrome are present at any given time.

PRESENTING SIGNS AND SYMPTOMS

The oral ulcers of Behçet's syndrome resemble typical aphthous ulcers with a painful, white, pseudomembrane ulcer base surrounded by an erythematous halo. They are often the initial sign of the disease, which typically affects young adults, especially males. These ulcers extend into the pharynx or esophagus, resulting in dysphagia.

CLINICAL COURSE AND COMPLICATIONS

This syndrome is characterized by a tendency to recur, often several times annually. Joint, cutaneous, neurologic and gastrointestinal complications are not uncommon.

LABORATORY AIDS

There are none.

CYCLIC NEUTROPENIA

DEFINITION

Cyclic neutropenia is a possibly inherited defect of early hematopoietic stem cells that manifests as periodic decreases of neutrophilic leukocytes in the peripheral blood. Clinical disease appears and regresses spontaneously according to the altering leukocyte count.

PRESENTING SIGNS AND SYMPTOMS

Cyclic neutropenia presents orally as multiple shallow ulcerations (with or without erythematous rimming) and severe ulcerative gingivitis that leads to alveolar bone loss or premature periodontitis. The gingivitis and ulcerations typically recur every 3 to 4 weeks and persist for 5 to 8 days before healing; these recurrences correspond to depressions in the leukocyte count, and healing occurs as these counts return to normal. Mild fever, malaise, otitis media, headache, joint pain, and sore throat are often present during neutropenic episodes.

CLINICAL COURSE AND COMPLICATIONS

The disease lasts throughout life, although spontaneous improvement in adulthood has been occasionally reported. Early loss of dentition from periodontitis is common.

LABORATORY AIDS

Hematologic examination may have to be repeated weekly until a depression or complete absence of neutrophils is noted in peripheral blood. Biopsy of oral ulcers shows them to be agranulocytic, but this is not necessarily diagnostic.

AGRANULOCYTOSIS

SYNONYMS

Malignant neutropenia, agranulocytic angina.

DEFINITION

Agranulocytosis is an acute disease characterized by marked leukopenia and most often occurs as a cytotoxic sensitivity response to a wide variety of drugs.

PRESENTING SIGNS AND SYMPTOMS

The lowered resistance to infections seen in agranulocytosis leads to typical ulcerative lesions of the gingiva and buccal or palatal mucosae or both. The lesions are well defined with a gray-brown to yellow-green base and are without erythematous periphery. The patient complains particularly of sore throat and dysphagia, and regional lymph nodes may be enlarged. Gingival ulceration and necrosis are commonly seen.

CLINICAL COURSE AND COMPLICATIONS

Oral lesions of this disease tend to worsen continually as long as the leukopenia persists untreated; periodontal involvement may lead to loosening of teeth and sequestration of alveolar bone. Secondary infection may lead to a fatal outcome.

LABORATORY AIDS

The hemogram shows a marked decrease or complete absence of mature granulocytes. The reader is referred to the agranulocytosis article for more detail.

NECROTIZING ULCERATIVE GINGIVOSTOMATITIS

SYNONYMS

Vincent's disease, trench mouth, fusospirochetal infection, acute necrotizing ulceromembranous gingivitis.

DEFINITION

Necrotizing ulcerative gingivostomatitis is an acute or subacute gingival inflammation of young adults probably caused by a combination of vibrios, hemolytic streptococci, certain viruses, and poor oral hygiene.

PRESENTING SIGNS AND SYMPTOMS

This disease, with its marked predilection for males in their early twenties, is characterized by tender, swollen, red gingival papillae that rapidly undergo painful ulceration, producing almost pathognomonic punched-out erosions of these papillae. The free gingiva becomes covered with a gray pseudomembrane, while pain, tenderness, and bleeding cause great difficulty in eating. Halitosis (fetor ex ore) and excessive salivation are marked, as is regional lymphadenitis. Low-grade fever, headache, and malaise are common. The condition may spread to the pharynx or other oral sites if the patient's resistance is low.

CLINICAL COURSE AND COMPLICATIONS

With treatment the condition subsides within 48 hours; without treatment it can continue for months or lead to septicemia, cancrum oris (noma) or death in debilitated patients. Spontaneous remission and healing also may occur in 1 to 3 weeks. Recurrences are common.

LABORATORY AIDS

The diagnosis is made clinically, but peripheral blood will show a mild leukocytosis with a relative lymphomonocytosis. Microscopic demonstration of fusobacteria or spirella is of no value because they may normally be found in the mouth.

VESICLES AND BULLAE

MUCOCELE

SYNONYMS

Mucus retention phenomenon, mucus retention cyst, ranula.

DEFINITION

A mucocele is a subepithelial pooling of mucus resulting from the traumatic rupture of a salivary gland duct. Occasionally, obstruction of such a duct results in distention and subsequent epithelial-lined cyst formation without the escape of mucus into connective tissues. When the large ducts of the sublingual or submandibular glands are involved, ranula is the term used for the resultant oral floor lesion.

PRESENTING SIGNS AND SYMPTOMS

A mucocele usually appears suddenly on the lower lip mucosa as a soft, fluctuant, transparent or blue "blister" of 2 to 10 mm in diameter. The lesions are occasionally tender, occasionally multiple, and have a characteristic history of disappearing after rupture only to reappear several hours to several weeks later. The ranulas of the oral floor are large, often displacing an entire side of the floor; they tend to be more painful than their smaller counterparts on the lips, and they are often associated with pain and enlargement during or after meals.

CLINICAL COURSE AND COMPLICATIONS

Recurrences are common unless the causative salivary gland is removed surgically. Occasionally a small mucocele will become transformed into a pyogenic granuloma and subsequently sclerose into an irritation fibroma.

LABORATORY AIDS

Biopsy will demonstrate pools of mucus within a fibrovascular connective tissue with mild sialadenitis of adjacent salivary glands.

EPIDERMOID CYST

SYNONYMS

Epidermal cyst, dermoid cyst, epidermoid inclusion cyst.

PRESENTING SIGNS AND SYMPTOMS

Epidermoid or dermoid cysts of the mouth are usually located in the floor and are typically sessile or somewhat pedunculated yellow-white painless nodules, 2 to 8 mm in diameter. The thinness of the overlying mucosa often imparts a semitransparent, cystic appearance to these lesions that is reminiscent of pustules. While young adults most frequently present with these cysts, no age is exempt.

CLINICAL COURSE AND COMPLICATIONS

Most epidermoid cysts of the mouth remain small and innocuous indefinitely. Occasional deep-seated lesions of the oral floor will reach the size of an egg and may interfere with speech and swallowing.

LABORATORY AIDS

Biopsy will show a keratin-filled cyst lined by mature stratified squamous epithelium with or without skin appendages.

HERPES SIMPLEX, PRIMARY AND SECONDARY

SYNONYMS

Acute herpetic gingivostomatitis, herpetic stomatitis, recurrent herpes simplex, herpes labialis, fever blisters, cold sores.

DEFINITION

This is an acute vesicular infection by the herpes simplex ectodermotropic virus, a virus that belongs in the common group with that of herpes zoster, chickenpox, and probably cytomegalic inclusion virus. *Herpes hominus* type 1 produces oral and paraoral lesions and is pantropic in affected newborn infants, while *Herpes hominus* type 2 produces genital disease (herpes genitalis). The primary attack, or herpetic gingivostomatitis, usually occurs in early life, although clinical disease is seldom severe enough to be called to the attention of a parent or physician. Regardless of whether the primary infection is clinical or subclinical, recurrent (secondary) herpetic lesions develop later in many persons; it has been estimated that up to 90 per cent of the adult population are carriers of the virus.

PRESENTING SIGNS AND SYMPTOMS

Primary infection with *Herpes hominus* type 1 occurs between 1 and 5 years of age and is characterized by multiple vesicular eruptions of the gingival, labial, and buccal mucosa that rupture rapidly, leaving painful raw or yellow-white pseudomembranous erosions with red inflammatory halos. There is considerable gingival swelling, halitosis, and increased salivation with frequent yellow crusting of the vermilion border of the lips. Systemic involvement includes high fever, irritability, dehydration, malaise, headache, dysphagia, and regional lymphadenitis.

Recurrent herpes simplex (herpes labialis) almost invariably presents as multiple and coalescing clear vesicles at the vermilion border of the lips. These painful vesicles rapidly rupture, becoming covered with a yellow-brown crust, but for 1 or 2 days before their formation the patient is often aware of a tingling or burning sensation in the area. Recurrences generally are quite self-limiting and occur at the same sites; rarely, intraoral recurrent herpes is noted on the gingiva or hard palate. Regional lymphadenitis and fever are absent in recurrent disease. A variety of stimuli may precipitate recurrent herpes simplex, including fever, respiratory infection, sunlight, nonspecific gastroenteritis, food allergy, menstruation, or mechanical trauma.

CLINICAL COURSE AND COMPLICATIONS

Primary herpes simplex heals spontaneously without scarring within 10 to 14 days. Recurrence of the primary form is extremely rare, and when occurring in older patients, should lead to a suspicion of leukemia or an immunodeficient condition. Recurrent herpes simplex is self-limiting and lesions heal without scar formation within 4 to 15 days.

Complications of infection by herpes simplex virus are numerous and varied. Herpetic meningoencephalitis or generalized herpes simplex of the newborn infant, characterized by central nervous system and visceral involvement, commonly is fatal. Eczema herpeticum (Kaposi's varicelliform eruption) is a herpetic infection of a primary eczema, is most often seen in infants and young children and may terminate fatally. Herpetic conjunctivitis may produce edema and hyperemia of the palpebral conjunctiva, keratitis, corneal ulceration, and vesicles of the eyelids. Inoculation herpes simplex is a primary form of the infection that is most often seen on the fingers of dentists, physicians, and dental hygienists who have examined patients with clinical disease.

LABORATORY AIDS

Late in the course of a primary herpes simplex infection the antiherpes antibody titer is elevated; this is noted earlier in secondary infections. Paul's test, inoculation of an affected patient's saliva onto a rabbit cornea, will produce typical dendritic keratitis within 24 to 48 hours. A biopsy of an intact vesicle or a smear of a ruptured lesion demonstrates characteristic cells with ballooning degeneration, multinucleation, or the presence of eosinophilic intra-nuclear inclusions (Lipschütz bodies), but such cells can also be seen in herpes zoster and varicella vesicles.

HERPANGINA

SYNONYMS

Aphthous pharyngitis, Coxsackievirus group A infection.

PRESENTING SIGNS AND SYMPTOMS

Herpangina, produced by group A and B Coxsackieviruses, is limited to the soft palate and oropharynx in children; extension anteriorly is rare. After a 2 to 9 day incubation period the disease presents with rapid onset of sore throat, fever, malaise, headache, muscle ache, and cervical lymphadenitis. The clinical findings in the mouth and pharynx significantly aid diagnosis, presenting as fewer than a dozen small reddish vesicles of the soft palate, uvula and fauces, usually painful, symmetrical, and rapidly ruptured.

CLINICAL COURSE AND COMPLICATIONS

The disease usually resolves in 2 to 6 days; rarely, acute parotitis, meningitis, or hemolytic anemia may result.

LABORATORY AIDS

Herpangina is usually distinctive enough to be diagnosed clinically; however, serologic tests for virus-neutralizing and complement-fixing antibodies may be performed. The virus can be isolated from hamsters or mice after inoculation of scrapings from the ruptured vesicles.

HAND-FOOT-AND-MOUTH DISEASE

SYNONYM

Aphthous fever.

PRESENTING SIGNS AND SYMPTOMS

This acute, contagious infection, caused by several coxsackieviruses, almost invariably occurs in children and produces lesions with a pathognomonic distribution oral cavity, hands, and feet. The virus has an estimated incubation period of 2 to 6 days; a subfebrile stage and mild malaise are common. The oral lesions are located primarily on the lips and buccal mucosa, sparing the posterior mouth and oropharynx. Initial lesions are red papules 2 to 10 mm in diameter, which become gray-white vesicles within 1 or 2 days; total numbers of mucosal and skin vesicles range from 20 to 100, with only 5 to 10 in the mouth. After the vesicles rupture, painful ulcers with white or gray pseudomembranous bases remain. Regional lymphadenitis is rare.

CLINICAL COURSE AND COMPLICATIONS

Spontaneous healing of all lesions occurs within 1 to 2 weeks.

LABORATORY AIDS

This disease is usually diagnosed clinically; however, complement fixation and inoculation of guinea pigs or suckling mice may be used for isolation and diagnosis of the virus. Smears from ruptured vesicles may demonstrate intracytoplasmic eosinophilic inclusion bodies.

ERYTHEMA MULTIFORME

SYNONYMS

Erythema multiforme exudativum, Stevens-Johnson syndrome, ectodermosis erosiva pluriorifacialis.

DEFINITION

Erythema multiforme is a dermatologic disorder that is probably a hypersensitivity reaction and is often, but not invariably, precipitated by allergens such as antibiotics and viruses, especially the herpes simplex virus. Infection or initial drug intake might precede erythema multiforme by 1 to 3 weeks.

PRESENTING SIGNS AND SYMPTOMS

This disease usually is seen in young adults, and a variety of skin and mucosal lesions are found, often on a single individual. Upper respiratory tract infection, fever, malaise, and arthralgia may be early features. Typical oral lesions consist of erosions and bullae that rapidly burst to leave large, painful ulcerations with white pseudomembranous bases. Although any oral membrane may be affected, the lips are almost constantly affected, often producing a thick hemorrhagic crusting. Skin lesions may be bullae, solid macules, or target-like macules (pathognomonic, if present); occasionally oral

lesions are seen without skin manifestations. Severe involvement of skin, oral mucosa, conjunctival mucosa, and genital mucosa, with a tendency toward leukopenia, is known as Stevens-Johnson syndrome.

CLINICAL COURSE AND COMPLICATIONS

This disease runs its course in 2 to 5 weeks and recurrences are uncommon. Once there is recurrence, however, the patient may suffer periodic bouts for a decade or more. Rarely, a fulminating course, complicated by secondary infection, may lead to a fatal outcome.

LABORATORY AIDS

The diagnosis is made on the basis of clinical information. A microscopic examination of a bullous lesion will generally show the bulla to be subepithelial, thereby ruling out pemphigus vulgaris, but biopsy is otherwise nonspecific.

PEMPHIGUS VULGARIS

DEFINITION

Pemphigus vulgaris is an autoimmune dermatologic disorder of middle-aged and older individuals, especially those of Jewish extraction.

PRESENTING SIGNS AND SYMPTOMS

Oral lesions are invariably present during the course of the disease and often precede the development of skin lesions by several years. The typical oral and skin lesions are bullae of varying sizes that rupture rapidly to leave painful ulcers with gray-white pseudomembranous bases. These bullae tend to arise from clinically normal skin or mucosa and, in fact, may be produced on normal surfaces by lateral pressure or friction (Nikolsky's sign). Eye and genital mucosae tend to be spared in the early stages of this disease, as opposed to erythema multiforme or benign mucous membrane pemphigoid.

CLINICAL COURSE AND COMPLICATIONS

The disease becomes more severe at varying rates, with or without spontaneous remissions and exacerbations. Long-term systemic steroid therapy usually controls the disease; if left untreated, it progresses to death resulting from dehydration, septicemia, or cachexia toxicity.

LABORATORY AIDS

Biopsy of skin or oral bullae will reveal intra-epithelial blister formation immediately above the basal cell layer. Smears of intraoral bullae may demonstrate detached acantholytic epithelial cells with characteristically enlarged, hyperchromatic nuclei (Tzanck cells). Antibodies against the epithelial cells of the skin or oral mucosae can be found in vivo in the intercellular cement regions or circulating in the blood. Direct or indirect immunofluorescent procedures will demonstrate binding of IgG and complement to the cell membranes of the spinous epithelial layer.

BENIGN MUCOUS MEMBRANE PEMPHIGOID (BMMP)

SYNONYMS

Pemphigoid, mucous membrane pemphigoid, cicatricial pemphigoid.

DEFINITION

BMMP is a chronic, nonfatal autoimmune disorder of middle-aged and elderly persons that resembles bullous pemphigoid except that its lesions have a strong predilection for mucous membranes.

PRESENTING SIGNS AND SYMPTOMS

BMMP is characterized by bullous lesions of the oral, conjunctival, and genital mucous membranes. The oral bullae are usually few in number and may last for 1 to 2 days before rupturing to leave slightly tender ulcerations with white-gray pseudomembranous bases. Erythema of the oral mucosa is a constant feature, often persisting for several weeks after the ulcers have healed. The eye erythema and bullous formation are found on both bulbar and palpebral conjunctivae and, unlike the oral lesions, tend to heal with scarring (symblepharon or synechiae formation). Occasionally, skin, pharyngeal, laryngeal, esophageal, nasal, and anal lesions are noted. Oral lesions usually precede those of the conjunctiva or genitalia.

CLINICAL COURSE AND COMPLICATIONS

This disease follows a protracted course characterized by periods of exacerbation and remission. Individual oral lesions heal without scarring within 2 to 4 weeks, but repeated conjunctival involvement may lead to corneal cloudings, loss of cilia, and cicatricial fibrous bands. The major complication of this disease is entropion with blindness in about 30 per cent of patients with uncontrolled lesions.

LABORATORY AIDS

Biopsy reveals subepithelial bullous formation that is nonspecific but does rule out pemphigus vulgaris. Antibasement membrane antibodies in serum can be detected and direct immunofluorescence demonstrates that immunoglobulins and complement are bound to the epithelial basement membrane.

SOFT TISSUE MASSES

PYOGENIC GRANULOMA

SYNONYMS

Granuloma pyogenicum, proud flesh, pregnancy tumor, hormonal tumor, epulis granulomatosum (if developing in tooth socket).

DEFINITION

Pyogenic granuloma is a common type of inflammatory hyperplasia in the mouth or on the skin. It is essentially exuberant overgrowth of granulation tissue in response to local trauma or infection. These growths are especially common in a tooth socket after recent extraction and in the later stages of pregnancy, in which they may be multiple and associated with prominent gingivitis. Puberty and birth control medications may produce lesions similar to those seen in pregnancy.

PRESENTING SIGNS AND SYMPTOMS

The lesions typically present as soft, painless, ulcerated, easily bleeding polypoid masses with broad bases. They usually are quite vascular in appearance but the necrotic surface areas are often covered by a white, sloughing pseudomembrane that resembles pus, hence the "pyogenic" terminology. Pus is seldom, however, a feature of this lesion. Pyogenic granulomas may occur at any age, being especially prone to occur in young adults and to females.

CLINICAL COURSE AND COMPLICATIONS

While these lesions often have an alarmingly rapid onset, may become 2 cm or more in diameter, and commonly recur after conservative surgical removal, they have no malignant potential. Pyogenic granulomas of pregnancy

(pregnancy tumors) are especially known for their dramatic diminution in size postpartum; more typically, pyogenic granulomas tend to fibrose with time, eventuating in typical irritation fibromas.

LABORATORY AIDS

Biopsy will be diagnostic, showing marked neocapillary proliferation, edema, and inflammatory cells of both the acute and chronic types.

PERIPHERAL GIANT CELL GRANULOMA

SYNONYMS

Peripheral giant cell reparative granuloma, peripheral giant cell tumor, giant cell epulis, epulis granulomatosum (if developing in a tooth socket).

DEFINITION

Peripheral giant cell granulomas are common inflammatory hyperplasias of the mucoperiosteum, and by definition, therefore, must arise on the gingival tissues or from a tooth socket. The exact cause of this entity is unknown, but appears to be local trauma or infection.

PRESENTING SIGNS AND SYMPTOMS

These lesions are typically deep red, easily bleeding, painless, often ulcerated, and usually nodular polyps or broad-based masses on the gingiva of middle-aged persons, especially women. Unlike pyogenic granulomas, they do not tend to be multiple, are not more common in pregnancy, and occasionally become 4 to 5 cm in diameter, but clinical resemblance to pyogenic granulomas is otherwise remarkable. Peripheral giant cell granulomas may form palpable and radiographically visible bone deep in their bulk. Occasionally a peripheral lesion is contiguous with its intraosseous counterpart, the central giant cell granuloma.

CLINICAL COURSE AND COMPLICATIONS

After a rapid onset, these lesions become quiescent and may eventually diminish in size and fibrose into a typical irritation fibroma. Because of the deep periodontal origin of peripheral giant cell granulomas, they have an even greater recurrence tendency than pyogenic granulomas, but malignant transformation has not been reported.

LABORATORY AIDS

Biopsy will be diagnostic, showing numerous multinucleated giant cells scattered throughout a cellular connective tissue stroma. Large, multiple, or actively recurring lesions should lead the clinician to check the patient's serum calcium, phosphorus, and alkaline phosphatase levels, as peripheral giant cell granulomas are clinically and microscopically indistinguishable from the "brown tumors" of hyperparathyroidism.

IRRITATION FIBROMA

SYNONYMS

Inflammatory fibrous hyperplasia, traumatic fibroma, fibrous epulis, fibroepithelial polyp.

DEFINITION

Irritation fibromas are very common inflammatory hyperplasias of fibrous connective tissue in response to acute or chronic mechanical trauma or infection. Several oral lesions gradually fibrose and are transformed into irritation fibromas — e.g., mucoceles, pyogenic granulomas, and peripheral giant cell granulomas — but more commonly the lesions are firm and fibrous from their early stages.

PRESENTING SIGNS AND SYMPTOMS

Irritation fibromas are typically firm, nonhemorrhagic, nontender polypoid masses of the buccal, labial, or other mucosal surfaces. They are usually smooth-surfaced and of normal coloration, but may be lobulated and may be white from keratinization of the surface. While they occasionally reach 3 to 4 cm in diameter, the great majority are less than a centimeter in diameter.

CLINICAL COURSE AND COMPLICATIONS

These lesions grow slowly and growth stops as they mature. There is no malignant potential and recurrence after conservative surgical removal is uncommon.

LABORATORY AIDS

Biopsy will be diagnostic, showing densely collagenic connective tissue covered by a normal mucosal epithelium.

DENTURE HYPERPLASIA

SYNONYMS

Epulis fissuratum, denture injury tumor, inflammatory fibrous hyperplasia.

DEFINITION

This common oral lesion is an inflammatory hyperplasia of fibrous connective tissues resulting from the chronic inflammation or mechanical irritation or both caused by ill-fitting dentures.

PRESENTING SIGNS AND SYMPTOMS

Denture hyperplasias are typically elongated, firm, nonhemorrhagic, nontender folds of tissue located along the edge of a loose-fitting denture; several redundant folds may be present. While they are usually of normal coloration, acute trauma or superimposed inflammation may produce an erythematous and ulcerated surface. Similar folds of fibrous tissue occur on the crest of an alveolus that has undergone marked bone resorption. Occasionally, leaf-shaped hyperplasias occur under the denture base, and these may produce a bony concavity in the palate owing to pressure atrophy of palatal bone.

CLINICAL COURSE AND COMPLICATIONS

Denture hyperplasias develop slowly and have a limited growth potential. After maturation the lesions remain indefinitely and even after surgical removal they tend to recur unless the offending denture is corrected or replaced. While these lesions may look alarming clinically, they are not considered to be premalignant.

LABORATORY AIDS

The clinical appearance of denture hyperplasia is usually diagnostic, but biopsy will show characteristic fibrous and collagenic hyperplasia.

PAPILLOMA

SYNONYM

Squamous papilloma.

DEFINITION

The papilloma is a relatively common, benign neoplastic proliferation of mucosal epithelium that is similar clinically and microscopically to the common wart (verruca vulgaris) of the skin. It may be initiated by a virus, as are warts, but such a virus has not been yet isolated.

PRESENTING SIGNS AND SYMPTOMS

The papilloma is typically a single soft, nonhemorrhagic, nontender, papillomatous or cauliflower-like growth on a stalk. Typically small and white (keratinized surface), they may reach several centimeters in size and may be normal or red in color with a pebbled, rather than papillary surface. These lesions are most frequently seen on the tongue and soft palate of a middle-aged or older person; they are occasionally multiple.

CLINICAL COURSE AND COMPLICATIONS

After initial slow growth, papillomas remain unchanged indefinitely; there is no tendency toward malignant transformation.

LABORATORY AIDS

Biopsy is diagnostic, demonstrating numerous finger-like projections with connective tissue cores running to the stalk of the lesion. White lesions show hyperkeratosis of the covering epithelium.

PHENYTOIN GINGIVAL HYPERPLASIA

SYNONYMS

Phenytoin gingivitis, phenytoin gingival fibromatosis, diphenylhydantoin hyperplasia.

DEFINITION

Phenytoin gingival hyperplasia is a fibrous hyperplasia of the gingivae arising as a side effect of phenytoin used in the control of epileptic convulsions and other neurologic disorders.

PRESENTING SIGNS AND SYMPTOMS

Phenytoin intake often results in a firm, nonhemorrhagic, nontender, fibrous enlargement of all gingival tissues, occasionally to the point of completely covering the teeth with fibrous tissue. Unless secondarily inflamed, phenytoin gingivae are of normal coloration.

CLINICAL COURSE AND COMPLICATIONS

This fibrous gingival overgrowth continues slowly while the patient is taking the drug, and recurrence after surgical removal is common. The severity of the condition is usually related to the patient's oral hygiene and the duration of therapy; gingival hyperplasia may be avoided in patients with excellent oral hygiene.

LABORATORY AIDS

History and clinical appearance offer the best diagnostic potential, but biopsy will demonstrate a uniform, avascular proliferation of collagenic connective tissues.

PREMALIGNANT AND MALIGNANT LESIONS OF THE MOUTH

By J. RICHARD ALLISON, JR., M.D.
Columbia, South Carolina

Oral cancers comprise 5 to 6 per cent of all cancers in the United States and up to 40 per cent in areas such as Southeast Asia. Prevention and early detection are then the sine qua non of any good medical care, which begins with a complete and thorough examination of the oral cavity. Benign oral tumors, diseases, and infectious conditions must be recognized and differentiated from premalignant and malignant lesions. Suspicious lesions should be biopsied and if found to be benign should be watched and rebiopsied if there is either continued clinical suspicion or any variation in the lesion. An adequate specimen is important for pathologic diagnosis. Intraoral and extraoral palpation may aid in this regard. Exfoliative cytologic studies or staining and Wood's light fluorescence may be helpful if positive, but negative results should not be relied on when there is clinical suspicion. Table 1 lists the types of lesions in the categories of premalignant and malignant lesions.

PREVENTION

Alcohol intake predisposes to a tenfold increase in oral cancer. Smoking, chewing tobacco, and snuff dipping also are very important contributing factors. In Southeast Asia the 40 per cent prevalence of oral cancer in all types of cancer is thought to be due to chewing tobacco. Betel nut chewing is also a contributing factor. Sunlight exposure is responsible for the increased frequency of cancer of the lower lip.

PREMALIGNANT LESIONS

Leukoplakia refers to any white patch and is a general and otherwise nonspecific term. It may be a benign reactive hyperplasia, or it may atrophy and remain so. It may be premalignant from an early stage or become premalignant only after being present in a benign stage for years. It is characterized by gray or white patches, adherent or fibrous, flat, thick, or verrucous, in patches or plaques. It is found more often in men and those over 40, more often in smokers or snuff users. On the lips, the lower lip is more often involved as ultraviolet radiation is a prime cause. When irritation — mechanical, chemical, infectious, or secondary to nutritional or a disease state — is present, it should be corrected as part of the diagnostic work-up in distinguishing between benign and premalignant leukoplakia. With the clinical diagnosis of leukoplakia, 3 to 5 per cent of biopsies on the average will show invasive squamous cell cancer.

Arsenical keratoses generally are more common on the skin, usually appearing 10 to 20 years after the intake of arsenic. They may be present on the mucous membrane and look like atypical leukoplakia or Bowen's disease. Usually there are atypical warty keratoses on the palms and soles and frequently also bowenoid-like lesions on the trunk. Biopsy will confirm the diagnosis of this premalignant lesion that can eventuate into a squamous cell cancer.

Solar cheilitis is a mixture of actinic keratotic change and leukoplakia characterized by crust, scale, erosions, fissures, and white-on-gray patches. Recurrent herpes simplex is present frequently. It is most commonly found on the lower lip because ultraviolet radiation plays a major causative role. It may be confused with lupus erythematosus with secondary photosensitivity. It can degenerate into squamous cell cancer.

Cheilitis glandularis is characterized by enlargement and inflammatory changes with crusts and scales covering the heterotopic salivary glands of the lips, usually the lower one. Squamous cell cancer may develop, possibly

Table 1. *Types of Premalignant and Malignant Lesions*

Premalignant
1. Leukoplakia
2. Arsenical keratosis
3. Solar cheilitis
4. Cheilitis glandularis
5. Mixed tumors of the palate
6. Lichen planus
7. Chronic irritation

Malignant
1. Erythroplasia of Querat⎱ Carcinomas in situ
2. Bowen's disease   ⎰
3. Squamous cell carcinoma
4. Adenocarcinoma
5. Sarcoma: fibrosarcoma, osteogenic sarcoma, reticulum cell sarcoma, lymphosarcoma, chondrosarcoma, giant cell sarcoma, neurofibrosarcoma, leiomyosarcoma, liposarcoma, and malignant neurilemoma and Kaposi's
6. Melanoma
7. Lymphoepithelioma (transitional cell carcinoma)
8. Metastatic: less than 1 per cent spread to oral structures (most are adenocarcinomas from breast, lungs, or kidneys)

secondary to chronic inflammation and ultraviolet radiation.

Mixed tumors of the palate occasionally undergo malignant degeneration or arise as malignant mixed tumors. They are small to large, papular to nodular tumors. Any with unusual growth or appearance must be biopsied or totally excised.

Lichen planus. Squamous cell cancers may develop in as many as 10 per cent of cases of oral lichen planus. When lichen planus is present on the skin, 10 to 50 per cent of the patients will have oral involvement. Generally the malignant degeneration takes place only in cases of long-term involvement, particularly the atrophic type.

Chronic irritation seems to play a more predisposing role in the development of carcinoma of the oral mucosa than of the skin. Therefore all such areas need to be watched, treated, or biopsied. The conditions involved include papillary hyperplasia of the palate secondary to dental plate trauma, burns and chronic stomatitis, gingivitis secondary to poor hygiene or traumatic erosion, and chronic infections such as tuberculosis, syphilis, Vincent's disease, and lupus erythematosus.

KERATOACANTHOMAS

These rapidly growing, usually self-healing tumors of the skin may occur within the oral cavity, although more often are found on the junction of the lips and skin or mucous membranes. They do not fit clearly into the categories of premalignant or malignant lesions because they are benign. They are discussed here because neither the clinical nor the pathologic picture can be relied on for enough diagnostic validity to safely assume their benign condition. When the lesion is within the oral cavity, the characteristic central keratin plug is usually missing as a result of the moisture soaking it out. Although the growth of the tumor in 4 to 6 weeks, which would take 3 to 6 months in a squamous cell cancer, is a helpful clue in the diagnosis, there is no absolute clinical or pathologic difference between a keratoacanthoma and a squamous cell cancer. Expert clinical and pathologic coordination are needed for the diagnosis.

MALIGNANT LESIONS

Oral malignancies have a poor prognosis, with only a 30 per cent survival rate. Almost 90 per cent are squamous cell cancers that metastasize earlier than their counterparts on the skin. Since late detection is a contributing factor, adequate examination of the lips and oral cavity is very important. Salivary gland carcinomas of various types make up most of the other cancers. Sarcomas, lymphomas, and melanomas and other cancers do occur, including metastatic cancers.

Presenting Signs and Symptoms. They are insidious, easily overlooked, and may start as precancers or carcinomas in situ, or de novo, or degenerative changes as secondary to tertiary luetic glossitis. They may be symptomless or not, depending on the location, degree of invasion and destruction, and pressure on adjacent tissue. Ulceration and bleeding usually precede pain. When adenocarcinoma of a salivary gland is present, paresthesia, paralysis, trismus, and dysphagia may occur. Melanomas of the palate occur more often in black people.

FUNCTIONAL DISORDERS OF THE GASTROINTESTINAL TRACT

By RAY E. CLOUSE, M.D.,
and DAVID H. ALPERS, M.D.

St. Louis, Missouri

SYNONYMS

The gastrointestinal tract is a common site for the expression of symptoms that arise in an apparently normal organ, and practically no part of the intestine is free from this problem. Certain particular complaints or syndromes are more common than others and have been better recognized. Names that these disorders are given are usually descriptive and include globus hystericus, primary esophageal spasm, functional nausea and vomiting, nervous stomach, irritable bowel syndrome, proctalgia fugax, and pruritus ani. As one might expect, there are many other common names for some of the less well-defined and more variable symptom complexes (Table 1). Irritable bowel syndrome is the preferred designation for the largest group of such symptoms, since this title reflects lack of restriction to the colon and does not suggest an inflammatory process.

DEFINITION

As the word functional implies, these disorders occur in organs without detectable structural abnormality. But this is not to suggest that there is nothing wrong; often a derangement lies in the function of an organ. In general, the definition of any one of these problems reflects an abnormal or uncomfortable sensation appearing to arise in or from a structurally normal organ. Thus, globus hystericus defines a feeling of a persistent lump in the throat, and pruritus ani implies a sensation of itching in the anal canal or on the perianal skin without any local pathology. Although excluding structural abnormalities is inherent to the pure diagnosis of the functional gastrointestinal disturbances, this is not to say they cannot occur along with other diseases, and at such times the functional diagnosis is more difficult to make. Because these disorders are not characterized by structural

abnormalities, the inclination is to define them strictly by exclusion and to imply a totally emotional or nonorganic basis of the disorders. However, specific derangements of gastrointestinal physiology have been recognized, in particular with the irritable bowel syndrome and esophageal spasm, emphasizing the true abnormalities of function that may be present.

The irritable bowel syndrome deserves separate attention, since it represents one of the most common gastrointestinal disorders seen by practicing physicians. Many symptom complexes have been grouped under this title and many definitions have been proposed. As mentioned in the following section, the syndrome can be subdivided into more specific clinical pictures, but an acceptable inclusive definition would be: a chronic disorder involving mainly the colon and rectum, but sparing no part of the tubular gastrointestinal tract, manifested by daily patterned irregularity of bowel function with or without abdominal pain. The disorder takes a relapsing and remitting course that sometimes parallels psychologic stress and often is associated with a definite psychiatric disorder. This broad definition allows for the variability seen in clinical presentations and should suggest to the physician the comprehensive nature of the disorder.

CLINICAL FEATURES

Patients may present with functional disorders at any age and the duration of complaints is greatly variable. Often the same problem will have recurred many times, possibly with less severity, before a patient will make it known to his physician. Careful searching for such a history is usually necessary. The possible symptom complexes are innumerable and generally have in common only the production of unpleasant sensations (nausea, flatus, etc.) or pain.

IRRITABLE BOWEL SYNDROME

Various recognizable patterns have been noted in the irritable bowel syndrome. Patients with this disorder have daily symptoms that are chronic (more than 3 to 6 months) and unchanging. Weight loss is not usually a feature nor are systemic symptoms of disease. Complaints are not limited to the colon, and patients may have nausea, vomiting, and dyspepsia in addition to other abdominal symptoms. Although there are multiple variations, three major clinical presentations will describe most patients with this syndrome.

1. Constipation and Pain. Usually these

Table 1. *Common Symptomatic Disorders of the Anatomically Normal GI Tract*

I. Primarily esophageal location
  A. Globus hystericus
  B. Primary esophageal spasm
  C. Aerophagia
II. Primarily gastric location
  A. Nausea and vomiting
  B. Epigastric pain
III. Primarily colorectal location
  A. Stress-induced symptoms (nervous stomach, nervous diarrhea)
  B. Irritable bowel syndrome (functional bowel disease, irritable colon, spastic colon, spastic colitis, mucous colitis)
  C. Proctalgia fugax
IV. Primarily anal location
  A. Incontinence
  B. Pruritus ani

symptoms have been present for years before the patient seeks medical attention. Laxative abuse may surface in the history, as might the frequent use of enemas. The accompanying abdominal pain can be severe; at times these patients will appear in emergency rooms, receive surgical evaluation, and occasionally even end up undergoing laparotomy. Usually the pain is of a dull aching nature, present much of the day, does not interfere with sleep, and may or may not be relieved by a bowel movement or expulsion of flatus. When these actions do relieve the pain, it is quite helpful in localizing the source of pain to the colon. In the same way, belching that relieves pain points to the esophagus as the source. The discomfort in the syndrome is usually located in the hypogastrium, lower quadrants, and not infrequently over the entire abdomen and may even be in bizarre locations radiating or originating outside the abdomen. Radiation into the rectum when it occurs is differentiated from other diseases with rectal pathology in which radiation proceeds into the abdomen from the rectum. An important exception to this is the pain of proctalgia fugax, which also radiates from the rectum into the abdomen, but there is no structural abnormality. Characteristically, as can be seen from the description, the discomfort in IBS does not fit the pain pattern of any recognizable organic abdominal disorder and often may not be of intestinal origin.

Patients can present with abdominal pain alone, with no changes in bowel pattern, but this presentation is not considered part of the irritable bowel syndrome. In this setting one often finds an emotional disturbance, such as an obsessive compulsive pattern or depression. In interviewing, one must be alert to eliciting appropriate symptoms of depression including insomnia, loss of appetite, crying spells, and feelings of worthlessness.

2. Alternating Constipation and Diarrhea. These patients will also have chronic histories, and they may be able to identify particular changes in psychologic mood or anxiety levels paralleling the swing in the bowel habit. Motility studies have identified mechanisms whereby these alternating habits might be explained. Classically, depression is associated with constipation, and this can be explained on the basis of a generalized decrease in motility of the colon. However, in some patients there appears to be localized decreased motility in the distal colon allowing for less resistance to mass movement contractions. In these patients, depression might be associated with diarrhea. In the same way, heightened anxiety can be associated with either a generalized increase in contractions producing increased mucus and watery diarrhea or localized spasm in the distal colon producing hard pellet-like stools. Consequently, at times patients will be able to describe changes in emotional symptoms that will parallel in a particular way changes in bowel habits. This kind of correlation is not frequent, however, and, at any rate, is not necessary for the diagnosis. Usually a crampy abdominal pain in the left lower quadrant or more generalized discomfort will be associated with this altered bowel habit. The pain is more apt to be relieved by bowel movement or passage of flatus and seems to originate in the distal colon. Gaseousness and bloating are prominent and a large amount of mucus is noticed in the stool.

3. Diarrhea. A careful history is necessary to avoid embarking on a major work-up in a patient with irritable bowel syndrome and diarrhea alone. Abdominal pain similar to that seen in patients with alternating bowel habits may be seen and is helpful in localizing the disorder largely to the colon. Weight loss or any other signs of malabsorption are generally not seen. The stool can be watery but usually is soft and amounts to less than 500 ml per 24 hours. Most frequently, bowel movements occur after meals and often are clustered in the morning and evening. Although nocturnal diarrhea is not the rule, patients may report late-night or early-morning bowel movements. Careful history, however, often reveals a concomitant sleep disturbance, the bowel movements not actually awakening the patient from sleep. Copious amounts of mucus may be noted, but blood is not acceptable on the basis of the syndrome alone. Often a history of excessive caffeine ingestion (cola, tea, or coffee) or sensitivity to milk products may be elicited. Such dietary factors may exacerbate but do not cause the underlying disorder of motility.

Few patients are able to recognize a relationship between emotional symptoms and alterations in their bowel habits or exacerbations of pain or diarrhea. Clear-cut associations of emotional crises and the onset of symptoms, especially in a recurring fashion, certainly lead the physician to suspect an emotional basis for the symptoms. The history may uncover striking parallels that had been unsuspected by the patient. Some authors feel that correlations between life stresses and exacerbations of functional bowel complaints, and in particular exacerbations of the irritable bowel syndrome, can be drawn in almost all cases. We do not agree that the correlations are frequent or close. However, emotional disorders do often occur in the IBS and frequently predate the gastrointestinal symptoms.

Since the IBS has been better defined than many of the other functional gastrointestinal disturbances, more attention has been paid to the psychiatric make-up of these patients, and there is no question of the marked prevalence of psychiatric disorders in this population. However, definable psychiatric abnormalities probably are also frequent in other chronic gastrointestinal syndromes. Recognized psychiatric disturbances have been noted in up to 75 per cent of referred IBS patients, with depression, hysteria, and anxiety neurosis being common, while schizophrenia and mania are rarely seen. Serious psychiatric derangements are probably less prevalent in a general practice population. The psychiatric symptoms generally antedate the gastrointestinal symptoms. Consequently a careful psychiatric history is mandatory when a functional gastrointestinal complaint is suspected. Not only is this history helpful in supporting a positive diagnosis, but it is extremely helpful in establishing successful therapeutic regimens and reasonable prognoses.

Determining the significance of an emotional disturbance when evaluating a gastrointestinal complaint requires an aware, sensitive, and patient physician. Multiple interviews may be needed to obtain a thorough psychiatric profile without repelling the patient. In difficult cases, after satisfactory rapport is established, referral to a psychiatrist for a diagnostic interview may be necessary. Keep in mind, however, that at least a fourth of these patients lack such identifiable abnormalities and that a psychiatric disorder is not a criterion for diagnosis. Even when one is present, treatment by a psychiatrist is usually not so helpful as attentive follow-up by the primary physician.

STRESS-INDUCED SYMPTOMS

Not covered under the descriptions of the various forms of the irritable bowel syndrome is the large number of patients with transient abdominal symptoms that appear with stressful situations in everyday life. These patients may present with diarrhea, constipation, or abdominal pain similar to that seen in chronic irritable bowel syndrome, but the symptoms may not occur daily, their duration is short, and pain is more likely of colonic origin. These complaints are clearly related to particular stresses such as death of a relative, periods of examination in school, or difficulty in marriage, and generally abate with removal of these stresses. As would be expected, underlying psychiatric disturbances are much less common in this large group and a chronic course is unlikely, although relapses of the same symptoms in future stressful situations can occur.

Three other chronic symptom complexes are seen less frequently than the irritable bowel syndrome, but occur with regularity in practice. These include esophageal spasm, nausea and vomiting, and pruritus ani.

ESOPHAGEAL SPASM

The major symptoms are pain and dysphagia. The pain may have the same distribution as coronary pain but is usually not associated with sweating, nausea, or generalized weakness, and is precipitated by meals but not by exertion or cold surroundings. The dysphagia is striking because it occurs equally for liquids and for solids. As with the irritable bowel syndrome these symptoms are unchanging and chronic. Anxiety is a frequent complaint, with or without actual anxiety neurosis.

NAUSEA AND VOMITING

These symptoms occur over a long time, occasionally with associated abdominal pain, and are remarkably unassociated with weight loss. Depression is a frequent accompanying illness and in fact is often the cause of the complaints. This symptom complex is rarely seen in men.

PRURITUS ANI

This name includes all causes of perianal itching. Once organic lesions have been excluded, the emotional basis of the pruritus can be established. The itching that occurs is constant, often worse at night, and truly perianal. Anxiety is a very frequent symptom in such patients.

PHYSICAL EXAMINATION

Physical examination in this group of disorders is usually remarkable only for its normalcy. Patients with the irritable bowel syndrome may have diffuse abdominal tenderness or tenderness over the sigmoid colon, but the amount of pain might seem out of proportion to objective physical findings. Occasionally the pain will improve with constant pressure in contrast with the pain from structural lesions, which usually worsens under the same conditions. Proctoscopic examination may produce significant spasm and pain, especially with minimal air insufflation, and an increased amount of mucus might also be noted. Melanosis coli, an accumulation of pigment in the mucosa and submucosa of the colon and rectum, is sometimes found and reflects long-standing laxative use. Perianal erythema and excoriation are seen in pruritus ani with lichenification and hyperpigmentation of perianal skin in very chronic cases.

COURSE AND COMPLICATIONS

The courses of the functional disorders can be predicted from the descriptions of the various syndromes. Chronic syndromes tend to remain chronic and somewhat refractory to therapeutic maneuvers. Improvement in an underlying psychiatric disturbance might antedate or parallel improvements in the gastrointestinal disorder. Intermittent symptoms strictly related to emotional stress improve with resolution of the stress.

The disorders themselves are quite slowly progressive with age, with symptoms worsening after the age of 50. This fact is important to recognize, because the long-standing symptoms associated with physiologic disturbances can worsen at the time of life when the physician is concerned about superimposed organic disease such as cancer. The onset of truly new symptoms or findings becomes crucial then in determining the extent of the work-up.

Complications can result from these functional abnormalities. Prolonged vomiting can lead to esophagitis, improperly managed pain can lead to drug addiction, and possibly irritable bowel syndrome can result in diverticulosis. Other potential problems include electrolyte imbalance from protracted vomiting or diarrhea, and enema or laxative abuse from long-standing constipation.

DIAGNOSIS

Although functional disorders are often diagnosed by exclusion, the extent of the work-up usually reflects the confidence of the physician in his diagnosis as established by a careful history. A thorough history is the cornerstone of diagnosing these disorders, for a superficial discussion of the complaints will only lead to multiple unnecessary and unrevealing diagnostic studies. It is justified to first consider the possibility of a functional problem when evaluating anyone with a gastrointestinal symptom, since the gastrointestinal tract is such a common focus for these complaints. One should be cautious, however, in making the diagnosis of a functional disorder, particularly the irritable bowel syndrome, appearing for the first time in a patient over the age of 50. A careful history will reveal the features inconsistent with a structural lesion or features typical of the syndromes mentioned. The psychiatric history might uncover a recognizable disorder (e.g., hysteria) that together with the other historical points would allow a physician confidence to make the diagnosis on these positive grounds rather than by laborious exclusion.

Besides a thorough physical examination, proctoscopy should be performed on patients with bowel complaints referable to the colon, looking for the findings mentioned earlier. Fresh stool during proctoscopy can be examined for mucus, ova and parasites, and blood. Stool guaiacs should be negative, although other causes of guaiac-positive stools, such as hemorrhoids, can coexist with functional disorders. Routine laboratory data are normal. An erythrocyte sedimentation rate can be obtained if there is no other reason for it to be elevated, although this test is occasionally misleading. Endocrinopathies, in particular hyperthyroidism and hypothyroidism, should be excluded by appropriate laboratory tests if there are suggestive features. In patients with bloating and diarrhea, lactose intolerance should be ruled out; lactase deficiency is a common finding occuring in as much as 10 to 20 per cent of the adult white population and up to 75 per cent of the adult black population. Although lactase deficiency is responsible for the symptoms in some patients, intolerance to lactose might simply be exacerbating underlying irritable bowel syndrome. In such cases elimination of milk products from the diet as a diagnostic maneuver will result in improvement but not resolution of the symptoms. Appropriate barium x-rays are necessary, especially in patients over 40, but once initial adequate studies are obtained repeated examinations for the same chronic complaints should be avoided. The point at which no more tests are ordered depends on the confidence of the physician in identifying and caring for the disorder. In certain situations, therapeutic trials directed toward the underlying psychiatric disturbance (e.g., depression) or the underlying physiologic disturbance (e.g., esophageal spasm) may help secure the diagnosis.

More specific diagnostic tests are needed to establish the diagnosis of certain disorders. With esophageal spasm a barium swallow showing the classic corkscrew picture is diagnostic but relatively uncommon. A motility study is sometimes required to make the diagnosis. In addition to a motility study, however, each patient with dysphagia as a symptom of esophageal spasm should have esophagoscopy to rule out lesions such as carcinoma or esophagitis that can produce secondary esophageal spasm. In the initial investigation of prolonged nausea and vomiting, fiberoptic endoscopy is also recommended. This sensitive technique can detect unexpected peptic disease or other less common lesions missed on upper gastrointestinal x-rays that may be responsible, at least in part, for the symptoms. It is important, however, that an experienced endoscopist correlate any abnormalities noted during endoscopy with the magnitude and type of symptoms before assuming a causal relationship. Evaluation of pruritus ani requires, in addition to careful anoscopy-proctoscopy, scraping of the perianal area for potassium hydroxide (KOH) examination to exclude yeast and fungi and performance of the "Scotch Tape test" to exclude pinworm. This test is performed by placing a piece of cellophane tape on the perianal skin (preferably in the early morning before cleansing, scratching, or a bowel movement), removing it, and placing it directly onto a glass slide for examination under the microscope. The test should be repeated on several different days if the suspicion of pinworm remains.

PITFALLS IN DIAGNOSIS

Functional disorders can occur concomitantly with structural disorders and neither can be overlooked. Patients followed for years with chronic complaints need the same periodic routine evaluation given an asymptomatic patient to avoid missing a new structural development masked by the chronic symptoms. This includes a careful history and selected laboratory tests. The development of objective laboratory abnormalities or physical findings not readily explained should immediately alert the physician to this possibility. Early malignancies or inflammatory bowel disease may present with apparently functional symptoms when extensive evaluations fail to demonstrate the lesions. Consequently, even the confident physician should remain open-minded and vigilant.

Another potential error is failure to recognize a psychiatric disturbance associated with the functional gastrointestinal disorder. The outcome of such an oversight is not usually serious but can be so if hysteria is undiagnosed and surgery is performed. Such a patient may fail to respond to therapeutic endeavors and becomes an unpleasant burden. If another physician sought by the patient also fails to recognize the psychiatric disturbance, the cycle continues.

AEROPHAGIA

By J. ALFRED RIDER, M.D., Ph.D.
San Francisco, California

The word *aerophagia* comes from the Greek, *aero* and *phagein*, which literally means to eat air; thus patients afflicted with aerophagia are referred to as air swallowers. It has been estimated that approximately 70 per cent of the gas present in the intestinal tract occurs because of this mechanism. Strictly speaking, when aerophagia is discussed, other causes of gastrointestinal gas would not be considered. However, for completeness and because of common usage, gastrointestinal gas from any cause is lumped under this term. Consequently, other causes of gastrointestinal gas, as well as those directly related to the swallowing of air, are discussed in this article.

Such terms as bloating, gas, flatulence, cramping, meteorism, tympanites, and *magenblase* (from the German, meaning a "stomach bubble") have been used to describe the clinical symptoms associated with gastrointestinal gas. Swallowed air is, obviously, of the same composition as the atmosphere and consists primarily of nitrogen. Normally, one has approximately 150 ml of gas present in the gastrointestinal tract at all times. It is normal to swallow some air each time one eats or drinks. Moreover, one will swallow additional air by chewing gum, smoking, or sucking on candies.

SOURCES OF GAS

As just mentioned, swallowed air is the primary cause of gastrointestinal gas. This may occur in nervously tense persons as a neurotic habit. Some other causes of aerophagia are lesions of the oral pharynx, ill-fitting dentures, chronic sinusitis with "postnasal drip," and chronic bronchitis with coughing and swallowing of sputum. Some patients swallow air during ordinary breathing apparently by involuntary relaxation of the upper esophageal sphincter. A nasogastric tube, used postoperatively, is a constant source of irritation and promotes air swallowing; if the evacuation tube is not working properly, excess gas accumulates in the stomach and intestinal tract.

Another source of gastrointestinal gas is carbon dioxide, which is liberated when gastric juices come in contact with alkaline or effervescent beverages. In the small intestine, carbon dioxide is also formed from the carbonates of intestinal juices when the acid chyme is neutralized. If raw food enters the colon, there is production of gas, such as methane, hydrogen, and carbon dioxide, through the fermentation of the undigested food. Hydrogen sulfide may be present in small quantities and, if present, is responsible for malodorous flatus. The other gases are nonodorous. The formation of gas is especially increased if raw carbohydrates reach the colon. Food with a high cellulose content is unaffected by human digestion, in contrast to the digestion of herbivorous animals, and this leads to the production of gas through bacterial action in the colon. In the case of the often maligned bean, the cellulose acts as a protective coating and does not allow complete digestion of the carbohydrate particles so coated.

Another cause of gastrointestinal gas is intestinal obstruction from any cause such as carcinoma or adhesions, or intestinal ileus, which is commonly seen postoperatively.

A rare type of gas production results from extreme atmospheric pressure changes or from breathing abnormal gases. This is of little clinical importance at the moment, but may become more significant in future space travel. It also occurs in deep underwater diving. This type of gas exchange takes place in the direction that will create an equilibrium between partial tensions in individual gases in the blood and those in the intestines.

Achlorhydria has been indicated as a cause of gastrointestinal gas. This is the absence of hydrochloric acid and may result in the presence in the upper gastrointestinal tract of bacteria from the colon that, when acting on food, contribute to gas formation. Yeast may also be present and will contribute to the production of gas.

Rarely, mesenteric artery insufficiency, secondary to atherosclerosis, may result in increased gastrointestinal gas, and this disease must be considered in the elderly. Carcinoma anywhere in the gastrointestinal tract may cause symptoms of gastrointestinal gas such as bloating.

Other causes of gastrointestinal gas are malabsorption syndromes, secondary to pancreatic or biliary disease, and finally specific enzyme deficiencies, such as sucrase and lactase insufficiency.

SYMPTOMS

The symptoms of gastrointestinal gas vary considerably and are caused by distention of the gastrointestinal tract with air. This distention or stretching of the gastrointestinal tract may cause pain, which is often of a cramping or colicky nature. The gas per se may not cause symptoms unless there is associated spasm of the bowel musculature. It may be that these symptoms are caused by abnormal amounts of gas. On the other hand, similar symptoms may be caused by an abnormal response to relatively normal amounts of gas. Other symptoms are simply those of distention, often called bloating, and vague abdominal pressure. Additional frequent complaints are belching, passing flatus, and rumbling and gurgling sounds (borborygmi).

Splenic and hepatic flexure syndromes, caused by distention of the colonic flexures, may cause radiation of pain into the chest. The hepatic flexure syndrome may simulate biliary colic. The splenic flexure syndrome is characterized by pain in the left upper quadrant or into the chest, and even into the neck, occurring as a direct result of dilatation of the splenic flexure of the colon with gas, causing pressure on the diaphragm. There may be associated difficulty in taking a deep breath. The pain may be so severe that it may simulate myocardial infarction or angina. These patients usually have an irritable colon and often complain of intermittent constipation or diarrhea or both. The symptoms can be reproduced by insufflation of air into the splenic flexure via the colonoscope.

With pyloric obstruction, there is usually belching, hiccupping, or distention of the stomach.

Acute gastric dilatation, a rare condition occurring after surgery, may be lethal if unrecognized. The tremendous distention of the stomach compromises the respiratory process by inhibiting motion of the diaphragm, as well as interfering with cardiac venous return.

DIAGNOSIS

Diagnosis of gastrointestinal gas per se is not difficult. Essentially, one resorts to the history of excessive flatus, belching, complaints of bloating, and distention. The presence of gas can be confirmed by demonstration of abdominal tympany, and auscultation frequently will enable one to hear borborygmi (rumbling noises caused by the propulsion of gas through the intestines). Finally, a flat film of the abdomen will confirm gas. It is more important, however, to determine the cause of the gastrointestinal gas and, if possible, the amount and type of gas produced in the flatus.

HISTORY

A clinical history is important in determining if the patient has increased symptoms after eating or drinking. In air swallowing the patient will indicate that the symptoms are worse after eating, drinking, or chewing gum, or when he is nervous. In the case of an organic condition, such as enzyme deficiency, the history may bring out, for example, that the patient cannot tolerate milk. In the case of malabsorption syndrome, fats cannot be tolerated. In short, a complete history and dietary background must be obtained, including a record of the patient's operations.

PHYSICAL EXAMINATION

Obviously, a complete physical examination is necessary to rule out organic diseases such as abdominal tumor and rectal lesions. Careful percussion of the abdomen will indicate increased tympany, which will be generalized or confined to one area or another of the abdomen.

SPECIALIZED DIAGNOSTIC STUDIES

A flat film of the abdomen will show increased gas in the stomach, small bowel, and colon. This examination is important to rule out or determine whether intestinal obstruction is present. Furthermore, the flat film of the abdomen may be used to follow results of treatment.

It is important to rule out other organic disease, and a laboratory work-up should usually include x-ray of the colon, upper gastrointestinal tract, small bowel, and gallbladder. In patients with suspected mesenteric artery insufficiency, angiography is essential. An upper gastrointestinal endoscopy may be indicated. A proctoscopic examination is essential to determine the presence of rectal disease. A gastric analysis is important, as is a stool examination for parasites, undigested food particles, fat, starch, and occult blood. A small bowel biopsy is frequently indicated for ruling out sprue, Whipple's disease, giardiasis, malignancy, and Crohn's disease, and, of course, for direct determination of lactase and sucrase activity. Lactose and sucrose tolerance tests are important to give further proof of disaccharide intolerance.

Techniques for analysis of the amount and composition of flatus are now available in specialized laboratories. For example, sophisticated methods of determination utilize rectal balloons and analyses of the type of gas produced. If the flatus consists primarily of nitrogen and oxygen, then the gas comes from swallowing air. If it contains large quantities of methane, carbon dioxide, or hydrogen, then obviously these gases are generated within the bowel.

PITFALLS OF DIAGNOSIS

Although the majority of patients with symptoms of gastrointestinal gas are air swallowers, one must consider and rule out the other various causes. It is too easy to pass off patients with abdominal bloating or distention as neurotic, when in reality they may have a carcinoma of the bowel or a disaccharidase enzyme deficiency.

DYSPHAGIA

By JOEL E. RICHTER, M.D.,
and DONALD O. CASTELL, M.D.
Bethesda, Maryland

DEFINITION

Dysphagia, from the Greek phagia (to eat) and dys (with difficulty), is a broad term that refers to the category of symptoms including either difficulty with the initiation of a swallow or the sensation that food is being hindered or is stopping in its passage from mouth to stomach. Strictly speaking, this symptom should not be confused with odynophagia (pain with swallowing), although it is often difficult to clearly separate these two symptoms. In addition, the patient with a "lump in the throat" usually has the entirely different symptom complex of globus hystericus, which is discussed later and in the article on Functional Disorders of the Gastrointestinal Tract. The true dysphagia usually signifies the presence of organic disease, the cause of which can usually be identified with a proper understanding of the subtleties of clinical presentation of this symptom complex and with the careful documentation of the patient's medical history. In approaching a patient with dysphagia, specifics of the presenting history are crucial and should lead to a strong suspicion of the correct diagnosis in the majority of cases.

It is helpful in discussing dysphagia to divide the causes into two broad categories: *pre-esophageal* or oropharyngeal dysphagia, produced by those lesions that interfere with the coordinated neuromuscular complex controlling the initiation of swallowing, and *esophageal* dysphagia, produced by those lesions that actually interfere with transport of food through the esophagus.

PREESOPHAGEAL (OROPHARYNGEAL) DYSPHAGIA

A great variety of neural or muscular abnormalities can produce this form of dysphagia. A list of those entities more likely to produce this symptom is shown in Table 1. It is uncommon for these patients to present with an initial complaint of dysphagia, but rather they have this symptom as a part of a much greater total abnormality secondary to the disease. Usually, dysphagia does not present a difficult diagnostic problem in the patient with preesophageal dysphagia since the basic disease process is readily recognized. However, on occasion dysphagia may be the first manifestation of disease. Typically, these patients present with difficulty *initiating* a swallow. The patient will note that food does not follow the normal passage, but may regurgitate into the nasopharynx or into the trachea, with the resultant associated symptoms of sneezing or coughing frequently occurring

Table 1. *Major Causes of Pre-esophageal Dysphagia*

A. Disorders of striated muscle
  1. Polymyositis–Dermatomyositis
  2. Myasthenia gravis (m⁻ neural junction)
  3. Myotonic dystrophy
  4. Muscular dystrophy
  5 Miscellaneous (thyroid disorders, drugs)
B. Disorders of the nervous system
  1. Cerebrovascular disease
  2. Pseudobulbar palsy
  3 Amyotrophic lateral sclerosis
  4. Multiple sclerosis
  5. Parkinson's disease
  6. CNS tumor
  7 Other neurologic defects
C. Motor disorders of the upper esophageal sphincter (UES)
  1. Hypertensive UES (globus, spasm)
  2. Hypotensive UES (esophagopharyngeal regurgitation)
  3. Abnormal UES relaxation
    a. Incomplete relaxation (Cricopharyngeal achalasia? CNS lymphoma)
    b. Premature closure (Cricopharyngeal bar, Zenker's?)
    c. Delayed relaxation (Familial dysautonomia?)

when swallowing. In addition, these patients may notice that they have their greatest difficulty with liquids, which are more likely to move in the wrong direction.

ESOPHAGEAL DYSPHAGIA

This is a *transport* problem. Since one of the major functions of the esophagus is the transport of food from mouth to stomach, any organic abnormality of this structure will result in a delay of this normal transport process, commonly described by the patient as the sensation of food "hanging up," or "sticking" behind the sternum.

GLOBUS HYSTERICUS

Although globus hystericus is not a true form of dysphagia, it warrants separate discussion. True dysphagia occurs during or within seconds of swallowing. In contrast, globus hystericus is a tightness, fullness, discomfort, or lump in the throat that is more often present between or unrelated to swallowing. In fact, the sensation may be relieved by swallowing. True globus hystericus is usually, but not necessarily, confined to tense and neurotic persons; characteristically it does not disturb food ingestion or nutritional state; and it is an overworked, overdiagnosed, and an infrequently occurring condition. The real danger is for the clinician not to recognize true oropharyngeal dysphagia and, instead, to issue a hasty but erroneous diagnosis of globus hystericus.

It has been suggested that the sensation experienced by patients with globus hystericus can be duplicated by anyone attempting repetitive dry swallows. The classic sensation of globus hystericus will normally appear between the seventh and eleventh swallows. It has been proposed that the unconscious and frequent swallowing of saliva or dry swallowing by tense or neurotic patients leads to this sensation. Some patients have also been reported to have elevated upper esophageal sphincter pressure but have normal relaxation of this sphincter.

DIFFERENTIAL DIAGNOSIS

The site to which the patient refers his symptom may have value in localizing the specific lesion. If the patient identifies the dysphagia as causing a sensation referred to the suprasternal notch, there is little localizing value, since an abnormality in any portion of the esophagus may result in referred sensation to this area. In contrast, if the patient localizes his symptom at some point farther down the sternum, it is reasonable to expect that he is identifying the area where the organic obstruction occurs. This is particularly true if the sensation is identified at the lower end of the sternum, in which case a distal esophageal lesion is to be expected.

Lesions causing esophageal dysphagia are conveniently divided into categories: *mechanical obstruction* and *neuromuscular disturbances*. In each of these two categories there are a variety of causes but three major problems cause the majority of abnormalities in each of these two subsets (Table 2). As just mentioned, understanding the mode of presentation of these more common causes of dysphagia and organizing the taking of the medical history around this knowledge can often lead to a strong suspicion of a correct diagnosis. Figure 1 represents a flow diagram for the differential diagnosis of these lesions based on the presenting history.

The type of food that is causing symptoms is often of great assistance; the important differential point is that neuromuscular disorders may cause dysphagia for either liquids or solid food (Fig. 1A), whereas mechanical obstructing lesions will only cause dysphagia for solid foods initially (Fig. 1B). It is true that as the mechanical obstruction becomes almost complete, even liquids will not pass through the esophagus, and that the patient with a mechanically obstructing lesion can impact a solid bolus in the esophagus and secondarily have dysphagia for liquids. However, careful taking of the history should allow the beginning of the differentiation between these two broad categories of dysphagia.

In the patient with an apparent mechanical obstruction it is important to ascertain whether the symptom is progressive or has occurred only intermittently, for intermittent dysphagia for solid food is the hallmark of the patient with a Schatzki's ring. Patients with peptic stricture or carcinoma usually have progressive dysphagia. An important differential feature in these patients is the long-standing history of heartburn and frequent antacid use usually present in the patient with a peptic stricture. This is an important part of the historical differential since patients in both of these categories may be in an older age group and have progressive dysphagia and weight loss. In addition, because of their frequent association, heavy chronic alcohol intake and smoking should lead to a strong suspicion of esophageal cancer.

Separation of the three major neuromuscular abnormalities causing dysphagia also lends itself well to careful history-taking. Again, the presence of progressive or intermittent symptoms may be helpful. In the patient with progressive dysphagia, the presence of associated heartburn and free acid regurgitation should lead to a strong suspicion of a diagnosis of scleroderma. Patients with achalasia usually have had dysphagia for many months to years, with this history only becoming obvious with careful questioning because of the slow and insidious progression of this abnormality. True heartburn is unusual in patients with achalasia. A classic historical feature is the presence of nocturnal symptoms, that is, coughing or regurgitation of liquid into the mouth at night secondary to overflow from the dilated, fluid-filled esophagus. In the patient with intermittent symptoms, associated chest pain is the historical feature that should strongly arouse suspicion of a diagnosis of diffuse esophageal spasm.

DIAGNOSTIC TESTS

Following the taking of the history, the next most important diagnostic evaluation in these patients is the barium swallow. In patients with preesophageal dysphagia, the barium may flow in a variety of abnormal directions, either up into the nasopharynx, into the pyriform sinuses, or clearly into the trachea. In addition, in the patient with a Zenker's diverticulum, a well-defined pouch filled with barium is usually identified. A median bar or a bony osteophyte or upper esophageal web is often seen impinging on the barium column. Mechanical obstructing lesions to the esophagus are usually quite evident. Both the peptic stricture and esophageal carcinoma are identified as areas of fixed narrowing, with carcinoma usually showing a much more irregular appearance secondary to destruction of the normal mucosal pattern. A

Table 2. *Major Causes of Esophageal Dysphagia*

I. Neuromuscular (motility) disorders
  A. Most common
    1. Achalasia
    2. Scleroderma
    3. Diffuse esophageal spasm
  B. Other
    1. Other collagen disorders
    2. Chagas' disease
II. Mechanical obstruction
  A. Most common
    1. Peptic stricture
    2. Lower esophageal (Schatzki's) ring
    3 Carcinoma
  B. Other
    1. Esophageal web
    2. Esophageal diverticula
    3 Vascular compression
      a. Dysphagia lusoria
      b. Dysphagia aortica
    4. Mediastinal abnormalities
    5. Cervical osteoarthritis

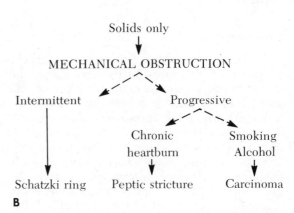

Figure 1A. Symptom differential of neuromuscular (motility) disorders causing dysphagia.

Figure 1B. Symptom differential of mechanically obstructing lesions causing dysphagia.

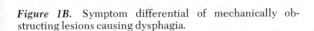

stricture in the mid or upper esophagus should suggest the presence of a Barrett's esophagus.

The lower esophageal (Schatzki's) ring is usually readily identified as a narrow invaginated area in the distal esophagus. It is important to note, however, that such a ring can be readily missed if barium is allowed to flow in a thin liquid column through the distal esophagus. The suspicious radiologist will ensure the distention of the phrenic ampulla with barium by having the patient do a Valsalva maneuver at the appropriate time, thus readily identifying the presence of this mucosal ring.

There are "typical" appearances of the major esophageal motility disturbances in the barium-filled esophagus. In achalasia the esophagus is classically widely dilated, but with the presence of a smooth symmetrical tapering at the distal end. With the patient standing, a fluid level is often apparent in the dilated esophagus.

This is in contrast to the patient with scleroderma in whom the esophagus may also be widely dilated, but the distal segment is also widely patent and shows rapid emptying of the esophagus (no fluid level) in the standing position. The barium-filled esophagus may take many forms in the patient with diffuse esophageal spasm. Localized areas of tertiary contractions may present with mild serrations of the barium column or with extreme abnormalities, giving the appearance of the so-called corkscrew esophagus, or with the presence of multiple pockets of barium, the "rosary bead esophagus." Esophageal dilatation is unusual in diffuse spasm.

Endoscopy with biopsy is usually the next procedure of importance in the differential diagnosis of mechanically obstructing lesions, as is discussed in the separate sections. Esophageal manometric studies are crucial to the specific diagnosis of the neuromuscular abnormalities. These motility defects represent the major clinical entities in which the esophageal manometric laboratory may be of assistance to the clinician. Characteristic manometric features for each of the major abnormalities are discussed in the appropriate sections.

ESOPHAGEAL DIVERTICULA

DEFINITION

Esophageal diverticula are sacculations extending outward from the lumen of the esophagus that usually contain all layers of the esophageal wall (true diverticulum), as opposed to those without a muscular wall (false diverticulum). These outpouchings occur at three main areas: (1) immediately above the upper esophageal sphincter (Zenker's diverticulum), (2) near the midpoint of the esophagus (traction diverticulum), and (3) immediately above the lower esophageal sphincter (epiphrenic diverticulum).

SYMPTOMS

Zenker's diverticulum presents the most classic group of symptoms. In its early stage when the sac is perpendicular to the neck and of small size, it rarely causes symptoms other than a fullness in the neck or transient preesophageal dysphagia. However, when the sac becomes large enough to retain food contents, symptoms increase. Patients may complain of worsening dysphagia, nocturnal pulmonary aspiration, gurgling in the throat, and regurgitation of undigested sweet or putrid food particles. These sacs may become so large that the retained contents may push anteriorly on the esophagus and completely obstruct it. These diverticula rarely bleed or perforate.

The midesophageal diverticula are generally found in totally asymptomatic patients. Occasionally patients with such diverticula will complain of mild dysphagia, regurgitation of undigested food, and rarely of esophageal obstruction.

It is difficult to tell whether the symptoms of an epiphrenic diverticulum are caused by the diverticulum itself or by the associated esophageal motor disorder. Nocturnal regurgitation or regurgitation of undigested food 3 to 4 hours after a meal may be reported. Patients have also complained of substernal fullness and discomfort on eating, which might be related to distension of the sac. One symptom is fairly unique to the presence of this diverticulum: the regurgitation of massive amounts of fluid, primarily at night. Presumably this fluid accumulates in the sac during the daytime hours spent upright and is regurgitated during periods of recumbency.

DIAGNOSIS

The diagnoses of esophageal and hypopharyngeal diverticula are usually made with a barium swallow. Occasionally the entire first glass of barium taken will disappear into spacious confines of an especially large diverticulum. Small diverticula can easily be missed if the hypopharyngeal area is not well examined or lateral views of the esophagus are not obtained. Another possible source of confusion might occur in the esophagus with many tertiary contractions. This may give a temporary appearance of numerous diverticula, but the changing pattern of subsequent swallows will eliminate the source of confusion.

Esophageal diverticula represent one reason why upper gastrointestinal series should be obtained before elective endoscopic procedures. The unwary endoscopist might easily enter and perforate a Zenker's diverticulum while blindly passing the endoscope past the hypopharyngeal area. The role of endoscopy in relationship to diverticula is primarily to exclude other lesions that might adversely affect or be related to the diverticulum formation. All patients should have complete manometric studies before any surgical repair. This is particularly true of epiphrenic diverticulum, which frequently will recur after simple resection if the associated motility disorder is not corrected.

STRICTURES, RINGS, AND WEBS

DEFINITION

A stricture is a benign narrowing of the esophagus caused by either edema and inflammation (reversible stricture), or fibrous scar tissue (true stricture) that has been produced by a previous injury. Most commonly, benign strictures are secondary to reflux esophagitis. These are located in the lower portion of the esophagus near the lower esophageal sphincter. They may be quite short or extend to the aortic arch. Strictures associated with Barrett's esophagus or corrosive injuries are more commonly located in midesophagus and are of variable length.

A mucosal ring is a thin membranous ring of mucosa projecting into the lumen of the esophagus. The most common rings occur at the distal esophageal squamocolumnar mucosal junction and are called Schatzki's rings, or "B" rings.

Webs are thin projections of benign hyperkeratotic squamous mucosa projecting into the lumen as a small shelf. Although they may be found anywhere in the esophagus, they are usually located immediately below the cricopharyngeus. Cervical webs have been associated with iron deficiency anemia (Plummer-Vinson or Paterson-Kelly syndrome) and pernicious anemia. An association between hypopharyngeal cancers and webs has also been noted.

SYMPTOMS

Intermittent dysphagia for solid food is the most common symptom associated with webs and rings, but the majority of patients are asymptomatic. Variable lumen narrowing results in symptoms in patients with Schatzki's ring, but all patients have dysphagia when the lumen is narrowed to 12 mm or less.

Patients having a Schatzki's ring of small diameter classically have *intermittent* dysphagia for solid food only. In addition, there is often a history of dysphagia occurring only during situations of excess tension, probably the result of failure of a patient to chew his food adequately at these times. The intermittent nature and the relationship to tension often lead to the assumption that the patient has a functional disorder. Absolute confirmation that the patient's symptoms are produced by the lower esophageal ring can be obtained in the fluoroscopic unit by having the patient swallow a barium-soaked marshmallow and verifying that retention of this bolus reproduces the patient's symptoms. Dysphagia that occurs daily or is associated with odynophagia is unlikely to be caused by an esophageal ring. Another classic presentation of lower esophageal ring is sudden, total esophageal obstruction caused by meat impaction. Frequently these patients undergo endoscopy, and during the dislodgement of the bolus of meat, the esophageal ring may be unknowingly ruptured. The endoscopist usually comments that the esophagus is normal and this is confirmed by the barium swallow.

Strictures will cause obstructive symptoms of variable severity, dependent upon the degree of luminal narrowing and length of the stricture. Dysphagia caused by a stricture is usually progressive, in both frequency of occurrence and decrease in the size of the bolus that can be passed. Patients may gradually change their diet so that they avoid solid, then semisolid foods. As stated previously, these patients classically have a long-standing history of chronic indigestion or heartburn and antacid usage. Occasionally, however, there is no history of heartburn and the development of the stricture

may be the first manifestation of chronic reflux in the patient with a nonsensitive esophagus. In the heartburn patient, with the development of the stricture and associated dysphagia, there is often relief of the previous reflux symptoms. Occasionally, dysphagia will be the presenting symptom of a stricture, thus causing concern about a cancer.

DIAGNOSIS

Radiologic techniques are the best method for the diagnosis of both webs and rings. Cineesophagrams will most often detect cervical webs. Since the webs are usually located on the anterior surface of the esophagus, lateral and oblique films are often necessary to make the diagnosis. The lower esophageal ring is best demonstrated when the lower segment of the esophagus is distended. This can best be accomplished by the patient's taking a deep breath and holding it as the peristaltic wave approaches the distal esophagus. It is important to note that the lower esophageal ring usually appears as a thin symmetrical narrowing 3 to 5 cm above the esophagogastric junction. If asymmetry is seen, a web is the most likely cause. If a thick ring is seen, then the cause is more likely a localized ring stricture resulting from reflux esophagitis.

Radiologic techniques are helpful, but a definitive diagnosis of a stricture requires endoscopy, especially if benign strictures are to be differentiated from carcinoma. Multiple biopsies and brush cytologies should be obtained during the endoscopic evaluation of all strictures. Bougienage before biopsies may be necessary to evaluate strictures thoroughly when the esophageal lumen is markedly narrowed. Occasionally, endoscopy can help differentiate a true lower esophageal ring from an annular stricture. A stricture will usually resist passage of the endoscope and will often be associated with mucosal changes of reflux esophagitis such as ulceration and bleeding.

INTRINSIC LESIONS

DEFINITION

Lesions of the wall of the esophagus that may cause obstruction include congenital cysts, reduplication, benign tumors, and malignant tumors. The most common benign tumor is the leiomyoma, although it occurs one tenth as frequently as malignant tumors. Other less infrequent benign lesions include lipomas, squamous papillomas, epithelial cysts, and inflammatory pseudotumors. Benign tumors of the esophagus are usually an incidental finding at autopsy and rarely cause any major clinical manifestations.

SYMPTOMS

Benign tumors and cysts are usually asymptomatic and are discovered by serendipity during the course of a routine barium swallow or upper gastrointestinal series for totally unrelated symptoms. Bleeding rarely has been reported secondary to leiomyomas.

Progressive dysphagia is the most common clinical presentation of carcinoma of the esophagus. Dysphagia in an individual over 40 years of age should always be assumed to be due to cancer until proven otherwise. These patients usually describe progressive dysphagia of relatively short duration, typically beginning only with solid foods, but eventually progressing to affect liquids and even swallowed secretions. There is usually weight loss, although this is not a specific symptom, since all patients with dysphagia tend to lose weight because of their difficulty in eating.

Pain is also a classic manifestation of carcinoma of the esophagus and represents an unfavorable sign, because it usually signifies extension of the tumor outside the confines of the esophagus. The pain is usually steady, located substernally, and gradually increases to the point that many patients require narcotics for pain relief. As the esophageal obstruction increases and food intake is decreased, weight loss will ensue. This appears to occur surprisingly late, in view of the degree of esophageal obstruction that is found at the time of demonstrable weight loss. In most cases of obstruction, the potential lumen size must be reduced to around 10 to 13 mm before persistent severe dysphagia will occur.

Late in the course, pulmonary complications become a major problem. These patients often expectorate continuously to avoid aspiration of their saliva. Severe cough, dyspnea, infections, and aspiration pneumonia may result secondary to severe esophageal obstruction, or acquired tracheoesophageal fistula secondary to tumor eroding into a bronchus. Excessive bleeding is rare, but more commonly the patient suffers from slow blood loss manifested by symptoms of iron deficiency anemia. Other rare symptoms are hoarseness caused by involvement of the recurrent laryngeal nerve and hiccups denoting spread of the tumor to the diaphragm or invasion of the phrenic nerve.

DIAGNOSIS

Intrinsic lesions of the esophagus will be suspected on the basis of history and usually first confirmed by a barium esophagram. Malignant tumors of the esophagus usually demonstrate irregular luminal encroachment with a shelf or ridge noted at the superior portion of the tumor. Unfortunately, tumor can present as merely a smooth narrowing, making differentiation from a benign stricture almost impossible by radiologic criteria. A helpful point is that dilatation of the esophagus is not common above a malignant stenosing lesion. The cardia and fundus should be well evaluated. Distortion of the normal contour or displacement of the fundus away from the diaphragm may suggest an adenocarcinoma in the cardia invading the lower esophagus. Occasionally one may see evidence of mediastinal or hilar tumor masses in a patient with esophageal carcinoma.

X-rays can also be of use in staging the tumor and evaluating its potential extent and resectability. If the tumor is greater than 5 cm in length, 90 per cent of patients will have extensive metastases. Marked deviation of the longitudinal axis of the esophagus usually implies tumor extension through the wall of the esophagus and fixation to the mediastinal structures. Benign tumors of the esophagus usually bulge into the barium column with a sharp smooth surface, indicating their subepithelial or intramural location. Leiomyomas occasionally are calcified and may appear to encircle the esophagus.

Endoscopy should be regularly performed after x-ray studies to investigate mucosal alteration, obtain biopsy specimens, or aid in the dilatation of the obstructive segment. The extent of the tumor may be better assessed at direct visualization and, if possible, the endoscope should be retroflexed in the stomach and the cardia thoroughly evaluated. Primary adenocarcinoma of the stomach may mimic both esophageal carcinoma and achalasia. Brush cytologies and multiple small mucosal pinch biopsies should routinely be obtained. Careful attention to obtaining good cytologies is especially important in esophageal carcinoma, as adequate tissue by mucosal biopsy may be difficult to obtain. With the combination of these two methods, a pathologic diagnosis may be made in more than 90 per cent of patients. If the esophagus is markedly obstructed, esophageal dilatation may be necessary before adequate visualization and biopsies of the tumor can be obtained. Endoscopic evaluation of benign tumors usually demonstrates elevation of normal mucosa over a soft, pliable mass. Endoscopic biopsy is not recommended because of the inability to obtain diagnostic tissue and the theoretical possibility of creating an esophageal fistula through the mucosal defect after a surgical resection.

EXTRINSIC LESIONS

SYMPTOMS

External compression and displacement of the esophagus may be produced by a multitude of lesions that do not actually invade the esophageal wall. Ironically, some extrinsic lesions may produce marked deviation of the esophagus yet cause few symptoms. A classic example is the distortion created by a massive left atrial enlargement secondary to mitral stenosis. In the elderly, large cervical osteophytes are not an uncommon cause of intermittent upper esophageal dysphagia. Vascular lesions such as an aberrant right subclavian artery compressing the esophageal lumen (dysphagia lusoria) or dilated aneurysmic aorta compressing the esophagus (dysphagia aortica) may rarely cause dysphagia. Any mediastinal lesion, either primary or metastatic, may encroach upon the esophagus from the posterior mediastinum, causing dysphagia. Severe infection, a large retrosternal thyroid, postsurgical conditions, or idiopathic mediastinitis with fibrosis may also cause dysphagia.

DIAGNOSIS

Radiographic studies utilizing a well-distended esophagus usually confirms external esophageal compression with displacement, preservation of a normal mucosal pattern, and evidence of a paraesophageal mass. Further studies including mediastinoscopy, thyroid scan, and angiography usually are necessary to confirm the specific diagnosis. Osteophytic spurs of the cervical spine can be easily diagnosed on lateral views of the neck. The demonstration of hang-up of a barium-impregnated marshmallow at the point of bony prominence may help to ensure that the osteophytes are related to the symptomatology.

Esophagoscopy will help to confirm the extramucosal location of the compressing lesion but is primarily indicated to rule out associated intrinsic lesions of the esophagus. Gentle probing of the protrusion under direct visualization may be helpful. Cystic and vascular lesions may often be indented, whereas solid tumors are firm and nonindentable. Vascular lesions may pulsate, but care must be taken to differentiate true pulsation of such a lesion from transmitted pulsation from vascular structures behind nonvascular lesions.

FOREIGN BODIES

DEFINITION

Most ingested foreign bodies that become impacted consist of poorly chewed food masses, animal bones, or nonorganic objects. Most foreign objects that can be started down the esophagus do not linger but proceed down into the stomach and then usually end in the feces. Coins are the major exception to this rule. These usually tend to lodge high in the esophagus around the level of T_1 vertebrae. Infants, the senile elderly, alcoholics, the mentally deranged, and patients with constricting lesions of the esophagus are most likely victims of esophageal obstruction. Food masses that tend to impact include meat, vegetable matter, and citrus fruit.

Obstruction most commonly occurs in the elderly secondary to incomplete mastication as a result of either carelessness or dental and gum disease. Ingestion of foreign bodies by infants and children is often related to parental carelessness. Recently, aluminum "pop-top" tabs from beverage containers have become a particular hazard. These shiny objects, which commonly litter recreational areas, are irresistible to toddlers. Institutionalized mental patients are probably the largest group of foreign body swallowers. Patients with benign and malignant constricting lesions of the esophagus may note intermittent obstruction. Patients with esophageal rings (Schatzki's rings) not uncommonly will initially present with acute obstruction secondary to meat impaction.

SYMPTOMS

Foreign body ingestion and retention in the esophagus may cause acute pain, dysphagia, coughing paroxysms, gagging, and choking. The victim usually attempts to clear the foreign body by vomiting or washing it through with water. If complete esophageal obstruction occurs, the patient may note severe pain secondary to muscular spasm and drooling, as his salivary secretions overflow. This can be very distressing, may result in aspiration, and does not resolve until the obstruction is cleared. If damage to the mucosa or submucosa without perforation has occurred, a sensation of an impacted object may persist long after the object has actually been passed.

If perforation has occurred, the patient generally will note severe mid sternal and epigastric pain that may radiate through between the shoulder blades. The patient may become dyspneic, cyanotic, and diaphoretic. On examination, he may appear pale and sweaty, have tachycardia, and may be in shock. The epigastric pain may be so severe as to suggest acute pancreatitis or a perforated duodenal ulcer.

Acute glottic obstruction, frequently secondary to a large bolus of meat, is associated with marked distress, cyanosis, and obvious choking. The patient cannot speak to summon help and may die in minutes as a result of asphyxiation. Known as the "cafe coronary syndrome," as it frequently occurs in restaurants, the acute obstruction may be relieved by the Heimlich maneuver.

DIAGNOSIS

The history and the presence or absence of symptoms cannot always be relied on in diagnosing either the ingestion or retention of foreign bodies in the esophagus. Plain films of the neck, including lateral views, chest x-rays, and abdominal films, may be particularly helpful.

Some objects, such as aluminum pull tabs and bones, may be only faintly visible on radiographic studies, so careful analysis of the films is essential. Food, dental components, plastic, glass, or wood may be radiolucent and thus not detectable by radiologic means; therefore, foreign body ingestion is not excluded by a negative x-ray survey. Flat objects, particularly coins, may lodge in the esophagus or tracheobronchial tree, creating a particular diagnostic problem.

Chest x-ray may be especially helpful, as a coin will usually lie in the frontal plane if it lies in the esophagus and in the sagittal plane if in the tracheobronchial tree. When food impaction occurs in the esophagus, a barium swallow is safe and usually diagnostic. If perforation is suspected, water-soluble contrast material (Gastrografin) is preferable to barium for initial examination. Gastrografin causes no significant mediastinal reaction but it also may be too radiolucent to define the site of perforation and spillage. If this initial examination does not allow recognition of perforation, barium then can be used for its better resolving power.

Esophagoscopy may be necessary as a diagnostic procedure, especially in dealing with radiolucent objects. It is imperative after the relief of foreign body impactions that the esophagus be studied thoroughly by barium esophagram, endoscopy, and motility studies to exclude anatomic and motor disorders as the cause of the obstruction.

ESOPHAGITIS

DEFINITION

True esophagitis refers to histologic changes of inflammation that may or may not be associated with macroscopic changes in the esophageal mucosa, or with clinical symptoms. Heartburn is a major symptom of esophagitis, although the two are not always synonymous. There are many forms of esophagitis, but this discussion will emphasize gastroesophageal reflux disease (reflux esophagitis), which is a common clinical problem. Other rare causes of esophagitis include alkaline reflux, postradiation, trauma, corrosive injuries, stasis, and infections primarily related to monilia and herpes simplex.

Reflux occurs when gastric or duodenal contents escape into the esophagus without associated belching or vomiting. This process may or may not produce symptoms. Regurgitation implies that the patient has become aware of reflux that has passed not only the lower esophageal sphincter but also the upper esophageal sphincter. It may be manifested by the appearance of fluid on the pillow at night, by filling of the mouth with fluid, or by aspiration and coughing. Broadly defined, reflux esophagitis is the constellation of symptoms and consequences to the esophagus that results from contact of gastric or intestinal contents with the esophageal mucosa.

The terms hiatal hernia and esophageal reflux are often firmly linked in a cause-and-effect relationship. Recent studies refute this association and suggest that the formation of a hiatal hernia may be a natural part of the aging process. The vast majority of patients with a hiatal hernia do not have reflux. When a hiatal hernia is associated with reflux esophagitis, primary attention should be focused on the esophageal reflux and not upon the hernia. Failure to do so may lead to unnecessary surgical intervention that, though correcting the anatomic structure, may not prevent further gastroesophageal reflux.

SYMPTOMS

The hallmark of gastroesophageal reflux disease is heartburn. Heartburn is usually not described as a pain but rather as an uncomfortable burning sensation located behind the sternum, tending to move into the neck, and waxing and waning in intensity. Heartburn tends to occur approximately 1 hour after meals and can be induced by the ingestion of citrus juices, greasy foods, spicy foods, chocolate, alcohol, and by smoking. Heartburn is more common when the patient is recumbent or bending over. Patients typically complain that their heartburn awakens them soon after they fall asleep as compared with patients with duodenal ulcer who are more likely to awaken in the early morning with a burning sensation. The correlation of severity of heartburn with histologic or macroscopic evidence of esophagitis is not consistent. Many patients with histologic proof of esophagitis have mild or no symptoms, while, in contrast, some patients with severe symptoms have only mild histologic mucosal changes.

The pain associated with esophagitis may mimic angina. Features that favor esophagitis are (1) pain occurring predominantly at rest, when supine, or after meals; (2) chest pain having a delayed or no response to sublingual nitroglycerine; (3) pain, predominantly awakening the patient at night, without associated diaphoresis, nausea, or tachycardia; (4) precipitation of pain by the ingestion of various foods; and (5) repeatedly normal electrocardiogram and stress tests despite frequent episodes of "angina." The differentiation of esophageal from cardiac pain is frequently challenging, but of obvious therapeutic importance.

An unequivocal symptom of esophageal reflux is the regurgitation of food into the mouth, usually at night or upon bending over. The patient may state that he awakens at night with a mouth full of acid or because of coughing or a strangling sensation. Regurgitation reflects rather severe reflux.

Another less common symptom of esophageal reflux is "water brash." Although some individuals use this term synonymously with heartburn, it actually refers to the filling of the mouth suddenly with a clear, slightly salty fluid that comes in extremely large quantities. It seems unlikely that this material is brought up from the stomach and probably is secreted by the salivary glands.

Dysphagia, though uncommon, may be associated with esophageal reflux. The dysphagia is usually with solid foods only, and arrest of the bolus is usually transitory. If dysphagia is a persistent or progressive complaint, one should suspect an esophageal stricture secondary to prolonged reflux. Odynophagia and weight loss are uncommon unless associated with severe esophagitis or mechanical obstruction. Chronic iron deficiency anemia is occasionally associated with reflux esophagitis. However, it is unwise to attribute significant blood loss to esoph-

agitis until the entire gastrointestinal tract has been thoroughly evaluated by radiologic and endoscopic studies. Acute hemorrhage esophagitis is possible and can be severe, but is an infrequent source of upper gastrointestinal hemorrhage. Intermittent wheezing, hoarseness, or "asthma" may be the only clinical manifestation of reflux, especially in children. Many of these patients will have minimal or no heartburn and may well not be aware of nocturnal regurgitation.

DIAGNOSIS

Esophagitis may often be correctly diagnosed by history alone, making fancy diagnostic studies unnecessary and expensive. If there is some doubt about the diagnosis or atypical symptoms, then the initial study should be a barium swallow and upper gastrointestinal series. The study is done not to support the diagnosis of reflux or to demonstrate a hiatal hernia but rather to rule out other possible abnormalities such as peptic ulcer disease and also to exclude complications of chronic reflux such as a peptic stricture or esophageal ulceration. Normal x-ray findings never rule out esophagitis or reflux, nor does the presence of reflux during the barium study give strong evidence that this is the cause of the patient's symptoms. Although hiatal hernia was once considered to be of major importance in the production of reflux, its finding has little importance in predicting whether a patient's symptoms are secondary to reflux.

Following the upper gastrointestinal series, it is reasonable to give most patients a trial of antireflux therapy, including antacids. Only after failure of this approach and certainly before considering any surgical intervention is it necessary to pursue more aggressive diagnostic studies. The flow diagram (Fig. 2) illustrates our diagnostic approach to the patient with gastroesophageal reflux disease.

Tests of esophageal reflux are helpfully divided into three categories (1) those indicating possible reflux; (2) those measuring the results or effect of reflux; and (3) tests that actually measure reflux. *Esophageal manometry* with measurement of the lower esophageal sphincter pressure may indicate possible reflux. Although a lower esophageal sphincter pressure of less than 10 mm Hg is typical of patients with esophageal reflux, there is much variation in this value. Many patients with well-documented esophagitis will have sphincter pressures greater than 10 mm Hg and some asymptomatic subjects have been studied with pressure below this value. Consequently, lower esophageal sphincter pressure in a given pa-

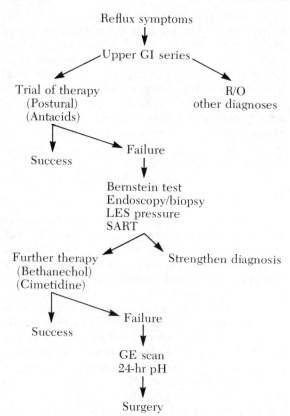

Reflux symptoms

Upper GI series

Trial of therapy
(Postural)
(Antacids)

R/O
other diagnoses

Success   Failure

Bernstein test
Endoscopy/biopsy
LES pressure
SART

Further therapy
(Bethanechol)
(Cimetidine)

Strengthen diagnosis

Success   Failure

GE scan
24-hr pH

Surgery

Figure 2. Approach to the heartburn patient.

tient is often too imprecise to identify a potential for reflux. However, as a more useful clinical tool in the diagnosis of esophageal reflux, a pressure less than 6 mm Hg correlates well with abnormal reflux, and pressure above 20 mm Hg indicates low probability of reflux. Abnormality of esophageal motor activity in the esophageal body may also contribute to esophageal irritation by interfering in the acid clearance from the esophagus. Recognition of decreased esophageal peristalsis during manometric study is important as these patients do particularly poorly after antireflux surgery owing to acid stasis in the esophagus.

Tests measuring results or effects of reflux include the *acid perfusion (Bernstein) test, endoscopy,* and *esophageal mucosal biopsy.* The acid perfusion test if performed in a blinded fashion has been reported to be positive in up to 90 per cent of patients with esophageal reflux. The test demonstrates sensitivity of the distal esophagus to acid and provides no information on the degree of reflux. Direct endoscopic observation of erythema, friability, erosions, or ulcerations of the esophageal mucosa are reliable signs of esophagitis. The findings are definitive when clearly present, but unfortunately are often quite subtle or absent, even in the presence of specific histologic abnormalities on

mucosal biopsy. For this reason biopsies are necessary for the accurate diagnosis of esophagitis in many patients. Biopsy forceps, available with most fiberoptic endoscopes, usually do not yield tissue specimens of sufficient size and depth to allow accurate interpretation. Some physicians therefore prefer suction biopsies taken from the lower esophagus 2 to 10 cm above the esophagogastric mucosal junction. Biopsy tubes can be positioned fluoroscopically, or preferably under endoscopic visualization.

Modern histologic criteria for reflux esophagitis include (1) hyperplasia of the basal cell layer of the epithelium, (2) thinning of the epithelial layer and relative elongation of the papillae (rete pegs), (3) neutrophils infiltrating the lamina propria, and (4) exudates and erosions of the surface epithelium.

Although the barium swallow may occasionally demonstrate actual reflux, better tests include the *standard acid reflux test, gastroesophageal scintiscan* and *24-hour pH monitoring.* The standard acid reflux test is performed using a pH probe positioned 5 cm above the lower esophageal sphincter. With the patient in different positions, various breathing maneuvers are performed. A drop in intraesophageal pH to less than 4 is considered evidence of reflux. Eighty per cent of patients with reflux will have an abnormal test. This study when combined with esophageal biopsies provides the most sensitive and specific tests for reflux esophagitis.

A radioisotope scintiscan has been recently employed to document reflux and also to give a quantitative assessment of the amount of reflux. This scintiscan employs a radioisotope (^{99m}Tc-sulfur colloid; 100 uC$_1$) as the marker of reflux. In addition, increasing abdominal compression is used as the stress to unmask incompetence of the reflux barrier. Although a very sensitive test, it requires a well-equipped radioisotope laboratory with facilities for computerized gamma counting over the esophagus and stomach, and should be used only for those patients in whom a diagnosis of reflux is not clarified by other studies.

Twenty-four hour pH monitoring measures exposure time of the distal esophageal mucosa to acid gastric juices via a pH probe placed 5 cm above the lower esophageal sphincter. Continuous recording are made during modified daily activity, eating, and sleeping. This test records reflux during physiologic activity and does not stress the antireflux mechanism with unnatural respiratory maneuvers or unphysiologic abdominal compression. The principal disadvantage of this test is the requirement for overnight hospitalization. Like the scintiscan, this test should be reserved for the patient with a difficult diagnostic problem not responding to treatment or in a preoperative evaluation before antireflux surgery.

BARRETT'S ESOPHAGUS

DEFINITION

Barrett's esophagus is a disorder that is either congenital or acquired, and consists of columnar epithelium replacing the normal squamous epithelium of the lower esophagus. It is usually associated with a hiatal hernia and chronic reflux of gastric contents into the esophagus. The extent of this mucosal change may occur over variable lengths of the esophagus proximally, often extending as high as the mid or upper third of the esophagus. It may be associated with ulcerations (most commonly just below the squamocolumnar junction), bleeding, and stricture. Patients with Barrett's esophagus are also known to have a propensity to develop adenocarcinoma of the esophageal body, with a reported incidence of 3 to 9 per cent.

SYMPTOMS

Patients with Barrett's esophagus usually experience long-standing symptoms of gastroesophageal reflux. In addition, if a stricture is present, the patient may complain of progressive dysphagia. Other frequent symptoms are epigastric pain, eructation, weight loss, indigestion, and hematemesis.

DIAGNOSIS

The barium esophagram is almost always abnormal. The characteristic findings include a hiatal hernia, patulous esophagogastric junction, and mid esophageal stricture. Other findings may include the presence of an esophageal ulceration or irregular mid esophageal narrowing, suggesting carcinoma.

Endoscopic examination with biopsies is diagnostic of Barrett's esophagus. The proximal squamous mucosa may be friable, erythematous, or completely normal in appearance. Stricture, when present, is located at the junction of the squamous and columnar mucosa. Esophageal ulceration, if present, is found just below this level in the columnar mucosa. Definitive diagnosis demands the histologic presence of columnar epithelium within the esophagus (not within a hiatal hernia pouch). Biopsies taken at several levels using a multipurpose biopsy tube are most helpful and often demonstrate the transition from squamous to columnar epithelium.

Esophageal manometric studies have consistently demonstrated peristaltic activity in both the squamous and columnar segments of the Barrett's esophagus. The resting lower esophageal sphincter pressure is usually decreased. Pertechnetate esophageal scintiscans have recently been used for diagnosis but are only helpful if the columnar epithelium contains acid-secreting parietal cells.

ACHALASIA

DEFINITION

Achalasia was one of the first motor disorders of the esophagus to be recognized clinically. Although the age of onset is usually between 20 and 40, cases in infants have been reported. The disease may be familial and adult onset in parent and offspring has been reported. There are two main defects in achalasia: (1) obstruction at the esophagogastric junction, and (2) abnormal esophageal peristalsis. Obstruction was initially attributed to spasm of the cardia or lower esophageal sphincter, and the condition was called cardiospasm. Subsequently, manometric techniques revealed that the lower esophageal sphincter had abnormally high resting pressures and showed absence or incomplete relaxation with swallowing, hence the term achalasia, which literally means "failure of relaxation." The defect in the esophageal body is emphasized by two more terms that have been used to refer to this disease, namely, "megaesophagus," because of the striking dilatation that may occur, and "aperistalsis," to describe the absence of normal peristaltic contractions in the lower two thirds of the body of the esophagus.

Chronic Chagas' disease caused by *Trypanosoma cruzi* infection may be associated with megaesophagus, which displays clinical and manometric findings identical to those seen in idiopathic achalasia. Carcinomas, primarily adenocarcinoma of the stomach, may present with clinical, radiologic, and manometric findings resembling idiopathic achalasia. Distinctive differential features include the older age of the patients, brief duration of symptoms, marked weight loss, and absence of esophageal dilatation.

SYMPTOMS

The insidious development of this motor abnormality is often relatively imperceptible to the patient. With careful questioning, it becomes apparent that there has been difficulty with eating over many months to years, with the patient learning to adapt. Typically, these patients will find that it takes much longer for them to eat the normal meal than it does their companions, or that they have developed a variety of associated maneuvers such as the ingestion of water or a Valsalva type of maneuver to aid in swallowing.

Dysphagia for both solids and liquids is the classic symptom that brings most patients to medical attention. Ironically, those patients with minimal esophageal dilatation tend to have more dysphagia than those with a widely dilated tortuous esophagus. The dysphagia is usually painless, progressive, and frequently worse during periods of emotional stress, or when the patient is trying to eat rapidly. Regurgitation of retained material is another common symptom. This may be provoked by change in position or exercise and is particularly troublesome at night. The material brought up from the esophagus is often recognized as food that has been eaten many hours previously. It tends not to have an acid taste. In fact, true heartburn is an uncommon manifestation of achalasia.

Because of frequent regurgitation of liquid material from the dilated esophagus, pulmonary symptoms may be prominent and not uncommonly the patient may seek medical help primarily because of wheezing, coughing, choking, or recurrent aspiration pneumonias. Weight loss is common in patients with achalasia and therefore does not always suggest the possibility of a carcinoma.

Patients with achalasia may display ingenious and bizarre techniques to compensate for their disease. Certain postural maneuvers, such as throwing the shoulders back, lifting the neck, and performing a rapid Valsalva maneuver, help retained food to pass into the stomach. These techniques aid the transmission of hydraulic forces down the esophageal lumen and help partially to overcome the elevated lower esophageal sphincter pressures. Patients may learn to eat less later in the day and some develop a ritual of induced regurgitation before bedtime to prevent the bothersome nocturnal symptoms.

DIAGNOSIS

The diagnosis of achalasia can occasionally be made by examining a routine chest film. One may see (1) a fluid level within the esophagus, (2) absence of a gastric air bubble, (3) a widened mediastinum, (4) a double density overlying the cardiac shadow, or (5) a thin curving line of the dilated esophageal wall in the right upper mediastinum.

Barium examination of the esophagus is the most common and easily available form of diagnostic aid. Characteristic features include a smoothly tapered narrowing at the distal end of the esophagus (parrot's beak), the presence of a fluid level in the upper part of the esophagus owing to retained esophageal secretions and ingested material and esophageal dilatation, which in advanced disease produces the classic "sigmoid" esophagus. Cineradiographic studies reveal a lack of peristalsis in the lower two thirds of the esophagus. The break-like symmetrical narrowing of the distal end of the esophagus helps to differentiate achalasia from the more ragged appearance of carcinoma involving the cardia. Proximal dilatation is also unusual in carcinoma and common in achalasia. The persistent fluid level helps to separate achalasia radiographically from scleroderma, in which barium is retained with the patient supine but empties readily fron the esophagus in the upright position. In scleroderma, there is also no distal narrowing unless reflux esophagitis has lead to a stricture.

Panendoscopy with biopsy and cytologic examination should be performed in every patient with achalasia to exclude other causes of obstruction, particularly carcinoma. Several days of clear liquids followed by intubation and cleansing of the esophagus just prior to endoscopy will prevent aspiration during the procedure and allow better visualization of the esophageal mucosa. The lumen of the esophagus is usually dilated, whereas the lower esophageal sphincter is closed and fails to open for prolonged periods despite the introduction of air. There may be evidence of stasis esophagitis and no peristaltic waves are seen. The closed lower sphincter should open easily with gentle pressure by the endoscope. If firm resistance is experienced, an organic stricture or malignancy should be suspected. Once the stomach is entered, particular attention should be paid to the cardia. This should include retroflexion of the tip of the endoscope to allow better visualization of the cardia to help rule out an adenocarcinoma causing secondary achalasia. With the endoscope in the stomach, a guide wire may be passed through the endoscopic biopsy channel to aid in the passage of therapeutic dilatators or motility catheters.

The diagnosis of achalasia should always be established by esophageal manometry. Using perfused recording catheters, the characteristic manometric features include: (1) absence of peristalsis in the body of the esophagus; (2) elevated resting intraesophageal pressure; (3) a

Table 3. *Manometric Features of Achalasia*

Absent peristalsis
Elevated intraesophageal pressure (>gastric)
Hypertensive lower esophageal sphincter (>30 mm Hg)
Incomplete sphincter relaxation

hypertensive lower esophageal sphincter (usually greater than 30 mm Hg); and (4) incomplete relaxation of the sphincter with swallowing (Table 3). Early in the course, low amplitude, spontaneous, nonprogressive, nonperistaltic waves may be recorded within the body of the esophagus, but later there is usually a total absence of pressure response.

This combination of manometric features usually allows precise diagnosis of achalasia. Methacholine (Mecholyl), 2 to 10 mg subcutaneously, or bethanechol (Urecholine), 2.5 to 5.0 mg subcutaneously, may be helpful in variant cases. A positive response is indicated by a sustained increase in intraluminal pressure to greater than 25 mm Hg above baseline values. Positive tests have also been reported in diffuse spasm and carcinoma infiltrating the lower esophagus and thereby decreasing the diagnostic usefulness of the agent.

DIFFUSE ESOPHAGEAL SPASM

DEFINITION

Diffuse esophageal spasm is a clinical syndrome characterized by the triad of (1) episodic chest pain and dysphagia, (2) tertiary contractions on x-ray, and (3) a manometric pattern characterized by repetitive simultaneous contractions as well as intermittent normal peristalsis. Striking abnormalities of the barium esophagram are often associated with this condition and have prompted the introduction of a variety of colorful synonyms, including curling, beading, corkscrew esophagus, rosary bead esophagus, functional diverticulosis, pseudodiverticulosis, segmental spasm, elevator esophagus, knuckle duster, and tertiary contractions. Similar changes in the barium-filled esophagus also occur in asymptomatic people, particularly the elderly, resulting in considerable confusion in precise definition of the syndrome on the basis of x-ray findings. The diagnosis of "symptomatic" diffuse esophageal spasm should be reserved for those patients having characteristic abnormalities of esophageal manometrics or barium esophagram associated with chest pain or dysphagia.

SYMPTOMS

The pain of diffuse esophageal spasm may be quite variable. It may be dull to colicky, mild or severe, and extremely brief to persistent. It is usually substernal but may radiate into the jaws and neck, down the arms, or through to the back. It may appear during or after a meal or awaken the patient at night, and it may occur alone or during the episodes of dysphagia, or both. The appearance of this symptom complex in older patients may mimic angina pectoris, and the known relief of diffuse esophageal spasm by sublingual nitroglycerin may make the differential diagnosis next to impossible without the aid of an electrocardiogram or treadmill stress test.

Dysphagia may also be quite variable. It may be precipitated by emotion or the ingestion of cold, hot, or carbonated beverages. The patient may note painful or painless sticking of food, both liquids and solids. Unlike achalasia, dysphagia is typically intermittent in occurrence and rarely progressive in severity. Syncope on swallowing has been reported with esophageal spasm probably secondary to a vagal reflex. Weight loss is rare.

DIAGNOSIS

A plain film of the chest reveals no characteristic findings. Abnormalities on barium esophagram are characterized by the presence of simultaneous, nonperistaltic contractions that result in segmentation of the barium in the lower half of the esophagram. The appearance may vary from mild serrations of the margin of the barium-filled esophagus to subdivisions or outpouching of the esophageal outline. A bolus of barium, observed cineradiographically, may become trapped, be pushed back and forth, or forced orad. In contrast to achalasia, the esophagus does not become dilated.

The diagnosis of diffuse esophageal spasm should not be made without definite manometric evidence of esophageal motor abnormality, although the specific defects are less well defined because of the numerous manometric variations that may compose this syndrome. The manometric hallmark of this condition is the occurrence of *repetitive nonperistaltic contractions* in the lower portion of the esophagus. These nonperistaltic contractions frequently follow a swallow but often occur spontaneously through the esophagus. Peristaltic contraction waves may also be seen intermittently. High amplitude and increased duration of the contraction waves are also manometric features often seen in patients with diffuse esophageal spasm (Table 4). Amplitudes exceeding 140 mm Hg are commonly seen and occasionally a sustained "tetanic" contraction may be seen with reproduction of the patient's chest pain. Generally, the lower esophageal sphincter pressures are normal and complete relaxation occurs. The resting pressure in the body of the esophagus is also normal in patients with diffuse spasm. Recently, it has been reported that these patients have a supersensitive muscular response of the esophagus to subcutaneous or intravenous pentagastrin. This response is similar to the exaggerated response to methacholine (Mecholyl) that can also be seen in patients with diffuse esophageal spasm.

The role of endoscopy in this disorder is to exclude all other lesions that may cause spasm, dysphagia, or odynophagia, and hence mimic diffuse esophageal spasm.

NONSPECIFIC ESOPHAGEAL MOTOR DYSFUNCTION

It is important to recognize that many patients with dysphagia or chest pain or both have motility abnormalities not meeting accepted definitions of achalasia or esophageal spasm. Part of this problem relates to definitions: achalasia seems fairly well defined by abnormalities of lower esophageal sphincter relaxation and absence of peristalsis. However, spasm is less clearly defined and a variety of manometric phenomena such as repetitive contractions, high amplitude contractions, and prolonged duration of contractions are included in this diagnosis. Many patients with occasional repetitive contractions, spontaneous contractions, impaired sphincter relaxation, or increased sphincter pressure do not have manometric patterns diagnostic of either spasm or achalasia. It has been proposed that perhaps achalasia and diffuse esophageal spasm constitute two ends of a spectrum of a broader category of esophageal motility disorders, with predominant sphincter dysfunction and aperistalsis at one end (achalasia) and predominant esophageal activity at the other (spasm). There is considerable evidence that these two diseases are interrelated and have overlapping manifestations with increasing numbers of cases of transition from spasm to achalasia being recognized. Other evidence

Table 4. *Manometric Features of Diffuse Esophageal Spasm*

Repetitive, nonperistaltic (simultaneous) contractions
Spontaneous motor activity
Intermittent normal peristalsis
Increased amplitude or duration of contraction

---

that achalasia and esophageal spasm represent the ends of the spectrum of esophageal motor disorders includes the presence of a positive methacholine response in both entities, and the manometric aspects of the condition termed "vigorous achalasia," which demonstrates features of both diseases.

The gray area between the two more clearly defined motor disorders of achalasia and spasm includes abnormalities conveniently classified as nonspecific esophageal motor dysfunction. Included in this category should be patients with symptoms of dysphagia or chest pain or both, having abnormal esophageal motility other than typical diffuse spasm, achalasia, or scleroderma, and with no systemic disease associated with abnormal esophageal motility.

GASTRITIS

By ANGELO E. DAGRADI, M.D.
Garden Grove, California

The inflammatory diseases of the stomach may be acute or chronic in nature. Although they vary greatly in degree of severity, they have serious implications because of the functional (interference with secretion of acid-pepsin and intrinsic factor) and structural alterations (mucosal atrophy) that they are prone to elicit, and the complications that may ensue, such as hemorrhage, ulceration, pernicious anemia, mucosal polyps, or carcinoma.

The inflammation may be localized to a certain area of the stomach or may involve it diffusely; all layers of the gastric wall may be affected or the disorder may be restricted to the superficial strata alone, the mucosa and submucosa. Bleeding may occur and may be occult or torrential. It usually derives from multiple, punctate erosions in the mucosa. (The term *erosion* indicates a defect that does not penetrate more deeply than the muscularis mucosa.) Destruction of the glandular structures by the inflammatory process eventuates in their replacement by an intestinal type of epithelium that is mucus-secreting (atrophic mucosa) and is subject to complications (ulceration and neoplastic degeneration) as just indicated.

A broad spectrum of causative factors can occasion this disease. These include exogenous (corrosive poisons, certain medications, ethanol, etc.) and endogenous (bile-trypsin reflux) chemical agents; bacterial, fungus, viral, or protozoan infections (affecting the stomach by

direct invasion or by toxins that they elaborate);
physical agents (x-irradiation, thermal injury);
metabolic (vitamin deficiencies, endocrinopathies) and genetic (pernicious anemia) disorders.

In common with all other diseases, gastric
inflammation may be symptomatic or may exist
in the absence of symptoms. When present,
symptoms are usually nonspecific in nature and
include nausea, vomiting, anorexia, weight loss,
dyspepsia, weakness, epigastric pain and tenderness, hematemesis or melena or both, and
diarrhea. Epigastric pain or distress is associated usually with ingestion of food and derives
from stretching and distention of the inflamed
wall. Diarrhea and iron deficiency anemia may
occur in consequence of achlorhydria resulting
from destruction of the gastric glandular apparatus.

The diagnosis of gastritis derives tentatively
from the anamnesis, symptoms, and physical
findings. These are developed from, and are
predicated upon, an understanding of the factors that have been elucidated and described.
This is usually sufficient for the diagnosis of
acute gastritis, such as that resulting from food
poisoning, since this is generally a self-limiting
disorder. Invasive diagnostic modalities are seldom required in this condition and are merely
of academic value.

A definitive diagnosis of gastritis is established by gastroscopy (occasionally by surgery
or autopsy) with microscopic confirmation of
tissue specimens obtained by visually targeted
biopsy. This procedure is performed commonly
(1) when gastric mucosal inflammation occasions upper gastrointestinal bleeding severe
enough that identification of the nature and
location of the source is required for proper
management, and (2) when the cause for persistent upper gastrointestinal symptoms is
sought in patients in whom the radiographic
findings are nonrevealing. Gastroscopy may
also reveal the existence of gastritis, as an additional finding, when the primary purpose of the
examination is for other indications (peptic
ulcer disease, gastric cancer, hiatal hernia,
etc.).

Because the relatively hidden location of gastric inflammatory processes requires the use of
highly specialized techniques for their detection, there exists a strong tendency to minimize
their symptomatic proclivities and long-range
implications. Interestingly, however, when inflammatory lesions similar in nature and appearance to those encountered in the stomach
are observed to involve the mucosa of a visually
accessible area such as the buccal mucosa, clinicians do not hesitate to acknowledge their presence and relate to them any local symptoms that
may be present.

PEPTIC ULCER

By BENNETT E. ROTH, M.D.
Burbank, California

Peptic ulcer disease is due to the combined
effects of acid and pepsin resulting in the digestion of the mucosal surface of the stomach or
duodenum. Histologically these lesions are
similar, with signs of disruption of surface epithelium and the extension of inflammatory granulation tissue to at least the muscularis mucosa.

The incidence of duodenal ulcer and gastric
ulcer is 1.3 per cent and 0.5 per cent per year,
respectively, in the population of the United
States. Approximately 10 per cent of the population have had or will have the diagnosis of
peptic ulcer disease made during their lifetime.

In order to properly diagnose ulcer disease,
the physician must take a careful history and be
aware of the variety of ways in which it may
present.

SYMPTOMS AND SIGNS

The classic symptom of uncomplicated peptic
ulcer disease is gnawing, burning, or boring-
like pain in the epigastrium occurring 1 to 3
hours after eating or awakening and is generally
relieved by eating or the use of antacids. The
pain often occurs in a cluster of several days or
weeks and then may spontaneously abate only
to occur at some later date. At times it is described as a hunger sensation or feeling of
nausea. This classic sequence of eating, pain,
and relief by eating is most suggestive of ulcer
disease. However, other conditions may mimic
this entity, such as esophagitis, functional
bowel syndrome, drug-induced dyspepsia, or
rare conditions of the stomach such as Crohn's
disease, Menetrier's disease, and occasionally
the early stages of carcinoma of the stomach or
pancreas. Furthermore, the classic pattern described occurs in only approximately 50 per
cent of the patients with ulcer disease. There
are many patients with ulcers who are asymptomatic and whose lesions are diagnosed only
when complications arise or at the time of an
upper gastrointestinal series done for other purposes. Patients with gastric ulcers may complain shortly after eating. Those with pyloric
channel ulcers often complain of pain with
meals associated with vomiting and less relief
with antacids. Therefore, the physician cannot
rely solely on the history in making the diagnosis.

Physical examination is oftentimes nonspecific. There may be epigastric tenderness on palpation of the abdomen. A succussion splash may be found in the presence of gastric outlet obstruction. However, it is apparent that at the time of the initial presentation of dyspeptic symptoms the physician must proceed with a complete work-up to delineate the underlying process.

The upper GI series represents the most commonly used diagnostic study for the initial diagnosis of peptic ulcer disease. When performed by a skilled radiologist, the diagnosis can be made in 80 to 85 per cent of cases. If an uncomplicated duodenal ulcer crater is identified, one can institute therapy. If evidence of marked gastric hypersecretion is noted — e.g., excessive intraluminal fluid, ulcers in atypical locations, gastric hyper-rugosity — then the possibility of the Zollinger-Ellison syndrome must be considered and a fasting serum gastrin level obtained. This will be discussed more fully later. Most physicians think that a patient with gastric ulcer seen on radiographic examination should undergo endoscopic examination with biopsy to exclude the presence of malignancy. This should be carried out, even if the ulcer appears benign, since 4 per cent of such lesions eventually turn out to harbor malignancy. Certainly, if the radiologist suggests the possibility of malignant ulceration, endoscopy, biopsy, and brush cytology are indicated.

If the radiographic study is inconclusive or negative, endoscopic examination is needed. This procedure is safe and highly accurate both in locating ulcers and in defining the presence of other diseases that may mimic peptic ulcer disease. In a patient with a history of previous gastric surgery for peptic ulcer disease, endoscopy is the first diagnostic procedure of choice. If at the time of endoscopy for peptic ulcer disease no ulcer crater can be identified, but there is evidence of friability and mucosal disruption of the gastric or duodenal mucosa, then one should consider the diagnosis of gastritis or erosive duodenitis. If the mucosa appears erythematous but nonfriable, then this diagnosis is not applied to such patients and they should not be considered as having acid-peptic disease. The presence of gastritis or duodenitis should probably be considered part of the spectrum of ulcer disease and treated in a similar fashion. Caution should be exercised before considering any surgical procedures for such patients.

LABORATORY STUDIES

As just mentioned, the fasting serum gastrin is of value in evaluating a patient with suspected Zollinger-Ellison syndrome. It should also be obtained in a patient with peptic ulcer disease and hypercalcemia, patients with family histories of multiple endocrine adenomatosis, with recurrent ulcers following surgery, and in all patients prior to elective ulcer surgery.

The gastric analysis is of limited usefulness. In many situations it has been supplanted by serum gastrin determinations. These are cheaper and easier to obtain. Furthermore, the great overlap in the level of basal and maximal acid secretion among patients with duodenal ulcers, gastric ulcers, and normals is significant. The gastric analysis, however, should be done in all patients with recurrent ulcer following surgery to investigate the possibilities of incomplete vagotomy or Zollinger-Ellison syndrome. Serum calcium determinations should be obtained in all patients with ulcer disease. If this is elevated, the presence of hyperparathyroidism should be suspected. Often, the patients with combined ulcer disease and hyperparathyroidism will be found to have a form of multiple endocrine adenomatosis and have Zollinger-Ellison syndrome.

COMPLICATIONS

Bleeding from ulcers occurs in 10 to 20 per cent of patients who have been followed over long periods of time. A history of melena, iron deficiency anemia or the presence of occult blood in the stool should prompt a thorough investigation into the possibility of bleeding duodenal or gastric ulcer. The presence of overt gastrointestinal hemorrhage manifested as hematemesis with hypovolemia requires prompt diagnostic evaluation. Once this patient's condition is stabilized, a large-bore nasogastric tube is placed and the stomach lavaged with iced saline solution to remove blood and clots and ascertain the rate of ongoing bleeding. Following this, the best diagnostic tool is endoscopic examination. Optimally this should be carried out within the first 6 to 12 hours following hospitalization. The timing depends on the rapidity of bleeding, the stability of the patient's condition, and the consideration of therapeutic maneuvers such as surgery.

Gastric outlet obstruction may be seen in association with pyloric channel ulcers or acute and chronic ulcer disease of the duodenal bulb or distal gastric antrum. This may be suggested at the time of upper gastrointestinal x-ray examination by the presence of foodstuff and secretions, or the slow rate of emptying of the stomach. The saline load test is more accurate and will define abnormalities of gastric emptying even when the x-ray examination fails to suggest its presence. This is carried out by placing a nasogastric tube in the gastric antrum, emptying the stomach completely and instilling 750 ml of isotonic saline solution rapidly. The tube is then clamped for 30 minutes, after which the stomach is aspirated again as much as possible. The presence of greater than 350 ml of saline following this 30-minute period suggests an abnormality in gastric emptying. The use of radioactive-labeled meals with scanning is another means of demonstrating obstruction with delayed emptying but is more expensive and is not universally available.

The presence of perforated duodenal or gastric ulcer is generally associated with signs of an acute abdomen and the presence of free intra-abdominal air visible beneath the diaphragm on chest and abdominal x-ray. Many such patients may be treated medically. The decision regarding surgery and its timing is dependent on the history of previous ulcer disease or symptoms and the signs of potential peritonitis.

FOLLOW-UP

Duodenal ulcer is a chronic disease with a strong potential for recurrence and periods of exacerbation and remission. A patient with history of previous duodenal ulcer who experiences recurrent symptoms can be re-treated in the absence of complications without the need for additional x-ray or endoscopic study. However, should complicating factors occur or should the patient fail to respond to routine management, upper GI series or endoscopy are needed to ensure the validity of the diagnosis.

Gastric ulcers should be followed serially at 4 to 6 week intervals to ensure complete healing. An ulcer that is initially found to be benign via endoscopic examination and that is visible on x-ray can be followed by this technique until it appears to be healed. At that time a follow-up endoscopy is recommended to ensure that complete mucosal healing has occurred and to rule out the possibility of occult carcinoma.

NEOPLASMS OF THE STOMACH

By WILLIAM D. SEYBOLD, M.D.
Houston, Texas

A variety of tumors arise in the stomach: the epithelial ones — polyps and carcinoma —from its lining; and mesenchymal ones — leiomyomas, leiomyosarcomas, and lymphosar-comas — from its wall. Carcinoma surpasses all others in importance because it is the most common and the most lethal. It is a deadly disease but not a hopeless one. Its incidence is diminishing, and it can be cured by current means. The problem is to recognize the presence of cancer so that a timely and well-performed operation may be done to eradicate it. For those who come to operation before the disease has spread beyond the walls of the stomach, the probability of cure approaches 50 per cent. For those who do not, medicine has nothing curative to offer.

CANCER OF THE STOMACH

There are two bright spots in the present scene. The first is the decline in incidence of gastric cancer in the United States during the past 50 years, for reasons unknown. In 1930 cancer of the stomach was the most frequent cause of death from cancer among American males. The age-adjusted death rate was 29 per 100,000. In 1976, that rate had fallen to 7 per 100,000, and was exceeded by that of cancer of the lung (53 per 100,000), colon and rectum (19 per 100,000), prostate (13 per 100,000), and pancreas (9 per 100,000).

The second encouraging fact is that diagnostic means are available to almost eliminate the guesswork about the nature of an ulcerating lesion of the stomach. For many years the response of an ulcer to medical treatment was an accepted means of distinguishing a benign from a malignant lesion of the stomach in doubtful cases. Such a clinical trial is no longer an acceptable option. Now, immediate recognition of the malignant lesion is possible in 95 per cent of cases with a combination of radiologic, endoscopic, cytologic, and biopsy studies.

Cancer of the stomach is more common in the male than in the female (1.5 to 1.0). As with cancer generally, the peak incidence is in the sixth and seventh decades.

Those people with pernicious anemia, achlorhydria, or gastric atrophy are at greater risk than others of developing gastric cancer. Therefore, special attention should be paid them.

SYMPTOMS

The problem in early diagnosis is that gastric cancer, like visceral cancer in general, often produces no symptoms or signs until it has become locally extensive. By that time it has usually spread to regional lymph nodes or beyond, and the opportunity for surgical excision has passed.

Symptoms may be absent or minimal and are often mild. They are anorexia, epigastric distress, and early satiety; appearing in middle-aged or older persons, they should alert the physician to look for gastric cancer. Weight loss, obstructive symptoms, anemia secondary to chronic blood loss, weakness, and easy fatigue are usually manifestations of long-standing disease. Massive bleeding is rare, but the presence of occult blood in the stool or gastric aspirate is common.

PHYSICAL SIGNS

Pallor, evidence of weight loss, a palpable scalene node (Virchow's), an epigastric mass, or a mass in the pelvic cul-de-sac are late developments. The goal of the physician is the detection of the gastric lesion before these signs appear. After they appear, prospects of cure are poor.

LABORATORY AIDS IN DIAGNOSIS

Unexplained anemia should lead to the search for a gastrointestinal source of occult bleeding. The stomach is a good place to start. It is an accepted fact that people with pernicious anemia are at increased risk of developing gastric cancer. It is also true that achlorhydria is a factor that is related to gastric cancer. Fifty per cent of patients with gastric cancer have free hydrochloric acid in their stomach, but, in people with achlorhydria, the incidence of gastric cancer is higher than in comparable groups with free acid present.

There are no other useful chemical tests and no immunologic tests that are helpful in establishing the diagnosis.

RADIOLOGIC DIAGNOSIS

Radiologic examination of the stomach by a skilled radiologist is the first and most important procedure that can lead to an early diagnosis.

Cancer of the stomach may appear as an ulcer, as a mass, or as an area of rigidity in the stomach wall that is normally pliable. Whereas the radiologist cannot always distinguish between a benign and a malignant lesion, there are certain radiographic features of gastric cancer that enable him to give a positive opinion with confidence when they are present: a mass with ulceration, rigidity of the wall, and fixed narrowing of the antrum or body of the stomach.

ENDOSCOPIC EXAMINATION, BIOPSY, AND CYTOLOGY

Perhaps in the young patient with a small benign-appearing ulcer at the angle on the lesser curvature, endoscopic examination is unnecessary. Certainly in patients with large tumors, obstruction, or obvious cancer, diagnosed on the basis of radiographic and clinical evidence, it may sometimes be omitted. But endoscopic examination with biopsy or cytologic studies or both makes accurate diagnosis possible in 95 per cent of the patients with gastric cancer. The recent development of improved fiberoptic endoscopes has made these techniques quite safe and accurate in expert hands.

In a 1977 report from the University of Chicago Medical Center, a correct positive cytologic report was obtained in 85 per cent of 183 proven cancers and a correct positive histologic report was obtained in 80 per cent. By one or both techniques a correct positive report was received in 95 per cent.

Tumors of the cardia are difficult for the endoscopist as well as for the radiologist. Stenosis at the esophagogastric junction by submucosal spread of the fundal gastric tumors into the distal esophagus makes interpretation and tissue recovery or exfoliated-cell recovery difficult. But, by using clinical, radiographic, and endoscopic evidence, the physician should make few errors in mistaking a benign fibrous stricture at the cardia for a cancer.

SARCOMAS

Lymphosarcomas account for less than 10 per cent of malignancies of the stomach. They are of two varieties: lymphomatous and reticulum cell. The former has a better prognosis than adenocarcinoma of the stomach, and radiation therapy as a complement to resection seems to contribute to improved survival. By contrast, roentgen therapy has no significant role in the control of gastric carcinoma.

The clinical manifestations of lymphosarcoma of the stomach are the same as those of carcinoma. Sometimes the tumor attains much greater volume (bulk) than adenocarcinoma before the diagnosis of gastric malignancy is made, and this fact, in addition to the presence of unusually large rugal folds, may lead the radiologist to suspect the lymphomatous nature of the lesion. In the University of Chicago study, previously cited, cytology or biopsy with the gastroscope or both permitted a positive diagnosis in all 13 patients with lymphosarcoma.

Leiomyosarcomas are rare. In a group of sarcomas of the stomach reported by Remine from the Mayo Clinic, there were 55 leiomyosarcomas and 224 lymphosarcomas. They arise from smooth muscle of the wall of the stomach, but ulceration of the overlying mucosa may give rise to severe bleeding. These tumors may become quite large before being discovered. Resection is the only effective treatment.

BENIGN TUMORS

Ninety-five per cent of gastric tumors are malignant. In the 5 per cent that are benign, polyps and leiomyomas make up the majority. Current opinion holds that 75 to 80 per cent of the polypoid lesions are hyperplastic and not neoplastic, but in some series as many as 20 per cent have been found to be malignant. Therefore, the consensus is that gastric polyps should be removed. This can often be accomplished with the modern fiberoptic instruments. As a practical matter, polyps larger than 2 cm in diameter are likely to be cancer.

Symptoms. Benign tumors can produce pain, obstructive symptoms, or bleeding. Small polypoid lesions are more often seen by the endoscopist than by the radiologist, but it is usually the presence of some abnormality observed by the radiologist that leads to endoscopic examination.

SCREENING FOR GASTRIC NEOPLASMS

Screening for gastric neoplasms for the whole population is impractical and unwarranted. There are some who recommend regular periodic screening for members of families in which cancer of the stomach has occurred, but the facts do not support this policy. An increase of cancer has not been reported in a large group so studied. There is a consensus, however, that patients with pernicious anemia, achlorhydria and hypochlorhydria, and gastric atrophy should be examined for gastric lesions annually. They constitute a relatively high-risk group.

So while we await better understanding of gastric cancer and better methods to control it, the physician is obligated to apply the best that current knowledge and technique provides; these are a high index of suspicion, prompt and thorough study if gastric malignancy is suspected, an early diagnosis, and a well-performed operation. This is the best there is to offer.

TUMORS OF THE SMALL INTESTINE

By GLEN A. LEHMAN, M.D.,
and ROBERT A. RANKIN, M.D.

Indianapolis, Indiana

Small intestinal tumors are rare and comprise approximately 1 per cent of all clinically detected gastrointestinal neoplasms. In most cases the clinician must have a high index of suspicion to diagnose such tumors. Many small intestinal tumors are asymptomatic and are not discovered during life. Although most of these quiescent tumors are benign, 60 to 75 per cent of all symptomatic tumors prove to be malignant. Such tumors may arise from the epithelium or develop from the subepithelial structures. The benign tumors include adenomas, leiomyomas, villous adenomas, lipomas, angiomas, fibromas, and inflammatory polyps. The adenocarcinomas, lymphomas, and various sarcomas, most of which are leiomyosarcomas, make up the malignant tumors. Carcinoid tumors may be malignant or benign. Tumors are found in all age groups but are much more frequent after age 40.

PRESENTING SIGNS AND SYMPTOMS

Small intestinal tumors give rise largely to nonspecific symptoms. Crampy abdominal pain, nausea, vomiting, and distention may occur as the tumors cause intestinal obstruction by intussusception or primary mass effect. Tumor ulceration or necrosis may produce gastrointestinal bleeding that is occult (iron deficiency anemia or stool occult blood or both) or overt (melena most commonly). Fever and weight loss may occur with malignant lesions.

The physical examination is often normal, especially in benign lesions. Abdominal distention and high-pitched, tinkling bowel sounds suggest intestinal obstruction. A palpable mass is rare with benign lesions and occurs in approximately one third of malignant tumors.

SPECIAL SYNDROMES ASSOCIATED WITH SMALL INTESTINAL TUMORS

Carcinoid tumors (argentaffinomas) are most commonly asymptomatic and found coincidentally at laparotomy for other causes. Ileal and appendiceal carcinoids are most frequent. These tumors secrete 5-hydroxytryptamine (serotonin), which is inactivated by the liver. In the presence of hepatic metastases, the typical syndrome of flushing, diarrhea, and right-sided valvular heart lesions occurs. Serotonin is metabolized into 5-hydroxyindolacetic acid (5-HIAA), producing abnormal urinary elevations of the latter compound. False-positive elevations of 5-HIAA may occur from ingestion of glycerol guaiacolate, mephenesin, acetanilid, and methocarbamol as well as pineapples, bananas, and nuts. Patients with gluten enteropathy may also have elevated 5-HIAA levels.

Patients with gluten enteropathy are at increased risk for developing small bowel tumors, with lymphomas being the most common type. Such tumors occur more commonly in patients with a long history of celiac disease, especially if dietary gluten restriction has not been strict.

There are several hereditary syndromes in which those patients affected have an increased incidence of small intestinal tumors. In Peutz-Jeghers syndrome (autosomal dominant), hamartomatous polyps of the small intestine, stomach, or colon are associated with melanin spots of the buccal mucosa, lips, and fingers. Such polyps are only rarely associated with malignancy. In Gardner's syndrome (autosomal dominant), subcutaneous benign tumors and osteomas are associated with adenomas and adenocarcinomas of the entire gastrointestinal tract. Such small bowel carcinomas are most commonly periampullary. In Cronkhite-Canada syndrome, diffuse gastrointestinal polyposis (inflammatory polyps) is associated with alopecia, nail dystrophy, and cutaneous hyperpigmentation. In von Recklinghausen's disease, neurofibromas of the central and peripheral nervous systems are associated with multiple café au lait spots. Neurofibromas may develop anywhere along the entire gastrointestinal tract in such patients and, rarely, sarcomatous degeneration may occur.

DIAGNOSTIC TESTS

Laboratory studies are generally of little help, except for stool occult blood testing, blood hemoglobin level, and 5-HIAA for metastatic carcinoid. Up to 20 per cent of patients with small intestinal tumors will have a hemoglobin of less than 10 grams per dl (100 ml). Radiographic studies are the major nonoperative methods we have to detect these tumors. Supine and upright abdominal plain films evaluate for signs of obstruction and soft tissue mass. Standard upper gastrointestinal and antegrade small bowel series should be performed first and will demonstrate large tumors if present. If clinical suspicion demands further definition of small intestinal anatomy, any of four specialized barium small bowel studies may be chosen (Table 1). The duodenum is best visualized by hypotonic duodenography. If small intestinal obstruction exists requiring Miller-Abbott tube decompression, barium may be injected once the tube tip has progressed to the obstructing lesion. The most detailed small intestinal mucosal views are obtained with enteroclysis and the retrograde small bowel series. Enteroclysis involves distal duodenal intubation and rapid instillation of a barium suspension followed by water or air. Careful fluoroscopy of the entire small intestine is performed and excellent mucosal detail of individual loops is obtained. The retrograde small bowel series is an extension of the full column barium enema, during which glucagon is given to relax the ileocecal valve and small bowel. The retrograde flow of barium throughout the entire small intestine is carefully monitored fluoroscopically. The common x-ray findings with small intestinal tumors are a mucosal filling defect, dilatation proximal to a lesion, or rigidity or irregularity of the bowel wall.

Current gastrointestinal endoscopes that are accessible to most medical communities can readily visualize the entire duodenum and sometimes the proximal 10 to 20 cm of jejunum. Lesions in these areas can usually be specifically defined and biopsied. Endoscopes that view the entire small bowel are still largely experimental. Ultrasound or computerized axial tomography are not good screening tools for these tumors. Both methods can evaluate the liver and retroperitoneum for tumor metastases or determine if a mass is cystic or solid.

Visceral angiography is indicated for rapid gastrointestinal bleeding greater than 1 ml per minute. Even if bleeding is not demonstrated by intraluminal dye extravasation, tumor neo-

vascularity may be seen. Up to 10 per cent of patients with chronic gastrointestinal blood loss may have small bowel tumors as a source of the bleeding.

Less rapid bleeding may be identified by the fluorescein string test. A radiopaque string is passed by mouth and peristalsis is permitted to carry the tip into the ileum. The string position is documented by a plain abdominal x-ray. Twenty ml of fluorescein is injected intravenously and the string is removed in 5 minutes. The string is examined grossly and with ultraviolet light for blood. The string is laid on the abdominal film to determine the anatomic site of bleeding. Administration of intravenous technetium-99m sulfur colloid with subsequent total abdominal scanning has recently been advocated for detection of slow, continuous gastrointestinal bleeding. Efficacy of the test is still unknown.

TUMOR CHARACTERISTICS

Of malignant tumors, approximately 46 per cent are adenocarcinomas, 23 per cent are carcinoids, 18 per cent are lymphomas, and 13 per cent are sarcomas (most of which are leiomyosarcomas). At the time of discovery well over half are already metastatic, and this approaches 80 to 90 per cent of adenocarcinoma. By definition, malignant carcinoids show evidence of metastases, but even with metastases survival rates are good. Of small bowel tumors, the leiomyosarcoma is most likely to be palpable on physical examination (50 to 60 per cent). Adenocarcinomas are largely limited to the duodenum. Lymphomas and carcinoid tumors are more common in the ileum. Metastatic lesions to the small intestine most commonly arise from breast carcinomas, melanomas, renal cell carcinomas, choriocarcinomas, or bronchogenic car-

Table 1. *Small Bowel Barium Studies*

Study	When to Use	Best Defined Area	Discomfort°
Antegrade small bowel series	Generally first study for any suspected small bowel lesion	Modest view of entire small bowel but duodenum and jejunum best	0
Hypotonic duodenography	Questionable duodenal lesions by ASBS	Duodenum	1
Miller-Abbott tube study	Partial small bowel obstruction requiring decompression	Specific area of obstruction	2
Enteroclysis	Previous studies negative or non-diagnostic and lesion still suspected	Jejunum slightly better than ileum	3
Retrograde small bowel series	Suspected ileal disease (especially terminal ileum)	Ileum better than jejunum	4

°0 = none; 4 = most.

cinomas. Endometriomas will rarely "metastasize" to the ileum. Benign tumors are more randomly scattered along the small bowel. Leiomyomas and hemangiomas have the greatest tendency to bleed.

Small intestinal tumors are uncommon lesions. With more widespread application of sensitive diagnostic tools, nonoperative or preoperative definition of these lesions is now possible.

INTESTINAL OBSTRUCTION

By PAUL R. HASTINGS, M.D., *and* ISIDORE COHN, JR., M.D.

New Orleans, Louisiana

DEFINITIONS

Intestinal obstruction is a general term that refers to any interference with the normal passage of air, liquid, or solid material from the mouth to the anus. It can be further defined as *complete* or *partial*. A *simple obstruction* is one in which interference with the passage of the intestinal contents is the only problem. A *closed loop* obstruction is one in which both ends of a segment of bowel are occluded. *Strangulation obstruction* refers to that condition in which there is compromise of the vascular supply to at least a portion of the bowel wall.

An etiologic classification further defines this entity. The various causes or mechanisms are outlined below. The broad subdivisions are mechanical (dynamic), paralytic (nonmechanical, adynamic), and vascular obstruction. The term *ileus* refers to any form of intestinal obstruction. Many misuse this term to signify a paralytic or adynamic mechanism. The appropriate modifier(s), such as simple, mechanical ileus or paralytic ileus secondary to peritonitis, should be added for clarity and to avoid confusion.

The location of an intestinal obstruction further clarifies the diagnosis (esophageal, gastric, duodenal, small intestinal, colonic, and rectal).

CAUSES

I. Mechanical obstruction (dynamic)
  A. Narrowing of lumen, intrinsic lesions
    1. Congenital
      a. Atresia
      b. Stenosis
      c. Imperforate anus, malformations of anus and rectum
      d. Malrotations
      e. Cysts and reduplications
      f. Meckel's diverticulum
    2. Acquired
      a. Inflammatory
        (1) Enteritis
        (2) Granulomatous disease, specific and nonspecific
        (3) Diverticulitis
      b. Traumatic
      c. Ischemic — secondary stricture
      d. Neoplastic
        (1) Benign tumors, small or large bowel
        (2) Malignant tumors, small or large bowel
        (3) Endometriosis
  B. Adhesive bands
    1. Congenital
    2. Inflammatory
    3. Traumatic
    4. Neoplastic
  C. Hernia
    1. External
    2. Internal
  D. Extraintestinal masses or structures
    1. Abscess
    2. Tumor
    3. Pregnancy
    4. Annular pancreas
    5. Superior mesenteric artery syndrome
  E. Stomal or anastomotic obstruction
    1. Edema
    2. Stricture
  F. Volvulus
  G. Intussusception
  H. Obturation
    1. Gallstones
    2. Foreign bodies
    3. Worms
    4. Bezoars
    5. Meconium
    6. Fecal impaction
  I. Congenital defects, Hirschsprung's disease
  J. Radiation stenosis
II. Paralytic or adynamic ileus
  A. Peritonitis
  B. Toxic
    1. Pneumonia
    2. Uremia
    3. Generalized infection
  C. Electrolyte imbalance
  D. Neurogenic
    1. Spinal cord lesion

2. Fracture of spine, pelvis, femur, etc.
3. Plumbism
4. Retroperitoneal hematoma or operation
E. Megacolon
III. Vascular obstruction
    A. Thrombosis of mesenteric vessels
    B. Embolism of mesenteric vessels

CLINICAL MANIFESTATIONS

The symptoms and signs as well as the physical findings will depend to a large extent on the cause and on the location of the obstruction. The age of the patient may also provide diagnostic clues. Mechanical obstructions in the newborn are usually due to defects in development or heredity. The older infant will more likely have an obstruction owing to a hernia, an intussusception, or a volvulus. Patients of intermediate age are most likely to develop an intestinal obstruction from adhesions or hernias, and older patients have a progressive tendency to have neoplasms as their cause for obstruction.

Symptoms. The key symptoms in patients with intestinal obstruction are pain, vomiting, and obstipation.

Pain is the most characteristic feature of intestinal obstruction for patients with obstruction located below the ligament of Trietz. Pain may be absent in those patients with esophageal, gastric, or duodenal obstruction. Classically, the pain in simple obstruction is episodic and colicky. It results from bowel distention and the efforts of intestinal peristalsis to push the bowel contents past the obstructing point. In upper small bowel obstruction the pain may be located primarily in the upper abdomen. The pain may be located in the mid abdomen with lower small bowel obstruction, and in the lower abdomen with colon obstruction. However, these findings are not constant. The colicky character of the pain often causes the patient to move about in an attempt to find a more comfortable position. The interval between attacks of colic is generally shorter (4 to 5 minutes) for mid to upper small bowel obstruction and longer (10 to 15 minutes) for lower obstructions.

Patients with an adynamic ileus usually do not have colicky episodic abdominal pain — they frequently have steady generalized abdominal discomfort. If the pain becomes constant after initial symptoms of episodic pain, strangulation or perforation is quite likely.

Vomiting is another key feature in the symptom complex. The timing in relationship to the pain, the frequency, the amount, and the character are important guides to the diagnosis.

Reflex vomiting may occur almost immediately after the obstruction occurs. This may be followed by a variable period of quiescence. Vomiting may resume in a short interval of time with higher obstructions or may reappear after 1 to 2 days or not at all in lower gastrointestinal obstructions. Generally, higher obstructions are associated with vomitus that occurs more frequently and is of larger quantity. The character of the vomitus may give an important clue to the location of the obstruction. Gastric obstruction may produce clear gastric juice or recently ingested foodstuffs in the vomitus or aspirate. Duodenal obstructions may be bilious in character. With a progressively lower location in the gastrointestinal tract, the resultant bacterial overgrowth in the distended, stagnant, obstructed segment will produce the so-called *feculent vomitus.*

Obstipation is an important symptom that can provide valuable information regarding the location and the completeness of the obstruction. In partial obstructions the patient may mention intermittent stooling and flatulence or there may be alternating diarrhea and constipation. With complete obstruction the cessation of expelling of fecal contents may be abrupt. It should be remembered, however, that the intestinal contents distal to the point of obstruction may continue to be expelled for some time after a complete obstruction, and abdominal x-rays taken early may still show air or feces or both in the colon!

The history may also include complaints of abdominal distention, fever, thirst, palpitations, weight loss, weakness, and anorexia. Specific questioning as to diuretic use, known hernias, previous abdominal surgery, or previous similar episodes is mandatory.

Course. The course of patients with intestinal obstruction is extremely variable. Patients with partial obstruction may have intermittent symptoms or less intense symptoms and signs for a protracted period. Higher obstructions generally produce a more rapid progression of symptoms than lower obstructions. When perforation or strangulation complicates the illness, the course will be fulminant.

The pattern for patients with an adynamic or functional ileus also will be variable; it depends to a large extent upon the underlying mechanism of the obstruction. If peritonitis is the underlying cause, normal peristaltic progression of the gastrointestinal contents will not take place until the cause of the peritonitis is controlled. An obstruction related to an electrolyte imbalance will require appropriate correction of the imbalance before intestinal function returns. The dysfunction related to such conditions as retroperitoneal hematomas, fractures, renal stones, uremia, and sepsis will depend on the many inter-related factors that each encompasses.

Physical Examination. The physical examination should extend from an examination for scleral icterus to an assessment of peripheral pulses. Rectal and pelvic examination, stool and nasogastric aspirate, guaiac test, and proctosigmoidoscopic examination should be included routinely.

Inspection will allow a determination of hydration by examination of skin turgor and mucous membrane moisture. Obvious hernias and abdominal scars should be noted. Distention may be quite marked in lower obstructions and in long-standing obstructions. It may be absent in high intestinal obstructions. In sigmoid volvulus the degree of distention is out of proportion to the duration of the obstruction.

Auscultation of the chest may elicit arrhythmias or murmurs that could be associated with mesenteric emboli. Auscultation will usually reveal a relatively quiet abdomen if the ileus is secondary to an adynamic or paralytic ileus or if there is strangulation or perforation present. The bowel sounds in a mechanical ileus are characteristically high-pitched, metallic, or tinkling in quality, and associated with episodic rushes. The bowel sounds between the rushes usually are active or hyperactive initially. The interval between rushes is generally shorter with higher obstructions than it is with lower obstructions. With obstructions of longer duration the initially active interval between rushes may be replaced by hypoactive bowel sounds. Percussion will usually elicit a tympanitic note with most obstructions.

Palpation in simple obstruction usually reveals only mild tenderness or none. Muscle guarding or tenderness or both are suggestive of the presence of strangulation or perforation. If these findings are accompanied by tachycardia, elevated temperature, and elevated white blood cell (WBC) count, then strangulation obstruction or bowel perforation must be considered. A palpable mass may indicate a neoplastic cause for the obstruction. Occasionally with strangulation obstruction a mass can be palpated that has been caused by an attempt by the omentum and loops of bowel to "wall off" the strangulated segment.

Physical findings of weight loss, jaundice, hepatomegaly, abdominal nodules, rectal shelf, and lymphadenopathy might point to neoplasia as cause of the obstruction. Generalized or localized atherosclerotic disease, with or without cardiac arrhythmia, may support a vascular occlusion cause. An increased pulse rate indicates hypovolemia or sepsis or both. Hypotension can be present with either extreme hypovolemia or sepsis.

COMPLICATIONS

Strangulation of the bowel wall is a common complication. This may be caused by arterial embolus or thrombosis, mesenteric venous thrombosis, or by "end vessel" disease such as with systemic lupus erythematosus or with ischemic colitis. The mesenteric vascular supply to a bowel segment can be interrupted by adhesions, hernia rings, or the occlusive "kink" of the vasculature that can occur with a volvulus.

Perforation can result from strangulation or it can occur from progressive distention of the bowel. Progressive bowel distention leading to perforation is particularly common with closed loop obstructions and with colonic obstructions with a competent ileocecal valve.

The systemic effects that are seen with intestinal obstructions are primarily due to dehydration, electrolyte imbalance, and/or sepsis. Significant hypovolemia can occur rapidly with any obstruction. Loss of plasma volume occurs by sequestration of fluid, colloid, electrolytes, and even red cells into the gut lumen, bowel wall, or peritoneal cavity. Hypotension and tachycardia can be the result. Sepsis with shock, tachycardia, elevated WBC count, and fever is seen with strangulation, perforation, and/or aspiration of vomited gastrointestinal contents.

LABORATORY FINDINGS

The diagnosis of intestinal obstruction cannot be made on the basis of laboratory studies, but supportive data and information relative to the important reparative efforts are essential. The specific laboratory findings may vary from normal to a marked derangement, depending on the duration of the disease and the presence or absence of the specific complications as just outlined. The battery of laboratory determinations discussed in the following paragraphs is essential for proper evaluation of all patients suspected of having an intestinal obstruction.

Hematocrit and hemoglobin determinations can serve as a guide to the relative hydration of a patient, particularly if followed serially. With significant loss of plasma volume into the gut wall, bowel lumen, or peritoneal cavity, marked hemoconcentration will be evident. However, if sepsis or bleeding accompanies this disease, the hematocrit may be quite low. The WBC count may be elevated with advanced simple obstruction or with strangulation and perforation. Elevation of the WBC count in the range of 10,000 to 20,000 per cu mm cannot by itself be used to differentiate between simple and complicated obstructions. WBC counts greater than 20,000 per cu mm are commonly seen with mesenteric vascular occlusion.

Urinalysis will usually be normal with early

uncomplicated obstructions. In the absence of acute or chronic renal failure, dehydration will lead to elevated urine specific gravity and osmolality. The actual urine output is an important guide for fluid and electrolyte therapy in the presence of normal kidneys. Mild to moderate ketonuria, mild proteinuria, and mild glucosuria may be seen, reflecting the metabolic and endocrine derangements of starvation and systemic trauma that can accompany this disease entity.

A serum electrolyte determination is essential to guide reparative therapy. If the obstruction is gastric in location, prolonged vomiting or nasogastric suction or both usually lead to hyponatremic, hypochloremic, hypokalemic metabolic alkalosis. Obstruction in other locations will give variable results, depending on the relative loss of alkaline versus acid secretions. A significant metabolic acidosis indicates either prolonged starvation with alkaline gastrointestinal content loss or strangulation and/or perforation. The combined effects of hypovolemia and sepsis as seen with either strangulation or perforation can produce systemic alterations of cardiovascular performance, regional perfusion, or cellular level defects in aerobic metabolism. The result may be profound acidosis. Arterial blood gases as well as the electrolyte profile are important to assess this derangement.

Arterial blood gases are also important to assess oxygenation and ventilation that may be seriously impaired with aspiration or diaphragmatic elevation or both.

Elevated amylase levels may be produced in these patients by several mechanisms. Strangulated bowel may irritate the pancreas. The passage of toxic components from a strangulated loop into the peritoneal cavity can result in amylase absorption. Increased pressure within the bowel may be transmitted to the pancreatic ducts and cause a secondary pancreatitis. There also may be amylase release from other parts of the alimentary tract. However, only about 20 per cent of patients with strangulation obstruction have an elevated amylase level.

Blood urea nitrogen levels may be elevated with dehydration, with blood in the lumen of the bowel, or with acute or chronic renal failure.

A stool specimen should be examined for both gross and occult blood. Gross blood is frequently present in intussusception and appears late in strangulation secondary to vascular occlusion. Occult blood may be seen in other types of strangulation obstruction.

X-Ray Examination

X-ray studies are the most important adjunct to the carefully performed history and physical examination. Careful interpretation by the clinician *and* radiologist frequently can aid in determining the location and the etiology of the obstruction, and the presence or absence of perforation. Initial plain films of the abdomen in both the supine and erect positions are mandatory. If the patient's condition is such that erect films cannot be obtained, then lateral decubitus x-rays should be performed. Erect and lateral chest x-rays are also helpful to detect the presence of associated pulmonary disease or aspiration, and to give evidence of diaphragmatic elevation or free air under the diaphragm or both.

The distribution of gas and fluid within the bowel is the key to appropriate interpretation. Normally there is gas in both the stomach and the colon in healthy persons. Small bowel gas can be seen in normal infants and occasionally in patients with severe gastroenteritis, extreme aerophagia, and extreme constipation. If the obstruction is located in the upper small bowel, duodenum, stomach, or esophagus, the plain film of the abdomen may be normal. With more distal obstructions there will be a progressive dilatation of the bowel with accumulation of liquid and air that separates into the classic air-fluid levels in the upright film. Small bowel can usually be distinguished from colon by the size of distended loops, by the more central location of the small bowel loops, by the stepladder configuration, and by the appearance of valvulae conniventes in the small bowel in contrast to the haustral markings in the colon.

Large bowel obstructions usually can be detected by demonstration of dilated proximal colon with the typical haustral markings visualized. If the ileocecal valve is competent, there may be only large bowel visualized with a varying degree of distention. If the ileocecal valve is incompetent, there may be varying small bowel x-ray findings along with the colon distention. A competent ileocecal valve may lead to perforation at the cecum because the closed loop obstruction thus created does not allow "decompression" proximal into the small bowel.

There is usually marked abdominal distention with a volvulus of the colon. Plain x-rays will confirm this and will additionally show displacement of the bowel from its normal location, the double air-fluid levels, and the sharp cut-off at the point of torsion, with distended loops of proximal bowel. A barium enema will confirm the diagnosis by demonstrating the characteristic "bird's beak" deformity.

The presence of air in the biliary tree may be seen in patients with an intestinal obstruction secondary to the obturator effect of an impacted gallstone, classically located intraluminally in the distal ileum.

A barium enema examination is helpful when the clinical picture and plain x-rays suggest colon obstruction. The type of obstruction and the specific location often can be determined. A barium enema is also helpful when there is difficulty in differentiating between small and large bowel gas patterns. Additionally, a carefully administered barium enema can be therapeutic for some intussusceptions and for a sigmoid volvulus, provided that there is no evidence of strangulation or perforation.

The potential dangers of a barium enema are many. If a perforation is present but unrecognized, barium peritonitis can be produced; if inflammatory bowel lesions are present, the hydrostatic pressure effects of a barium enema could lead to a perforation; and if there is a partial obstruction and barium is forced past the point of obstruction, the partial obstruction can be converted to a complete obstruction.

Plain films of the abdomen obtained on patients with adynamic or paralytic ileus usually reveal diffuse dilatation of all or part of the gastrointestinal tract, depending on the cause and the location of the underlying process. Careful correlation with other clinical and laboratory findings is essential for differentiation.

Contrast studies of the upper gastrointestinal tract are occasionally useful. Differentiation between an adynamic ileus and a mechanical obstruction sometimes can be made by seeing if the contrast material traverses the length of the gastrointestinal tract in the adynamic ileus or by revealing the point of obstruction in the dynamic ileus. Water-soluble contrast material generally is unsatisfactory unless a very high obstruction is present or unless it is administered through a long intestinal tube. Rapid dilution and dispersion of the water-soluble contrast material precludes satisfactory visualization. Most surgeons condemn the routine use of barium for the differential diagnosis of upper gastrointestinal tract obstructions because of the difficulty in ridding the bowel of the accumulated barium and because of the potential for converting a partial obstruction into a complete one.

PITFALLS IN DIAGNOSIS

The greatest pitfall in diagnosis is the failure to differentiate between uncomplicated simple obstructions and complicated obstructions with a closed loop, strangulation, or perforation. Frequently, inordinate delays in therapy occur because of unnecessary diagnostic maneuvers, prolonged resuscitation, or the dangerous reliance on one's supposed clinical ability to differentiate complicated from uncomplicated ob-

structions. Frequently the diagnosis of strangulation is not made until laparotomy is performed. The classic findings of tachycardia, leukocytosis, fever, and abdominal tenderness are not always present with strangulation obstruction or perforation. If observation is allowed until *all* these findings are present, an unnecessary increase in morbidity and mortality will result.

ACUTE APPENDICITIS

By WILLIAM WARREN BABSON, M.D., *and* ALEXANDER N. GUNN II, M.D.

Gloucester, Massachusetts

Acute appendicitis remains a common surgical emergency, and the incidence of perforation continues at a steady rate. An estimated 7 per cent of the population will at some time develop appendicitis. Its greatest incidence is in those in late childhood and in younger adults. When the condition is diagnosed and the patient operated upon before perforation, it is highly curable, the morbidity is almost nil, and the hospital stay and loss of activity are minimal. A 15 per cent error in diagnosis may be acceptable in the removal of normal appendices, but it certainly presents a challenge for improvement. On the other hand, failure to operate before perforation on 15 per cent of patients with acute appendicitis should not be acceptable, as it results in great morbidity, threat of mortality, and extended hospital stay and disability.

Since Dr. Reginald Fitz presented his landmark paper "Acute Appendicitis and Its Clinical Pathological Significance" on June 17, 1886, there have been volumes written on the subject. The diagnosis of *typical* appendicitis has been well documented and is well understood. However, it is the *atypical* appendicitis that is largely responsible for errors in diagnosis, delayed surgery, perforation, and the vast majority of complications.

PRESENTING SYMPTOMS AND SIGNS

Pain, the salient complaint, is typically periumbilical, comes on rather gradually, and is steady, with variations in degree. Frequently, the pain occurs as a cramping sensation with urge to defecate, but should defecation occur, there is only temporary, if any, relief. Some patients may describe the pain as "gas" or "pressure," and may not admit to pain as such. The site of the pain may be high enough in the epigastrium to point to upper abdominal pathology and even coronary occlusion. Sudden onset of pain will suggest a perforation of an organ rather than appendicitis. Nausea and vomiting, once or twice, follow the onset of pain. If careful history indicates that they preceded the pain, the diagnosis of appendicitis is unlikely.

After several hours, pain shifts to the right lower abdomen and tenderness localizes at the site of the appendix. It is unlikely, indeed, for the onset of pain to occur in the appendix area. Exceptions to this include a fairly recent previous attack or one beginning during heavy sleep or other narcosis, so that initial pain is not noted. On the other hand, steady general abdominal pain shifting to the right lower abdomen with local tenderness is almost always caused by appendicitis.

There is low-grade fever that may be elevated to 101 F (38.3 C), and the pulse rate increases after several hours. Higher values suggest complications. The patient prefers to lie quietly, frequently with his right thigh and knee flexed, in contrast with the restless patient who has smooth muscle spasm from a ureteral calculus. After the patient has indicated the point of maximum pain and tenderness, examination should commence at the opposite side of the abdomen, with light percussion by a single finger used. This technique will often help identify the point of greatest inflammation. Loops of bowel with gas and irritating contents often appear tender, but with gentle percussion this tenderness is not consistent.

Peristalsis is usually decreased and may be absent in later stages. Very active peristalsis strongly suggests gastroenteritis. Gentle pressure with the stethoscope while listening for bowel sounds is another excellent method of searching for localized and rebound tenderness. Detection of involuntary spasm may be best accomplished when the patient is relaxed and the right thigh flexed. If abdominal palpation is done during the pelvic and rectal examination, with the patient's attention diverted away from the abdomen, a more accurate assessment of abdominal findings may be made.

LABORATORY FINDINGS

The white blood cell (WBC) count and percentage of polys are usually increased in appendicitis. However, normal values by no means rule out the disease. Their presence, like fever, indicates an acute process. A very high WBC, 20,000 per cu mm and higher, raises some doubt as to the diagnosis of uncomplicated appendicitis. Sometimes the WBC is normal, but with an elevated poly count.

The urine examination may reveal white and red blood cells in the urine owing to close proximity of the appendix to the ureter. However, the RBC could suggest a ureteral calculus. Ketosis may be found in the presence of vomiting and dehydration, particularly in the young. Blood cultures are important in late cases and in the presence of a chill.

RADIOLOGY OF APPENDICITIS

Plain films may demonstrate appendicolith. This is a laminated oval appendiceal calculus, 0.5 to 2.0 cm, occurring singly in 70 per cent of cases. It may be confused with gallstones, ureteral calculus, mesenteric nodes, and bone islands. The calculus is seen in only 1 per cent of normal persons, but has been reported in 12 per cent of patients with appendicitis. A patient presenting with abdominal pain and appendicolith has a 90 per cent likelihood of having appendicitis.

Localized ileus and loss of tissue lines point to an inflammatory process in the abdomen.

The barium enema is achieving an increasingly important role in the diagnosis of appendicitis in a patient whose condition is difficult to diagnose. Studies of many patients have been reported without complication. Experienced radiologists have reported only 3 per cent false-positive results and 7 per cent false-negative ones. This test is helpful in correlating the appendiceal site with the area of tenderness and in demonstrating other pathologic entities. Flattening and filling defects of the cecal wall are characteristics of appendicitis, and larger defects — cecal, right colon, or rectosigmoid — may be caused by appendiceal abscesses. A negative study with good filling of appendix may allow the surgeon an opportunity for further watchful waiting. However, 15 per cent of normal persons have nonfilling appendices and filling of the appendix in a patient with acute appendicitis may occur.

COMPLICATIONS

Perforation and peritonitis, abscess, severe ileus, fecal fistula, and wound infection are all immediate complications. A chill and early spiking fever may herald septic pylephlebitis. Late complications include residual abscesses in the pelvis, abdomen, and subhepatic and subphrenic areas and small bowel obstructions and hernias.

PITFALLS

Fifteen to 20 per cent of patients with appendicitis present an atypical clinical picture that produces difficulties in diagnosis. Contributing factors include position of the appendix; occurrence of the disease in the very young, the elderly, and pregnant women; and severe obstructing gangrenous appendicitis that may not be recognized before perforation. Patients with concomitant pathologic states such as obesity and severe diabetes, and the patient on steroids present additional difficulties.

APPENDICITIS IN INFANCY AND CHILDHOOD

Although rare in patients under 2 years of age and infrequent before age 5, it is the most common condition requiring surgery in childhood. Its symptoms are variable and the course is brief, with perforation occurring in 6 to 12 hours. The omentum is short and the appendix long; this decreases the walling-off process. The frequency of fecaliths is great. The systemic and local resistance is poor, and incidence of perforation is especially high in those under age 2 (70 per cent).

A fussy, sick child rejects the pacifier and is unhappy and in apparent pain. The examiner must use great care and warm hands; he approaches the abdomen first with greatest gentleness in areas where there is less pain. Use of a suppository containing 2.5 mg pentobarbital per lb will help relax the child. Abdominal pain, vomiting (90 per cent), and slight fever with persistent local tenderness are of great significance in pointing to appendicitis.

The conditions in differential diagnosis in infancy and childhood include constipation, gastroenteritis, mesenteric adenitis, primary peritonitis, pyelonephritis, and pneumonia.

Constipation may be relieved by enema. This is safe in the early stages and when the child is not toxic. In *gastroenteritis* the pain is intermittent, accompanied usually by diarrhea. Tenderness is more general and with percussion is not constant. *Mesenteric adenitis* at times follows respiratory infection. The abdominal pain does not have the usual shift, vomiting is less common, and tenderness is not constant. The child with *primary peritonitis* is toxic early in the illness and the course is more rapid. There is generalized tenderness and guarding with early distention and a quiet abdomen. In *pyelonephritis*, the tenderness relates more to the kidney area and the urine examination is definitive. *Pneumonia* is accompanied by higher fever, leukocytosis, cough, and increased grunting respirations. There is little or no percussion tenderness and peristalsis is present. Upper abdominal muscle guarding is voluntary. Chest x-ray may not show an early pneumonia. Chest examination may be diagnostic.

APPENDICITIS IN THE ELDERLY

Five per cent of cases of appendicitis occur in those over 60 years of age, and perforation may approximate 60 per cent. Symptoms are not as pronounced, the fever is less, and the white blood cell count and percentage of polys may be normal.

The frequent presence of fecaliths and prior disease of the appendix, both of which foster early rupture, are factors making appendicitis a serious challenge in the elderly. Increased frequency of concomitant disease adds to the difficulty of diagnosis.

Appendicitis often presents in an occult fashion, and the most salient finding may be a tender mass in the right abdomen, present for a number of days or more. This is usually a retrocecal abscess. However, when walling-off has not occurred, the patient is in danger of free perforation. Unfortunately, vague symptoms and lesser findings may allay the concern of patient and physician alike.

APPENDICITIS IN PREGNANCY

Its frequency matches that in nonpregnant women, and it is the commonest extrauterine condition requiring abdominal surgery. During the latter stages of pregnancy, the enlarging uterus displaces the cecum and appendix superiorly, laterally, and frequently posteriorly, with resulting shifting of localization of pain and tenderness.

When the patient with acute appendicitis changes position, the tenderness usually does not move with the uterus.

Psoas and obturator signs have significant diagnostic value because of their commonly close relationship to the appendix. Early operation is essential. It is well tolerated; complications are not.

RETROCECAL APPENDICITIS

The appendix is not infrequently found in the retroperitoneal area behind the cecum or right colon. When there is a considerable degree of malrotation, it may be found in almost any position in the abdomen, even in a diaphragmatic hernia in the left chest.

In retrocecal appendicitis, onset may be accompanied by vague and mild discomfort and lesser physical findings. The peritoneum may show little or no reaction, with rebound absent and peristalsis normal.

PELVIC APPENDICITIS

The history will be reasonably typical, but the findings may be more difficult to assess. There may be diarrhea and bladder symptoms. Mucus with diarrhea in a patient without previous history of this, is strong evidence of pelvic appendicitis with phlegmon or abscess or both. Abdominal signs develop later in the course of the disease. The rectal and pelvic examination are of great importance. Careful gentle examination is carried out with the finger palpating first on the left and then on the right. Fullness and tenderness in the cul-de-sac will occur as phlegmon or abscess develops.

ASSOCIATED WITH HERNIA

When the appendix is in a hernia sac, appendicits will present with atypical findings. Again the symptoms will follow the expected pattern, but the localization of tenderness may be masked.

A small femoral hernia containing a necrotic appendix may be overlooked because of little or no peritoneal reaction and location of pain high in the abdomen.

GANGRENOUS APPENDICITIS WITH OBSTRUCTION FROM FECALITH

There will usually be more severe pain initially with more vomiting. When gangrene has developed (6 to 8 hours), the pain may relent to a large degree and in addition, there may be little inflammatory reaction to create local tenderness. After the latent period of 10 to 12 hours, the organ may perforate into the free peritoneal cavity and the resulting release of pressure, for a short time, again is felt as a period of relief. However, from that time on there is return of abdominal pain, vomiting, and distention of peritonitis. The pathology in this situation results from blocking of the appendiceal lumen by a fecalith, increase in the intraluminal pressure, and thrombosis of vessels with loss of nerve and blood supply.

The majority of patients with acute appendicitis have mixed pathology: some degree of fecalith obstruction and suppuration from a mucosal ulceration. These appendices develop periappendicitis with fibrin and often early walling-off, giving earlier localization of tenderness and guarding. Pure suppurative appendicitis without obstruction follows this pattern as well. But the estimated 10 to 15 per cent of cases involving obstructive gangrenous appendicitis and little peritoneal reaction in the pre-perforation phase are serious indeed.

The general abdominal pain is mediated through the autonomic nervous system, whereas the pain from localized inflammatory process is mediated via parietal peritoneum and the somatic intercostal nerves.

One of the most insidious and dangerous forms of appendicitis may occur in a member of a family or community in which there are a number of patients ill with *gastroenteritis*. One of this number remains ill, diarrhea ceases, distention occurs, and a delayed diagnosis of late appendicitis and peritonitis is made. The pathology may have been aggravated by administration of a laxative and violent peristalsis responsible for the initiation of appendicitis.

The patient on *prolonged steroid therapy* who develops appendicitis may present with minimal symptoms and signs, yet be gravely ill. Early perforation and extremely poor resistance to infection make this a hazardous situation.

The *diabetic with ketosis* and acute appendicitis may also have fewer symptoms and signs. Semicoma may preclude the finding of usual signs.

Acute appendicitis as well as cholecystitis and pancreatitis may become evident in the *postoperative course* of abdominal surgery more often than one would anticipate. Because of this timing, it may present a confusing picture. Smooth muscle contraction about a fecalith or gallstone may result from the use of morphine.

History of prior appendectomy should not completely negate possibility of appendicitis. The history may be in error or an unrecognized segment may have been left behind.

DIFFERENTIAL DIAGNOSIS

Many pathologic entities have features resembling appendicitis and need consideration in the patient with abdominal pain.

Pain and sensitivity of skin may be the result of prevesicle herpes zoster. Strain, tear, or hematoma of an abdominal wall muscle may present with local tenderness and even guarding. Lidocaine infiltration is an excellent therapeutic test in this situation.

Only laparotomy may distinguish a correct diagnosis from among the many conditions that produce an acute abdomen. Included are cecal, Meckel's, and sigmoid diverticulitis, foreign body perforation, and mesenteric adenitis.

Inflammatory, neoplastic, obstructive, and vascular disorders of the bowel may be distinguished by various x-ray and other diagnostic aids. Cancer of the cecum and the left colon creates confusion; left colon cancer causes back pressure on the cecum with development of pain, tenderness, and distention.

The female organs need careful consideration in diagnosis. Acute salpingitis usually creates a spreading pelvic inflammation with high fever and white blood cell count and tenderness. The cervical Gram stain may be helpful. The pain in ruptured follicle cyst is sudden in onset, with rapid development of signs in the pelvis and rather early abatement. This condition is related to the menstrual cycle. Torsion of the pedicle gives rapid onset of pain but findings lag. Ruptured tubal pregnancy is associated with hemorrhage. All of these conditions have individual characteristics and symptoms and signs. Laparoscopy may prove to be a valuable diagnostic tool.

In perforated peptic ulcer and acute pancreatitis, irritating fluids may run down the right gutter, mimicking the shift of pain in appendicitis. In the elderly, an acutely inflamed gallbladder can present at a level below the navel.

Calculus in the right ureter will give sudden onset of severe, sharp, intermittent pain, with restlessness, sweating, and vomiting. Percussion tenderness over the right kidney is significant. Intravenous pyelogram and urine studies are essential.

Medical conditions that may be accompanied by abdominal pain include hepatitis, gastroenteritis, pneumonia, and diabetes with ketosis. Various spinal nerve lesions, lead poisoning, malaria, black widow spider bite, and acute porphyria are conditions that occasionally have been considered in the differential diagnosis.

CONCLUSION

Careful history and physical examination, repeated as often as needed (usually in the hospital setting) during the first 18 to 20 hours with such diagnostic techniques as are deemed helpful, are the greatest aids in avoiding the pitfalls that dangerous appendicitis may present.

When this point in time has been reached and the threat of appendicitis still exists, especially in the vulnerable patient, surgical exploration should be performed.

CROHN'S DISEASE

By CHARLES A. FLOOD, M.D.
New York, New York

Synonyms

Crohn, Ginsberg, and Oppenheimer first described this disease in 1932 under the name regional ileitis. As it became evident that the disorder can affect any level of the gastrointestinal tract, other names were devised. It is now commonly referred to as regional enteritis or Crohn's disease. Other names are based on the site of involvement, such as terminal ileitis, regional jejunitis, ileitis or colitis, ileocolitis and right-sided colitis. Still other names are based upon pathologic characteristics, such as granulomatous enteritis, transmural colitis, and chronic cicatrizing enteritis. Perhaps because of the diversity of sites of involvement, the current trend is to refer to the entity as Crohn's disease. Inflammatory bowel disease is another useful and more general term that includes "Crohn's disease" and "ulcerative colitis" under one simplified heading.

Definitions

Crohn's disease is an inflammatory process of unknown cause. The inflammation is transmural, involving both the mucous membrane and the deeper layers of the gut. Noncaseating granulomas are found on histologic examination in about 50 per cent of patients.

There is some evidence that Crohn's disease is caused by a filtrable agent. There is also some evidence for the concept that it is an autoimmune disorder.

Crohn's disease and ulcerative colitis are more common in Jews than in non-Jews and in whites as compared with nonwhites. There is an increased familial incidence. Emotional disorders are frequently present in patients with inflammatory bowel disease and exacerbations are related, at times, to emotional upsets.

Presenting Signs and Symptoms

Crohn's disease appears at any age but most commonly starts in youth. Involvement of the small bowel results in abdominal discomfort and loose stools. The onset of symptoms is usually insidious and the patient has often been ill for a year or two before the diagnosis is established. The abdominal discomfort is typically located in the mid abdomen and right lower quadrant, and may be described as bloating, a sense of fullness, "gas," pain after meals, cramping, or sensations of borborygmi. The distress is sometimes associated with passage of gas or stool but usually it is not. While most patients have brief periods of distress, some complain of more steady pain.

In small bowel involvement the diarrhea is mild. The stools are soft or semisoft without gross blood. Periods of fever may occur and occasionally the disease presents as fever of unknown origin. Fistula-in-ano is so common that its mere presence suggests the possibility of small bowel disease, even in patients with no intestinal complaints.

Abdominal examination is usually of little diagnostic assistance. There may be right lower quadrant tenderness and a mass may be felt in this region. Distended loops of bowel suggest the presence of obstruction.

Colonic Involvement

Crohn's disease of the colon presents a different pattern of symptoms, varying with the extent of disease. Extensive involvement of the colon produces symptoms that are commonly indistinguishable from those of ulcerative colitis. Watery diarrhea with or without bleeding is the major complaint. Severe exacerbations are accompanied by fever.

Extraintestinal Manifestations

Joint pain without objective findings is the commonest extraintestinal manifestation of Crohn's disease. Ankylosing spondylitis, involving especially the sacroiliac joints, is quite frequent. Occasionally, joint effusions occur. The rheumatoid factor is absent.

Cutaneous manifestations include erythema nodosum and pyoderma gangrenosum.

The hepatic abnormalities in Crohn's disease range from fatty liver to cirrhosis. Mild hepatic disease is asymptomatic and may be manifested only by enzyme changes. Sclerosing cholangitis is a rare complication.

Various types of ocular inflammation such as iritis and iridocyclitis occasionally occur.

Acute Crohn's Disease

Acute inflammation of the terminal ileum is a disorder that is discovered in patients who are explored for suspected acute appendicitis without a history of pre-existing disease. The relation between this clinical entity and the usual picture of Crohn's disease is problematic. Many patients recover completely and permanently.

COMPLICATIONS

Perforation. The transmural character of the disease process often leads to gradual perforation of the bowel wall. Internal fistulization between bowel loops or other abdominal viscera is associated with abdominal pain, fever, or leukocytosis. Free perforation of the small bowel into the peritoneal cavity is unusual.

Fistulization in Crohn's disease is typified by the frequently occurring fistula-in-ano. This process often results in perirectal abscess and rectovaginal fistula.

Obstruction. Narrowing of the small bowel lumen may result in colicky pain, nausea, and vomiting. Acute obstruction occurs from impaction of food particles, stenosis, or intestinal adhesions.

Hemorrhage. A massive upper gastrointestinal type of blood loss, similar to that of duodenal ulcer, may occur in Crohn's disease of the small bowel. Emergency surgical intervention is rarely required, but a bleeding ulcer must, at times, be ruled out by endoscopy. Massive blood loss from Crohn's disease of the colon is rare.

Malnutrition and Malabsorption. Various avitaminoses occur in extensive Crohn's disease of the small bowel. Steatorrhea and deficient absorption of vitamin B_{12} and bile salts are found in patients with involvement of more than 100 cm of distal ileum. Gallstones are a common complication in patients with small bowel disease and are perhaps attributable to impaired absorption of bile salts with a resultant lithogenic bile. There is also an increased incidence of renal calculi. This has been attributed to fat malabsorption with binding of calcium to fatty acids in the gut and a resultant increased absorption of oxalates that would otherwise be bound to calcium and excreted in the stool.

Crohn's disease in children before and at puberty may cause a delay in growth and in sexual maturation. Treatment with steroids can aggravate the growth problem.

Toxic Megacolon. Toxic megacolon occurs in Crohn's disease of the colon as it does in ulcerative colitis. Patients with inflammatory bowel disease involving the colon who are seriously ill require monitoring for the development of this serious complication.

Carcinoma. Although it has been thought that colonic malignancy is less common in Crohn's disease of the colon than in ulcerative colitis, both diseases are currently regarded as predisposing to malignancy.

LABORATORY AND X-RAY FINDINGS

Anemia is usually a result of iron deficiency or occasionally of other causes, including reduced absorption of vitamin B_{12}. During acute exacerbations, elevations of the white blood cell count and sedimentation rate occur, but these tests are not sensitive indicators of disease activity. The stools may contain occult blood. Hypoalbuminemia, associated with excessive loss of plasma protein into the intestine, occurs in sicker patients. Hepatic involvement may be manifested by elevations of alkaline phosphatase and serum transaminases.

The diagnosis of Crohn's disease of the small bowel is based mainly on x-ray study. Mucosal damage is manifested by irregularities in the mucosal outline. The lumen of the bowel is often narrowed, the wall stiffened, and there may be separation of intestinal loops. Roentgenograms taken at half-hourly intervals and spot films of the ileocecal area are essential for adequate study. Fistulas and diseased areas alternating with normal-appearing bowel may be encountered.

In Crohn's disease of the colon, the rectum and sigmoid are usually not involved. The barium enema outlines small shadows that suggest discrete ulcers in the bowel wall. Unilateral spiculations that resemble diverticular disease or the presence of a stricture also suggest Crohn's disease. However, x-ray changes are often diffuse, nonspecific, and indistinguishable from the changes seen in ulcerative colitis.

ENDOSCOPY

Sigmoidoscopy or colonoscopy is also of major importance in the diagnosis of Crohn's disease of the colon. The rectal mucosa usually appears normal. If a fistula-in-ano is present, one may see pus extruded through the fistulous opening. If the disease involves the rectum, it may present as multiple superficial scattered ulcers. However, there is often diffuse mucosal involvement with edema, granularity, and friability indistinguishable from ulcerative colitis. Biopsy of the rectal mucosa sometimes reveals the granulomas of Crohn's disease.

Colonoscopy is necessary when inflammatory changes are not apparent on radiologic and sigmoidoscopic examination. The gross changes that are characteristic are discrete and often serpiginous ulcers with a relatively normal intervening mucosa. Sometimes the changes are unilateral. However, the inflammatory changes may be diffuse. Biopsy of the mucosa obtained through the colonoscope sometimes shows the presence of granulomata.

COURSE OF THE DISEASE

Crohn's disease is a chronic illness characterized by exacerbations and remissions. The exacerbations occur at irregular, unpredictable intervals. Remissions may be brief or may last for many years. Laboratory studies are of little value in the estimation of disease activity, and management must be guided chiefly by the symptomatic course.

The clinical picture may be completely controlled by intermittent drug therapy or may require continued treatment. Surgical intervention in patients with Crohn's disease of the small bowel is commonly followed by recurrence after an interval of freedom from disease activity.

PITFALLS IN DIAGNOSIS

Among the many patients who present with a prolonged history of abdominal discomfort and loose stools that may be classified as irritable bowel syndrome, a few will be found to have Crohn's disease of the small intestine. This diagnosis will be overlooked if radiologic studies are not performed. Conversely, misinterpretation of x-ray changes in the small bowel occasionally results in an erroneous diagnosis of Crohn's disease. At times this is due to overzealous emphasis on minor abnormalities or to a technically inadequate study.

Other diseases of the small bowel can be confused with Crohn's disease radiologically. These include lymphosarcoma and occasionally nontropical sprue or tuberculosis of the ileum.

Crohn's disease of the large bowel may be difficult or impossible to distinguish radiologically from nonspecific ulcerative colitis, especially if there is no associated ileal involvement. Diverticulitis can also be radiologically indistinguishable from Crohn's disease. Ischemic colitis results in a radiologic pattern of "thumb printing" that can also resemble Crohn's disease.

Colonoscopy is very useful in distinguishing Crohn's disease from ulcerative colitis. In the former the mucosal changes are often of the spotty or unilateral type with large ulcerations and intervening areas of relatively normal mucosa. In the latter, the mucosal changes are diffuse. Colonoscopic biopsy is often too superficial to be diagnostic.

It should be emphasized that Crohn's disease of the colon and nonspecific ulcerative colitis are overlapping diagnostic entities. At times they are indistinguishable. Both the pathologist and the endoscopist depend partly upon the distribution of the disease in the classification of these disorders. However, the pathologic examination of resected specimens of the large bowel sometimes reveals a picture that is intermediate or is subject to differing interpretations. Fortunately at the present time the conservative programs for management of Crohn's

disease of the colon and of ulcerative colitis are essentially the same and the results of conservative therapy are similar. A strict differentiation is not essential for medical treatment, although the outlook after surgical therapy, in the experience of some observers, is somewhat different.

CHRONIC ULCERATIVE COLITIS

By JOHN R. GAMBLE, M.D.
San Francisco, California

INTRODUCTION AND DEFINITION

Chronic ulcerative colitis is an inflammatory disease of the colon of uncertain cause and is manifested by bloody diarrhea of varying degrees and severity. It may be mild and involve only the rectum or severe enough to be a medical emergency. The peak incidence of onset is in early adult life, the same period in which occurs the most serious complication — carcinoma. Prompt and accurate diagnosis is thus necessary, no matter what the stage of illness.

PRESENTING SYMPTOMS AND SIGNS

Rectal Bleeding. The symptom most frequently leading to the discovery of chronic ulcerative colitis is rectal bleeding. If physicians use good judgment in thoroughly investigating all patients who have this symptom by a digital examination of the rectum, a proctoscopic examination, and roentgenogram of the colon, the diagnosis of chronic ulcerative colitis, as well as that of other important causes of rectal bleeding, will be made promptly. It is important to realize that the patient with ulcerative colitis confined to the rectum (common in patients in the early stages of the disease and in half of the patients with well-established disease) may not have diarrhea and complains only of rectal bleeding with or without tenesmus. The patient who has more extensive or total colonic involvement usually presents with bloody diarrhea, fever, nausea, and abdominal cramping.

Diarrhea. When ulcerative colitis presents with diarrhea, the fecal material is usually, but not always, bloody — the converse being true in Crohn's disease of the colon. The diarrhea will, additionally, have organic features such as nocturnal stools and urgency incontinence, and will be associated with weight loss. Occasionally, however, the diarrhea may be so mild as to suggest a functional cause, but the experienced clinician realizes that the irritable bowel syndrome is a diagnosis of exclusion and will not dismiss any history of diarrhea as nonorganic without appropriate investigation.

Toxic Dilatation. Chronic ulcerative colitis may present as an overwhelming, acute illness with severe diarrhea, fever, and colonic dilatation. The absence of a previous history of inflammatory bowel disease should not negate ulcerative colitis as a diagnostic consideration in such a patient. It is a medical emergency and its early recognition is imperative.

Nonspecific Symptoms. Occasionally, chronic ulcerative colitis will involve no history of diarrhea or bleeding and may be overlooked as a diagnostic consideration in a patient who has only weight loss, iron deficiency anemia, anorexia, abdominal pain, growth retardation, or fever of undetermined origin. The possibility of inflammatory bowel disease should, however, always be a consideration in this situation.

Presentation with Extracolonic Manifestations. Chronic ulcerative colitis may be a systemic disease involving many other organs and systems, and one should be alert to the possibility that its presenting symptoms may not be those of bowel disease at all. When examining a patient with rheumatoid spondylitis, nondeforming seronegative peripheral arthritis of major joints, iritis or episcleritis, cholestatic liver disease, sclerosing cholangitis, pyoderma gangrenosum, erythema nodosum, or unexplained thromboembolic phenomena, the clinician must always search for possible underlying inflammatory bowel disease.

PHYSICAL FINDINGS

The patient who has limited disease (proctitis) usually is not ill or debilitated and may have no positive physical findings or only granularity on digital rectal examination. The patient with total colonic involvement whose disease is in remission may also have no abnormalities on physical examination, but when the disease is active the patient is typically very ill and pale with evidence of weight loss, dehydration, malnutrition, or retardation of growth and development. Additionally, if the presentation is that of toxic dilatation of the colon, there may be rebound tenderness, abdominal distention, fever, absent bowel sounds — an obviously ill patient. Thus the physical findings are a function of the extent and activity of the disease, and there is no constant or typical pattern. Additional physi-

cal findings related to the extracolonic manifestations may be noted as previously outlined.

LOCAL COMPLICATIONS

Chronic ulcerative colitis, during its long course of activity, may be complicated by local inflammatory strictures, carcinoma, and adenomatous polyps or pseudopolyps, as well as toxic dilatation. Occasionally, it is difficult to distinguish between a benign stricture and a carcinoma, or between a pseudopolyp and a true adenomatous polyp. Newer diagnostic techniques are helpful in both differentiations.

COURSE

Most frequently, chronic ulcerative colitis is a disease of remissions and exacerbations of unpredictable duration. The patient with proctitis alone may be well for long periods and then experience flares of rectal bleeding and tenesmus lasting days or weeks. Patients who have more extensive colonic involvement also have periods of activity alternating with periods in which there are no symptoms or perhaps only mild diarrhea.

Ulcerative colitis usually begins in the rectum and may be confined to that area permanently in about half of the involved patients. In others, the disease spreads proximally over a period of weeks or months to involve some or all of the colon in a uniform fashion. One is not able to predict, early in the course of the disease, which patients will have limited involvement; but as a general rule, patients whose disease does not extend beyond the proctosigmoidoscopic level for a 2-year period have a less than 10 per cent chance of future extension of their disease. Extracolonic manifestations may be seen in patients who have limited or total involvement.

DIFFERENTIAL DIAGNOSIS

In the usual presentation with bloody diarrhea of recent onset, the clinician must carefully exclude other similarly presenting conditions such as acute bacillary dysentery, amebic colitis, ischemic colitis, Crohn's disease of the colon, radiation-induced colitis, drug-induced colitis, and colonic neoplasms. A stool culture and examination of the stool for parasites are always indicated and the patient should be questioned about the use of drugs, especially lincomycin and clindamycin, both of which may result in ulcerative proctitis or colitis. Only when the aforementioned possibilities have been eliminated and when diagnostic studies are otherwise typical of chronic ulcerative colitis may one be reasonably certain of the diagnosis and plan therapy accordingly.

DIAGNOSTIC METHODS

The Proctosigmoidoscopic Examination. Positive findings are present on proctoscopic examination in over 90 per cent of patients with active chronic ulcerative colitis. This procedure definitively confirms the diagnosis rapidly and simply in the vast majority of patients. Typically, one will see diffusely granular, friable mucosa, and the normal fine submucosal vascular pattern will be lacking. In more advanced disease, pseudopolyps may be seen. The finding of large ulcerations with normal intervening mucosa, or of extensive perianal disease, is suggestive of Crohn's disease rather than of chronic ulcerative colitis. When the disease is inactive, there may be evidence of mucosal bridging or strapping, or the examination may be entirely negative. The proctoscopic examination will also allow some definition of the extent of the disease if the abnormality is limited to the rectum or rectosigmoid with normal mucosa evident at higher levels. Proctoscopy also affords the opportunity of biopsying the mucosa, which can aid in the more positive identification of the disease or, on the other hand, confirm an alternative diagnosis such as amebic colitis or Crohn's disease.

Roentgenographic Findings. In early ulcerative colitis, the only roentgenologic abnormality on barium enema may be a serrated appearance of the bowel wall corresponding to the fine, superficial ulcerations present. The extent of the disease can usually be determined roentgenologically. As the disease progresses, the colon may become shortened and without haustral markings.

The significant difference between ulcerative colitis and Crohn's disease as seen by barium enema is the uniformity of appearance of the bowel affected by ulcerative colitis. Crohn's disease of the colon, roentgenographically, is characterized by skip areas of intervening normal appearance.

COLONOSCOPY

In ulcerative colitis per se, colonoscopy is not indicated. It may be helpful in diagnosing carcinoma, but it has little other use in diagnosing ulcerative colitis because a proctoscopic appearance combined with barium enema will provide all the necessary information for reaching a diagnosis.

BIOPSY

Biopsy of the rectal mucosa may distinguish ulcerative colitis in over 90 per cent of patients. Biopsy studies showing metaplasia of the mucosa may be helpful in predicting those who will develop carcinoma. This pathologic diagnosis should be made only by an experienced pathologist. Other features, such as age of onset (before 20) and persistence and severity of symptoms, must also be taken into consideration as risk factors in development of carcinoma.

One of the more frequent conditions mistaken for chronic ulcerative colitis is the "laxative abuse" colon. As radiologists may not be able to distinguish this condition, proctoscopy with biopsy may be important.

CELIAC DISEASE

By O. DHODANAND KOWLESSAR, M.D.
Philadelphia, Pennsylvania

SYNONYMS

Nontropical sprue, celiac sprue, sprue syndrome, idiopathic sprue, idiopathic steatorrhea, primary malabsorption, gluten-induced enteropathy, and Gee-Thaysen disease.

DEFINITION

Celiac disease is a disease of intestinal malabsorption of a wide variety of nutrients, resulting from characteristic if not specific pathologic alterations of the small intestinal mucosa, which are produced by the ingestion of certain gluten-containing cereal grains by susceptible persons. Prompt clinical, biochemical, and histologic improvement follows the withdrawal of gluten-containing cereal grains from the diet. Its prevalence is not known. The incidence varies considerably in different parts of the world, and is highest in West Ireland (1 in 300). The disease is worldwide in its distribution.

Two theories of the mechanism of gluten-gliadin toxicity in celiac disease have been proposed. One states that the intestinal absorptive cell is deficient in one or more enzymes that normally break down gliadin peptides, and that residual polypeptides not affected by this action injure the epithelial absorbing cell. The other major theory suggests that the morphologic changes seen in the small intestinal mucosa are due to the interaction of gluten with the immunocytes in the lamina propria, in which the immunocytes are sensitized. This interaction results in the formation of various immune products. These products interact with the absorptive cell to cause lysis and premature cell death with compensatory increase in crypt cell proliferation and a flat mucosal lesion. The presence of specific immune response in the intestinal mucosa of celiac patients suggested the existence of a genetically determined ability to produce such a response. Indeed, histocompatibility antigen determination revealed an incidence of HL-A B8 of 88 per cent in those with the condition compared to controls without the disease. More recently an even greater incidence of the presence of the HL-A DW3 antigen has been found in patients with celiac disease (27 of 28 patients), suggesting that this antigen may be the primary determinant. Although the evidence for an immunologic process is substantial, it is not yet conclusive. Further research is needed to define either the antigen or the substrate derived from gluten proteins.

A fascinating and unusual relationship exists between celiac disease and dermatitis herpetiformis. Almost all patients with dermatitis herpetiformis have a mild mucosal lesion of the proximal jejunum responsive to a low-gluten diet, while their skin lesions improve with sulfone administration. Of note, only a few patients with celiac disease have dermatitis herpetiformis. It is of further interest that the prevalence of the histocompatibility antigens HL-A B8 and HL-A DW3 in dermatitis herpetiformis patients is much higher than in normal persons.

PRESENTING SIGNS AND SYMPTOMS

The clinical manifestations of celiac disease vary tremendously from patient to patient. The dominant features in the clinical presentations can be divided into two broad categories: abdominal signs and symptoms and those related to the wide variety of deficiencies that occur in this disease. Classically, diarrhea and weight loss dominate the clinical picture. In most cases the diarrhea consists of frequent, glistening, bulky, foul-smelling stools, which vary from watery to loose to semisolid. Crampy abdominal pain with distention and increased flatulence contribute to the abdominal symptoms. Anorexia, nausea, and vomiting occur with less frequency than diarrhea. It should be remembered that a patient with celiac disease can have only one bowel movement daily, but it is usually large, bulky, and foul-smelling.

The signs and symptoms created by the various deficiencies can be directly traced to the abnormal small intestinal mucosal cells and their brush borders. Thus the malabsorption of fats results in loss of calories in the stool, followed by weight loss, weakness, and fatigue. Anemia with associated breathlessness, easy fatigability, cheilosis and glossitis, and numbness and tingling of the fingers and toes is secondary to the malabsorption of iron, folic acid, and vitamin B_{12}. Tetany, diffuse bone pain, and susceptibility to fractures are secondary to calcium and vitamin D malabsorption. Easy bruising, ecchymoses, bleeding gums, and occasionally hematuria and hemarthrosis are caused by vitamin K malabsorption and secondary hypoprothrombinemia. Peripheral edema is due to hypoalbuminemia that is secondary to amino acid malabsorption and protein weeping from the damaged intestinal mucosa.

Electrolyte losses secondary to diarrhea, vomiting, and malabsorption lead to dehydration with dry pigmented skin and muscle cramps. Other signs and symptoms include emotional lability, nocturia, irregular menses, impaired vibration sense, low blood pressure, hyperkeratosis follicularis, and clubbing of the fingers.

COURSE

The insidious onset of symptoms after introduction of cereals is characteristic of this disease, with an age distribution of 6 to 18 months in pediatric patients. The child with celiac disease is often miserable, negativistic, and depressed. He is characterized by protuberant abdomen, muscle wasting (especially of the buttocks and extremities), and hypotonia with retrogression in standing and walking. He has pale, soft, malodorous, frequent, occasionally constipated stools and failure to thrive; occasionally, effortless vomiting of large volume is also characteristic.

The gradual response (well under way in a few weeks) to a low-gluten diet and the maintenance of perfect health while on a strict diet, with slow and insidious relapses when the diet is relaxed, is typical. If these children are not maintained on a strict low-gluten diet, even though not overtly ill, their growth and development throughout adolescence is slower than normal. The condition of some patients remains in remission without overt relapses, whereas others have a return of many of their symptoms in the third and fourth decade. In approximately half of the adult patients, the clinical manifestations of malabsorption develop during the third to the seventh decade, without an antecedent history of the childhood disease. In some, the disease becomes clinically manifest after gastric surgery or in association with hypoglobulinemia and agammaglobulinemia, or after megaloblastic anemia of pregnancy, diabetes mellitus, emotional problems, or an episode of viral or bacterial enteritis.

The symptoms and signs tend to be intermittent, with frequent episodes of partial, spontaneous, albeit incomplete, remissions. In view of the chronicity of the diarrhea, many of these patients have been diagnosed as having the irritable bowel syndrome. In some patients the iron deficiency anemia, osteoporosis, osteomalacia, hemorrhagic tendencies, and peripheral neuropathy overshadow any problem with bowel movements, which may be regular.

PHYSICAL EXAMINATION

Physical findings vary among patients. Some patients exhibit no physical abnormalities. The physical signs depend on the secondary deficiencies created by the malabsorption of various food substances. As are the children, infants are usually miserable, negativistic, and depressed. They may have abdominal distention, muscle wasting of limbs and buttocks, hypotonia, and thinness with evident weight loss. Adults appear chronically ill, emaciated, with pale mucous membranes and dry, scaly skin, which is occasionally hyperpigmented. The blood pressure is low or normal. The hair may be thin and sparse. There are usually glossitis and cheilosis. The striking finding is abdominal distention with hyperactive bowel sounds. Peripheral edema is often present. There may be clubbing of the fingers. Other findings include positive Trousseau and Chvostek signs, ecchymoses, hematomas, skeletal deformities secondary to osteoporosis and osteomalacia, and in some cases, short stature.

COMPLICATIONS

The majority of complications are secondary to the prolonged intestinal malabsorption and are invariably the patient's presenting complaints. These include peripheral edema, symptoms and signs of iron deficiency or megaloblastic anemia, tetany, hemarthrosis, massive hematuria, multiple bone fractures, osteomalacia and osteoporosis, peripheral neuropathy, subacute combined degeneration, pancreatic insufficiency, small intestinal intussusception, and volvulus of the sigmoid colon.

Among the most dreaded complications of this disease are lymphomas of the mixed cell or histiocytic type (reticulum cell sarcoma), Hodgkin's disease, or lymphosarcoma. Carcinoma of the esophagus, stomach, small intestine, and colon have also been described as complicating this disorder. It has been suggested that patients with a long history of steatorrhea secondary to undiagnosed celiac disease are more prone to develop these complications. A number of complications can occur while the patient is on a gluten-free diet. These include progressive muscular atrophy, progressive myeloradiculoneuropathy, and acute jejunal and ileal ulcerations with stricture, intestinal obstruction, and perforation with peritonitis.

DIAGNOSIS

The diagnosis is based upon (1) typical history; (2) laboratory findings, suggestive of malabsorption, generally including steatorrhea; (3) characteristic histologic changes in a peroral jejunal mucosal biopsy; (4) dramatic and eventually complete improvement in the clinical, biochemical, and radiologic abnormalities, with near-complete improvement in the histology of the small intestinal mucosa after the institution of a low-gluten diet; and (5) clinical and biochemical relapse or worsening of the jejunal biopsy with a gluten or gliadin challenge, which may be necessary in a rare, questionable case.

A specific diagnosis is necessary because of the availability of effective therapy in the form of a low-gluten diet.

LABORATORY FINDINGS

Fat Malabsorption. Fat malabsorption is present in the majority of patients. The weight of a 24-hour stool collection is over 150 to 200 grams. Microscopic examination with Sudan III stain may demonstrate an increase in fat droplets (*N. Engl. J. Med., 264*:85–87, 1961). A 3 to 6 day stool collection is made while the patient is on a 100-gram fat diet or a regular diet containing between 80 and 100 grams of fat. The average daily excretion is determined chemically. The patients will show a fat excretion of 10 to 40 grams per 24 hours (normal <6 grams per 24 hours). In the near future the ^{14}C-labeled triolein breath test may be available and become extremely valuable for the documentation of steatorrhea because of its sensitivity and specificity.

Carbohydrate Absorption. The disturbance of carbohydrate metabolism and absorption is multifaceted. A flat oral glucose test is characteristic, but either a normal response or hyperglycemia can also occur. Diabetes mellitus has been estimated to occur in 2 per cent of patients with celiac disease and is probably a coincidental finding. The incidence of secondary pancreatic insufficiency is not known, but it does occur in a small number of patients. Thus, the bicarbonate, volume, and enzyme response in the pancreatic juice after the intravenous injection of 1 clinical unit of secretin per kg of body weight should be determined in celiac patients with high fecal nitrogen, low fecal excretion of trypsin and chymotrypsin, fat excretion greater than 40 grams per 24 hours, and hyperglycemia. The distinction of celiac disease from pancreatic insufficiency is aided by the determination of absorption and subsequent urinary excretion of orally administered D-xylose. In untreated celiac disease, the 5-hour excretion of D-xylose is less than 4.2 grams (usually 0.5 to 2.5 grams) after the oral administration of 25 grams of D-xylose. A low urinary excretion of D-xylose is characteristic of disease with diffuse mucosal abnormalities in the duodenum and jejunum. In addition, myxedema, renal disease, ascites, and acute alcoholism may cause low levels of urinary excretion. Hepatic disease results in increased values. Patients with pancreatic insufficiency with normal kidney function absorb and excrete normal quantities of D-xylose (over 4.2 grams per 5 hours).

Hematologic. Iron-deficiency anemia with hypochromia, microcytosis on blood smear, and low serum iron may be observed. The white blood cell count varies between 5000 and 8000 per cu mm. Granulopenia around 500 per cu mm occurs rarely. Other patients have a megaloblastic anemia secondary to folic acid or have vitamin B_{12} deficiency or both. Serum folate ranges between 0.7 and 3.5 nanograms per ml (normal >3.5 nanograms per ml) in the majority of patients, when determined. The Schilling test in patients with severe ileal disease reveals an excretion of less than 5 per cent and is uncorrected by the addition of intrinsic factor and broad-spectrum antibiotics, thus differentiating it from pernicious anemia and blind loop variants, respectively.

Other Absorptive Defects. The serum carotene is a useful screening test and levels below 50 micrograms per dl (100 ml) are invariably seen. Low serum albumin, cholesterol, vitamin A, and prothrombin (corrected by administration of vitamin K) may occur. In patients with osteomalacia, the serum calcium is low, with normal or low serum phosphorus and elevated bone alkaline phosphatase. A bone biopsy is necessary to make the diagnosis of osteomalacia and should reveal increases in the number of osteoid foci and widening of the osteoid seams. A generalized deficiency of intestinal disaccharidase activity occurs secondary to epithelial cell damage. Lactase is most affected. A lactose tolerance test with 75 grams of lactose produces abdominal cramps and diarrhea with a blood glucose rise of less than 22 mg per dl. Quantitative assay of lactase in a jejunal biopsy will show depressed levels in all untreated patients. A hydrogen breath test after lactose ingestion will show an increase in breath hydrogen.

SMALL INTESTINAL RADIOGRAPHS

Radiographs of the small intestine cannot establish a diagnosis of celiac disease but are helpful in eliminating other possible causes of malabsorption or diarrhea. The small bowel series usually reveals a nonspecific malabsorption pattern. The abnormal findings, when they occur, include dilatation of the small intestine, marked coarsening or complete obliteration of the mucosal folds, and fragmentation and flocculation of the barium meal within the lumen of the gut. In mild or moderate disease, the mucosal pattern is distorted in the proximal small intestine. In patients with severe disease, the mucosal pattern is abnormal throughout the small intestine up to and including the ileum.

BIOPSY OF THE SMALL INTESTINE

Biopsy of the distal duodenum by means of the duodenoscope or proximal jejunum with any of the available peroral suction instruments or biopsy capsules reveals characteristic alterations in mucosal tissue. The appearance of the tissue in celiac disease contrasts sharply with normal tissue under the light microscope, showing complete loss of villous architecture, while the intestinal crypts are markedly elongated and open onto a flat, absorptive surface. The luminal epithelial cells are cuboidal rather than columnar, with loss of nuclear polarity, mucosal cryptoplasmic basophilia, and vacuolization. The brush or striated border is markedly attenuated. There is an apparent increase in intraepithelial lymphocytes (IEL), but in a recent study the number of IEL was the same as in normal tissue before or after treatment. The undifferentiated crypt cells are markedly increased in number with an increase in the number of mitoses. The cellularity of the lamina propria is regularly increased and consists largely of immunoglobulin-producing plasma cells (IgM), lymphocytes, and some eosinophils and polymorphonuclear leukocytes. Classically, the abnormal cells are confined to the proximal small intestine, while in severe cases the mucosa of the entire small bowel is involved. Although the lesion is not entirely specific for celiac disease, in the temperate zone most patients with these changes have celiac disease and respond to a low-gluten diet. More than one normal jejunal biopsy excludes untreated celiac disease.

THERAPEUTIC TRIAL

The treatment of choice is a low-gluten diet, which excludes all cereal grains except rice and corn. To follow this diet strictly, all labels must be carefully read to eliminate completely those products containing wheat, rye, barley, and probably oats. Early in the course of therapy, milk and milk products may have to be excluded in view of the striking number of celiac patients with secondary lactase deficiency. The vast majority of these patients will respond to the low-gluten diet clinically, biochemically, and histologically. Striking symptomatic improvement can occur within 48 hours to a week. A few patients may require as much as 6 months before a striking weight gain is made and a sense of well-being recurs. The surface epithelium becomes tall and columnar within 2 weeks, but even on a strict diet, it may take many years before the villous pattern approaches normalcy.

Lack of response to a low-gluten diet suggests an incorrect diagnosis, failure to adhere strictly to the diet, or a complication such as intestinal ulceration, reticulum cell sarcoma, or pancreatic insufficiency. Minor dietary indiscretions while the patient is in remission may be tolerated without symptoms; but with continued indiscretion, mucosal damage and malabsorption will ensue.

PITFALLS IN DIAGNOSIS

Although the histologic changes of the peroral jejunal biopsy are highly suggestive of celiac disease, they may be seen in other diseases that cause malabsorption, such as tropical sprue, intestinal lymphoma, giardiasis, and rarely small intestinal stasis with bacterial overgrowth, strongyloidiasis, eosinophilic gastroenteritis, refractory sprue, and diffuse ileojejunitis. Tropical sprue is seen only in endemic areas or in patients coming from endemic areas. *Giardia lamblia*, if suspected, should be sought in duodenal aspirates, proximal jejunal biopsies, and in stool specimens. Malabsorption and an abnormal biopsy may be associated with agammaglobulinemias or hypogammaglobulinemias.

The differentiation of celiac disease from intestinal lymphoma presenting with malabsorption and a flat biopsy may be very difficult. The presence of fever, severe abdominal pain, striking hypoalbuminemia, and failure to respond to a low-gluten diet should suggest the correct diagnosis. It should be remembered that intestinal lymphoma may complicate celiac disease, in which case the patient may experience an exacerbation of symptoms despite rigid adherence to a low-gluten diet.

The condition in a very small percentage of patients with a flat mucosal lesion of the proximal small intestine is refractory to the low-gluten diet from the time of diagnosis. Some of these patients may respond to treatment with corticosteroids, others may respond to azathioprine or cyclophosphamide. Others who appear to have refractory disease develop the syndrome of chronic, ulcerative, nongranulomatous jejunitis, which may have patchy mucosal lesions histologically indistinguishable from the flat mucosa of celiac disease. The prognosis in this group of patients is usually poor.

It is possible that the new technique of organ culture of peroral biopsies may aid in differentiating celiac diseases from other causes of a flat intestinal mucosa.

VASCULAR DISEASE OF THE MESENTERY

By KENNETH L. MATTOX, M.D.,
and ARTHUR C. BEALL, JR., M.D.
Houston, Texas

SYNONYMS

Mesenteric vascular insufficiency, intestinal angina, abdominal angina, mesenteric infarction, nonocclusive mesenteric ischemia, mesenteric arteriovenous occlusive disease.

DEFINITION

Vascular disease of the mesentery is present when there is a decreased flow through the mesenteric vessels secondary to occlusion, embolus, ligature, external trauma, or low perfusion conditions and is manifest by malfunction of the involved congested, ischemic, or infarcted bowel.

Presenting Signs, Symptoms, and Physical Findings

The presenting condition of the patient is dependent upon the rate of onset, the integrity of collateral circulation, and the extent of occlusion or perfusion. Complete occlusion of one or even two of the major visceral arteries may occasionally be seen at autopsy in a patient who was completely asymptomatic. Portal vein ligation or complete occlusion may not result in bowel infarction or insufficiency. Chronic insufficiency may be manifest by weight loss and postprandial abdominal pain. Such a patient is anorexic and malnourished. In prolonged nutritional deprivation, glossitis, cheilosis, and dependent edema may be present. A midabdominal bruit may be heard. There may be signs of portal hypertension. In patients with arteritis and small arterial occlusion, there may be systemic manifestations of one of the collagen diseases.

The patient with frank mesenteric infarction has severe abdominal pain and may be devoid of any significant objective abdominal findings. Very early and briefly the abdominal pain may be cramping in nature with hyperactive bowel sounds. Fifty per cent of these patients have nonocclusive mesenteric ischemia; therefore low cardiac output, congestive heart failure, hypovolemia, septic shock, or a history of digitalis medication is occasionally present. The patient may be seriously ill and poorly responsive, with abdominal distention, absent bowel sounds, bloody diarrhea, fever, and subsequently hypothermia, tachycardia, and shock.

Course

The patient with "intestinal angina" becomes progressively more malnourished and may subsequently develop frank intestinal infarction if revascularization is not performed. There is no medical therapy for frank intestinal infarction, regardless of the cause. The survival rate for persons having emergency resection for intestinal infarction secondary to vascular compromise has been reportedly less than 10 per cent.

Common Complications

Complications of chronic mesenteric vascular insufficiency include weight loss, cachexia, and malnutrition. Patients surviving resection of infarcted bowel may develop diarrhea, malabsorption, or the "short bowel syndrome." Despite adequate resection of nonviable bowel

and reanastomosis at healthy tissue, progression of the ischemic zones and anastomotic disruption prompt the concept of a "second look" operation 24 to 72 hours after the first operation. The usual infectious complications that follow a perforated viscus should be considered.

Laboratory Findings

Laboratory determinations are of little value in the differential diagnosis. Acute occlusion may be associated with moderate to severe leukocytosis. The functional extracellular fluid deficits associated with bowel infarction may be manifested with rising blood urea nitrogen and hematocrit determinations. Serum electrolytes usually document a metabolic acidosis. More than likely, the laboratory values will reflect those changes associated with the pre-existing disease process.

In progressive subtotal mesenteric arterial occlusion, laboratory studies may document intestinal malabsorption consistent with the clinical state. Fat absorption first is impaired with an increase in fecal fat and diminished ^{131}I triolein absorption. Later, carbohydrate and protein absorption are impaired and the D-xylose and cobalt-labeled B_{12} absorption tests are indicative of abnormal absorption. Serum albumin, cholesterol, carotene, and calcium may be diminished. If hypovitaminosis has not been corrected, a hypochromic macrocytic anemia is present and the prothrombin time is prolonged.

Roentgenographic Examination

In acute situations, often only a portable x-ray supine film of the abdomen is available. These usually demonstrate diffuse dilatation of the small and large bowel, occasionally with air-fluid levels. No diagnostic pattern appears consistently, and the usual interpretation is that of adynamic ileus. In chronic, incomplete occlusion, roentgenographic studies are of more value. The plain films usually are normal but a barium meal with small bowel follow-through reveals abnormal progression of barium with "puddling" in some areas and apparent segmental narrowing in others. The mucosal pattern may appear coarsened.

With necrosis of the bowel wall, air that has entered into the subserosal plane may appear as a string or a ring of gas outside the lumen of the bowel. Air appearing in the portal venous system is usually a preterminal sign and is indicative of a grave prognosis.

Although rarely indicated in the acute bowel necrosis, angiographic demonstration of the abdominal aorta is the only definitive diagnostic examination among patients suspected of having chronic intestinal ischemia. Lateral aortography often is adequate, but selective angiography with frontal and lateral views after injection of contrast material into the celiac and superior mesenteric arteries is preferable. Occasionally, remarkable collateralization is seen from the branches of the inferior mesenteric artery to the superior mesenteric arterial system. Occlusion of the inferior mesenteric artery usually is not associated with symptoms unless the celiac and superior mesenteric arteries are involved by the atheromatous process. At least a 50 per cent narrowing of the celiac and superior mesenteric arteries is required before a significant reduction in arterial flow to the intestine occurs.

EXPLORATORY CELIOTOMY

Operation should only await resuscitative measures to correct fluid, electrolyte, acid/base, and hemodynamic abnormalities. In the acutely ill patient, exploratory celiotomy is the only conclusive procedure available to the clinician. Unfortunately, the majority of these patients are so desperately ill that this diagnostic procedure is delayed until a stage when it is of little therapeutic benefit. Final confirmation of the diagnosis of chronic obstructive disease involving the mesenteric arteries requires exploration with measurement of gradients across the areas of obstruction. Arterial reconstructive procedures are applicable if bowel necrosis is not present.

PITFALLS IN DIAGNOSIS

Celiotomy in patients with ischemic bowel may be delayed because the abdomen is nontender and there are systemic symptoms of congestive heart failure, hypovolemia, or shock, thus prompting an erroneous diagnosis of ileus. Since 50 per cent of patients with mesenteric infarction have nonocclusive mesenteric ischemia, adequate hydration and mesenteric perfusion are required rather than further dehydration brought about through forced diuresis. Even in the patient with chronic mesenteric ischemia, the physician may be diverted to more common diagnostic differentials, such as carcinomatosis, pancreatic insufficiency, and malabsorption states.

INTESTINAL DISACCHARIDASE DEFICIENCY

By CONSTANTINE ARVANITAKIS, M.D., *and* SANDA NOUSIA-ARVANITAKIS, M.D.

Kansas City, Kansas

SYNONYMS

Lactase deficiency, lactose intolerance, sucrase-isomaltase deficiency, sucrose intolerance, trehalose intolerance, disaccharide intolerance.

DEFINITION

The disaccharides lactose, sucrose, maltose, and trehalose are hydrolyzed to their constituent monosaccharides before they are absorbed from the small intestinal mucosa. The brush border of the small intestinal mucosa contains specific digestive enzymes that are located at the microvillus membrane of the mature columnar epithelial cell and split the disaccharides to glucose, galactose, and fructose. Glucose and galactose are absorbed by an active transport process requiring sodium and energy, whereas fructose is absorbed by facilitated diffusion.

Lactase hydrolyzes lactose to glucose and galactose; *sucrase* hydrolyzes sucrose to glucose and fructose; *maltase* and *trehalase* hydrolyze maltose and trehalose, respectively, to two molecules of glucose. Disaccharide intolerance following the ingestion of the offending dietary disaccharide results from a deficiency in intestinal disaccharidases. This deficiency in the enzymatic activity of disaccharidases is either (1) primary, as a result of an isolated defect of a digestive enzyme, or (2) secondary, owing to small intestinal disease, reduction of the brush border surface, malnutrition, or drugs.

The most common disaccharidase deficiency is lactase deficiency. Primary lactase deficiency may be either congenital, which is a rare form, or acquired (adult hypolactasia), which usually develops in adulthood with the progressive reduction of lactase activity after infancy. This form of lactase deficiency is prevalent in certain ethnic groups such as black Americans, Jews, Greeks, Eskimos, Asians, Latin Americans, and black Africans. The incidence of lactase deficiency in these groups may be as high as 50 to 90 per cent. By contrast, lactase deficiency is uncommon in Northern Europeans and Northern Americans. From a teleological point of view it can be argued that lactase deficiency represents a normal biological process, since lactase activity is decreased with age corresponding to the lessened consumption of milk in adult life.

Epidemiologic studies have shown a good correlation between lactase activity and milk consumption per capita — lactase deficiency is prevalent in countries where milk is not ingested in large quantities.

The congenital form of lactase deficiency is present at birth, usually occurs in siblings, and is probably inherited as an autosomal recessive gene.

Secondary lactase deficiency, both in children and adults, is a common problem in clinical practice. It occurs in any disease that causes damage of the small intestinal mucosa (celiac sprue, tropical sprue, viral or bacterial gastroenteritis, inflammatory bowel disease), in nutritional deficiency states (prolonged starvation, protein malnutrition), in short bowel syndrome, and following the administration of drugs (colchicine, aminoglycosides). Lactase activity may be restored to normal following the successful treatment of the primary disease and the improvement in the damage of the small intestinal mucosa.

Sucrase-isomaltase deficiency is an isolated enzymatic deficiency inherited as an autosomal recessive gene. Immunochemical studies in the brush border have shown that subjects with this deficiency completely lack sucrase and isomaltase. Finally, another unusual form of disaccharidase deficiency is trehalase deficiency. Trehalase hydrolyzes trehalose, a glucosidoglucoside found in mushrooms, to two molecules of glucose-trehalose — thus the rarity of trehalose intolerance, since symptoms do not occur with the ingestion of any other food.

PRESENTING SYMPTOMS AND SIGNS

The severity of the clinical manifestations of disaccharidase deficiency depends on the degree of enzymatic deficiency and the amount of disaccharide (substrate) presented to the brush border for hydrolysis. Some patients may tolerate 1 to 2 glasses of milk, equivalent to 12 to 24 grams of lactose (240 ml of milk are equivalent to 12 grams of lactose). Others with low levels of lactase may develop symptoms with the ingestion of small amounts of lactose (3 to 8 grams). Common presenting symptoms and signs are diarrhea, borborygmi, flatulence, bloating, and abdominal cramps. The pathogenesis of these manifestations is due to the following factors:

1. The unhydrolyzed disaccharide entering the lumen of the small intestine with its high osmotic activity causes movement of fluid from the plasma to lumen, resulting in excessive secretion in the bowel.

2. Because of increased volume of intraluminal fluid, transit time is shortened and as a result, the absorption of excessive fluid is impaired.

3. The unhydrolyzed disaccharide that enters the colonic lumen is subject to fermentation by the colonic flora, with the release of lactic acid, short chain fatty acids, carbon dioxide, and hydrogen. These acid substances alter the pH of the colonic lumen and, as a result, sodium and water absorption from the colonic mucosa is impaired and diarrhea occurs.

Symptoms become manifest within half an hour to 1 hour after the ingestion of the offending disaccharide. Excessive consumption of milk, for example, in pregnancy or in patients with peptic ulcer disease, may unmask the existence of lactase deficiency. Disaccharidase deficiency is not a serious disease in adults, but in infants it constitutes an entirely different entity. Disaccharidase deficiency in infancy and childhood presents with failure to thrive, vomiting, diarrhea, metabolic acidosis, dehydration, aminoaciduria, steatorrhea, and malnutrition. Symptoms usually develop during the first weeks of life with the ingestion of the offending disaccharide; the symptoms are resolved with the elimination of the sugar from the diet.

PHYSICAL EXAMINATION FINDINGS

There are no significant findings in disaccharidase deficiency unless it is secondary to another disease, in which case clinical manifestations of this condition may be present.

LABORATORY FINDINGS

The establishment of the diagnosis of disaccharidase deficiency is significant for two reasons. First, elimination of the dietary disaccharides that cause symptoms results in resolution of symptoms. Second, the clinical manifestations of disaccharidase deficiency frequently simulate other gastrointestinal disorders or, conversely, the coexistence of disaccharidase deficiency with other digestive diseases aggravates these conditions. The diagnostic tests of disaccharidase deficiency are the following:

Small Intestinal Mucosal Biopsy and Disaccharidase Assay. This is the most accurate and definitive test. Small intestinal mucosal biopsy is obtained at the area of the ligament of

Treitz and specific activity of disaccharidase is measured in the mucosal homogenate. In addition to the diagnostic value in disaccharidase deficiency, intestinal biopsy provides information on the histologic appearance of the small intestinal mucosa in malabsorptive syndromes.

Small intestinal biopsy is a safe procedure, but it poses considerable practical difficulties in that it requires intestinal intubation, fluoroscopy, and the availability of laboratory methods for disaccharidase assay. Accordingly, it is reasonable to state that this procedure is usually reserved for special cases in which the diagnosis cannot be established by other means. It is especially important in infants or children for the diagnosis of sucrase-isomaltase deficiency.

Disaccharide Tolerance Test. This is an indirect diagnostic test based on the measurement of hydrolytic products of disaccharides in the blood, mainly glucose, following the oral administration of disaccharides. The most commonly performed test is the lactose tolerance test (LTT) for the diagnosis of lactase deficiency. It is generally acceptable to give 50 grams of lactose (2 grams per kg body weight in children) in 400 ml of water and draw blood samples for glucose at 0, 15, 30, 60, 90, and 120 minutes. Measurement of glucose in capillary blood is more accurate than in venous blood. A rise of blood sugar above 20 mg per dl (100 ml) is considered a normal LTT. If the rise in blood glucose is less than 20 mg per dl, the test should be considered abnormal. The possibility of hexose malabsorption, however, should be excluded in order to establish accurately the diagnosis of lactase deficiency. In this case, the test is repeated with the administration of 25 grams of glucose-galactose mixture and measurement of blood glucose. One modification of LTT that provides a higher degree of accuracy is administration of lactose with alcohol and measurement of blood galactose. Alcohol is given to block the conversion of galactose to glucose in the liver. The use of alcohol, however, limits the application of the test in children and in patients with liver disease.

During the performance of the LTT the patient is observed for clinical manifestations of lactase deficiency. It should be noted that the presence or absence of symptoms alone does not constitute a reliable index of lactase deficiency. Symptoms depend on the degree of lactase deficiency, and the tolerance to lactose ingestion varies a great deal. The results of LTT taken together with the clinical observation provide a more reliable combination in the diagnosis of lactase deficiency.

Despite the wide application of LTT and disaccharide tolerance test in general, there are important limitations in the diagnostic value of the method. It has been reported in several studies that the rate of false-positive results, that is, flat curve of LTT with normal lactase, can be as high as 20 to 30 per cent. This is mainly due to the fact that blood glucose levels are not determined only by the rate of lactose hydrolysis but also they are influenced by other factors. These include the rate of gastric emptying, the rate of intestinal absorption, the rate of glucose clearing from the blood, and a host of hormonal and metabolic interactions. Some of these limitations may be overcome — for example, the effect of gastric emptying can be eliminated by infusing the disaccharide intraduodenally —but this modification limits the practicality of the test. In summary, the accumulated clinical experience indicates that LTT is a useful test but the results should be interpreted with caution and in the light of clinical manifestations.

^{14}C-lactose Breath Test. Radioactive isotopes in breath tests have been increasingly used in the diagnosis of malabsorptive syndromes. ^{14}C-lactose breath test has been evaluated in the diagnosis of lactase deficiency with satisfactory results. The test is based on the principle that ^{14}C-lactose is hydrolyzed to galactose and ^{14}C-glucose, which is further metabolized via the glycolytic and phosphogluconate oxidative pathway to form $^{14}CO_2$. Radioactive CO_2 is exhaled in the breath, whereby measurement of the specific activity of $^{14}CO_2$ provides an indirect index of lactase activity.

The test is performed as follows: 50 grams of cold lactose are given with 5 μCi of ^{14}C-lactose; breath is collected at 0, 30 minutes, and 1, 2, 3, and 4 hours; and $^{14}CO_2$ activity is calculated. A single breath collection obtained at 2 hours is sufficient to separate normal subjects from lactase-deficient subjects. Normal controls excrete 25 per cent of the administered dose, whereas patients with lactase deficiency excrete 10 per cent or less. The surface under the curve correlates well with lactase activity in intestinal mucosal homogenates.

The test is practical and simple, easy to administer, reliable, and obviates the need for the venipunctures of LTT. Comparative studies have shown that the ^{14}C-lactose breath test is more accurate than LTT, with a significantly lower incidence of false-positive or false-negative results. The main disadvantage of the test is its inclusion of radioactive isotope, which limits it use in children and pregnant women. The radiation exposure, however, is very low. It has been estimated that 5 μCi of ^{14}C-lactose results in a whole-body radiation exposure of 3 $\times$ 10^{-4} rads, which is less than the radiation exposure from a routine chest x-ray. Moreover, the effective half-life of radiolabeled carbon is relatively short (6 to 24 hours) with the bulk of the administered dose eliminated in 24 hours. Another disadvantage of the test is that the results of $^{14}CO_2$ are influenced by diabetes mellitus characterized by a decrease of ^{14}C-glucose conversion to $^{14}CO_2$.

Hydrogen Breath Test. Another indirect but reliable approach in the diagnosis of disaccharidase deficiency is the measurement of hydrogen in the breath following the oral administration of the offending disaccharide. In subjects with normal lactase activity, the amount of breath hydrogen is extremely small and does not increase with administration of lactose. By contrast, the amount of excreted hydrogen in the breath is significantly increased with lactose or other disaccharides that are not hydrolyzed, reach the colon and are fermented to form carbon dioxide, lactic acid, and hydrogen.

The distinct advantage of the hydrogen breath test besides its high degree of accuracy is that radioactive isotopes are not used. Therefore it finds a wide application in children and pregnant women. In addition, the presence of other metabolic factors does not influence hydrogen production. The disadvantages of the test are the requirement of a bulky apparatus for breath collection, and the availability of gas liquid chromatography, a more complex and specialized procedure compared with liquid scintillation for $^{14}CO_2$ measurement. The results of the test may be influenced by antibiotics, which alter the colonic flora and hence hydrogen production. Comparative studies evaluating indirect tests of lactase deficiency have shown that the hydrogen breath test and ^{14}C-lactose breath test are superior to the standard LTT in terms of specificity and compare favorably with lactase assay in intestinal mucosal homogenates. It can be predicted that these tests will become popular because they combine simplicity and a high degree of accuracy.

Stool Examination. In children with diarrhea due to disaccharidase deficiency, the measurement of stool pH is a helpful screening test. As a general rule, stool pH is 6 or less in children with disaccharidase deficiency owing to fermentation of the unhydrolyzed disaccharide in the colon to acid compounds, lactic acid, and short-chain fatty acids. Another more reliable screening test is the quantitative measurement of reducing substances in the stool. Following the oral administration of the disaccharide, stool is diluted with water and placed in a test tube with a Clinitest tablet. The color of the mixture turns to red in the presence of reducing substances. In the case of sucrose intolerance, the sample should be first hydro-lyzed with 1 N HCl and then boiled because sucrose is not a reducing substance.

These tests, which are helpful in infants and children, have limited diagnostic value in adults.

THERAPEUTIC TESTS

Resolution of clinical manifestations of disaccharide intolerance as a result of elimination of the offending disaccharide from the diet can be used as a diagnostic indicator of disaccharidase deficiency.

PITFALLS IN DIAGNOSIS

Indirect tests of disaccharidase deficiency are influenced by the rate of gastric emptying and metabolic conditions such as diabetes mellitus, which affect glucose metabolism. In these patients, the most accurate and definitive diagnostic test remains the small intestinal biopsy and disaccharidase assay in the mucosal homogenate.

DIVERTICULAR DISEASE OF THE COLON

By MICHAEL W. KIMBALL, M.D., F.A.C.G.
Solana Beach, California

DIVERTICULOSIS

SYNONYMS

Diverticulosis coli; diverticulae.

DEFINITION

Diverticulosis of the colon is a term used to describe the condition that includes the spectrum from prediverticular disease to diverticulosis itself and finally the complications of diverticulitis and diverticular hemorrhage. The first condition, prediverticular disease, relates to the pathophysiologic development of abnormalities within the colonic musculature. The teniae coli become thickened, as does the circular muscle, and unusually high pressures are generated within the lumen. Recent evidence suggests that diets that are deficient in fiber (bran, etc.) allow for development of localized areas of extensive segmentation of intraluminal pressure. As these areas of extensive pressure develop, herniation of small pouches of the mucosa and muscularis protrude through the musculature onto the serosal surface. This, then, is the stage at which the diverticula are present.

Diverticulosis is most common in the elderly, in whom the incidence approximates 50 per cent of the population in Western civilization by the age of 80. It is interesting to note that the incidence is much less in developing countries, where dietary fiber is more abundant. The incidence in females exceeds slightly that in males. One form of the disease is probably hereditary, in that it occurs at a younger age and is associated with more significant complications.

The complex of emotional stress and functional bowel syndrome (spastic colon) is difficult to correlate with this condition.

PRESENTING SIGNS AND SYMPTOMS

The initial diagnosis of diverticulosis is often made on a barium enema x-ray examination. The diverticula may be single or innumerable. They may occur anywhere from the sigmoid colon to the cecum. Contributing symptoms to diverticulosis may be difficult to diagnose, particularly in the early prediverticular phase, because of the nonspecific nature of lower abdominal cramping, a minor change in bowel habits, and a sensation of incomplete evacuation or fullness and nonspecific tenderness. These symptoms may simply be related to changes in tone within the colon musculature and may not be due to the anatomic development of the condition itself. Simple functional bowel and prediverticular disease certainly overlap. As will be seen from the discussion on diverticulitis, the signs and symptoms become those of inflammation rather than of the condition itself.

On physical examination, one may be able to palpate some tenderness over the colon, particularly the sigmoid area. Sometimes a thickened or spastic colon may be palpable. At the time of sigmoidoscopic or colonoscopic examination, the diverticular orifices may be noted. Tiny fecaliths may be extruded into the lumen, suggesting the presence of diverticula as well. On occasion, excessive spasm at the rectosigmoid junction may be encountered.

DIAGNOSTIC FINDINGS

X-ray examination of the colon revealing the diverticulosis is the main method of diagnosis. On occasion, prediverticular disease may be diagnosed by x-ray, if a corrugated sawtooth configuration of hypertrophied muscles is noted.

COURSE AND COMPLICATIONS

With progressive age, increasing morbidity in the form of diverticulitis and diverticular hemorrhage occurs. In addition, progressive functional constipation may be noted. The increased incidence of other conditions include cholelithiasis, esophageal hiatal hernia, and hemorrhoids. These all may be related to dietary fiber deficiencies. The incidence of carcinoma of the colon in these patients is probably no greater than in the general population. However, the two may be found coincidentally together. In fact, one of the pitfalls of diagnosis lies in the interpretation of barium enema examination — there is difficulty in adequately visualizing the colonic mucosa for polyps or carcinomas. One of the more common indications for colonoscopic examinations today is the possibility of polyps or carcinoma or both in the presence of diverticular disease.

In summary, the development of increased pressures in the sigmoid colon with muscular thickening leads to the prediverticular state, which then may progress to increased muscular spasticity and herniation of the mucous membrane and development of the diverticula. Nonspecific lower bowel complaints may be found in these patients and generally the diagnosis is made by barium enema x-ray. Many people do not have signs or symptoms referable to diverticulosis, and only when one of the complications occurs does the condition become a true disease.

DIVERTICULITIS

SYNONYMS

Acute diverticular disease of the colon; acute diverticulitis; left-sided appendicitis.

DEFINITION

If one of the diverticula becomes obstructed owing to inspissated fecal material, a closed space may develop. Bacterial invasion of the abraded mucosal surface gives rise to an acute inflammatory process. *Escherichia coli* is in the majority among the intestinal flora. With development of the inflammatory process bacterial invasion of adjacent stuctures, a number of problems may occur. These include local containment with simple involvement of the serosal surface, the pericolic fat, and a localized peritonitis. If the process spreads, free perforation or fistulization may occur into surrounding organs such as the bladder or an adjacent diverticulum. Pus and necrotic debris, as well as a reaction within regional lymph nodes, develop.

PRESENTING SIGNS AND SYMPTOMS

Depending on the extent of inflammation, the patient's symptoms may include low-grade temperature, localized pain and tenderness, peritonitis and frank sepsis, and/or septic shock. Many patients are totally asymptomatic until just before the acute attack; however, some will report recent changes in bowel habits, particularly constipation. Bleeding is generally not a complication of acute diverticulitis. Other signs and symptoms relate to fistulization into the bladder, causing pneumaturia or recurrent pyuria. Fecal discharge through the vagina in case of fistulization into this space might be noted. Chronic diverticulitis relates to more long-standing inflammation of a milder nature. The symptoms here would involve change in bowel habits such as constipation, some chronic left lower quadrant pain, possible pain upon defecation, and the awareness of a fullness or tenderness in the left lower quadrant of the abdomen. A spectrum exists ranging from a patient with mild contained inflammatory process to an obviously acutely ill individual with findings of diffuse peritonitis.

PHYSICAL EXAMINATION FINDINGS

Again depending upon the acuteness and severity of the attack, one would expect to find localized tenderness with guarding, rigidity, and rebound up to and including diffuse peritoneal signs. Temperature from the range of 100 to 103 F (37.8 to 39.4 C), generalized toxicity, and sepsis may be found. Specific findings within the abdomen generally are on the left side. The presence of a vaginal discharge and/or pyuria and hematuria might be observed as well. Rectal examination itself is generally unremarkable unless a pericolic abscess is present, whereupon a tender mass might be noted.

COURSE

The course is variable. Many attacks of diverticulitis are relatively mild and respond to conservative management of antibiotics and bowel rest. Some of these may be treated on an outpatient basis. However, in patients of increasing age and with other associated diseases, a more severe attack necessitating hospitalization may be encountered. There appears to be little relationship between the severity or frequency of attacks and the number or location of the diverticula, although 90 per cent of surgery for diverticulitis is performed with involvement of the sigmoid colon. Approximately 50 per cent of patients who survive the first attack of diverticulitis will remain symptom free. Approximately 25 per cent will be readmitted for recurrence within a few months and a fourth of these will need surgery. It is apparent that once recurrences have developed, further difficulty will necessitate more aggressive surgical therapy. Mortality ranges from 3 per cent during the first hospitalization to 12 per cent over a 5-year follow-up, again depending on the severity and the association with other significant disease processes in the elderly.

LABORATORY FINDINGS

In acute attacks the most common findings are those of leukocytosis with a shift to the left. Sedimentation rate is elevated. Involvement of the bladder would be reflected in pyuria and hematuria, as well as a positive urine culture. X-ray examination again is the main diagnostic tool. An initial acute abdomen series is indicated to rule out perforation manifested by free intraperitoneal air. In the face of acute diverticulitis, meglumine diatrizoate (Gastrografin) should be used rather than barium because of the possibility of extravasation of the barium. In a mild case barium may be used and here the findings of a localized area of tenderness, spasticity, spiculation, and contained perforation would be noted. Also, a demonstration of a fistula, a sinus tract, or a pericolic abscess is diagnostic. Use of a flexible sigmoidoscope or colonoscope may be difficult because of colon spasm or sharp angulation and fixation of the sigmoid colon. In the face of an acute attack of diverticulitis this procedure is contraindicated. However, if one were to perform this procedure, a diverticular orifice might be visualized with areas of surrounding erythema and edema. Pelvic echography or computed tomography (CT) scanning or both could be utilized to demonstrate abscesses.

PITFALLS IN DIAGNOSIS

The main differential lies in any inflammatory process in the lower abdomen, including involvement of the bladder or kidney with cystitis and/or pyelonephritis, and the ovaries or uterus with cysts and tumors. A free perforation without localized findings would be difficult to differentiate preoperatively from such conditions as perforated appendix or perforated ulcer. Carcinoma of the colon must be ruled out. As previously noted, there may be difficulty in interpretation of a barium enema in the presence of diverticular disease. Colonoscopy may be used to resolve this question. Other conditions include Crohn's disease of the colon (granulomatous colitis), ulcerative colitis, amebic colitis, acute bacterial colitis such as that caused by Salmonella and Shigella, and ischemic colitis. They all cause lower abdominal pain and inflammation of the colon and adjacent structures.

In summary, diverticulitis is the common complication of diverticulosis manifested by inflammation and bacterial invasion with its acute localizing symptoms and signs of fever and tenderness. More drastic complications of fistulization and perforation may occur.

DIVERTICULAR BLEEDING

SYNONYM

Lower gastrointestinal bleeding.

DEFINITION

Hemorrhage is the other common problem of diverticular disease. It should be noted that diverticular bleeding and diverticulitis do not necessarily occur together. The erosion into small vessels within the diverticulae is generally venous in origin. The bleeding may be massive or it may be recurrent or chronic low-grade oozing.

PRESENTING SIGNS AND SYMPTOMS

Depending upon the magnitude of the bleeding, one may simply report hematochezia up to and including gross bloody diarrhea with clots. If the latter occurs, symptoms of hypotension and acute anemia, tachycardia, and diaphoresis may be present. There may be some lower abdominal cramping or the desire to defecate, or the bleeding may occur totally asymptomatic.

COURSE

The majority of the patients stop bleeding spontaneously even if the bleeding is massive.

The amount of blood lost is then the main determinant in terms of morbidity. Approximately one third of the patients will rebleed in a matter of months to years. An occasional patient will continue to bleed vigorously enough to warrant immediate surgery.

The accompanying complications are related to the problems of acute anemia, such as transfusion reactions, hypotension, and cardiovascular collapse.

LABORATORY FINDINGS

The only specific laboratory finding is anemia with hemoglobin and hematocrit values of 3 and 10 grams per dl (100 ml) to 15 and 45 volumes per cent, depending on the magnitude of blood loss.

PITFALLS IN DIAGNOSIS

The main difficulty lies with identifying the site of the bleeding. Recent evidence indicates that although the sigmoid colon is most commonly affected with diverticulosis, the bleeding still more frequently occurs from the right side or ascending colon. Therefore the need to identify the site of the bleeding becomes most important, particularly if surgical intervention is required. Colonoscopic examination may be performed and blood may be seen trickling from the orifices of the diverticula. The difficulty in colonoscopic interpretation, however, lies in cleansing the bowel adequately on a rapid basis, so that the lumen will be visible. Arteriography is of value if the bleeding is brisk enough to allow for extravasation of material at the rate of a 0.5 ml per minute. A barium x-ray is of value only in demonstrating the diverticula and ruling out other conditions but will not allow for visualization of the site of bleeding. A barium enema x-ray is often touted as a therapeutic test if the bleeding stops; however, the bleeding may stop spontaneously without barium.

Other causes of bleeding that may be coincident with diverticulosis and must be differentiated include, as I have already mentioned, carcinoma, ischemic colitis, other forms of acute colitis including ulcerative and granulomatous, and infections as well as hemorrhoids. Upper gastrointestinal bleeding such as from gastritis or duodenal ulceration may present with bleeding brisk enough to cause the stool to change from the black of melena to more reddish or purple color. In evaluating lower gastrointestinal bleeding it is always important to rule out upper gastrointestinal bleeding, either by a negative nasogastric aspiration or, more desirably, upper gastrointestinal endoscopy. Angiodysplasia is another cause of acute lower gastrointestinal bleeding.

Chronic occult bleeding is less commonly associated with diverticulosis. In the face of recurrent positive stool guaiac tests, one must look carefully for the occult carcinoma by x-ray or colonoscopic examination.

In summary, the erosion of small blood vessels into diverticulae may give rise to lower chronic bleeding, which can be relatively mild or more massive bleeding with associated acute blood loss and hypotension. Both types may stop spontaneously.

TUMORS OF THE COLON AND RECTUM

By WILLIAM W. H. RUDD, M.D.
Toronto, Ontario, Canada

INCIDENCE

Colorectal cancer is the most common major cancer diagnosed in both men and women. Its incidence in North America is rising steadily. There were about 100,000 new cases diagnosed last year and only 86,000 new cases 5 years ago. The rate of colorectal cancer has climbed from 39.3 per 100,000 in 1947, to 43 per 100,000 in 1968, and is now at 46 per 100,000.

It is obvious that, with only about a 50 per cent survival rate, half of the colorectal cancers were discovered too late. Even with recent advances in surgery, radiotherapy, and chemotherapy, the survival rate for colon and rectal cancer has changed little in the last 20 years. Our only hope for improving these grim statistics is in finding better techniques and applying them clinically to make the diagnosis earlier and then the treatment more effective.

ETIOLOGY

A great deal of effort, time, and money is currently being spent on research in an effort to find the cause of colorectal cancer. Recent evidence implicates the adverse effects of the affluent American diet, especially overconsumption of beef, fat, and unrefined sugar and lack of fiber. There is some evidence that these factors may influence the concentration of carcinogens within the colon. It is believed that these carcinogens create mucosal cellular dysplasia, then polyps, and finally malignant tumors.

The work of Dr. Basil Morson in London, England has elucidated this transition and made us more aware of the importance of the adenomatous polyp. He has shown quite clearly that a gradual transition usually is made from normal mucosa to mild, moderate, and then severe dysplasia, which then evolves into the adenomatous polyp. If it is left long enough, the polyp will probably advance to an adenocarcinoma. Dr. Morson's point is that we should be much more concerned about benign polyps than we have been in the past. If they were all removed, a dramatic drop would occur in the incidence of adenocarcinoma.

EARLY DIAGNOSIS

A striking example in support of the removal of adenomatous polyps is the clinical study carried out by Dr. Victor A. Gilbertsen at the University of Minnesota Medical Center in Minneapolis. His group now has a 31-year-old study of over 20,000 patients in whom a total of over 120,000 proctosigmoidoscopies were done. In this number of patient years, one would expect to find about 90 cancers of the rectum. Because all polyps were removed, in the ongoing series (after the initial examination), only 13 patients were found to have adenocarcinomas: of these 13, 8 had carcinoma in situ, 4 had extension into the submucosa and only 1, who had refused excision for a period of 2 years, had extension into the muscularis. Most of these patients required only local excision of the tumor through the rectum; two had an abdominal perineal resection which, in retrospect, was probably unnecessary. There have been no deaths in this entire series from rectal cancer. This confirms that early diagnosis and excision of benign polyps will almost eradicate cancer within the reach of the sigmoidoscope.

It behooves the family physician to carry out routine sigmoidoscopies on patients. This fairly simple procedure requires only moderate expertise; my colleagues and I believe strongly that every family physician should become proficient in this important diagnostic procedure. We recommend that sigmoidoscopy be done biannually on asymptomatic patients over 45 years of age, and annually in older patients and in those who are in a high-risk category. There is strong support in the work of both Morson and Gilbertsen for the removal of all polyps. If sigmoidoscopy and polypectomy of benign polyps were carried out universally, the incidence of rectal cancer would drop dramatically.

Another area of promise in the early diagnosis of colorectal cancer has been the mass screening of asymptomatic people for blood in the stool. This is shown best by the study by Dr. Greegor of Columbus, Ohio. The technique is based on the assumption that most colorectal cancers would, if scraped by coarse foods, bleed at least minimally. If one could then use an extremely sensitive test for blood (one part in 5000 detected), a positive result from this mass screening test would indicate those patients in whom more extensive and costly investigation was indicated.

This guaiac test, which costs only about $1.00 per patient, has given promising results in situations in which both doctor and patient are well motivated. Dr. Greegor had tested over 1000 patients and found that approximately 5 per cent tested had positive results for blood. Further investigation revealed that a total of 2 per cent had a neoplasm; half of these lesions were benign polyps and the other half were malignant.

One problem with this test is that it picks up blood from other sources such as consumed meat; we are looking forward to the day when only human blood will be detected. The diet must therefore exclude meat and the patient must brush his teeth lightly in order to avoid a false-positive result. Also, for a few days, the diet must be high in roughage (such as popcorn and nuts) to try to scrape the lesion, so it will bleed. Another problem is that many patients are unwilling to collect their stool sample and still another is that some are afraid to do the test because they fear a positive result. Even in our highly motivated situation, out of 1000 possible patients, we successfully completed the analysis of only 350. Still, this is one of the best, most inexpensive mass screening tests we have. It could help to make an earlier diagnosis of colorectal tumors.

COLON X-RAYS

In a busy referral practice of colon and rectal surgery, one has the opportunity to compare colon x-rays carried out at many different centers. All too often these x-rays must be repeated because of poor preparation. How many early colon lesions are missed because of poor preparation? This time-honored procedure would show more lesions earlier if the bowel preparation would be uniformly improved.

The ideal laxative has yet to be discovered.

On the one hand, we would like to make it as easy as possible for patients to avoid nausea, cramps, and the required fasting about which they complain so bitterly. Yet on the other hand, the colon must be clean for a proper examination. Also, we believe that some flexibility should be built into the laxative routine because these products do affect patients differently.

We have found a liquifying oral product such as sodium biphosphate–sodium phosphate (Phospho-Soda) to be both superior and better tolerated than irritating and cramp-producing products such as castor oil. We ask our patients to go on clear fluids at noon and take Phospho-Soda that evening. If the patients do not have at least six bowel movements, the last one being clear, they are then asked to take Phospho-Soda again on the morning of the x-ray. This gives the extra flexibility we think is important and catches most of those patients in whom the one dose would have been inadequate and the x-ray examination useless.

For inpatients, high colonic washouts in the x-ray department with special tilt tables and collection containers are excellent but expensive: they use up valuable space and time, so that fewer studies can be done. However, this is the routine followed in the Malmo technique and it certainly gives the best pictures; you reap the rewards of your efforts in picking up smaller lesions earlier.

Another inpatient technique that works quite well is the instillation of several liters of electrolyte solution through a Levin tube into the stomach. This results in the very thorough flushing of the entire small and large bowel. The only problem is, of course, that many patients object to the tube and almost none will take the fluid without it.

Several good methods are available for effectively cleansing the colon in preparation for colon x-ray. If it is done well the first time, it will save the cost of a repeated study. Meticulous preparation does result in the diagnosis of earlier lesions. It is worth the extra trouble.

HIGH-RISK PATIENTS

In the absence of the widespread use of a reliable screening test for the detection of early lesions of the colon and rectum, we must concentrate our efforts on identifying and then investigating those patients who are at higher risk. It is vital that we always keep in mind those features that put patients in this group. Their investigation will yield higher returns and be more cost effective.

Many of the symptoms commonly taught,

such as abdominal cramps, change in bowel habits, and loss of appetite and weight, are indicative of fairly advanced colon lesions. In our experience, the one sign in the history that may suggest a neoplasm at an earlier stage is streaking of blood, especially if it is darker red or clotted, on the surface of the stool. This should suggest a neoplasm until proven otherwise by more extensive investigation. Streaking of blood should not be confused with that which results from hemorrhoids or proctitis and which is usually seen in the toilet water or at the end of the bowel movement. Patients with this symptom should be investigated, but those with streaking of blood on the surface of the stool automatically require sigmoidoscopy, air contrast colon x-ray, and even colonoscopy.

There are several other groups of patients who are at higher risk. Any patient with a polyp seen on sigmoidoscopy has a greater chance of having a second polyp proximally in the colon. Dr. Frank Theuerkauf of Erie, Pennsylvania has shown that patients who have one or more polyps seen on sigmoidoscopy have a 50 per cent chance of having a polyp found on colonoscopy when this examination is done carefully, all the way to the cecum. Many of these polyps in his series were missed on colon x-ray examinations, often because of poor bowel preparation. Our experience tends to support his findings. Surely the implications of the study done by Gilbertsen on sigmoidoscopy and removal of all polyps in the rectum would suggest a similar reasoning for polypectomy on colonoscopy. Could the results he had on repeat sigmoidoscopy not be duplicated with colonoscopy?

Patients with a previous colon polyp should similarly be considered in this higher risk group and followed as will be described.

The incidence of metachronous cancer of the colon is indication enough to recommend a careful follow-up on patients who have had surgery for colon cancer in the past.

Studies have shown that patients with a positive family history of colon cancer are at higher risk and should be investigated earlier or even more routinely, since the yield will be much greater in them, too.

Finally, the patient with long-term ulcerative colitis is in a much higher risk situation. This group can now be followed much better with new techniques using colonoscopy.

COLONOSCOPY

The greatest single advance in the early diagnosis and even prevention of cancer of the colon in the past few years may well be colonoscopy. It is true that this procedure is a highly technical one that requires a fair amount of skill not only for the diagnostic procedure but even more for the removal of polyps. The instrument is quite expensive, and the procedure in the past has been done only in larger centers. However, with the realization of its true value, colonoscopy is being used more widely now and also in smaller centers, especially for diagnosis. Complications tend to occur with inexperienced operators but are still quite infrequent. The most severe of these, of course, is perforation, but this can be avoided by sticking to the proper indication for colonoscopy and observing the contraindications (such as acute ulcerative colitis). Of course, technique is important and one must avoid forcible insertion of the scope. The other major complication is bleeding, especially after a polypectomy: this occurs mostly in villous-type tumors because the wire snare will cut through this soft tumor more quickly and not allow adequate coagulation of the base.

Colonoscopy is easier now with the third generation scopes than it was a few years ago; I am sure this method will continue to be used. It still must be done meticulously by a physician who is willing to take the time to do it carefully. This is because lesions can also be missed with the colonoscope, especially in the so-called blind areas. However, this should occur much less frequently than it does in colon x-ray examinations and hence the value of the combined approach, using both colonoscopy and barium enema alternately.

There is no doubt in our practice that many adenocarcinomas, missed by x-ray, have been found early with the colonoscope and cured by surgery. I am sure that this experience has been duplicated many times throughout the world and that in 10 years' time we may note a significant drop in the death rate from colon cancer. It is obvious that not everyone could routinely have a colonoscopy examination even though this would be ideal, as shown by the work of Gilbertsen and Morson. The removal of all polyps would certainly be a giant step forward. However, in this day of high cost of medical care, cost effectiveness must be considered and the difficult problem of selecting which patients should have this examination becomes important.

INDICATIONS FOR COLONOSCOPY

The most common indication for colonoscopy is a suspected polyp seen on the colon x-ray examination. This is an absolute indication for colonoscopy examination, biopsy, and attempted snare excision of the polyp, unless the patient has an extremely broad-based tumor and one is concerned about the possibility of perforation. Removal of the polyps serves two purposes: one, it prevents them from becoming malignant in due course, and two, occasionally one will diagnose a cancer at an early stage of development; this allows surgical excision and cure.

The next commonest indication for colonoscopy is a tumor of the colon suspected from x-ray. Colonoscopy will then make a definite diagnosis in most cases either by a biopsy or brush cytology. False-positive x-ray results from poor preparation involving stool and gas or from segmental spasm of the colon can be ruled out by colonoscopy examination; unnecessary surgery can thus be avoided. Furthermore, when a carcinoma distal to the ascending colon is confirmed at biopsy, colonoscopy should be carried out all the way to the cecum, provided there is no significant stenosis and force is not required to push the scope through the tumor. This is to rule out synchronous cancers that may be detected only on colonoscopy; they may be too small to palpate through the wall of the colon even at the time of laparotomy. Furthermore, their preoperative discovery will prevent a great deal of postoperative embarrassment.

A third indication for colonoscopy is the finding of polyps on sigmoidoscopy as suggested by Dr. Theuerkauf. He has found in his practice that 50 per cent of those patients who had one or more polyps disclosed on sigmoidoscopy had another polyp found proximally on total colonoscopy to the cecum. Findings by my colleagues and me tend to support this statement; we believe that the more adenomatous polyps that are seen on sigmoidoscopy, the greater the likelihood that more will be found on colonoscopy. The findings of Morson also seem to be supported here, in that the more polyps that are found on sigmoidoscopy or colonoscopy, the more likely it is that a carcinoma will also be found. Therefore, whenever a polyp is found, the index of suspicion should immediately be raised. Colonoscopy should probably be recommended in the patient with one polyp found on sigmoidoscopy. It should definitely be done, in my opinion, if the polyp is a villous tumor, if two or more adenomatous polyps are found on sigmoidoscopy, or if one polyp plus other indications, such as rectal bleeding, a history of a previous polyp, and positive family history of polyps or colon cancer, are present.

The fourth indication is the patient with a history of bright or dark red blood streaking on the surface of the stool when no lesion is found on anoscopy, sigmoidoscopy, or x-ray. Diverticula may or may not have been found on enema examination. This indication also applies to patients with any bleeding per rectum without any obvious cause on proctosigmoidoscopy and also in those in whom blood was seen coming from proximal to the sigmoidoscope, with no blood source seen distally.

A fifth indication for colonoscopy is the follow-up of those with previously resected cancers of the colon. We all know that metachronous cancers occur in a much higher frequency than normal and therefore this is a high-risk group of patients requiring repeat studies in the future. We would follow the routine to be described.

Another indication for colonoscopy is the high-risk patient. The group includes those with polyps previously removed by colonoscopy, those whose siblings or parents have a strong history of polyps or a history of colon cancer, and those patients with a previous carcinoma. In these patients, we recommend a sigmoidoscopy every year, a colonoscopy (if it was done well the last time) every 2 to 3 years, with barium enema air contrast colon x-ray halfway in between.

The last common indication for colonoscopy is the follow-up of patients with long-term ulcerative colitis. There are two quite significant advantages in this situation. The first is that colonoscopy will determine much more accurately than radiologic examination how far proximally in the colon the disease extends. The importance of determining this is simply that carcinoma of the colon, in patients with long-term ulcerative colitis, occurs infrequently unless the disease involves the entire colon. The second important advantage is that multiple biopsies can be taken throughout the colon in an effort to predict which patients are more likely to develop an adenocarcinoma in the future. The mucosal biopsies are examined under the microscope for the degree of dysplasia, according to the criteria of Morson. Unfortunately, the interpretation of the slides requires an expert pathologist with a special interest in this field. Nevertheless, this new diagnostic technique is of considerable value when we are faced with the difficult decision as to whether to recommend colectomy in a patient who has few symptoms but who has had the disease for 10 years or more.

If there is no significant dysplasia, we would be much happier to continue watching the patient for another year. However, if severe dysplasia is present, it suggests precancerous changes and a colectomy is indicated. Morson has found that a number of patients with microscopic precancerous changes, when a colectomy was carried out, already had a cancer in the resected specimen. It must also be remembered that cancer is more difficult to discover in patients with inflammatory bowel disease, even with colonoscopy.

ANGIOGRAPHY

Selective angiography of the mesenteric vessels may give a characteristic tumor blush of the venous phase in certain tumors and is of value in the differential diagnosis, especially if the tumor is intramural or vascular.

NEW EXPERIMENTAL METHODS OF DETECTING EARLY COLON CANCER

A great deal of research is being channeled into the search for better means of making an earlier diagnosis of colon cancer. A few will be mentioned.

The most widely known at the moment is the carcinoembryonic antigen (CEA) detected by Gold in 1965. This antigen was detected in saline extracts of an adenocarcinoma and other entodermally derived tumors. It was first thought to be quite specific, but the result could not be duplicated as successfully by others. This test is not as reliable for making the original diagnosis as was originally hoped. However, studies have shown that if the CEA level was below 2.5 nanograms per ml preoperatively, the prognosis was much better in that there was only a 5 per cent recurrence rate at 2 years. This compares with those patients with a CEA level of greater than 7 nanograms per ml, who had a 75 per cent recurrence rate in 2 years. It has also been shown that, if the CEA is done at regular intervals postoperatively, and there is a sudden elevation, one can be pretty sure there is recurrent tumor, even though clinical evidence usually takes another 6 months to become apparent. Unfortunately, the test is fairly expensive and the results may vary.

A newer test is claimed by Dr. Frank DeLand to have an accuracy of 90 per cent in CEA-producing tumors. He has used a purified[131]I radiolabeled antibody to the specific antigen (CEA) and then identified the neoplasm in more than 200 patients by external scintillation imaging at 48 hours. This technique shows not only primary but secondary tumors and probably shows them at an earlier stage in their development.

A computerized tube leukocyte adherence inhibition test (LAI) is also suggested to be more accurate than the serum CEA analysis, especially in earlier lesions. The test depends upon the observation that leukocytes from cancer patients, when incubated with extracts of cancer of the same organ, lose their property of adherence to a glass surface. Few false-positive tests were encountered, which was encouraging. However, further refinement of this test is required.

In these tests, the aim has been to diagnose a tumor already present. Dr. W. R. Bruce of Toronto, Canada, and others have developed a means of determining carcinogens in the stool. They think that if one could do this on a mass scale, those patients with a high positive result might be prevented from developing a neoplasm by medication or alteration of their diet or both. This, of course, would be the ultimate diagnosis: one made even before the development of a cancer. Prevention would then come into its own.

DIFFERENTIAL DIAGNOSIS

Although this discussion has covered mainly polyps and adenocarcinoma of the colon and rectum, the same techniques apply to the diagnosis of other lesions of the colon. History, physical, anal digital examination, anoscopy, and sigmoidoscopy as well as barium enema and colonoscopy all have their place. One must exclude such conditions as diverticular disease and associated complications in the differential diagnosis. Juvenile and metaplastic polyps are of no consequence and need not be considered. In a differential diagnosis, there are a number of tumors that occur quite infrequently and arise deep to the mucosa, and in the wall of the colon. Some of these include lipoma, leiomyoma, sarcoma, malignant lymphoma, hemangioma, and carcinoid tumor. In most cases, these do not penetrate through the mucosa and cannot be seen by colonoscopy. However, on radiologic examination, the typical malignant "overhanging shoulders" picture is not present and instead, the appearance is one of a space-occupying lesion. For the most part, bleeding is rare in these mural-type tumors. Carcinoids usually involve the submucosa and may be evident only if they are malignant, in which case such systemic symptoms as intermittent hypertension, palpitations, and flushing may be present. The laboratory finding of increased amounts of 5-hydroxyindoleacetic acid in the urine is diagnostic. Malignant melanoma is more commonly mucosal or submucosal and occasionally polypoid. Its texture is much firmer than that of an adenoma.

ANORECTAL AND PERIANAL DISORDERS

By CLYDE E. CULP, M.D.
Rochester, Minnesota

Most patients with an anorectal or a perianal problem consider the lesion to be "hemorrhoids." During the period from self-diagnosis to seeking of professional advice, considerable suffering and possible damage to the related anatomic structures may occur.

TERMINOLOGY

The nomenclature given to the anorectal region by various authors is cause for confusion. In this article, the anorectum and the surgical anal canal will be considered to be synonymous. This structure, which includes about 2 cm of the rectum, extends distally from the readily palpable puborectalis portion of the levator ani muscle (anorectal ring) to the anal verge (anal margin).

The anatomic anal canal is about 3 cm long and extends distally from the dentate line or margin (pectinate line, anorectal line) to the anal verge. In the remainder of this discussion, the term *anal canal* will refer to the anatomic anal canal. The proximal one third of the canal has been called the *pecten*. This region is of great proctologic importance because it represents a zone of transition. Its integument is a modified squamous epithelium, which becomes transitional and finally changes into rectal mucosa proximally from the dentate line. For this covering of the pecten, Gorsch suggested the term *anoderm*. The pecten contains an anastomotic zone between the internal and the skin-covered external hemorrhoids. The lymphatic drainage of the region divides into a proximal and a distal component. The nerve supply changes from that of somatic response to that of the visceral system above the dentate line. The cryptoglandular apparatus, which extends into the pecten below the dentate margin, may be the site of an infective process involving an anal crypt and gland, thus leading to the development of a fistulous abscess.

PATIENT HISTORY

An adequate patient history is necessary and will provide the diagnostic insight for successful management.

The discomfort experienced by the patient may range from pain to "an irritated feeling." The relationship of this discomfort to defecation and its duration (intermittent or constant) and type (throbbing or sharp jabbing) are important. When does the pain appear? Does it awaken the patient? Can sleep be attained in the presence of the discomfort? Is medication necessary to control the problem? If so, what drugs are used? Have the patient place the finger on the site in question in order that each of you is evaluating the identical site. Pruritus is frequently interpreted as pain and must be defined.

Previous anorectal, gastrointestinal, or pelvic operations, as well as other types of treatment to the region, should be recorded.

Discomfort is often endured, but when blood is noted by the patient, an immediate consultation is requested. What is causing the bleeding? Is it related to defecation? The consistency of the stool at the time of the bleeding is helpful to know. Is blood present only when undue straining is necessary? What is the color of the blood? Are clots present? Is the discomfort associated with the bleeding? The appearance of pink or slightly blood-tinged mucus is suggestive of neoplasia. Bleeding may need to be confirmed by having the patient strain while seated on the toilet.

The type and frequency of the stool is helpful information. What is the patient's interpretation of the term "diarrhea" or "constipation"? Is a large or small stool passed when diarrhea is present? Is blood present, and if so, is it mixed with or on the surface of the fecal mass? Do the feces appear to be "greasy" or float on the surface of the water? In persistent diarrhea, one should ascertain if the patient needs to defecate during the night. If so, how many times? One should learn if abdominal cramping is present and if defecation relieves the cramping.

RECORD OF PERTINENT FINDINGS

Frequently, the location of a lesion is documented by reference to a clock face. In order to provide accurate records, the position of the patient at the time of that particular examination also must be designated. A more precise method refers to anatomic quadrants. Whereas 6 o'clock becomes 12 o'clock as the patient is shifted from the lithotomy to the prone position, reference to a lesion located in the right anterior quadrant will never change the site.

The anal verge (margin) serves as an excellent reference point for perianal lesions, for example, a draining sinus, left posterior, 3 cm from the anal verge.

In recording the level of a rectal or an anal canal lesion, either the dentate line or anal verge can be used as a reference. If the dentate line is used, the 3 cm length of the average anal canal is subtracted from the level noted on the proctosigmoidoscope.

PHYSICAL EXAMINATION

Adequate illumination and exposure of the perianal region and anal canal can be best obtained with the patient in the knee-chest position. A hydraulic tilt table is an asset but not a necessity for examination.

Inspection. A patient with an anorectal complaint is often apprehensive not only because of the problem but also because of the various stories that have been circulated regarding the "procto" examination. The "undignified" position and inability to see the examiner add to the situation.

During assessment of the anal region, "vocal anesthesia" is begun by the practitioner to allay the patient's fears by alerting the patient to each maneuver and to anticipate any cause for discomfort. Maintaining a constant "play-by-play" conversation diverts the patient's personal preoccupation and increases the attention to the instructions of the examiner.

The anogenital integument is evaluated for skin abnormalities. The thickened, whitish skin resulting from pruritus should be differentiated from Paget's disease or the whitish patches of thin, wrinkled skin of lichen sclerosus et atrophicus. Crohn's disease affecting the perianal skin may cause a dusky or cyanotic discoloration and an intense pruritus. The acutely inflamed skin of a yeast infection should be differentiated from that due to excessive sweating. Psoriasis may be present, as may other common skin disorders. Basal and squamous cell carcinomas are not infrequent. Rarely, a malignant melanoma will be seen, and its presence should be considered when an unusual "thrombotic" external hemorrhoid is seen. Condyloma acuminatum (venereal wart), either discrete or conglomerate, is seen as macerated whitish excrescences involving the perianal area, anal canal, and frequently the rectal mucosa. These warty lesions are readily distinguished from the moist flat areas of luetic condyloma latum.

A draining sinus is suggestive of a fistula-in-ano, but hidradenitis suppurativa should be differentiated, as should Crohn's disease and actinomycosis. Although anal tags of skin may result from an untreated para-anal hematoma (thrombotic hemorrhoid) or a surgical procedure, the presence of an anal ulcer (fissure-in-ano, fissure ulcer) or anal Crohn's disease should be considered.

The anal skin folds are gently separated to expose the anal canal. Discomfort produced by this maneuver is suggestive of an anal ulcer, which is usually located on the posterior wall. Again, the indolent ulcer of Crohn's disease must be distinguished from a fissure ulcer. A skin depression or sinus located in the postanal region, particularly if the protruding hair is attached, indicates a developmental cyst in the precoccygeal or presacral space. At this time, the activity of the voluntary sphincter can be assessed for the degree and force of the anal closure. Finally, the intergluteal cleft is inspected for pilonidal dimple(s) or sinuses, hidradenitis suppurativa, or the "pinking" of psoriasis.

Digital Examination. A carefully conducted, gentle digital examination is frequently more rewarding than is endoscopic visualization of the anal canal. The examiner should develop a routine by which the same structures are felt by the same manner of digital insertion and extraction at each examination. Such familiarity allows even tiny abnormalities to be appreciated by the finger pad.

Standing on the patient's left, the examiner slowly inserts a well-lubricated, finger-cotted left first digit into the anal canal. In this manner, the "blind area" posteriorly and above the anorectal ring can be evaluated with the pad of the finger. Vocal anesthesia stresses the importance of sphincter relaxation. Because the sphincter muscles fatigue easily, the digit should be inserted by maintaining a steady pressure for a short time. Often stroking the anal margins several times causes muscular relaxation and allows penetration of the digit. Finally, the taking of a deep breath by the patient often allows the finger to be fully inserted.

As the finger enters the anal canal, an annular depression is often noted. As the name implies, the intersphincter groove represents the boundary between the lower border of the internal sphincter and the external voluntary sphincter muscle. The pecten and the narrowest portion of the canal are encountered next as the finger is advanced proximally. One must distinguish the resistance of a pathologic narrowing (contracture) from that provided by the patient voluntarily. Again, a deep breath by the examinee generally allows the necessary relaxation, if an abnormality is not present. The contracture may be related to a previous surgical procedure, chronic laxative use, or inflammatory bowel disease.

When a painful lesion is present in the anal canal, the use of topical anesthetic agents has been suggested; however, I am not impressed with the efficacy of such preparations. In the cooperative patient, digital examination can be done utilizing the fifth digit if necessary; this gently distends the anal canal opposite the site of the lesion. The digital pressure on the muscular structures is away from the lesion, and the edges of the ulcer undergo little or no separation, thus preventing abrasion of the ulcer base. The examinee should be informed not to contract the sphincter while the examiner's finger is slowly being withdrawn, because muscle spasm may be provoked.

With penetration of the digit, the consistency of the canal tissues is acknowledged, as well as any other abnormalities of the walls. A depressed or scarred area at the level of the dentate line or the pecten is suggestive of the primary source of a fistula. Enlarged anal papillae are encountered, but their location and visualization of a whitish skin-covered projection exclude the possibility of an adenomatous polyp.

As the finger moves into the rectal ampulla, the prostate and often the seminal vesicles are identified anteriorly, as is the internal genitalia in the female. The rectal mucosa is assessed, and any departure from its usual smooth nature suggests the possibility of inflammatory bowel disease, polyp formation, or primary malignancy.

The lateral walls and adjacent tissues are evaluated, as is the cul-de-sac. The latter extrarectal region may have tender irregularities due to endometriosis. Tenderness with an induration or a mass is usually related to an inflammatory response — diverticulitis in particular. Metastatic seeding or a mass may be present. Fixation provided by a mass constitutes a rectal shelf (Blumer). An extrinsic mass can be differentiated from a mass arising within the rectal lumen by determining the mobility of the rectal wall and mucosa. When invasion of the rectal wall by an extrinsic process occurs, the examiner's finger usually can delineate whether the mucosal infiltration is of intrinsic origin.

Radiation therapy may have caused an intense fibrotic response with fixation of the rectal wall or extrarectal tissues (or both), making the differentiation of recurrent neoplasia difficult.

Bidigital manipulation of the sphincter musculature often will identify a deeply situated process and usually an early abscess formation. Rectovaginal examination may be used to locate a fistulous communication betweeen these organs. Added information regarding a cul-de-sac mass or an inflammatory process involving the rectovaginal septum or sphincter musculature is obtained from the bimanual examination.

The finger covering should be examined for evidence of gross bleeding or purulent material.

The perianal area should be scrutinized for evidence of purulent material caused by the milking action of the withdrawal of the finger.

Proctosigmoidoscopy. Direct visualization of the rectum and adjacent sigmoid should always precede the barium study of the large intestine. Because of the confines of the bony pelvis and the overlying loops of bowel, one cannot depend on the radiologic survey to rule out disease in the rectum or the rectosigmoid.

The terminal portion of the bowel is prepared for endoscopy by means of prepared disposable or warm tapwater enemas, which should be taken 30 to 60 minutes before the examination.

Again, vocal anesthesia is important in completing a successful examination. The patient is informed that the instrument will pass into the rectum without difficulty because it is of a smaller diameter than the examiner's index finger. Mouth breathing at the examinee's usual rate abets sphincter relaxation. As the instrument passes into the rectum, its obturator is withdrawn, and the remainder of the examination is carried out under direct vision of the lumen.

Approximately 12 cm from the anal verge, the rectosigmoidal angulation, which appears to lead into a blind loop, is encountered. A feeling of discomfort or impending defecation is experienced by the examinee. The examiner should anticipate these sensations and warn the patient of this possibility. "Sagging" of the patient's back is helpful, as well as relaxation of the abdominal muscles, in preventing straining and allows the passage of the sigmoidoscope through the rectosigmoidal segment into the sigmoid.

Solving the blind-loop problem requires experience. A helpful maneuver is to withdraw the endoscope a short distance until a mucosal fold comes into view. When this occurs, the end of the sigmoidoscope is manipulated in the same direction, and the lumen soon becomes visible.

The sigmoidoscope cannot be inserted to 25 cm in every patient. Persistent attempts to accomplish this cause undue discomfort and probable alienation of the patient for future examination. Perforation of the intestinal wall is always a possibility, and forceful attempts to gain an additional few centimeters of visualization make this possibility a probability.

Insufflation of air adds to the patient's discomfort and seldom provides visualization of the lumen ahead. Buie often said, "*Talk* the scope into the patient's sigmoid but *blow* it out." A small amount of air from the bulb, plus that gained by equalization of atmospheric pressure on withdrawal of the obturator, separates the mucosal folds of the lumen for optimal visualization. The instrument is withdrawn distally in a rotatory manner, and the folds are flattened so that each surface can be assessed.

Coloration of the rectal mucosa is a variable and an undependable finding. The type of enema taken may cause changes in color. Mucus production, unless the mucus is pink or blood-tinged, has little meaning. Mucosa that can be made to bleed from the minimal trauma of a cotton-tipped applicator has significance. Obliteration of the underlying vascular network is suggestive of mucosal edema and an abnormal state.

The pattern of ulcerative colitis of the mucosal type is one of generalized mucosal granularity in which various degrees of bleeding (pink sandpaper) are seen. A mucopurulent exudate may be present, as well as denudation of areas of mucosa, which may be associated with inflammatory polyps or "pseudopolyps." Crohn's disease is seen as a discontinuous process in the small bowel. Similar findings are seen in the terminal portion of the bowel and are characterized by shallow ulcers that have irregular, undermined edges, with normal mucosa between. Longitudinally directed (bear claw or rake) ulcers may be seen, but as in the other example the intervening mucosa is free of disease. Some antibiotics cause a persistent diarrhea. Endoscopic visualization may reveal dirty white to tannish areas on the mucosa which may coalesce in varying degrees. Attempts to sweep away these areas result in some bleeding from the underlying mucosa. Such findings are consistent with pseudomembranous colitis.

Mucosal elevations or projections may be of submucosal origin. These "polyps" are usually due to lymphoid hyperplasia; their multiplicity might cause confusion with multiple polyposis. The relative uniformity in size and submucosal origin should differentiate them from adenomatous polyps. Biopsy study will provide the final diagnosis.

Mammillations, excrescences, or polyps less than 0.5 cm may be destroyed when they are found, unless extenuating circumstances exist. Studies have demonstrated that, with polyps of this size, the incidence of malignancy is nil. Attempts to remove a specimen of tissue from these small growths may be an exercise in futility, and the attendant bleeding may necessitate fulguration of a large area for control. When first visualized, small lesions should be destroyed by means of a suitable electrocautery unit. Referral of a patient for treatment of a small polyp may result in a fruitless search by the examiner because the "polyp" may have been of lymphoid origin or metaplastic and may

have regressed spontaneously during the time interval between visits to the physician.

The soft "carpeting" effect often noted adjacent to the main mass of a low rectal villous adenoma is frequently overlooked on digital examination. Samples from firm or ulcerated areas noted in the main tumor mass should be submitted for biopsy study, as well as specimens from the softer adjacent tissue. If there is no evidence of invasive malignancy, the entire growth can be excised transanally and submitted for complete histopathologic analysis.

The level and the quadrant affected by any of the previously mentioned lesions should be documented. In the assessment of a malignant lesion, the degree of involvement of the bowel circumference is necessary. Barium study of the colon should not be attempted if an annular lesion is visualized. Likewise, a lesion that prevents visualization of the lumen proximal to the lesion should not be evaluated by a contrast radiograph. The unevacuated barium may obstruct the bowel at the strictured site. Fixation of the bowel by the malignancy is assessed, because this finding is an indication of the extension of the process.

After the gross characteristics of a probable malignant tumor are evaluated, biopsy specimens are removed for study. Tissue is removed from both the edge and the center or areas of ulceration. Although bleeding occurs, it is usually minor, especially if a blunt-cupped type of instrument has been used and if the sample is twisted free from the lesion. Biopsy forceps with long, narrow "alligator jaws" may penetrate too deeply, gathering some of the muscularis propria in its grasp, and thus lead to excessive bleeding when the specimen is withdrawn. This is particularly true if small lesions, ulcers, or the mucosa is to be sampled.

RADIOGRAPHY

Barium study of the colon using fluoroscopy with an image-intensifier, as well as the use of "spot" films, is an important adjunct to the usual preevacuation and postevacuation films in search of colonic lesions. Air contrast studies are useful in locating small polyps and for ascertaining whether a pedicle is present in polypoid growths.

Occasionally, the proctosigmoidoscopic examination and barium studies fail to demonstrate the source of the continued bleeding. A narrowed segment of sigmoid associated with diverticular disease is cause for concern when the results of radiographic studies are equivocal. In both instances, the use of the flexible colonoscope may solve the problem.

LABORATORY EXAMINATION

The examination of the stool for parasites and ova depends on the patient population. However, because of worldwide travel of our populations, stool examination and culture have become routine study. If properly conducted, a search for occult blood is a worthwhile routine procedure and may have as its reward the discovery of the so-called "silent" carcinoma of the colon.

ANAL ABRASION

The integument of the anal canal is frequently split or torn by the passage of a large, hard fecal mass. Explosive or frequent loose stools may have a similar effect. Scarring of the anal canal decreases the elasticity of the tissues, thus making the structure susceptible to trauma from the stool. Occasionally, sharp-edged undigestible material (for example, bone, grain husks) may disrupt the epithelial continuity of the anal canal.

These insults to the anal canal result in an abrasion that usually heals spontaneously within a few days. The pain is a sharp, stinging sensation that usually occurs as the fecal mass begins to pass through the anal canal. The pain does not persist for any appreciable time, although a sense of discomfort may be present for several days. Bleeding is present and may be sufficient to color the water of the toilet bowl, particularly if a small external hemorrhoid varix has been lacerated.

If the patient is examined within 48 hours, a shallow, linear defect is noted in the anal skin. The edges are often irregular or jagged and may contain clotted blood. Frequently, the defect is located anteriorly in the female, but when in either quadrant, the defect is generally just off the midline. Frequently, healing has taken place but stretching the skin demonstrates its inherent fragility, with the appearance of one or more superficial linear defects on its surface. This condition often explains the complaint of repeated "fissure" formation and "the acute fissures" that heal spontaneously or with medical treatment. Establishment of an improved bowel pattern usually eliminates the problem.

ANAL ULCER (FISSURE-IN-ANO, FISSURE ULCER)

An anal ulcer probably results from anal abrasion that cannot heal spontaneously because of the inflammation. Most of these ulcers are located posteriorly in or adjacent to the midline. The predominance of the posterior location may be related to anatomic factors that predispose the region to trauma during the passage of feces.

The margins of the defect become indurated and elevated, thus preventing spontaneous healing. The attendant lymphatic stasis causes an elevated tab of skin to develop at the distal extremity of the ulcer and an enlarged (hypertrophic) anal papilla at the dentate margin. Such findings are classed as the "fissure triad": sentinel skin tag, ulcer, and enlarged anal papilla.

Adjustments of the bowel habit may allow the ulcer to heal, only to recur later during an abnormal and injurious fecal passage. Explosive loose stool can be as traumatic as the hard, large stool mass. The scarring produced by the chronicity of the defect causes additional fixation and narrowing of the anal canal, thus increasing the susceptibility to trauma.

Extreme pain associated with defecation is the main complaint. The discomfort begins as the anal canal becomes dilated by the fecal mass and continues with gradual abatement during the ensuing few hours. Bleeding is usually limited to a few drops or none at all. An intense, intermittent pruritus, which cannot be treated in the usual manner because of the painful area, may appear.

Constipation may be present because of the postponement of defecation by a fearful and apprehensive patient. Some patients find it necessary to have additional formed stools each day. Normally, the internal sphincter relaxes at defecation. When an ulcer exists, the base is split by the dilating effect of the passage of the fecal mass, exposing muscle fibers in the ulcer base and causing spasm of the internal sphincter. A voluntary component is added by the patient who attempts to maintain a small anal caliber and who completes defecation in the shortest time possible. The voluntary activity impedes complete evacuation of the rectum because of the ultimate closure of the anal canal by the activated external sphincter muscle.

If frequent loose stools are associated with an anal ulcer, inflammatory bowel disease (ulcerative colitis, Crohn's disease) should be ruled out.

Disturbances of urinary bladder function are seen and may be the main complaint of a stoic patient. It is difficult to appreciate the excruciating discomfort that can be caused by a relatively small ulcer in the anal canal.

Squamous cell carcinoma, extramammary Paget's disease, and metastatic spread from a rectal cancer give symptoms similar to those of an anal ulcer.

CROHN'S DISEASE

Ulceration of the anal canal may be the first evidence of Crohn's disease. Ulcers are present in about 25 per cent of patients with small bowel involvement and in almost 80 per cent when the colon or rectum (or both) is affected.

Whereas the midline area of the anal canal is involved by the ulcer of fissure-in-ano, the lateral quadrants are often the site of the ulcerations of Crohn's disease. These indolent ulcers may be multiple, affecting several quadrants at one time. Satellite ulcers may be located in the perianal skin. The skin tags associated with the ulcer are often very large. The perianal skin has a dusky discoloration and a peculiar, almost wooden induration. It is not difficult to postulate that the anal alterations are related to the obstruction of the lymphatic channels, as is found in Crohn's disease of the small intestine. Dilated lymphatic vessels of the skin are often found on histopathologic study. Lymph stasis is not conducive to normal healing. An anal abrasion caused by the trauma of an increased number of stools could display delayed healing under these circumstances. The hyperplastic skin tag, skin discoloration, and skin induration also could be explained on the basis of the reduction of lymphatic drainage.

Occasionally, a small postoperative mucosal ectropion is suggestive of an anal ulcer. The appearance of the surgically misplaced rectal mucosa suggests the presence of granulation tissue.

Children are likely to develop anal "fissures," most being abrasions. Many children pass a stool of tremendous size without particular or prolonged difficulty. Response to an increase of dietary bulk or proprietary bulk preparations, as in adults, is gratifying. Adequate intake of fluid, particularly water, is a necessity. Fluid intake can be assured if the patient drinks a full glass of water each time that the urinary bladder is emptied. This combination produces a softer stool mass to sustain the anal caliber by its dilating effect.

When a fissure ulcer is associated with narrowing due to scarring or when frequent abrasions are associated with a prominent (spastic) internal sphincter muscle, surgical management may be recommended if conservative measures fail. Wide surgical excision of the fissure, with release of the scarring to provide adequate anal caliber and a resulting thin, flat, pliable scar, is indicated. Internal sphincterotomy done in the lateral quadrant usually provides relief for the recurrent deep abrasions without appreciable anal narrowing. In either instance, consumption of adequate bulk and fluids should be advised to maintain the new anal caliber by the dilating effect of the softer, malleable stool mass.

THE FISTULOUS ABSCESS

The anorectal abscess and fistula-in-ano cannot be discussed as separate entities because one is the continuance of the other. A fistula is the persistence (chronic) of a contracted cavity of an acute anorectal abscess. Eisenhammer has used the cognomen "fistulous abscess" to identify this chain of events.

The nidus of infection involves the cryptoglandular apparatus associated with the dentate line. "Cryptitis" is an evanescent event, and its chronic state is unlikely. The pyogenic process develops in an anal intramuscular gland, which in turn may perforate the internal sphincter muscle, or the gland may actually occupy the space between the circular (internal sphincter) and the longitudinal muscle of the anorectum — the intermuscular space. Some studies have demonstrated extension of the gland through the longitudinal muscle, which may explain the cause of some "complicated" abscesses.

Most anorectal fistulous abscesses extend distally from the intermuscular space and into the perianal tissues. The intersphincter groove may be obliterated by the bulk of developing abscess. The disposition of the fascial planes, the musculo-fibro-elastic extensions, and the lymphatic distribution contribute to the depth and degree of involvement of the subcutaneous tissues by the abscess. The primary opening of the fistulous abscess is the point of its origin and is usually found at the dentate margin. The secondary opening is in the perianal skin, being the site of spontaneous rupture or the result of a surgical drainage wound.

Pain associated with an anorectal abscess is constant, throbbing, and intensified with defecation. Digital examination demonstrates filling of the intersphincteric groove and tender induration of the area around the point of origin. Visualization by endoscopy may reveal little but a suggestive swelling or possibly a drop of purulent material at the dentate line. Bidigital examination is helpful in localizing an early purulent collection. More frequently, the patient is seen after localization and fluctuation of the abscess have occurred.

Although the main consideration in this discussion is diagnosis, a few words regarding office management of an anorectal abscess are in order. Antibiotic therapy at any stage in the development of an anorectal abscess is unwise. The patient may have to be protected from complications because of other body impairments, but antibiotics should not be used as the primary agent for treatment of the abscess. An abscess in this location should be considered as an emergency and prompt surgical drainage instituted. If mild constitutional symptoms are present and the process is localized, drainage can be done as an office procedure with local infiltration anesthesia. The incision should be placed as near the anal margin as possible to reduce the length of the fistulous tract. An incision of the cruciate or criss-cross type is utilized. When the "ears" of the wound are trimmed away, adequate drainage is maintained, and this makes packing of the wound or the use of drains unnecessary. The wound should allow the fingertip to be introduced to gently explore the cavity and to break up any loculations that might be present. In a series of patients, about 33 per cent of perianal abscesses did not result in fistula formation. When a large or deeply placed process is present and particularly if constitutional symptoms appear, hospitalization is necessary. The abscess thus can be evaluated under regional anesthesia and drainage established.

Often the patient seeks advice because of continued discharge or "a hemorrhoidal condition." Examination demonstrates a draining perianal sinus whose history as an abscess may be difficult to obtain. Most of these patients have a fistulous abscess, as defined by a palpable cord of tissue extending from a secondary opening to the primary opening at the level of the dentate line.

Two fistulous conditions should be detailed because the commonly applied surgical treatment plan may lead to disastrous results. Admittedly, the final proof of the cause of the fistula may require examination with muscular relaxation provided by regional anesthesia.

Hidradenitis suppurativa may involve the apocrine glands in the integument of the distal two thirds of the anal canal. The skin of the proximal one third of the canal usually lacks hair with its appendages. Characteristic scarring is usually present and varies from small pits to flattened depressed areas, often with overhanging edges or skin bridges between adjacent areas of scarring. Although epithelialization is suggestive of a quiescent appearance, palpation proximally from the draining sinus may cause watery purulent material to appear within scarred areas. Gentle passage of a malleable probe (ethmoid) often defines the communication and demonstrates that its course in the tissues is above the internal sphincter muscle. Frequently, the draining sinus is located relatively far from the anal verge (scrotal base, distal perineum, buttock) and is suggestive of a complicated fistula-in-ano. Further evaluation demonstrates the superficial involvement of extension along the dermal tissue plane, permitting surgical exteriorization without sphincter damage. The perineal region also may contain characteristic scarring that may communicate with the sinus tract in question. Additional diagnostic aids are gained from a history of chronicity, axillary involvement, "blind boils," and recurrence with extension after a simple drainage procedure.

Involvement of the terminal portion of the bowel by Crohn's disease may result in extensive fistulization of the anorectum. These fistulas should be distinguished from the common fistulous abscess originating in the cryptoglandular structures. Fistulotomy will compound the problems by adding a large indolent wound and will compromise an already precarious continence. The primary opening is in a mucosal ulcer of the rectum, usually near but proximal to the dentate line. The extension does not follow the usual pattern of fascial planes but often progresses through the rectal wall and associated muscular elements on a relatively deep plane.

The tendency for fistulization is probably on the same basis as that noted in the enteritis of Crohn's disease. The "fissuring" of an ulcerated area is a pathologic characteristic of the disease. The defect involves all layers of the intestinal wall, allowing subsequent fistulization into an adjacent loop of bowel or to the skin surface. A similar process undoubtedly occurs from an ulcer of the rectum and would explain the extensive and deep fistulization as well as the presence of several primary sites that are independent of one another. Multiple secondary openings are common, with evidence that some have traversed the midline of the perianal region. A rectovaginal fistula is not rare in the female patient. The cyanotic discoloration of the adjacent perianal skin, associated bowel habit changes, and visualization of the shallow, irregular, or longitudinal ulcers of the mucosa will properly identify this condition.

Utilizing the internal sphincter for the point of reference, several general statements may be made regarding fistulas. First, the fistulous abscess, which has its origin in an anal crypt and associated gland, occurs most frequently. The abscess occupies the space (intermuscular) between the internal sphincter and the longitudinal fibroelastic muscular elements that constitute the rectal wall. The tract of the fistula lies below the internal sphincter muscle. Second, hidradenitis suppurativa begins in an apocrine gland, and the process extends intradermally to rupture on the skin surface. The tract lies above the internal sphincter muscle. Third, fistulas associated with Crohn's disease have their origin in an ulcer (or ulcers) of the rectal mucosa, which often perforates the entire rectal wall. The tract not only is below the internal sphincter muscle but also is often deep (extrarectal) as well.

HEMORRHOIDAL DISEASE

Varicosities and dilatation of the internal hemorrhoidal plexus of veins account for the primary symptoms of bleeding and protrusion (prolapse) of hemorrhoids. Usually, there is an associated enlargement of the external hemorrhoidal group of veins as well, but bleeding seldom occurs from these skin-covered veins. The dentate margin demarcates one plexus from the other.

The submucosal fibromuscular attachments become progressively attenuated and weakened, allowing prolapse of the venous complexes and the overlying mucosa distally into the anal canal. Early in the course of the condition, protrusion or bleeding (or both) is noted only during the straining of defecation. Spontaneous reduction of the prolapsus follows passage of the feces. As the integrity of the fibromuscular tissue becomes further compromised, prolapse may occur when only slight intra-abdominal pressure is exerted, for example, during bending over to pick up an object from the floor.

With this ease of protrusion, a small area may "pop out," even while sitting, and the trauma of the underclothing causes bleeding, which at times may be sufficient to soak through the outer garments. Examination may demonstrate pink skin-colored areas replacing the mucosa proximal to the dentate line. Microscopic examination confirms the squamous metaplasia, which is probably a protective mechanism.

The bright red blood begins as a slight stain on the toilet tissue. As the condition worsens, bleeding may color the water of the toilet bowl and in some patients may actually "squirt out" with defecation.

By having the patient strain on the stool for several minutes, then inspecting the anal area with the patient in a half-erect position, the bleeding or prolapse (or both) can be verified. The patient's description of "prolapsing piles" may be a filling of the external plexus. "Rectal prolapse" usually is an extreme degree of hemorrhoidal protrusion. The protruded tissue is composed of segments, whereas a prolapsed rectum has concentric rings of mucosa on its surface and the lumen is displaced posteriorly. A patulous anus or one with very little tone is suggestive of a complete rectal prolapse.

Pain is not a primary symptom of hemorrhoidal disease. However, a thrombosis or a hematoma of the external hemorrhoidal veins is discomforting and incapacitating, depending on the extent of involvement.

When pruritus, low-back pain, and rectal "pains" are a patient's main problem, whether or not they are associated with the primary symptoms of hemorrhoidal disease, surgical treatment will only ameliorate the bleeding or protrusion.

PERITONITIS AND INTRA-ABDOMINAL INFECTION*

By CLEON W. GOODWIN, JR., M.D.,
WILLIAM F. McMANUS, M.D.,
and BASIL A. PRUITT, JR., M.D.
Fort Sam Houston, Texas

The peritoneal cavity is a freely communicating space covered with a serous lining of mesothelial cells. These cells cover a large surface and display remarkable physiologic and regenerative properties after injury and inflammation. Clinically, the response to irritation presents as peritonitis, which may be localized, especially in the adult, and present with discrete symptoms and minimal physiologic derangements, or it may be generalized with nonspecific clinical signs of massive fluid loss and overwhelming infection. Untreated peritonitis may result in abscess formation and death.

PRIMARY PERITONITIS

Primary peritonitis is rare and is not generally caused by an operatively correctable lesion. The signs and symptoms are indistinguishable from those caused by diseases requiring operative intervention, and patients with primary peritonitis may be first diagnosed at the time of celiotomy. In spite of a typical inflammatory response and identification of bacterial organisms, no visceral disease is present. Primary

*The opinions or assertions contained herein are the private views of the authors and are not to be construed as official or as reflecting the views of the Department of the Army or the Department of Defense.

peritonitis is not a specific entity with a common cause but is rather a group of diseases. Young children are most commonly involved and frequently have associated chronic diseases, especially postnecrotic cirrhosis and the nephrotic syndrome. Before 1950, gram-positive bacteria were almost exclusively isolated from infected peritoneal fluid. Pneumococcal peritonitis occurs most frequently and often follows pneumococcal pneumonia or otitis media. Peritonitis caused by streptococcal infection occasionally follows erysipelas, and that caused by staphylococci is usually preceded by an extra-abdominal abscess. Primary tuberculous peritonitis without an adjacent focus of disease is exceedingly rare.

Since 1950, the incidence of primary peritonitis caused by gram-negative bacteria has increased. This has paralleled increasing availability and use of antibiotics, which have eradicated chronic infections of the upper respiratory and urinary tracts and pulmonary infections. Although a prior extra-abdominal infection may precede primary peritonitis, spread by hematogenous, lymphatic, and female genital tract routes has not been documented.

The usual clinical presentation of patients with primary peritonitis may be indistinguishable from that of secondary peritonitis. Additional information suggesting primary peritonitis includes young age and a history of nephrosis or postnecrotic cirrhosis, especially if ascites is present. Given these particular circumstances, it is acceptable to proceed with abdominal paracentesis, followed by immediate Gram stain of the peritoneal aspirate. If gram-positive organisms are present, the patient should be treated with appropriate antibiotics. If gram-negative organisms are identified, secondary contamination from an intra-abdominal source is more likely than de novo infection, and celiotomy should be performed promptly. If no acute visceral disease is found after careful inspection of the abdominal contents, the peritoneal exudate should be evaluated by Gram stain and culture. The appendix should be removed, the incision closed without drains, and appropriate antibiotics begun in adequate doses. Following recovery, children should have evaluation of renal and immunologic function.

SECONDARY PERITONITIS

Secondary peritonitis is more common than primary peritonitis and should be the prime consideration in a patient with signs of intra-abdominal infection. Secondary peritonitis affects all ages and almost always reflects underlying abnormalities requiring urgent operative intervention. Many classic texts detail the differential diagnosis of the "acute abdomen," and only the common categories will be mentioned. Diseases of the gastrointestinal tract may cause peritonitis by perforation of a viscus, by contiguous spread from infected viscera, or by direct trauma. Perforation of an acutely inflamed appendix or diverticulum disseminates bacteria, which have proved already to be virulent by virtue of their initiation of the basic disease. An initially sterile chemical peritonitis can arise from leakage of gastric acid, bile, blood, meconium, or urine. Causes of this type of peritonitis include perforated peptic ulcer, perforated meconium ileus, and rupture of the urinary bladder or gallbladder. The patients may demonstrate vague symptoms until the parietal peritoneum becomes inflamed.

Retroperitoneal disease may also cause intra-abdominal infection. Acute pyelonephritis, perinephric abscesses, and pancreatic abscesses may extend into the peritoneal cavity. Primary pelvic infections, such as salpingitis and ruptured tubo-ovarian abscess, may present as intra-abdominal infections. A particularly difficult form of peritonitis to evaluate occurs in the postoperative period. Pain from the abdominal incision and from serosal reaction may be confused with that caused by drainage of bile from an open cystic duct or by intestinal contents from an anastomotic leak. Unless the abnormal peritoneal fluid drains externally, the cause often remains obscure.

HISTORY

A careful history is most useful for determining the cause of peritonitis rather than the actual diagnosis, which is evident from the physical findings. Since peritonitis usually arises from pre-existing visceral disease, specific symptom complexes often suggest the involved organ system. A past history of similar episodes, such as with cholelithiasis or renal calculi, may help determine the necessity for and timing of surgical intervention.

Abdominal pain is the single most important symptom of peritonitis. Its location, quality, radiation, and progression provide the most accurate clues to the cause of abdominal pain. Usually the pain of peritoneal irritation is preceded by pain caused by the primary visceral disease process. Because the intra-abdominal organs contain no somatic nerve supply, visceral pain is poorly localized and often reflects the embryologic origins of the organ involved. Early inflammation may present with diffuse, ill-defined pain; however, with involvement of the adjacent parietal peritoneum, the location of the pain often becomes specific for the organ involved and its character may reflect the progress of the inflammatory process. Thus, lower quadrant pain on the right most often reflects acute appendicitis, while that involving the left usually arises from acute diverticulitis of the sigmoid colon. Right upper quadrant pain is seen with biliary tract disease and perforated peptic ulcer, although the latter may first present with right lower quadrant pain generated by the dependent drainage of duodenal contents down the pericolic gutter. Generalized abdominal pain suggests an advanced stage of peritonitis, especially in children, who have diminished ability to contain intra-abdominal infection.

Abdominal pain may be cramping or constant in character. The waxing and waning nature of cramping pain suggests obstruction of a hollow viscus, such as the biliary tract, ureter, or intestine. This type of pain reflects an early stage of disease before mural necrosis and subsequent peritoneal involvement occur. Timely surgical intervention may prevent visceral destruction, as in intestinal obstruction, or may not be required, as with a spontaneously passed ureteral calculus. On the other hand, constant, steady abdominal pain indicates continuing involvement of a solid organ, such as the pancreas, or progression to necrosis, such as strangulated obstruction, and peritoneal irritation confirms the advanced nature of the process.

Occasionally, involvement of certain organs will cause pain in areas distant from the primary inflammatory process. Thus, acute cholecystitis with irritation of the nearby diaphragm may generate right shoulder pain, while a calculus in a ureter will cause pain in the scrotum. Pelvic inflammatory disease may cause right upper quadrant pain, presumably by formation of fibrinous adhesions between the liver capsule and abdominal wall.

PHYSICAL EXAMINATION

The physical findings of peritonitis depend on the patient's state of health. Advanced age, impaired mentation, hypovolemia, severe sepsis, and medications such as opiates or steroids may attenuate or obliterate physical signs of infection. Most patients with peritonitis are febrile (up to 40 C [104 F]) and have tachycardia. Breathing is often shallow and rapid. Observation of the patient's spontaneous movements in response to pain may provide important information about the nature and progression of the disease process. Patients with pancreatitis and other diseases still confined to the involved organ are constantly moving, searching for a position of comfort. In contrast, once peritoneal irritation has occurred, patients lie quietly, avoiding any movement and consequent stimulation of the inflamed peritoneum. Jaundice, when present, may indicate biliary tract disease, but it may also be a nonspecific manifestation of sepsis. A distended abdomen suggests bowel obstruction or massive gas leak through a gastrointestinal perforation, especially if air overlies the liver. Ascites suggests chronic liver disease or the nephrotic syndrome. Infection below the diaphragms may be associated with pleural effusion or basilar pneumonitis. Bowel sounds may be hypoactive or absent.

Abdominal tenderness is the most prominent and informative physical sign of peritonitis. If the tenderness is localized, additional information is provided that may help identify the organ system involved and aid in planning the operative approach. Generalized tenderness establishes only that peritonitis is present, often advanced. Tenderness by direct palpation, performed in a systematic and gentle manner, is the most reliable indicator of the presence of peritonitis. If rebound tenderness is elicited, the patient will likely not permit additional examination, although it may be the only sign present in early stages of the disease. A variant and more acceptable sign is percussion rebound tenderness; this is often an effective method of eliciting evidence of peritonitis in patients complaining of extreme abdominal pain. Referred tenderness, such as that generated by acute appendicitis by palpation of the left lower quadrant, is helpful when present.

Voluntary guarding can be minimized with gentle palpation and is usually present over the region of the abdomen directly involved with the acute inflammatory process. However, as the process becomes more generalized, voluntary guarding will give way to generalized rigidity, the so-called "board-like surgical abdomen."

Rectal examination is essential in the evaluation of the patient with peritonitis. Although signs of appendicitis or of a low-lying diverticular abscess can occasionally be detected, rectal examination is most useful for excluding pelvic inflammatory disease. Posterior parietal peritoneal irritation, usually by appendicitis, can be detected by appearance of pain caused by external rotation of the fully flexed thigh (obturator sign). Likewise, inflammation along the psoas muscle in the retroperitoneum is confirmed by the onset of pain elicited by having the patient elevate his fully extended leg.

LABORATORY AND ROENTGENOLOGIC STUDIES

Although the diagnosis of peritonitis can be established in the majority of occasions on the basis of clinical findings, certain laboratory studies lend credence to this diagnosis and rarely may be the only means of determining whether a surgically correctable disease exists. A hemogram, including hemoglobin concentration, white blood cell count, and differential, points not only to the diagnosis but also to the patient's physiologic response to the insult. Hemoconcentration in the face of long-standing signs of peritoneal irritation indicates intravascular volume contraction and the need for plasma volume restitution. Most patients with peritonitis have an elevated polymorphonuclear white cell count, usually in the range of 10,000 to 16,000 cells per ml of blood. Higher counts may indicate the presence of an untoward complication, such as bowel infarction or abscess formation, or nonoperative disease, such as primary peritonitis or any of the leukemoid reactions. A preponderance of lymphocytes helps differentiate gastrointestinal manifestations of viral infections from acute surgical diseases. Subnormal white blood cell counts, especially with many immature forms, indicate overwhelming sepsis, or may occur immediately after a visceral perforation. Leukopenia may also be seen in patients who are taking chronic steroid medication, which may obscure the physical signs of an intra-abdominal catastrophe.

The next most important laboratory aid is a urinalysis to differentiate urinary tract disease from an intra-abdominal process. Although an inflamed organ, such as the appendix, lying near the ureter or bladder can generate white cells in the urine, pyuria generally indicates acute pyelonephritis (white cell casts) or acute cystitis (clumps of white cells). Hematuria, in the absence of trauma, most commonly is associated with ureterolithiasis or renal tuberculosis. The presence of glucose, bile, and albumin provides important information about the cause of abdominal pain and tenderness. Proteinuria with signs of peritonitis in children should suggest primary peritonitis. Finally, the presence of bacteria in the microscopic sediment is diagnostic of urinary tract infection.

Occasionally, other ancillary studies yield important information about the nature of intraperitoneal disease. Of these, the serum amylase is helpful. Although not specific, hyperamylasemia usually denotes acute pancreatitis; however, acute salpingitis and infarcted bowel will also cause elevated serum amylase concentrations, as may intestinal obstruction. Liver function studies will occasionally differentiate calculous biliary tract disease from hepatitis. An electrocardiogram may be needed to separate the pain of an acute myocardial infarction from that of primary abdominal disease. Most other laboratory studies, such as blood gases and serum electrolytes, serve only to define the patient's general response to disease.

Important roentgenograms include posterior-anterior and lateral views of the chest and supine and upright films of the abdomen. Thus, certain intrathoracic disease such as pneumonitis, pneumothorax, or rib fracture, which can present with abdominal signs, can be eliminated. The abdominal films must be carefully searched for evidence of calculi, suggesting biliary or urinary tract disease, or for abnormal distribution of air. Air under the diaphragms usually originates from a perforated ulcer or colonic diverticulum; only rarely is a ruptured appendix associated with extraluminal air. Ancillary signs suggesting the location of intra-abdominal disease include obliteration of structures, such as the psoas shadow by an adjacent appendicitis. Radiologic contrast studies are seldom necessary when the diagnosis of peritonitis has been established.

If the well-established guidelines are followed, peritoneal paracentesis is a valuable diagnostic aid, especially in children with suspected primary peritonitis and in patients with abdominal trauma. Any fluid obtained is examined by Gram stain, cell count, amylase determination, and culture and sensitivity studies. The presence of purulence in the abdominal cavity usually indicates secondary peritonitis. Conversely, failure to find any fluid, or a "negative tap," does not mean that such disease is absent. Finally, if all these studies and repeated physical examination by the same observers still leave the diagnosis of peritonitis in doubt, celiotomy is justified. The morbidity and mortality of celiotomy in which no surgical disease is found is small compared with that of an ignored intra-abdominal infection.

COURSE

If diagnosed in an accurate and timely fashion, primary peritonitis usually responds to antibiotic therapy. Treatment is then directed toward any underlying disease, which determines the ultimate prognosis.

Celiotomy both confirms the diagnosis of secondary peritonitis and permits direct treatment of the primary disease. If detected early, peritonitis may be well localized by surrounding viscera and omentum, and removal and drainage of the infectious focus usually results in complete recovery. If peritonitis has been present for a prolonged period of time and has spread throughout the abdominal cavity, the infection may be sequestered in multiloculated abscesses, which may be difficult to identify or approach because of dense inflammatory adhesions.

COMPLICATIONS OF PERITONITIS

Early complications of peritonitis are inseparable from those of the immediate postoperative state, namely decreased respiratory capacity predisposing to atelectasis, fluid shifts resulting in hypovolemia, and paralytic ileus leading to intestinal distention. If infection is adequately controlled by the operative procedure, the disturbances soon relent.

If infection remains undetected or is inadequately controlled, a number of potentially fatal complications can occur. Infection within the peritoneal cavity may seed the blood and result in lethal septic shock. As the peritoneum and retroperitoneum become more intensely involved with the septic process, spread to the portal venous system may produce pylephlebitis, a complication now made rare by the philosophy prevailing in the medical community of early operative intervention. Dense peritoneal adhesions and inflammatory masses may produce intestinal obstruction. Furthermore, these masses will on occasion erode into adjacent structures, producing fistulas to skin, bladder, vagina, and other segments of the gastrointestinal tract.

Perhaps the most life-threatening complication of peritonitis is an intra-abdominal abscess. Usually the result of long-standing infection, the intra-abdominal abscess may be localized and easily drained, or may be multifocal and involve most of the peritoneal space. In order to initiate treatment of such abscesses, an appreciation of the anatomy of the peritoneal spaces, a thorough history and physical examination, and knowledge of available diagnostic aids are required. This discussion includes retroperitoneal abscesses because the signs, symptoms, diagnostic studies, and clinical course are similar to those of intraperitoneal abscesses.

The peritoneal cavity is a fully enclosed space completely surrounded by a mesothelial membrane. The retroperitoneum can be conveniently divided into two parts. The anterior retroperitoneal space lies between the posterior peritoneum and the transversalis fascia. Infection in this space, such as from diverticulitis of the colon, may present not only with abdominal findings but also with complaints localized to the back, hip, or thigh. The posterior retroperitoneum lies behind the transversalis fascia and forms a potential space from the mediastinum to the upper thigh, which explains the extensive and bizarre migration of some peripancreatic and perinephric abscesses. Abscesses in either of the potential spaces may communicate directly with the peritoneal cavity. The intraperitoneal space is a freely communicating cavity partially partitioned by multiple serous membranes. Barnard's classic description, that the coronary ligaments suspend the liver from the diaphragm, has been demonstrated to be incorrect. In fact, the coronary ligaments are attached to the posterior abdominal wall, and no true division of the various subphrenic spaces exists.

The right subphrenic space is composed of three relatively well-defined areas. The suprahepatic, or subdiaphragmatic, space lies between the liver and the diaphragm. The subhepatic space lies beneath the inferior surface of the liver. The hepatorenal pouch of Morison is merely the posterior portion of the right subhepatic space. An extraperitoneal space lies between the bare area of the liver and the diaphragm and is enclosed by the coronary ligaments. The falciform ligament divides the right from the left subphrenic space. Because of the small size of the left lobe of the liver, the left suprahepatic space and the anterior portion of the subhepatic space combine to form a single recognizable space. The posterior subhepatic space forms the lesser sac, or omental bursa, and communicates with the right subhepatic space through the foramen of Winslow.

All four major subphrenic spaces (excluding the extraperitoneal potential space over the bare area of the liver) open freely into the free peritoneal cavity. Surrounding viscera and other membranes, such as the greater omentum and the reflections of the peritoneum from posterior organs onto the abdominal wall, may adhere to one another and form potential spaces for interloop pericolic and iliac abscesses. Drainage to positions of greatest dependency, such as the pouch of Douglas in females and the rectovesical pouch in males, explains the high incidence of pelvic abscesses. Abscess formation may involve all of these spaces in continuity, forming a giant horseshoe abscess.

The etiology of abscesses in a particular location depends on both the surrounding anatomy and the dynamics of gravity drainage. Abscesses of the right subhepatic space most commonly are secondary to inflammatory disease of the right kidney, gallbladder, duodenum, the right and transverse colon, and the appendix. Lesser sac abscesses arise most often from pancreatitis or a perforated ulcer. Infection in the left subphrenic space is most frequently associated with trauma and gastric, splenic, and pancreatic surgery. Interloop abscesses arise both from primary inflammatory bowel disease, such as regional enteritis, and from loculations arising from the body's attempt to wall off foci of infection. Abscesses in the pericolic areas can arise from adjacent infections, such as diverticulitis or appendicitis, or from dependent drainage of perforated organs, as occurs with the drainage of duodenal contents to the right lower quadrant with perforated peptic ulcer disease. Finally, purulence from any location in the abdomen can find its way into the pelvis.

The patient harboring an intra-abdominal abscess usually presents with symptoms of serious systemic infection, and often gives a history of repeated bouts of chills and fever. If no specific localizing signs are obvious, it is often difficult to establish that an occult abscess is responsible for the patient's sepsis. A careful history should include details of previous trauma, peritonitis, or surgical procedures. Uncontrolled abdominal sepsis in a young patient most likely follows acute appendicitis, while in elderly patients, acute diverticulitis is a more likely source. If the abscess lies against the abdominal wall, localization is usually easy and requires minimal diagnostic studies. However, deep abscesses may produce vague and seemingly peculiar symptoms. Subphrenic abscesses can produce hiccoughs or pain along the costal margin or in the shoulder. Interloop abscesses can cause bowel obstruction or diarrhea. Bladder dysfunction may arise from pelvic abscesses.

Fever, chills, and tachycardia reflect the patient's systemic response to sepsis. Discrete physical signs depend on the location of the intra-abdominal abscess. Subphrenic abscesses usually demonstrate at least one of the following: upper quadrant tenderness, signs of a pleural effusion or elevated hemidiaphragm, a palpable mass, or jaundice. Direct tenderness or a palpable mass may reveal an interloop or pericolic abscess. A careful rectal examination, combined with a bimanual pelvic examination in female patients, is required to detect pelvic collections.

In spite of a careful history and meticulous, repeated physical examinations, the presence and location of an intra-abdominal abscess may be unclear. Positive blood cultures and an elevated white blood cell count lend support to the diagnosis. The simplest and most rewarding diagnostic aids are plain roentgenograms of the chest and abdomen. Pulmonic infiltrates are evident on chest x-ray in up to 90 per cent of patients with subphrenic abscesses and are often accompanied by a pleural effusion. Unusual gas patterns are present in 25 per cent of patients with abscesses. Scoliosis due to ipsilateral splinting of flank muscles or displacement of an organ also aids in localizing the abscess. Fluoroscopy documents a fixed diaphragm in over half of patients with peritonitis. A subdiaphragmatic abscess appears on combined technetium 99m liver-lung scan as a gap between the dome of the liver and the diaphragm.

Gray-scale ultrasonography offers an accurate and economical method to localize intra-abdominal abscesses and should be employed if standard roentgenograms are unrevealing. Both transverse and longitudinal scans should be carried out so that collections in remote locations, such as the pouch of Douglas or the rectovesical pouch, will not be overlooked. An abscess appears as a relatively echo-free area surrounded by highly reflective irregular walls. Within the cavity are multiple internal echoes, rising from cellular debris. However, not all fluid collections are abscesses. Loculated ascites, fluid-filled loops of bowel, and ovarian cysts present an appearance similar to an abscess but can be distinguished from the latter by smooth thin walls and the absence of internal echoes.

Gallium 67 citrate has a relatively high affinity for inflammatory tissue and has been used to localize abscesses. However, a significant percentage of false-positive and false-negative results limit its usefulness. Furthermore, some patients may not be able to tolerate the bowel preparation required for a readable scan. Local accumulations of autogenous leukocytes labeled with indium 111 can also be detected in abscesses by gamma counter scanning and imaging. The use of this isotope to localize abscesses is presently preferred to that of gallium 67 because of its higher abscess-to-blood activity ratios, its physical characteristics, its lesser elution, and the lesser occurrence of falsely positive and falsely negative tests.

Computerized tomography (CT) also is a rapidly developing and highly accurate diagnostic modality and is especially useful for localizing abscesses in the retroperitoneum, liver, pancreas, and kidney. Its accuracy is probably equal to gray-scale ultrasonography in delineating subphrenic and pelvic abscesses. Most techniques utilize a radiopaque contrast agent, and with the more recent software programs, the intrinsic nature of a mass lesion is often indicated. The greatest disadvantage of CT scanning is its significant cost. It is likely that 90 to 95 per cent of intra-abdominal abscesses can be identified by a careful review of the patient's history, repeated physical examinations, roentgenograms of the chest and abdomen, and gray-scale ultrasonography. Occasionally, addition of more expensive modalities will be necessary. In a few cases, all diagnostic maneuvers fail, and celiotomy is indicated.

PITFALLS IN DIAGNOSIS

Most errors in the diagnostic evaluation of a patient with suspected peritonitis or intra-abdominal abscess arise from inadequate consideration of the many nonsurgical diseases that stimulate these processes. Most of these diseases can be eliminated from consideration by a complete history, a physical examination, and preliminary laboratory tests. Thus, pneumonia, acute myocardial infarction, herpes zoster, diabetes mellitus, rib fracture, pleuritis, pericarditis, and pancreatitis are usually apparent if present. Less common diseases that may deceive the physician are pulmonary embolism, tabes dorsalis, porphyria, lead colic, epilepsy, and hemolytic crises. Complications from ureterolithiasis and acute pancreatitis may necessitate surgical intervention later in the clinical course. All of these diseases may so closely mimic an acute intraperitoneal infection that laparotomy is indicated to exclude peritonitis from further consideration.

HEPATIC AND PERIHEPATIC ABSCESS

By CHARLES F. FREY, M.D.,
W. LANE VERLENDEN, III, M.D.,
Davis, California

and GREGORY M. GRAVES, M.D.
New York, New York

A diagnosis not considered is seldom made. This aphorism is highly applicable to the diagnosis of hepatic and perihepatic abscesses. The systemic and local manifestations of both pyogenic and amebic abscesses of liver and perihepatic spaces are quite variable, and may be mistaken for those of cholangitis, perforated viscus, mesenteric artery thrombosis, embolus, pneumonia, pancreatitis, hepatitis, or associated diseases. The most important element in the diagnosis of these abscesses is the physician who suspects their presence despite a wide range of clinical presentations. In the absence of a diagnosis and appropriate therapy, these abscesses are invariably lethal. Early diagnosis and appropriate treatment of hepatic and perihepatic abscesses on the other hand will result in a low patient mortality and morbidity. Once the clinician's suspicion of a hepatic or perihepatic abscess is aroused, powerful diagnostic tools such as ultrasound, radioisotopic scintillation, scanning of the liver and lung, and celiac angiography are available to confirm their presence or absence.

HEPATIC ABSCESS

Recent reports from hospitals in Boston, New York, Chicago, and Detroit indicate that 90 per cent or more of hepatic abscesses are pyogenic, most of the remainder resulting from *Entamoeba histolytica*, or, rarely, fungal (usually actinomycosis). In many areas of the world outside the United States, the incidence of amebic abscess exceeds that of pyogenic abscess; therefore, in patients not native to the United States or those who have traveled widely, the incidence of amebic abscesses will be higher.

PYOGENIC ABSCESS

Hepatic abscesses of pyogenic origin can be subclassified on the basis of the route of bacterial invasion of the liver, e.g., ascending infection through the biliary tract, hematogenous spread via the portal venous system, seeding through the hepatic artery from a bacteremia or by direct extension from a gastric ulcer perforating into the liver, or gangrenous cholecystitis. Recent reports indicate that the incidence of hepatic abscess of the liver has not changed, but the frequency of invasion by the biliary and portal routes has decreased, and spread through the hepatic artery has increased.

Ascending infection through the biliary tract from cholangitis resulting from extrahepatic biliary obstruction from a calculus, neoplasm, or stricture was the most frequently reported cause of parenchymal hepatic abscesses during the 1940s and 1950s. Since then, the incidence of ascending infection among patients with pyogenic hepatic abscesses has fallen from 50 to 25 per cent of the total number of abscesses according to some reports, although it still remains the most common source of infection in other reports.

Hematogenous spread from intra-abdominal infection through tributaries of the portal vein occurs in 20 to 45 per cent of all patients with pyogenic hepatic abscesses. The foci of infection are most often associated with disease of the gastrointestinal tract. Seeding of the portal tributaries is thought to occur from infections such as diverticulitis, perforating carcinoma of the colon, appendicitis, or pancreatic abscesses. A small percentage of these patients may develop pyelophlebitis (a suppurative thrombophlebitis).

Over the past 10 years, there has been a progressive increase in the number of liver abscesses seeded by pathogenetic bacteria through the hepatic artery. More often than not, no preceding evidence of localized infection or bacteremia exists. Such abscesses are often referred to as cryptogenic and now represent over

50 per cent of all pyogenic abscesses of the liver seen in some institutions.

Aside from the intra-abdominal infection or bacteremia, hepatic injury is the most frequent factor (5 to 10 per cent) predisposing to abscess formation. The injury may not have to be penetrating to introduce infection. Blunt trauma to the liver causing a subcapsular hematoma or infarcts secondary to thromboembolic disease produce necrotic liver and collections of blood and bile that are subject to secondary infection by bowel organisms, including anaerobes.

Pyogenic abscesses may be solitary, multiple, or multilobular, and microscopic or macroscopic. Twenty to 30 per cent of hepatic abscesses are microscopic. Microscopic abscesses most frequently result from biliary infection secondary to acute obstructive suppurative cholangitis or bacteremia associated with serious underlying disease.

About 40 per cent of macroscopic pyogenic hepatic abscesses are multiple. The most common organism recovered from both single and multiple abscesses is *Escherichia coli*. A mixed bowel flora, including Enterobacteriacea, anaerobes, and gram-positive cocci, is found in about 25 per cent of hepatic abscesses. The incidence of anaerobes grown on culture is directly related to use of anaerobic transport culture media. In as many as one third of all pyogenic hepatic abscesses, anaerobes may be the only isolate, and their recovery in abscesses with mixed flora may be even higher. The use of improved culture techniques, particularly the anaerobic transport media, has markedly diminished the number of so-called sterile abscesses. Repeating Gram stains of the abscess fluid is a means of determining the presence of anaerobic organisms, which may be identified only on stain and not on culture.

Pyogenic gram-positive cocci, either group A streptococci or *Staphylococcus aureus*, are likely to be recovered from the abscesses and blood in children, most of whom have altered defense mechanisms from leukemia or chronic debilitating disease.

Growth is reported in blood cultures in about 30 per cent of all patients with abscesses. Although all ages and both sexes are subject to pyogenic hepatic abscesses, the overall predilection seems to be shifting, moving up the average age of those afflicted from the fourth to the sixth decade.

The symptoms are most severe and their onset most rapid in those patients with multiple microscopic and macroscopic abscesses of the liver. Patients with cholangitis or bacteremia tend to have a rapid onset of symptoms with chills, high fever, and prostration, and those with acute obstructive suppurative cholangitis

are jaundiced. Anemia, leukocytosis, hypoalbuminemia and a 50 per cent chance of positive blood cultures are characteristic of patients with multiple hepatic abscess.

Patients with large solitary hepatic abscesses often have a more insidious course evolving over 4 to 5 weeks before the diagnosis is established. The presenting symptom is most often fever, often accompanied by chills, anorexia, nausea and vomiting, right upper quadrant pain, malaise, weakness, and weight loss. Pulmonary symptoms, including cough, shoulder pain, hemoptysis, or pleurisy, may be prominent, indicating penetration or adherence of the abscess to the diaphragm.

Right upper quadrant tenderness and hepatomegaly occur in half the patients. Jaundice is seen principally in those patients with obstructive biliary disease. Less frequently, abdominal distention and evidence of pleural effusion or ascites may be noted. Fixation of the diaphragm, pleural effusion, or a right lower lobe infiltrate may be noted on radiologic examination of the chest. Marked leukocytosis of about 18,000 per cu mm is the most frequently noted laboratory abnormality. Increased values of alkaline phosphatase, bilirubin, and serum glutamic oxaloacetic transaminase (SGOT) and depressed levels of albumin are frequently detected on liver function studies.

Untreated pyogenic abscesses of the liver are fatal. Death usually occurs from septicemia or rupture into the chest or abdominal cavity, with consequent empyema, lung abscess, or generalized peritonitis.

AMEBIC ABSCESS

The incidence of amebic abscess of the liver, although less than 10 per cent of all hepatic abscesses in the northern United States, is significantly more common in the South. Young adult males are most commonly afflicted by this complication of intestinal amebiasis. The disease is acquired by man through ingestion of the cysts of *Entamoeba histolytica*, which, in the large intestine, develop into trophozoites. The trophozoites responsible for hepatic abscesses migrate through the intestinal mucosa and enter the portal venous channels to the liver. However, only 10 per cent of patients with amebic liver abscesses can recall any symptoms suggestive of an intestinal infestation, and trophozoites are even less frequently recovered in the stool.

The clinical presentation and predilection of the amebic abscesses for the superior aspect of the right lobe of the liver are of some help in differentiating the amebic from the pyogenic abscess. Making the distinction between a pyogenic and an amebic abscess is essential to proper treatment. Pyogenic liver abscesses must be drained, but not amebic abscesses.

Although the presenting symptoms and signs of amebic abscesses are similar to those of pyogenic abscesses, the degree of fever, elevation of white blood cell count, and progression of systemic manifestations tend to be less marked in patients with an amebic abscess. Pulmonary changes are much more likely to be associated with an amebic than a pyogenic abscess. On radiologic examination, as many as 70 per cent of patients with amebic abscesses have an elevated or fixed right diaphragm, 30 per cent a pleural effusion, and 24 per cent a pneumonitis. Penetration of the right diaphragm by direct extension of the amebic abscess located in the superior aspect of the right lobe of the liver occurs in 20 per cent of the patients with amebic abscess of the liver. The changes in the right lower lung lobe are quite characteristic, producing a triangular opacity based on the diaphragm often associated with a pleural effusion or pneumonitis. Rupture into the bronchus may be one of the early signs of pulmonary extension.

Secondary infection of amebic abscesses of the liver is uncommon in this country, but is reported to be as high as 30 per cent by investigators in Korea. Should operative intervention be undertaken by mistake, secondary infection often develops.

Aspiration of the hepatic abscess often produces the anchovy-colored pus characteristic of an amebic abscess. Recovery of the amebas in the aspirated pus is successful in only 30 per cent of cases. However, the most reliable test for the presence of amebic abscess of the liver is the indirect hemagglutination test as performed at the National Center for Disease Control in Atlanta, Georgia, free of charge. The test is particularly helpful in that it gives positive results only with liver or lung or other systemic involvement, and negative results when the infestation is limited to the intestine. Unfortunately, time and distance create delays of 3 to 4 weeks in reporting of results. Serologic testing for amebiasis is becoming more available locally with manufacturers providing latex agglutination (Ames), countercurrent-immunoelectrophoretic agglutination (Cardio), and now indirect hemagglutination IHA kits (Cal Biochebering). Each of the kits, which vary in cost from $15 to $150, can be used to test 5 to 10 separate sera. Short shelf life of the reconstituted agents is a major drawback.

PERIHEPATIC ABSCESS

Perihepatic abscesses frequently follow an intra-abdominal operation (90 per cent) but can also occur de novo (e.g., as a complication of pancreatitis, or rupture of a hepatic abscess). These perihepatic abscesses are most frequently described by their anatomic location beneath the diaphragm (subdiaphragmatic) or beneath the liver (subhepatic). These spaces are further subdivided into right and left, and, in the case of subdiaphragmatic abscesses, into anterior and posterior and intraperitoneal and extraperitoneal. There are a total of three extensions of the subdiaphragmatic space bilaterally.

SUBPHRENIC OR SUBHEPATIC ABSCESS

Subphrenic or subhepatic abscesses most often result from direct extension of an infection from elsewhere in the abdominal cavity or from perforation of a hollow viscus, or after operative intervention on the stomach or biliary tract.

Rupture of a gangrenous gallbladder, a liver, or pancreatic abscess are examples of infections that frequently extend into the subhepatic and subphrenic spaces. Perforated duodenal or gastric ulcers, perforated appendicitis, and duodenal rupture from trauma are frequent causes of subhepatic or subphrenic abscesses. However, by far the most frequent causes of subphrenic or subhepatic abscesses are previous operations, particularly those involving the stomach and biliary tract, appendix, and small bowel.

The enteric organisms are most frequently grown from cultures of these abscesses. The

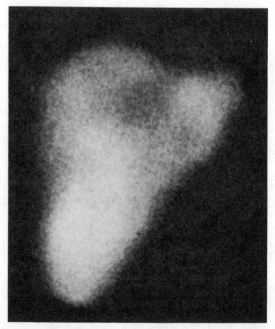

Figure 1. Sixty-two-year-old white male developed fever and abdominal pain 1 year after removal of a retained common duct stone. 3.5 mCi. ^{99m}Tc sulfur-colloid shows cold defect in right lobe of liver.

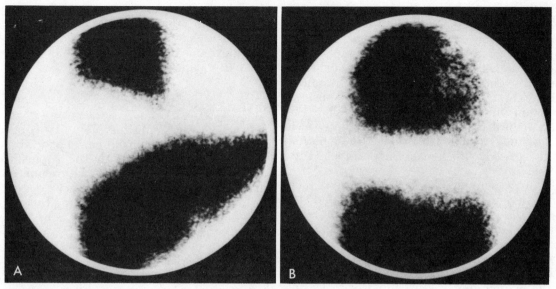

Figure 2. Subphrenic abscess in 46-year-old male alcoholic with complications after pancreatitis. The large abscess, visualized as an increased separation between liver and lung on the combined liver/lung scan, is seen on both anterior (A) and lateral (B) views.

incidence of anaerobic organisms is reported to be higher as a result of increased use of anaerobic transport media.

After an operation in which an intra-abdominal abscess develops, physical examination of the abdomen may be made difficult because of the presence of a recent incision, tubes, drains, and dressings. In perihepatic abscesses fever is usually, but not invariably, present. Patients least likely to be febrile are those who are elderly or who have suffered a prolonged debilitating illness. Anorexia is almost invariably present. Right upper quadrant pain and tenderness when present are helpful in localizing the abscess, but more often than not are absent. Radiologic examination often shows a pleural effusion, a fixed diaphragm, and occasionally an air-fluid level outside the gastrointestinal tract. Few alterations in liver function are present. The white cell count is usually elevated above 10,000 per cu mm, except in the elderly.

DIAGNOSTIC PROCEDURES

Once the physician suspects the presence of a hepatic or perihepatic abscess, he now has the tools to identify not only their presence but also the location of macroscopic abscesses of over 1 to 2 cm in diameter with a high degree of reliability. The clinical course, signs, and symptoms with or without elevation or fixation of the hemidiaphragm or evidence of a pleural effusion on conventional roentgenographic studies

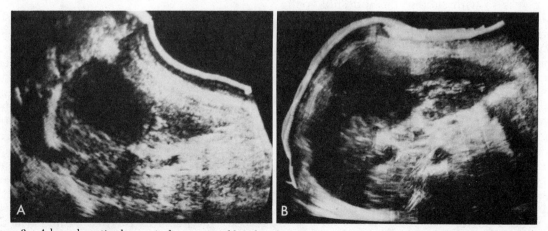

Figure 3. A large hepatic abscess is demonstrated by ultrasonography on both transverse (A) and longitudinal (B) scans.

should raise the possibility of a hepatic or perihepatic abscess. With the use of the new diagnostic techniques consisting of radioisotope scan of the liver, ultrasonography, and arteriography, the feasibility of establishing a diagnosis and initiating therapy promptly exists. The average interval from the onset of symptoms until diagnosis has been reduced by over a third since the advent of these techniques and is a major factor in declining mortality associated with hepatic or perihepatic abscesses.

In liver scintigraphy, a noninvasive technique, liver anatomy can be demonstrated simply by the intravenous injection of technetium 99m-labeled sulfur colloid particles that are phagocytized by the Kupffer cells. Abscesses or other space-occupying lesions appear as a cold defect in the liver (Fig. 1). A sequential flow study, using either sulfur colloid or ^{99m}Tc pertechnetate, helps differentiate vascular tumors from avascular abscesses or cysts. Gallium 67 citrate, which labels polymorphonuclear cells, can be utilized to differentiate abscesses from cysts, but the gallium will also label hepatic malignancies. These techniques are useful in differentiating abscesses from other space-occupying lesions of the liver. Of particular usefulness in the identification of subphrenic abscesses is the combined lung and liver scan (Fig. 2). Right lateral and anterior views in the presence of an abscess demonstrate a separation between the lung base and superior border of the liver. ^{99m}Tc MAA macroaggregates of albumin are used to delineate the lung and ^{99m}Tc sulfur colloid the liver.

Ultrasonography is another relatively new noninvasive procedure combining the echo techniques of sonar and the two-dimensional visualization of radar, making it possible to bounce high frequency sound off tissue interfaces (Fig. 3). The technique appears to be most effective in identifying hepatic abscesses, and much less so with subphrenic and subhepatic abscesses. Left subphrenic abscesses are particularly hard to identify.

Arteriography is an invasive procedure that should be employed only after use of the radioisotope scan and ultrasonography. Celiac and superior mesenteric artery injections are performed through percutaneous femoral artery catheterization. Some reports indicate that arteriography provides more precise localization of liver abscesses than scintiscans. Significant features seen on arteriography in the presence of an abscess are stretching of the hepatic vessels, an absence of vasculature within the abscess, and a capillary blush around the abscess during the venous phase.

Computerized tomography (CT) is a noninvasive procedure that, while more expensive than ultrasonography, is highly effective in the identification and localization of both hepatic and perihepatic abscesses.

PITFALLS IN DIAGNOSIS

Crucial to reducing the mortality associated with pyogenic hepatic and perihepatic abscesses is early drainage. With the sophisticated techniques now available to help confirm the diagnosis of an abscess, failure by the clinician to include hepatic or perihepatic abscesses in his admitting differential diagnosis has become the chief factor in delay.

Patients with a hepatic or perihepatic abscess are often misdiagnosed as having fever of unknown origin, perforated viscus, mesenteric artery occlusion, pneumonia, bacteremia, metastatic carcinoma, pulmonary emboli, hepatitis, or pancreatitis.

HEPATITIS

By ALLEN L. GINSBERG, M.D.
Washington, D.C.

The term hepatitis means inflammation of the liver. It implies hepatocellular necrosis. Hepatic injury can be caused by viruses, a wide variety of medications and hepatotoxins such as alcohol, by ischemia, and by metabolic disorders such as Wilson's disease. Hepatitis may be acute or chronic. It may be mild or moderate, or in rare instances can be fulminant and fatal.

ACUTE VIRAL HEPATITIS

At least three groups of viruses — termed A, B, and non-A, non-B — as well as the Epstein-Barr virus and cytomegalovirus, commonly produce hepatitis. For many years the term hepatitis A was used interchangeably with the term "infectious hepatitis" and the term hepatitis B was used interchangeably with the term "serum hepatitis." Use of the old terms "infectious" and "serum" hepatitis has caused much confusion and they have been abandoned, although they are important from a historic perspective.

These terms were abandoned because, when tests for the hepatitis B virus became available, it was found that many cases of sporadic hepatitis not involving a history of transfusions or parenteral exposure that were previously thought to be "infectious hepatitis" were caused by the hepatitis B virus. Furthermore, once blood used for transfusions was pretested for the hepatitis B surface antigen, most post-transfusion hepatitis B was eliminated. Ninety per cent of post-transfusion hepatitis is today caused by non-A, non-B hepatitis. The term "non-A, non-B" is used rather than hepatitis C because it is suspected that more than one viral agent is responsible for this disease.

SYMPTOMS AND SIGNS

Many patients have inapparent hepatitis, detectable only by elevation of serum transaminase activity (either serum glutamic oxaloacetic transaminase [SGOT] or serum glutamic pyruvic transaminase [SGPT]), and development of immunologic markers of viral infection. Estimates vary widely as to the number of inapparent cases (1 to 10) for every icteric case. Symptomatic cases may be anicteric or icteric. The symptoms are flu-like and anicteric cases can easily be mistaken for influenza if appropriate tests are not performed. It is thought by many investigators that patients with anicteric hepatitis are statistically more likely to develop chronic hepatitis.

Most of the symptoms of hepatitis A, B, and "non-A, non-B" hepatitis are similar; however, there are some noteworthy differences. Hepatitis A usually has an abrupt onset with a rapid transition (within a period of hours) from health to acute illness. Onset is typically heralded by temperature of 100 to 104 F (37.8 to 40 C), chills, headache, and myalgias. This preicteric phase of illness usually lasts 2 to 5 days. In contrast, in hepatitis B the onset is usually insidious and is characterized by several days or weeks of easy fatigability. A frank arthritis and serum sickness–like picture occurs during this preicteric stage in 20 per cent of patients with hepatitis B and is related to the formation of immune complexes. This syndrome disappears before the onset of clinical hepatitis with jaundice and has not been reported in non-B viral hepatitis.

Patients with symptomatic viral hepatitis usually become nauseated and lose their appetite and taste for cigarettes. Urine darkens when serum bilirubin is between 2 and 3 mg per dl (100 ml). A few days following this, patients note that their eyes have turned yellow. Clinical jaundice, which is best observed using direct sunlight, usually cannot be detected by the astute physician until the serum bilirubin exceeds 3 mg per dl. In hepatitis A it is common

for the onset of jaundice to be associated with a rapid improvement of symptoms. About half of the patients will have mild itching and note that their stools are pale. Abdominal pain is unusual except for some mild tenderness to percussion and palpation of the distended liver and a vague right upper quadrant discomfort, presumably caused by stretching of the liver capsule. The liver is commonly enlarged to 12 to 14 cm and is often palpable 2 to 5 cm below the costal margin. The spleen is palpable in 10 to 20 per cent of patients and mild posterior cervical adenopathy may be present. If there is sore throat, adenopathy, or persistent fever, mononucleosis and cytomegalovirus infection should be ruled out, particularly if atypical monocytes are seen on peripheral smear. Hematomas and ecchymoses may be present in more severe cases and reversible spider angiomas and palmar erythema may occur but are unusual. Edema or ascites should suggest a more chronic disease process.

Hepatitis A usually resolves in 2 to 4 weeks, whereas hepatitis B commonly takes 2 to 3 months to resolve. Acute mortality from fulminant hepatitis is less than 1 per cent. Hepatitis A does not become chronic; however, 5 to 10 per cent of patients with hepatitis B become chronic carriers of the virus and many of these have either chronic persistent or chronic active hepatitis. It appears that as many as 25 per cent of patients with post-transfusion non-A, non-B hepatitis may develop chronic liver disease.

LABORATORY FINDINGS

Classically, the SGOT and SGPT are markedly elevated (values over 1000 units) and the serum alkaline phosphatase is minimally elevated. The serum bilirubin is usually less than 10 mg per dl. Marked icterus (bilirubin > 20 mg per dl) that is out of proportion to the degree of clinical illness or transaminase elevation should suggest associated hemolysis. Serum albumin, globulin, and prothrombin time are usually normal. A prolonged prothrombin time and low blood glucose levels may be ominous signs heralding hepatic failure.

EPIDEMIOLOGY AND SPECIFIC SEROLOGIC TESTS

Viral hepatitis usually develops in specific epidemiologic settings. A knowledge of the epidemiology of these viruses is therefore necessary for appropriate clinical suspicion and accurate diagnosis.

HEPATITIS A

Virus A infection has a short incubation period (25 to 40 days), is highly contagious, and often occurs in epidemics. Hepatitis A was described by Hippocrates as "infectious icterus" more than 2000 years ago. The disease has long been a major military problem. Napoleon's soldiers suffered from hepatitis, as did more than 70,000 union troops during the Civil War and innumerable soldiers in both the Korean War and the Vietnam conflict. There have been several epidemics related to ingestion of contaminated shellfish. Food and water-borne epidemics and epidemics originating in child care centers still occur on a regular basis.

The hepatitis A virus (HAV) has recently been isolated from stool of patients in the incubation period of hepatitis A. Assays of acute and convalescent sera for antibodies to HAV have been utilized to confirm hepatitis A viral infection in some research laboratories. Radioimmune assays for HAV have been developed and have been used to document HAV in stool, liver, spleen, lymph nodes, bile, and glomerular basement membranes. Using such assays, HAV is found in the stool as early as 14 days before the onset of symptoms. Maximal shedding of virus usually peaks at the onset of SGOT elevations, which is often when fever and chills are occurring at the onset of clinical illness. Shedding rapidly falls off and usually disappears or becomes insignificant a few days later, when SGOT peaks and jaundice occurs. This fits well with the epidemiologic observation that patients with hepatitis A are usually not infectious after the onset of jaundice. No chronic shedders of HAV have yet been found and the HAV does not appear to be a cause of chronic hepatitis or of post-transfusion hepatitis. Recently a radioimmune assay for IgM antibodies to the HAV has been developed that allows the diagnosis of hepatitis A infection from a single acute phase serum. It is likely that such an assay will be commercially available within the foreseeable future.

HEPATITIS B

Hepatitis B has an incubation period of 50 to 180 days and is classically transmitted by the parenteral route. Our understanding of hepatitis B has increased logarithmically since Blumberg's discovery of the Australia antigen. This antigen is a lipoprotein found on the surface of the hepatitis B virus, which is produced in great excess. It has been renamed hepatitis B surface antigen (HB_sAg). HB_sAg is a marker of both acute and chronic infections with the hepatitis B virus. Approximately 0.1 per cent of the

United States population are asymptomatic carriers of HB_sAg. In some parts of the world such as Southeast Asia as many as 10 per cent of the population are positive for HB_sAg and many have chronic hepatitis.

Antibody to the surface antigen (anti-HB_s) usually develops after recovery from hepatitis and is a marker of past infection. It affords some protection against infection and can be administered passively in either standard or hyperimmune globulin in an effort to protect individuals exposed to the hepatitis B virus. Other markers of hepatitis B infection are hepatitis B core antigen (HB_cAg), which is found in the nuclei of hepatocytes, and antibody to the core (anti-HB_c), which can be found in serum. E antigen and DNA polymerase are other markers of hepatitis B infection and appear to be associated with increased infectivity.

Hepatitis B is spread by sexual contact, and currently the majority of patients seen in the United States with hepatitis B are male homosexuals. Five per cent of male homosexuals are carriers of HB_sAg and 69 per cent have one or more serologic markers of past or present infection. Outbreaks of hepatitis B are common in hemodialysis and oncology units. Drug abusers that share needles also commonly develop hepatitis B. Medical and dental professionals are also at higher risk than the general population.

NON-A, NON-B HEPATITIS

Non-A, non-B hepatitis tends to occur in the same settings as hepatitis B. Because blood utilized for transfusion is screened for HB_sAg, post-transfusion hepatitis B has been virtually eliminated and 90 per cent of post-transfusion hepatitis in the United States today is caused by non-A, non-B hepatitis. Many of these cases progress to chronic active hepatitis. Features of hepatitis A, B, and non-A, non-B hepatitis are compared in Table 1.

PATHOLOGY

Liver biopsy is not usually required for diagnosis. Typical biopsy shows swollen hepatocytes (balloon cells). As cells degenerate, cytoplasm may stain dark red with eosin, and the nucleus becomes pyknotic or is extruded. These hyalinized cells are called acidophilic bodies or Councilman-like bodies. Inflammatory cells, predominantly mononuclear, accumulate in portal tracts and around central veins in areas from which hepatocytes have vanished.

Mild features of acute hepatitis associated with chronic inflammatory infiltration, predomi-

Table 1. *Comparison of Features of Viral Hepatitis*

	A	B	Non-A, Non-B
Agent identified	+	+	Not yet
Tissue culture	−	−	−
Susceptible animals	Marmoset Chimpanzee	Chimpanzee Rhesus monkey	Chimpanzee
Incubation period	15–40 days	50–180 days	Usually 6–7 weeks 2–20 week range
CLINICAL			
Onset	Abrupt	Often insidious	Abrupt or insidious
Prodrome fever	+	−	−
Arthritis	−	+	?
Course	Brief	Prolonged	Prolonged
LABORATORY			
IgM	++++	+	?
SGOT/GPT	Transient (1–3 wk)	Prolonged	Prolonged
HB_sAg	−	+	−
PROGNOSIS			
Mortality	0.2–0.4% (rare)	2–10%	(2–10%)
CAH, cirrhosis	−	+	+
Hepatoma	−	+	?
Polyarteritis nodosa	−	+	−
Renal	−	+	−
TRANSMISSION			
Food-borne	+	−	Not yet
Water-borne	+	−	Not yet
Shellfish related	+	−	Not yet
Primate handler	+	−	−
Parenteral inoculation	+	+	+
Transfusion	−	+	+
Hemodialysis related	−	+	+
Oral	+	+	Not yet
Vertical (maternal-fetal)	−	+	Not yet
Sporadic	+	+	+
Sexual transmission	+	+	+

nantly portal, may persist. If the limiting plate around the portal area remains intact (no piecemeal necrosis), if there is little or no fibrosis, and if the lobular architecture is preserved, this is called chronic persistent hepatitis. It is considered benign and requires no therapy. Alternatively, chronic inflammatory infiltration involving portal tracts may extend into the parenchyma, with piecemeal necrosis. Complete lobules or parts of adjacent lobules may be destroyed, with broad strands of collapsed reticulum "bridging" adjacent portal tracts. These changes have been termed chronic active hepatitis. In general, in acute viral hepatitis it is wise to postpone liver biopsy until liver functions have been abnormal for at least three months, because prior to this time a self-limited histologic picture identical to chronic active hepatitis may be seen.

DIFFERENTIAL DIAGNOSIS

Toxic Hepatitis. In all patients with evidence of hepatocellular damage (acute or chronic) the possibility that the liver cell abnormality is caused or aggravated by a reaction to a drug or toxin should be seriously considered. It is a wise policy to withdraw all but absolutely essential medications from the patient with hepatitis.

Some drugs are intrinsically toxic to the liver, while in other cases injury results from host idiosyncrasy. Intrinsically toxic substances such as carbon tetrachloride (CCl_4), poisonous mushrooms, or acetaminophen produce a predictable injury in everyone. The injury is dose related and reproducible. Host idiosyncrasy can result either from an allergic hypersensitivity (halothane, phenytoin, sulfonamide) or from a metabolic idiosyncrasy in which a toxic metabolite is produced (isoniazid). Hypersensitivity reactions are characterized by (1) low incidence of reaction; (2) dose independence; (3) injury after a fixed period of exposure (period of sensitization); (4) prompt recurrence on challenge; (5) accompanying systemic manifestations of rash, fever, and eosinophilia; and (6) tissue eosinophilia or granulomas.

Table 2.   *Common Drugs That Can Cause Hepatitis*

Drug	Type of Injury	Mechanism
ANTIBIOTICS		
Isoniazid (INH)	Cytotoxic	Metabolic idiosyncrasy
Sulfonamides	Cytotoxic, mixed	Hypersensitivity
Erythromycin estolate	Cholestatic	—
Tetracycline	Toxic steatosis	Intrinsically toxic
Nitrofurantoin	Chronic hepatitis	Hypersensitivity
	Cholestasis, mixed	
ANESTHETICS		
Halothane	Cytotoxic	Hypersensitivity
Methoxyflurane	Cytotoxic	Hypersensitivity
ANALGESICS, ANTIPYRETICS,		
ANTINFLAMMATORY AGENTS		
Acetaminophen	Cytotoxic	Intrinsically toxic
Salicylates	Cytotoxic	Intrinsically toxic
Phenylbutazone	Mixed	Hypersensitivity
		Intrinsically toxic
ANTIHYPERTENSIVES		
Alpha methyldopa	Mixed	Hypersensitivity
	Chronic active hepatitis	
HORMONES		
Oral contraceptives	Cholestatic and tumorigenic	Metabolic idiosyncrasy
Anabolic steroids	Cholestatic and tumorigenic	Metabolic idiosyncrasy
TRANQUILIZERS AND SEDATIVES		
Phenothiazine drugs	Cholestatic	—
Benzodiazepine drugs	Cholestatic	—
ANTIDEPRESSANTS		
Iproniazid	Cytotoxic	Metabolic idiosyncrasy
Tri-cycle compounds	Cholestatic, mixed	—
MISCELLANEOUS		
Phenytoin	Cytotoxic, mixed	Hypersensitivity
Quinidine	Mixed	Hypersensitivity

Drug hepatitis may be predominantly cytotoxic, closely mimicking viral hepatitis histologically. The SGOT is very high, while the alkaline phosphatase elevations are only modest. Isoniazid and halothane are good examples. Injury may also be in the form of toxic steatosis in which microvesicular fat is seen. Parenteral tetracycline causes this type of injury. Transaminases are not as high as with toxic necrosis or viral hepatitis. Some drugs such as chlorpromazine and anabolic steroids may produce cholestatic changes that may mimic obstructive jaundice more than hepatitis. Serum alkaline phosphatase is often markedly elevated in the presence of only minimal transaminase elevations. Some drugs produce a mixed cytotoxic-cholestatic picture and others such as alpha methyldopa and oxyphenisatin will clinically and histologically mimic chronic active hepatitis. Common drugs that can cause hepatitis are listed is Table 2.

ALCOHOLIC HEPATITIS

Alcoholic hepatitis, which is the most common form of toxic hepatitis, deserves special note. Alcoholic hepatitis, also referred to as alcoholic steatonecrosis, is an acute syndrome that results from severe and prolonged alcoholism. It is often but not always associated with malnutrition. Symptoms include weakness, anorexia, nausea, jaundice (60 per cent), fever (60 per cent), and ascites (50 per cent). Ninety per cent have hepatomegaly and 50 per cent have spider angiomata. Collateral veins and splenomegaly indicative of portal hypertension are frequently present. Patients with more severe cases may have asterixis and hepatic encephalopathy. Laboratory studies commonly reveal an anemia and a leukocytosis that at times may be marked. Serum bilirubin is elevated in 80 per cent of patients. The SGOT is almost always elevated; however, it is less than 300 units in over 95 per cent of patients. SGPT abnormalities are almost always less prominent and rarely exceed 100 units. A ratio of SGOT to SGPT in excess of 2:1 should always raise the clinical suspicion of alcohol-induced liver injury. Other common laboratory abnormalities include alkaline phosphatase elevation usually less than three times normal values, depressed serum albumin, elevated serum globulin, and prolonged prothrombin time.

OTHER CAUSES OF HEPATOCELLULAR INJURY

A variety of other entities can mimic either acute or chronic hepatitis. Many of these conditions are either reactions to infections or related to ischemia or both. Bacterial infections ranging from leptospirosis to gram-negative sepsis, parasitic infections (malaria, *Entamoeba histolytica*, and toxoplasmosis), and rickettsial infections (Q fever and typhus) can all produce hepatocellular injury. Ischemic changes leading to centrolobular necrosis can also mimic hepatitis. They can be produced by severe congestive heart failure or by hypotensive or anoxic episodes. It is important to consider these possibilities in the appropriate clinical setting.

CIRRHOSIS OF THE LIVER

By THOMAS W. KIERNAN, M.D.,
and ARUN SAMANTA, M.D.

East Orange, New Jersey

The liver architecture in cirrhosis is, by definition, distorted by parenchymal nodules separated by fibrous bands. The clinical manifestations of this disease are partly due to the etiologic mechanisms that ultimately result in cirrhosis. However, disordered hepatocyte function due to these disorders and the deranged hepatic hemodynamics that result from lobular distortion are the main reasons for the general nonspecific symptoms and signs characteristic of cirrhosis.

PATHOGENESIS

Cirrhosis always results from a precursor lesion characterized by liver cell necrosis and often leukocyte infiltration. A variety of causes are responsible (Table 1). Alcoholic hepatitis, for example, results in cirrhosis in nearly one third of those afflicted. The direct effect of ethanol or acetaldehyde (its first metabolite) and/or cell-mediated immune mechanisms reactive to alcoholic hyaline have been implicated in the pathogenesis of this hepatitis. Sensitized lymphocytes to the hyaline appear to elaborate a fibrogenic factor, resultant in the increased fibrogenic activity of hepatic fibroblasts. These cells deposit collagen in areas of injury, subsequently leading to hepatic fibrosis (centrilobular) and cirrhosis.

In chronic active hepatitis, continued injury around the limiting plate of the portal triad leads to fibrosis in portal-portal and portal-central areas of the hepatic lobule. A cell-mediated immune response to liver specific

Table 1. *Etiologic Disorders in Cirrhosis*

Alcoholic hepatitis

Chronic active hepatitis
  1. Hepatitis virus, type B
  2. Hepatitis virus, type non-A, non-B
  3. Idiopathic

Drug-induced hepatitis
  1. Predictable agents, e.g., methotrexate
  2. Unpredictable agents, e.g., halothane

Congestive cirrhosis
  1. Congestive heart failure
  2. Budd-Chiari syndrome
  3. Venoclusive hepatitic venous disease
  4. Sickle cell disease

Secondary biliary cirrhosis (i.e., chronic biliary tract obstruction)

Incomplete biliary cirrhosis following cystic fibrosis

Congenital syphilis

Hereditary hemorrhagic telangiectasia

Inborn errors of metabolism
  1. Iron storage disease
  2. Wilson's disease (copper storage disease)
  3. Type IV glycogen storage disease
  4. Alpha-1-antitrypsin deficiency
  5. Galactosemia
  6. Tyrosinosis
  7. Hereditary fructose intolerance
  8. Thalassemia
  9. Hypermethioninemia

Unknown causes
  1. Primary biliary cirrhosis
  2. Cryptogenic cirrhosis
  3. Sarcoid cirrhosis
  4. Indian childhood cirrhosis

Intestinal bypass surgery

Table 2. *Drugs Associated with Cirrhosis*

Cinchophen (and derivatives)
Phenylbutazone
Arsenicals
Methotrexate
6-mercaptopurine
Chlorpromazine
Oxyphenisatin
Monoamine oxidase inhibitors
Halothane

lipoprotein may be responsible for continued liver cell necrosis and subsequent fibrosis. Common causes of chronic hepatitis include the hepatitis viruses type B and type non-A, non-B.

Other hepatic disorders characterized by cirrhosis, and for which the exact mechanisms of injury are less clear, include cryptogenic cirrhosis, primary biliary cirrhosis, Indian childhood cirrhosis, and sarcoid cirrhosis.

Congestive cirrhosis has resulted from prolonged congestive heart failure, diseases of the hepatic veins (Budd-Chiari and veno-occlusive disease), and sickle cell disease. Secondary biliary cirrhosis is due to prolonged obstruction of the extrahepatic biliary ducts. Cystic fibrosis has been associated with cirrhosis because of bile ductular obstruction by mucus. Cirrhosis may characterize congenital syphilis or hereditary hemorrhagic telangiectasia.

Drugs and chemicals have induced cirrhosis. Cirrhosis may follow use of some drugs predictably (e.g., methotrexate). Halothane and monaminoxidase inhibitors are some common drugs that commonly and unpredictably result in cirrhosis (Table 2).

Abnormalities of inborn metabolism are clearly implicated in cirrhosis. Wilson's disease (copper storage) and iron overload (hemochromatosis) are examples. Galactosemia, type IV glycogen storage disease, tyrosinosis, hereditary fructose intolerance, alpha-1 antitrypsin deficiency, hypermethioninemia, and thalassemia are others. Intestinal bypass surgery for obesity commonly leads to fatty liver degeneration; but it may also occasionally lead to cirrhosis. The list of causes is obviously long and broadly based. However, a careful clinical understanding of these predisposing disorders is essential, since treatment is directed at the mechanism leading to cirrhosis.

NOMENCLATURE

The varieties of cirrhosis have been classified using anatomic description or specific cause. The liver has been described anatomically using the terms macronodular (when nodules are generally larger than 1 cm in diameter), micronodular (when nodules are generally smaller) and mixed nodular. Many specific disorders may, however, be manifested by one or more of these three anatomic types. Attempts at defining cirrhosis according to cause have led to long lists of names for specific entities. Cirrhosis due to viral hepatitis type B, for example, has been called posthepatitic cirrhosis, postcollapse cirrhosis, and postnecrotic cirrhosis, among other names. The Fogarty International Congress on Nomenclature of Diseases of the Liver and Biliary Tract (1975) has advocated defining each cirrhotic entity according to its specific cause (Table 1).

CLINICAL ASPECT

History. Constitutional symptoms caused by cirrhosis are usually reflective of abnormal liver cell function. Nonspecific entities such as malaise, fatigue, lethargy, anorexia, and nausea are common. Other symptoms reflect the activity of concomitant inflammation. Fever, chills, and abdominal pain are examples. Other more specific symptoms may result from liver cell dysfunction: jaundice, pruritus, diarrhea, dark urine, and light acholic stools. Hematemesis, melena, and abdominal swelling (ascites) may be associated with aberrant hepatic hemodynamics attendant on cirrhosis.

Specific symptoms may reflect the unique clinical entity leading to cirrhosis. Wilson's disease, for example, may present with its neurologic symptoms. Iron storage disease may have symptoms related to the complicating diabetes mellitus or cardiomyopathy. An accurate knowledge of the extrahepatic manifestations of the many preceding disorders leading to cirrhosis is helpful (Table 3).

The factors of age and sex may direct the clinician's attention to specific causes. Wilson's disease, for example, is more commonly symptomatic during adolescence, whereas primary biliary cirrhosis is characteristically a disease of middle-aged women.

Alcohol consumption and medication use are important historical clues. Awareness of the patient's occupation and his responsibilities may lead to discovery of toxin or chemical exposures (e.g., a person working in the rubber industry may be exposed to the hepatotoxin vinyl chloride).

A family history of liver disease is common in Wilson's disease and iron storage disease. A history of hepatitis or exposure to parenterally

Table 3. Clinical Clues to Etiology of Cirrhosis*

Etiology	History	Physical	Investigations†
Alcoholic hepatitis	Alcohol consumption	Large parotids; myopathy; Dupuytren's contracture; testicular atrophy; neuropathy	SGOT > SGPT; polymorphonuclear leukocytosis
Chronic active hepatitis	Illicit drugs; transfusions; previous acute hepatitis	Multi-organ involvement: rash, arthritis, thyroiditis, colitis, etc. Endocrine: hypercorticism, hirsutism	Positive HB$_S$Ag; elevated gamma globulin
Primary biliary cirrhosis	Female sex; middle age; pruritus before icterus	Xanthomata; CRST syndrome; finger clubbing	Elevated IgM; antimitochondrial antibody
Iron storage disease	Positive family history	Signs of pseudogout; cardiomyopathy; diabetes; bronze skin; testicular atrophy	Elevated serum ferritin
Wilson's disease	Family history of liver or neurologic disease; childhood or adolescence onset	Kayser-Fleischer rings; osteochondritis dessicans; CNS and basal ganglia disorder	Low serum ceruloplasmin
Cryptogenic cirrhosis	Affects mostly women	Associated diseases: arthritis, thyroiditis, nephritis, etc.	Elevated gamma globulin; positive anti-nuclear antibodies

*Partial assessment of selected etiologies.
†Excluding biopsy.

administered illicit drugs might uncover the cause for chronic hepatitis. Arthralgia, and a history of hives, hematuria, or rash may suggest chronic active hepatitis.

Patients with cirrhosis, on occasion, are totally asymptomatic. The clinician must have a high index of suspicion in order to uncover it.

Physical Examination. The clinician has three goals in his physical examination of the patient with cirrhosis: (1) to define the character of the liver, (2) to identify its nonspecific complications, and (3) to identify the extrahepatic manifestations of its causative mechanisms.

The cirrhotic liver is frequently enlarged because of concomitant progressive hepatocellular necrosis and degeneration, reactive edema, and leukocytic infiltration. When the causative disorder has become quiescent or arrested (naturally or through definitive treatment), liver size will decrease. (Usual liver size in the adult is defined by percussion, with relative dullness demarcating the upper and lower borders of the liver. Percussion is performed in the right midclavicular line [RMCL] and midsternal line [MSL]. The normal sizes are 15±2 cm RMCL and 4±2 cm MSL.) The cirrhotic liver has a fine to grossly nodular surface. This latter characteristic may not be well elicited in obese patients or in patients with large ascites. A bruit may be heard over the liver. It is best heard just to the right of the xiphoid process. Alcoholic hepatitis, hepatocellular carcinoma, and arteriovenous fistulas may also be associated with this sign.

Extrahepatic findings owing to cirrhosis involve many systems. Jaundice may be noted on careful inspection of the conjunctivae, sclerae, underside of the tongue, soft palate, and skin. Gynecomastia, facial hair loss, a female escutcheon, and testicular atrophy are due in part to abnormalities in sex hormone metabolism. Peripheral cyanosis, clubbing, abdominal collateral veins, palmar erythema, arterial spider veins, and tachycardia are due to disordered pulmonary, splanchnic, and cardiovascular hemodynamics. Peripheral edema and ascites (characterized by flank bulging, shifting dullness, or a fluid wave) demonstrate disordered splanchnic hemodynamics and abnormal sodium and water clearance. Acholic stools may be due to biliary duct gallstones. Melena or a bloody nasogastric aspirate may reflect bleeding esophageal varices. Altered mentation, asterixis, lethargy, stupor, and coma characterize portasystemic encephalopathy. White nailbeds seem to reflect low serum albumin levels.

Specific attention to the physical clues for the underlying mechanisms for cirrhosis is essential. Kayser-Fleischer corneal rings, a grossly flapping tremor, and a spastic gait should alert the clinician to Wilson's disease. The other entities causing cirrhosis can be identified similarly by examining the patient for specific telltale signs suggestive of the diseases (Table 3).

LABORATORY PROFILES

Biochemical Tests. Enzyme assays such as SGOT (aspartate aminotransferase) or SGPT (alanine aminotransferase) are nonspecific assays of cellular injury. Alkaline phosphatases may vary from normal to markedly abnormal (twofold to sevenfold elevation) in the absence of biliary obstruction. This test suffers, however, by its lack of hepatic specificity. Serum protein determinations demonstrate ordinarily a high gamma globulin and a normal or low serum albumin. Specific abnormalities of immunoglobulins may be helpful in primary biliary cirrhosis, in which a marked elevation of IgM is noted. Specific tests reflective of collagen turnover, such as urinary hydroxyproline levels, are too unreliable to be of assistance. Serum bile acids (fasting or 2-hour postprandial levels) and indocyanine green dye clearance may assist the clinician when biochemical tests are equivocally abnormal and cellular function is to be assessed. Serum cholesterol levels are high in primary biliary cirrhosis and obstructive biliary disease. These findings are also too nonspecific to be very useful. Ceruloplasmin levels are low in Wilson's disease. Ferritin levels are elevated in iron storage disease.

Serologic Tests. Serologic tests are helpful only in defining causative mechanisms of cirrhosis. Specific tests for hepatitis B surface antigen and alcoholic hyaline are useful for defining specific entities. Cellular (organelle-specific) antibodies, like smooth muscle and antinuclear antibodies, are noted in chronic active hepatitis, but none are pathognomonic. An antimitochondrial antibody is found in 90 per cent of patients with primary biliary cirrhosis, although it may be found in chronic active hepatitis and obstructive biliary disease less commonly.

LIVER BIOPSY

Liver biopsy is required for the definitive diagnosis of cirrhosis. Blind percutaneous biopsies with the Menghini needle are frequently misleading because of shattered biopsy specimens. Better samples are cut with the Vim-Silverman needle. Random sampling error may prevent the pathologist from diagnosing cirrhosis in 10 per cent of patients. Specific biopsy can be done incidentally during laparotomy for other conditions, or with the assistance of the peritoneoscope. Regenerative nodules or pseudolobules or both characterize cirrhosis. Specific stains for iron, copper, viral antigens, and cellular inclusions may assist in defining the cause.

RADIOLOGY

Routine radiologic procedures are usually not of benefit in the evaluation of the cirrhotic liver (see Complications).

RADIONUCLIDE SCANNING

Liver scanning with technetium 99m sulfur colloid shows a diffuse patchy uptake over the liver, which is often difficult to distinguish from multiple small defects of the liver. Usually the spleen is notably enlarged. Uptake of hepatic-bypassed colloid is noted in the vertebral spine.

HEMATOLOGY

Peripheral smears may demonstrate microcytic, normocytic, or macrocytic red cells. Iron deficiency may characterize the alcoholic who has recurrent gastrointestinal bleeding. Depleted folic acid stores in alcoholic cirrhosis may result in a macrocytic anemia with megaloblastic changes in the bone marrow. Ringed sideroblasts may be seen on occasion.

Macrocytes and "spur" cells may also be noted on a blood smear. Disordered cholesterol-lecithin relationships in the red cell stroma are accountable. At times hemolytic anemia may result because of high ratio of red cell cholesterol to lecithin. Hemolytic anemia has been noted for other reasons in Wilson's disease and primary biliary cirrhosis.

Pancytopenia may be a reflection of hypersplenism, the effect of iron or folate deficiencies, or the direct effect of alcohol.

Cirrhotic patients are prone to ecchymoses and bleeding. Impaired protein synthesis results in decreased levels of Factors II, V, VII, IX, and X. Diminished platelet counts may be due to hypersplenism or the effects of alcohol. Fibrin split products are elevated in the blood of cirrhotics because of impaired extraction by the liver. Clinical coagulopathy caused by these latter products is often not clinically apparent. Cirrhotic ascites has been shown to have elevated levels. The displacement of this fluid into the systemic circulation through a peritoneo-jugular surgical shunt, however, may result in increased systemic levels leading to disseminated intravascular coagulopathy.

URINALYSIS

Urinalysis is not ordinarily abnormal in cirrhotics. One third may have a "proximal" renal tubular acidosis with a persistently alkaline urine pH. Urine potassium and calcium levels may be elevated in this condition.

COMPLICATIONS

Jaundice in cirrhosis is ordinarily due to impaired hepatocellular function. Cirrhotics are prone to pigmented (calcium bilirubinate) stones, which may cause biliary obstruction. Ultrasound of the gallbladder and biliary tract and a flat plate of the abdomen may be helpful screening techniques. Often a careful evaluation using percutaneous transhepatic cholangiography or endoscopic retrograde cholangiopancreatography is indicated. Alteration in bile composition may also lead to steatorrhea in cirrhosis.

Gastrointestinal bleeding in a cirrhotic patient is commonly due to bleeding esophageal varices. In alcoholic cirrhotics acute gastritis, peptic ulcer, esophagitis, and esophageal mucosal tears need to be considered. Early upper gastrointestinal fiberoptic endoscopy or celiac angiography or both may help to define the bleeding lesion. Hepatic vein cannulation may be helpful afterward in assessing portal hypertension. The wedge pressure is frequently a reflection of portal pressure in patients with postsinusoidal portal hypertension. Direct cannulation of the portal vein by umbilical catheterization is feasible for this evaluation in some large centers. Direct portography can then be carried out.

Ascites is characteristic of severe cirrhosis. Peritoneal fluid should be routinely assessed for bacteria, mycobacteria, fungi, and neoplastic cells. The fluid is ordinarily transudative (specific gravity less than 1.015 and fluid protein less than 2.5 grams per dl [100 ml]). In 10 per cent of patients the fluid may be exudative. Peritoneoscopy with peritoneal biopsy may be indicated for fluid of uncertain origin.

Portasystemic encephalopathy is characterized in cirrhosis by a disordered mentation subsequently evolving into stupor and coma. Asterixis is noted in one phase only of the staging of this problem. Hepatic fetor is irregularly present. A careful evaluation for an inciting cause such as infection, gastrointestinal bleeding, use of sedatives, or hypokalemia must be made for definitive treatment. Treatment of the underlying causes of the liver disease is also pertinent. Hypophosphatemia may aggravate this disorder.

Functional failure of the kidneys can be seen in cirrhosis. Sodium retention may be noted in the low daily output of urine sodium. As free water clearance becomes further impaired, urine volume and serum sodium decrease, as creatinine and blood urea nitrogen (BUN) progressively rise. When kidney failure is due to hepatocellular disease alone, the prognosis is poor. When an aggravating problem such as a treatable infection can be defined, the prognosis is still poor, but less grave.

Serum electrolyte patterns are commonly abnormal in cirrhosis. Impaired sodium and free water clearance may lead to hyponatremia. Hypokalemia is a complication of the secondary elevations of aldosterone. Magnesium and zinc depletion syndromes may result from an increased clearance of these electrolytes before functional renal failure ensues.

Cirrhosis may lead to disordered systemic as well as splanchnic hemodynamics. Cirrhosis results in intrapulmonary shunts leading to low arterial PO_2. A decrease in perhipheral resistance may lead to resting tachycardia and low systolic and a wide pulse pressure. High output cardiac failure may complicate cirrhosis, especially in patients undergoing portasystemic shunts.

Osteomalacia may complicate primary biliary cirrhosis. In the same patients an alteration in 25 hydroxylation of vitamin D_3 may play a part, but malabsorption of vitamin D may occur because of disordered bile composition. Vitamin A deficiency may be noted at times.

Cirrhotic patients are prone to systemic bacterial infections. Deranged humoral and cell-mediated immune responses are the likely causes. Infection may result in fever or hypothermia. Coliform bacteria, pneumococci, and *M. tuberculosis* are common agents. Spontaneous septicemia and peritonitis are two complications carrying a grave prognosis.

The hepatic biotransformation of many drugs is impaired in cirrhosis, as a result of decreased functional parenchymal mass and intrahepatic shunting of splanchnic blood bypassing the liver cell. Toxic levels of drugs, such as theophylline and lidocaine, can occur with routine dosage. The central nervous system is also peculiarly sensitive to the depressant effects of sedatives, narcotics, and analgesics.

Whenever a cirrhotic patient's condition begins to deteriorate (e.g., weight loss, apathy, progressive jaundice), the clinician should be suspicious of an underlying hepatocellular carcinoma. This neoplasm has been described in patients with cirrhosis owing to hemochromatosis, chronic active hepatitis, and alcoholism. Hypercalcemia, inappropriate erythrocytosis, and hypoglycemia are some of the extraheptic manifestations of this cancer that should raise the clinician's index of suspicion. Hepatic arteriography may allow a vascular blush to demarcate this lesion.

DISEASES OF THE GALLBLADDER AND BILIARY TRACT

By ROBERT J. BOLT, M.D.

Sacramento, California

INTRODUCTION

Table 1 lists the rather limited spectrum of clinical syndromes that are seen in patients with gallbladder or biliary tract disease or both. The clinician's first objective is to recognize, on the basis of the patient's complaints and physical findings, whether he is dealing with cholecystitis (gallbladder inflammation), cholangitis (inflammation of the biliary tree), obstruction within the ducts (cystic duct or common duct) of the biliary tree, with hematobilia, or with a combination of these.

Cholecystitis is suggested when fever, leukocytosis, epigastric pain, nausea and/or vomiting and right upper quadrant tenderness are present. The condition may be secondary to obstruction (stones, sclerosis, neoplasm, etc.) within the ducts or biliary tract or it may be primary (acalculous) such as that seen in systemic infection (typhoid fever) or vascular insufficiency (polyarteritis nodosum).

Cholangitis is suggested if any or all of the symptoms just mentioned are accompanied by shaking chills, hypotension, onset of jaundice, tender palpable liver, and even shock.

Obstruction is heralded by biliary colic and the onset of jaundice.

Hematobilia manifests itself by occult bleeding in stools when it is mild or frank melena in more severe cases. The underlying cause of hematobilia is usually neoplasia.

The clinician's second objective is to determine the underlying anatomic defect or pathologic lesion causing the symptoms. Table 2 lists the abnormalities that usually result in clinical symptoms. Table 3 lists abnormalities of the gallbladder that, in the absence of complications, cause no symptoms or, at best, may be associated with nonspecific symptoms. These nonspecific symptoms, although traditionally accepted as a part of gallbladder disease, are seen as often in the absence of gallbladder abnormalities as they are in the presence of disease.

It must be emphasized that many, perhaps most, abnormalities of the gallbladder exist without causing *disease* (symptoms). It is for this reason that Table 4 is divided into two sections: section A, nonspecific (nondefinitive) symptoms and section B, definitive symptoms. This differentiation requires emphasis, since a significant number of investigative studies are carried out on the basis of nonspecific symptoms. When abnormalities are discovered, the clinician tends to equate the abnormality found with disease of which the patient complains. Unfortunately, cholecystectomy rarely results in ablation of symptoms in these situations, particularly if the strong placebo effect of surgery is taken into account. This is not unique to gallbladder abnormalities but, for reasons unknown, it has not been accorded the same prominence as in other parts of the gastrointestinal tract. For example, clinicians are well aware that many persons have diverticulosis without diverticulitis, and many have hiatal hernias without significant regurgitation or esophagitis or both. In the same manner gallbladder abnormalities listed in Table 3 commonly exist in the absence of such factors as cholecystitis and obstruction of the biliary tree. Stated differently, a significant number of patients, perhaps a majority, with gallstones, cholecystoses, or congenital abnormalities of the gallbladder have no symptoms at all or nonspecific symptoms that will not be relieved by operative intervention (Table 4–A). Thus, the clinician in making these diagnoses is diagnosing an abnormality but not a disease.

As stated, specific symptoms and signs of gallbladder or biliary tract disease (Table 4–B, C) result from either inflammation (cholecystitis, cholangitis) or obstruction (cystic duct, common duct, biliary radicals) or both. Rarely, gastrointestinal bleeding may result from erosions or ulcer within the gallbladder or biliary tree.

Table 1. *Clinical Syndromes of Patients with Gallbladder or Biliary Tract Disease*

I. Gallbladder
  A. Cholecystitis, acute
    1. Acalculous
    2. Calculous
    3. Unique types
      a. Emphysematous
      b. Hydrops
      c. Empyema
  B. Cholecystitis, chronic
    1. Acalculous
    2. Calculous
II. Biliary Tract
  A. Cholangitis
    1. Acute
    2. Chronic
  B. Obstructive
  C. Hematobilia

Table 2. *Abnormalities of Gallbladder and Biliary Tract Usually Resulting in Symptoms*

I. Biliary Tract
   A. Impacted stones in cystic duct, common duct, or biliary tree
   B. Sclerosis of duct system–localized or diffuse
   C. Neoplasia of gallbladder, biliary ducts, or biliary tract
   D. Congenital abnormalities of ductule system
II. Gallbladder
   1. Systemic infections resulting in inflammation of wall
   2. Vascular insufficiency and necrosis of wall

Most commonly, bleeding is the result of neoplasm. In diagnosing, the clinician must separate gallbladder *abnormalities* from gallbladder and biliary tract *disease*. The first are asymptomatic; the second are symptomatic. Subsequent discussion in this article concerns in more detail the diagnosis of and determination of the basic lesion causing one of the three previously mentioned syndromes, that is, cholecystitis, cholangitis, or obstruction of the biliary tree.

ACUTE CHOLECYSTITIS WITHOUT JAUNDICE

Inflammation of the gallbladder may result from obstruction of the cystic duct, most commonly by stones, and secondary infection or infection of the gallbladder associated with such systemic disease as typhoid fever. It may also occur as a result of decreased blood supply to the gallbladder (vasculitis; e.g., polyarteritis nodosum). In the absence of common duct or biliary tract involvement, jaundice does not occur. Symptoms in an acute case consist of varying combinations of epigastric pain — biliary colic, fever, nausea, and vomiting. Vomiting has been said to occur only in common duct obstruction but in my experience it is common in cholecystitis of any type. The syndrome of epigastric pain and biliary colic is

Table 3. *Abnormalities of Gallbladder without Definitive Symptoms (no dis-ease) or with Nonspecific Symptoms*

1. Uncomplicated cholelithiasis
2. Uncomplicated cholecystoses
   a. Cholesterolosis (strawberry gallbladder)
   b. Adenomyomatosis (intramural diverticulosis)
      (1) Diffuse
      (2) Annular
      (3) Localized
3. Congenital
   a. Agenesis
   b. Double
   c. Displaced
   d. Shape abnormalities

Table 4. *Symptoms and Signs of Gallbladder or Biliary Tract Disease*

A. Nonspecific symptoms
   1. Fat intolerance
   2. Indigestion
   3. Pyrosis, flatulence
B. Definitive symptoms
   1. Epigastric pain–biliary colic
   2. Nausea and vomiting
   3. Chills/fever
   4. Pruritus
   5. Jaundice–urine and stool color changes
   6. Weight loss
C. Signs
   1. Tenderness (RUQ)
   2. Palpable liver
   3. Jaundice
   4. Rebound and rigidity
   5. Palpable gallbladder

strongly suggestive of gallbladder disease, particularly when cystic duct obstruction is present. Since it is highly specific, it must be clearly defined. Table 5 enumerates its characteristics.

The term "colic" is, unfortunately, firmly established by tradition, although in the true sense of the word the pain is not "colicky." Fever in the acute stage is highly variable: in the acalculous type, as in typhoid fever and periarteritis nodosum, it predominates. In the calculous group, obstruction of the cystic duct may result in biliary colic as the predominant symptom and fever may be absent to minimal. Physical examination in the acute stage reveals an anxious patient in obvious pain. Abdominal examination shows moderate to marked right upper quadrant tenderness even though the patient may complain of epigastric pain. Rebound and rigidity are absent unless perforation is impending or has already occurred.

Laboratory findings are helpful in a negative sense. They are normal except for variable elevation of the white blood cell count and moderate left shift depending on the degree of infection and the underlying cause (e.g., stone in duct, systemic infection, or vasculitis). Use of the investigative methods necessary to confirm

Table 5. *Biliary "Colic"*

1. Onset is abrupt.
2. Onset is anytime of night or day but characteristically from midnight to 6 A.M.
3. The pain is not "colicky" but reaches a peak rapidly and plateaus.
4. Pain typically lasts from 6 to 12 hours.
5. Pain begins in the epigastrium, then becomes localized to the right upper quadrant with referral to the scapula.
6. Associated symptoms are nausea usually, and vomiting, particularly if common duct obstruction occurs.

the diagnosis and elucidate the basic cause has changed in recent years with the development of intravenous cholangiography, intravenous technetium 99m pyridoxilidine glutamate (^{99m}Tc PG), ultrasound, and computerized axial tomography. Choice of tests varies with the clinical situation, particularly the urgency and the presence of jaundice. In an acute cholecystitis without jaundice the following tests should be selected in the indicated order:

1. Plain film of abdomen
2. Intravenous cholangiography (dye or ^{99m}Tc PG)
3. Ultrasound
4. Computerized tomography
5. Oral cholecystography

Step one should always be a plain film of the abdomen. Approximately 10 to 15 per cent of gallstones are radiopaque and can be visualized. Again one must be cautious in attaching a causal relationship when stones are visualized on a plain film since a significant number of asymptomatic persons harbor stones (10 to 15 per cent whites, 5 to 10 per cent blacks, 70 to 80 per cent native Americans). Their presence may be coincidental rather than causal. Occasionally an enlarged gallbladder (hydrops, empyema) may be demonstrated. On rare occasions emphysematous cholecystitis may be diagnosed on the basis of gas visualized within the gallbladder wall.

Oral cholecystography is usually not possible in the acute situation. Many patients are too nauseated to tolerate the contrast material. Moreover, the situation frequently demands more rapid clarification than can be obtained with oral cholecystogram. Thus, intravenous cholangiography is the most commonly ordered second test. It presents the liver with a large amount of dye in a short period of time. The dye is rapidly excreted by the liver, filling the gallbladder and bile ducts. Normally the entire extrahepatic biliary tree is visualized, especially when tomography is used. Cholangiography carries some risk. Hepatic damage and acute renal failure owing to tubular necrosis have been reported. Less serious reactions include nausea, vomiting, and fall in blood pressure. Slow injection may prevent or alleviate these complications. Ioglycamide (Biligram) is reported to result in fewer toxic reactions than iodipamide (Biligrafin). Similarly, drip infusion rather than bolus injection is preferable. Intravenous ^{99m}Tc PG has the same indication and interpretation as intravenous dye administration. It is particularly useful when dye hypersensitivity is suspected. Because of its cost, its use is not advised as a routine alternative to the use of contrast media. In both these procedures a normally visualizing gallbladder virtually

rules out acute cholecystitis. A well visualizing common duct and nonvisualizing gallbladder, on the other hand, is virtually pathognomonic of cystic duct obstruction. If neither gallbladder nor common duct is visible, the cause may be other than acute cholecystitis.

Summary. When dealing with the possibility of acute cholecystitis without common duct obstruction, appropriate values assigned to the patient's symptoms, signs found on physical examination, laboratory values, and intelligent interpretation of findings on plain film and intravenous cholangiography will establish the diagnosis in the majority of cases. Other tests such as gray-scale ultrasound, computer-assisted tomography, and biliary drainage are rarely necessary. The latter is of more use in chronic cholecystitis without jaundice and will be discussed under that topic. Invasive methods should never be necessary to establish the diagnosis of acute cholecystitis in the absence of jaundice. Thus ultrasound and tomography are the only potentially useful procedures if the diagnosis remains unclear. Gray-scale ultrasonography may be helpful but its diagnostic accuracy is variable and is reported to be in the range of 82 per cent by Mosley. Infusion tomography appears to have the most promise but is rarely necessary in the nonjaundiced patient. It is discussed under acute cholecystitis with jaundice.

CHRONIC CHOLECYSTITIS WITHOUT JAUNDICE

Again we are concerned with those patients having symptoms and signs suggestive of gallbladder disease without common duct or biliary tract obstruction: that is, without jaundice. The clinical picture here is one of recurrent episodes of acute cholecystitis, usually consisting of episodes of short duration and relatively mild attacks with spontaneous recovery. Physical findings during any given episode are similar to those described under acute cholecystitis but somewhat less obvious. Between attacks patients are usually free of symptoms and in good health. Diagnosis is dependent on demonstration of gallbladder stones in the presence of rather typical clinical symptoms. The stones may be demonstrated again by plain film as with acute cholecystitis. The finding of a nonfunctioning gallbladder or a gallbladder containing stones on oral cholecystography in the presence of typical, recurrent symptoms is diagnostic. In contrast to the urgency of dealing with acute cholecystitis, there is, under usual circumstances, no urgency in the chronic cholecystitis group. Since oral cholecystography is associated with less risk and visualizes the gallbladder stones better than intravenous cholangiography, it is traditional under ordinary circumstances to utilize this procedure as the initial method of investigation following the plain film of the abdomen. This assumes:

1. No urgency
2. Absence of jaundice
3. Absence of nausea and vomiting
4. Intact absorptive mechanisms (no diarrhea, malabsorption, or pancreatic disease)
5. Normal liver function or minimal dysfunction
6. A cooperative patient

Drugs presently used for oral cholecystography are all substituted triiodobenzoic acid compounds. Those excreted by the liver and used to evaluate the gallbladder are of high molecular weight and have at least one side chain at the 5 position of the benzene ring. They are moderately lipid-soluble and when absorbed from the small bowel become tightly bound to plasma albumin and are transported to the liver. Within the liver they are conjugated with glycuronic acid, which renders them water-soluble, and then are excreted into the biliary tree. When given orally they are administered 12 hours before radiograms are taken and fatty foods are prohibited to prevent emptying of the gallbladder. Normally, the gallbladder mucosa is impermeable to the drug. Absorption does not occur through the gallbladder mucosa and thus visualization of the gallbladder results.

If one knows that the patient took the tablets but the gallbladder fails to visualize, there is 95 per cent certainty that either the gallbladder is inflamed or the cystic duct is blocked or both. Normal visualization without demonstration of stones carries the similar probability, that is, 95 per cent chance that the gallbladder is normal.

A problem not uncommonly faced is the presence of typical symptoms (particularly biliary colic) and normal gallbladder visualization on oral cholecystography. A number of additional steps have been suggested in this situation. Most are controversial at best. Use of gray-scale ultrasonography and tomography may demonstrate sludge or small stones not visualized by oral cholangiography. Intravenous cholangiography is generally not helpful in this situation, being less reliable than the oral cholecystogram in demonstrating gallbladder stones. Examination of bile for cholesterol crystals or pigment casts or both before and after cholecystokinin stimulation may be helpful. In my experience and in the experience of the majority of radiologists, timed gallbladder emptying of orally administered contrast media is highly variable and does not lend itself to accurate quantitative measurement or clear differentiation of the abnormal from the normal. Inflammation of the gallbladder wall is only one of multiple factors determining the rate of gallbladder emptying. Factors include:

1. Compliance of gallbladder wall
2. Rate of gastric emptying*
3. Sensitivity of the duodenal receptors*
4. Quantitation of CCK output from the duodenum*
5. Sensitivity of gallbladder receptors (evidence for increased CCK but delayed gallbladder response in diabetics, for example)
6. The degree of enterohepatic circulation
7. Abnormalities of gallbladder, cystic, or common duct sphincter mechanisms
8. Sphincter of Oddi responsiveness

Summary. The diagnosis of chronic cholecystitis relies heavily on the presence of typical symptoms and signs with confirmation by plain film of the abdomen or oral cholecystography or both. When such radiologic confirmation is lacking, one can resort to ultrasound or tomography or both of the abdomen, biliary drainage, and/or evaluation of motor activity of the gallbladder. The latter is perhaps the least reliable as a confirmatory test. When symptoms and signs are typical but confirmation is totally lacking, the likelihood of gallbladder disease is remote. The diagnosis in reported cases has generally been based on typical symptoms and repeated normal oral cholecystograms without additional testing. How much clarification the additional tests described provide is undetermined at this time.

CHOLANGITIS OR OBSTRUCTIVE JAUNDICE OR BOTH

Diseases of the gallbladder or biliary tree or both, as indicated in the introductory portion of this article, manifest themselves in any one or combination of the following: cholecystitis, cholangitis, jaundice, or bleeding (hematobilia). Most cases of cholecystitis present without jaundice (without obstruction of the common duct). On the other hand, cholangitis is more commonly associated with obstruction of the biliary tree and hence jaundice. Cholangitis, in the acute form, is a serious complication. Shaking chills are common and hypotension and shock may follow. In the aged, clouding of the sensorium and disorientation are common.

Just as acute or chronic cholecystitis commonly exists without jaundice, obstruction and jaundice may exist without either cholecystitis or cholangitis. Thus, symptoms in obstructive

---

*If fat meal or oil is used.

jaundice vary with the presence or absence of "-itis" — either cholecystitis or cholangitis. Causes of obstruction of the biliary tree include stones, neoplasms, sclerosis, or congenital anomalies of the biliary tract such as hypoplasia or aplasia. Symptoms depend on the site of obstruction, completeness of obstruction, the rapidity of onset, and whether infection and inflammation of the gallbladder or biliary tree results. Because neoplasia and sclerosis of the ductal system may be incipient in their progression, intraductal pressure accommodations occur and pain is absent or minimal despite progressive jaundice.

Acute impaction of the common duct by stones, on the other hand, is almost invariably accompanied by pain. Nevertheless it will, on rare occasions, simulate the relative painless jaundice of neoplasia. When the gallbladder or biliary tree becomes infected and inflamed secondary to obstruction, all the symptoms in Table 4–B will be present. When infection and inflammation are minimal or absent, jaundice along with changes in urine and stool color may be the only complaints. The degree of symptomatology overlaps among these multiple causes of obstruction. *The diagnosis of the underlying lesion on the basis of symptoms or signs is, at best, uncertain.* It is in this situation that invasive diagnostic techniques must be utilized. The following signs must be regarded as suggestive only.

Palpable gallbladder. Courvoisier's law still has validity. It is the result of distention of a normal gallbladder wall — usually, but not always, the result of neoplastic blockage of the common duct. The gallbladder wall is not infrequently inflamed and fibrosed in the presence of stones and hence not distensible. Rarely, a firm, irregular gallbladder is palpated as the result of primary gallbladder neoplasm.

Palpable liver. Common duct obstruction frequently results in a minimally enlarged liver. The edge is smooth, sharp, and only minimally tender. Rarely is it palpable more than one or two finger breadths below the right costal margin. A large, nontender, hard, nodular liver is, of course, suggestive of primary or metastatic neoplasm.

Liver function tests in obstructive jaundice include the spectrum from entirely normal to distinctly abnormal. Hepatocellular dysfunction is not a reliable indicator of the degree of obstruction. Indeed, complete obstruction is frequently unaccompanied by liver dysfunction, while minimal partial obstruction may be accompanied by severe hepatic dysfunction. Alkaline phosphatase and cholesterol levels (especially the former) are consistently elevated in obstructive jaundice, particularly when the

obstruction is prolonged. Marked elevation of cholesterol levels is most commonly seen when the cause of obstruction is intrahepatic. It may occasionally be present in extrahepatic obstruction as well. Bilirubin increase is marked by corresponding increase of the esterified fraction (1 minute direct) but liver dysfunction resulting from the obstruction makes this criterion unreliable at times.

Under usual circumstances the use of noninvasive methods is to be preferred to invasive methods. Use of one of the invasive methods is frequently necessary as an initial step, particularly under the following circumstances:

1. To definitively differentiate extrahepatic obstruction from parenchymatous or intrahepatic obstructive jaundice.

2. To localize the site of the obstruction in the bile duct system.

3. In an urgent situation when signs of impending catastrophe (shaking chills, hypotension, etc.) suggest the need for immediate surgery.

Certain noninvasive tools are of no value in the presence of jaundice (TSB>3.0). To request them is not only a waste of the radiologist's time but is costly to the patient, carries some risk, and may result in delay in definitive diagnosis. These procedures are (1) oral cholecystography, (2) intravenous cholangiography, and (3) intravenous ^{99m}Tc PG.

Fortunately, other newer noninvasive methods may establish the diagnosis in the presence of jaundice. These include gray-scale ultrasound, computerized axial tomography, and infusion tomography. As with the nonjaundiced patient, the initial step should be a plain film of the abdomen. Again one must be cautious in attaching a causal relationship when stones are visualized.

Gray-scale ultrasonography has been used to demonstrate gallstones and may have a particular use in the jaundiced patient. Reports of its accuracy vary widely. Nevertheless, it is a safe, relatively inexpensive procedure that may provide a rapid and accurate answer in 80 to 90 per cent of patients.

Perhaps the most promising of the noninvasive methods in the presence of jaundice is the use of infusion tomography. First reported by Genereux and Tchang in 1970, it has been used in only limited trials in the United States. The method involves the intravenous administration of 150 ml of 60 per cent Urographin (meglumine diatrizoate) and 150 ml of 5 per cent dextrose and water. During rapid infusion, linear tomograms of the anterior third of the right upper quadrant are obtained. A thickened gallbladder wall visualizes as an opacified ring indicating cholecystitis. Diagnostic accuracy has been re-

Table 6. *Cost Effectiveness of Procedures*

		Nonjaundice			Obstructive Jaundice	
Diagnostic Procedure	COST	ACUTE CHOLECYSTITIS	CHRONIC CHOLECYSTITIS	CHRONIC CHOLE-CYSTITIS°	ACUTE	CHRONIC
Noninvasive						
Plain film	1.0	+	+	+	+	+
Oral cholecystography	2.5	0	+++	−	NI	NI
Motor function (CCK)	4.5	NI	+	+	NI	NI
IV cholangiogram	4.5	++++	+	+	NI	NI
IV Te⁹⁹ PG	8.7	+++	NI	NI	NI	NI
Ultrasound	2.5	++	++	++	++	++
Infusion tomography	?	?	?	?	++++	++++
Biliary drainage	4.5	NI	+	+	NI	NI
Invasive						
Percutaneous cholangiogram	7.0 ⎫					
Retrograde cholangiogram	11.0 ⎬	NI	NI	NI	++++	++++
Transjugular cholangiogram	? ⎭					

Cost is relative to plain film as base; that is, if plain film costs $25, oral cholecystography would cost 2.5 × $25.00 or $62.50. Actual figures will vary with hospital or clinic.

°Normal oral chol.

NI = not indicated.

1 – 4+ = increasing efficacy.

0 = usually not possible during acute episode. Used after the acute episode has subsided, the rating of 3–4+ is given.

? = cost or effectiveness not determined at this time.

ported in as many as 96 per cent of positive cases and 94 per cent of histologically proven negative cases.

Biliary drainage is of little value in the jaundiced patient, since little or no bile is obtained. Moreover, use of cholecystokinin in this situation is hazardous.

A precise diagnosis may require use of an invasive method. Invasive cholangiography can be accomplished by one of three approaches: transjugular, retrograde, and percutaneous. Of the three, the percutaneous approach is most generally available, most cost effective, lowest in morbidity, and accurate. Transjugular approach is a specialized technique and not widely available. Moreover, it provides direct access of the infected bile to the venous system.

Retrograde cholangiography, like transjugular, requires a specialized technique, may require a prolonged time to complete successfully, and often entails retrograde injection into infected bile with a potential for inducing cholangitis. It is the most costly of the three approaches. In my experience it is most useful in the nonjaundiced postcholecystectomy syndrome patients in whom stones, sclerosis, or other obstructing lesions may be visualized in the intrahepatic portion of the biliary tree.

When the percutaneous route is used, the patient should be prescheduled for surgery in the event that markedly dilated bile ducts under high pressure are encountered. However, using the "skinny" needle, Pereiras et al.

reported visualization in 95.6 per cent of 45 cases of nondilated biliary tree and visualization in 100 per cent of patients with dilated biliary tree. This is an overall visualization rate of 98.5 per cent. They reported no morbidity or mortality in 131 consecutive patients.

Summary. When obstructive symptoms such as jaundice are predominant, standard tests — oral cholecystography, intravenous cholangiography, and intravenous ⁹⁹ᵐTc PG — *are of no value.* The only noninvasive tests of potential value are ultrasound, computerized tomography, and, in particular, infusion tomography. Invasive methods must be resorted to in many of these patients. Selection of the route for cholangiography depends on specific circumstances and availability of the experienced personnel.

Finally, a word about the abnormalities listed in Table 3. If one of these is discovered as a result of typical symptoms (Table 4–B, C) one may assume that complications such as intermittent ductal obstruction by stones and inflammation of the gallbladder wall have probably occurred. In the absence of typical symptoms (Table 4–A), one should look elsewhere for a cause of symptoms, particularly in the functional category. Congenital abnormalities of the gallbladder, in particular, are rarely the cause of symptoms unless stone formation and impaction or inflammation of the wall or both have occurred.

One must, in this cost-conscious era, take into

account the cost effectiveness of procedures available to the clinician. Table 6 summarizes this.

ACUTE AND CHRONIC PANCREATITIS

By GEORGE R. McSWAIN, M.D.,
and MARION C. ANDERSON, M.D.

Charleston, South Carolina

Pancreatitis is a highly variable inflammatory process that may range from a simple self-limited edema to an overwhelming hemorrhagic necrosis. In the United States the cause of pancreatitis can be traced to the chronic consumption of excessive amounts of alcohol or to chronic biliary tract inflammation with cholelithiasis, in a high proportion of patients. Other less common associated conditions include trauma, metabolic abnormalities such as hyperparathyroidism and hyperlipidemia, familial disorders, nutritional deficiencies, and toxic reactions to drugs and other commercial products.

Regardless of the underlying causes, the severe forms of acute pancreatitis are characterized by marked reductions of the effective circulating blood volume, the potential risk of local vascular and parenchymatous necrosis in and adjacent to the gland, and the development of functional impairment of other vital organ systems that may result in serious complications and even death.

ACUTE PANCREATITIS

CLINICAL FINDINGS

Acute pancreatitis begins with the development of upper abdominal pain, usually severe in character, located in the epigastrium and subcostal areas and frequently radiating to the lower dorsal area of the back. Nausea and vomiting are common.

On physical examination there is often a vague sensation of fullness in the epigastric region, but rarely a well-defined mass. Tenderness is present throughout the upper abdomen and moderate to severe distention is a common finding. Jaundice may occur in 15 to 25 per cent of patients. In some cases this results from a stone impacted in the ampulla of Vater. Other causes include inflammatory compression of the terminal bile duct as it passes through the pancreas en route to the ampulla and hepatocellular dysfunction secondary to the toxic effects of products produced in the inflamed gland and carried to the liver by the portal circulation. Serosanguineous fluid originating from the severely inflamed pancreas may dissect into the muscular planes of the posterior abdomen and present as ecchymoses in the flanks (Grey Turner's sign) or periumbilical area (Cullen's sign). Hypocalcemia may result in tetany, although in our experience this is a rare manifestation. Fat necrosis may occur in the subcutaneous tissues and present as tender areas of nodularity over the trunk and proximal extremities. When fluid loss is pronounced, hypovolemia is manifested by hypotension and tachycardia.

In a high proportion of patients (80 to 90 per cent), the inflammatory process responds to simple therapeutic measures including bed rest, pain control, fluid and electrolyte replacement, and suppression of exocrine secretion with nasogastric suction.

The remainder of patients are not so fortunate, and the magnitude of the illness is much more intense. Circulating blood volume may be reduced by as much as 30 to 40 per cent and this results in hemoconcentration, decreased urinary output, and hypotension. Marked elevations of the leukocyte count strongly suggest the development of pancreatic and peripancreatic necrosis. Pancreatic abscess formation is usually a late manifestation. Other vital organ systems begin to show evidence of functional impairment. Table 1 summarizes the systemic complications that frequently accompany severe forms of acute pancreatitis.

LABORATORY FINDINGS

Unfortunately, there is no laboratory test that will specifically and unequivocally identify the patient with acute pancreatitis. The serum amylase is elevated in approximately 70 per cent of cases; however, hyperamylasemia may occur in a number of other acute abdominal conditions, including cholecystitis, perforated ulcer, and intestinal infarction, which are frequently confused with acute pancreatitis. Persistent elevations of amylase may indicate the development of a pseudocyst or abscess. Serial variations in amylase are difficult to interpret. Decreasing levels may indicate improvement

Table 1. *Systemic Complications of Acute Pancreatitis*

Pulmonary
   Pleural effusion
   Atelectasis
   Pneumonia
   Acute respiratory distress syndrome

Renal
   Oliguria
   Anuria

Hepatic
   Jaundice
   Hepatic insufficiency

Cardiac
   ECG changes suggesting ischemia
   Arrhythmias

CNS
   Confusion
   Disorientation
   Coma

Gastrointestinal
   Peritonitis
   Ileus

Coagulation
   Disseminated intravascular coagulation
   Thrombosis/embolism

but also may occur with severe necrotizing forms of the disease. Normal levels also occur in cases associated with lipemic serum because high lipid levels inhibit the enzyme assay technique. In contrast, very high amylase values, especially if over 1000 Somogyi units, are not necessarily a poor prognostic indicator and in fact have been inversely related to the severity of pancreatitis.

The urinary amylase remains elevated for longer intervals following the onset of the attack. Quantitative determination of the amylase content of a 2-hour urinary collection is helpful in the patient with adequate renal function.

Recently, the amylase-to-creatinine ratio has been recommended as a more definitive test. The calculation of the ratio between renal amylase clearance and creatinine clearance has been found to have a high specificity.

$$\frac{C_{am}}{C_{cr}}\ \% = \frac{\text{amylase urine}}{\text{amylase serum}} \times \frac{\text{creatinine serum}}{\text{creatinine urine}} \times 100$$

This simple calculation can be made with a single post collection of simultaneously obtained samples of blood and urine, thus avoiding the time, labor, and errors involved in timed urine collections. Normal values are reliably from 1 to 5 per cent. Patients with acute pancreatitis usually have values of greater than 6 per cent. Those with macroamylasemia are identified by values of less than 1 per cent.

The enzyme lipase is not found in salivary glands, and elevated levels tend to be more reliable than amylase in diagnosing acute pancreatitis. Unfortunately, the test is not as useful clinically as the amylase test because the assay is more difficult, requires a longer period of time, and the results are not readily available in an acute situation.

Elevated levels of amylase or lipase in ascitic or pleural fluid obtained by needle aspiration are reliable indicators of pancreatitis. The absolute values are generally higher than those found in serum, especially if greater than 1000 Somogyi units per 100 ml and if found in serosanguineous fluid. With perforated peptic ulcer, bile is usually present in the peritoneal fluid in addition to pancreatic enzymes.

Hyperglycemia is frequently observed during the acute stages of the disease, and when present in conjunction with an elevated amylase, increases the probability that the problem is, indeed, pancreatitis. Glucose tolerance tests may remain abnormal well after the serum glucose levels have returned to normal.

Hypocalcemia may occur, particularly in the severe forms of pancreatitis, and levels below 7.5 mg per 100 ml are considered to indicate a poor prognosis. In the rare cases of pancreatitis secondary to hyperparathyroidism, a normal serum ionized calcium may reflect significant reduction in levels that existed before the attack. Several theories have been proposed to explain the development of hypocalcemia, including the deposition of ionized calcium in areas of fat necrosis and the impairment of calcium mobilization from bone secondary to excessive glucagon secretion by the inflamed gland.

Abnormal lipid metabolism may occur in the course of pancreatitis. Lactescence occurs when the triglyceride levels exceed 300 mg per dl (100 ml). Lipemic serum interferes with the serum amylase assay, and recent findings have implicated high lipid levels in the pathogenesis of respiratory failure associated with severe pancreatitis. Hyperlipoproteinemia of types I, IV, and V are also associated with acute pancreatitis either as a result of the attack or as an etiologic agent. The latter is established following recovery if hyperlipoproteinemia persists.

Patients with severe pancreatitis reflect the vascular impairment, hemorrhage, parenchymatous necrosis, and systemic complications in a variety of laboratory tests. The leukocyte count often exceeds 20,000. The hemoglobin and hematocrit, which are elevated initially because of hemoconcentration, fall precipitously following fluid and electrolyte replacement. These

Table 2. *Laboratory Studies Indicating Severe Pancreatitis*

HGB/HCT–Initial	– > 14/50
HGB/HCT–After hydration	– < 8/30
WBC	– > 20,000
Urine volume	– < 20 ml/hr
Urine Sp. Gr.	– > 1.025
Blood glucose	– > 200 mg%
Serum Ca^{++}	– < 7.5 mg/%
Pulmonary function	
PaO$_2$	– < 60 mmHg
PaCO$_2$	– > 45 mmHg
pH	– < 7.4
Renal function	
BUN	– > 30 mg%
Creatinine	– > 2.0 mg%
Hepatic function	
Bilirubin	– > 4.0 mg%
Albumin	– < 3.0 mg%
Prothrombin time	– > 14.0 sec.
SGOT	– > 250 mu/ml
LDH	– > 350 Iu
Coagulation	
Platelets	– ↓
Fibrinogen	– ↓
Fibrin split products	– ↑

characteristics of severe acute pancreatitis are summarized in Table 2. It should be emphasized at this point that similar laboratory findings also accompany a number of other acute abdominal conditions that may be confused with severe pancreatitis. These include gangrenous cholecystitis, suppurative cholangitis, perforated viscus, strangulation obstruction, mesenteric arterial or venous occlusion, and leaking abdominal aneurysm. Since most of these conditions demand early surgical correction, it is imperative to establish an accurate diagnosis at the earliest possible hour. Failure of the patient to improve or evidence of deterioration in spite of adequate restorative therapy is an indication for surgical exploration to establish a definitive diagnosis.

Radiographic Studies

X-ray studies may be helpful in establishing the diagnosis. Pleural effusion and lower lobe atelectasis or pneumonitis may occur, usually in the left hemithorax. Severe pancreatitis often is associated with the development of findings consistent with the acute respiratory distress syndrome, including diffuse patchy infiltrates throughout both lung fields.

In the abdomen, ileus is a common finding, with segmental dilatation of the small intestine, the "sentinel loop" sign. Alcoholics often show evidence of calcification in the region of the pancreas. Spasm in the transverse colon with proximal distention, the so-called "colon cutoff" sign, is said to occur as a consequence of the inflammatory process involving the transverse mesocolon and colon.

An edematous pancreas may cause widening of the duodenal C-loop on barium meal studies; mucosal edema and spasm of the antrum and proximal duodenum also may occur. The presence of a pseudocyst often causes displacement of adjacent segments of the stomach and duodenum.

Other Studies

Gray-scale ultrasonography may be of considerable value in demonstrating pancreatic enlargement, cystic collections, and the presence of gallstones.

Pancreas scanning utilizing selenium, which is incorporated into proteins produced by the acinar cells, shows poor uptake during pancreatitis and therefore offers little information. Gallium scans have been shown to visualize the inflamed pancreas and the isotope appears to localize particularly well in acute pseudocysts.

In the acute phase peritoneal lavage may be of help in establishing a high enzyme value in the peritoneal fluid and in determining the presence or absence of bacteria. The latter are more likely to be present in other conditions such as perforated viscus or intestinal infarction, which may be confused with severe pancreatitis.

For the great majority of patients who respond promptly to conservative management, improvement occurs rapidly. Following recovery, additional diagnostic studies should be undertaken to determine the cause for the attack. The studies that are employed in this assessment are listed in Table 3. It should be emphasized that gallbladder function may be abnormal for several weeks following an attack of acute pancreatitis, and therefore nonvisualization with either oral or intravenous cholangiography does not necessarily indicate intrinsic biliary disease. Surgically remediable conditions such as gallstones and hyperparathyroidism should be corrected without delay to avoid recurrences.

Table 3. *Diagnostic Studies During Recovery Phase*

Glucose tolerance test
Calcium and phosphorus
Parathyroid hormone
Lipids:
  Triglycerides
  Lipoprotein electrophoresis (Types I, IV, V)
Cholecystography
Barium meal study
  Hypotonic duodenography
Endoscopy
Ultrasonography

CHRONIC PANCREATITIS

Chronic pancreatitis develops as a consequence of repeated acute attacks. The pathologic changes vary, depending upon the underlying cause.

In gallstone-induced pancreatitis, recurrent acute attacks may occur; however, as the acute phase subsides the gland usually recovers its normal consistency rather rapidly and there is little evidence of permanent damage either to the parenchyma or the ductal system. Complete eradication of the gallstones and surgical correction of stenosis, which may occur at the ampullary level, result in permanent cure in a high proportion of cases (> 95 per cent).

In contrast, the chronic pancreatitis associated with chronic alcoholism is a slowly progressive process, punctuated with acute exacerbations that tend to become more frequent and less intense with time. This reduction in the severity of attacks is probably due to a decrease in the amount of enzyme produced by the damaged exocrine pancreas. As the disease advances, the gland becomes increasingly fibrotic and atrophic, and the ductal system is obstructed by multiple sites of stricture. Obstruction is often associated with the development of calcium-containing calculi. Ultimately, both endocrine and exocrine function deteriorate and the patients develop diabetes and steatorrhea with marked weight loss. Narcotic addiction can occur as a consequence of the chronic, increasingly intense upper abdominal and back pain that characterizes the disease.

Although pseudocysts may develop in association with any form of pancreatitis, they are particularly common in patients with chronic alcoholism, probably because of the high-grade exocrine obstruction that accompanies this form of the disease. Our personal surgical experience indicates that nearly 70 per cent of patients with chronic alcoholic pancreatitis have one or more pseudocysts that may occur anywhere within the substance of the gland.

LABORATORY STUDIES

Serum and urinary enzymes may be normal or elevated. Prolonged elevations of the amylase may indicate exocrine obstruction or the presence of a pseudocyst or both.

In advanced disease diabetes develops with associated hyperglycemia, glycosuria, abnormal glucose tolerance tests, and reduced serum insulin levels.

Steatorrhea is manifested by weight loss and microscopic evidence of increased fat and meat fibers in stool specimens stained with sudan and eosin. The finding of more than 10 meat fibers per low-power field or more than 100 fat globules per high-power field indicates significant malabsorption. Quantitative analysis of a 72-hour stool specimen for fat content can be performed when the patient is receiving a standard 100 gram per day fat diet. Excretion of more than 6 grams of fat per 24 hours indicates significant steatorrhea. Administration of enteric pancreatic enzyme preparations will correct the defect if the steatorrhea originates from exocrine insufficiency. Quantitative analysis for nitrogen and pancreatic enzymes also can be performed on the stool.

Hepatic function may be abnormal in chronic pancreatitis because of either the toxic effects of alcohol on the liver or the malnutrition associated with exocrine insufficiency.

DUODENAL INTUBATION

Direct measurement of basal and stimulated pancreatic secretion can be obtained utilizing a double-lumened (Drieling) tube, which permits continuous aspiration of both gastric and duodenal contents. The *Lundh test* meal consists of a formulated meal that includes fat, carbohydrate, and protein, and is used to stimulate pancreatic secretion. The sample is analyzed for the enzyme trypsin. *Pancreozymin-cholecystokinin* given intravenously in a dose of 75 IDU simulates the presence of protein and fat in the duodenum and causes secretion of enzymes by the acinar cells. Samples are analyzed for trypsin and compared with established normal values. *Secretin*, given intravenously in a dose of 1 to 4 CU per kg, simulates the presence of hydrochloric acid in the duodenum and causes the secretion of electrolytes and water by the centroacinar and intercalated duct cells of the pancreas. The specimen is analyzed for volume (normal >2 ml per kg in 80 minutes), bicarbonate concentration (normal > 80 mEq per liter) and bicarbonate output (normal >10 mEq in 30 minutes).

CYTOLOGIC STUDIES

Cytologic studies can be performed on specimens obtained by duodenal drainage or aspiration from an endoscopically placed pancreatic duct cannula. Cytological examination is helpful in the differential diagnosis of pancreatic masses.

Recently, samples have also been obtained for aspiration cytology using a 15-cm long, 23-gauge spinal needle guided into the mass by fluoroscopy or ultrasonography. Complications of this technique have been reported to be rare, even though the thin needle undoubtedly passes through multiple intra-abdominal structures. Aspiration biopsy also may be performed at operation by passing a 22-gauge needle into the pancreatic mass through the wall of the duodenum. It should be noted that a negative cytology report on samples obtained by any of these methods does not reliably rule out carcinoma.

RADIOGRAPHIC FINDINGS

Plain films of the abdomen may show calcifications in the region of the pancreas. This usually occurs in association with obstruction secondary to ductal strictures and is almost always a manifestation of alcoholism. *Cholecystography* is indicated to exclude the presence of gallstones. Oral cholecystography may fail to visualize the gallbladder early in the course of recovery from an acute exacerbation. Intravenous cholangiography may provide information regarding the presence of common duct stones or stenosis in the lower portion of the common duct as it traverses the head of the pancreas. The latter is a frequent finding in alcoholic pancreatitis.

Endoscopic retrograde cholangiography and pancreatography (ERCP), when successful, provides direct radiographic demonstration of the biliary and pancreatic ducts and is particularly helpful in assessing the degree of stenosis in the terminal common duct and changes in the duct of Wirsung. The normal pancreatic duct has a sigmoid configuration, measuring about 3 mm in diameter in the head, 2.0 mm in the body, and 1.0 mm in the tail. A duct greater than 5.0 mm is considered to be dilated and probably involved in obstruction. Other findings include the presence of strictures, which may produce a "chain of lakes" configuration and intraductal calculi. Occasionally a pseudocyst that connects with the duct system also will visualize. Tumors involving the ductal system also may be identified with this technique.

Barium meal studies may show displacement of the stomach or duodenum by the pancreas or an associated pseudocyst. Antral and proximal duodenal spasm are common findings in patients with chronic pancreatitis. Occasionally a large cyst in the body or tail of the gland may cause displacement of the adjacent colon on *barium enema.*

Angiography is helpful in identifying vascular anomalies that are common in the region of the biliary tract and pancreas and is valuable information in planning various surgical procedures used to treat chronic pancreatitis. Displacement of vessels and vascular encasement may occur with either chronic pancreatitis or cancer of the pancreas. Tumors also may show either hypovascularity or hypervascularity. Superselective or magnification techniques and injection of epinephrine and tolazoline (Priscoline) may improve accuracy.

OTHER STUDIES

Gray-scale ultrasonography is helpful by identifying calculi and in the localization of cystic or solid masses in the pancreas. *Computerized tomography* (CT) also is useful in demonstrating stones and cystic or solid masses affecting the pancreas. The quality of tomograms is poor in thin patients who lack peripancreatic fat that affords accurate discrimination of the pancreas and in patients with multiple loops of air-filled intestine.

The objective of evaluation in chronic pancreatitis is to identify various endocrine and exocrine deficiencies. The latter usually can be corrected with appropriate medical management. The principal indication for surgical intervention is unrelenting upper abdominal and back pain that fails to respond to medical measures and subjects the patient to the risk of narcotic addiction. Pain usually is caused by ductal obstruction or persistent pseudocysts that develop secondary to strictures involving the major pancreatic ducts. Surgical decompression of the obstructed ducts and pseudocysts will relieve the pain; however, continued consumption of alcohol in the postoperative period ultimately results in progressive chronic pancreatitis and recurrence of symptoms.

PANCREATIC CYSTS AND NEOPLASMS

By AVRAM M. COOPERMAN, M.D., and ROBERT E. HERMANN, M.D.
Cleveland, Ohio

Pancreatic cysts and neoplasms include a variety of benign and malignant cysts and tumors with multiple presentations and causes. Pancreatic cysts include pseudocysts, retention cysts, congenital cysts, and cystadenomas. Solid tumors include carcinoma and both functional and nonfunctional islet cell tumors.

PSEUDOCYSTS

Cystic accumulations of fluid rich in pancreatic enzymes that develop after pancreatitis, carcinoma, and trauma describe the nonepithelial-lined pancreatic pseudocyst.

SYMPTOMS AND SIGNS

Regardless of the cause of pseudocysts, the presenting symptoms and signs are similar. Epigastric pain or fullness, anorexia, and weight loss are most common. In 30 to 50 per cent of patients, the pseudocyst is palpable and detected by the patient as well as the examiner. In 10 per cent of patients, atypical features exist. These include jaundice (from compression of the bile duct or associated pancreatitis in the head of the gland), gastrointestinal hemorrhage (from varices secondary to splenic vein thromboses or erosion into adjacent viscera), and *pancreatic* ascites (secondary to leakage of the cyst or pancreatic duct). Unusual locations and presentation may occur and include mediastinal, cervical, or intrasplenic location.

COURSE

Until recently the natural history of pseudocysts has been difficult to plot because small lesions are difficult to detect and follow. Using ultrasound, 50 per cent of patients with severe bouts of pancreatitis have cystic collections of fluid in the lesser sac. Many are asymptomatic. Approximately 25 to 40 per cent of pseudocysts resolve spontaneously, usually within 6 weeks after diagnosis.

DIAGNOSIS

A number of tests are available to diagnose pseudocysts. A plain roentgenogram of the abdomen may show displacement of contiguous viscera (secondary to fluid in the cyst). Indirect evidence may be further provided by a barium roentgenogram of the stomach or an intravenous pyelogram, both of which are of less necessity today. Direct visualization of the pseudocyst is provided by ultrasound (US) or computerized tomography (CT). Cost alone favors using ultrasound if personnel with expertise are available to correctly interpret the scan. A further advantage of these techniques is that the cyst may be followed to maturation or resolution. In some instances, particularly when pain is out of proportion to the findings or when chronic pancreatitis is present, endoscopic retrograde cholangiopancreatography (ERCP) may define associated duct abnormalities should surgery be contemplated. Since sepsis and rarely death secondary to infection of the pseudocyst have been reported, this test should be used infrequently and only when it may alter or affect planned treatment.

TRUE CYSTS

Benign cystic lesions that have columnar or cuboidal epithelium (retention or congenital) are very uncommon and are definitely diagnosed only at surgery. They may be suspected when pancreatitis or trauma does not precede the development of a mass or when associated hepatic and renal cysts coexist in children.

CYSTADENOMA OR CYSTADENOCARCINOMA OF THE PANCREAS

Approximately 10 per cent of cystic lesions of the pancreas are neoplastic cysts — most frequently cystadenoma or cystadenocarcinoma.

SYMPTOMS AND SIGNS

In the absence of abdominal pain or pancreatitis, the insidious onset of abdominal discomfort, fullness, and a mass suggests cystadenoma or cystadenocarcinoma. About 400 cases have been reported with a striking predominance in women (nine times as common) compared to men. A palpable epigastric mass or left upper quadrant fullness is the most common finding.

DIAGNOSIS

As with pancreatic pseudocysts, a variety of indirect tests are available to establish the diagnosis of a cystic lesion. Cost efficiency limits indiscriminate use of all these examinations. Availability and expertise dictate what is possible at each institution. US or CT may establish the size of the cyst, the relationship to contiguous organs, the part of the pancreas involved (head, body, tail), and the presence of both solid and cystic components.

Barium studies to delineate gastric, duodenal, and transverse colon anatomy may confirm the US or CT images and help the surgeon determine his operative approach.

COURSE

Slow, progressive increase in size of the mass is common. Hepatic metastases occur late and usually after multiple attempts to remove the cyst.

SOLID PANCREATIC NEOPLASMS

Solid pancreatic neoplasms unfortunately mean cancer in over 90 per cent of patients. This neoplasm is now the fourth most common malignant tumor and is increasing in frequency for unknown reasons. Since 90 per cent of patients will succumb within 48 months after the condition is diagnosed, it is important to establish a diagnosis rapidly and with a minimum of tests.

Adenocarcinoma arising from ductular epithelium accounts for over 90 per cent of the lesions. It arises in the head of the gland in 70 per cent, the body in 20 per cent, and the tail of the pancreas in 10 per cent.

Lesions in the head of the pancreas produce jaundice or gastrointestinal hemorrhage, while lesions in the body and tail cause pain (retroperitoneal nerve invasion) and, much less frequently, jaundice.

Since four lesions arising at or near the ampulla of Vater may mimic each other, differentiation between them is frequently difficult, both preoperatively and intraoperatively. These tumors include cancer of the head of the pancreas, distal common bile duct, duodenum, or ampulla of Vater and have similar presenting symptoms and signs. Persistent and progressive jaundice is the hallmark of cancer of the head of the pancreas, usually accompanied by pain and significant weight loss (15 lbs [7 kg] or more). Less frequently, gastrointestinal hemorrhage secondary to duodenal ulceration or duodenal obstruction are associated features.

SIGNS

Nonspecific Signs. Aside from icterus, nonspecific signs are frequently found. A dilated and palpable gallbladder (Courvoisier's sign) implies obstruction below the cystic duct, usually owing to a periampullary malignancy. A palpable, enlarged liver may indicate nonspecific enlargement or intrahepatic metastases. Signs of metastases, including periumbilical nodules (Sister Mary Joseph's sign) or left supraclavicular nodes (Virchow's node), indicate distant metastases.

LABORATORY TESTS

Because jaundice is progressive and intense, the level of serum bilirubin is frequently greater than 10 mg per dl(100 ml) at the time of diagnosis. Almost all of this is conjugated. Proportionate or at times significantly higher levels of alkaline phosphatase denote biliary obstruction. Modest elevations of transaminase may also be occasionally seen.

DIAGNOSTIC TESTS

When jaundice is the presenting sign, diagnostic tests must be carefully selected to demonstrate the site of obstruction and the presence or absence of metastases. A number of tests are available to directly and indirectly enable this diagnosis to be made. A number of studies have attempted to compare and analyze these but comparison is limited because many of these tests are dependent on individual skills.

Endoscopic examination of the stomach and duodenum is essential to exclude an ampullary or duodenal tumor. Encroachment of the medial duodenal wall may indicate a pancreatic lesion. Since endoscopy is available, reasonably inexpensive, and valuable, we favor it as an early test.

US or CT to visualize the pancreas, liver (to exclude metastasis), and bile ducts is next done. The value is obvious.

In many patients these tests suffice before surgery. In a few patients further definition of bile duct anatomy is necessary. This may be done by percutaneous transhepatic cholangiography (PTC) or endoscopic retrograde cholangiopancreatography (ERCP). Availability, expertise, and experience will determine which will be used, and when.

Upper gastrointestinal studies with barium will help exclude impending obstruction, but this can also be determined at surgery. Liver scans are of little help, since laparotomy will invariably be needed to relieve jaundice. Arteriography (particularly splenic) and hepatic catheterization are less often needed today, particularly with noninvasive scanning so available.

COURSE

The natural course of cancer of the head of the pancreas is progressive and inexorable. Less than 10 per cent of patients undergo pancreaticoduodenal resection because regional, distant, or contiguous spread of tumor precludes attempts at curative resection. Decompression of an obstructed bile duct and liver by a biliary enteric bypass relieves jaundice but it is unclear whether survival is significantly prolonged by these operations. Hepatic metastases, ascites, anorexia, or gastrointestinal hemorrhage secondary to obstructed mesenteric and portal veins are the usual causes of death — almost always within 5 years. Resection of the head of the pancreas, distal bile duct, duodenum, gallbladder, and distal stomach (Whipple operation) can be done in less than 10 per cent of patients, with an operative mortality that ranges from 5 to 30 per cent. This mortality rate makes it important to accurately diagnose the tumor by biopsy or cytologic diagnosis.

CANCER OF THE BODY AND TAIL OF THE PANCREAS

Malignant tumors of the body and tail of the pancreas are fatal in 100 per cent of cases unless discovered by serendipity at surgery done for other reasons.

SYMPTOMS

Weight loss and midepigastric pain boring through or radiating into the back are the hallmarks of cancer of the body and tail of the pancreas. Deep vein phlebitis of the lower extremity, which may be recurrent and migratory, is frequently associated with adenocarcinoma of the body of the pancreas. Pain relieved by leaning forward is characteristic of retroperitoneal involvement.

SIGNS

Cancer of the body of the pancreas is non-palpable in nearly all patients. Since metastases are frequent, hepatomegaly and cervical nodes should be sought. Arterial bruits or venous hums in the left upper quadrant denote compression of the splenic artery and vein.

DIAGNOSES

US or CT provides direct imaging of the pancreas, bile ducts, and liver and in time should prove to be the most sensitive, noninvasive test to establish the diagnosis. Angiography (encasement of vessels) and ERCP (abrupt blockage of mid duct) may help in atypical presentations and provide strong indirect evidence of cancer.

Peritoneoscopy with biopsy of metastases or laparotomy will establish the diagnosis and determine resectability (an unfortunately rare circumstance).

COURSE

Treated or untreated cancer of the body and tail of the pancreas runs an inexorable course leading to death within months to years. Ascites, jaundice (frequently owing to liver metastases), and back pain (secondary to retroperitoneal perineural invasion) are ominous late signs. Resectability is quite uncommon unless the tumor is discovered by chance at the time of laparotomy done for other reasons. We have never encountered a resectable lesion when a laparotomy with the preoperative diagnosis of cancer of the body or tail of the pancreas has been done.

ISLET CELL TUMORS

A third type of pancreatic neoplasm, usually solid and only rarely cystic, is the islet cell tumor. This tumor most often presents because of overproduction of one or more hormones or causes hypoglycemia (excess insulin), duodenal or marginal ulcers (gastrin), or watery diarrhea (vasoactive intestinal polypeptide or other members of the secretin family).

HYPERINSULINISM

Overproduction of insulin by benign (90 per cent), malignant (10 per cent), or hyperplastic (less than 2 per cent) islet cell tumors frequently causes considerable confusion for patients who suffer from hypoglycemia and for physicians trying to establish the diagnosis.

SYMPTOMS

Dizziness, weakness, palpitations, sweating, confusion, convulsions, and coma are the spectrum of symptoms experienced by hypoglycemic patients. As suggested by Whipple and Frantz, symptoms may be caused by exercise or fasting; the sugar level at the time of symptoms is 50 mg per dl or less and symptoms abate with administration of glucose.

DIAGNOSIS

Today the diagnosis of hyperinsulinism is facilitated by techniques that measure serum insulin by radioimmunoassay. Elevated levels or inappropriately elevated levels proportionate to plasma glucose have eased the diagnosis in most patients. A fast for 48 to 72 hours under observation still remains a reliable method for inducing symptoms. Provocative tests using leucine, tolbutamide, glucagon, and arginine are infrequently used. Measurement of proinsulin and C peptide are newer assays that help establish the diagnosis of organic hyperinsulinism. Proinsulin levels are elevated in insulinoma patients even when total insulin levels are normal. C-peptide concentrations of insulin reflect endogenous pancreatic output and may be used to exclude exogenous causes of hyperinsulinism.

PREOPERATIVE LOCALIZATION

Having established a diagnosis of hyperinsulinism, preoperative localization by angiography reassures physicians, surgeons, and patients that a tumor may be found. Selective splenic artery catheterization with magnification views of the pancreas is available in most hospitals. Accurate localization is possible in 50 to 85 per cent of cases. More recently in a few institutions, transhepatic catheterization of the splenic vein with determination of insulin concentrations can localize the hyperfunctioning segment of pancreas.

COURSE

Since 90 per cent of insulin-producing lesions are benign and single, symptoms are usually due to excess production of insulin and not to metastases. While some individuals, not suspecting the diagnosis, eat frequently to avoid hypoglycemic episodes, the risks of central nervous damage from hypoglycemia are real in most patients and surgery is the wisest treatment.

GASTRINOMA (ZOLLINGER-ELLISON SYNDROME)

Some islet cell tumors produce gastrin, a hormone that causes excessive and significant quantities of gastric acid and pepsin. As a result, duodenal mechanisms that neutralize acid are overcome and ulcerations of the duodenum and jejunum are produced.

SYMPTOMS AND SIGNS

When first described in 1955 in patients with recurrent or ectopic ulcerations, marked gastric acid secretion in patients with nonbeta cell tumors established the diagnosis. Today, nearly 30 per cent of these patients present with ordinary symptoms of duodenal ulcer disease present for one or more years and 20 per cent have ulcer symptoms of more than 5 years' duration. One third have associated endocrine abnormalities such as hyperparathyroidism, renal stones, and adrenal or pituitary tumors.

DIAGNOSIS

Elevated basal levels of serum gastrin two or more times normal or basal acid output greater than 15 mEq per hour make the diagnosis. In uncertain cases, secretin (1 mg per kg) or calcium (5 mg per kg) infusion should result in doubling of serum gastrin. Angiography may localize the lesion if present in the pancreas.

Unfortunately, the test is of less value than with hyperinsulinism, since 50 per cent of benign lesions are multiple and two thirds of the malignant lesions have metastasized before diagnosis.

COURSE

Untreated or incorrectly treated, the disease terminates fatally from surgical complications or complications of the ulcer. The efficacy of such histamine receptor antagonists as cimetidine (Tagamet) has been documented in about 25 per cent of patients treated for periods of up to 3 years. If metastases are present, half the patients will succumb within 5 years.

WATERY DIARRHEA SYNDROME

Even less frequent than insulinoma and gastrinoma is the syndrome known as pancreatic cholera, watery diarrhea, or Verner-Morrison syndrome.

SYMPTOMS AND SIGNS

Although this too is a spectrum of a disease presentation, nearly half the patients have profuse watery diarrhea in excess of 4 to 6 liters per day, hypokalemia, and hyperglycemia. Less frequently, hypercalcemia and flushing are associated findings.

DIAGNOSIS

Common causes of diarrhea must be excluded. Inflammatory bowel disease (Crohn's disease and ulcerative colitis), laxative abuse, and functional diarrhea should be sought, as they are most common. Sigmoidoscopy and barium studies of the gastrointestinal tract help exclude some of these. Angiography may localize a pancreatic or extraperitoneal tumor. Perhaps the best diagnostic tests are serum radioimmunoassays for peptides of the "secretin" family.

If elevated levels of secretin, glucagon, and vasoactive intestinal polypeptide (VIP) are documented by reliable radioimmunoassay, this diagnosis must be strongly suspected.

COURSE

Untreated and undiagnosed, the metabolic effects of uncontrolled diarrhea may be fatal. Excision of benign or malignant pancreatic or extrapancreatic tumors may cure or relieve the diarrhea. Malignant tumors prove fatal, usually because of hypokalemia, dehydration, or uncontrolled electrolyte and fluid disturbances.

DIAPHRAGMATIC HERNIAS

By DAVID B. SKINNER, M.D.

Chicago, Illinois

Defects in the diaphragmatic muscle and tendon may occur at the natural orifices in the diaphragm, at sites of developmental failure, or secondary to trauma. Such defects permit abdominal contents to enter the less than atmospheric pressure environment of the thorax as diaphragmatic hernias. The most common diaphragmatic hernia is protrusion of the stomach through the esophageal hiatus, or hiatal hernia. A classification of diaphragmatic hernias is presented in Table 1.

The type I, sliding, or axial hiatal hernia is caused by a generalized weakening of the phrenoesophageal membrane, which is a fusion of the abdominal and endothoracic fascia on the diaphragm inserting into the submucosal layers of the esophagus several centimeters above the esophagogastric junction. Weakening of this membrane is common in the fifth, sixth, and seventh decades of life and allows a cephalad migration of the gastroesophageal junction. Anteriorly the stomach is covered by a reflection of peritoneum, whereas posteriorly the retroperitoneal attachments of the stomach are maintained — hence the designation sliding hernia. These hernias are extremely common in the United States population and are clinically without significance unless accompanied by abnormal degrees of gastroesophageal reflux.

The type II, rolling, or paraesophageal hernia is caused by a localized weakness in the phrenoesophageal membrane at the point where the peritoneum is reflected off the membrane anteriorly and laterally. Generally the posterior retroperitoneal attachments of the cardia remain intact. A portion of the gastric fundus herniates through the weakness into the thorax. Because of the constant abdominal to thoracic pressure gradients, there is a tendency for these hernias to enlarge. In doing so, more and more of the stomach herniates into the chest and the entire circumferential attachments of the phrenoesophageal membrane may weaken, allowing a combined type I and type II hernia to occur. Eventually the entire stomach may migrate into the chest in an upside down and rotated position. Adjacent organs, including colon, spleen, and small intestine, may be found in giant combined hiatal hernia sacs.

The parahiatal hernia, in which a portion of stomach herniates through a separate opening in the diaphragm adjacent to the esophageal hiatus, is rare. Attenuation of the narrow margin of diaphragm muscle between the esophagus and stomach generally occurs and causes this type of hernia in advanced form to be similar to the paraesophageal hernia.

Traumatic diaphragmatic hernias may occur anywhere in the diaphragm from penetrating injuries or from dehiscence of surgical incisions and closures. Spontaneous rupture of the diaphragm from blunt trauma most commonly occurs posteriorly and in the left diaphragm.

The congenital diaphragmatic hernia through the foramen of Bochdalek normally presents as a surgical emergency in the newborn and is most common in the left chest. The defect is in the posterior lateral portion of the diaphragm, where the central process fails to fuse with the chest wall component of the diaphragmatic development. Less severe forms of congenital herniation through the foramen of Bochdalek may take the form of a diaphragmatic eventration and may be discovered at any time in life as an incidental finding on a chest x-ray. The foramen of Morgagni hernia more commonly develops later in life and rarely presents as a surgical emergency. The transverse colon and omentum are the organs normally in the hernia.

HIATAL HERNIA

Hiatal hernia is one of the most common abnormalities detected in adults. The incidence of a type I hiatal hernia observed during barium swallow radiographs varies between 10 and 90 per cent, depending upon the aggressiveness of the radiologist in attempting to demonstrate a hernia. Type I hiatal hernia is of no clinical signficance unless accompanied by abnormal gastroesophageal reflux. Reflux, not hiatal hernia, causes symptoms and complications. Reflux may occur in the absence of a detectable hiatal

---

Table 1. *Diaphragmatic Hernias — Classification*

I. Hiatal hernia
   A. Type I, sliding, or axial
   B. Type II, rolling, or paraesophageal
   C. Combined types
II. Parahiatal hernia
III. Traumatic diaphragmatic hernia
   A. Iatrogenic
   B. Spontaneous
IV. Congenital diaphragmatic hernias
   A. Pleuroperitoneal canal (Bochdalek's foramen hernia)
   B. Retrocostal-sternal (foramen of Morgagni hernia)

hernia, and abnormal reflux does not commonly accompany the majority of asymptomatic radiographically identified type I hiatal hernias.

SYMPTOMS AND SIGNS

There are no specific symptoms caused by a type I hiatal hernia. When abnormal reflux accompanies a hiatal hernia, the typical symptoms are those of heartburn and regurgitation of gastric contents aggravated by postural maneuvers such as stooping and lying flat, and relieved by standing erect. Other symptoms caused by reflux include dysphagia resulting from reflux-induced spasms or stricture of the esophagus, globus hystericus or difficulty in initiating swallowing related to irritation of the cervical esophagus from advanced reflux, gastrointestinal bleeding from esophagitis, and chronic cough with recurring pneumonias caused by aspiration of regurgitated gastric contents.

The rare type II hiatal hernia in its pure form is generally not accompanied by reflux. Symptoms are frequently vague and nonspecific unless a complication of the hernia develops. Often the patient notes a postprandial fullness and distention or pressure in the chest. Gurgling sounds from the chest may be heard. When the hernia is complicated, symptoms may include massive or mild gastrointestinal bleeding, total obstruction to swallowing, dyspnea, cyanosis, air hunger, fever, and collapse.

CLINICAL COURSE

The fate of the asymptomatic radiographically identified type I hiatal hernia is unknown, but probably most remain asymptomatic and uncomplicated. When abnormal gastroesophageal reflux accompanies a hiatal hernia, symptoms may develop and complications ensue. From 24-hour esophageal pH observations, patterns of abnormal reflux are identifiable. Patients having daytime upright reflux frequently note symptoms of heartburn, aerophagia, bloating, and indigestion. It appears that this type of reflux by itself rarely leads to serious complications, as the upright position and repeated swallowing rapidly empty gastric contents from the esophagus. When there is prolonged contact of regurgitated gastric secretion with the esophageal mucosa, such as occurs after nocturnal reflux while the patient is asleep in the horizontal position, severe esophagitis may develop, leading to chronic or massive bleeding, stricture, ulceration, development of columnar-lined epithelium in the esophagus, or nocturnal aspiration. In patients who develop ulcerative esophagitis from reflux, progression to stricture with or without bleeding occurs. In patients with minimal or no esophagitis in spite of marked symptoms of heartburn and regurgitation, there is no evidence to suggest that they will develop esophagitis and its complications.

The course of the type II hiatal hernia is one of gradual enlargement of the hernia sac with eventual transposition of the entire stomach into the thorax. The gastroesophageal junction remains relatively fixed at the level of the diaphragm, and the pylorus is gradually drawn up toward the diaphragm. This places the two fixed points at the upper and lower end of the stomach adjacent to each other and creates the setting in which gastric volvulus with resulting obstruction and infarction can occur. This in turn can be a fatal event. Inexorable enlargement with increasing risk of fatal mechanical complications is the typical course of the type II hiatal hernia.

COMPLICATIONS

The complications of type I hiatal hernia are entirely related to the degree and pattern of gastroesophageal reflux. Reflux causes the complications of esophagitis, bleeding, stricture, and aspiration. The presence of these complications should be detected in the diagnostic workup of the patient as a guide for therapy. In patients with long-standing gastroesophageal reflux, repeated bouts of esophagitis followed by healing of the mucosa lead to a gradual cephalad migration of columnar epithelium termed Barrett's esophagus. Gastric ulcers may develop in this abnormal epithelium, and an increased risk of adenocarcinoma of the esophagus occurs in such patients.

The type II hiatal hernia is complicated by intrathoracic gastric distention with resulting decrease in lung volume, and the possibility of gastric volvulus, obstruction, strangulation, and infarction. In combined types of hiatal hernia the complications of both types may occur. Massive bleeding from a gastric ulcer in the stomach pouch or from severe esophagitis may occur.

PHYSICAL FINDINGS

The diagnosis of the type I hiatal hernia is made primarily from a pattern of typical symptoms and is confirmed by appropriate radiographic and esophageal function tests. There are no specific physical findings. In patients with a type II hiatal hernia, the physical findings relate to the size of the hernia. There may be changes in breath sounds in the left chest, and the presence of intestinal sounds may be heard during chest auscultation if the patient is asked to swallow a glass of water during the examination. Otherwise, there are no other direct physical findings of the hiatal hernia.

Similarly, there are no specific biochemical or hematologic laboratory findings caused by hiatal hernia. Bleeding complications cause an iron deficiency anemia. Evaluation of the electrocardiogram and pulmonary function tests are both important. Many patients with reflux complain of chest pain often thought to be a component of the heartburn, but which must be differentiated from ischemic heart disease. Similarly, patients with reflux or a large type II hiatal hernia may have abnormal pulmonary function caused by aspiration of gastric contents or by the compression of adjacent lung by the large hiatal hernia.

RADIOGRAPHY

Radiology is the primary method to diagnose hiatal hernia. This is an anatomic defect that requires anatomic demonstration by radiographic findings or by surgical or autopsy dissection. Generally the type II paraesophageal hernia is easily diagnosed on barium swallow examination. The concept of incarceration of the stomach in the hiatal hernia sac is not particularly useful, because the abdominal to thoracic pressure gradient holds the stomach within the hernia sac most of the time even though it may be easily reducible by appropriate posturing or by surgical dissection. Evaluation of the type I hiatal hernia is a more difficult problem for the radiologist. By pressing hard on the abdomen while the patient is taking deep breaths, and by placing the patient in various body positions, a type I hiatal hernia may be demonstrated in a number of patients with no symptoms or disease whatsoever. The real challenge to the radiologist is diagnosing abnormal degrees of gastroesophageal reflux.

Abnormal reflux is seen spontaneously by the radiologist in 40 per cent or less of those patients who ultimately prove to have this diagnosis. Several methods are used in an effort to improve the value of the barium swallow examination in detecting reflux. To date, none of these are uniformly successful. The so-called water sipping test or asking the patient to swallow water while the cardia is observed and while pressure is applied to the abdomen is claimed by some to improve the accuracy of diagnosing an incompetent cardia. However, reflux under these conditions is a physiologic event. When a human being swallows, the distal esophageal segment relaxes its normal high pressure zone, which represents a barrier to reflux. If pressure is applied to the abdomen at the same time, reflux can be induced in normal subjects by this test. It is not a reliable guide to pathologic degrees of gastroesophageal reflux.

The use of cine barium swallow studies is of value in patients with suspected reflux and hiatal hernia. Unfortunately the short time available for observation of the cardia frequently precludes observation of the reflux event. Nevertheless, many patients with esophageal disorders have motor disturbances of the esophagus, and these are better evaluated by cine barium swallows than by conventional radiographic techniques. When dysphagia is part of the symptom complex, it is useful to ask the patient to swallow barium-impregnated marshmallows of varying sizes to calibrate the diameter of the obstruction. The cine acid barium swallow has value in demonstrating acid-induced motor disorders of the esophagus and may have a higher correlation with reflux-induced symptoms than any of the other radiographic techniques.

The value of the barium swallow examination is in the detection of the type II and combined hiatal hernias, in the observation of obstructing lesions of the esophagus, including motor disorders, and in the identification of the type I hiatal hernia that may be associated with abnormal reflux. If the radiologist sees reflux spontaneously, this is almost always a significant finding. However, the failure of the radiologist to observe reflux does not exclude this as the primary diagnosis.

ESOPHAGEAL FUNCTION TESTS

Because of dissatisfaction with the ability of radiographic studies to diagnose abnormal gastroesophageal reflux, esophageal function tests are employed. The first of these is esophageal manometry, by which pressures are measured at various levels in the esophagus using pressure transducers and a multichannel recorder. Conventional manometry uses three open tip water-filled tubes with the openings spaced 5 cm apart. Electronic transducers introduced in a bundle with the levels 5 cm apart may be used alternatively. The manometry catheter is inserted like a nasogastric tube into the stomach, and gastric pressures are recorded. The train of catheters is slowly withdrawn across the gastroesophageal junction into the esophagus. In normal persons a high pressure zone extending over 2.5 to 4 cm is observed at the gastroesophageal junction. The amplitude of this high pressure zone is 8 to 18 mm Hg, depending somewhat upon the method of measurement employed. The pressure drops to gastric levels when the patient swallows. The point of respiratory reversal during the breathing cycle is normally identified midway in the high pressure zone. During inhalation, abdominal pressure rises and thoracic pressure falls. The point at which this respiratory pressure inversion occurs is taken as the physiologic level of the diaphragm. Dissociation between this level and the high pressure zone identifies a hiatal hernia of significant size. After passing through the high pressure zone the manometry catheter is withdrawn through the esophagus, where normal peristalsis is observed. Cricopharyngeal sphincter pressures are measured as the tube is withdrawn.

Although there is a general statistical correlation between the amplitude of the distal esophageal high pressure zone and the presence or absence of abnormal reflux, the correlation between the absolute value of the high pressure zone in an individual patient and the presence or absence of reflux is not exact enough to permit manometry to be a useful diagnostic test for an incompetent cardia. Manometry is essential for locating the gastroesophageal junction for the subsequent placement of a pH electrode, and is most useful in ruling out other disorders such as achalasia, scleroderma, or diffuse esophageal spasm and other motor disorders.

For the direct measurement of reflux, a pH electrode is employed in the performance of a standard acid-reflux test. Manometry is done first to identify the high pressure zone. A long pH electrode is introduced as a nasogastric tube into the stomach, and the presence of gastric acid is verified. The pH probe is withdrawn so that its tip lies 5 cm above the high pressure zone. An acid load is placed in the stomach via the manometry catheter. The patient is asked to perform a standard set of respiratory and postural maneuvers, including deep breathing, coughing, the Valsalva maneuver, and the Muller maneuver, while lying in a supine, right side down, left side down, and head down position. Drops of pH to less than 4 are taken as direct evidence of reflux. Normal human beings may reflux up to two times under these conditions, whereas patients with abnormal degrees of reflux have repeated and prolonged drops in pH. A score is based upon the number of times reflux occurs during the various positions and respiratory maneuvers.

In difficult or complicated cases, 24-hour pH monitoring of the distal esophagus 5 cm above the high pressure zone is remarkably useful. The patient records on a strip chart recorder any symptoms or activities during the 24-hour period. There is often a marked correlation between symptoms and activities with a drop in pH in the esophagus or a persistent low pH. This highly sensitive test provides the baseline upon which evaluation of other diagnostic tests is made.

For esophagitis to occur, prolonged contact between regurgitated acid peptic materials and the esophageal mucosa is important. The acid-clearing test evaluates the ability of the esophagus to empty regurgitated gastric contents. A 15-ml bolus of 0.1 N hydrochloric acid is placed in the mid esophagus, and pH is monitored in the distal esophagus while the patient is asked to swallow at intervals. Normally acid is cleared from the esophagus by peristaltic waves initiated by swallowing, and pH is restored to neutral in 10 swallows or less. Patients at risk of developing esophagitis frequently have prolonged acid clearing and may not raise the pH during the course of 30 or more swallows.

Pain of esophageal origin is frequently difficult to differentiate from pain of cardiac, gastroduodenal, pancreatic, or biliary tract origin. For this reason the acid perfusion test was developed. In this test a nasoesophageal tube is placed midway down the esophagus. 0.1 N hydrochloric acid and isotonic saline solutions are alternately infused into the esophagus for periods of 10 minutes each without the patient's knowing which is being infused. A positive test occurs when the patient's spontaneous symptoms are induced by acid perfusion and relieved by saline perfusion. This technique has value in linking atypical symptoms to esophageal origin, but does not in itself prove the presence of abnormal reflux or esophagitis.

Abnormal esophageal mucosa can be detected by measuring the potential difference of the mucosal lining. Normally the gastric epithelium has a markedly different potential difference from normal squamous epithelium, malignant epithelium, and ulcerative areas. Measurement of the potential difference in the esophagus related to the manometry and pH electrode findings may be useful in detecting complications such as the esophagus lined with columnar epithelium or ulcerative esophagitis. These findings must be verified by esophagoscopy.

The most frequent and serious complication of reflux accompanying a hiatal hernia is esophagitis. This term literally means inflammation of the esophagus, so diagnosis depends upon gross and microscopic observation of the esophagus, usually accomplished by esophagoscopy. The flexible fiberoptic esophagoscope is preferred in patients without an obstructing lesion of the esophagus, as the optical system permits magnification of the mucosa and the flexible esophagoscope reduces the risk associated with a rigid esophagoscope. Endoscopy is indicated in any patient in whom symptoms and esophageal function tests suggest abnormal gastroesophageal reflux and the possibility of esophagitis. It is indicated in any patient complaining of dysphagia or in whom an abnormality of the esophagus is seen by barium swallow.

At endoscopy, the visual findings are used to grade the severity of the esophagitis. No esophagitis is recorded when no reddening or ulceration is seen. Reddening of the distal esophagus without ulceration is scored as Grade I esophagitis. When visible ulcers through the mucosa are seen, Grade II esophagitis is recorded. Stiffening and fibrosis in the wall gives a different appearance to the endoscopist and is scored as Grade III esophagitis. Frank narrowing to the degree to which an esophagoscope cannot be passed is Grade IV esophagitis or reflux-induced stricture. Great care must be taken to differentiate this from carcinoma. The biopsies obtainable through the flexible fiberoptic esophagoscope are shallow, and may not be sufficient to exclude a carcinoma. For esophageal strictures, an open rigid esophagoscope is used through which bougies can be passed to dilate the channel and large biopsy forceps can be introduced to take deep biopsies into the submucosa in an effort to exclude neoplastic change.

Early changes in the esophageal mucosa induced by reflux cause the appearance of reddening without ulceration. If the biopsy is taken from these areas, the ratio of penetration of the rete pegs to the surface epithelium is greater than 60 per cent. Hyperplasia of the basal layer is often seen, and neovascularization of the epithelium may be observed. Although these findings are thought to account for the reddened appearance of the distal esophagus, they do not indicate the presence of true esophagitis and do not imply that further ulceration and stricture may occur. When the esophagoscopic findings suggest the presence of Barrett's esophagus based upon the distinctive coloration of the mucosa, it is important that multiple biopsies be taken. Dysplasia of the columnar cells may be observed, and some patients may have carcinoma in situ or frank invasive carcinoma arising in a Barrett epithelium. Neoplastic changes may be focal and scattered, so it is important that multiple biopsies be obtained.

Based upon multiple diagnostic studies, of which radiographic barium swallow, esophageal manometry and pH measurements, and endoscopic observation are most important, information is obtained by which the significance of hiatal hernia is determined, and reflux-induced changes may be differentiated from other esophageal disorders such as achalasia, spasm, neoplasm, and motor disturbances. Indi-cations for therapy are based upon the findings.

TRAUMATIC DIAPHRAGMATIC HERNIA

Traumatic diaphragmatic hernia from penetrating or blunt injury may be immediately apparent upon examination of the patient and inspection of a chest x-ray. On the other hand, this diagnosis is frequently missed for several days or longer until such time as extensive translocation of abdominal contents into the chest occurs with resulting risk of intestinal obstruction and volvulus. Spontaneous rupture of the diaphragm should be suspected in any patient who sustains significant blunt chest and upper abdominal trauma. Since the rupture from blunt trauma frequently occurs posteriorly, the diagnosis is best made by a lateral chest film that may not have been obtained in the emergency setting. If there is posterior blunting of the costophrenic angle and the appearance of fluid in the chest, this injury should be suspected. Bloody fluid may be obtained on thoracentesis. After stabilization of the patient's other injuries, radiographic evaluation of the upper and lower intestinal tract may confirm the diagnosis if there is doubt. These diagnostic procedures should be performed promptly before migration of a large amount of abdominal contents into the chest.

CONGENITAL DIAPHRAGMATIC HERNIA

Herniation of abdominal contents through the pleuroperitoneal canal in the newborn may present as a surgical emergency. Within the first hours of life the infant may appear short of breath, be tachypneic, have attacks of cyanosis, and be hypotensive. The trachea may be in the midline or shifted to the opposite side. The diagnosis is generally made by chest x-ray showing multiple air-filled viscera in the hemithorax. If the diagnosis is in doubt, instillation of a small amount of contrast material into the gastrointestinal tract should lead to ready confirmation of the diagnosis, but usually this test is not needed or advisable.

Later in life, eventration of the diaphragm related to a congenital defect may be difficult to differentiate from phrenic paralysis. This differentiation is made by careful review of the history to determine whether there is any illness that might cause phrenic nerve injury and by review of older x-rays when available to determine if the lesion is of long standing. Generally this disorder causes no significant abnormality and does not require a repair unless a significant amount of the hemithorax is occupied by the abdominal viscera.

Congenital hernia through the foramen of Morgagni is also not normally detected until later in life. It usually presents as an asymptomatic mass seen in the anterior lower mediastinum on chest x-ray. The diagnosis is most readily confirmed by a barium enema examinaton that shows cephalad displacement of the midtransverse colon either into the hernia sac or near it if omentum is incarcerated in the hernia sac. Complications of this hernia occur only if intestine is caught in the hernia. In such cases intestinal obstruction may develop, and the hernia should be repaired.

Section 9

DISORDERS OF
METABOLISM

RICKETS

By D. E. C. COLE, M.D.,
and C. R. SCRIVER, M.D.

Montreal, Quebec, Canada

Rickets is a disorder of mineral deposition in preosseous cartilage of epiphyseal growth plates and in matrix of growing bone; in osteomalacia, the disorder is confined to endosteal remodeling sites of mature bone matrix. Thus, it is the stage of bone growth and development that determines whether the combined process of rickets and osteomalacia, or osteomalacia alone, will occur when mineral metabolism is disturbed.

Inadequate mineralization follows those disturbances of metabolism that primarily affect either calcium availability (calciopenic causes) or phosphate availability (phosphopenic causes). It is understood, of course, that availability of phosphorus is the major ultimate determinant of clinical rickets or osteomalacia or both, and the calciopenic causes of rickets have their effect through phosphorus depletion secondary to the action of parathyroid hormone, whereas the phosphopenic forms reflect primary abnormalities of phosphate availability or conservation.

The role of vitamin D itself in the pathogenesis of rickets is still uncertain. It is now clearly evident that vitamin D through its hormonal derivative 1,25-(OH)$_2$D stimulates net intestinal absorption of calcium. However, there is recent, albeit tentative, evidence that another derivative, 24,25-(OH)$_2$D, may be directly involved in bone mineralization per se. Thus deficiencies of vitamin D or its hydroxylated derivatives could lead to impairment of both calcium availability and bone mineralization.

Vitamin D can be considered a "prohormone." In man, it has two environmental sources: one in the diet, as vitamin D$_2$ (ergocalciferol) or vitamin D$_3$ (cholecalciferol); the other in skin, where photolysis of 7-dehydrocholesterol by 296 to 310 nm ultraviolet radiation yields cholecalciferol. Thus diet, skin pigmentation, climate, and geographic latitude each contribute to human vitamin D homeostasis. Vitamin D (D$_2$ or D$_3$) is transported in the blood from skin to liver on a serum α-globulin called group-specific component (Gc). In hepatocytes the side chain is hydroxylated at the 25 position by a mixed function oxidase; 25-OH vitamin D is then transported by the Gc protein to the kidney, where 1α- or 24-hydroxylation takes place in mitochondria. 1α,25-(OH)$_2$D acts as a hormone exerting feedback regulation of 1-hydroxylase activity. The mechanism of regulation is a matter of continuing research; apparently, calcium and phosphate ions and parathyroid hormone are each involved. Up to now, 24,25-(OH)$_2$D biosynthesis has been viewed as a reciprocal function of 1-hydroxylation. The normal requirement for vitamin D is 400 units per day or about 50 nanograms per kg per day (1 IU = 25 nanograms vitamin D). The relative requirement ratios for vitamin D: 25-OH-D: 1,25-(OH)$_2$D are about 10:3:1.

DIAGNOSIS OF RICKETS AND ALLIED BONE DISEASE

A careful clinical history (for environmental events and clinical course) and an equally careful family history (for hereditary aspects) are the starting points in diagnosis. Accurate measurements of total serum calcium, phosphorus, and alkaline phosphatase are required. X-ray examination to confirm the rachitic (or osteomalacic) process or to identify nonrachitic forms of bone disease is also essential. Supplementary analyses of urine metabolites, serum immunoreactive parathyroid hormone (iPTH), and serum vitamin D metabolites can be quite useful adjuncts in diagnosis.

Normal Values. The mean total serum calcium level falls about 0.5 mg per dl (100 ml) between infancy and late adolescence from 10.2 mg per dl to 9.7 mg per dl (Arnaud, S., and Stickler, G.); two standard deviations are approximately $\pm$ 0.5 mg per dl at all ages. Total serum calcium must be corrected for variation in serum protein and specific gravity. The correction for protein is: measured [Ca]$_s$ $-$ (0.689 $\times$ total proteins) + 5.06. The correction for specific gravity is: measured [Ca]$_s$ = [(SG$_{obs}$ $-1.027) \times 250$]. The mean fasting serum phosphorus level falls from 5.7 mg per dl to 4.8 mg per dl between infancy and late adolescence. It falls further to 4.0 mg per dl in adults; two standard deviations is at least $\pm$ 1.0 mg per dl at all ages. The mean serum alkaline phosphatase value again falls with age from 102 IU to 53 IU in late adolescence and to 24 IU in adults. Two standard deviations is at least half the mean value. Serum iPTH should be less than 40 μlEq per ml for the C-terminal peptide assay. Normal serum vitamin D values are not widely established. They are probably influenced by age, geographic location, climate, and regional dietary practices. The range for 25-OH-D is 25 to 35 nanograms per ml; for 1,25-(OH)$_2$D it is 20 to 60 picograms per ml. Higher values are usually found in the younger subjects.

CLASSIFICATION OF RICKETS

The origins of rickets (and osteomalacia) are understandably complex. Certainly there can be no "final" classification as long as our knowledge about vitamin D metabolism is still evolving and many aspects of mineral metabolism have yet to be discovered. Table 1 is an interim classification. The calciopenic and phosphopenic groupings are merely attempts to recognize primary origins of the relevant forms of rickets.

However, they have implications for treatment: calciopenic forms require vitamin D hormone or calcium replacement, and phosphopenic forms require phosphate replacement and vitamin D. Special attention is paid to the changing clinical and biochemical features of

Table 1. *Causes of Rickets and Osteomalacia*

I. Origin in Calciopenia
  A. Inadequate calcium intake
  B. Inadequate intake of vitamin D
    1. Environmental deficiency (diet; sunlight)
    2. Malabsorption
  C. Disturbances of vitamin D metabolism
    1. Decreased formation of 25-OH-D
      (a) Hepatocellular disease
      (b) Anticonvulsant medications
    2. Decreased formation of 1,25-$(OH)_2D$ or target organ resistance
      (a) Autosomal recessive vitamin D dependency (type I)
      (b) Renal osteodystrophy (see below)
      (c) Hypoparathyroidism and pseudohypoparathyroidism (see below)
      (d) Vitamin D dependency (type II)

II. Origin in phosphopenia
  A. Inadequate intake of phosphorus
    1. Dietary deficiency
    2. Symptomatic deficiency (antacid medication, etc.)
  B. Deficient renal reabsorption
    1. Specific phosphate transport defects
      (a) X-linked hypophosphatemia
      (b) Autosomal hypophosphatemic bone disease
    2 Multiple dysfunctions (Fanconi syndrome): Idiopathic and symptomatic forms
    3. Renal tubular acidosis
    4. Miscellaneous causes
      (a) Neurofibromatosis
      (b) Fibrous dysplasia
      (c) Tumors (see below)

III. Complex origin
  A. Renal osteodystrophy
  B. States of decreased parathyroid function
  C. Tumors
  D. Neonatal rickets

IV. Diseases with skeletal manifestations resembling rickets
  A. Hypophosphatasia (and pseudohypophosphatasia)
  B. Metaphyseal dysplasia
  C. Fibrogenesis imperfecta ossium

---

vitamin D deficiency (Table 2) during evolution of the stages of calciopenia. A compensatory parathyroid gland response with emergence of hypophosphatemia secondary to inhibition of renal tubular reabsorption accounts for the staging. The importance of (secondary) phosphopenia in the pathogenesis of rickets is revealed in the evolution of vitamin D deficiency.

CALCIOPENIC RICKETS

INADEQUATE CALCIUM INTAKE

Rickets can occur in the rapidly growing infant receiving adequate vitamin D nutrition if the calcium intake is insufficient to meet requirements. This can be the case in the premature infant and in the breast-fed infant, and also in the occasional infant exposed to an unusual diet poor in calcium. The normal serum level of 25-OH-D and the dietary history will reveal the origin of this genuine form of calciopenia relative to phosphorus. The biochemical signs resemble vitamin D deficiency.

DEFICIENCY OF VITAMIN D

Simple (Nutrition)

In infants, the manifestations of vitamin D deficiency rickets (Table 2) are most likely to be observed during the period of rapid growth. Contributing factors include antepartum maternal nutrition, prematurity, the adequacy of mineral and vitamin D nutrition after birth, and the extent of postpartum exposure to sunlight. Human milk, once thought to be a marginal source of vitamin D, contains a water-soluble sulfated form of the vitamin that can be utilized by the newborn. When the maternal vitamin D status is suboptimal, as is the case with socioeconomic deprivation or limited exposure to sunlight in winter months, nutritional rickets may appear in the breast-fed newborn. Macrobiotic and vegetarian dietary regimens that avoid fortified cow's milk may be deficient in vitamin D. A careful dietary history is always indicated in those dietary practices inconsistent with normal bone growth and should indicate appropriate preventive measures.

Three progressive clinical and biochemical stages of vitamin D deficiency may be distinguished on clinical, biochemical, and radiologic grounds (Table 2). Stage 1 is characterized by manifestations of hypocalcemia; typical skeletal signs appear in stage 2 or 3. The latter (in advancing order of severity) include craniotabes; costochondral beading; enlarged wrists, knees and ankles; Harrison's groove; frontal and parietal bossing of skull (caput quadratum);

Table 2. *Stages of Vitamin D Deficiency in Children*

	Stage I	*Stage II*	*Stage III*
A. Clinical features			
Typical age/onset (mo)	3–7 mo.	5–12 mo	6 mo. and older
Usual clinical presentation	Convulsions, tetany	Skeletal signs bronchopneumonia	More advanced skeletal signs; convulsions and tetany
Principal physical signs	± craniotabes	Moderate clinical rickets, pulmonary changes, some classic bony signs; deformities may not be present	Severe clinical rickets usually with bony deformities; pulmonary changes
B. Radiologic features	Minimal changes best seen in skull	Early to moderate classic skeletal changes	Moderate to advanced skeletal changes; signs of hyperparathyroidism
C. Biochemical features (Normal values for infants)			
1. Serum Ca (>9 mg/dl)	↓	Normal	↓
2. Serum Pi (>4.5 mg/dl)	Normal	↓	↓
3. Alkaline phosphatase	Normal to sl ↑	↑	↑
4. Serum iPTH (<40 μlEq/ml)	Normal or sl ↑	↑	↑↑
5. Urine amino acids	Normal	Increased generalized aminoaciduria	Increased generalized aminoaciduria

long bone and spinal deformities: genu valgum (knock-knees) or genu varum (bowlegs); lordosis and scoliosis; "dwarfism" (when severe); delayed and defective dentition; pathologic fractures.

Rachitic changes in the bony thorax may be responsible for the well-known clinical association of rickets with respiratory system disease.

Neuromuscular features are usually due to hypocalcemia; these include tetany, laryngeal stridor, positive Chvostek and Trousseau signs, and generalized convulsions. Decreased muscle tone and fatigue owing to hypophosphatemia may be present in stages 2 and 3. Vitamin D deficiency rickets should respond in 1 or 2 weeks to replacement therapy with oral vitamin D (50 micrograms per kg per day).

When the epiphyses have fused, nutritional vitamin D deficiency causes osteomalacia. Two groups at increased risk for osteomalacia are women whose vitamin D depletion may manifest itself in their offspring, and the elderly person with inadequate exposure to sunlight or poor dietary habits. Significantly decreased plasma 25-OH-D (<10 nanograms per ml) has been found in one third of the elderly patients with femoral neck fractures.

Vitamin D Malabsorption

Vitamin D is a fat-soluble substance. Rickets or osteomalacia secondary to steatorrhea is well documented. Intestinal malabsorption or the interruption of enterohepatic circulation that accompanies cholestasis impairs vitamin D absorption. The clinical history should suggest the primary condition; however, the physician should be alert to signs of malabsorption in infants with active rickets "resistant" to normal supplemental doses of vitamin D. The radiologic picture is usually complicated by osteoporosis resulting from impaired general nutrition. Malabsorption syndromes are often very resistant to oral vitamin D therapy and, if calcium absorption is greatly impaired, even parenteral vitamin therapy will be inadequate. Treatment of the primary condition is mandatory.

DISTURBANCES OF VITAMIN D HORMONE BIOSYNTHESIS

Decreased Formation of 25-OH-Vitamin D

Hepatocellular Disease. Severe hepatocellular disease can cause rickets or osteomalacia. Decreased hepatic hydroxylation of parent vitamin D and interruption of enterohepatic circulation are possible causes; in any event, serum 25-OH-D levels are depressed. Treatment with vitamin D hormone is usually indicated.

Anticonvulsant Medications. Chronic administration of phenytoin (diphenylhydantoin), phenobarbital, or primidone may impair 25-hydroxylation of vitamin D. Ambulant patients treated with anticonvulsants are usually at lower risk; institutionalized and bedridden patients tend to have a higher incidence of symptomatic vitamin D metabolite deficiency. The problem may be pharmacogenetic in origin, intrinsic factors in the presence of anticonvulsant drugs determining appearance of the syndrome in specific patients. Patients on a combination of drugs are more likely to be affected. The normal daily requirement for vitamin D (400 IU per day) is elevated; however, no universal "prophylactic" dosage (2000 to 5000 IU per day) can be recommended because of the risk of hypercalcemia, particularly in inactive patients. Careful monitoring of the patient is mandatory whenever prophylaxis is attempted. A persistently elevated alkaline phosphatase should be interpreted with caution since anticonvulsant drugs may alter hepatic metabolism and affect alkaline phosphatase levels. Special analytic methods that selectively measure alkaline phosphatase of hepatic or intestinal origin may be a useful adjunct in diagnosis.

Decreased 1α-Hydroxylation Activity or Target Organ Resistance

Vitamin D Dependency (Pseudodeficiency Rickets) (Type I). Early postnatal appearance of "deficiency" rickets in an infant with adequate dietary intake should suggest vitamin D dependency, particularly when the rachitic condition fails to respond to normal requirement for vitamin D. The condition is inherited as an autosomal recessive: it is presumed to be a deficiency of 1α-hydroxylase activity.

Florid skeletal changes resembling stage 3 of the deficiency syndrome are apparent (see Table 2). Enamel hypoplasia of teeth that calcify postnatally is often apparent in late-diagnosed patients.

Serum 25-OH-D is usually elevated while serum 1,25-(OH)$_2$D concentrations are well below normal. Patients with type I autosomal recessive vitamin D dependency (ARVDD) are not "resistant" to treatment. Vitamin D in doses from 40,000 to 100,000 IU per day promotes healing of the calciopenia. A prompt response to "physiologic" amounts (1 to 2 micrograms per day) of 1α-hydroxylated forms of vitamin D [1,25-(OH)$_2$D or 1α-OH-Vitamin D] is a diagnostic clinical test.

Vitamin D Dependency (Type II) (Target Organ Resistance to Vitamin D). Late-appearing osteomalacia, chronic hypocalcemia, increased serum iPTH, and increased serum levels of 1,25-(OH)$_2$D are found in this newly reported condition. The failure of 1,25-(OH)$_2$D supplements (up to 7 micrograms per day) to repair the condition indicates some form of target organ resistance. Patients reported so far with this form of vitamin D dependency are adult and most commonly female.

PHOSPHOPENIC RICKETS

INADEQUATE INTAKE

Although most diets meet phosphorus requirements, total parenteral nutrition (TPN) can provoke symptomatic hypophosphatemia. In adults, bone mass is not normally affected by TPN-induced hypophosphatemia.

Chronic oral administration of antacid gels that form insoluble phosphate complexes can cause phosphopenia and osteomalacia. In growing children, and particularly in neonates receiving TPN, associated hypophosphatemia may be a rachitogenic factor.

DEFICIENT RENAL REABSORPTION OF PHOSPHATE

Isolated Defects of Phosphate Reabsorption

X-linked Hypophosphatemic Rickets: Familial Vitamin D Resistant Rickets. X-linked hypophosphatemia can be considered the prototype of phosphopenic rickets. A selective transport defect in the brush border (luminal) membrane of renal tubular epithelium is the origin of impaired phosphate reabsorption and hypophosphatemia.

Hypophosphatemia appears soon after birth in male hemizygotes and severely affected female heterozygotes. Rickets is usually apparent 3 to 6 months after birth. Linear growth is severely impaired, particularly in the lower body segment (growth is below the 3rd percentile).

Biochemical features include severe hypophosphatemia and normal serum calcium, elevated alkaline phosphatase, essentially normal serum iPTH, and normal tubular function with the exception of the phosphate transport defect. Serum levels of 25-OH-D are normal; the 1,25-(OH)$_2$D level is modestly below normal for reasons that are unclear.

The disease is inherited as an X-linked dominant and female carriers are hypophosphatemic; their bone disease is not expressed in direct proportion to their hypophosphatemia. There is an increased requirement for phosphorus; accordingly, the prevention of rickets involves dietary phosphorus supplementation of 1 to 4 grams per day. Phosphate-induced hypocalcemia and hyperparathyroidism are suppressed by vitamin D therapy [about 1 to 2 micrograms 1,25-(OH)$_2$D per day.]

Hypophosphatemic Bone Disease (HBD). An autosomal condition, inherited as a dominant, HBD is essentially nonrachitic even in infancy and childhood, despite serum phosphorus levels equivalent to those observed in X-linked hypophosphatemia. Osteomalacic changes are found in the metaphyses of long bones. Serum 1,25-(OH)$_2$D and iPTH levels are normal. A selective defect in tubular conservation of phosphate has been demonstrated, which is independent of that controlled by the X-linked gene. The presenting clinical feature is genu varum in the second year of life and modest attentuation of linear growth (3rd to 10th percentile).

The Fanconi Syndrome and Allied Disorders (Multiple Abnormalities of Tubular Reabsorption)

The Fanconi syndrome is distinguished by coexistent hyperphosphatemia, glucosuria, and generalized hyperaminoaciduria. It is usually accompanied by: (1) acidosis, due to an inability to reabsorb HCO_3^-; (2) polyuria and dehydration, due to inability to conserve H_2O; and (3) hypokalemia and hypercalciuria.

The syndrome is either idiopathic or symptomatic. Most forms are inherited as autosomal recessives, although one variant (Lowe's syndrome) is an X-linked recessive. Autosomal dominant and sporadic forms of the idiopathic syndrome also occur. The symptomatic forms are secondary to either a primary event —such as exposure to heavy metals, outdated tetracyclines, and other toxins — or other hereditary disease such as galactosemia, hereditary fructose intolerance, glycogenosis, cystinosis, hereditary tyrosinemia, Wilson's disease (hepatolenticular degeneration), and hepatorenal syndrome. The oculocerebrorenal syndrome of Lowe-Terry-Machlachan has characteristic clinical features that include areflexia and muscular hypotonia, congenital cataract and glaucoma, and buphthalmos.

Diagnosis involves identification of the primary causes of symptomatic forms of the Fanconi syndrome; treatment in such cases is usually directed toward the primary condition (e.g., galactose restriction in galactosemia). If the syndrome is idiopathic or an untreatable symptomatic form, then compensatory replacement of solutes, electrolytes, and water is required. Phosphate replacement, correction of acidosis, and modest amounts of vitamin D (5000 IU per day) may be necessary (in various combinations and in accordance with the nature of the syndrome phenotype) to heal rickets.

Progressive loss of glomerular function — a complication of cystinosis and in some cases of the idiopathic form — requires the appropriate tailoring of phosphate intake to match progressive phosphate retention.

The Renal Tubular Acidoses (RTA) and Allied Disorders

Rickets may occur in chronic acidosis; the pathogenesis is often complex. The hyperchloremic acidosis associated with ureterocolic anastomosis can cause phosphopenia. Repair of the acidosis corrects phosphopenia and heals the rickets. Of the primary forms of renal tubular acidosis associated with defective bicarbon-

ate transport (proximal RTA) or defective H^+ excretion (distal RTA), only the latter manifests rickets. In addition to the male predominance of this hereditary condition and the signs of distal RTA, there is prominent hypercalcuria (>10 mg per kg per day versus normal of 0.3 to 8 mg per kg per day and additional disturbances of mineral metabolism. Correction of the acidosis (1 to 2 mEq HCO_3^- per kg per day) corrects the disturbances of calcium and phosphate metabolism and heals the rickets.

Miscellaneous Causes

Increased phosphate excretion and relative phosphopenia may complicate neurofibromatosis (von Recklinghausen disease) and polyostotic fibrous dysplasia. Since bony changes are usually mild and slow to develop, diagnosis depends on examination of serum phosphate and phosphate reabsorption index.

COMPLEX ORIGIN

RENAL OSTEODYSTROPHY

Uremic bone pathology is the result of several complex and interrelated events that both reduce renal hydroxylation reactions and decrease sensitivity of target organs (intestine and bone) to the biologic effects of vitamin D hormones(s). Decreased renal clearance of phosphate with hyperphosphatemia, hypocalcemia, and hyperparathyroidism are related in various ways to reduction of renal mass and impaired 25-OH-D hydroxylation activity. The specific rachitic component of uremic osteodystrophy is a variable aspect of the total picture and is related to the linear growth rate in the patient. The radiologic and clinical features of renal osteodystrophy are usually distinctive and diagnostic. Management must involve careful monitoring of therapy for the hypocalcemic component beyond restriction of phosphate intake, since levels of 1,25-$(OH)_2$D are frequently low. This metabolite will ameliorate the effects of hyperparathyroidism on the skeleton more than the rickets and osteomalacia; 25-OH-D appears to be more efficacious in the healing of "renal rickets." This finding suggests that 24,25-$(OH)_2$D may be important in skeletal mineralization. The so-called target organ resistance to vitamin D may reflect this facet of the problem.

STATES OF DECREASED PARATHYROID FUNCTION

Deficiency of parathyroid hormone (PTH) or decreased renal responsiveness to PTH (pseudohypoparathyroidism) have both been associated with altered vitamin D metabolism. There is some evidence for decreased formation of 1,25-$(OH)_2D$ and for resistance to 1,25-$(OH)_2D$ present in serum. The resistance is not complete, since patients demonstrate only mild skeletal changes consistent with osteomalacia and may become normocalcemic with 1,25-$(OH)_2D$ administration.

TUMORS

Rickets and osteomalacia are recognized as infrequently occurring but important paraneoplastic syndromes. They appear to accompany tumors of mesenchymal origin; viz., hemangiopericytomas, hemangiomas, and giant cell tumors of bone. Both phosphopenic (increased phosphate excretion) and calciopenic causes [decreased 1,25-$(OH)_2D$ levels] have been advanced. Cure is effected by removal of the tumor.

NEONATAL RICKETS

As with all aspects of neonatal nutrition, maintenance of an adequate environment for normal mineralization in premature newborns is a difficult task. There is evidence for decreased absorption of calcium and phosphorus; decreased 25-hydroxylation of vitamin D by the liver; "decreased" serum levels of 1,25-$(OH)_2D$; and resistance to exogenously administered 1,25-$(OH)_2D$. Furthermore, appropriate norms for biochemical parameters at various gestational ages are not yet widely established.

Factors that are known to lead to severe osteopenia with a substantial rachitic component include prolonged parenteral nutrition, chronic acidosis, restricted mineral intake (associated with exclusive feeding of human breast milk), and cholestasis (often accompanying parenteral nutrition). Skeletal changes may be similar to those described earlier, but radiologic findings such as metaphyseal widening and severe demineralization are likely to be more prominent than actual physical signs. There is some evidence that severe rachitic demineralization of the bony thorax contributes substantially to chronic respiratory distress such as that seen in Mikity-Wilson syndrome. Finally, hypophosphatemia results in relative muscle weakness that may exacerbate marginal pulmonary or cardiac function. The careful monitoring and maintenance of serum calcium and phosphorus during chronic parenteral or oral alimentation in premature intensive care is the key to prevention; supplementation of 1,25-$(OH)_2D$ may be required in some cases.

DISEASES WITH SKELETAL MANIFESTATIONS RESEMBLING RICKETS

Primary disorders of bone matrix formation may result in decreased mineralization and hence a radiologic picture resembling rickets or osteomalacia.

In *hypophosphatasia*, a deficiency of bone alkaline phosphatase is associated with an autosomal recessive syndrome of severe osteopenia. Serum calcium and phosphorus are not significantly lowered but the presence of large amounts of phosphoethanolamine in the urine on amino acid chromatography is diagnostic. In most cases, the skeletal fraction of serum alkaline phosphatase is greatly depressed, but in some (pseudo-hypophosphatasia) it may be normal.

Metaphyseal dysostosis is radiologically similar to rickets but the absence of any biochemical evidence of a mineralization defect implies that the primary problem resides in matrix formation. It is inherited in an autosomal recessive manner.

Fibrogenesis imperfecta ossium is a rare adult disorder of bone collagen fibril formation that results in a radiologic picture of osteomalacia without any abnormality of mineral metabolism. Diagnosis is confirmed by typical findings on bone biopsy.

HYPERLIPIDEMIA

By WILLIAM E. CONNOR, M.D.
Portland, Oregon

By any definition, primary hyperlipidemia is one of the most common conditions seen in the practice of medicine and certainly the most frequent genetic abnormality. Patients of any age and of either sex may have or develop hyperlipidemia. With the widespread use of chemical screening tests, more and more patients with asymptomatic hyperlipidemia will now be identified and specific diagnoses required.

Hyperlipidemia is important clinically for four reasons: (1) it is causative of coronary heart disease and atherosclerosis generally; (2) profound hypertriglyceridemia is associated with episodes of abdominal pain and with acute pancreatitis; (3) xanthomas of the skin and tendons develop, which are external hallmarks of the underlying hyperlipidemia; and (4) hyperlipidemia may be secondary to another disease process and thus may point the way for the eventual diagnosis of that disease, e.g., the hyperlipidemia of hypothyroidism.

CRITERIA FOR DIAGNOSIS

Primary hyperlipidemia occurs when the plasma cholesterol or triglyceride levels or both are at or above those elevations associated with certain diseases (e.g., coronary heart disease, xanthomas, pancreatitis). Currently accepted lower levels for the diagnosis of hyperlipidemia are shown in Table 1.

The blood for diagnosis should ideally be obtained after a 12- to 14-hour fast when the patient is consuming his customary diet, is not losing weight, and is not suffering from a concurrent severe or stressful illness. The ultimate diagnosis of hyperlipidemia must rest upon at least two, and preferably three, plasma lipid determinations taken a week or more apart. The diagnosis should be approached with considerable care, because primary hyperlipidemia is likely to be a permanent problem necessitating a lifetime of attention. The criteria for hyperlipidemia in children are listed, because hyperlipidemia is usually familial and because it is common in children. The diagnosis of primary hyperlipidemia is always on firmer ground if hyperlipidemia is also detected in one or more first degree relatives.

Early in the work-up, it is necessary to establish that the hyperlipidemia is primary or secondary. Prominent secondary causes that must be eliminated include (1) uncontrolled diabetes mellitus, (2) hypothyroidism, (3) nephrotic syndrome, (4) renal dialysis and transplantation, (5) steroid therapy (corticoids, oral contraceptives), (6) mid or late pregnancy, (7) biliary obstruction, (8) glycogen storage disease, and (9) dysglobulinemia or autoimmune disease.

CLASSIFICATION

A given patient will readily fall into one of three categories: (1) those patients with primarily hypercholesterolemia, (2) those with hypertriglyceridemia without chylomicrons, and (3) those with hypertriglyceridemia and chylomicrons. With only hypercholesterolemia, the plasma will be clear, whereas plasma containing high triglyceride concentrations will generally be cloudy or even lactescent. If chylomicrons are present, a diagnostic point of great

Table 1.

	Plasma Cholesterol	Plasma Triglyceride
For children	200 mg/dl (100 ml) and above	140 mg/dl (100 ml) and above
For adults	220 mg/dl (100 ml) and above	180 mg/dl (100 ml) and above

significance, a lactescent sample of plasma allowed to sit overnight will form a layer of "cream" at the top of the tube. A pragmatic and useful approach to treatment may be developed on the basis of this preliminary classification.

It is now appropriate to pinpoint the specific hyperlipidemic disorders in terms of clinical symptomatology and lipoprotein disorders. These diseases can be grouped into three main categories. They are listed in order of frequency and clinical importance.

FAMILIAL HYPERCHOLESTEROLEMIA (XANTHOMATOUS HYPERCHOLESTEROLEMIA, TYPES II-a AND II-b HYPERLIPOPROTEINEMIA, HYPERBETALIPOPROTEINEMIA)

DEFINITION

This condition is characterized by increased low density of beta lipoproteins, which are the chief carriers of cholesterol in the plasma. Consequently, the plasma cholesterol is moderately to profoundly elevated, with plasma triglyceride levels usually but not always normal. The cause of the hypercholesterolemia may be impairment of low density lipoprotein removal from the plasma.

CLINICAL FINDINGS

Inherited as an autosomal dominant, familial hypercholesterolemia may be found at any age and in either sex. Xanthelasma and tuberous and tendon xanthoma occur in many patients, especially when plasma cholesterol levels are above 300 mg per dl (100 ml). Atherosclerosis is greatly accelerated, many patients having developed overt coronary heart disease before the age of 40. Women with familial hypercholesterolemia lose their usual protection against the development of coronary heart disease during the menstruating years. Children with the uncommon homozygous form are severely afflicted with both vascular disease and xanthomas. Other children and adults with the very common heterozygous form may have a long latency period without clinical manifestations other than hypercholesterolemia. Obesity is not related to this form of hyperlipidemia except in those patients with concomitant mild hypertriglyceridemia (type II-b, combined hyperlipidemia) who are usually overweight. Patients with familial hypercholesterolemia have an unremitting, life-long problem.

LABORATORY FINDINGS

The plasma cholesterol elevation ranges from 220 to 800 mg per dl or more in adults and from 200 to 800 mg per dl. in children. The plasma cholesterol level is directly correlated with the concentration of low density lipoprotein. The plasma is characteristically clear and the triglyceride content normal or even low (type II-a). However, some patients have an additional lipoprotein abnormality, increased very low density lipoprotein (VLDL) or pre-betalipoprotein (type II-b). They have both hypercholesterolemia and mild hypertriglyceridemia (usually under 300 mg per dl).

Based upon the plasma cholesterol level and clinical findings, familial hypercholesterolemia may be subclassified as mild heterozygous (220 to 270 mg per dl), severe heterozygous (270 to 600 mg per dl), and homozygous (above 600 mg per dl). The diagnosis of familial hypercholesterolemia is not helped by the use of lipoprotein electrophoresis.

PITFALLS IN DIAGNOSIS

There is seldom confusion once secondary causes of hyperlipidemia have been ruled out unless the plasma triglyceride level is also elevated (type II-b). A strong family history of hypercholesterolemia will help differentiate II-b from other hypertriglyceridemic states. In type II-b, the patient's plasma cholesterol level is generally higher than his triglyceride elevation — cholesterol, 350 mg per dl; triglyceride, 270 mg per dl.

HYPERTRIGLYCERIDEMIA WITHOUT CHYLOMICRONS (HYPERPREBETALIPO-PROTEINEMIA; TYPE IV HYPERLIPO-PROTEINEMIA—COMMON; TYPE III HYPERLIPOPROTEINEMIA—RARE)

DEFINITION

Hypertriglyceridemia is common and usually results from an increase in triglyceride-rich very low density (VLDL) or prebetalipoprotein.

It is commonly known as type IV hyperlipoproteinemia. The synthesis of VLDL is increased (from increased caloric substrate) and its catabolism is impaired (possibly from concurrent adiposity). The rare type III hyperlipoproteinemia is considered similarly because of common clinical and therapeutic features. It results from the presence of large quantities of an intermediate lipoprotein (IDL) that carries large quantities of both triglyceride and cholesterol. IDL accumulates because of a presumed catabolic block in the usual conversion of VLDL to low density lipoprotein. It is also called an abnormal VLDL and a floating betalipoprotein.

CLINICAL FEATURES

These diseases are familial but usually occur only in adult life. Patients with hypertriglyceridemia are commonly overweight and have impaired glucose tolerance tests or else are overtly diabetic. Xanthomas are a hallmark of the type III patient, especially large yellow-red tuberous xanthomas, yellow-orange planar xanthomas of the palmar surface of the hands, and tendon xanthomas. Vascular disease is probably more common in the type IV patient than in normals. However, premature vascular disease is much less frequent than in familial hypercholesterolemia. Atherosclerosis is even more accelerated in the type III patient. Especially remarkable is the extensive peripheral vascular disease of type III disease.

LABORATORY FINDINGS

The hypertriglyceridemia of these patients may range from slight to moderate elevation. The plasma cholesterol level is elevated as well, with rare exceptions. The plasma is cloudy, even lactescent, usually without chylomicrons. Typically, the type IV patient has cholesterol levels of 200 to 300 mg per dl and triglyceride concentrations of 200 to 1000 mg per dl). The type III patient has a higher cholesterol level, 300 to 500 mg per dl, and a lower triglyceride, 300 to 700 mg per dl. Triglyceride may be only slightly higher than cholesterol. Electrophoresis is not clinically helpful or reliable. Ultracentrifugation may be used for further clarification of the diagnosis. If the ratio of VLDL cholesterol to total plasma triglyceride is 0.3 or greater, the impression of type III hyperlipidemia is further substantiated.

DIAGNOSTIC PITFALLS

These hypertriglyceridemic patients are frequently confused with patients with familial hypercholesterolemia, who may also have concomitant hypertriglyceridemia (type II-b). Familial patterns of hyperlipidemia may clarify the diagnosis. Fortunately, initial therapies are similar for all three of these conditions (types IV, III, and II-b). It is crucial to clarify the issue of secondary hyperlipidemia, because most of the patients with secondary hyperlipidemia will fall into this hypertriglyceridemic group. Although the vast majority of these patients are overweight, a few may be slender.

HYPERTRIGLYCERIDEMIA WITH CHYLOMICRONS (TYPES I AND V HYPERLIPOPROTEINEMIA)

DEFINITION

The hallmark of this condition is the presence of large quantities of chylomicrons resulting from an absence or deficiency of lipoprotein lipase. This enzyme is responsible for clearing from the blood recently absorbed dietary fat being transported in chylomicrons. Chylomicron retention occurs in both types I and V. In addition, the type V patient has a second lipoprotein abnormality, an excess of very low density lipoproteins (VLDL) which further augments the profound degree of hypertriglyceridemia.

CLINICAL FEATURES

The type I patient is extremely rare and clinically resembles the type V patient who is seen more commonly. Both these disorders are frequently detected in infancy and childhood because of the occurrence of episodes of severe abdominal pain and of acute pancreatitis during hyperlipidemic crises. In addition, the profound lactescence of their plasmas calls attention to the underlying hyperlipidemic problem whenever blood is being analyzed for other purposes. Other clinical features include lipemia retinalis and eruptive xanthoma (yellow-red lesions) widely distributed in the skin, and appearing and disappearing in weeks as the chylomicronemia waxes and wanes. Excessive alcohol intake may contribute to the problem in the type V patient. Some patients may be overweight and have abnormal glucose tolerance tests. Others, especially the children, are slender. The incidence of atherosclerotic vascular disease is increased in type V patients, whereas data from a limited number of patients indicate no enhancement in type I disease. The response to a fat-free formula or very low fat diet (5 per cent of total calories) is diagnostic. Chylomicron formation is lessened and triglyceride levels fall by 50 per cent or more after 3 to 5 days of the low fat diet.

LABORATORY FINDINGS

Chylomicrons are invariably identified from the layer of "cream" that floats to the top of a lactescent plasma specimen allowed to sit in the refrigerator overnight.

These patients have profound hypertriglyceridemia, up to 10,000 mg per dl from the triglyceride-rich chylomicrons present in the fasting state. Cholesterol levels are also elevated, but secondarily, up to 600 to 1000 mg per dl. For example, a typical type V patient might have 7000 mg per dl of triglyceride and 650 mg per dl of cholesterol circulating in the plasma. Spuriously depressed are water-soluble substances, especially electrolytes, because of the dilution effect from the high triglyceride that may occupy up to 10 per cent of the usual plasma water.

DIAGNOSTIC PITFALLS

"Hypertriglyceridemia with chylomicrons" may be seen in uncontrolled diabetics, especially with ketosis. Insulin produces dramatic improvement. The diagnosis of hyperchylomicronemia is crucial for the prescription of the appropriate dietary therapy (an extremely low fat diet). Thus confusion with "hypertriglyceridemia *without* chylomicrons" must be avoided, because that condition has a different dietary therapy, that may further injure the type V patient. When the type V patient is treated with the very low fat diet, chylomicrons largely disappear but the VLDL abnormality remains. The plasma lipids may then resemble those of some type IV patients (triglyceride, 700 mg per dl; cholesterol, 180 mg per dl).

GOUT

By BERNARD F. GERMAIN, M.D.,
FRANK B. VASEY, M.D.,
and LUIS R. ESPINOZA, M.D.

Tampa, Florida

DEFINITION

Gout is caused by the formation and deposition of monosodium urate crystals within body fluids and tissues. Articular gout is caused by urate crystals in the joints. Tophaceous gout results from massive deposition of urate crystals in tissue. Renal deposition of urate and uric acid crystals causes urate nephropathy, uric acid nephropathy, and uric acid stones. The occurrence of gout correlates with an elevated serum uric acid level (hyperuricemia), although hyperuricemia may not always be present during an episode of gout. Conversely, hyperuricemia is frequently present in the absence of gout. Uric acid renal stones and urate nephropathy correlate with an increased urinary excretion of uric acid.

PRESENTING SIGNS AND SYMPTOMS

Acute articular gout is the most common form of gout. Early in the course of gout the attacks are usually characteristic, and the diagnosis can be suspected from the description of the attacks. Acute articular gout begins suddenly, usually in one or two joints (a monarticular or pauciarticular onset). A lower extremity joint is usually involved first, the first metatarsophalangeal joint (the big toe), the ankle, or the knee. The elbow or olecranon bursa is another early site of gouty involvement. About half the time gout begins in the first metatarsophalangeal joint (podagra). Almost all patients with repeated attacks of gout have had an episode of podagra; thus a history of acute podagra strongly suggests gout and should be asked of all arthritis patients. Gout rarely if ever occurs in the spine.

The attack of gout is marked by severe pain, tenderness, swelling, heat, and redness. The severity of the pain is often characteristic. The patient will describe it as the worst pain he or she has ever experienced. Often the patient will not tolerate anything to touch the affected joint, and weight bearing is not tolerated. Frequently the patient will describe going to bed well and awakening with severe pain and swelling in the joint. A precipitating factor can sometimes be identified — trauma to the joint, acute alcohol intake, dietary excess, surgery, or rapid weight loss. The attack usually increases in intensity over the next 24 hours then gradually subsides over the next 6 to 7 days. Subsequent attacks are intermittent at varying intervals of weeks to years. Between attacks the joints are normal.

Gout is primarily a disease of men, beginning for the most part in the fourth and fifth decades. Gout in women is distinctly uncommon before the menopause.

If the gouty attacks continue without treatment that lowers the serum uric acid level, chronic gout may supervene. Rather than the characteristic pattern of acute episodic attacks, a chronic symmetrical arthritis of multiple peripheral joints develops. The patient will usually have had episodic gout for many years before chronic gouty arthritis supervenes. Chronic gout often occurs simultaneously with massive deposition of urate crystals in soft tissue (tophi). Tophi may be found on the ears, in the olecranon bursae, over the extensor surface of the elbows, along the Achilles tendons, and over the joints.

Uric acid renal stones present in a similar fashion to renal stones in general: acute flank pain, hematuria, repeated urinary tract infections, or urinary obstruction. Uric acid renal stones may on occasion occur before articular gout. Gout and hyperuricemia are also associated with an increased prevalence of calcium renal stones. Urate nephropathy causes a gradual deterioration of renal function. Uric acid nephropathy presents as acute renal failure in the face of marked uricaciduria usually secondary to chemotherapy in patients with leukemia or lymphoma.

COURSE

The course of gout is quite variable. The patient may have only one episode of gout, or episodes separated by many years. More commonly the attacks will occur with increasing frequency. The attacks tend to last longer as time passes and more joints are involved. In some patients chronic tophaceous gout supervenes. Uric acid renal stones may occur during the course of the disease and with or without urate nephropathy lead to gradual loss of renal function.

PHYSICAL EXAMINATION

Early in the acute attack the joint is tender, swollen, warm, and red. Palpation or movement of the joint is very painful. Often the attack will begin with involvement of the first metatarsophalangeal joint, but the inflammation will spread to the tarsus and ankle so that the entire foot is involved. As the attack continues, the skin becomes thickened and wrinkled (tree bark effect). The skin often desquamates, creating a clinical picture that may mimic septic cellulitis. The inflammation may be along tendon sheaths and present as a tenosynovitis of the dorsum of the hands or feet.

In chronic gout, tophi may be found on the helix and antihelix of the ear, within the olecranon bursae, on the extensor surface of the forearm, on the Achilles tendons, and over joints. These are usually nodular deposits; they may drain white chalky material that can be identified as urate crystals.

If chronic gouty arthritis is present, the patient may have synovitis of multiple joints in a symmetrical pattern.

Associated conditions such as hypertension, obesity, arteriosclerotic heart disease, and evidence of alcohol excess should be looked for during the physical examination.

COMPLICATIONS

Gout itself is a complication of hyperuricemia. The incidence of gout increases with the magnitude and duration of the hyperuricemia. Hyperuricemia may be primary, owing to an unknown metabolic defect leading to overproduction of uric acid or to renal underexcretion of uric acid or both, or hyperuricemia and gout may be secondary to another underlying disease. Consequently, each patient with gout must be carefully examined to rule out an underlying disease. This will be discussed further under Pitfalls in Diagnosis.

Chronic persistent gouty arthritis and tophaceous gout are complications of untreated episodic articular gout. Renal uric acid stones and urate nephropathy are also complications of untreated hyperuricemia, although these statements should not be interpreted to mean all patients with asymptomatic hyperuricemia should be treated.

In time, articular gout may, with the deposition of large quantities of urate crystals, cause severe destructive changes in the soft tissue structures, cartilage, and periarticular bone of the joints, leading to deformities and crippling. Soft tissue swelling can cause compression of adjacent nerves leading to compression neuropathies such as carpal tunnel syndrome. Tophi may drain and may become secondarily infected.

Uric acid stones may cause urinary obstruction with secondary pyelonephritis, hydronephrosis, or hydroureter. These conditions may lead to chronic renal failure. Urate nephropathy results from deposition of urate crystals within the renal interstitial tissue that in turn leads to chronic interstitial nephritis and gradual renal failure. Acute massive hyperuricemia as may occur in the treatment of leukemia or lymphoma causes a massive uric acid excretion in the urine and uric acid crystal deposition in the renal tubules, renal pelvis, and ureters. This may cause acute renal failure and is termed uric acid nephropathy.

Gout is associated with an increased incidence of hypertriglyceridemia, obesity, excessive alcohol consumption, hypertension, and arteriosclerotic coronary artery disease. The exact relationship of these conditions to gout is unknown, but the clinical associations are clear, and gouty patients should be screened for these problems.

LABORATORY STUDIES

Most patients with gout have an increased serum uric acid level (hyperuricemia), although occasionally the serum uric acid level may be normal during an acute attack. Hyperuricemia is arbitrarily defined as serum uric acid levels outside of the central 95 per cent distribution of serum uric acid values in the healthy population. Using the uricase-spectrophotometric method of determining serum uric acid, 7.0 mg per 100 ml is considered the upper limit of normal in men and 6.0 mg per 100 ml in females. Using the more common phosphotungstic acid reduction employed in automated multiple analyzers, normal values are approximately 1 mg per 100 ml higher.

During an acute attack of gout the white blood cell count may be elevated with a shift of the differential white cell count to the left (increased polymorphonuclear leukocytes). The erythrocyte sedimentation rate may also be elevated during acute episodes. The key to the diagnosis of gout is the identification of urate crystals in the synovial fluid. Excepting perhaps for the most classic attack of podagra, urate crystals should always be identified to confirm the diagnosis of gout. The synovial fluid is aspirated from the joint using conventional techniques and then crystals are searched for, using an ordinary light microscope, followed by the use of polarized light and, if possible, the use of a first-order red compensator. Urate crystals are needle-shaped and are found during the acute attack, both intracellular (within polymorphonuclear leukocytes) and extracellular. Between acute attacks in a chronic gouty effusion the crystals may be predominantly extracellular. Occasionally only a few crystals will be present and a prolonged, careful search of the synovial fluid will be necessary to find the crystals. The crystals may be easier to find using polarized light. Urate crystals are birefringent; they shine brightly under polarized light. This characteristic helps to distinguish urate crystals.

A second form of crystal-induced arthritis, called calcium pyrophosphate deposition disease, may mimic gout clinically. These crystals are usually rhomboid in shape and weakly birefringent, but on occasion they may be needle-shaped and simulate urate crystals. Urate crystals and calcium pyrophosphate crystals behave differently under a first-order red compensator. Urate crystals are yellow parallel to the optic axis of the first-order red compensator and blue perpendicular to it. This is termed negative birefringence. Calcium pyrophosphate crystals are just the opposite, blue when parallel and yellow when perpendicular (positive birefringence).

An inexpensive system can be substituted for the special microscope required for this procedure. A polarizing lens can be placed over the light source of an ordinary light microscope and a second polarizing lens placed in the barrel of the microscope above the objective. The first polarizing lens is rotated until a dark field is obtained. The first-order red compensator is substituted by the use of an ordinary microscope slide with two pieces of superimposed clear cellophane tape. The slide is placed over the bottom polarizing lens and rotated until a red or violet background is obtained. Urate crystals will then appear yellow parallel to the long axis of the slide and blue perpendicular to it; the opposite occurs with calcium pyrophosphate crystals.

The aspirated synovial fluid has the characteristics of an inflammatory fluid. The white cell count is high, usually above 5000 white cells per cu mm with a slight predominance of polymorphonuclear leukocytes (greater than 60 per cent). The fluid is turbid, often a milky white color. The viscosity may be poor with a poor mucin clot test and string test. The synovial fluid glucose is usually within 10 per cent of a simultaneous serum glucose. Gram stain of the synovial fluid and cultures of the synovial fluid should, of course, be negative for infectious organisms.

Serum glucose and triglycerides should be checked in patients with gout to rule out the clinical associates of glucose intolerance and hyperlipidemia.

Evaluation of renal function is important in gouty patients. Evidence of renal stones and secondary infection should be searched for — hematuria, pyuria, and bacteriuria. Urinalysis, blood urea nitrogen (BUN), serum creatinine

and creatinine clearance should be obtained to rule out embarrassed renal function, which may be due to urate nephropathy or the frequent clinical associate, hypertension. These studies are also necessary as baseline values to follow the urinary function of gouty patients at yearly intervals. Albuminuria and decreased maximal urinary concentrating ability are early signs of urate nephropathy.

X-ray examinations of involved joints are usually normal in acute episodic articular gout except for soft tissue swelling. In chronic tophaceous gout, cartilage destruction leads to narrowed joint spaces, and bony deposition of urate crystals causes punched-out areas of subchondral bone on the phalanges of the feet and hands. A characteristic overhanging margin is often seen on the gouty erosion. In tophaceous gout the large soft tissue masses can be seen on the x-ray. Considerable bony destruction may be present in long-standing tophaceous gout.

THERAPEUTIC TESTS

Colchicine, the traditional treatment for acute gouty attacks, has been supplanted to some extent by nonsteroidal anti-inflammatory agents such as phenylbutazone and indomethacin that relieve the acute inflammation but do not produce the gastrointestinal side effects of colchicine. However, colchicine has a degree of specificity that may be diagnostically helpful. Colchicine would rarely be expected to relieve the symptoms of other types of arthritis. Prompt response to oral or intravenous colchicine is very suggestive of gout.

DIAGNOSTIC PITFALLS

The most common pitfall is to assume that the laboratory finding of hyperuricemia means the patient with arthritis has gout. Hyperuricemia is a commonly found abnormality and may be present unrelated to the patient's arthritis. Identification of urate crystals in the synovial fluid positively diagnoses gout, although a classic attack of podagra relieved by colchicine would certainly be highly suggestive of gout and would be a reasonable clinical diagnosis.

The next pitfall to avoid is the failure to diagnose the primary disease in secondary gout. Hyperuricemia may be primary; that is, the cause is unknown. Patients with primary hyperuricemia may be overproducers of uric acid, underexcreters of uric acid, or may represent a combination of the two processes. But there are a number of recognizable disorders that lead to secondary hyperuricemia and, as a result, to secondary gout.

Overproduction of uric acid and resultant hyperuricemia may occur in diseases or conditions characterized by increased nucleic acid catabolism. These are (1) hematologic disorders: primary polycythemia vera, secondary polycythemia, leukemia, multiple myeloma, myeloid metaplasia, lymphoma, Hodgkin's disease, sickle cell anemia, pernicious anemia under treatment, hemolytic anemias, and radiation or chemotherapy of lymphoma, leukemia, or polycythemia; and (2) psoriasis.

Hyperuricemia may be caused by decreased renal excretion of uric acid secondary to a correctable or at least identifiable cause. (1) Lead poisoning may be due to industrial exposure or to the consumption of lead-containing moonshine whiskey: saturnine gout. (2) Low-dose salicylates (less than 2 grams per day) cause renal retention of uric acid. (3) Starvation or crash diets induce ketosis that reduces tubular excretion of uric acid. (4) Acute alcohol consumption. (5) Diabetic ketoacidosis. (6) Contraction of extracellular volume secondary to dehydration, salt loss, or diuretics. (7) Chronic renal insufficiency of any cause, although gouty arthritis rarely occurs in this setting. (8) Type I glycogen storage disease. (9) Eclampsia. (10) Diuretics other than spironolactone and triamterene (the thiazide diuretics, ethacrynic acid, and furosemide). (11) Other drugs such as pyrazinamide, ethambutol, acetazolamide, diphenylhydantoin, nicotinic acid, and levodopa. Certain endocrinopathies have been associated with hyperuricemia: congenital vasopressin-resistant diabetes insipidus, hyperparathyroidism and hypoparathyroidism, hypothyroidism, and idiopathic hypercalciuria. Hyperuricemia has also been associated with sarcoidosis, chronic beryllium poisoning, Down's syndrome, Paget's disease of bone, and a high dietary intake of yeast.

Certain drugs will interfere with the colorimetric method of determining serum uric acid levels and give spuriously high results: theophylline, theobromine, methyldopa, ascorbic acid, and methylated xanthines in coffee, tea, or cocoa.

Certain drugs will cause a low serum uric acid level and potentially confuse the diagnosis: bishydroxycoumarin (Dicumarol, Dicoumarin), chlorprothixene (Taractin), phenylbutazone (Butazolidin), high dose salicylates (greater than 2 to 3 grams per day), glycopyrrolate (Robinul), guaifenesin (Robitussin), acetohexamide (Dymelor), meprobamate and tridihexethyl chloride (Milpath), oral cholecystographic agents, and, of course, allopurinal (Zyloprim), probenecid (Benemid, Colbenemid), and sulfinpyrazone (Anturane).

A bunion, or hallux valgus deformity, of the big toe may be mistaken for gout. A bunion is often associated with osteoarthritis of the first metatarsophalangeal joint leading to chronic pain and swelling of that joint and not uncommonly an overlying bursitis. This may be confused with gout. The pain and swelling is insidious in onset and chronic rather than the episodic, severe attacks of gout. X-ray examination shows osteoarthritis of the first metatarsophalangeal joint.

A prolonged attack of gout in the foot and ankle may mimic a septic cellulitis. The entire foot may be swollen, warm, and the overlying skin may look very much like that seen in a bacterial cellulitis.

Most physicians assume that an attack of gout will respond rapidly to appropriate treatment with colchicine or a nonsteroidal anti-inflammatory drug. If the attack has been untreated for a week or more, the resolution of the attack may be slow, that is, several weeks.

The crystal-induced arthritis caused by calcium pyrophosphate crystals may mimic acute gouty arthritis (pseudogout). Differentiation of the two crystals, urate and calcium pyrophosphate, by first-order red compensator and the x-ray finding of chondrocalcinosis in pseudogout makes this distinction.

Occasionally an acute attack of gout will occur in a patient with a normal serum uric acid level. This may be initially confusing but repeat serum uric acid determinations will usually be elevated.

THE PORPHYRIAS

By G. H. ELDER, M.D.
Cardiff, United Kingdom

INTRODUCTION AND CLASSIFICATION

The porphyrias are disorders of heme synthesis in which characteristic clinical features are accompanied by overproduction of porphyrins or porphyrin precursors or both. The clinical features are of two types: skin lesions caused by photosensitization by porphyrins; and acute attacks of porphyria, typically with severe abdominal pain accompanied by neuropathy and mental disturbances, which are often precipitated by drugs such as the barbiturates.

Table 1. *Classification of the Porphyrias*

Site of Heme Precursor Overproduction	Type of Porphyria	Synonyms	Over-production of PBG and Acute Attacks	Over-production of Porphyrins and Skin Lesions
Erythropoietic	Erythropoietic porphyria (EP)	Congenital erythropoietic porphyria, Günther's disease, porphyria congenita	0	+
Erythrohepatic	Protoporphyria (PP)	Erythropoietic protoporphyria, erythrohepatic porphyria	0	+
Hepatic	Acute intermittent porphyria (AIP)		+	0
	Variegate porphyria (VP)	Mixed, or South African genetic, porphyria; porphyria cutanea tarda hereditaria	+	+
	Hereditary coproporphyria (HC)		+	+
	Porphyria cutanea tarda (PCT)	Symptomatic, symptomatic cutaneous hepatic, or chronic hepatic porphyria; porphyria cutanea tarda symptomatica	0	+

The porphyrias can be classified according to the sites of overproduction of porphyrins and porphyrin precursors within the body (Table 1). In erythropoietic porphyria and protoporphyria, porphyrins accumulate within erythroid cells, and thus these types can be distinguished from the purely hepatic porphyrias in which erythrocyte porphyrin concentrations are always normal. Photosensitization occurs in all the porphyrias in which there is overproduction of porphyrins ("the cutaneous porphyrias"), that is, in all types except acute intermittent porphyria. Acute attacks of porphyria are always associated with overproduction of the porphyrin precursor, porphobilinogen (PBG), and do not occur in the erythropoietic and erythrohepatic porphyrias, or in porphyria cutanea tarda (PCT), in all of which the excretion of PBG is always normal. PCT is probably the most common porphyria, whereas the next most likely to be encountered, except in South Africa,

are acute intermittent porphyria (AIP) and protoporphyria (PP). In South Africa, both variegate porphyria (VP), among those of Dutch descent, and PCT, among the Bantu, are frequent.

Figure 1 outlines the pathway of heme biosynthesis. Only porphyrinogens belonging to the type III isomer series are converted to heme. Under normal conditions less than 1 per cent of the porphyrinogens formed are type I isomers. Apart from protoporphyrin IX, porphyrins are not intermediates but are formed by oxidation of porphyrinogens, both within the body and after excretion. Current techniques for the measurement of porphyrins in urine and feces include oxidation of porphyrinogens so that any present are estimated as porphyrins.

It is now clear that the porphyrias are the clinical consequence of enzyme defects in this pathway (Fig. 1). Heme synthesis — either in the bone marrow or in the liver — is maintained

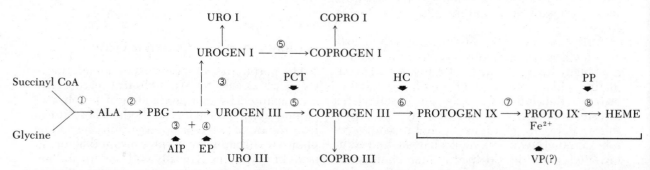

Figure 1. The heme biosynthetic pathway, showing sites of enzyme defects in the porphyrias. ① 5-Aminolevulinate (ALA) synthase. ② Porphobilinogen (PBG) synthase. ③ Uroporphyrinogen (UROGEN)-I-synthase. ④ (UROGEN-III) cosynthase. ⑤ UROGEN-decarboxylase. ⑥ Coproporphyrinogen (COPROGEN)-oxidase. ⑦ Protoporphyrinogen (PROTOGEN)-oxidase. ⑧ Ferrochelatase. Other abbreviations are as in Table 1.

by compensatory increases in substrate concentration that are brought about through an increase in the activity of the first, and rate-limiting, enzyme of the pathway, ALA-synthase, which is under negative feedback control by the end-product, heme. Thus each enzyme defect leads to a specific pattern of substrate accumulation, which can be recognized by measurements of porphyrins and porphyrin precursors in urine, feces, and erythrocytes (Table 2).

With the exception of PCT, all the porphyrias show clear-cut patterns of inheritance. Erythropoietic porphyria (EP) is inherited as an autosomal recessive, whereas PP and the three forms of hepatic porphyria in which acute attacks occur (Table 1) are autosomal dominants. Clinical expression of the autosomal dominant types of porphyria is variable, and persons who have inherited the enzyme defect but have never had symptoms attributable to porphyria — latent porphyrics — are common in affected families. In the inherited hepatic porphyrias, every effort should be made to detect latent porphyrics in order to warn them against drugs that are known to precipitate acute attacks. PCT is a syndrome that occurs most frequently as an uncommon associate of a number of conditions, in most of which there is evidence of hepatocellular damage. The most common of these is liver damage caused by alcohol; but the syndrome may complicate other types of chronic liver disease; follow the administration of estrogens, including oral contraceptive preparations; occur in connective tissue disorders, particularly systemic lupus erythematosus; or be caused by poisoning with certain hepatotoxic polychlorinated aromatic hydrocarbons, notably hexachlorobenzene and 2,3,7,8-tetrachlorodibenzo-p-dioxin. PCT is particularly common in areas where both alcoholism and hepatic siderosis are frequent, as among the Bantu, but is uncommon in hemochromatosis and other disorders of iron storage. Less than 10 per cent of patients have relatives with latent or clinically overt PCT.

Diagnosis of the Porphyrias. The diagnosis of any type of porphyria depends on the clinical features, on family studies, and on the pattern of overproduction of porphyrins or porphyrin precursors or both. The clinical features alone are never sufficiently specific to be diagnostic, and a history of proved porphyria in a relative is often absent. Thus the diagnosis ultimately depends on laboratory measurements of porphyrins and their precursors. In order to avoid diagnostic errors these tests must be carried out on samples of urine, feces, and erythrocytes from every patient suspected of having porphyria.

Although the screening tests described below are usually adequate to exclude the diagnosis of porphyria, the precise diagnosis of a particular type requires quantitative measurements of porphyrins and porphyrin precursors. The techniques that are most widely used at present depend on solvent extraction and partition. These divide porphyrins into fractions — uroporphyrin, coproporphyrin, and protoporphyrin — depending on their physicochemical properties, which usually, but not always, consist mainly of the porphyrin after which they are named. Type I and III isomers are not separated by these techniques. With the advent of thin-layer chromatography (TLC) and high-performance liquid chromatography (HPLC), methods for the measurement of individual porphyrins have been introduced, but these offer

Table 2. *Porphyrin Precursors and Porphyrin Fractions in the Porphyrias*

Condition	ALA (mg/24 hr)	PBG (mg/24 hr)	Urine (μg/24 hrs)		Feces (μg/g dry wt)		
			COPRO	URO	COPRO	PROTO	ETHER INSOL ("X-FRACTION")
Erythropoietic porphyria	N	N	800–3000°	2600–10,400°	5700°	340	Often increased (uroporphyrin)
Protoporphyria	N	N	N	N	Usually N	N–350	N
Acute intermittent porphyria	5–80	10–120		From PBG in vitro	Usually N	Usually N	Usually N
Hereditary coproporphyria (remission)	N	N	150–600	N	1000–4000	Usually N	
Variegate porphyria (acute attack)	10–150	15–200	300–5000	From PBG in vitro	80–1500	200–2000	42–900 (X-porphyrin)
Porphyria cutanea tarda	N	N	150–600	1500–12,000	25–260	20–260	12–360 (7-carboxyl porphyrin)
Reference values	<6.0	<2.0	0–160	5–30	0–27	0–75	0–21

Representative values or ranges are shown. N = normal.
° Mainly isomer type I.

Table 3. *Porphyrin and Porphyrin Precursor Abnormalities in Conditions Other Than the Porphyrias*

Condition	Erythrocytes	Urine	Feces
Porphyrinurias			
Lead poisoning	Increased proto	ALA and copro III increased; PBG usually N	Usually N
Alcohol abuse	Increased proto, copro°	Increased copro III	N
Impaired biliary excretion (hepatocellular disease, cholestasis, etc.)	N	Increased copro (mainly I)	N
Miscellaneous systemic disorders: severe infection, reticuloses			
Hematologic disorders			
Iron deficiency anemia	Increased proto	N	N
Sideroblastic and hemolytic anemias	Increased proto, copro	N	N
Miscellaneous			
Gastrointestinal hemorrhage	N	N	Increased proto fraction

N = normal.
°If sideroblasts are present.

few advantages over solvent-partition techniques for diagnostic use.

Increased concentrations of heme precursors in red cells, urine, and feces may occur in conditions other than the porphyrias. The most important of these are listed in Table 3.

ERYTHROPOIETIC PORPHYRIA (EP)

CLINICAL FEATURES

Most patients with this very rare condition have presented before the age of 3, either when red urine is noticed in early infancy or with severe photosensitivity of sun-exposed skin. Acute skin lesions and chronic skin changes are similar to those described later for the cutaneous hepatic porphyrias; but since photosensitization persists throughout life, much more severe and mutilating scarring occurs. Both the deciduous and permanent teeth may be colored brownish-red by porphyrin ("erythrodontia") and show red fluorescence in ultraviolet light (Wood's filter). Hemolytic anemia and splenomegaly are common.

LABORATORY DIAGNOSIS

Urine and feces contain large amounts of isomer type I porphyrins, predominantly uroporphyrin in the urine and coproporphyrin in the feces (Table 2). Uroporphyrin and coproporphyrin concentrations are increased in erythrocytes and plasma (Table 4). Normoblasts in the bone marrow and circulating erythroid cells show red fluorescence owing to porphyrins when examined in ultraviolet light.

PITFALLS IN DIAGNOSIS

Erythropoietic porphyria (EP) may be confused with porphyria cutanea tarda (PCT), because both PCT in young children and EP presenting in adult life have been described.

PROTOPORPHYRIA (PP)

CLINICAL FEATURES

Most patients present during childhood with symptoms of photosensitivity — burning, itching, and a painful pricking sensation in sun-exposed skin — which usually start within 30 minutes of exposure. The symptoms may be provoked by sunlight that has passed through glass, which is uncommon in other types of photosensitivity and is due to porphyrin-induced photosensitization to wavelengths longer than 400 nm. Onset of symptoms after adolescence is very unusual, and about two thirds of the patients have a family history of photosensitivity. Accompanying edema and erythema are usual, but in some patients there

Table 4. *Erythrocyte Porphyrins in the Porphyrias*

Condition	Proto°	Copro°	Uro°
Erythropoietic porphyria	50	140	300
Protoporphyria	400–3000	Often increased (less than proto)	N
Reference values	4–52	0–4	0

°Representative values in µg/100 ml packed red cells.

may be no objective signs of photosensitivity. Blisters, which are common in the other cutaneous porphyrias, are infrequent in PP. White nails, which are painful and may eventually be lost, petechiae, and hirsutism are other uncommon features.

Acute skin changes may be followed by crusting and the formation of shallow scars, particularly on the nose and cheeks. Eventually the skin may become coarse and lichenoid, especially around the eyes, on the bridge of the nose, and on the backs of the hands. The pale, waxy appearance of some areas of thickened skin may resemble the changes of lipoid proteinosis.

Photosensitivity caused by protoporphyria persists throughout life, usually with exacerbations in the spring and summer. In the majority of patients, there is no improvement with age. The main complications are the formation of protoporphyrin-containing gallstones and the development of liver disease. Although almost all patients have normal biochemical tests of liver function, it is probable that most store protoporphyrin in their livers, where it is visible as crystals when needle biopsy samples are examined histologically. A small number of patients (less than 20 have been reported) develop hepatic cirrhosis with cholestatic jaundice and liver failure that progresses rapidly to death in hepatic coma. During this stage severe photosensitivity, occasionally with bullae resembling these in the cutaneous hepatic porphyrias, may develop.

Patients with polymorphic light eruption and all cases of unexplained photosensitivity should be screened for PP by appropriate laboratory investigations.

Laboratory Diagnosis

The diagnosis of PP is confirmed by demonstrating an increased concentration of protoporphyrin in erythrocytes (Table 4). Less constant findings are increased plasma and fecal protoporphyrin concentrations (Table 2). Urinary porphyrin excretion is normal in uncomplicated PP. In patients with cholestasis and liver disease there may be coproporphyrinuria, as in other types of liver disease (Table 3). Recently a urinary porphyrin pattern, similar to that of PCT, has been reported in one patient with terminal liver failure.

Screening Tests for Increased Erythrocyte Porphyrin Concentration. Two screening tests are in use:

1. Extraction of red cell porphyrins into acid. In this test, 0.1 ml of fresh, heparinized blood, collected into a container giving protection from light, is added to 2.5 ml of peroxide-free ether:acetic acid (5:1, by volume) and macerated with a glass rod. The supernatant is transferred to a thin-walled glass tube and shaken with 0.5 ml of 3 M-HCl. After separation of the phases, the lower acid layer is examined in ultraviolet light (Wood's filter). The presence of a faint pink to bright red fluorescence indicates excess porphyrin. The test is positive in PP and the eythropoietic porphyrias and may be positive in iron deficiency anemia, in other anemias, and in lead poisoning (Table 3). Asymptomatic relatives of patients with PP may also have increased erythrocyte protoporphyrin levels. Although erythrocyte porphyrins are always normal in the hepatic porphyrias, the test may be positive in some patients with active skin lesions, owing to the presence of porphyrins in plasma.

2. Fluorescence microscopy. In normal blood only occasional erythrocytes show red fluorescence. In PP and other conditions in which red cell porphyrin levels are raised (Tables 3 and 4), numerous fluorescent cells are seen. Protoporphyrin in erythrocytes is stable for at least a minute, when a saline-diluted unfixed blood smear is viewed in light (380 to 500 nm) from an iodine tungsten 100-watt quartz lamp, but disappears rapidly and may be missed when the more usual mercury-vapor lamp is used.

Either of these tests will detect patients with PP, but fluorescence microscopy is the more reliable, as occasional false negatives occur with the extraction test. All positive screening tests require confirmation by quantitative measurements in which red cells are separated from plasma.

In lead poisoning, and in iron deficiency and other anemias, protoporphyrin levels tend to be lower than in PP and plasma porphyrin concentrations are normal. These conditions should not cause confusion, because photosensitivity is absent, whereas the clinically insignificant anemia that is common in PP is normochromic and microcytic. In lead poisoning, iron deficiency and other anemias, the red cells contain Zn-protoporphyrin, whereas in PP they contain protoporphyrin. Acid extraction methods for the measurement of erythrocyte porphyrins convert the zinc complex to protoporphyrin dication but, if neutral extraction or dilution is used, the two forms of porphyrin can be distinguished by fluorescence emission spectroscopy. This distinction may help differentiation.

Pitfalls in Diagnosis

Photosensitivity in PP may be unaccompanied by any objective signs and dismissed as functional unless biochemical investigations are carried out. In only two thirds of patients can porphyrin-type photosensitization be demonstrated by irradiation monochromator testing. Increased red cell protoporphyrin may be missed by tests that measure Zn-protoporphyrin.

THE HEPATIC PORPHYRIAS

The hepatic porphyrias rarely present before puberty. Presymptomatic diagnosis of the types inherited as autosomal dominants by measuring porphyrin and porphyrin precursor excretion is not possible in children, because heme precursor excretion usually does not become abnormal until after puberty.

CLINICAL PRESENTATION

The hepatic porphyrias present in one of three ways: with an acute attack alone, with skin lesions alone, or with an acute attack accompanied by skin lesions. In acute intermittent porphyria (AIP) acute attacks are the only clinical feature, whereas in porphyria cutanea tarda (PCT) only skin lesions occur. Some 60 per cent of patients with variegate porphyria (VP) present with acute attacks; three quarters of these have skin lesions. The remaining 40 per cent present with skin lesions alone. Hereditary coproporphyria (HC) almost always presents with an acute attack which may occasionally, especially if there is accompanying cholestasis, be accompanied by skin lesions. The clinical features of the acute attack are the same in AIP, VP, and HC. The skin lesions of VP, HC, and PCT are, likewise, clinically indistinguishable. These two types of clinical manifestations, as well as some special features of PCT, are described later.

THE ACUTE ATTACK

The capacity of acute attacks of porphyria to mimic a wide variety of clinical conditions is well known, and the diagnosis depends essentially on clinical awareness that a particular patient might have porphyria coupled with correct performance of an appropriate test to demonstrate increased levels of PBG in the urine.

Acute attacks are more common in females (sex ration about 3:1) and usually occur in the second to fourth decades. Barbiturates have been implicated in the precipitation of over 70 per cent of acute attacks. These and other provoking factors are listed in Table 5. The most common presenting symptom is abdominal pain. Less commonly, patients may present with psychiatric disturbances, or with symp-

Table 5. *Precipitating Factors in Acute Porphyria*

Drugs°
Barbiturates
Sulfonamides
Glutethimide
Dichloralphenazone
Estrogens/progestogens
Griseofulvin
Chlordiazepoxide
Hydantoin and succinimide anticonvulsants
Meprobamate
Tolbutamide
Methyldopa
Other factors
Alcohol
Infection
Cyclic-menstrual
Low-calorie diet
Emotional stress

°Only the more important drugs are shown.

toms caused by a predominantly motor neuropathy.

The typical clinical picture is one of abdominal pain, accompanied by pain in the limbs, often with paresthesia, constipation, and mental confusion. Muscular weakness, which may not be present at the outset, develops rapidly in about two thirds of the patients. Many of these features are present in severe lead poisoning, which is also associated with abnormalities of heme precursor excretion (Table 3). The type of abdominal pain varies. It may be a severe, lower abdominal colic or a persistent, dull ache and is sometimes accompanied by lumbar back pain or chest pain. It is often so severe and unremitting that patients become markedly distressed, restless, and anxious for analgesics, to an extent that may suggest "over reaction." Vomiting and constipation are frequent.

The neuropathy is usually preceded by abdominal pain or mental disturbances or both. It follows no fixed pattern, but is predominantly motor in type. Pain and tenderness of affected muscles, with paresthesia, may precede the development of weakness. Limb involvement tends to be symmetrical and to affect proximal muscle groups more than distal and the upper limbs more than the lower. Less frequently the trunk muscles and sphincters may be involved. The muscular weakness may be widespread and progress to respiratory paralysis, or it may involve a single limb or group of muscles. Advanced stages may resemble the Guillain-Barré syndrome. The cranial nerves may be affected, paralysis of the facial nerves and ocular disturbances being prominent. Patterns of sensory loss are variable. Convulsions may occur. Mental changes are nonspecific and include confusion, hallucinations, emotional lability, and depression, which may be prominent after recovery.

There are few physical findings. Patients are usually apyrexial. On examination, the abdomen is soft and marked tenderness is unusual. The liver is not palpable. Sinus tachycardia, which is present in most patients during the acute phase, is a useful physical sign, particularly in the differential diagnosis of the neuropathy, and may be accompanied by moderate hypertension.

Acute attacks, which may persist for days or weeks, are eventually followed by remission, but often recur after months or years. Neuropathy is the complication that threatens life. Its course is unpredictable, and death may occur either suddenly or after prolonged respiratory paralysis and coma. Recovery from paralysis is usual, but may take months or years, the rate being, to some extent, related to severity.

The assessment of abdominal pain, without other features of the acute attack, in a patient known to have an inherited form of hepatic porphyria is often a difficult clinical problem. Although in individual patients PBG levels are high during acute attacks, the likelihood of abdominal symptoms in AIP being due to porphyria cannot be predicted from the amount of PBG in the urine.

Laboratory Findings. Routine investigations help exclude other causes of abdominal pain and neuropathy. X-rays of the abdomen may show distended loops of bowel proximal to segments contracted by spasm. The cerebrospinal fluid is characteristically normal, but minor increases in protein concentration have been reported (less than 100 mg per 100 ml). Anemia is not a feature of the hepatic porphyrias. Leukocytosis is unusual and related to coexisting infection. Conventional liver function tests are frequently normal, apart from retention of Bromsulphalein, which is found in most patients during the acute phase. Hyponatremia, caused by water intoxication secondary to abnormalities of renal function or inappropriate antidiuretic hormone (ADH) secretion, is common and may be severe enough to cause disturbances of consciousness during the acute attacks. Hypocalcemia, hypomagnesemia, hypokalemia, azotemia, and alkalosis, often associated with severe vomiting, have been described. Increases in serum thyroxine-binding globulin, cholesterol, and β-lipoprotein, as well as various asymptomatic endocrine abnormalities, have also been reported.

The Skin Lesions

The most frequent and important skin changes in the hepatic porphyrias are increased mechanical fragility of the skin, so that trivial trauma leads to erosions, and the formation of vesicles and bullae. These changes are restricted to sun-exposed areas of skin, particularly the backs of the hands and forearms, the forehead, and the scalp. The bullae are subepidermal and may occasionally be hemorrhagic. The erosions formed by rupturing the bullae and by mechanical removal of the skin surface are followed by crusts and scabs that eventually heal, often with scar formation. Erosions may become infected and cause extensive scarring with contractures and atrophy of the terminal phalanges. The symptoms of photosensitivity, which are so prominent in PP and EP, are often absent in the cutaneous hepatic porphyrias.

Other chronic skin lesions occur in addition to scarring. The most important are milia, hirsutism, and pigmentation. Facial hirsutism may be striking in women and was a notable feature in the children who developed porphyria caused by hexachlorobenzene poisoning in Turkey between 1956 and 1960. Patchy pigmentation on the backs of the hands, the forearms, and the face is common and may intermingle with areas of depigmentation. Less commonly, scleroderma-like plaques occur, particularly on the face, and may invade the hairline, producing a characteristic receding alopecia that rarely becomes total. When hair loss occurs, skin lesions on the scalp may be particularly severe. The more severe chronic lesions are more common in PCT than in VP. However, in the absence of features of an acute attack or a family history of VP or both, these conditions cannot be distinguished clinically.

The skin lesions of the hepatic porphyrias are sufficiently characteristic for laboratory confirmation of the diagnosis of porphyria to be predicted with considerable accuracy. However, identical bullous lesions have been reported on rare occasions in patients taking certain drugs — nalidixic acid and tetracyclines — and in some patients undergoing chronic hemodialysis.

Porphyria Cutanea Tarda

Skin lesions, appearing most frequently in the second half of the summer, are the sole clinical manifestation of this syndrome, which is now the most common form of porphyria. The syndrome is essentially a cutaneous indicator of underlying liver cell disease, and it is this which determines the prognosis. Patients who present with skin lesions frequently have no clinical evidence of liver disease. In most series about 60 to 70 per cent of the patients have been middle-aged men who consume large amounts of alcohol but who, at least in Europe, are not usually socially incapacitated alcoholics. On occasion cryptogenic cirrhosis and other types of nonalcoholic liver disease may present as PCT. Less commonly the skin lesions of porphyria are noticed as an incidental finding in a patient with clinical liver disease or a connective tissue disorder. Recently the number of young women presenting with PCT, apparently precipitated by oral contraceptive agents, has increased. This reaction does not usually appear until these compounds have been taken for at least 3 months and does not invariably disappear when they are stopped. It must not be confused with the severe skin lesions that occur when cholestatic jaundice, resulting from these compounds (or any other cause), occurs in VP and diverts porphyrins from biliary excretion into the systemic circulation.

Without treatment, PCT usually runs a chronic course with exacerbation of the skin lesions during the summer months. Administration of chloroquine may produce a hepatotoxic reaction with fever and malaise, associated with massive porphyrinuria. Treatment with low doses of chloroquine, or by repeated venesection, produces prolonged remission, which may also occur either after withdrawal of alcohol or spontaneously.

Laboratory Findings. Biochemical tests of liver function may be abnormal, the most frequent findings being an increase in the aspartate or alanine aminotransferases and increased Bromsulphalein retention. Plasma iron concentrations are frequently increased, but the total iron-binding capacity (TIBC) is usually normal. Routine hematologic tests are normal.

The liver in PCT contains high concentrations of uroporphyrin (often 300 to 1000 micrograms per gram wet weight). Most needle biopsy samples show a brilliant red fluorescence when viewed in ultraviolet light, whereas fluorescence microscopy of smear or crushed cell preparations reveals porphyrin storage in all, provided contact with formalin is avoided. Histologic abnormalities of the liver are present in almost all patients, including both those with normal liver function tests and those with PCT caused by oral contraceptives. Patchy hepatic cell necrosis with associated inflammatory changes and fibrosis, often with fatty infiltration, is the most common finding, but an established cirrhosis has been present in as many as a third of the patients in some series. Hepatic siderosis is present in virtually all patients. It has been claimed that the incidence of adenocarcinoma of the liver is higher in patients with PCT and cirrhosis than in nonporphyric cirrhotics. Four patients have been described in whom cutaneous hepatic porphyria was due to

the presence of a porphyrin-producing hepatoma — either benign or malignant — in an otherwise normal liver. All patients with PCT should be carefully examined for the presence of a hepatic tumor.

BIOCHEMICAL DIAGNOSIS OF THE HEPATIC PORPHYRIAS

The precise diagnosis of any form of hepatic porphyria depends on establishing the presence of its characteristic pattern of heme precursor excretion (Table 2), by measuring porphyrin precursors in urine and porphyrins in both urine and feces. Omission of fecal analyses is an important source of diagnostic error.

Screening Tests. Quantitative measurements are time consuming, and a number of screening tests are in widespread use.

Porphobilinogen (PBG) in Urine. PBG rapidly polymerizes in urine, especially under acid conditions, to form both porphobilin and uroporphyrin. These reactions underlie the change in the color of the urine on standing from normal, when fresh, to a dark brown-red, which is characteristic of acute porphyria. A random specimen of urine should therefore be used for screening for PBG and should be tested as soon as possible after collection. Equal volumes of urine and Ehrlich's reagent (0.28 per cent [w/v] p-dimethylaminobenzaldehyde in 7 M-HCl in the Watson-Schwartz and the Rimington tests) are mixed. PBG reacts immediately to give a red color, whereas the identical color given by urobilinogen takes up to 2 minutes to reach maximum intensity. Other compounds giving a red color in this test are listed in Table 6. After neutralization

Table 6. *Substances Giving a Red Color in the Screening Test for PBG*

Substances reacting with Ehrlich's reagent
  Porphobilinogen
  Urobilinogen
  Metabolites of
    Levomepromazine
    Cascara sagrada bark extract
    Sedormid
  Phylloerythrinogen
  Pyrrole mono- and dicarboxylic acids
  Indoles
Indicators° — red in acid solution
  Methyl red
  Phenazopyridinium chloride
  Urosein

°Can be detected by adding acid without p-dimethylaminobenzaldehyde to urine.

with saturated sodium acetate, the urobilinogen-color complex can be extracted into organic solvents, whereas the PBG complex remains in the aqueous phase. If butanol, or an amylbenzyl alcohol mixture, is used for the extraction rather than chloroform (with which there are occasional false positives), this test distinguishes PBG from other Ehrlich-reactors (Table 6). Even fresh urines containing PBG frequently contain some porphyrin produced by polymerization in vitro. This process can be accelerated by acidifying the urine to pH 2 and heating to 37 C, which may help substantiate the presence of PBG.

This test is positive during an acute attack of porphyria. The lower limit of detection of PBG is about 10 mg per liter, which is higher than the upper limit of normal (see Table 2). PBG levels may be much lower in remission than during acute attacks, and this test should therefore never be used to exclude porphobilinogenuria during remission or in family studies. The same limitation applies to a more sensitive screening test, in which PBG is concentrated and partially purified by anion exchange chromatography, which will detect about 5 mg PBG per liter. All positive screening tests for PBG must be confirmed by a reliable quantitative technique.

Porphyrins in Urine. Porphyrins are extracted into amyl alcohol and concentrated by shaking 4 ml fresh urine, adjusted to pH 3.5 with glacial acetic acid, with 1 ml amyl alcohol. The phases are separated by centrifugation and examined in ultraviolet light (Wood's filter). Pink or red fluorescence in the upper organic layer indicates the presence of porphyrins. This test extracts both uroporphyrin and coproporphyrin but is less prone to error than screening tests in which separation of these porphyrins is attempted. A positive result — which may be due to any cause of increased urinary porphyrin (Tables 2 and 3) — must be confirmed by a quantitative technique that measures both uroporphyrin and coproporphyrin fractions. False negatives are uncommon but may occur owing to extraction of compounds which either fluoresce intensely themselves or quench the fluorescence of porphyrins.

The color of the urine is an unreliable guide to the presence of porphyrins, especially in patients with liver disease. Urines containing more than 5 to 10 mg per liter of porphyrin are often reddish-brown and fluoresce when examined in ultraviolet light.

Porphyrins in Feces. A button of feces (about 1 cm in diameter) and 0.5 ml glacial acetic acid are ground together with a glass rod. Five ml of peroxide-free ether is added and mixed thoroughly with the fecal suspension. The supernatant is decanted and extracted with 1.4 M-HCl (0.5 ml). A faint pink to bright red fluorescence in the lower aqueous layer indicates the presence of porphyrins of potentially clinical significance. Any red fluorescence in the upper organic layer is due to chlorophyll-derived pigments from the diet and is unimportant. This test is difficult to interpret. The intensity of fluorescence is proportional to the porphyrin content of the sample, and some normal samples, especially from constipated patients, may show porphyrin fluorescence. In addition, the protoporphyrin fraction of normal feces is largely derived from sources other than the protoporphyrin excreted in the bile, particularly from the action of bacteria on heme compounds in the diet. Alimentary tract bleeding is an important cause of an increased fecal protoporphyrin fraction (Table 3), which is not invariably accompanied by a positive test for occult blood. This screening test does not detect increases in fecal ether-insoluble porphyrins. Quantitative porphyrin measurements should be carried out on all samples that show definite porphyrin fluorescence.

Confirmatory Tests. Quantitative estimations of PBG and ALA in urine and of porphyrin fractions in urine and feces will confirm the diagnosis of a particular type of porphyria in most patients. Measurement of individual porphyrins by chromatographic techniques and other specialized investigations may help resolve diagnostic problems.

Acute Intermittent Porphyria. Urinary PBG excretion is increased during acute attacks and, in almost all patients, remains increased during clinical remission. The urine usually contains excess uroporphyrin formed by condensation in vitro of PBG. Urinary ALA levels are also elevated but are lower than those of PBG except when delay in testing has allowed the much less stable PBG to polymerize. In lead poisoning, ALA levels are always much greater than those of PBG, which only increase in severe poisoning, and coproporphyrin III excretion is increased (Table 3). Fecal porphyrin concentrations are usually normal, in contrast to VP and HC (Table 2).

Measurement of PBG and ALA in urine will detect most relatives with latent acute intermittent porphyria, but adult latent cases with normal porphyrin precursor excretion do occur. The activity of uroporphyrinogen-I-synthase in red cells from persons carrying the gene for acute intermittent porphyria is close to 50 per cent of the activity in red cells from unaffected members of the same family. In normal and porphyric subjects enzyme activity is affected by various factors, notably red cell age and genetic variation, so there is some overlap between the range of activities found in these two groups. Although this limits the predictive value of the method in individual patients, study of enzyme activity within families is a useful adjunct to urine measurements and enables at least some latent porphyrics — including prepubertal children — with normal precursor excretion to be detected. Enzyme levels are high and variable in cord blood and in newborn children, and diagnosis may be difficult before the age of 4 months.

Variegate Porphyria. During acute attacks, urinary PBG and ALA are increased as in acute intermittent porphyria. Urinary coproporphyrin levels are usually increased, the proportion of coproporphyrin to uroporphyrin being variable and dependent on the degree of condensation of PBG. The important diagnostic findings which differentiate this condition from AIP and HC are the increases in fecal protoporphyrin and ether-insoluble (X-porphyrin) porphyrin fractions, with protoporphyrin usually exceeding coproporphyrin by about twofold (Table 2). The ether-insoluble porphyrin fraction, which is obtained by extracting the fecal residue with 45 per cent urea–4 per cent Triton X-100 solution after ether-soluble porphyrins have been removed, contains a group of water-soluble porphyrin conjugates (probably peptides) known as X-porphyrins. Current methods for the identification of the porphyrins in this fraction as "X-porphyrins" are not suitable for routine use.

Fecal porphyrin excretion is similar in patients who present with skin lesions alone, but urinary PBG and ALA excretion is often normal, the only urinary abnormality being an increase in coproporphyrin excretion. In clinical remission and in latent cases the urine may be normal, and diagnosis depends on demonstrating abnormal fecal porphyrin excretion. In family studies, all three porphyrin fractions should be measured on at least two separate samples. Even so, it is probable that not all latent cases will be detected.

Hereditary Coproporphyria. This condition is characterized by increased excretion of coproporphyrin III in the feces and, during clinical activity, in the urine (Table 2). Porphyrin precursor excretion is increased during acute attacks. For family studies, both fecal coproporphyrin excretion and coproporphyrinogen oxidase activity in lymphocytes or fibroblasts should be measured, as porphyrin excretion may occasionally be normal in latent HC.

Porphyria Cutanea Tarda. The characteristic abnormality is an increase in the urinary uroporphyrin fraction, the porphyrin being excreted as such and not coming from polymerization of PBG (Table 2). PBG excretion is always normal, as, with rare exceptions, is that of ALA. The urinary coproporphyrin fraction may be increased but is always less than the uroporphyrin fraction (Table 2). Fecal porphyrin excretion is variable. Typically there are moderate increases in both the coproporphyrin and ether-insoluble (X-porphyrin) fractions, with the coproporphyrin fraction either equaling or exceeding the protoporphyrin fraction (Table 2). There is some overlap between the values for fecal porphyrin fractions obtained in PCT and VP (Table 2).

In clinical remission both urinary and fecal porphyrin excretion decrease and may eventually return to normal if remission is prolonged. Uncommonly, patients with alcoholic and other types of liver disease, or relatives of patients with PCT, have porphyrin excretion patterns identical to those seen in PCT in remission, and so have been described as having latent PCT.

The increases in the urinary and fecal porphyrin fractions are due to the excretion of uroporphyrins I and III (about 70 per cent I), porphyrins with 7, 6, and 5 carboxyl groups, and porphyrins of the isocoproporphyrin series, which are derived from intermediates of the reaction catalyzed by uroporphyrinogen decarboxylase (Fig. 1), as well as coproporphyrins I and III (about 60 per cent III). Measurement of the individual components of this complex mixture provides a number of techniques for distinguishing PCT that are useful in difficult cases. Thus thin-layer chromatography (TLC), or high-performance-liquid chromatography (HPLC) of the methyl esters of urinary and fecal porphyrins reveals typical patterns with the percentages of uroporphyrin and 7-carboxyl porphyrin in the urine (45 to 80 per cent and 15 to 35 per cent of the total porphyrin, respectively) and the isocoproporphyrin:coproporphyrin ratio in the feces (greater than 0.5 in patients with active skin lesions) being of particular value. The ether-insoluble (X-porphyrin) fraction in the feces consists largely of 7-carboxyl porphyrin, true X-porphyrin probably being within normal limits.

PITFALLS IN DIAGNOSIS

The diagnosis of the hepatic porphyrias is usually straightforward, provided that urine tests are carried out on fresh specimens and both urine and feces are examined. The porphyrinurias (Table 3) are due to increased coproporphyrin excretion and should not cause confusion if fecal specimens are also tested (compare Tables 2 and 3). When the associated constipation makes it difficult to obtain samples of feces during the acute attack, they should be tested when available after recovery. Failure to do this may lead to misdiagnosis of VP and AIP.

PCT and VP presenting with skin lesions alone cannot be distinguished clinically when there is no family history of the latter, particularly when the patient is a young woman taking an oral contraceptive preparation. Episodes of abdominal pain, perhaps caused by pancreatitis, and neuropathies may occur in alcoholics with PCT and also cause confusion. In most of these patients the laboratory diagnosis is straightforward. In a few, biochemical findings may be misleading. Condensation of PBG to uroporphyrin may leave normal PBG levels so that the urinary findings in cutaneous VP resemble those in PCT. Rarely, intercurrent cholestasis in a patient with VP may lead to a decrease in fecal porphyrin excretion, with an increase in X-porphyrin in the urine. Since this is estimated as part of the uroporphyrin fraction, biochemical findings may resemble PCT. Urinary and fecal investigations should always be repeated, family studies carried out, and, if possible, one of the special confirmatory tests depending on the measurement of individual porphyrins performed, in any clinically or biochemically atypical case of "porphyria cutanea tarda" — particularly those with fecal porphyrin concentrations similar to those of VP or with jaundice. Very rarely, EP may present in adult life. Confusion with PCT is avoided if erythrocyte porphyrin concentrations are measured.

HEPATOLENTICULAR DEGENERATION

(Wilson's Disease)

By SEAN O'REILLY, M.D.
Washington, D.C.

SYNONYMS

Progressive lenticular degeneration, tetanoid chorea, pseudosclerosis of Westphal-Strümpell, familial hepatocerebral degeneration.

DEFINITION

Wilson's disease is heredofamilial and therefore primarily genetically determined. The exact nature of the abnormal gene or genes is unknown and it is not possible to state with certainty what the *primary* genetically determined defect might be. The genetic defect is inherited in an autosomal recessive manner. This means that each parent must contribute at least one of a pair of abnormal alleles and be heterozygous for the abnormal gene. It also implies that there is one chance in four that any other sibling in a family in which the diagnosis has been confirmed will be homozygously normal or homozygously abnormal, and one chance in two that the sib will be a heterozygote or carrier. It is very uncommon to find abnormal homozygotes in more than one generation unless there has been a great deal of intermarriage, and hence consanguinity, in the family. Although the precise nature of the primary genetically determined defect is not known, it is clearly related to abnormal physiology of an essential trace element, copper; this abnormality has been demonstrated in both homozygotes and heterozygotes for the defective gene or genes.

It is possible to state that the abnormal allele in the carrier determines somehow a relatively minor pathophysiology of copper, characterized by prolongation of retention of copper in the whole body with corresponding reduction in the amount excreted. This disturbance can be documented by appropriate studies that are described later, but it does not appear to be associated with any tissue damage or clinical symptoms. The double dose in the homozygously abnormal subject, however, determines a much more serious defect in the absorption, distribution, and excretion of copper and results in abnormal deposits of copper in various organs, notably liver, brain, kidneys, and cornea. In liver, brain, and kidneys, the abnormal deposits lead to tissue damage, biochemical abnormalities, and a rather protean although stereotyped spectrum of clinical phenomena. In the cornea, copper deposition produces a characteristic and almost pathognomonic sign of the disease, the Kayser-Fleischer ring.

PRESENTING SIGNS AND SYMPTOMS

The protean nature of the phenotypic clinical manifestations of Wilson's disease has been alluded to in the preceding paragraph. Although it was put on the map, so to speak, by a neurologist, it is by no means an exclusive preserve of neurologists. Indeed, it is a disease "for all seasons." Patients may seek help from a wide assortment of medical and other professionals other than neurologists — pediatricians, internists, gastroenterologists, hematologists, ophthalmologists, psychiatrists, even clinical psychologists and school counselors.

There is, in fact, a good deal of evidence, anecdotal as well as in the medical literature, to suggest that behavioral disturbance, psychiatric symptoms, and difficulties in school may be the earliest symptomatic presentation in the majority of patients. There is nothing specific or characteristic about such symptoms, unfortunately, but in most cases they do result in referral of the child for a medical evaluation. It is too much to expect, perhaps, that Wilson's disease be considered in the differential diagnosis of every obscure symptom complex in childhood, adolescence, or early adult life. Since, however, it is a treatable disease, and a missed diagnosis or a diagnosis long delayed may allow irreversible organ damage to occur, physicians should think of the possibility of this disease in the work-up of at least four groups of patients:

1. Young subjects with a tentative diagnosis of childhood autism.

2. Those thought to have idiopathic juvenile cirrhosis.

3. Children and adolescents with progressive basal ganglia disorders, an unexplained hemolytic anemia, renal osteodystrophy, renal tubular acidosis, or a Fanconi-like syndrome.

4. Adults thought to have atypical multiple sclerosis or nonspecific hepatocerebral degeneration.

The cardinal sign to be looked for in all cases is occasionally present in asymptomatic homozygotes and certainly should be sought in sibs of known patients. It is a pigmented ring on the cornea known as the Kayser-Fleischer ring after the ophthalmologists who described it. It is of interest that it was first found in patients labeled as having Westphal-Strümpel pseudosclerosis, an entity which for some years Kinnier Wilson refused to accept as a variety of "his disease!"

The Kayser-Fleischer ring is an artifact, a sort of optical illusion produced on the cornea by light scattered and reflected from deposits of copper on Descemet's membrane in the cornea itself. These deposits are discrete and granular and can be stained in biopsy or autopsy sections by means of a variety of histochemical stains for copper. In addition, there is a rather diffuse deposition of copper throughout the substantia propria of the cornea.

The ring usually has a smoky brown appearance but may be grayish-green or gray, especially against the background of the dark-brown iris, as in orientals and blacks. When fully developed it extends around the entire periphery of the cornea, although it is most dense at the upper and lower poles, and in early stages it may be seen only at the upper pole as a crescent. It is distinguished from arcus senilis, which is commonly seen in young black adults, by the fact that it extends to the limbus of the cornea, whereas there is seen to be a clear zone between arcus senilis and the limbus.

It is, of course, easiest to see against the background of a light blue or blue iris, but it can be seen by the naked eye in most patients if one looks carefully from above or laterally with oblique illumination. A useful maneuver is use of a short-acting mydriatic to dilate the pupil and get the iris out of the way. However, there are patients in whom it is not possible to see a Kayser-Fleischer ring without slit-lamp microscopy and gonioscopy; one cannot say it has been excluded until such an instrumental examination has been made by an experienced examiner. If present, it is diagnostic. But it is not completely pathognomonic, since a Kayser-Fleischer–like ring has been described in patients with cryptogenic cirrhosis, active chronic hepatitis, and neonatal hepatitis. It is true that the patients described apparently did not have as marked an increase in liver copper or biochemical findings related to other organ involvement as do patients with Wilson's disease. Nevertheless, it could be difficult to differentiate the two conditions without extensive studies including radiolabeled copper studies, as described later, in other sibs and the parents.

COURSE

I have stressed the protean nature of the phenotypic clinical manifestations and variable clinical presentation of Wilson's disease. Overall, the course is equally variable. Nonetheless, the presentation, clinical findings, and course in those patients with predominant neurologic features are more stereotyped. These patients can be divided into two groups:

1. Those with classic Wilson's disease, presenting with impaired skill performance in the first decade of life or early adolescence. This most frequently is noticed in school as a deterioration in writing and other manual skills, often attributed to laziness or to mental illness if there is, in addition, some personality or behavioral change. Over the course of a few months to a year or so there is obvious neurologic deterioration: development of choreiform involuntary movements, dysarthria, flapping tremor, rigidity, and akinesia, progressing to bilateral dystonia. At first the dystonia may be segmental, most frequently involving the facial muscles and producing a rather characteristic vacuous or silly dystonic grin. Occasionally, there is asso-

ciated with this a raucous crowing laugh and spastic dysarthria. Sooner or later, the dystonia progresses in hemiplegic fashion, leading to an immobile mute state with remarkable bilateral extensor dystonia. The course may be as short as 6 months in occasional patients; most commonly it is several years. It should be stressed that even if the diagnosis is not established until the neurologic disorder is well advanced, appropriate treatment with penicillamine or other copper-chelating agent should be begun and persevered with. Remarkable improvement can occur over the space of a couple of years even in apparently hopeless cases.

2. A larger group whose neurologic symptoms do not begin until adult life, frequently in the twenties, but sometimes as late as the fourth or fifth decade. In these patients tremor or other involuntary movement such as chorea, ballism, or ataxia is the presenting symptom. These symptoms are frequently mistaken for those of early Parkinsonism, Huntington's disease, nonfamilial chorea, biballismus, torsion dystonia, spinocerebellar degeneration, or multiple sclerosis. This mistake is perhaps understandable, given a patient with clinical signs of a lesion at several levels — spinocerebellar system, basal ganglia, and frontal lobes — and a somewhat variable course. It is true that there are no remissions in this variety of Wilson's disease, but some spontaneous improvement may occur, or a plateau may be reached with no obvious deterioration for a year or more.

The course of patients with these late onset cases, which are frequently similar to those in patients described in the European literature as having pseudosclerosis of Westphal and Strümpell, is quite chronic and drawn out, even if untreated. Survival for 10 years or more is not uncommon. Nevertheless, if untreated, Wilson's disease is invariably fatal, sooner or later — sooner, as a rule, in those patients with an early onset in infancy or early childhood, whether the onset be hepatic, hematologic, or neurologic. In general the prognosis is worse for those children presenting with subacute hepatic damage. The prognosis is similar to that of any other variety of severe and fatal hepatitis or toxic hepatic necrosis, and death may occur in 2 months or less. The course and prognosis is not much better in infants or young children presenting with a severe and rapidly progressive bilateral striatal syndrome or bilateral hemiplegic extensor dystonia, suggestive of necrotic degeneration of the lentiform nuclei. Death has occurred as early as 6 months from onset, but the more common course in the untreated patient is 2 or 3 years.

An early episode of hepatic damage with jaundice may appear to resolve spontaneously, with recovery of adequate liver function for a few years. Most such patients, however, have postnecrotic cirrhosis, and repeated damage eventually results in a scarred shrunken liver with portal hypertension, enlarged spleen, and esophageal varices. Hemorrhage from the latter may terminate the illness and the patient's life.

By contrast, those patients whose disease is not manifested until later in life, especially those with neurologic features described as typical of pseudosclerosis of Westphal-Strümpell and notably those with little or no evidence of serious hepatic or renal dysfunction, have a more benign, chronic, and drawn-out course. This is evident from case reports and reviews of the natural history of the untreated disease. The introduction of effective therapy has significantly altered the prognosis and the course of the disease in all its varieties. This fact, which is well documented, simply emphasizes the necessity for early diagnosis and adequate investigation of all siblings of the patient who has first come to diagnosis in a given family.

Physical Findings

From what has been already said, it is evident that the findings on clinical examination may be quite variable. There may be *none* in asymptomatic sibs of a known patient, one or more of whom may nonetheless be homozygously abnormal. Occasionally such asymptomatic homozygotes may have a Kayser-Fleischer corneal ring that is readily seen even by the nonprofessional observer, as happened in the case of one of the families that I have studied. In another of our patients whose condition was far advanced, unfortunately, when first seen and diagnosed, it was possible to see a fully developed Kayser-Fleischer ring in a photograph of the child taken 2 years before she had any symptoms whatever.

It may be possible, however, to see a ring *only* on slit-lamp microscopy and gonioscopy, which should, therefore, be regarded as an essential examination in the work-up of sibs no less than in the case of symptomatic suspects for the disease. In the predominantly hepatic form of the disease, the clinical findings may be those associated with cirrhosis from any cause — jaundice, spider nevi, palmar erythema, ascites, or gynecomastia in the male. Occasionally, a patient will present with an acute hemolytic crisis and the only physical finding may be pallor and some jaundice. Hyperpigmentation owing to excess melanin deposition is common over the anterior aspect of the lower legs. It is uncommon to find any physical signs referable to the renal lesions, but a very occasional patient may present with spontaneous fractures. Exceptionally, the findings may be those of renal rickets or of the nephrotic syndrome.

The neurologic clinical findings will depend on the age of onset, the stage, and the type of neurologic form of the disease. In the childhood subacute form the physical findings may be limited to choreiform involuntary movements, grimacing in a silly dystonic fashion, segmental dystonia somewhat reminiscent of torsion dystonia, or there may be found bilateral extensor dystonia in a hemiplegic distribution and akinetic mutism, with the mouth open in a dystonic grin. There may be signs of hypothalamic lesions, such as fever of unexplained etiology, sweating, tachycardia, hypotension.

In the more benign chronic neurologic form of late onset, the physical findings may be involuntary movements of choreic, ballistic, or athetotic type; tremor may be parkinson-like but more commonly it is a flapping or wing-beating tremor, with asterixis quite similar to that seen in hepatic pre-coma or carbon dioxide narcosis.

One can frequently demonstrate a mild striatal syndrome even when the extensor rigidity of the classic subacute cases is not present. The minimal sign of this is a tactile avoidance reaction on stroking lightly the distal hand or foot on its palmar or dorsal surface.

The patient may have cerebellar ataxia and dysarthria, but nystagmus is uncommon. There may be frontal lobe release signs such as the snouting or sucking reflexes, grasp reflexes, an increased jaw jerk; there is occasionally dementia, but the commonest finding on mental status examination in these chronic cases is a peculiarly facile jocose affect. Such patients are frequently prone to playing pranks on others — usually childish and obvious ones, with the patient laughing and crowing dystonically the while. "Sunflower" cataract and azure lunulae have been described in patients with well-established disease, but they are extremely rare and cannot be said to be restricted to Wilson's disease.

In summary, one can only agree with Walshe's statement that there is no such thing in practice as a "typical" case of Wilson's disease. In the last analysis, diagnosis will depend on a high index of suspicion, the detection of Kayser-Fleischer rings, and documentation of other abnormalities in the handling of copper.

COMPLICATIONS

Although the abnormal metabolism of copper just alluded to is fundamental in this disease and is probably fairly close to the primary genetically determined defect, it is evident from personal experience and from the literature that not all organs are equally affected by the abnormal disposition of copper that ensues. The complications to be expected, therefore, are as varied as the phenotypic clinical manifestations. Thus the patient whose liver is predominantly affected may die of progressive liver failure, hepatic coma, a bleeding tendency, esophageal varices, and hemorrhage; namely, the inevitable complications seen in progressive liver disease from any other cause.

The patient with the more chronic hepatic disease may develop hypersplenism with leukopenia, thrombocytopenia, hemorrhage, and rarely, splenic infarction. Generalized osteoporosis is common and may lead to fractures or pseudofractures, particularly in those patients with osteomalacia and renal osteodystrophy. Renal damage may lead to metabolic acidosis and hypercalciuria, which can be complicated by nephrolithiasis. The progressive downhill course of untreated patients, or of patients with disease so advanced that organ damage is irreversible even with optimal therapy is punctuated by those complications common to any chronic debilitating illness: dysphagia leading to malnutrition or inhalation pneumona, bed sores, and urinary tract infection consequent on incontinence and catheterization.

Although psychiatric symptoms are common, as previously noted, it is of interest that frank psychosis is a rare event. Occasionally, however, the combination of behavioral disturbance and progressive immobilizing extensor dystonia may lead to a misdiagnosis of catatonic schizophrenia. The iatrogenic complications of such a mistaken diagnosis—for example, phenothiazine intoxication, tardive dyskinesia—may further hamper diagnosis.

LABORATORY FINDINGS

In a disease so variable in the age of onset of clinical symptoms and in distribution of organ damage, one could expect the laboratory findings to be equally protean and unpredictable at a given point in time. This is indeed found to be true in many patients, at least so far as routine clinical laboratory investigation is concerned. In the classic neurologic form of the disease, for instance, there may be no symptoms or clinical signs referable to any organ other than the central nervous system. In some of these patients routine hematologic values, routine urinalysis, and routine liver function tests may all be within normal limits.

Conversely, in patients with the primary "abdominal" form of the disease, routine laboratory tests of nervous system function, such as the electroencephalogram (EEG), may be normal. Nonetheless, in many patients, even presymptomatic ones, a fairly characteristic spectrum of laboratory findings may be found and should be sought. Most of these are related, directly or indirectly, to the abnormal metabolism of copper that can be demonstrated by appropriate specialized investigation in all patients, both symptomatic and asymptomatic, and in the heterozygote to a lesser degree.

Thus, in most homozygotes, ceruloplasmin will be found to be reduced or even absent in the plasma or serum. Normal values for this copper protein vary from one laboratory to the next depending on the method of measurement and on the quality control exercised in the laboratory. In general, immunochemical determination using specific antibody, whether by radial immunodiffusion, immunoprecipitation, or immunoelectrophoresis or electroimmunodiffusion, gives the highest values, ranging in normal control sera from 20 to 45 or 48 mg per dl (100 ml). Spectrophotometric measurement of the cupric copper signal, if properly carried out, can be equally reliable, but it is a reference rather than a routine method. Most clinical laboratories rely on a variety of methods that measure the enzymatic activity of ceruloplasmin against a variety of nonphysiologic substrates, notably paraphenylene diamine or its dimethyl derivative. With such methods the levels in normal subjects are somewhat lower than with the immunochemical ones, the range being 15 to 35 mg per dl. Various factors can affect the enzymatic activity, either depressing it (e.g., ascorbic acid) or enhancing it (e.g., ferrous ion), so that false-positive or false-negative results may occur.

Similarly, levels of ceruloplasmin measured immunochemically may occasionally be misleading, as in the case of those families in which asymptomatic homozygotes and heterozygotes have apparently normal or near-normal levels of ceruloplasmin by immunochemical determination, whereas on further investigation, this is found to be apoprotein or ceruloplasmin devoid of copper. For these reasons it is wiser to request ceruloplasmin determination by more than one method. The results can be double checked also by measuring the total serum copper by a reliable modern method such as atomic absorption spectrophotometry or neutron activation. Since in normal subjects 94 or 95 per cent of the total serum copper is bound in ceruloplasmin, there should be good correspondence between total serum copper and ceruloplasmin levels in normal subjects: a significant discrepancy such as finding the total serum copper to be higher than expected, on the basis

of the ceruloplasmin level reported in the same specimen, would raise the suspicion of a larger than normal amount of "free" serum copper that is the usual situation in the typical case of Wilson's disease. Since the copper content of normal ceruloplasmin is 0.34 per cent, a level of, say, 30 mg of ceruloplasmin would correspond to about 102 micrograms of copper per dl. The range of normal serum copper reported from various laboratories in the United States is fairly wide, from 100 micrograms to 180 micrograms per dl, with reported means varying from 105 to 130 micrograms and standard deviations of from 2 to 4 micrograms per dl.

In normal subjects, therefore, serum copper determination provides a reliable check on ceruloplasmin levels and vice versa. The usual finding in most patients with Wilson's disease is a ceruloplasmin level of 0 to 10 micrograms or so and a serum copper of 20 to 40 micrograms per dl.

Urinary copper is usually increased in homozygotes of Wilson's disease. Depending on the method and the care taken in collecting the urine to avoid contamination with extraneous copper, the 24-hour excretion of copper in normal subjects is under 100 micrograms. By contrast, most wilsonian homozygotes show a resting urinary excretion of 150 micrograms or more per 24-hour period.

Wilsonian patients with significant renal tubular pathology may show an aminoaciduria, which is usually generalized and associated with normal plasma aminoacids; phosphaturia and uricosuria may be present with consequent hypophosphatemia and hypouricemia. Of the latter, low serum uric acid (2 mg or less per dl) is perhaps the most common routine laboratory finding. Difficulty in acidifying the urine, usually because of a proximal tubular defect, is usually not picked up unless it is looked for by appropriate tests such as ammonium chloride loading.

Those patients with a history of hemolytic episodes may show appropriate laboratory findings such as anemia, increased reticulocyte count, low serum iron, and normal, low, or increased total iron-binding capacity, but in such patients the routine hematologic picture may be surprisingly normal. In all such patients, however, and even in those with no history of hemolytic crises, one finds consistently low serum iron, some increase in iron-binding capacity — although not the levels found in hemolytic anemia of other causes — bone marrow with no stainable iron, and iron kinetic studies showing typical findings of iron deficiency, including a red cell lifespan reduced to 20 or 30 days. The iron deficiency could be corrected by use of iron dextran (Imferon), but the shortened red cell lifespan remained unaffected.

Total red cell copper and levels of the red cell copper-zinc protein erythrocuprein (superoxide dismutase) are normal in this disease. Nevertheless, as will be mentioned later, the metabolism of copper in the red blood cell is not normal in Wilson's disease.

Any or all of the usual laboratory tests of liver function may be abnormal, even in those patients with no history or clinical findings to suggest liver disease. Thus some presymptomatic homozygotes may have abnormal liver function tests, especially elevated liver enzymes or isozymes in the serum. If in addition they have Kayser-Fleischer rings, the diagnosis is made. But in some patients, especially those with the predominant neurologic form, all liver function tests may be normal.

Radiologic tests may show generalized skeletal demineralization, joint degenerative changes, multiple growth lines in long bones, and fractures or pseudofractures. Computerized tomography (CT) of the head in the neurologic patients may show changes only now beginning to be described in the literature. They range from signs of rarefaction and minimal tissue loss in the region of the caudate and lenticular nuclei in early disease to frank bilateral cavitation in the same basal ganglia regions in advanced disease. One could expect to see lesions in the frontal lobes, cerebellum (especially dentate nucleus region), and the pons in the chronic pseudosclerotic variety of the disease, but it is difficult to see how such lesions could be distinguished from demyelinating plaques or multiple cystic infarcts resulting from inflammatory or degenerative vascular disease.

Biopsy of the liver or of the kidney in patients with symptoms related to these organs may be diagnostic, if the copper content of the samples is measured by a reliable method such as atomic absorption spectrophotometry, neutron activation, or established biochemical procedures. Histochemical demonstration of increased copper deposition may be possible but the methods are not always reliable. Electron probe microanalysis can show the increased deposits and their location at the cellular level, but even in centers with advanced equipment this is scarcely a routine tool! The histologic or ultramicroscopic findings in liver or kidney biopsy specimens are nonspecific and not diagnostic.

Radiochemical investigation of the metabolism of copper using radioactive copper provides the most sensitive and reliable means of identifying homozygotes — whether symptomatic or not — and heterozygotes, and distinguishing them from normal subjects.

If the longer-lived radionuclide ^{67}copper (with physical half-life of 61 hours approximately) is available, the maximum amount of information can be obtained from such studies. Using ^{67}copper, either alone or in combination with ^{64}copper (physical half-life of 12 hours approximately), it has been shown that:

1. Copper absorption from the gut is increased in homozygotes as compared with heterozygotes and normal subjects.

2. Retention of copper is prolonged in the whole body in both homozygotes and heterozygotes, greater in the former.

3. Retention of copper in the liver is prolonged in both, most marked in homozygotes.

4. In both, excretion of copper into the intestine is decreased, as manifested by decreased biliary and stool radioactive copper following intravenous administration of the tracer.

5. Urinary excretion of radioactive copper is usually increased significantly in the homozygote; in the heterozygote it is usually normal (cumulative 10-day excretion less than 1 per cent) or only very slightly increased.

6. Plasma clearance of radioactive copper may be a little slower than normal in homozygotes; it is usually normal in heterozygotes.

7. Ceruloplasmin biosynthesis, as manifested by feedback to plasma of radioactive copper associated with newly synthesized ceruloplasmin, is much diminished or not demonstrable in most homozygotes; it is more or less normal in heterozygotes. A subpopulation of wilsonian homozygotes alluded to earlier has normal or even increased ceruloplasmin biosynthesis.

8. Uptake of radioactive copper is increased into red blood cells in homozygotes as compared with heterozygotes, normal, or other control subjects. In addition, in the homozygote, although levels of the red cell copper-zinc protein (erythrocuprein, cytocuprein, superoxide dismutase) are normal, uptake of radioactive copper in this protein is impaired.

The only control patients in whom some or more of these eight abnormalities were found were patients with advanced hepatocellular failure. However, the absence of Kayser-Fleischer rings in the latter and its presence in wilsonian homozygotes served to distinguish them.

It is true that such detailed studies may be beyond the scope of most medical centers. Nevertheless, diagnosing Wilson's disease in its earliest, even presymptomatic stages is so important that we should emphasize that the most consistent abnormality of the metabolism of copper in homozygotes demonstrated by adequate radioactive copper studies is considerable reduction in the biliary excretion, and consequently in the stool content, of an intravenous tracer dose of ^{67}copper. Collecting stool for 10 to 12 days after such a dose (50 to 100 microcuries), homogenizing it, mixing it with a thixotropic agent, and measuring the radioactivity in a large sample gamma ray counter may be sufficient to show that a patient suspected of having Wilson's disease is normal. Such a limited study, although expensive, is feasible for the ordinary well-equipped nuclear medicine laboratory. Borderline or slightly abnormal results would indicate the necessity of further more detailed investigation or referral. Finally, in doubtful or borderline cases, a therapeutic test may be helpful.

The cupriuresis produced in homozygotes over a 12 to 24 hour period by a single test dose of penicillamine is usually much greater in homozygotes than in heterozygotes and normal subjects. In the latter it seldom exceeds 400 to 500 micrograms; in the former it usually ranges from 800 to several thousand micrograms, depending on the concentration of nonceruloplasmin (loosely bound) copper in the plasma. Such a therapeutic test may be positive even in those homozygotes with normal plasma levels of ceruloplasmin, but the occasional false-negative results must be expected in such patients.

Pitfalls in Diagnosis

From what has been said about the variability in the age of onset and type of clinical symptoms and even in the biochemical manifestations of Wilson's disease, a number of pitfalls in diagnosis are evident. The first is failure to think of the disease in the differential diagnosis of hepatic, hematologic, neurologic, renal, or psychiatric disorders in young children, adolescents, and young adults. A second pitfall is failure to see the Kayser-Fleischer ring on naked-eye inspection, and failure to use or to request slit lamp microscopy in such patients to confirm its absence. Even so it may be missed in its early stages of development and should be looked for repeatedly in patients about whom the index of suspicion is high.

The third source of error is to mistake a pigmented premature arcus senilis or pigmentary anomaly of the anterior chamber for a Kayser-Fleischer ring. In such patients, as with those in whom a Kayser-Fleischer ring is missed, the error lies in relying on just one manifestation, albeit an important one, of the deranged copper metabolism. Biochemical and even radioactive copper studies are necessary in order to avoid this pitfall, as well as the rare error that occurs when the condition of a patient with biliary cirrhosis is confidently diagnosed as Wilson's disease because a Kayser-Fleischer ring was present.

A similar mistake was more common when it was thought that a low level or absence of ceruloplasmin in serum or plasma was an invariable manifestation of the genetic defect, but the error is still made. Low ceruloplasmin values are found occasionally in patients with severe hepatocellular damage from any cause, and in patients with malabsorption, protein-losing gastroenteropathy, the nephrotic syndrome, and almost invariably in the first few months of life. Hypercupriuria and increased liver copper may be found in infants and in biliary cirrhosis, thus compounding the problem and resulting in a false-positive diagnosis.

The more common error has been, however, to exclude the diagnosis of Wilson's disease because ceruloplasmin or serum copper levels were normal, or because urinary excretion of copper was not very much increased.

IRON STORAGE DISEASES

By WARD D. NOYES, M.D.
Gainesville, Florida

Synonyms

Hemochromatosis, hemosiderosis, bronze diabetes, pigmentary cirrhosis.

Definition and Classification

Iron in excess causes damage principally to the liver, the pancreas, and the heart with clinical manifestations of cirrhosis, diabetes, and myocardial failure. This excess may develop from a rare heritable defect in which an undue amount of iron is absorbed from the diet with a gradual accumulation over years that finally becomes toxic. More frequently, iron overload develops via chronic transfusion therapy, an acquired change in iron absorption, or excessive dietary or medicinal iron intake. The initial tissue pattern of iron deposition differs in the hereditary and acquired forms, but the resulting clinical manifestations are similar. The synonyms noted frequently cause confusion about the cause, making it preferable to term the condition iron storage disease qualified by the express cause if known, e.g., transfusional.

Iron is a crucial element in body economy, and is conserved and recycled to minimize the development of iron deficiency. Body mechanisms are ill equipped to deal with excess iron; if the normal storage mechanisms fail, iron escapes to cells unaccustomed to high concentrations, where it becomes cytotoxic. Particularly vulnerable are the hepatocytes, myocardium, and cells of various endocrine organs. In the heritable form, the leak of iron through the intestinal mucosa over many years permits an overload from normal dietary sources. In addition, the storage cells of the reticuloendothelial system hold proportionately less of the iron so that early in the course excess amounts may be seen in hepatocytes. Eventually, iron stores may total 20 or more grams, contrasting to the usual 2 to 4 grams. This defect is frequently evident as an autosomal recessive, but clinically the disease is seen in a 4:1 predominance in males, possibly owing to the natural loss of iron through menstrual blood flow in women. Symptoms appear in the fourth to sixth decade but may be arrested with treatment if the tissue damage is not permanent.

Acquired changes in iron absorption are seen in chronic iron-loading anemias such as thalassemia and sideroblastic anemias, in patients with portal cirrhosis, and in porphyria cutanea tarda. Unusually large amounts of iron may be ingested by dietary or medicinal means and accumulate over several decades to produce the same clinical picture. Lastly, when chronic transfusions have breached the 100-unit mark without concomitant blood loss, iron toxicity may appear. In most of the acquired cases, the iron overload will be of a lesser degree — in the 10- to 20-gram range. This description does not include acute iron toxicity or localized iron deposits as seen in pulmonary hemosiderosis or in the kidney in association with hemoglobinuria.

Presenting Signs and Symptoms

The discovery of hepatomegaly, evidence of liver failure, a dark hue to the skin, and diabetes mellitus are the hallmarks of advanced disease. In younger patients, cardiac arrhythmia or unexplained myocardial failure may precede other signs. Occasionally weakness, abdominal pain, or peripheral neuropathy is present. Arthritis involving both large and small joints results from associated chondrocalcinosis as well as iron deposits. The hepatomegaly may be confirmed on abdominal flat-plate with an unusually dense hepatic shadow as a reflection of

the iron deposited there. Computerized axial tomography may show qualitatively enhanced density of the liver from these iron stores. Ascites, splenomegaly, spider angiomas, gynecomastia, palmar erythema, and jaundice may all be evident in advanced stages as a result of hepatic failure. The darkening or slate-gray color of the skin is most often related to melanin deposition, perhaps as a reflection of altered adrenal-pituitary balance, but iron deposits may also be found on biopsy. Diabetes, frequently requiring insulin, is correlated with iron deposits in islet cells and acinar cells of the pancreas. Vascular changes in the fundi and renal glomeruli may develop as they do in the usual diabetes mellitus. Despite extensive deposits in thyroid, adrenal, pituitary, testes, and many other tissues, clinical problems with these organs are usually not evident. Hepatomas occur three times as frequently in this disease as they do in other forms of cirrhosis and may be heralded by a painful nodular enlargement of the liver.

Laboratory Diagnosis

High serum iron values reflect the large body stores and usually are >200 micrograms per 100 ml. Serum iron-binding capacity is nearly saturated, frequently >90 per cent. A liver biopsy is most helpful in confirming the pathologic amounts of iron present and in providing a demonstration of the degree of liver damage. Biopsy of the bone marrow may show similar changes in iron deposits but is less helpful than examination of the liver. No satisfactory means of quantitating iron stores is available, but an indication can be gained by measuring the urinary iron excretion during 24 hours after a parenteral injection (0.5 gram) of deferoxamine. Normal persons will excrete less than 2 mg, whereas those with iron overload frequently excrete 5 mg and more. Lastly, serum ferritin levels that normally are under 350 nanograms per ml are almost always in excess of 500 nanograms per ml in iron storage disease. High values may also be found with liver cell necrosis or severe inflammatory states.

The evaluation should include not only confirmation of iron storage but, if possible, determination of the basic cause. This is critical in preventing further progression of the disease from acquired factors or, if the disease is heritable, initiation of treatment in other family members who have subclinical disease that may be detected upon close scrutiny. Chronic anemia, transfusions, and medicinal intake can be determined by history. Careful questioning can elicit data about unusual dietary intake, and well water should be analyzed for iron content if suspect. Differentiating between alcoholic cirrhosis complicated by iron overload and heritable disease in a person who imbibes heavily may be impossible. Measurements of serum iron and ferritin levels in siblings or other close relatives may help in suggesting the familial disease. Further, if the overload is remedied by as few as 50 phlebotomy units, the acquired form is likely, whereas the heritable disease may require 100 or more phlebotomies to achieve a normal serum iron value. Many patients who are untreated die from cardiac or hepatic complications within 2 to 5 years of onset of symptoms so that removal of the excess iron by phlebotomy is imperative.

DIABETES MELLITUS

By RICHARD A. GUTHRIE, M.D.,
and M. HUSAIN JAWADI, M.D.
Wichita, Kansas

DEFINITION

Diabetes mellitus is not a single disease but a syndrome characterized by hyperglycemia, glycosuria, and effects on other facets of metabolism, e.g., protein, lipid, and vascular (micro and macro) abnormalities.

CLASSIFICATION

Diabetes mellitus can be classified into two categories: idiopathic and secondary. Secondary causes of diabetes mellitus include acromegaly, Cushing's syndrome, pheochromocytoma, pancreatectomy, pancreatitis, hemochromatosis, and thyrotoxicosis. Idiopathic diabetes mellitus subdivides into two groups: juvenile or insulin-dependent diabetes mellitus (IDDM or Type I) and adult-onset or noninsulin-dependent diabetes mellitus (NIDDM or Type II). The NIDDM group includes maturity-onset diabetes in the young (MODY), a recently described group of children with glucose and insulin abnormalities similar to those of adults (NIDDM). NIDDM can be further classified to nonobese NIDDM and obese NIDDM, on the basis of whether the patient is less than or more than 120 per cent of ideal body weight. Table 1 shows general characteristics of these groups.

Recently, diabetologists gathered under the auspices of the National Institutes of Health (NIH) to discuss recommendations in regard to the classification of the disease. They were of the view that previous nomenclature for the early stages of diabetes mellitus, viz., chemical diabetes, subclinical diabetes, borderline diabetes, latent diabetes, and stress diabetes, was so confusing that even the experts disagree over the interpretation of these terms. The NIH conference recommended that these terms be abandoned in favor of the proposed term *impaired glucose tolerance* (IGT).

They also introduced two new terms: (1) *previous abnormality of glucose tolerance*

Table 1. *General Characteristics in Two Groups of Idiopathic Diabetes*

	IDDM	NIDDM
Synonyms	Juvenile or ketosis-prone DM	Adult or ketosis-resistant onset DM
Age of onset	*Usually* below 25	*Usually* over 40
Type of onset	Sudden	Insidious
Time of onset	Peak at 12–14 years of age	Peak at 65 years of age
Prevalence	0.5%	2%
Presentation	Polyuria, polydypsia, polyphagia, ketoacidosis	Asymptomatic or nonketotic; hyperosmolar coma
Nutrition	Often thin	Usually overweight
Ketosis	Frequent	Seldom
Control by diet	Never helps	Often helps
Control by oral agents	Infrequent	Often helps
Complication	Microvascular	Macrovascular

(Prev AGT) and (2) *potential abnormality of glucose tolerance (Pot AGT)*. The first category is restricted to those persons who have previously had either impaired oral glucose tolerance test (OGTT) or diabetic hyperglycemia. Stress diabetes and gestational diabetes are included in this class.

The second term describes a statistical-risk type of person who has never exhibited glucose intolerance but is at increased risk over that of the general population: family history, history of mothers who have had high birth weight babies, positive islet cell antibody, positive HLA B_8 BW_{15}, DW_3, and BW_4, and obesity. The previously used class of prediabetic is included in this category.

The results of the NIH conference have now been completed and have been disseminated to experts in the field for comment. We believe that the new classification categories are of value. The advantage to such a classification is that it removes the term diabetes from use in persons who are asymptomatic but have abnormal carbohydrate tolerance based on arbitrary criteria. The dilemma in the past has been overutilization of the term diabetes; this term can have adverse psychologic or other effects (insurability or employability), while the abnormality may be mild and the patient asymptomatic. For example, if the criteria for diagnosis of "chemical diabetes" were a normal fasting blood sugar (FBS) and a blood sugar (BS) during the oral glucose tolerance test (OGTT) above 165 mg per dl (100 ml), what about the person who has a high normal FBS and a BS on OGTT of 164 mg per dl? Is that person at any less risk than a person with a lower FBS and a BS on OGTT of 165 mg per dl? Even though the answers at present are not known, it makes little sense to jeopardize the insurability or employability of one and not the other. Thus, the new terminology of impaired glucose tolerance has been established without reference to diabetes. Long-term studies are needed to validate the concepts behind the classification and such studies are being done. Until such studies determine whether people with mild glucose intolerance have progression to definitive diabetes mellitus or develop the vascular complications of diabetes mellitus, it is best to avoid the diabetes mellitus label with all that it implies.

The NIH classification did not address the problem in the young; stating, in effect, that not enough data were available to do so. Studies in our laboratory indicate that the young may fall into five categories:

(1) *Overt diabetes mellitus*. This class includes symptomatic insulin-dependent diabetics who present with classic symptoms of polydipsia, polyuria, polyphagia, and weight loss with or without diabetic ketoacidosis (DKA) and with hyperglycemia (usually marked) and hypoinsulinemia. Glucose tolerance testing is usually not necessary in this group because of the presence of symptoms, diabetic ketoacidosis, or fasting hyperglycemia.

(2) *Maturity-onset diabetes in the young (MODY)*. This form of diabetes mellitus was described by Fajans at the University of Michigan. These children are usually obese and may or may not have symptoms. The children do have an elevated fasting blood sugar, abnormal postprandial sugars, and have abnormal oral glucose tolerance tests. Serum insulin levels are usually elevated. There is usually a family history of NIDDM. Response to treatment is much like that of maturity-onset diabetes or NIDDM.

(3) *Impaired glucose tolerance (IGT) with hypoinsulinemia*. These individuals are asymptomatic, may or may not (though usually do with stress) have glycosuria, a normal fasting blood sugar, and abnormal oral glucose tolerance test. In this group, insulin secretion during the oral glucose tolerance test is markedly impaired and may be low to other provocative tests as well. In our experience over the past 20 years, the condition of most of these individuals progresses rapidly to overt diabetes mellitus (IDDM) within a short period of time, usually only a few months.

(4) *Impaired glucose tolerance (IGT) with normal or elevated serum insulin*. These individuals are asymptomatic, may or may not be obese, usually do not have glycosuria except in extreme stress, have a normal fasting blood sugar, and their condition tends not to progress. These children probably represent an early form of MODY, but have not yet reached a stage of symptoms or an elevated fasting blood sugar to be so classified.

(5) *Potential abnormality of glucose tolerance (Pot AGT)*. This includes those who are genetically susceptible (Table 2) but have no signs, symptoms, or abnormal chemistry (previously called prediabetes).

A sixth classification consisting of those whose condition is described as *previous abnormality of glucose tolerance* (Prev AGT) may also exist. The most common stresses in childhood that might cause transient glycosuria and an impaired oral glucose tolerance test are infection, burns, and emotional upheaval. Later glucose tolerance testing may be normal once the stress is past.

The laboratory basis for these classifications is discussed later.

Table 2. *Genetic Disorders Associated with Glucose Intolerance/Tolerance and/or Insulin Resistance*

Alström syndrome
Ataxia telangiectasia
Cockayne syndrome
Cystic fibrosis
Fanconi anemia
Friedreich ataxia
Glucose-6-phosphate dehydrogenase deficiency
Type 1 glycogen storage disease
Gout
Hemochromatosis
Huntington disease
Hutchinson-Gilford (progeria) syndrome
Hyperlipidemia, diabetes, hypogonadism, and short stature syndrome
Hyperlipoproteinemia III, IV, and V
Laurence-Moon-Biedl syndrome
Lipoatrophic diabetes
Muscular dystrophy
Myotonic dystrophy
Ocular hypertension induced by dexamethasone
Optic atrophy and diabetes
Hereditary relapsing pancreatitis
Photomyoclonus, diabetes, deafness, neuropathy, and cerebral dysfunction
Pineal hyperplasia and diabetes
Acute intermittent porphyria
Pheochromocytoma
Prader-Willi syndrome
Refsum syndrome
Retinitis pigmentosa, neuropathy, ataxia, and diabetes
Rothmund-Thomson syndrome
Schmidt syndrome
Werner syndrome

CLINICAL FEATURES OF DIABETES MELLITUS

Arataeus described the clinical features of diabetes mellitus in the second century A.D. The description of these clinical features holds true even today. We quote: "Diabetes is a wonderful affection — being a melting down of the flesh and limbs into urine.... The patient never stops making water.... The patients are short-lived for the melting is rapid and death speedy."

Depending upon the age and sex of the patient, diabetes mellitus can present in different forms. In the pediatric age group, the patient may have a variety of symptoms including polyuria, enuresis, polydipsia, weight loss, and failure to thrive; in women of childbearing years, the patient may have a history of delivering large babies. Female subjects may present with symptoms and signs of postprandial hypoglycemia; male subjects may present with phimosis or nonhealing ulcers. Besides having the classic symptoms of polyuria, polydipsia, polyphagia, and weight loss as seen in all age groups, elderly patients may develop life-threatening dehydration and hyperosmolar coma with or without ketoacidosis. These are a few of the clues in the history, physical examination, and routine laboratory studies that necessitate a consideration of the diagnosis of diabetes mellitus. The usual symptoms and signs of diabetes mellitus are outlined in Table 3. The physical findings in diabetes mellitus depend upon the severity and duration of the hyperglycemia. Nonhealing wounds, rapid fluctuations in visual acuity, and infections of the mouth, vagina, and genitourinary tract are seen in hyperglycemia of even short duration, whereas atherosclerosis, myocardial infarction, peripheral neuropathy, nephrotic syndrome, cataract, and autonomic instability are seen in patients with long-standing hyperglycemia.

Table 3. *Usual Symptoms and Signs of Diabetes Mellitus*

History	Physical Examination	Laboratory Studies
Family history	Obesity	Plasma glucose mg/dl
Large babies	Orthostatic hypotension	Fasting 140
Pregnancy	Eye	2 hr 160–200
Abortions	Change in acuity	Glycosuria
Toxemias	Cataract	Hyperlipoproteinemia
Hydramnios	Retinopathy	
Stillbirth	Hepatosplenomegaly	
Congenital defects	Genitourinary	
Hypoglycemia	Nephrotic syndrome	
Vascular disease	Infection	
Pruritus	Bladder, spincter disturbances	
Impotence	Vulvovaginitis	
	Gastrointestinal	
	Nocturnal diarrhea	
	Delayed gastric emptying	
	Malabsorption syndrome	
	Neuromuscular	
	Vascular disease	
	Xanthomatosis	
	Charcot joints	

LABORATORY DIAGNOSIS OF DIABETES MELLITUS

If subjects present with any of these symptoms and signs, we obtain a double-voided urine specimen for the presence of sugar and also obtain a fasting plasma glucose. If patients have a fasting plasma glucose greater than 140 mg per dl on two different occasions, we conclude that they have diabetes mellitus. The presence of hyperglycemia is a sine qua non for the diagnosis of diabetes mellitus. If the fasting glucose values are equivocal, we obtain a 2-hour postprandial plasma glucose after a heavy lunch. If the 2-hour postprandial plasma glucose is over 180 mg per dl, we make a similar interpretation even though the 2-hour postprandial plasma glucose values are less accurate for diagnosis of diabetes mellitus than are the fasting values. In patients with equivocal results, we perform an oral glucose tolerance test.

ORAL GLUCOSE TOLERANCE TEST (OGTT)

We instruct the patient to consume an unrestricted diet (at least 300 grams carbohydrate in adults and 65 per cent carbohydrates in children) for at least 3 days before the test. The high carbohydrate diet is provided to sensitize the beta-cells to the glucose stimulus. In most individuals, it is not necessary to give the carbohydrate supplement because their diets are already adequate in carbohydrates, but it should be done since many individuals in our society may be on low carbohydrate diets (fad diets of various kinds often are high in protein and low in carbohydrate), which may modify OGTT results. The subject is asked to fast for 10 hours before the test. The test is performed in the morning. The subject is asked not to smoke throughout the test and to remain seated. The dose of glucose administered is 1.75 grams per kg ideal body weight for height to a maximum

Table 4. *Criteria for Diagnosis of Chemical Diabetes by Oral Glucose Tolerance*

Fajans and Conn[1] — 1.75 grams/kg	1–hr > 185 1½–hr > 160 2–hr > 140	All three values abnormal
United States Public Health Service (USPHS), Wilkerson[2] — 100 grams	Fasting > 130 = 1 point 1–hr > 195 = ½ point 2–hr > 140 = ½ point 3–hr > 130 = 1 point	Two points or more
O'Sullivan and Mahon[3] (for use in pregnancy) — 100 grams	Fasting > 110 1–hr > 195 2–hr > 175 3–hr > 150	Two or more values abnormal
ADA (American Diabetes Association)[4] — 40 grams/m²	Fasting > 115 1–hr > 185 1½–hr > 165 2–hr > 140	Elevated fasting or all three post-test values abnormal
Danowski: Glucose tolerance sum[5] — 1.75 grams/kg	*Venous whole blood*	Sum = fasting + 1 hr + 2 hr + 3 hr

	Adults	Children
Normal	< 450	< 450
Borderline	450–700	450–650
Diabetic	> 700	> 650

Seltzer[6]: for children — 1.75 grams/kg	*Capillary whole blood* Fasting > 115 1–hr > 175 2–hr > 140 3–hr > 125	Elevated fasting or 2 of 3 post-test values abnormal

1. Ann. N.Y. Acad. Sci. 82:208, 1959.
2. J. Chronic Dis. 13:6, 1961.
3. Diabetes 13:278, 1964.
4. Diabetes 18:299, 1969.
5. Metabolism 22:295, 1973.
6. Ellenberg and Rifkin (eds.): *Diabetes Mellitus: Theory and Practice.* New York, McGraw-Hill Book Co., 1979, p. 480.

dose of 75 grams. After a fasting blood and a urine specimen are collected, the calculated amount of glucose is administered orally. The blood sample is collected at 30 minutes and every hour for 3 hours and is analyzed for both glucose and insulin. If we suspect late hypoglycemia, we prolong this test to 5 or 6 hours. Urine is obtained simultaneously and tested by two-drop Clinitest. Plasma glucose values are usually determined using automated true glucose methods. In children, we often use capillary whole blood obtained by finger stick because of the problem of repeated venipunctures. Insulins are done by radioimmunoassay.

Interpretation of OGTT. Simultaneously obtained urine glucose values give us an idea about renal threshold for glucose. Various investigators have developed different criteria for the interpretation of the OGTT (Table 4). One test therefore could be abnormal with one person's criteria but could be normal with other criteria. The NIH-sponsored diabetes committee has recommended a new interpretation of the results of OGTT (Table 5).

In children, we prefer the values of Pickens and Burkeholder (Oral Glucose Tolerance Tests in Normal Children. Diabetes *16*:11, 1967) for

Table 5. *Criteria from NIH Conference for Diagnosis of Diabetes Mellitus*

1. *Criteria for diagnosing DM on the basis of FBS*
   FBS > 140 mg/dl on more than one occasion

2. *Criteria for normal glucose tolerance*
   FBS < 115 mg/dl and 2 hr plasma glucose > 140 mg/dl but no value between zero time and 2 hrs > 200 mg/dl

3. *Criteria for diagnosing DM on the basis of OGTT* (not required if FBS is >140 mg/dl on more than one occasion):
   a. DM
      2 hr plasma glucose >200 mg/dl and at least one value between zero time and 2 hrs >200 mg/dl
   b. Impaired glucose tolerance
      2 hr plasma glucose > 140 mg/dl and < 200 mg/dl and at least one value between zero time and 2 hrs > 200 mg/dl

4. *Gestational DM*
   a. Gestational DM is diagnosed when two or more of the following plasma glucose values are met or exceeded (after 100 gram glucose dose) in a pregnant woman:
      Fasting–105 mg/dl
      1 hour–190 mg/dl
      2 hours–165 mg/dl
      3 hours–145 mg/dl
   b. Impaired gestational GTT
      2 hr plasma glucose 120–164 mg/dl

DM = Diabetes mellitus.
FBS = Fasting blood sugar.
OGTT = Oral glucose tolerance test.
GTT = Glucose tolerance test.

interpretation of the OGTT. These norms are based upon values obtained in 200 nondiabetic children with no family history of diabetes and no physical disease. The children were ambulatory. Jackson, Guthrie, and Murthy added 200 more children to the Pickens and Burkeholder norms and obtained insulin values in this group. This total group then constitutes the largest group of children tested (400 children for glucose values and 200 children for insulin), anywhere in the world. The values are for a Somogyi filtrate of capillary whole blood but are very close to values of Drash and Rosenbloom, which were obtained on venous plasma.

Overt diabetes mellitus is diagnosed if fasting glucose values are above the 97th percentile of the Pickens and Burkeholder norms (Fig. 1). If the fasting blood sugar value is below the 97th percentile but other values are elevated we may have a diagnosis of impaired glucose tolerance, according to the following criteria: (1) if two or more values, exclusive of the half-hour value, are above the 97th percentile on two or more tests separated by at least 1 month; (2) if two or more values, exclusive of the half-hour value, are above the 90th percentile on two or more tests as just noted, we would make a diagnosis of probable impaired glucose tolerance (IGT), (3) if two or more values, exclusive of the half-hour value, are above the 84th percentile but below the 90th percentile on two or more tests, we would make a diagnosis of possible IGT.

The serum insulin values increase the sensitivity of the OGTT. The serum insulin values, however, are not used to establish a diagnosis of diabetes but rather are used to increase the sensitivity of the testing and to guide therapy. For example, observation of children in our clinic who had very low serum insulin values confirmed that these children progress rapidly to overt insulin-dependent diabetes mellitus (IDDM) even when their glucose values showed only mild impairment. On the other hand, children with high serum insulin values even in the presence of very abnormal glucose values show only very slow or no progression of their abnormality.

Factors That Influence the OGTT. Before making a definite interpretation of OGTT, we make sure that the patient does not have the following environmental factors or clinical states that might result in a high plasma glucose value (Tables 6, 7).

1. *Diet.* If the patient did not consume liberal, adequate carbohydrates before testing, decreased insulin secretion may result.

2. *Drugs.* Various therapeutic agents influence either insulin secretion or carbohydrate

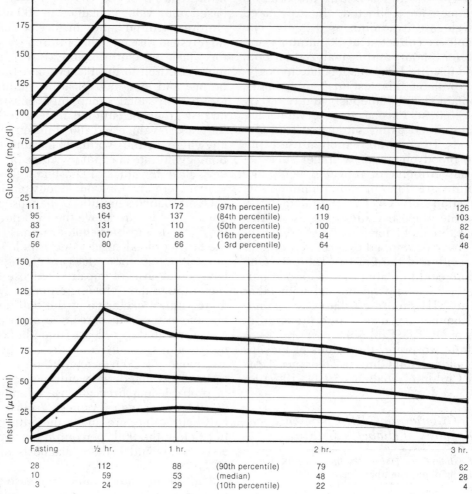

111	183	172	(97th percentile)	140	126
95	164	137	(84th percentile)	119	103
83	131	110	(50th percentile)	100	82
67	107	86	(16th percentile)	84	64
56	80	66	(3rd percentile)	64	48

Fasting	½ hr.	1 hr.		2 hr.	3 hr.
28	112	88	(90th percentile)	79	62
10	59	53	(median)	48	28
3	24	29	(10th percentile)	22	4

Figure 1. Normal percentiles for glucose and insulin for the oral glucose tolerance test in children (5 to 7).

Table 6. *Environmental Factors in Diabetes Mellitus*

1. Diet
2. Drugs
   a. Diuretics (especially thiazides)
   b. Glucocorticoids
   c. Oral contraceptives
   d. Phenytoin
   e. Xanthines (no coffee or tea)
   f. Nicotine (no smoking)
   g. Sympathomimetic amines (most decongestants)
3. Age
4. Stress
   a. Infection
   b. Acute myocardial infarction
   c. Fever
   d. Severe emotional stress
   e. Burns
5. Physical inactivity
6. Pregnancy
7. Gastrointestinal abnormality
8. Other systemic illness

turnover rates. If the subject was taking these drugs, it is wise to discontinue them before the OGTT.

3. *Age.* Carbohydrate tolerance deteriorates with age even though fasting plasma values have changed very little. A reasonable rule of

Table 7. *Clinical Disorders That Influence Carbohydrate Tolerance*

Hormonal Factors	Pancreatic
1. Acromegaly	1. Pancreatectomy
2. Pheochromocytoma	2. Acute and chronic pancreatitis
3. Cushing disease	3. Hemochromotosis
4. Aldosteronoma	
5. Somatostatinoma	
6. Glucagonoma	

thumb is to add 10 mg per dl to 1 hour and 2 hour values for each decade above age 50.

4. *Stress.* Any stress, physical or emotional, results in increased secretion of catecholamines, which influence carbohydrate metabolism.

5. *Gastrointestinal abnormalities.* In partial alimentary tract surgery or in peptic ulcer disease, one may get a flat glucose tolerance test. Occasionally the subject shows 1-hour postglucose hyperglycemia followed by hypoglycemia (the so-called dumping syndrome).

6. *Other systemic illness.* Liver disease, renal insufficiency, and potassium deficiency may result in carbohydrate intolerance.

The presence of these abnormal factors and other associated clinical disorders listed in Table 7 that influence carbohydrate tolerance must be considered before OGTT is performed.

OTHER TESTS

1. *Urine glucose.* We prefer the two-drop Clinitest method with results expressed in percentage.

2. *Glycosylated hemoglobin (Hb A_1C).* We perform Hb A_1C routinely as a measure of diabetic control once diagnosis is established. The patient is started on insulin therapy. Some authors are advocating this test for diagnosis. Hb A_1C may have value in the diagnosis of diabetes, but further standardization of the test methods and norms for diagnosis are needed before widespread adoption for this purpose.

3. *HLA antigen and basement membrane thickness (BMT).* These are not done as a routine; we perform these tests as we include the subjects into our research protocol. We repeat BMT once a year as a measure of diabetic complications. BMT is *not* a prerequisite for the diagnosis of DM.

4. *Other tests,* including an intravenous glucose tolerance test, and cortisone glucose tolerance test, are no longer performed for diagnosis. Extensive use of the intravenous glucose tolerance test in our laboratory has shown it to be less sensitive than the OGTT for diagnosis. It is used only as a research tool to test insulin responsiveness. The cortisone glucose tolerance test is not well standardized and offers no advantages over the standard oral glucose tolerance test for diagnosis.

NATURAL HISTORY OF IDIOPATHIC DIABETES MELLITUS

Our knowledge in regard to the course of asymptomatic diabetes mellitus is scanty. The best data available are from the long-term studies of Fajan et al. In their studies a majority of young diabetics who had abnormality of the glucose tolerance test did not have progression to frank diabetes. In some persons, an abnormal glucose tolerance test reverted to normal.

In our population of diabetic children there is a small group of patients with an abnormal glucose tolerance test with low serum insulin levels. The condition of patients in this group will frequently deteriorate rapidly to insulin-dependent diabetes mellitus. Overall in our experience about 12 per cent of children with impaired glucose tolerance became overt diabetics. In the group with low insulin secretion, the number was much higher (about 30 per cent in 1 to 2 years), but in the group with elevated serum insulin values only 3 to 5 per cent deteriorated over 3 to 5 years. Thus, we believe that the serum insulin values can be helpful, especially in children, in determining prognosis, and perhaps therapy. Data from our program indicate that the early institution of insulin therapy in insulin-dependent diabetes mellitus may prolong the remission or "honeymoon" phase of the disease. Perhaps then the institution of insulin therapy during the early or chemical diabetic phase (IGT) in children with low insulin-secreting capacity may also prolong the period during which there is some remaining beta-cell function, although this remains to be proved.

Our studies indicate that in uncontrolled diabetes, capillary basement membrane thickness increases, whereas with tight metabolic control, the thickened basement membrane may revert to normal. Since thickened capillary basement membranes are the pathologic lesion of diabetic microvascular disease, it would seem to be prudent to attain and maintain as high a level of metabolic control as is possible to achieve and to do so as early in the disease process as is feasible. The best possible control of diabetes mellitus is achieved through the internal secretion of insulin by the beta cells. Since early treatment may preserve beta-cell function and thus enhance control, we think it should be instituted in individuals with low insulin secreting ability as early as possible.

DISORDERS OF PROTEIN METABOLISM

By WALTER J. K. TANNENBERG, M.D.
Chestnut Hill, Massachusetts

AGAMMAGLOBULINEMIA

DEFINITION

This includes a large group of syndromes characterized by deficiencies of one or more immunoglobulins and manifested by severe recurrent infections. These are listed in rough order of decreasing frequency in the population.

1. *Dysgammaglobulinemia (selective immunoglobulin deficiency).* Defects include IgA alone, IgA with IgG, and IgA with IgM, the remaining immunoglobulins being normal. Isolated IgA deficiency occurs with a frequency of 1 per 600 to 700 people.

2. *Acquired.* This is due to malignant disease of the lymphoid system; the degree of deficiency varies.

3. *Common variable (late onset).* Defects of IgG and IgA, occurring in the second to sixth decade and often associated with autoimmune diseases, various malignancies, and familial clustering.

4. *X-linked agammaglobulinemia (Bruton).* Male infants have marked defects in IgG, IgA, and IgM.

5. *Severe combined immunodeficiency (SCID, Swiss type, thymic alymphoplasia).* Rapidly fatal in infants born with neither immunoglobulins nor lymphoid tissue. Some also lack adenosine deaminase, allowing prenatal diagnosis.

6. *Ataxia-telangiectasia.* Children exhibit ataxia, oculocutaneous telangiectasia, autosomal recessive inheritance, and recurrent respiratory infections related to IgA deficiency.

7. *Wiskott-Aldrich.* X-linked with eczema, thrombocytopenia, and frequent infections related to IgM deficiency.

PRESENTING SIGNS AND SYMPTOMS

The history invariably reveals recurrent lingering infections of the upper and lower respiratory tract. The gut may be affected by diarrhea, malabsorption, and protein-losing enteropathy. Hemolytic anemia, neutropenia, thrombocytopenia, nephritis, rashes, and arthritis may occur, probably on an autoimmune basis.

COURSE

This is highly variable depending on the type of defect. Isolated absence of IgA may not produce symptoms, while SCID leads to death only weeks after birth. Many patients with acquired, common variable, dysgammaglobulinemia or X-linked forms can be readily managed with replacement therapy and antibiotics as needed. The course of the more severe congenital forms is generally downhill; death from infections or malignancy is common. Experimental methods of lymphoid tissue transplantation have met with some success.

LABORATORY FINDINGS

In the congenital forms, the serum contains less than 100 mg per dl (100 ml) of IgG; IgA and IgM may be barely detectable. IgG levels of up to 500 mg per dl may be seen in the milder acquired and common variable forms. Isoantibodies to type A and B red blood cell antigens may be absent. No antibodies may be found against antigens used in childhood immunization (DPT). There may be an absolute lymphocytopenia in the blood. Plasma cells are absent from the bone marrow and lymphoid tissue. Classification is aided by special assays for B and T lymphocytes.

COMPLICATIONS

Iatrogenic complications may be avoided by not immunizing patients with vaccines containing living viruses.

MACROGLOBULINEMIA

SYNONYMS

Waldenström's macroglobulinemia, Waldenström's hyperglobulinemic purpura.

DEFINITION

This is a B-cell lymphoma characterized by plasmacytoid lymphocytic infiltrates and an IgM monoclonal gammopathy.

PRESENTING SIGNS AND SYMPTOMS

Anemia, purpura, or the hyperviscosity syndrome predominates.

PHYSICAL EXAMINATION

Lymphadenopathy and hepatosplenomegaly occur in one half of the patients. Purpura and mucosal bleeding are also frequent. Hyperviscosity of the blood is revealed by "sausage-like" engorgement of the retinal veins, central nervous system defects, peripheral neuropathy, and vascular embarrassment of the extremities.

COURSE

The course is progressive with a fatal outcome, usually 1 to 10 years after diagnosis.

LABORATORY FINDINGS

Peripheral Blood. Anemia is always present, owing to bleeding, hemolysis, or low production. Thrombocytopenia occurs, and platelet function may be altered by IgM coating. Coagulation factors may function poorly because of complexes formed with IgM.

Bone Marrow. There is a diffuse pleomorphic infiltrate predominantly of plasmacytoid lymphocytes with lymphocytes and plasma cells. Mast cells are occasionally and characteristically prominent.

BIOCHEMICAL FINDINGS

Total serum globulins are elevated. Serum electrophoresis shows a monoclonal gammopathy. Immunoelectrophoresis and immunodiffusion assays reveal IgM levels usually above 100 mg per dl. Bence Jones proteinuria is found in one third of patients. Monitoring of the serum viscosity is a useful guide to therapy, as neurologic symptoms do not occur until the viscosity relative to water exceeds 4 (normal relative serum viscosity is 1.8).

COMPLICATIONS

Central nervous system (CNS) dysfunction due to hyperviscosity of the blood is most serious. Renal function may be impaired. About 5 per cent of patients develop cryoglobulins. Amyloidosis may occur.

CRYOGLOBULINEMIA

SYNONYM

Cryoglobulinemic purpura.

DEFINITION

This is a chronic disturbance of circulation, most often of cutaneous and peripheral vessels, caused by intravascular precipitation of certain immunoglobulins below 37 C. It may precede ("idiopathic") or accompany plasma cell dyscrasias characterized by monoclonal gammopathies as well as various inflammatory diseases.

PRESENTING SIGNS AND SYMPTOMS

Cold intolerance may produce Raynaud's phenomenon, purpura, epistaxis, urticaria, neuropathy, or ulcerations of the extremities. These may draw attention to signs of an underlying disease, such as multiple myeloma, macroglobulinemia, lymphoma, systemic lupus erythematosus (SLE), or chronic inflammatory disorders.

COURSE

The course is that of the underlying disease. The determinant of cold symptoms is the temperature at which the cryoglobulin becomes insoluble, not the protein's serum concentration.

PHYSICAL EXAMINATION

The skin of the extremities exhibits large petechiae, vasculitis, or ulcers. Petechiae can be produced by cooling the skin briefly with ice. Retinal hemorrhages, CNS dysfunction, or peripheral neuropathy may be present.

LABORATORY FINDINGS

The blood must be kept warm during collection, clotting, and serum separation. When serum is incubated at 4 C between 24 and 96 hours, a cryoglobulin precipitate or gel will form, and it will dissolve when warmed to 37 C. Urinalysis usually reveals proteinuria and microscopic hematuria.

Serum or urine electrophoresis often shows a monoclonal gammopathy or Bence Jones protein. A polyclonal gammopathy is usually seen in SLE or inflammatory disorders. Immunoelectrophoresis of the isolated cryoglobulin will identify its components, most commonly IgM or IgG. IgA, Bence Jones protein, and complexes between a monoclonal and a normal immunoglobulin may also be seen.

HEAVY CHAIN DISEASES

SYNONYMS

Franklin's disease; α-chain disease; γ-chain disease; μ-chain disease.

DEFINITION

This disease is a malignant plasma cell dyscrasia producing excess immunoglobulin heavy chains of either α, γ, or μ types. About 100 cases have been reported.

PRESENTING SIGNS AND SYMPTOMS

α-Chain disease is most common and is seen most often in Sephardic Jews and Arabs under age 40. It presents as a lymphoma of the small bowel with diarrhea and malabsorption. γ-Chain disease presents with lymphadenopathy, hepatosplenomegaly, edema and erythema of the soft palate, and recurrent infections. Only about a dozen cases of μ-chain disease have been reported, mostly in patients with long-standing chronic lymphocytic leukemia.

PHYSICAL EXAMINATION

Abdominal masses are often palpable in α-chain disease; hepatosplenomegaly is occasionally present. Lymphadenopathy is generally present in γ- and μ-chain diseases.

COMPLICATIONS

α-Chain disease often leads to malabsorption syndromes, electrolyte imbalances owing to diarrhea, and recurrent respiratory tract infections.

LABORATORY FINDINGS

Serum and urine electrophoresis show an abnormal protein peak, usually in the β region, often broader and smaller than a typical monoclonal gammopathy, and with diminished normal immunoglobulins. Immunoelectrophoresis is diagnostic when appropriate antisera are used to demonstrate heavy chains not associated with light chains.

There is generally pancytopenia of the blood. The bone marrow has increased numbers of plasma cells and lymphocytes. Large cytoplasmic vacuoles in plasma cells are often seen in μ-chain disease. Bowel x-rays in α-chain disease show malabsorption signs.

COURSE

While these diseases are usually fatal in months or years, too few patients are known to describe accurately their natural history.

AMYLOIDOSIS

DEFINITION

This is a group of progressive diseases in which the function of blood vessels and other tissues is compromised by the extracellular deposition of a poorly soluble, eosinophilic, fibrillar protein. This protein, amyloid, is composed of the degradation products of a number of serum proteins, all of which have in common a structure that lends itself to arrangement in a β-pleated sheet conformation. Amyloidosis can be classified into three types based on its major protein component, neglecting the minor components.

1. Primary amyloidosis, occurring in a variety of immunoglobulin-producing plasma cell tumors, and composed of portions of the variable region of immunoglobulin light chain.

2. Secondary amyloidosis, occurring in many chronic inflammatory diseases including infections, rheumatoid arthritis, and familial Mediterranean fever, and composed of portions of an acute-phase serum reactant protein termed serum protein AA (SAA).

3. Hereditary amyloidosis involving nerves, kidney, or heart in which the source of amyloid protein is not clear.

PRESENTING SIGNS AND SYMPTOMS

None are specific, since amyloidosis mimics a host of diseases. Common diagnostic clues include unexplained weakness and weight loss, macroglossia, the carpal tunnel syndrome, neuropathy, skin nodules, heart failure, the nephrotic syndrome, and purpura.

PHYSICAL EXAMINATION

As noted, nothing is specific. Findings may include smooth, firm hepatosplenomegaly, ascites, pleural effusions, cardiomegaly, as well as abnormalities owing to any of the underlying diseases.

LABORATORY FINDINGS

Nothing is specific. Evidence may include the hypoalbuminemia, hypercholesterolemia, and proteinuria of the nephrotic syndrome. Microscopic hematuria is common. Retention of bromsulfalein in the serum is often 0 per cent even in the presence of evident liver disease, owing to adsorption of the dye by amyloid.

Serum electrophoresis may show the monoclonal gammopathy of a plasma cell dyscrasia or the diffuse hyperglobulinemia of a chronic inflammatory disease.

COURSE

Progressive dysfunction of affected organ systems is the rule. Sometimes secondary amyloidosis can be ameliorated by cure of the underlying disease.

DIAGNOSIS

The diagnosis must be given consideration, utilizing only the vague clues just noted. Biopsy demonstration of amyloid with Congo red staining and birefringence is required. The rectal mucosa yields best results. The gingivae, skin, bone marrow, or other involved areas are often useful. Liver biopsy is probably safe if a "skinny needle" technique is used. Amyloid can almost always be demonstrated in the blood vessels of the aged.

HEREDITARY DEFICIENCIES OF COMPLEMENT COMPONENTS

DEFINITION

More than 13 plasma proteins compose the classic and alternate complement system. Hereditary deficiencies have been reported for all except C1q, C9, and the alternate pathway. Except for C1 inhibitor deficiency, all are inherited as autosomal recessive traits. Disease appears only in homozygotes, who usually have less than 1 per cent of normal of the affected component present, other components generally being normal.

Complement defects and their associated diseases are outlined in Table 1. Only the deficiency of C1 inhibitor is described in detail.

DIAGNOSIS

This depends on a high degree of suspicion during the evaluation of severe, recurrent infections and variants of immunologically mediated diseases such as systemic lupus erythematosus.

HEREDITARY ANGIOEDEMA

SYNONYM

Hereditary angioneurotic edema (Osler).

DEFINITION

This disease is manifested by repeated attacks of nonpruritic edema of any part of the body. It is caused by deficient synthesis or function of the plasma inhibitor of the first component of complement (C1INH; C1 esterase inhibitor). It is an autosomal dominant trait.

PRESENTING SIGNS AND SYMPTOMS

Mild trauma, especially dental work, may initiate attacks in more than half the patients. Local subjective discomfort may be felt before the appearance of edema. Recurrent attacks of mild to massive edema may affect the airway, face, and extremities. Edema of the gastrointestinal tract is reflected by crampy abdominal pain and diarrhea.

COURSE

Acute attacks are self-limited, lasting hours to several days. The disease is lifelong, with attacks at irregular intervals of days to years. Death from airway obstruction can occur.

PHYSICAL EXAMINATION

The patient may be mildly affected or near collapse. Brawny, nonpitting edema affects the

Table 1. *Diseases Associated with Complement Component Deficiency*

Component	No. Cases Reported	Associated Disease
C1q	0	
C1r	3	SLE°; chronic glomerulonephritis
C1s	5	SLE
C2	>40	None; SLE; discoid LE; anaphylactoid purpura; vasculitis; infections; dermatomyositis; nephritis; Hodgkin's
C3	4	Infections
C4	2	SLE
C5	2	SLE; infections
C5 dysfunction	2	Infections and eczema
C6	2	Infections
C7	8	None; infections; Raynaud's; Sclerodactyly; SLE
C8	2	Infections; SLE
C9	0	
C1 INH	Many	Hereditary angioedema; SLE; partial lipidodystrophy
C3b Inact	1	Infections; Klinefelter's

°Systemic lupus erythematosus.

face or one or more extremities. Pharyngeal edema with stridor heralds airway obstruction. Bowel edema may lead to a moderately tender abdomen, but signs of peritoneal irritation are usually absent. Hypotension is due to loss of fluid into the bowel. Occasionally a transient erythematous or seripiginous rash appears on the edematous area or elsewhere. Urticaria never occurs. Old tracheostomy or laparotomy scars may be present.

COMMON COMPLICATIONS

Airway obstruction leads to a significant mortality rate and tracheostomy may be needed. Cerebral edema may result in seizures and hemiparesis. Abdominal pain may lead to unnecessary laparotomy. Partial lipidodystrophy and systemic lupus erythematosus are occasionally associated with the disease.

LABORATORY FINDINGS

The serum level of C1 inhibitor is always low, ranging from 0 to 7 mg per dl with a mean of about 2 mg per dl (N = 15 to 18 mg per dl). The serum level of C2 and C4 is always low during an attack but may rise to nearly normal during remission.

Fifteen to 20 per cent of patients have a variant disease in which C1INH levels are normal but the protein is inactive. This may be suspected by the typical syndrome and low C2 or C4 levels. Functional C1INH assays must be done in specialized laboratories.

Peripheral blood. The hematocrit, white blood cell (WBC) count, and serum sodium level may be elevated during an attack due to fluid sequestration.

PITFALLS IN DIAGNOSIS

Diagnosis may be unsuspected and overlooked for decades. The absence of pruritus and urticaria distinguishes hereditary angioedema from allergic angioedema. The recurrent history and absence of peritoneal signs weighs against a surgical abdominal emergency.

Interpretation of laboratory results may be difficult. C4 and C2 levels may be low in many disorders in which complement activation plays a role. Assays of other complement components, such as C3 (β 1C) and total hemolytic complement activities (CH_{50}) are useless; they are usually normal in hereditary angioedema and low in a wide variety of other diseases.

PROTEIN-LOSING ENTEROPATHY

SYNONYMS

Idiopathic hypoproteinemia, essential hypoproteinemia, idiopathic hypercatabolic hypoproteinemia, idiopathic hypoalbuminemia.

DEFINITION

This disorder is manifested by decreased levels of all serum proteins, which are lost through the gut in excessive amounts. A wide variety of diseases of the gastrointestinal tract and the heart appear to be responsible.

PRESENTING SIGNS AND SYMPTOMS

Dependent edema or anasarca is present. Signs of the underlying disease must then be sought.

COURSE

The course is chronic, much depending on the nature of the basic disease. Low immunoglobulin levels may predispose to severe bacterial infections.

PHYSICAL EXAMINATION

The only characteristic finding is edema.

LABORATORY FINDINGS

There is marked hypoproteinemia with all protein fractions more or less reduced.

MEASUREMENT OF GASTROINTESTINAL PROTEIN LOSS

Ten to 30 μCi of ^{131}I-labeled polyvinylpyrrolidone are given intravenously and the total radioactivity is measured in a 4-day stool collection. Normal people excrete less than 1.5 per cent of the total initial radioactivity, while those with excessive losses into the gut excrete between 2.9 and 32.5 per cent. If ^{51}Cr-labeled albumin is used, normals excrete less than 0.7 per cent, while patients with the disorder lose between 2 and 40 per cent.

UNDERLYING DISEASES

Some of the more common associations are listed in Table 2.

Table 2. *Underlying Conditions in Protein-Losing Enteropathy*

Esophageal carcinoma
Gastric carcinoma
Giant hypertrophy of the gastric mucosa
Atrophic gastritis
Postgastrectomy syndrome
Nontropical sprue
Tropical sprue
Regional enteritis
Whipple's disease
Lymphoma of the bowel
Gastrointestinal tuberculosis
Intestinal lymphangiectasia
Ulcerative colitis
Colon neoplasm
Congestive heart failure
Constrictive pericarditis
Agammaglobulinemia
Nephrosis
Angioneurotic edema
Allergic gastroenteropathy

ANALBUMINEMIA

DEFINITION

Analbuminemia is a benign condition in which serum albumin is nearly absent, probably owing to an autosomal recessive genetic defect in albumin synthesis. Less than a dozen cases have been reported.

PRESENTING SIGNS AND SYMPTOMS

Patients are generally in good health. Mild pedal edema may be the only complaint.

COURSE

Good health is enjoyed during a normal lifespan.

PHYSICAL EXAMINATION

This is normal except for mild vespertine pedal edema and mild hypotension.

LABORATORY FINDINGS

Serum electrophoresis reveals the absence of the usual albumin peak. Small amounts of normal albumin, between 1 and 24 mg per dl, can be detected by immunochemical methods. Serum globulins, especially gamma globulins, are somewhat increased. The osmotic pressure of the serum is reduced to less than one half normal. Serum cholesterol is elevated, triglyceride levels are normal, and serum calcium may

be low. The erythrocyte sedimentation rate is elevated, while the formed blood elements are normal. Individuals thought to be heterozygous for this trait have normal albumin levels.

BISALBUMINEMIA

DEFINITION

The hereditary form is a benign condition in which a person possesses equal amounts of two electrophoretically distinct species of serum albumin. A second hereditary form exhibits small amounts of albumin dimers. Acquired forms show shifts in albumin electrophoretic mobility when the protein is complexed to antibiotics or is partially degraded by proteolytic enzymes in the course of pancreatitis.

PRESENTING SIGNS AND SYMPTOMS

None. This abnormality is discovered when affected sera are fortuitously subjected to electrophoresis.

COURSE

The hereditary forms affect neither health nor disease. Bisalbuminemia in the course of pancreatitis is a diagnostic clue to the presence of a pancreatic duct fistula.

LABORATORY FINDINGS

Hereditary. Serum electrophoresis reveals two albumin peaks of equal size. The second peak may have a faster or slower mobility than the normal albumin, depending on the buffer system used; at least 28 variants have been observed. The two albumins are also found in other body fluids, including the cerebrospinal fluid. A second variant is revealed as a small, slow albumin peak on electrophoresis, composed of stable dimers and comprising but 10 to 15 per cent of the total albumin.

Acquired. Variable amounts of albumin with faster than normal mobility are seen, the peaks being more diffuse than normal albumin.

GENETICS

The trait is inherited as an autosomal codominant, usually in heterozygous form, although homozygotes have been observed. The abnormal albumin locus is genetically linked to that of another serum protein, the group-specific component (Gc). The gene frequency in European populations is roughly 0.0007, while that in certain Canadian Indian tribes such as the Naskapi is 0.13.

BIOCHEMISTRY

In the few cases analyzed, a single amino acid substitution has been found in the inherited abnormal albumin. In acquired forms, massive doses of β-lactam antibiotics are found complexed to normal albumin. Pancreatic enzymes that enter the circulation, including chymotrypsin and carboxy-peptidase A and B, have been shown to alter the electrophoretic mobility of albumin by partial degradation.

CONGENITAL TRANSCOBALAMINE I DEFICIENCY

SYNONYMS

Deficiency of R-type binder, deficiency of cobalophilin.

DEFINITION

This is a benign condition, inherited probably as an autosomal recessive, in which transcobalamine I (TC I) is absent from the blood.

PRESENTING SIGNS AND SYMPTOMS

None. The condition is discovered fortuitously during investigations of low serum vitamin B_{12} levels.

COURSE

No morbidity that might be associated with any aspect of vitamin B_{12} metabolism has been described. Only two patients have been reported.

LABORATORY FINDINGS

Total serum vitamin B_{12} is low (90 nanograms per liter; N 150 to 800 nanograms per liter). Specific radioimmunoassay for TC I reveals a small amount of immunoreactive material in the serum, but no vitamin B_{12} is bound to it. Vitamin B_{12}-binding proteins immunologically identical to TC I (but electrophoretically different owing to varying carbohydrate content) are found normally in saliva, cerebrospinal fluid (CSF), gastric juice, and granulocytes. In this disorder, these proteins (sometimes called R-type binding proteins) are absent from all these sources.

PITFALLS IN DIAGNOSIS

Since about three fourths of all serum vitamin B_{12} is normally bound to TC 1, the absence of this protein is reflected by a low serum vitamin B_{12} level. The vitamin B_{12} assayed is that bound to TC II. A false diagnosis of vitamin B_{12} deficiency can be avoided by observing a normal Schilling test, absence of megaloblastic changes of blood and bone marrow, and absence of neurologic signs.

CONGENITAL TRANSCOBALAMINE II DEFICIENCY

DEFINITION

This is a disease caused by a congenital absence from the plasma of transcobalamine II (TC II) and manifested by a rapidly fatal course unless treated.

PRESENTING SIGNS AND SYMPTOMS

After a few weeks of life, infants rapidly develop a debilitating illness with severe megaloblastic anemia, oral ulcerations, vomiting, and diarrhea.

COURSE

The course in the three reported cases was that of a rapid decline, fortunately interrupted by proper diagnosis and treatment. Otherwise, it might be expected to be fatal; two siblings of one patient had died of severe infections in early infancy.

PHYSICAL EXAMINATION

Infants are very sick, having oral ulcers, signs of anemia, infection, bleeding, and malnourishment.

LABORATORY FINDINGS

The peripheral blood develops macrocytic anemia, granulocytopenia, thrombocytopenia, and reticulocytopenia. The bone marrow exhibits typical and profound megaloblastic changes. Agammaglobulinemia with an inability to synthesize antibody to a challenge even at 3 months of age has been seen. Cell-mediated immunity is normal.

Serum vitamin B_{12} and folate levels are normal. The diagnosis is made by showing the complete absence of TC II (N is 25 micrograms per liter) by polyacrylamide gel electrophoresis or by the use of specific antiserum to TC II.

PITFALLS IN DIAGNOSIS

The presence of severe megaloblastic anemia in an infant whose serum levels of vitamin B_{12} and folate are normal is unique and puzzling. The serum vitamin B_{12} assayed is bound to transcobalamine I, which normally accounts for 75 per cent of the total serum vitamin B_{12}. However, TC I appears neither to play a vital role in the vitamin's metabolism nor to be able to substitute for the apparent essential functions of TC II.

ISOLATED ABSENCE OF TRANSFERRIN

SYNONYMS

Atransferrinemia, asiderophilinemia.

DEFINITION

Iron cannot be transported through the plasma to the bone marrow when transferrin is absent, resulting in a profound iron-deficiency anemia. The condition is rare, occurring preterminally in fatal diseases or as a congenital defect.

PRESENTING SIGNS AND SYMPTOMS

In acquired forms, severe anemia occurs in the course of an underlying terminal disease. In the untreated congenital form, anemia produces weakness and pallor. Presentation after transfusion therapy reveals signs of hemochromatosis.

COURSE

Although iron absorption is normal, iron is not utilized by the bone marrow and anemia must be corrected by transfusion. The course is prolonged but generally fatal owing to complications of iron overload.

PHYSICAL EXAMINATION

Transfusion hemochromatosis produces bronze skin pigmentation, cardiac failure, and hepatosplenomegaly.

LABORATORY FINDINGS

There is a profound hypochromic microcytic anemia. Serum iron content is low, 14 to 65 micrograms per dl, and iron-binding capacity is fully saturated. Immunoelectrophoresis is diagnostic, demonstrating the absence of transferrin.

HYPOGLYCEMIA

By JESSE D. IBARRA, JR., M.D., F.A.C.P.
Temple, Texas

Recent publicity in the popular press has led the public to believe that symptomatic hypoglycemia is commonly a cause of many psychic and physical ailments. The physician frequently meets problem patients who come to him with a self-diagnosis or misdiagnosis by other physicians who have not used appropriately rigid diagnostic criteria. Having a misdiagnosis of hypoglycemia provides a reason for symptoms but subjects the patient to long-term incapacity and unnecessary regimens. Therefore, the physician confronted with the problem of "hypoglycemia" needs to be familiar with the symptoms and disturbed physiology of the disease to rule out or confirm the diagnosis.

Man benefits from a refined, integrated system for maintaining circulating plasma glucose levels at a remarkably constant level, ranging from 60 to 160 mg per 100 ml during fasting and fed states. When this well-synchronized system is deranged by functional or organic illnesses, abnormal glucose levels result and symptoms appear. Hypoglycemia refers to a group of physiologic derangements that disturb the normal glucose homeostasis.

SYNONYMS

Reactive hypoglycemia, anxiety hypoglycemia, alimentary hypoglycemia, functional hyperinsulinism, and dysinsulinism are synonyms of the entity recognized as functional hypoglycemia.

DEFINITION

Hypoglycemia as a diagnosis implies that blood sugar concentration is depressed below the accepted normal concentration in plasma and manifested clinically by a characteristic symptom complex. The level of plasma glucose depression necessary to induce symptoms is quite variable. Many studies have shown that frequently blood sugars can be measured at levels below 50 mg in asymptomatic individuals in fasting states and during glucose tolerance tests. Therefore for any measured level of glucose to be significant, a correlation with the clinical symptom complex must be established.

The rate of fall in the glucose level may be a factor in the evolution of symptoms, but current evidence suggests that a critical low level of

Table 1. *Symptoms of Hypoglycemia*

Symptoms due to catecholamine release
  (Sympathetic discharge, hyperepinephrinemia)
  Sweating
  Trembling (shakiness)
  Tachycardia
  Nervousness and anxiety
  Weakness
  Hunger
  Nausea and vomiting

Symptoms due to inadequate delivery of glucose to brain
  Headache
  Slow cerebration
  Irritability
  Personality changes (bizarre behavior)
  Speech and gait disorders
  Mental confusion
  Convulsions (coma)
  Permanent mental and neurologic damage

glucose is the only important precipitant of the chain of clinical events.

The symptoms of hypoglycemia are similar regardless of the cause, and their presence or absence should be determined by careful interrogation of the patient. The manifestations of the symptom complex can be remembered easily if classified according to the pathologic physiology (Table 1). Hypoglycemia causes catecholamine release, which in turn activates the autonomic nervous system to produce sweating, trembling (shakiness), tachycardia, nervousness and anxiety, weakness, hunger, nausea, and vomiting. A subnormal blood sugar alone may produce central nervous system disturbances secondary to decreased cerebral glucose and oxygen utilization. The symptoms induced are nonspecific headache, slow cerebration, irritability, personality changes (bizarre behavior), and disorders of speech and gait. Severe and persistent glucose deprivation of the central nervous system may produce mental confusion, convulsions (coma), and permanent mental and neurologic damage.

After a symptom complex suggestive of hypoglycemia has been elicited, it is important to prove that a low blood sugar is indeed the cause. Prompt subsidence of symptoms following ingestion of food or administration of glucose is indirect proof of low glucose concentration in the blood, and a blood glucose level lower than 50 mg per 100 ml (during an episode of symptoms) strongly suggests the diagnosis of hypoglycemia. Because patients often are symptom-free when seen, various diagnostic maneuvers may be needed to confirm the presence of hypoglycemia.

ETIOLOGY

Once the clinician confirms a suspected diagnosis of hypoglycemia by documenting low blood sugars, the cause must be investigated. Table 2 outlines a simplified classification of the most frequent causes. A more extensive classification of the etiologic classification of hypoglycemia was published by Conn and Pek.

The numerous causes of hypoglycemia can be divided into functional and organic. Of the various types of functional derangement, idiopathic hypoglycemia is the most common and reflects an excessive islet cell response to a normal stimulus for the secretion of insulin. Symptoms never occur in a fasting state but appear 90 to 180 minutes after meals and subside within 15 to 20 minutes. Loss of consciousness or convulsions are never seen. However, obtunded mentation and a staring expression may lead to a misdiagnosis of petit mal seizures. These appear more often in individuals who are tense, driven, and perfectionist.

In contrast to idiopathic hypoglycemia, ali-

Table 2. *Causes of Hypoglycemia*

Functional hypoglycemia
Postprandial
  Idiopathic hypoglycemia
  Alimentary hypoglycemia (postgastrectomy)
  Reactive delayed hyperinsulinism (early diabetes)
Fasting
  Excessive muscular activity
  Severe undernutrition or starvation
  Lactation
  Renal glycosuria
  Malabsorption
Organic hypoglycemia
Pancreatic
  Islet cell tumor (carcinoma or adenoma)
  Islet cell hyperplasia
Nonislet cell tumors
Hepatic disease
  Hepatic enzyme defects (galactosemia, glycogen storage disease, fructose intolerance)
  Cirrhosis
  Alcoholism (with starvation)
Endocrine disorders
  Hypopituitarism
  Adrenal cortical insufficiency
  Hypothyroidism
Pediatric
  Idiopathic familial hypoglycemia
  Leucine hypoglycemia
  Hypoglycemia in newborn infants of diabetic mothers
Pharmacogenic
  Factitious
  Iatrogenic (insulin or sulfonylurea)
  Miscellaneous (many amino acids, nicotinic acid, iproniazid, propranolol)

mentary hypoglycemia is produced by excessive stimulation. Due to rapid absorption of glucose from the intestine, such as may occur in patients after partial gastrectomy, the blood sugar concentration increases to higher than normal levels. The increased level produces a greater than normal release of insulin with subsequent excessive lowering of the blood sugar.

Patients with early diabetes mellitus may present with postprandial hypoglycemia as their initial symptom. This is due to delayed but excessive insulin release after a meal. As time passes, the pancreatic beta cells lose their ability to overrespond and the hypoglycemic episodes subside.

Excessive utilization or loss of carbohydrates owing to strenuous exercise, lactation, or renal glycosuria may produce hypoglycemia, or a lower blood glucose may occur from decreased or deficient absorption, as in starvation or malabsorption syndromes. In these circumstances, the hypoglycemic episodes usually occur during periods of decreased food intake or fasting and are neither abrupt nor severe.

The causes of organic hypoglycemia are many. Symptoms usually are more severe than those of the functional variety and are not necessarily triggered by a carbohydrate stimulus. Insulin production independent of stimulus or need can occur in the presence of hyperplasia or tumors of the islet cells of the pancreas. In recent years nonpancreatic tumors have been reported in association with hypoglycemia. Lipsett and co-workers have reviewed 100 cases of nonpancreatic tumors that produced hypoglycemia, and Unger has reviewed the causative mechanisms.

Hepatic disease owing to specific enzyme defects such as galactosemia, glycogen storage disease, and fructose intolerance may produce hypoglycemia. Cirrhosis and alcoholism, associated with starvation, may also cause hypoglycemia. Although hypoglycemia may occur in patients with these diseases, it usually is not the outstanding feature; however, in some predisposed persons, hypoglycemia following alcoholic intoxication may be severe and cause coma. Arky, Veverbrants, and Abramson reported five patients with insulin-dependent diabetes with irreversible hypoglycemia following ingestion of alcohol. Galactosemia and fructose intolerance occur early in infancy, and hypoglycemia may be severe. Diagnosis of these conditions usually is not difficult.

Hypopituitarism as well as adrenal and thyroid deficiencies may produce varying degrees of hypoglycemia but usually there is an associated inadequate or delayed food intake. While the symptoms of hypoglycemia in these conditions are usually minor, severe or even fatal hypoglycemia may ensue if pituitary or adrenal insufficiency remains untreated. The underlying endocrine disorder is quite obvious when hypoglycemia occurs in patients with these diseases.

Hypoglycemia in a child less than 2 years of age is frequently difficult to explain. Familial idiopathic hypoglycemia of infancy generally undergoes spontaneous remission by the age of 6 to 10 years. Most patients with idiopathic hypoglycemia have a family history of diabetes mellitus.

In infants, leucine sensitivity produces hypoglycemia. It has been proved that leucine induces increased production of insulin by the pancreas. In newborn infants of diabetic mothers, hypoglycemia frequently is transient but at times serious. Awareness of this possibility is extremely important. The mechanism is transient overactivity of the infant's pancreas (beta cells) in response to maternal hyperglycemia before birth.

Factitious hypoglycemia is encountered occasionally. This can be caused by self-administration of excessive insulin in diabetics or nondiabetics. Oral hypoglycemics can cause excessive beta-cell stimulation and produce symptomatic hypoglycemia.

Once the symptom complex of hypoglycemia has been established, the physician must prove the diagnosis chemically and determine the reason for the low blood sugar level.

DIAGNOSIS

Frequently the symptomatology is unclear and the diagnosis already applied, making it mandatory for the physician to prove or disprove the diagnosis of hypoglycemia. To encompass all possible etiologies following a protocol for investigation has proven quite satisfactory (Table 3).

If a patient is having frequent and/or vague symptoms, hospitalization for close observation and detection of recurrences of symptoms may be quite helpful. During the first 3 days in the hospital a high carbohydrate diet (250 to 300 grams daily) is prescribed. Only three meals are scheduled, prohibiting food between meals and at bedtime. This allows adequate periods of time for functional hypoglycemia to occur. The urine is tested by Diastix four times each day before meals and at bedtime, and blood sugar measurements are made daily in the fasting state and at midafternoon. Orders are given for immediate withdrawal of a blood sample for glucose and immunoreactive insulin (IRI) lev-

Table 3. *Investigation of Hypoglycemia*

Hospital Days	
1, 2, 3	High-carbohydrate diet (300 grams) Daily fasting blood sugar determination Diastix four times a day (before meals and at bedtime) 3 P.M. blood sugar
4	5-hour glucose tolerance test
5	Tolbutamide test 72-hour fast begins (fifth day)
6, 7	72-hour fast continues (only unsweetened tea and coffee) Daily blood sugar and immunoreactive insulin determinations 7 A.M. and 3 P.M.
8	Fast completed — 7 A.M.; blood sugar and immunoreactive insulin determinations (before breakfast)

els whenever symptoms suggesting hypoglycemia occur.

During this 3-day period the patient is observed closely and the hospital staff alerted to the possibilities of symptomatic episodes occurring. This observation period offers an opportunity to question the patient further and elucidate possible psychologic causes producing emotional symptoms that can mimic hypoglycemia. If these are suspected and rapport has been established, psychologic evaluation can be obtained and termination of further investigation may be possible.

Following patient preparation with a high-carbohydrate diet for 3 days, a 5-hour glucose tolerance test (GTT) is performed on the fourth day. During this test the patient should be observed carefully and any appearance of symptoms noted and correlated with the blood sugar levels drawn at that time. Orders are given to draw blood for glucose level any time symptoms appear.

If the physician still suspects hypoglycemia and wants to rule out organic disease, further investigation is necessary. On the fifth day an intravenous tolbutamide test is performed. After dissolving a diagnostic ampule of tolbutamide (Orinase), 1 gram in 20 ml of sterile saline, the solution is injected intravenously over a 2-minute period. Blood samples for plasma insulin are drawn at 0, 2, 5, 15, 30, 60, and 180 minutes. At 15, 30, 60, 90, 120, 150, and 180 minutes, blood sugar is measured.

The tolbutamide test is performed in a fasting state. The fasting period can begin on this test day and be prolonged for 72 hours. During this period of fasting, blood sugar and immunoreactive insulin are measured daily and whenever symptoms suggest hypoglycemia. The last blood sugar and insulin measurements are taken at the end of the 72-hour fast, before breakfast on the eighth day.

INTERPRETATION OF TESTS

Fasting Plasma Glucose and Insulin. During fasting, decreased plasma glucose associated with elevated plasma insulin is an abnormal finding that indicates inappropriately increased secretion of insulin. This abnormal combination may be seen in patients with insulinoma, idiopathic hypoglycemia of infancy, leucine sensitivity, in patients receiving sulfonyluria, or following administration of exogenous insulin.

Five-Hour Oral Glucose Tolerance Test. A glucose tolerance test is valuable for confirming functional or reactive hypoglycemia, alimentary hypoglycemia, and late reactive hypoglycemia in patients with early diabetes mellitus. A characteristic glucose tolerance curve identifies each of these types of hypoglycemia (Fig. 1). This test may not be useful in detecting insulinoma. In a patient with insulinoma the response to glucose varies, even when the test is repeated.

Intravenous Tolbutamide Test. A normal plasma insulin response to the injection of tolbutamide will be maximal at the 2- or 5-minute point, with a rather prompt decrease recorded during the next hour. In patients with insulinoma the response usually will be supernormal with plasma insulin values exceeding 150 microunits per milliliter and at times surpassing 1000 microunits. Insulin levels also tend to remain higher longer following the injection of tolbutamide in patients with insulinoma.

The blood glucose response to tolbutamide provides rapid assessment of the results of the

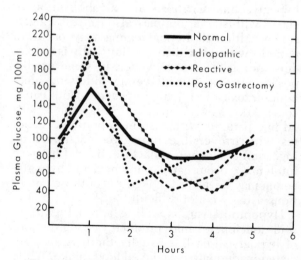

Figure 1. Representative plasma glucose curves.

test. The normal response is a fall in plasma glucose, the lowest level occurring at about the 30-minute point with a return to the fasting level during the rest of the 3-hour test period. In patients with insulinoma the maximal fall in blood sugar will occur somewhat earlier, and characteristically the measurement will remain below the basal level for the entire 3 hours (Fig. 2). In the first hour it has been found that there is a fair amount of overlap between normals and patients with hyperinsulinism, and false positives and negatives may be found. However, in the second and third hour, this overlap is considerably decreased and the interrelationship of the glucose and insulin levels can be more discriminatory. The response to the tolbutamide test has not been uniformly positive in all patients with proved insulinoma, and if this diagnosis is strongly suspected the test should be repeated or followed by a 72-hour fasting period.

72-Hour Fasting Period. During this period, simultaneous plasma glucose and immunoreactive insulin (IRI) levels are obtained twice daily (Table 3). The glucose usually will drop below 60 mg per 100 ml and frequently below 50 mg per 100 ml while patients may remain asymptomatic. The correlation of the insulin with the glucose level is very important since the inappropriate secretion of insulin is indicative of insulinoma or hyperplasia of islet cell tissue. When blood glucose decreases to 50 or 60 mg per 100 ml or below, insulin levels usually measure below 20 units per ml. Therefore, a glucose measurement below 60 mg per 100 ml with a simultaneous immunoreactive insulin level of 50 microunits per ml or above is quite suspicious for inappropriate secretion of insulin. Glucose-to-IRI ratios have been reported by several investigators as quite helpful in diagnosis.

Other Tests. Leucine or glucagon has been administered intravenously to stimulate plasma insulin release. At times testing with these substances is valuable in distinguishing normal from abnormal insulin-release states. Glucagon, when given intravenously or subcutaneously, mobilizes glycogen from the liver and helps to rule out the presence of glycogen storage disease. Epinephrine may be used for the same purpose. Fructose and galactose tolerance tests may confirm the presence of disorders involv-

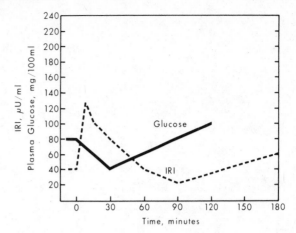

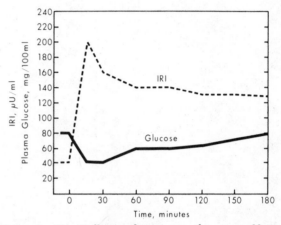

Figure 2. Top, Tolbutamide test, normal response. Notice the "double cross" of the glucose-IRI curves. Bottom, Abnormal response. Notice the persistent elevated IRI and low glucose and no crossing of these curves.

ing metabolism of these sugars. The measurement of free C peptide, free insulin, and circulatory antibodies directed against insulin provides a good discriminatory approach for the detection of factitious hypoglycemia.

In view of the relationship between insulin-producing tumors of the pancreas and other endocrine tumors occurring in a familial pattern, patients with a diagnosis of insulinoma and their immediate kin should be studied to rule out familial multiple endocrine adenomatosis. The clinical survey should include a roentgenogram of the skull, measurements of calcium and phosphorus concentrations in serum, and plasma and urine cortisol determinations.

Section 10

DISORDERS OF THE ENDOCRINE SYSTEM

HYPOPITUITARISM

By ALEXANDER TAYLOR, M.D.,
and ROBERTO F. ESCAMILLA, M.D.

San Francisco, California

NAME OF DISEASE

Several clinical pictures belong in this category, depending on age of onset, the degree and type of pituitary insufficiency, and the underlying pathology. If the onset is in childhood and the insufficiency is of moderate degree, the condition is called *hypophyseal infantilism*. If the condition occurs during adult years and pituitary insufficiency is extreme, *Simmonds' disease* will be the diagnosis. If onset follows a complicated pregnancy and is due to infarction and necrosis in the anterior pituitary, *Sheehan's syndrome* is the descriptive term. This can be of varying severity. If the patient presents a decidedly myxedematous appearance and the marked thyroid deficiency is secondary to pituitary insufficiency, the proper diagnosis would be *pituitary myxedema*. If adrenal cortical insufficiency is most prominent in the presenting picture, *secondary adrenal cortical insufficiency* would be the diagnosis, whereas if eunuchoid features are most prominent, the diagnosis *secondary eunuchoidism* would be appropriate.

SYNONYMS

Synonyms for hypopituitarism are: *hypophyseal infantilism* (pituitary dwarfism, Levi-Lorain infantilism, ateliosis, preadolescent anterior pituitary deficiency); *Simmonds' disease* (extreme insufficiency of the adenohypophysis, hypophyseal cachexia, and Sheehan's syndrome); *Sheehan's syndrome* (postpartum hypopituitarism); *pituitary myxedema* (secondary myxedema); *secondary adrenal cortical insufficiency* (hypoadrenotropic Addison's disease); and *secondary eunuchoidism* (hypogonadotropic eunuchoidism).

Sheehan's syndrome is of variable severity and may present the complete picture of Simmonds' disease, or at the opposite extreme, only failure to lactate.

DEFINITION

These types of anterior pituitary insufficiency result from deficient production of one or several of the tropic hormones by the adenohypophysis, with concomitant insufficiency of the target organs. These tropic hormones have been identified and comprise the following: adenocorticotropic hormone (ACTH), growth hormone (GH), thyroid-stimulating hormone (TSH), follicle-stimulating hormone (FSH), luteinizing hormone (LH) (also known as interstitial cell stimulating hormone [ICSH] in the male), and prolactin or lactogenic hormone. FSH causes stimulation of spermatogenesis in the male.

Pathologic causes of decreased function of the anterior pituitary include nonsecretory pituitary tumors, metastatic tumors, cysts, granulomas, infarction, infection, trauma, irradiation, hemorrhage, aneurysm, hemochromatosis, and occasionally, "idiopathic." It has been estimated that over 75 per cent of the anterior pituitary is destroyed when there is severe hypopituitarism. In recent years the influence of hypothalamic centers on anterior pituitary function has been demonstrated. Lesions in the hypothalamus can cause definite changes in anterior pituitary function.

PRESENTING SIGNS AND SYMPTOMS

Hypophyseal Infantilism. A history of failure to grow and failure to mature sexually are the two most common findings. If a pituitary tumor is the causative agent, headaches and changes in vision occur. Mental development is usually normal. If diabetes insipidus is part of the clinical picture, increased thirst and polyuria may be prominent. Patients are generally shy with some feeling of inferiority.

Simmonds' Disease. Loss of sexual function is usually an early sign with amenorrhea in women and loss of sexual potency in men. Loss of weight may progress to cachexia. Asthenia and weakness are prominent. Loss or thinning of axillary and pubic hair, psychic changes, apathy, and somnolence may occur. Anorexia is frequent.

Sheehan's Syndrome. The onset is postpartum; this condition frequently follows a delivery complicated by hemorrhage and shock. Varying degrees of hypopituitarism then develop, depending on the size of the pituitary infarction. Failure of lactation is a frequent early sign.

Pituitary Myxedema. Loss of sexual function is usually early and bloating and myxedema of features develop. However, the patient may not lose weight and actually can gain. Weakness, sensitivity to cold, loss of sexual hair, and drowsiness and apathy are apparent. Some patients with Sheehan's syndrome develop this condition.

Secondary Adrenal Cortical Insufficiency. Loss of sexual function is an early symptom followed by weight loss, asthenia, and mild pigmentation. Emergency treatment for adrenal cortical insufficiency may be necessary.

Secondary Eunuchoidism. Delayed sexual development and diminished or absent sexual function are the indicators.

COURSE

In hypophyseal infantilism the young patient sees his peers "grow away from him" and he is unable to keep up in physical or social spheres. The general condition is dependent on the cause and severity of the hypopituitarism.

With the adult forms of hypopituitarism the course may be prolonged, with gradual development of the symptoms and signs over a period of many years. Exceptions to this occur when the hypopituitarism is severe or is suddenly aggravated by activity of the pathologic process. Adrenal cortical insufficiency is a hazard when ACTH secretion is impaired and emergency corticosteroid therapy may be necessary. With tumors, deficiencies of the pituitary hormones usually occur in the following order: gonadotropins (FSH and LH) in adults and growth hormone in children; thyrotropic hormone (TSH); and adrenocorticotropic hormone. In Sheehan's syndrome deficiency of prolactin becomes apparent. Isolated hormone deficiences are seen.

PHYSICAL FINDINGS

Hypophyseal Infantilism. Short stature is usually obvious and retardation of development of the primary sex organs may be marked. Secondary sexual characteristics such as axillary and pubic hair and breast enlargement in girls do not occur and the patient may have a youthful, childish appearance.

Simmonds' Disease. If severe and prolonged, patients are cachectic and prematurely aged. Skin and hair are dry, the former showing fine wrinkling and occasional mild pigmentation. Axillary and pubic hair are sparse or absent. The patient appears apathetic and depressed, and occasionally somnolent. Atrophic changes are apparent in the external and internal genitalia and in females the breasts are atrophic. Blood pressure is generally low.

Sheehan's Syndrome. Physical findings in these women may be those of Simmonds' disease or pituitary myxedema or may be minimal with minor changes, depending on the degree of hypopituitarism.

Pituitary Myxedema. These patients look decidedly myxedematous and either lose little weight or actually may gain. Features are puffy and bloated and the skin is dry and scaly. A pale, slightly yellowish tinge may be apparent due to carotinemia. There is usually thinning or absence of the axillary and pubic hair and also thinning of the scalp and eyebrow hair. Also, there is atrophy of the external and internal genitalia. Asthenia and somnolence are evident and either apathy or a depressed attitude is usual. Occasionally there is premature or rapid aging. Blood pressure is low. Orthostatic hypotension is common.

Secondary Adrenal Cortical Deficiency. The patient may appear to have true Addison's disease, although little or no pigmentation is present and the skin does not tan. Blood pressure is low. Weight loss is frequent and atrophy of external and internal genitalia may be apparent.

Secondary Eunuchoidism. These patients may resemble primary hypogonadal eunuchoids but can be distinguished from them by laboratory means (low levels of gonadotropins). The patients may be of normal height or slightly tall with relatively long arms and legs (eunuchoid proportions). Genitalia are small and atrophic and secondary sexual characteristics are poorly developed or absent with sparse axillary and pubic hair growth and little breast development in females. Fine wrinkling of the skin occurs, especially around the mouth.

Patients with any of these conditions should be studied for signs of pituitary tumor, including careful checks of vision and visual fields. Increasing pressure from an enlarging tumor can cause blindness or convulsions and hallucinations.

COMMON COMPLICATIONS

The most dangerous complication in any of these patients is the occurrence of acute adrenal cortical insufficiency with hypotensive shock and coma. This can be part of the illness or the result of an exacerbation of the hypopituitarism with loss of ACTH. Emergency treatment with corticosteroids can be lifesaving.

Hypoglycemia is an occasional complication of hypopituitarism and hypoadrenocorticism. Since this diagnosis is now being made with increasing frequency, it would seem prudent to check pituitary function in patients with hypoglycemia. Such investigations will occasionally reveal an unsuspected pituitary tumor.

Anemia occurs with some frequency in moderate to severe hypopituitarism. It is usually of the microcytic type but is often unresponsive to iron therapy until hormones (thyroid, androgens) are added to the therapeutic regimen.

Carotinemia has been found frequently in severe hypopituitarism, as well as in untreated myxedema. It may result in a yellowish pallor of the skin.

Atrophic vaginitis is frequent in female patients with severe hypopituitarism. It responds well to treatment with estrogens.

LABORATORY FINDINGS

Since hypopituitarism can result from deficiencies of one or several of the tropic hormones, there may be considerable variation in laboratory findings. There is no "simple test" for pituitary function. Function of the pituitary itself and also of the glands secondarily affected is usually tested. Hypothalamic-releasing factors also may be investigated. Functional tests using stimulative or suppressive maneuvers also give helpful information. These are catalogued at the various levels.

First, however, the patient should be investigated for enlargement of the gland. A simple x-ray of the sella turcica can reveal an enlargement, deformity, or erosion by a growing tumor. Calcification is frequently seen in suprasellar cysts, and with pituitary stones. More detailed information can be elicited by x-ray tomography of the sella, which also can reveal microadenomata of the gland. Still further information can be obtained from a computerized axial tomography scan, particularly in ruling out the empty sella syndrome. Occasionally, pneumoencephalograms are necessary to document extension of the tumor above the sella. Measurements of blood levels of pituitary hormones are now available, including those of ACTH, GH, FSH, LH, TSH, and prolactin. Prolactin (normal ranges 0 to 40 nanograms per ml) measurements have proven particularly valuable and should be done whenever a pituitary tumor is suspected. Elevation indicates overactivity, but it should be low or unmeasurable in hypopituitarism.

Thyroid function can be evaluated in the usual way by measurements of T_3 and T_4. In hypopituitarism they should be low and, since the hypothyroidism is "secondary," the TSH also should be low. In order to differentiate between hypothalamic and pituitary origin of the disease, a measurement of thyrotropin-releasing hormone (TRH) of the hypothalamus is helpful. A low level would indicate hypothalamic origin, and a high level would place the primary disease in the pituitary.

Adrenal cortical function has been tested for years by measuring the urinary output of 17-ketosteroids (normal 5 to 20 mg per 24 hours) or 17-hydroxycorticoids (normal 3 to 11 mg per 24 hours). These are low in hypopituitarism. Adrenal functional capacity has been measured by noting the effect of stimulation with ACTH. More recently, blood cortisol is measured (normal, fasting, 6 to 26 micrograms per 100 ml). This also would be low in hypopituitarism. Functional capacity is more easily measured by administering 0.25 mg. of cosyntropin (Cortrosyn) intravenously and retesting the level of blood cortisol in 1 hour. Normally this should be at least twice the fasting level. When low levels are found, a measurement of blood ACTH would indicate pituitary origin if the value is low.

Insulin tolerance tests have been used in the diagnosis of hypopituitarism and show an exaggerated response with low levels of blood glucose. If a tendency to hypoglycemia is present, this test carries some risk and must be performed under careful observation, as severe or even fatal hypoglycemia can occur.

In investigating gonadal function, plasma testosterone has been helpful in men (normal 400 to 1000 micrograms per 100 ml), being low in hypopituitarism. In women, measurement of plasma estrogens also would be low (normal estradiol 12 to 186 picograms per ml). A helpful screening test is the level of cornification in cells in a vaginal smear. Results of all these tests are usually combined with the measurement of blood FSH (normal 3 to 15 milli-international units per ml) or LH (normal same), or both FSH and LH would be low in hypopituitarism.

Growth hormone can be measured in blood (normal 0 to 20 nanograms per ml) and functional capacity of the pituitary for this has been measured by several stimulation maneuvers, including insulin-induced hypoglycemia, arginine infusion, brisk exercise, and use of levodopa. Arginine infusion seems preferable but usually requires hospitalization. The metyrapone test has been used for a number of years to measure pituitary corticotropin (ACTH) reserve and involves measuring 17-hydroxycorticoids in 24-hour urine samples before and after administering metyrapone either orally or intravenously. Normally the 17 OHCS level in the urine should at least double, owing to an enzyme inhibition. This test may still be helpful in patients with borderline deficiency.

In a test suggested by Watts and Keffer (Watts, N. B. and Keffer, J. H.: Practical Endocrine Diagnosis. Philadelphia, Lea & Febiger, 1978), the patient's growth hormone and prolactin reserve and the adenopituitary-hypothalamic axis may be elevated simultaneously. It involves measurements of blood sugar, cortisol, growth hormone, prolactin, and ACTH before and after a dose of regular insulin given intravenously. The patient is observed with great caution during the test.

A practical approach in most patients would seem to be x-ray studies of the sellar region; measurements of blood growth hormone, prolactin, and FSH; and measurements of thyroid function (T_3, T_4), adrenal function with cosyntropin test (with blood cortisols), and gonadal function by blood testosterone or estrogens and vaginal smear. Blood glucose can be measured, fasting and after eating, or a 5-hour glucose tolerance test can be run.

The other tests generally are more complicated; they can be set up if indicated by the clinical situation.

As previously stated, blood counts may show a microcytic anemia and routine urinalysis is usually normal.

PITFALLS IN DIAGNOSIS

Differential diagnosis is important in several of the clinical pictures.

Hypophyseal Infantilism. This condition differs from hypothyroid dwarfism in that the latter condition is characterized by shorter stature, characteristic puffy features, and a protruding umbilical hernia. Bone age is usually quite retarded (compared to moderately in hypopituitarism). TSH may be elevated, as may be thyrotropin-releasing hormone (TRH).

Gonadal Dysgenesis (Turner's Syndrome). Most patients are girls and are moderately short. They average 4 feet 8 inches (142 cm) as adults. Build is stocky with "shield chest" and wide carrying angle of arms. The patients may have webbed neck and other anomalies. An important diagnostic point is that their blood or urine FSH is elevated compared with low levels in hypopituitarism.

Simmonds' Disease. The cachectic form of this condition may be very similar to anorexia nervosa, which also is characterized by marked loss of weight and loss of sexual function. However, with anorexia nervosa, the patients generally are unconcerned by loss of weight and continue to be active physically. There may be some hair loss, but not specifically the sexual hair as in the hypopituitary state. Hormone measurements may be low, from both the primary and secondary glands but, surprisingly, the cortisol and growth hormone levels can be elevated. A history of onset following a complicated pregnancy and delivery indicates organic cause (Sheehan's syndrome).

Pituitary Myxedema. It is important to differentiate this condition from primary myxedema. Early loss of sex function favors pituitary disease. Measurements of TSH usually are elevated in primary myxedema and show an exaggerated increase following administration of hypothalamic thyrotropin-releasing hormone (TRH) from the hypothalamus. In pituitary myxedema, associated adrenal cortical insufficiency is a hazard and may be apparent in tests or in clinical course. Onset following a pregnancy and complicated delivery favors pituitary disease.

Secondary Adrenal Cortical Insufficiency. This condition is differentiated from true Addison's disease by early loss of sexual function and early loss of weight. Pigmentation is much less or absent. Blood levels of ACTH will be low; these tend to be high in Addison's disease. X-ray evidence of a pituitary tumor indicates pituitary origin.

ACROMEGALY

By RAYMOND V. RANDALL, M.D.
Rochester, Minnesota

SYNONYMS

Adult hypersomatotropism, adult hyperpituitarism, Marie's disease.

DEFINITION

Acromegaly (from Greek "akros," extremity, and "megale," great) is a disease characterized by enlargement of the soft tissues of the hands, feet, and face, including the ears, nose, lips, and tongue; thickening, and sometimes darkening and hirsutism, of the skin; enlargement of the mandible and frontal sinuses; thickening of the calvarium; deepening of the voice; widening of the cortical bones of the hands and feet and elongation of the ribs; hyperhidrosis; and, sometimes, splanchnomegaly. This condition is caused by excessive and inappropriate secretion of growth hormone by a tumor of the anterior pituitary gland. Such tumors, when stained by conventional dyes used for light microscopy, may be composed of well-granulated eosinophilic cells, poorly granulated eosinophilic cells, a mixture of eosinophilic and chromophobe cells, or only chromophobe cells, and are almost invariably benign. Eosinophilic hyperplasia of the anterior pituitary as a cause of acromegaly must be exceedingly rare, if, indeed, it occurs at all. Although many students of acromegaly, myself included, believe that acromegaly is basically a hypothalamic disorder resulting from (1) an excessive production of growth hormone–releasing factor by the hypothalamus, (2) a decreased production of growth hormone–inhibiting hormone (somatostatin) by the hypothalamus, or (3) an imbalance between these two hypothalamic regulatory substances, others believe that growth hormone–producing tumors of the anterior pituitary grow and function independently of influences from the hypothalamus. Ectopic growth hormone–producing tumors, especially carcinoid tumors of the lung, have been seen in association with acromegaly, but their causal relationship to the acromegaly is not clear at this time. Recently, several reports were published on ectopic tumors that produced a growth hormone–releasing substance, and that were associated with acromegaly that regressed when the tumor was removed.

Acromegaly usually begins about the time of or after the closure of the epiphyses of the long bones in early adulthood toward the end of the second decade, or during the third or fourth decades of life, and, if not treated, continues as an active process for 20 to 30 years or longer. If excessive secretion of growth hormone begins much before closure of the epiphyses of the long bones, then gigantism results, and with continued excessive secretion of growth hormone, acromegaly eventually ensues, resulting in a combination of gigantism and acromegaly.

Presenting Signs and Symptoms

As acromegaly becomes manifest, the patient develops puffiness of the soft tissues of the face, hands, and feet, with a corresponding need for an increase in the size of hats, gloves, rings, and shoes. The hands and fingers feel tight, stiff, and clumsy. The eyelids become thick and puffy. The lips, ears, and nose increase in size, and as the tongue, larynx, and paranasal sinuses enlarge, the voice becomes deeper and more resonant, with the voice of the acromegalic female often being mistaken for a male voice. The patient develops perpetual hyperhidrosis, the facial complexion is marred by an oiliness and increase in size of the pores, the skin over the entire body becomes thickened, the nasolabial folds and wrinkles on the forehead become accentuated, and the scalp may be thrown into deep folds (cutis verticis gyrata). Generalized melanosis is common, and this is often accompanied by acanthosis nigricans. The body hair, including that of the scalp, grows coarser, and hirsutism may emerge, especially in the females. The fat pads of the feet thicken, and a deep longitudinal groove may develop in the plantar surface (plantar groove).

As the disease progresses, the mandible enlarges and elongates, and the lower jaw may protrude beyond the upper jaw, causing malocclusion and underbite. Concomitantly, the spacing between the teeth may increase. If the patient is edentulous, the dentures no longer fit. The frontal sinuses enlarge, and the brows protrude. The zygomatic arches increase in size, causing prominent cheek bones and a relative hollowness of the temporal muscles. There gradually ensues a marked change in appearance. Some patients with acromegaly become depressed, and this is especially true of females, who tend to be upset by their change in countenance and body image. These feelings are enhanced by the startling effect their appearance often has on strangers.

Early in the course of the disease, patients often develop lethargy, weakness, and nonspecific musculoskeletal aches. An occasional patient, especially males, will, to the contrary, have an increase in strength, endurance, and sexual drive, although decreased libido and, in females, irregular menses and amenorrhea are usual. Headaches are common, often severe, but do not have any characteristics specific for acromegaly. Acroparesthesias from bilateral median nerve entrapment (carpal tunnel syndrome) are present in about 30 per cent of patients and may become troublesome and even disabling. Lactation in females, but rarely in males, is occasionally present.

The epiphyses of the ribs do not close in the third decade of life as they normally do, and, hence, the ribs continue to grow in length and the thorax acquires an increased anteroposterior dimension. This, along with the development of dorsal kyphosis, gives a barrel-shaped appearance to the chest.

The pituitary tumor responsible for the acromegaly usually grows slowly, but it can grow large enough to give rise to any of the various findings associated with encroachment of tumor on adjacent structures, such as enlargement of the sella, anterior pituitary failure, visual field defects, hypothalamic disorders, headaches, III, IV, and VI nerve palsies, and cerebrospinal rhinorrhea. Rarely do these tumors grow large enough to cause increased intracranial pressure or diabetes insipidus.

The earliest manifestations of acromegaly — especially the soft tissue changes — are subtle and insidious and almost invariably escape notice by the patient, the patient's family, and even the patient's physician; the disease is usually not recognized until fairly marked bony changes have taken place. This is unfortunate, because although the soft tissue changes are readily reversed by any treatment that halts the overproduction of growth hormone by the pituitary tumor, the bony changes are permanent.

COURSE

The course of acromegaly is varied. The usual history of the disease is to remain hormonally active, that is, to maintain overproduction of growth hormone indefinitely, unless successful treatment is directed to the pituitary tumor. Hence, it is not uncommon to study untreated acromegalic patients who have had acromegaly for 20 or 30 years or more, and find that they still have excessive secretion of growth hormone. Such patients do not give a history of continued, unrelenting enlargement of the afflicted parts of the body. This is because such enlargement reaches a plateau after a number of years, and the hands, for example, reach a maximal size that is not exceeded even though they continue to be exposed to excessive amounts of growth hormone for many more years. Also, interestingly enough, various parts of the body are affected differently in different persons. For example, some acromegalics develop marked prognathism, whereas others do not, even though the acromegalic process remains active for years. Some patients develop cutis verticis gyrata, melanosis, hirsutism, or plantar grooves; others never do. This presumably reflects variability in end-organ sensitivity, but for reasons that are not known.

Some patients with untreated, long-standing acromegaly present with "burned out" acromegaly. What this term implies depends upon the author using it, but in general it connotes a patient with partial or complete anterior pituitary failure and acromegaly that has spontaneously become hormonally inactive; that is, the pituitary tumor is no longer producing excessive amounts of growth hormone. In actuality, most such patients, even though having anterior pituitary failure of variable degrees, will have overproduction of growth hormone. It is the exceptional patient who has spontaneous cessation of growth hormone, probably secondary to a hemorrhage or infarction of the pituitary tumor.

Radiation therapy or surgery directed to the pituitary tumor is not always completely successful. Although such treatment may reduce the mass or function of the tumor enough to result in partial regression of the soft tissue and other changes associated with active acromegaly, in such instances, this reversal of symptoms is not synonymous with a cure.

COMPLICATIONS AND ASSOCIATED ENDOCRINE DISORDERS

Hypertension and arteriosclerosis with cardiovascular and renal complications are common, and congestive heart failure, myocardial infarction, or stroke is often the cause of death. Renal failure may also occur.

Diabetes mellitus is frequent, with different series of acromegalic patients showing a prevalence of 20 to 60 per cent. There are not as yet enough statistical data to be able to state whether hypertensive and arteriosclerotic cardiovascular renal complications are more frequent in those acromegalic patients who have diabetes mellitus. In my experience, the diabetes is usually mild in the sense of being readily controlled by diet alone or diet plus small doses of insulin; insulin resistance, although it does occur, is rare; and diabetic retinopathy is infrequently seen. Diabetes mellitus, when defined as hyperglycemia or abnormal glucose tolerance, frequently disappears when the acromegaly becomes hormonally inactive, but the prevalence of diabetes mellitus recurring in later years in such patients is not known.

Acromegaly may be associated with other endocrine diseases. The most common is nontoxic nodular goiter. Occasionally, a toxic nodular goiter (Plummer's disease) or Graves' disease may be found in a patient with acromegaly, but there seems to be no definite causal relationship between acromegaly and these thyroid disorders.

Acromegaly is seen as part of type I or Wermer's familial multiple endocrine neoplasia (MEN or MEA) syndrome, and as such may be associated with primary hyperparathyroidism from chief cell adenomatosis, benign or malignant insulin-producing islet cell adenomas of the pancreas, and the Zollinger-Ellison syndrome with duodenal or gastric ulcers. Aside from its role as part of the MEN syndrome, acromegaly is not regarded as an inherited disease. Primary hyperparathyroidism from a parathyroid tumor, not a part of the MEN syndrome, is also seen in association with acromegaly. Although hypercalciuria may be secondary to hormonally active acromegaly alone, renal stones on this basis are relatively rare, and the finding of renal stones should alert the physician to the possibility of coexisting primary hyperparathyroidism. A few cases of Cushing's syndrome, pheochromocytoma, or primary hyperaldosteronism have been reported in patients with acromegaly, and, again, no causal relationship has been identified.

Osteoarthritis, especially of the spine, shoulders, hips, and knees, seems to be more prevalent in acromegalic patients than in the general population, and may be disabling.

Hemorrhage into the pituitary tumor of acromegaly may occur, resulting in severe headache, sudden third, fourth or sixth nerve palsy, findings of a subarachnoid hemorrhage when bleeding extends beyond the tumor, pituitary apoplexy, and even death.

PHYSICAL EXAMINATION

General. The physiognomy of advanced acromegaly is characterized by its coarse, puffy features; prominent supraorbital ridges; prognathism; puffy eyelids; large ears, lips, and nose accentuated by heavy nasolabial folds; heavy cheek bones and temporal hollowness; and furrowed brow and scalp. The voice is deep and resonant, and speech is often slurred by the large tongue that fills the mouth, and which may have deep indentations along its edges from the opposed teeth. The teeth may be widely spaced and the lower incisors often jut forward of the upper incisors with resulting malocclusion. Many acromegalic patients are taller than average, reflecting the fact that acromegaly often begins in the second decade of life as the epiphyses are beginning to close, but not early enough to lead to gigantism. These features, along with the large hands and feet, often make acromegaly diagnosable at a glance and constitute the "typical acromegalic appearance."

Skin. The skin is thick, oily, and excessively moist from hyperhidrosis, and that over the face is coarsened by enlarged pores. The skin is frequently hypermelanotic and hirsute. Acanthosis nigricans may be present, and the pressure areas, nipples, and genitalia are usually hyperpigmented, even in the absence of acanthosis nigricans. The body is frequently covered with countless nevi and fibromata mollusca, which have a predilection for the moist axillae and areas beneath the female breasts. The forehead is often heavily wrinkled, the scalp may be furrowed by cutis verticis gyrata, and the plantar surfaces may be partially divided by a deep, longitudinal groove.

Joints. Advanced osteoarthritic changes may be evident in the large joints such as the shoulders, hips, and knees — less frequently in the elbows, wrists, ankles, fingers, and toes, although the spine, especially the lumbar area, is often involved.

Extremities. In addition to the large, broad, fleshy hands and feet with sausage-like fingers and toes, one may find the sensory changes and muscular atrophy associated with a carpal tunnel syndrome.

Eyes. Aside from the puffy lids, one should look for possible extraocular motor palsies, visual field defects, optic nerve atrophy, diabetic retinopathy, and hypertensive changes. It is unusual to find papilledema from increased intracranial pressure, because the pituitary tumor rarely grows large enough to obstruct the ventricular system.

Thyroid. The physician should look for multinodular goiter. The thyroid may be difficult to palpate, because the overlying neck muscles are often large. Enlargement of the underlying laryngeal cartilages may lead the examiner to estimate the size of the thyroid to be larger than it actually is, and irregularities in the cartilages may be mistaken for thyroid nodules.

Breasts. Galactorrhea may be present, less often in males than females. Adequate examination may reveal galactorrhea, previously unknown to the patient.

Cardiovascular System. Hypertension may be present, as may cardiomegaly, even in the absence of hypertension. Acromegalic cardiomyopathy with a loud mitral systolic murmur and left ventricular failure is occasionally present.

Abdomen. The splanchnomegaly of acromegaly is responsible for the liver being readily palpable in many acromegalic patients. It is less common for the spleen to be palpable.

Genitalia. The external genitalia are usually hyperpigmented in both sexes. The male genitalia are often larger than average, unless anterior pituitary failure supervenes. The uterus is frequently larger than average.

Anterior Pituitary Failure. If the acromegalic patient is seen after anterior pituitary failure has taken place, one will find a widespread paleness and loss of body hair, aside from scalp hair, superimposed on the classic acromegalic features — a striking contrast to the hirsute, melanotic acromegalic patient in full bloom.

LABORATORY EXAMINATION

Currently, the single most important laboratory test for the diagnosis of hormonally active acromegaly is the finding of an increased value for fasting serum or plasma growth hormone (hGH) as measured by radioimmunoassay. In our laboratories the normal range of hGH for females is 0 to 10 nanograms per ml and 0 to 5 nanograms per ml for males. The normal range varies with different laboratories. Normally with hyperglycemia, as during a glucose tolerance test, the value for hGH will fall to zero or near zero (<1 nanogram per ml) in 30 to 60 minutes. In the hormonally active acromegalic patient, the response of hGH during a glucose tolerance test varies. The value for hGH may fall toward but not reach the normal range, remain unchanged, rise, or vary in a random fashion during the glucose tolerance test. Likewise, any of these patterns may occur during insulin-induced hypoglycemia (insulin tolerance test) in contrast to the expected rise in hGH in the normal person, in whom the values for glucose fall during the test by 50 per cent of the baseline value or more.

In hormonally quiescent acromegaly, the fasting serum or plasma hGH values will be within the normal range, but they do not always suppress normally with hyperglycemia during a glucose tolerance test.

It is important to realize that the level of serum or plasma hGH is often not indicative of the intensity of the activity and progression of the acromegalic process, as judged by rapidity of change in the soft tissues, bony growth, and other biochemical abnormalities.

Other laboratory findings helpful in arriving at a diagnosis of hormonally active acromegaly are as follows:

1. *Phosphorus.* Prior to the advent of the radioimmunoassay of hGH, an elevated serum inorganic phosphorus was the most helpful test. However, many patients with hormonally active acromegaly have a normal serum phosphorus. Also, the development of primary hyperparathyroidism will decrease an elevated serum phosphorus into but rarely below the normal range. When the value for serum phosphorus is increased, coexisting renal failure must be excluded before attributing the elevation to active acromegaly.

2. *Hypercalciuria and hypercalcemia.* Hypercalciuria of 450 to 700 mg per 24 hours is not uncommon in hormonally active acromegaly, and these values are greater than those expected in uncomplicated primary hyperparathyroidism. If the 24-hour urinary calcium is greater than 900 mg, one should expect the presence of primary hyperparathyroidism in addition to active acromegaly. Active acromegaly alone can elevate the serum calcium 0.5 to 1.0 mg per dl (100 ml) above the normal range, but with higher values concomitant primary hyperparathyroidism must be suspected. In a small series of patients, we found that the assay for parathormone readily distinguished those patients with hormonally active acromegaly and primary hyperparathyroidism from those with hypercalcemia secondary to hormonally active acromegaly alone.

3. *Serum alkaline phosphatase.* In the absence of coexisting primary hyperparathyroidism with bony involvement, elevation of the isoenzymes of bone alkaline phosphatase usually signifies highly active acromegaly.

4. *Hyperglycemia and abnormal glucose tolerance.* As indicated earlier, the incidence of diabetes mellitus varies in different reports. Hypoglycemia will be found if there are coexisting insulin-producing islet cell adenomas of the pancreas.

5. *Basal metabolic rate.* Hormonally active acromegaly can elevate the basal metabolic rate by as much as +50 to +70 per cent. The reason for this is not known, but the basal metabolic rate (BMR) falls in unison with the hGH level after successful treatment. In acromegaly, an elevated BMR almost invariably means hormonally active acromegaly rather than the presence of hyperthyroidism.

6. *Urinary 17-ketosteroids and 17-hydroxycorticosteroids (or 17-ketogenic steroids).* Although the values for urinary 17-ketosteroids and 17-hydroxycorticosteroids (or 17-ketogenic steroids) are usually normal, they may be elevated by 50 to 100 per cent in hormonally active acromegaly, although interestingly enough the plasma corticosteroids are normal. Such acromegalic patients do not show evidence of corticosteroid excess, the adrenals respond normally to metyrapone and dexamethasone testing, and the abnormal values return to normal when the acromegaly is rendered quiescent.

7. *Prolactin.* In the presence of galactorrhea in acromegaly, the value for serum prolactin by radioimmunoassay is usually elevated. However, we have had patients with hormonally active acromegaly and galactorrhea in whom the values for serum prolactin were normal. The galactorrhea disappeared after successful treatment of the acromegaly.

8. *Costochondral epiphyses.* Since the epiphyses of the ribs do not normally close in the third decade of life in active acromegaly, biopsy of the costochondral junction will show active endochondral bone formation greater than expected for the chronologic age of the patient. This was used as an autobioassay of hGH activity before the radioimmunoassay for hGH was developed. The costochondral junction closes and becomes quiescent as the acromegaly becomes quiescent.

The standard laboratory studies such as routine blood counts, sedimentation rate, electrolytes, serum protein electrophoresis, and urinalysis are normal. The electrocardiogram may be normal or may show left ventricular hypertrophy or other findings expected in hypertensive and arteriosclerotic heart disease — there are no ECG findings unique to acromegaly.

X-Ray Findings. Roentgenograms of the skull typically show increase in the size of the frontal and other paranasal sinuses, thickening of the calvarium, prominence of the occipital tuberosity, enlargement of the mandible, and accentuation of hyperostosis frontalis, if such be present, especially in females. The sella may be enlarged and eroded. It is important to realize that a normal sella does not exclude the possibility of acromegaly or an intrasellar tumor, and that hormonal hyperactivity and tumor growth do not parallel one another. An acromegalic pituitary tumor can remain the same size for years and yet be highly active insofar as production of growth hormone is concerned. Conversely, an acromegalic pituitary tumor can be growing quite rapidly and yet not be very active insofar as hormone production is concerned. A small intrasellar pituitary tumor may not be seen on standard views of the skull and yet be readily detected with special anteroposterior and lateral views of the sella taken serially every 3 mm with spiral tomographic or polytomographic techniques. Bilateral carotid angiography *with* magnification and subtraction views may reveal tumors as small as 3 or 4 mm in diameter, not seen otherwise. An adequate search for a pituitary tumor may require all these techniques. Pneumoencephalography is of little value in demonstrating a pituitary tumor unless there is suprasellar extension of the tumor. Occasionally pneumoencephalography in acromegalic patients will show a partially empty sella (see pp. 787 to 788). An empty sella syndrome does not rule out the presence of a pituitary tumor — there are well-documented instances, including patients among my series, wherein a pituitary tumor was removed from a partially empty sella.

Roentgenograms of the hands show bony and soft tissue enlargement with arrowhead configuration of the terminal bony phalanges. If the patient has primary hyperparathyroidism in addition, the bones may show subperiosteal resorption and bony cysts. Roentgenograms of the feet show enlargement of the bones and soft tissues, and increase in thickness of the fatty heel pad beyond the upper normal thickness of 21 mm.

Visual Fields. The visual fields should be charted accurately by tangential screen or perimetric examination. Typically, the earliest field change from a pituitary tumor associated with acromegaly is a loss of vision in the upper, outer quadrant of each eye. As the tumor enlarges, bitemporal hemianopia will develop, and finally only an islet of vision will remain in the nasal portion of each eye before complete loss of vision occurs. The optic nerves will show progressive atrophy as the visual fields slowly deteriorate.

Electroencephalogram and Echoencephalogram. In general, electroencephalography and echoencephalography are of little help in demonstrating a pituitary tumor.

Computerized Tomography (CT Scan). Suprasellar extension of a pituitary tumor is readily detected by CT scanning. However, in general, to date such scanning has been disappointing in revealing the presence of intrasellar tumors without suprasellar extension.

Spinal Fluid Examination. In the presence of suprasellar extension of a hormonally active pituitary tumor of acromegaly, the value for cerebrospinal fluid hGH will be well above 1 nanogram per ml, and such elevated values can be considered diagnostic of suprasellar extension.

PITFALLS IN DIAGNOSIS

There are three major pitfalls in dealing with patients who have or are suspected of having acromegaly.

1. *Failure to identify the tumor.* A normal-appearing sella on standard roentgenographic views of the skull does not rule out a pituitary tumor. The increased amount of bone in the calvarium and the enlarged paranasal and mastoid sinuses in the acromegalic skull make it difficult to identify the bony limits of the sella. It may take spiral tomographic or polytomographic AP and lateral views of the sella with serial cuts every 3 mm to demonstrate a small pituitary tumor. If these studies are not diagnostic, bilateral carotid angiography with magnification and subtraction views are indicated in an attempt to demonstrate the tumor. The physician should assume that all patients with acromegaly have a pituitary tumor, and no effort should be spared to demonstrate the tumor if other studies show the acromegaly to be hormonally active, because, barring extenuating circumstances, it is usually desirable to treat the tumor in an attempt to render it hormonally inactive. Currently, successful treatment implies a direct attack on the pituitary tumor by surgery or radiation therapy, because adequate chemotherapy of acromegaly is not available on a routine clinical basis, in this country, at the time of this writing.

Instances of ectopic production of hGH and eosinophilic hyperplasia of the pituitary (if indeed, it exists at all) are exceedingly rare.

2. *Failure to appreciate the hormonal activity of the acromegaly.* In general, hormonally active acromegaly is associated with abnormally elevated values for serum or plasma hGH that do not suppress with hyperglycemia. It is well recognized that the activity of the acromegalic process is not directly proportional to the level of hGH. Likewise, it is possible to have hormonally active acromegaly, as judged by other biologic criteria, in the presence of normal serum or plasma values for hGH, and the acromegaly will become quiescent with appropriate treatment. This reflects the fact that the pituitary tumor is probably making a biologically

active GH that is not completely identical to normally occurring hGH and, hence, is not well detected by the radioimmunoassay for hGH, which utilizes antibodies against normally occurring hGH. Hence, the physician must use other criteria when values for serum or plasma hGH do not confirm the clinical impression of hormonally active acromegaly.

3. *Failure to recognize early acromegaly.* This is the most difficult pitfall of all to avoid, and one for which there is no satisfactory answer. It is logical to assume that there is a spectrum of acromegaly from frank, obvious acromegaly to subclinical acromegaly, wherein hGH values are elevated, but there has not been time for the recognizable stigmata of acromegaly to have developed. There are no good criteria for detecting subclinical or early clinical acromegaly. In the absence of adequate guidelines, it would seem appropriate to screen by serum or plasma hGH determinations all patients with newly diagnosed pituitary tumors and all patients suspected of having acromegaly. If, under such circumstances, an elevated hGH value is found, one cannot automatically assume that hormonally active acromegaly is present. Some normal females, patients of either sex taking estrogens or L-dopa, patients not basal (especially if just physically active), or patients with hypoglycemia may have elevated values for hGH. These values will suppress with hyperglycemia, and hence, a glucose tolerance test is indicated. Food deprivation, imposed or self-induced, may also elevate hGH values. Indeed, some patients with advanced anorexia nervosa will have values for plasma or serum hGH two to three times greater than those seen with hormonally active acromegaly.

DIFFERENTIAL DIAGNOSIS

Fortunately only a few diseases can be mistaken for acromegaly. The most frequent problem is the rare, inheritable condition of pachydermoperiostosis. The thick skin, wrinkled forehead, enlarged hands, wrists, feet, and ankles, and marked hyperhidrosis associated with this disease almost invariably lead to a mistaken diagnosis of acromegaly unless the physician is familiar with the syndrome of pachydermoperiostosis. Roentgenograms of the hands and wrists readily show the typical changes of osteoarthropathy, which should point to the proper diagnosis of pachydermoperiostosis. Roentgenograms will also identify the rare patient with pulmonary osteoarthropathy advanced enough to be mistaken for acromegaly.

Normal large-boned and muscular persons, females with masculinization, or patients with simple prognathism or cerebral gigantism may be mistakenly diagnosed as having acromegaly. Measurement of serum or plasma hGH should readily exclude a diagnosis of acromegaly in such patients.

DIABETES INSIPIDUS*

By DAVID H. P. STREETEN, M.B., D.Phil., *and* ARNOLD M. MOSES, M.D.

Syracuse, New York

DEFINITION

Diabetes insipidus is a disorder associated with excessive water intake and output, which results from subnormal release or action of vasopressin (antidiuretic hormone [ADH], arginine vasopressin [AVP]).

CLINICAL MANIFESTATIONS

Diabetes insipidus commonly presents with polyuria — the passage of large volumes of dilute urine at frequent intervals — and a seemingly insatiable thirst leading to the intake of large volumes of fluids, usually iced drinks. When the disorder is severe, patients may urinate and drink as often as every 20 minutes during the day and several times at night. In milder forms of diabetes insipidus the excessive turnover of fluids may be slight and only barely noticeable. Enuresis is common in children with diabetes insipidus. Evidence of dehydration is usually absent unless or until fluid intake is restricted because of unconsciousness, derangements of the thirst mechanisms, unavailability of water, or infancy.

Additional clinical findings may result from associated manifestations of the responsible lesion(s).

Central Diabetes Insipidus
1. *Tumors* (craniopharyngioma, chromophobe adenoma, glioma, metastatic carcinoma)

*Supported by a Research Grant (HL 22051) from the National Heart, Lung and Blood Institute, a Graduate Training Grant in Endocrinology (AM 07146) from the National Institute of Arthritis, Metabolism and Digestive Diseases and a Grant (RR–229) from the General Clinical Research Centers Program of the Division of Research Resources, U.S. Public Health Services.

and *infiltrative disorders* (Hand-Schüller-Christian disease, sarcoidosis, tuberculosis) may cause (1) symptoms and signs of a space-occupying mass, such as bitemporal or other forms of hemianopsia, optic atrophy, headaches, cranial nerve lesions, hypothalamic features (narcolepsy, cataplexy, sham rage, fever, obesity); and (2) features resulting from deficiency or excess of the pituitary hormones, ACTH, growth hormone, thyrotropin, gonadotropin, prolactin.

2. *Trauma* to the head, usually severe, and often causing basal skull fractures.

3. *Neurosurgical* hypophysectomies and hypothalamic procedures.

4. *Hereditary* forms of diabetes insipidus may result from autosomal dominant or X-linked recessive transmission of malformation of the ganglion cells in the supraoptic nuclei.

5. *Idiopathic* insufficiency of vasopressin release is usually associated with no anterior pituitary deficiencies but may occasionally occur together with unitropic or multiple hormone deficiencies.

Nephrogenic Diabetes Insipidus

1. *Hereditary* tubular disorder with dominant X-linked transmission.

2. *Chronic renal diseases*: pyelonephritis, medullary cystic disease, myeloma, obstructive uropathy, Sjögren's syndrome, after renal transplantation.

3. *Drugs* that impair tubular response to ADH: lithium, demeclocycline.

4. Biochemical impairment of ADH responsiveness: hypercalcemia, hypokalemia.

5. Sickle cell disease.

Diabetes insipidus can be distinguished clinically and/or by special tests (discussed under Diagnostic Tests) from (1) the *urinary frequency* that results from cystitis, pyelonephritis, and other irritative causes that are usually not associated with excessive urine volumes, with the passage of dilute urine (specific gravity 1.000 to 1.003), or with polydipsia, and from (2) *primary polydipsia* resulting from psychologic causes, drugs such as thioridazine (Mellaril), and presumed lesions of the thirst center. The dehydration test is usually conclusive in differentiating diabetes insipidus from these conditions.

COURSE

Post-traumatic and surgically induced diabetes insipidus are frequently transient, lasting from a few hours to several months. Remissions seldom occur more than 6 months after the initiating event. When tumor is the cause, progressive loss of anterior pituitary function with growth of the tumor may result in the appearance of other manifestations of the tumor. Concomitant reduction of ACTH production may result in amelioration of the polyuria and polydipsia until cortisol deficiency is corrected. Treatment of the tumor with drugs or irradiation may also reduce the severity of central diabetes insipidus. The other types of central diabetes insipidus are usually permanent, changing little in severity or in therapeutic requirements with the passage of time. However, drug-induced nephrogenic diabetes insipidus disappears shortly after use of the offending drug has been terminated.

COMPLICATIONS

Complications of diabetes insipidus are of three types:

1. Severe bladder distension, hydroureter, hydronephrosis, and renal insufficiency resulting from inadequate therapy, and not uncommonly seen in patients with the nephrogenic type.

2. Serious dehydration caused by inadequate fluid intake in patients who are unconscious or suffering from impaired thirst, or infants whose physical and mental growth may be retarded in consequence.

3. Side effects of therapy, such as allergic reactions or infections following vasopressin injections, and hypoglycemia during chlorpropamide administration.

DIAGNOSTIC TESTS

Diagnostic tests are all intended to determine whether a specific stimulus to ADH release such as dehydration, hypertonic saline infusion, or spontaneous plasma hyperosmolality induces appropriate ADH release as reflected in measurements of plasma ADH concentrations (when available) or the effects of released ADH on urinary osmolality. Three procedures are recommended: correlation of serum and urinary osmolality, dehydration test, and tests of osmoreceptor function.

Correlation of Serum and Urinary Osmolality

There is a well-defined relationship between serum and urinary osmolality in normal subjects, which is depicted in Figure 1. Plotting the results of simultaneous osmolality measurements in serum and urine on this figure will give a rapid indication of whether the patient is likely to have diabetes insipidus or not. When equivocal or borderline results are obtained (coordinates on or near the right side of the shaded area), a curve of these serum-to-urinary osmolality relationships during a period of fluid deprivation for a few hours will usually indicate

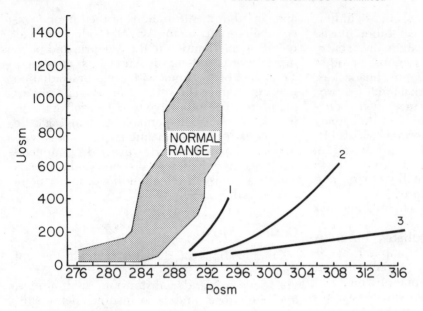

Figure 1. Diagnosis of diabetes insipidus (DI) by concurrent serum and urinary osmolality measurements. By plotting the results of serial determinations on these axes, severe DI (3) may be differentiated from mild DI (2) and from DI resulting from an elevated osmotic threshold for vasopressin release (1).

clearly the presence of the disease, reflected by a subnormal rise in urinary osmolality with increasing serum osmolality. This procedure usually enables one to differentiate severe diabetes insipidus (curve 3) from the partial or mild type (curve 2) and from diabetes insipidus resulting from an elevation of the osmotic threshold for vasopressin release (curve 1). It is simple, safe, and can be performed postoperatively by reducing the rate of an intravenous infusion to determine whether urinary osmolality is increased normally with rising serum osmolality. The possibility that diabetes insipidus diagnosed in this way may be of the nephrogenic type should usually be tested by determining whether vasopressin administration (aqueous Pitressin, 5 units subcutaneously or desmopressin DDAVP 20 micrograms intranasally) raises urinary osmolality by more than 50 per cent in the first hour after its administration, as will not happen in nephrogenic diabetes insipidus. In occasional patients, the measurement of plasma ADH concentration is of help in differentiating the central from the nephrogenic type.

Dehydration Test

Vasopressin deficiency is demonstrated in this procedure by the finding that urinary osmolality is raised significantly further by exogenous vasopressin administration than by endogenous vasopressin released after dehydration for several hours. After fluid deprivation for 16 hours (or for shorter periods in patients whose 24-hour urine excretion is above 10 liters), it is found that measurements of urinary osmolality become constant, rising less than 30 mOsm per kg in successive hours. In the presence of adequate ADH, this urinary osmolality is a reflection of the osmolality of the interstitium at

the apices of the renal papillae. When ADH deficiency exists, the urinary osmolality can be strikingly elevated above this "plateau" by vasopressin administration. The test is performed as follows:

1. Weigh patient at start of total fluid and food deprivation (6 P.M. or 4 A.M.).

2. Collect urine hourly from 6 A.M. for measurements of volume and osmolality.

3. When two or three successive urinary osmolalities have increased by less than 30 mOsm per kg or after 17 hours of fluid deprivation, measure serum osmolality, weigh patient, and administer aqueous vasopressin (Pitressin), 5 units subcutaneously or DDAVP 20 micrograms intranasally.

4. Measure urinary volume and osmolality in the following hour.

Serum osmolality after dehydration should exceed 288 mOsm per kg (the usual osmotic threshold for vasopressin release). If it is well below this level, the patient may have been inadequately dehydrated because of antecedent overhydration resulting from compulsive water drinking, and the test should be prolonged or repeated with a longer period of fluid deprivation. If urinary osmolality increases by more than 50 per cent after the vasopressin administration, central diabetes insipidus is present and may be severe (if urinary osmolality before ADH administration was less than serum osmolality) or mild (if Uosm is more than Sosm before ADH administration). If urinary osmolality is higher than serum osmolality after dehydration and falls or rises by less than 9 per cent after vasopressin administration, the disease is absent. If urinary osmolality fails to exceed serum osmolality after dehydration and fails to rise more than 50 per cent after vasopressin administration, the patient has nephrogenic diabetes insipidus. In this event, renal function studies, serum calcium and potassium measurements, and other determinations should be made to ascertain which type of nephrogenic diabetes insipidus is present (see p. 723).

Occasional patients who have diabetes insipidus because of "high-set" osmoreceptors are found to show a "normal" response to the dehydration test. However, serum osmolality after fluid deprivation for 17 hours is above normal levels, usually 294 to 304 mOsm per kg, reflecting their elevated osmotic thresholds for vasopressin release. If the thirst mechanism is impaired, these patients might be said to have "essential" hypernatremia.

Tests of Osmoreceptor Function

Observation of responses in urinary osmolality or serum ADH concentration to hypertonic saline infusions in waterloaded subjects provides direct evidence of the integrity or deficiency of osmoreceptor function. A waterload, 20 ml per kg of ideal body weight, is administered and maintained with further water intake in volumes equal to those of the urine voided every 15 minutes. With the patient recumbent between voidings and with a needle filled with heparin (1:1000) in a vein in each forearm, 5 per cent NaCl solution is infused through one needle, starting when urinary excretion has been stable for four to eight 15-minute periods. In the modified Hickey-Hare test, 5 per cent NaCl is infused at 0.125 ml per kg per minute for 45 minutes with 15-minute urine collections for volume and osmolality measurements during and for 45 minutes after this infusion, and with serum osmolality measurements before and after the infusion. Diabetes insipidus is present if there is no saline-induced fall in free water clearance:

$$\frac{\text{urine flow}}{\text{rate}} = \frac{\text{urine osmolality} \times \text{urine flow rate}}{\text{serum osmolality}}$$

The osmotic threshold for vasopressin release may be determined by infusing the 5 per cent NaCl by pump at 0.05 ml per kg per minute and measuring serum and urinary osmolality every 15 minutes until (1) 45 minutes after an abrupt and continuing decrease in urine flow-rate, or (2) 5 per cent NaCl has been infused for more than 2 hours, or (3) severe discomfort or headache is experienced by the patient. Serum osmolality will be found to rise linearly with time during the NaCl infusion. The serum osmolality that is calculated by interpolation to be present when free water clearance first falls two standard deviations below the mean preinfusion level is the osmotic threshold for vasopressin release. In diabetes insipidus this threshold is usually absent but may be present and elevated above the normal range (285 to 292 mOsm per kg) in patients with high-set osmoreceptors. If used to diagnose the disease, the hypertonic saline infusion procedures should always be followed by determination of renal responsiveness to ADH administration in the form of vasopressin (Pitressin) 5 units subcutaneously or DDAVP 20 micrograms intranasally.

In patients with central diabetes insipidus, a fall in 24-hour urine volume to below 2 liters usually occurs after the first subcutaneous injection of vasopressin tannate (Pitressin tannate in oil), 5 units, or after DDAVP, 20 micrograms intranasally every 12 hours. Such a therapeutic response confirms the presence of central diabetes insipidus but should not be relied upon as a diagnostic procedure, since it may be present in compulsive water drinkers and may be absent if the Pitressin is incorrectly administered or if rhinitis interferes with the absorption of DDAVP.

MEASUREMENTS OF PLASMA ADH CONCENTRATIONS

When these become more generally available they may be used to diagnose central diabetes insipidus by finding a subnormal rise in plasma ADH level after dehydration or after hypertonic saline infusion, or by finding that plasma ADH concentration is inappropriately low at the prevailing level of serum osmolality.

HYPERPROLACTI-NEMIA

By RAYMOND V. RANDALL, M.D.

Rochester, Minnesota

DEFINITION

Hyperprolactinemia means an abnormal increase in values for serum prolactin and it may or may not be associated with the signs and symptoms that are discussed later.

CAUSES

Hyperprolactinemia may be associated with a large number of conditions listed in Table 1. The formation and release of prolactin by prolactin-producing cells in the anterior pitu-

Table 1. *Conditions Associated With Hyperprolactinemia*

1. *CNS Disorders and Disturbances*
   Tumor
       Pituitary tumor
           Chromophobe
           Eosinophil (acidophil)
           Basophil
       Craniopharyngioma
       Pinealoma
       Astrocytoma
       Meningioma
       Hemangioma
       Other primary tumors
       Metastasis to hypothalamus
   Hyperplasia of prolactin-producing pituitary cells
   Surgical procedures
       Stalk section
       Resection of intrasellar or suprasellar tumor
   Sheehan's syndrome
   Empty sella syndrome
   Pseudotumor cerebri
   Arachnoiditis and encephalitis
   Tabes dorsalis
   Syringomyelia
   Pneumoencephalography
   Psychiatric illness
   Pseudocyesis
   Sarcoidosis
   Histiocytosis X

2. *Other Endocrine Relationships*
   Primary hypothyroidism
       Without sellar enlargement
       With sellar enlargement
   Hyperthyroidism
   Adrenal carcinoma
   Adrenal cortical hyperplasia
   Polycystic ovaries
   Chorionepithelioma of testis
   Multiple endocrine adenomatosis (neoplasias)
   Ovarian resection
   Hysterectomy
   Dilation and curettage
   Ectopic tumor production of prolactin
       Hypernephroma
       Bronchogenic carcinoma

3. *Disturbances of Thoracic Wall*
   Stimulation of nonpuerperal female or of male breasts
   Unilateral mastectomy
   Mammoplasty
   Thoracic surgery
   Trauma
   Atopic dermatitis
   Herpes zoster

4. *Hepatic Cirrhosis*

5. *Renal Failure*

6. *Drug Related*
   Hormones
       Estrogen-progesterone combination
           During administration
           After withdrawal
       Progesterone
       Androgen
   Psychotropic drugs
       Phenothiazines
           Chlorpromazine (Thorazine, Largactil)
           Thioridazine (Mellaril)
           Methotrimeprazine (Levoprone)
           Trimeprazine (Temaril)
           Piperazine nucleus
               Prochlorperazine (Compazine)
               Thiopropazate (Dartal)
               Fluphenazine (Prolixin, Sevinol)
               Perphenazine (Trilafon)
               Thioproperazine (Mayeptil)
               Trifluoperazine (Stelazine)
       Tricyclic antidepressants
           Imipramine (Tofranil)
           Amitriptyline (Elavil, Tryptizol)
       Butyrophenones
           Haloperidol (Haldol, Aloperidine)
           Droperidol (Innovar)
       Chlorprothixene (Taractan, Truxal)
   Anti-anxiety drugs
       Meprobamate (Equanil, Miltown)
       Chlordiazepoxide (Librium)
   Antihypertensive drugs
       Methyldopa (Aldomet)
       Reserpine (Serpasil)
   Histamine H_2 receptor antagonists
       Cimetidine (Tagamet)

Adapted from Table 2–II, Gould, B. K., Randall, R. V., Kempers, R. D., Ryan, R. J.: Galactorrhea. Courtesy of Charles C Thomas, Publisher, Springfield, Ill., 1974.

itary is controlled by the hypothalamus. In contrast to other anterior pituitary hormones, hypothalamic control of prolactin production and release seems to be primarily one of inhibition. The hypothalamus secretes prolactin-inhibiting factor (PIF) into the long portal blood system, which runs from the hypothalamus down the pituitary stalk to the anterior pituitary, where PIF acts on the prolactin-producing cells of the pituitary. Although PIF has been demonstrated in hypothalamic extracts, it has not yet been purified and characterized. A prolactin-releasing factor (PRF) has also been demon-

strated and it too has not been purified or characterized. It is of interest that thyrotropin-releasing hormone (TRH) is a potent prolactin-releasing substance, but it is not thought to be the normally occurring PRF. It is believed that PIF rather than PRF is the dominant hormone in the control of prolactin production and release.

The tumors in and around the pituitary can cause hyperprolactinemia in one of three ways. Many primary pituitary tumors are prolactin-secreting tumors. Tumors that do not secrete prolactin can cause hyperprolactinemia either by impinging upon the area of the hypothalamus that produces PIF and hence preventing the production or release or both of PIF, or by impinging upon the long portal blood system and preventing PIF from flowing from the hypothalamus to the anterior pituitary.

It is thought that hyperactivity and hyperplasia of the prolactin-producing cells of the anterior pituitary can result from failure of PIF to exert its inhibitory effects on these cells. Prolactin cell hyperplasia is also caused by estrogens, many of the psychotropic drugs, and other drugs. Although several ectopic tumors have been shown to produce excessive prolactin, to date no one has demonstrated the production of a PRF substance or an anti-PIF substance by an ectopic tumor.

In the past, the terms Del Castillo, Chiari-Frommel, and Forbes-Albright syndromes have been used to describe certain situations in which patients had amenorrhea and galactorrhea. The term Del Castillo syndrome has been used to refer to amenorrhea and galactorrhea in a nulliparous female without evidence of a pituitary tumor. The Chiari-Frommel syndrome was defined as amenorrhea and galactorrhea occurring in the postpartum female without evidence of a pituitary tumor. The Forbes-Albright syndrome was the presence of amenorrhea and galactorrhea in a female with a pituitary tumor without relation to parity. It is now evident that most if not all of the patients with these conditions have a prolactin-producing pituitary tumor; some of these tumors may be as small as 3 to 4 mm and detected only by special procedures to be described later. However, there is evidence to suggest that an occasional patient may have hyperplasia of the prolactin-producing cells, causing the so-called Del Castillo or Chiari-Frommel syndromes. I have also seen several patients who have had amenorrhea and galactorrhea without evident cause that disappeared spontaneously after a year or so. It is presumed, but not known, that these patients had transient hyperfunction of the prolactin-producing cells for reasons that are not clear.

Presenting Signs and Symptoms

Many patients with hyperprolactinemia have no signs or symptoms related to excessive prolactin, but others do. In addition to galactorrhea, there may be hormonal dysfunction. In females there may be: galactorrhea without changes in menses or fertility; anovulatory regular menses with or without galactorrhea; ovulatory or anovulatory irregular menses with or without galactorrhea; or amenorrhea with or without galactorrhea. In males there may be galactorrhea with no change in libido or potentia; decreased libido and potentia with or without galactorrhea; and oligospermia or azoospermia.

It is not known why galactorrhea occurs in some persons who have hyperprolactinemia while it does not in many others. A person with hyperprolactinemia and galactorrhea can have all the same hormonal measurements as another person who has hyperprolactinemia but no galactorrhea. Galactorrhea is more commonly found in females than in males and when it occurs in males, it is generally not associated with gynecomastia. Indeed, patients who have gynecomastia without galactorrhea rarely have hyperprolactinemia.

It is also not clear how hyperprolactinemia causes disturbances in menses and ovulation. Such patients, in general, have a normal serum follicle-stimulating hormone (FSH) that is in the lower portion of the normal range, low normal or decreased luteinizing hormone (LH), and low normal or decreased estrogen values, but interestingly enough, a normal or exaggerated response following the administration of gonadotropin-releasing hormone (GnRH). Prolactin in excess suppresses the normal pulsatile secretion of follicle-stimulating (FSH) and luteinizing hormones (LH) by the pituitary and prevents or diminishes the normal, midcycle LH surge that results in ovulation. It has also been shown that physiologic amounts of prolactin are essential for the secretion of progesterone by the granulosa cells of the Graafian follicle but increased concentrations of prolactin suppress secretion of progesterone, which can result in amenorrhea. When normal females are given estrogens they respond by releasing LH, a response that is absent in patients with hyperprolactinemia who are given estrogens.

The mechanisms whereby hyperprolactinemia effects male libido, potentia, and sperm production are equally unclear. However, it has been shown that prolactin inhibits the enzyme 5-alpha reductase that converts hormonally inert testosterone to hormonally active dihydrotestosterone. Hyperprolactinemia by this mechanism could result not only in hypoandrogenism but also in oligospermia or azoospermia, because a high concentration of dihydrotestosterone in the tubules is essential for normal spermatogenesis.

In view of these facts, one cannot always ascribe gonadal dysfunction in patients with pituitary tumors to destruction of the normal gonadotropin-producing cells of the pituitary, as we used to think, but rather one should look for hyperprolactinemia in all patients with gonadal dysfunction who have a tumor in the pituitary or in the suprasellar area.

COURSE

As hyperprolactinemia develops, patients not only may develop galactorrhea and the hormonal dysfunctions as described, but also may have effects related to the course of the underlying cause of the hyperprolactinemia, if it is secondary to some cause other than the drugs that cause hyperprolactinemia.

ASSOCIATED ENDOCRINE DISORDERS

As seen in Table 1, there are many endocrine disorders that may be seen in association with hyperprolactinemia. Two warrant further comment. (1) Prolactin-producing pituitary tumors may be seen in association with the syndrome of multiple endocrine adenomatosis (MEA syndrome), also known as multiple endocrine neoplasias (MEN syndrome). Too few patients with this syndrome have been studied to know how often the associated pituitary tumor, when it occurs as part of the syndrome, is prolactin-producing. (2) There are numerous reports of the empty sella syndrome being associated with hyperprolactinemia. I have treated several patients who have had a small prolactin-producing pituitary microadenoma* in association with an empty sella syndrome and similar patients have been reported by others. At this point it is not clear whether all patients with an empty sella syndrome and hyperprolactinemia have such a microadenoma, since many of the reported cases have not been adequately investigated to rule out the presence of a prolactin-producing microadenoma. It is my practice to do bilateral carotid angiography with magnification and subtraction views in all patients who have an empty sella syndrome and hyperprolactinemia.

PHYSICAL EXAMINATION

Female patients with hyperprolactinemia may have galactorrhea. Usually the breasts look normal, but some patients with galactorrhea may have turgid, full breasts that look like the breasts of a nursing mother. The physician should not only ask whether galactorrhea is present but also should check for galactorrhea by pressing on the breasts and nipples because many patients who have galactorrhea are unaware of its presence until it is found by the examining physician. It is also interesting that many patients who know they have galactorrhea will not volunteer this information because they think it is a normal process. When examining a

---

* A microadenoma is defined as a tumor 10 mm or less in diameter.

breast for galactorrhea, the physician should be aware of the fact that the first secretions to issue from the nipple of a galactorrheic breast may be serous rather than milky appearing and then as pressing continues the fluid assumes a milky color. If there be any doubt as to whether the expressed material is galactorrhea, the secretions should be smeared on a glass slide and stained with Sudan IV. Galactorrhea contains fatty droplets that stain vividly with Sudan IV. Females with hypoestrogenism from hyperprolactinemia may have an estrogen-deficient vaginal mucosa and a small uterus.

Males with hyperprolactinemia, in addition to galactorrhea, may have a small prostate and testes that are slightly smaller and softer than normal.

LABORATORY FINDINGS

By definition, hyperprolactinemia means an elevation in the level of circulating prolactin that is measured as serum prolactin. In our laboratories the normal basal range for females is up to 23 nanograms per ml and for males up to 20 nanograms per ml of serum. Exercise and stress will elevate the serum prolactin. Serum prolactin is also normally increased during sleep and may not fall to normal basal levels until 30 minutes or so after awakening. Hence, blood should not be drawn immediately upon the patient's awakening for measurements of serum prolactin. Patients who are taking estrogenic substances, including birth control pills that contain estrogenic materials, may have an increase in basal prolactin values slightly above the normal range. Patients who are taking psychotropic drugs may have prolactin values up to several hundred nanograms per ml. Prolactin-producing pituitary tumors may result in serum prolactin values as great as 10,000 nanograms per ml or more. There are numerous statements in the literature that various prolactin values such as greater than 100, 150, or 200 nanograms per ml are diagnostic of a prolactin-producing pituitary tumor, assuming that there is no other cause that could elevate the serum prolactin, such as psychotropic drugs. This certainly has been true in my experience, but it should be emphasized that many patients with a proven prolactin-producing pituitary tumor have had prolactin values under 100 and I have seen many patients whose values were less than 50. In a few instances patients with proven prolactin-producing pituitary tumors have had normal values for serum prolactin. It is assumed, but not proven, that in such instances the tumor was making biologically active fragments or an analogue of normal prolactin that was not fully measured by the assay designed to measure normal prolactin.

A number of inhibition and stimulation tests have been used in attempts to differentiate hyperprolactinemia secondary to prolactin-producing pituitary tumors from other causes of hyperprolactinemia, but none has proven to be completely reliable. The test that I have found to be the most helpful is the thyrotropin-releasing hormone (TRH) test. Blood for a basal serum prolactin is obtained, the patient is given 400 micrograms of TRH intravenously and blood for serum prolactin is obtained 30 and 60 minutes later. Normally, TRH given in this manner will result in a 50 to 300 per cent rise in serum prolactin, and this is true in many instances in which hyperprolactinemia is not secondary to a prolactin-producing pituitary tumor. On the other hand, in the presence of a prolactin-producing pituitary, the serum prolactin should not rise after TRH. However, some tumors do respond to TRH, and hence the test is strongly suggestive, but not diagnostic, of a tumor if there is no response to TRH, but a good response to TRH definitely does not rule out the presence of a tumor.

Hyperprolactinemia in females can result in low normal values for FSH, low normal or below normal values for LH, and low normal or below normal values for estrogens. As a general rule the values for LH will be lower than those for FSH, the reverse of the polycystic ovary syndrome, in which frequently the values for LH are higher than those for FSH. In males, hyperprolactinemia can lead to low values for serum testosterone and oligospermia or azoospermia.

When a prolactin-producing pituitary tumor or a suprasellar tumor is suspected, the following studies are useful and each procedure will be discussed along with its advantages and disadvantages.

Roentgenograms of the Skull. Roentgenograms of the skull are obtained with standard AP, PA, and stereoscopic lateral views. If a pituitary tumor is present, there may be an increase in sellar size, bulging or a double contour of the floor of the sella, erosion of the anterior clinoids and posterior clinoids, or erosion and displacement of the dorsum of the sella. In rare instances, primary pituitary tumors may contain calcification, probably secondary to an old hemorrhage. Suprasellar tumors may be detected by the fact that they contain calcification or because they have eroded the dorsum and posterior clinoids of the sella. When a pituitary microadenoma is present, the diagnostic changes may not be noted on standard views of the skull.

Polycyclic Tomography. Polycyclic tomograms of the sella taken every 2 to 3 mm from right to left along the frontal plane (lateral views) and anteroposteriorly along the sagittal plane of the sella will often show changes diagnostic of a pituitary microadenoma that cannot be appreciated on standard roentgenographic views of the skull. These tumors may cause small inferior bulging of the floor of the sella, along with thinning or erosion of the floor. In some instances rather than a bulge, the floor of the sella when seen in the PA views will slope downward in a straight line from one side to the other. Fortunately, most microadenomas of the pituitary begin in the inferior portion of the pituitary and hence will be evident on polycyclic tomograms long before they grow large enough to cause significant enlargement of the sella or changes in the clinoids or dorsum.

Visual Fields. Perimetric visual field determinations should be made on all patients suspected of having an intrasellar or suprasellar tumor. Most patients with a pituitary microadenoma will have normal visual fields because the tumor is not large enough to impinge upon the optic chiasm or nerves. On the other hand, suprasellar lesions, which may not be seen in standard roentgenograms of the skull or polycyclic tomograms of the sella, may cause impairment of the visual fields.

Computerized Tomography. Computed tomographic (CT) views, both with and without contrast medium, are to be obtained only when the visual fields are abnormal or when a suprasellar lesion is suspected. Most intrasellar microadenomas of the pituitary, with rare exceptions, will not show on CT scans. However, a new generation of CT scanners is now available and capable of showing small tumors within the sella. It is important that contrast medium be used in all such studies, since we occasionally see suprasellar extension of an intrasellar tumor or a suprasellar tumor that is not well seen with plain CT views but that shows up well when contrast medium is used. Downward extension of a pituitary tumor through the floor of the sella into the sphenoid sinus can often be detected by CT scans or polycyclic tomograms.

Carotid Angiography. Bilateral carotid angiography with magnification and subtraction views is helpful in revealing not only the presence of pituitary tumors but also their extent. By the techniques used at our institution it is possible to identify pituitary microadenomas as small as 3 to 4 mm in diameter. Such angiograms also give the neurosurgeon helpful information about the location of the carotids and whether an aneurysm is present. Knowing the location of the internal carotid arteries is particularly helpful when a transsphenoidal approach to a pituitary tumor is planned, because we have occasionally seen a patient whose internal carotids were so close together in the region of the sella that it was not possible to use the transsphenoidal route.

Pneumoencephalography. Because pneumoencephalography will not show a tumor that is totally within the sella, this procedure was abandoned by us in favor of bilateral carotid angiography when the transsphenoidal route became the preferred approach to pituitary tumors. However, pneumoencephalography is still used in our institution when an empty sella syndrome is suspected or when a hypothalamic, suprasellar lesion is suspected but not detected by CT scanning.

Cerebrospinal Fluid Prolactin. Examination of the cerebrospinal fluid (CSF) for excessive GH, ACTH, TSH, FSH, and LH has been helpful in detecting suprasellar extension of intrasellar tumors producing these hormones in excess. The finding of excessive CSF prolactin was initially thought to be an indicator of suprasellar extension of prolactin-producing tumors. However, it is now recognized that increased values for CSF prolactin may be present in patients with prolactin-producing tumors that do not extend above the sella and hence the finding of excessive prolactin in the CSF is not always indicative of suprasellar extension of a prolactin-producing tumor.

PITFALLS IN DIAGNOSIS

The presence of galactorrhea is often the first clue to hyperprolactinemia. As noted, the physician should not only ask patients whether galactorrhea is present but also should check for it during the physical examination since many patients with galactorrhea are unaware of its presence until it is found by the examining physician. Galactorrhea that is unexplained on physiologic grounds (recent childbirth, nursing, etc.) should always be investigated if questioning the patient does not reveal an obvious cause such as the use of psychotropic drugs. Measurement of serum prolactin should then be done and the patient should be questioned about irregular menses, infertility, and loss of libido. Conversely, all patients, both male and female, who have infertility problems should have a determination of serum prolactin as part of their examination. If the serum prolactin is increased above the normal range, an intrasellar or suprasellar tumor must be ruled out. It should be pointed out that, despite the present-day roentgenographic techniques that are helpful in detecting almost all pituitary tumors and supra-

sellar tumors, an occasional tumor may be too small to be detected initially and hence patients who are suspected of having such a tumor should be re-examined periodically.

HYPERTHYROIDISM

By IAN D. HAY, M.B., PH.D.,
and COLUM A. GORMAN, M.B., PH.D.
Rochester, Minnesota

SYNONYM

Thyrotoxicosis.

DEFINITION

Hyperthyroidism may be defined as a complex clinical syndrome resulting from excess concentrations of circulating and tissue thyroid hormones. In most cases, both thyroxine (T_4) and triiodothyronine (T_3) circulate in excess but in recent years examples of isolated hormonal excess, so-called T_3- and T_4-toxicosis, have been recognized. In individual patients the clinical manifestations may range from subtle to florid; the intensity of signs and symptoms varies, depending on the duration of disease and the cause of the hyperthyroidism.

Of the causes of hyperthyroidism listed in Table 1, Graves' disease is by far the most common. Occurring at any age in life (including

Table 1. *Etiology of Hyperthyroidism*

A. Due to autonomous thyroid overactivity
   1. Graves' disease, toxic diffuse goiter (TDG)
   2. Hashimoto's thyroiditis with persistent hyperthyroidism
   3. Plummer's disease, toxic multinodular goiter (TMNG)
   4. Toxic autonomously functioning thyroid adenoma (AFTA)
B. Due to hormonal discharge during thyroiditis
   1. Granulomatous thyroiditis — painful or silent
   2. Lymphocytic thyroiditis with transient hyperthyroidism
C. Due to exogenous thyroid hormone
   1. Iatrogenic hyperthyroidism
   2 Factitious hyperthyroidism
D. Due to exogenous iodide (Job-Basedow)
   1. With thyroid autonomy (TDG, TMNG, or AFTA)
   2. With previously normal thyroid function

the neonatal period) but predominantly in females under 40 years, it is characterized by diffuse thyroid involvement wherein all of the functioning tissue is hyperactive. Pituitary thyroid-stimulating hormone (TSH) does not appear to be responsible for the thyroid stimulation but a family of immunoglobulins with thyroid-stimulating properties, variably termed long-acting thyroid stimulator protector (LATS-P), human thyroid stimulator (HTS), thyroid-stimulating immunoglobulins (TSI), and thyroid-stimulating antibodies (TSAb), are thought by many investigators to play a central role in the pathogenesis of the disease. The goiter and hyperthyroidism comprise only one element of the syndrome of Graves' disease, which includes ophthalmopathy, a unique dermopathy (localized myxedema), nail changes, and acropachy. All of these associated features may precede, accompany, or follow the expression of the hyperthyroidism, and restoration of the euthyroid state does not regularly influence the course of the associated phenomena. Occasionally, patients with Hashimoto's (goitrous autoimmune) thyroiditis may also have persistent hyperthyroidism. This subgroup of patients is said to have "hashitoxicosis."

Plummer's disease, by contrast, is not accompanied by associated phenomena. Characteristically, the hyperthyroidism commences gradually, typically in an elderly patient with multinodular goiter for many years. It is theorized that in toxic multinodular goiter, multiple areas in a long-standing goiter assume autonomous functional capabilities, while other nodular portions within the gland may be functionless owing to previous degeneration. In the less common situation of autonomous functioning thyroid adenoma, a solitary autonomous nodule, usually at least 3 cm in diameter, suppresses TSH to such an extent that on thyroid scan the nodule is seen to be the only tissue concentrating isotope.

The second main group of thyrotoxic patients are those who develop a transient hyperthyroidism during the active inflammatory phase of thyroiditis. The clinical sequence of thyroid hormone discharge, accompanied by mild hyperthyroidism followed by temporary hypothyroidism and subsequent recovery was first recognized in the subacute (granulomatous) type of thyroiditis. Since 1975 an increasing number of cases of spontaneously resolving hyperthyroidism have been recognized in which thyroid biopsy showed the appearance of lymphocytic thyroiditis. In contrast to the cases of "hashitoxicosis," such patients have low values of radioactive iodine uptake (RAIU). Regardless of the histological variety of thyroiditis, however, the important feature of this type of hyperthyroidism is that the disease tends to be self-limiting and only rarely requires more than symptomatic treatment.

The thyroid diseases classified under categories A and B in Table 1 represent the common primary thyroid conditions causing hyperthyroidism. Exogenous hyperthyroidism does, however, also exist and can be caused either by the administration of excess thyroid hormone or by the ingestion of large doses of iodine (Jod-Basedow disease). The hyperthyroidism seen with thyroid hormone ingestion is often iatrogenic but may also be self-induced, sometimes surreptitiously (thyrotoxicosis factitia). Jod-Basedow, first recognized in endemic goitrous areas, has also been seen in iodide-sufficient areas in patients with preexisting thyroid autonomy and recently was reported to have occurred in some patients with apparently previously normal thyroid glands, living in a relatively iodine-deficient area.

For completeness, Table 2 lists further causes of hyperthyroidism but these particular types of thyrotoxicosis are in practice so rare that they will not be further considered in this section.

Presenting Signs and Symptoms

The variety of complaints with which a hyperthyroid patient may present reflects the multiple sites of action of excess thyroid hormone. Often first symptoms may be related to increased heat production owing to an increase in basal metabolic rate but occasionally psychologic symptoms predominate and may accurately mimic an anxiety state. Most thyrotoxic patients on direct questioning will, however, admit to characteristic thyroid-mediated effects on the cardiovascular, gastrointestinal, and neuromuscular systems.

Hyperthyroid patients typically complain of "feeling warm all the time." They are heat intolerant, tend to prefer the cooler weather, and many, particularly women, will complain of noticing an increase in their sweating.

Often thyrotoxic patients complain of difficulty in concentration and tend to be irritable,

Table 2. *Rare Causes of Hyperthyroidism*

A. Due to pituitary TSH hypersecretion
  1. TSH-producing pituitary adenoma
  2. Inappropriate TSH regulation by hypothalamus
B. Due to ectopic thyroid stimulators
  1. Benign and malignant trophoblastic tumors
  2. Other nonthyroid malignancies, e.g., of testis
C. Due to mass of functioning tumor in metastatic follicular thyroid carcinoma
D. Due to adenomatous transformation of thyroid tissue in ovarian teratoma (struma ovarii)

jittery, and restless. Emotional lability may lead to a situation wherein the patient may at one moment be jovial and laughing and at another, for no apparent reason, be depressed, agitated, and tearful. Many thyrotoxics complain of tiredness and easy fatiguability but some, on the other hand, are never apparently tired and find it impossible to stop and relax.

Effects on the cardiovascular system result in the frequent complaints of palpitations and shortness of breath on exertion. Angina may appear for the first time or may be exacerbated in a patient with pre-existing coronary heart disease. Cardiovascular symptoms tend to predominate in the elderly thyrotoxic who may present with high output heart failure accompanied by paroxysmal atrial fibrillation. In this fairly common situation, failure of digoxin in normal dosage to control the tachycardia may alert the physician to the possibility of hyperthyroidism.

The gastrointestinal symptom seen typically in hyperthyroidism is weight loss despite increases in both appetite and food intake. Occasionally, however, in older patients appetite may be decreased and in younger patients weight may actually increase owing to overcompensated appetite stimulation. Increased frequency of bowel movement is common in hyperthyroidism.

The neuromuscular manifestations of thyrotoxicosis are many and variable but the most common are the nonspecific tremor, particularly during purposeful movements of the hands, and the sometimes profound proximal muscular weakness. Typical myopathic complaints are of difficulty in climbing stairs, getting up from sitting or from a bathtub, and shaving and combing hair. More unusual are the rare associations of thyrotoxicosis with either myasthenia gravis or hypokalemic periodic paralysis.

In addition to the symptoms common to all types of hyperthyroidism that result from excessive circulating thyroid hormone, patients with Graves' disease may show the ophthalmopathy, acropachy, or localized myxedema that are specific characteristics of that disease. Typical symptoms include eye pain, swelling, lacrimation, photophobia, blurring of vision, or double vision.

Hidden or "masked" hyperthyroidism refers to those not uncommon elderly patients who present with unexplained atrial fibrillation, palpitations, angina of effort, or heart failure. Other atypical presentations are: apparent choreoathetosis in children, tremor in adults, fever of unknown origin, and generalized edema. Occasional patients show the reverse of the usual hyperkinetic state, the so-called "apathetic hyperthyroidism." Such patients may be depressed with an emotionally flat affect and hypokinesis and the diagnosis may be easily overlooked because of the absence of the classical features of hyperthyroidism.

COURSE

In the era before effective therapy was available, about 10 per cent of patients with Graves' disease died because of hyperthyroidism. Mild cases were expected to remit spontaneously but patients with the more severe cases did not recover. About 25 per cent of mild cases were considered spontaneously cured within months or years while another 15 to 30 per cent, although improving with time, did not completely resolve.

Low-grade hyperthyroidism may persist relatively unchanged for up to 25 years or the course may be punctuated by frequent remissions and relapses. More severe grades of thyrotoxicosis may occasionally end fatally and the cause of death may vary from cardiac failure through extreme wasting and malnutrition, advanced myopathy or myasthenia, to liver failure.

PHYSICAL EXAMINATION AND FINDINGS

Physical examination of a hyperthyroid patient may reveal a wide range of clinical signs that not only reflect the vulnerability of different organ systems to the effects of excess thyroid hormone but are also dependent on the rate of onset and severity of the disease. Many of the physical findings may be directly attributed to the excess tissue concentrations of thyroid hormone but others, e.g., the findings on thyroid palpation or the associated phenomena of Graves' disease, may reflect the specific disease process responsible for causing the hyperthyroidism. In the past, attempts were made to develop from the variety of findings encountered a composite "thyrotoxicosis index" that would correlate well with the presence or absence of hyperthyroidism. Signs that showed a high correlation with thyrotoxicosis included weight loss, thyroid enlargement, hyperkinesis, fine finger tremor, and tachycardia or atrial fibrillation.

In the hyperthyroid patient careful examination of the extremities can often yield valuable clinical information. Typically, the skin in thyrotoxicosis is fine-textured, velvety in consistency, soft, warm, and moist. The nails may show onycholysis (separation of the nail from the nail bed), particularly affecting the fourth and fifth fingers, and examination of the legs can sometimes reveal peripheral edema or pretibial myxedema. This latter feature, seen in less than 5 per cent of patients with Graves' disease, consists of raised, firm plaques, usually on the anterolateral aspects of the lower leg, and the overlying skin, generally darker in color than adjacent normal tissue, has an orange peel or pigskin appearance. An even rarer finding in a minority of patients with Graves' disease is so-called "thyroid acropachy," which in its fully developed form consists of clubbing of the fingers and toes, periosteal new bone formation principally involving the phalanges, and soft tissue swelling, particularly overlying the affected bones.

Examination of the thyroid will usually differentiate between the diffuse, often firm, goiter of Graves' disease and the toxic multinodular goiter (TMNG) or solitary autonomously functioning thyroid adenoma (AFTA). The thyroid enlargement in Graves' disease is typically symmetrical but is occasionally nodular and may vary from a barely palpable normal-sized gland (15 to 20 grams) to an enlargement of five times (100 grams) or, rarely, even more. In the more florid expressions of Graves' disease, a bruit is frequently audible over the thyroid. Patients with TMNG usually have large, firm, multinodular glands that may extend substernally or be almost entirely substernal, making palpation difficult. The solitary AFTA causing hyperthyroidism is typically more than 2.5 to 3.0 cm in diameter and is almost invariably palpable, sometimes representing the only palpable thyroid tissue because of involution of adjacent thyroid parenchyma.

Examination of the cardiovascular system in a hyperthyroid patient usually reveals a rapid and bounding pulse that may be either regular owing to sinus tachycardia or irregular due to frequent extrasystoles or atrial fibrillation. Characteristically, the elevated systolic and decreased diastolic blood pressure leads to an elevation in pulse pressure and on auscultation the heart sounds are loud and ringing. Carotid pulsations are frequently particularly vigorous. Often a systolic murmur is heard over the entire precordium and occasionally a grunting pulmonary systolic sound (Lerman-Means murmur), best heard over the sternum in the second left intercostal space, is also present. Thyrotoxicosis should always be suspected if an elderly female patient develops atrial fibrillation and congestive cardiac failure in the absence of either ischemic or rheumatic heart disease.

Of all the signs of thyrotoxicosis the psychiatric and neuromuscular ones are perhaps the most varied. In many patients the emotional pattern is that of hypomania or pathologic well-being (euphoria), but in others hyperactivity has produced a state of exhaustion and a profound fatigue or asthenia results. In most patients reflexes are hyperkinetic and hypermetric, reaction is shortened, and a fine tremor of low amplitude and high frequency (about 6 per second) is characteristic. Proximal muscular weakness (thyrotoxic myopathy) is detectable in the majority of patients and in the more severe cases this is accompanied by muscular atrophy, which is particularly well seen in the muscles of the shoulder girdle.

The eye findings in hyperthyroidism are of particular interest and may be classified into two groups, sometimes described as noninfiltrative and infiltrative ophthalmopathy. The first of these are ophthalmic phenomena reflecting thyrotoxicosis per se and apparently resulting from sympathetic overactivity. The second group are those phenomena unique for Graves' disease and caused by specific pathologic changes in the orbit and its contents.

In the first group reflecting hyperthyroidism from any cause, there may be retraction of the upper eyelids, a finding that probably represents excessive sympathetic nervous system activity, producing spasm of Müller's muscle, an integral part of the retractile mechanism of the upper eyelid. This change is regularly reversible with restoration of the euthyroid state and should not be confused with the permanent, sometimes asymmetric, lid retraction seen in the infiltrative disease as a result of fibrous shortening of the levator palpebrae superioris. Other findings that may be features of the noninfiltrative disease include a widening of the palpebral aperture, lid lag, a staring or frightened expression, infrequent blinking, and absence of forehead wrinkling on upward gaze.

The finding of infiltrative ophthalmopathy is generally considered pathognomonic of Graves' disease. Basic features include vascular hyperemia of the conjunctivae and over the insertions of the rectus muscles, periorbital and conjunctival edema (chemosis), inability of the upper lid to cover the globe, weakness and imbalance of the extraocular muscles, and exophthalmos (proptosis). Often the first indication of ophthalmoplegia is the complaint that during upward gaze the patient feels an uncomfortable strain. If paresis develops, it may cause an imbalance in the coordinated movement of the eyes, resulting either in poor convergence or diplopia. The inferior rectus is the most common muscle involved, followed closely in frequency by the lateral rectus.

The protrusion of the globes seen in Graves' ophthalmopathy is caused by infiltration and swelling of retrobulbar tissue and extraocular muscles by edema, fluid, fat, an acid mucopolysaccharide substance, and various inflammatory cells. Exophthalmos is usually bilateral but may be asymmetric or even unilateral. The Krahn exophthalmometer allows accurate measurement of the distance between the anterior surface of the globe and the lateral orbital rim. Normal measurements in Caucasians are 18 to 20 mm or less and up to 3 mm of asymmetry is acceptable as a normal finding.

In addition to the cosmetic problems caused by proptosis, serious complications may occur that may lead to eventual loss of vision. These may result either as a consequence of exposure of the globe leading to corneal ulceration and panophthalmitis or from optic nerve injury, either from traction or from compression at the optic foramen. Interference with orbital venous drainage will commonly cause periorbital edema and chemosis but in severe cases it may also cause orbital pain and occasionally raised intraocular pressure.

COMMON COMPLICATIONS

Complications generally occur in hyperthyroidism as a consequence of prolonged exposure of organ systems to excessive concentrations of thyroid hormones. They may affect particularly the cardiovascular, gastrointestinal, and neuromuscular systems and, as described, may include high output cardiac failure; arrhythmias, particularly atrial fibrillation; and rarely heart block, malabsorption, and severe myopathy that occasionally involves the bulbar muscles. In Graves' disease the ophthalmopathy may progress to such a degree that vision itself may be threatened.

Fortunately, the most severe complication of hyperthyroidism, toxic crisis or "thyroid storm," is fast becoming a rare occurrence. Formerly a frequent occurrence after surgery on the incompletely prepared patient, it is now considered a disease of neglect and seen only in those patients with severe untreated disease or those whose thyrotoxicosis is complicated by an additional acute medical problem, for example, an acute infection or the development of diabetic ketoacidosis. Clinically, it can be considered as a sudden and violent exacerbation of the signs and symptoms of thyrotoxicosis and it is characterized by fever, usually over 39 C (102 F), extreme tachycardia, varied disorders of heart rhythm, and nervous hyperirritability rapidly progressing to exhaustion and often to coma. Prompt medical therapy can usually reverse the condition within hours, but despite the use of antithyroid drugs, adrenergic blocking agents, and occasionally adrenocortical steroids, the mortality from thyroid storm is still probably in the range of 10 to 15 per cent.

LABORATORY FINDINGS

Since the clinical syndrome of hyperthyroidism results from excess concentrations of circulating and tissue thyroid hormones, it seems logical that the first line of confirmatory laboratory tests should be direct measurements of circulating thyroid hormones.

Serum Total Thyroxine (T_4). This is the most important and widely available thyroid function test. It is measured either by radioimmunoassay (RIA) or the now less popular competitive protein-binding (CPB) technique. Both of these methods are sensitive, specific, and inexpensive and neither is affected by recent iodide contamination. Results are usually available in 24 hours and a normal value is typically in the range of 5.0 to 13.5 micrograms per dl (100 ml). A T_4 value of greater than 13.5 micrograms per dl is usually an indication of thyrotoxicosis but because T_4 is largely (99.95 per cent) bound to thyroid hormone-binding protein, principally thyroxine-binding globulin (TBG), then such a value may be due to an increased concentration of binding protein. Elevations of TBG that result in a secondary elevation of total serum T_4 levels occur in pregnancy, liver disease, as a result of estrogen therapy or chronic narcotic drug usage, and on a genetic basis. It is therefore essential in these circumstances to obtain a measure of thyroid hormone binding before making a diagnosis of hyperthyroidism on the basis of T_4 alone.

If patients with thyroid hormone-binding protein (THBP) abnormalities are excluded, the total serum T_4 concentration does show good discrimination between euthyroid and hyperthyroid individuals. However, a normal T_4 level does not exclude a diagnosis of thyrotoxicosis because of the preferential T_3 secretion seen in the 5 to 25 per cent of thyrotoxics who have so-called "T_3-toxicosis." The converse and much rarer situation of elevated T_4 levels with normal T_3 concentrations (T_4-toxicosis) has also been described, particularly in elderly sick patients usually with multiple and complicated nonthyroid illnesses.

Thyroid-Binding Proteins and the Free T_4 Index (FTI). The most commonly employed method for assessing thyroid hormone binding is the T_3-resin uptake test. This procedure determines the number of unoccupied thyroid hormone-binding sites in serum. It consists of adding radioiodine-labeled T_3 to the patient's serum and incubating this with a second binder (e.g., red cells or a resin), which competes for labeled T_3 with the unoccupied binding sites in the patient's serum. The T_3 resin uptake varies inversely with the number of unoccupied thyroid hormone binding sites in the patient's serum. Thus, when there are excess binding sites in the patient's serum owing to a high TBG level, the T_3 uptake will be low, while with diminished binding sites owing to either TBG deficiency or hyperthyroidism with consequent saturation of sites, the T_3 uptake will be high.

From separate measurements of serum T_4 and T_3-resin uptake, a free T_4 index (FTI) may be calculated by multiplication. Such an index is directly proportional to the free T_4 concentration in the serum and is a means of correcting total T_4 levels for changes in thyroid hormone binding. Recently, two tests, the effective thyroxine ratio and the normalized serum thyroxine, have been developed to eliminate the need for a separate T_3 uptake test. They depend upon an internal correction to compensate for binding protein anomalies. They have the potential advantage of convenience but no improvement in accuracy has been demonstrated over the use of serum T_4 and T_3 resin in combination.

Serum Free Thyroxine (FT$_4$). This test is rarely performed routinely but does estimate that fraction of serum T_4 which is not bound to THBP, viz., the putative active portion of the hormone. In the procedure, labeled T_4 added to the patient's serum equilibrates with the free and bound hormone. The free fraction is estimated by determining the dialysable portion of the added label and is then multiplied by the total T_4 (as determined by conventional methods) to yield the FT$_4$ level. The normal range for the serum FT$_4$ concentration is approximately 1 to 3 nanograms per ml and in most instances there is good linear correlation between the FT$_4$ and the FTI when plotted against each other in patients with thyroid-binding protein variations and those who have thyroid dysfunction.

Serum Total Triiodothyronine (T$_3$). Serum total T_3 concentration can be measured by radioimmunoassay and is an increasingly available test of thyroid function. In view of the disproportionate increase in T_3 secretion in most cases of thyrotoxicosis, little overlap has been observed in total T_3 levels between euthyroid and hyperthyroid patients. Borderline high levels of T_3, however, may be found in euthyroid Graves' disease (ophthalmopathy without hyperthyroidism) and in euthyroid patients with AFTA. The incidence of T_3 toxicosis among patients presenting with hyperthyroidism for the first time varies from 5 to 25 per cent and in general is higher in those areas where dietary iodine intake is suboptimal. The T_3 values in euthyroid subjects fall typically in the 90 to 230 nanograms per dl range. Serum T_3 levels tend to decrease with age and often are reduced as a consequence of acute or chronic nonthyroidal illness, malnutrition, or acute loss in body weight. The total T_3 is considered to be the most consistently abnormal test of thyroid function in the investigation of patients with suspected hyperthyroidism. However, in clinical practice most centers prefer to confirm the presence of hyperthyroidism by means of a total or free serum thyroxine test or both, reserving the use of the T_3 RIA to those few patients who do not have elevated serum T_4 concentrations but in whom the clinical suspicion of hyperthyroidism persists.

OTHER LABORATORY TESTS

In the laboratory assessment of patients with a clinical diagnosis of hyperthyroidism, the first investigations should be a serum T_4 concentration and a T_3 resin uptake or some other direct or indirect measurement of free T_4 or TBG concentration. If these studies indicate high concentrations of both total and free T_4, then the diagnosis is confirmed. However, if the levels are normal or equivocal, the possibility of T_3-toxicosis should be considered and a serum T_3 concentration determined. If both T_4 and T_3 levels are within the normal range, it becomes necessary to demonstrate that the thyroid is operating independently of endogenous TSH and such autonomy can best be demonstrated by a thyroid suppression test.

Thyroid Suppression Test. This test usually consists of the determination of thyroidal radioactive iodine uptake (RAIU) before and after the administration of 75 or 100 micrograms oral T_3 daily for 4 to 7 days. However, it may also be performed by determining RAIU before and 7 days after a single oral dose of 3 mg of T_4, a regimen that appears to be better tolerated by most patients. The test relies on the premise that if thyroid hormone levels are raised above normal by administration of T_3 or T_4, pituitary TSH output is suppressed and in normal patients this will be evident by a reduction in thyroid ^{131}I uptake to 50 per cent or less of pretreatment levels. In patients with Graves' disease or autonomously functioning nodules, thyroid function is independent of TSH and administration of thyroid hormone results in little or no change in ^{131}I uptake. This test has now been largely supplanted by the TRH stimulation test, which depends on a different premise.

TRH (Protirelin) Stimulation Test. This test employs synthetic TRH to stimulate the release of TSH from the pituitary gland. It is effective with intravenous TRH doses of 200 to 500 micrograms and serum TSH is determined before and again after 20 or 30 minutes. In euthyroidism, the rise in serum TSH is generally greater than 4 microunits per ml and the 20 or 30 minute level is usually at least 100 per cent more than the baseline value. By contrast, in hyperthyroid patients there is no increase in serum TSH. It must be realized that the serum TSH response may also be blunted or absent in euthyroid patients with ophthalmic Graves' disease, autonomously functioning thyroid adenoma, or multinodular goiter, and in about 5 per cent of the normal population.

At present, most clinicians use the TRH test to exclude rather than to positively diagnose hyperthyroidism. A normal increment in serum TSH after TRH administration is inconsistent with the hyperthyroid state. For the reasons stated, an absent response cannot be considered proof of thyrotoxicosis.

Thyroid RAIU and Imaging Procedures. With the advent of reliable and specific techniques for the measurement of circulating thyroid hormones, the need for determination of the thyroidal RAIU in the investigation of hyperthyroidism has greatly diminished. However, the 24-hour RAIU test, measuring uptake of ^{131}I after the oral administration of a 2 to 5 mCi dose, continues to have a significant role to play in two specific circumstances: (1) in determining the cause of the hyperthyroidism in order to institute appropriate therapy, and (2) in demonstrating satisfactory iodine trapping before the administration of a therapeutic dose of radioiodine. It has been found useful to subdivide hyperthyroid patients into those patients with relatively high RAIU and those with very low RAIU. Causes of hyperthyroidism with a 24-hour RAIU greater than 12 to 15 per cent include Graves' disease, toxic multinodular goiter, toxic autonomously functioning thyroid adenoma, TSH-producing pituitary adenoma, and trophoblastic tumors. By contrast, a 24-hour RAIU of less than 3 per cent is characteristic of silent thyroiditis, the hyperthyroidism owing to exogenous thyroid hormone or iodine, struma ovarii, and metastatic follicular thyroid carcinoma.

Thyroid imaging procedures with ^{123}I, technetium-99m, or ^{131}I are of value only when the distribution of functioning tissue within the thyroid is suspected to be abnormal, as in toxic multinodular goiter and autonomously functioning thyroid adenoma. In the typical patient with Graves' disease, who has a diffuse symmetric thyroid enlargement, the scan is redundant, expensive, and exposes the patient to unnecessary radiation. Scans may be helpful in the extremely rare circumstances of hyperthyroidism owing to struma ovarii or metastatic functioning follicular thyroid carcinoma.

TSH Stimulation Test. This test, consisting of the determination of RAIU before and after the administration of exogenous bovine TSH and formerly used to differentiate primary from secondary hypothyroidism, has recently been introduced into the spectrum of laboratory tests used in the evaluation of hyperthyroidism. Specifically, its usefulness lies in the differentiation of patients with the spontaneously resolving hyperthyroidism due to silent thyroiditis from those patients who surreptitiously ingest thyroid hormone (thyrotoxicosis factitia). In silent thyroiditis the administration of exogenous TSH fails to increase the RAIU while in thyrotoxicosis factitia, the TSH injections will markedly increase the RAIU provided that the patient's thyroid does not have fibrous atrophy that makes it unresponsive to TSH stimulation.

PITFALLS IN DIAGNOSIS

Difficulty in making a clinical diagnosis of thyrotoxicosis may be encountered when the disease is not florid, when it seems limited to one organ system, or when the symptoms are unusual. Such problems can be encountered at any age but often occur in the elderly population. Cardiac failure or an arrhythmia that is insensitive to digoxin treatment may be the only ostensible difficulty until a careful workup reveals the true nature of the problem. The finding of myasthenia gravis, diabetes mellitus that is particularly hard to regulate, or unexplained wasting should suggest hyperthyroidism as a possible underlying disorder. Occasionally, marked edema dependent in nature, uncontrollable diarrhea, or severe itching without evident cause may be the sole presenting manifestation of Graves' disease.

The laboratory diagnosis of hyperthyroidism becomes more difficult when patients have anomalies of thyroxine-binding protein usually related to treatment with estrogen or to liver disease. Serum T_3 levels are lower in patients who have been fasting or in those with chronic disease. Serum T_4 levels may be spuriously elevated during heparin therapy. The best protection against an incorrect diagnosis is to obtain thyroid function tests on hospitalized patients only when a clinical suspicion of thyrotoxicosis exists; to test in clearly defined circumstances in which the patient's recent medications are known; and to rely on combinations of tests rather than a single test for the definitive diagnosis of hyperthyroidism.

HYPOTHYROIDISM

By JAY D. H. SILVERBERG, M.D.,
and GERARD N. BURROW, M.D.

Toronto, Ontario, Canada

DEFINITIONS

Normal thyroid hormone secretion depends on a functioning hypothalamic–pituitary–thyroid axis that operates as a classic negative feedback system. Hypothyroidism may occur when any part of the systems fails to function adequately.

Hypothyroidism may be defined as failure of the thyroid gland to secrete enough thyroxine (T_4) and triiodothyronine (T_3) to maintain normal metabolic function. Primary hypothyroidism represents a pathologic lesion in the thyroid gland and is characterized by a compensatory increase in thyrotropin (TSH) secretion in addition to low circulating levels of thyroid hormones. Secondary hypothyroidism results from inadequate pituitary gland function and is characterized by low circulating levels of TSH that result in low concentration of circulating thyroid hormones. Tertiary hypothyroidism presumably results from inadequate thyrotropin-releasing hormone (TRH). As a consequence, TSH secretion is decreased, resulting again in low levels of circulating thyroid hormones. Tertiary hypothyroidism is thought to occur, but as yet decreased concentrations of TRH have not been determined. All three types of hypothyroidism may be caused by a variety of pathologic conditions (Table 1).

Hypothyroidism may be classified by the age of onset. Thyroid failure in infancy is known as cretinism. In childhood or adolescence thyroid failure is known as juvenile hypothyroidism, while in the postadolescent period the term adult hypothyroidism is used.

Advanced hypothyroidism, often termed myxedema, is characterized by the deposition of glycosaminoglycans, hyaluronic acid, and chondroitin sulfate in tissues. However, many authors use the terms myxedema and hypothyroidism synonymously.

ETIOLOGY

Ablation of the thyroid gland by surgery or by radioactive iodine (^{131}I) is the most common cause of hypothyroidism today.

Postsurgical hypothyroidism is usually manifested in the first year following surgery but the onset may occasionally be prolonged beyond this period. Recurrent laryngeal nerve paralysis and hypoparathyroidism are often associated with surgically induced hypothyroidism. After surgery for Graves' disease, transient hypothyroidism may occur in the first few weeks postoperatively. In this situation expectant observation rather than early treatment may be warranted, provided the hypothyroidism is mild.

Hypothyroidism following treatment with radioactive iodine is even more common than following surgery. The incidence of thyroid failure following radioactive iodine treatment depends upon the dose and uptake of the radioisotope by the thyroid gland, and individual variation (possible concomitant immune destruction). About 10 per cent of patients will develop hypothyroidism in the first year following treatment. In subsequent years 2 to 4 per cent of patients will become hypothyroid per annum, giving an incidence of hypothyroidism of about 40 per cent 10 years after treatment. The likelihood of thyroid failure is increased by multiple therapeutic doses of radioiodine. Transient hypothyroidism with full recovery may also follow radioiodine therapy.

Another frequently seen cause of primary hypothyroidism is autoimmune thyroiditis (Hashimoto's thyroiditis, chronic lymphocytic thyroiditis, struma lymphomatosa). This condition occurs more frequently in women, usually in the 40 to 60 age group; however, cases occur from childhood to old age. Currently, thyroid destruction is thought to result from immune mechanisms, with both humoral and cell-mediated immunity playing a role. Antibodies to various thyroid antigens are found circulating in the serum of most patients. Pathologically, the thyroid shows eosinophilic changes in some parenchymal cells (Askenazy cells) along with infiltration of the gland with lymphocytes and monocytes.

Other causes of primary hypothyroidism are rare. Developmental defects such as aplasia or maldescent of the thyroid as well as genetically determined defects in thyroid hormone synthesis occur with a frequency of less than 1 in 4000 births in most series. A host of drugs have been implicated in bringing about primary hypothyroidism (phenylbutazone, cobalt, lithium, paraminosalicylic acid [PAS], topical resorcinal, thioureas, perchlorate). Interestingly, iodine when given in sufficient doses will transiently inhibit thyroid hormone synthesis (Wolff-Chaikoff effect) and release. Unless the thyroid gland is damaged, for example, by radioactive iodine or Hashimoto's thyroiditis, most individuals will escape from this inhibitory effect. Iodine deficiency, once a common cause of hypothyroidism in many areas, is uncommon in developed countries.

Table 1. *Etiology of Hypothyroidism*

Primary hypothyroidism
  Albative
    Postsurgery
    Postradioactive iodine
  Autoimmune
  Congenital
    Agenesis and maldevelopment
    Maldescent
    Dyshormonogenesis
  Drugs
    Thionamides
    Iodine
    Phenylbutazone
    Cobalt
    Paraminosalicylic acid
    Resorcinol
    Thioureas
    Perchlorate
  Iodine deficiency
  Goitrogens, e.g., plants of class Cruciferae
  Riedel's struma
  Infiltrative disease, e.g., sarcoidosis
  Hypothyroid phase of subacute thyroiditis
Secondary hypothyroidism
  Adenoma
  Craniopharyngioma
  Vascular accidents
  Trauma
  Metastases
  Congenital aplasia
  Absence of thyrotrophs
Tertiary hypothyroidism
  Trauma
  Tumors
  Irradiation
  Developmental defects
Peripheral (rare)
  Insensitivity to thyroid hormone

A more complete summary of the causes of hypothyroidism is shown in Table 1.

Clinical Presentation. Recent studies have indicated that congenital hypothyroidism occurs as often as one in 4000 births. Untreated, many of these children will develop cretinism with severe mental retardation. Prompt treatment with thyroid hormone may prevent cretinism, making early diagnosis imperative. The classic clinical signs of acretin, such as a large tongue and umbilical hernia, are relatively late signs.

The clinical presentation of congenital hypothyroidism in the first few days of life is often quite subtle and nonspecific. In an effort to pinpoint some clinical clues that would alert physicians to the presence of congenital hypothyroidism, the early records of infants with hypothyroidism have been tabulated in a retrospective fashion and early clinical features compiled from hypothyroid children detected through screening programs. Clinical indicators that should arouse suspicion include: (1) diminished fetal activity prenatally; (2) a history of postmaturity with the gestational period prolonged beyond 42 weeks and increased birth weight (infant heavier than 4 kg in weight); (3) evidence of delayed skeletal maturation with retarded ossification centers (clinically this may present as a large posterior fontanel, greater than 1 square centimeter in diameter, less specifically as a low nasal ridge and "mongoloid features"); (4) a history of respiratory distress syndrome (RDS), especially in an infant with a birth weight of more than 2.5 kg; (5) evidence of poor tissue perfusion characterized by peripheral cyanosis and possibly a delay in the closure of the ductus arteriosus; (6) hypothermia with rectal temperatures of less than 95 F (35 C); (7) infants that are often seen to be floppy, lethargic, and feeding poorly; (8) evidence of mucoprotein deposition such as edema of the feet, labia, and eyelids; upper respiratory tract deposition of mucoprotein gives these infants a large tongue and a coarse cry; (9) prolongation of the period of physiologic jaundice beyond 3 days, occasionally as long as 3 weeks (part of the icterus may be explained by hypercarotinemia); (10) a delay in the onset of stooling beyond 20 hours, occasionally up to 4 days, with concomitant abdominal distention. A summary of these signs compiled by Guyda et al. is listed in Table 2.

If the diagnosis of thyroid insufficiency should be missed in a child in the neonatal period, the classic features of cretinism will appear at about 6 to 12 months postpartum. Often, at this time, irreversible damage has been done to the central nervous system, resulting in impaired intellectual development. These infants have a narrow forehead, puffy eyes and cheeks, a narrow nasal bridge with a pug nose and a large, thick, protruding tongue. The neck is thick and the abdomen is distended, often with an umbilical hernia. General growth is retarded, with shortened legs. Hair is

Table 2. *Early Clinical Clues of Congenital Hypothyroidism*

H	ernia, umbilical
Y	chromosome absent (i.e., female)
P	allor, coldness, hypothermia
O	edematous or typical facies
T	ongue enlarged
H	ypotonia
Y	ellow (prolongation of physiologic jaundice)
R	ough, dry skin
O	pen posterior fontanel
I	nactive defecation
D	uration of gestation prolonged

Five or more criteria favor hypothyroidism. Courtesy of Dr. Harvey Guyda.

sparse and dry, and the skin is cool and rough. The child is lethargic and hypotonic, and has delayed milestones. Hopefully, with the aid of neonatal screening for hypothyroidism, classic congenital cretinism will soon disappear.

ADULTS

In adults the clinical presentation of hypothyroidism is often insidious in onset, variable as to the degree of severity, and nonspecific in nature. Hypothyroid patients may present with cardiovascular, musculoskeletal, neurologic, or even psychiatric complaints. Often considerable time elapses before appropriate attention is directed toward the thyroid.

In general, adult patients with hypothyroidism will complain of fatigue, intellectual slowing, loss of initiative, generalized cold intolerance, as well as somnolence and lethargy. Patients also have anorexia, mild weight gain, and constipation. Vague muscle stiffness and aching associated with tingling paresthesias are commonplace. Hearing loss and night blindness are occasionally encountered. Female patients may have irregular and excessively heavy menstrual periods sometimes associated with galactorrhea; males often have loss of libido and occasionally oligospermia.

On clinical inspection hypothyroid patients appear sluggish and dull. Mucoproteinaceous infiltrates are responsible for the puffy face, nonpitting edema about the hands, feet, and supraclavicular area, macroglossia, the croaky, hoarse voice, and the nerve entrapment syndromes (e.g., carpal tunnel syndrome). The skin is cool, pale, dry, and often has a yellowish tinge. The hair is brittle, lusterless, and lost in significant amounts from the scalp and eyebrows. The nails are brittle and slow growing. The resting pulse rate is slow and arterial pulses are weak. There may be a mild decrease in systolic blood pressure with a concomitant increase in diastolic blood pressure. The precordium is silent, the heart sounds are distant, and cardiomegaly may be present. Pericardial effusion may be responsible for the cardiomegaly. Evidence of effusion may also be found in the pleural spaces, the peritoneal cavity, and in large joints. Classically, the relaxation phase of the deep tendon reflexes is slowed.

Patients with flagrant hypothyroidism are seldom difficult to recognize, but as noted, the presentation can be variable. Efforts have therefore been made to examine whether certain features are more meaningful than others in arriving at a diagnosis. Billewicz (1969) surveyed hypothyroid and euthyroid populations to ascertain the frequency of various signs and symptoms. Items with the largest discriminant factor were diminished sweating, cold intolerance, hoarseness, paresthesias, slow movements, coarse skin, periorbital puffiness, a slow pulse rate, and a delay in the relaxation phase of the ankle jerks. Items weighted as zero with respect to their discriminant value were mental lethargy, muscle pain, puffiness of the wrists, and supraclavicular puffiness.

MYXEDEMA COMA

Patients with neglected or undiagnosed hypothyroidism are at risk for myxedema coma, the end stage form of severe thyroid failure. This condition is usually seen in elderly patients with coronary artery disease or other systemic illnesses. The triggering events that may catapult hypothyroid patients into this life-threatening form of the illness are poor household heating in winter, the administration of central nervous system depressants, especially barbiturates, and infection, especially pneumonia. Patients with myxedema coma along with the classic features of severe hypothyroidism show progressive stupor until frank loss of consciousness develops. Hypoventilation may be present along with respiratory acidosis as well as a raised serum lactate level secondary to poor tissue perfusion. In addition, hypothermia, paralytic ileus, urinary retention, and hypotension that is poorly responsive to vasopressors are found. Prompt recognition of myxedema coma is mandatory, for even with the best medical management, survival is often no better than 50 per cent.

LABORATORY DIAGNOSIS

The most frequently used laboratory procedures for establishing the diagnosis of hypothyroidism are measurements of circulating thyroid hormone levels, test of hypothalmic-pituitary function, and tests measuring the effect of thyroid hormones on peripheral tissues.

The single most important laboratory test in documenting hypothyroidism is a determination of the serum thyroxine level. Today serum T_4 is measured directly and accurately either by competitive protein-binding assay or radioimmunoassay. Thyroid hormones are carried in serum bound to proteins and an estimate of thyroxine-binding proteins is essential in the interpretation of a total serum T_4 value. The most commonly used index of thyroxine protein binding is the resin T_3 uptake (RT_3U), which should not be confused with serum triiodothyronine (T_3RIA). The total serum T_4 and T_3 resin uptake may be combined into a free thyroxine index (FTI). The FTI correlates well with the free thyroxine concentration, which is the metabolically active fraction and is for the most part low in patients with clinical hypothyroidism. The serum T_3 concentration is less helpful than the serum T_4 or FTI in confirming the diagnosis of hypothyroidism. Quite often T_3 levels are in the normal range in hypothyroid patients with low serum T_4 values; conversely, serum T_3 concentrations may be frankly low in euthyroid patients with systemic illness.

In primary hypothyroidism elevations in the serum TSH concentration are often found before changes are noted in the other thyroid function tests. The TSH determination is the most sensitive thyroid function test commonly available to diagnose primary hypothyroidism. Occasionally clinically euthyroid patients are found who have an elevated serum TSH determination but have normal values for serum T_4 and the FTI. These patients have often been treated for thyrotoxicosis or have autoimmune thyroiditis. Such patients have a decreased functioning thyroid mass and may have subclinical hypothyroidism. Careful observation and follow-up are required to be certain they do not become overtly hypothyroid.

Thyroid antibodies do not aid in establishing the presence of hypothyroidism but they do offer help in determining the cause. In clinical practice antibodies to thyroglobulin and thyroid microsomal antigen are measured. High titers of antibodies are usually present in autoimmune thyroiditis and postablative hypothyroidism (i.e., treated patients with Graves' disease).

When secondary hypothyroidism is suspected in a patient, a single TSH determination is of little value. Standard radioimmunoassays for TSH are quite insensitive at the lower end of the normal range and a substantial proportion of healthy people may have "undetectable" levels of TSH. To determine whether a serum TSH is inappropriately low, a stimulation test with TRH may be employed. TRH is a tripeptide synthesized by neurons in the hypothalamus that is released into the hypophyseal-portal system and stimulates the thyrotrophs of the anterior pituitary. In secondary hypothyroidism, the TSH response to TRH is blunted; in tertiary hypothyroidism the TSH response to TRH may be present, absent, or delayed. In practice it is often difficult to distinguish secondary from possible tertiary causes of hypothyroidism using TRH testing.

Measurements of the serum TSH level and the TRH stimulation test, when indicated, have supplanted the cumbersome and often inaccurate TSH stimulation test (viz., measurement of the radioactive iodine uptake before and after TSH injection) in distinguishing primary from secondary hypothyroidism.

Once the diagnosis of primary or secondary hypothyroidism has been established, the clinician must be convinced that the hypothalamic-pituitary-adrenal axis is intact before thyroid hormone therapy is instituted. Thyroid hormone replacement in the presence of adrenal or corticotroph insufficiency may result in an adrenal crisis.

ROUTINE LABORATORY TESTS IN HYPOTHYROIDISM

Since thyroid hormones have such an important function in maintaining normal metabolism, it is not surprising that a deficiency of thyroid hormones would have a profound effect on many hematologic and serologic tests. It is important to know the effects of hypothyroidism on routine laboratory studies to prevent the misinterpretation of laboratory data.

Table 3 displays a summary of the effects of hypothyroidism upon routine laboratory tests.

PITFALLS IN DIAGNOSIS

Children with hypothyroidism occasionally present with short stature and a delayed bone age. Such children may have an enlarged sella turcica on skull x-ray. This does not necessarily imply secondary hypothyroidism caused by a pituitary tumor. In all likelihood the sellar enlargement is caused by hypertrophy of the thyrotrophs of the anterior pituitary. In this situation a determination of the serum TSH level should establish whether primary or secondary hypothyroidism is present.

Table 3. *Effect of Hypothyroidism on Routine Laboratory Tests*

Hematologic tests
  Hemoglobin: Anemia present in 1/3 of patients
  WBC: Normal
  Platelets: Normal
  ESR: Elevated

Biochemical tests
  Electrolytes: Occasionally serum sodium decreased
  Uric Acid: Elevated
  SGOT, CPK, LDH: All may be elevated
  Serum cholesterol: Elevated
  Serum triglycerides: Often elevated
  17-ketosteroids and 17-hydroxycorticoids: Low; ACTH stimulation test and metapyrone test often low in eucorticoid hypothyroid patients.

Other
  ECG: Low voltage, nonspecific ST and T wave changes
  Chest x-ray: Occasionally, evidence of pleural and pericardial effusion.

Another atypical presentation of hypothyroidism in children is with the onset of isosexual true precocious puberty. This syndrome occurs more frequently with female patients. Why such patients have premature maturation of the "gonadostat" is unclear. Interestingly, regression of secondary sexual characteristics takes place upon return to the euthyroid state with treatment.

In clinical practice, many patients are found who have been started on thyroid hormone replacement for vague complaints without adequate laboratory documentation to determine whether hypothyroidism had indeed been present. When confronted with a patient taking thyroid hormone (thyroxine), the clinician often must decide whether therapy is justified. Therapy must be stopped for at least 35 days in order to confirm the presence of hypothyroidism. Premature reassessment of the patient prior to 5 weeks off therapy may be insufficient for full recovery of the hypothalamic-pituitary-thyroid axis from chronic suppression. In children under the age of 3, thyroid hormone therapy should never be withheld, since 5 weeks without therapy in a truly hypothyroid infant may have permanent effects on central nervous system development.

THYROIDITIS

By JOHN T. DUNN, M.D.
Charlottesville, Virginia

"Thyroiditis" is a term used for several types of inflammatory or infiltrative lesions of the thyroid. The varieties to be considered here have the thyroid as the chief or sole focus of the disease. They will be classified as (1) acute (suppurative), (2) subacute, (3) Hashimoto's, or (4) Riedel's. These four are discussed individually.

Thyroiditis may rarely occur as part of systemic diseases such as syphilis, tuberculosis, sarcoidosis, mycoses, or amyloidosis. The involvement in these instances seldom produces symptoms, and diagnosis will depend on histologic examination. Inflammation of the thyroid can be seen following strangulation or other acute trauma, or occasionally following ^{131}I therapy for thyrotoxicosis or carcinoma. In these situations the diagnosis is apparent from the history, and interference with thyroid function is rare.

ACUTE SUPPURATIVE THYROIDITIS

DEFINITION

This is a bacterial infection of the thyroid, following either septicemia or direct extension of a septic process from neighboring tissues. Never common, it has virtually disappeared since the introduction of antibiotics.

SIGNS AND SYMPTOMS

The onset is acute. Pain in the thyroid region is the outstanding symptom. It may be increased by movement of the head and by swallowing. Otalgia is frequent. The patient has symptoms of an acute bacterial infection, including fever, chills, and malaise. While the thyroid may be the first organ attacked by the septic process, suppurative thyroiditis will frequently be preceded symptomatically by infection elsewhere, making its diagnosis more obvious. Occasionally it will be the first manifestation of defective host immune defenses, as in leukemia.

COURSE AND COMPLICATIONS

With adequate antibiotic therapy the thyroiditis may be expected to heal with no permanent impairment of thyroid function. Local complications include tracheal compression and abscess formation. If not treated, the infection may spread to adjacent tissue, destroying tracheal and laryngeal cartilage, causing mediastinitis or pharyngitis followed by bronchopneumonia, or promoting cellulitis and abscess formation elsewhere in the neck. Untreated suppurative thyroiditis may also damage enough of the gland to effect permanent hypothyroidism.

PHYSICAL EXAMINATION FINDINGS

The patient is febrile and acutely ill. The anterior neck is swollen, hot, red, and quite tender. Typically, the entire thyroid is involved. A primary source of bacterial infection should be sought by a careful general examination of the patient.

LABORATORY FINDINGS

Granulocytosis and an elevation of the sedimentation rate will be found, as in most pyogenic infections. The serum thyroxine (T_4), triiodothyronine (T_3), T_3 resin uptake, and ^{131}I uptake should all be normal unless massive destruction of thyroid tissue has occurred. Bacteriologic diagnosis can be obtained by needle aspiration of the thyroid, but this procedure carries the hazard of spreading the infection. Careful examination for more accessible foci of infection such as draining abscesses, pharyngitis, or septicemia should yield material satisfactory for organism identification and antibiotic sensitivity.

PITFALLS IN DIAGNOSIS

Acute suppurative thyroiditis is not always easy to distinguish from subacute nonsuppurative thyroiditis. In the latter, pain and tenderness are usually less severe and signs of local or systemic bacterial infection will not be present. Occasionally, hemorrhage into a thyroid nodule or cyst may produce acute pain and tenderness; this possibility can usually be differentiated from acute suppurative thyroiditis by the sudden onset of pain, by its localization, by prior evidence of a nodular gland, and by the absence of signs of infection.

SUBACUTE THYROIDITIS

SYNONYMS

De Quervain's thyroiditis, granulomatous thyroiditis, giant cell thyroiditis, pseudotuberculous thyroiditis.

DEFINITION

An inflammation of the thyroid characterized histologically by the presence of giant cells and clinically by its self-limiting course and abnormalities in iodine metabolism. It is frequently found in association with viral illness, particularly mumps and Coxsackie virus infections. Current opinion favors a viral cause in most cases, although this has been proved by direct culture on only a few occasions.

PRESENTING SIGNS AND SYMPTOMS

The typical patient will show swelling of the neck, tenderness over the thyroid, sore throat, pain on swallowing, otalgia, mild fever, and malaise. These symptoms usually develop over several weeks and may vary greatly in severity. Occasionally, there will be no pain or tenderness, and the rapid goiter formation is attributed erroneously to cancer. At other times the onset is acute, with chills, high fever, and prostration. Initially the inflammation may be restricted to one lobe of the thyroid, but eventual involvement of the entire gland is to be expected. In the early stages mild symptoms of hyperthyroidism may be encountered; these are attributed to release of stored hormone by the inflamed thyroid.

COURSE AND COMPLICATIONS

Active thyroiditis usually continues for 2 to 8 weeks and then regresses spontaneously. Recurrences are common and may occur several times over the ensuing year. Complete recovery is the rule, and permanent hypothyroidism is limited to approximately 10 per cent of patients.

PHYSICAL EXAMINATION FINDINGS

Characteristically the thyroid is tender, often strikingly so, and moderately enlarged (two to three times normal size). In texture it is firm, occasionally stony hard. Infrequently, the inflammation will be localized and suggest an adenoma or malignancy. Mild fever and malaise are common.

LABORATORY STUDIES

The two most useful laboratory tests are the sedimentation rate and the radioiodine uptake. The former will usually be markedly elevated, with a value of over 50 mm by the Westergren method. The uptake of radioiodine is greatly depressed or absent over the affected portion of the gland. This should aid in distinguishing it from other causes of hyperthyroidism. During the recovery phase the ^{131}I uptake may rise to levels above normal and remain elevated for several weeks.

The serum T_4, T_3, and T_3 resin uptake may all be increased in the early stages of the disease, reflecting the transient hyperthyroidism that comes with disruption of thyroid follicles and discharge of stored hormone into the circulation. During recovery these tests may be in the hypothyroid range and the serum thyroid-stimulating hormone (TSH) may be elevated. Test for serum antibodies to thyroid antigens may be transiently positive, usually at low titers.

In most instances, the clinical course and laboratory findings will make the diagnosis clear-cut. Occasionally, needle biopsy of the thyroid may be useful if the diagnosis remains in doubt.

HASHIMOTO'S THYROIDITIS

SYNONYMS

Autoimmune thyroiditis, chronic thyroiditis, struma lymphomatosa, lymphadenoid goiter, lymphocytic thyroiditis.

DEFINITION AND PATHOGENESIS

This is a disorder characterized histologically by diffuse lymphocytic infiltration and fibrotic replacement of acinar tissue in the thyroid, and immunologically by circulating antibodies to one or several distinct antigens from thyroid tissue. It is by far the most common form of thyroiditis and one of the most frequent causes of goiter.

Its pathogenesis is unknown, but autoimmune phenomena play a prominent role. There is a close relationship between Graves' disease and Hashimoto's thyroiditis. Both may show lymphocytic infiltration histologically, have antibodies to the same thyroid antigens, and occur within the same families.

As with most thyroid diseases, Hashimoto's disease is much more common in females than males, by a ratio of 5 to 1 or greater. In the United States the disease appears to have increased in frequency over the past several decades. It has been suggested that this may be related to an increase in the iodine content of the diet, since patients with Hashimoto's frequently show impairment of iodine utilization in hormone biosynthesis.

PRESENTING SIGNS AND SYMPTOMS

The usual initial symptom is swelling of the thyroid. Rarely is it painful. Slow enlargement may be observed over many months or years without other symptoms. When the thyroid increases sufficiently to impinge upon neighboring structures, symptoms of choking, dysphagia, and dyspnea may appear.

An alternative presentation is the appearance of hypothyroidism, with or without evidence of a goiter. Indeed, Hashimoto's thyroiditis is the usual cause of primary hypothyroidism in adults.

COURSE

This will be variable. The goiter may remain stationary for many years or continue to enlarge gradually. As normal acinar tissue is replaced by fibrosis, hypothyroidism may ensue without disappearance of the goiter. When hypothyroidism without goiter is the presenting symptom, the course will be that of progressive severity of the hypothyroidism until corrected by replacement therapy.

PHYSICAL EXAMINATION FINDINGS

The most prominent feature is the goiter. Characteristically, the thyroid is diffusely and symmetrically enlarged, often exhibiting a prominent pyramidal lobe. In texture it is firm, as in untreated Graves' disease. Frank nodularity is unusual, although slight diffuse irregularity of the surface is common. Hypothyroidism, when it occurs, is as described elsewhere in this book.

Hashimoto's thyroiditis occasionally accompanies other diseases with immunologic manifestations, most notably pernicious anemia, Addison's disease, and juvenile-onset diabetes. Evidence of such disorders may help in the diagnosis of the thyroiditis. Contrariwise, in patients with established Hashimoto's thyroiditis, the possibility of other autoimmune diseases should be considered.

COMMON COMPLICATIONS

The two most frequent sequelae are hypothyroidism and compression of adjacent structures by the goiter. Available evidence does not favor an alleged increase in thyroid carcinoma.

LABORATORY FINDINGS

The useful laboratory examinations in autoimmune thyroiditis are chiefly limited to indices of thyroid function and specific immunologic reactions. The serum TSH level is the most sensitive indicator of hypothyroidism. The serum T_4 and T_3 resin uptake will usually be in the low or low normal range. The ^{131}I uptake may vary from low to high; it is frequently higher than expected from other measures of thyroid function.

Two simple tests for circulating antibodies to specific thyroid antigens may be of great value in the diagnosis. The more sensitive of these is the detection of an antibody to a microsomal antigen. Depending on the titer arbitrarily designated as significant in a given laboratory, the test will be positive for from 60 to 90 per cent of patients. Sustained elevated titers are not found in other thyroid diseases except Graves' disease, which has a close immunological relationship to Hashimoto's. Another immunologic test for serum antibodies to thyroglobulin will also frequently be positive, and in some laboratories has been more sensitive as a detector than the microsomal antibody. In general, it is worth doing both tests, since some patients will be positive to one and not to the other.

A thyroid scan may be of value in showing a patchy uptake of radioactivity, although a similar pattern may be seen in multinodular goiter. Needle biopsy or needle aspiration can be done when a definitive diagnosis is required.

PITFALLS IN DIAGNOSIS

Under most circumstances the diagnosis can be made easily by the combination of a diffuse, slightly irregular, firm goiter, with or without hypothyroidism, and positive antibody titers. If the antibodies are negative it may be difficult to distinguish Hashimoto's from the diffuse or multinodular goiter associated with familial thyroidal defects. Practically, such a distinction is not always necessary, since the treatment for both conditions is thyroid hormone replacement, and both have a favorable prognosis when so treated.

RIEDEL'S THYROIDITIS

SYMPTOMS

Ligneous thyroiditis, fibrous thyroiditis, chronic sclerosing thyroiditis.

DEFINITION

The disease is a chronic progressive fibrosis of the thyroid with destruction of normal tissue and fibrotic extension to neighboring structures. The cause is unknown and the condition is extremely rare.

PRESENTING SIGNS AND SYMPTOMS

The first symptom is usually thyroidal enlargement, frequently asymmetric. Pain is commonly present over the thyroid or referred to the ear or posterior neck. Symptoms of local pressure appear early, particularly dyspnea; others frequently encountered are dysphagia and dysphonia.

COURSE AND COMPLICATIONS

The outcome is unpredictable. In some instances the fibrotic process halts spontaneously and may even regress. More often, there is gradual and relentless progression to invade an increasing portion of perithyroidal tissue. Eventually, all the structures of the anterior neck may be glued together by dense fibrous bands. The most frequent complications are from compression of neighboring structures in the neck, particularly the trachea, the recurrent laryngeal nerve, and the major vessels. Uncommonly, the destruction of the thyroid may be extensive enough to produce hypothyroidism.

PHYSICAL EXAMINATION FINDINGS

The thyroid is usually stony hard to palpation. It is enlarged but seldom more than two to three times normal size. It is fixed to neighboring tissue and does not move with swallowing. The gland surface is fairly regular, in contrast to most cancers. The absence of tracheal deviation and of enlarged lymph nodes may also help to distinguish Riedel's thyroiditis from thyroid carcinoma. The effects of compression are much more marked than would be expected from the goiter size. Despite these features, surgical inspection will usually be necessary to establish the diagnosis.

LABORATORY FINDINGS

Tests of thyroid function will be normal, unless hypothyroidism has appeared. Antithyroglobulin antibodies have been found only at low serum dilutions in the few patients tested.

THYROID TUMORS

By BROWN DOBYNS, M.D., Ph.D.
Cleveland, Ohio

Any palpable mass in the thyroid deserves diagnostic attention. Such a lesion may be malignant or the site of potential malignancy. It may be the cause of thyrotoxicosis either when discovered or in the future.

HISTOLOGIC TYPES OF MALIGNANT TUMORS OF THE THYROID

Malignant lesions of the thyroid represent the widest possible range of malignant behavior.

PAPILLARY AND MIXED PAPILLARY AND FOLLICULAR CARCINOMA

Many observers are inclined to classify all malignant neoplasms as papillary if a papillary configuration is found in any area of the lesion. If looked upon in this manner the group as a whole represents 70 or 75 per cent of all thyroid carcinomas. Because of differences in capacity for hormone production and biological aggressiveness, it is appropriate to subdivide this large group when considering diagnosis and management.

Pure papillary carcinoma occurs almost exclusively in younger persons. It is extremely slow growing. Survival may be expected for many years with lingering disease present. It takes up no radioiodine. The metastases are confined to lymph nodes and lung. The lesions are often cystic and sometimes histologically confused with papillary cystadenomas, which have excessive radioiodine uptake. Occasionally, death may occur under the age of 40.

Mixed papillary and follicular lesions represent a spectrum of papillary with various amounts of follicular structure containing some colloid. This is a considerably more aggressive lesion than the pure papillary lesion. It spreads to lymph nodes and lung but may also appear in the follicular form silently in bone. There is a wide spectrum of uptake of radioiodine from case to case and metastasis to metastasis. There may be none or there may be enough uptake to be of therapeutic value, but there is almost always less than 1/100th (gram for gram) of the uptake in normal thyroid tissue in the same individual.

When a papillary structure is found in the neoplasm in older patients, a search through multiple samples of the mass usually reveals occasional small undifferentiated areas. It is a serious mistake to apply the connotation of behavior that accompanies papillary lesions and to assume that the lesion has low-grade malignancy, for such lesions may be expected to behave in a manner characteristic of the most undifferentiated part.

Follicular Carcinoma

This lesion usually starts as a discrete encapsulated mass with some but relatively little affinity for radioiodine. It often poses a diagnostic problem when small because it may resemble normal thyroid tissue and has not yet declared its potential for metastasis. By the time it has reached clinically significant size, it will, after thorough search, show areas of blood vessel or capsular invasion, a criterion for making the diagnosis of malignancy. There may be widespread metastases with a predilection for bones and lung. The lesions occur in middle and later life and are most often asymptomatic. The uptake of radioiodine is better than with other malignant lesions, but even in the most favorable cases (for radioiodine therapy) the lesion takes up far less than the accompanying normal thyroid tissue. Although a very few of these tumors have been reported to be hyperfunctioning, the documentation based on actual counts has not been reported to substantiate the claims. However, hyperthyroidism associated with this lesion can be demonstrated on rare occasions in which an enormous total volume of functioning metastatic tissue scattered throughout the body may be autonomously producing hormone. The metastatic sites are often controlled with radioiodine for many years but ultimately all patients develop neoplastic variants that take up no radioiodine and when lodged in a vital site are lethal.

ANAPLASTIC CARCINOMA

These lesions are among the most rapidly growing of all malignant neoplasms. They represent about 15 per cent of carcinomas and usually occur in older individuals as a single rapidly growing mass or may appear as a diffuse rapid enlargement of the whole thyroid. Histologically they show all forms of rapidly multiplying malignant cells resembling sarcoma and carcinoma. Unfortunately, days and weeks elapse before patients seek advice, or there is diagnostic delay. More unfortunately, a hopeless attitude has persisted toward surgical intervention when the nature of the lesion is suspected and only a biopsy is obtained. However, surgical cures have occurred in which the true thyroid capsule had not yet been invaded (the author has had three such cases), as when a small, cold, rapidly growing mass was carefully removed without violating the capsule. The clue to operability for possible cure of such lesions is the absence of recurrent laryngeal nerve paralysis.

MEDULLARY CARCINOMA

This lesion represents approximately 3 to 5 per cent of thyroid carcinomas. It may occur as a familial trait among certain families or as an isolated sporadic event. A surprising number of the familial type of this rare tumor have been found in recent years because of interest in screening all family members by serum calcitonin assays. Radioimmunoassay for calcitonin has not only served to screen individuals thought to be at risk but it has served also as a method for detecting recurrence of disease in patients presumably cured by surgical removal.

Approximately 30 per cent of sporadic lesions have been found to have metastasized to lymph nodes when the histologic diagnosis is made. Very minute nonpalpable lesions may be found during the course of screening families. When these lesions come to light in younger patients they usually can be cured by removal. The medullary carcinomas usually are located at the junction of the upper and middle third of the lobe and as a rule are bilateral. The lesion may be accompanied by pheochromocytoma and hyperplasia or adenomas of the parathyroids. This combination of lesions is known as multiple endocrine adenomas (MEA, type II). Submucosal neuromas may also be found on the tongue, lips, and eyelids in the familial type of disease. If a lesion is present, the release of calcitonin may be stimulated by the intravenous administration of calcium chloride or pentagastrin.

LYMPHOMA AND SMALL CELL CARCINOMA

In the past the distinction between lymphoma and small cell carcinoma has been most difficult to make with the usual histologic preparations. More recently the electron microscope has permitted distinction between the two types of cells. Either of these lesions may be encountered in a diffusely enlarging thyroid. The lymphoma is often confused with or associated with Hashimoto's thyroiditis. In the past the distinction between the two diseases was made retrospectively. The survival of the patient with small cell carcinoma is similar to that of patients with anaplastic carcinoma. It was rarely cured and rapidly lethal. The lymphoma following incomplete removal responded to external irradiation and indeed appeared to be cured in 20 per cent of patients.

HISTORY

Certain features in the history may raise the suspicion that a lesion of the thyroid is malignant. When the lesion appears later in life, especially in males, it should be suspected of being malignant. Observed growth should heighten suspicion. A change in the quality of the voice suggests recurrent laryngeal nerve involvement and paralysis, resulting in malfunction of one vocal cord. It should be kept in mind that recurrent nerve involvement may occur so insidiously that the movement of the opposite vocal cord may compensate and make the patient less aware of impairment. Those who are accomplished singers are acutely aware of the change. The development of dysphagia is not the only indication of growth; adherence of the mass to surrounding structures can be, also. Onset of pain associated with acute appearance of a sizeable mass suggests hemorrhage, which is most common in the hyperfunctioning adenomas but may occur in papillary carcinomas and lead to cyst formation. Pain of a steady nature is more often associated with thyroiditis, but on rare occasions pain accompanied by massive growth may represent malignancy. A history of the presence of a goiter or a mass for many years is no basis for reassurance regarding the possibility of malignancy.

A history of radiation treatment for thymic enlargement in infancy, for recurrent tonsillitis or pharyngitis in children, for acne of the neck or face in adolescence, or for tuberculous cervical lymph adenitis in young adults may be followed by the development of carcinoma of the thyroid.

Such radiation-related lesions evolve very slowly and most often appear 10 to 25 years following exposure. Any individual who has had such exposure should be examined by careful palpation annually by an experienced examiner. Scans are done only if there is a suspicion of a mass.

The history associated with hyperfunctioning adenoma(s) is usually quite subtle (by hyperfunctioning we mean functioning in excess of the remaining extranodular thyroid tissue). The symptoms produced by the hyperfunctioning adenoma(s) are usually significantly different from those of Graves' disease and are far less evident to the patient. Although the metabolism of the person is elevated as in Graves' disease, there is relatively little restlessness, nervousness, or irritability, and eye signs are absent. A relatively long interval of time (usually years) elapses between the appearance of a mass or masses and the time when the compensating decline of function in the extranodular tissue has approached zero and the lesion has begun to overproduce the bodily need for hormone. Such an autonomously functioning adenoma is usually reliably demonstrable by its greater uptake of ^{131}I. This finding does not necessarily mean that the patient has yet become thyrotoxic. Only about 25 per cent of hyperfunctioning adenomas are accompanied by clinical thyrotoxicosis at the time the mass is discovered or shortly after.

The most common clinical complaint relates to cardiac function, usually arrhythmia. Since necrosis and hemorrhage are prone to develop in such hyperfunctioning lesions, the mass often enlarges rather acutely and leads to discovery. This is occasionally accompanied by some vague soreness. The increase in size develops over several days and is caused by effu-

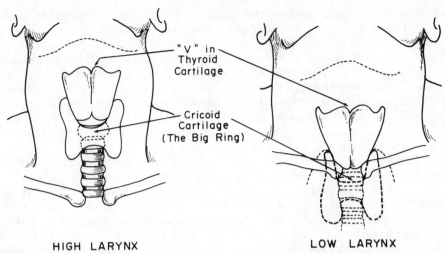

HIGH LARYNX   **LOW LARYNX**

Figure 1. A diagrammatic representation of variations in the position of the thyroid gland with respect to the superior thoracic inlet. The position of the thyroid isthmus bears a constant relationship to the larynx. Identification of the position of the larynx directs the examiner to the position of the thyroid which in some cases may be so low it is only palpable with special effort.

sion of fluid into the area of necrosis. Slow spontaneous resorption results in shrinkage, which is sometimes credited to the giving of thyroid hormone and occurs over several weeks.

PHYSICAL EXAMINATION

A great deal is to be learned from the physical examination of a nodular goiter. The findings contribute more to the plan for management than any other source of data. Certain steps in the examination of the thyroid should be followed in developing an understanding of the anatomic relationships and the character of the pathology in a given case. Whether the examiner should stand in front of or behind the subject has been debated. An examiner must have a clear mental image of the thyroid. Experience is gained by seeing the thyroid exposed after a physical examination has been made and the examiner has made up his mind what probably exists under his examining fingers. Many nodular goiters do not require surgical exploration, depending on what is meant by "nodular goiter." The physical examination is particularly important for the surgeon, because his decision to explore or not to explore a so-called "nodular goiter" is usually based on the accuracy of such an examination. He is in a particularly advantageous position because, if the condition is one that requires operation, he has an opportunity to repeatedly check his examinations and improve on his accuracy. It has been of particular interest to observe that most surgeons examine from the front of the neck because so many features are missed from the

back. The visual examination of the thyroid before and during palpation often gives much information.

There is considerable variation in the position of structures within the neck (Fig. 1). Orientation with respect to the position of the larynx is the first step in determining where the thyroid is. The normal thyroid isthmus always bears the same relationship to the cricoid cartilage, viz., upper edge of isthmus at the lower edge of the cricoid cartilage. The top of the larynx is easily identified by the "V" in the midline of the thyroid cartilage. The cricoid cartilage is palpated at the base of the larynx just below the thyroid cartilage and appears as a very large, thick first ring of the trachea. Irrespective of the size or position of the lateral lobes of the thyroid, this cartilage identifies the upper margin of a normal isthmus, where it is firmly attached. Thus, by knowing exactly where the lateral lobes must be as they relate to the isthmus, the examiner knows precisely where to look for the thyroid and masses in it. In some patients, such as those with a long neck, the larynx usually lies high in the neck; in individuals with a short thick neck, the lower part of the larynx (and most of the thyroid) may actually lie within the superior thoracic inlet. Being forewarned of the possibility of a very low-lying thyroid, the examiner will realize that the only way a mass in such a thyroid will be found is by palpation with the fingers as low as possible and only when the patient swallows and raises the larynx and thyroid lobes with it. Many so-called substernal masses are discovered only by a clear appreciation of the anatomic relationships in each patient.

After the position of the larynx is determined, the size and regularity of the thyroid are appraised. Asymmetry is usually a clue to the presence of a mass in one lobe. A clue to the presence of asymmetry is deviation of the larynx. An imaginary line drawn through the "V" of the thyroid cartilage and the center of the cricoid cartilage will give an idea as to the tilt of the larynx. Deviation of the trachea leads to a search for the mass that is causing it. The asymmetry and the size of the lobes prompts suspicion that there may be a mass buried in the larger lobe.

Aggressive palpation is necessary to find a mass and judge its nature. It is generally conceded that an experienced examiner can feel almost any mass 1 cm or larger and can feel any mass that is detectable by scanning or imaging. The fingers or thumb pushes the sternocleidomastoid muscle backward and laterally so that the fingers lie medial to it. This permits the fingers to forcefully rub the lobe against the lateral side of the trachea and larynx. The fingers are searching for variations in consistency or localization of tenderness in the lobe. The approximate normal location of the upper limit of the superior pole and the lower edge of the lobe can be anticipated quite precisely from having identified the upper and lower limits of the isthmus. With this technique, the limits of a normal thyroid can usually be felt. The examiner can recognize the presence of the mass either by moving the fingers up and down over the lobe, or by applying steady pressure with the fingers over the upper part of the lobe while asking the patient to swallow; thus the lobe containing the mass is moved up and down under the fingers (the thyroid always moves with the larynx).

If a mass is suspected as a result of these maneuvers, then the object of the next maneuver is to catch the mass by inserting the finger under the lower edge of the mass at the height of a swallow. Following the act of swallowing, the larynx will tend to drop back to its normal position but the mass is still forcibly elevated on the tip of the finger. The restraining pressure is then gradually released just enough to let the mass squeeze under the finger. The mass is thus quite apparent and several questions about it can be answered: Is it spherical as a discrete neoplasm that in the mind's eye might be surrounded by a capsule? Is the consistency of the mass quite different from (harder than) the remainder of the lobe? If it is very hard, it is more likely to be a malignant process. Can the mass be moved on the trachea or larynx? If there is a sense of fixation, it may represent an infiltration of a malignant process invading surrounding tissues or an inflammatory reaction around a necrotic adenoma. By such aggressive, objective palpation, the examiner may single out each of several existing masses and characterize them, especially a dominant one. A tendency toward adherence, hardness, or a sense of fine roughness on the surface of the mass are all characteristics that prompt suspicion that a mass is malignant. Malignancy is found in 12 to 18 per cent of single masses and in 5 to 7 per cent among multiple masses.

In the case of any nodular goiter, a search for significant lymphadenopathy is important. Lymphatic spread from the thyroid occurs in five possible directions. The most common is from the middle and lower part of the lobe backward to minute nodes lying immediately along the tracheoesophageal groove and from this point downward into the mediastinum. These are usually not palpable. Direct lateral spread to the jugular chain produces nodes that are most easily palpable. Sometimes spread in this direction is discovered only far lateral in the posterior triangle of the neck. A primary lesion near the superior pole often spreads upward along the superior thyroid artery to produce palpable nodes high in the jugular chain. There are minute nodes lying along the upper and lower margins of the isthmus. These may be the first to be involved. Although these nodes may be minute, they are easily felt by quite superficial palpation as tiny hard masses the size of a BB shot. Unfortunately in lymphocytic thyroiditis these nodes also become easily palpable. From this area the spread may be upward to additional tiny nodes on each side of the thyroglossal tract. It should be kept in mind that, except for the nodes at the isthmus, lymph nodes do not move up and down on swallowing, while nodules that lie in the lateral part of the lobe and that are sometimes confused with lymph nodes in the jugular chain do move up and down.

Indirect laryngoscopy to appraise the function of the vocal cords is an important part of any examination of a nodular goiter, especially when malignancy is suspected. If there is any suggestion of change in the character of the voice, the examination is obligatory. Normally the vocal cords adduct to the midline on phonation and abduct widely so that inhalation can take place. Malignant infiltration of the recurrent laryngeal nerve results in neither abduction nor adduction. The cord lies midway in a cadaveric position and does not move. Slight movement of the cord resulting from air flowing by should not be interpreted as movement. The cadaveric position should not be misinterpreted by mild degrees of rotation of the whole larynx created by a mass lying outside the larynx. In the case of traumatic injury to the recurrent nerve (surgical injury), the paralysis results in an adducted cord, fixed in the midline position. This often causes some stridor. These distinctive findings of position are most important in the patient who has had previous thyroid surgery for an adenomatous goiter and subsequently is found to have nerve paralysis. The presence of a cadaveric cord prompts re-evaluation of the original pathologic findings. The presence of a midline cord prompts suspicion that there was previous injury to the nerve.

OTHER PHASES OF EXAMINATION

LABORATORY TESTS

Laboratory tests are of relatively little value in distinguishing benign and malignant diseases in nodular goiter. Measuring serum thyroxine or free thyroxine level may be quite useful when there is a suspicion of thyrotoxicosis or when a hyperfunctioning adenoma has been found on radioisotope scanning. It may also be of some value in detecting hypothyroidism associated with a lobulated, deficiency type of gland or Hashimoto's thyroiditis. However, it does not shed much light on the nature of a cold nodule. The radioimmunoassay for thyroid-stimulating hormone (TSH) is preferred if hypothyroidism is a consideration.

THYROID SCANNING OR IMAGING

Scanning or imaging of the thyroid is a most important part of the examination of the thyroid because it gives a rough idea of the functional nature of certain masses that have been found by palpation. It is of little value in detecting small lesions that experienced fingers cannot feel. Radioiodine ^{131}I or ^{123}I is used for scanning. The thyroid takes up this isotope just as it does ordinary iodine. In most cases, that uptake represents utilization of iodine in the production of thyroid hormone. ^{131}I was originally used. Technetium was used by many because of its short half-life and because of the minimal radiation to the patient, but this isotope does not become organically bound as does iodine and therefore is not a reliable measure of the function of the tissue in question. More recently ^{123}I has been used because of its short half-life. Any scanning, imaging, or uptakes should be done with one of the isotopes of iodine.

It is most important that the person who carries out the scanning or imaging procedures is not only a physician but one with experience and skill in palpation of the thyroid and with knowledge of the physical features that represent various pathologic processes in the thyroid.

He must indicate on the picture that is produced the exact location of the cricoid and thyroid cartilage, the isthmus, and the location and size of each mass with respect to those structures and the areas of blackening. The functional quality of the mass must be related to the *particular* nodule that is drawing primary attention.

The identification of the hyperfunctioning adenoma is quite precise, since the increased concentration of the isotope in such a lesion stands out and is not masked by superimposed paranodular tissue. The more hormone the lesion contributes to bodily need, the more the remainder of the gland is suppressed, until an excess of hormone is produced and the patient is thyrotoxic.

At best, imaging or rectolinear scanning of cold nodules is rather imprecise (1) because neoplasms are buried within the "normal" thyroid tissue (which takes up the isotope) lying in front of and behind the mass, (2) because there may be superimposition of masses, and (3) because the center of a lesion may be necrotic and not take up iodine as does the viable part of the lesion. Just how cold a mass may be is not only based on the relative lack of blackening of the image coinciding with the mass compared to the normal part of the gland but also is based on an appreciation of the relative size of the mass (thickness — from the physical examination) and the anticipated volume of normal thyroid tissue stretched out over the front of and behind the mass. The smaller the mass or the more voluminous the overlying parenchyma, the more difficult it will be to judge the degree of coldness of the mass. Thus, the accuracy of the physical examination at the time the image is produced is of great importance. A cold mass less than 1 cm in diameter is not reliably detected by scanning or imaging. When the actual amount of radioiodine is measured in a small sample of neoplasm and separately measured in an equal weight of paranodular thyroid tissue in the laboratory, 90 per cent of all carcinomas prove to have taken up less than 1/100th of the ^{131}I of the normal thyroid tissue. Distinctly cold masses must be suspected of being malignant, but functional tumors with a necrotic center or a mass of lymphocytic thyroiditis will take up very little or no radioiodine and may be confused with cold neoplasms.

ULTRASONOGRAPHY OF THYROID NODULES

Use of ultrasonography has been explored increasingly to distinguish between solid and cystic neoplasms. Cysts may be readily identified. Unfortunately, a considerable number of papillary adenocarcinomas of the thyroid are cystic so that the recognition of a cyst does not rule out the presence of a malignant lesion.

The identification of a cyst has prompted some to attempt needle aspiration. Collapse of the cyst without the recovery of diagnostic cells or tissue may give a false sense of security and delay the removal of a malignant lesion. Ultrasonography yields interesting information but contributes little to the management of a cold nodule that should be removed for a definitive diagnosis.

NEEDLE BIOPSY

The use of fine needle aspiration (needle biopsy) of thyroid nodules has received increasing trial. It requires the diagnostic skill of a pathologist who has had a great deal of experience with pathology of the thyroid. Reports based on work of highly experienced investigators have indicated that many carcinomas can be detected by this technique. The method seems to be reliable only when carcinoma is found. Negative findings may be considered encouraging but not completely reassuring. Some high degrees of accuracy have been reported from data that included many lesions that were removed surgically to be sure. Most thyroid carcinomas grow quite slowly (years), so that some lesions that were considered benign at biopsy may not yet have declared themselves as clinically malignant. Pathologists sometimes have difficulty reaching a firm decision regarding malignancy among many of the "atypical lesions" when they have the whole specimen in hand or find after a search of many microscopic preparations that there is capsular or blood vessel invasion. In light of this fact, it seems unreasonable to base judgment on a minute sample of tissue that may be far from representative and often may not include some of the capsule. At times the needle does not strike the tissue desired or there is considerable fluid obtained, suggesting that the sample of tissue may be undergoing necrosis and is not representative. It should be noted that a surprising number of cystic lesions prove to be papillary carcinomas. In view of these uncertainties and the relative simplicity (in experienced hands) of removing a mass after careful physical examination and scanning, surgical removal is the best way to treat cold nodules. The abundance of vital structures in the relatively small areas of the neck requires that those who do attempt needle biopsy should be thoroughly acquainted with the anatomy of the thyroid area. Puncture of the trachea or esophagus or the formation of hematomas is not unheard of, even in experienced hands.

THYROID CYSTS

True epithelial-lined cysts of the thyroid, other than thyroglossal duct cysts, are rare but degenerating cystic adenomas are quite common. They are cold to isotope scan unless there is a rind of hyperfunctioning tissue surrounding the liquid but within a capsule. Aspiration or needle biopsy may not answer the question of malignancy in the individual patient. There is little point in finding out whether or not a lesion is cystic, because if it is negative the situation demands more inquiry and if it is positive prompt surgical exploration is required.

HASHIMOTO'S THYROIDITIS

Hashimoto's thyroiditis is an unusually common disease. Early in its development there are often localized areas of lymphocytic infiltration that take the form of a firm nodule. These pose a diagnostic problem compared to the more obvious diagnosis when the disease is diffuse, lobulated and firm. Since the nodule of Hashimoto's disease replaces normal thyroid tissue, the area is cold on scan. The slightly irregular margins and firmness prompt suspicion that it may be an infiltrating carcinoma. Needle biopsy may be helpful, but mild degrees of diffuse lymphocytic infiltration in what seems to be a normal thyroid may give reassuring but misleading results if the point of the needle should miss the mass. Local surgical excision may be the only safe way to rule out carcinoma. Various specific thyroid antibody tests may be helpful here if the titer is high and the observation is in younger individuals. The presence of antibodies may also be misleading. If the sample of tissue is inadequate or the histologic appearance is inconclusive, formal biopsy is advisable.

The diffuse lobulated firm type of Hashimoto's thyroiditis is a less serious diagnostic problem. The physical examination reveals no dominant area that commands attention. The scan usually shows a diffusely mottled pattern of uptake.

The chronic phase of granulomatous thyroiditis may be confused with a neoplastic process. The hardness and irregularity arouse suspicion. There is often a mild to moderate degree of hypothyroidism. Here the "nodules" found on palpation represent compensatory hypertrophy of less involved areas of the gland. The scan, when precisely related to nodules in the gland, is reassuring and the administration of thyroxine causes those hypertrophied areas to shrink. The hypertrophied areas are not true neoplasms.

TREATMENT OF THYROID NODULES WITH THYROID HORMONE AS A DIAGNOSTIC PROCEDURE

The administration of thyroid hormone has been advocated by some as a diagnostic maneuver for thyroid nodules. There are two types of "nodular goiter." A distinction between the two, primarily on the basis of physical examination, is used for deciding whether thyroid hormone should be tried in a patient with a lumpy goiter. One is the diffusely lobulated or bosselated gland that is a manifestation of a low-grade chronic hormone deficiency state (not detectable by usual laboratory tests) in which case the entire gland is responding to a stimulus to fulfill a need. The entire gland slowly develops chronic hypertrophy. The gland becomes lobulated. On light palpation a sense of masses may be obtained but on deep aggressive palpation there is no asymmetry and no discrete spherical mass stands out. The patient with this gland should be given a diagnostic trial of thyroxine, which amounts to suppressive therapy. If this course is chosen, the physician has two obligations: (1) enough hormone must be given to suppress activity of the gland, usually 0.3 mg of levothyroxine a day; and (2) the same physician who started the trial should reexamine the gland after 6 or 8 weeks to make sure that the gland has decreased in size and that no discrete masses previously buried in the enlarged gland have become evident.

The other type of "nodular goiter" contains one or more discrete areas that stand out as masses. These seem to have margins and display a different consistency than the remaining parenchyma of the gland. These lesions are usually neoplasms, adenomas or possibly carcinomas. If the mass(es) drawing attention is shown by scanning to be functionally different from the remainder of the gland, the evidence for a neoplasm (benign or malignant) is increased. Neoplasms are not benefited by giving thyroid hormone. It has been argued that such neoplasms may shrink, and the evidence seems overwhelming to some observers that they do shrink. The dramatic shrinkage observed is either attributable to resorption of necrotic debris and fluid secondary to spontaneous necrosis or due to shrinkage of the extranodular tissue that seemed to make the goiter smaller but on careful examination did not make the masses smaller. It is usually the occurrence of necrosis in an adenoma that causes swelling and takes the patient to the doctor. This sets the stage for misinterpretation, if thyroid hormone is given. The author has never seen a true adenoma shrink significantly or disappear (only to regrow in time) that could not be shown upon removal to be caused by recent spontaneous necrosis and resorption. Cold lesions should be excised by a surgeon experienced with thyroid surgery. It is useless to give a trial of thyroid hormone therapy for discrete masses.

THE DIAGNOSTIC SURGICAL APPROACH TO THE THYROID MASS

The surgical approach to a thyroid mass is based on the suspicion that the lesion may be malignant. A careful physical examination should set the tone of thinking regarding the probable course to be taken. The surgical objective is to make a diagnosis and to accomplish all that is necessary at a single operation.

First consideration is whether the lesion represents a lobulated gland or a gland bearing a single mass or a dominant mass among others of less significance. The single mass usually deserves more prompt action than multiple masses. If the mass is not cold on scan and not a discrete lesion that is different from the rest of the gland, then suppression therapy with thyroxine may be tried. If the mass is cold on scan, surgical removal, not just biopsy, must be strongly considered.

The hot nodule (on scan) is preferably removed surgically with preservation of all extra nodular tissue that is possible. The hot nodule is not malignant but occasionally another separate mass that is malignant may exist in the same gland. There is no place for thyroxine therapy in the case of the hot nodule; its removal is simple and definitive. Radioiodine may be given. The radiation preferentially is delivered to the mass; however, it requires a larger dose of the isotope than Graves' disease and the mass, although diminished in function, often remains physically present.

Cold nodules should be removed or a good reason found for not doing so. Growth, hardness, and fixation of the lesion; voice change; sense of pressure; and solitary nature of the lesion in a male suggest urgency in that order. Thyroxine supplement will not make discrete neoplasms go away. Its use in the cold nodule may waste valuable time.

Complete surgical excision is the most effective method of cure of carcinoma of the thyroid. At least it is the first step in the use of other forms of therapy. Although "cure" rate for most of the carcinomas is quite high in experienced hands, a prompt and definite diagnosis enhances that success.

The removal of lesions that prove to be simple adenomas is accomplished with minimal risk in the hands of surgeons with experience. There is little sacrifice of normal tissue and subsequent thyroid supplement is seldom required.

A logical surgical approach is as follows. All patients with thyroid masses should receive a trace amount of radioiodine before surgery (often the residual from a scan). A small incision is used in the hope that simple removal is all that will be required, but the incision should be large enough for examination of both lobes so that no other masses are left behind. A search is made for any suspicious lymph nodes lying immediately adjacent to the lesion. Unless there is a gross hint of malignancy, the mass is excised without violation of the capsule and with preservation of all normal tissue possible. Frozen section diagnosis and a radioiodine assay of the tumor is performed during surgery. If the frozen section shows the lesion to be malignant, the remainder of the entire lobe and isthmus are removed. If by chance the diagnosis is inconclusive and the sample of tumor contains very little radioiodine on assay, the entire lobe is removed completely, regardless of the histologic uncertainty because the final diagnosis may be positive. The adjacent lymph nodes that drain the area of the tumor are removed and examined. It is a foregone conclusion that the recurrent laryngeal nerve is meticulously traced and preserved, as are both parathyroids adjacent to that lobe. If the lesion is malignant and contains minute amounts of radioiodine on assay and at least some follicular structure is present, then all normal thyroid tissue is completely removed in preparation for radioiodine therapy, if metastases should subsequently appear. (The assay of function of the lesion will already be available in case it is needed.)

If lymph nodes are involved, wide excision of nodes within the lymphatic drainage area is carried out as indicated by sampling of nodes by frozen section. In experienced hands, damage to the recurrent laryngeal nerve is extremely rare (unless it is deliberately sacrificed because of the proximity of the disease). Postoperative parathyroid insufficiency is rare if the parathyroids are carefully identified and saved on their vascular pedicles. If deficiency should occur, it is only temporary, even if transplantation of parathyroid tissue is necessary. If total thyroidectomy was intended in anticipation of future use of radioiodine, the operative field is surveyed for residual radioactivity while the wound remains open. This is done to be sure that absolutely all functioning thyroid tissue has been removed before the wound is closed. There will then never be a question of whether subsequent uptake of radioiodine in the area is attributable to residual normal tissue or to recurrent disease. Although all lymph node–bearing tissue is meticulously removed, extend-

ing down into the upper mediastinum, gross mutilation does not result. The sternocleidomastoid that was disconnected from the sternum to permit wide dissection is reattached to preserve the normal contour of the neck. Thus each step of the surgical procedure is a diagnostic maneuver to accomplish eradication of the disease at that operation.

HYPERPARA-THYROIDISM

by GIRAUD V. FOSTER, M.D., Ph.D., and TAH HSIUNG HSU, M.D.

Baltimore, Maryland

Hyperparathyroidism is a condition of increased activity of the parathyroid glands characterized by hypersecretion of parathyroid hormone. Once thought of as a rare disease usually associated with striking manifestations, it is now detected by demonstration of hypercalcemia by multichannel screening methods as frequently as in one in a thousand patients. In many of these, the disease begins insidiously, follows a benign course, and is only manifested by subtle symptoms.

Classically a distinction is made between primary, secondary, and tertiary hyperparathyroidism. Primary hyperparathyroidism arises de novo from unknown causes. In 92 per cent of patients it is due to adenoma, in 6 per cent it is secondary to hyperplasia, and in 2 per cent it is caused by carcinoma of the parathyroids. In an unselected population, the incidence of primary hyperparathyroidism far exceeds that of secondary or tertiary disease. Secondary hyperparathyroidism arises as a consequence of hypocalcemic stimulation of the parathyroid glands. Most frequently this is secondary to renal failure but can be induced by any condition with low levels of serum calcium that are often accompanied by hyperphosphatemia or caused by it. In a small percentage of these patients, it is thought that the secretory activity of one or more parathyroid glands becomes independent of the serum calcium concentration. This state of autonomy is referred to as tertiary hyperparathyroidism. While this is a useful concept, present methods of diagnosis are insufficiently refined to identify with assurance those patients with true autonomous secretion.

Since the clinical features of secondary hyperparathyroidism are usually dominated by the underlying disease, the following discussion is restricted to primary hyperparathyroidism and to neoplasms that secrete a substance that is either immunologically or biologically similar or identical to parathyroid hormone.

CLINICAL PRESENTATION AND CONSIDERATIONS AFFECTING INDEX OF SUSPICION

Suspicion that hyperparathyroidism is present should always be entertained whenever one of the following factors is present: (1) relatively asymptomic hypercalcemia, (2) clinical evidence of excess parathyroid hormone or hypercalcemia or both, (3) family history of hyperparathyroidism, and (4) conditions associated with an increased incidence of hyperparathyroidism, inclusive of multiple endocrine adenoma syndromes and malignant tumors that secrete biologically active polypeptides. The mode of presentation of hyperparathyroidism is largely determined by the association with one or more of the forementioned.

Relatively Asymptomic Hypercalcemia. The majority of these patients are brought to the attention of a physician because of the fortuitous discovery of previously unsuspected hypercalcemia. When documented to have been present for more than 1 year, hypercalcemia is less likely to be due to a cause that is difficult to exclude. Many of these patients are either asymptomatic or have nonspecific complaints. The most frequent symptoms, when present, are lethargy, loss of ability to perform simple calculations, and a general failure to function normally, both intellectually and physically. These frequently can only be appreciated in retrospect following correction of hypercalcemia.

Clinical Evidence of Hypercalcemia or Excess Parathyroid Hormone. Patients with chronic hypercalcemia commonly present with a history of renal colic or stones. About 6 to 15 per cent of all patients with renal stones eventually are found to have hyperparathyroidism. Before present-day screening of blood biochemical parameters by multichannel analysis, many patients were first seen with bone pain, progressive kyphosis, or fractures as a result of osteitis fibrosa cystica. Today, advanced bone disease is less often seen. Some clinicians believe that hyperparathyroidism presenting with renal lithiasis and hyperparathyroidism with skeletal involvement constitute separate disease entities, since the concomitant occurrence of both complications is relatively rare. While this generalization holds true in adults, it does not in children, in whom more often than not both kidney and bone problems are present in the same patient.

Other signs and symptoms associated with excess parathyroid hormone production and hypercalcemia are listed in Table 1. Hyperparathyroidism should always be considered in the differential diagnosis of unexplained gastrointestinal complaints, osteoporosis, muscle weakness, or changes in sensorium or intellect.

Physical findings associated with hyperparathyroidism are usually secondary to acute or chronic hypercalcemia and are most often too nonspecific to be of diagnostic value. Only a few cases of parathyroid adenoma presenting as a palpable neck tumor have been reported. Band keratopathy, a result of chronic hypercalcemia, is a useful diagnostic sign but rarely present. Roentgenologic changes observed in bone are frequently important in suggesting the disease and are summarized in Table 2. The most useful sign is subperiosteal resorption of the phalanges.

Family History of Hyperparathyroidism. In the absence of polyglandular disease, less than 1 per cent of patients appear to have inherited their condition. When present, familial hyperparathyroidism usually declares itself in childhood as an autosomal dominant disease, frequently runs a stormy course, and can be

Table 1. *Signs and Symptoms of Hyperparathyroidism*

Ocular
  Calcium deposits in cornea, palpebral fissures, (conjunctiva, sclera, lens, and uveal tract)°
Neuromuscular
  Vague to overt changes in mentation, apathy, anxiety, depression, confusion, psychosis; hypoactive deep tendon reflexes, diminished vibratory appreciation, paresthesias (long tract signs, deafness, visual impairment, papilledema); muscle fatigue, tongue fasciculation, hypotonia, proximal muscle weakness, muscle wasting (muscle pain, abnormalities of gait, paresis, dysphagia, hoarseness, dysphonia, aphasia)
Cardiovascular
  Hypertension, increased sensitivity to digitalis, conduction disturbances (especially supraventricular arrhythmias)
Gastrointestinal
  Anorexia, nausea, vomiting, weight loss, epigastric distress, peptic ulcer disease, constipation, pancreatitis (pancreatic insufficiency)
Renal
  Renal colic, stones, polydipsia, polyuria, symptoms of renal failure
Skeletal, Dental, and Rheumatologic
  (Bone pain; loose teeth, epulis, arthritis, arthralgias)
Dermal
  (Pruritus, recurrent ecchymosis, gangrene)

°Those that are rarely observed are indicated in parentheses.

Table 2. *Common Radiologic Changes in Primary Hyperparathyroidism*

Osteopenia
Early and often subtle erosive changes observed in metacarpals: best demonstrated using fine grain industrial film. In more advanced disease shortening of the terminal phalanges, generalized evidence of demineralization, bone deformities, and pathologic fractures can be seen.

Bone Cysts
Most commonly found in clavicles, ribs, and mandible and less commonly in skull and long bones.

Calcification of Soft Tissues
Structures most often affected include walls of great arteries and renal parenchyma (nephrocalcinosis). Lungs, pancreas, stomach, and subcutaneous tissues infrequently affected.

Stones
Stones in kidney, bladder, prostate, and gallbladder are occasionally observed.

Loss of Lamina Dura
Dental abnormalities rarely occur in absence of skeletal changes.

Metaphyseal Sclerosis
More commonly seen in association with secondary hyperparathyroidism. When present, changes are most apparent in vertebrae.

Table 3. *Causes of Hypercalcemia*

Common
Malignancies (especially breast and lung, with or without osseous metastases)
Hyperparathyroidism

Less Common
Milk-alkali syndrome
Sarcoidosis
Multiple myeloma
Hypervitaminosis D
Drug-induced (thiazides, estrogens, vitamin A)

Rare
Thyrotoxicosis
Addison's disease
Immobilization
Hypercalcemia of infancy
Pheochromocytoma

---

associated with other endocrinopathies. The diagnosis is usually made by close observance of serum calcium over a period of years. Primarily because of early detection, most patients are without symptoms when the condition is first recognized.

Conditions Associated with an Increased Incidence of Hyperparathyroidism. Parathyroid adenomas are suspected in all patients with multiple endocrine adenoma (MEA) syndromes inclusive of MEA I (adenomas of the pituitary, pancreas, adrenal, thyroid, parathyroid, and gastrin-secreting cells), MEA II (medullary carcinoma of the thyroid, parathyroid adenoma, and pheochromocytoma), and MEA III (medullary carcinoma of the thyroid, parathyroid adenoma, pheochromocytoma, marfanoid habitus, mucosal neuromas, medullated corneal nerve fibers, ganglioneuromatosis, and skin lesions of the von Recklinghausen variety), as well as in patients with malignancies known or thought to secrete a parathyroid hormone–like substance. Of these neoplasms the most common are those of kidney or lung. In every patient with proven elevations of parathyroid hormone, a diligent search must be carried out to exclude tumors of these organs.

Recently as many as 30 per cent of all patients with hyperparathyroidism have been reported to have had radiation to the head or neck for benign disease in childhood. Parathyroid hyperfunction is associated with doses as low as 300 rads, occurs concomitantly in some in-stances with thyroid carcinoma, and has a peak incidence 20 to 30 years after initial exposure.

DIAGNOSTIC APPROACH

The cornerstones of the diagnosis of hyperparathyroidism in a patient under suspicion are: (1) confirmation of hypercalcemia, (2) exclusion of other causes of elevated serum calcium (Table 3), (3) verification of inappropriately high levels of parathyroid hormone, and (4) localization of the source of excessive parathyroid hormone secretion. Since few medical facilities are able to provide the results of serum parathyroid hormone (PTH) in less than a few weeks and because inherent problems in current radioimmunoassays of PTH have not as yet been resolved, assessment of PTH-related biochemical changes and exclusion of nonparathyroid hormone causes of hypercalcemia are still essential in practice.

Confirmation of Hypercalcemia. The cardinal manifestation of hyperparathyroidism is hypercalcemia, which is usually present at least at some time during the course of the disease. In those few patients in whom it is not observed, ionic calcium is most likely elevated. Determination of ionic calcium, however, is technically difficult, subject to errors from inappropriate collection of specimens, and is generally not available to most clinicians.

Because demonstration of hypercalcemia is pivotal to the diagnosis, before further testing is done, elevated serum calcium levels should be confirmed in two or more blood samples obtained on different occasions. Collection of blood should be made without venous stasis, which can spuriously elevate the concentration of calcium. Furthermore, since approximately 30 per cent of serum calcium is bound to albumin, aberrations in the serum albumin can effect changes in total serum calcium. If albumin concentrations are subnormal, the calcium level can be corrected by adding 0.8 mg per dl (100 ml) for each 1 gram of albumin per dl below the normal limit.

Exclusion of Other Causes of Hypercalcemia. Once hypercalcemia is firmly established, its cause should be determined. The diagnosis of hyperparathyroidism often can be inferred by exclusion of other causes of hypercalcemia (Table 3). This can usually be done by taking a thorough history and performing a complete physical examination and, indirectly, by searching for biochemical changes other than hypercalcemia that are induced by excessive parathyroid hormone.

An exacting history is obtained to exclude intake of thiazide diuretics, excessive calcium concurrently with alkali, and supraphysiologic amounts of vitamin A or D as well as symptoms of any underlying disease known to produce hypercalcemia. When possible, family members should be questioned, since hypercalcemia can adversely alter the patient's memory. A complete physical examination and appropriate x-rays are required to exclude malignancy or sarcoidosis. Likewise, serum electrophoresis is necessary to exclude multiple myeloma. Unless there is a history of immobilization or an elevated alkaline phosphatase, a bone survey to rule out Paget's disease is seldom warranted. Similarly, diagnostic investigations to exclude Addison's disease, thyrotoxicosis, and pheochromocytoma are not required unless these conditions are suspected on clinical grounds. In special instances in which hypercalcemia might be caused by hyperabsorption of calcium by the gut, as in sarcoid, milk-alkali syndrome, or vitamin D intoxication, a cortisone suppression test is frequently useful. This is carried out by measuring the blood calcium levels before, during, and after daily administration of 120 mg of cortisone acetate for 7 to 10 days.

Concomitant primary hyperparathyroidism has been reported in patients with thyrotoxicosis, sarcoid, Paget's disease, and a variety of malignancies. Association with these conditions is rare but important since hyperparathyroidism must, on occasion, be excluded even in patients with apparent nonparathyroid-related causes of hypercalcemia.

Confirmatory Laboratory Findings. Other laboratory findings that may help to support the diagnosis of primary hyperparathyroidism include hypophosphatemia, which is present in 50 per cent of patients, and hyperchloremic acidosis, present in 30 per cent. These abnormalities are consequences of enhanced urinary excretion of phosphate and bicarbonate, respectively. In the absence of renal insufficiency, urinary calcium excretion is increased in proportion to the magnitude of hypercalcemia. However, since parathyroid hormone enhances calcium reabsorption by the renal tubules, excretion of calcium is less in hyperparathyroidism than in hypercalcemia from other causes. Consequently, in hyperparathyroidism, urinary calcium excretion rarely exceeds 400 mg per day.

Other laboratory tests, inclusive of renal tubular reabsorption of phosphate, urinary excretion of hydroxyproline, serum uric acid, and serum alkaline phosphatase, are insufficiently specific to be diagnostically useful.

Recently, urinary cyclic AMP has been demonstrated to be a sensitive, albeit nonspecific, indirect index of hyperparathyroidism. It is elevated in about 95 per cent of patients with the disease, even in those who do not have consistently elevated levels of parathyroid hormone. While this is not diagnostic of hyperparathyroidism, patients with hypercalcemia due to other causes have normal values with the exception of thyrotoxicosis and pheochromocytoma. These can readily be excluded by appropriate studies if indicated.

Verification of Inappropriately High Blood Levels of Parathyroid Hormone. Concurrent with carrying out laboratory studies to support the diagnosis of hyperparathyroidism and exclude other causes of hypercalcemia, it is present practice to measure parathyroid hormone if the clinical index of suspicion is high. The diagnosis of hyperparathyroidism is confirmed by demonstrating supranormal levels or levels that are inappropriately high with respect to the ambient plasma calcium. In the absence of the disease, hypercalcemia should suppress parathyroid hormone secretion. Consequently, an elevated or normal level of parathyroid hormone in the presence of hypercalcemia should theoretically indicate hyperparathyroidism and low levels exclude the disease. Despite the availability of reasonably reliable radioimmunoassays for parathyroid hormone, confirmation of the diagnosis may be fraught with difficulties. Among these may be the following:

1. Levels of parathyroid hormone may not accurately reflect secretion rate. Parathyroid hormone is heterogeneous in serum. Characteristically, biologically intact hormone and active fragments containing the N–terminal portion of the molecule are short-lived and, when detectable, are found only in low concentrations. The predominant and most readily measured form is the biologically inert carboxy-terminal fragment. It is against this carboxy-terminal portion of the molecule that most antisera used in currently available radio-

immunoassays are directed. As a consequence, most commercially available radioimmuno-assays measure predominantly biologically inactive fragments.

2. Small adenomas may only intermittently be associated with elevated parathyroid hormone levels, since elevations of parathyroid hormone and calcium are usually related to tumor size. For this reason serial determinations of plasma calcium may be required, with only those specimens with demonstrated elevated levels being submitted for parathyroid hormone determination.

3. Measurement of parathyroid hormone cannot differentiate between primary hyperparathyroidism and parathyroid hormone-secreting neoplasms. The problem has three elements. First, the magnitude of the levels is not helpful in distinguishing between these two conditions. Second, demonstration of immunologically active hormone does not preclude the possibility of a biologically inert or partially inert circulating substance, be it prohormone or otherwise. Third, if recent reports are to be believed, a high percentage of patients with malignancies may have, in fact, concomitant primary hyperparathyroidism.

4. Serum parathyroid hormone levels are frequently elevated in renal insufficiency. The diagnosis of primary hyperparathyroidism in a patient with coexistent renal failure or with renal failure as a result of chronic hyperparathyroidism is therefore not possible unless hypercalcemia has been documented before the onset of renal failure.

5. Factors other than serum calcium can affect the secretion of parathyroid hormone. Parathyroid hormone levels are occasionally elevated in patients following lithium treatment, ingestion of supraphysiologic amounts of vitamin A, and prolonged immobilization. In contrast, excessive secretion of hormone by parathyroid tumors can be inhibited by hypomagnesemia. It is therefore imperative to obtain a relevant history and measure serum magnesium in all patients in whom hyperparathyroidism is suspected.

Localization of Parathyroid Tumors. In the hands of experienced parathyroid surgeons, 95 per cent of parathyroid tumors are found during initial exploration of the neck. The remainder, however, may not be readily located, especially if they are small, imbedded in the thyroid, or are within the mediastinum. Differential venous catheterization of the neck veins coupled with concomitant measurement of parathyroid hormone from multiple sites (using, if possible, an assay in which the antibody is directed against the intact or N–terminal portion of the hormone) is recommended in these latter pa-

tients. The success rate of this procedure, however, may be impaired by previous neck exploration, since postoperative scar tissue may cause anatomic distortion of major vessels. For this reason localization of a tumor can be anticipated in only about half the patients studied. It is the general opinion that this test is not warranted before the initial operation, since the probability of the surgeon finding the tumor exceeds the probability that it will be discovered using the method and false-positive results may be misleading. Other tests to localize parathyroid tumors — inclusive of massage of the neck followed by measurement of peripheral parathyroid hormone, ultrasound, 75-seleno-methionine scanning, and thermography — are probably of little use. Only selective arteriography, when carried out in conjunction with differential neck vein catherization, can be of help.

Figure 1 summarizes our approach for distinguishing primary hyperparathyroidism from other causes of hypercalcemia in patients in whom parathyroid hormone has been measured.

CLINICAL COURSE

Since the pattern of presentation of hyperparathyroidism is changing with more asymptomatic or mildly symptomatic patients being discovered serendipitously, prospective studies are urgently needed to re-evaluate the clinical course of the disease. At the present time only the following points warrant comment. First, it would appear that only approximately 20 per cent of patients initially diagnosed when asymptomatic require surgery within a 5-year period. Second, hyperparathyroidism is more likely to be more severe in children than in adults. Third, adenomatous changes may occur in more than one parathyroid gland in approximately 6 per cent of patients. Fourth, hypercalcemic crises can occur suddenly. Symptoms associated with hypercalcemic crises may include sudden onset of anorexia, nausea, vomiting, hypotension, polydipsia, polyuria, confusion, coma, and even death. Usually serum calcium levels exceed 16 mg per dl. In most instances of testing no precipitating event is found, but in some patients dehydration, immobilization, thiazide therapy, phosphate depletion commonly induced by antacids, and onset of menopause precede the development of symptoms.

COMPLICATIONS

The principal complications of hyperparathyroidism in terms of both severity and frequency

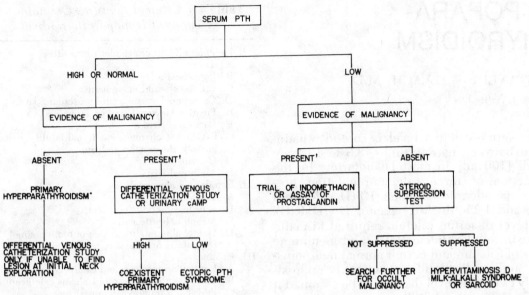

Figure 1. Flow chart for distinguishing primary hyperparathyroidism from other causes of hypercalcemia in patients in whom thyroid hormone has been measured.

are (1) changes induced by hypercalcemia, (2) renal diseases inclusive of nephrolithiasis, nephrocalcinosis, and renal failure, and (3) bone diseases inclusive of osteitis fibrosa cystica, osteoporosis, and metaphyseal sclerosis. Other complications are implicit in the signs and symptoms listed in Table 1. Of special clinical importance are dehydration, mental obtundation, and increased sensitivity to digitalis, since they contribute to mortality.

HYPERCALCEMIA ASSOCIATED WITH MALIGNANT DISEASE

Hypercalcemia is a common complication of malignant disease. In a survey of 450 patients admitted to a general hospital for radiotherapy of cancer, 9 per cent had hypercalcemia. In most instances the hypercalcemia appears abruptly and late in the course of the disease when the diagnosis is already obvious. In some patients, however, the tumor may be occult, and an extensive search for the neoplasm is necessary. The elevated serum calcium may be due to (1) production of parathyroid hormone or a parathyroid hormone–like substance (ectopic hyperparathyroidism); (2) secretion by the tumor of prostaglandins, osteoclast-activating factor or a vitamin D–like sterol; or (3) coexistent primary hyperparathyroidism. Of these, the

first and the last entities are associated with high serum parathyroid hormone levels. Therefore whenever hyperparathyroidism is confirmed by radioimmunoassay of parathyroid hormone, cognizance must be given to the possibility that abnormal levels are due to a parathyroid hormone-secreting neoplasm. Since the majority of these are either lung or renal cell carcinomas, chest films and intravenous pyelograms should be obtained to exclude their presence.

Osteoclastic activating factor is often produced by myeloma cells, while in other tumors hypercalcemia may be mediated by prostaglandins. Patients with both conditions usually have low serum parathyroid hormone levels. If prostaglandin assays are unavailable, excessive prostaglandin activity can often be inferred by the lowering of serum calcium produced by a therapeutic trial of indomethacin or salicylates.

Extensive diagnostic investigation of hypercalcemia in patients with well-documented, far-advanced incurable malignancies is usually not encouraged unless aggressive treatment is intended. The ultimate decision to pursue a vigorous search for the cause should depend upon the relative advantages and disadvantages of palliative therapy as an alternative to surgery and upon the patient's immediate prognosis.

HYPOPARA-THYROIDISM

By STANLEY WALLACH, M.D.

Albany, New York

The serum calcium level is carefully maintained between narrow limits (8.6 to 10.4 mg per dl [100 ml] in most laboratories) by the interaction of three calcium-regulating hormones, parathyroid hormone (PTH), calcitonin (CT), and 1,25-dihydroxyvitamin D_3 (DHCC). The level of serum calcium required to maintain extracellular, intracellular, and membrane levels of calcium and permit normal neuromuscular and cardiovascular function is approximately twice the level that would be assumed if physicochemical solubility characteristics prevailed and no hormonal control were present. In that event, the serum calcium level would decline to levels of 3.5 to 5.0 mg per dl.

Any trend toward hypocalcemia generates compensory secretion of PTH and decreases the stimulus for CT secretion. The increase in the plasma PTH level, in turn, stimulates the renal tubular cells to augment their 1-hydroxylase activity and a larger amount of DHCC is thereby produced from its circulating precursor, 25-hydroxyvitamin D_3. The physiologic adjustments that occur as a result of these changes in hormonal secretion are an increase in calcium absorption ($\uparrow$ DHCC), an increase in renal tubular reabsorption of filtered calcium ($\uparrow$ PTH, $\downarrow$ CT), and most importantly, an increase in bone resorption ($\uparrow$ PTH, $\downarrow$ CT, $\uparrow$ DHCC). All three adjustments will correct the initial hypocalcemic stimulus and once this is accomplished, hormone secretion may return to basal levels. It is therefore evident that PTH is the major hormone involved in this aspect of calcium homeostasis and a loss of parathyroid function will lead to hypocalcemia and a derangement in physiologic functions dependent on normocalcemia.

Permanent deficiency of parathyroid function may result from (1) spontaneous degeneration of the parathyroid glands (idiopathic hypoparathyroidism), (2) infarctive degeneration or removal of the parathyroid glands secondary to surgical procedures of the neck (postoperative hypoparathyroidism), and (3) a defect in end-organ (skeleton, kidney) responses to secreted parathyroid hormone (pseudohypoparathyroidism). Physical findings and routine laboratory data common to all three types of hypoparathyroidism are shown in Table 1. The severity of these physical findings and laboratory abnor-

Table 1. *Clinical Features Common to All Types of Hypoparathyroidism*

I. Heightened neuromuscular irritability
  A. Tremor
  B. Paresthesias
  C. Choreoathetoid movements
  D. Carpopedal spasm, other muscular spasms
  E. Positive Chvostek and/or Trousseau's sign
  F. Laryngeal stridor
  G. Psychiatric changes: emotional lability, irritability, anxiety, depression, delirium
  H. Convulsions
  I. Abnormal EEG
II. Ectodermal abnormalities
  A. Coarse skin
  B. Hair loss on body and scalp
  C. Atrophic, brittle nails
  D. Dental abnormalities: lack of tooth enamel; hypoplasia or aplasia of teeth
III. Calcinosis
  A. Lenticular opacities and cataracts
  B. Basal ganglia and choroid plexus calcification
  C. Peripheral tendon calcinosis
IV. Biochemical abnormalities
  A. Hypocalcemia
  B. High normal to high serum PO_4
  C. Decreased urine calcium and phosphate excretion
  D. Low or normal plasma iPTH level
  E. Low or normal cyclic AMP excretion
V. Other
  A. Abnormal ECG: prolonged QT interval, slurred QRS complex, ST and T wave changes
  B. Skeletal x-rays: osteosclerosis or osteopenia; absence of rachitic changes
  C. Increased spinal fluid pressure and/or papilledema

malities depend not only on the degree of parathyroid hypofunction and resultant hypocalcemia but also on the duration of the hypofunction and resultant hypocalcemia before appropriate treatment is given. The physical findings involving heightened neuromuscular irritability range from tremor through choreiform movements and carpopedal spasm to grand mal seizures. Calcium is required to maintain the stability of neural and muscle fiber membranes and when hypocalcemia occurs, loss of calcium from critical neuromuscular membrane loci causes impulses to flow too easily through the system, leading to inappropriate tetanic manifestations. Peculiarly, there is wide variability among patients as to which of the manifestations indicated in Table 1 will occur. In general, the more severe and sudden the hypocalcemia, the more neuromuscular irritability will be observed. However, there are many exceptions to this rule and patients with total serum calcium levels of 5 mg per dl may have no manifestations of increased neuromuscular irritability, spontaneous or provoked.

Patients with prolonged hypocalcemia, especially if it is caused by hypoparathyroidism, will frequently develop lenticular opacities that may progress to mature cataract formation. Less frequently, they may develop calcinosis of the basal ganglia and/or choroid plexus of the brain and of peripheral tendons. The reason for calcium deposition despite hypocalcemia is unknown but may be a peculiar sensitivity of these structures to deposit amorphous calcium phosphate when the serum PO_4 is markedly elevated. Brain calcinosis is usually asymptomatic, although there have been sporadic reports of extrapyramidal manifestations in such patients. Tendon calcinosis may cause acute episodes of calcific tendinitis.

Table 2 outlines the features of each of the three types of hypoparathyroidism that are unique to that particular type. Except for occasional pseudohypoparathyroid patients who may show none of the physical stigmata of that type and also may have partial responses to injected parathyroid hormone, confusion between the three types should not occur. Rarely, pseudohypoparathyroid patients may shuttle back and forth between hypocalcemia and normocalcemia, indicating that there is a variable defect in end-organ sensitivity to PTH. They may also remain permanently hypocalcemic or normocalcemic and in the latter instance (pseudopseudohypoparathyroidism), the diagnosis requires that some physical stigmata of the condition be present. If there is a family history of pseudo- or

Table 2. *Distinguishing Clinical Features of Various Types of Hypoparathyroidism*

I. Idiopathic hypoparathyroidism
   A. Autoantibodies to parathyroid cells, other endocrine organs, intrinsic factor, gastric parietal cells, etc.
   B. Associated endocrine deficiencies, pernicious anemia, vitiligo, mucocutaneous moniliasis, etc.
   C. Positive modified Ellsworth-Howard test (increase in urinary cyclic AMP and phosphate excretion); positive calcemic response to prolonged administration of parathyroid extract
II. Postoperative hypoparathyroidism
   A. History of neck surgery with onset of clinical features of hypoparathyroidism 1 day to several years after surgery
   B. Positive modified Ellsworth-Howard test as per above
III. Pseudohypoparathyroidism
   A. Short stature
   B. Rounded face
   C. Mental retardation variable
   D. Shortened metacarpal, metatarsal, and/or phalangeal bones
   E. Ectopic bone formation, calcinosis, and/or skeletal exostoses
   F. Normal or high plasma iPTH level
   G. Subnormal response to modified Ellsworth-Howard test and/or discordant results between renal and skeletal responses to administered parathyroid extract

---

pseudopseudohypoparathyroidism, this may also be of diagnostic value.

The major differential diagnostic problem is to distinguish hypoparathyroid patients from among a larger group of hypocalcemic patients. As indicated in Table 3, there are relatively few conditions in which hypocalcemia can occur, and distinguishing characteristics will usually point to the correct diagnosis. The severity of the decrease in the serum calcium is not often helpful, since any of the diagnoses in Table 3 can cause profound hypocalcemia. In general, however, idiopathic and pseudohypoparathyroidism tend to cause very low serum calcium levels (3.5 to 6.0 mg per dl), whereas in postoperative hypoparathyroidism and other hypocalcemic conditions, serum calcium levels of 6.5 to 8.0 mg per dl are more usual. The serum PO_4 level may also be helpful because in hypoparathyroidism, the serum PO_4 ranges from high normal to very high levels (4.5 to 10.0 mg per dl), whereas in hypocalcemic conditions other than renal insufficiency, serum PO_4 levels are usually normal or low. However, there are notable exceptions to this rule. Finally, the plasma PTH level, determined by a radioimmunoassay that is somewhat insensitive (iPTH), is usually not helpful because normal subjects may have nondetectable iPTH levels and hypoparathyroid patients may have detectable circulating iPTH within the low to mid-normal range. However, hypocalcemic patients with normal parathyroid function should theoretically have stimulation of their parathyroid glands to greater than normal secretion.

The finding of a high iPTH level in a hypocalcemic patient rules out idiopathic and postoperative hypoparathyroidism but not pseudohypoparathyroidism. The latter type of patients have normal parathyroid gland secretory ability and may react to hypocalcemia with increased levels of iPTH that do not trigger expected end-organ responses. There is also one reported case of a hypocalcemic patient with an increased iPTH level in whom normal responses to injected PTH were observed, suggesting that the patient secreted a "counterfeit" PTH that was immunologically similar to authentic PTH but was biologically inactive.

In summary, the diagnosis of hypoparathyroidism requires a low serum calcium level and a high normal to distinctly high serum PO_4 with normal serum protein levels and no evidence of renal insufficiency. Clinical findings of heightened neuromuscular irritability and brain or tendon calcinosis are compatible clinical features, but cannot be used to make a diagnosis in the absence of hypocalcemia, since they may occur on an idiopathic basis. The neuromuscular abnormalities can also be produced by al-

Table 3. *Other Causes of Hypocalcemia*

Common Causes	*Distinguishing Features*
1. Pseudohypocalcemia (normal ionic Ca^{++} with low serum protein bound Ca moiety)	No signs or symptoms of hypocalcemia, low serum albumin, normal ionic Ca^{++} (if available).
2. Renal insufficiency	Increased BUN and serum creatinine.
3. Malabsorption	Steatorrhea, multiple mineral and vitamin deficiencies, decreased serum Mg, other characteristics of the particular type of malabsorption present.
4. Alcoholism	History of alcohol abuse, signs of cirrhosis of the liver, decreased serum PO_4 and Mg.
5. Malnutrition	Evidence of cachexia and inadequate food intake, multiple mineral and vitamin deficiencies.
Unusual Causes	
1. High-dose glucocorticoid administration	History of glucocorticoid treatment, evidence of Cushing's syndrome.
2. Acute pancreatitis	Severe abdominal pain, fever, hypotension, increased serum amylase.
3. Vitamin D–dependent or resistant rickets	Skeletal deformities and pain, x-ray evidence of osteomalacia, increased serum alkaline phosphatase.
4. Osteoblastic metastases	Abnormal skeletal x-rays.
5. Medullary carcinoma of the thyroid	Thyromegaly, abnormal thyroid scan, increased serum calcitonin level.

kalosis and by hypomagnesemia as readily as by hypocalcemia.

The second requirement is that other causes of hypocalcemia are ruled out using the discordant features outlined in Table 3. Thirdly, if there has not been prior surgery of the neck, an attempt should be made to distinguish idiopathic from pseudohypoparathyroidism. Pseudohypoparathyroidism is often hereditary and when afflicted families are identified, screening programs can be instituted to accomplish earlier diagnosis and treatment. A very helpful diagnostic feature is a family history of similar problems, especially of the co-associated somatic abnormalities, which may be variable in an afflicted family. If this approach is not fruitful, it may be necessary to do a modified Ellsworth-Howard test to determine whether the kidney and skeleton are sensitive to PTH. Although purified PTH and its active amino-terminal peptide have been prepared, they are not approved for human use; it is necessary to use the parathyroid extract prepared and marketed by Eli Lilly and Co. A short test to measure renal responsiveness to PTH can be used in which hourly urine levels of PO_4 and cyclic adenosine monophosphate (AMP) are determined for 3 hours before and 3 hours after intravenous injection of 200 units of parathyroid extract. A longer test is also in use in which 200 units of

the parathyroid extract is injected intramuscularly 4 times a day for 3 days and the serum calcium measured twice a day to determine whether there is a significant increase in serum calcium levels indicating skeletal responsiveness to PTH. Since parathyroid extract sometimes loses its potency before the expiration date, it is prudent to order the extract only when the tests just mentioned are to be done. Even so, if the patient fails to respond to parathyroid extract, it is then necessary to do a short test on a normal volunteer using the same preparation of parathyroid extract to prove potency.

Idiopathic hypoparathyroidism is usually an acquired disease, presumably secondary to idiopathic parathyroid destruction. Some cases appear to be autoimmune in nature since circulating antibodies to parathyroid cell components can be demonstrated by specialized techniques. Although there are a few case reports suggesting otherwise, external x-irradiation and high-dose ^{131}I administration for thyroid disease do not cause parathyroid dysfunction. On rare occasions idiopathic hypoparathyroidism may be familial, especially when it occurs in association with an assortment of endocrine deficiencies including diabetes mellitus, Addison's disease, and hypothyroidism and nonendocrine manifestations such as pernicious anemia, vitiligo, mucocutaneous moniliasis, etc., in other family members. Individuals within such families can be shown to have antibodies to cellular components of various endocrine organs, to intrinsic factor, gastric parietal cells, and so forth. These patients will respond to parathyroid extract in a manner similar to control subjects.

States of transient hypoparathyroidism have also been described after surgery on the neck in infants born of hypercalcemic (usually hyperparathyroid) mothers and in patients with correctable magnesium deficiency. It is very common for hypocalcemia to be present for the first 24 hours after neck surgery. However, this event is usually ascribed to sudden calcitonin release stimulated by manipulation of the thyroid. When hypocalcemia persists or appears later, it is usually due to surgical damage to the parathyroids. If the parathyroid injury is not too severe the hypocalcemia may be transient with eventual full recovery of function. It may take only a week or as long as 18 months for the recovery of partially injured parathyroids, and it may be necessary to treat such patients in the interim.

Neonatal hypocalcemia due to placental transfer of calcium from hypercalcemic mothers and consequent inhibition of fetal parathyroid function usually disappears within 2 weeks of delivery. However, such infants may be severely hypocalcemic and have convulsions in the interim, requiring treatment.

Magnesium deficiency impairs parathyroid function by inhibiting parathyroid secretion and also by rendering the end organs less responsive to PTH. Magnesium deficiency most often occurs in malabsorptive states and in alcoholics. The response of such patients' hypocalcemia to magnesium replacement is unpredictable because they may have independent calcium and vitamin D metabolite deficiency as well.

CHRONIC ADRENAL INSUFFICIENCY

By ROBERT D. ZIPSER, M.D.,
and JOHN E. BETHUNE, M.D.

Los Angeles, California

In 1849 Thomas Addison elegantly described the pigmentation and fatal asthenia with destruction of the adrenal glands. In recent years, primarily with the reduced incidence of tuberculosis, this classic form of Addison's disease has become a rare disorder. However, there is increasing recognition of those secondary forms of chronic adrenal insufficiency that result from dysfunction of the hypothalamic-pituitary and the renin-aldosterone axes. In contrast to Addison's disease, these other syndromes are more subtle in presentation.

DEFINITIONS

Primary adrenal insufficiency (Addison's disease): Absolute or partial deficiency of glucocorticoids (principally cortisol), mineralocorticoids (aldosterone), and adrenal androgens results from direct destruction of the adrenal cortex. Cortisol (hydrocortisone) deficiency is responsible for the pigmentation, weakness, and life-threatening intolerance to stress. Aldosterone deficiency causes hyperkalemia and to a lesser degree sodium wasting. Loss of adrenal androgens is clinically apparent only in women, in whom sexual hair may be reduced.

Secondary adrenal insufficiency: Loss of cortisol and adrenal androgen production, but with preservation of aldosterone, is the result of prolonged reduction in ACTH. Reversible atrophy of the adrenal cortex results.

Hypoaldosteronism: Selective deficiency of aldosterone due to an adrenal enzyme defect is exceedingly rare. Hypoaldosteronism associated with low plasma renin activity, mild renal impairment, and hyperkalemia are the characteristics of hyporeninemic hypoaldosteronism. This acquired syndrome was first characterized in 1957 by Hudson and is now recognized as a major cause of hyperkalemia.

Congenital adrenal hyperplasia: Inborn errors in adrenal enzymes result in a variety of uncommon syndromes of cortisol deficiency and varying degrees of salt wasting and androgenization.

PATHOGENESIS

Primary. Idiopathic (autoimmune) adrenal atrophy accounts for over two thirds of the cases of Addison's disease. Tuberculosis is becoming less common but is still the second leading cause. Histoplasmosis, blastomycosis, and coccidioidomycosis are important causes in some geographic regions. Other causes include hemochromatosis, sarcoidosis, and adrenal hemorrhage. Malignancies frequently metastasize to the adrenal glands but uncommonly destroy enough of the glands to cause adrenal insufficiency.

Autoimmune adrenal atrophy is sometimes familial and associated with a specific human histocompatibility antigen (HLA–B8). Inheritance may be autosomal recessive or autosomal dominant. Other autoimmune diseases are frequently associated, including Hashimoto's thyroiditis (this association is termed Schmidt's syndrome), Graves' disease, pernicious anemia, diabetes mellitus, hypoparathyroidism, gonadal failure, and vitiligo. Both cell-mediated and humoral immune systems are involved in adrenal destruction, and adrenal antibodies are frequently present. These antibodies rarely, if ever, occur in patients with adrenal insufficiency secondary to tuberculosis or with pituitary failure. Also in contrast to tuberculous Addison's disease, autoimmune destruction tends to spare the adrenal medulla. Thus stimulated epinephrine excretion remains normal. However, aldosterone and adrenal androgens are deficient in both autoimmune and tuberculous diseases.

Congenital adrenal hyperplasia is a form of primary adrenal insufficiency, although incomplete enzyme deficiencies with a secondary increase in ACTH secretion may result in production of adequate life-sustaining quantities of cortisol. In the most common enzyme deficiency (21-hydroxylase) cortisol secretion is maintained at the expense of increased ACTH secretion with subsequent increased adrenal androgen production. Female infants may develop ambiguous genitalia and males may undergo precocious androgenization. Approximately half of these children also have inadequate aldosterone secretion and salt wasting, and dehydration may be their presenting symptom. With more complete deficiency in cortisol production, hydrocortisone replacement may be life-sustaining. Other enzyme deficiencies may be manifest with hypertension (11-hydroxylase deficiency) or incomplete sexual development (17-hydroxylase). Inheritance is autosomal recessive.

Secondary. Within a few days of loss of ACTH secretion, the adrenal cortex begins to atrophy. Pituitary and hypothalmic diseases including tumors, vascular insufficiency such as postpartum necrosis (Sheehan's syndrome), metastatic disease, or granulomatous disease may result in complete loss of ACTH secretion or impaired reserve that may be inadequate during times of stress. Multiple pituitary hormones are usually deficient, although occasionally there is an isolated loss of ACTH.

ACTH suppression from pharmacologic administration of glucocorticoids is probably the most common cause of secondary adrenal insufficiency. The patient may not be aware that injections of medicine for arthritis or that dermatologic preparations for chronic skin disease may contain steroids. Long-acting preparations such as dexamethasone and multiple daily doses of the shorter-acting prednisone and prednisolone are particularly likely to suppress ACTH secretion. If suppression continues for several weeks ACTH-secreting ability also becomes impaired. With cessation of exogenous steroid administration, the pituitary-adrenal axis may take 9 to 12 months to resume normal function. In the first few days and weeks of this interval patients may spontaneously manifest signs of adrenal insufficiency. Severe stress any time during the 9 to 12 month period may elicit acute adrenal insufficiency. Aldosterone secretion is controlled primarily by the renin-angiotensin axis and is maintained during secondary adrenal insufficiency.

Hypoaldosteronism. Congenital deficiency in corticosterone methyloxidase results in isolated deficiency of aldosterone and is manifest in infancy as severe hyperkalemia and salt wasting. Congenital deficiency in renal receptors for aldosterone (pseudohypoaldosteronism) results in similar manifestations. In adults aldosterone deficiency is not uncommon. This acquired deficiency is associated with impaired secretion of renin from the kidney. Diabetic nephropathy or chronic pyelonephritis is the most common underlying cause. Occasionally amyloidosis, lead poisoning, or nephrosclerosis is the cause. Renin deficiency may not be a complete explanation because aldosterone secretion is also impaired in response to hyperkalemia and to infusions of ACTH. In its severest form hyporeninemic hypoaldosteronism leads to life-threatening hyperkalemia and cardiac arrhythmias.

PRESENTING SIGNS AND SYMPTOMS

It is difficult to improve upon Thomas Addison's clinical description from 1855: "The leading and characteristic features of the morbid state to which I would direct attention are anaemia, general languor and debility, remarkable feebleness of the heart's action, irritability of the stomach, and a peculiar change in color in the skin, occurring in connection with a diseased condition of the supra-renal capsules." In modern times the presentation is essentially identical. With rare exceptions all patients present with weakness, weight loss, anorexia, hypotension, and pigmentation. Exceptions occur when the disease is diagnosed early in its course as in the first few weeks following abdominal surgery or retroperitoneal hemorrhage or in the familial disorder following diagnosis of the proband.

The symptoms develop insidiously over several weeks and postural dizziness may be the presenting complaint. An occasional patient with previous hypertension presents with normal blood pressure. However, pigmentation is usually the sign that evokes the clinician's suspicion. Pigmentation increases not only in sun-exposed areas but also in the creases of the hands, axillae, and abdomen. The face is pigmented and blotches of pigmentation occur on the tongue and gums. Vitiligo may interrupt the pigmentation in autoimmune disease. Melanocyte-stimulating hormone (β-MSH) was initially thought to cause the pigmentation but it is now established that β-MSH does not circulate in man and is a fragment of a larger protein, β-lipotropin. It is not clear if ACTH or β-lipotropin or another pituitary factor causes the pigmentation, but in patients with secondary adrenal insufficiency and diminished ACTH secretion pigmentation is not present.

The cellular mechanisms by which cortisol exerts its permissive actions on body function include both direct cell membrane effects and new protein synthesis. Multiple organ systems are disrupted by cortisol deficiency. Mental changes range from fatigue to psychosis. Decreased cardiac output is compounded by salt wasting and dehydration from aldosterone deficiency and is manifest as postural hypotension. There are prerenal azotemia and impaired ability to excrete a water load. Gastrointestinal manifestations include anorexia, vomiting, diarrhea, and, occasionally, abdominal pain. Some patients note altered taste perception and salt craving. Menstrual irregularity, especially amenorrhea, is common, and both men and women have reduced libido.

With secondary adrenal insufficiency the presenting signs may reflect loss of other pituitary hormones. Patients may appear myxedematous or present with headache, visual impairment, and other signs of pituitary tumor. With autoimmune polyglandular failure involving the gonads, and the thyroid and adrenal glands, the syndrome may resemble pituitary failure, and hypopituitarism may be incorrectly diagnosed. However, with secondary adrenal failure there is no hyperpigmentation and aldosterone maintains normal serum potassium concentration.

Isolated hypoaldosteronism is usually suggested by otherwise unexplained hyperkalemia. Cardiac arrhythmias may prompt the initial measurement of electrolytes. The clinical setting is usually in long-standing diabetes mellitus with mild renal impairment and occasionally with autonomic neuropathy. Chronic pyelonephritis is the most common cause in nondiabetics. The initial recognition of hyperkalemia may follow glucose administration to the diabetic or initiation of sodium restriction or potassium-sparing diuretics. These maneuvers would aggravate the underlying aldosterone impairment in potassium excretion.

LABORATORY FINDINGS

Hyperkalemia, hyponatremia, and prerenal azotemia are characteristics of Addison's disease. Serum potassium may reach 9 mEq per liter, but a normal concentration may result from diarrhea and vomiting and does not exclude the diagnosis. Sodium is lost through the kidney and urine sodium excretion remains abnormally high despite dehydration. Serum sodium may fall to as low as 110 or 120 mEq per liter. In rare instances serum calcium is increased. The dehydration may also account for the small heart size on chest x-ray. Despite hemoconcentration from dehydration, there is usually mild anemia. In autoimmune Addison's disease, pernicious anemia may also be present. Fasting hypoglycemia may result from impaired gluconeogenesis.

Secondary adrenal insufficiency is often associated with hyponatremia despite normal aldosterone production. Unexplained hyponatremia as low as 110 to 130 mEq per liter should always suggest hypopituitarism. In isolated hypoaldosteronism, serum potassium may reach 9 mEq per liter, but serum sodium is only slightly reduced to 130 to 140 mEq per liter. Thus, in the adult, cortisol and aldosterone may be equally important in sodium balance.

Endocrinologic testing to confirm the diagnosis of Addison's disease requires documentation that the adrenal cortex will not respond to ACTH. A simple screening test is the administration of 0.25 mg (25 units) of synthetic αl-24 ACTH intravenously. Normal subjects increase plasma cortisol to greater than 18 to 20 micrograms per dl (100 ml) within 60 minutes. Chronic ACTH deficiency with secondary adrenal atrophy may blunt the ACTH response, so the definitive diagnosis requires 3 days of intravenous ACTH (25 units over 8 hours daily) or of intramuscular depot ACTH (80 units daily). Persistently suppressed plasma cortisol (less than 20 micrograms per dl) confirms primary failure. Utilization of urinary 17-hydroxysteroids or 17-ketogenic steroids as a test for cortisol insufficiency or 17-ketosteroids as a measure of adrenal androgen insufficiency has generally been replaced by the blood studies, although 17-hydroxysteroids are occasionally measured during the 3-day ACTH test. Measurement of random plasma cortisol concentration without the ACTH provocative test may be misleading because of normal variations in secretion and no indication of reserve.

Simultaneous measurement of plasma ACTH and cortisol may eventually replace ACTH stimulation tests. Addison's disease is the only situation in which ACTH is markedly elevated and cortisol is markedly deficient. However, at the time of this writing the variability of ACTH measurements limits its usefulness to confirming the dynamic tests. ACTH concentration is elevated with primary disease and low or low normal with secondary failure.

With suspected pituitary insufficiency a variety of unstimulated and provocative tests may be used. Thyroid function tests may reveal depressed serum T_4 and thyroid-stimulating hormone (TSH). In postmenopausal females, luteinizing hormone (LH) and follicle-stimulating hormone (FSH) are normally elevated, and documentation of low LH and FSH concentration is particularly suggestive. In premenopausal women and in men, low LH and FSH concentration are diagnostic only if combined with documentation of low estrogen or testosterone concentration. Evaluation of the hypothalamic-pituitary adrenal axis utilizes either metyrapone administration or the insulin tolerance test. Metyrapone blocks adrenal 11-hydroxylase, lowers plasma cortisol, and increases ACTH and other adrenal steroids. As a screening test, 2 or 3 grams of metyrapone orally at 11 or 12 P.M. will suppress 8 A.M. cortisol to less than 2 micrograms per dl and stimulate its immediate precursor, 11-deoxycortisol (compound S), to greater than 7 micrograms per dl. Definitive metyrapone testing requires 3-day administration in the hospital with measurement of urinary 17-hydroxysteroids.

The insulin tolerance test using 0.05 to 0.15 unit per kg of body weight (regular insulin) should also be done in the hospital setting with careful monitoring of symptoms of hypoglycemia. Blood sugar should fall to less than 40 mg per dl or by 50 per cent of basal within 30 minutes. Both growth hormone and cortisol are stimulated in normal subjects. The patient should never be left unattended during this test. The metyrapone or insulin tolerance tests may also be used to test the recovery of pituitary-adrenal responsiveness in patients with prolonged treatment with synthetic steroids. In this situation a normally elevated morning plasma cortisol concentration may also be suggestive of normal return of adrenal function. However, it is more prudent to continue to treat all susceptible patients with steroids during periods of stress for 9 to 12 months after cessation of steroid therapy.

In suspected hyporeninemic hypoaldosteronism it is essential to exclude Addison's disease as the cause of the hyperkalemia. The ACTH screening test is usually sufficient. Suppressed plasma renin activity (PRA) and plasma or urinary aldosterone are confirmed by either several days of a sodium-restricted diet or, more commonly, by documenting impaired response of both PRA and aldosterone to 60 mg of furosemide intravenously followed by 2 hours of upright posture. About 20 per cent of normal subjects fail to normally increase PRA by this maneuver, so it is essential to document suppressed plasma or urinary aldosterone as well. The diagnosis is confirmed by a therapeutic trial of a synthetic mineralocorticoid such as fludrocortisone (0.1 mg daily), which should normalize the serum potassium within 3 to 5 days.

The unusual disorders of congenital adrenal hyperplasia are suspected by elevated urinary 17-ketosteroid excretion and, in the female, by increased plasma testosterone. The 21-hydroxylase defect is confirmed by increased plasma 17-hydroxyprogesterone or urinary pregnenatriol. The 11-hydroxylase deficiency is associated with increased plasma 11-deoxycortisol concentration.

PITFALLS IN DIAGNOSIS

The most common pitfall in diagnosing Addison's disease is not to consider the diagnosis or to summarily attribute hyperkalemia, hyponatremia, or hyperpigmentation to other causes. Nor should the diagnosis be excluded if serum potassium or serum sodium concentration is normal. With endocrinologic testing, unstimulated plasma cortisol concentration and urinary steroid excretion are generally inadequate and should be supplemented with provocative ACTH testing. The syndrome of hyporeninemic hypoaldosteronism is most frequently missed because hyperkalemia is attributed to the mild renal failure. However, with aroused suspicion and the use of short screening tests to exclude normal adrenal function, the correct diagnosis is rapidly established.

ACUTE ADRENOCORTICAL INSUFFICIENCY

By CHARLES E. BIRD, M.D.
Kingston, Ontario, Canada

SYNONYMS

Acute adrenal failure, acute adrenal insufficiency, addisonian crisis, acute adrenal hypocorticism.

DEFINITION

This is a life-threatening medical emergency resulting from an inadequate supply of glucocorticoid and mineralocorticoid steroid hormones to the body. The normally functioning adrenal cortex produces adequate amounts of cortisol (hydrocortisone) and aldosterone as the necessary glucocorticoid and mineralocorticoid hormone. The endogenous production of these hormones may be impaired owing to primary adrenocortical disease (see article on chronic adrenal insufficiency) or as a secondary result of disease in the hypothalamus or pituitary (see article on hypopituitarism). Sudden severe stress such as infection, acute myocardial infarction, general anesthesia, or trauma will create a demand for steroid production that the adrenal cannot meet.

The more common cause of acute adrenocortical insufficiency is seen in the patient who is taking a glucocorticoid in either physiologic doses (replacement following endocrine ablative therapy for breast cancer) or pharmacologic doses for specific disease states such as rheumatoid arthritis, collagen vascular disease, or hematologic disorders. Owing to intercurrent illness, the glucocorticoid is either omitted or not increased sufficiently to meet the body needs.

CLINICAL PICTURE

The presenting signs and symptoms are non-specific and common to many acute illnesses. The patient notes marked muscle weakness and fatigue; anorexia, nausea, vomiting, and diarrhea are common. While a fever may occur early, it is not always found. Patients with pituitary insufficiency may present with hypoglycemia and actually show hypothermia. The mental state may vary from mild confusion to frank psychosis. On examination the patient will show evidence of moderate to severe dehydration. The blood pressure will be low and the heart rate will be rapid. There may be evidence of previous adrenal surgery, the cushingoid changes of glucocorticoid replacement therapy, or signs of pituitary insufficiency as reflected in hypothyroidism and hypogonadism. The typical pigmentation of chronic adrenocortical insufficiency may be accentuated.

There may be focal signs of the disease process that precipitated the episode of acute adrenocortical insufficiency. Bronchopneumonia, genitourinary infections, and myocardial disease may be found.

If unrecognized or untreated, the dehydration and hypotension progressively worsen and death results.

LABORATORY FINDINGS

The peripheral blood may not show a significant anemia because this can be masked by the dehydration. Following therapy, however, patients who have had acute or chronic adrenocortical insufficiency show a normocytic normochromic anemia. There may be a mild lymphocytosis and eosinophilia.

The dehydration produces prerenal azotemia with an increase in creatinine. The combined gastrointestinal fluid losses and impaired renal function result in hyponatremia and hyperkalemia. Hypercalcemia is also common. The blood sugar may be normal or low.

The life-threatening nature of the disease does not allow time for definitive adrenocortical diagnostic tests before therapy. If the diagnosis is considered, therapy with glucocorticoids and intravenous saline should be recommended. It is helpful to obtain blood for a later serum cortisol determination before starting therapy. This may turn out to be in the low normal range (<12 micrograms per dl [100 ml]). In acute stressful illness the serum cortisol is nearly always greater than 25 micrograms per dl.

The specific diagnostic tests are discussed in the article dealing with chronic adrenal insufficiency.

Patients who were previously taking exogenous glucocorticoids in physiologic or pharmacologic doses may show few if any hematologic changes in the acute illness. Within 24 to 48 hours, however, they will show the electrolyte and creatine changes.

THERAPEUTIC TEST

If the diagnosis of acute adrenocortical insufficiency is considered, the combined administration of cortisol and intravenous fluids often results in a dramatic clinical improvement within an hour. This response gives strong support to the diagnosis.

PITFALLS IN DIAGNOSIS

As the clinical picture is common to nearly all acute illnesses, it is easy to miss the diagnosis. This is a major error, as specific therapy is life-saving. Making this diagnosis when it does not apply is much less serious because a therapeutic test in general will not cause serious harm.

CUSHING'S SYNDROME

By ROBERTO FRANCO-SAENZ, M.D., *and* PATRICK J. MULROW, M.D.

Toledo, Ohio

DEFINITION

Cushing's syndrome is the result of chronic overproduction of glucocorticoids by the adrenal cortex, or it can be produced iatrogenically by the prolonged administration of glucocorticoids or ACTH. The syndrome, first described by Harvey Cushing in 1932, is characterized by truncal obesity, hypertension, glucosuria, and decreased glucose tolerance, amenorrhea, hirsutism, purplish cutaneous striae, and osteoporosis. In Cushing's original description, he suggested that the syndrome was due to "pituitary basophilism," but soon after it was found that neoplasms of the adrenal cortex could also produce the syndrome. More recently, it was recognized that a large variety of nonendocrine tumors can secrete an ACTH-like peptide similar to pituitary ACTH, leading to severe degrees of adrenal hyperplasia and Cushing's syndrome. The term ectopic ACTH syndrome is now widely used for this variant.

INCIDENCE

Spontaneous Cushing's syndrome is rare. The incidence has been estimated as 1:5000 hospital admissions or 1:1000 postmortem examinations. Cushing's syndrome occurs in all races and is more frequent in patients between the ages of 20 and 60, but it can also occur in children, although less frequently. Cushing's syndrome

associated with pituitary-dependent adrenal cortical hyperplasia and adrenal tumors is four times more frequent in females than in males. However, Cushing's syndrome secondary to ectopic production of ACTH by nonendocrine tumors is more common in males.

CLASSIFICATION

The term Cushing's syndrome refers to the clinical manifestations of hypercortisolism independent of its cause; the term Cushing's disease is reserved only for hypercortisolism and bilateral adrenal hyperplasia from ACTH excess of pituitary origin. The causes of Cushing's syndrome can be classified according to the pathophysiology, as seen in Table 1. Because of widespread use of glucocorticoids for nonendocrine diseases, the most common cause of Cushing's syndrome seen in clinical practice is iatrogenic. As patients with iatrogenic Cushing's syndrome usually do not present a diagnostic problem, the discussion to follow refers primarily to endogenous or spontaneous Cushing's syndrome.

Bilateral adrenal hyperplasia with ACTH excess of pituitary origin and no demonstrable evidence of pituitary tumor is the most common cause of Cushing's syndrome and comprises approximately 60 to 70 per cent of the cases. Cushing's disease caused by bilateral adrenal hyperplasia, secondary to pituitary tumors with sellar enlargement, occurs in approximately 10 per cent of the cases. Some cases of bilateral adrenal cortical hyperplasia without overt evidence of pituitary tumor may be due to hypothalamic dysfunction, whereby the "set point" for negative feedback by plasma cortisol at the hypothalamo-pituitary ACTH-releasing center is abnormally high, leading to excess of pituitary ACTH — hypercortisolism — and adrenal hyperplasia. Abnormalities of the central neurotransmitter regulation of corticotropin-releasing factor (CRF) and ACTH have recently been suggested as a causative factor in Cushing's disease. However, the possibility that the ma-

Table 1.   *Causes of Cushing's Syndrome*

I. *ACTH-dependent*
  A. Adrenal hyperplasia
    1. Secondary to ACTH-producing pituitary tumor
    2. Secondary to hypothalamic dysfunction
    3. Ectopic ACTH syndrome
    4. Prolonged use of ACTH
II. *ACTH-independent*
  A. Adrenal neoplasia
    1. Adenoma
    2. Carcinoma
    3 Nodular "adenomatous" hyperplasia
  B. Prolonged use of glucocorticoids

jority of cases of Cushing's disease are due to small microadenomas of the pituitary gland, undetectable by present diagnostic techniques, cannot be excluded, especially as a significant number of these patients develop pituitary tumors after bilateral adrenalectomy. Furthermore, with the advances made in pituitary surgery by the introduction of the operating microscope and the development of microdissection techniques, a significant number of patients with Cushing's disease and a normal-size sella turcica have been found to have centrally located intrapituitary microadenomas varying in size from 3 to 10 mm. When the syndrome is produced by a pituitary tumor, the tumor is more frequently a chromophobe adenoma and less often a basophilic adenoma. Although the tumors are usually benign, they may protrude outside the sella and produce compression of the optic chiasma and hypothalamus.

The ectopic ACTH syndrome is produced by a variety of nonendocrine neoplasms. These tumors are usually malignant, but benign bronchial adenomas may produce the syndrome. The tumors reported as being most commonly associated with the ectopic ACTH syndrome are oat cell carcinoma of the bronchus, pancreatic islet cell tumors, and thymic tumors.

Recent observations suggest that such neoplasms synthetize and release biologically and immunologically active ACTH as well as a larger common precursor for ACTH and β-lipotropin (β-LPH). Also, these tumors have been reported to produce β-MSH, which was thought to be responsible for the frequent hyperpigmentation seen in these patients. However, it has now been shown that β-MSH is probably an artifact derived from β-LPH during extraction and purification procedures. In addition, some pancreatic and lung tumors produce corticotropin-releasing factor (CRF-like material) besides ACTH. Patients with ectopic ACTH have high circulating levels of ACTH and complete remission of the syndrome has been reported after successful removal of these tumors.

Recent evidence shows that over half of the patients with carcinoma of the lung without clinical evidence of the ectopic ACTH syndrome have high plasma levels of ACTH and that nearly all tumor extracts from lung cancer, regardless of the histologic type, contain significant concentrations of ACTH that consist primarily of the larger precursor peptide ("big-ACTH") of lesser biological activity. However, clinical evidence of the ectopic ACTH syndrome develops in only 2 per cent of patients with lung cancer. The expression of the clinical syndrome appears to depend on the enzymatic ability of these tumors to convert "big-ACTH" to biologically active ACTH.

Adrenal adenomas are responsible for the development of Cushing's syndrome in approximately 10 per cent of patients. In some adenomas, the primary secretion of the tumor is cortisol and the clinical picture is dominated by the hypercatabolic effects of excess glucocorticoids. However, some adrenal adenomas may show excess androgen production as well as glucocorticoid excess, and the clinical picture may be a mixture of hypercortisolism and virilization. Adrenal adenomas are more frequent in females, and are more common on the left than the right, but can be bilateral. When unilateral adenomas are present, the contralateral adrenal is usually atrophic. Multiple microadenomas involving both adrenals are sometimes found, and this condition has been called "nodular cortical hyperplasia" or "adenomatous hyperplasia of the adrenals." The adrenal tissue outside the adenomas is either hyperplastic or atrophic. Endogenous ACTH levels are usually low, but in some patients they may be inappropriately high for the levels of plasma cortisol. After bilateral adrenalectomy, a number of patients with nodular cortical hyperplasia show supranormal levels of plasma ACTH and some patients develop pituitary tumors, following a course similar to that of patients with bilateral adrenal hyperplasia secondary to ACTH excess of pituitary origin. Patients with nodular cortical hyperplasia of the adrenals may combine features of bilateral hyperplasia with those of adrenal adenomas. The diagnosis of the cause of Cushing's syndrome in these patients may be difficult, as they may show hyperresponsiveness to exogenous ACTH or metyrapone, similar to that seen in patients with Cushing's disease, but with failure to suppress with the high dexamethasone dose (8 mg per day) as is seen in autonomous adrenal adenomas or carcinomas.

Adrenal carcinomas are as common as adenomas, and they are the most frequent cause of Cushing's syndrome in children. Carcinomas may vary in size from a few centimeters to large tumor masses that can be palpated through the abdominal wall. In some well-differentiated carcinomas, the histologic appearance may resemble that of an adenoma, and only the subsequent clinical course and long-term follow-up will determine the correct diagnosis. Patients with Cushing's syndrome resulting from adrenal carcinoma may develop virilization in females or gynecomastia and feminization in males. Occasionally, Cushing's syndrome can be produced by tumors originating in embryologic remnants of adrenal cortical tissue located in the perirenal area, ovaries, or testicles.

PRESENTING SIGNS AND SYMPTOMS

The initial complaints are usually related to weight gain, menstrual irregularities, hirsutism, fatigue, and muscle weakness. Personality changes and frequent mood swings are common. Also, symptoms attributable to hypertension or carbohydrate intolerance such as polyuria and polydipsia are common. In children, the most frequent presenting sign is progressive weight gain with stunted linear growth. Unusual presenting signs are osteoporosis or hypertension. In view of the high prevalence of obesity, hypertension, diabetes, and menstrual irregularities in the general population, the physician is often confronted with a patient with several of the features of Cushing's syndrome and must determine the extent of the investigations to be performed. A very careful history and physical examination with special attention to the typical signs of hypercortisolism plus careful analysis of some of the routine laboratory tests and the overnight dexamethasone suppression test will help to determine the need for further evaluation.

COURSE

The course of Cushing's syndrome is usually progressive, and it has been estimated that, if the condition is untreated, the 5-year mortality rate is approximately 50 per cent. However, the course more accurately will reflect the underlying cause of the syndrome. Patients with Cushing's disease may have a fluctuating clinical course with exacerbations and remissions, whereas patients with adrenal carcinomas and those with the ectopic ACTH syndrome may have a rapid downhill course leading to early death.

PHYSICAL EXAMINATION AND FINDINGS

The frequency of symptoms and signs of Cushing's syndrome is shown in Table 2. The most common manifestation of Cushing's syndrome is obesity. Central redistribution of fat pads leads to the typical accumulation of fat in the trunk and face. This is particularly obvious in the lateral aspects of the face, leading to the classic "moon" facies, and in the cervicodorsal region, leading to "buffalo hump" and fullness of the supraclavicular fossae. The abdomen is often protuberant and pendulous, and the extremities are thin owing to muscle wasting. Obesity may also be general without the typical centripetal distribution. On the other hand, truncal obesity can occur without the presence of Cushing's syndrome. Extreme obesity is uncommon in Cushing's syndrome. The face is

Table 2. *Incidence of Clinical Manifestations of Cushing's Syndrome*

Obesity	95%
Hypertension	82%
Glucosuria and decreased glucose tolerance	81%
Menstrual and sexual dysfunction	76%
Weakness	72%
Hirsutism and acne	69%
Striae	60%
Easy bruising	59%
Osteoporosis	57%
Psychiatric disturbances	57%
Edema	49%
Polyuria	20%
Ocular changes	9%

frequently plethoric. The skin is atrophic with thinning of the stratum corneum and increased transparency, permitting the underlying capillary plexus to be seen. These skin changes are especially apparent in the dorsum of the hands and forearms, where minor trauma may produce easy bruising. Ecchymosis or purpuric lesions in these regions as well as in the legs are frequently seen. Wide purple striae are noted, especially around the abdomen, hips, and upper portion of the thighs. The striae are usually over 1 cm in width. The presence of white or pink striae is not important for the diagnosis. Fungal infections and tinea versicolor may be seen. Weakness and muscle atrophy are commonly found, especially involving the proximal muscles. This is most marked in the muscles of the pelvic girdle, and often the patients are unable to stand from a low-sitting or squatting position without assistance. Back pain is a common complaint, and it is usually due to osteoporosis of the spine. Osteoporosis can be generalized, but the more vulnerable places are the spinal column and the rib cage. Compression fractures of the vertebrae, with loss of height and kyphosis and rib fractures after minor trauma, are seen in advanced disease. Hirsutism and acne are equally prevalent, but true virilization such as temporal balding, deepening of the voice, and clitoral enlargement are rare; when present, they should alert the physician to the possibility of adrenal carcinoma, because frequently carcinomas may have a coexistent excess of adrenal androgens. Mild to moderate hypertension is seen in approximately 85 per cent of the patients, and evidence of left ventricular hypertrophy is common. Polyuria and polydipsia may be present, but overt diabetes occurs in only 20 per cent of the patients. Personality changes, irritability, depression, or even frank psychotic episodes may be seen. Exophthalmos and puffiness of the eyelids occur in less than 10 per cent of the patients, and nephrolithiasis occurs in approximately 20 per cent. In patients with Cushing's syndrome and pituitary tumors, headaches and signs of compression of the optic chiasma with progressive loss of vision may be present but are rare in the untreated patient. Patients with Cushing's syndrome caused by ectopic ACTH may lack most of the clinical features of Cushing's syndrome. Weight loss secondary to the underlying malignant process is common. Often the patients become markedly pigmented. Muscle weakness, edema, and unexplained hypokalemic metabolic alkalosis or severe diabetes of rapid onset are important clinical clues to Cushing's syndrome caused by ectopic ACTH.

LABORATORY FINDINGS

Routine laboratory findings suggestive but not diagnostic of Cushing's syndrome include mild neutrophilic leukocytosis with a decrease in the percentage of lymphocytes to below 20 per cent. Eosinophils are usually absent in the differential white count, and the absolute eosinophil count is below 100 per cu mm in 90 per cent of the patients. The hematocrit is usually normal in spite of the plethoric appearance of the patients, but in approximately 10 per cent of the patients mild erythrocytosis may be present. The fasting blood sugar is frequently normal. In 20 per cent of the patients, overt diabetes with persistent fasting hyperglycemia and glycosuria may be present, but the glucose tolerance test is abnormal in approximately 80 per cent of the patients. Serum electrolytes are usually normal, but mild hypokalemia and metabolic alkalosis occur in a minority of patients. However, as stated before, persistent hypokalemic alkalosis in a patient not taking diuretics may be an important clue to the presence of the ectopic ACTH syndrome or adrenal carcinoma. Mild hypercalciuria is common in patients with Cushing's syndrome.

SPECIFIC LABORATORY TESTS

In patients in whom the history and physical findings are highly suggestive of Cushing's syndrome, laboratory evaluation is necessary and specific tests are indicated to answer two questions: (1) Does the patient have Cushing's syndrome? (2) What is the cause of adrenocortical overactivity?

As an important preliminary step, *all drugs should be stopped* if possible during the diagnostic period. This is of particular importance, as a large number of analgesics, tranquilizers, diuretics, and antimicrobial agents are known to interfere with the technique for determination of 17-hydroxycorticosteroids (17-OHCS, Porter-Silber chromogens) and 17-ketosteroids (17-KS). Also, some drugs may induce changes in cortisol secretion, metabolism, or excretion, or they may interfere with the metabolism of drugs used for diagnostic purposes such as dexamethasone or metyrapone. For the diagnosis of Cushing's syndrome, the following sequence of tests is helpful (Fig. 1).

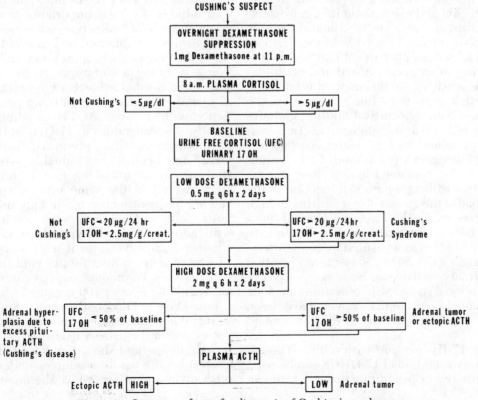

Figure 1. Sequence of tests for diagnosis of Cushing's syndrome.

Overnight Dexamethasone Suppression. As an outpatient screening test, the overnight dexamethasone is the simplest, most reliable test. This test has been found to be abnormal in 97 per cent of patients with proved Cushing's syndrome. In this test, 1 mg of dexamethasone is administered orally at 11 P.M., and the plasma cortisol is measured between 8 and 9 A.M. the following morning. In normal persons the early morning surge of ACTH secretion is obliterated by this dose of dexamethasone, and the 8 A.M. plasma cortisol is generally 5 micrograms per 100 ml or less. In patients with Cushing's syndrome, cortisol secretion is not suppressed, and the 8 A.M. plasma cortisol usually exceeds 10 micrograms per 100 ml. False-positive results can be seen in patients with hyperthyroidism in whom there is a high metabolic clearance of dexamethasone, or in patients receiving medications which induce liver enzymes that rapidly metabolize dexamethasone. Also, some obese patients and patients receiving estrogens may not show a normal suppression. Because of the high reliability of the test and the very low incidence of false-negative results, any patient who shows lack of suppression should undergo further evaluation; in our experience, the determination of free urinary cortisol is the most specific and reliable subsequent step.

Urinary Free Cortisol. This test is considered by many as the single most important test for the diagnosis of hypercortisolism. Urinary free cortisol is increased in over 90 per cent of the patients with Cushing's syndrome and in only 8 per cent of those without it. A consistently normal urinary free cortisol should exclude the diagnosis of Cushing's syndrome. Urinary free cortisol represents cortisol that is excreted in the urine in an unconjugated and unaltered form. The sensitivity of this method is based on the fact that only the "free" cortisol in the plasma (not bound to cortisol-binding globulin [CBG]) is filtrable at the glomerulus. In hypercortisolism, when the total plasma cortisol exceeds 20 micrograms per 100 ml, CBG is saturated and the concentration of free plasma cortisol rises with a proportional increase in the filtered load at the glomerulus, resulting in high urinary free cortisol excretion. Normal nonstressed persons excrete less than 100 micrograms per 24 hours as measured by competitive-binding analysis. A 50 to 250 per cent elevation of free urinary cortisol can be seen after physical or emotional stress. Mild elevations are seen in pregnancy, and normal values have been reported in obese patients with "cushingoid obesity."

Urinary 17-Hydroxycorticosteroids. The 24-hour urinary excretion of 17-OHCS can be used as an alternative or in addition to the determination of free urinary cortisol. However, it should be noted that 15 per cent of the patients with Cushing's syndrome excrete normal amounts of 17-OHCS, and many patients with diseases other than Cushing's syndrome excrete increased amounts of 17-OHCS. Also, there are large differences between individual subjects and wide variations in the same subject from day to day. The 17-OHCS are measured by a colorimetric technique, and a large number of commonly used drugs interfere with the technique, leading to spurious results. The 17-OHCS measure tetrahydrocortisol and tetrahydrocortisone, the major metabolic products of cortisol. Also, they measure the metabolic product of 11-desoxycortisol (compound S), the immediate percursor of cortisol, which under normal conditions is present in small amounts. Normal values for 17-OHCS vary from laboratory to laboratory. Cortisol secretion rate and urinary excretion of 17-OHCS are proportional to body mass. Obese normal subjects may have high urinary 17-OHCS indistinguishable from those of patients with Cushing's syndrome. As urinary creatinine excretion is roughly proportional to lean body mass, it is important to measure the creatinine content of all 24-hour urine specimens. By expressing the 17-OHCS per gram of creatinine, a better discrimination between normal subjects and patients with Cushing's syndrome is shown. Creatinine excretion is relatively constant, and day-to-day variations in an individual subject should not exceed 20 per cent. Determination of urinary creatinine is of critical importance to assess the completeness of collection when several 24-hour urines are obtained and to avoid errors of interpretation of the suppression and stimulation test owing to improper collection of the specimen. Normal subjects excrete 3 to 7 mg of 17-OHCS per gram of creatinine per day. Patients with ectopic ACTH syndrome show greatly elevated values of 17-OHCS. In spite of its shortcomings, the determination of the 17-OHCS has been a very valuable asset for the study of adrenocortical function. 17-KS may also be measured in the same urinary specimens, and are frequently elevated but are not of diagnostic value in Cushing's syndrome in patients with adrenal cortical hyperplasia or adrenal adenoma. However, great elevations of the 17-KS are seen in over 50 per cent of patients with adrenal carcinoma, with values ranging between 50 and over 100 mg per 24 hours.

Low-Dose Dexamethasone Suppression Test. When the baseline urinary free cortisol is elevated or the urinary excretion of 17-OHCS is high, the patient should be hospitalized, and after collecting baseline samples under the hospital environment for 2 days the *low-dose dex-*

amethasone suppression test is performed. Dexamethasone, 0.5 mg, is administered orally every 6 hours for 2 days, and daily 24-hour urine samples are collected for urinary free cortisol, 17-OHCS, and creatinine. Failure of suppression of the urinary free cortisol below 20 micrograms per 24 hours or failure to suppress the 17-OHCS to less than 2.5 mg per gram of creatinine during the second day of dexamethasone administration will definitely establish the diagnosis of Cushing's syndrome. This test, if properly performed, is the most discriminating test for the diagnosis of Cushing's syndrome and is abnormal in 99 per cent of the patients with Cushing's syndrome. Abnormal responses are found in only 15 per cent of patients without Cushing's syndrome.

High-Dose Dexamethasone Suppression Test. The low-dose dexamethasone test should be immediately followed by the *high-dose dexamethasone test*, in which 2 mg of dexamethasone is administered orally every 6 hours for 2 days. Daily 24-hour urine samples are collected for urinary free cortisol, 17-OHCS, and creatinine. This test is the most valuable one for identifying the lesion responsible for Cushing's syndrome. Failure of suppression of the urinary free cortisol or the urinary 17-OHCS during the second day of the high-dose dexamethasone is suggestive of an autonomously functioning adrenal adenoma or carcinoma, or the ectopic ACTH syndrome. Failure to suppress with the low-dose dexamethasone but suppression to less than 50 per cent of the baseline values of urinary free cortisol of 17-OHCS with the high-dose dexamethasone test is suggestive of Cushing's disease, that is, bilateral adrenal hyperplasia caused by excess pituitary ACTH, and has been noted in 82 per cent of the patients. Further differentiation can be accomplished by the determination of plasma ACTH and the metyrapone test.

Plasma ACTH Measurements. The determination of plasma ACTH by radioimmunoassay, although still technically difficult, helps differentiate patients with Cushing's syndrome caused by adrenal adenoma or carcinoma from those who have the ectopic ACTH syndrome. Patients with adrenal adenomas or carcinomas have either low or undetectable plasma ACTH levels, whereas patients with the ectopic ACTH syndrome have very high levels of plasma ACTH. Patients with bilateral adrenal hyperplasia caused by an excess of pituitary ACTH may have normal or high levels of ACTH, but even normal levels are "inappropriately" high for the levels of plasma cortisol and lack the diurnal periodicity of ACTH secretion.

Metyrapone Test. Metyrapone is a powerful inhibitor of adrenocortical 11β-hydroxylase and blocks the synthesis of cortisol at the level of 11-desoxycortisol (compound S). By lowering the plasma levels of cortisol, metyrapone causes the release of corticotropin-releasing factor (CRF) from the hypothalamus and ACTH from the pituitary, which in turn increases the synthesis of steroids by the adrenal to the step of 11-desoxycortisol (compound S). The increased production of compound S can be measured by the determination of 17-OHCS in the urine. The test consists in the administration of 750 mg of metyrapone orally every 4 hours for 6 doses; 24-hour urine is collected for 17-OHCS and creatinine on the day of administration of metyrapone and the day after. Normal persons show a twofold to fourfold increase in the urinary excretion of 17-OHCS on the day of metyrapone administration or the following day. Patients with pituitary dependent bilateral adrenal hyperplasia show hyperresponsiveness to metyrapone. Patients with adrenal adenoma or carcinoma show either no change or a slight fall in the excretion of 17-OHCS, and patients with ectopic ACTH syndrome show either no change or a slight increase in the excretion of 17-OHCS (Table 3).

The diurnal variation of plasma cortisol should also be obtained in patients suspected of having Cushing's syndrome. Plasma cortisol is measured at 8 A.M. and 8 P.M. Lack of diurnal variation is observed in 80 to 90 per cent of patients with Cushing's syndrome. However, a large number of normal persons may show lack of diurnal variation. As cortisol secretion is episodic and wide fluctuations in the levels may occur within a short period of time, false-positive results may be seen.

In our experience, the ACTH stimulation test does not add any significant information to the diagnosis of the cause of Cushing's syndrome. Most patients with pituitary-dependent bilateral adrenal hyperplasia usually show hyperresponsiveness to exogenous ACTH, patients with adrenal carcinoma rarely respond to ACTH, and half the patients with adrenal adenomas may show a response.

Radiologic Findings and Other Tests. X-rays of the skull may reveal enlargement of the sella turcica with erosion of the posterior clinoid processes in patients with Cushing's disease and pituitary tumors. Polytomograms of the sellar region are necessary to evaluate minor erosions or irregularities of the floor of the sella. Pneumoencephalograms are most helpful in outlining suprasellar extension of the tumor and in ruling out an "empty sella." Carotid angiograms are useful in outlining lateral extension of the tumor, excluding the presence of aneurysms, and may indicate the degree of vascularity of the tumor. Computerized axial

Table 3. Laboratory Tests in the Differential Diagnosis of Cushing's Syndrome

| | Plasma Cortisol | | Plasma ACTH | Baseline Urinary Steroids | | Low-Dose Dexamethasone Test | | High-Dose Dexamethasone Test | | Metyrapone Test (17-OHCS) |
	OVERNIGHT DEXAMETHASONE SUPPRESSION	DIURNAL RHYTHM		URINARY FREE CORTISOL μg/24 hr	17-OHCS, mg/gram CREATININE	URINARY FREE CORTISOL μg/24 hr	17-OHCS, mg/gram CREATININE	URINARY FREE CORTISOL μg/24 hr	17-OHCS, mg/gram CREATININE	
Normal	<5 μg/100 ml	N	N	<100	3–7	<20	<2.5	<20	<2.5	2–4 × baseline
Pituitary-dependent adrenal hyperplasia	↑	A	N° or ↑	↑	↑	↑	↑	<50% baseline	<50% baseline	3–6 × baseline
Autonomous adrenal tumor	↑	A	↓ or U	↑	↑	↑	↑	↑	↑	NC or ↓
Ectopic ACTH	↑	A	↑↑	↑↑	↑↑	↑	↑	↑	↑	NC or ↑

A = Absent.
N = Normal.
NC = No change.
U = Undetectable.
° = "Inappropriately" high for levels of plasma cortisol.

tomography may be valuable to show clinically unsuspected extrasellar extension.

Visual fields and perimetry are sensitive indicators of compression to the optic chiasma. Roentgenograms of the chest may reveal evidence of cardiomegaly caused by hypertension, or they may reveal the presence of a bronchogenic or mediastinal tumor responsible for the ectopic ACTH syndrome. X-rays of the dorsolumbar spine may show varying degrees of osteoporosis. Intravenous pyelograms are usually of no help, but when they reveal a large suprarenal mass displacing one of the kidneys, adrenal carcinoma is present. Adrenal arteriograms or venograms may be of help in outlining the adrenal pathology, but they require a great deal of expertise and are rarely necessary. Venograms should be done only by an experienced radiologist. Complications of adrenal venography are relatively common. Adrenal hemorrhage may occur in approximately 10 per cent of the patients. Failure of visualization of the right adrenal, even under expert hands, occurs in 15 per cent of the patients. All patients undergoing adrenal venography experience significant pain during the procedure.

The development and increased availability of ^{131}I-19 cholesterol adrenal scan appears to be a promising noninvasive tool for the diagnosis of Cushing's syndrome, but careful evaluation of the technique over a period of time is necessary to establish the final role of adrenal scanning.

DIFFERENTIAL DIAGNOSIS

Obesity is the most common factor to be clinically confused with Cushing's syndrome, especially in those patients who are also hypertensive and diabetic and may be hirsute. Some normal obese patients may show a "cushingoid habitus" and may have menstrual irregularities. The urinary excretion of 17-OHCS may be high owing to the increased cortisol secretion rate present in obesity. These patients occasionally show a lack of normal suppression with the overnight dexamethasone, but the urinary free cortisol has been reported to be normal, and they suppress normally with the low-dose dexamethasone test. The plasma ACTH and plasma cortisol are usually normal and show a diurnal variation.

Patients with severe mental depression may show several of the biochemical abnormalities of Cushing's syndrome. In depressed patients most of the clinical manifestations of Cushing's syndrome are absent, but they may have increased 17-OHCS, lack of suppression with dexamethasone, and lack of diurnal rhythm of plasma ACTH and cortisol. Distinction between depressed patients and those with ectopic ACTH syndrome may be difficult. Patients with the ectopic ACTH syndrome usually have much higher levels of 17-OHCS, plasma cortisol, and plasma ACTH than depressed patients. Also, hypokalemic alkalosis, edema, and hyperpigmentation are common in the ectopic ACTH syndrome and rare in depression.

Patients surreptitiously taking glucocorticoids may present a diagnostic problem. This rare situation is more common in mentally disturbed nurses, medical students, and other medical and paramedical personnel. These patients may display most of the clinical features of Cushing's syndrome, but hirsutism is usually absent. Careful surveillance in a hospital environment and, if one is successful in eliminating the intake of steroids, the administration of 1 mg of dexamethasone daily with determination of urinary 17-OHCS and 17-KS over a few days may lead to the diagnosis. Patients with exogenous Cushing's syndrome will have chronic suppression of the hypothalamic-pituitary-adrenal axis and will have low levels of excretion of 17-OHCS while on this dose of dexamethasone, whereas patients with endogenous Cushing's syndrome will have elevated urinary 17-OHCS.

COMPLICATIONS

The most frequent complications of Cushing's syndrome are poor wound healing, tendency to infections, congestive heart failure, arteriosclerosis, and compression fractures of the spinal column. Pituitary tumors, visual disturbances, and hyperpigmentation (Nelson's syndrome) develop in approximately 10 per cent of patients with bilateral adrenal hyperplasia after total adrenalectomy.

PITFALLS IN DIAGNOSIS

Drug interference with the laboratory test, incompleteness of urine collections, and failure to perform the tests in a standardized manner are frequent causes of misdiagnosis. Physical or emotional stress or intercurrent illness at the time the evaluation is done are common causes of erroneous diagnosis. In patients with Cushing's disease without evidence of pituitary tumor, or when there is no obvious evidence for the cause of the syndrome, re-evaluation is mandatory *after* a few weeks, and *absolute certainty* of the diagnosis is necessary before any therapeutic maneuvers are contemplated.

HYPERALDO-STERONISM

By CHARLES R. ROST, M.D.,
and MORRIS SCHAMBELAN, M.D.

San Francisco, California

Aldosterone is the principal mineralocorticoid hormone secreted by the adrenal cortex. Normally, the renin-angiotensin system is the major factor controlling aldosterone secretion. Renin is released from the juxtaglomerular cells of the kidney primarily in response to a reduction in renal perfusion pressure or a decrease in effective circulating volume, or both. Renin enzymatically cleaves the hepatic α_2-globulin renin substrate liberating the decapeptide angiotensin I. Removal of the carboxy-terminal dipeptide by an endothelial converting enzyme produces the octapeptide angiotensin II. Angiotensin II and the heptapeptide des-Aspartyl[1]-angiotensin II (angiotensin III) stimulate directly the zona glomerulosa of the adrenal gland to increase aldosterone secretion. Aldosterone, by its action in the kidney, increases transepithelial transport of sodium, and the resultant sodium retention tends to ameliorate the initial stimulus for renin secretion. In addition, aldosterone secretion is influenced by adrenocorticotropin (ACTH) and potassium. When stimulation by the renin-angiotensin system is reduced during prolonged periods of recumbency, plasma aldosterone concentrations can be shown to correlate with those of cortisol, suggesting ACTH control of secretion. Increases in plasma potassium concentration normally increase aldosterone secretion, whereas hypokalemia will suppress it. Although greatly oversimplified, this scheme provides an adequate framework for understanding the pathophysiology and clinical aspects of the syndromes of hyperaldosteronism.

Hypersecretion of aldosterone can occur as a primary adrenal disorder or in response to increased stimulation by the renin-angiotensin system or ACTH. The syndrome of primary aldosteronism is an adrenal disorder characterized by autonomous production of mineralocorticoid hormone. The syndrome of secondary aldosteronism results from the overstimulation of an otherwise normal adrenal gland by the renin-angiotensin system. This article considers the diagnosis of hyperaldosteronism from the standpoint of the pathophysiologic characteristics of these two syndromes.

PRIMARY ALDOSTERONISM

PATHOPHYSIOLOGY

In the syndrome of primary aldosteronism, autonomous overproduction of aldosterone by the adrenal gland can be due to a benign adenoma, a carcinoma, or diffuse bilateral nodular hyperplasia. By far the most commonly seen cause is an adenoma, accounting for 75 to 85 per cent of cases. Less than 1 per cent are due to a functioning carcinoma, and the remaining 15 to 25 per cent result from bilateral hyperplasia. The extremely rare cases of so-called glucocorticoid-remediable hyperaldosteronism are believed to result from excessive stimulation of the adrenal cortex by ACTH. The patterns of mineralocorticoid secretion and the degree of autonomy from the renin-angiotensin system vary between the different entities.

Primary aldosteronism resulting from an aldosterone-producing adenoma is generally associated with distinctly elevated aldosterone excretion rates that show a great degree of autonomy from the renin-angiotensin system. Variations in plasma aldosterone concentration correlate with those of cortisol and are usually not influenced by changes in posture. This finding suggests that the tumor is no longer responsive to the small changes in plasma renin activity that occur with upright posture but has retained its sensitivity to ACTH. Aldosterone excretion rates in patients with primary aldosteronism owing to bilateral hyperplasia may be close to, and sometimes fall within, the normal range. Plasma aldosterone concentration increases with postural stimulation and these changes correlate with changes in plasma renin activity, suggesting that hyperplastic tissue has retained its sensitivity to angiotensin. Markedly elevated aldosterone excretion rates are seen in patients with primary aldosteronism from a functioning adrenal carcinoma. Plasma aldosterone concentrations do not correlate with those of cortisol or with plasma renin activity. Elevated levels of other adrenal steroids may also be found in these patients.

Primary overproduction of aldosterone or exogenous administration of large doses of mineralocorticoid hormones results in increased sodium reabsorption in the distal nephron. As a consequence, the extracellular fluid volume is expanded until approximately 1.5 to 2.5 kg of excess fluid has been retained. At this point, there is a marked reduction of proximal tubular sodium reabsorption. The resultant increased delivery of sodium to the distal tubule supersedes the increased capacity for distal sodium reabsorption, so that a new steady state of sodium balance is achieved. This phenomenon is referred to as "renal escape" or "mineralocorticoid escape." Further expansion of extracellular fluid volume does not occur despite continued hypersecretion or exogenous administration of mineralocorticoid hormone. An administered sodium load will actually be excreted more rapidly than in normal subjects. Two of the cardinal findings of the syndrome of primary aldosteronism, hypertension and suppressed plasma renin activity, probably result from this expansion of extracellular fluid volume.

The mineralocorticoid hormone–enhanced sodium reabsorption in the distal tubule and collecting duct results in increased secretion of potassium and hydrogen ion in these portions of the nephron. Even when the renal escape mechanism has allowed a new steady state of sodium balance to develop, mineralocorticoid-dependent potassium secretion and hydrogen ion secretion continue. The increased delivery of sodium to the distal nephron may actually augment the potassium secretion.

CLINICAL FINDINGS

Patients with primary aldosteronism usually are detected during evaluation of hypertension. Although the recognition of primary aldosteronism is important because it is a potentially curable form of hypertension, less than 1 per cent of unselected hypertensive patients have this disorder. The syndrome is found in women more often than in men by a 2:1 margin. The patients are usually between 30 and 50 years of age.

The hypertension may be associated with frontal headaches. Blood pressure elevation is generally moderate to severe, although the hypertension may be labile. True malignant hypertension develops very rarely, but pressure elevations up to 280 mm Hg systolic and 140 mm Hg diastolic can occur. Most of the major complications of hypertension can occur. Hypertensive retinopathy occurs in about 50 per cent of patients, but papilledema is rare. Cardiomegaly is present in about 40 per cent of patients. As with other forms of hypertension, there is an increased incidence of cerebrovascular disease and of myocardial infarction in patients with primary aldosteronism. Of particular note is the typical absence of peripheral edema and the lack of pathologic changes of necrotizing arteriolitis.

Aside from headache, the majority of presenting symptoms are related to hypokalemia and therefore their presence or severity depends on the degree of potassium depletion. In the mildly hypokalemic patient, complaints of muscle weakness, polyuria (especially nocturia), poly-

dipsia, and paresthesias are frequently encountered. If the hypokalemia is more severe, the patient may experience intermittent paralysis of the legs and arms or even tetany. In patients with marked hypokalemia, autonomic dysfunction presenting as orthostatic hypotension without reflex tachycardia may be seen.

Mild hypernatremia, hypokalemia, and metabolic alkalosis characterize the electrolyte profile. A dilute urine may be found because hypokalemia impairs the renal-concentrating mechanism. The electrocardiogram may show left ventricular hypertrophy with or without signs of strain, and in severe hypokalemia, U waves will be present. The chest roentgenogram may show an increased cardiac silhouette with or without signs of congestive failure. Urinary 17-hydroxysteroids and 17-ketosteroids are within normal limits except in patients with functioning adrenal carcinoma. The pathognomonic laboratory abnormalities in cases of primary aldosteronism are an elevated aldosterone excretion rate with suppressed and nonstimulable peripheral plasma renin activity (see Diagnosis).

Hypertension may not always be present and the severity of the hypokalemia is variable. Who, then, should be evaluated for primary aldosteronism? Any patient who has hypertension and hypokalemia in the absence of diuretic therapy should be evaluated. Patients with hypertension and profound sensitivity to the hypokalemic effects of diuretics, those with unexplained hypokalemia and no hypertension, and those with hypertension who demonstrate prompt lowering of blood pressure with a trial of spironolactone should also be suspected of possibly having primary aldosteronism.

DIAGNOSIS

Hyperaldosteronism may be documented by showing an increased secretion rate, an increased excretion rate, or an elevated plasma concentration of the hormone. Secretion rate determinations require the administration of radiolabeled aldosterone and such studies are available only at research centers. Single measurements of plasma aldosterone concentration may be misleading because even patients with markedly increased secretion rates show diurnal variations in plasma levels and a single sample may not reflect the hyperaldosteronism. The measurement of the 24-hour urinary excretion of the 18-glucuronide metabolite of aldosterone has been shown to reflect aldosterone production accurately. The urine should be collected while the patient consumes a normal sodium intake (120 to 180 mEq per day).

Demonstration of suppressed and nonstimulable plasma renin activity in a patient with elevated plasma or urinary aldosterone levels establishes the diagnosis of *primary* aldosteronism. Blood samples for plasma renin activity should be obtained while the patient is supine and after several hours of quiet ambulation. Ingestion of a low-sodium diet (10 mEq per day) for 3 days will not increase plasma renin activity. Shorter stimulation protocols using either oral or intravenous administration of furosemide (40 mg intravenously or 60 mg orally) with or without ambulation have also been in vogue. However, the measurement of plasma renin activity while the patient is in the recumbent and upright positions and is consuming a normal sodium intake will demonstrate suppression of the renin-angiotensin system in almost all cases of primary aldosteronism. Blood samples can be obtained at the same time for the measurement of plasma aldosterone concentration and the concentrations of other adrenal steroids. These determinations may help confirm the diagnosis or aid in differentiating an adrenal adenoma from hyperplasia.

Autonomy of aldosterone production can be confirmed by demonstrating failure of suppression of the hormone levels by maneuvers that normally suppress the renin-angiotensin-aldosterone axis. Proposed methods include (1) the intramuscular administration of 10 mg of deoxycorticosterone acetate every 12 hours for 3 days, (2) the oral administration of 0.2 mg fludrocortisone 3 times a day for 3 days, and (3) the intravenous infusion of 2 liters of isotonic saline solution over 4 hours. The normal person will respond to these maneuvers by suppressing renin production, thereby decreasing angiotensin II formation, and subsequently, suppressing aldosterone production. These maneuvers will usually not suppress aldosterone levels in patients with primary aldosteronism.

The principal reason for attempting to differentiate between aldosterone-producing adenoma and bilateral hyperplasia is to select the most appropriate therapy. Although the hypertension, hypokalemia, and metabolic alkalosis can be controlled in most patients by spironolactone therapy, surgical therapy may be indicated. For example, unilateral adrenalectomy will result in long-term cure in approximately 70 per cent of patients whose condition is due to an adenoma, whereas even bilateral adrenalectomy in most patients with hyperplasia does not ameliorate the effects of the hypertension.

Several biochemical determinations have been proposed to differentiate adenoma from hyperplasia. Patients with an adenoma generally have lower supine plasma renin activity values and plasma potassium concentrations with higher supine plasma aldosterone concentrations than patients with hyperplasia. Most patients with adenoma have supine plasma aldosterone concentrations greater than 20 nanograms per dl (100 ml); the responses to posture are also different. The plasma aldosterone concentration usually is unchanged or decreases with assumption of the upright posture (comparing 0800-hour to 1200-hour values) in patients with an adenoma, whereas it usually increases with upright posture in patients with hyperplasia. Specific procedures for locating an aldosterone-producing adenoma (see the next section) will also aid in differentiating a tumor from hyperplasia.

Excess secretion of other mineralocorticoid hormones or ingestion of substances with mineralocorticoid hormone–like properties can also result in hypertension, hypokalemia, metabolic alkalosis, and suppressed plasma renin activity. Several congenital syndromes have been described in which deoxycorticosterone levels are elevated (for example, 11β- and 17α-hydroxylase deficiency syndromes). Excessive ingestion of licorice or carbenoxalone has been reported to produce a similar syndrome. However, in all of these syndromes aldosterone secretion is suppressed.

It is estimated that about 25 per cent of patients with essential hypertension also have suppressed plasma renin activity but aldosterone levels are normal or low. The pathophysiology of low-renin essential hypertension is unknown. Some investigators believe that these patients have excessive amounts of an unidentified mineralocorticoid hormone–like substance. This substance, whether originating from the adrenal gland or some other tissue, produces the hypertensive syndrome. However, another possible explanation for the low-renin state is that the adrenal cortex has increased sensitivity to angiotensin. This concept would explain normal aldosterone production in the presence of low plasma renin activity.

Location of an Aldosterone-Producing Adenoma

Once the diagnosis of primary aldosteronism is established and before a costly and potentially hazardous work-up for differential diagnosis and determination of the location of a tumor is begun, a question must be answered: If an adenoma is present, should surgical excision be recommended? In an elderly patient who may have other medical problems that would contraindicate all but absolutely necessary surgery, attempts at diagnosis should end once high aldosterone excretion and suppressed plasma renin activity have been demonstrated. On the other hand, a young, otherwise healthy patient, facing a lifetime of treatment for hypertension, should receive a complete work-up including, if indicated, exploratory surgery.

Almost all adenomas are unilateral and proper preoperative locating procedures can help minimize the surgical procedure and thus reduce perioperative morbidity. Although biochemical studies can strongly suggest the presence of an adenoma, specific localization procedures should be carried out to confirm its presence. Plain abdominal roentgenographic studies or an intravenous pyelogram may indirectly show an adenoma by a mass effect on the kidney; only large adenomas and carcinomas can be seen this way. Because the average aldosterone-producing adenoma is only 1.5 to 2.0 cm in size, more refined techniques are needed for visualization.

Because of variable arterial supply to the adrenal gland and fairly normal vascularity of adrenal adenomas, arteriography is not a high-yield procedure. Larger tumors can usually be identified by abdominal ultrasonography. However, the size of the majority of adenomas is below the resolution of present technology. Computerized axial tomography of the adrenal glands provides better resolution of smaller adenomas. Adenomas less than 1 cm in size have been identified. The greater the amount of periadrenal fat, the greater the contrast of the outline of the adrenal gland and the better the chances of recognizing a small adenoma. On a good-quality scan, hyperplasia can be diagnosed. As experience with more sophisticated ultrasound and tomography equipment grows, these techniques will probably become the methods of choice for locating adrenal tumors.

Visualization of the adrenal glands by scintillation scanning after intravenous injection of ^{131}I-19-iodocholesterol or ^{131}I-6β-iodomethyl-19-norcholesterol may locate unilateral disease. The characteristic finding of high uptake of radioactivity in one gland with little or no uptake in the contralateral gland is considered to indicate the presence of an adenoma in the "hot" gland. Some false-positive scans have been reported. In some patients neither adrenal gland will visualize. The labeled cholesterol compounds are also taken up by other steroid hormone–producing glands such as the ovaries and testes. Long-term effects of such radiation exposure have not been fully evaluated.

Sampling of the venous drainage from the adrenal glands may demonstrate differential secretion of aldosterone in patients with an adenoma. High aldosterone levels are found in the effluent from the gland containing the adenoma, whereas values comparable to those in peripheral plasma will be seen on the contralateral side. In patients with hyperplasia the venous effluent from both glands should show similarly elevated concentrations of aldosterone. The technique of adrenal vein catheterization is difficult and requires an experienced radiologist. Once the adrenal vein is catheterized, an adenoma can sometimes be identified by retrograde injection of contrast medium. However, hyperplastic glands with large nodules can give false-positive venography results. Also, the adrenal gland is friable and adrenal infarction with subsequent adrenal insufficiency following venography has been reported.

Occasionally, patients will be seen who have biochemical evidence that strongly suggests an adenoma but in whom all of the above tests have failed to locate a tumor. If the clinical situation dictates, surgical exploration of both adrenal glands may be necessary.

SECONDARY ALDOSTERONISM

PATHOPHYSIOLOGY AND CLINICAL FINDINGS

In contrast with the syndromes of primary aldosteronism, in patients with the syndrome of secondary aldosteronism the adrenal cortex responds appropriately to physiologic stimuli. The increased secretion of aldosterone results from excessive stimulation of the zona glomerulosa by the renin-angiotensin system. To date, no clinical syndromes of increased angiotensin II production without increased plasma renin activity have been described. Therefore, secondary aldosteronism is always associated with hyperreninemia. There are a variety of clinical entities that are associated with such hyperreninemia. These syndromes vary in their clinical presentation and may be conveniently subdivided on the basis of the presence or absence of hypertension.

In some of these conditions, the hyperreninemia and hyperaldosteronism can be considered to be physiologically appropriate responses to alterations in the effective circulating blood volume. For example, patients with essential hypertension receiving diuretic therapy often have elevated levels of plasma renin activity because of the effects of the diuretics. Similarly, in patients with salt-losing nephritis, renin secretion will increase in an attempt to conserve sodium, whereas in patients with congestive heart failure, renin secretion will increase in an attempt to preserve effective circulating blood volume.

In other conditions, the hyperreninemia may be physiologic or pathologic. For example, in pregnant women the increased level of estrogens results in increased production of renin substrate by the liver. As a result, plasma renin activity and aldosterone secretion increase. This can be considered a physiologic response to counteract the mineralocorticoid-antagonist effects of the progestins. The administration of exogenous estrogens to otherwise healthy persons occasionally produces hypertension. These patients have increased plasma renin activity, presumably as a consequence of estrogen-induced increased renin substrate levels. However, a causal role of the renin-angiotensin system in estrogen-induced hypertension has not been proved.

In the other conditions, the hyperreninemia is clearly pathologic. The rare syndrome of a renin-producing tumor, and renin secretion from a Wilms' tumor together with accelerated hypertension, necrotizing vasculitis, and renovascular hypertension are all examples of diseases in which the hyperreninemia causes the hypertension. The first two are examples of primary overproduction of renin. The last three examples of overproduction of renin presumably are a result of decreased perfusion of the kidneys. Some patients with essential hypertension may exhibit elevated plasma renin activity and hyperaldosteronism without evidence of renal or vascular disease. Whether or not the activation of the renin-angiotensin system is responsible for the hypertension is not known.

Edematous states such as nephrosis, congestive heart failure, and cirrhosis of the liver are associated with secondary aldosteronism as a result of physiologic activation of the renin-angiotensin system. Other edematous states such as idiopathic edema and localized edema may also be associated with hyperaldosteronism. The increased secretion of aldosterone appears to correlate with the accumulation of edema fluid. Once a stable weight is achieved, plasma and urinary aldosterone values may be normal.

The clinical manifestations of primary aldosteronism can for the most part be explained on the basis of the mineralocorticoid-induced alterations in renal sodium, potassium, and hydrogen ion homeostasis. With secondary aldosteronism, however, clinical manifestations depend to a large extent on the underlying disease and the contribution from mineralocorticoid hormone excess is variable. In conditions associated with primary overproduction of renin, such as renin-producing tumors, the triad of hypertension, hypokalemia, and metabolic alkalosis may be prominent. However, in conditions such as congestive heart failure, the mineralocorticoid hormone excess may produce different findings, e.g., edema, and these findings contribute to a lesser extent to the overall clinical presentation. The pathophysiology of the mineralocorticoid hormone–induced manifestations has been discussed previously.

DIAGNOSIS

The diagnosis of *secondary* aldosteronism is made by demonstrating excessive secretion of aldosterone coupled with elevated levels of plasma renin activity. In many patients, such as those with the edematous states, the clinical setting will be such that a presumptive diagnosis of secondary aldosteronism is all that is needed before therapy is initiated. In others a more definitive diagnosis is required. The conditions for collection of samples for the measurement of aldosterone excretion and plasma renin activity are the same as described in the section on primary aldosteronism. Because overproduction of renin is suspected, all studies should be carried out while the patient consumes a normal-to-high-sodium diet. There is no need to measure stimulated renin activity.

Certain pharmocologic agents have been used to confirm that hypertension or hyperaldosteronism is secondary to overactivity of the renin-angiotensin system. Saralasin (Investigative) is a competitive antagonist of angiotensin II. Intravenous infusion of this agent will result in significant reduction of blood pressure in patients with hyperreninemic states. Peptides isolated from snake venom have been shown to inhibit the angiotensin-converting enzyme, and thus decrease angiotensin II generation; both oral and intravenous preparations have been used on a research basis. Patients with secondary aldosteronism will have a decrease in aldosterone excretion and blood pressure. However, patients with nonhyperreninemic hypertension may also have a reduction in blood pressure. This may be related to simultaneous inhibition of bradykinin metabolism, a function closely related to angiotensin-converting enzyme activity.

PHEOCHROMO-CYTOMA

By NORMAN H. ERTEL, M.D.,
and MICHAEL GUTKIN, M.D.

Newark, New Jersey

DEFINITION

Pheochromocytomas are chromaffin cell tumors, derived from neurectoderm. Eighty-five per cent or more occur in the adrenal medulla. Most extra-adrenal tumors are found within the abdomen, occurring in either the superior para-aortic area or in the organ of Zuckerkandl at the bifurcation of the aorta. They are rarely seen in the posterior mediastinum, urinary bladder, neck, and brain. Pheochromocytomas are most likely to present in the fourth to sixth decades, but they are an important source of hypertension in children under 15 years of age, when hypertension is usually of the secondary type. About 10 per cent of pheochromocytomas occur in children and 10 per cent are familial, bilateral, multiple, malignant, or extra-adrenal.

This uncommon disease is important because it is one of the curable causes of severe hypertension. Hypertension-screening programs reveal an incidence of 0.1 to 0.7 per cent, and 1000 deaths per year have been attributed to pheochromocytoma in the United States alone.

FAMILIAL PHEOCHROMOCYTOMA

The tumor is familial in 10 per cent of cases and bilateral in 50 per cent of familial disease. Adrenal medullary hyperplasia (diffuse or multinodular) has been described in two large kindreds both as a precursor of pheochromocytoma and an early form of clinical disease. The familial disorder usually exists in association with other hereditary features, such as the phakomatoses (von Recklinghausen's disease, von Hippel-Lindau's disease) or multiple endocrine neoplasia (MEN) syndromes, types 2 and 3. The most common components of MEN type 2 (Sipple's syndrome) are medullary carcinoma of the thyroid, pheochromocytoma, and parathyroid hyperplasia. MEN type 3 also features medullary carcinoma of the thyroid and pheochromocytoma but differs from type 2 in the absence of hyperparathyroidism and the presence of mucosal neuromas, thickened corneal nerves, marfanoid habitus, and alimentary tract ganglio-neuromatosis. Incomplete manifestations of these familial syndromes, such as café au lait spots or medullary carcinoma of the thyroid, may signal an undetected pheochromocytoma in an individual patient. Asymptomatic members of families with multiple endocrine neoplasia should be screened for latent pheochromocytoma. As many as 30 per cent of deaths in MEN type 2 may be attributed to pheochromocytoma.

PRESENTING SIGNS AND SYMPTOMS

Most cases of pheochromocytoma are detected as a result of finding either sustained hypertension or a history of paroxysms or both. Forceful palpitation with or without tachycardia, severe headache, and fear of impending doom are the most dramatic features of the paroxysm. Nausea and vomiting, tremor, pallor or flushing, chest pain, weakness, nervousness, epigastric pain, and dyspnea are noted with some frequency. Unfortunately, there are no symptoms specific for pheochromocytoma in the interval between attacks, even when hypertension is sustained. Furthermore, the labile pulse and headache of essential hypertension overlap with the symptoms of the acute paroxysm. Therefore the few physical signs that are suggestive of pheochromocytoma should be sought vigorously by the examining physician. The most important of these are postural hypotension, profuse diaphoresis, dilated pupils, evidence of weight loss, unexplained fever, and prolonged tachycardia. A paroxysmal attack provoked by anesthesia, change in position, palpation of abdominal mass, compression of the abdomen as by a tight girdle, or a sudden change in temperature while showering is of particular diagnostic value. When a paroxysm is provoked by micturition or swallowing a large bolus of food, the physician should suspect a tumor in the bladder or posterior mediastinum, respectively. A paradoxic hypertensive response to drugs that release stored catecholamines, such as guanethidine, parenteral reserpine, alpha-methyldopa, imipramine, saralasin, or general anesthesia should strongly suggest pheochromocytoma. When this occurs, prompt treatment with the short-acting alpha-adrenergic blocker phentolamine may be lifesaving. Exceptionally severe and prolonged hypotension after a single dose of prazosin has been noted. In patients whose pheochromocytoma is a part of multiple endocrine neoplasia, the signs and symptoms of the associated disease, such as the enlarged thyroid and diarrhea of medullary carcinoma of the thyroid, may predominate.

COURSE

The untreated hypertensive patient with pheochromocytoma is liable to develop any of the complications of severe essential hypertension, including nephropathy, stroke, cardiac failure, retinopathy, and accelerated atherosclerosis. Catecholamine-secreting tumors may be present for many years before hypertension is detectable. Patients who are normotensive between paroxysms may not manifest chronic hypertensive vascular disease. During the acute attack, the patient is in danger of developing sudden severe retinopathy, pulmonary edema, and cerebral hemorrhage. The paroxysmal form of the disease may evolve into sustained hypertension after a variable span of up to 35 years. Sustained hypertension is found in 50 to 60 per cent of adults and 90 per cent of children. Pheochromocytoma occurring during pregnancy bears an unusually grave prognosis for both mother and child. The severe antepartum symptoms are usually attributed to toxemia of pregnancy. Catastrophic episodes of shock, hyperpyrexia up to 110 F (43.3 C), arrhythmias, pulmonary edema, and cerebral hemorrhage frequently lead to death.

PHYSICAL EXAMINATION FINDINGS

An abdominal mass is palpable in only 15 per cent of patients. Therefore the physical findings are primarily related to peripheral effects of excessive catecholamine secretion. The hallmark of the disease is sustained or intermittent hypertension, but pheochromocytoma may produce hypertension for decades without recurrent vasomotor paroxysms. Therefore the presence of long-standing sustained hypertension should not eliminate suspicion of pheochromocytoma. In Sipple's syndrome, a thyroidal mass is frequently palpable for many years before pheochromocytoma becomes clinically manifest. It was once stated that pheochromocytoma is not seen in obese patients. However, weight loss and hypermetabolism are mainly seen in patients with marked elevations of serum-free fatty acids; an increase in body weight of 10 per cent or more is seen in about one third of patients.

COMPLICATIONS: COMMON AND UNCOMMON

The most common complications related to sustained or paroxysmal hypertension have been detailed under Course. Chemical or frank clinical diabetes is present in most patients with pheochromocytoma owing to increased glycogenolysis and suppression of insulin release by circulating catecholamines. Diabetic ketoacidosis is rare and may indicate an underlying true genetic diabetes mellitus. Cholelithiasis is found in 20 per cent of patients with pheochromocytoma. Renal artery stenosis owing to compression by tumor, fibromuscular dysplasia, or atherosclerosis is an uncommon but important complicaton of pheochromocytoma since both conditions may contribute to the hypertension.

In tumors that secrete epinephrine predominantly, catastrophic hypotensive episodes may alternate with hypertension. Abdominal pain, nausea and vomiting, ileus, fever, leukocytosis, tachycardia, and profuse sweating may lead to the mistaken diagnosis of a surgical abdomen or sepsis. Tumors secreting large quantities of catecholamines may present as paralytic ileus, and this complication is usually lethal.

Congestive heart failure that is resistant to the usual therapeutic maneuvers may suggest the presence of catecholamine-induced cardiomyopathy, especially when long-standing hypertension has not been documented. Pheochromocytoma may also present as an acute noncardiogenic pulmonary edema in patients with previously normal lungs ("adult respiratory distress syndrome").

ROENTGENOGRAPHY

A plain abdominal x-ray will locate the tumor in about 15 to 20 per cent of patients and may show "eggshell" calcification in the area of the adrenal. In about 50 per cent of patients, localization is aided by intravenous pyelography with nephrotomography. The most important advance in the localization of both intra- and extra-adrenal pheochromocytomas has been the recognition of the usefulness of computerized axial tomography (CT scan) and ultrasonography). Most pheochromocytomas are larger than 1 to 2 cm and therefore are frequently defined by one of these noninvasive procedures. If they are not, then radionuclide scanning, using either negative imaging with iodocholesterol or positive imaging with technetium (99 TC^m-Sn-DTPA) may be useful, but these procedures should still be considered experimental. Invasive procedures such as aortography, selective adrenal arteriography, or venography, and vena caval catheterization for plasma catecholamines are hazardous and often misleading in the localization of tumors. We recommend, therefore, that such procedures be reserved for unusual cases, such as the patient who has had an unsuccessful exploration, and that the patient be pretreated with phenoxybenzamine before they are undertaken. The rare intrathoracic tumor is almost always seen on a routine chest x-ray, particularly when oblique views are obtained.

SPECIFIC LABORATORY FINDINGS

A high hematocrit is occasionally found and may be due to a decreased plasma volume, a true increase in red blood cell mass, or both. Plasma volume is low in less than one third of cases. High plasma renin activity has been noted in this disease and may be the reason for the mild hypokalemia noted by some authors. Plasma insulin levels are inappropriately low for the simultaneous blood glucose, and free fatty acids are correspondingly high. Gross or microscopic hematuria may be the first clue to the presence of an associated hypernephroma or a pheochromocytoma of the urinary tract. Hypercalcemia and hypophosphatemia may be due to ectopic parathormone production in a few patients but is usually due to associated parathyroid hyperplasia in the familial cases.

Measurement of urinary catecholamines and their major metabolites is the principal laboratory method for the diagnosis of pheochromocytoma. The major metabolites of norepinephrine are normetanephrine and vanillylmandelic acid (VMA); of epinephrine, metanephrine and VMA; of dopamine, homovanillic acid (HVA). The tests most commonly used are of urinary total catecholamines, metanephrines, and VMA. Any one of these will be elevated in over 90 per cent of patients with pheochromocytoma. When a normal value is returned in a patient strongly suspected of harboring this tumor, repeated assays of the same substance or measurement of another excretion product will invariably secure the diagnosis. In the rare event that repeated determinations yield normal values, two possibilities should be considered: (1) the chemical determinations are inaccurate and specimens should be sent to a reference laboratory, and (2) elevated urinary catecholamines or metabolites are present only intermittently and samples should be collected during a paroxysm if possible.

There are several methods for the measurement of catecholamines and their metabolites. The clinician should be acquainted with the instructions of his laboratory concerning collection of the specimen and interference by drugs. Urine is collected in a brown bottle containing 15 ml of 6N HCl and stored in the cold. When VMA is assayed by a nonspecific screening method or by chromatographic techniques, the patient should be on a diet devoid of tea, coffee, vanillin-flavored foods, bananas, and fruits for three days before the urine collection. Fortunately, the method of choice, in which VMA is converted to vanillin, is not affected by antecedent diet. Normal values for 24-hour excretion in adults are:

Total catecholamines	$< 150 \ \mu g$
Norepinephrine	$< 70 \ \mu g$
Epinephrine	$< 20 \ \mu g$
Total metanephrines	< 1.3 mg
VMA (vanillin method)	< 7 mg
HVA (homovanillic acid)	< 10 mg
Dopamine	$< 200 \ \mu g$

Alpha-methyldopa (Aldomet) is excreted in part as alpha-methylnorepinephrine and will lead to very high results in the urinary catecholamine determination but will not significantly affect metanephrines or VMA. Other medications, such as tetracyclines, vitamin B complex, and epinephrine and its congeners used in treatment of asthma or allergic disorders, may lead to spurious elevations of urinary catecholamines. MAO inhibitors may lead to increased excretion of the metanephrines and increased excretion of VMA by altering catecholamine catabolism. Clofibrate (Atromid-S) may lead to a false decrease in VMA levels, and nalidixic acid (NegGram) may lead to a false increase. When levodopa is given at high-dose levels, homovanillic acid is excreted in gram amounts, and there is slight elevation of urinary VMA.

There are some clinical situations in which measurement of a different metabolite may be helpful:

1. In cases in which urinary values are borderline or clinically unexpected, further testing is mandatory before subjecting the patient to surgery.

2. Analysis of a urine sample collected during a paroxysm is more likely to show an acute rise in the catecholamines as compared with metanephrines or VMA.

3. Separate determination of norepinephrine and epinephrine has limited value in localizing the tumor. Although the enzyme for the conversion of norepinephrine to epinephrine is normally present only in the adrenal medulla and the organ of Zuckerkandl, some pheochromocytomas in intrathoracic sites have been found to secrete significant quantities of epinephrine.

4. Benign pheochromocytoma in adults rarely results in increased excretion of the norepinephrine precursor, dopamine, and its major metabolite homovanillic acid (HVA). However, almost half of malignant pheochromocytomas result in increased urinary levels of dopamine or HVA or both. Since it is difficult to ascertain whether a pheochromocytoma is benign or malignant by the usual pathologic criteria, measurement of these compounds may be of important prognostic value.

Sensitive and accurate isotope derivative techniques have been developed for plasma catecholamines. Normal values are:

Norepinephrine   100–300 pg/ml
Epinephrine   0–90 pg/ml
Dopamine   0–50 pg/ml

The plasma catecholamine assay has not been as useful as the urinary procedures for the following reasons:

1. It is technically more difficult and expensive to perform.

2. There may be wide variations from minute to minute in patients, particularly those under stress.

3. Elevations may be noted upon standing or with cigarette smoking.

4. Elevated values may be found in some patients with essential hypertension or with depression.

PHARMACOLOGIC TESTS

The availability of reliable and diagnostic urinary assay methods has lessened the need for potentially dangerous and often misleading pharmacologic tests. When such tests are deemed necessary, some basic precautions will safeguard the patient and increase their diagnostic value. A reproducible baseline blood pressure must be obtained. Two physicians should be present to administer the drug and record the pulse and condition of the patient. A sham test using 1 ml of isotonic saline is necessary to test the response of the patient to the stress of the procedure. The test drug is injected into one line, while the second is available for administration of phentolamine mesylate (Regitine) for hypertensive crisis, or norepinephrine bitartrate (Levophed) for severe hypotension.

Phentolamine Test. When blood pressure is consistently elevated, the rapid injection of 5 mg of the alpha adrenergic blocking agent phentolamine mesylate will cause a fall in blood pressure greater than 35/25 mm Hg in a patient with pheochromocytoma. When clinical suspicion is high, it is prudent to use a preliminary dose of 1 mg. Blood pressures are recorded every minute for 5 minutes before the drug is given, and every minute for 10 minutes afterward. Unfortunately, many false-positive results have been obtained in patients with uremia, strokes, and malignant hypertension as well as in patients taking drugs commonly used in the treatment of hypertension. This test has recently been modified with the knowledge that catecholamines inhibit the release of insulin. An intravenous infusion of 10 per cent glucose in water is given at a rate of 2 ml per minute for 30 minutes before and after the

injection of 5 mg phentolamine. Blood is taken before and at 1-minute intervals for 5 minutes after the drug is given. A diagnostic fall in blood pressure accompanied by a rise in insulin exceeding 13 microunits per ml and a fall in glucose of 18 or more mg per 100 ml has been seen only in patients with pheochromocytoma or patients with severe hyperthyroidism.

The major usefulness of this test is in clinical situations in which immediate diagnosis and treatment of a hypertensive emergency due to suspected pheochromocytoma is necessary.

Phenoxybenzamine Therapeutic Trial. In some patients with very brief, recurring attacks, all tests may be within normal limits. Complete cessation of these attacks with chronic oral phenoxybenzamine may establish the correct diagnosis.

Glucagon Stimulation Test. Histamine, tyramine, and glucagon have been used to provoke a sudden rise in blood pressure in normotensive patients suspected of harboring a pheochromocytoma. Since the histamine test may be hazardous, leading to complications and death owing to stroke or myocardial infarction, we recommend that this test be abandoned. The tyramine test is not recommended because of frequent falsely positive and negative results. When a provocative test is indicated, we recommend the glucagon test. It is relatively safe and falsely positive only in patients with severe hyperthyroidism but may be negative in one third of patients with proven pheochromocytoma. Inject 1 mg crystalline glucagon in 1 ml of diluent rapidly intravenously and record blood pressures every 30 seconds for 5 minutes, then every minute for the following 5 minutes. A positive response is a rise of 35/25 mm Hg over the baseline. The rise is usually noted in the first 3 minutes. Occasionally, there is a major pressor response to 1 mg glucagon. If a pheochromocytoma is strongly suspected, a preliminary dose of 0.5 mg should be used.

PITFALLS IN DIAGNOSIS

The greatest difficulty in the diagnosis of pheochromocytoma is the failure to consider this disease in a patient with apparently clear-cut essential hypertension, anxiety neurosis, diabetes mellitus, or hyperthyroidism. The surgeon or internist who is surprised by an unexpected paroxysmal crisis will never forget the experience. Since sustained hypertension is so frequently the only sign of the disease, at least one 24-hour urine specimen should be assayed for VMA or total metanephrines in every newly detected hypertensive patient.

Hyperthyroidism is particularly important to consider in the differential diagnosis. Increased basal metabolic rate (BMR), weight loss, tachycardia, arrhythmias, palpitation, diaphoresis, tremulousness, and increased neck girth and goiter may be seen in both diseases. The glucagon and phentolamine tests may be positive. Except in those rare instances in which the two diseases coexist, thyroid function tests are not abnormal in patients with pheochromocytoma, while urinary VMA and metanephrines are not significantly elevated in most patients with thyrotoxicosis.

Certain patients with a hyperdynamic circulatory state have recurrent attacks of forceful or rapid palpitation and anxiety, accompanied by a rise in blood pressure. Urinary VMA and metanephrines are normal in these patients, but slightly elevated urinary catecholamines at the time of an attack may present a diagnostic problem.

Patients treated with MAO inhibitors are subject to hypertensive crises and flushing when they ingest foods rich in tyramine or drugs that release endogenous catecholamines. Major reactions to foods (aged cheese, wine, beer, pickled herring, and chicken livers) and drugs (amphetamine, ephedrine and metaraminol) have been reported. Recognition of this syndrome is critical, since administration of phentolamine effectively aborts the attack.

Brain tumors, particularly in the posterior fossa, may cause sustained or intermittent hypertension and elevated levels of urinary catecholamines and metabolites. Careful neurologic examination should define the lesion in all such patients.

When paroxysmal attacks are seen in nurses, medical students, or other medical and paramedical personnel, particularly those with a history of psychiatric disorder, surreptitious self-administration of norepinephrine, ephedrine, or isoproterenol should be suspected ("pseudopheochromocytoma"). Urinary catecholamines and metabolites may be elevated. Provocative tests will be negative, but phentolamine given during an "attack" will lower the blood pressure.

Hypertensive episodes partially relieved by phentolamine may be seen in association with chest pain, or in the premonitory period before myocardial infarction, in patients with coronary artery disease. Urinary catecholamine excretion may be moderately increased during the attack, but metanephrine and VMA levels are usually normal.

Hypertensive patients treated with clonidine in whom the drug is suddenly discontinued may have a hypertensive crisis within the next 1 to 2 days associated with signs of sympathetic hyperactivity and elevated plasma and urinary catecholamines. Similar evidence of "sympathetic rebound" may be seen when other sympathetic blocking agents are precipitously withdrawn. Such situations may be treated by either reinstitution of the drug or by phentolamine.

CARCINOID TUMOR AND CARCINOID SYNDROME

By FRANK E. SMITH, M.D.,
and MONTAGUE LANE, M.D.
Houston, Texas

Synonym

Argentaffinoma.

Definition and Pathology

Carcinoid tumors arise in endodermal tissues most commonly from sites throughout the gastrointestinal tract and less frequently from bronchi and endodermal components of teratomas. Primary locations include appendix, ileum, colon, rectum, stomach, duodenum, jejunum, pancreas, biliary ducts, gallbladder, esophagus, Meckel's diverticulum, bronchus, larynx, and ovarian and testicular teratomas.

In the gut, the carcinoids begin in the Kulchitsky cells of the crypts of Lieberkühn. Intracytoplasmic granules of these cells reduce silver salts, resulting in a positive "argentaffin reaction." The term "argyrophilic reaction" pertains to "argentaffin-negative" carcinoids, which stain with silver after the addition of a reducing substance. Hence, the argentaffin reaction is not a constant feature of carcinoids and is therefore not an absolute requirement to establish a pathologic diagnosis.

Carcinoids represent less than 1 per cent of all gastrointestinal tumors. Grossly, carcinoids may be yellow to light gray and often appear to originate submucously because of their predilection to invade rather than to extend intraluminally from their true beginning sites in the mucosa. It is rare for lesions to encroach on the bowel lumen, and only occasionally do annular lesions occur. Gastric and duodenal lesions bleed frequently and are associated with ulcers or ulcerative masses. Intussusception may occur with small bowel carcinoids, but more commonly mesenteric fibrosis, kinking, and matted bowel loops are the pathogenesis of obstruction. Multicentricity has been reported in up to 40 per cent of jejunoileal tumors and in 8 per cent of rectal carcinoids, but not in other sites.

Several histologic patterns of carcinoid tumors exist but do not correlate with prognosis or course of disease. Tumors arising in the foregut and midgut are commonly argentaffin or argyrophil positive and may be associated with carcinoid syndrome, whereas hindgut carcinoids are argentaffin negative and are not associated with the syndrome.

Important clinicopathologic features relating unfavorably to prognosis include (1) size of primary greater than 1 to 2 cm, (2) involvement of the muscularis, (3) nodal involvement, and (4) distant metastases (lymphatic and hematogenous) most commonly to the liver and only rarely to lung, bone, or brain.

The carcinoid syndrome results from release of one or more bioactive tumor products into the systemic circulation and is described subsequently in this article.

Since Oberndorfer's introduction of the term "carcinoid" in 1909, approximately 4000 cases of the tumor have been described.

PRESENTING SIGNS AND SYMPTOMS

General. The majority of carcinoid patients are asymptomatic. Fatigue, weakness, anorexia, weight loss, and edema are late systemic features of disease and are usually associated with liver involvement, chronic cardiac decompensation, and/or nutritional compromise.

Gastrointestinal. Appendiceal, gastroduodenal, and rectal lesions are usually asymptomatic. Small bowel and colonic carcinoids may be associated with acute abdominal pain, e.g., intussusception, but more often cause chronic partial obstructive symptoms resulting from kinking or fibrosis within the mesentery adjoining the bowel. Annular obstructing tumors are rare. Melena and iron deficiency anemia are most common with ulcerative, gastric, or duodenal lesions.

Right lower quadrant pain mimicking appendicitis occurs in over half the patients with symptomatic appendiceal carcinoids.

Generalized abdominal pain, which may be extremely severe and is often associated with disabling, frequent, explosive watery diarrhea, is an important symptom complex of the carcinoid syndrome. The intestinal hypermotility is a pharmacologic effect of serotonin and kinins present in biochemically active carcinoids most frequently when liver metastases are present. Cutaneous flushing may coincide with the attacks of diarrhea. Gastric carcinoids may cause symptoms of peptic ulceration perhaps related to increased histamine production from tumors in this location.

Hepatomegaly resulting from metastases may be massive and can cause right upper quadrant discomfort or the sharper pain of hepatic capsular pressure effects and/or a dragging heaviness reflecting the large bulk of the organ. These symptoms can precede the carcinoid syndrome by years. Jaundice, hypoglycemia, and other symptoms of liver dysfunction are absent early in the course of disease, but may occur in the terminal stages.

Vascular Effects. Cutaneous flushing is a typical feature of carcinoid syndrome. Bradykinin levels are almost uniformly elevated and may be mediated in part by discharges of catecholamines, pentagastrin, or histamine. Injected bradykinin will reproduce flushing. Flushing in some patients may be almost completely blocked by concomitant administration of H_1 and H_2 blockers, (antihistamines and cimetidine). Pentagastrin-induced flushing can be blocked by somatostatin, which inhibits the release and action of gastrin in those patients in whom this biochemical pathway is responsible for the carcinoid flush. Prostaglandins have also been isolated from carcinoid tumors and produce flushing when injected into normal persons. They may be responsible for flushing in some patients who do not have elevated kinin levels. Patients may describe flushing attacks as "spells," during which the color of the skin of the head and neck followed by the trunk and extremities changes to pink, bright red, or a violaceous blue-red hue, lasting from 1 to 10 minutes and recurring in some persons up to 25 to 30 times per day.

Patients may associate carcinoid flush with physical exertion, emotion, tumor manipulation, catecholamine administration, alcohol ingestion, vagal stimulation, or various foods. Symptoms coincident with flushing may include itching, sweating, palpitations, anxiety, facial swelling, and syncope because of hypotension caused by marked vasodilation in response to kinin release.

Shortness of breath and wheezing as a consequence of bronchospasm are seen in about half the patients with carcinoid syndrome. Shortness of breath, cough, wheezing, ankle swelling, and other cardiac symptoms may also be expressions of valvular disease, usually pulmonary stenosis and tricuspid insufficiency, caused by endocardial plaque depositions that are most marked on the distal portion of the valves. Left-sided lesions are less usual and involve the mitral valve leaflets and chordae tendineae. Occasionally, lesions are seen in the atria, superior and inferior vena cava, systemic veins, and coronary sinus. Carcinoid heart disease occurs in approximately half the patients with the carcinoid syndrome.

Miscellaneous. Symptoms may originate from a variety of endocrinologic abnormalities associated with carcinoid tumors; for example, ectopic production of ACTH, growth hormone, or parathormone may all produce weakness. Muscular weakness has been a major symptom in a few recently reported patients with carcinoid myopathy. Impotence and decrease in libido have been suspected to be related to increased luteinizing hormone production in some patients, but data are inconclusive. Mental, gastrointestinal, and cutaneous symptoms may result from a pellagrinous syndrome caused by shunting of tryptophan from the niacin pathway to be used in serotonin synthesis. Usually less than 3 per cent of tryptophan is converted to serotonin. Carcinoid tumors may utilize as much as 70 per cent of available tryptophan for serotonin production.

COURSE

The traditional view that carcinoids are associated with a long course must be tempered by the realization that symptomatic patients with lesions over 2 cm have only a 5 per cent 5-year survival rate. The high incidence of appendiceal lesions relative to other primary sites favorably shifts overall survival for the total group of carcinoid patients, as patients with appendiceal lesions rarely die of their disease. Nevertheless, persons with advanced tumors have long been known to survive 5 to 25 years, and one author recently observed 5 of 24 patients with hepatic metastases surviving 5 years and 4 patients, 10 years.

Prognosis by primary site is most favorable for appendix, intermediate for ileum and stomach, and worst for bronchial and colonic tumors.

The immediate cause of death may be hepatic failure, bowel obstruction, vascular collapse and shock, respiratory failure with bronchoconstriction, congestive heart failure, or cachexia.

PHYSICAL EXAMINATION

Vital Signs. These may be entirely normal. During a flush, tachycardia, tachypnea, hypotension, and shock may be present.

General Appearance. This may vary from normal to cachectic. Edema related to hypoalbuminemia and/or heart failure may be prominent.

Skin. The carcinoid flush ranges in color from pink to deep red to violaceous in the skin over the neck and head, and later may involve the trunk and extremities. Sweating, tearing, anxiety, and facial edema can accompany a flush. Gastric carcinoids may cause a distinctive flush with a well demarcated undulating border, bright red in hue. In patients with disease of long duration telangiectases appear, and facial skin may assume a permanent bluish discoloration. Hyperpigmentation of the face, neck, and areas of the extremities exposed to solar radiation occurs in patients with the pellagra-like syndrome.

Cardiopulmonary. Patients may be dyspneic and cyanotic from bronchospasm, with asthma-like auscultatory findings, or from congestive failure, with rales and peripheral edema; right-sided failure patterns predominate. S4 and S3 gallops may be prominent. The most frequent murmurs of carcinoid syndrome are those of pulmonary stenosis and tricuspid insufficiency. Only occasionally are mitral murmurs heard. Prominent "a" or "v" waves are seen in the neck when significant stenotic or insufficiency lesions are present. A pulsatile liver suggests tricuspid insufficiency. Bruits over the liver may also be heard.

Gastrointestinal. Abdominal tenderness may be found in the right lower quadrant in appendiceal carcinoid patients, in the right upper quadrant when hepatomegaly is present, and may be generalized, mimicking the acute abdomen, during hyperperistaltic "crises." Nodular hepatomegaly is common, and friction rubs may be heard over areas of capsular involvement. The systemic physical evidences of hepatic insufficiency occur late in the course of disease. Palpable masses denoting a primary intra-abdominal lesion occur in as many as one third of patients. Rectal, ovarian, and testicular carcinoids may be palpated, and detectable blood on the examining finger occurs in only a minority of patients.

Bowel sounds can be extremely prominent when hyperperistalsis arises from bioactive tumor products or when mechanical obstruction (up to two thirds of patients) is present.

Other. Carcinoid myopathy is marked by prominent proximal muscle group weakness.

Common Complications. These have been described under Presenting Signs and Symptoms and Physical Examination.

LABORATORY FINDINGS

General laboratory tests may be completely normal when limited disease is present. In patients with more advanced malignancy the anemias of chronic disease, blood loss, liver disease, and gastrointestinal rapid transit may be seen. During carcinoid crises, leukocytosis and thrombocytosis are common. In patients with advanced disease, abnormalities of hepatocellular function, including hypoalbuminemia, may be prominent. Hypoalbuminemia may also result from excessive watery diarrhea. Hypokalemia and salt wasting from inordinate gastrointestinal losses may be seen as well as dilutional abnormalities of serum electrolytes in patients with anasarca, hepatic insufficiency, or congestive heart failure. Rarely, hypokalemic alkalosis indicates Cushing's syndrome associated with carcinoid, and hypercalcemia with hypophosphatemia may indicate hyperparathyroidism. Steatorrhea and malabsorption have been noted as unusual findings in some patients with carcinoid. The most critical laboratory determination in carcinoid syndrome is the measurement of 5-hydroxyindoleacetic acid (5-HIAA) in the urine. This substance is the metabolite of serotonin (5-hydroxytryptophan or 5-HT) through the action of monoamine oxidase aldehyde dehydrogenase. Normally, the 24-hour urine 5-HIAA is 2 to 10 mg. Carcinoid patients excrete 30 to 600 mg per 24 hours. Hyperserotoninemia is also present in carcinoid syndrome, but serotonin is not usually assayed in general hospital laboratories. Occasional patients with carcinoid have low urinary 5-HIAA, but they may excrete large amounts of 5-hydroxytryptophan and 5-hydroxytryptamine, enabling diagnosis to be made chromatographically. The radiographic appearance of gastrointestinal carcinoids is not distinctive, but small bowel polypoid lesions, particularly if multiple and if associated with angulation of intestinal loops because of paraintestinal involvement, may increase the index of suspicion for this tumor.

BIOCHEMICAL FINDINGS

Kinins. These physiologically active amines play an important role in many features of carcinoid syndrome. Plasma levels are elevated in almost all patients during a flush. Kallikrein, present in the primary tumor but more commonly in hepatic metastases, becomes activated possibly by sympathomimetic amines, resulting in conversion of plasma kininogen to bradykinin. Bronchoconstriction, vasodilation, intestinal hypermotility, and increased capillary permeability occur as the kinins are activated.

Catecholamines. Catecholamines are postulated to act as mediators of the kinin system. Administration of catecholamines causes a flush associated with a rise in kinin levels. This phenomenon has been employed in a limited sense as a provocative test. Five micrograms of epinephrine given intravenously induces a flush in 1 to 2 minutes. The reliability of this test is unknown.

Histamine. Serotonin may mediate the release of histamine in some patients with carcinoid, and increased serum and urinary histamine may be detected. The pharmacologic effects of histamine closely mimic those of the kinins but have the additional capacity to increase the output of gastric acid. This may be responsible for the increased incidence of peptic ulceration in gastric carcinoids.

Prostaglandins. The observation of prostaglandin activity in patients with carcinoids, mentioned earlier, suggests the possibility of a role of these substances in the pathogenesis of flushing when kinins are nondetectable.

Endocrine Abnormalities. In recent years a growing interest in the endocrine relationships of carcinoid tumors has evolved.

Adrenal Dysfunction. Cushing's syndrome has been reported associated with carcinoids producing ACTH. Of current interest is the observation that serotonin antagonists have effects on adrenal function in patients with carcinoid, suggesting serotoninergic control of cortisol secretion.

Growth Hormone. Increased levels of growth hormone have been correlated with high serum serotonin, and urinary 5-HIAA and hormone levels decrease toward normal upon treatment with serotonin antagonists.

Gonadal Hormones. Although results must be considered as currently inconclusive, data imply that luteinizing hormone secretion may be high in males with carcinoid and might account for decrease in libido and/or impotence in affected patients.

Calcitonin. Carcinoid patients with increased serum calcium and low serum phosphorus have been shown to have elevated serum immunoreactive calcitonin, without higher concentrations in neck venous catheter samples, suggesting that calcitonin originated in tumor rather than the thyroid gland. In addition, elevated levels of calcitonin have been documented in carcinoid tumor extracts. The thesis advanced is that hyperparathyroidism in these carcinoid patients may be a compensatory response to high circulating calcitonin.

PITFALLS IN DIAGNOSIS

The major differential diagnoses include intra-abdominal malignancies; carcinoma of the lung, ovary, or testicle; asthma; non-carcinoid valvular heart disease; and allergic states, including angioneurotic edema and anaphylactoid reactions. Non-carcinoid bases for minimal increases in 5-HIAA excretion (10 to 20 mg per 24 hours) include several malabsorption states, which actually cause increased excretion of other indoles that can be identified chromatographically.

Ingestion of foods high in serotonin content (avocados, bananas, pineapples, tomatoes, and walnuts) will result in falsely elevated urinary 5-HIAA. Antipyretics (phenacetin), muscle relaxants (methocarbamol), and glyceryl guaiacolate cause urinary chromophores to be misinterpreted as 5-HIAA. False negative results caused by interference with the colorimetric reaction occur with phenothiazines and mandelic acid derivatives (methenamine mandelate).

EMPTY SELLA SYNDROME

By STEPHEN F. HODGSON, M.D.,
and RAYMOND V. RANDALL, M.D.

Rochester, Minnesota

DEFINITION

The term "empty sella turcica" describes a sella turcica whose anatomic features include an incomplete diaphragma sellae through which a pouch of arachnoid filled with cerebrospinal fluid descends into the sella and flattens and compresses the pituitary gland, and may enlarge the bony sella turcica. Gross anatomic inspection gives one the impression that the sella is empty, and radiographically the sella may be enlarged and the intrasellar subarachnoid space may contain contrast medium, as from a previous myelogram, or air, during pneumoencephalographic examination.

An empty sella can exist for two reasons: (1) An anatomic variation occurs in which the diaphragma sellae is incompletely formed, allowing the suprasellar arachnoid membrane to herniate through the diaphragmatic opening. In time, the hydrostatic pressure of the cerebrospinal fluid may cause enlargement of the intrasellar arachnoid pouch, which, in turn, may result in compression of the pituitary gland and enlargement and demineralization of the bony sella. This type of empty sella is common,

occurring with a prevalence of approximately 6 per cent, and is referred to as the "idiopathic" or "primary" empty sella syndrome. (2) Tissue loss occurs within the sella after surgical or radiotherapeutic ablation of an expanding intrasellar mass, or after spontaneous infarction of a pituitary tumor. Structures which are normally suprasellar in position, including the optic chiasm, may herniate downward into the sella or become drawn into the sella by contracting scar tissue. This type is referred to as the "secondary" empty sella syndrome.

PRESENTING SIGNS AND SYMPTOMS

The idiopathic empty sella is probably a relatively common condition, its prevalence being masked by its usually small degree of sellar enlargement and generally asymptomatic course. It occurs approximately five times more frequently in women than in men. Complaints that lead to the diagnosis are often nonspecific, and the majority of cases are discovered serendipitously during investigations for conditions unrelated to the pituitary. The patients who are found to have the idiopathic empty sella syndrome are usually middle-aged, multiparous women with complaints that vary from headaches and sinus trouble to mild menstrual disorders. However, the syndrome has been found in both sexes at all ages. Physical examination reveals a high prevalence of obesity, and often mild hypertension. Visual field abnormalities and physical evidence of endocrine disorders are conspicuously absent. Nontraumatic spinal fluid rhinorrhea can result from extensive erosion of the bony sella. Pseudotumor cerebri has been reported in association with the empty sella syndrome, and hence examination of the optic discs must not be omitted.

DIAGNOSIS

Standard roentgenograms of the head and sellar tomography reveal a globular and usually symmetrical enlargement of the sella. However, asymmetric enlargement of the sella may occur, especially if there are infrasellar septa in the sphenoid sinus. Demineralization of cortical bone may be present. Pneumoencephalography with the patient's head placed in the brow-up position demonstrates air within the sella. Computerized axial tomography and pituitary angiography, although useful at times, may be of no help in the diagnosis and have not replaced pneumoencephalography as the definitive diagnostic procedure.

Routine laboratory tests are unaffected by this condition. Endocrine abnormalities are rare and, when present, are usually due to endocrine end-organ disease, unrelated to the empty sella. Pituitary function is normal in the great majority of patients, but isolated instances of presumed associated pituitary dysfunction have been recorded, and minor abnormalities in pituitary reserve and pituitary-hypothalamic relationships have been observed. Thus it is not entirely clear at this time whether the idiopathic empty sella syndrome can lead to clinically significant endocrine deficiencies, and thorough endocrine investigation is therefore essential in the clinical investigation and assessment of these patients.

COMPLICATIONS

Rarely, nontraumatic cerebrospinal fluid rhinorrhea has been reported in association with the empty sella syndrome. This is considered to be due to the opening of embryonic vestigial channels during transient increases in cerebrospinal fluid pressure, such as occurs during coughing or sneezing. Several instances of empty sella in association with pseudotumor cerebri have also been reported — the pathophysiology of this association is not well defined. Since the pituitary, although distorted in shape, remains a normally functioning organ, its susceptibility to other pathologic entities remains unchanged. Hence the scattered reports of the chance association of empty sella with a functioning pituitary microadenoma are not surprising.

DIFFERENTIAL DIAGNOSIS

The importance of recognition of the empty sella syndrome lies in its differentiation from an expanding tumor within the sella, such as a pituitary adenoma, and thereby the avoidance of therapeutic error. This is especially true when there are progressive visual field defects, which can occur with the secondary empty sella syndrome as well as with expanding tumors within the sella. Visual field defects occurring after operation or irradiation of a pituitary tumor are usually considered evidence of a recurrent or persistent tumor. However, identical changes in the visual fields occurring months or years after therapy can be caused by the development of a secondary empty sella syndrome.

Pneumoencephalography with tomography during placement of the head in the brow-up position is currently the procedure of choice to establish the diagnosis in both the idiopathic and the secondary empty sella syndromes. In our experience, computerized tomography (EMI scan) has been of limited value in making the diagnosis in either syndrome. We have made a diagnosis of idiopathic empty sella syndrome in a few patients in whom roentgenograms of the head unexpectedly revealed myelographic dye within the sella.

TREATMENT AND FOLLOW-UP EXAMINATION

Idiopathic and secondary empty sella syndromes require no treatment except in two situations. The occurrence of cerebrospinal fluid rhinorrhea warrants transsphenoidal operation to stop the leak, thus precluding possible ascending infection and meningitis. The secondary empty sella syndrome may lead to progressive visual field defects from herniation of the optic chiasm into the sella. If the defects become extensive, operation will be required to return the chiasm to its customary position.

All patients with an empty sella syndrome, idiopathic or secondary, should be examined periodically. Examination should include roentgenograms of the head for comparison of sellar size, endocrine evaluation, funduscopic examination, inquiry about possible cerebrospinal fluid rhinorrhea, and, in patients with secondary empty sella syndrome, plotting of the visual fields.

Section 11

DISEASES OF THE UROGENITAL TRACT

ACUTE RENAL FAILURE

By JOSEPH M. MALIN, JR., M.D.
Richland, Washington

DEFINITION

Acute renal failure is characterized by the acute onset of anuria or oliguria (24-hour urinary output of less than 400 ml) that, if untreated, leads to azotemia, uremia, and death.

PRESENTING SIGNS AND SYMPTOMS

The presenting signs and symptoms are stated in the definition. More specific symptoms are directly related to the cause of renal failure, and therefore the single most important factor in establishing the etiology is the antecedent history. The history also determines the choice and number of diagnostic procedures that will be necessary.

ETIOLOGY

The cause of acute renal failure may be categorized into prerenal (decreased renal blood flow), renal, or postrenal (obstruction) groups. The changes that occur in the renal parenchyma are often reversible, and therefore it is important to establish and correct the cause of acute renal failure early in the course of the disease.

Prerenal Causes. Prerenal causes of acute renal failure are related to decreased renal blood flow. A history of *shock,* severe *congestive heart failure,* or *dehydration* preceding the onset of the oliguric state suggests that a temporary restriction of renal blood flow has led to acute tubular necrosis. The sudden onset of bilateral or unilateral flank pain with associated anuria may indicate *renal artery occlusion.* A history of severe atherosclerosis and hypertension suggests possible renal artery stenosis with superimposed acute occlusion, whereas a history of subacute bacterial endocarditis suggests renal artery emboli. Major *trauma,* especially with destruction of large amounts of muscular tissue, may cause precipitation of myoglobin in the proximal nephron. *Burns, hemolytic reactions, eclampsia,* and *mismatched transfusions* are other possible causative factors.

Renal Causes. *Renal glomerulopathy* or *vasculitis* might be suspected if the patient has had glomerulonephritis, recent streptococcal infection, or a history of drug sensitivity with recent exposure. *Nephrotoxins* such as ethylene glycol, carbon tetrachloride, or bichloride of mercury as well as many unknown nephrotoxins that are found in heroin and other abused drugs may produce oliguria or anuria secondary to renal vascular or tubular damage.

Postrenal Obstruction. Of all the causes of acute renal failure, obstruction is most easily diagnosed and readily corrected. A history of difficulty in voiding and acute suprapubic pain may represent acute urinary retention secondary to some form of bladder outlet obstruction. *Benign prostatic hypertrophy, carcinoma of the prostate,* and severe *urethral stricture* disease are the most common reasons for obstruction.

Acute urinary retention is an obvious cause of anuria and is easily relieved by catheter drainage of the urinary bladder. Oliguria or anuria in a patient with renal colic and a history of kidney stones or gout suggests *ureteral calculi.* A history of phenacetin ingestion suggests *papillary necrosis,* whereas methysergide ingestion suggests *retroperitoneal fibrosis* as a possible cause of ureteral obstruction. Complete anuria immediately following difficult pelvic surgery strongly suggests the possibility of *ureteral injury.*

LABORATORY STUDIES

Urinalysis. A low, fixed specific gravity indicates tubular damage; proteinuria and granular casts suggest chronic parenchymal renal disease, whereas red blood cell casts are associated with active glomerulonephritis. Microscopic examination may demonstrate a renal papilla, uric acid, cystine, or calcium oxylate crystals. Free hemoglobin may appear in the urine of a patient with intravascular hemolysis or myoglobin in trauma.

Chemical Studies. Elevation of the serum creatinine or blood urea nitrogen will be found in azotemia. The ratio of urine urea to blood urea nitrogen will be less than 10 in most patients with acute tubular necrosis, whereas prerenal and glomerular diseases do not usually lower this ratio. In acute tubular necrosis the kidney loses its ability to reabsorb sodium, and an increased concentration of urine sodium with a relative decrease in urine potassium will be noted. Urine osmolality to blood osmolality ratios of less than 1 suggest impaired tubular concentration.

THERAPEUTIC TESTS

In patients whose oliguric state is secondary to electrolyte imbalance, severe dehydration, or depleted intravascular volume, the intravenous infusion of 25 grams of mannitol or 80 mg of furosemide will temporarily increase urinary output. Intravenous infusion of hypertonic saline may be used but must be administered cautiously to avoid acute pulmonary edema.

RADIOLOGIC STUDIES

A high-dose infusion intravenous pyelogram, using 1 ml of contrast material per lb of body weight with a maximum dose of 150 ml may give useful information in oliguric patients with a blood urea nitrogen level of less than 75 mg per 100 ml. In any case, the plain film of the abdomen alone may demonstrate the cause of anuria, i.e., urinary tract calculi. Retrograde urography should be performed on all patients who have had a sudden onset of total anuria or persistent oliguria when the history suggests obstruction or when a history is not available. Renal venography and renal arteriography should be performed in those patients whose history suggests vascular occlusion.

RENAL BIOPSY

Percutaneous renal biopsy should be performed when parenchymal renal disease is suspected. Proper histologic classification of disease will indicate proper therapy when a reversible condition is demonstrated.

GLOMERULO-NEPHRITIS

By STEPHEN I. RIFKIN, M.D.,
and DANA L. SHIRES, JR., M.D.
Tampa, Florida

Glomerulonephritis encompasses a large number of diseases whose common denominator is glomerular injury. The pathogenesis of this injury involves at least two immunologic mechanisms: immune complex disease and antiglomerular basement membrane antibody disease. These mechanisms produce many patterns of damage that can be characterized by clinical features, laboratory evaluation, and examination of renal biopsy specimens. Although clinical and laboratory presentations vary, the response of the kidney to glomerular injury is stereotyped to the extent that biopsy confirmation is mandatory for accurate diagnosis.

Analysis of renal biopsies and laboratory findings requires understanding of normal renal histology and function. The nephron is the functioning unit of the kidney, and the glomerulus is the filtering component of the nephron. The glomerulus has two basic areas, the capillary loop and the mesangium, and three basic cell types, endothelial, epithelial, and mesangial cells. The actual filtering process occurs in the capillary loop. The loop is lined on its inner aspect by an endothelial cell. A basement membrane surrounds most of the endothelial cell, and epithelial cells form an outer lining about the basement membrane. Discrete foot processes from the epithelial cells are in contact with the basement membrane. The mesangial area can be thought of as the inner support structure of the glomerulus. It is composed of mesangial cells and mesangial matrix. The mesangial cells also have significant reticuloendothelial cell functions.

Adequate renal biopsy analysis should include examination by light microscopy, immunofluorescent microscopy, and electron microscopy. Light microscopy is the classic method and gives information about cellularity and can be used to make a gross estimate of glomerular basement membrane thickness. Immunofluorescent microscopy is performed by staining glomeruli with fluorescent antisera to various factors involved in glomerular injury, such as the immunoglobulins and components of the complement system. If any of these components are present, a fluorescent pattern will be seen when the appropriate antiserum is used. Electron microscopy, by means of its tremendous magnifying ability, gives a close view of the glomerular basement membrane, the epithelial foot processes, and will generally demonstrate, if they are present in the glomerulus, electron-dense deposits thought to be immune complexes.

In immune complex disease, the kidney appears to be an innocent bystander, inundated by circulating antigen-antibody complexes. The classic prototype of this is serum sickness. In serum sickness a foreign protein, unrelated to the kidney, is administered. The antibodies made against the protein couple with it, forming complexes. When complexes of the appropriate size are formed at the stage of moderate antigen excess, deposition occurs in the glomeruli.

Complement is fixed and activates a variety of noxious agents, producing glomerular damage. If the antigen is given in a single large injection, the process is self-limited; but if it is given in small daily doses over a period of weeks, chronic, progressive disease occurs. Recently, a second mechanism for immune complex deposition has been suggested. This theory proposes that complexes may also form by combination of antibody and antigen in situ within the glomerulus.

Multiple patterns of immune complex injury can be seen on light microscopy. Immunofluorescent studies show deposition of complement and immunoglobulins. The deposits are irregularly distributed and discrete, appearing under immunofluorescence in what has been described as a lumpy, bumpy distribution. Electron microscopy demonstrates the presence and distribution of immune complexes and any abnormalities of cell proliferation.

In contrast, in antiglomerular basement membrane antibody disease, antibodies to glomerular basement membrane are produced. The antibodies fix complement and set off the same mediators of membrane damage as in immune complex disease. Light microscopy reveals a variety of nonspecific types of glomerular damage, often with associated epithelial crescent formation. Immunofluorescence shows a linear, ribbon-like staining for immunoglobulins. Electron microscopy fails to show any electron-dense deposits.

Laboratory investigation of glomerular injury begins with the urinalysis. A dipstick evaluation gives gross estimates of proteinuria and hematuria. Microscopic examination of fresh urine allows for better quantification of hematuria. Two to three red cells per high-power field is accepted as normal. The presence of red cell casts implicates the kidney as the source of the hematuria. These casts, however, do not persist in alkaline or hypotonic urine and repeated examinations may be necessary to rule out their presence when one is searching for a glomerular lesion. Blood urea nitrogen (BUN) and serum creatinine are used as a rough measure of renal function. Creatinine is the normal end product of muscle metabolism and is produced at a relatively constant rate. It is primarily filtered and not reabsorbed. The production rate of urea, however, may vary significantly, depending upon the patient's rate of catabolism. Substantial amounts are reabsorbed in the renal tubules in patients with a diminished effective intravascular volume. Of the two, serum creatinine is the more reliable indicator of renal function. Unfortunately, a substantial decrease in renal function is necessary before

clear-cut abnormalities of blood urea nitrogen (BUN) or serum creatinine are seen. A timed urine collection for calculation of the creatinine clearance is necessary for a more precise quantification of the glomerular filtration rate and urine protein losses. The clearance ratio of a relatively small and a relatively large protein molecule, e.g., transferrin and IgG, is used in estimating the degree of selectivity of proteinuria, which aids in defining the leakiness of the glomerular basement membrane. A higher degree of selectivity, that is, excretion of primarily small protein molecules, is interpreted as reflecting a less porous glomerular basement membrane.

More sophisticated laboratory studies include the fluorescent antinuclear antibody test for collagen vascular disease, various screening tests for the presence of recent streptococcal infection, and a test to determine the profile of the complement system. Complement is composed of a series of factors found in normal serum that are activated in a sequential fashion. Activation of complement can lead to cellular injury. Complement is activated by either the classic or alternate pathways, each producing different serum complement profiles. Classic pathway activation, generally initiated by immune complexes, goes through C1, C4, C2 to activate C3 and then the remainder of the complement cascade. This tends to produce low serum levels of C1q, C4, and C3. Alternate pathway activation bypasses C1, C4, and C2, directly cleaving C3, and is caused by such agents as immunoglobulin aggregates, polysaccharides (inulin and zymosan), endotoxins, and properdin. This results in a normal serum C1q and C4 with a low serum C3. Thus precise complement profiles vary with different glomerular diseases.

Table 1 presents a convenient classification of glomerulonephritis based on immunologic mechanisms and subdivides according to biopsy characteristics. Following the outline of Table 1, the immune complex diseases are discussed first, followed by antiglomerular antibody disease and then several miscellaneous diseases. It needs to be emphasized that, although generalizations can and will be made about specific diseases, there may be wide individual variations in laboratory findings, chemical presentations, course, and outcome.

PROLIFERATIVE GLOMERULONEPHRITIS

The prototype of proliferative glomerulonephritis is acute poststreptococcal glomerulonephritis, a sequela of infection with a ne-

Table 1. *Classification of Glomerulonephritis*

A. Immune complex disease
  1. Proliferative
  2. Membranous
  3. Membranoproliferative
    a. Type I
    b. Type II–dense deposit disease
  4. Focal glomerulonephritis
B. Antiglomerular basement antibody disease with or
  without pulmonary hemorrhage
C. Miscellaneous
  1. Rapidly progressive glomerulonephritis
  2. Lipoid nephrosis
  3. Focal glomerulosclerosis

phritogenic strain of streptococcus. Acute glomerulonephritis has also been reported in such diverse entities as viral infections, subacute bacterial endocarditis, and the Guillain-Barré syndrome. Cellular proliferation is evident on light microscopy. Immunofluorescence demonstrates deposition of immunoglobulins and complement in a lumpy, bumpy fashion. Electron microscopy confirms immune complex deposition in a subepithelial distribution very much as in acute serum sickness.

Acute poststreptococcal glomerulonephritis has a classic presentation. From 9 to 21 days after streptococcal infection, after initial symptoms of the infection have completely subsided, weakness and anorexia return. Quite short latent periods of only a few days suggest an exacerbation of pre-existing disease. The streptococcal infection may have been a pharyngitis in the usual sporadic case or a skin infection in epidemic nephritis. The patient notices periorbital and ankle edema and frequently dyspnea. Urine volume decreases and the urine looks like tea or a cola drink because of hematuria. Abdominal pain, nausea, and vomiting may be present. Hypertension is frequent and may present with headache or convulsions. The oliguria or anuria usually lasts only a few days. Hematuria and red cell casts are the classic findings of the urinalysis. Proteinuria is characteristically present but uncommonly exceeds 3.5 grams per day. The anti-streptolysin-O titer (ASO titer) becomes elevated in 1 to 3 weeks, peaks in 3 to 5 weeks, and, in 50 per cent of patients, returns to normal within 6 months. However, only 70 to 80 per cent of patients have an elevated ASO titer, and if the patient has been treated with antibiotics, the percentage decreases to 10 to 15 per cent. Streptococcal skin infections may not be associated with substantial rises in the ASO titer, so other serologic evidence for preceding streptococcal infection is necessary. Although complement levels vary, a common profile demonstrates substan-

tial depression of C3 accompanied by depression of C1q or C4 or both.

Microscopic hematuria may persist for several years. Proteinuria has been reported to persist for more than 12 months in 61 per cent of the patients and for more than 24 months in 36 per cent. The urinalysis can remain abnormal long after the patient's symptoms subside. A poor prognostic indicator is an initial presentation with severe renal dysfunction and the presence of numerous epithelial crescents on biopsy. Adults fare substantially worse than children, and preschool children fare the best. The incidence and overall outcome of acute poststreptococcal glomerulonephritis are still matters of substantial controversy. Studies have recently demonstrated that many, if not most, people with acute poststreptococcal glomerulonephritis are asymptomatic and their condition is discovered only when large groups are systematically screened by urinalysis and serum complement levels. These findings cast into doubt our past ideas on the incidence of the disease and suggest that past data on the natural history were based on inadequate samples. Recently reported long-term studies indicate that acute poststreptococcal glomerulonephritis may cause more residual damage than previously supposed.

MEMBRANOUS GLOMERULONEPHRITIS

Membranous glomerulonephritis (MGN) is the most common cause of the idiopathic nephrotic syndrome in adults. Seventy-five to 80 per cent of patients with idiopathic membranous glomerulonephritis present with the nephrotic syndrome. It is associated with a variety of underlying diseases including carcinomas, lymphomas, heavy metal intoxication, hepatitis B antigenemia, and malaria. There is a wide age range for the onset of this disease process, but the majority of patients are more than 40 years old. They are more often male, usually have nonselective proteinuria, and often have microscopic hematuria. Serum complement levels are normal. On biopsy, subepithelial immune complexes are seen without evidence of cellular proliferation. The complexes are gradually incorporated into the glomerular basement membrane. Spikes of glomerular basement membrane between deposits are seen with light microscopy and a silver stain. Immunofluorescence shows granular deposition of IgG and C3. Approximately 30 per cent of patients have deposits of IgM or IgA or both, and 20 per cent have deposition of early complement components. Electron microscopy confirms the findings of subepithelial immune complex deposition. The course of MGN is extremely variable, making evaluation of any therapy difficult. Estimates are that approximately 25 per cent of patients have a spontaneous remission while 40 per cent have progression to some degree of chronic renal insufficiency. Patients without the nephrotic syndrome have the more benign course and rarely progress to end-stage renal disease. Children also appear to do somewhat better than adults, with a better remission rate and a slower progression of the disease. Recurrence of the disease in renal allografts is rare.

MEMBRANOPROLIFERATIVE GLOMERULONEPHRITIS

This disease is also called mesangiocapillary glomerulonephritis or hypocomplementemic glomerulonephritis. The majority of patients are between the ages of 5 and 15 years. It may be subdivided pathologically into types I and II. In type I, there are subendothelial and mesangial immune complex deposits, an increase in mesangial matrix, and mesangial cell proliferation with intrusion of the mesangial cell matrix between the glomerular basement membrane and the endothelial cells. Duplication of the glomerular basement membrane or "splitting" of the glomerular basement membrane in association with the deposition of immunoglobulins and C3 is often present. Deposition of early-acting complement components C1q and C4 also occurs.

Type II membranoproliferative glomerulonephritis is referred to as dense-deposit disease. It has a striking biopsy picture with the glomerular basement membrane greatly thickened and partially or totally replaced by an amorphous, homogenous, highly electron-dense material. It has been suggested that this density may represent an intrinsic alteration of the glomerular basement membrane structure. All glomeruli are involved to a variable extent. Intramembranous deposition occurs in the tubular basement membranes in a segmental fashion. There is usually an associated mesangial cell proliferation and occasional crescent formation. Immunofluorescence shows granular or pseudolinear staining for C3 in a distribution identical to that of the intramembranous deposits and mesangial staining. Immunoglobulins, C1q, and C4 are either scanty or absent.

Complement profiles are abnormal but vary considerably. C3 is depressed but may fluctuate greatly during the course of the illness. Type I is most often associated with classic pathway activation of complement with low C3, C4, and C1q; type II with alternate pathway activation of complement, low levels of C3, normal C4, and normal C1q. In addition, C3NeF, a heat-stable nonimmunoglobulin gamma globulin capable of activating complement at the C3 level, is often found in the plasma of patients with membranoproliferative glomerulonephritis. C3NeF is more commonly found in type II than in type I.

Although there is an association between type II disease and partial lipodystrophy in a small number of patients, the clinical presentation and clinical course, as well as the outcome, are similar for both disease types. Membranoproliferative glomerulonephritis is the cause of 5 to 10 per cent of the idiopathic nephrotic syndrome of childhood. The presentation varies: according to one estimate approximately 50 per cent of the patients present with the nephrotic syndrome, 30 per cent present with asymptomatic proteinuria and recurrent hematuria, and 20 per cent present with an acute nephritic syndrome. Mild hypertension occurs in approximately one third of patients and depressed renal function is common. The prognosis is poor. Five-year survival rates were 87 per cent in one large study, with 44 per cent of patients developing chronic renal insufficiency within 5 years. An actuarial analysis of patients with type II MPGN suggests that 50 per cent develop end-stage renal disease by the tenth year. Membranoproliferative glomerulonephritis may recur in renal allografts and current evidence suggests that type II disease will recur in virtually all grafts.

FOCAL GLOMERULONEPHRITIS

The pathologic picture of focal glomerulonephritis is found in many diseases including systemic lupus erythematosus, Henoch-Schönlein purpura, and idiopathic benign essential hematuria. The distinction between these diseases is made on clinical and laboratory grounds.

One form of idiopathic benign essential hematuria is called IgA nephropathy or "Berger's disease." It commonly presents in children or young adults as persistent microscopic or intermittent gross hematuria. The hematuria is often exacerbated by strenuous exercise or upper respiratory tract infections. Renal function is usually normal at time of diagnosis, and proteinuria mild, if present at all. Hypertension is not common until late in the disease. Serum complement levels are normal. An elevated serum IgA is usually present.

Renal biopsy reveals focal mesangial matrix increase, some mesangial cell proliferation, and mesangial immune complex deposits. The predominant immunofluorescent staining is for IgA in a mesangial distribution. There may be varying intensities of staining for IgG, IgM, and C3. C1q and C4 are usually not present.

This disease generally follows an indolent course, but up to 50 per cent of patients have been reported to develop end-stage renal disease over a 15 to 20 year period following diagnosis. Poor prognostic indicators are the presence of hypertension, proteinuria above 2 grams per 24 hours, and decreased glomerular filtration rate at the time of biopsy. Recurrent disease is a risk in renal allografts.

ANTIGLOMERLULAR BASEMENT MEMBRANE ANTIBODY DISEASE

This is an uncommon disease with an estimated incidence of approximately 5 per cent of all cases of glomerulonephritis. Its hallmark is the presence of circulating glomerular basement membrane antibodies, in contrast to their absence in immune complex disease. In lieu of the demonstration of circulating antibodies, the presence of a linear immunofluorescent pattern for IgG is extremely strong evidence. A weak linear pattern may be seen in patients with diabetes mellitus; an extremely densely packed granular pattern can be mistaken for a linear pattern. Ten per cent of normal biopsies have been reported to have a linear "accentuation" of the glomerular basement membrane when stained for IgG; occasionally with quite advanced disease, no glomeruli with typical linear deposits are observed. Therefore the immunofluorescent study alone can at times be misleading. The presence of linear tubular basement membrane antibody staining occurs in approximately 70 per cent of patients and supports the diagnosis. Electron microscopic findings are helpful in that they fail to reveal evidence of immune complexes. There are no light microscopy findings that are pathognomonic of glomerular injury induced by antiglomerular basement membrane antibody.

When associated with pulmonary hemorrhage, this disease is called Goodpasture's syndrome. Pulmonary disease precedes or is coincident with the onset of renal dysfunction in more than 70 per cent of patients with an average delay of approximately 3 months between the onset of the two symptoms. There is a striking preponderance of young adult males. Serum complement levels are normal. The renal disease is generally quite severe, but milder cases with remissions are now being reported. The diagnosis is strongly suggested by the combination of renal failure and pulmonary hemorrhage, but a similar picture may also occur with the vasculitides and immune complex forms of glomerular injury.

Current data suggest that the antiglomerular basement membrane antibody production is self-limited, with titers falling to undetectable levels over an average period of 7 to 8 months. If therapy can prevent irreversible renal damage during the period of antibody production, the prognosis should be substantially altered for the better. The disease may recur in renal transplants, but if the recipient has no detectable circulating antibodies before grafting, the recurrence is generally mild. Present policy is to defer transplantation until the disappearance of circulating antiglomerular basement membrane antibodies.

RAPIDLY PROGRESSIVE GLOMERULONEPHRITIS

Rapidly progressive glomerulonephritis (RPGN) appears to have a wide variety of causes cutting across the immunologic classification given in Table 1. Therefore, it has been classified under the Miscellaneous heading. This process is also called extracapillary proliferative glomerulonephritis, crescentic glomerulonephritis, subacute glomerulonephritis, or malignant glomerulonephritis. It is distinguished by its rapid downhill course and a striking biopsy picture. Causes include streptococcal infections, the vasculitides, systemic lupus erythematosus, antiglomerular basement antibody disease, and idiopathic disease. The clinical course is that of progressive loss of renal function occurring over weeks to months. There are extracapillary epithelial crescents in the majority of glomeruli. These crescents are formed by the cells lining Bowman's capsule that become hyperplastic and literally crush the glomerular capillaries. Findings typical of immune complexes are seen in those cases associated with immune complex disease, and linear staining for IgG is seen in those cases associated with antiglomerular basement antibody disease. An additional subdivision of patients with rapidly progressive glomerulonephritis without immune complexes or only sparse deposits and no evidence of antiglomerular basement membrane antibody disease has recently been described. Substantial incidence figures have not been recorded to date; however, those available suggest that 20 to 30 per cent of patients may fall into this category, with the remainder being divided between antiglomerular basement membrane antibody disease and immune complex disease.

The clinical features and prognosis appear to be similar for all three types of RPGN. There is a slight male preponderance, an insidious onset with nonspecific signs and symptoms. The overall patient survival is 30 to 50 per cent without dialysis or transplantation. Serum complement levels are usually normal. The chances for recovery are slim if more than 70 per cent of glomeruli are extensively involved with crescents.

LIPOID NEPHROSIS

Other names for this include minimal change disease, nil disease, and no change by light microscopy disease. It is by far the most common cause of the idiopathic nephrotic syndrome of childhood and accounts for 10 to 30 per cent of the nephrotic syndrome in adults. The patients generally present with highly selective proteinuria, normal or near normal renal function, an unremarkable urinary sediment, normal blood pressure, and normal serum complement levels. Occasional patients may have microscopic hematuria, and in adults poorly selective proteinuria is more often found. The glomeruli show little or no changes on light microscopy and immunofluorescence is negative. Electron microscopy reveals fusion of the epithelial cell foot processes but is otherwise negative. There is no clear-cut evidence for either an antiglomerular basement membrane antibody or an immune complex etiology. It has been suggested that lipoid nephrosis results from an abnormality of T-cell function, but this is still speculative. An association exists between lipoid nephrosis and Hodgkin's disease, and there are reports of patients developing lipoid nephrosis in association with exposure to allergens.

This is a rather indolent disease in children, lasting for many years with periods of remission and relapse. An occasional patient may have progression to chronic renal failure. In adults, the prognosis does not appear to be nearly as good, and considerable numbers have progression to chronic renal failure. Because up to 90 per cent of children respond promptly to steroid therapy, a therapeutic and diagnostic trial with steroids is often attempted in lieu of a renal biopsy. This is less frequently done in adults because of the much lower incidence of lipoid nephrosis. Initial steroid response rates for adults are fairly close to that for children. Approximately two thirds of patients responding to steroids will have relapse and require additional treatment, and 5 to 10 per cent of patients have primary steroid resistance. Cyclophospha-

mide therapy has been beneficial in patients failing to respond to or having relapse following steroid therapy. (This specific use of cyclophosphamide is not listed in the manufacturer's official directive.) This disease has been reported to recur in renal allografts.

FOCAL GLOMERULOSCLEROSIS

Focal glomerulosclerosis occurs in 5 to 15 per cent of children with the nephrotic syndrome and has been reported to occur in a similar or slightly higher percentage of adults. Differentiation between this syndrome and lipoid nephrosis is necessary because long-term prognosis may be quite different. Distinguishing features include a higher incidence of (1) microscopic hematuria, (2) nonselective proteinuria, (3) renal dysfunction at the time of initial diagnosis, (4) hypertension, and (5) a much lower incidence (less than 15 per cent) of steroid responsiveness. In spite of these differences, a recent report of the International Study of Kidney Disease in Children, in which a multivariate analysis of clinical and laboratory evaluation of children with the idiopathic nephrotic syndrome was used, failed to demonstrate a good discrimination between these two diseases. Thus, biopsy is mandatory for a firm diagnosis. Focal segmental areas of sclerosis without evidence of inflammation are seen in the glomeruli. There are no proliferative or membranous changes. Positive immunofluorescence for IgM and C3 in the affected lobules has been consistently reported. Occasional electron-dense deposits are seen in the same areas by electron microscopy. These changes are thought to first occur in the juxtamedullary glomeruli, and it is possible, if the biopsy specimen does not include this area, to miss the diagnosis. Focal segmental scarring is not specific for a single disease entity and may be simulated by glomerular scarring following proliferative glomerulonephritis. To further complicate the picture, this histologic picture may also occur in patients with relapsing steroid-responsive lipoid nephrosis after the disease has been present for some 2 to 15 years. This overlap between the two entities complicates both our ability to diagnose and to prognosticate. Although occasional remissions occur, focal glomerulosclerosis has a much poorer prognosis than lipoid nephrosis, with an actuarial survival in one large series of 75 per cent at 5 years, 60 per cent in 10 years, and 38 per cent in 15 years. This disease may recur in renal allografts.

NEPHROTIC SYNDROME

By ALAN M. ROBSON, M.D.,
and LINDA C. LONEY, M.D.

St. Louis, Missouri

DEFINITION

The nephrotic syndrome represents a clinical entity characterized by proteinuria, hypoproteinemia (predominantly hypoalbuminemia), edema, and hyperlipidemia. To require any arbitrary level of abnormality in one of these determinants before accepting a diagnosis of nephrotic syndrome is inappropriate. For example, in patients with nephrotic syndrome, urinary protein excretion usually exceeds 3.5 grams per day per 1.73 square meters of body surface area. However, in children with minimal change nephrotic syndrome, proteinuria may amount to less than 1 gram per day per 1.73 square meters of body surface area, especially if severe hypoalbuminemia is present; yet the existence of a nephrotic syndrome in these children cannot be denied.

There are numerous causes of the nephrotic syndrome, some of the more common ones being listed in Tables 1 and 2. Thus, once the presence of a nephrotic syndrome has been established, it is essential to undertake the

Table 1. *Diseases Associated with the Nephrotic Syndrome*

1. Glomerulopathies not associated with known systemic disease (see Table 2 for more detail)
2. Malignancies: Hodgkin's disease, leukemia, carcinomas, multiple myeloma
3. Diabetes mellitus
4. Infectious diseases: syphilis, malaria, subacute bacterial endocarditis, cytomegalic inclusion disease, toxoplasmosis, schistosomiasis, pyelonephritis
5. Collagen vascular diseases: systemic lupus erythematosus, periarteritis, dermatomyositis
6. Cardiovascular diseases: renal vein thrombosis, inferior vena caval thrombosis, constrictive pericarditis, congestive heart failure
7. Nephrotoxins: organic and inorganic mercury, gold, bismuth
8. Allergens and drugs: bee stings, poison oak and ivy, milk allergy, snake bites; trimethadione, paramethadione, penicillamine, probenecid, heroin use
9. Congenital (Finnish and other types) nephrotic syndrome, hereditary nephritis
10. Miscellaneous diseases: amyloidosis, renal transplantation, pregnancy, obesity, sickle cell anemia

Table 2. *Approximate Incidences of Diseases Found in Pediatric and Adult Patients with Nephrotic Syndrome**

Disease Entity	Relative Incidence (%)	
	CHILDREN	ADULTS
Minimal change (nil lesion)	66	15
Focal glomerular sclerosis	9	10
Glomerulonephritis:		
Membranous	3	22
Membranoproliferative	8	7
Other†	9	23
Other diseases‡	5	23
Total	100%	100%

*Figures averaged from selected, published series. Figures meant only as a guide. Comparable values in individual centers will vary depending on patterns of patient referral.
†Includes all other proliferative glomerulonephritides.
‡For example, diabetes mellitus, systemic lupus erythematosus, amyloid, anaphylactoid purpura.

equally important and often more difficult task of defining the underlying cause. This often can be accomplished from a careful history, a thorough physical examination, and laboratory tests. If these findings indicate that the nephrotic syndrome is secondary to a glomerulopathy (Table 2), a complete histologic diagnosis should be established in most patients by renal biopsy. The resulting information is helpful in determining prognosis and in managing the patient. This approach is preferable to that sometimes advocated, of labeling all nephrotic patients with glomerulopathies as having "idiopathic nephrotic syndrome." This term is misleading. In these disease states the cause of the immune complex deposition in the kidneys may be unknown or idiopathic, but the cause of the nephrotic syndrome is not.

PRESENTING SIGNS AND SYMPTOMS

Diseases that cause the nephrotic syndrome have varying incidences at different ages (Table 2). Thus minimal change disease has a much higher incidence in children than in adults. In contrast, membranous glomerulonephritis and diseases such as diabetes mellitus are much more commonly the cause of nephrotic syndrome in adults. Since the underlying cause modifies the patient's mode of presentation, signs and symptoms of the syndrome often differ in the child and in the adult.

The peak age of onset of minimal change nephrotic syndrome is at the third year of life, although it may present at any age. In childhood the incidence in males is approximately 2.5 times that in females, but in the adult age group, equal numbers of males and females are affected. There may be a positive family history for nephrotic syndrome: the incidence of the disease in a relative of an affected patient is approximately 100 times the incidence in the general population. Edema is the predominant symptom or sign, with dependent edema usually being the first abnormality noted. It is more marked in the lower extremities after a period of exercise or standing but is predominantly in the periorbital or lumbosacral areas after sleeping. Although variable in amount, periorbital edema may be sufficiently severe to interfere with vision, pedal edema may prevent the wearing of a normal size shoe, ascites may cause clothes to be too tight or result in respiratory difficulty, and either scrotal or labial edema may be incapacitating. After diagnosis, a patient frequently realizes that dependent or periorbital edema had been variably present for several weeks or months previously. Not infrequently, an upper respiratory tract infection or other viral infection precedes by 2 or 3 days the appearance of the edema. Similarly, an allergic response to pollen, to bee stings, or to poison oak or ivy may appear to be a precipitating factor. Indeed, 40 per cent or more of children with minimal change nephrotic syndrome may have atopy.

Sometimes the existence of the nephrotic syndrome may be first suspected from the finding of proteinuria on a routine urinalysis or patients may mention excessive foaming of the urine, a consequence of massive proteinuria. Such patients may have mild degrees of edema that are difficult to detect clinically, since an adult patient usually has to accumulate 2 or more liters of additional extracellular fluid before it can be detected as pitting edema. Nonspecific vague symptoms of the nephrotic syndrome include malaise, fatigability, irascibility, depression, and loss of the feeling of well-being. These symptoms rarely dominate the clinical picture and are not the usual presenting ones. The pallor resulting from edema may be misinterpreted as indicating the presence of anemia. Rarely, the development of cellulitis, peritonitis, or pneumonia may be the first sign that eventually results in the diagnosis of an underlying nephrotic syndrome.

In patients with a nephrotic syndrome resulting from one of the glomerulonephritides, the initial abnormalities that prompt the patient to seek medical advice include hematuria, hypertension, or the symptoms of renal insufficiency. Alternatively, the extrarenal signs of a systemic disease such as systemic lupus erythematosus or of the precipitating cause of the nephrotic syndrome such as diabetes mellitus may be the initial and dominant features of the patient's disease.

PHYSICAL FINDINGS

The presence of dependent edema is usually the most notable abnormal physical finding and when fluid retention is severe, anasarca is obvious. Ascites and pleural effusions should be looked for and may be sufficiently marked to embarrass respiration. The retina has a characteristic "wet" appearance. The normally white lunulae of the fingernails may be pink, whereas the remainder of the nail bed may be white secondary to subungual edema. Paired white lines (Mees' lines) may be seen on both the fingernails and toenails. Inguinal or umbilical hernias may be found, especially with severe or prolonged ascites. The elasticity of the auricular cartilage appears decreased.

Blood pressure in patients with minimal change nephrotic syndrome is usually normal, but mild hypertension may be found in up to 20 per cent of children and in up to 45 per cent of adults. Growth failure in children may be significant, especially in those who have had multiple relapses of the syndrome requiring long courses of steroids in high dosages. The presence of cellulitis may be readily apparent; less obvious infections such as peritonitis or pneumonia should be sought, especially in patients with fever or leukocytosis and who are taking steroids, since these drugs may mask the usual symptoms. Pallor consequent upon the edema and the clinical features of apparent hypothyroidism may also be noted on occasion, although characteristically patients are euthyroid. Patients often are irritable or may have depressive symptoms, especially when they have anasarca.

If glomerulonephritis is the underlying cause for the nephrotic syndrome, severe hypertension is found more frequently and may be associated with secondary changes such as a hypertensive retinopathy. Patients with glomerulonephritis may manifest the physical findings of azotemia such as the characteristic earthen skin color or even asterixis. If a systemic disease is the underlying cause of the nephrotic syndrome, the clinical features of this disease may be readily apparent.

LABORATORY FINDINGS

Urine. Many urinary abnormalities are common to nephrotic patients irrespective of the underlying cause. Proteinuria, usually 3 to 4+ by dipstick, varies from less than 1 to more than 25 grams per 1.73 square meter of body surface area per day. The values for adult patients are usually in excess of 3 grams per day. Pediatric patients frequently spill less protein even when corrections are made for the differences in body size. In part as a consequence of this proteinuria, the urine specific gravity is characteristically high, being in excess of 1.025 and not infrequently being 1.035.

The urine sediment often contains oval fat bodies. Lipiduria is better diagnosed, however, using a microscope equipped with polarized light and demonstrating doubly refractile fat bodies ("Maltese crosses") in degenerative fatty vacuoles in the cytoplasm of desquamated renal epithelial cells or free in the urine as neutral fat droplets. Characteristically, urines with heavy proteinuria also contain hyaline casts.

Other urinary findings vary depending upon the cause of the disease. In patients with minimal change nephrotic syndrome, macroscopic hematuria is unusual, although mild microscopic hematuria, e.g., 10 red blood cells (RBC) per high power field in a centrifuged urine sample, may be found in up to one third of patients. In contrast, in patients with the nephrotic syndrome secondary to glomerulonephritis, the urine sediment tends to show a greater abnormality, with more cellular elements and casts including granular, cellular, and mixed hyaline casts being present. Unfortunately, one cannot always differentiate patients with a minimal change lesion from those with glomerulonephritis on the basis of urine sediment abnormalities alone. One exception to this general rule is the presence of a "telescoped" urine sediment, which indicates the presence of systemic lupus erythematosus or, less frequently, some other progressive glomerulonephritis.

Peripheral Blood. Hypoalbuminemia is common to all nephrotic patients, and marked hyperlipidemia occurs in most. Total serum protein is characteristically reduced to between 4.5 and 5.5 grams per 100 ml; serum albumin concentrations usually fall below 2 grams per 100 ml and not infrequently to below 1 gram per 100 ml. However, in some patients the concentrations of these proteins are remarkably well preserved despite massive proteinuria. Serum α_1-globulin concentrations are usually normal or slightly decreased, whereas levels of serum α_2- and β-globulins are characteristically increased. Although the concentration of gamma globulin determined by electrophoresis is normal or reduced, the levels of individual components vary. Serum IgG levels average approximately 20 per cent of normal, whereas IgA levels are less severely reduced and IgM and IgE levels are increased, particularly in minimal change nephrotic syndrome.

Serum total cholesterol concentration is almost always elevated. The average level is increased to approximately 400 mg per 100 ml, with values in excess of 1000 mg per 100 ml having been recorded. Phospholipid may also be increased, but the cholesterol-to-phospholipid ratio is almost invariably elevated, as are serum triglyceride levels. Despite these changes the plasma of patients with nephrotic syndrome usually does not become lactescent until triglyceride levels exceed 400 mg per 100 ml or four times their normal level. The lipoprotein profiles characteristic of the nephrotic syndrome are types II and V in contrast to the type IV profiles that are seen in uremic patients. Low and very low density lipoprotein levels are elevated early in the course of the disease; high density lipoprotein levels may be moderately elevated but tend to fall to subnormal levels with severe hypoalbuminemia.

Despite massive amounts of edema, the serum electrolytes are usually within the normal range. The serum sodium may be low (e.g., to 130 mEq per liter) in the presence of marked hyperlipidemia. This artifact results from the high concentrations of blood lipid that contains no sodium, and thus plasma osmolality remains unchanged. Such pseudohyponatremia requires no treatment, in contrast to true hyponatremia, in which both plasma sodium and osmolality are reduced. Serum calcium may be low, owing in part to the hypoproteinemia and resulting reduction of bound calcium. The hypocalcemia, however, may be out of proportion to the hypoalbuminemia, and ionized calcium levels may be reduced by 15 to 20 per cent as well, probably owing to reduced blood levels of 25-hydroxy vitamin D found in nephrotic syndrome. Symptoms of hypocalcemia rarely occur. Total and ionized serum calcium levels return to normal with remission of the nephrotic syndrome. Serum phosphorus is normal unless the nephrotic sydnrome is associated with renal insufficiency.

In minimal change nephrotic syndrome, blood urea nitrogen and serum creatinine values are characteristically normal even though glomerular filtration rates measured by inulin clearance average only 80 per cent of normal. However, occasional patients with this syndrome may have their glomerular filtration rates reduced unexpectedly to 20 or 30 per cent of normal, perhaps representing the development of acute renal failure secondary to severe hypovolemia. Azotemia, however, more often results when the nephrotic syndrome is secondary to a glomerulonephritis or a systemic disease that is associated with nephron damage and loss. Unfortunately, the presence or absence of azotemia cannot be used as a reliable indicator in the differential diagnosis of the nephrotic syndrome.

Hemoglobin levels and hematocrits may be

normal or even increased if there is hemoconcentration consequent upon hypoproteinemia. This may help to differentiate patients with minimal change disease from those with severe renal insufficiency, who usually have anemia.

Serum complement and its components are normal in minimal change nephrotic syndrome. Reduced levels of the third component of complement (β-1-C globulin) indicate that a glomerulonephritis underlies the nephrotic syndrome but do not occur invariably with glomerulonephritis.

Plasma renin activity and urine excretion of catechols are increased in the nephrotic patient. Abnormal plasma levels of binding proteins for hormones and metals may be accounted for by urinary loss. This is the proposed explanation for the decreased plasma 25-hydroxy vitamin D_3 and ionized calcium concentrations found in the nephrotic patient. Similarly, urinary loss of thyroid-binding globulin and prealbumin probably results in the decreased half-life of thyroxine and makes interpretation of the studies of thyroid function difficult in the nephrotic patient. These patients often appear hypothyroid but usually are euthyroid despite low values for serum protein–bound iodine and increased uptake of iodine by the thyroid gland. If an iron deficiency anemia develops in the nephrotic syndrome it may well be due to urinary loss of transferrin. Urinary loss of Factor B may result in decreased opsonization of *Escherichia coli* and may contribute to the susceptibility of nephrotic patients to infections.

Special Studies. *Renal Biopsy.* Virtually every patient with the nephrotic syndrome warrants a renal biopsy to diagnose the underlying renal pathology, to help in selecting the appropriate therapeutic approach, and to determine prognosis. The exception to this rule is the patient under 5 years of age with the typical clinical features of minimal change nephrotic syndrome. As detailed in the succeeding paragraphs, such a patient may be given a therapeutic trial of steroids and needs a biopsy only if there is no response to this therapy or if multiple relapses occur.

Renal biopsy is a specialized technique and should be done only in centers whose personnel are familiar with the technique and where adequate facilities for examination using light microscopy, immunofluorescent microscopy, and electron microscopy are available. The following are the more common pathologic findings:

1. *Minimal change lesion.* This is characterized by no remarkable glomerular findings on light or immunofluorescent microscopy, although electron microscopy demonstrates fusion of the podocytes (epithelial cell foot processes) in the glomerulus. Apparent vacuolization in the cells of the proximal convoluted tubules is characteristic. Prognosis is very good in both children and adults.

A similar picture complicated by mildly increased cellularity in the mesangial regions and by moderate deposition of IgM in the glomeruli has been described. It remains to be determined whether this represents a variant of the minimal change lesion or is a separate clinical entity.

2. *Focal glomerulosclerosis.* Light microscopic examination of renal tissue from patients with focal glomerulosclerosis demonstrates portions of glomeruli that are sclerotic. Characteristically, superficial nephrons obtained on renal biopsy are less severely involved, and the lesion may be missed by sampling error. Immunofluorescent microscopy may demonstrate no abnormality or nonspecific glomerular deposition of several plasma proteins, including albumin, fibrinogen, immunoglobulins, and complement in the sclerotic lesions. Electron microscopy shows foot process fusion but has not helped elucidate the nature of the sclerotic lesions. In the adult, prognosis is not favorable; progressive renal failure not responsive to steroid therapy is to be expected. In children the prognosis is not always so bleak, 40 per cent of patients showing partial or complete remission of the nephrotic syndrome when treated with steroids.

3. *Glomerulonephritis.* Common to all forms of glomerulonephritis is the glomerular localization of immunoglobulin or complement as demonstrated by immunofluorescent microscopy. Discussion of proposed pathologic classifications is not appropriate here. However, two diagnoses should be mentioned: (a) *Membranous glomerulonephritis*, which is characterized by glomerular capillary basement membrane thickening, usually without a remarkable increase in the number of cells in the glomerulus. Electron microscopy demonstrates abnormal electron-dense deposits on the epithelial side of the basement membrane. The clinical course of this disease is highly variable, with 25 per cent of all patients having spontaneous remission and an equal number developing progressive renal failure in addition to the nephrotic syndrome. The remaining 50 per cent of patients have persistent proteinuria but relatively stable, although reduced, renal function for many years. (b) *Membranoproliferative glomerulonephritis*, which is now a well-described clinicopathologic entity. By light microscopy these patients have glomerular basement membrane thickening. An increased number of mesangial deposits of immunoglobulin or complement or both are seen on immunofluorescent

microscopy. Two types are discernible by electron microscopy. Type 1 has predominantly subendothelial and mesangial immune complex deposits, whereas type 2 has unusually electron-dense deposits within the basement membrane ("dense-deposit disease"). The two pathologic types are remarkably similar clinically, with patients having nephrotic syndrome, progressive renal failure, hypertension, and low serum concentrations of the third component of complement. Prognosis is variable, and thus therapy must be individualized.

There remains a group of patients whose renal biopsies are diagnosed as "glomerulonephritis" but who do not fit into the aforementioned categories. The glomeruli in the biopsies of these patients are usually characterized by increased numbers of mesangial cells, leukocytic infiltration, or increased numbers of other glomerular cells (proliferation). Sometimes this is associated with glomerular crescents, glomerular necrosis, or mesangial expansion. In general, it may be stated that the presentation of necrosis in glomerular tufts or of crescents about the capillary tuft is an unfavorable pathologic feature.

Selectivity of Proteinuria. In minimal change nephrotic syndrome the urinary clearance of albumin or transferrin is great when compared with clearance of larger proteins such as IgG (highly selective proteinuria). In contrast, patients with membranous or proliferative glomerular changes usually have disproportionately greater clearances of the larger proteins (nonselective proteinuria). While measurements of protein selectivity will separate groups of patients with different disease entities from one another, measurements from individual patients do not provide a basis for diagnosis of the type of renal disease present. In addition, a variety of technical problems has limited the usefulness of measuring selectivity of proteinuria as a clinical tool.

Coagulation Changes. Patients with the nephrotic syndrome have been shown to have significant elevations of Factors V and VIII, fibrinogen, plasminogen, and α_2-macroglobulin, with reduction in levels of fibrinolytic activity, antiplasmin activity, and α_1-antitrypsin. These changes probably result from increased protein synthesis and, along with hemoconcentration, account for the increased tendency to thrombosis observed in the nephrotic syndrome. Urinary loss of the smaller molecular weight coagulation Factors II, VII, IX, X, and possibly XI and XII, may account for the hypocoagulable state that has been described in occasional nephrotic patients.

Other. Circulating soluble immune complexes have been found in significantly higher titers in patients in relapse from steroid-responsive minimal change nephrotic syndrome than in control populations. The pathophysiologic or clinical significance of this observation remains to be elucidated. There is a significantly higher incidence of minimal change nephrotic syndrome in patients with the HLA antigen B12. The presence of congenital nephrotic syndrome of the Finnish type can be diagnosed accurately prenatally by the finding of elevated concentrations of α-fetoprotein in the amniotic fluid, although neural tube defects are also associated with elevated amniotic concentrations of this protein. Finally, it should be remembered that 10 per cent of adult patients with a nephrotic syndrome have an underlying malignancy.

THERAPEUTIC TESTS

Under certain circumstances, rather than performing a renal biopsy before treatment is started (see under Renal Biopsy), it is acceptable to determine the patient's responsiveness to steroids. For such a therapeutic test we recommend prednisone in a dose of at least 60 mg per day per 1.73 square meters of body surface area given as a single morning dose. A diuresis with loss of edema and disappearance of proteinuria is considered confirmatory evidence for a minimal change renal lesion in young children. However, a patient should not be considered unresponsive unless treatment has been given for 28 days without remission. In adults, steroid treatment without a renal biopsy is not recommended.

COMPLICATIONS

The patient with nephrotic syndrome is particularly susceptible to develop infections. Pneumococcal peritonitis occurs less frequently now than it did previously, but it still should be considered as a potential hazard and should be recognized early before treatment with steroids is begun. The use of pneumococcal vaccine (Pneumovax) will not necessarily prevent future pneumococcal infections in the nephrotic patient. The administration of other immunizations may precipitate a relapse of minimal change disease. Gram-negative septicemia, periorbital cellulitis, cellulitis in the legs, erysipeloid eruptions, pneumonia, pneumonitis, and septicemia are other infections that may be seen.

There is a significantly higher incidence of both arterial and venous thrombosis in patients with the nephrotic syndrome. This may involve the leg veins and axillary and subclavian veins as well as the pulmonary, femoral, coronary, and mesenteric arteries. Thrombosis of the renal veins may be a complication of the nephrotic syndrome secondary to immune complex glomerulonephritis or amyloidosis.

An occasional nephrotic patient may develop hypovolemia, shock, and even acute renal failure, especially at the time of a steroid-induced diuresis. Because this potential complication can be fatal, we prefer to keep nephrotic patients hospitalized under close observation until the diuresis has been completed, the urine output has returned to normal, and body weight has stabilized.

Patients with prolonged, massive proteinuria may develop negative nitrogen balance, and malnutrition has been described. We have never seen this complication in a *pediatric* patient with a minimal change lesion but we advocate a high-protein diet in an attempt to replace urinary protein losses.

Progressive azotemia is not expected in a patient with minimal change lesion, although it is common in patients with focal glomerulosclerosis or of an underlying glomerulonephritis. Despite the lipidemia, only an occasional patient has been shown to develop atherosclerosis as a complication of the nephrotic syndrome. The complications of steroid therapy, including hypokalemia, weakness, obesity, osteopenia, and cataracts, may be striking in those patients treated with these drugs for prolonged periods.

DIFFERENTIAL DIAGNOSIS

The diagnosis of nephrotic syndrome usually is not difficult, but other causes of hypoalbuminemia and generalized edema must be included in the differential diagnosis. These include heart failure, liver disease, malabsorption and malnutrition, protein-losing enteropathy or cystic fibrosis in infants, as well as local causes of edema such as lymphatic occlusion. Absence of significant proteinuria is helpful in separating most of these entities from the nephrotic syndrome.

COURSE

Both the course taken by the patient and the prognosis depend on the underlying cause of the nephrotic syndrome.

Minimal Change Nephrotic Syndrome. In the preantibiotic, presteroid era two thirds of the patients with nephrotic syndrome died. The introduction of sulfonamides as antibacterial agents reduced this figure drastically to approximately 20 per cent, and the prognosis has been improved even further by the introduction of newer drugs. The use of steroids has improved morbidity dramatically, although it has had little effect on mortality.

Although an occasional patient will show a spontaneous remission, the majority require treatment with steroids; up to 90 per cent of patients respond to steroids with loss of edema and proteinuria. (These patients are referred to as being "steroid responsive.") The onset of response is usually heralded by a diuresis and progressive loss of edema that may begin within 6 days of commencing prednisone but more often is seen after 2 weeks of treatment; occasional patients do not respond for up to 28 days. The diuresis usually persists for 3 or 4 days with daily urine volumes of up to 2 liters or more. Urine protein concentration falls as urine volume increases, but proteinuria usually persists for several days after the diuresis has begun. The hypoproteinemia and hypercholesterolemia persist for several weeks or months, but values do return to normal.

Approximately 50 per cent of patients will have relapse, the majority responding once again to a further course of steroids. A significant number will have multiple relapses, and if there are more than three relapses per year, such patients are referred to as "frequent relapsers." Patients who relapse as steroid therapy is being withdrawn are labeled as being "steroid dependent."

Despite the frustrating course taken by many of the patients with frequent relapses, the long-term prognosis remains good. In one large series of pediatric patients almost 70 per cent entered adult life in prolonged and presumed permanent remission with no evidence of any residual renal disease. Quite often relapses stopped when the patient entered puberty. In this same series an additional 20 per cent of the children were alive and well at the end of the follow-up period but spilled protein in their urine; 9 per cent of the patients had died. As not all of these patients had the diagnosis of minimal change disease confirmed by histology, the prognosis for minimal change disease may be shown subsequently to be even better than this.

It has been recognized only recently that adult patients with minimal change disease entity have similar courses to those taken by children with the same pathologic diagnosis. In a series of 49 adult patients with proven minimal change glomerular lesions, follow-up extended for up to 19 years. Of the nine patients who died only one was uremic; three deaths were probably related to complications of treatment. Eleven of the patients were still relapsing at the time follow-up was complete, but 29 patients were well and off all treatment.

Other Causes. The long-term prognosis for patients with nephrotic syndrome secondary to glomerulonephritis varies and depends on the nature of the renal disease, as well as on the stage in the disease course at which diagnosis is made. Many of the patients develop progressing azotemia and eventually require chronic hemodialysis. If renal transplantation is performed in these patients, the underlying disease may recur in the transplanted kidney. However, it is important to emphasize that with appropriate therapy edema can be controlled in the majority of patients, and that this combined with other symptomatic treatment will often improve the patient's well-being, permitting a return to a more normal life.

NEOPLASMS AND CYSTIC DISEASE OF THE KIDNEY

By RUSSELL V. TAYLOR, M.D.,
and KENNETH A. KROPP, M.D.
Toledo, Ohio

NEOPLASMS

Neoplasms and the various cystic diseases of the kidney comprise the majority of renal masses in both symptomatic and asymptomatic patients. More than 8 per cent of all patients examined by intravenous urography will show evidence of a renal mass. This figure rises to 16 to 18 per cent in a group of older men with primarily prostatic symptoms who receive an intravenous urogram as part of their routine investigation. A combination of clinical, laboratory, and radiographic examination should give a diagnostic accuracy of greater than 95 per cent in the evaluation of renal masses.

EMBRYONAL TUMORS

Wilms' tumor, also known as embryonal adenomyosarcoma or nephroblastoma, is the only common embryonal tumor and the most common of the intra-abdominal malignancies in children. The incidence is around 0.5 per 100,000 in children under 14 years of age with no evident sex predominance. Sixty-five per cent of patients are less than 4 years of age at the time of diagnosis, but they are rare in children less than 1 year of age.

A palpable flank or abdominal mass is the principal clue to diagnosis in most patients. Abdominal pain, fatigue, malaise, and weight loss are also seen, but hematuria is uncommon. Hypertension is stated to be common, but the true incidence is difficult to determine, primarily owing to technical problems in accurately measuring blood pressure in young children. Hydronephrosis, multicystic dysplastic kidney, and neuroblastoma are the common differential considerations.

LABORATORY AND RADIOLOGIC FEATURES

There are no characteristic laboratory abnormalities, although anemia can be found in up to one third of patients. Baseline liver function studies should be obtained, as well as tests of urine, homovanillic, and vanillylmandelic acids to aid in the differentiation from neuroblastoma. The intravenous urogram is the single most useful test and is often diagnostic. Eighty to 90 per cent of kidneys with Wilms' tumor will show good function on the intravenous pyelogram (IVP), in contrast to hydronephrotic or multicystic dysplastic kidneys that often do not function. The tumor tends to distort the calyceal architecture rather than displace the kidney. Neuroblastoma, on the other hand, displaces the kidney downward, giving the characteristic "drooping lily" sign on the IVP. With Wilms' tumor, elongation and stretching of the calyces are commonly seen. Calcification, always subtle and not extensive, is seen in 10 to 15 per cent of Wilms' tumors, whereas it is seen in about 30 per cent of neuroblastomas and is generally dense and mottled.

Wilms' tumor is bilateral in 5 per cent of patients, so careful examination of the opposite kidney both radiographically and by the surgeon is mandatory. Arteriography is not necessary and carries a definite morbidity in young children, but is sometimes useful in combination with venacavography in difficult cases. Five per cent of patients suspected of having a Wilms' tumor prove to have a different lesion at exploration; half of these are benign. The most common site of metastases is the lungs, so tomograms should be done preoperatively as a staging procedure.

TUMORS OF THE RENAL PELVIS

Cancer of the renal pelvis constitutes about 5 per cent of all renal tumors. About 90 per cent of these are transitional cell carcinomas. The much less common squamous cell carcinoma and the rare adenocarcinoma are generally associated with long-standing infection, obstruction, and stones. Transitional cell carcinomas are most common in the sixth or seventh decade and men predominate two or three to one.

A high percentage of patients will have a previous history of transitional cell carcinoma of the bladder, and 30 to 50 per cent of those who present with a renal pelvic tumor will have a transitional cell cancer elsewhere in the genitourinary tract. Tumors will be found in the opposite pelvis or ureter in 3 to 4 per cent.

Patients afflicted with the Balkan nephropathy and those who abuse phenacetin-containing analgesics have a much higher incidence of renal pelvic tumors. The cause of the Balkan nephropathy is unknown, but the tumors tend to be multiple and low grade. In the case of analgesic nephropathy it is rare for those without papillary necrosis to develop tumors. The role of chemical carcinogens, which have been implicated in transitional cell carcinoma of the bladder, is unclear in renal pelvic tumors.

CLINICAL PRESENTATION

Hematuria, either gross or microscopic, is the presenting sign in 80 to 90 per cent of cases. It is usually painless but may be associated with colicky pain when the ureter is transiently obstructed by clots. In these cases, the hematuria may be terminal and the patient can be seen to pass worm-like clots. A flank mass may be palpable if there is hydronephrosis owing to obstruction of the ureteropelvic junction or if the tumor has extended beyond the kidney. It is an ominous clinical sign. Because of the frequently associated bladder carcinomas, irritative symptoms of frequency and dysuria may predominate in the clinical presentation.

DIAGNOSTIC EVALUATION

Intravenous urography most often demonstrates a negative filling defect in an otherwise fairly normal renal pelvis. This must be differentiated from nonopaque stones, blood clots, various inflammatory lesions such as pyelitis cystica, and extrinsic lesions such as vascular imprints or parapelvic cysts.

Sometimes the filling defect is seen to have a papillary surface on the IVP, but retrograde pyelography with diluted contrast material and air contrast is most often necessary to demonstrate this finding. Stones and clots can sometimes be seen to change position during retrograde pyelography and extrinsic imprints on the renal pelvis can usually be filled out with gentle pressure. The retrograde pyelogram will also allow the collection of urine for culture and cytology, as these tumors commonly shed neoplastic cells. Cells can also be collected by brushing the lesion, a technique which is similar to bronchial brushing. Another important role of the retrograde pyelogram is to delineate additional tumors in the ureter of a nonfunctioning kidney.

The kidney may fail to visualize in 25 to 30 per cent of patients and a renal parenchymal mass is seen in about 10 per cent. In those patients, angiography may prove useful. Findings on angiography can include an enlarged pelviureteric artery, fine neovascularity, vascular encasement, and pruning of intrarenal vessels, especially in extensive tumors. The florid neovascularity and arteriovenous stunting characteristic of a renal adenocarcinoma are not seen. Evidence of extensive tumor may preclude surgery in some patients, but in general, the role of angiography is to rule out renal adenocarcinoma. Angiography is also useful in demonstrating vascular impressions on the renal pelvis, a frequent cause of a benign filling defect.

Metastases commonly occur in the lungs, bones, and liver, with about one third of patients presenting with widespread disease. Low-grade tumors confined to the pelvis offer good survival following nephroureterectomy with excision of a bladder cuff or local excision of the lesion.

For high-stage or high-grade tumors, the survival is dismal; most patients are dead within 2 years. Because of the high incidence of bladder tumors in these patients, all should have frequent follow-up cystoscopies.

ADENOCARCINOMA

Clear cell or renal cell adenocarcinoma was thought by Grawitz in the late 19th Century to arise from adrenal nests in the kidney. Early synonyms were Grawitz's tumor or hypernephroma, but recent studies point to the proximal tubular epithelial cell as the cell of origin and renal cell adenocarcinoma is the more appropriate terminology. These tumors comprise 90 per cent of all adult kidney tumors. The incidence of renal cell adenocarcinoma in the United States is about 5 per 100,000 and there is a 2 to 1 male predominence. The peak incidence is in the sixth decade but the tumor has been reported in all age groups. As with other adenocarcinomas there is no solid clue to the etiology of renal adenocarcinoma, but cigarette smoking is a positive risk factor.

A variety of histologic types are reported with several cell types often seen in the same tumor. Reports of improved survival based on cell type are conflicting, but nuclear grade does seem to have some prognostic value. Pathologic stage has the most direct bearing on ultimate outcome, with patients who have tumors confined within Gerota's fascia (Stages I and II) having approximately 50 per cent 5-year survival when treated with radical nephrectomy and regional lymph node dissection. Extension into the renal vein or vena cava only (Stage IIIA) offers a much better prognosis than metastases to local lymph nodes (Stage IIIB). Patients presenting with distant metastases (Stage IV) have poor survival and most die within 2 years. Nephrectomy is sometimes done in Stage IV disease to palliate local symptoms but has no bearing on survival. There appears to be a higher than expected incidence of asymptomatic renal adenocarcinomas in end-stage kidneys removed as a preliminary to renal transplantation. These tumors tend to be small and metastases have not been noted after several years of careful follow-up.

CLINICAL AND LABORATORY FEATURES

Up to 50 per cent of patients with renal adenocarcinoma present with vague constitutional or primarily nonurinary symptoms. This makes the diagnosis a challenging exercise. The classic triad of flank pain, renal mass, and hematuria is of interest only for its scarcity and is more often found in advanced disease. Hematuria alone, however, is found in over 50 per cent of patients. Extrarenal manifestations are common and may be divided into two categories: those arising from the systemic effects of the disease and those arising from hormones produced by the tumor.

Anemia is found in up to one quarter of the patients and is the most common hematologic abnormality noted. The anemia is hypochromic with low serum iron and total iron-binding capacity. It is thought to be due to bone marrow depression secondary to the tumor, although occasionally the hematuria can be of sufficient magnitude to cause an anemia.

Fever is found in about 10 per cent of patients and in 3 per cent, fever is the only initial presenting symptom. An endogenous pyrogen has been demonstrated in some patients. Vague gastrointestinal symptoms are frequently seen and if primary gastrointestinal studies fail to disclose any abnormalities, excretory urography must be performed.

The syndrome of hepatic dysfunction is seen in up to 40 per cent of patients with renal adenocarcinoma. Liver biopsies have shown only a reactive hepatitis, and the laboratory abnormalities commonly revert to normal following nephrectomy. Failure to do so, even in the absence of demonstrable metastatic disease, has an ominous prognosis; conversely, solely biochemical liver abnormalities should not preclude surgery. Occlusion of the renal vein and vena cava can produce acute varicocele and lower extremity edema.

Erythrocytosis is seen in 1 to 5 per cent and erythropoietin has been isolated from some tumors. Hypercalcemia is another common hormonally mediated abnormality. Elevated parathormone levels have been found in some, but not all patients. Elevated prostaglandin-like factors have been isolated in association with hypercalcemia. Hypertension is common and elevated renin levels are sometimes found. Many other rare clinical endocrine syndromes have also been described.

RADIOLOGIC FEATURES

The diagnosis of most renal adenocarcinomas is suggested on excretory urography by the presence of a renal mass. High dose techniques and nephrotomography, when used in the investigation of hematuria, will increase the yield, but generally other radiologic techniques must be used to confirm the diagnosis.

Ultrasonography can be useful in differentiating cystic from solid renal masses with a high degree of accuracy if strict criteria are followed. However, some masses will exhibit an indeterminate pattern and ultrasonography alone cannot be relied upon to differentiate cyst from tumor. Selective renal angiography provides the best method of confirming the diagnosis of renal adenocarcinoma.

The tumor is usually highly vascular with arteriovenous fistulas, venous lakes, and microaneurysms commonly seen. Up to 22 per cent of tumors either are avascular or show minimal vascularity, but careful attention to the nephrogram phase of the renal angiogram may show poor definition of tumor margins, in contrast to the sharp "beak sign" seen in simple renal cysts.

If a tumor is demonstrated by renal angiography, hepatic arteriograms should be done as well as an inferior venacavogram as part of a staging procedure. Lung, liver, and bone are the primary sites of metastases, so full lung tomograms, radionucleotide liver scan, and bone scan should be performed as well.

Computerized tomography (CT) is emerging as a valuable tool in assessing the degree of local disease but is unlikely to replace the older modalities in the assessment of renal masses.

OTHER MALIGNANT TUMORS

The kidney may be involved uncommonly by other malignant processes. Sarcomas comprise 1 to 3 per cent of all primary renal malignancies. Because of their large size and rapid growth, it is often difficult to determine whether the kidney is the primary site or is involved secondarily. They may occur at any age, but are most common in the fifth and sixth decades. The most common presentation is a flank mass. Radiologic studies show a relatively hypovascular mass suggesting renal adenocarcinoma, and final diagnosis generally rests on pathologic findings.

The lymphoma-leukemia group of malignancies is sometimes found to involve the kidney. Leukemia is an infiltrative process and the pyelogram can sometimes resemble that in adult polycystic disease, with stretched and thinned calyces. Peripheral blood smears will always show evidence of this systemic disease, however. Lymphoma may be primarily localized to the kidney and present as a renal mass.

The kidney is often the site of clinically inapparent metastatic disease. Lung cancers are the most common primary. As many as 20 per cent of patients dying of primary lung cancer exhibit renal metastases at autopsy. Although the majority of these tumors are silent, occasionally a symptomatic renal mass is the first presenting sign of a primary lung cancer.

BENIGN RENAL TUMORS

The simple cyst is the most common benign renal tumor or mass and is considered in a later section. Benign solid tumors are uncommon and usually silent, unless they produce symptoms owing to their size.

Cortical adenoma is the most common benign solid tumor. These are found most commonly in the fourth decade and are three to four times more common in men. The relationship of adenomas to adenocarcinoma is not clear, but it is generally of little practical significance, as the two are often indistinguishable by radiographic means. Nephrectomy is often carried out because of the possibility of neoplasm.

Angiomyolipoma, or renal hamartoma, is an interesting benign tumor composed of vascular, muscular, and lipomatous tissue. It is found most frequently in association with the tuberous sclerosis complex but can be seen as an isolated lesion within or on the kidney. Excretory urography will disclose a mass that may reach considerable size. Angiography will show a bizarre vascular pattern that is often confused with renal adenocarcinoma. The tumor is more common in women and sometimes the diagnosis may be suspected when the renal mass is seen to show patchy and irregular areas of decreased density; these represent the fatty components of the tumor. Spontaneous rupture may occur, with patients presenting in shock. Nephrectomy is commonly performed owing to the difficulty in differentiating this tumor from renal adenocarcinoma.

The renal oncocytoma is another interesting benign tumor. It is clinically and radiologically indistinguishable from renal adenocarcinoma. Formerly the cause of much confusion, it is now a well recognized pathologic entity.

Many other benign solid renal tumors have been described, including fibromas and lipomas. These are all decidedly uncommon and generally cannot be diagnosed short of surgical exploration. Table 1 summarizes the important clinical features of the most common renal neoplasms and cysts.

Table 1. *Clinical and Radiologic Features of Renal Neoplasms and Cysts*

Criteria	Adenocarcinoma	Transitional CA of Pelvis	Simple Cyst
Age	50 to 70	60 to 70	50+
Male:Female ratio	2:1	2:1	1:1
Hematuria	50%	80 to 90%	Rare
Constitutional symptoms	Common (50%)	Rare	Rare
Other tumors	No	Other transitional ca common	No
IVP	Mass Indeterminate borders	Filling defect	Mass Sharp borders
Ultrasound	Solid or indeterminate with internal echoes	Not helpful	Echo-free with shadowing
Arteriogram	80% hypervascular tumors	Generally normal	Avascular mass

CYSTIC DISEASES

LOCALIZED AND SEGMENTAL (SIMPLE) CYSTS

The most common cystic abnormality of the kidney and indeed the most common renal mass is the simple cyst. These may be large or small, unilateral or bilateral. They are rarely singular, being accompanied in most cases by a number of clinically inapparent smaller cysts. They are commonly found in the older age group. The cysts are characteristically unilocular and do not communicate with the renal pelvis. They do not contain urine, but do contain a clear serous fluid with a low specific gravity and small amounts of chloride, albumin, and cholesterol.

CLINICAL AND LABORATORY FEATURES

Most cysts are discovered incidentally on excretory urography, although some may present as an abdominal or flank mass. Bleeding into cysts is uncommon, but it may be responsible for flank pain or hematuria. Infection is likewise uncommon but may be the cause for presentation. Cysts are also occasionally associated with polycythemia. There are no characteristic laboratory abnormalities, most patients demonstrating normal renal function and urine sediment.

RADIOLOGIC FEATURES

The differentiation of cyst from tumor when a renal mass is suspected is done primarily by radiologic criteria, although sometimes exploration will be needed for definitive diagnosis. Nephrotomography can provide valuable clues. Cysts tend to grow away from the periphery of the kidney, although some will distort the calyceal system. When the cyst is on the periphery of the kidney, the characteristic "beak" or "lip" sign will be seen, especially in the nephrogram phase, as the cyst is sharply differentiated from the surrounding normal parenchyma.

Ultrasonography is also of value if an echo-free area is demonstrated, especially if it remains free of echoes over a wide range of gain settings. Cysts usually also show a "shadowing" effect with an accumulation of echoes on the side of the cyst farthest from the ultrasonic transducer.

Arteriography will show vessels stretched over an avascular area corresponding to that seen in the nephrogram phase of the excretory urogram.

One of the most useful diagnostic tools is percutaneous cyst puncture performed under ultrasonic or fluoroscopic control. Any fluid obtained is sent for cytology, as well as bio-chemical tests for lactic dehydrogenase (LDH), cholesterol, and fat. The cyst is then filled with contrast material and air, and multiple radiographs are taken in various projections so that the entire wall of the cyst is visualized. A simple cyst will show a smooth wall throughout. Failure to obtain fluid, the finding of bloody or cloudy fluid, or any elevation of lipids or LDH suggests neoplasm and requires surgical exploration. Cystic renal adenocarcinomas, which comprise about 7 per cent of all renal adenocarcinomas, will show irregularities in the wall. Proper application of these techniques gives a high diagnostic accuracy, but if any doubt exists, surgical exploration should be undertaken.

ADULT POLYCYSTIC KIDNEY DISEASE

Adult polycystic kidney disease (APCD) is the most common cystic disease in humans, with an estimated incidence of 1 in 500 people. It is transmitted as an autosomal dominant trait, affects males and females with equal frequency, and is the third most common cause of renal failure leading to transplantation. The disease usually presents during the fourth decade of life, although it has been reported in all age groups. There is remarkable similarity in the age of onset of symptoms for each family group. This fact is of clinical importance, because if a patient has no evidence of disease when he is 10 years beyond his family's mean age of onset of symptoms, he has a less than 5 per cent chance of possessing the gene for APCD. The cause is unknown, but microdissection studies show that the cystic nephrons — unlike simple cysts — communicate with the glomerulus and with the collecting system. Micropuncture studies show two populations of cysts: one group filled with fluid that has the electrolyte composition of proximal tubular fluid and one group filled with distal tubular fluid.

CLINICAL AND LABORATORY FEATURES

Early in the disease there may be no clinical signs or demonstrable laboratory abnormalities. Flank discomfort is often the presenting complaint. Failure to show maximum urine concentration with water deprivation in the face of normal creatinine clearance is said to be the first clinical sign. In reality, however, the diagnosis is most often suggested by excretory urography.

Fifty per cent or more of patients present with palpable bilateral flank masses; 50 per cent have hematuria and 50 per cent are hypertensive. The combination of uremia, bilateral flank masses, and hypertension should make one very suspicious of APCD. Hepatic cysts are common and 50 per cent of patients with APCD will have berry aneurysms of the circle of Willis. Conversely, 6 per cent of those presenting with a subarachnoid hemorrhage from a ruptured berry aneurysm will show APCD when investigated.

RADIOLOGIC FEATURES

The excretory urogram will characteristically show large, although still approximately reniform, kidneys with the calyces stretched and distorted from the cysts. Cysts may also obstruct the pelvis. The disease is always bilateral but may be asynchronous in presentation.

Ultrasonography will confirm the presence of clusters of cysts, and computerized tomography (CT) scans show the cysts outlined by thin parenchyma in beautiful detail. Retrograde pyelography is not generally necessary to make the diagnosis and instrumentation should be avoided, for infection is a leading cause of death. The diagnosis should not be made lightly, in view of the profound genetic implications. Children and siblings of an afflicted patient should be followed carefully for the appearance of the disease.

INFANTILE POLYCYSTIC KIDNEY DISEASE

Infantile polycystic kidney disease is an uncommon autosomal recessive disorder that may present at any age. There is a strong association with congenital hepatic fibrosis and portal hypertension. This is a spectrum disease with varying degrees of severity.

Clinically, the patients seem to fall into two groups. One group of patients will present at birth with oliguric renal failure, large kidneys that do not transilluminate, and pulmonary hypoplasia. These all die from pulmonary failure within the first few days of life. Autopsy shows huge reniform kidneys with ectasia of the collecting ducts and small cortical cysts. Fibrosis of the smaller bile ducts is also seen. The other group may present later in childhood or early adulthood with varying degrees of renal or hepatic insufficiency, hypertension, hepatosplenomegaly, and growth retardation. Generally, portal hypertension is the primary problem with the renal disease secondary. The kidneys may be large or small and an IVP can show either a mottled pattern from contrast puddling in cysts or a sunburst pattern from ductal ectasia. If an adult with known hepatic fibrosis

shows ductal ectasia on an IVP, he should be considered to have IPCD and followed closely for the development of renal failure.

MEDULLARY SPONGE KIDNEY

Medullary sponge kidney (MSK) is a relatively common disorder with an estimated incidence of one in 50,000 to one in 20,000 in the general population. The cause is unknown, but it is thought to be a heritable syndrome, although the genetics must be complex. It may present at any age, generally with one of the three major complications of this otherwise benign disorder.

About 50 per cent of patients with MSK will have nephrolithiasis. The stones are generally calcium phosphate; this is a relatively uncommon type of stone otherwise. Twenty per cent will show hematuria and about 30 per cent will have pyelonephritis.

The diagnosis is made almost exclusively from the excretory urogram. Plain films of the abdomen may show multiple linear calcifications that represent stones within the dilated collecting tubules of the renal papillae. The IVP will show normal or slightly enlarged kidneys with an absence of cortical cysts or calcifications. The ectatic tubules fill with contrast before the calyces and because of stasis they remain opacified after the calyces are empty of contrast medium. The pattern is consistent in repeated examinations, in contrast to the transient pyramidal blush often seen on otherwise normal IVP.

Uncomplicated MSK is a benign disease. Unfortunately, most patients experience colic, hematuria, or infection at some time during their lives. However, the prognosis remains excellent; only 10 per cent of patients with MSK do poorly as a result of the complications of the disease.

THE UREMIC MEDULLARY CYSTIC DISEASE COMPLEX

The uremic medullary cystic disease complex may comprise more than one disease. The complex is uncommon, however, and currently is best thought of as a single entity. Genetic studies suggest a small number of sporadic cases and a rare autosomal dominant variant, with most cases showing autosomal recessive inheritance. The autosomal recessive group is often labeled familial juvenile nephronophthisis and is sometimes associated with retinal-renal dysplasia or retinitis pigmentosa.

As the name suggests, these patients present with uremia. At autopsy the kidney is shrunken, scarred, and pale. There is a thick cortex with

Table 2. *Clinical Differences Among Three Common Cystic Disorders of the Kidney*

Criteria	Nephronophthisis Uremic Medullary Disease	Polycystic Disease	Medullary Sponge Kidney
Flank pain	Usually absent	Usually present	With complications
Hypertension	Unusual	Frequent	Unusual
Hematuria	Absent	Often present	With complications
X-ray	Small kidneys	Large kidneys with cysts	Normal kidneys
Age at death	10–40 years	5 or 50 years	Normal
Familial incidence	75%	75%	20%

multiple small medullary cysts. Salt wasting is frequently seen. This salt wasting combined with the absence of hypertension and the absence of infection with a positive family history of renal failure should suggest the diagnosis. Radiologic studies are not generally helpful; small kidneys without cysts or calcifications are shown.

Table 2 summarizes the important clinical features of the three more common cystic diseases of the kidney.

HEREDITARY SYNDROMES

Renal cysts and dysplasia are commonly seen in a variety of hereditary syndromes. Two of the most common are tuberous sclerosis and von Hippel-Lindau disease. Both of these are autosomal dominant diseases with variable ages of onset. The renal cysts may antedate any other clinical features of the diseases and are characteristically lined with an extremely hyperplastic epithelium. Patients with either syndrome are at very high risk for renal adenocarcinomas that are often multiple or bilateral and associated with other cysts. Benign renal tumors, most commonly angiomyolipomas, are also seen in a wide variety of hereditary syndromes.

PYELONEPHRITIS

By WILLIAM L. MCGUFFIN, JR., M.D.,
Houston, Texas

and J. CAULIE GUNNELLS, JR., M.D.
Durham, North Carolina

Pyelonephritis is a clinical syndrome secondary to bacterial infection of the renal parenchyma and pelviocalyceal system. The pathologic findings in this disorder may be consistent with the diagnosis but not entirely diagnostic; therefore, in order to establish the diagnosis, one must demonstrate either active bacterial growth or the fact that bacteria have been present in the renal parenchyma. The mere presence of a urinary tract infection or even repeated infections does not establish the diagnosis of pyelonephritis. As the clear demonstration of bacteria in the genitourinary system constitutes the major laboratory confirmation in the search for pyelonephritis, it is important at the outset to define what is considered to be significant bacterial growth in urine cultures. Significant bacteriuria is defined as the presence of more than 100,000 organisms per ml of urine.

CLINICAL PRESENTATION

History. The clinical picture or presentation of acute pyelonephritis is variable. The typical patient with acute pyelonephritis usually presents with symptoms of lower tract disease characterized by urgency, frequency, dysuria, double voiding, and suprapubic pressure or discomfort along with a history of some associated change in color or odor of the urine. With extension of the infection beyond the confines of the lower genitourinary tract to the kidney parenchyma, the sudden onset of shaking chills, diaphoresis, fever, or flank or back discomfort will usually be observed. It is not unusual for these latter symptoms to appear without prior lower tract symptoms. Often with the development of systemic signs, associated gastrointestinal symptoms of anorexia, nausea, vomiting, or even paralytic ileus may be evident and are at times misinterpreted as an acute intraabdominal event. In the rare patient with hematogenous dissemination of bacteria, foci of infection elsewhere will affect the kidney before the lower urinary tract is involved, thereby producing predominant symptoms of retroperitoneal infection, such as perinephric abscess.

Patients at the extremes of age tend to be atypical, with children often presenting with failure to thrive, refusal to eat, fever of undetermined origin, and enuresis, whereas the elderly patient may present with gram-negative sepsis.

It should be noted here that only half the patients seen with symptoms of urinary tract infection have bacteriuria. Also the correlation between symptoms and site of infection is not good, as many patients with pyelonephritis have no chills or fever or flank pain, whereas a significant number of patients with those symptoms will have only lower urinary tract infection.

The clinical history of chronic pyelonephritis is also variable. As chronic pyelonephritis almost never occurs in the absence of associated functional or anatomic abnormalities of the genitourinary tract, a history of instrumentation and recurrent urinary tract irritative or obstructive symptoms should be carefully sought. Evidence of structural defects may be rather obvious, as exemplified by primary neurologic disease or benign prostatic hypertrophy in an elderly male. However, the clinical presentation may be quite subtle, such as childhood urinary incontinence, spraying of the urinary stream, infrequent but massive voidings (megalocystis), or enuresis. In many patients, the entire course is most insidious and the disease is detected during a routine examination for symptoms of malaise, lethargy, anemia, weight loss, or hypertension. These symptoms may reflect just coexistent renal insufficiency.

Physical Examination. The findings on physical examination in acute pyelonephritis are generally nonspecific and variable, reflecting for the most part the systemic response to any infectious process. The majority of the patients will be febrile, usually in the range of 103 to 105 F (39.4 to 40.5 C), and there may be associated tenderness to percussion over one or both costovertebral areas or to deep palpation in the upper abdominal quadrants. However, extremes of age and associated coexistent systemic illnesses may blunt these sparse physical findings. The more obvious features on physical examination may be those representing a complication of the infection (the hypotension of volume contraction to overt shock of gram-negative sepsis or clinical conditions in which there should be a high index of suspicion of concomitant urinary tract infection, such as renal colic and bladder distention secondary to lower urinary tract obstruction, or an indwelling catheter).

It should be mentioned that careful examination of the external genitalia for the detection of congenital anomalies, such as hypospadias, may reveal a clue to the presence of coexistent upper tract developmental anomalies.

As the disease progresses, there are no characteristic or diagnostic physical findings except in patients who present with severe depression of renal function and the multiple physical findings of increasing azotemia such as pallor, anemia, uremic fetor, weight loss, weakness, anorexia, nausea, vomiting, hypertension, possible asterixis, and mental changes of encephalopathy. The variable expression of these abnormalities reflects not only the level of decreased renal function but also, at times, the rapidity of change with an acute exacerbation or recurrence of renal parenchymal infection with the predominant findings similar to those outlined earlier for acute pyelonephritis.

LABORATORY FINDINGS

The presence or absence of pyuria or bacteriuria is of utmost importance as the first step in the laboratory diagnosis of acute pyelonephritis. The natural sequence thereafter is urine culture on appropriate media for the precise identification of the infecting organism(s), followed by antibiotic sensitivities to aid in the selection of antimicrobial therapy.

Urine Collection. Proper collection of the urine sample for analysis and culture is a prime consideration if one is to accurately diagnose the presence of urinary tract infection. The clean midstream technique is the most widely used method of collecting urine for culture and is the method of choice. Scrupulous attention to cleansing of the external genitalia, careful patient and nursing staff instructions, and immediate examination and culture of the urine are required. Urethral catheterization is rarely necessary except in the special circumstances usually found in seriously ill and/or elderly bedridden patients. Sterile procedures must be observed with this method to avoid contamination of the specimen and the introduction of bacteria into the urinary tract. Suprapubic bladder puncture has also been used widely to collect specimens from patients, particularly infants, with whom problems exist.

Urinalysis. The color of the urine may be entirely normal; however, grossly infected urine may be cloudy, containing variable amounts of blood and on rare occasion fragments of calculi or renal tissue. The odor may be unpleasant, but this change may be produced by urinary stasis either before or after collection. The specific gravity or osmolality of the urine more often reflects the state of hydration, but the presence of a dilute urine has been used to support a diagnosis of parenchymal bacterial infection. The urine pH is usually acid but may be alkaline as a reflection of ammonia production by infection with urea-splitting organisms (Proteus). Qualitative proteinuria is often present but minimal in degree. Quantitative protein excretion, when measured, is usually less than 1 to 2 grams per 24 hours; when present in greater amounts, it should raise some question as to the presence of coexistent glomerular or systemic disease.

A careful microscopic examination of the urinary sediment by the physician cannot be overemphasized. If the urine cannot be examined immediately after collection, it should be refrigerated, possibly with an added preservative (formalin). Unless the sediment is unusually heavy, the urine should be centrifuged in the usual manner, and the small button of sediment remaining after the supernate is decanted is transferred to a clean slide for microscopic examination in a stained or unstained state.

A procedure of diagnostic importance is the examination of the noncentrifuged Gram-stained urine. If bacteria (a single organism) are seen under these conditions, a presumptive diagnosis of significant bacteriuria (colony count greater than 10^5 organisms per ml of urine on quantitative culture) can be made. A similar diagnosis may be invoked if more than 20 bacterial organisms per high power field are visualized in an unstained but centrifuged urine sediment. The accurate identification or detection of bacteria in spun or unspun urine sediments may be facilitated by the use of phase contrast microscopy.

The presence of pyuria, either singly or in clumps, suggests inflammation, and although a frequent finding in urinary tract infection, it is nonspecific and must be evaluated in relation to the entire clinical picture as well as to other associated urinary sediment abnormalities. Of greater diagnostic value is the demonstration of a leukocyte cast, which is generally interpreted as indicative of renal parenchymal inflammation and which in the absence of other types of cellular casts provides strong support for a diagnosis of pyelonephritis.

The finding of gross or microscopic hematuria is variable but not uncommon. Evidence of additional sediment abnormalities such as fragments of renal tissue is helpful, but they are infrequently found. The presence of crystalluria has no diagnostic value in this clinical setting.

The utilization of a number of special stains and techniques to improve identification of bacteria and pus cells has been advocated, but these tests are rarely useful.

A note of caution: Acute pyelonephritis may exist in the absence of both pyuria and bacteriuria. This may occur in the patient with hematogenous dissemination of infection to the renal parenchyma without communication to urinary drainage, as in renal carbuncle or perinephric abscess. In addition, with patients in whom there is parenchymal infection behind obstructing lesions, the urinary sediment may be amazingly benign.

The urinalysis in patients with chronic pyelonephritis may reveal all the features just discussed. The demonstration of significant bacteriuria is infrequent in this disorder, as often the culture will be negative, demonstrate multiple organisms of low colony count or doubtful pathogenesis, or reveal less than 10^5 organisms of a single pathogen. In addition, one may observe granular, hyaline, or broad waxy casts that are nonspecific and usually reflect some degree of general parenchymal renal damage.

Urine Culture. Quantitative bacteriologic examination of properly collected and processed clean-voided samples of urine provides the cornerstone of laboratory diagnosis and future antimicrobial therapy in the patient with acute pyelonephritis. Significant bacteriuria is said to exist when the growth of bacteria is greater than 10^5 organisms per ml of urine; using this criterion, one is able to reduce significantly the confusion that often exists in the differentiation between contamination and true bacteriuria. With the use of a single urine culture, a confidence limit of 80 per cent is achieved; this can be increased to 95 per cent with the use of two consecutive culture samples that demonstrate the same organism. Inconsistent urine cultures showing more than one organism and an associated low colony count should be suspected of contamination and repeated. It is in this clinical setting that the appropriate and judicious use of invasive techniques (suprapubic aspirate or bladder catheterization) may be helpful. In addition, bacterial flora such as diphtheroids, staphylococci, and microaerophilic streptococci should be considered contaminants except in unusual circumstances.

In chronic pyelonephritis when the disease may be quiescent, the urine culture is often sterile or reveals low bacterial counts (less than 10^5 organisms per ml of urine) with varied and multiple organisms. In this setting, the *repeated* demonstration of such findings is clinically significant and is considered sufficient evidence for treatment with specific bactericidal antimicrobials. However, when symptoms are present, a higher yield of significant bacteriuria will be observed. The bacterial flora is similar to that seen in acute pyelonephritis, with the exception that organisms of the Enterobacter, Klebsiella, Proteus, Pseudomonas, and enterococcal species are found more often than is *Escherichia coli* in this disease, with the frequent emergence of drug resistance on antibiotic sensitivity testing.

There are several new methods for obtaining culture information that compare favorably with the aforementioned more standard techniques, and these can be done in the office or home.

The first is the dip-inoculum method, which enables on-the-spot inoculation, thus avoiding multiplication of contaminants in the urine during transportation to the laboratory. A glass slide is coated on one side with a medium that supports the growth of most aerobic organisms. The other side is coated with a selective medium that allows only gram-negative bacteria to grow. The slide is inoculated by dipping it into the urine or having the patient void directly onto the slide. The reliability of this technique is excellent and about equal to the more standard techniques. Most urinary pathogens have been shown to grow satisfactorily at room temperature on the dip slides.

Pad culture media have been introduced (Microstix, Ames Co.). The medium pad contains colorless tetrazolium, which, when reduced in the presence of bacterial growth, produces discrete red spots on the pad. The density of the spots correlates with the number of bacteria in the urine specimen. These can be used at home and incubated for 48 to 72 hours in a warm place and in careful studies have given results comparable to those obtained in the laboratory. This only documents the presence of bacteriuria and does not identify the organism.

These two methods are especially helpful for patients with recurrent urinary tract infections who have been completely evaluated and in whom the physician may have decided to treat symptomatic urinary tract infections with a short course of antibiotics.

Many indirect tests for bacteriuria have been devised, including Griess' nitrite test (reduction of nitrate to nitrite by bacteria), glucose reduction test, catalase test, and endotoxin assay. None of these tests have replaced bacterial counts, and the high incidence of false positive and/or negative results has made them unreliable as screening procedures.

Although selection of antimicrobial therapy is not difficult in the absence of complications, the need for initial antibiotic sensitivity studies must be emphasized.

Peripheral Blood. In acute pyelonephritis most patients exhibit a leukocytosis of 15,000 to 20,000 per cu mm with an increase of immature neutrophils in the differential count. In addition, the neutrophils may display toxic granulation or vacuolization. Anemia is not usual in the patient with acute pyelonephritis, and its presence should suggest underlying coexistent disease.

In chronic pyelonephritis the total leukocyte count and differential blood count are normal in the absence of acute infection. A normocytic normochromic anemia may be present as in other forms of renal insufficiency. The anemia may be more severe, because chronic infection will act synergistically with renal insufficiency to depress bone marrow function.

Biochemical Findings. The patient with uncomplicated acute pyelonephritis does not characteristically exhibit evidence of renal insufficiency; however, a nonspecific elevation of blood urea nitrogen may be a reflection of volume contraction and dehydration. It may be of value to obtain a biochemical profile in these patients to detect the coexistence of underlying predisposing diseases that may alter initial therapy and eventual prognosis.

In chronic pyelonephritis the only specific biochemical changes are those related to progressive loss of nephron function with resultant azotemia. The well-known laboratory alterations of renal failure will not be outlined in detail. It should be pointed out that it is not unusual for the patient to present with laboratory evidence of rather far advanced renal failure but relatively few associated symptoms unless an intercurrent reversible exacerbation of renal insufficiency occurs, as may be seen with dehydration, congestive heart failure, electrolyte imbalance, or the hypercatabolism of an unrelated febrile illness. Such potentially correctable causes of increased renal insufficiency should always be sought and appropriately treated when present.

Three characteristic but not necessarily diagnostic features of chronic interstitial nephritis (chronic pyelonephritis) have been said to be helpful in the evaluation and treatment of these patients:

1. Inability to maximally concentrate the urine leads to symptoms of polyuria and polydipsia. In contrast to other forms of chronic parenchymal renal disease, this defect may occur early in chronic pyelonephritis before the development of severe filtration rate depression. Functionally, the nephron is resistant to vasopressin and water deprivation; however, attempts to demonstrate this defect by means of the latter maneuver should be resisted because of the well-known resultant decrease in renal blood flow and filtration rate associated with volume contraction.

2. Hyperchloremic acidosis can be differentiated from classic renal tubular acidosis by evidence of decreased renal function and an acid urine. The early appearance of this tubular dysfunction may be associated with other tubular defects, such as an exaggerated urinary calcium loss. This may lead to an earlier appearance of renal osteodystrophy in certain patients.

3. Altered tubular and medullary function leads to exaggerated sodium loss; therefore, inappropriate sodium restriction in the absence of severe hypertension and congestive heart failure should be avoided. This tendency to-

ward sodium wasting is believed by some to explain in part the lower incidence of hypertension in this disease. In a normally hydrated patient, the measurement of a 24-hour urinary sodium excretion after maintenance of a fixed, but not restricted, dietary sodium intake for 5 to 7 days will provide an accurate estimate of the necessary level of dietary or other sources (alkali) of sodium for replacement losses.

These fundamental alterations reflect the early and preferential involvement of the medulla and interstitium in these diseases; however, it should be stressed that as the disease progresses, a simultaneous deterioration of glomerular and tubular function may be present, leading to blood chemistry values that are no different from those of any other type of renal insufficiency.

ROENTGENOLOGIC AND/OR UROGRAPHIC STUDIES

Various types of radiologic and urologic procedures are available for the evaluation of the patient who presents with initial or recurrent urinary tract infection compatible with pyelonephritis. In general, most physicians agree that, in the female who presents an uncomplicated course responding immediately to the usual antimicrobial therapy, further investigation might well be delayed until a second episode unless there is a high degree of clinical suspicion of underlying congenital abnormalities or coexistent systemic illness. In contrast, the presence of an isolated episode of acute pyelonephritis in all males and children should be followed by appropriate radiologic and urologic evaluation to reveal correctable obstructing defects or additional systemic disease.

In patients requiring further evaluation, the following studies should be included: intravenous urography with or without nephrotomography, cystoscopy, and a voiding cystourethrogram. In patients suspected of having obstruction but in whom standard intravenous pyelography is contraindicated or fails to reveal obstruction, renal ultrasound examination or computerized tomography (CT) will establish the presence or absence of obstruction. The need for retrograde urography would be determined by the finding of obstruction demonstrated on the previously mentioned studies.

The routine use of the plain film of the abdomen (KUB) in all patients with acute pyelonephritis should be considered. This noninvasive study often enables one to assess the presence or absence of normal renal outlines, thereby supporting the need for additional studies. It may also demonstrate radiopaque renal or ureteral stones as well as nephrocalcinosis. The presence of a poorly outlined psoas stripe may suggest the presence of a retroperitoneal mass or perinephric abscess.

In chronic pyelonephritis, the plain film of the abdomen (KUB) as just outlined is equally applicable. Intravenous urography utilizing the drip infusion or bolus technique seems to provide the most useful information in the average patient, as it affords better visualization of the renal parenchyma and collecting system in the azotemic patient. Likewise, there is no necessity for overnight dehydration, a procedure that should be avoided in all patients with renal insufficiency. In the patient with more severe renal insufficiency, the addition of nephrotomography at the time of administration of contrast medium may be advantageous. One should avoid intravenous pyelography in patients with very severe renal failure (creatinine >12). An assessment of renal size can be obtained via ultrasound or on occasion plain abdominal tomography.

In chronic pyelonephritis the radiographic changes are usually an overall decrease in renal size, often with disproportionate involvement between the two kidneys. The cortical outlines are often irregular, with numerous depressions and associated blunting, irregularity, and dilatation of the pelviocalyceal systems. It has been reported that the radiographic change most specific for this disease is cortical scarring and thinning with blunting of the *corresponding* papillae. The presence of hydronephrosis or hydroureter suggesting obstruction or the failure to visualize the genitourinary tract may be considered indication for instrumentation with retrograde urography. The addition of a postvoiding bladder film after studies to visualize the upper urinary tract may be helpful in assessing the presence or absence of obstructive lesions distal to the urinary bladder sphincter.

SPECIFIC DIAGNOSTIC PROCEDURES

The demonstration of true bacteriuria with a positive urine culture is the sine qua non of acute pyelonephritis. However, this finding does not differentiate pyelonephritis from lower tract infection. The site of infection has possible important implications regarding the long-term course and treatment. Although renal bacteriuria has been associated with frequent relapse of the infection (same organism), bladder bacteriuria has been associated with less frequent recurrence of infection, and when it occurred it was usually reinfection (new infection with new pathogen), not relapse.

Utilizing these criteria, it has been suggested that in a relapse (recurrent disease with the same organisms) the infection usually rose from one or both kidneys, and in these patients a more prolonged course of specific antimicrobial therapy might prove beneficial; reinfection more likely indicates that infections are confined to the bladder and that the future course of the disease is not altered by the prolonged duration of initial treatment for the individual infection. These observations again stress the importance of precise definition of the bacteriologic flora responsible for the initial infection together with careful antibiotic sensitivity testing, followed by the use of appropriate antibiotics.

Other important observations include the fact that patients with lower tract symptoms who have less than 10,000 counts per ml are more likely to have renal bacteriuria. Proteus organisms in the urine also point strongly to renal infection. Patients with renal infection show more than 20,000 leukocytes per ml of urine, but most of those who have bladder infections have less than 20,000 leukocytes per ml.

The most reliable technique for distinguishing renal from bladder bacteriuria is that of bilateral ureteral catheterization with separate cultures of ureteral and bladder urine. However, as this procedure is followed by a low but definite incidence of complications and the possible transfer of infection from the lower to the upper tract, attempts have been made to develop equally effective but more benign techniques.

A bladder washout technique has been devised for obtaining ureteral urine without catheterizing the ureters. A triple lumen Foley catheter is inserted and a specimen of bladder urine obtained. The bladder is emptied, and 100 ml of sterile saline containing 5 mg of gentamicin (or 2 mg of neomycin) and 125,000 units of topical streptokinase-streptodornase or 2 ampules of bovine fibrinolysin and desoxyribonuclease (Elase) is injected into the bladder and allowed to remain for 30 to 45 minutes. The bladder is again emptied and washed out with 2 liters of sterile saline and the last few milliliters saved for postwashout culture. Urine collections are made every 10 minutes until three additional specimens are collected with bacterial counts performed on all specimens. Patients are classified as having lower tract infection if all cultures after the bladder washout are negative. Patients are classified as having upper tract infection if both of the following criteria are met: (1) bacterial counts of greater than 10^2 organisms per ml are present in the ureteral samples and (2) there is at least a 10-fold increase between the postwashout sample and the ureteral specimens.

Other, more indirect methods for localizing the site of bacterial infection have been devised. The most widely used is the measurement of antibodies in the patient's serum against the O antigen of the bacteria causing the infection. When the infection involves the renal parenchyma, antibodies are present in significant titers but are absent or present only in low titers when infection is confined to the lower urinary tract.

Another method utilizes the detection of antibody-coated bacteria in the urine sediment. It has been demonstrated that the presence of antibody-coated bacteria correlates well with renal localization in women; however, in men with prostatic infection, antibody-coated bacteria may be detected in the absence of renal bacterial involvement.

Renal parenchymal involvement has also been defined on the basis of impairment in the capacity to produce a concentrated urine; the nonspecificity and potential hazards of this technique have already been reviewed.

Percutaneous renal biopsy has not been useful in patients with acute pyelonephritis, and in our opinion it is contraindicated if there is acute bacterial infection of renal parenchyma.

COURSE AND COMPLICATIONS

In the majority of patients with acute pyelonephritis, the symptoms and signs resolve in 3 to 5 days, often in the untreated as well as treated patients. However, most untreated patients will continue to have asymptomatic bacteriuria and frequently suffer a relapse of symptomatic infection. It is unusual for the patient with uncomplicated acute pyelonephritis to develop rapid and progressive destruction of the renal parenchyma of life-threatening proportions, although a significant number of patients will have coexistent bacteremia or septicemia. It should be recognized that the disappearance of symptoms cannot be relied upon to indicate bacteriologic cure. It is most important to obtain appropriate urine cultures during and after the completed course of therapy. As mentioned previously, patients with continuous bacteriuria or recurrent urinary tract infection in the absence of anatomic abnormalities or coexistent underlying systemic disease will rarely, if ever, develop "chronic pyelonephritis" with resultant renal insufficiency and the uremic syndrome. The primary goal of treatment in these patients would be for symptomatic relief or to prevent sepsis, especially in the elderly.

DIFFERENTIAL DIAGNOSIS AND COMPLICATIONS

Patients with renal infarction may present with symptoms suggesting a urinary tract infection, and an intravenous pyelogram (IVP) at later stages may show scarring similar to that seen in chronic pyelonephritis. Acute glomerulonephritis in its early stages may be confused with acute pyelonephritis, especially in the few patients who have predominantly pyuria in the urinary sediment. Patients with polyarteritis may also have predominantly pyuria. In the late stages, chronic glomerulonephritis with bilateral shrunken kidneys may be difficult to distinguish from chronic pyelonephritis.

Papillary necrosis is an uncommon complication in pyelonephritis and occurs more often in diabetic patients. It may also occur in analgesic abuse interstitial nephritis as well as in sickle cell disease without infection. Perinephritic abscess is a rare complication of pyelonephritis. When it occurs, it is usually in association with ureteral obstruction, most commonly renal calculi, with Proteus and *E. coli* being the most frequently cultured organisms. The symptoms may range from those typical of acute pyelonephritis to fever of unknown origin. Extravasation of contrast media into the perirenal area is the only specific radiographic feature of perinephritic abscess. In this situation the kidney will not exhibit the characteristic movement with respiration when viewed under fluoroscopy during intravenous pyelography. The presence of a perinephritic abscess may also be detected by renal ultrasound examination or CT scanning.

Later in the course of chronic pyelonephritis hypertension may become evident. The presence of hypertension commonly occurs with the onset of renal insufficiency and may accelerate the progression of renal insufficiency.

PITFALLS IN DIAGNOSIS

The majority of patients present with classic signs and symptoms, and there is little diagnostic difficulty. The major pitfall is often overdiagnosis and treatment. To diagnose pyelonephritis as a specific form of urinary tract infection, one should demonstrate the presence of renal parenchymal infection by one or more of the methods previously described. Also, if leukocytes or bacteria are not seen in the urinary sediment but the clinical features are suggestive of pyelonephritis, one should investigate

the patient for intrarenal or perirenal abscess as well as urinary tract obstruction.

The most common error is the misdiagnosis of other kidney diseases as pyelonephritis. Chronic interstitial nephritis caused by a variety of agents can produce all the changes attributed to chronic pyelonephritis except for the demonstration of specific bacteria within renal tissue, a rare phenomenon in clinical practice. In fact, it has been demonstrated recently in a large group of patients with chronic interstitial nephritis that infection could rarely be implicated as the primary causative factor in its pathogenesis. The primary causative factors were anatomic abnormalities, analgesic abuse, hyperuricemia, nephrosclerosis, and renal stone disease, with bacterial infection playing a secondary role in only 27 per cent.

HYDRONEPHROSIS

By JOHN W. BEST, M.D.
York, Pennsylvania

Hydronephrosis is defined as the dilatation of the renal pelvis and calyceal system of the kidney with retained urine. This condition is most commonly caused by obstruction to urinary drainage and results in pressure atrophy and destruction of the functioning renal tissue. The degree of dilatation may vary from a slightly enlarged kidney to an immense, urine-distended sac that completely fills the abdominal cavity. The hydronephrosis may be unilateral or bilateral, depending upon the site of the urinary tract obstruction. The condition affects members of both sexes and is encountered in all age groups from infancy to old age.

ETIOLOGY

The most common underlying cause of hydronephrosis is some form of obstructive uropathy. It is therefore not a disease entity in itself but rather a pathologic physiologic response to partial or intermittent blockage of urinary drainage. The basis may be mechanical or neuromuscular dysfunction. The factors causing mechanical obstruction are multitudinous and may present anywhere in the urinary tract from the external urethral meatus to the ureteropelvic junction. The obstruction in certain instances may be produced by extrinsic pressure arising outside the urinary tract itself. Following is a listing of the most common anatomic or mechanical factors causing obstructive uropathy:

Urethra
  Atresia or pinpoint meatus
  Calculus
  Stricture
  Tumor
  Congenital posterior valves
  Congenital anomalies
Bladder and bladder neck
  Contracture of bladder neck
  Prostatic hyperplasia
  Prostatic neoplasm
  Prolapse of ureterocele
  Diverticulum of bladder
  Tumor
  Calculus
Ureter
  Stenosis of orifice
  Stricture
  Ureterocele
  Pregnancy
  Periureteritis
  Calculus
  Tumor (intrinsic or extrinsic)
  Retroperitoneal fibrosis or
  Ormond's disease
  Congenital anomaly
Renal pelvis or ureteropelvic junction
  Aberrant renal vessels
  Stricture or stenosis
  Angulation or kinks of ureter
  Periureteral or peripelvic fibrosis
  Calculus
  Tumor
  Anomalies of ureteral insertion

In most instances the underlying cause of hydronephrosis is demonstrable obstruction, but an ill-defined group of disorders related to congenital neuromuscular dysfunction cause megaloureter and hydronephrosis. These kidneys and ureters may reach huge size, ultimately resulting in renal atrophy and loss of renal function. Also, a variable group of congenital anomalies such as horseshoe kidney, pelvic ectopic kidney, and anomalies of the ureter, bladder, and urethra may contribute to or result in congenital hydronephrosis.

Pathologic Physiology

The continued production of urine is necessary for the establishment of hydronephrosis. Sudden complete occlusion of the ureter such as experimental ligation or the accidental ligation during surgery in most instances does not lead to hydronephrosis. In these cases the production of urine continues only until the intrarenal pressure of the tubules, calyces, and pelvis equals the filtration pressure. The kidney then becomes functionless, urine production ceases, and primary atrophy, not hydronephrosis, develops.

In the partial or incomplete obstruction, however, compensatory backflow of urine occurs. At first this is pyelovenous and later tubulovenous, so that a pressure gradient is maintained, permitting glomerular filtration to continue, and hydronephrotic dilatation of the pelvis and kidney will develop. The progressive dilatation and thinning of the renal pelvis with retained urine increases intrarenal pressure, ultimately resulting in tissue atrophy and compression of the vascular structures with diminution of the nutrient blood supply to the renal and intrarenal parenchyma. The dilatation is not confined to the pelvis but extends to the tubules and collecting systems with compression of the nutritive arterioles, adding still further to the atrophy and deterioration of renal function, and resulting in ultimate destruction of the kidney as an excretory unit.

The location of the obstruction determines the type and extent of the hydronephrosis. A single obstruction at or above the level of the ureterovesical junction (supravesical) produces unilateral hydronephrosis; obstruction below this level will produce bilateral hydronephrosis.

Hydronephrotic kidneys may be encountered in the newborn or in older infants. Among the common conditions that produce hydronephrosis in the young are congenital valves of the posterior urethra, atresia of the urethral meatus, congenital stricture of the urethra, contracture of the bladder neck, bilateral or unilateral ureteral stricture or stenosis, and neuromuscular dysfunction, which is often associated with spina bifida and congenital anomalies of the kidney and ureter. Calculi may be a factor but are usually rare in children.

Obstruction at the bladder neck or distal to it may occur in any age group. The principal causes of infravesical obstruction are lesions of the bladder neck, prostatic hyperplasia, prostatic neoplasm, contractures, or stricture. Obstruction may also be caused by calculus or bladder neoplasm as well as lesions distal to the bladder neck such as stricture, congenital valves of the urethra, tumor, calculus, or atresia of the urethral meatus. Early in the process the bladder may be able to compensate by hypertrophy of its musculature and will continue to empty its contents; but as the obstruction persists, the bladder musculature decompensates, urine is retained, back pressure develops, the ureters dilate, urine retention occurs within the renal pelves and hydroureters, and hydronephrosis develops. The mechanism of the obstructive process is the same in a child 4 years of age with congenital posterior urethral valves as in a patriarch 84 years of age with obstructive benign prostatic hypertrophy.

The principal causes of supravesical obstruction with blockage at or above the level of the ureterovesical junction are calculi (ureteral or renal), stricture, aberrant vessels, fibrous bands, and periureteral or pelvic adhesions. The most common site is the ureteropelvic junction where the cause may be a congenital narrowing or atresia of the junction or obstruction owing to blockage by an aberrant or anomalous blood vessel, calculus, or tumor. The ureter, however, may be involved at any level, and calculus or stricture is the most common cause. Ureteral obstruction can occur either unilaterally or bilaterally from extrinsic pressure or retroperitoneal masses or neoplasm. Extension of carcinoma of the cervix is a common cause of ureteral compression in women, and carcinoma of the prostate in men may produce secondary ureteral occlusion. Neoplasms such as sarcoma and lymphoma may secondarily involve the lower ureteral segments. Retroperitoneal fibrosis or Ormond's disease may present symptoms of bilateral ureteral occlusion.

The hydronephrosis of pregnancy is well documented. During pregnancy the upper urinary tract undergoes dilatation in as many as 80 per cent of patients during gestation, and the changes must be considered as physiologic. The enlarging pregnant uterus displaces and compresses the ureters, and the maximum dilatation is superior to the brim of the bony pelvis. The degree of dilatation is most marked on the right, although both kidneys are frequently involved. In addition to the mechanical factors of obstruction it has been suggested that a hormonal effect with loss of smooth muscle tone may be a factor, but it would appear that the pressure of the enlarging uterus is the most logical explanation of this physiologic hydronephrosis of pregnancy. The changes are manifested toward the end of the first trimester and achieve a maximum at about the seventh month. After delivery, regression occurs and is usually complete by 2 months.

COURSE

The clinical and pathologic course of hydronephrosis is that of progressive increasing dilatation with atrophy and loss of renal function until the kidneys are completely destroyed as functional units. If the condition is unilateral, there will be destruction of the affected kidney,

but in bilateral hydronephrosis the end result is progressive renal failure, uremia, and death. Fortunately in a large percentage of cases the condition may be reversible if severe renal damage has not occurred. Marked improvement or a return to normal function may be expected upon the surgical removal of the obstruction to urinary drainage. The prognosis will depend upon the stage at which the diagnosis is established and proper corrective treatment instituted. Hence, the earlier the diagnosis is established and proper treatment instituted, the better the prognosis for conservation and restoration of renal function.

PRESENTING SIGNS AND SYMPTOMS

In most instances progressive chronic hydronephrosis presents very little in the way of pathognomonic subjective symptoms. Usually the symptoms are those of the principal underlying cause of the obstruction, i.e., calculus, stricture, prostatic hypertrophy, and ureteropelvic obstruction. In many instances the patient may be asymptomatic until the onset of secondary infection. In some the condition is completely silent, and the diagnosis is established during the course of a complete routine urologic examination or upon investigation by pyelograms of a hypertensive state. In certain instances the condition is unsuspected until general disability and cachexia associated with renal insufficiency and uremia draw attention to a far advanced bilateral hydronephrosis with irreparable renal damage.

Pain. The chief presenting symptom of all hydronephrosis, regardless of cause, is lumbar back pain. The pain may be dull and constant or, with stone and acute obstruction, colicky in nature. Perhaps the most severe and excruciating pain occurs in those rare instances of intermittent obstruction associated with a sudden filling and overdistention of the renal pelvis. This may correspond to the so-called "Dietl's crisis" and is usually on the basis of a congenital high insertion of the ureter at the ureteropelvic junction or a sudden obstructive kinking in a redundant ureter and hypermobile kidney. The obstruction may relieve itself only to recur at intervals. Studies must be made at the time of the attack, or the diagnosis may be missed. The onset may be initiated by overhydration and sudden overfilling of the renal pelvis. I recall a patient whose severe, recurrent colic was initiated by bouts of heavy beer drinking; the diagnosis was not made until intravenous pyelograms were taken during an acute attack and the presence of hydronephrosis was established.

The pain is usually located in the costovertebral angle of the affected side and may radiate anteriorly. If it is associated with the passage of a stone, the pain may radiate to the loin or to the genitalia of the affected side.

Mass. A renal mass may or may not be palpable. In many instances, despite a moderate-sized hydronephrosis, no definite tumor can be elicited on physical examination. However, in infants the only sign may be the palpation of an abdominal mass, indicating a far advanced congenital hydronephrotic kidney.

Urinary symptoms are often lacking unless associated with obstruction by stricture or obstructive bladder neck syndrome. Hematuria may be associated with colic caused by stones or tumor. On rare occasions trauma may compound previously unsuspected hydronephrosis, causing hematuria from contusion or trauma to the dilated kidney.

Often the only presenting symptom is the onset of secondary infection when chills, fever, malaise, and generalized sepsis point to the underlying obstruction and hydronephrosis.

Gastrointestinal Symptoms. The pressure exerted by a large hydronephrotic kidney on adjacent organs may produce gastrointestinal symptoms such as nausea, ill-defined abdominal distress, and vomiting. In instances when vague and ill-defined gastrointestinal symptoms persist with negative gastrointestinal findings, investigation of the urinary tract by intravenous pyelogram may prove fruitful in demonstrating an underlying obstructive hydronephrosis as the cause.

DIAGNOSIS

As may be noted from the wide variety of obstructive factors causing hydronephrosis, the diagnosis depends upon careful consideration of the entire urinary tract. It is essential to determine not only the presence of hydronephrosis but the location of the obstruction, nature of the lesion, and the extent of renal damage. This requires complete urologic investigation including careful history, physical examination, intravenous pyelography, and the use of cystoscopy, endoscopy, ureteral catheterization, cystograms, bacteriologic examination of the urine, and blood studies as necessary to establish the exact diagnosis.

Ordinary physical examination, as previously noted, may or may not be helpful. A palpable mass in the renal or perirenal area must be differentiated from renal tumor, cyst, or retroperitoneal or abdominal mass. Excretory urography will prove diagnostic in most instances. In the past 5 years advances in intravenous urography have permitted much greater accuracy of diagnosis. The utilization of larger amounts and greater concentration of the contrast medium in combination with tomography, if indicated in routine excretory urography, has greatly increased the accuracy of diagnosis by this method.

The plain film may reveal a suspected renal mass, but the visualization of the urinary tract by contrast medium is necessary for diagnosis. Standard intravenous urograms are usually sufficient, but the double-dose technique may be necessary in obese patients. In instances of diminished renal function, the infusion drip technique together with tomography may be diagnostic and may obviate the necessity of retrograde pyelograms. It must be borne in mind that there are certain dangers associated with excretory urographic media, but these fortunately are rare and can be anticipated by any experienced radiologist.

When visualization by excretory urography is inadequate because of renal insufficiency or when the nature of the obstruction requires visualization, all the instrumental skills of the urologist, including cystoscopy, endoscopy, and retrograde pyelograms, may be necessary to establish the mechanics and nature of the obstructive lesion.

Lesions of the urethra, posterior urethral channel, and bladder neck require endoscopy for exact diagnosis. Retrograde pyelograms performed by introduction of a ureteral catheter or bulb ureterogram to fill the upper urinary tract with opaque dye may be necessary, particularly in cases of far advanced renal damage or obstruction by stone or stricture. Such studies are necessary to plan the surgical approach to relieve the obstruction.

Cystograms are necessary, particularly in children when ureteral reflux may be present and complicates the obstructive process. However, reflux can also develop in adults with bladder neck lesions, and this possibility must not be overlooked.

Urethrograms may be helpful in demonstrating intraluminal lesions of the urethra such as strictures, posterior valves, diverticula, or false passages essential in proper diagnosis of lower tract lesions.

Thus the entire armamentarium of the radiologist and the urologist must be utilized to arrive at a definitive diagnosis of the obstructive uropathy and to determine necessary treatment and prognosis.

LABORATORY TESTS

Urine. In uninfected hydronephrosis the urine is negative. If infection supervenes, white blood cells and albumin are noted.

Blood. There are no diagnostic hematologic findings in hydronephrosis. Should secondary infection be present, leukocytosis may be seen. In cases of advanced renal damage elevation of the blood urea nitrogen and secondary anemia may be noted secondary to the uremia.

COMPLICATIONS

The most common complication is the development of secondary infection. The retention and stasis of urine in hydronephrosis present an ideal situation for secondary infection, and it is this development that frequently leads to the investigation necessary to establish the diagnosis.

Calculus formation is common in hydronephrosis. As previously noted, calculi may be the primary cause of obstruction, but in other instances when infection has occurred, calculi may form secondarily in the already established hydronephrotic renal pelvis or calyces.

The most serious complication is the progressive loss of renal function. When unilateral, it may lead to the loss of a kidney; if bilateral, progressive deterioration of the renal function results in renal failure and uremia.

PITFALLS IN DIAGNOSIS

As is usual in medicine our diagnostic sins are usually those of omission rather than commission. The serious significance and disastrous complications of obstructive uropathy must constantly be borne in mind in all instances of urinary tract infection or dysfunction. All too frequently, repeated bouts of infection of the urinary tract are treated medically and specific diagnostic studies are delayed too long. Two repeated infections in the male and three in the female within a period of 1 year mandate complete diagnostic studies of the urinary tract. In those instances of vague abdominal and gastrointestinal symptoms an intravenous urogram should be an integral part of the diagnostic survey. A high index of suspicion is essential for the early diagnosis of hydronephrosis and to allow institution of proper therapy to conserve and preserve renal function.

URINARY INFECTIONS

By JOSEPH H. KIEFER, M.D.,
and THOMAS C. MALVAR, M.D.

Chicago, Illinois

DEFINITION AND GENERAL CONSIDERATIONS

Urinary tract infections constitute a major problem in clinical practice. They involve a significant portion of the general population and the immeasurable morbidity that results from them cannot be overemphasized. Accurate diagnosis is not always easy and treatment is often quite as challenging.

Urinary tract infections are caused by the active growth of a significant number of bacteria in the urinary tract. These infections are either acute, chronic, or asymptomatic. The site of infection may be the lower urinary tract, such as in cystitis and prostatitis, or the upper urinary tract, or both. Complicating structural abnormalities are sometimes present.

INCIDENCE

The incidence of urinary tract infections varies with age and sex. It is found in about 1 per cent of school girls and about 0.03 per cent of boys of the same age. The figure increases with age and is said to be as high as 7 to 12 per cent in females over the age of 60. In males, the incidence is also higher beyond the age of 50 but considerably less than that of women. Approximately 3 to 4 per cent of women of child-bearing age are involved.

Certain other factors are known to increase the incidence of urinary infections. Foremost among these are diabetes, pregnancy, urethral instrumentations and catheterizations, and the presence of structural abnormalities in the urinary tract. About 6 per cent of pregnant females are noted to have bacteriuria on initial examination. This increases to 7 per cent by the third trimester. An increase in the number of females showing positive cultures among the indigent population as noted by some authors suggests that socioeconomic factors may also play a role in the frequency of urinary infections. Lastly, the increased use of urethral instruments and catheters has become one of the leading causes of nosocomial infections. The incidence of infection with an indwelling Foley catheter is about 50 per cent after the first 24 hours and almost 100 per cent by 96 hours if no preventive measures are used.

CLINICAL MANIFESTATIONS

Urinary tract infection presents itself in varied ways. The most easily recognizable symptom complex is that of the lower urinary tract syndrome commonly referred to as cystitis. Frequency, urgency, dysuria and suprapubic discomfort or pain are usually present. Hematuria is sometimes found. This condition is predominantly a disease of women and young girls. A comparable condition occurs in men in the form of prostatitis.

When systemic symptoms such as chills, fever, prostration, nausea, and vomiting are prominent or when there is pain in one or both lumbar regions, renal parenchymal involvement is suspected. No one really knows how often the kidneys themselves are involved in lower urinary tract infections.

COURSE

An acute infection may subside with or without treatment. The symptoms disappear and the urine becomes sterile. The condition may never return again or there may be recurrent bouts of infection interspersed with symptom-free intervals. If a recurrent infection occurs within 2 weeks after the cessation of therapy and the same species and type-specific strain of bacterium present originally is found, the condition is called a relapse. If a new pathogen is identified, the recurrence is called a reinfection. In 80 per cent of circumstances, relapsing infections signify a renal source of infection. Among the other causes, chronic bacterial prostatitis is now recognized as probably the most common relapsing infection in males. A reinfection is usually associated with recurrent bacteriuria.

COMMON COMPLICATIONS

One of the most feared complications of urinary tract infection is gram-negative bacteremia with resultant endotoxic shock. Gram-negative bacteremia probably occurs more frequently than we would like to believe and is the most common serious complication of urinary tract infections. Fortunately, most cases are transient and produce few or no symptoms. Bacteremia often occurs during manipulation of infected tissues such as may occur during urethral instrumentation or prostatic massage, particularly in the acute stage. It also occurs in the presence of obstruction of the urinary tract such as ureteral obstruction from stones or in acute urinary retention from an enlarged prostate gland. In transient bacteremia, a subsequent bacterial endocarditis may occur if a previously damaged heart valve is present. In occasional and unpredictable circumstances, the gram-negative bacteremia progresses into the shock stage with its resultant high mortality rate.

Other sequelae of urinary tract infections include perinephric or renal cortical abscesses, ureterovesical reflux, and subsequent permanent renal damage that may lead to renal failure.

Small cortical abscesses may occur with pyelonephritis, particularly the acute type. Renal carbuncle may also occur and is usually hematogenously acquired from a distant focus of infection.

Ureterovesical reflux is commonly found in association with urinary tract infections, particularly in children. In the past, numerous operations were performed on these patients in the belief that the infection of the upper tracts could be eliminated by eliminating the reflux. However, the reflux was often noted to disappear spontaneously with adequate antibacterial therapy. This latter fact suggests that the majority of cases of ureterovesical reflux are the result rather than the cause of the infections. Presently, only patients with the more severe cases of ureterovesical reflux and those whose cases are associated with other structural abnormalities are being operated upon.

LABORATORY FINDINGS

The diagnosis of urinary tract infections is based on laboratory findings. This is also the only means to identify the large group of asymptomatic patients with bacteriuria. Quantitative cultures of 100,000 or more bacteria per ml of properly collected urine is virtually diagnostic of a urinary tract infection.

The clean-catch midstream technique of collecting urine is the most widely used method. When a urine specimen is carefully collected in this manner under supervision, patients who do not have infections will have fewer than 1000 organisms per ml of urine. As much as 95 per cent correlation with the clinical condition is attainable using this technique. However, this percentage of reliability is not always obtainable in clinical practice. This is due to the fact that the ideal conditions for a proper collection of urine are not always present. Under such circumstances, the reliability index of a single midstream urine specimen that is sent for bacteriologic studies is probably only 80 per cent.

Correlation with the clinical picture and repeated cultures may be necessary to enhance the diagnostic accuracy. In certain instances, urethral catheterizations may be employed. Suprapubic needle aspiration is used in special circumstances but should be performed only by physicians who are familiar with the technique.

If the urine culture shows less than 100,000 colonies per ml but the clinical picture is typical, presence of infection should be assumed. If the urine culture is less than 100,000 colonies per ml of urine but more than 10,000, a repeat culture must be done. Infection is present if the same bacterium as originally present is found in the second or third cultures. If the subsequent cultures reveal a different species of bacteria, the organisms are considered as contaminants. In males, a properly collected specimen showing 10,000 bacteria per ml is considered significant.

A number of methods for differentiating renal involvement in bacteriuria are being used at present. Measurement of O-specific hemagglutinating and other antibody titers, tests of maximal concentrating ability, detection of antibody-coated bacteria, differentiation between relapsing and reinfection type of recurrence and other methods are being used. Presently, only bilateral ureteral catheterizations can localize infection with certainty and so the search continues for a noninvasive technique of localization. It should be pointed out, however, that the detection of antibody-coated bacteria in the urine is gaining wide acceptance as a reliable noninvasive tool in detecting kidney involvement.

Escherichia coli is responsible for 50 to 75 per cent of all urinary infections. The Proteus group is next in frequency, then Klebsiella, Pseudomonas, and cocci; *Mycobacterium tuberculosis*, various fungi, and others are less common. Resistant infections are usually associated with previous antibiotic treatment, instrumentation, or presence of structural abnormalities. In the overwhelming majority of patients with first infections, *E. coli* is the organism isolated. If any other type of bacteria is found, a search for structural abnormalities should be started.

PERIPHERAL BLOOD

In acute infections, a peripheral polymorphonuclear leukocytosis is common. In febrile patients, particularly during or shortly after a chill, the offending bacteria may be isolated from the blood using proper bacteriologic techniques.

URINALYSIS

The findings on microscopic examination of the urine are quite helpful to the physician when dealing with urinary tract infections.

Pyuria. The commonest cause of cloudy urine is not pyuria but phosphaturia. Usually, the presence of significant pyuria (more than 5 pus cells per high power field [HPF]) indicates the presence of urinary infection. However, pyuria can occur in the absence of infection and infection can occur without pyuria. Determining the presence or absence of pyuria is therefore a convenient but not entirely accurate method of screening for urinary tract infection. A number of simple quantitative bacteriologic (dip-slide method, filter paper method) and chemical (Griess test) methods are now available and are suitable for office and survey work.

Bacteriuria. If bacteria are seen in a stained or unstained sediment of centrifuged urine, a presumptive diagnosis of urinary tract infection can be made since it has been shown that this finding equates well with the presence of 100,000 bacteria per ml and over. A stained specimen is necessary when ruling out cocci, since they are not readily recognized in unstained smears.

Hematuria. The presence of gross or persistent microscopic hematuria may indicate the presence of calculi or tumors and usually demands prompt urologic evaluation.

A low specific gravity may connote overhydration with subsequent diuresis and bacterial dilution; therefore, a urine culture done on the same urine sample that shows less than 100,000 bacteria per ml should not be construed as evidence of the absence of infection.

UROLOGIC EVALUATION

Evaluation of the genitourinary tract is usually indicated for patients with urinary tract infections that fail to respond to the usual antibacterials and those who have recurrent episodes of bacteriuria. It should also be done if the medical history suggests the possible presence of a structural abnormality of the urinary tract and as a general rule for all male patients with urinary tract infection.

The urologic evaluation usually consists of an intravenous urogram and a cystoscopic examination. Urethral calibration, cystometry, ureteral catheterization with or without retrograde pyelography, cystography and voiding cystourethrography, nephrotomography, and various other procedures may be done as indicated.

In addition, a search for any possible extraurinary sources of infection may be necessary. The physician should pay particular attention to certain gynecologic conditions such as vaginitis and cervicitis, since they are quite often associated with urinary infections. The presence of certain gastrointestinal conditions such as diverticulitis and biliary tract infections should not be overlooked.

PITFALLS IN DIAGNOSIS

Errors in the diagnosis of urinary infections are often due to false-positive culture findings. The latter result from errors in the technique of collection and handling of the urine specimen, such as poor preparation of the patient, inadequate instruction and supervision during the process of collection, and delays between collection and culture. Difficulties encountered in obtaining specimens from children and uncooperative elderly patients and urine collection in patients who are menstruating or those with heavy vaginal discharge all contribute to the likelihood of a false-positive result.

False-negative results are not as frequent but equally important. These occur when the infected area is isolated from the rest of the urinary tract as in pyelonephritis associated with ureteral obstruction owing to stones, tumor, or stricture, in which the urine from the involved kidney does not get through to the bladder. This situation may also be found in renal cortical infections that do not communicate with the renal pelvis or in prostatitis in which the urine may be sterile in spite of a continued infection of the prostate.

A truly negative urine culture, however, occurs in some women with symptoms simulating cystitis. Functional and structural abnormalities are sometimes found. However, in a significant number of these women, the cause is not readily apparent in spite of a thorough urologic work-up. Suffice it to say that in over 50 per cent of the latter, the patient either will have a history of previous urinary tract infection or will eventually have a subsequent positive urine culture.

One cannot always make an absolutely accurate diagnosis in dealing with urinary infections. Observance of proper technique in the collection and handling of the urine specimens, the use of a catheter when necessary, or even suprapubic needle aspiration, combined with proper attention to details in the history and physical examination and repeat cultures when in doubt, will help increase the accuracy of diagnosis.

TUMORS OF THE URINARY BLADDER

By RANDALL G. ROWLAND, M.D., PH.D.,
and ROBERT A. GARRETT, M.D.
Indianapolis, Indiana

INTRODUCTION

The genesis of bladder cancer is that of multifocal urethelial changes beginning with cellular atypia and hyperplasia progressing to dysplasia and subsequently to carcinoma. The lesions may remain sessile or become papillary in form. Some become invasive in adjacent tissue and metastasize to local and regional lymph nodes, bones, and other viscera in turn. The rate of progression along this spectrum is dependent on the biological potential of each lesion. At any given time, individual tumors in a patient may be at variable stages of the natural history. The clinical evaluation of bladder tumors centers on an attempt to determine the stage of the natural history that exists when the patient is first seen and is an effort to gather information that will assist in judging the future behavior of the tumor.

Approximately 90 per cent of all bladder tumors are transitional cell carcinoma. The majority of the remainder is composed of squamous cell carcinoma, adenocarcinoma, and mixed tumors. In addition to these epithelial tumors, mesenchymal tumors of the bladder occur but are exceedingly rare. Sarcomatous tumors of childhood are not discussed here.

PRESENTING SIGNS AND SYMPTOMS

Although gross hematuria is a common presenting complaint, recognition of the importance of accompanying or independent symptoms of vesical irritation such as frequency, urgency, and dysuria is essential to prompt recognition of patients with bladder tumors. Occasionally, a tumor mass in a strategic location may result in bladder outlet obstruction with its attendant symptoms of hesitancy or obstruction. The possibility that irritative bladder symptoms in the aging male population may be due to neoplastic changes such as carcinoma in situ should not be dismissed despite the prevalence of symptoms caused by bladder neck obstruction from benign prostatic hyperplasia.

Occasionally, patients with bladder tumor will have no clinical symptoms. In these patients, the diagnosis of bladder tumors is made by evaluation of abnormal laboratory findings such as microscopic hematuria or incidental abnormalities noted on radiologic studies. In the majority of patients, symptomatic or epidemiologic history will prompt consideration of the diagnosis of bladder tumor. Physical findings such as lower abdominal or rectal masses or renal enlargement are found only in patients with far-advanced lesions. Bimanual examination is the most helpful maneuver of the physical examination; however, it is best performed under anesthesia at the time of bladder biopsy. If a mass is palpable, the size, consistency, location (including apparent involvement of other organs), and mobility should be noted.

LABORATORY FINDINGS

Routine urinalysis including microscopic evaluation of freshly voided, centrifuged urine is essential in the evaluation of patients with symptoms suggestive of bladder tumor. Eighty per cent of all patients with bladder tumor will have gross or microscopic hematuria. The findings of pyuria and bacteriuria can help identify those patients whose symptoms are most likely due to infection; however, caution must be exercised in these cases, since bladder tumors can be secondarily infected. The findings on urinalysis are not specific for bladder tumors, with the exception of the rare instance in which tumor fragments may be recognized in the urinary sediment. Investigation of the causes of abnormalities on routine urinalysis, particularly microscopic hematuria, can lead to the diagnosis of an asymptomatic bladder tumor.

Urinary cytology is a sensitive, specific technique for making the initial diagnosis and for following patients with the history of bladder tumors. The reliability of cytology depends upon the adequacy of collection of specimens as well as the skill of the individual cytopathologist evaluating the smears. In the best of hands, the false-negative rate may exceed that of direct cystoscopic examination for the diagnosis of bladder tumors.

Hematologic findings are not specific for bladder cancer; however, in cases of far-advanced bladder tumor, anemia may be present. Also, an elevation of blood urea nitrogen (BUN) and serum creatinine will be noted if there is significant obstruction of the upper urinary tracts by bladder tumors.

CYSTOSCOPY

Cystoscopy is essential to evaluate the bladder and urethra accurately when a bladder tumor is suspected. In addition to looking for overt papillary and sessile lesions, the examiner should regard with suspicion any mucosal abnormalities, particularly encrusted or apparently inflammatory areas.

If a tumor or a suspicious area is seen, transurethral biopsies are made to establish the diagnosis and provide information about the grade, extent, depth, and biological potential of bladder tumors. Biopsied sites should be carefully recorded for future reference with regard to treatment and recurrences.

A bimanual examination should be performed both before and after tumors are resected or biopsies are done. If a mass is noted, the size, location, extent of involvement, and fixation of surrounding tissue should be recorded. Particular attention should be paid to the persistence of a mass or residual induration and fixation after removal of the bladder tumor.

Biopsy specimens can be taken by aspirating tissue samples with an open-end blunt-tipped urethral catheter, a cold cup biopsy forceps, or a standard resectoscope. Each of these instruments has specific advantages and limitations. Biopsy specimen collection by either aspiration or cold cup can be performed without anesthesia and is particularly valuable for use in outpatients. The resectoscope is required for doing biopsies when muscle sections are needed to assess the extent of tumor invasion.

Both papillary and sessile lesions should be removed to the level of the bladder wall. The base of the tumor should be resected into the muscle and submitted separately for histologic study. If the size or location of the tumor(s) makes complete resection inadvisable, the tumor margin and base should be biopsied for accurate assessment of the extent of the tumor.

Studies have shown a high incidence of carcinoma in situ or severe atypia of the epithelium both adjacent to overt bladder tumors and in areas that are apparently uninvolved distant from overt tumors. The most frequent sites of unapparent mucosal change are the left lateral, right lateral, and posterior walls, while the dome and trigone are relatively spared. In addition to biopsies of obvious and questionable lesions, random biopsies are performed to assess the status of the epithelium in the other frequently involved areas.

HISTOLOGIC STUDIES

Careful histologic examination of step sections of the tissue biopsies is essential. From these studies, the cell type is identified and the grade of tumor or degree of differentiation is assigned (Table 1). The depth of invasion is used to assign an initial clinical stage using the

Table 1. *Grading of Bladder Tumors*

I–Well differentiated
II–Moderately well differentiated
III–Poorly differentiated
IV–Anaplastic

terminology of Jewett or the International Union Against Cancer (UICC) (Table 2).

A close correlation between tumor grade and the likelihood of invasion has been observed. Of low-grade lesions (Grade I) approximately 6 per cent are invasive, while of high-grade lesions (Grade III) 82 per cent are invasive. If multiple lesions are noted at a given time or if frequent recurrences are observed, the lesions are more likely to become invasive. Chromosomal analysis and the deletion of normally present ABO-isoantigens are currently being investigated as means of measuring the biological potential of bladder tumors.

ADDITIONAL TECHNIQUES FOR STAGING

Cystoscopic examination and transurethral biopsies even with information provided on bimanual examination have definite limitations in distinguishing Stage B from Stage C lesions. Also, these techniques cannot identify Stage D disease unequivocally.

Information regarding higher stages of a bladder tumor can be obtained from intravenous pyelograms. Distal ureteral obstruction in the presence of a bladder tumor indicates an invasive lesion in approximately 98 per cent of patients. Also, maintenance of a fixed shape of the bladder wall at different bladder volumes seen during an intravenous pyelogram is indicative of an invasive lesion.

Double and triple contrast cystography with angiography have been developed to improve the accuracy of staging. Bilateral hypogastric angiography has been used successfully by some to delineate margins of high-grade lesions. Lymphangiography has not been successful in most series in identifying patients with lymphatic involvement. Chest roentgenograms

Table 2. *Staging of Bladder Tumors*

Depth of Invasion	Jewett Stage	UICC Stage
Mucosa	O	TIS
Submucosa	A	T1
Superficial muscle	B$_1$	T2
Deep muscle	B$_2$	T3
Perivesical fat	C	T3
Metastases	D	T4

other than routine admission films have not generally been useful. Bone surveys, bone scans, and bone marrow studies are commonly used but have rarely provided useful information in our experiences. Ultrasonography and computerized axial tomography both have promise as techniques that can delineate the depth of invasion of a bladder tumor as well as the presence of metastatic disease.

PITFALLS IN DIAGNOSIS

One of the most common errors in diagnosing bladder tumors is overlooking the incidental finding of microscopic hematuria on urinalysis. Another error is not considering bladder tumor as a diagnosis when treating irritative bladder symptoms. Cystoscopically the greatest errors in diagnosing and staging bladder tumors come from taking biopsy material that is inadequate for judging the depth of the tumor and for detecting random involvement of the bladder epithelium. Until recent times, the significance of severe dysplasia or carcinoma in situ was not recognized.

The early and correct diagnosis of bladder cancer requires suspicion of bladder tumor in patients with hematuria or voiding symptoms as well as in the patient who is asymptomatic but has microscopic hematuria. Accurate staging, coupled with information regarding grade, extent, and biological potential, is critical to the rational management and assessment of results. Although the laboratory and x-ray examinations described and the cystoscopic findings and biopsies provide valuable presumptive information, open surgical staging including lymph node resection is frequently required to obtain the desirable degree of accuracy in staging bladder tumors.

PROSTATITIS

By ALAN J. WEIN, M.D.,
and PAUL R. LEBERMAN, M.D.
Philadelphia, Pennsylvania

DEFINITION

Prostatitis denotes an inflammation of the prostatic acini and their surrounding stroma. True infection is most often caused by gram-negative bacteria (*Escherichia coli*, Proteus, Klebsiella, Pseudomonas) and less commonly by gram-positive organisms (enterococci and possibly *Staphylococcus albus*). Unusual causes of infection include viruses, fungi, Mycoplasma, Chlamydia, Trichomonas, and tubercle bacilli. Routes of infection include (1) ascending, from the urethra; (2) antegrade passage of infected bladder urine; (3) hematogenous dissemination; and (4) lymphatic spread. Granulomatous prostatitis is an entity of unknown cause characterized by chronic inflammatory cells and lipid-laden macrophages. Such a gland may present a hard, nodular posterior surface, often confused with that of carcinoma.

ACUTE BACTERIAL PROSTATITIS

This is an easily recognized entity characterized by a fulminant bacterial infection involving most of the gland. Symptoms include urinary urgency, dysuria, diurnal and nocturnal frequency, and low back and/or perineal pain. The onset is sudden. Chills, fever, myalgia, and arthralgia are often present. Varying degrees of bladder outlet obstruction and its attendant symptoms may occur, depending on the degree of enlargement of the gland. A urethral discharge often occurs.

The diagnosis is generally made on the basis of the history and a rectal examination that reveals an acutely tender, edematous, warm prostate gland. Areas of induration alternating with softer areas may represent abscess formation. The pathogen can be identified by culture of the urethral discharge or a midstream urine specimen, because the bladder urine is usually infected also. If acute prostatitis is strongly suspected, manipulation of the gland should be avoided because of the danger of septicemia.

Antibiotic treatment generally results in improvement within several days. Possible complications include urinary retention, cystitis, epididymitis, prostatic abscess, pyelonephritis, and chronic prostatitis. A thorough urologic work-up should be done after full recovery to exclude any predisposing factor.

CHRONIC BACTERIAL PROSTATITIS

This entity is probably the most common cause of relapsing urinary infections in men. It is difficult to diagnose precisely. The condition may be generalized or localized to a small area of the gland. The symptoms, which vary, may include frequency, urgency, dysuria (especially terminal), difficult or poor urination, occasional low-grade fever, and pain in the lower back, suprapubic, and/or perineal area. A urethral discharge may occur. Malaise, various genital aches and pains, painful ejaculation, and a decrease in libido and potency may be a part of the symptomatology or may represent a functional psychoneurotic overlay.

The rectal examination may be normal or may demonstrate prostatic tenderness. The gland may be enlarged, and areas of induration may be enlarged and palpable. Pressure on the gland may reproduce a part or all of the patient's pain pattern.

An accurate diagnosis is possible only by bacteriologic localization studies such as those promoted by Meares and Stamey. The urine and prostatic secretions are divided as follows: (1) the first voided 10 ml, termed VB1; (2) an aliquot of midstream urine (VB2); (3) the expressed prostatic secretions, if any, after prostatic massage (EPS); and (4) an aliquot of urine voided after prostatic massage (VB3). If the bladder urine is sterile, bacterial prostatitis may be diagnosed if the colony count is significantly higher in EPS and VB3 than in VB1. If the bladder urine is infected, the localization test cannot be used, because all specimens will show a heavy growth of organisms. In such patients, treatment for 3 to 4 days will generally sterilize the bladder urine but not the prostate, so that cultures of EPS and VB3 are likely to remain positive.

Clinically, chronic bacterial prostatitis may be mimicked by chronic abacterial prostatitis, malignancy of the bladder or prostate, urethral stricture, obstructive prostatic hypertrophy, bladder calculi, and inflammatory disease of an area adjacent to the prostate or the bladder. Possible complications include relapsing lower urinary tract infection and pyelonephritis.

Antibiotic treatment may be successful in relieving the initial symptoms, but because of the difficulty in achieving an adequate antibiotic concentration in prostatic tissue, eradication is very difficult and relapses are common.

CHRONIC ABACTERIAL PROSTATITIS

Many patients complain of symptoms similar to those of chronic bacterial prostatitis, but no pathogen is found by bacterial localization studies or by special isolation techniques for other known causative agents. This condition may be referred to as nonspecific prostatitis, abacterial prostatitis, or prostatosis. Commonly, these patients have no chills or fever and complain of vaguer, more subjective symptoms than the previous group. They often, however, exhibit greater than 10 white blood cells per high power field in their expressed prostatic secretions. It is unclear whether the complaints of such patients represent an as yet undefined clinical entity or a psychosomatic illness, or both.

Antibiotic treatment is least successful in this group, and the course of the disease tends to be one of exacerbation and remission, often associated with the patient's emotional status.

BENIGN PROSTATIC HYPERTROPHY

By R. H. HARRISON, M.D.
Bryan, Texas

INTRODUCTION

The *pathogenesis* of prostatic hypertrophy is postulated to result from the proliferation of periurethral glands surrounding the prostatic urethra. This proliferation begins at puberty, stimulated by the increasing ratio of testosterone to estrogen through the fourth decade, causing adenoma formation. With the decreasing ratio of male hormones to female hormones after age 40, the adenomas may increase in number and size to compress the bladder neck and prostatic urethra, producing urinary obstructive symptoms in an estimated 5 to 10 per cent of men out of the 25 per cent who have digitally palpable enlarged prostates during the fifth decade. With each additional decade the percentage with obstructive symptoms increases by an additional 15 until by age 100, 85 to 90 per cent of all men will have sufficient obstructive symptoms to necessitate surgery.

The normal prostate has traditionally been described as the size of a Spanish chestnut, 4 to 5 cm in length, 3 to 4 cm in width, 15 to 20 grams in weight, with a palpable texture approximating the consistency of the thenar eminence of the hand. With hypertrophy the gland may symmetrically enlarge or there may be asymmetrically enlargement of one or more of the five lobes of the prostate. This assists the clinician in appreciating the occasional benign nodularity and irregularity of hypertrophy yet the conspicuous absence of overall hypertrophy when the middle lobe has enlarged, causing a "ball-valve" phenomenon with obstructive symptoms that are often advanced. The adenomas are predominantly glandular, although some prostates have considerable fibrous stroma. This fact explains the variance in descriptions of the normal consistency of benign prostatic hypertrophy.

SYMPTOMS

Men with hypertrophy of the prostate may have no symptoms so long as the bladder is able to compensate and overcome the progressively obstructing infravesical prostate. With obstruction, the subjective symptoms of hesitancy in initiating voiding, straining, intermittency with dribbling, and often the sensation of incomplete emptying begin. Frequency, small-quantity voidings and nocturia announce bladder decompensation. Men often initially complain of a weak stream with decreased size and force and of having to stand very close to the urinal and occasionally having to sit to gain relief.

Symptoms often develop so insidiously a man may not realize he has a remediable problem until there is advanced bladder decompensation with or without secondary "back pressure" changes in the kidneys, with azotemia progressing to uremia if not corrected. Clinically, this is referred to as *silent prostatism*. These patients may have overflow incontinence with a distended bladder that is percussable. They will tell the examiner that they have had to let their belt out several notches. Complete urinary retention is the sine qua non of obstruction. As the obstruction usually develops progressively over a period of years, the bladder muscles hypertrophy and thicken. Herniations (cellules) may enlarge to form diverticuli between the muscle bundles. On occasion these diverticuli reach sizes as large as the bladder itself. Long-standing elevations of bladder pressure can cause decompensation of the uretero-vesical junction, permitting reflux. The thickened bladder wall can compress and obstruct either or both ureters. Thus "J"ing is produced at the ureterovesical junction, as are ureterectasis and hydroureteronephrosis. Prolonged obstruction may lead to renal insufficiency.

Patients may present with symptoms of chronic illness such as nausea, vomiting, anorexia, apathy, weakness, weight loss, and even symptoms of right-sided congestive heart failure as a result of the effects of long-standing back pressure on the upper urinary system. Those men with long-term chronic obstruction may have superimposed urinary infections and calculus disease. Treatment results are quicker in the noninfected urinary system; morbidity is decreased if the bladder has not decompensated to an atonic state. The morbidity and mortality rates are directly related to the degree of azotemia and uremia. Infection from residual urine causes dysuria, stranguria, tenesmus, and chills and fever of varying degrees. Bleeding from surface vessels of the prostate is not uncommon.

PHYSICAL DIAGNOSIS

Gentle rectal examination with the examiner carefully evaluating the prostate from the bladder to the apex, side to side, is the first step. If congestion of the seminal vesicles and prostate is present, the soft bogginess is apparent, sometimes loculated. Without massage per se, several drops of the milky fluid will be emitted from the external meatus. In benign prostatic hypertrophy (BPH) the prostate is soft to rubbery in consistency, usually smooth and movable. The degree of tenderness depends on variations among individuals and their pain thresholds as well as on the vigor of the examiner. If the prostate is tense and the feel to palpation is similar to that of the tip of one's nose, acute prostatitis is likely and excessive digital pressure with massage is ill advised. More complete prostatic examination is deferred until a follow-up visit after specific treatment.

Numerous positions for rectal examination have been described. The least traumatic to the patient is obviously the superior technique, as cooperation is of the essence. Flexing the patient over the examination table with both elbows supporting the trunk, knees straight, toes together with heels apart, the patient clasping the four fingers of each hand and pulling (reinforcement technique) often will allow maximum anal sphincter relaxation. Another "trick" is to instruct the man to bear down as in defecation. This will permit easier introduction of a well-lubricated forefinger with rapid evaluation of the prostate gland and seminal vesicles.

Although the normal-sized benign prostate in the adult male is easy to reach over, the prostate can become so large that the examiner's finger cannot reach over the top. The physician is interested in the "feel" or texture of the prostate and in estimating the degree of enlargement (size). Arbitrarily the clinician refers to the enlargement in grades 1+ to 4+: 1+ is spoken of as between 25 and 35 grams; 2+, 40 and 50 grams; 3+, 60 and 90 grams; and 4+, over 100 grams. The tip of the forefinger of a glove size 9 hand reaches the base of the prostate in 2+ (40 to 50 grams) benign prostatic hypertrophy. Prostatic examination should be done after the patient has voided to avoid overestimating prostatic hypertrophy. It is disconcerting to the medical student who has examined a man with urinary retention and estimated a 4+ gland to discover that the patient has no more than a 1+ to 2+ gland after a few days of urinary bladder catheter drainage. Allowing the large distended bladder to recompensate and the renal function to return to maximum is accomplished with urethral Foley catheter drainage or suprapubic drainage if a catheter cannot be introduced into the urethra.

The size of the prostate does not necessarily correlate with the severity of obstruction, as many men with large prostates can empty their bladders with a relatively good stream. Conversely, a small amount of benign prostatic hypertrophy may produce severe obstruction, as in middle lobe hypertrophy, even though palpation indicates a prostate of normal size and consistency. One of the most reliable evaluations of obstructive prostatism is the so-called fisherman's test. If the patient is a fisherman, ask if he uses a coffee can to urinate in or if he can urinate over the side of a boat. His wife may volunteer that it takes him a long time to get out of the bathroom, as occasionally men downgrade their symptoms. When possible, observing the patient void is the easiest way to determine if he has difficulty. If his face turns red, the veins in his neck stand out, the urine dribbles out rather than in a full uninterrupted stream, and if he passes flatus and/or his underclothes demonstrate fecal stains, the clinician knows the man has obstructive disease. Fortunately, if urethral bleeding or hematuria occurs, the patient will seek medical attention more promptly.

There are various medications that can worsen the symptoms of obstructive prostatism that may precipitate urinary retention. Smooth muscle relaxants such as propantheline and antihistamines can inhibit bladder contractility. The use of diuretics may produce "bladder fatigue." Cold weather with less water loss through perspiration may precipitate retention of urine. One of the most common causes of urinary retention develops when an elderly man with borderline prostatic obstruction is put to bed because of illness or surgery. The urinary system of some of these patients will recompensate once they are ambulatory, in others it will not. Certain conditions such as cerebrovascular accidents (strokes) will precipitate retention because of compromised detrussor function. Combined abdominoperineal resection, hemorrhoidectomy, and herniorrhaphy often precipitate urinary retention.

SUPPORTIVE DIAGNOSTIC EXAMINATION AND TESTS

Routine *complete urinalysis* including microscopic examination is the premier diagnostic method in that it often determines the diagnostic and therapeutic events to follow; also, it may be routinely done in most doctors' offices and is inexpensive.

A *residual urine measurement* is used by many in determining bladder compensation and to collect a specimen for culture, although many urologists are satisfied with a midvoided collection for study. They prefer not to use instruments on the urethra unless the patient is azotemic, to prevent the possibility of introducing infection into a sterile system probably already compromised by varying degrees of obstruction.

If the urine is infected and does not clear with a chemotherapeutic agent, *urine culture* and sensitivity studies should be undertaken to aid in choosing antibiotics before, during, and after surgery.

The complete blood count (CBC) is essential to evaluate the overall general condition of the patient. Anemia may be present in patients with renal deterioration and this condition should be treated. An elevated white blood cell (WBC) count may herald more serious disease.

The *blood urea nitrogen* (BUN) and *creatinine* determinations are the simplest and least expensive crude evaluations of renal function. If these are significantly elevated, the urinary system must be drained until the maximum renal function is reached and has stabilized, at which time the future management will be determined.

The kidney, ureter, and bladder (KUB) x-ray is usually all that is necessary to tell the examiner that there are two kidneys and there are no urinary calculi. The incidence of upper urinary tract abnormality is insignificant if the CBC, BUN, and creatinine are normal. At an additional $50 to $100 cost, the *excretory urogram* (IVP) may detect the presence of upper tract obstruction, the degree of hydroureteronephrosis, the location of calculi, and ureterectasis, renal masses, significant residual urine, and bladder diverticuli. It also gives a crude measurement of intravesical intrusion from below by the prostate.

Normal *retrograde urethrograms* rule out urethral stricture disease and can give some information as to the size of the prostate but is not a study routinely utilized in evaluation of benign prostatic hypertrophy (BPH). *Uroflometry* translates subjective feelings of urine flow into objective measurements. It is not essential and is considered an academic research tool that adds little to observation of the voided stream and does little for the patient other than add nonessential data and additional cost to the workup.

Panendoscopy and *cystoscopy* are usually done under anesthesia preliminary to actual urologic surgery. Endoscopy without anesthesia in the office is often traumatic and will only serve to "stir things up." It adds little in evaluating benign prostatic hypertrophy (BPH) except to reaffirm the clinical impression and measure the side effects from obstruction such as bladder trabeculation, bladder calculi, and diverticuli. Endoscopy will detect unsuspected bladder tumors. When performed immediately prior to the transurethral resection (TUR), the cost is included in the resection charge.

Those physicians who send their laboratory work out of the office have observed that the *sequential multiple analysis* (SMA) profile provides considerable additional biochemical information. The clinician should remember to collect blood for acid and alkaline phosphatase analysis before vigorous prostatic digital examination lest occasional false-positive elevations be obtained.

DIFFERENTIAL DIAGNOSIS

Carcinoma of the prostate is one of the most common malignancies in men. The prostate may feel woody hard and irregular on rectal examination. Carcinoma should be suspected when there is rapid onset of obstructive symptoms. When suspected, immediate referral to a urologist for proper histopathologic grading and staging is suggested so that proper treatment may be initiated to ensure that the maximum in life expectancy may be obtained.

Acute prostatitis in men is usually accompanied by perineal pain, varying degrees of urgency, frequency, and burning, and the usual symptoms of toxicity with chills and fever. The prostate will be firm and tense to palpation. It is more prevalent in younger men and may accompany acute urethritis with urethral discharge. Ejaculation is painful and should be discouraged until the acute process has resolved. Men with *subacute prostatitis* will present with less severe symptoms than those with acute prostatitis. Rectal digital examination will reveal areas of tenseness perhaps loculated and other areas less involved. In men with *chronic prostatitis*, the prostate and seminal vesicles are more indurated and thickened. Often there will be significant areas of bogginess and fullness that may be massaged out of the prostate into the urethra, producing dramatic relief of perineal fullness (prostadynia) with an improved urinary stream. This is referred to as *congestive prostatovesiculitis* or *prostatosis*. Frequent ejaculation is encouraged.

Urethral strictures are suspected when there is an antecedent history of trauma, instrumentation, gonorrhea, or recurrent urethral discharge. The urinary stream may be split or forked. The pressure may be somewhat adequate, but the size is greatly diminished. Retrograde urethrogram, urethral calibration and/or panendoscopy under direct vision will make the diagnosis.

Prostatic calculi may feel gritty on palpation, giving the clinician a crepitation impression. If large, they may be noted on a KUB. They may mimic adenocarcinoma of the prostate. There is a 10 per cent incidence of cancer in patients with prostatic calculi. Corpora amylacea are commonly seen in the acini on histology slides. Black submucosal studding in the prostatic urethra is characteristic. The symptoms of chronic prostatitis may be present, although often the man will be asymptomatic and the calculi will be noted on routine annual rectal examination, which is recommended for all men age 40 and over.

Varying degrees of *neurogenic bladder* in the older man with generalized arteriosclerosis must be considered. Hyperactive reflexia with urgency and precipitate voiding may be alleviated with anticholinergic drugs. Some neurologic lesions, such as those caused by diabetes mellitus, may weaken bladder contractions and produce symptoms similar to those caused by benign prostatic hypertrophy. Bladder atonicity will be demonstrated with filling to large capacity without any objective sensation of urgency or pain or increase in pressure, which may be recorded by simple office cystometry. Because the chronically obstructed, dilated bladder with atony from benign prostatic hypertrophy may produce a similar cystometrogram, the clinician should rule out neurologic disease.

Various *medications* and *drugs* used in the treatment of sinusitis, peptic ulcer, parkinsonism, and heart disease may cause urinary difficulties. The urinary system in these men may have adequately compensated for benign prostatic hypertrophy but they experience detrusor weakness from the medication. If the drugs are discontinued or modified, usually the former urinary status will return.

Bladder neck contracture, which may occur at any age, is thought to be a congenital disorder that is not recognized until enough time has elapsed for the bladder to decompensate. It is characterized by hyperplasia of muscle and fibrous tissue around the bladder neck.

PROSTATIC CANCER

By GENE ROSENBERG, M.D.,
New York, New York

and HARRY GRABSTALD, M.D.
Gainesville, Florida

INTRODUCTION

Prostatic cancer is the most common cancer in men over 50 years of age. It has been estimated that there were more than 36,000 new cases of prostatic cancer in the United States during 1979, with approximately 18,000 deaths from this disease annually. It is the leading cause of cancer deaths in older men.

The autopsy incidence varies with age and with the care and diligence with which prostatic cancer is sought. The incidence of cancer varies in various age groups from 14 to 80 per cent. The high, 80 per cent, is in men in their ninth decade.

The incidence of prostatic cancer found at autopsy is significantly higher than the incidence discovered clinically. A similar discrepancy exists between the incidence of latent prostatic cancer and the mortality rate from cancer of the prostate. This latter discrepancy suggests that the natural history of latent prostatic carcinoma is such that the patient dies with the disease rather than because of it.

Table 1 shows equivalencies of classification in two cancer grading systems, the Jewett classification and the TNM system. Table 2 explains the TNM system. In this system, latent carcinoma is defined as a Stage T0 neoplasm. Occult carcinoma refers to a neoplasm not detectable on rectal examination. Occult prostatic

Table 1. *Conversion Table: Jewett Classification and TNM System*

Jewett Classification (1975)	TNM System (1978)
A₁	T0 N0 M0
A₂	T1 N0 M0
B₁ B₂	T2 N0 M0
C	T3 N0 M0
D₁	T0-4 N1, 2, 3 M0
D₂	T0-4 N0-4 M1 T0-4 N4 M0

Table 2. *Explanation of TNM* System*

Primary Tumor

T0 No tumor palpable; includes incidental findings of cancer in a biopsy or operative specimen.

T1 Tumor intracapsular surrounded by normal gland.

T2 Tumor confined to gland, deforming contour, and invading capsule, but lateral sulci and seminal vesicle are not involved.

T3 Tumor extends beyond capsule with or without involvement of lateral sulci and/or seminal vesicles.

T4 Tumor fixed or involving neighboring structures.

Nodal Involvement

N0 No involvement of regional nodes.

N1 Involvement of a single regional lymph node.

N2 Involvement of multiple regional lymph nodes.

N3 Free space between tumor and fixed pelvic wall mass.

N4 Involvement of juxtaregional nodes.

Distant Metastases

M0 No (known) metastasis

M1 Distant metastasis present. Specify location.

*Tumor, node, metastasis.

cancers are frequently of advanced stage when clinical manifestations occur.

PRESENTING SIGNS AND SYMPTOMS

The prostate is the organ most frequently removed for what is thought to be benign disease and in which the highest incidence of latent cancer is subsequently found. For this reason, its removal affords an unusual opportunity for the accidental diagnosis of incidental cancer. Thus the finding of unsuspected cancer in the "benign prostate," removed because of obstructive uropathy, may be considered a method of early diagnosis. By definition the patient with Stage T0 cancer of the prostate has no symptoms attributable to the cancer itself. If urinary symptoms exist, they result from associated disease. Often there are a few microscopic foci of adenocarcinoma found in the surgical specimen that confirm the diagnosis. The reported incidence of cancer in prostates removed for "benign" disease varies from 5 to 25 per cent, depending on how thoroughly the surgical specimen is examined.

Patients with Stage T1 prostatic cancer are also among those whose condition is diagnosed at the removal of glands thought to be "benign." Usually there are multiple foci (>5) of prostatic adenocarcinoma in the surgical specimen. Not infrequently these patients describe the relatively sudden onset (<6 weeks) of lower tract symptoms. These symptoms are usually those of prostatism.

The patient with Stage T2 prostatic cancer is often asymptomatic. If he has symptoms, they are related to associated disease, as benign prostatic hyperplasia, or other disorders of the kidney, bladder, or urethra. The diagnosis is merely suspected when a hard nodule is palpated on rectal examination. There are no confirmatory blood or x-ray studies that will diagnose a Stage T2 prostatic cancer. The diagnosis depends on biopsy of the prostate gland when a suspicious area of induration is found on rectal examination. Highly experienced surgeons have understaged the T2 cancers. One investigator notes that almost 15 per cent of these tumors thought to be T2 clinically were pathologically T3. Furthermore, 7 to 27 per cent of the patients whose lesions were thought to be N0 were really N1 or N2.

Stage T3 neoplasms of the prostate are more likely to call attention to themselves by causing obstructive uropathy. Approximately 40 per cent of prostatic cancers will be Stage T3 when first diagnosed. Prostatism or hematuria or both may be seen in such patients. As many as 80 per cent of patients in clinical Stage T3N0 will be found in Stage T3N1, 2, or 3.

Patients with Stage T4 adenocarcinoma of the prostate will generally experience the lower urinary symptoms mentioned earlier as a consequence of the primary tumor. Infiltration into the bladder neck may result in urgency and, with further growth, urinary retention. Extension behind the bladder neck may result in unilateral or bilateral hydronephrosis. Patients may describe fever, flank pain, or uremic symptoms as well as rectal symptoms. Pelvic or perineal pains may occur in cases in which the prostatic tumor involves the periosteum of the pelvic bones by direct extension.

The medical history is of no value in indicating early nodal involvement. Patients in nodal stage N1 will generally not have referable symptoms. When multiple regional lymph nodes are involved (Stage N2), patients may be asymptomatic or may experience radicular pain from nerve compression. Most common among these types are lumbar pain, sciatica, obturator neuralgia, and spinal cord compression syndromes. When lymphatic metastases result in hydronephrosis, the spectrum of symptoms ranges from none to flank pain, fever, or uremia.

Patients in nodal Stage N3 have lymphatic metastases forming a fixed pelvic mass. These patients may complain of pelvic pain related to periosteal irritation. There may be increasing abdominal girth or supraclavicular metastases in patients in whom marked lymphatic involvement beyond the pelvis is found (nodal Stage N4).

The medical history may, in certain instances,

point quite accurately to the osseous metastases of prostatic cancer. Osseous metastases are the next most common type after lymphatic metastases. Complaints of bone pain are commonly associated with prostatic cancer metastatic to the lumbar and thoracic vertebrae, pelvis, ribs, skull, and extremities. Pathologic fractures may be presenting complaints. This is especially true when vertebral fractures result in spinal cord compression. Complaints of "arthritis" of recent onset should be considered as metastases until proven otherwise in this population.

Pulmonary metastases are usually of the lymphangitic type. These patients may present with a nonproductive cough or exertional dyspnea. Hepatic metastases are usually a late finding and these patients will usually complain of a right upper quadrant pain or jaundice. Pleuritic chest pain may result from pleural metastases. Intracranial and cutaneous metastases are rarely seen.

PHYSICAL EXAMINATION FINDINGS

A complete general physical examination is mandatory for the proper diagnosis of prostatic cancer. There are specific findings in the urologic examination that further refine the diagnosis. The rectal examination is of central importance in the diagnosis of prostatic malignancy. In one study, careful rectal examination can be credited with suggesting prostatic cancer in the 15 per cent of patients asymptomatic for their disease whose lesion was picked up on screening examination.

There are no palpable rectal findings in patients with stage T0 disease. The prostate gland has a benign consistency. Anatomic staging suggests that the disease in patients with multifocal prostatic carcinomas not evident on rectal examination be labeled T1. The biopsy would then be used to determine that the prostatic capsule remains intact. Stage T1 prostatic tumors show an intracapsular area of carcinoma surrounded by a normal capsule. The overall prostatic contour is unchanged, although the cancer is not necessarily restricted to one lobe.

Stage T2 prostatic carcinomas deform the glandular contour. Although involving the prostatic capsule, they remain confined by it. This stage includes the common prostatic "nodule." Stage T3 prostatic neoplasms extend beyond the capsule, often with involvement of the seminal vesicles, lateral sulci, or bladder neck. Seminal vesicles are not normally palpable. Their identification on rectal examination in this setting suggests malignant extension.

Patients with Stage T4 carcinoma of the prostate may demonstrate fixation to the pelvic wall or rectum. While the anterior rectal wall may be sufficiently deformed to result in straining at stool, it is rarely invaded. Denonvilliers' fascia, formed by two obliterated peritoneal reflections, forms a barrier against neoplastic extension. On occasion, prostatic cancer may involve the membranous urethra or corpora cavernosa. Malignant priapism is seen in cases in which gross invasion of the corpora cavernosa has occurred. Only two other pelvic tumors will invade or metastasize to the penis with any regularity: bladder and rectal cancers.

Involvement of the regional lymph nodes is not usually appreciable on physical examination (Stages N1, 2). When multiple regional nodes are involved (Stage N2) causing upper tract obstruction, a hydronephrotic kidney may be palpable. The regional lymph nodes themselves would not be accessible to palpation ordinarily. Examination under anesthesia may allow discovery of these nodes. If massive metastasis to the pelvic lymphatics has occurred, a lower abdominal mass may be felt (nodal Stage N3).

Nodal Stage N4 may rarely allow palpation of a para-aortic abdominal mass or involved cervical lymph nodes or both. Osseous metastases may be associated with local tenderness, especially when the periosteum is involved or when marrow space is expanded. More frequently, metastases are nontender on palpation.

LABORATORY FINDINGS: PERIPHERAL BLOOD

Localized prostatic carcinoma is rarely associated with anemia. If osseous metastases are extensive, a myelophthisic anemia may result. The peripheral smear from such patients will demonstrate abnormal erythrocytic morphologies, including "teardrop" cells.

Routine blood chemistries will not show alterations until late in the course of disease. Azotemia, resulting from bilateral ureteral obstruction, is found in very advanced disease. A creatinine level greater than 2.0 mg per 100 ml in this setting usually implies severe bilateral hydronephrosis.

The determination of serum acid phosphatase has proved to be a valuable serologic test for the diagnosis and staging of prostatic tumors. The serum acid phosphatase (by enzyme assay) is elevated in 70 to 80 per cent of the patients with metastatic cancer of the prostate. It is also elevated in 10 to 15 per cent of "localized" carcinomas and almost never in benign prostatic diseases. Most studies claiming such eleva-

tions have not had the benefits of surgical staging.

Several methods have been used for the determination of serum acid phosphatase. The enzymatic assays have been the most widely employed. The Gutman method uses disodium monophenyl phosphate as the substrate. Another enzymatic assay uses beta-glycerophosphate as the substrate (Bodanksy). The Bodansky technique has fewer false-positives, making it more specific.

Modification of these enzymatic assays has been attempted. L-Tartrate has been found to inhibit preferentially the prostatic fraction of the total serum acid phosphatase activity. Results have shown that the number of false fractional elevations is reduced; however, L-tartrate also reduces the assay's added sensitivity and raises the number of false-negatives.

Rectal examination very rarely elevates serum acid phosphatase. Accordingly, it has been recommended that this determination be done before rectal examination.

Enzymatic assays have shown 4 per cent of patients with elevated serum acid phosphatase levels in clinical Stages T0, 1, and 2. These same assays have demonstrated 46 per cent with elevations in stages T3 and T4, N0-4 and M0-1. False elevations have been noted in 3.5 per cent of the control group, with other diseases.

The radioimmunoassay (RIA) has shown elevated levels of serum acid phosphatase in 43 per cent of stages T0, T1, and T2, and elevations in 94 per cent of Stages T3 and T4, N0-4 and M0-1.

False elevations were reported in 6 per cent of patients with other diseases.

The far greater sensitivity of the radioimmunoassay has prompted some to consider it as a screening test. This approach has been shown to be untenable. Both high cost and large numbers of false-positive results sharply limit its value as a screening examination.

Recent efforts have led to development of the counterimmunoelectrophoresis technique (CIEP). This technique is as sensitive as RIA, simple to perform, and much less expensive in cost and time.

Both RIA and CIEP may shortly be surpassed as the solid phase immunofluorometric assay (SPIF) is perfected. This technique has about 1000 times greater sensitivity than RIA or CIEP. Values as low as 60 picograms per ml of acid phosphatase in the serum may be easily detected. If the promise of low cost is borne out, then the era of routine screening for prostatic carcinoma may be at hand.

Finding of increased serum acid phosphatase

activity has been noted in several nonprostatic diseases. These include: (1) bone diseases including Paget's disease, multiple myeloma, osteogenic sarcoma, and rheumatoid arthritis with osteoporosis; (2) carcinoma with osseous or hepatic metastases, including breasts, colon, adrenal, lung, and kidney neoplasms; (3) disease affecting the liver, including Gaucher's disease, Niemann-Pick disease, extrahepatic biliary obstruction, cirrhosis, and others. It is hoped that the newer assays (RIA, CIEP, SPIF) will help distinguish many of these diseases from prostatic carcinoma. Elevated serum acid phosphatase generally implies prostatic cancer metastases.

Elevations of serum alkaline phosphatase values may occur in patients with prostatic cancer with osseous metastases and have been reported in approximately 90 per cent of such patients. This test is useful mainly in following the course of patients with osseous metastases from prostatic carcinoma. It is not useful in diagnosis, since elevations are seen in a variety of liver diseases, Paget's disease of bone, skeletal fractures, and hyperparathyroidism.

Other serologic determinations have been found helpful in diagnosing prostatic carcinoma. Isoenzymes of serum lactate dehydrogenase (LDH) have been studied. It has been shown that LDH4 often increases, whereas LDH5 often decreases.

Similarly, serum carcinoembryonic antigen levels (CEA) have been found elevated in almost 35 per cent of all patients with proven prostatic cancer. Serum ribonuclease values have been found increased in a majority of patients with prostatic cancer. These additional serologic tests are all nonspecific and of limited value clinically.

BONE MARROW

Bone marrow acid phosphatase study has limited value. False-positive values are found in up to 60 per cent. Hemolysis has been identified as a significant factor in such spurious elevations.

Bone marrow biopsy and aspiration have been occasionally helpful when they are performed as follow-up to an abnormal bone scan or x-ray study.

OTHER LABORATORY TESTS

Prostatic fluid has been thought to represent a sampling of the gland's epithelial lining. Lactate dehydrogenase isoenzymes have been evaluated for their diagnostic information. Specifically, LDH1 and LDH5 were assayed in prostatic fluid to distinguish prostatic hyperplasia from carcinoma. These isoenzymes were found to be nonspecific, since prostatitis yielded the same pattern. Subsequently, C3 complement and transferrin levels in prostatic fluid were assayed. These tests seem to possess discriminatory abilities in preliminary evaluations. In one study, all the patients with prostatic carcinoma showed elevated activities of C3 and transferrin and none of the other prostatic diseases. Patients with prostatitis did not show any such elevations.

Cytologic smears of expressed prostatic fluid may rarely be of value. Authors of several series report accuracies of 40 to 80 per cent, falsely positive values in 4 to 22 per cent, and falsely negative values in 1 to 30 per cent. When used as an isolated screening technique, cytology has not offered any significant advantage over rectal examination in diagnosing occult or unsuspected prostatic neoplasms, as it has in the lung, bladder, or cervix.

Ultrasonography has been used as a transrectal scan for the evaluation of prostatic cancer. It is most helpful in patients with prostatic nodules and especially in identifying those patients whose conditions warrant repeat studies or open biopsy. Prostatic tumors may be accurately staged by ultrasonic scanning once the initial diagnosis has been established. The role of ultrasound in this disease remains to be defined.

URINARY FINDINGS

The routine urine analysis is not helpful in the diagnosis of prostatic malignancy. Hematuria may be found in patients with numerous diseases besides prostatic cancer. Hematuria occurs especially when the tumor is locally advanced, involving the prostatic mucosal lining. Hematuria may be of significance in following the course of prostatic carcinoma but by itself is not of help in diagnosis.

Urinary cytology is similarly of little value in diagnosis or management of prostatic adenocarcinoma. It may be of considerable value in transitional cell carcinoma of the prostate. This unusual tumor will not be further considered here and is mentioned only for completeness.

RADIOGRAPHY

Skeletal x-rays can identify metastases from prostatic carcinoma with a great reliability. The plain abdominal x-ray (KUB) will demonstrate metastatic carcinoma of the prostate when 30 to 50 per cent of a given area is replaced by tumor cells. The radiographic pattern is usually mixed osteoblastic-osteolytic in the majority, with the remainder osteoblastic. A pure osteolytic pattern is rare. Bone tomography or special views are often informative in demonstrating metastatic disease. Osseous lesions are most commonly seen in the body pelvis, lumbar vertebrae, and proximal femurs, respectively. They may, however, involve any part of the skeletal system. The orderly bony trabeculae are replaced by a snowball type of appearance. The radiographic appearance may at times suggest Paget's disease of bone, chronic fluoride ingestion, or a bone island. Distinguishing features are usually present, although a bone biopsy may be indispensable at times. For completeness, the skeletal survey should include two views of all vertebrae, long bones, and skull.

In addition, the plain film (KUB) may demonstrate soft tissue metastases. Lymph node metastases may result in loss of the psoas shadows, displaced gas pattern, or renal enlargement from hydronephrosis.

The intravenous urogram is quite helpful in patients with prostatic carcinoma. The earliest obstruction with hydronephrosis is well seen on such examination. Lymphatic metastases are strongly suggested when the ureters are deviated from their usual position. The bladder and bladder neck may be pushed superiorly by an enlarged prostatic neoplasm. Increased postvoiding residual urine and even urinary retention may be seen when bladder outlet obstruction exists.

Bipedal lymphangiography has been recommended to detect lymphatic metastases from prostatic carcinoma. As a staging procedure, it is intended to provide information about the pelvic lymph nodes draining the prostate. Generally, lymph nodes involved with metastases will appear enlarged and contain irregular nonopacifying areas. Normal lymph nodes may vary widely in shape and size, although they usually have a regular contour. The diameter of most lymph nodes outside the inguinal region usually does not exceed 1.5 cm. The pattern of opacification is normally homogenous. Irregular patterns of opacification may indicate fibrous or adipose tissue replacement as well as metastatic disease. Practically, a nodal metastasis must be at least 3 mm in size before radiographic detection is possible. Non-neoplastic filling defects are especially common in the inguinal and inferior group of external iliac nodes. As a rule, filling defects 10 mm or more in size can be considered suggestive of tumor. Overall, the bipedal lymphangiogram will diagnose 70 per cent of nodal metastases from prostatic carcinoma.

Prostatic lymphography has recently been suggested. Injection into the prostate has been shown to be a less time-consuming and more direct procedure and may outline the internal iliac and deep pelvic nodes. Prostatic lymphography currently has a role yet to be defined in the diagnosis of prostatic carcinoma.

Directed lymph node aspiration by the "skinny needle" technique has been suggested to increase the reliability of the conclusions based on bipedal lymphangiography. Because of the relative inexperience with this technique, its role is also currently undefined. Many urologists will recommend a staging pelvic lymphadenectomy with or without a lymphangiogram. Only certainty about the nodal status will allow a rational decision for or against a given modality of treatment.

RADIOISOTOPE STUDIES

Developments in nuclear medicine have allowed the detection of osseous metastases at an earlier stage than possible with the skeletal survey. Scintiscans have generally been performed with technetium^{99m} pyrophosphate and have been found to demonstrate metastases weeks or months before x-ray changes are apparent. In many centers, skeletal surveys are no longer done routinely. Rather, a scintiscan is performed in a patient with clinically suspected or proven carcinoma of the prostate. Subsequently, x-rays of the positive areas of isotope uptake are performed, including tomographic views if required. The x-rays will usually confirm the diagnosis of metastatic disease.

The bone scan is unfortunately quite sensitive to any osseous abnormalities. Increased isotopic uptake is mostly related to increased vascularity and may be seen in Paget's disease of bone, healing fractures, osteomyelitis, arthritis, and blunt skeletal trauma. It has been shown that osseous metastases from prostatic carcinoma will generally fall into three isotopic patterns: (1) asymmetric skeletal uptake, normal renal imaging (84 per cent); (2) symmetric uptake, faint renal imaging (8 per cent); and (3) symmetric uptake, normal renal imaging (8 per cent). The first pattern will not cause much difficulty in interpretation. The second and third patterns show a generalized homogeneous eburnation that is quite striking on plain x-ray. The distinction of the second type suggests a rather short prognosis compared with the third type.

PROSTATE BIOPSY

Prostate biopsy is the cornerstone of diagnosis. A tissue diagnosis must be unequivocally obtained before any therapeutic maneuvers are planned. Prostatic biopsy is indicated whenever clinical suspicion is high and subsequent therapy will be planned accordingly. Perineal punch and transrectal biopsy are the two most frequently used approaches. What is generally said about the accuracy of the perineal punch biopsy technique is, in reality, applicable to all needle biopsy techniques, namely, that a positive diagnosis is meaningful, but a negative one does not rule out cancer. In skilled hands, either technique will yield over 90 per cent in accuracy.

The accuracy of the procedure in an individual patient depends upon the experience of the examiner and the stage of the disease. Additional advantages are that tissue can be studied on permanent rather than frozen sections and that repeat biopsy is easily accomplished when necessary. The fact that local anesthesia is generally sufficient is also a great advantage, as is the fact that there is little, if any, risk of impotence, incontinence, rectal injury, or tumor seeding. There has been a 7 to 15 per cent morbidity, with hematuria, hematoma, and infection as the most common.

Transurethral prostatic biopsy has limited use for diagnostic purposes, since most tumors originate in the posterior lobe, away from the periurethral portion. Advanced prostatic cancers (Stages T3 and T4) may be approached easily by this technique, especially with periurethral involvement.

Stage T0 tumors are currently followed by transurethral biopsy at many centers. The greatest tendency in these low-stage tumors is for local recurrence. Transurethral prostatic biopsy is generally of no assistance in the diagnosis of prostatic cancer initially. It may well provide the most accurate follow-up in patients with known Stage T0 cancer.

Cystourethroscopy has an important role in the staging of the primary tumor. It is ideally suited to determine whether there is tumor extension into the urethra, the bladder neck, or the trigone.

TUMOR GRADE

In general, poorly differentiated prostatic adenocarcinoma has a worse prognosis than the more differentiated tumors. Several authors have demonstrated a direct correlation between tumor grade and prognosis. Many pathologists will accordingly grade the tissue submitted to them from I to IV. Grade I tumors are the most differentiated cancers and Grade IV the least differentiated. As expected, the overall prognosis is most closely associated with the least differentiated cancers. The biochemical differentiation follows a similar pattern, with almost all Grade I tumors elaborating acid phosphatase and almost 20 per cent of Grade IV tumors showing an absence of this enzyme.

There are several histologic varieties of prostatic cancer, including adenocarcinoma (96 per cent), squamous cell carcinoma (1 to 2 per cent), transitional cell carcinoma (1 to 2 per cent), carcinoma of the prostatic utricle (endometrioid), and carcinosarcoma. Only adenocarcinomas will elaborate acid phosphatase and only these are hormonally responsive.

PITFALLS IN DIAGNOSIS

It is easy to be misled by induration of the prostate on rectal examination. Biopsy is mandatory. Differential diagnosis includes granulomatous prostatitis, calculi, chronic prostatitis, fibrosis and benign hyperplasia.

INTRASCROTAL MASSES AND TUMORS

By MELVIN C. KADESKY, M.D.
Dallas, Texas

The nature of masses within the scrotum generally can be determined by history, physical examination, and a few simple laboratory tests. A careful history regarding systemic disease and abnormalities relating to the urinary tract is of particular importance. Previous urinary tract infection or instrumentation or both suggest an infectious process rather than tumor. The physical examination brings into play all the classic arts of physical diagnosis — inspection, palpation, and auscultation. A urinalysis, complete blood count, and intravenous pyelograms are about the only laboratory tests required.

The primary concern when dealing with scrotal masses is the advisability of surgical intervention. A value judgment is required as to whether the swelling represents an acute inflammatory process, tumor, or obstruction of the blood supply to the testicle. If the last of these is the case, then immediate exploration is in order.

LESIONS OF THE TESTICLE

Although scrotal swellings are usually referred to as a knot on the testicle, most intrascrotal masses are associated with the appendages. We deal with three conditions causing swelling of the testicle per se: (1) inflammatory (orchitis), (2) mechanical (torsion), and (3) neoplastic.

INFLAMMATORY

ACUTE ORCHITIS

The onset of an acute orchitis is usually sudden and is accompanied by fever and its systemic effects. The testicular pain varies from slight discomfort and sense of weight to excruciating pain radiating to the perineum or inguinal or sacroiliac regions. The testicle swells rapidly, is firm, and is exquisitely tender. The skin of the scrotum is red, edematous, warm, and sensitive to the touch. The epididymis and spermatic cord may be involved in a bacterial infection. However, the most common orchitis, mumps, usually involves only the testicle. An acute swelling of the testicle associated with parotitis or a history of exposure to mumps within 4 to 5 days is probably mumps orchitis. This condition is uncommon before puberty.

CHRONIC ORCHITIS

1. Tuberculous orchitis results from the direct extension of the infection from an involved epididymis. The diagnosis is made by proving genitourinary tract tuberculosis by culturing the urine and microscopic sections of the testicle and epididymis.

2. Luetic orchitis is seldom seen by the present-day physician. It attacks the testicle per se. The pathologic changes are essentially microscopic and belong to the tertiary stage. Luetic orchitis usually manifests itself in middle and later life, and the most frequent complaint is diminution or loss of sexual power. The onset is insidious and painless, with the testicle moderately enlarged, globular, smooth, and indurated. The final test is a positive serology and response to antiluetic therapy.

MECHANICAL

Torsion of the testicle (spermatic cord) is a medical emergency. Proper diagnosis is essential, for only immediate correction, by either external manipulation or surgical intervention, will save the testicle. This condition is actually an axial rotation or twisting of the spermatic cord upon itself, with cutting off of the blood supply to the testicle, epididymis, and other strangulated structures. The onset is sudden with excruciating pain in the testicle, followed by extreme tenderness. This pain may radiate along the inguinal cord but is often localized within the scrotum. A patient with intermittent torsion will give a history of sudden pain with just as sudden relief after self-palpation or manipulation of the testicle. The gonad is tender and the epididymis cannot be palpated in its usual posterior position. Shortly after onset, edema and hyperemia of the overlying skin appear. This edema often has the appearance of an orange peel (peau d'orange) edema. Such appearance should alert one to the possibility of torsion. The testicle is characteristically elevated to the upper part of the scrotum by shortening of the cord and spasm of the cremasteric muscles. If untreated, the scrotal contents gradually swell and fluid forms in the tunica vaginalis, making it impossible to delineate any of the intrascrotal structures.

DIFFERENTIAL DIAGNOSIS

Torsion of the testicle is most frequently confused with acute epididymitis. The latter is more common after puberty and is often accompanied by pyuria. Torsion occurs predominantly in childhood or adolescence, and pyuria is rarely present in the initial stages. The pain associated with torsion is usually more sudden in onset and intially more excruciating than that of epididymitis. Elevation of the testis in patients with torsion fails to relieve the pain (Prehn's sign), which is contrary to the case in epididymitis. This sign is not infallible. Strangulated hernia, trauma, testicular tumor with hemorrhage into the tumor, and insect bites of the scrotum are other conditions that must be considered. Early diagnosis of torsion of the testicle is imperative, for if the condition persists for more than 8 hours, infarction or complete gangrene of the testicle results. If there is any question as to the possibility of torsion of the spermatic cord, immediate exploration is indicated to establish the diagnosis.

NEOPLASIA

Testicular tumor is a disease that usually affects young adults but may be seen at any age. This is the most common neoplasm in males in the third and fourth decades. Early diagnosis and treatment are essential, for chances of a favorable prognosis decrease rapidly once the tumor has spread beyond the confines of the testicle. Benign tumors of the testicle are uncommon and can be differentiated from malignant tumors only by microscopic examination.

In all cases of testicular swelling, the rule "If there is any doubt, explore" holds true.

There are several different types of testicular tumors, and the following classification is presented for completeness. Although the initial therapy is the same, the continuing treatment depends upon microscopic appraisal.

I. Germinal tumors: 97 per cent of all testicular tumors
   A. Seminoma: 40 per cent of germinal tumors
     1. Typical — 90 per cent
     2. Spermatocytic — 10 per cent
   B. Embryonal carcinoma: 15 to 20 per cent of germinal tumors
   C. Teratocarcinoma (teratoma with malignant areas): 20 to 25 per cent of germinal tumors
   D. Teratoma: 1 to 5 per cent of germinal tumors
   E. Choriocarcinoma: 1 per cent
   F. Combined tumors; including seminoma combinations: 15 to 20 per cent
II. Nongerminal tumors: 3 per cent of all testicular tumors
   A. Interstitial tumors
   B. Gonadostromal tumors
   C. Miscellaneous tumors; sarcomas, lymphomas, etc.

Although a specific cause cannot be implicated, certain clinical observations are noteworthy. The relationship of maldescent of the testes and neoplasm is well known, as the cryptorchid testicle is 20 times more prone to become neoplastic than the normal descended testicle. Orchidopexy does not change the propensity to malignant change but at least gets the testicle into a more accessible position for self-examination. It is important to emphasize this self-examination to the patient who has had an orchidopexy.

Trauma is described as a preceding event in about 10 per cent of all testicular tumors. This is more likely a fortuitous discovery than a true causative factor.

Signs and Symptoms

The presenting symptom is generally swelling or heaviness of the testicle, a "knot" on the testicle, or both. On physical examination, there may be a discrete nodule or a diffuse nontender enlargement of the testicle. The remainder of the examination is usually unremarkable. The left supraclavicular nodes should be examined, as they are often the first to show metastatic carcinoma from the testicle.

Laboratory Tests

The complete blood count (CBC) and urinalysis are usually within normal limits. Urinary chorionic gonadotropin values may be increased, particularly with choriocarcinoma. An intravenous pyelogram gives a rough evaluation as to possible retroperitoneal node involvement. Chest x-rays should be taken to look for pulmonary metastases.

Differential Diagnosis

On occasion (10 to 15 per cent), a testicular tumor presents as an acute swelling with sudden onset of pain, and palpation is all but impossible. Epididymitis per se is associated with testicular tumor in about 25 per cent of the patients. Hemorrhage into a neoplasm can mimic epididymitis. In such instances, treatment for epididymitis is instituted. However, if there is no improvement within 3 to 5 days, exploration is then indicated. If any doubt exists as to the certainty of the diagnosis in an instance of intrascrotal mass, exploration is mandated. This exploration should be through an inguinal incision with control of the spermatic vessels before the testicle is delivered into the wound.

LESIONS OF THE EPIDIDYMIS

NEOPLASIA

Malignant neoplasms of the epididymis are quite rare, with carcinoma and sarcoma occurring with about equal frequency. The most common neoplasm is an adenomatoid tumor, which is a benign localized tumor of mesothelial origin occurring more often in the globus minor or tail of the epididymis. The usual complaint is of a hard, nontender mass in the epididymis causing neither particular discomfort nor other symptoms. On physical examination, a firm to hard mass is felt in the epididymis, but the findings do not suggest the presence of an inflammatory lesion. Laboratory studies are not significant. The diagnosis is made by exploration.

INFECTION

The most common intrascrotal mass is the result of infection of the epididymis; it is most often caused by bacterial invasion of the epididymis and occurs much more frequently than orchitis. Before the use of antibiotics, the gonococcus was a very common cause. Now, specific infections are relatively infrequent. The invasion may be ascending by way of the vas deferens from foci of infection in the urethra, prostate, and/or seminal vesicles, or the epididymal involvement may be blood-borne from a focus of infection elsewhere in the body. Involvement of the epididymis in an acute lower urinary tract infection may result from urethral instrumentation, physical exertion, sexual or alcoholic excess, or rectal examination with too vigorous massage of the acutely inflamed prostate.

SIGNS AND SYMPTOMS

The onset of acute epididymitis is usually sudden, with pain, tenderness, and swelling of the epididymis often accompanied by chills, fever, nausea, and prostration. The pain may radiate to the rectum, lower back, or suprapubic region. Frequently there is inguinal discomfort and pain along the spermatic cord. Motion aggravates the discomfort, and the patient will walk into the office with a rather typical gait.

Early in the course of the disease the epididymis may be palpated separately from the testicle. This is of utmost importance, for to be unable to make this distinction dictates exploration. The tenderness often makes examination extremely difficult. Injection of the cord structures with a local anesthetic agent will facilitate this examination and usually reduces the overall morbidity associated with epididymitis, as well as giving the patient temporary pain relief.

An inflammatory hydrocele often appears within 24 to 48 hours of onset. The scrotum becomes tense with a globular, exquisitely tender mass, which may or may not transilluminate. Examination of the testicle and epididymis is impossible, because the hydrocele surrounds the testicle and, in addition, exerts a constant unremitting pressure on the gonad. Occasionally, needling of the hydrocele to remove fluid will allow a more thorough examination, but usually operative intervention is required to establish the exact nature of the problem and to control the pain.

LABORATORY TESTS

Complete Blood Count. The complete blood count (CBC) reveals elevation of the white count, with the appearance of less mature forms of neutrophils indicative of an acute infection.

Urinalysis. Usually there is an associated pyuria. However, epididymitis may result from reflux of sterile urine through the vas deferens or from blood-borne infection; thus a sterile urine does not rule out epididymitis.

Prostatic Secretion. There is usually an increase in the number of white blood cells.

X-Ray. Epididymitis often is associated with a urinary tract infection or bacilluria, which in turn is commonly associated with abnormalities of the urinary tract. Therefore any patient with epididymitis should have an intravenous pyelogram and, after the acute infection has subsided, evaluation of the posterior urethra and bladder neck by urethrogram, calibration or cystoscopy.

DIFFERENTIAL DIAGNOSIS

In establishing the diagnosis of acute epididymitis, it is important to rule out testicular tumor and torsion of the spermatic cord. These have been discussed previously. If the suspected epididymitis is not typical or fails to respond to therapy, or if there is any question as to the exact diagnosis, exploration is indicated.

OTHER LESIONS OF THE EPIDIDYMIS

SPERMATOCELE

This is a rupture of the rete testes with the formation of a nontender mass attached to the head of the epididymis. Usually spermatoceles are asymptomatic but may cause discomfort because of their size. Examination reveals a cystic mass that transilluminates. The diagnosis can be confirmed by needling and obtaining milky fluid which contains sperm. However, this is rarely necessary.

CYST OF THE EPIDIDYMIS

These small, round, firm, and moderately tender masses often follow an episode of acute epididymitis and may be located anywhere in the epididymis. Sometimes they will transilluminate.

SPERM GRANULOMA

These are small, tender, discrete masses within the epididymis that persist over a period of time and usually do not transilluminate. The exact diagnosis is made by exploration and excision.

LESIONS OF THE SPERMATIC CORD

HYDROCELE

There is a potential space between the tunica vaginalis and the testicle which usually contains a few milliliters of serous fluid. When, for some reason, absorption of the fluid by the tunica vaginalis is inadequate, a hydrocele develops. This is an accumulation of a fluid within a serous sac, usually the tunica vaginalis testis or the vaginal process of the spermatic cord. Hydroceles may occur at any age.

TYPES OF HYDROCELE

1. Congenital hydrocele occurs before the closure of the funicular process so that the sac communicates with the peritoneal cavity.

2. Infantile hydrocele occurs when the funicular process is closed at its upper outlet.

3. Hydrocele of the spermatic cord may be a diffuse serous effusion in the loose connective tissues of the cord, or it may be encysted.

4. Simple hydrocele is the collection of fluid within the tunica vaginalis.

SIGNS AND SYMPTOMS

The chief complaint is usually inconvenience caused by the size and weight of the mass. At other times, the finding of a nontender mass with the resulting concern about neoplasm is the presenting complaint. Pain is not a usual part of the symptom complex. The physical examination reveals a scrotal mass, usually of pyriform or globular shape, with the larger end above. Above this smooth, elastic tumor the normal spermatic cord can be palpated and the margin of the external ring defined, thus demonstrating that the swelling is not a hernia. In a true uncomplicated hydrocele, transillumination will cause the whole tumor to glow with a pinkish light. As the testicle, which is usually situated at the posterior inferior aspect of the tumor, casts a shadow, its location is readily ascertained. During transillumination, the hand that is used to render the hydrocele and skin tight should also keep the fluid from collecting at the bottom or back of the scrotum by squeezing it above the testicle where the translucency can be demonstrated.

DIFFERENTIAL DIAGNOSIS

Hernia. Hernia can be excluded as the spermatic cord can be grasped above the swelling and the unobscured margin of the inguinal ring palpated. Furthermore, a hernia is not translucent, gives an impulse on coughing, and usually can be reduced into the inguinal canal.

Hematocele. Usually there is a history of trauma. The mass is less elastic, often tender, painful, and heavy, and does not transilluminate.

Spermatocele. This is a smooth-walled mass attached to the upper pole of the epididymis which does not surround the testicle but transilluminates.

VARICOCELE

Varicocele is an elongation, dilatation, and tortuosity of the veins of the pampiniform plexus. The vessels most commonly affected are the spermatic veins, although not infrequently the deferential or cremasteric veins will be involved. The condition usually occurs on the left (97 per cent), but may be bilateral. The cause of varicocele is probably the incompetence of the valve at the right angle point of entry of the left spermatic vein into the left renal vein. However, chronic passive congestion induced by unrelieved sexual stimulation has been suggested as a cause.

SIGNS AND SYMPTOMS

The complaint may be that of a "dragging" feeling or just a presence of a mass that can cause discomfort because of size. The enlarged tortuous veins characteristically feel like a "bag of worms." The testicle on the affected side hangs lower, and the scrotum itself may be pendulous and irregular. Lifting the scrotum with the patient supine will cause the varicocele to empty, but as soon as he stands erect it will refill.

The acute onset of a varicocele on the left or the presence of a varicocele on the right requires evaluation to be certain that the spermatic vein is not obstructed by a renal or retroperitoneal tumor.

MISCELLANEOUS

Other causes of masses of the spermatic cord are rare. Malignant tumors do occur, the most common being of sarcomatous origin. Fibroadenomas and lipomas are other conditions that may present themselves. These are localized, nontender firm to hard masses which do not transilluminate. The exact diagnosis is made by exploration.

Section 12

ALLERGY

HAY FEVER, ALIAS SEASONAL ALLERGIC RHINITIS, SEASONAL POLLINOSIS

By JOHN A. CARLSTON, M.D.,
and HARVEY D. DAVIS, M.D.

Virginia Beach, Virginia

DEFINITION AND SYMPTOMS

Hay fever has nothing to do with hay or fever but is a misnomer originally describing ragweed allergic rhinitis during the haying season. The term "hay fever" has now come to mean any seasonal allergic rhinitis. It may be defined as a disease of the ears, nose, and throat, characterized by sneezing, rhinorrhea, postnasal drainage, nasal congestion, and itching of the nose, palate, throat, ears, and eyes with lacrimation. Besides upper respiratory symptoms, seasonal asthma may be present and seasonal eczema and urticaria may occur occasionally. Ragweed-sensitive patients are symptomatic from August 15th through September in many areas of the United States. Similarly, rose fever is grass pollen "hay fever" that is most prevalent in late May and June. Lilac fever is tree pollen "hay fever," present when trees are pollinating in March and April. Tree and grass pollen hay fever seasons may vary more than the ragweed hay fever season, depending upon the regional climate. Weed pollen other than ragweed may also cause symptoms. Allergic rhinitis to mold spores also occurs with a peak in the late fall.

Hay fever, or seasonal pollinosis, occurs in the atopic population only after exposure to the pollen to which the patient is specifically sensitive. Seasonal rhinitis may progress to asthma or to perennial allergic rhinitis with seasonal exacerbations. Symptoms usually increase in severity as the season progresses. The course of hay fever with treatment is usually improved after three years of hyposensitization. Nonimmunized patients do not "outgrow their allergies." However, they may improve when they move to an area that has less of the specific pollen to which they are sensitive. They may also improve if they decrease their exposure with environmental controls such as air conditioning or removal of such other antigens from their environment, as pets, feather pillows, or mattress dust.

PHYSICAL EXAMINATION

Physical examination reveals pale, boggy nasal membranes and a profuse thin, watery nasal secretion. Lymphoid hypertrophy on the posterior oropharynx is often present from prolonged postnasal drainage. The conjunctivae are frequently injected and occasionally swollen. Infraorbital edema and discoloration may give the appearance of "allergic shiners." A transverse nasal crease may be present from prolonged rubbing of the nose. Serous otitis media may be evident and if unilateral, a positive Weber test is elicited. The anterior nasal membranes may be red from the use of decongestant nasal sprays or drops. They may also be red from infectious rhinitis or from rubbing of the nose. Another distinguishing sign of allergy versus coryza is chapping of the upper lip. This is frequently found in infectious rhinitis and rarely found in allergic rhinitis.

LABORATORY STUDIES

Laboratory findings include eosinophilia over 5 per cent with elevated total eosinophil counts over 300 cells per cu mm. A nasal smear will demonstrate chiefly eosinophils as opposed to the predominant neutrophils in infectious rhinitis. IgE levels are usually elevated. Confirmation of the diagnosis is made by skin testing. In most patients, scratch tests or prick tests give an impressive wheal and flare in 15 to 20 minutes. Some less sensitive patients react only to the intradermal tests. Testing strengths, and interpretations of these tests, is best left to one who is experienced and does this frequently. Fresh dilutions of the proper testing strengths are required as these solutions may deteriorate rapidly. Other tests that may be done are conjunctival and nasal provocative tests. These are not done routinely because they may be dangerous and are expensive because of the time involved. Confirmation of the diagnosis by the radioallergosorbent test (RAST) is accurate but is less sensitive and much more expensive. Consequently, this particular test is inappropriate outside of the research setting, even though it is now being offered by some commercial laboratories.

The culprit in hay fever is IgE-specific antibodies to pollen. These antibodies may decrease in hyposensitization, which is the gradual injection of increasing amounts of specific antigens over a specified time sequence. Some patients actually have elevated IgE levels after hyposensitization. Their clinical improvement may be attributed to a significant increase in IgG, blocking antibody. Another explanation for improvement is decreased leukocyte histamine release to challenge with antigens.

DIFFERENTIAL DIAGNOSIS

A history plus corroborative skin tests are usually sufficient for diagnosis. However, if vasomotor rhinitis is suspected, a therapeutic trial on an antihistamine without decongestant will often distinguish allergy from the over-reactive nasal mucosa of vasomotor rhinitis. Pitfalls in this diagnosis may be: (1) eosinophilia and eosinophils in nasal secretions are not always present, (2) skin tests that are impressive in size do not appear in some patients, and (3) some patients may have lower respiratory involvement during the pollen season. Rhinitis medicamentosa is rarely a diagnostic problem. This type of rebound allergic membrane occurs from the overuse of local decongestant sprays and drops. Sometimes rhinitis medicamentosa may be due to rauwolfia serpentina or reserpine. Nasal congestion may be aggravated by a beta-blocking drug such as propranolol.

THE ASTHMAS IN ADULTS

By ARTHUR BERGNER, M.D., *and* RENEE K. BERGNER, M.D.

Burlington, Vermont

SYNONYMS

Asthma, reactive airways disease, increased bronchial reactivity, reversible obstructive airways disease, twitchy lung syndrome.

DEFINITION

The asthmas (the plural is being used to emphasize that multiple entities are included under this title) are characterized by: (1) increased bronchial reactivity, that is, bronchi and bronchial mucosa that overreact to stimulation resulting in airways obstruction; and (2) heterogeneity (variability) of almost all aspects of the condition.

Increased bronchial reactivity implies that reversibility is also a characteristic, but wheezing is not. "All that wheezes is not asthma." Conversely, all asthma does not wheeze. The bronchi react by constriction of the peribronchial musculature that narrows the lumen, by edema and swelling of the mucous membranes that also narrow the lumen, and by hypersecretion of mucus into the lumen. All three elements cause obstruction of the airways. Excessive emphasis on bronchoconstriction (admittedly important because of our ability to therapeutically bronchodilate) may result in relative neglect of edema and secretions. Appreciation of the important roles of edema and hypersecretion is critical to diagnosis and therapy, since these factors contribute substantially to the nature, severity, and persistence of the presenting signs and symptoms, pulmonary function test results, complications, course, and prognosis. The increased bronchial reactivity that characterizes the asthmas is also commonly found in patients who have been defined as having bronchitis. Clinically, the fuzzy lines of demarcation between asthma, bronchitis, and "asthmatic bronchitis" may well depend on what proportional contributions are being made by edema and secretions as compared with bronchoconstriction. The lines of definition are likely to remain indistinct until we improve our diagnostic techniques for identifying mechanisms that cause pulmonary pathology. According to current thinking, bronchitis is characterized by inflammation of the bronchi, a characteristic almost invariably found in the asthmas as well.

In a patient with increased bronchial reactivity, the bronchi may respond to: mechanical stimuli, chemical stimuli, infectious (usually viral) stimuli, specific allergenic stimuli, unknown or unidentified stimuli, and combinations of these. Although in years past it had been frequently but erroneously said that "if you have asthma, you must be allergic to *something,*" some recent studies suggest that (antigen-IgE antibody) allergy may not account for even 50 per cent of the asthmas. Moreover, anxiety and emotional factors have not been documented as the cause of a bronchial reactivity syndrome nor have there been compelling data to demonstrate these factors as clinically significant stimuli of reactive airways. Consequently, focus on allergy alone or consideration of emotions as a major factor in asthma may deter the clinician from appropriate investigation and detract from his accuracy in defining the causes and nature of his patient's airways obstruction.

Heterogeneity is a hallmark of the asthmas and should serve as a constant reminder that it is not a single disease. Heterogeneity is manifested with respect to etiology, severity, frequency and duration of exacerbations, predominant mechanism, variability of inciting agents, and response to therapy. Increased bronchial reactivity may be primary; that is, it may exist alone as an independent entity, or it may be secondary to, or associated with, another disease or condition, for example, as a concomitant of chronic (irreversible) obstructive pulmonary disease. Recognizing hyperresponsive airways does not provide a final diagnosis. Causes and mechanisms should be identified, if possible, and other pulmonary or systemic processes should be identified or ruled out.

Allergic Asthma. The old classification of extrinsic and intrinsic asthma is gradually falling into disfavor as immunologic and pathophysiologic sophistication increases. Extrinsic asthma — which we now know as "IgE-mediated asthma" resulting from exogenous antigen, usually inhaled, reacting with IgE antibody (reagin or homocytotropic antibody) — may well be identified as "allergic asthma." For clarity of diagnosis and because of therapeutic implications, the "allergic asthma" label should be reserved for the IgE mechanism.

Immunologic Asthma. There is evidence that exogenous antigens may also react with classes of antibody other than IgE and at times with lymphocytes to cause reversible airways obstruction. Asthma mediated by immunologic mechanisms other than IgE would appropriately be classified as "immunologic asthma," with refinement of definition into further subsets depending upon development and use of newer diagnostic techniques.

Non-immunologic Asthma. The third major category is the largest category. It includes asthmas caused by all mechanisms other than antigen-antibody or antigen-lymphocyte. The number of subsets of asthma within this category seems to be so great that we may expect this category to be divided and redivided as research progresses. Currently, it would include, for example, such entities as exercise-induced asthma, aspirin-induced asthma (not antigen-antibody, therefore not "allergic"), late onset asthma, "cardiac asthma," and idiopathic asthma, the latter probably being the largest subcategory.

Recent improved care and evolving definitions and diagnostic techniques make it difficult to place any credence on prevalence, morbidity, or mortality statistics available at this time.

PRESENTING SIGNS AND SYMPTOMS

The physician may see the patient initially at a time when no signs or symptoms are present.

This should not be surprising since asthma may be episodic with symptom-free periods. On the other hand, some patients present stating that they have "asthma" while lacking understanding of the term, sometimes even confusing the symptoms of wheezing and shortness of breath with sneezing and nasal congestion.

The initial presentation of asthma is highly variable. Symptoms are chiefly direct manifestations of airway obstruction or inflammation such as dyspnea, wheezing, cough, and tightness. Considerable anxiety is often present, but this should be considered to be a consequence of the airway obstruction rather than a cause of it. More subtle symptoms include those of fatigue, irritability, or manifestations of hyperventilation, representing results of airway obstruction. The history is critical to making a diagnosis as to the cause and precipitating factors. It is helpful to recognize patterns of asthma that suggest airborne allergens or other nonallergic precipitants, for it may be possible by appropriate environmental control to minimize the patient's exposure to these precipitants. In addition to a general medical history that may reveal cardiac, systemic, or other primary pulmonary diseases, the following major areas should be pursued:

1. *Earliest age of onset.* Patients often initially report the onset as the beginning of the most recent series of exacerbations, for example the past year, while neglecting to mention that they had asthma in childhood. A history of asthma "since birth" should be pursued, because if the onset of asthma was in the first several weeks one must consider hereditary or congenital conditions. If by onset "since birth" the patient means later infancy or childhood, then cause, course, and prognosis may be quite different. Onset after the age of 35 is not commonly due to IgE-mediated allergy, if the patient had never truly experienced asthma prior to that.

2. *Pattern of seasonality.* If a pattern of seasonality is identified over several years, diagnosis is facilitated. However, familiarity with allergens and exacerbating factors that vary with seasons is necessary to make even a presumptive diagnosis. Patients who are sensitive to domestic animal danders seem to have greater difficulty in the winter than the summer, presumably owing to the increased concentration of antigen in the confined indoor home environment. Some of these patients become completely asymptomatic during the summer months and believe falsely that they have "outgrown their asthma." Patients with IgE-mediated responses to alternaria or other mold spores prevalent outdoors during the warm weather months should give a history of exacerbation during the

appropriate season. Heavy outdoor concentrations of certain mold spores are a more likely cause of seasonal asthma than are pollens. New evidence suggests that the role of pollens as a cause of asthma has been overemphasized in the past. Making use of the seasonal history requires knowledge of seasonal patterns within the geographic area of the patient's residence.

3. *Precipitating factors.* A great deal of skepticism must be exercised when the patient offers a history of "allergy" to one or more items. It requires experience and sophistication to distinguish between those items that are capable of reacting with IgE antibody from those conditions that are irritating to a hyperreactive tracheobronchial tree. Some agents are capable of being both allergen and irritant in the same patient or allergen in one patient while an irritant in another.

Whether or not an allergic or immunologic mechanism is operative, such nonspecific stimuli as odors, dusts, smoke, and aerosols, as well as a great variety of other mechanical and chemical irritants, can play an important role in precipitating airway obstruction. Temperature, temperature changes, humidity or lack of it, wind, weather changes, and barometric pressure are frequently implicated clinically as precipitating causes. However, hard data to confirm this are lacking, except that cold, dry air has been demonstrated to cause airway obstruction and to augment exercise-induced asthma.

Rhinitis, sneezing, and nasal itching may precede allergic asthma, but these symptoms are end-organ effects that may also precede asthma induced by irritants or infection. Recent evidence indicates that certain strains of viruses are capable of precipitating asthma, whereas most bacterial respiratory infections will not. Thus if asthma is accompanied by an apparent respiratory tract infection, it is almost always a viral infection (with exceptions). It has been conjectured that many cases of nonallergic asthma may be the result of permanent damage to the tracheobronchial tree inflicted by certain viruses.

In any patient who has active asthma or who has had recent asthma, the capacity for exertion will be limited, and exercise will generally aggravate asthma that is poorly controlled. Pure exercise-induced asthma seems rare, and nearly always suggests the existence of an underlying inflammatory process as the cause of hyperresponsiveness to exertion.

4. *Environment.* The details of an environmental history are essential to interpret allergy skin tests and may give strong indications for the primary cause or main precipitating factors. Exacerbations during the week with remissions on weekends or vice versa may suggest that a major precipitating factor may be at work or at home. Animal dander (skin flakes) seems to be a strong and common cause of allergic asthma. Therefore exposure to animals or to animal epidermal products such as feathers or horsehair should raise a suspicion of an allergic response to them. Some heating systems favor particularly heavy exposures to dust and mold. Humidifiers, air conditioning, and indoor plant soil may also serve as heavy mold spore sources.

The causative antigens in dust, if any, have not yet been definitively identified, although mites (microscopic insects) are believed to be responsible for an antigen-antibody reaction at least in some patients. However, because dust is also an irritant, it is difficult to conclude whether symptoms arising from dust in any given patient are due to an allergenic component within it, or due to its irritant ability to stimulate the vagal reflex pathway.

5. *Timing.* Recurrent asthma is frequently nocturnal. In contrast with paroxysmal nocturnal dyspnea of congestive heart failure, relief does not immediately follow rising, but comes only with the passage of time or the mobilization of obstructing pulmonary secretions. Even when there is no evidence to suggest congestive heart failure, asthma frequently tends to be worse with recumbency. Exposure to airborne allergens frequently may cause symptoms within minutes, but the development of symptoms may also be delayed by several hours. In particular, asthma precipitated by IgG mechanisms, often a result of occupational exposures to an antigen, may result in symptoms consistently appearing many hours later, while away from the work exposure.

6. *Family history.* The word atopy is not well defined in the medical literature and its use is gradually being abandoned. In the past, it had been used to indicate a family history of "allergy" or a medical condition characterized by features believed to be "allergic." However, although allergic asthma tends to run in families and be associated with allergic rhinitis, so does nonallergic asthma tend to run in families and be associated with nonallergic rhinitis. Consequently, the finding of a family history of asthma or rhinitis does not confirm the presence of an IgE-mediated mechanism in the patient under investigation. Patients often report that a relative has "allergies," without sufficient information to distinguish between an IgE-mediated mechanism and an adverse or irritant mechanism causing respiratory symptoms. History of positive skin tests must also be viewed with some skepticism (see Laboratory Examination)

because of the limitations of allergy skin testing. On the other hand, a family history may be helpful if it reveals cystic fibrosis or suggests familial bronchiectasis or emphysema (alpha-1-antitrypsin deficiency).

7. *Food and medication reactions.* Although current information seems to indicate that, at least in adults, food is a rare cause of reactive airways disease, acute precipitous airway obstruction undoubtedly can follow ingestion of peanuts, nuts, fish, and shellfish in some patients. These patients usually do not require medical expertise to diagnose their condition or pinpoint the cause. Considerable doubt exists as to whether foods can cause chronic or persistent reversible obstructive airways disease. Acute wheezing may occur as an allergic response to the administration of some medications. Immediate acute, delayed acute, or chronic symptoms of nonallergic airways obstruction may follow the ingestion of aspirin, other antiarthritic medication, or tartrazine in some food and drugs (FD&C Yellow Dye no. 5). Airways obstruction following ingestion of these substances is more prevalent than was previously thought, but the cause may not be recognized by the patient. Laboratory challenge may be necessary to define this idiosyncrasy.

Course

Recent accumulation of information from a variety of sources provides us with new insights into the course of asthma. The insights revolve around the findings that many patients do not perceive that they have airways obstruction until several of their pulmonary function tests indicate that they are 30 to 50 per cent compromised. The implication is that one cannot rely on the patient's history to determine accurately the time of onset or the time of resolution of an asthmatic episode. The onset, severity, recovery from or persistence of obstructed airways cannot be determined by a patient's perception or even a physician's physical examination. The majority of severe asthmatic episodes, with few exceptions, develop gradually and resolve gradually, whether therapy was required or not.

Incomplete resolution or chronic stimuli result in a chronic inflammatory state, often *asymptomatic*, that is manifested by abnormal pulmonary function tests, abnormal arterial blood gases, and, perhaps most importantly, by continued hyperresponsiveness to further asthmagenic insults. As long as airways obstruction and inflammation remain, the airways of an asthmatic patient exist in a compromised, "pushover" state, making those airways more hyperreactive and more susceptible to further exacerbation on exposure to offending stimuli.

Evidence now indicates that "attacks" do not usually come on suddenly and that episodes are not usually resolved and reversed completely when they *appear* to be "broken" by therapeutic intervention. Appreciating the limitations of signs and symptoms and understanding that asthma episodes do not attack sharply and do not get broken sharply leads to the conclusion that asthma does not "attack." Continued use of the phrase "asthma attack" and "break the attack" will not only perpetuate misunderstanding of the course of most asthma episodes but will also interfere with both accurate diagnosis and appropriate, timely therapy.

In many asthmatics, pulmonary functions do not return to normal even when the patient has been asymptomatic for months. The course of a given patient may appear quite different, depending upon whether symptoms or pulmonary function studies are followed. Regardless of the parameters followed, the course of asthma is highly variable, in a given patient and from patient to patient. The frequency, duration, and severity of episodes, the length of symptom-free periods, and the long-term course of the condition cannot be described or predicted with generalizations because of the heterogeneity of the asthmas. However, a patient who experiences exacerbations primarily or exclusively owing to an occupational precipitating factor or animal in the home may gradually achieve a dramatic and persisting remission after the precipitant and patient are separated and so long as avoidance is continued. After an animal is removed, it appears that particles with animal antigen may linger in some homes for months, in spite of vigorous cleaning efforts. A single short exposure to an antigenic stimulus may cause waxing and waning symptomatic airways obstruction for several days after that exposure.

Persistent or high-dose antigen exposure, some aspirin-induced and viral-induced exacerbations, and chronic or excessive use of sympathomimetic aerosols have been associated with some severe, persistent, and progressive episodes of asthma. Whatever the cause, when asthma does progress and continue for an extended period of time, it may become refractory to the usual therapeutic measures ("status asthmaticus") and can result in respiratory failure. With new modalities of therapy and monitoring, asthma fatalities are expected to decrease significantly.

PHYSICAL EXAMINATION

Many asthmatic patients when asymptomatic may show no abnormalities on physical examination. Some of these patients without signs or symptoms will have impairment of their pulmonary function. Other patients who deny symptoms will have audible wheezes or prolonged expiration or both. On the other hand, a patient may be in severe distress owing to airway obstruction and manifest no audible wheezing.

The differences between wheezes and rhonchi are subjective. Nevertheless, auscultation with the goal of detecting sound produced by mucus rattling as compared with air passing through narrowed airways may enable a rough clinical judgment of the relative role of secretions in the patient being examined. Many patients with active asthma "learn" to breathe in the sometimes wheeze-free or less wheezy midtidal volume, presumably because they are, at least subconsciously, aware that full inspiration and expiration may precipitate end-inspiratory or end-expiratory discomfort, cough, or increased wheeze. Consequently, failure of the physician to elicit the patient's *full* vital capacity during auscultation may result in a flagrantly inaccurate assessment of physical findings. Cough, without wheeze, may be the only physical sign of airway obstruction and may be apparent only with full inspirations. Laughter, cough, forced breathing, hyperventilation, or exertion may demonstrate the irritable state of the airways by inducing further reflex bronchospasm. Cough, wheeze, and tachypnea are certainly to be noted, but their presence, absence, or appearance is not a reliable indicator of the presence, absence, or severity of reversible obstructive airways disease.

As respiratory difficulties increase, blood pressure and heart rate are frequently increased, but a history of medications in the past 8 hours is crucial since these findings may represent excessive use of inhaled or other sympathomimetics. If sympathomimetics are not the cause of the tachycardia and hypertension, then judicious use of sympathomimetics or other therapy that relieves obstruction may result in reduction of pulse rate and blood pressure.

With increasing severity, the accessory muscles of respiration are used, the shoulders are held in an elevated position, the chest appears hyperinflated and wheezing may be heard throughout both inspiration and expiration. Severity cannot be judged by wheezing, rhonchi, or the inspiration-expiration ratio. Good clinical correlation with severity is seen with pulsus paradoxus, sternocleidomastoid contraction, and to a lesser degree with supraclavicular indrawing, but absence of these signs does not assure absence of severity. Other danger signals on examination include silent chest, cyanosis, disturbance of consciousness, supraclavicular subcutaneous crepitations, cervical crepitations, or other signs suggesting pneumomediastinum or pneumothorax.

COMMON COMPLICATIONS

Asthma does not itself cause fever. If fever is present, a complicating infection or a complicated hypersensitivity disease must be considered. If the asthma had exacerbated during the course of an infection, it is far more likely to be viral rather than bacterial and antibiotics are not usually required. Whether or not asthmatics get more respiratory infections than non-asthmatics is not yet a settled question. Patchy atelectasis is not uncommon in severe asthma; however, any indication of consolidation, infiltrate, density, or parenchymal process suggests consideration of a complication or secondary unrelated pathologic process.

Two specific sequelae of severe asthma, often seen in adolescents, are pneumothorax and pneumomediastinum. Although intermittent positive-pressure breathing machines have been implicated in some cases, these complications may occur without the use of such apparatus.

Hypoxemia predisposes the asthmatic patient to dysrhythmias, especially, but not exclusively, in the elderly. Medications with arrhythmogenic potential, particularly the Freon-propelled sympathomimetics, are a special threat to the irritable myocardium. Patients frequently do not consider aerosols as medications. They therefore use them to excess without fear of overdose and do not report their use when a history of medications is taken. Consequently, if an asthmatic is seen acutely and is not *specifically* asked about aerosol use in the previous 24 hours, the physician may unwittingly precipitate a serious, if not fatal, arrhythmia by administering additional excessive sympathomimetics by injection, inhalation, or ingestion. With the recent increase in the pharmacologic armamentarium of asthma medications, the physician treating asthma must be constantly vigilant for the complications that may be caused by therapy. A complication of any chronic disease is anxiety. A victim of chronic asthma is likely to suffer the same consequence unless (1) misconceptions are removed by patient education, (2) cause of the asthma is identified and eliminated, when possible, and (3) when not possible, chronic therapy promotes functional normality.

As for long-term complications associated with chronic asthma, there is little evidence that uncomplicated allergic asthma, even of very long standing, is associated with any irreversible deterioration of lung function. It has not been demonstrated whether other subsets of asthmatics develop permanent pulmonary damage, but this may well depend on the causative or associated mechanisms yet to be identified.

LABORATORY EXAMINATION

The laboratory examinations useful in the assessment of acute asthma will be considered first. The white blood cell count is normal or slightly elevated. Marked leukocytosis or left shift should raise suspicion of infection provided the patient did not receive recent treatment with a sympathomimetic. The eosinophil count may or may not be elevated, but eosinophilia or its absence does not prove or rule out an allergic mechanism. A very high elevation, more than 1000 per cu mm, should raise suspicion of neoplasia, allergic bronchopulmonary aspergillosis, vasculitis, parasitism or some other hypereosinophilic process. The old adage that "eosinophilia means either allergy or parasites" is inaccurate and may be misleading.

The chest x-ray is important to exclude complicating disorders of the heart and lungs, especially pneumonia, congestive heart failure, pneumothorax, and pneumomediastinum. As the patient with acute asthma is commonly dehydrated, a second chest x-ray taken after rehydration may occasionally reveal an infiltrate not seen on the first one.

The electrocardiogram will regularly reveal sinus tachycardia and will often show right axis deviation and sometimes right ventricular or right atrial enlargement, abnormalities that frequently revert to normal as the acute illness is controlled.

The most important laboratory examination in the acutely ill asthmatic patient is arterial blood gas analysis. The earliest abnormalities seen in asthma are diminution in the partial pressures of oxygen (PO_2) and carbon dioxide (PCO_2) with a respiratory alkalosis. With increasing severity of asthma, the PO_2 may fall to levels associated with considerable desaturation of hemoglobin while the PCO_2 remains low and the respiratory alkalosis persists. Occasionally, a mixed respiratory alkalosis and metabolic acidosis is seen; unless there is sufficient arterial deoxygenation to explain the metabolic acidosis on the basis of inadequate oxygen delivery for metabolic needs, an intercurrent basis for the metabolic acidosis must be sought. Retention of carbon dioxide with respiratory acidosis is seen only in the severest uncomplicated asthma. Since the PCO_2 is usually depressed in acute asthma, a normal or elevated PCO_2 in such a patient must be considered as an indication of severe asthma. In patients whose asthma is complicated by chronic bronchitis, however, marked reduction in PCO_2 is less likely to be seen, and a normal or slightly elevated PCO_2 does not necessarily indicate as grave a state of affairs as it does in a patient with uncomplicated asthma. The diminution in PO_2 is due to regional mismatch of ventilation with perfusion, and is the most important index to the patient's clinical state. As PO_2 drops to 50 torr, intubation must be considered. So far as possible, patients should be maintained on a known inspired oxygen concentration so that serial determinations of the alveolar-arterial oxygen gradient can be made.

Measurements of forced vital capacity, 1-second forced expiratory volume, and peak expiratory flow rate can be made at the bedside with simple equipment and are useful in the assessment of acute asthma and in following its course. A fall in the vital capacity below 1 liter or in the 1-second forced expiratory volume below 0.5 liter without improvement on administration of a bronchodilator is a grave sign. More extensive pulmonary function testing is better postponed and used to assess residual abnormalities remaining after maximal response to treatment. Simple office spirometry as an objective method of assessing the status of asthmatics during follow-up is gradually becoming the standard practice in many communities since clinical evaluations of severity have demonstrated poor reliability.

The sputum of patients with acute asthma will vary in quantity, consistency, and color with the mechanism inducing the asthma, the degree of inflammation as compared with bronchospasm, the duration of this episode, the presence of complicating infection, and the state of hydration. Examination of the sputum for mucus plugs may suggest such diagnoses as bronchiectasis, broncholithiasis, and if the plugs are brown, allergic bronchopulmonary aspergillosis (ABPA). This latter diagnosis may have further support if fungal hyphae are seen on fungal smear or if aspergillus grows in fungal culture. Sputum and peripheral eosinophilia in ABPA tends to be higher than in simple allergic asthma, but sputum eosinophilia may be seen in pulmonary diseases other than ABPA and allergic asthma. Other fungi and organic dusts may also cause obstructive airways disease and eosinophilia.

The elective diagnostic evaluation of an asthmatic patient should include a detailed history regarding allergic background and specific precipitating factors, a complete evaluation of pulmonary function, and specific testing to elucidate the role of suspected precipitants.

Complete evaluation of pulmonary function should include spirometry and determination of lung volumes before and after the administration of an inhaled bronchodilator. Spirometry should include measurement of late-expiratory flow rates — for example, the maximum mid-expiration flow rate — which are more sensitive to small airway obstruction than are peak expiratory flow or 1-second forced expiration volume, and which are less dependent on the patient's effort. In contrast to other diseases causing dyspnea, the asthmatic patient's pulmonary function will typically improve after the administration of a bronchodilator; however, failure to observe such improvement must not be taken as unequivocal evidence of irreversible disease. The patient may already be saturated with bronchodilators or, if inflammatory edema and secretions are the predominant cause of obstruction, he may not respond to bronchodilators but may still show improvement after the administration of corticosteroids or after the mobilization of secretions.

Routine testing for suspected environmental precipitants will consist chiefly of skin testing with extracts of suspected inhalant allergens. Meticulous allergy skin testing may be extremely valuable in that it may provide the identification of allergenic precipitants in allergic asthma and may help to establish whether the cause of the asthma is allergy or not. On the other hand, if the testing is not done well or if the limitations of testing are not recognized, the patient and the involved physician may be hopelessly diverted from actual predominant causes and instead may immerse themselves with concerns and therapy that will yield no beneficial result. A positive skin test to a particular allergen, to be clinically significant, must have its validity confirmed. It is confirmed by a correlating history that exposure to that allergen regularly results in the development or exacerbation of asthma symptoms. Additional limitations of skin tests are that results will vary depending on the concentration of the extract used, the dose administered, the method of administration (scratch, intracutaneous, puncture, prick, etc.), the subjective interpretation and grading of the reaction, the antigenicity of a given lot of an extract (because extracts are neither antigenically pure nor standardized by antigenicity), the technique of administration (e.g., needle depth), local blood flow, and integrity of autonomic innervation of cutaneous vessels. Positive allergy skin tests are found in people without allergic disease. Some extracts in some concentrations may give nonspecific irritative reactions indistinguishable from positive skin tests. IgE skin reactivity does not prove IgE bronchial reactivity; therefore, a positive allergy skin test in an asthmatic patient does not establish that the antigen tested is the cause of the asthma.

The radioallergosorbent test (RAST), a test for *specific* IgE antibodies, may be a useful alternative to skin testing under special circumstances, but this in vitro test has been demonstrated to be no more accurate than skin testing. RAST is subject to many of the same limitations as skin testing — for example, purity and standardization of the extract used. The most notable limitation is that a positive RAST result must also have its clinical validity confirmed by a correlating history that exposure to that allergen regularly results in the development or exacerbation of asthma symptoms.

Total serum IgE shows some correlation with IgE-mediated disease; but this is merely a statistical statement. Since total IgE may be elevated in normals and in association with other conditions, and since it may be within normal limits in patients with allergic disease, it cannot be relied upon to definitely separate allergic from nonallergic asthma.

Bronchoprovocation (inhalation challenge) with aerosols of antigens, pharmacologic mediators, or other suspected precipitants, and direct provocational testing with treadmill exercise or substances such as aspirin or tartrazine may be of value in individual patients, but are best done in a laboratory whose personnel are experienced in such procedures.

PITFALLS IN DIAGNOSIS

The differential diagnosis of asthma includes nearly every disease affecting the lungs and tracheobronchial tree. Even diseases that do not ordinarily cause manifestations of asthma may do so in asthmatics. It is not unusual to find asthma secondary to, or concomitant with, another pulmonary or systemic condition. Perhaps the two most common pitfalls are: (1) assuming "asthma" is a diagnosis, when actually it may be a symptom or syndrome of one or many possible causes and (2) assuming an allergic cause with insufficient evidence. Asthma may be *nonallergic* and may nevertheless be associated with peripheral, sputum or nasal eosinophilia, chronic nasal symptoms, sinusitis, nasal polyposis, elevated total serum IgE levels, positive allergy skin tests, or favorable response to steroids.

Unilateral pathology or obstruction may result in bilateral findings on examination. Extrathoracic (e.g., laryngotracheal) airway obstruction can also result in obstructive sounds transmitted throughout the chest. In considering the differential diagnosis, it is particularly important to exclude congestive heart failure ("cardiac asthma") and enlarged thyroid or foreign body. Other disorders that can mimic asthma include emphysema, chronic bronchitis, bronchiectasis, cystic fibrosis, tuberculosis, vasculitis, pulmonary embolism, lymphatic carcinomatosis, pulmonary fibrosis, and the carcinoid syndrome; but no such list can pretend to be exhaustive. Many pitfalls in diagnosis may be avoided by adopting the recommendation of Dr. Richard S. Farr that asthma should be considered "reversible obstructive airways disease of unknown etiology until proven otherwise."

ASTHMA IN CHILDHOOD

By E. M. HEIMLICH, M.D.
Skokie, Illinois

DEFINITION

Despite great progress in the understanding of the immunologic and pathophysiologic mechanisms associated with this disorder, there is still no generally accepted definition of asthma. To many it appears reasonable to consider it as a hereditarily conditioned constitutional predisposition to the acquisition of a state of hyper-reactivity of airways, particularly the bronchi. A wide variety of stimuli (allergic, infectious, immunologic, physical, chemical, psychological, climatic) impinge on this reactive state to provoke variable, episodic, and frequently paroxysmal airways obstruction that is expressed symptomatically as wheezing or respiratory distress or both.

The basic constitutional disorder is probably biochemical. It is manifest immunologically as exaggerated antibody response (particularly IgE) and lymphocyte dysfunction, and physiologically as a relative degree of beta-adrenergic blockade. This blockade renders the airways susceptible to bronchial smooth muscle contraction associated with varying degrees of increased and thickened mucous secretion, edema of the bronchial mucosa, and vascular engorgement — all frequently with concomitant eosinophilia. The exact mechanism of in-

heritance is unknown, but the familial tendency to this and other associated "atopic" disorders such as allergic rhinitis, hay fever, eczema, and urticaria is a useful indicator to this diagnosis.

SYNONYMS

Asthmatic bronchitis, allergic bronchiolitis, and pseudoasthma are terms that have been applied when symptoms suggesting upper or lower respiratory infection precede or are associated with attacks.

COURSE

The course of the disease is characterized by a high degree of variability and a very broad clinical spectrum. Onset may occur in early infancy, first episodes often being diagnosed as infectious (probably viral) bronchiolitis. These may recur one or more times to age 2 or 3, to then abate without further repetition. Wheezing episodes, with or without premonitory or accompanying indications of respiratory infection, may, however, persist into later childhood, frequently after allergen exposure, physical or psychological stress, or exercise.

First attacks usually occur before age 8, and diagnosed asthma usually subsides at or during puberty. In many instances of early childhood onset, regression is either spontaneously or therapeutically achieved. In a minority of about 10 per cent of children attacks are progressively more frequent and severe, and in some cases are quasi continuous (intractable asthma), with increased risk of episodes of status asthmaticus and respiratory failure.

Persistence of attacks through adolescence usually indicates a high degree of severity and probable continued adult morbidity. Many children whose asthma abates at adolescence may experience adult re-exacerbation at or after climacteric.

The disease is potentially reversible and in the absence of secondary complications does not lead to permanent structural damage of lung, airways, or thoracic cage.

PRESENTING SIGNS AND SYMPTOMS

Given the variable course and the spectrum of the disease, signs and symptoms are also very variable, and depend on the state of the disorder at the time the patient presents. The airways obstruction causes cough, particularly nocturnal, which may be the only presenting symptom. Wheezing, more pronounced in the expiratory phase of respiration than in the inspiratory phase but usually audible during both, is the usual presenting symptom and sign. Dyspnea is commonly present, as evidenced by the use of accessory muscles of respiration, flaring alae nasi, orthopneic posture, and anxiety; in severe stages there may be hypoxia with or without cyanosis.

Just as all that wheezes is not asthma (see Pitfalls in Diagnosis), all asthma does not wheeze. The absence or disappearance of wheezing in a child during a severe episode, indicating fairly complete airways obstruction to significant segments of lung, is a serious symptom that may indicate impending respiratory failure.

PHYSICAL EXAMINATION AND FINDINGS

On auscultation there is prolongation of the expiratory phase of respiration with widespread wheezing and scattered course and fine muscle rales. Mild to moderate tachycardia and tachypnea are usually present, and mild temperature elevations are not uncommon. There may be abdominal pain, particularly when coughing is severe. Breath sounds may be suppressed and tidal airflow so restricted that breath sounds are barely audible. In moderate to severe asthma of some duration and chronicity one finds a hyperinflated chest with increased anteroposterior diameter, hyperresonant to percussion. In severe asthma there are depressed flattened diaphragms, and liver and spleen may be palpable.

COMPLICATIONS

Those complications that are acute and related to severe episodes are status asthmaticus, a term used to describe severe attacks resistant to the usual therapeutic modalities and persisting over 12 or more hours. Status asthmaticus requires hospitalization and intensive care. Atelectasis, pneumothorax, and pneumomediastinum can all ensue during episodes of acute airways obstruction, either spontaneously or as complications of assisted ventilation.

Complications related to chronicity may be both physical and psychological. There is a tendency to deficient growth and development secondary to inadequate nutrition and physical activity when the disease has not been adequately controlled. As in other chronic distressing diseases, secondary psychological pathology, especially in parent-child and child-environment relations, may become a major

problem and even a predominant pathogenetic mechanism in the disease process. Evidence that psychological factors may be primary in the pathogenesis of the disorder is not convincing.

LABORATORY FINDINGS

Blood. Apart from eosinophilia, there are no relevant or consistent blood abnormalities. Total blood eosinophil counts are usually mildly elevated even in quiescent periods, rise sharply with exacerbations, and fall rapidly (sometimes to subnormal levels) as attacks subside or chronic symptoms are controlled. Immunoglobulin E concentrations are frequently, but not invariably, elevated. Blood gases, pH, and biochemistry are within normal limits except in very severe episodes.

Pulmonary Findings. Chest x-rays are rarely diagnostic in the absence of acute complications, usually revealing nonspecific increased bronchial markings, signs of hyperinflation, and minimal patchy atelectasis.

Simple spirometry or peak-flow meter determinations usually reveal decreased timed vital capacity (FEV_1) and peak expiratory flow rate (PEFR) even during periods of subjective well-being. More sophisticated pulmonary function examinations will reveal an increase in functional residual capacity, total lung capacity, maximum breathing capacity, and pulmonary resistance and compliance — all reflecting airways obstruction and chronic hyperinflation. During acute episodes measures of pulmonary function may drop to below 50 per cent of predicted norms for height, weight, and age.

The hyperreactivity of the bronchial tree of asthmatic children renders most of them sensitive to exercise-induced bronchospasm. Exercise testing by treadmill, bicycle ergometer, or simple running for 6 to 8 minutes (sufficient to raise pulse rate to 140 to 150) induces significant measurable decreases in pulmonary function in the 5- to 20-minute postexercise period. Such exercise testing is a valuable adjunct to diagnosis.

ALLERGY TESTS

A great majority of asthmatic children become sensitized to a limited spectrum of exogenous allergens (grass, tree, and weed pollens; house dust and house dust mite; animal and bird epithelial detritus; foods) producing IgE (and sometimes IgG) antibodies. Such sensitization can be revealed by classic techniques of skin testing or by specialized in vitro immunologic techniques (RAST or its modifications, leukocyte histamine release, etc.). Provocation tests may be used as well to identify specific inhalant allergens, measured doses of allergen extract being administered by inhalation and response measured by pulmonary function testing. Asthmatics are bronchially hyperresponsive to aerosol administration of cholinergic drugs, and provocation testing with them has been used also as an adjunct to diagnosis.

THERAPEUTIC TESTS

During relatively quiescent phases, beta-adrenergic stimulant bronchodilators may be administered by injection or inhalation with pre- and postadministration pulmonary function control to establish the presence and degree of bronchoconstriction. During acute phases symptomatic response to beta-agonists is frequently of diagnostic as well as of therapeutic utility. Bronchial asthma is so commonly steroid responsive that this quality has been considered essential to its definition. A therapeutic trial of response to corticosteroids may be useful when diagnosis remains uncertain.

PITFALLS IN DIAGNOSIS

Moderate to severe bronchial asthma is rarely misdiagnosed. Despite the variability and broad spectrum of the disease, the history, physical examination, and chest x-ray usually give reliable indications of the diagnosis and exclude differential diagnoses. When bronchiolitis occurs for the first time in an infant, the diagnosis may remain obscure pending further evolution. Any obstructive process, whether endogenous or exogenous, in the respiratory tree can produce wheezing. The differential diagnosis must include such disorders as aspirated foreign body, cystic fibrosis, cystic disease of the lung, tracheitis, congenital malformations, tumors, lymphomas, and reticuloendotheliosis, for which pathognomonic or highly suggestive symptoms, signs, and laboratory findings are discernible.

It is important to establish the diagnosis of bronchial asthma in children as early as possible so that appropriate therapy can be instituted in timely fashion to abort progress of the disorder, prevent potential complications, and ensure optimal physical and psychologic growth and development.

DRUG REACTIONS

By SIDNEY FRIEDLAENDER, M.D.
Southfield, Michigan

INTRODUCTION

Adverse reactions to drugs are increasingly frequent occurrences as the number of active pharmacologic agents proliferate. Limited understanding of the genesis of such untoward responses adds to confusion in diagnosis, and often leads to erroneous conclusions and unwarranted limitations in therapy. Whether the symptoms observed are due to a drug or to the illness for which the drug is given is a common dilemma faced by every clinician, and not easily resolved. Beyond this problem is the tendency to regard each and every adverse effect reasonably related to drug therapy as an "allergic reaction," which implies involvement of an immunologic mechanism. Such assumptions are frequently incorrect. It is well at the outset of this discussion to clarify the terminology used to describe drug reactions, and then to examine the mechanisms involved in their production, insofar as they are presently understood.

CLASSIFICATION OF DRUG REACTIONS

Toxicity. Such symptoms are dose-related, caused by the direct action on the tissue of the host which may be related to overdosage, or to failure to metabolize, detoxify, or excrete the drug. Examples are bleeding from overuse of anticoagulants, or nephrosis after mercury ingestion. In the presence of liver disease, failure to metabolize and detoxify drugs at a normal rate may result in increased toxicity. In renal failure, many drugs that are normally excreted by kidney accumulate and produce toxic reactions.

Side Effects. These are undesirable but unavoidable pharmacologic effects of the drug. Side effects occur after normal doses, and are more intense in some people than in others. Drowsiness from antihistaminics and excessive central nervous system stimulation from ephedrine are common examples. Many drugs have multiple pharmacologic actions, of which only one may be desirable as far as the patient is concerned. All others would be classed as side effects.

Secondary Effects. These are indirect but not inevitable results of the primary action of the drug. For example, development of fungal infection in patients receiving antibiotics, resulting from ecologic disturbance of normal relationships among organisms, or the development of gout after treatment with antimetabolites would be considered secondary effects.

Drug Interactions. These are actions of one drug on the toxicity of another when administered together or in some temporal relationship. Two drugs may compete for identical protein-binding sites, with the result that one with the greater affinity for binding can replace the other. For example, the drug warfarin may be displaced by phenylbutazone, with the result of increased bleeding induced by a large amount of unbound warfarin in the serum. Other drugs with the capacity of displacing anticoagulants from their binding sites are clofibrate, diphenylhydantoin, mefenamic acid, and salicylates, among others. Interference with drug metabolism through their actions on hepatic microsomes located in the hepatic endoplasmic reticulum may also lead to untoward effects. Drugs such as barbiturates, griseofulvin, and meprobamates lead to rapid metabolism of warfarin. Decreased synthesis of vitamin K by antibiotics may also increase the risk of bleeding in patients on anticoagulants. Oral hypoglycemic agents are also affected by other drugs. Tolbutamide can induce protracted hypoglycemia when drugs such as phenylbutazone, salicylates, and propranolol are being given. Oral hypoglycemic agents may also be antagonized by diuretics and phenothiazines. Electrolyte disturbances produced by one drug often influence the toxic effect of another. The common example is combined digitalis and diuretic therapy, in which resultant potassium loss from diuretic action makes the patient more susceptible to digitalis intoxication.

Intolerance. Intolerance is defined as exaggerated pharmacologic effects from small amounts of a drug mimicking symptoms of overdosage; for example, vertigo or tinnitus from a standard dose of aspirin, or swollen glands and rash from small doses of iodides.

Idiosyncrasy. Such reactions represent qualitatively abnormal responses, not dependent on the pharmacology or dosage of the drug. Such symptoms differ from overdosage, and are sometimes difficult to classify. They are not mediated immunologically. The underlying mechanism in many cases is unknown, but in some instances may be due to an inherited enzyme abnormality, which becomes evident only after administration of certain drugs. Hemolytic anemia occurring in patients receiving oxidant drugs may be related to deficiency in glucose-6-phosphate dehydrogenase (G-6-PD) enzyme necessary for metabolism of glucose. Primaquine was the original drug recognized in this syndrome, but it is now realized that many oxidant drugs can induce hemolysis in such patients, including sulfonamides, nitrofurans, phenacetin, phenylhydrazine, and vitamin K. Other examples are peripheral neuritis after isoniazid in patients lacking acetyltransferase, or the development of hemolysis and methemoglobinemia among patients with a rare hemoglobin (hemoglobin Zurich).

Allergy or Hypersensitivity. Such reactions represent the most frequent and important causes of drug reactions, presenting symptoms qualitatively unlike those of normal drug action or overdosage. They differ from idiosyncrasy in that they result from an immunologic mechanism. Allergic reactions are frequently confused with idiosyncrasy, which they can mimic closely, and in some cases years of investigation have failed to clearly differentiate the mechanism involved. For instance, aspirin may induce reactions with symptoms characteristic of most allergic responses, yet lack a proved immunologic mechanism. It has been theorized that aspirin in such cases stimulates altered kinin receptors in the lungs and capillaries.

The classification of Gell and Coombs may be applied to drug-induced allergic reactions, as follows:

Anaphylactic (Type I). These are the most serious, potentially fatal reactions, occurring within moments of administration of the drug. Symptoms are characterized by urticaria, hypotension, and shock. Such reactions are mediated primarily by IgE antibodies, and complement is not involved. Accelerated reactions may occur from 1 to 72 hours after drug administration, and are usually manifested by urticaria, asthma, and occasionally morbilliform eruptions and laryngeal edema.

Cytolytic or Cytotoxic (Type II). Antibody (IgG or IgM) reacts with antigen that is attached to the cell wall, or is part of the cell wall itself. Complement is involved, and generally results in cell destruction. The most common examples of this type of reaction are drug-induced immune hemolytic anemia and transfusion reactions from incompatible blood.

Immune or Toxic Complex (Type III). These reactions involve the complexing of antigen and antibody within the circulation to form soluble complexes that are deposited in the microvasculature, evoking inflammatory reactions. They are complement mediated, and generally involve IgG. Serum sickness is the most typical example of this reaction. The nephritis of systemic lupus erythematosus is mediated through this mechanism.

Cell-Mediated or Delayed Hypersensitivity (Type IV). Humoral antibody is not involved in this type of response, and depends on specifically altered or sensitized lymphocytes. Contact-type sensitivity is the prime example of this type of reaction, and would include many drugs that produce cutaneous reactions on direct contact with the suspected drug.

FACTORS PREDISPOSING TO DRUG REACTIONS

There are no consistent patterns of age or sex helpful to the physician. Genetic factors may be involved, with the tendency for allergic (atopic) persons to develop skin-sensitizing antibodies to a drug such as penicillin to a greater degree than nonatopic persons. A genetic basis is suggested by the observation that aplastic anemia from chloramphenicol is apparently very low in certain countries of the world where it is used extensively. The possibility that infection predisposes to development of drug hypersensitivity has also been considered. The high incidence of exanthematic rashes caused by ampicillin in patients with infectious mononucleosis has been cited as a possible example. Evidence that such reactions are due to immunologic mechanisms is open to doubt. An abnormally high incidence of hypersensitivity reactions to drugs in patients with systemic lupus erythematosus has also been noted, although, again, convincing evidence for an immunologic mechanism has not been established.

It has been known for years that certain drugs have a greater sensitizing potential than others. Drugs, or their metabolic breakdown products, act as haptens, combining covalently with protein to become immunogenic.

Although it has been shown that with halogenated dinitrobenzene compounds a correlation exists between their rate of reactivity with protein and the potency for producing sensitivity, such a mechanism has not been demonstrated for most drugs. Penicillin represents the most notable instance, in which metabolites are responsible for the reactions. Penicillin is a low-molecular-weight substance that does not combine firmly with serum protein to form an antigenic complex. Degradation to chemically reactive metabolites that combine with protein to form benzylpenicilloyl (BPO) haptenic groups is the way penicillin is handled to a great extent. The BPO group is referred to as the "major" antigenic determinant. BPO conjugates may be formed by reacting with a nonimmunogenic synthetic polypeptide such as polylysine to form a new reagent, penicilloyl-polylysine (PPL). Direct skin testing with PPL is much safer, and evidence suggests that a positive PPL skin test in patients not already on penicillin therapy is predictive of an urticarial reaction if penicillin is given. A mixture of highly reactive penicillin metabolites known as the "minor determinant mixture" (MDM) has been used in clinical studies with the finding that a positive skin test with MDM indicates a significant risk of anaphylactic reaction. MDM is still a research tool, whereas PPL is commercially available.

Cross-sensitization is also of great clinical importance. A patient who develops allergic symptoms to one compound sometimes reacts to related compounds. For example, cross-reactivity occurs between all the penicillins and between penicillin and cephalosporin derivates. Cross-reactions between phenothiazines are common. Neomycin cross-reacts with streptomycin. A patient sensitized to benzocaine may react to paraphenylenediamine and hair dye.

The appearance of the drug in a hidden or unfamiliar form is also a possibility. Penicillin in milk products is an example often cited for the persistence of urticaria in those who have previously experienced a reaction to penicillin. There is also evidence that tartrazine, a coal-tar dye (FD&C Yellow no. 5) found in yellow-colored medicine, candies, and food products, should be avoided by aspirin-sensitive patients.

HISTORY

History is the most important step in diagnosis of drug reactions. It is essential that the physician obtain detailed information concerning all drugs that the patient is currently taking or has taken in the weeks or months prior to the onset of the presenting symptoms. Direct questioning concerning specific medications, which the patient himself may not consider as actual "drugs," is required. Patients frequently do not regard aspirin, analgesics, anovulatory agents, or vitamins as drugs. Suspicion must also be directed toward foods that may contain drugs, such as quinine in tonic water, or penicillin in milk products. The occurrence of a reaction several days or weeks after drug ingestion is possible, and such information can be elicited only by careful questioning. The recognition of a drug reaction is frequently possible when the symptoms are those more characteristic of an allergic response, such as urticaria, or when the patient has experienced such a reaction before from the same or similar drug. Unfortunately, the manifestations of the drug reaction may resemble those of the illness for which the drug was taken, and evaluation becomes more diffi-

cult. When a drug reaction is suspected, all drug therapy should be stopped if possible. If symptoms disappear, the drugs can be reintroduced singly, starting with the drug least likely to be involved. Use of a substitute drug that does not cross-react with one already taken should be sought. When the drugs already in use are essential to the well-being of the patient, some additional diagnostic efforts are required, as well as appropriate therapy to control the symptoms of the reaction. Frequently it becomes a matter of the physician's judgment to determine which course constitutes the least risk to the patient. In most patients, a high index of suspicion, together with knowledge concerning the reaction potential of the drugs involved, will lead to a satisfactory outcome.

CLINICAL MANIFESTATIONS

Drugs may produce a wide spectrum of clinical signs and symptoms, and more than one type of reaction may be seen simultaneously in the same patient. Symptoms may be cutaneous or systemic, and may mimic other disease. Reactions of a particular type may be related to certain drugs.

Cutaneous Reactions. *Pruritus* is a common feature, but it is rarely the only symptom. *Urticaria* is the most frequent reaction, and may occur alone or as a component of a serum sickness-type reaction. Although it may subside when the offending drug is withdrawn, in some cases, especially those caused by penicillin, it may continue for some time after the medication has been withdrawn. *Exanthematic eruptions* may occur and closely simulate those resulting from infection, and at times progress to an exfoliative dermatitis. Erythematous rashes are common in patients with infectious mononucleosis who are treated with ampicillin. *Exfoliative dermatitis* may be associated with heavy metals, barbiturates, and sulfonamides. *Bullae* are associated with iodides or bromides. *Erythema multiforme* and its severe variant, Stevens-Johnson syndrome, are manifestations of drug hypersensitivity reported from sulfonamides, barbiturates, and many other drugs. *Lichenoid eruptions* resembling lichen planus may be caused by drugs such as gold salts, thiazides, and antimalarials. *Fixed drug eruptions*, which present characteristic single or multiple plaque-like lesions recurring at the same site each time the drug is taken, are most often seen after the use of phenolphthalein, barbiturates, and sulfonamides. *Contact dermatitis* is often produced by neomycin, streptomycin, penicillin, and local anesthetics containing benzocaine and procaine, as well as ointment bases, especially those containing lanolin. *Drug-induced eczematous reactions related to cross-sensitivity* may occur in patients sensitized locally who subsequently ingest the drug in a different form. For example, a patient sensitized to quinine in hair tonic may develop a generalized eczematous reaction when quinine is taken by mouth. Those sensitized to balsam of Peru in cosmetics may experience an eruption after ingestion of cinnamon.

Photosensitization reactions are generally classified into *phototoxic* and *photoallergic*. The former are not immunologically mediated, and involve the type of reaction in which a drug may increase the degree of sunburn caused by exposure to ultraviolet light. Demethylchlortetracycline is the most commonly recognized cause of this reaction. On the other hand, *photoallergic* reactions are immune responses, and may be eczematous, urticarial, papular, bullous, or lichenoid. Such skin eruptions develop while the patient is taking the drug and is exposed to sunlight. The reaction may recur for some time after the drug has been discontinued, whenever exposure to light occurs. Sulfonamides, thiazides, tolbutamide, chlorpromazine, and related compounds have been implicated in this type of response.

Nonthrombocytopenic purpura may be caused by drugs. Thiazides, iodides, gold salts, sulfonamides, barbiturates, and the hypnotic carbromal have been implicated. More recently tartrazine (FD&C Yellow no. 5) has been reported as a cause.

Systemic Reactions. *Fever* is a common manifestation, and may accompany any type of drug sensitivity reaction. *Anaphylaxis* is the most important, and potentially fatal, reaction occurring within minutes of drug administration. Pallor, apprehension, chest pain, difficulty in breathing, unconsciousness, and sometimes death constitute this most profound occurrence. All these symptoms also occur in nonfatal cases, frequently associated with erythema and urticaria, and may be accompanied by severe abdominal pain. Fortunately the majority of patients recover with the aid of parenteral epinephrine, intravenous theophylline, antihistamines, pressor agents, and parenteral corticosteroids. Penicillin, local anesthetics, pollen extracts, and foreign sera are the most common causes, and many diverse medications have been implicated.

Bronchial asthma is frequently a part of the anaphylactic reaction, associated with other symptoms, notably urticaria. Aspirin appears to be the most common cause, especially in patients who have pre-existing asthma associated with nasal polyps. For some reason not yet understood, the triad of aspirin sensitivity, nasal polyps, and severe asthma is often observed. The supposition that aspirin is involved in an antigen-antibody reaction has not been proved, and speculation concerning the mechanism involved still exists. The clinical manifestations of such aspirin reactions are indistinguishable from classic immune reactions of the anaphylactic type. Some patients who react in this manner to aspirin also exhibit similar responses to other analgesics, including indomethacin and mefenamic acid. Tartrazine has also been described in this relationship.

The serum sickness reaction, a term applied to all reactions of this type regardless of inciting cause, consists of fever, joint pain, and urticaria, occurring from 3 to 21 days after administration of a drug or serum. It may follow a primary injection or administration of the drug, and persist for weeks or months after its discontinuation, subsiding spontaneously in most cases. Penicillin is the most common cause, although a wide variety of drugs have been implicated.

Vasculitis is often associated with drug hypersensitivity, and it may not be possible to learn whether vasculitis is due to the drug or is a manifestation of the underlying disease itself. Present evidence indicates that vasculitis is an immune-complex reaction (Type III) in the blood vessel wall. Recently it has been observed that certain cases of chronic urticaria, especially those associated with elevated sedimentation rates, are manifestations of vasculitis.

Anaphylactoid purpura (Henoch-Schönlein syndrome) is a form of vasculitis associated with nonthrombocytopenic purpura and articular and gastrointestinal involvement. A drug cause should be suspected in adults. Salicylates, chlorothiazide, quinine, and azo dyes have been implicated.

Systemic lupus erythematosus (SLE) syndrome occurs in patients taking certain drugs, most frequently hydralazine and procainamide. All the manifestations of SLE are seen in such patients, including the LE cell phenomenon. Discontinuation of the drug generally results in clinical improvement. Other drugs, including isonicotinic acid and penicillamine, have been implicated. Although antibodies to a suspected drug are demonstrated in some patients, it has not been proved that these are indeed the actual cause of the reaction. It has been suggested that there are patients with a "lupus diathesis" who metabolize drugs in such a way that they are prone to react with nucleoprotein.

Hepatic Manifestations. Toxic liver damage produced by direct injury to liver cells is probably more common than hypersensitivity mechanisms. Carbon tetrachloride, chloroform, gold salts, 6-mercaptopurine, and tetracycline are some of the drugs known to produce toxic reactions. Certain drugs, such as C-17 alkyl-substituted testosterones, produce hepatic damage in almost all patients who use the drug over a long period of time. Hypersensitivity reactions involving the liver are encountered in only a small proportion of those taking the drug, and may be associated with eosinophilia, fever, and skin rashes, which improve after discontinuation of the drug. Among the drugs most frequently involved are the phenothiazines, chlorpropamide, and phenylbutazone. A more serious type of hypersensitivity with hepatocellular damage and death caused by liver failure has occurred after use of many drugs, including sulfonamides, cinchophen, methyldopa, and halothane. Although there is strong evidence that an immunologic mechanism is operating, no immunologic test has been of any proved value in diagnosis.

Nephropathy. Although many drugs cause renal damage, the mechanism is frequently other than immunologic. Sulfonamides cause obstructive nephropathy owing to deposition of crystals in the renal tubules. Methoxyflurane anesthesia is associated with the accumulation of oxalate crystals in the tubules and interstitium of the kidney. Direct toxic effects on the kidney have been described from bacitracin and amphotericin. Many renal lesions have been ascribed to drug hypersensitivity with features similar to those observed in serum sickness. Sulfonamides, mercury compounds, gold salts, and penicillin have all been described in connection with immunologic reactions in the kidney. Penicillins are the most important cause of interstitial nephritis and tubular damage. Nephropathy after prolonged use of analgesics, notably phenacetin, is suspected to be a hypersensitivity reaction to the drug.

Pulmonary Manifestations. Although bronchial asthma is the most common pulmonary manifestation of drug reactions, hypersensitivity lung disease (extrinsic allergic alveolitis) has been associated with the inhalation of powdered extracts of bovine or porcine pituitary glands for treatment of diabetes insipidus. The prototype for the mechanism involved would be so-called "farmer's lung," caused by inhalation of organic dusts. Another pulmonary reaction has been reported after the use of nitrofurantoin. Initial symptoms develop several days after the drug is started, consisting of fever, cough, dyspnea, pleuritic chest pains, and occasionally cyanosis. Interstitial changes may be observed on chest x-ray, and pleural effusion may be present. Recovery follows promptly when the drug is stopped, and recurs upon readministration. Similar reactions have been recently reported in some patients from inhalation of the new prophylactic antiasthmatic drug disodium cromoglycate. Pulmonary infiltrates with eosinophilia (Löffler's syndrome) have been noted after use of penicillin, sulfonamides, and other drugs.

Hematologic Manifestations. Blood dyscrasias caused by drugs through toxicity on bone marrow or through inborn metabolic errors are recognized mechanisms. Drug reactions involving immunologic mechanisms are generally classed into three types, and more than one type may be involved: (1) *Drug-hapten type*, in which the drug reacts with body protein to produce a complete antigen with resulting antigen-antibody interaction. (2) *Innocent-bystander type*, in which the interaction of drug and specific antibody results in damage to cells that are not actively involved in the binding of antigen and antibody. Quinidine-induced thrombocytopenia and chlorpropamide-induced hemolysis are examples. (3) *Autoimmune reactions* producing some change in the red blood cell membrane that renders it autoantigenic. This is a mechanism by which alpha-methyldopa is thought to produce hemolytic anemia. About 20 per cent of those receiving the drug have serologic evidence of autoimmune reaction, although fewer than 1 per cent develop hemolytic anemia. Hemolysis may persist for some time after the drug is withdrawn. Other drugs are reported to be involved in similar reactions. Drug-induced thrombocytopenia, hemolytic anemia, agranulocytosis, and aplastic anemia are common manifestations related to direct drug toxicity, genetic errors, or hypersensitivity mechanisms. (See manufacturer's official directive for specific information for all aforementioned drugs.)

DIAGNOSTIC TESTS

It should be realized that skin tests and serologic tests in the diagnosis of drug hypersensitivity are of limited value. Frequently, many tests are positive in patients who are subsequently found able to tolerate full doses of a suspected drug. The ultimate in determining the relationship of a drug to a patient's symptoms is test-dosing after recovery. This is fraught with danger, and unless the need for the drug is of compelling urgency, a search for an alternative drug should be made.

Scratch or *intradermal skin tests* to determine immediate-type hypersensitivity (IgE) are occasionally useful. It should be recalled that most drugs are simple chemical compounds, which require conjugation to a protein to make them complete antigens. The ability to elicit whealing skin reactions is ordinarily limited to such protein agents as antisera, ACTH, insulin, liver extract, and egg vaccines. The value of skin testing in penicillin sensitivity has been discussed. Many allergists are aware that testing with benzyl-penicillin is too dangerous for routine use, as fatal anaphylactic reactions have occurred in very sensitive patients. A strong history of previous anaphylactic reaction should preclude skin testing with benzyl-penicillin, or, if undertaken, should be performed in a setting in which resuscitation is possible. Skin testing with penicilloyl-polylysine (PPL) is safer, but the correlation of a positive response with clinical sensitivity to penicillin is not as close. The use of the minor determinant mixture (MDM) is still a research procedure, as the mixture is not commercially available. A recent study indicates that both tests must be administered to detect the maximal number of hypersensitive persons. It has been suggested that a scratch test with 10,000 units per ml of penicillin G may be used in the absence of MDM preparation.

Patch testing is useful in the prediction of contact dermatitis, through elicitation of cellular or delayed type (Type IV) reaction when the suspected antigen is applied directly to the skin for a 24- to 48-hour period.

In the *skin window technique*, a drop of drug solution is applied to an abraded area of skin and covered with a cover-glass for a period of time. The cover-glass is subsequently stained for the presence of cells, and is occasionally informative. This technique has not achieved widespread use.

In vitro tests, which are dependent on the demonstration of *histamine release* from *the patient's leukocytes* or from *passively sensitized lung tissue*, are research procedures that can be performed only in special laboratories. Most in vitro tests have been found to be of limited clinical value, except those designed specifically for investigation of reactions involving formed elements of the blood. In some cases the tests are subject to variations in technique that influence their validity, and the results from most laboratories provide very little guidance for the physician.

The *basophil degranulation test* has been extensively studied by various investigators, with reports varying from enthusiastic endorsement to total condemnation. The test is not sufficiently reliable to make the results of diagnostic value.

The *lymphocyte transformation test*, which involves blast transformation of patient lymphocytes when cultured in the presence of the suspected antigen, has been used in the inves-

tigation of drug hypersensitivity. Again, the test is not consistent enough to be of value diagnostically.

The *leukocyte-migration inhibition test* is another technique adapted from the research laboratory. The complexities involved have not allowed it to become a clinically feasible test for the average clinician.

Detection of hemagglutinating antibodies (IgG), which depends on agglutination of red cells by antibody in the patient's serum, has been applied to many different drugs. As a diagnostic tool it has limited value, because a positive result indicates only that the patient has developed antibody to the drug, and does not necessarily mean that the drug is responsible for symptoms. Almost all patients receiving a drug may develop hemagglutinating antibodies to that drug, without any relationship to any untoward reaction.

In the case of drug reactions involving formed elements of the blood, the value of diagnostic in vitro tests is greater. In the evaluation of thrombocytopenia, a battery of in vitro tests has been used to determine drug-dependent antibody. Such testing must be performed as early as possible, as antibody may disappear in just a few days. A *complement-fixation test with antibody concentration* is considered to be the most reliable and most sensitive of these tests. In drug-induced hemolytic anemia, the *antiglobulin (Coombs) test* is the most useful procedure. This consists of the addition of an antibody directed against gamma globulin that provides a bridge between two antibody-coated cells. The *direct Coombs test* consists of suspending the patient's own washed red cells in a broad-spectrum antiglobulin serum. Agglutination of these cells indicates that they were coated in vivo with immunoglobulin, complement, or both. The *indirect Coombs test* is performed with red cells suspended in the patient's serum in the presence of drug. If agglutination or lysis does not occur, the cells are washed and resuspended in antiglobulin serum. If this causes agglutination, indications are that the cells were coated with gamma globulin or complement. In agranulocytosis, tests involving *leukocyte agglutination* and *complement fixation* have been used.

The *radioallergosorbent test (RAST)* is a more recent method of detecting reaginic antibodies to allergens, and has already been utilized in the case of drug reactions. The RAST technique may be employed to detect circulating IgE antibodies directed against the major penicillin antigen determinant, the penicilloyl group. The penicilloyl RAST correlates quite well with a positive PPL skin test, and is of sufficient sensitivity to detect patients at risk for anaphylactic reaction mediated by penicilloyl-specific IgE. This technique has not yet been applied to the detection of the minor determinants (MDM), which leaves a considerable void in the accurate prediction of penicillin reactions.

SUMMARY

The most satisfactory approach to the diagnosis of drug reactions is a high index of suspicion concerning the drugs being taken, or previously taken, and an adequate understanding of the mechanisms involved. It is necessary to be aware that laboratory tests for drug reactions are of limited value, and require careful interpretation. The time the test is performed, the period elapsed since the reaction, and the degree of sensitivity of the test are all involved in proper evaluation of diagnostic usefulness. Until such time as a battery of in vitro tests becomes available that has a greater degree of reliability and specificity, one must rely on a careful history and clinical judgment in evaluating those suspected of having drug reactions. The absolute need to determine whether a drug is involved in any particular symptom complex must be considered in the light of what the drug offers the patient if it is continued. It must be realized that at times it is impossible to determine the relationship of drug to symptoms, or to separate it from symptoms that may be due to the patient's illness. It is quite possible that rapidly developing knowledge in this field will provide more reliable in vitro techniques that will have greater meaning in the diagnosis of drug reactions.

Section 13

DISEASES OF THE NERVOUS SYSTEM

CEREBROVASCULAR DISEASE

By B. H. EIDELMAN, M.D., D. PHIL., M.R.C.P.

and O. M. REINMUTH, M.D.

Pittsburgh, Pennsylvania

The diagnosis of cerebrovascular disorders is made primarily on the clinical features. There is no substitution for a thorough history and careful examination. In addition to the standard neurologic evaluation, a detailed assessment of the patient's vascular status must be made. The arteries of the head, neck, and extremities are examined for delayed or absent pulsations. Careful auscultation of the cervical vessels must be carried out to determine the presence of bruits. It is of importance not to compress the vessel under examination as this may create a spurious murmur. Cervical bruits may arise from causes other than arterial stenosis and may occur with severe anemia, hyperthyroidism, and fever. Bruits low in the neck can be heard in young adults in the absence of vascular disease. A bruit heard under the angle of the mandible suggests stenosis at the bifurcation or in the proximal internal carotid artery. Bruits in the supraclavicular region may be indicative of subclavian or vertebral arterial disease. Absence of a bruit does not imply that the underlying vessels are patent.

In addition to auscultation, the vascular examination includes measurement of the blood pressure in the supine and erect positions and comparison of blood pressure recordings in both arms. Assessment of the cardiac status is also an essential part of the examination. Ophthalmoscopic examination should be carried out to assess the status of the retinal vessels. Examination of the fundi may yield important information concerning the presence of embolic disease and can provide clues to the diagnosis of systemic conditions such as polycythemia, dysproteinemia, and collagen vascular disease.

On completion of the physical examination, further investigation is dictated by the need to confirm the diagnosis and to determine whether any treatable cause or contributing factors are present. In general terms, investigations aimed toward discovering surgically treatable arterial disease should not be pursued if other factors forbid surgical repair.

The purposes for investigation of patients with vascular disease are as follows:

1. To establish that the patient's neurologic problem has a vascular basis and to exclude different pathologic entities.
2. To determine the nature of the vascular incident, e.g., to distinguish an infarct from a hematoma.
3. To determine whether the occlusion is intracranial or extracranial and to exclude the heart and great vessels as a source of emboli.
4. To assess whether the condition is stable or progressing.
5. To identify possible risk factors that may lead to worsening or recurrence of the stroke.

LABORATORY STUDIES

Routine laboratory studies may reveal important abnormalities. Blood sugar levels may indicate diabetes or hypoglycemia. The hemoglobin and hematocrit would show anemia and polycythemia, the complete blood count (CBC) the evidence of blood dyscrasias. An erythrocyte sedimentation rate should be carried out as this may be elevated in the presence of collagen vascular disease or temporal arteritis. The blood serology is obtained to exclude syphilis. A chest x-ray is valuable in detecting heart and chronic lung disease. An electrocardiogram is useful to detect heart disease that may have a direct bearing on the cause of the stroke and also may be of importance in relation to the subsequent rehabilitation.

NEUROLOGIC STUDIES

Plain x-rays of the skull have a place in the investigation of strokes; their main function is to exclude a fracture arising from an unsuspected head injury.

A lumbar puncture in the stroke patient need not be carried out as a routine measure. Examination of the cerebrospinal fluid (CSF) is indicated when there is diagnostic doubt. The presence of blood in the CSF strongly suggests hemorrhage. If the stroke is embolic, anticoagulant therapy may be interdicted when excessive numbers of red blood cells (RBC) are present in CSF.

Brain scanning is a noninvasive procedure that is of value in the evaluation of patients with an acute stroke. Brain scans map the cerebral distribution of an intravenously administered tracer. Abnormal uptake of the isotope occurs in regions where the blood-brain barrier has been disrupted. In the case of an ischemic episode, the brain scan becomes positive 1 to 7 days after the acute event. The typical picture of an infarct is a wedge-shaped area of increased uptake in the regional distribution of the middle cerebral artery. Abnormal areas of activity may be seen in the anterior and posterior distributions with occlusions of the anterior posterior cerebral arteries, respectively. An intracerebral hematoma may also produce a positive scan, but the uptake of the isotope usually does not include the cortex. Neoplasms produce positive areas of uptake that may be difficult to distinguish from the area of an infarct. Serial scanning may be of use in differentiating vascular disease from neoplasms.

Computerized tomography (CT), which relies on the measurement of the attenuation by the cerebral structures of multiple x-ray beams, has proved to be an extremely valuable adjunct in the diagnosis of vascular disease. CT is particularly useful in the diagnosis of intracerebral hemorrhage and it is possible to detect the occurrence, location, and extent of the hemorrhage within a few minutes of the extravasation of blood. CT is the investigation of choice in the diagnosis of acute intracerebral hematoma. The CT appearance of an acute intracerebral hematoma is one of a well-defined area of increased density surrounded by decreased density owing to edema. The lesion decreases in size and density with time. The rate of resolution depends on the size of the hematoma, with a large hemorrhage taking several months to resolve. CT is also useful in detecting infarcts that appear as an area of decreased density that may show contrast enhancement.

NONINVASIVE TECHNIQUES FOR DETECTING EXTRACRANIAL VASCULAR DISEASE

A number of techniques have been devised for the detection of occult cerebrovascular disease. These tests have limitations and at best serve as screening tests. Nonetheless they can provide useful information concerning the state of the extracranial vascular system and deserve mention. These investigations include ophthalmodynamometry, ocular plethysmography. Doppler imaging, and Doppler directional flow tests.

Ophthalmodynamometry measures differences in retinal artery pressure of the two eyes. Graded pressure is applied to the eyeball and the retinal arteries are observed. As pressure is applied, pulsations appear in the retinal arteries and this point signifies the diastolic end-point. With further application of pressure, the pulsations disappear; this signifies a systolic end-point. If there is more than 20 per cent difference in pressure between the eyes, internal carotid artery disease is implied on the side with the lower pressure.

Ocular plethysmography measures and records ocular pulsations. Each ocular pulse represents the change in the volume flow of the globe produced by pulsatile arterial flow. The pulses are obtained simultaneously from both eyes and the lagging of one ocular pulse behind the other indicates pathology of the internal carotid artery on the delayed side.

Doppler imaging utilizes a continuous wave Doppler flowmeter to obtain the two-dimensional image of the region from which the sound pattern is generated. From the localization of sound waves, it is possible to build up a graphic display of the region under study and in this way the anatomic configuration of the vessel can be obtained. The usefulness of this technique lies in its ability to provide noninvasive anatomic details and it may be of more value at present for following a lesion than for original definitive diagnostic use.

Doppler directional flow studies are used to provide information concerning the direction of flow in branches in the external carotid artery. Vessels that may be studied in this way are the superficial temporal, facial, and angular arteries. Normally, blood flows from the intracranial to extracranial circulations in these branches. Reversal of flow indicates stenosis or obstruction of the internal carotid artery.

The noninvasive techniques are able to detect occlusions or major stenosis of extracranial vessels. As yet, they are not reliable in the demonstration of nonocclusive atheromatous plaques that may be an important source of emboli. For this reason, angiography remains the investigation of choice in the demonstration of pathology involving the major cerebral vessels. The principal indications for angiography are:

1. In the investigation of patients with transient neurologic symptoms referable to the carotid circulation when cardiac or other causes for such symptoms have been excluded. Transient ischemic episodes referable to the vertebral-basilar system have a more benign outlook. In general, they do not merit further study except when clinical evidence suggests a subclavian steal phenomenon or if the episodes are persistently related to head turning, which may indicate external compression of the vertebral artery.

2. In instances of subarachnoid hemorrhage when investigation is essential for the demonstration and localization of aneurysms or arteriovenous abnormalities. Arteriography has little place in the investigation of a completed stroke except for cases in which diagnostic doubt exists, such as in the case of arteritis or aneurysm, or when bypass is contemplated for changing symptoms.

Modern practice has changed rapidly to favor considered use of CT scanning. The nature and reliability of the information to be gained appears time and again to justify the moderately higher economic cost.

METABOLIC ENCEPHALOPATHY

By SIMON HORENSTEIN, M.D.

St. Louis, Missouri

INTRODUCTION

The terms metabolic encephalopathy, exogenous or secondary encephalopathy, and metabolic coma are applied to brain disorders of diverse origin that are all characterized by some alteration of consciousness, impaired mental function, disordered posture and movement, released cerebral automatisms, and recently acquired biochemical and electrophysiologic abnormalities. These conditions result from exogenous intoxications, reactions to drugs, or diseases that alter metabolism of parts of the body outside the central nervous system, affecting it secondarily. Endogenous derangements of cerebral metabolism resulting from disordered nerve cell metabolism independent of changes in the functions of extraneural organs are not considered here. This article emphasizes common disorders that may be lethal or require urgent treatment. Table 1 lists the common forms of metabolic encephalopathy and the approaches to their diagnosis.

CLINICAL CONSIDERATIONS

The major features of metabolic encephalopathy are disturbance of consciousness, impairment of mental function, release of cerebral automatisms, disorder of posture and movement, and abnormality of body chemistry. They are present to varying degrees in each patient. Except for the acute confusional disorder leading to coma within 7 to 9 seconds following abrupt and complete anoxia, these conditions usually begin slowly and evolve over the course of minutes (e.g., hypoglycemia), hours (e.g., hepatic stupor), or days (e.g., uremic encephalopathy) rather than developing within a few seconds. In this way, therefore, they can usually be separated from epileptic disorders or their consequences, which are most often abrupt in onset. Metabolic encephalopathy almost always emerges from a background of clear-cut, previously known, and easily recognized systemic disease. When it does not, the history is likely to be defective. It frequently occurs while the patient is under medical observation and often is the direct result of drugs or other treatments administered in the hospital. As a general rule, the appearance of a neurologic syndrome in a patient suffering from a non-neurologic disease should suggest that the syndrome results from the pre-existent disease or its treatment.

The most important causes of metabolic brain disease are (1) exposure to exogenous poisons, in particular, sedative or tranquilizing drugs medically or self-prescribed; (2) metabolic acidosis regardless of origin; (3) disease of liver, kidney, lung, or endocrine organs; (4) hypoxia or anoxia of any type; (5) ischemia; (6) hypoglycemia; or (7) derangements of ionic equilibrium or serum osmolality.

The ease with which any given patient may develop any form of metabolic encephalopathy and the rate of its evolution are not uniform but appear to depend upon the nature, progression, and degree of change of the basic disorder. They seem also to be proportional to the age of the patient, the quality of his general health, the nature, severity, and duration of pre-existing or associated brain lesions, the concomitant administration of medication, the nature of the environment in which the illness is evolving, and the exogenous stress to which he is exposed.

Rapid change in acid-base equilibrium may result in asymmetric fluid shifts in various body compartments; in turn, these shifts help create, maintain, or enhance confusion. This is likely to complicate the treatment of renal disease and the mental disorder may indicate the development of secondary water intoxication. Extreme youth may be a factor that affords some protection against hypoxia. Alternatively, elderly patients often develop symptoms of drug intoxication at relatively lower doses and blood levels than do younger people (e.g., carbamazepine or digitalis). It is believed that derangements associated with congestive heart failure, chronic obstructive pulmonary disease, or diabetes mellitus may be additive to those induced by biochemical abnormalities or endocrine organ failure. Such a concatenation of events compounds the effects of each, thus causing encephalopathy earlier or to a greater degree than might have occurred in a person suffering a less complex illness.

In any disorder that might affect behavior, a

nervous system that has been compromised by intrinsic or endogenous disease has less "behavioral reserve." A common example is the ease with which patients with senile dementia may become severely confused when subjected to minor degrees of fever, hypotension, or dehydration. Of manageable and hence therapeutically significant factors, the administration of sedative, hypnotic, analgesic, anticholinergic, or stimulant drugs may worsen other effects of metabolic derangement. The occurrence of progressive confusion and stupor in a hospitalized patient who was alert at admission often reflects adverse reaction to medication.

The environment in which a potentially confusional illness is proceeding determines to an important degree the extent of the mental disorder. A silent room in which the patient sees little more than bare walls and hears little save indistinct or muffled sounds alone may result in "perceptual isolation," hallucinosis, disorientation, and often prolonged periods of sleeping. In patients recovering from drug withdrawal delirium or hepatic or uremic encephalopathy, the provision of a light, frequent visitors, familiar objects to look at or handle, and protection from indistinct sounds may lessen the confusion and materially reduce the mental disorder. Alternatively, an environment that prevents normal wake and sleep patterns may enhance or cause one.

The disturbance of consciousness that occurs in metabolic brain disease may be expressed as delirium, stupor, or alternation between them and appears to result from affection of the cerebral cortex, the reticular formation, or both. Environmental factors often determine moment-to-moment changes in the severity of the delirium or stupor independently of any change in the underlying metabolic disorder. Thus it often happens that in the same patient, and with little if any change in body chemistry, rapid fluctuations between delirium and stupor occur as the patient is stimulated, examined, or subjected to nursing procedures.

Confusion is the common denominator of delirium and stupor. This term is applied to any mental disturbance in which an individual's orientation to himself and his environment has become grossly altered despite the relative preservation of other mental or intellectual functions, including the ability to speak, read, calculate, or abstract. It usually is acute and transient. The senses of time (including knowledge of the date and the ability to estimate elapsed time) and full orientation for place are usually first and most severely affected. Personal disorientation occurs later and represents a more extreme aspect of confusion, which may

be so severe that the patient does not know whether he is dressed. It is rare that patients forget their own names. Loss of memory for one's own name with preservation of other aspects of orientation and mental function is highly suggestive of a psychogenic disorder or malingering.

When confusion is accompanied by drowsiness or lethargy, the patient is said to be *stuporous*. He may often be found asleep and difficult to arouse. Once alerted, he may be unable to maintain an attentive state and may repeatedly doze. Occasionally the stuporous patient will become agitated when aroused. Such fluctuation appears more common than a steadily maintained state.

Confusion accompanied by restlessness, sustained sleeplessness, and excessive attentiveness to any novel stimulus is called *delirium*. In this "hypermetabolic" state the patient is usually sweaty, wide-eyed, tremulous, readily startled, and often actively hallucinating. The hallucinations are usually auditory in drug withdrawal states, when their content is most likely to be offensive and obscene, provoking additional excitement and terror. Visual hallucinations may range from moving spots referred to the periphery of the visual field that the patient endlessly pursues but never quite catches to others that are highly organized, at which he stares fixedly. The former is characteristic of drug withdrawal delirium and the latter often accompanies drug intoxication. Somesthetic hallucinations such as the sensation that ants are crawling on or beneath the skin or that someone else is sharing the bed are common although less often described.

Stupor suggests a metabolic encephalopathy of hepatic or endocrinopathic origin, whereas delirium is more likely to be present with milder degrees of hypoxia, uremia, or withdrawal from drugs, especially alcohol. If the metabolic encephalopathy is associated with deficiency of a vitamin or other nutritional factor, the heightened energy requirements of delirium may seriously and rapidly deplete whatever stores remain of the cofactor and thus may cause new or heightened neurologic deficits. These are likely to be quite specific as they reflect neuronal failure, which is maximal in regions most dependent on the deficient substance. Thus, the distribution of lesions in the mamillary bodies, median dorsal thalamus, the floor of the fourth ventricle, and around the aqueduct of Sylvius in Wernicke-Korsakoff disease reflects the greater dependence of these structures on thiamine. Delirium or stupor may be followed by progressive impairment of consciousness, leading eventually to deep coma. In these states signs of decompensation of the brainstem (loss of pupillary and vestibular reflexes, respiratory failure, and decerebration or flaccidity) may be present.

The intellectual changes accompanying metabolic brain disease, especially when chronic or recurrent and mild enough to sustain detailed examination, are variable. They frequently become permanent and irreversible. The chief residual disorders are likely to impair memory, attention, and emotional control. Other intellectual parameters such as the ability to abstract and plan, calculate, reason, and use language may be affected, although not necessarily in proportion to the memory disorder. The latter may be so severe that recollection of past and present events is lost, leaving intact only very short-term memory. It may spare large segments of unrelated memoranda to which the patient has free access, but severely impair retrieval and hence serial memory. When the physician does not know the genesis of the disorder or the history of the illness, the finding of severe intellectual deficits may cause him to think that he is dealing with a primary dementing disorder. The diagnostic clue invariably resides in the fact that an acute systemic illness is present. Profound disorders of intellect without intense confusion are not features of acute metabolic encephalopathies.

Intense confusion may, however, mean that a recently acquired metabolic encephalopathy has been overlaid upon some other brain disorder, e.g., pre-existing senile dementia or the cumulative effects of multiple small infarcts. Although acute confusional states tend to subside, many who have suffered episodes of metabolic encephalopathy are left with permanent intellectual changes. This is particularly likely to occur after cofactor deficiency, metabolic acidosis, hypoglycemia, ischemia, and hypoxia. Moreover, since some confusional states tend to recur, cumulative damage may result in progressive dementia. In other conditions such as hepatic encephalopathy, the change in mental state fluctuates with variation in the concentration of toxic material present in the blood and hence the cells of the brain. Improvement in mental function after admission to the hospital despite lack of specific treatment may mean that the patient has been exposed to an exogenous or self-administered toxin such as industrial wastes, barbiturates, or scopolamine or has failed to comply with treatment, as may happen in thyroid disease with the development of myxedema encephalopathy. Lasting intellectual loss in chronic metabolic encephalopathy is likely to be subtle, variable, and marked by major disorders of conative function in which planning, execution, judgment, and abstracting capacities are impaired, while language functions, vision, and perception are better preserved.

The behavioral outcome in any patient appears to depend upon interaction among three sets of forces. The first of these is anatomic. Thus, lesions that involve the prefrontal regions, as in hypoxia, will cause severe impairment of planning and skilled performance. A second is the volume of the lesion. Therefore, the degree and extent of pathology affect the totality of behavioral change independent of its location. This may be seen by comparing the severity of behavioral disintegration after hypoglycemia with its preservation after capsular infarction. The third is the nature of the premorbid personality, including the patient's special skills, intelligence, and habitual reaction patterns.

Motor derangements regularly occur in chronic and acute forms of metabolic encephalopathy but are not present to the same degree in every patient. Their existence may often be a clue to the presence of metabolic brain disorder. They may be divided into those that impair the use of the limbs, face, and trunk and others that express themselves as autonomic abnormalities involving particularly sweating, the reactions of the pupils, and breathing.

The most common of the motor abnormalities are tremor and restlessness. The latter is seen in delirious or agitated patients who because of defective attention are attracted by each novel stimulus. The occurrence of unclear or indistinct events in the environment and the patient's inability to sustain interest in one of them while deferring responses to others appear to be necessary for hyperactivity.

Myoclonus is observed in nearly all forms of metabolic encephalopathy. It may be "bulbar" or abrupt, bilateral, symmetrical flexion of the neck, trunk, and limbs. These movements may occur singly or repeatedly. When they are repeated, they tend to be self-sustaining. They resemble the common and normal startle reaction that is seen when a preoccupied person is unexpectedly touched or spoken to, but differ as they do not habituate. Thus, the startle reaction can rarely be evoked more than twice, but stimulus-sensitive myoclonus may be elicited over and again. Focal, segmental, or isolated myoclonus is more common than the "bulbar" form and may involve multiple foci simultaneously. It is less likely to be provoked by sound, light, or touch but often bears a close relationship to muscle contraction, occurring as a quick jerk or twitch at the beginning or end of movement. Each focus generally remains restricted to a muscle or segment of one. Such myoclonus rarely becomes generalized and is only infrequently a precursor of a generalized convulsion. Multifocal myoclonus is quite common, and careful bedside evaluation should confirm that several foci are active simultaneously. Myoclonus may be seen as a gross duplicated or repeated contraction of very brief duration. Occasionally a whole muscle is involved, with joint displacement. Each twitch is quite brief, although occasionally a focus of myoclonus may become sustained, producing continuing localized contraction of a body segment, such as the pectoralis major or a quadrant of the abdominal wall. This is called status epilepticus partialis continua. A simultaneously recorded electroencephalogram may disclose multiphasic periodic bursts of high-amplitude sharp and slow activity, or conversely it may contain only low-amplitude slow activity. Isolated myoclonus often has no electroencephalographic counterpart. Myoclonus, including continuous forms, usually does not subside upon anticonvulsant drug administration, may be present when the patient is asleep as well as awake, and may persist into the recovery period. It is an early and frequent phenomenon of drug withdrawal, especially alcohol and barbiturates, and a relatively late although persistent one in conditions such as uremia. In many forms of chronic metabolic encephalopathy such as hepatic, its variations often provide a sensitive indication of fluctuations in the underlying process. Myoclonus appears to indicate disorganization in the pattern of neuronal activation of muscles. It is not an "epileptic" phenomenon in the ordinary sense of the term and may result from disease at any anatomic level, including the spinal cord.

Asterixis, also called liver or metabolic "flap," is an intermittent irregularity of sustained effort that complicates numerous metabolic encephalopathies. It is totally unrelated to any other disorder of movement and is involuntary rather than the result of inattentiveness. Most patients are unaware of its presence and cannot restrain it upon exhortation to do so. It represents a violation of the law of reciprocal innervation as for a brief time simultaneous inhibition of protagonistic and antagonistic muscles occurs. This event is seen clinically as the lapse of posture. The subsequent quick recovery of the erstwhile extended posture of the wrist, fingers, toes, or ankles completes the "flap." Asterixis may be seen in the tongue, face, or eyebrows. It may be asymmetric and is not present to the same extent in all affected areas or at all times. In uremia and hepatic insufficiency it appears early and is frequent. It is most readily evoked by asking the patient to maintain a part of his body in a fixed position, such as extending the wrist and fingers. Since many patients with asterixis are drowsy or stuporous, one must ensure that the patient is awake and alert enough to comply when his limbs are being examined, but it is possible to recognize the flapping tremors of asterixis even in a drowsy patient. If such a person is asked to squeeze the examiner's fingers firmly and steadily, an irregular relaxation and contraction may be felt. If alternatively the bulb of a sphygmomanometer is compressed, variations in pressure can be seen. These techniques are useful because they require less conscious effort. Asterixis may also be appreciated when the grasp reflex is tested.

Both static and kinetic tremor are common in metabolic encephalopathy and may persist after recovery. As they are usually rapid and of moderate amplitude, they are easily seen. They ordinarily appear on both sides of the body and tend to be symmetrical. The tremor in metabolic encephalopathy is hardly ever present at rest and hence is readily distinguished from that of paralysis agitans or that resulting from chronic exposure to phenothiazine drugs. It may occur during the active phase of movement (kinetic), or after movement has been completed and the limb is maintained in a fixed position (static), or both. Along with asterixis, it disappears in coma. When permanent, it indicates some fixed alteration of brain function. Pathologic studies have failed to implicate any single part of the brain, hence the tremor may represent either the result of diffuse structural effects or permanent impairment of some unidentified forebrain transmitter mechanism.

Persistent focal weakness, lateralized reflex abnormalities, or specific disorder such as aphasia are not parts of metabolic encephalopathy. However, when the onset of metabolic encephalopathy has been abrupt, transient focal changes may occur, especially in very young children. This is particularly so in hypoglycemia and, despite examples to the contrary, need not indicate associated cerebral vascular or structural brain pathology. Nevertheless, their persistence for more than a few hours in an adult patient who is presumed to have metabolic encephalopathy should alert the examiner to the possibility of an additional process, especially if the focal or lateralized defects are profound while the confusional or "encephalopathic" component is mild, or they persist while or after the metabolic irregularity is being or has been corrected. Disordered naming is a common feature of metabolic encephalopathies as well as numerous other brain disorders. This disorder of language function is identified by impairment of the capacity to recall or think of the names of objects, although the correct names are readily chosen from a list recited to the patient. Speech is fluent. Comprehension of spoken language and the ability to repeat test phrases are preserved. Other aphasic manifestations such as loss of fluency or auditory incomprehension are not seen in metabolic encephalopathy except when a focal lesion is also present.

Generalized weakness or asthenia may be found and there may be increased stretch reflexes. Spasticity, that is, exaggeration of shortening and lengthening reactions, does not occur. Grasp reflexes, perioral prehensile responses that are produced by tactile or visual stimulation of the lips or cheek, tonic foot (exaggerated plantar flexion and inversion of the foot after stroking the sole), or extensor plantar responses are common. Varying degrees of apparently willed resistance to passive limb manipulation (countermovements, or *gegenhalten*) may also be seen in the early stages of metabolic encephalopathy. Generalized tonic-clonic seizures fortunately are not terribly frequent. They are peculiar to no form of metabolic encephalopathy. While usually only one or two occur, occasional status epilepticus is encountered. Focal convulsions, especially when there is no derangement of the mental state, should raise the possibility of focal brain disease rather than metabolic encephalopathy. Decisions regarding additional diagnostic studies such as arteriography or computerized tomographic scanning should be based on the degree to which the issues requiring such definition are present.

With progressive disintegration of brain function, the patient will lapse more deeply into stupor. As he does so, the form of the clinical disorder becomes one in which cortical mechanisms are replaced by those that reflect activity of the diencephalon. The patient now is quiet and lies with his upper limbs flexed and the lower extended. Doll's head eye movements (oculocephalic reflexes) become exaggerated. These are readily elicited by turning the head smartly from side to side or up and down. The eyes seem to remain fixed on a point in space and thus appear to move opposite to the direction in which the head has been turned. The patient defends himself against painful or noxious stimulation by moving his hand toward it and attempting to remove it. As the encephalopathic process worsens, however, the patient may lapse into coma from which he cannot be aroused and may develop decerebrate postures in which his spine and limbs are extended firmly at the hips and shoulders. Lesser degrees of heightened muscle tone are found distally in the limbs, the fingers usually remaining loosely

flexed. Painful or noxious stimulation enhances the decerebrate state. Defense reactions are absent. As the patient further declines into coma, his limbs may become flaccid, and painful stimulation now leads to withdrawal of the leg. A characteristic feature of intoxication, especially with barbiturates, meprobamate, chloral hydrate, and glutethimide, is improvement in the neurologic examination upon handling. This may be documented by recording an electroencephalogram during stimulation and noting that diffuse slow waves are replaced by faster ones as the record becomes regionally different (desynchronization).

Autonomic function is affected to some extent in most patients with metabolic encephalopathy. The reactions of the pupils to light are preserved early in metabolic coma with the exception of states following the use of drugs that themselves affect the pupils. Morphine, heroin, and other opiates cause small or pinpoint, although still reactive, pupils that dilate upon the administration of an opiate antagonist. Glutethimide produces slightly dilated, usually fixed pupils. Scopolamine, atropine, or other anticholinergic drug poisoning is marked by dilated fixed pupils. Prolonged hypoxia may be associated with either very small or large, unreactive, and unequal pupils. The persistence of pupillary abnormalities of any sort following hypoxia usually indicates disorder of one or more portions of the brainstem, ordinarily adjacent to the aqueduct of Sylvius in the midbrain tegmentum. Body temperature regulation may also be altered. It is often reduced in hypothyroidism, after hypoglycemia, or after the ingestion or administration of barbiturates, anticholinergic drugs, salicylates, and combinations of antihistamines, phenothiazines, or meperidine. Agitated delirium, such as that associated with drug withdrawal, may result in marked increase in energy requirements and heat production. The hyperthermia is usually accompanied by some elevation of blood pressure, tachycardia, and profuse perspiration. Blood pressure regulation in many of the metabolic encephalopathies may be unstable, and in the case of agitated delirium, treatment designed to calm the patient may result in marked fall to levels that are inadequate for cerebral perfusion. Orthostatic postural or centrally mediated hypotension may accompany encephalopathy caused by drug ingestion, thiamine deficiency, hypoglycemia, or hypoxia. That following hypoxia may persist for several days and expose the patient to additional risk of ischemic brain damage. If the hypotension is of the "centrally" mediated variety, such compensatory phenomena as feeling faint and having dim vision, tingling lips and fingers, pallor, and tachycardia will be absent. There will be no warning.

Respiration is the most significant autonomic function affected in metabolic encephalopathy. A differential scheme of the respiratory abnormalities found in common clinical comas is found in Table 1. The usefulness of a respiratory disorder as a diagnostic aid is limited to those patients free of pre-existing disease of the lung or thoracic cage. The presence of the latter conditions or the simultaneous operation of multiple encephalopathic mechanisms further limit the utility of the scheme. In any approach to decompensation of brain function, respiratory patterns are likely to reflect physiologic derangements rather than specific disease states. The chief use of such a table is in helping identify encephalopathy resulting from metabolic acidosis, a potentially lethal state requiring prompt treatment.

The pattern of respiration in metabolic disorders depends on the degree to which systemic acid-base regulation has been disordered, the direction in which it is changing, the extent to which chemoreceptors are functioning, and the functional and structural integrity of the brainstem. Acidosis may occur in metabolic comas caused by uremia, diabetes (either ketoacidosis or lactic acidosis), hypoxia, or various forms of drug intoxication. Hyperventilation is its typical respiratory abnormality. In this condition the serum pH will be less than 7.3, the serum bicarbonate below 10 mEq per liter, and the $PaCO_2$ under 35 mm Hg. Hyperventilation may also result from respiratory alkalosis, but in that condition the serum pH is elevated and the bicarbonate between 15 and 30 mEq per liter. Respiratory alkalosis occurs in hepatic coma, certain forms of cardiopulmonary disease, salicylate poisoning, and bacterial endotoxic shock or sepsis and follows central neurogenic hyperventilation.

Hypoventilation may result from either metabolic alkalosis or respiratory acidosis. In the former state, the serum pH exceeds 7.45 and the serum bicarbonate 30 mEq per liter. It does not ordinarily cause severe encephalopathy. The conditions that cause it, including complications of diuretic therapy, hypokalemia of any cause, primary hyperaldosteronism, hyperadrenocorticism, and loss of gastric hydrochloric acid after prolonged vomiting, are usually self-evident or readily discovered. Respiratory acidosis is associated with serum pH of less than 7.35 but marked elevation of $PaCO_2$. The latter is invariably greater than 45 mm Hg and usually over 55. The serum bicarbonate is often elevated but this elevation cannot be relied upon; the level may be normal, especially after partial treatment. The PaO_2 is usually depressed. Re-

spiratory acidosis usually occurs in chronic pulmonary disease or peripheral respiratory failure secondary to acute or chronic neuromuscular disorder (infective polyneuritis or late muscular dystrophy), or poisoning with a depressant drug. When the former is the cause, the physical habitus and signs of chronic pulmonary disease or the pickwickian syndrome are usually present. The neuromuscular causes of peripheral failure should also be readily apparent. Hypoxia may complicate hypercarbia in cases of peripheral respiratory failure secondary to neuromuscular disorders or depressant drug poisoning.

DIFFERENTIATION FROM OTHER DISORDERS

Metabolic encephalopathy is usually obvious, as it develops in the context of general disease. It can generally be recognized quickly and accurately, although it may be confused with endogenous depression, mental retardation, primary dementia, endogenous encephalopathies, stroke, or intracranial mass lesions, especially bilateral subdural hematoma. It is usually readily distinguished from depression and mental retardation, because the thinking, behavior, and state of consciousness of the patient with metabolic encephalopathy have only recently become deranged, and the patient has earlier sought treatment for the underlying systemic disease. Neither depression nor retardation causes stupor. The mood of the patient with metabolic encephalopathy is usually labile rather than steadily depressed. There is evidence of prior mental attainment exceeding that to be expected in retardation. This may be established on mental state examination by noting the breadth of vocabulary, mental arithmetic ability, and a rich fund of information.

The adult retardate retains both the simplicity of affect and the intellect of the juvenile. He ordinarily cannot perform the operations of mental arithmetic. His fund of knowledge is limited to the features of his immediate environment. He usually cannot comprehend or comply with the command to reverse the order in which digits are spoken to him, though he may be able to repeat a series of up to 6 digits. The myoclonus and changes in reflexes, movement, posture, respiratory rate and rhythm, and size of pupils that are so likely to be part of metabolic encephalopathy do not occur in either case.

Conversely, the recent or recurrent decline in mood identifies the depressed patient. The onset of the disorder with a change in affect and mood is as important in the recognition of depression as is systemic disease in metabolic encephalopathy. Despite psychomotor retardation that may block responses, the depressed person is nevertheless clearly alert and without confusion or intellectual or neurologic abnormality. The retarded person is ordinarily alert and responsive although intellectually dull. The neurologic examination is normal except for evidence of ancient growth disturbance with or without movement disorder in the case of patients whose mental retardation arose from an encephaloclastic illness in childhood. This is not to say, however, that metabolic brain disorder cannot be superimposed upon either depression or mental retardation, especially when patients are given drugs aimed at modifying their behavior.

Stupor or coma attributable to hysteria is easily differentiated because of the patient's apparent state of well-being, history of emotional disorder or multiple mysterious illnesses, and ready response to suggestion. In hysterical, confusional, or amnestic states in which the patient remains responsive, the primary disorientation is for one's own name and location in space, leaving intact major intellectual functions. Metabolic parameters and the electroencephalogram are normal in unmedicated hysterical or other psychogenic states, although sustained hyperventilation may cause hypocapnia. The mental state in schizophrenia is marked by a sense of unreality, a thought disorder that is often paranoid, and somatic delusions. Hallucinations are highly systematized, continual, and often pleasurable. The neurologic examination in psychiatric disorders is either normal or marked by inconsistencies that help disclose the nature of the disorder. Asterixis and myoclonus are never present. If there is anxiety, some tremor may be seen, and schizophrenics may assume and maintain cataleptic postures or attitudes.

Dementing illnesses, such as Alzheimer's or Pick's disease, and endogenous disorders of brain metabolism that may or may not be associated with extraneural metabolic abnormalities (Wilson's disease, cerebral lipidoses) should be thought of as primary disorders of brain function or metabolism. Patients with these disorders can readily be separated from those patients in whom metabolic encephalopathy complicates disease that is primary outside the nervous system. The history is generally longer and often subtler. Stigmata such as the Kayser-Fleischer ring or sebaceous adenoma may be present. Grave acute biochemical disorders such as hypoglycemia, hypoxia, metabolic acidosis, or renal or liver failure are usually absent in the early part of the illness when neurologic manifestations are emerging. The demented patient ordinarily is alert and displays far more loss of intellect and much less agitation and

personal disorientation. His major defects are in memory, affect, language, and cognitive and conative function. Autonomic and respiratory disorders are absent in both types of primary brain disease. Motor disorders usually occur late in Alzheimer's disease and senile dementia, although they are prominent in Huntington's and Wilson's diseases. Myoclonus, although present, is usually less important than choreoathetosis, and asterixis is usually absent until late.

Stroke may be confused with metabolic encephalopathy when the effect has been to produce a short-lived disturbance that primarily affects behavior, such as transient global amnesia or cortical blindness. The sudden emergence of a highly characteristic disorder when the patient has otherwise been well and the finding of normal or only slightly altered blood chemistries serve to identify this type of disorder. Since most of these states are transient, their rapid resolution often answers the question of their nature. Seizures, myoclonus, and asterixis are unusual.

Chronic infections may present with myoclonus, loss of intellectual function, seizures, headache, and stiff neck. The frequency of the last three features and the absence of asterixis or autonomic abnormality should lead one away from metabolic encephalopathy. Spinal fluid examination usually settles the issue.

Intracranial mass lesions (abscess, hematoma, brain tumors, or normal pressure hydrocephalus) may produce serious problems in differentiation, especially when one is trying to identify a bilateral and more or less symmetric subdural hematoma in an elderly or alcoholic person. Patients with intracranial space-occupying lesions may be either stuporous or tremulous or display many of the postural and motor changes present in metabolic encephalopathy. They often suffer some metabolic derangement, especially if the brain lesion is metastatic and the primary tumor produces a false hormone, resulting in hyponatremia or hypoglycemia. Treatment of the latter may result in change, including worsening of the neurologic disorder. Autonomic and ventilatory irregularities and asterixis are usually absent, whereas focal seizures, lateralized neurologic deficits, headache, abnormalities seen in the computerized tomography (CT) scan, and raised spinal fluid pressure are common features of these progressive illnesses. There is often evidence of cancer elsewhere or a history of recent trauma followed by altered behavior. Signs of injury may be found on the body or head. If the intracranial mass lesion has arisen in the posterior fossa, there are usually abnormalities of eye movement or the lower cranial nerves, phenomena that are rarely encountered in metabolic disorders except in the context of chronic malnutrition and thiamine depletion with alcoholism. There is usually no evidence of significant or recently decompensated extrinsic disease except cancer, and the metabolic parameters in the blood and urine are usually normal or nearly so in intracranial mass lesions. The performance of diagnostic procedures such as a CT or nuclide scan or arteriogram may be required to resolve doubtful cases. In view of the importance of early application of appropriate treatment for subdural hematoma, diagnostic study should not be delayed once the suspicion has arisen.

Approach to Diagnosis

The successful diagnosis of metabolic encephalopathy requires thorough attention to the history and physical examination and a reasonable amount of shrewdness in using clinical clues. One should suspect drug ingestion if a previously physically well but psychologically disturbed patient has been brought to the hospital, having been discovered in stupor or coma. Since most patients with metabolic encephalopathy have developed the disease in the context of recognizable antecedent extraneural disease, diagnosis in such a known case is not difficult. The history and general physical examination in unknown cases should focus on data that might indicate underlying hepatic, renal, cardiac, endocrine, or pulmonary disease. In hepatic encephalopathy, for example, signs of present or past liver decompensation including jaundice, ascites, spider nevi, periumbilical venous distention or hum, hemorrhoids, and palmar erythema are evident. The uremic patient is likely to be hypertensive, may display some degree of albuminuric retinopathy, frequently has had one or several seizures, and may be without ankle reflexes. Patients with cerebral ischemia or hypoxia secondary to heart disease often have hypertensive stigmata, cardiac enlargement, bradyarrhythmia or tachyarrhythmia, or signs of congestive failure. Pulmonary disease is usually evident with rales, an abnormal chest configuration, cyanosis, or obesity.

The neurologic signs that are of most critical importance in diagnosis, differentiation among the clinical forms, and assessment of the risks to the brain are, in order of importance, (1) the pattern of respiration; (2) nature and depth of the disorder of consciousness and accompanying mental and intellectual abnormalities; (3) seizures, grasp reflexes, myoclonus, asterixis, focal neurologic deficit, and the posture of the limbs; and (4) the nature of the pupillary response to light. In metabolic encephalopathy the neurologic signs do not usually point to a single anatomic locus but do in focal diseases of the brain. Moreover, they rarely show the cause of the encephalopathy or coma. The hemogram, fasting blood sugar, bilirubin, blood urea nitrogen (BUN), serum bicarbonate, and electrolytes, including Na, K, Mg, CA, P, and Cl, should be drawn as soon as the patient is encountered and should be processed during his initial examination. Since many hospital laboratories now encompass these values in multiple serial determinations, the commonly used SMA12 and SMA6 are adequate. When there is evidence of liver disease on physical examination or the bilirubin is found elevated on SMA12, serum ammonia should be obtained. In the event that any respiratory abnormality is observed, especially in the presence of any form of hyperventilation, arterial blood gases and pH should be obtained.

Whenever there is the least suspicion that the patient has ingested a drug, blood and urine samples should be obtained for multiple drug screening, and the gastric content removed with a large-bore tube and inspected for drug or other toxic particles. Respiratory alkalosis combined with metabolic acidosis, especially in a child, may mean salicylate ingestion, which may be verified by adding $FeCl_3$ to boiled urine and observing purplish discoloration.

An electrocardiogram should be obtained in every patient. The chest, skull, and cervical spine should be examined by x-ray. Signs of possible head injury should be noted, but hypoxia secondary to traumatic pleural effusion or pulmonary contusion should not be confused with respiratory depression occurring as a primary effect of head injury or concomitant upper spinal cord injury. In the latter case only a good lateral film is needed. In head trauma with altered consciousness, a CT scan should be obtained. Urinalysis should be obtained in comatose patients, by intermittent catheterization if necessary. It is our practice to examine the cerebrospinal fluid in every patient whose case is nontraumatic without papilledema, especially when the patient is febrile, as the diagnosis and treatment of bacterial meningitis should not be delayed. Every deeply stuporous or comatose patient should receive 50 ml of 50 per cent glucose as soon as blood has been drawn and before detailed examination, as hypoglycemic coma should be reversed as quickly as possible. This amount of glucose will do nothing to obscure the diagnosis of any other condition.

The electroencephalogram may be useful because rather characteristic wave patterns are seen in some forms of metabolic stupor. Performing an electroencephalogram should not, however, take priority over examination of the blood, urine, or spinal fluid or such imaging procedures as chest x-ray. The electroencephalogram is not particularly helpful in establishing the diagnosis in acute metabolic disorders. It may, however, be useful in identifying more chronic states, in following the course of an illness, in identifying episodic phenomena, or in quantifying the effect of treatment.

The electroencephalogram in most forms of metabolic encephalopathy is characterized by generalized and more or less symmetric slow waves. As consciousness becomes degraded, the record becomes slower, and the activity increasingly synchronous. It is often quite severely affected in diabetic, hypoglycemic, and uremic and hepatic encephalopathies. Among these the electroencephalogram in the encephalopathies is most likely to be helpful. Triphasic periodic slow waves usually first appear symmetrically, bilaterally, and frontally, extending caudally as the process worsens. The distribution of such waves in the posterior parts of the head bears a direct relationship to the severity of the illness. There may be relatively well-preserved posterior alpha activity when the frontal region is quite abnormal. Uncommonly in hepatic encephalopathy the slow activity begins occipitally or temporally. In both hypoglycemic and diabetic acidosis the diffusely slow electroencephalogram becomes normal upon correction of the metabolic abnormality. In the former the resolution is usually so rapid that infusion of glucose during electroencephalographic recording results in reversion of the record to normal within less than a minute. In hypoadrenal, hyposmolar, and hyponatremic states the electroencephalogram is usually slow with little or no activity faster than 7 Hz. The finding of any waking rhythm greater than 12 Hz should make one doubt that the encephalopathy is of these causes. Myxedema and hypopituitarism with secondary myxedema are also associated with slowing to less than 7 Hz. Hypercalcemia and hypocalcemia may both cause slow patterns, the latter condition often causing paroxysmal discharges. The electroencephalogram may also be excessively slowed in other electrolyte disorders and porphyria. For the most part the electroencephalogram reflects a failure of cortical activation rather than a specific illness.

The CT and brain scans have little place in the diagnosis of acute metabolic encephalopathy, especially when the patient is comatose, but may be of great value in chronic cases, particularly when such conditions as tumor, subdural hematoma, or normal pressure hydrocephalus are considerations.

PARTICULAR FORMS OF METABOLIC ENCEPHALOPATHY

Metabolic encephalopathy associated with hypoxia results from reduced arterial oxygen partial pressure (anoxic anoxia), oxygen-carrying capacity of the blood (anemic anoxia), or the reduction of cerebral blood flow (stagnant or ischemic anoxia). When chronic, the condition is characterized by delirium or stupor, confusion, hallucination, and seizures. The pupils are usually small but reactive, and breathing is periodic. When acute and severe, consciousness may be lost within a few seconds, and seizures and myoclonus are common, along with "decerebrate" postures. The arterial oxygen tensions are low, as are the cerebral venous oxygen tensions, indicating maximal extraction of oxygen by the blood. Reduced or negligible arteriovenous oxygen differences occur with advanced neuronal loss and are an indication of "brain death." If hypoxia is the consequence of chest disease, the latter always requires specific treatment. This form of encephalopathy may complicate pneumonia, neuromuscular disease, spinal cord injury, contusion of the lung, and multiple rib fractures, among a broad variety of conditions. It often begins with headache, restlessness, and hallucinosis. Common causes of ischemia are reduced cardiac output or intracranial vaso-occlusive conditions, which reduce cerebral blood flow by raising cerebral vascular resistance. Raised intracranial pressure may also reduce cerebral blood flow.

Hypoglycemia as a cause of encephalopathy, stupor, or coma is often readily evident, as the patient frequently is a known diabetic who has been receiving insulin or, more often, an elderly person who has been using an oral agent. The long-acting insulins appear far more likely to cause trouble in patients who eat poorly and are ill nourished with inadequate carbohydrate reserves. The hypoglycemic patient is usually confused and displays delirium or stupor that may last several minutes or hours before the patient lapses into coma. The postures of "decortication" and the movements of athetosis may precede deeper coma, with its signs of "decerebration." Some patients with hypoglycemia develop sharply focal or lateralized neurologic signs. Others have either focal or general convulsions or develop myoclonus. Focal deficits or seizures often indicate pre-existing or associated structural brain disease.

Metabolic acidosis announces itself by the development of hyperventilation. Its presence

Table 1. *Differentiation of Common Forms of Metabolic Encephalopathy*

Type	Features	Respiration	Laboratory
I. Exogenous poisons	Known user; flask or container found		
	a. Stupor or coma—often "sleep-like"; pupils may be small and reactive (opiates) or fixed and large (glutethimide, anticholinergics); odor of alcohol may be present; hypothermia with barbiturates, phenothiazine; nystagmus, ocular palsy with thiamine deficiency in alcoholic	Depressed	Serum pH less than 7.35, $PaCO_2$ less than 45 mm Hg; serum bicarbonate 20–30 mEq/L; drug detected in blood or urine
	b. Methyl alcohol, ethylene glycol, decomposed paraldehyde odor on breath or body in a stuporous or comatose person	Hyperventilation	Serum pH less than 7.3, $PaCO_2$ less than 35 mm Hg; serum bicarbonate less than 10 mEq/L
	Salicylates		
	c. Fever; stupor or coma, often in a child; if awake, may complain of dizziness or ringing in ears; history of chronic salicylate usage	Hyperventilation	Purple color generated by adding $FeCl_3$ to boiled urine; features of respiratory alkalosis; serum pH over 7.45, $PaCO_2$ less than 30 mm Hg, and serum bicarbonate 10–15 mEq/L
II. Metabolic acidosis	Acute coma in a uremic, diabetic (ketoacidosis or lactic acidosis), anoxia intoxication (see b above)	Hyperventilation	Serum pH less than 7.3, $PaCO_2$ less than 35 mm Hg, and serum bicarbonate less than 10 mEq/L; PO_2 under 50 mm Hg separates anoxic from spontaneous lactic acidosis
III. Hepatic encephalopathy	Signs of liver disease marked; asterixis, myoclonus prominent; may be decerebrate in deep coma	Hyperventilation	Bilirubin, NH_3 raised; EEG shows triphasic slow complexes; bicarbonate between 15–25 mEq/L with pH over 7.45 and $PaCO_2$ less than 30 mm Hg
IV. Uremic encephalopathy	Known renal disease; reflexes often reduced; uremic odor and frost; asterixis, myoclonus, seizures prominent	Hyperventilation	BUN over 50 mg per 100 ml; albumin, casts in urine; metabolic acidosis present (q.v.)
V. CO_2 narcosis or hypercarbic encephalopathy	Deformed, emphysematous chest, rales; cyanosis; clubbed fingers; occasional papilledema; often obese; slow respiratory rate	Hypoventilation	Serum pH less than 7.35; $PaCO_2$ greater than 45 mm Hg; PO_2 less than 40 mm Hg; serum bicarbonate 20–40 mEq/L, higher values in chronic forms
VI. Endocrinopathies: pituitary, thyroid, parathyroid, adrenal, pancreatic	Deep coma possible, especially in myxedema, but not the rule; signs of primary endocrine disorder often prominent or known; usually not primary presentation of underlying disorder; common clinical causes are abandonment of replacement therapy; especially in myxedema and stress or steroid withdrawal in first- or second-degree adrenal insufficiency	Respiration usually normal except in adrenal insufficiency where hypoventilation prominent	Hormonal abnormality on specific testing; CT scan, skull x-ray abnormal in pituitary disease; renal stones in hyperparathyroidism; metabolic acidosis (pH over 7.45, $PaCO_2$ under 55 mm Hg, and serum bicarbonate over 30 mEq/L with hypokalemia) in hyperadrenocorticism
VII. Hypoxia or anoxia	Cyanotic; cherry red (CO poison); purplish lips (methemoglobinemia); occurs with pulmonary disease, oxygen-poor environment (anoxic form), anemia, or hemoglobin inactivation (CO poisoning or methemoglobinemia); often history of use of acetophenetidin (anemic form)	Hyperventilation	Anoxic form—PO_2, O_2 saturation low; anemic form—PO_2 normal, saturation low or normal; anemia—CO hemoglobin, methemoglobin in blood
VIII. Ischemia (defective oxygen delivery plus accumulation of metabolic by-products)	Results from any condition which may lower cerebral blood flow, especially cardiac arrhythmia, myocardial or pulmonary infarction, shock, sepsis, congestive heart failure, vasospasm in hypertensive or lead encephalopathy, fat embolism to lung	Usually hyperventilation, but breaths may be shallow; arrest of respiration may occur	PO_2, O_2 saturation may be normal; ECG abnormal; enzymes elevated in serum; PO_2, CO_2 decreased, lung scan positive in pulmonary embolism; raised intracranial pressure and CSF protein in lead, hypertension; fat globules in urine, sputum in fat embolism

Table 1. *Differentiation of Common Forms of Metabolic Encephalopathy* (Continued)

Type	Features	Respiration	Laboratory
IX. Hypoglycemia	Vast majority in diabetics receiving oral agents or insulin; may be abrupt or slow; usually recurrent; delirium-stupor, focal weakness, focal or generalized seizures, decerebration; reversed rapidly by 50 ml 50% glucose intravenously	Central neurogenic hyperventilation or Cheyne-Stokes respiration	Blood sugar less than 30 mg per 100 ml
X. Derangements of ionic equilibrium or serum osmolality	Delirium, stupor, weakness, seizures; may be seen following diuresis, excess water intake, and inadequate solute intake, especially after tap water enema or use of "water" diuresis, feeding of excess electrolyte, or hyperglycemia in diabetic or burned patients without ketosis; hypercalcemia may be seen in bone-destructive or chronic renal disease	Unaltered or hypoventilation	Na, K, Ca, Mg lowered or raised with appropriate abnormality of serum osmolality (less than 260 mOsm/L or more than 320); ECG in hypokalemia shows sagging ST segment, depressed T waves, elevated U waves

is readily confirmed by laboratory studies (Table 1). Although it is not the most frequent cause of metabolic encephalopathy, it requires urgent treatment as it can be lethal and delays permit increasingly severe cell injury and irreversible neuronal loss. Patients with metabolic coma of acute onset should be regarded as suffering hypoxia, hypoglycemia, and metabolic acidosis until proved otherwise. Physical examination, blood gas determination, and serum electrolyte measurement should lead quickly to the correct diagnosis and treatment.

Hepatic encephalopathy may appear as an apathetic stupor or agitated delirium and include any variety of abnormalities of consciousness, mental state, or posture, including "decerebration." Respiratory alkalosis with hyperventilation is seen commonly when such patients are stuporous. Grasp reflexes are usual, and the disorder is frequently marked by widespread asterixis. In chronic hepatocerebral disease gross and often irreversible abnormalities of mental state may be combined with chronic choreoathetosis. The serum ammonia in acute forms is usually raised, and the chemical changes of respiratory alkalosis are present. The serum ammonia level, however, does not always parallel the neurologic state. The cerebrospinal fluid is normal and does not contain bilirubin unless there has been an inflammatory meningeal disorder that alters the blood-brain barrier or the serum bilirubin has been over 5 mg per 100 ml for several days. Elevated spinal fluid protein may indicate alternative or additional pathology such as subdural hematoma.

Uremic encephalopathy may present as stupor or coma and is ordinarily associated with hyperventilation and metabolic acidosis. It is one form of metabolic encephalopathy in which the tendon reflexes may be diminished or absent owing to its common association with uremic polyneuropathy. The clinical signs are stupor proceeding to coma, shifting focal neurologic deficits, widespread myoclonus, and convulsions, although agitation and delirium may be present early. The common laboratory findings, in addition to those of serum acidosis, include varying degrees of azotemia. The level of azotemia and its rate of change appear to have little to do with the mental or neurologic disorder. It would seem that intracellular metabolic changes are not wholly reflected by fluctuations in the level of blood urea nitrogen. The cerebrospinal fluid appearance, pressure, and content are usually normal in uremia. Uremic meningitis occurs occasionally, the spinal fluid containing up to 500 cells of mixed type. Such patients may have a stiff neck. Elevation of spinal fluid pressure and papilledema are not part of uremic encephalopathy. Their presence usually indicates other processes such as hypertensive encephalopathy or water intoxication complicating renal dialysis. The latter may be inferred from the finding of hyponatremia or identified by serum osmolality of less than 260 mOsm per liter.

Since the uremic patient is usually hypertensive, the problem of differentiating uremic encephalopathy from that of hypertension is significant, as the therapies are quite different. Uremia is often associated with peripheral neuropathy and reduced reflexes. Hypertension is not. The reflexes in this state are likely to be exaggerated. The blood urea nitrogen (BUN) is nearly always quite high in uremia. This is less often so in hypertensive encephalopathy. Multifocal myoclonus and asterixis are common in uremia but unusual in hypertensive encephalopathy. Fleeting focal neurologic deficits, papilledema, unilateral or bilateral hemianopias, raised cerebrospinal fluid pressure and protein, and diastolic blood pressure over 120 mm Hg are the key features of hypertensive encephalopathy.

Hypercarbic encephalopathy or CO_2 narcosis ordinarily occurs against a background of chronic pulmonary disease. It frequently evolves slowly and runs a relapsing course characterized by marked hypoventilation, dull diffuse headache with or without intermittent drowsiness especially after meals, papilledema, and the blood chemical changes of respiratory acidosis. Most patients are cyanotic. Myoclonus, asterixis, and muscular irritability are common. Cerebrospinal fluid pressures may be very high, but the cell count and total protein are ordinarily normal. Acute decompensation of pulmonary function and the development of stupor are likely to follow pulmonary infection or the administration of sedative drugs. Many patients with chronic encephalopathy use bromides or other drugs that modify behavior or in other ways cause metabolic changes that obscure the clinical picture. Several other factors may be present, such as cerebral vascular disease or senility.

Alteration, especially when rapid, of the ionic environment or acid-base equilibrium may also alter the function of the nervous system, producing changes in alertness, muscle strength, orientation, and posture. When the ionic content of the serum has fallen, it is said to have become hypo-osmolar. Water flows into the electrolyte-rich brain from the ion-depleted serum in states of hypo-osmolality, thus resulting in brain swelling, with stupor, headache, disorientation, and eventually coma with brainstem decompensation. The reverse occurs when the serum electrolyte content becomes increased in relation to that of the brain, dehydration of which may be associated with delirium and agitation. If extreme, it can result in subpial hemorrhage, seizures, coma, and death. These events are more common in infants and are risks of the treatment of cerebral edema by osmolar diuresis. As a general rule, neurologic symptoms occur when there are sudden shifts in serum osmolality, regardless of the initial level, as slow shifts may be "compensated for" by incompletely understood mechanisms that enable the patient to tolerate quite abnormal levels of osmolality. Neurologic symptoms thus are more likely to result from abrupt shifts occurring during the course of treatment. Serum

osmolality may be calculated from clinical chemical data approximately as follows:

$$mOsm/liter = 2(Na + K) + \frac{glucose}{18} + \frac{BUN}{2.8}$$

The normal range is 285 to 295 mOsm per liter.

Hyperosmolar states result from water depletion, as in diarrhea, or from lower water intake than required by the amount of solutes consumed. They commonly reflect elevation of the serum sodium. The osmolality may exceed 320 to 330 mOsm per liter. "Hyperglycemic hyperosmolar nonketotic coma" occurs in elderly diabetics or those diabetics whose disease is untreated or neglected, or in patients after severe burns. The blood sugar may exceed 1000 mg per 100 ml and is always above 400 mg per 100 ml, thus adding 25 to 55 mOsm per liter to the serum values. The patients are usually stuporous rather than comatose. They often have convulsions. Symptoms remit upon hydration and use of isotonic saline solution followed by small amounts of insulin. Too rapid treatment may lead to cerebral water intoxication and may convert a stuporous confused state in a patient to lethal coma.

Hypo-osmolar states — "water intoxication" — may result from absolute or relative hyponatremia and may be the consequence of overzealous treatment of hyperosmolar states. The accumulation of fluid in the brain is followed by decreased intracellular potassium and extracellular sodium. When serum osmolality falls below 260 mOsm per liter, these ionic shifts enhance neuronal excitability, which is believed to result in seizures, delirium, and coma. The clinical conditions that result in this state include the replacement of sodium-containing body fluid by water, the use of diuretics, especially in the elderly, and severe renal disease. Tap water enemas in the preparation of infants or elderly patients for x-ray studies or the treatment of fecal impaction may be iatrogenic causes for water intoxication. Less commonly, inappropriate ADH production, adrenal insufficiency, hypothyroidism, excessive ingestion of water for psychic reasons, and renal dialysis are responsible.

Hypercalcemia occurring in chronic renal disease, sarcoid, metastases to bone, and other conditions may cause subacute dementia of nonspecific type, headache, and occasionally delusions of persecution. Moreover, in conditions that vary, as chronic renal disease, symptoms may remit and then return. Primary or secondary hypocalcemia may also present with a dementia, recurrent seizures, especially in children, and papilledema. Both these conditions should be identifiable through initial blood chemistry.

It often happens that the diagnosis of the specific form of metabolic encephalopathy is unclear, as the disorder in any given patient may result from multiple recurrent causes. This is especially likely when one is dealing with an elderly patient whose brain bears the changes of senile dementia or vascular disease and who suffers a degree of anoxia with the accumulation of tissue metabolites secondary to ischemia resulting from concurrent heart failure and whose restlessness has been treated inappropriately with diazepam or chlordiazepoxide and who has then acquired a diuretic-induced electrolyte disorder. The important rule in metabolic encephalopathy regardless of severity is to recognize that a neurologic disorder characterized by altered consciousness and impaired mental and motor function may belong to a class of illness that is metabolic and separate from structural disease. In each case the lethal factors that should receive first diagnostic and therapeutic consideration are hypoxia, hypoglycemia, and metabolic acidosis. In the presence of fever, intracranial infection must be excluded. When nystagmus or ocular palsy is present, thiamine deficiency should be considered. If these principles are kept in mind, the reversible lethal causes will be dealt with early, leaving adequate time to refine the diagnosis in safety.

BRAIN ABSCESSES

By EDWIN B. BOLDREY, M.D.
San Francisco, California

A brain abscess is a localized, more or less circumscribed collection of pus within the brain formed by disintegrated cerebral tissue, white blood cells, and the causative organisms. The abscess is usually encapsulated, although the degree of encapsulation varies widely, depending upon the virulence of the infecting organism and the resistance of the host. Focal brain injury, as from physical trauma, infected embolism, or septic thrombus, is essential to the development of the lesion. A nidus is thus provided in which may grow any of the pyogenic bacteria as well as yeasts, fungi, or, rarely, other organisms such as Protozoa.

The abscess may develop as the direct result of trauma such as that following a compound depressed skull fracture or in-driven foreign material — missiles, skin, hair, clothing, and dirt. The criteria of injured brain and contaminating pyogen are then fulfilled.

Head injury without fracture but resulting in subdural or epidural collections of blood may give rise to pyogenic empyema, usually through hematogenous conveyance from inadequately treated infected sites adjacent or elsewhere in the body. Pyogenic collections in this space also occur on occasion in association with meningitis — especially in children.

Although occurring less frequently now than in the past, infection from the accessory air sinuses of the skull, including the frontal, the ethmoid, the sphenoid, and the mastoid, may give rise to abscess. The usual sequence is that of septic venous thrombosis advancing retrograde into the brain — cerebrum or cerebellum — causing a focus of softening that contains bacteria and thus initiates the suppurative process. Direct extension of infection from an osteomyelitic skull may act similarly. In these situations the junction of the gray and white matter is the most common site of insult leading to abscess formation. No portion of the brain, however, is immune.

An infected embolism is the most common cause of abscess in the patient with congenital heart disease, pulmonary arteriovenous malformation, or any infection in the thoracic cage in which the filtering mechanism of the lung is bypassed. In this latter circumstance multiple abscesses are not uncommon.

Patients on an immunosuppressive regimen — for example, that following organ transplant — must be regarded as susceptible to brain abscess. The resistance of the host is then so impaired that even minor disruption of the blood-brain barrier may lead to a focal inflammatory process, which, if untreated, is followed by localized breakdown and suppuration.

The septic process having been initiated, the brain reacts by the development at a distance of a response involving capillaries and associated neuroglia and microglia, white blood cells, and fibroblasts. Brain tissue within this general and initially relatively indefinite perimeter soon reaches the stage in which it will be sacrificed. Generally in the cerebrum the process advances more rapidly into the white matter than into the gray, the gray having comparatively greater resistance probably because of its inherent vascularity. The gray matter is thinner at the depth of a sulcus than at the crown, and any breakthrough to the pia and the subarachnoid space is more likely to occur here.

Migration to the ventricular wall may occur; the abscess wall there is generally thinner than elsewhere. This is important because of the potential rupture of abscess contents into the ventricle following disruption of this wall after any environmental change, particularly that of reduced intraventricular pressure.

The brain's defense in the cerebellum is less, generally, than in the cerebrum and carries greater hazard to the patient because of the folial pattern with its crevices providing increased opportunity for spread of infection, because of a more delicately constituted pia and because of the vitally important adjacent brain stem, involvement of which by any inflammatory process carries a high morbidity and mortality.

There is generally some diffuse inflammation associated with the development of an abscess above or below the tentorium, and because of the relative size and importance of the contents this process is tolerated less satisfactorily in the posterior fossa.

The most common first sign of abscess is headache. However, in close subsequence are such items as convulsive seizures, drowsiness, personality change, disturbance in vision of both acuity and field, and all of these in association with current or recent potential source of infection under circumstances such as those delineated above, which, then, should lead to the suspicion of presence of a developing intracranial suppurative process. Unilateral motor or cortical sensory deficit should be included, as well as manifestations of cerebellar dysfunction. The condition is that of a space-occupying intracranial lesion, and the question of abscess is based upon a recognized potential source of pyogen. Particular emphasis must be placed upon the role of congenital heart disease or conditions of immunosuppression. Any disturbance of nervous system function in such a patient should lead to a thorough investigation relative to the possibility of abscess. These abscesses have been found to have reached tremendous size before making their presence known or, in the past, even suspected. The sudden appearance of a central nervous system disturbance in this group of patients must be regarded as being due to brain abscess until proved otherwise.

Headache as an early sign is usually lateralized or localized, and results from irritation of the adjacent meninges. Generalized headache is more commonly late and follows an increase of intracranial pressure.

Convulsive seizures result from the irritation of the brain cortex either from within or without, as in the case of subdural or even epidural empyema. The description of the seizure should lead one to the general vicinity of the lesion. The findings on clinical neurologic examination are those related to the locale. Later manifestations such as that of paralysis of function — motor, cortical, sensory, or visual — may be identified. Cerebellar abscess, particularly that following contiguous petrositis, may become manifest through disruption of coordination or of hearing.

The unattended abscess usually produces an increase in intracranial pressure early and will lead to imposition upon the aforementioned signs of such findings as papilledema, increasing drowsiness, stupor, or coma.

At times, abscess may be associated with meningitis, usually as a precursor, although also potentially as a result of the breakdown of encapsulation or the spread of pyogens into the ventricle or subarachnoid space. Under these circumstances resistance to cervical flexion or a positive Kernig sign may be present. The presence of either of these substantiates the suspicion that there is inflammatory craniospinal disease, but is of limited value in establishing a specific diagnosis of abscess. Spinal puncture should probably be withheld until other procedures, mentioned in the following paragraphs, have been utilized, if the clinical suspicion of the lesion has been raised.

A general history and physical examination is essential to the investigation of any clinical process, and that ultimately leading to the diagnosis of abscess is no exception.

Clinical laboratory studies such as blood counts are helpful if positive but may be misleading. Brain abscess may be present with a completely normal white blood cell count, and elevation usually means the presence of some other pathologic process in addition to the infection within the cranial cavity. The same may be said for the sedimentation rate. Seldom do these tests become a significantly determining factor in the diagnosis of the disease.

Plain skull films are usually obtained if the patient's condition is such as to allow time for this more deliberate approach to diagnosis. One would be searching for evidence then of infection in the accessory air sinuses or, rarely, over the convexity. Evidence of occult fracture in a patient incapable of giving an accurate history can also be found in plain skull x-rays. Manifestations of chronic intracranial pressure are uncommon with the usual acute abscess because of the speed of development of the disease process. The rare abscess of such chronicity as to permit erosion of the dorsum sellae will probably not be diagnosed properly until surgical intervention has been carried out.

The electroencephalogram may be helpful in the slowly progressing abscess, particularly when there has been a presenting symptom of localized headache or convulsive seizures. Focal electroencephalographic disturbance will help substantiate clinical manifestations of a local irritative process.

Pneumoencephalography — particularly by ventriculogram — has been helpful in the past. As the radioactive isotope scan or the computerized tomogram becomes more available, the use of pneumoencephalography will be progressively lessened. There may still be occasions when it will be required to identify precisely the location of a lesion so that the treatment with least morbidity may be planned. When turning to pneumography, however, it must be borne in mind that there is disruption of the balance of pressures within and outside the fluid-filled spaces that can lead to disruption of a thin-walled pus collection, soiling the adjacent fluid-filled space and potentially leading to complications or meningitis and/or even more particularly ventriculitis. Pneumography cannot be eliminated, but its value must be regarded as on a diminishing course.

Angiograms are helpful when these can be carried out without compromise of apparent increased intracranial pressure. In using this diagnostic device it must be remembered that the posterior fossa as well as the cerebral hemisphere and basal ganglia may contain this space-occupying lesion, that abscess may be multiple, and that therefore four vessel studies are in general indicated.

The radioactive isotope scan is a relatively innocuous procedure; it has become of particular value in identifying the presence of a focal space-occupying lesion that has disturbed the blood-brain barrier. This scan will not differentiate between abscess and neoplasm. Its value as a diagnostic tool, however, has progressively increased with sophistication of technique and interpretation of the findings.

The computerized tomogram (CT) has added tremendously to the early identification of abscess as well as any other space-occupying intracranial lesion. With time this complicated, expensive, but extremely valuable device will be used more and more frequently in situations in which the index of suspicion has heretofore been low. It has been of particular value in identifying multiple and multiloculated conditions. Undoubtedly it will add in a particular way to our knowledge of the natural history of the process.

Brain abscess must be preceded by focal cerebritis — that is, inflammation without actual breakdown of tissue leading to the accumulation of pus. The early consideration of this possibility in patients known to be carrying a high incidence of risk may, through the CT scan

or radioactive isotope scan, lead to recognition of early focal cerebritis and potentially to the institution of a therapeutic regimen that could block the development of tissue breakdown. When the probable source of infection permits, antibiotic therapy may be instituted and the otherwise potentially devastating sequelae of a developed abscess may be avoided.

The use of these techniques also has great value in following the results of therapy — surgical, medical, or a combination of the two.

In summary, a brain abscess is a space-occupying lesion within the cranium that entails an injury to the brain and is the source of pyogenic organism. Differential diagnosis must include neoplasm and hematoma as well as idiopathic intracranial hypertension and encephalitis.

There are certain patients in whom any evidence of progressive, acute or subacute, cerebral or cerebellar disease demands, at an early stage, a high index of suspicion that an abscess may be present. These include patients who have a history of physical trauma to, or infection involving, the skull or its air sinuses; those who have a known condition permitting elimination of the filtering mechanism of the lung; and those who have lowered tissue resistance such as that associated with immunosuppression.

ASEPTIC MENINGITIS AND VIRAL MENINGITIS

By DONALD M. McLEAN, M.D.
Vancouver, British Columbia, Canada

SYNONYMS

Acute lymphocytic meningitis, benign lymphocytic choriomeningitis, nonbacterial meningitis, serous meningitis, viral meningoencephalitis.

DEFINITION

Acute viral inflammation of the meninges, principally affecting the pia and arachnoid membranes, induces elaboration of excess cerebrospinal fluid (CSF), which is rich in leukocytes, principally lymphocytes, but the glucose and protein contents remain virtually unchanged. Headache and neck stiffness, usually accompanied by vomiting and fever, comprise the usual range of clinical manifestations. Mumps and enteroviruses are the common causative agents in aseptic meningitis.

Presenting Signs and Symptoms

There is sudden onset of severe frontal or parietal headache, usually accompanied by vomiting, and fever of 38 to 40 C (100 to 104 F). Neck and spine stiffness are noted shortly thereafter. Convulsions may signify the onset in about 15 per cent of children with mumps meningitis and in somewhat fewer patients with enteroviral meningitis. Usually medical attention is sought 12 to 24 hours after onset, at which time lumbar puncture is performed to reveal clear to cloudy CSF containing 30 to 3000 or more leukocytes per cu mm, the majority of which are lymphocytes.

Course

In mumps meningitis, temperature elevations above 38 C (100 F) usually persist for 2 to 4 days, but in 25 per cent of patients fever may persist 5 to 7 days. Abatement of symptoms, including headache, vomiting, and neck stiffness, often occurs within 6 hours of lumbar puncture when this is performed early in the illness. Enteroviral meningitis runs a similar course.

Mumps meningitis has been encountered during all months of the year, with an increased incidence during winter and spring. Enteroviral meningitis usually occurs only during summer and autumn.

Physical Examination Findings

Obvious neck stiffness is usually accompanied by the tripod sign. Kernig's and/or Brudzinski's signs are positive. Usually the skeletal musculature shows normal power and tone. In mumps meningitis, the incidence of illness in males exceeds that in females by 2:1 or greater, but in enteroviral meningitis the sex ratio is 1:1.

Common Complications

Mumps meningitis may develop from 6 days before to 14 days after the onset of swelling of the parotid or submandibular salivary glands or both, but 25 to 33 per cent of patients with virologically confirmed disease may exhibit meningitis without parotitis. Meningitis may be accompanied by other systemic manifestations of mumps virus infection, including pancreatitis when there is severe upper midline abdominal pain accompanied by a transient increase of serum amylase, unilateral or bilateral orchitis, or oophoritis manifested by lower abdominal pain. Hyperpyrexia may be accompanied by temporary mental confusion. Transient monoplegia or quadriplegia has been observed occasionally. Dehydration and electrolyte imbalance may result from protracted vomiting.

Enteroviral meningitis, especially that caused by echovirus-9, may be accompanied by a maculopapular rash in 33 per cent of patients. This rash shows a peripheral distribution, and is noted especially on the palms, but in contradistinction to measles it is not accompanied by nasal and conjunctival catarrh. Enteroviral meningitis caused by coxsackievirus group B may be accompanied by pleurodynia (sharp chest pain in deep inspiration plus a pleural friction rub), pericarditis (pericardial pain plus pericardial friction rub), serous peritonitis or mesenteric adenitis (severe generalized abdominal pain and tenderness), or severe myalgia affecting the skeletal musculature.

Clinical Laboratory Findings

Cerebrospinal fluid findings are pathognomonic of aseptic meningitis:

1. Total leukocyte count 30 to 3000 or more per cu mm, of which 70 to 99.9 per cent are lymphocytes. Many patients with mumps meningitis show CSF leukocyte counts above 500 per cu mm, but this is less common in enteroviral meningitis.

2. Sugar content normal (70 to 120 mg per dl [100 ml]).

3. Protein content usually normal at 30 to 40 mg per dl, but occasionally as high as 100 mg per dl.

4. Chloride content normal.

5. No microorganisms seen on Gram-stained smears.

6. Virions of mumps may be observed frequently in CSF, from patients with mumps meningitis, by electron microscopic examination after negative staining with phosphotungstic acid.

Additional findings in patients with complications may include the following:

1. Moderately diffusely abnormal electroencephalograms in patients with hyperpyrexia and temporary confusion or convulsions.

2. Inversion or flattening of the T waves in electrocardiographic leads V_3 to V_5 is noted regularly in pericarditis.

CAUSATIVE ORGANISMS

Most cases of aseptic meningitis are due to infections with two major groups of viruses, paramyxoviruses and picornaviruses. Within the paramyxovirus group, mumps virus is the sole virus serotype regularly associated with aseptic meningitis, but measles virus is an uncommon yet extremely important cause of encephalitis that may include meningeal involvement. Within the picornavirus group, comprising more than 60 serotypes, at least 14 virus serotypes are associated regularly with outbreaks of aseptic meningitis. These include echovirus types 4, 6, 9, 16, and 30, coxsackievirus types A9 and B1 through B5, and, less frequently, poliovirus types 1 through 3. Occasional cases of aseptic meningitis have resulted from infection with most of the other echovirus serotypes, particularly types 2, 3, 5, 7, 11, 14, 18, 19, 20, 21, 31, and 33, plus coxsackievirus B6. Usually during an epidemic, one enterovirus serotype becomes dominant, and a wide variety of other serotypes affect relatively few patients.

Viruses within other groups have been associated infrequently with aseptic meningitis. Adenovirus types 3 and 5 have been recovered from the CSF of patients with meningeal signs. Herpes simplex virus types 1 and 2 may occasionally induce disease of the central nervous system, which is usually manifested as encephalitis rather than meningitis. Arbovirus infections within the central nervous system usually induce encephalitis concomitantly with meningitis. North American arboviruses include infections by the alphaviruses (eastern and western equine encephalomyelitis), the flaviviruses (St. Louis encephalitis and Powassan virus), the Bunyaviruses (California encephalitis), and the orbiviruses (Colorado tick fever).

VIROLOGIC LABORATORY DIAGNOSIS

The cerebrospinal fluid constitutes the single most important specimen source for establishment of a definitive virologic diagnosis by laboratory techniques. Optimal rates of virus isolation or identification by other means are achieved when CSF is collected within 1 day after onset of meningitis. Virus isolation may be achieved in 33 per cent of cases of mumps meningitis and about 20 per cent of cases of enteroviral meningitis, by inoculation of primary monolayer tissue cultures of monkey kidney cells. Direct electron microscopic examination of uncentrifuged CSF after negative staining with phosphotungstic acid will reveal the pleomorphic enveloped mumps virions about 200 nm in diameter with helical nucleocapsids, in about the same proportion of cases of mumps meningitis whose CSF yields virus. Visualization of naked 27 nm icosahedral enterovirus virions in CSF of enteroviral meningitis is facilitated by addition of antiserum to the particular virus serotype before examination of negatively stained preparations, thereby also providing a rapid means of serologic identification of the causative virus. Enteroviruses attached to the surface of leukocytes in CSF have been identified serologically by specific immunofluorescence, after addition of homotypic fluorescein-labeled antiserum.

Since virus excretion occurs regularly in feces, and to a lesser extent in throats, of patients with enteroviral meningitis, isolation of virus from either of these specimens provides good presumptive evidence regarding the viral causation in at least 40 per cent of patients.

Collection of paired serum samples is essential for virologic diagnosis by serologic techniques. The first serum should be collected upon initial contact with the patient, and the second serum should be obtained not less than 24 hours after defervescence and abatement of meningeal signs. The interval between serum collections therefore is usually 3 to 7 days, but longer in some instances. In mumps meningitis, diagnosis is established by demonstration of rising antibody titers in hemagglutination inhibition (HI) tests using a recent CSF mumps virus isolate, or in complement fixation (CF) tests using the nucleocapsid or soluble (S) antigen. In enteroviral meningitis, rising antibody titers are demonstrated by tissue culture neutralization (NT) tests or by enzyme immunoassay (ELISA) tests.

PITFALLS IN DIAGNOSIS

Aseptic meningitis must be distinguished clearly from the following clinical conditions: (1) encephalitis, (2) purulent (bacterial) meningitis, (3) tuberculous meningitis, (4) leptospirosis, (5) leukemic infiltrations of the central nervous system, and (6) space-occupying lesions such as cerebral abscesses, neoplasms, or hydatid cysts.

1. *Encephalitis* is usually manifested by hyperpyrexia with temperatures of 40 to 42 C (104 to 107.5 F), accompanied by twitchings or convulsions, depression of the level of consciousness to stupor or coma, upgoing plantar reflexes, and occasionally spastic paresis of the skeletal muscles. This condition occurs rarely in mumps or enteroviral infections, but viruses found more commonly in association with encephalitis include herpes simplex, measles, and certain arboviruses.

2. *Purulent meningitis* has an equally sudden onset, accompanied by high fever and gross neck stiffness. The CSF contains numerous polymorphonuclear leukocytes, a grossly elevated protein level, and a glucose level from 0 to 50 mg per dl. Gram-stained smears may reveal bacteria intracellularly or extracellularly, and cultivation of bacteria such as *Neisseria meningitidis, Diplococcus pneumoniae,* or *Hemophilus influenzae* type B confirms the diagnosis.

3. *Tuberculous meningitis* may develop insidiously, and may present with clouding of consciousness, vomiting, and gross neck stiffness. Positive Mantoux reactions, together with lymphocytosis of CSF that shows a low sugar content, an elevated protein level, and a pellicle upon standing overnight, suggest the diagnosis of tuberculous meningitis, which is confirmed by cultivation of *Mycobacterium tuberculosis* or observation of acid-fast rods in smears of pellicles stained by the Ziehl-Neelsen method.

4. *Leptospirosis* is diagnosed by the isolation of Leptospira on appropriate artificial media, from CSF or blood of patients living in regions of high incidence of this infection in wild or domestic animals.

5. *Leukemic infiltrations* of the central nervous system usually show large numbers of abnormal leukocytes in CSF.

6. *Space-occupying lesions* are usually detected by a combination of diagnostic procedures, including electroencephalography, echoencephalography, x-ray of the skull, and air encephalography.

ACUTE BACTERIAL MENINGITIS

By MICHAEL DULLIGAN, M.D.,
and DAVID G. KLINE, M.D.

New Orleans, Louisiana

DEFINITION AND PATHOPHYSIOLOGY

Acute bacterial meningitis is an inflammation of the pia-arachnoid coverings of brain and spinal cord with purulent cerebrospinal fluid (CSF). Today, the most common pathogenesis for this disease is indirect or hematogenous spread of bacteria from nasopharynx, lungs, skin, and heart, respectively, to meninges. In preantibiotic days, the most common source of meningeal infection was direct extension intracranially from osteomyelitis of the petrous and mastoid portions of the temporal bone, secondary to suppurative otitis media. Other sources of direct spread include infected paranasal air sinuses, focal areas of osteomyelitis of the skull, brain abscess with rupture into ventricle or subarachnoid space, and congenital lesions with subarachnoid communication, such as dermal sinuses and weeping encephaloceles or myelomeningoceles.

Contamination of the subarachnoid space frequently occurs with trauma. This may arise from direct penetration of the brain or spinal subarachnoid space, or secondary to open fracture with dural tear and CSF leak.

Meningitis may result from neurosurgical procedures on the spine and skull in about 1 per cent of patients, particularly those in whom an air sinus or major CSF receptacle is transgressed. Ventriculomeningitis is currently being reported in 15 per cent of shunting procedures for hydrocephalus.

NEUROPATHOLOGY

Bacterial invasion of the subarachnoid space incites an intense inflammatory response, initiated by dilatation and congestion of the small pial blood vessels. Polymorphonuclear cells proliferate and pass through endothelial cell junctions along with plasma proteins to gain entry to the subarachnoid space. In 12 to 24 hours, frank pus covers the brain and spinal cord with heavy collections in the basal subarachnoid cisterns. Because of adhesions as well as pus, CSF flow is impeded at the level of the tentorial incisura. In addition, absorptive surfaces of the pacchionian granulations become coated, explaining hydrocephalus that is part of the syndrome of acute bacterial meningitis. With hematogenous spread, the vessels of the choroid plexus secrete bacteria into the ventricles; ventriculitis may ensue, depending upon the rate of flow of CSF from the ventricles.

BACTERIAL TYPES

Reasonably accurate prediction of organism type and thereby appropriate initial selection of an antibiotic may be made by knowing the patient's age and clinical history. *Escherichia coli* meningitis is seen in 35 per cent of neonatal patients (birth to 2 months of age). *Staphylococcus aureus* accounts for another 10 per cent, and should be suspected in babies with skin lesions.

From 2 months to 5 years of age, *Hemophilus influenzae* is the agent responsible for meningitis in 50 per cent of patients, and *Neisseria meningitidis* in 25 per cent. After age 5, an adult complement of antibodies to *Hemophilus influenzae* is present, making infection with this organism a rare event.

From age 5 to 40 years, *N. meningitidis* is cultured in 45 per cent of patients with spontaneous cases of meningitis. The disease occurs sporadically in the late winter and early spring, is associated with conditions of overcrowding and fatigue, and thus occurs in college dormitories and military training camps.

Over the age of 40 years, pneumococcus is responsible for about 50 per cent of cases of meningitis. Gram-negative species are found in 10 to 15 per cent of patients.

If the history is that of trauma with penetration of brain or subarachnoid space or a neurosurgical operation, *Staphylococcus aureus* is the organism in 80 per cent of patients. Pneumococcus is the agent in 80 per cent of patients with meningitis if there is a cerebrospinal fluid (CSF) leak. Meningitis associated with myelomeningocele is usually caused by *E. coli*, Pseudomonas, or *Staphylococcus aureus*. And finally, when meningitis occurs in patients with ventricular shunts, *Staphylococcus epidermidis* is by far the most common organism.

SIGNS AND SYMPTOMS

In the neonate, the symptoms may be vague. Irritability, lethargy, poor feeding, and convulsions are commonly found. Temperature may be normal or even hypothermic. Examination usually reveals a jittery state with high-pitched cry and a tense anterior fontanel. Physicians should not delay doing a lumbar puncture (LP) on an infant with the aforementioned signs, as the prognosis in bacterial meningitis is directly related to the rapidity of treatment.

Fever from 102 to 105 F (39 to 40.5 C) is usually present in children 2 to 5 years of age with meningitis. There is frequently a history of otitis media or respiratory tract infection. Seizures are common, and examination shows irritability, lethargy, vomiting, photophobia, meningismus, and increased reflexes. Older children complain of headache.

Patients over the age of 5 years present with the adult pattern of signs and symptoms, consisting of headache, chills, spiking fever, increased muscle tone, meningismus, frank organic dementia, and often papilledema.

DIAGNOSIS

Meningitis is diagnosed definitively by lumbar puncture and microscopic examination, as well as by culture of the CSF. The tap is made into the L3–4 subarachnoid space, and opening pressure is classically found to be above 180 mm H_2O. CSF is usually cloudy but may appear clear in the early stages, and yet may be teeming with organisms. There are typically 500 to 20,000 white blood cells with 90 per cent neutrophils. Spun sediment should always be Gram stained, and will show an organism in 75 per cent of cases, even though the patient is on antibiotics. When cultures fail, initial examination of the Gram-stained sediment may be the physician's only chance to identify an organism. CSF protein is generally elevated from 80 to 500 mg per 100 ml. CSF sugar is typically less than 35 mg per 100 ml if the serum sugar is normal. However, a concomitant serum sugar should always be obtained, as a diabetic with meningitis may show a "normal" CSF sugar, which is actually severely depressed when compared to serum levels. The CSF sugar should be one-half to two-thirds of the serum level.

Specimens should be carefully collected for culture and plated immediately on arrival in the laboratory on appropriate media to cover all possible species of bacteria seen in meningitis. Simultaneous cultures of blood, nasopharynx, urine, sputum, and skin lesions should be taken, as these may be of importance when CSF cultures are negative.

Recently Bland, Lister, and Ries reported the efficacy of increased CSF lactate and decreased CSF pH values in differentiating bacterial from viral meningitis. Such tests appear useful in separating partially treated bacterial meningitis from aseptic varieties. Also, cerebrospinal fluid lactic dehydrogenase values may be increased in partially treated bacterial meningitis, and this determination may be useful in atypical cases.

COMPLICATIONS

Death still occurs in 10 to 20 per cent of patients with acute bacterial meningitis. The death rate is especially high in the elderly and the very young. Severe neurologic deficit occurs in roughly 35 per cent of patients with meningitis, and includes hemiparesis, seizures, cranial nerve palsies, and mental deficiency. Hydrocephalus is a common sequela of bacterial meningitis, is usually of the communicating type, and may require a shunting operation.

Subdural effusion is found in 50 per cent of children under 18 months with bacterial meningitis, but is symptomatic in only 10 to 15 per cent. These effusions are, as a rule, bilateral, and are seen most frequently with *Hemophilus influenzae*.

Brain abscess may be a complication of meningitis, but it is often difficult to tell which was the initial process.

Cerebritis, or focal invasion of the cortex, may occur and should be considered in meningitis patients with lateralizing signs. Cortical vein thrombosis with cerebral infarction is the most common complication of meningitis associated with focal neurologic signs, such as third nerve palsy, hemiplegia, central seventh nerve palsy, and focal seizures.

DIFFERENTIAL DIAGNOSIS

Viral aseptic meningitis constitutes 30 to 40 per cent of all cases of meningitis and, in the early stages, may closely resemble bacterial infection. The symptoms and findings are less severe, however, and CSF shows less than 500 WBC's per ml, usually mononuclear cells but sometimes predominantly polymorphonuclear, a normal sugar, and no organisms.

Subarachnoid hemorrhage will present with headache, meningismus, confusion, and decreased level of consciousness, and there may also be low-grade fever owing to hypoventilation and atelectasis. The spiking fever and chills seen with meningitis are not present, and lumbar puncture (LP) should make the diagnosis.

Subdural empyema may give LP findings similar to meningitis, but there is usually a history of purulent rhinitis, and skull x-rays may show an opacified air sinus.

Brain abscess with rupture into the ventricle or subarachnoid space is classically associated with lateralizing signs and, in a desperately ill patient, papilledema. Technetium brain scan or computerized tomography scan, if available, is the initial diagnostic step. If the scans are impractical, an arteriogram should be done before the patient has spinal puncture, as the latter could prove disastrous if a brain abscess is present.

Posterior fossa tumors in children may present with low-grade fever, meningismus, and other signs somewhat suggestive of meningitis, but there will characteristically be papilledema and separated sutures on skull x-ray.

The subacute varieties of meningitis such as the tubercular and fungal forms give a protracted history and multiple cranial nerve palsies on examination. History of steroid therapy, hyperalimentation, diabetes mellitus, neoplasm, and immunosuppression for transplantation should alert the physician to look for fungal meningitis. Cultures should be made on Sabouraud's medium. CSF analysis in tubercular meningitis usually shows 25 to 500 lymphocytes, along with a low sugar and chloride and elevated protein. Cryptococcal meningitis has 40 to 400 polymorphonuclear cells with low sugar, high protein, and organisms on India ink stain in 50 per cent of patients. Chest x-ray may also corroborate both tubercular and cryptococcal disease as well as other fungal entities.

After posterior fossa surgery in children, especially for cerebellar astrocytoma, a picture of bacterial meningitis may be seen with high fever, stiff neck, and CSF with up to 2000 polymorphonuclear cells, as well as low sugar and high protein. However, Gram stain of the spun sediment and culture are negative for organisms. This form of aseptic meningitis results from blood or from some as yet unidentified product of the tumor that is irritating to the pia-arachnoid. Finally, it should be remembered that after pneumoencephalography or ventriculography there may be fever, meningismus, and several hundred polymorphonuclear cells in the CSF, as air is irritating to the ependymal surfaces.

VIRAL ENCEPHALITIS AND ENCEPHALOPATHY

By PAUL BROWN, M.D.
Bethesda, Maryland

DEFINITION

Viral encephalitis is a disease of the central nervous system characterized by an acutely altered state of consciousness that is usually accompanied by fever, headache, and a variety of neurologic signs, caused by a viral-induced process of inflammation and neuronal destruction.

Like all definitions, this one will not stand close examination without some qualification, but it is useful to indicate the most typical features of the disease. Strictly speaking, encephalitis refers to inflammation restricted to the brain, myelitis to inflammation of the spinal cord, and encephalomyelitis to combined brain and spinal cord inflammation. Since each of these descriptive illnesses can be caused by the same viruses, the term encephalitis will be understood throughout this article to represent these variants, as well as encephalitis associated with meningitic inflammation (meningoencephalitis).

Although the majority of viral encephalitides are acute, with a period of no more than a few days between onset and maximal expression of disease, many of the viruses can also produce a neurologic evolution extending over a week or more, and a few viruses are responsible for subacute or even frankly chronic neurologic diseases.

It must also be pointed out that the usual pathologic features of diffuse perivascular round cell infiltrates, microgliosis, and neuronal degeneration are not inflexible criteria of viral encephalitis, since the so-called postinfectious encephalitides, in which an immune mechanism rather than direct viral damage may be responsible for disease, are instead usually characterized by perivenular demyelination of the white matter.

The viral brain diseases of progressive multifocal leukoencephalopathy and Creutzfeldt-Jakob disease are more properly termed encephalopathies, since they are chronic processes in which inflammatory changes are either minimal or entirely absent.

CLINICAL PRESENTATION

Encephalitic illness may present as but one infrequent aspect of a systemic disease, such as measles or varicella, or it may be the sole manifestation of illness, as with herpes simplex and many arbovirus infections. When encephalitis complicates a systemic illness, it more often than not occurs after more characteristic features of the illness have become evident. When encephalitis is itself the major presenting illness, a minor, often influenza-like prodrome of headache, myalgia, malaise, and pharyngitis or upper respiratory symptoms may occur in the days or week before neurologic symptoms cause the patient to seek medical help.

The onset of neurologic symptoms is usually abrupt. These almost always include an altered state of consciousness — lethargy, drowsiness, or stupor — and often, if consciousness is not too depressed, confusion, disorientation, hallucinations, or some form of bizarre or at least uncharacteristic behavior. Fever, headache, stiffness of the neck, nausea, and vomiting are common complaints. Convulsions are especially frequent in children, in whom they can be the sole presenting symptom.

There may or may not be abnormalities other than those just described; what is seen will depend on the extent of inflammation and the areas of the central nervous system that are involved. Almost every neurologic sign, or combination of signs, has been described in individual case reports of patients with viral encephalitis; cerebral hemisphere involvement is evidenced by psychic abnormalities, disturbances of higher cortical function such as dysphasia, long-tract signs, and sensory losses; cerebellar or basal ganglia involvement by movement disorders; brain stem involvement by cranial nerve and long-tract signs and ataxia; and spinal cord involvement by flaccid paralyses, loss of tendon reflexes, bladder and bowel dysfunction, and variable sensory deficits.

DIFFERENTIAL DIAGNOSIS

To the patient who presents the clinical syndrome of acute viral encephalitis, diagnosis of a viral cause is of far less urgency than exclusion of nonviral causes, because most of the nonviral causes can be treated. To be misled by an imperfectly treated bacterial meningitis, a subdural hematoma resulting from inapparent head injury, or a case of salicylate intoxication can be one of the most costly mistakes in clinical medicine. Central nervous system damage is tragic under any circumstances, and preventable damage is inexcusable.

For this reason, discussion of viral encephalitis begins, rather than ends, with a consideration of differential diagnosis. In Table 1 are listed a number of conditions that can present a picture that is clinically indistinguishable from acute viral encephalitis. Many of these conditions can be conclusively diagnosed within an hour or two of the patient's admission, from careful attention to details of the history (even if obtained from others), physical examination, and appropriate laboratory studies. Close examination of the cerebrospinal fluid is particularly important, and should include, in addition to cellular enumeration and identification, both light and darkfield microscopy, India ink preparations, and smears of the centrifuged sediment stained by the Gram, Giemsa, and Ziehl-Neelsen methods. Fluid should also be cultured for anaerobic and aerobic bacteria, fungi, and mycobacteria.

Sometimes the patient will require further investigation as the clinical course unfolds, and the possibility of nonviral illness must be repeatedly questioned until a diagnosis of viral encephalitis has been established beyond any reasonable doubt. *The whole of the following discussion of particular viruses that cause encephalitis is of far less moment than the suc-*

Table 1. *Nonviral Conditions That Can Be Mistaken for Acute Viral Encephalitis*

Infections
    Bacterial: Especially very early or imperfectly treated meningitis or brain abscess, and parameningeal infections such as epidural abscess or petrositis; the ordinarily chronic illnesses caused by mycobacteria and spirochetes, especially leptospirosis, can also on occasion present acutely; Mycoplasma; endocarditis with embolization
    Fungi: Coccidioides, Cryptococcus, Blastomyces, Histoplasma, Nocardia, and Candida species
    Rickettsiae: Most species can produce CNS symptoms; Rocky Mountain spotted fever can be particularly difficult to distinguish from Colorado tick fever, especially when partially treated
    Protozoa: "Fresh water" amebiasis, increasingly common; *P. falciparum* malaria in travelers, which can be overlooked in temperate zones; Toxoplasma
    Metazoa: *Taenia solium* (cysticercosis), Echinococcus, Angiostrongylus, Trichinella, Schistosoma, Paragonimus (lung fluke), all typically chronic systemic diseases, can have unexpectedly abrupt onset of CNS symptoms, especially seizures; travel history essential
Intoxications
    Numerous causes, the most important of which are salicylates, barbiturates, and heavy metals, especially acute lead poisoning; tick paralysis (removal of tick is curative)
Endocrine/metabolic disorders
    Most important are acute sodium, calcium, or carbohydrate imbalance, especially in association with bacterial infection; porphyria; pheochromocytoma
Head trauma
Acute psychotic states and hysterias
Other causes
    Sarcoid, hyperglobulinemia, hypersensitivity syndromes, collagen diseases, and some neoplasms, including leukemia and lymphomas

cessful discrimination between viral encephalitis and other, treatable conditions.

LABORATORY TESTS

General laboratory studies, ordinarily of little diagnostic help in patients with viral encephalitis, can occasionally suggest the cause of illness in patients whose encephalitis represents but one manifestation of systemic disease. For example, examination of the blood will usually reveal atypical lymphocytes in patients with infectious mononucleosis; urinalysis can reveal characteristic cells of cytomegalic inclusion disease, and elevated amylase or transaminase levels can point to enteroviruses as the cause of associated encephalitis (amylase is almost never elevated in mumps in the absence of clinically apparent parotitis).

Lumbar puncture in most patients will reveal an opening pressure that is normal or slightly increased, a clear spinal fluid with increased numbers of white cells, most often in the range of 50 to 500 cells per cu mm, a slightly to moderately elevated protein concentration, and a normal glucose concentration. Occasionally, the initial spinal tap will yield entirely normal fluid, or only a marginal elevation of protein, but a repeat tap a day or two later will almost always be abnormal. Very early in the illness there is often a predominance of polymorphonuclear cells; but as the illness progresses, mononuclear cells become the dominant or exclusive cell type, and the protein level will often rise as the total cell count falls.

Certain findings can point to one or another viral cause: red cells as well as white cells in the cerebrospinal fluid suggest infection by either California encephalitis or herpes simplex viruses; persistence of significant numbers of polymorphonuclear cells with relatively high total cell counts is suggestive of Eastern equine encephalitis; and in encephalitis caused by infectious mononucleosis, a careful examination is occasionally rewarded by the discovery of atypical lymphocytes.

The *electroencephalogram* (EEG) is almost always abnormal in patients with encephalitis. A variety of alterations can occur, but usually there is seen a diffuse slow-wave activity, either delta or theta, with disruption of normal rhythms, and sometimes periodic high amplitude bursts, or spike and wave complexes. The special value of the EEG lies in its ability to demonstrate diffuse or bilateral pathology in patients who present clinically with a focal neurologic deficit: in the absence of severe depression of consciousness, generalized EEG dysrhythmias (with or without associated localized abnormalities) lead one away from alternative diagnoses such as tumor, abscess, or hematoma.

In exceptional circumstances, it may be necessary to obtain a brain scan, computerized cranial tomograms, pneumoencephalogram, or arteriogram, or even resort to surgical exploration to differentiate mass lesions from viral encephalitis presenting with a focal deficit.

CLINICAL COURSE

The evolution of viral encephalitis may run the gamut from a short-lived benign course to a devastating illness either leaving serious permanent neurologic deficits or ending in death. Although certain viruses ordinarily cause a very mild illness (mumps, California encephalitis) and others are notorious for their severity (herpes simplex, Eastern equine encephalitis), a complete spectrum of symptomatic disease has been described for every one of the viruses associated with encephalitis. Two complications that may occur during the course of the disease deserve special mention, as they may occur rapidly and unexpectedly and require immediate recognition to support or correct: a salt-wasting syndrome resulting from hypothalamic involvement, and interference with temperature or respiratory control centers owing to brain stem involvement.

The acute phase of encephalitic illness ordinarily lasts not more than a few days to a week, and its resolution can be either abrupt, as is characteristic of rubella and some of the arboviruses, or gradual, as often occurs in patients recovering from herpes simplex infections. Neurologic deficits may, however, continue to diminish over a period of weeks to months, so that patients who remain to some degree disabled on discharge from the hospital may be encouraged to expect further recovery in the future.

In Table 2 are listed the virus categories, reported case totals, and average mortality for acute viral encephalitis observed in the United States during the most recent 10-year period for which data are available (1968–1977). Looking down each column, it can be appreciated that (1) St. Louis encephalitis and mumps viruses have caused well over half the diagnosed cases of encephalitis during the past 10 years; (2) St. Louis encephalitis, herpes simplex, and varicella viruses have been responsible for over 80

per cent of the deaths; and (3) Eastern equine, herpes simplex, and herpes zoster encephalitis have had the worst prognosis. It can also be seen that in fewer than half of the reported cases of encephalitis has the specific viral cause been documented.

Not evident from the table are certain trends and year-by-year variability in cases over the past decade. For example, the number of cases of acute encephalitis caused by measles virus has, like varicella encephalitis, remained at about the same level throughout the decade, suggesting that the measles immunization program beginning in the mid 1960s had already achieved its maximum effect by 1970. In contrast, the more recent introduction of vaccines for mumps and rubella continues to reduce the incidence of both diseases, and in consequence the number of cases of encephalitis caused by these viruses has progressively decreased since 1970.

Characteristically, the incidence of arbovirus and enterovirus infections varies broadly from year to year. Some years there is but a handful of cases nationwide for one or another of the listed arboviruses or enteroviruses, whereas in other years encephalitic activity is epidemic. 1975 was a particularly severe year for several arboviruses (especially St. Louis encephalitis)

Table 2. *Reported Case Incidence and Mortality Rates of Acute Viral Encephalitis in the United States During the 10-Year Period 1968–1977* *

Virus Category		Number of Cases	Number of Deaths	Mortality (%)
Arboviruses	St. Louis	2538	179	7
	California	703	2	0.3
	Western equine	522	8	2
	Eastern equine	36	16	44
	Venezuelan	22	0	0.0
Herpesviruses	Simplex	497	150	30
	Zoster‡	40	14	35
	Epstein-Barr	25	3	12
	Cytomegalovirus	14	0	0.0
Enteroviruses	Echovirus	359†	3	1
	Coxsackievirus	87†	6	7
Viruses associated with childhood infections	Mumps	2030	31	2
	Varicella‡	605	124	20
	Measles	321	50	16
	Rubella	26	1	4
Viruses associated with other infections	Influenza	50	9	18
	Adenovirus	29	1	3
	LCM	8	0	0.0
TOTAL§		7912	597	8
Unspecified virus		12,662	1875	15
GRAND TOTAL§		20,574	2472	12

*Compiled from annual CDC surveillance reports with the assistance of Dr. Karl Kappus.

†An additional nearly equal number of possible cases, with enteroviral isolation only from the gastrointestinal tract, is included in the "unspecified virus" category.

‡Same virus, but distinct clinical syndromes.

§Not included are fewer than 5 cases each of encephalitis due to Powassan, parainfluenza, and respiratory syncytial viruses.

and also for echovirus encephalitis. California encephalitis and coxsackievirus encephalitis have generally shown the least yearly variability.

From an overall viewpoint of numbers of cases, numbers of deaths, and mortality rate, herpes simplex has been the most consistently occurring and gravest of all the acute viral encephalitides seen in the United States during the past decade. It is probably even more serious than the table would indicate, since the difficulty in establishing a specific diagnosis, together with the comparatively high mortality rate in the "unspecified virus" category, suggest that this group may contain a large additional number of herpes encephalitis cases.

This summary of the overall United States experience in recent years should be supplemented by current information obtained from the health department of the state where the physician is practicing, because an awareness of increased local activity of one or another virus can be useful to the clinician in balancing probabilities of viral diagnosis.

When combined with knowledge of the seasonal, geographic, and age group occurrence of disease, the clinical setting of an individual case of encephalitis can often furnish enough further information to make possible an informed guess about the correct viral etiology. For example, a Minnesota farmer's child who in August experienced the acute onset of fever and temporal lobe seizures would be most likely to have California (La Crosse) encephalitis. The same child seen in December would be suspected to have herpes simplex encephalitis. In a college student with pharyngitis, cervical adenopathy, and splenomegaly, encephalitis would probably be due to Epstein-Barr (EB) virus. Exposure to one of the childhood exanthems may be a clue to the cause of encephalitis in the adult for whom a history of past infection is uncertain.

Table 3 summarizes the distinctive features of the most commonly encountered viral encephalitides in the United States:

ST. LOUIS ENCEPHALITIS (SLE)
WESTERN EQUINE ENCEPHALITIS (WEE)
CALIFORNIA ENCEPHALITIS (CE)
HERPES SIMPLEX
ENTEROVIRUSES
MUMPS
MEASLES
VARICELLA

Less common types of encephalitis are described in the following paragraphs.

OTHER ARBOVIRUSES

Eastern equine encephalitis (EEE) occurs sporadically during the summer and fall along the Atlantic and Gulf coastal states, and as far south as Argentina. Limited epidemics have occurred in Louisiana, Massachusetts, New Jersey, Jamaica, and the Dominican Republic, usually in association with horse epizootics. The virus is transmitted by mosquitoes, has by far the highest rate of overt to subclinical infection (1 in 10 to 50 cases), and is characteristically the most devastating of all the arbovirus encephalitides, with a predilection for older adults and children, especially infants. Onset is sudden, with high fever, seizures, and frequent focal signs, progressing to coma and death within 3 to 5 days. A predominantly polymorphonuclear response is seen in both the cerebrospinal fluid and blood. Adults recover far more frequently than children, in whom survivors are usually left with neurologic sequelae.

Venezuelan equine encephalitis (VEE) occurs in South and Central America, and has been seen in the United States only in Texas, California, and Florida, where it is endemic in the Everglades. The virus is mosquito borne, affecting horses as well as man, and because of its tropical and subtropical distribution it may occur at almost any time of year. As with other equine encephalitides, the people most often affected are less than 15 or over 50 years of age. Prodromal febrile illness is not uncommon, and may show a biphasic course, with encephalitic symptoms appearing several days to a week after the prodrome. The severity of the illness has varied widely in different epidemics, as well as in sporadic cases.

Colorado tick fever occurs in the western United States in correspondence with the distribution of its vector, the wood tick. Disease is transmitted only in spring and summer, and has occasionally appeared in vacationers returning to their homes far from the endemic region. Typically, after an incubation period of 3 to 6 days, the illness presents a biphasic course of influenza-like symptoms, but with leukopenia and occasionally splenomegaly and rash. Encephalitis is an uncommon complication, occurring almost exclusively in children.

Powassan encephalitis has to date been described in only a few children living in eastern Canada and New York state. The disease is transmitted by ticks, occurs in the summer, and is not distinguished by any unusual clinical features. There have been two deaths, and in two of three other patients who recovered a dual infection with echoviruses was documented.

Other arbovirus infections that can cause encephalitis do not occur in North America, except in travelers who have been infected and then returned from endemic regions in other parts of the world. These include Japanese (Asia and the western Pacific), tick-borne (U.S.S.R.), Murray Valley (Australia and New Guinea), louping ill (Great Britain), West Nile (Egypt and the Near East), and yellow fever (South America and Africa).

OTHER HERPES VIRUSES

Epstein-Barr (EB) virus is responsible for classic, heterophil-positive infectious mononucleosis, which is occasionally complicated by neurologic disease. Encephalitis may supervene at any time during the course of illness, and rarely may be the presenting feature. EB virus may also cause encephalitis or transverse myelitis in patients without the clinical syndrome of infectious mononucleosis, and who may furthermore not have detectable heterophil antibody. The majority of patients are late adolescents or young adults, who acquire the virus of mononucleosis by oral contact. The incubation period is from 1 to 2 months in adults, and about half as long in children, and the clinical course is usually benign, although deaths have been reported. Diagnosis is simplified when the typical syndrome of infectious mononucleosis occurs in conjunction with an elevated heterophil antibody titer and atypical lymphocytes, particularly when they are also found in the cerebrospinal fluid. In their absence, diagnosis must be made by demonstration of fourfold or greater changes in antibodies to one or more of the EB virus antigens.

Cytomegalovirus (CMV) infection can be devastating, as in the congenital form, in which chronic encephalitis may produce microcephaly and developmental retardation or death; or it may be entirely asymptomatic, as is usual in acquired infection in children and adults. The virus can produce a heterophil-negative clinical syndrome of infectious mononucleosis, and is seen most often in a setting of altered immunity resulting from leukemia, lymphoma, or renal transplantation, and in postperfusion patients. Encephalitis in these patients is a distinctly rare complication with a usually benign outcome.

Herpes zoster is the same virus as that causing varicella, but is discussed separately because of the distinct clinical syndromes produced. The manifestations of herpes zoster represent reactivation of latent virus acquired during primary varicella infection, and, although seen occasionally in children and young adults, occur most often in middle and late adult life. Like CMV, herpes zoster shows a predisposition to affect patients with leukemia, lymphoma, and other immuno-altered states. The cutaneous eruption of segmentally distributed vesicles is distinctive, but may be preceded by several days of radicular dysesthesia or pain. Encephalitis is an unusual complication, which in the majority of cases begins 2 to 8 days after the onset of the cutaneous eruption, and is often serious or even fatal.

Herpesvirus simiae (B virus) is the monkey counterpart of herpes simplex in man, and exists as a latent infection in from 20 to 100 per cent of normal colonized monkeys. Its importance to man lies in the usually fatal encephalitis that follows infection from bites or, less commonly, simple exposure of traumatized skin to saliva or infected monkey tissue culture preparations. The incubation period is ordinarily between 10 and 20 days, and may be terminated by gastrointestinal symptoms or pneumonitis before the onset of neurologic signs. One case has been described in which encephalitis followed by a period of years the last contact with monkeys, and was preceded by a herpes zoster-like segmental vesicular eruption. The rare patient who recovers is almost always left with severe neurologic residua.

MISCELLANEOUS VIRUSES

Lymphocytic choriomeningitis (LCM) virus is endemic in certain smaller rodents, especially the common or house mouse, which through its secretions may contaminate human dwellings and, especially during the cooler months, result in inhalation infection. This is most often clinically inapparent, but after an incubation period of about a week, it can produce an influenzal or meningitic illness and, less commonly, encephalitis. An influenzal prodrome is seen in about half the patients with encephalitis, who may show a biphasic course with associated features of arthritis, orchitis, or pneumonitis. Recovery is usually complete, although a few deaths have been reported.

Rubella is associated with encephalitis in probably not more than 1 in every 5000 to 10,000 cases, and appears to complicate adolescent or adult infection more often than the usual childhood disease. As with other exanthems, neurologic signs usually appear a few days after onset of the rash, but may occur coincidentally or even precede it. Onset is usually abrupt and the clinical course rapid, with recovery or death occurring within a few days of onset. Delayed SSPE-like illness may rarely follow congenital or infantile infections (see below).

Rabies, smallpox, and *poliomyelitis,* discussed in separate articles of this book, have all but disappeared from the United States during the past decade.

LABORATORY VIRAL DIAGNOSIS

The physician who wishes to establish a precise viral cause in the patient with encephalitis must often be prepared to await the results of his labors until after the patient's illness has been resolved, and it may seem gratuitous to make the effort when the outcome will in all likelihood have no effect on his ability to care for the patient. Yet the interests of public health as well as the inherent satisfaction of establishing a diagnosis merit the additional attention required to collect and arrange for transportation of appropriate diagnostic specimens.

As quickly as possible after the patient is first seen, samples of heparinized or defibrinated blood, cerebrospinal fluid, urine, and nasopharyngeal and rectal swabs should be obtained for attempted viral isolation. (Not all these specimens may be needed in a particular case, but it is preferable to allow the laboratory to make that choice.) The swabs should be immersed in tissue culture media containing antibiotics and 10 per cent protein. (Infusion broth or even isotonic saline is a less than ideal substitute.) *All these specimens should be kept refrigerated and sent or, preferably, taken the same day to the nearest viral diagnostic laboratory, together with a very brief clinical summary.* If there is unavoidable delay of more than a day, all specimens except the whole blood should be stored frozen until delivery can be arranged.

A serum sample should also be obtained and kept frozen until a second sample can be obtained 2 to 3 weeks later. This may be done

Table 3. *Characteristics of the Most Frequently Encountered Viral Encephalitides in the United States*

Virus	Geographical Distribution	Seasonal Occurrence	Transmission	Ages Affected	Incubation Period	Distinctive Features
St. Louis encephalitis (SLE)	Sporadic cases nationwide; endemic in central and southwestern U.S. and in California; rural predominance in west, urban/suburban elsewhere	Summer/fall	Mosquitoes	Adults more often than children	5–15 days	Abrupt onset of prodromal illness followed by usually benign neurologic course, with often abrupt remission in 5–10 days; tends to be more severe in adults, with up to 30% mortality in epidemics
Western equine encephalitis (WEE)	Almost all U.S. cases occur west of Mississippi River; also occurs in Canada and Brazil	Summer/fall	Mosquitoes	Most often in young children and older adults	5–15 days	Clinically similar to SLE, but severity much greater in infants than adults; up to 15% mortality in epidemics
California encephalitis (CE)	Sporadic cases in North and South America and Europe; endemic in north-central and middle-Atlantic states; rural predominance	Summer/fall	Mosquitoes	Almost always under 15 yrs, especially in 5–9 yr age group	5–15 days	Prodrome is common; focal deficits (often fronto-temporal) in up to 40% of patients, and 50% present with seizures; sometimes red cells in CSF; fatalities are rare
Herpes simplex	Worldwide.	Year round	Direct human contact in primary infection; reactivation of latent herpes thereafter	All ages, but uncommon in 5–15 yr age group	?	Frequent URI prodrome, frontotemporal lobe localization with seizures, and red cells in CSF; usually severe, often prolonged clinical course

Enteroviruses (echovirus and coxsackievirus)	Worldwide	Year round, with summer-fall outbreaks	Human-to-human oral-fecal contamination	All ages, but somewhat more common in children	2–5 days	Usually benign course; often the only symptom, but can be associated with an array of systemic syndromes, including pleurodynia, peri- and myocarditis, orchitis, gastroenteritis, herpangina, exanthems
Mumps	Worldwide	Year round, with winter-spring outbreaks	Human-to-human air droplets	All ages, but mostly in children	Ca. 18 (12–26) days	Occurs about once per 400 cases, usually benign course; may precede, accompany, or follow parotitis (orchitis, pancreatitis in adults), or may be only symptom
Measles	Worldwide	Year round, with winter-spring outbreaks	Human-to-human air droplets	Mostly children	Ca. 10 (8–13) days	Occurs about once per 1000 cases, often serious illness; onset usually after rash, can occur coincidentally or even before; delayed, subacute form (SSPE)
Varicella	Worldwide	Year round, with winter-spring outbreaks	Human-to-human air droplets	Almost always in children	13–17 days	Occurs about once per 2000 cases, frequently serious illness; usually follows rash, but may accompany or precede it; transverse myelitis and cerebellar ataxia syndromes are distinctive

most conveniently on the occasion of a follow-up clinic visit. The pair of sera should then be sent to the laboratory, which will test them together for antibodies to appropriate viruses.

If all these things are done properly, an exact viral diagnosis may be expected in nearly three quarters of patients with viral encephalitis. Desultory efforts will be rewarded with correspondingly less success. The combination of viral isolation from cerebrospinal fluid or blood with demonstration of a fourfold or greater rise in serum antibody titers to the same virus provides the most secure basis for diagnosis. A rise in antibody, with or without viral isolation from elsewhere in the body, or viral isolation from the cerebrospinal fluid or blood in the absence of an antibody rise, provides a somewhat less certain but still probable diagnosis.

Should brain biopsy be indicated in the differential diagnosis of encephalitis, a portion of the tissue should be frozen and reserved for the laboratory, where attempts can be made to culture virus and look for viral antigen using fluorescent antibody microscopy. Some laboratories are also prepared to examine cerebrospinal fluid cells for viral antigen using fluorescent antibody methods. The centrifuged sediment is resuspended in a few drops of isotonic saline, and 1 drop is added to each of several slides, air dried, and fixed in acetone for 15 to 20 minutes. Slides should then be kept refrigerated or frozen until sent to the laboratory.

Virus has proved easiest to isolate from patients with encephalitis caused by enteroviral infections. Isolations from other encephalitides have been much less frequent, and serologic diagnosis therefore continues to be the most practical and often the only means by which specific viral causation can be established. Encephalitis resulting from herpes simplex presents a rather special diagnostic problem, as successful isolation of the virus from any other site than affected brain tissue is almost vanishingly rare, and a rise in antibody levels does not always occur even in proved cases; moreover, antibody fluctuations have been documented in association with encephalitis of other causes. Confirmed diagnoses of herpes simplex encephalitis are therefore most often described in biopsied or autopsied cases.

POSTINFECTIOUS ENCEPHALITIS

Certain viral infections, as well as vaccination and antirabic treatment, can result in a form of disease called postinfectious or postvaccinal encephalitis. Viruses most commonly implicated are those of measles, mumps, and varicella, whereas cases caused by smallpox, rubella, influenza, dengue, and yellow fever are comparatively rare.

A distinction between encephalitis resulting from direct viral invasion of the central nervous system and postinfectious encephalitis caused by an abnormal host-virus interaction is usually impossible to make on clinical grounds alone. Typically, onset of neurologic symptoms is abrupt and follows by several days the major systemic manifestations of the infection, but may occur simultaneously or, rarely, even before they have appeared. Postvaccinal encephalitis usually develops about 10 days after primary vaccination, with a range of from 2 to 24 days. Encephalitis occurring during the course of antirabic treatment usually appears from 1 to 3 weeks after the first dose of vaccine.

The clinical course of encephalitis is usually not distinctive, although cerebellar syndromes seem to occur more often in encephalitis associated with measles and chickenpox than with other viruses, and encephalomyelitic syndromes are frequent after antirabic treatment. Changes in the cerebrospinal fluid are similar to those described for acute viral encephalitis: lymphocytic pleocytosis, slightly increased protein, and normal glucose concentrations. Recovery or death usually occurs within 1 to 2 weeks after onset, with the mortality rate particularly high (40 to 60 per cent) in postvaccinal encephalitis.

Diagnosis depends on microscopic examination of central nervous system tissue, which reveals perivenular demyelination confined mainly to the white matter, variable thrombosis and hemorrhage, diffuse gliosis, and only minimal degeneration or necrosis of neurons.

SUBACUTE AND CHRONIC VIRAL ENCEPHALITIS AND ENCEPHALOPATHY

Subacute Sclerosing Panencephalitis (SSPE). Now recognized to be the result of a long-preceding infection with measles virus, SSPE is a rare disease of childhood and adolescence, usually occurring in patients between the ages of 5 and 15 (but, exceptionally, as late as 50 years of age), with an incubation period that is measured in years rather than in days or weeks. Over half the patients are found to have had an otherwise typical measles infection at less than 2 years of age. SSPE affects males twice as frequently as females, occurs all over the world, and is most prevalent in rural farming areas. However, fewer cases are being seen today than in the recent past, as measles itself is becoming a less common disease.

SSPE ordinarily evolves over a period of weeks to months, beginning with subtle changes in mentation or behavior, which slowly progress and combine with more obvious signs of brain damage, including myoclonic jerks, stumbling, movement disorders, and a variety of ocular abnormalities. Convulsions have occurred in a few patients. As the illness proceeds, mental deterioration becomes pronounced, disorders of speech, spasticity, and opisthotonos may be seen, and decerebrate rigidity signals impending coma and death, which usually occurs within 2 years of onset. About 5 per cent of patients have a prolonged course with long periods of stability or even remissions, and exceptional patients have survived for as long as 10 years. The disease has also been described in an acute fulminating form, with death occurring a month after onset.

An illness clinically indistinguishable from SSPE has also been described to follow by many years a congenital or infantile rubella infection. Usually beginning in late childhood or early adolescence, there appears a progressive neurologic syndrome consisting of mental deterioration, ataxia, spasticity, and myoclonus or seizures, with fatal termination in from several months to several years of onset.

Cerebrospinal fluid usually reveals an elevated IgG level with an oligocolonal pattern and paretic colloidal gold curve, but even in the rare acute form the cell count remains normal. The electroencephalogram (EEG) is invariably abnormal at some point during the illness, and a characteristic tracing of high amplitude delta waves in a "suppression burst" pattern is seen in some patients. Diagnosis can be confirmed by the demonstration of antibody to measles virus (or, in the case of rubella panencephalitis, to rubella virus) in the cerebrospinal fluid, or of unusually high titers in the serum. Brain biopsy is almost never required to establish the diagnosis.

At autopsy, a combination of demyelination, sclerosis, and mononuclear inflammatory changes is found throughout the brain. Type A inclusion bodies can be seen to contain viral particles by electron microscopy and viral antigen by fluorescent antibody staining; in some cases infectious virus has been isolated using co-cultivation tissue culture techniques.

Chronic Tick-Borne Encephalitis (TBE). The virus of tick-borne encephalitis, formerly known as Russian spring-summer encephalitis virus, usually causes an acute disease with an evolution similar to other acute viral encephalitides. However, in a proportion of patients (possibly as high as 20 per cent), symptoms of the acute infection may abate or even disappear, only to be followed in several months by the appearance of renewed disease characterized by (1) a chronic seizure disorder called epilepsia partialis continua or Kozhevnikov's epilepsy, or other movement abnormalities such as myoclonic epilepsy, chorea, choreoathetosis, dystonias, or tremors; (2) paralytic disorders resembling poliomyelitis; or (3) mixed types of syndromes.

The disease occurs in children and adults of both sexes but is most frequent in working-age males living in rural areas, who are at greatest risk to virus exposure from tick bites. The paralytic type of disease appears to terminate fatally more often than the chronic seizure syndromes, which in a significant number of patients stabilize or even remit, allowing a return to normal life.

The cerebrospinal fluid (CSF) may contain slightly increased cell and protein levels, and the EEG generally reflects the clinical picture, with seizure activity in epilepsy and slowing in paresis. Isolation of TBE virus from brain tissue or CSF obtained months after the onset of seizures (and long after the original acute illness) has been reported in only three patients. Diagnosis is therefore usually made on the basis of the clinical history, elevated serum or CSF antibody levels to TBE virus, and a neuropathologic picture of chronic panencephalitis.

The disease appears for the present to be limited to the U.S.S.R., although cases may be anticipated to occur in contiguous regions of Europe and southeast Asia, where viruses identical or closely similar to TBE virus have also been identified.

Progressive Multifocal Leukoencephalopathy (PML). First described in 1958, this rare demyelinating disease is now known to be caused by papovaviruses. Named after the patient from whom it was first isolated, JC virus has been responsible for nearly all of the cases from which virus isolations have been made; simian virus 40 (SV40) has been isolated in two cases.

The disease has been reported from many parts of the world. Males and females are about equally affected, and the great majority of cases occur in middle life. A striking feature of PML is its predilection for patients already suffering from a variety of diseases associated with immune deficiencies, most often leukemia or lymphoma, but also carcinomatosis, sarcoid, tuberculosis, systemic lupus erythematosus, rheumatoid arthritis, Whipple's disease, and renal transplantation followed by immunosuppressive therapy. In only a few patients has PML occurred in the absence of any associated clinically evident disorder (and in only one of these was the immune system studied and shown to be normal).

These pre-existing diseases are often present for many years before the onset of PML, which is usually insidious but relentlessly progressive. Mental deterioration, behavioral abnormalities, hemiparesis, aphasia, dysarthria, and visual impairment are the most frequently encountered complaints. Movement disorders and sensory deficits are less common, and headache is very unusual. Several patients have been found to have coincident CNS fungal infections, further complicating the clinical picture.

Cerebrospinal fluid is usually normal. In some patients, slight elevations in pressure, cells, or protein have been described as isolated abnormalities. The EEG is in contrast invariably abnormal, but the diffuse delta or theta slow wave patterns usually seen are not characteristic. Computerized cranial tomography has in some cases identified a distinctive pattern of asymmetrical patchy areas of low isotope uptake that has suggested the correct diagnosis.

Death usually occurs within 3 to 4 months, but rarely as early as 1 month or as late as several years after onset. Autopsy findings in the brain are characteristic: multiple areas of demyelination associated with abnormal, virus-laden oligodendrocytes and, often, giant astrocytes. Perivascular lymphocytic infiltration is uncommon, and when it occurs is usually confined to the foci of demyelination.

JC virus is nearly ubiquitous, with up to 75 per cent of cosmopolitan populations having acquired antibody from inapparent infection before adolescence. The virus evidently remains latent and, rarely, in a setting of altered immunity caused by chronic disease much later in life, invades and replicates in the central nervous system to produce PML. Further rises of antibody levels usually do not occur during the course of illness (reminiscent of latent herpes virus encephalitis, and unlike SSPE), so that serology is of no use in diagnosis, which is based on the clinical picture, typical pathology, and demonstration of viral antigen or infectious virus in the brain.

Creutzfeldt-Jakob Disease (CJD). Considered for decades as a chronic degeneration of the central nervous system, CJD has in recent years been reproduced in numerous subhuman primates as well as in rodents and the domestic cat, and is now appropriately classified as a transmissible virus dementia. It affects men and women equally, occurs most often between the ages of 55 and 75 years, but has been seen in persons as young as 17 and as old as 84 years of age.

Prodromal symptoms of asthenia, weight loss, or disordered sleep patterns, beginning weeks to months before the onset of neurologic signs,

can be elicited in nearly half of the patients. A gradually progressive mental deterioration is the most common neurologic presentation, but the sudden onset of vertigo, diplopia, ataxia, and even paralysis or paresthesia has been seen in up to 20 per cent of patients, often leading to a mistaken initial diagnosis of cerebrovascular accident.

As the illness progresses, a broad spectrum of clinical signs and symptoms may occur in association with the continuing mental deterioration. Myoclonus, with or without other types of movement disorders, occurs relatively late in the course of illness in nearly 90 per cent of patients. Cerebellar, visual, pyramidal, and extrapyramidal signs (especially severe oppositional rigidity) are also common, whereas lower motor neuron and sensory signs occur infrequently. Most patients are dead within 6 months of the onset of neurologic symptoms, but the clinical course can be as short as a month or as long as several years.

Cerebrospinal fluid is normal, except for an occasional slight elevation of protein concentration. The EEG, which initially may be normal, always deteriorates as the illness progresses, and in about half of patients shows a characteristic pattern of nearly regular high-voltage spikes at a frequency of 1 to 2 cycles per second. The combination of dementia, myoclonus, and this type of EEG pattern is extremely suggestive but not pathognomonic of CJD: exact imitations have been seen in the rare patient with Alzheimer's disease, metastatic carcinoma, and toxic or metabolic encephalopathies.

Serologic diagnosis is not possible, as no immune response to the virus has yet been demonstrated. Final diagnosis depends on the distinctive pathologic picture of astrocytosis, neuronal loss, and status spongiosus, and when possible, animal transmission studies.

It is not known how the disease is naturally acquired. Iatrogenic transmission has been documented to follow transplantation of an unsuspectedly infective cornea (1 case) and from contaminated stereotactic EEG electrodes used for deep brain recording (2 cases) after an interval of 16 to 20 months, but the maximum incubation period may be as long as 20 years. Although in the vast majority of cases no contact has been established between any one patient and another, approximately 10 per cent of cases occur in a familial pattern suggestive of autosomal dominant transmission, raising fascinating questions about the interplay of infectious and genetic determinants of the disease.

INTRACRANIAL NEOPLASMS

By ROBERT L. MARTUZA, M.D.,
and ROBERT G. OJEMANN, M.D.

Boston, Massachusetts

GENERAL CONSIDERATIONS

Intracranial neoplasms continue to be an important cause of morbidity and mortality. From infancy to age 15 brain tumors are second only to leukemia as a cause of cancer death, while in the 15 to 34 year age group, these tumors rank second in males and third in females. In patients over 35 years of age, these neoplasms are relatively less common than tumors of other organ systems, although still ranking fourth among causes of cancer mortality for males 35 to 54 years of age. Moreover, the importance of recognizing these lesions early in their course is underscored by the fact that a significant number of intracranial tumors are benign and as they enlarge they are associated with increasingly severe neurologic disability.

Primary neoplasms comprise the majority of intracranial tumors in patients up to 35 years of age and reach a peak incidence in the 40 to 60 year age range. Metastatic intracranial lesions are more common in the older population. The incidence of cerebral metastases appears to be increasing owing to the prolonged lifespan of many cancer patients and to the inability of some chemotherapeutic agents to penetrate the blood-brain barrier.

CLINICAL EVALUATION

A well-taken history is the most important part of the evaluation of a patient with a neurologic problem. Since an intracranial lesion may alter memory, it is important to ascertain the mental function of the patient early in the history-taking process, and, if function is impaired, to seek family members or friends for the details of the illness. After recording the account of the illness and noting its tempo of evolution, one should systematically inquire about neurologic symptoms not mentioned spontaneously.

The neurologic examination allows one to confirm the patient's complaints as well as to detect related areas of dysfunction in order to define the neuroanatomic location of the problem. Examination of the skull for exostoses, cutaneous abnormalities, tender areas, widened sutures, and proptosis should be done. A good general medical examination is, of course, essential to detect signs of metastatic disease as well as any systemic illness such as diabetes, coronary artery disease, or chronic pulmonary disease, which may be important in the overall management during medical and surgical therapy.

PRESENTING SYMPTOMS AND SIGNS

Headache is a common initial complaint of many patients with an intracranial tumor. Usually the headache is nonlocalizing and easily confused with a tension or sinus headache. Certain types of headache, however, are more commonly associated with an intracranial lesion. These include headaches that awaken the patient from sleep, recurrent morning headaches that may be associated with hydrocephalus, and headaches that are precipitated or relieved by changes in head position, which may be due to intermittent obstruction of cerebrospinal fluid flow. Pituitary tumors may be associated with midline retro-orbital headache. Midline cerebellar or foramen magnum tumors often cause severe occipital or upper cervical pain. If the patient describes the sudden onset of the worst headache he has ever had, the diagnosis of a subarachnoid hemorrhage from an aneurysm, arteriovenous malformation, or tumor must be the first consideration.

Seizures are the next most common symptom of an intracranial tumor, and headache or seizure or both are noted in over half of the patients with a primary intracranial tumor. A grand mal seizure may be the presenting complaint. Such seizures, however, are nonlocalizing and it is important to question the family about the initial motor focus or an initiating event such as staring, lip smacking, head turning, or eye deviation, since these may suggest the area of the brain where the seizure started. If the initiating event was not observed, the documentation of a focal postictal neurologic deficit such as weakness, sensory loss, or dysphasia may also be helpful in localizing the lesion.

Minor motor seizures, such as limb or facial twitching or even a frank jacksonian motor march, may seem unimportant to the patient and therefore such details must be specifically sought. This type of seizure localizes the lesion to the posterior frontal area. Sensory seizures may be described as a brief tingling of a limb or half of the face and in some cases may be associated with a jacksonian sensory march without a motor seizure; sensory seizures localize the lesion to the contralateral anterior parietal lobe. Visual seizures localize the lesion to the occipital lobe. Temporal lobe seizures are among the more difficult to diagnose and may go unnoticed by both the patient and the physician. Such seizures may vary from simple staring spells to automated motions (lip smacking, walking) or even to sudden episodes of rage. Some patients document olfactory or taste hallucinations or, less often, auditory sensations associated with vertigo. Others may note vague visceral complaints, unexplained alterations in the environment, or just feeling "unreal."

Symptoms associated with increased intracranial pressure may be present with tumors in any intracranial location. Headache, more common in the morning, is the most common symptom. Vomiting may occur and is often not associated with eating. Blurred vision or decreased acuity may be due to papilledema and in such cases a central scotoma or enlarged blind spot may be noted on examination. Later in the course of the illness, confusion, dulled mentation, or a short attention span may also ensue.

An intracranial tumor should also be considered in patients presenting with a hemispheric transient ischemic attack (TIA). Although most TIAs are due to cerebrovascular disease, such a presentation is found in some patients with a metastatic cerebral tumor and may represent a frank tumor embolus. The patient may then improve from this minor stroke, only to show a progressive downhill neurologic course months later as the metastatic tumor grows. Occasionally a malignant glioma or meningioma may be present as a TIA. In these cases the pathophysiology is unclear and at times the spell may be difficult to distinguish from a brief seizure.

LOCALIZATION IN RELATIONSHIP TO SYMPTOMS AND SIGNS

Symptoms or signs of progressive cortical dysfunction usually correlate well with the anatomic location of the lesion. *Prefrontal tumors* may produce personality change, loss of interest in daily activities or hobbies, and loss of social inhibitions, while examination may show primitive reflexes (grasp, suck). *Posterior frontal tumors* demonstrate contralateral spastic weakness and hyperreflexia and, if in the dominant hemisphere, Broca's dysphasia with an inability of the patient to express himself. *Anterior parietal lesions* may show contralateral sensory diminution or loss of cortical sensory functions such as position sense, two-point discrimination, double simultaneous stimulation, and graphesthesia. *Posterior parietal lesions* can cause a

contralateral inferior quadrantanopia. In the dominant (usually left) cerebral hemisphere, a Wernicke's dysphasia, with the inability to understand what is said or dyscalculia, may be present. Patients with nondominant (usually right) cerebral lesions may show constructional apraxia, right-left confusion, poor geographic localization, or diminished opticokinetic nystagmus to that side. *Temporal lobe lesions* are associated with a contralateral superior quadrantanopia and, in the dominant hemisphere, with a Wernicke's dysphasia. A contralateral hemianopia, usually congruous, is common with *occipital lobe lesions.*

Cerebellar tumors, if lateral in the hemisphere, typically produce ataxia, horizontal nystagmus, and ipsilateral incoordination and may be associated with localized cranial nerve dysfunction. *Midline cerebellar* (vermis) *lesions* are more often associated with truncal ataxia and vertical nystagmus. Such lesions may compress the outlets of cerebrospinal fluid (CSF) flow or the aqueduct of Sylvius and may present with a rapid progression of symptoms of hydrocephalus associated with increased intracranial pressure. This, if untreated, can progress to decerebrate spells (often misinterpreted as seizures) and eventually to cardiorespiratory arrest.

Symptoms or signs of *cranial nerve dysfunctions,* with the exception of isolated sixth nerve palsies, are quite useful in localizing a lesion.

I. Loss of olfaction can be detected using common items such as soap or talc and, when associated with a tumor, suggest an inferior medial frontal lesion. Elderly patients, heavy smokers, or patients with chronic sinusitis may have decreased olfaction without an intracranial process. Other causes of a recent onset of poor olfaction can include head trauma or a viral upper respiratory infection.

II. Because of its length within the cranium, the visual system may be compromised at one of several anatomic positions. A unilateral optic nerve lesion may cause decreased visual acuity, disc atrophy, a central scotoma, or a monocular field cut and may be associated with proptosis if the lesion extends into the orbit. Chiasmatic compression typically produces a bitemporal hemianopia, whereas compression of the optic tracts produces a contralateral hemianopia or quadrantanopia.

III, IV, VI. Abducens (VI) nerve dysfunction may be nonlocalizing and is often secondary to increased intracranial pressure. Oculomotor (III) dysfunction is seen in tumors of the cavernous sinus region or can be caused by medial temporal lobe (uncal) herniation in the late stages of a large cerebral mass. Involvement of more than one of the nerves of ocular motility strongly suggests a compressive lesion that may be located anywhere along their course.

V. Trigeminal hyperfunction (facial pain) or hypofunction (numbness) can be caused by tumors. The pain may be like that of "typical" tic douloureux or may present with features "atypical" in quality and duration. Hypalgesia may involve one or more of the trigeminal divisions if the lesion involves the nerve. An "onion skin" pattern with hypalgesia of the perioral region suggests compression of the trigeminal pathway in the brainstem.

VII. Facial nerve hyperfunction (hemifacial spasm) is occasionally caused by a tumor located in the posterior fossa where the facial nerve enters the brainstem. However, facial nerve hypofunction (weakness) is more common and the clinical examination can be useful in localizing the lesion. A central, or upper motor neuron, lesion will usually cause contralateral weakness with sparing of the upper face. Peripheral, or lower motor neuron, lesions generally cause weakness of the entire ipsilateral face. When such a lesion is proximal to the geniculate ganglion, there may also be diminished taste on the anterior tongue as well as a decrease in the production of tears.

VIII. The eighth cranial nerve is a combination of the cochlear nerve and the inferior and superior vestibular nerves. Vertigo, tinnitus, and deafness may all be caused by eighth nerve compression. Such details must be specifically sought because the vertigo is often transient and the hearing loss, even if profound, may go unnoticed by the patient.

IX, X. Dysfunction of these lower cranial nerves may cause hoarseness or dysphagia and on examination may be associated with palatal asymmetry or diminished pharyngeal sensation.

XI. The spinal accessory nerve is actually a cervical nerve that travels upward through the foramen magnum to exit with the ninth and tenth cranial nerves. Weakness of the sternocleidomastoid or trapezius may therefore be caused by tumors in the inferolateral posterior fossa, the foramen magnum, or the upper cervical canal.

XII. Weakness of half of the tongue can be demonstrated by noting ipsilateral tongue deviation or weak protrusion of the tongue into the cheek. With central (upper motor neuron) lesions, the contralateral tongue deviation may be associated with other signs of central dysfunction (central facial weakness, hemiparesis). Peripheral lesions may show ipsilateral hemiglossal atrophy or fasciculations and, in some cases, may be associated with other cranial nerve abnormalities.

DIAGNOSTIC STUDIES

The appropriate choice of diagnostic studies will depend upon the degree of suspicion one has that a patient harbors an intracerebral mass. For the patient with nonspecific intermittent headache without other signs or symptoms of neurologic dysfunction, it may be appropriate to evaluate for sinusitis and to probe into medical causes while treating the patient symptomatically. However, the patient with persisting headache or one or more of the aforementioned symptoms or signs of an intracranial mass lesion needs a further, more expedient, evaluation.

Previously, this usually included an initial skull series, electroencephalogram, a brain scan, and often a lumbar puncture. But, while the skull series can show effects of chronically elevated intracranial pressure or local bone erosions or exostoses associated with specific tumors, it is more often nondiagnostic. Similarly, while the electroencephalogram (EEG) may show focal slowing or spike formation, it does not give adequate anatomic detail to allow further therapy. Lumbar puncture does not give useful diagnostic information and on occasion may be dangerous, causing temporal lobe or cerebellar herniation.

For a patient with a suspected intracranial tumor, the first diagnostic procedure should be an unenhanced and a contrast-enhanced computerized tomographic (CT) scan. While the cost for scans is greater than for any of the other individual tests, it is less than that for the others combined; of most importance is the fact that it gives much more information. When positive, it may be, in some cases, the only radiographic study needed. In most situations, however, one needs to pursue further studies, usually cerebral angiography, as indicated by the presenting symptoms and the location of the suspected tumor.

SUPRATENTORIAL TUMORS

Gliomas (astrocytoma, oligodendroglioma, ependymoma) make up the majority of primary tumors of the cerebral hemispheres. Of these, about half are malignant (astrocytoma III or IV, or glioblastoma multiforme). The unenhanced CT scan typically shows a low-density lesion with surrounding edema and mass effect. The tumor may enhance diffusely with intravenous contrast injection or, as is common with the malignant lesions, the circumference of the tumor may enhance but the center will not, reflecting a central area of low metabolic rate or frank necrosis. Astrocytomas (grade I or II) or oligodendrogliomas may show calcific foci.

The CT picture of a supratentorial glioma may be difficult to distinguish from a metastatic tumor, an abscess, or a resolving stroke or hematoma (Fig. 1). At times, the injection of a double dose of contrast material may show additional foci suggesting metastatic disease. Angiography may be helpful by showing a pattern of fine irregular "tumor" vessels and early draining veins that are characteristic of the malignant gliomas. Metastases are often less vascular and an abscess may be entirely avascular or show only a rim of vascularity in its capsule on the angiogram.

Meningiomas are usually of higher density than surrounding brain on the unenhanced CT scan and may contain calcifications. Contrast enhancement is usually homogeneous (Fig. 2). Skull films may be helpful by showing local bone thickening. Since these tumors arise from the arachnoid cells, they will usually be found adjacent to the cranial vault and most commonly occur in specific locations: convexity, parasagittal, sphenoid ridge, olfactory groove, and tuberculum sella. The presenting symptoms and signs will reflect the tumor location. Convexity tumors present with seizures or one of the various modes of hemispheric cerebral dysfunction already mentioned. The parasagittal tumors affect lower extremity motor and sensory function. Sphenoid ridge lesions may present with visual loss, a field cut, extraocular dysfunction, seizures, or a change in mental function. Olfactory groove meningiomas typically show anosmia and bifrontal dysfunction. Tuberculum sella lesions cause decreasing vision and a bitemporal field cut. Since meningiomas grow slowly, they may reach enormous size before the patient seeks medical attention. Angiography is essential in almost all patients and should include both internal and external carotid injections. Meningiomas often show a vascular hilus supplying the lesion and a stellate vascular appearance within the tumor.

If the CT scan demonstrates a supratentorial intraventricular lesion, other tumors must be considered. A patient with a history of intermittent headache, especially if affected by postural changes, may have a *colloid cyst* of the third ventricle — a benign lesion attached to the posterior rim of the foramen of Monroe. The CT scan may show enlarged lateral ventricles but may not show the cyst. A double-contrast scan,

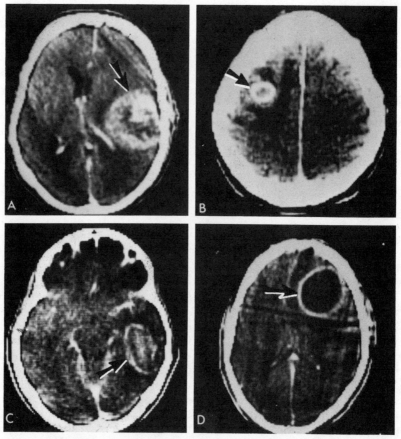

Figure 1. CT scans after contrast injection showing "ring-type" enhancement in four different types of pathology. The clinical history, angiography, and surgery are needed to clarify the diagnosis. (A) Astrocytoma, grade IV; (B) metastatic tumor; (C) resolving intracerebral hematoma; and (D) brain abscess.

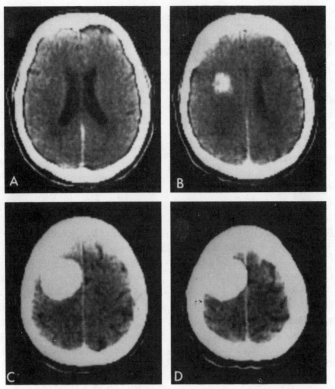

Figure 2. CT scans after contrast injection showing convexity meningioma. Some routine CT scans go only as high as scan A. It is important that higher scans be done in order not to miss important pathology. The diagnosis of meningioma is suggested by the well-circumscribed high density and the relationship to the inner table of the skull in scans C and D.

however, will often show the capsule and confirm the diagnosis. When there is doubt, however, angiography and, rarely, pneumoencephalography may have to be performed. Other intraventricular lesions include choroid plexus papillomas, ependymomas, astrocytomas, and, rarely, meningiomas.

POSTERIOR FOSSA TUMORS

Intrinsic lesions of the cerebellum will present with the symptoms previously described for lateral (hemispheric) cerebellar masses or for central (vermian) cerebellar masses. The CT scan is, again, the single most useful examination and will not only localize the lesion but may also demonstrate the degree of local distortion and associated hydrocephalus. Additionally, an enhanced scan may be helpful in suggesting the histologic diagnosis. A diffuse lesion, particularly if cystic, raises the possibility of an astrocytoma. An extremely vascular nodule with or without a cyst suggests hemangioblastoma; multiple lesions imply metastases. A low-density nonenhancing lesion could be an epidermoid; if calcium and fat are seen, a teratoma should be suspected. The age of the patient may also be helpful in that medulloblastomas and benign cerebellar astrocytomas are more common in the pediatric population, while older patients are more likely to have hemangioblastoma or metastatic tumors. If hemangioblastoma is suspected, retinal lesions of von Hippel-Lindau should be sought, renal function evaluated, and hematocrit obtained, since polycythemia has been associated with cerebellar hemangioblastomas. These patients will need a vertebral angiogram. Lumbar puncture should be avoided in patients suspected of having a posterior fossa tumor.

Patients with brainstem gliomas may present with a confusing pattern of unilateral or bilateral cranial nerve dysfunction that can appear to be either central or peripheral in nature. Moreover, while their overall course is one of downhill progression, it may be interspersed with periods of partial or complete remission, raising the possibility of a demyelinating illness. Skull films are usually not helpful. A CT scan may show posterior displacement of the fourth ventricle, a widened brainstem, or compression of the basal cisterns but, in many cases, this may be difficult to discern. Angiography usually reveals a brainstem widened by an avascular mass and a pneumoencephalogram is often needed for a final diagnosis.

Among the posterior fossa lesions extrinsic to the brain substance, *acoustic neuroma* is the most common. These Schwann cell tumors usually arise from the vestibular nerve within the internal auditory canal and initially expand the canal and grow medially to reside in the cerebellopontine angle. Early symptoms include unilateral hearing loss, vertigo, tinnitus, and difficulty with balance. Later, facial weakness, trigeminal dysfunction, cerebellar symptoms, or even hydrocephalus may ensue. When the history raises a suspicion of a cerebellopontine angle tumor or an internal auditory canal tumor, an audiogram, internal auditory canal tomograms, and a contrast enhanced CT scan are indicated. With a good history, an audiogram showing sensorineural hearing loss, an enlarged internal auditory canal, and a typical lesion on CT scan, no further preoperative studies are routinely needed (Fig. 3). However, if the history or CT scan is atypical, an angiogram may be important in diagnosing a meningioma or other tumor. Positive contrast cisternography of the cerebellopontine angle is now used only in those patients with a typical history and findings but a negative CT scan. In such patients, cisternography may demonstrate a small lesion at or within the canal. This is the ideal time to make the diagnosis, for the removal of such a small tumor is more likely to preserve facial function and occasionally hearing.

Other lesions at the base of the skull within the posterior fossa that may produce various patterns of cranial nerve disturbances include chordomas, epidermoids, meningiomas of the clivus or petrous ridge, metastases to the skull base, or nasopharyngeal carcinoma. The evaluation of such lesions will rely heavily upon the CT scan and tomograms of the skull base with angiography as indicated.

SELLAR OR PARASELLAR TUMORS

Endocrine hyperfunction or hypofunction and visual disturbances referable to the optic nerves, chiasm, tracts, or extraocular nerves can occur with lesions in the *sella* area. In addition to a thorough endocrinologic evaluation as discussed in the endocrinology chapters of this text, most patients will also need detailed neuro-ophthalmologic testing. Plain skull films and sella tomograms are essential to determine the sella size, the presence of asymmetry, or changes in the adjacent osseous structures. A CT scan can help to identify a suprasellar or intrasellar lesion (Fig. 4). A pneumoencephalogram has often been needed to delineate adequately the suprasellar anatomy in order to plan appropriate therapy. More recently, lumbar injection of metrizamide combined with CT scanning has shown adequate suprasellar detail,

replacing the pneumoencephalogram in some patients.

In the presence of endocrine hyperfunction a *pituitary adenoma* is virtually certain; however, hypofunction or normal function can be present with a nonfunctional pituitary adenoma, craniopharyngioma, suprasellar meningioma, or glioma of the optic or hypothalamic structures. On a CT scan, pituitary adenomas are contiguous with the sellar contents, usually contain no calcium, and may be either solid or cystic in nature. Craniopharyngiomas are often cystic and usually contain calcium. Meningiomas are typically solid and homogeneously enhancing; they may contain calcium, and may be associated with local hyperostoses. A thickened optic nerve or chiasm, often with a widened optic canal, suggests an optic glioma. For lesions that arise from within the sella, angiography may not be needed; however, lesions that are primarily suprasellar may require angiography to delineate vascular relationships, to evaluate vascular encasement, and to exclude a suprasellar giant aneurysm.

PINEAL AREA TUMORS

Because of their unique position with regard to the aqueduct of Sylvius and to the colliculi, *pineal area tumors* can present with hydrocephalus as well as ocular symptoms. Poor upgaze, difficulty with convergence, and pupils that constrict to accommodation but not to bright light (Parinaud's syndrome) are common. Vertical nystagmus, limb ataxia, or spastic weakness may also be present. A CT scan will usually define the lesion as well as allow evaluation of ventricular size. Arteriography will usually be needed to help in the differential diagnosis, to delineate the vascularity of the lesion and to demonstrate its relationship to the major midline veins. About half of these lesions are radiosensitive germinomas. The remainder include typical teratomas (which may show fat and calcium on CT scan), astrocytomas, pinealomas, and other rarer entities.

FORAMEN MAGNUM TUMORS

Although *foramen magnum tumors* comprise only a small percentage of all central nervous system tumors, their importance is underscored by the fact that most are benign and treatable, yet may be easily mistaken for other untreatable diseases. The most common symptom of a foramen magnum tumor is pain, which is usually posterior cervical or occipital, and often is made worse by coughing, sneezing, or neck motion. Most patients experience some sensory abnor-

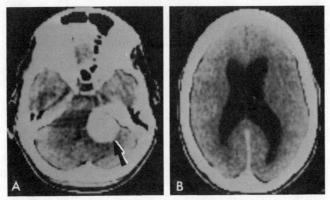

Figure 3. CT scans after contrast injection in a patient with symptoms and signs of an acoustic neuroma in the right cerebellopontine angle. (A) The tumor (arrow) is well circumscribed, adjacent to the petrous pyramid, and is compressing the brainstem and cerebellum. (B) Associated hydrocephalus is demonstrated by enlargement of the lateral ventricles.

mality during their course. This is most commonly upper extremity tingling, prickling, burning, or coldness. Posterior column dysfunction may appear early or late, depending upon the position of the tumor. Weakness had been classically described as progressing in a clockwise fashion (ipsilateral arm to ipsilateral leg to contralateral leg to contralateral arm). However, because the tumor may compress the pyramidal decussation at varying levels, all types of patterns of motor loss have been described, including bilateral upper limb weakness as well as crossed upper and lower limb weakness. Even weakness and atrophy of the hands can be present; this may falsely lead the physician to suspect a lower motor neuron lesion of the mid or lower cervical cord. The spinal accessory nerve is involved in about one third of patients, with less frequent involvement of the other cranial nerves.

The course of a patient with a foramen magnum tumor can extend over months or years and may be marked by periods of remission or partial remission, occasionally associated with steroid therapy. Some patients may therefore be followed for some period of time with an erroneous diagnosis of multiple sclerosis. The disease in other patients with slowly progressive upper extremity symptoms has been misdiagnosed as syringomyelia or amyotrophic lateral sclerosis (ALS). Still other patients with neck pain and motor symptoms have been diagnosed as having cervical cord compression from a degenerated disc. It is not uncommon for such a patient to undergo myelography and surgery at a lower cervical level.

Therefore, any patient with cervical symptoms attributed to multiple sclerosis, syringomyelia, or ALS, or any patient with a peculiar presentation of a cervical disc problem, particularly if he has not responded to appropriate therapy, should be suspected of having a foramen magnum tumor. Plain x-rays of the cervico-occipital junction may show foraminal enlarge-

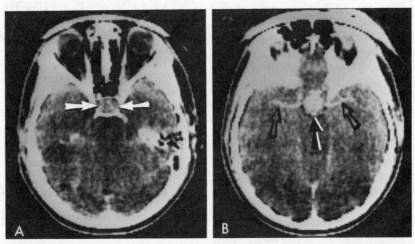

Figure 4. CT scans after contrast injection in a patient with symptoms and signs of a pituitary tumor. (A) The enhanced tumor is seen within the sella (arrow). (B) Suprasella extension of the tumor (solid arrow). Contrast material is seen in the middle cerebral arteries (open arrows).

ment from a neurofibroma but more often are not useful. The CT scan has also been misleading at times. The most important study is a myelogram with good visualization of both the anterior and posterior lips of the foramen magnum. If a tumor is found, vertebral angiography may be needed in order to plan the surgery.

SKULL LESIONS

Patients will occasionally present to the physician complaining of a skull deformity — usually a lump, less often a defect or tender area. At examination, the physician should note the location, size, and mobility of the lesion as well as whether or not it is compressible or is tender, and whether it changes with posture. Other lesions should be sought in order to exclude occipital or retromastoid adenopathy or multiple cranial metastases. A skull series is appropriate and may demonstrate either a blastic lesion, a lytic lesion, or mixed blastic and lytic lesions. Among the blastic lesions, osteomas are the most common benign neoplasms and are well-circumscribed, slowly enlarging outgrowths of either the inner or outer skull table. Typically, the diploe is preserved and there is no increase in vascular markings. Meningiomas, on the other hand, most extensively involve the inner table, obliterate the diploe, and may be associated with adjacent hyperostosis and increased vascular markings. Multiple blastic lesions suggest metastatic disease, commonly from tumors of the prostate, breast, or bladder.

Single lytic lesions may be due to a cranial epidermoid or dermoid. These often feel rubbery, are nontender, and are most commonly located in the supraorbital or anterior temporal area. Skull films reveal a sharply defined lucent area with sclerotic edges. A hemangioma of the skull can also present as a lytic lesion and may cause headache. Cavernous hemangiomas are the most common type and radiographically appear as an irregular lucent area with a "honeycombed" center. Metastatic lytic lesions may come from virtually any source. For the differential diagnosis of less common skull lesions, the reader is referred to one of the standard radiology texts.

PITFALLS IN DIAGNOSIS

When a well-taken history and a properly performed physical examination are combined with appropriately executed diagnostic tests, the diagnosis or exclusion of an intracerebral neoplasm can be made with a good degree of confidence. Exploratory neurosurgery is virtually a relic of the past. Yet, some pitfalls do exist at every stage of a patient's evaluation. A patient with a right parietal lobe lesion may neglect symptoms on his left side, or the subtleties of visual, auditory, or sensory loss may be overlooked by both the patient and the physician.

The CT scan has revolutionized the evaluation of the patient with cerebral disease, and, as we have pointed out, it has become the procedure of choice in the evaluation of many patients with a suspected intracranial neoplasm. However, it, too, may be misleading. A high convexity or parasagittal tumor may be missed entirely if the scans are not completed to the vertex (Fig. 2). Small lesions adjacent to bone may be difficult to visualize. Areas of acute demyelination or focal vasculitis may enhance with contrast and may be mistaken for tumors. Usually, however, they do not produce mass effect. Ring-like enhancement may be associated with tumor, abscess, or resolving infarction or hematoma (Fig. 1). The physician must be guided by the patient's general medical condition, the tempo of the illness, and whether or not the lesion is in a vascular distribution. When any lesion is noted on CT scan, it is important to compare a nonenhanced scan with a contrast-enhanced one; failure to do this has on several occasions led to an erroneous diagnosis. As already noted, it may even be necessary to give a double dose of contrast material in order to delineate a subtle lesion or to identify additional lesions. This tactic has, in some patients, eliminated the need for angiography or pneumoencephalography, thus reducing both risk and expense.

OPTIC NEURITIS

By GREGORY B. KROHEL, M.D.,
Albany, New York

and ROBERT S. HEPLER, M.D.
Los Angeles, California

SYNONYMS AND RELATED TERMS

Papillitis is optic neuritis in which ophthalmoscopic signs of disc swelling are visible. *Retrobulbar neuritis* is optic neuritis without visible ophthalmoscopic abnormalities. ("The patient sees nothing, and neither does the doctor.") *Neuroretinitis* is defined as papillitis with adjacent inflammation and edema of the retina. *Optic neuropathy* is a general term for optic nerve disease in the aforementioned categories. *Ischemic optic neuropathy* is a frequently encountered acute optic neuropathy in middle-aged and elderly persons with implications of interruption of blood supply to the optic nerve.

DEFINITION

Optic neuritis is most frequently encountered as an acute impairment of function of one optic nerve in a young adult. Fortunately, optic neuritis is frequently self-limited, with a strong tendency toward spontaneous improvement even though optic nerve function seldom returns to complete normality. Pathologic examination of involved optic nerve tissue is not generally possible, but the pathologic disorder is presumed to be optic nerve demyelination. The implication of actual inflammation or infection as derived from the term neuritis is probably incorrect in most cases, except for those rare events in which there is spread of inflammation from contiguous structures as in acute sinusitis, meningitis, or orbital cellulitis. Optic neuritis is associated with viral and postviral syndromes, intraocular inflammation, and in a statistically important manner, with multiple sclerosis.

PRESENTING SIGNS AND SYMPTOMS

The presenting complaint is usually acute loss of vision. The vision usually worsens over several days and the maximum impairment is reached within a week. Onset may be extremely rapid over the course of hours, and some patients may note beginning improvement in vision by the end of the first week. The adult form of optic neuritis usually presents unilaterally, while the childhood presentation may be bilateral and often may have systemic association with viral illness.

Pain commonly precedes visual loss by a day or two, and often the pain has stopped before maximal visual loss is reached. The pain is periorbital or retrobulbar in location and has a characteristic aggravation by eye movement. The severity of the pain is variable, but the accentuation by eye movement is so typical as to bring into doubt the diagnosis of optic neuritis when pain is totally absent. The globe may be tender to palpation. Some patients complain of mild photophobia, and they may note that they see better in a dimly lit environment. The patient may notice flashes of light while in a dark environment. These flashes, or "phosphenes," are precipitated by horizontal eye movement and usually last only several seconds.

Perceptive patients may note impairment of depth perception because of uniocular reduction in vision. Accordingly they may complain of particular difficulty in judging the distance of a moving object, such as a tennis ball. Color vision is profoundly reduced during and after an attack of optic neuritis, and a patient may complain subjectively of this aspect of impairment.

The recorded visual acuity during an attack of optic neuritis usually ranges between 20/60 and 20/400. Very profound visual loss, even at the point of loss of all light perception, is not rare during the acute phase. The occurrence of extremely mild attacks of this condition is suggested by observation of patients with electrophysiologic or ophthalmoscopic evidence of previous optic neuritis, who retain normal central acuity and have no history of previous visual loss.

The visual field abnormality in optic neuritis is usually a central scotoma, which may be demonstrated at the tangent screen by Goldmann perimetry, by confrontation, or by Amsler grid visual field testing. Less commonly, one may note arcuate, ring, or paracentral scotomas and enlargement of the physiologic blind spot. Such variations in the visual field defect, other than a simple central scotoma, should raise a question of other categories of optic neuropathy, such as ischemic optic neuropathy or optic nerve compression.

Either simple or complicated color vision testing can be used to document the usually profound color abnormality. Patients often note a difference in the brightness or saturation of a colored object when the object is presented alternately to each eye. In less sensitive color vision tests, such as the Ishihara or HRR pseudoisochromatic color plates, the patient may correctly identify all the plates. The patient, however, will report a difference in the brightness of the colors as perceived in the two eyes. More sensitive color testing such as the Farnsworth-Munsell 100 hue test may detect subtle defects in otherwise subclinical cases of optic neuritis. The color vision defects are seldom this difficult to demonstrate.

Light brightness is reduced in the involved eye, and the patient may notice spontaneously that everything viewed through the involved eye appears dark. One may test for this observation simply by swinging a penlight between both eyes and asking the patient on which side the light appears brighter. Occasionally, a patient with photophobia may report that the light in the involved eye is brighter. This confusing response is generated by reporting relative discomfort rather than relative brightness.

The most reliable objective sign of optic nerve function, and one that is particularly crucial in differentiating true optic neuritis from nonorganic visual complaints, is the afferent pupillary defect (Marcus Gunn) pupil sign. The impairment of nerve conduction in optic neuritis generates an imbalance in the amount of stimulation for pupillary light response. This imbalance is exquisitely sensitive. In clinical testing, the examiner swings a flashlight between both eyes, pausing momentarily with the light on either eye before swinging quickly to the opposite eye. On returning the light to the normal eye there is a bilateral pupillary constriction, in contrast to a bilateral dilatation of the pupil observed when the light returns to the involved eye. One cannot demonstrate this sign in patients with bilateral disease, unless there is a disparity in the amount of involvement of the two eyes. Also, patients with previous optic neuritis with residual optic atrophy may not display the afferent pupillary defect sign, as conduction is now abnormal in both eyes. The test is best performed in a semidarkened room, utilizing a bright penlight. The objective test for afferent pupillary defect correlates well with the subjective light brightness test.

Another objective, easily performed test of nerve conduction is the pupil cycle time. A thin, horizontal slit beam of moderate intensity is directed perpendicular to the iris at the inferior corneal scleral limbus. The beam is slowly elevated until it overlaps the pupillary margin. The pupil then constricts and the pupillary margin is moved away from the beam of light. As the pupil then spontaneously redilates, it encounters the light and again constricts as it comes into contact with the beam. The cycle of dilatation and constriction is timed. Runs of 30 cycles are timed for four runs, with the time to the nearest 0.1 second noted with a stopwatch. To obtain the pupil cycle time, the total time is divided by the total number of cycles. A conduction defect is present if the pupil cycle time is longer than 954 milliseconds, or if there is a difference of more than 70 milliseconds between the two eyes.

The Pulfrich stereophenomenon has been found by some examiners to be a useful test of optic nerve conduction. In performing this test, a long pendulum is swung at right angles to the patient's eyes at a distance of about 20 feet. The patient is directed to follow the motion of the pendulum and to describe it. A patient with a conduction defect of one eye will describe an elliptic path of the pendulum. The apparent depth of the elliptic pathway will be greater with more severe optic nerve dysfunction. The visual acuity must be at least 20/70 or better in the involved eye to perform this relatively subtle test.

The appearance of the fundus depends upon the cause of the optic neuritis and the stage at which the patient is examined. The postviral form of optic neuritis, which is more common in children, may show bilateral optic nerve swelling. Venous engorgement is present, but hemorrhages at the optic nerve margin are minimal if present at all. Adults with optic neuritis have either papillitis or retrobulbar neuritis. In the latter case there is no visible swelling of the disc, but some degree of optic atrophy is likely to become apparent on follow-up examination several weeks later. Patients with optic neuritis secondary to intraocular inflammation, or associated with multiple sclerosis, display sheathing of the retinal vessels. In some cases of papillitis, cells may be seen in the posterior vitreous space immediately anterior to the optic nerve. In the condition termed neuroretinitis, there is adjacent edema of the retina and exudates may be found in the macular region.

After acute optic neuritis has resolved, retrograde degeneration of axons in the optic nerve can produce grooved slit-like defects in the nerve fiber layer. These arcuate defects in the nerve fiber layer of the retina are best seen through a dilated pupil using a bright red-free light generated from a halogen ophthalmoscopic bulb. Therefore, it is possible to detect previous subtle attacks of optic neuritis by careful inspection of both the optic nerve and the nerve fiber layer. These grooves are not specific for optic neuritis, and they can result from other insults to the optic nerve such as ischemic optic neuropathy and glaucoma.

Visual evoked potentials (responses) (VEPs, VERs) can be useful in objectively documenting optic neuropathy. Such electrophysiologic testing can aid in detection of subclinical damage to an optic nerve, in conjunction with sophisticated color vision testing and careful inspection of the fundus for nerve fiber layer defects. VEPs are generated by exposing a patient to a patterned, repetitive visual stimulus. The occipital cortical activity is recorded with skin electrodes, and the summated cortical response constitutes the VEP. A delay of the VEP is characteristic, but not specific, for optic neuritis. An abnormal delay of the VEP, when combined with signs and symptoms of demyelination elsewhere in the nervous system, is highly suggestive of multiple sclerosis.

COURSE

Recovery of visual acuity is variable. Patients with idiopathic optic neuritis (the most common form) usually begin to improve in the second or third week. Acuity often returns to functionally good levels by the second month. Approximately 75 per cent of patients will have return to visual acuity in the 20/20 to 20/30 range, even though most patients will continue to report subtle abnormality in the central visual field and color vision defect, which they retain for the rest of their life. Of the remaining 25 per cent of patients, some improve initially but do not recover near normal acuity. An even smaller group of patients show little or no recovery, and in these individuals one must maintain some concern about the diagnosis. Repeated bouts of optic neuritis worsen the outlook for significant recovery. Approximately one sixth of patients with a single episode of optic neuritis will eventually develop multiple sclerosis. Prognostic factors significant in pointing toward future development of multiple sclerosis include positive typing for HLA antigen BT101 and winter onset of the initial attack in patients with this typing. Patients with recurrent attacks of optic neuritis involving the same eye also are more at risk. Patients who develop optic neuritis in the second eye have acquired a second presumably demyelinating lesion, and therefore may be considered as probably having multiple sclerosis.

A subsequent episode of optic neuritis in the same or opposite eye can be anticipated in approximately 20 per cent of patients. After recovery of good vision patients may notice transient deterioration of vision in the affected eye when exercising or taking a hot bath (Uhthoff's phenomenon). Vision returns to baseline levels when the exercise or hot bathing is stopped.

DIFFERENTIAL DIAGNOSIS

Acute ischemic optic neuropathy is often confused with optic neuritis. This ischemic disease usually occurs in an older age group (over 50 years of age) and often has a different pattern of visual loss. An altitudinal or arcuate scotoma suggests loss of blood supply to the involved optic nerve. The visual loss, predictably, is likely to be sudden and permanent. The associated swelling of the disc may be sectorial or complete, and superficial flame-shaped hemorrhages are prominent on the surface of the disc and the immediately adjacent retina. The optic nerve swelling is often pallid, in contrast to the hyperemic swelling of papillitis. The arterioles around the disc may be attenuated. Patients with ischemic optic neuropathy must be investigated for giant cell arteritis.

Leber's optic neuropathy may occur in either sex, but among white patients it is seen most often in young men. There may or may not be a positive family history. The fundus appearance is diagnostic, and it includes a distinctive swelling of the nerve fiber layer around the disc. Unlike papillitis, however, there is no leakage or staining observed on fluorescein angiography. In addition, one can observe circumpapillary telangiectatic vessels in the acute phase of Leber's optic neuropathy. Spontaneous recovery is poor, and visual loss is generally severe and permanent. Both eyes usually are involved sequentially, with a lapse of a few weeks or months between the first and second involvement.

Papilledema is usually a bilateral condition reflecting increased intracranial pressure. Normal central visual acuity is usually preserved, and the customary visual field abnormality is enlargement of the physiologic blind spot without central scotoma.

Central serous retinopathy can produce acute visual loss with a central scotoma. Pain is absent, and the pupil reacts normally. Fluorescein angiography reveals leakage of dye in the macular region, which shows a characteristic elevation of the retina on ophthalmoscopy. The optic nervehead should be inspected closely for signs of optic nerve pits, which are sometimes associated with central serous retinopathy. The macular dazzle test may be helpful in differentiating a subtle macular problem from retrobulbar neuritis. The patient is asked to stare at a bright penlight for 15 seconds after a baseline visual acuity is recorded. In optic nerve disease the acuity will return promptly to the pretest level. With macular disease such as central serous retinopathy, there is a delay in regeneration of photosynthetic elements, and the time required to return to pretest visual acuity is much greater than in optic nerve disease.

Compressive lesions of the optic nerve or chiasm are often mislabeled initially as optic neuritis. Any patient with presumed optic neuritis who does not have associated pain on ocular movement, who does not show evidence of visual recovery at 6 weeks, or who shows other atypical features, should be suspected of having a tumor. Improvement with steroids does not constitute a positive indication for optic neuritis, as patients with various compressive lesions often show initial improvement when treated with steroids. Also, it has been stressed in this review that spontaneous improvement in function is characteristic of optic neuritis. Therefore, it is difficult to evaluate treatment of optic neuritis, and one must not associate improvement in vision with confirmation of the diagnosis. Usually, but not always, the course of visual loss with space-occupying lesions will be slow and relentless without the episodes of exacerbation and remission so characteristic of optic neuritis.

FURTHER INVESTIGATION

Optic neuritis patients should have a complete blood count, sedimentation rate, and serologic testing for syphilis. Skull x-rays with views of the paranasal sinuses and optic foramina are also indicated. A careful ophthalmologic examination should rule out orbital or ocular inflammation. Most patients with optic neuritis should be referred for general neurologic evaluation. Examination of the cerebrospinal fluid may show elevations of IgG, which suggest multiple sclerosis. Spinal tap is not necessarily required in the evaluation of typical optic neuritis.

Atypical features or indications of progressive visual loss demand a complete radiologic evaluation including computerized tomography. Other causes of optic neuropathy (not ordinary optic neuritis) — such as B_{12} deficiency, tobacco and alcohol amblyopia, and exposure to toxins — should be considered if the optic neuropathy is bilateral and atypical. In general, the patient with an isolated episode of optic neuritis should *not* be warned about possible development of multiple sclerosis.

PITFALLS IN DIAGNOSIS

Compressive lesions (tumors), retinal disorders, and optic nerve disease secondary to orbital disorder (e.g., thyroid eye disease) are examples of major categories of disease that may be misinterpreted as optic neuritis. An extremely important additional category is that of nonorganic (hysterical or malingering) visual complaint. These potentially serious diagnostic pitfalls can be avoided by careful attention to historical analysis and physical examination of each patient with optic neuritis. Abnormal pupillary signs (afferent pupillary defect) are paramount in importance in confirming optic nerve dysfunction. Additional objective confirmation that organic disease is or is not present may be provided by VEP testing, although generally careful attention to pupillary signs will resolve this issue.

PAINFUL NEURALGIAS OF THE TRIGEMINAL, GLOSSOPHARYNGEAL, VAGUS, AND GENICULATE NERVES

By JOHN M. TEW, JR., M.D.
Cincinnati, Ohio

TRIGEMINAL NEURALGIA (TIC DOULOUREUX, FACIAL NEURALGIA)

DEFINITION

Trigeminal neuralgia is a condition of paroxysmal facial pain provoked by cutaneous stimuli to trigger points in the orofacial regions and radiating in the distribution of the trigeminal nerve.

PRESENTING SYMPTOMS

There are five features that distinguish tic douloureux from other painful conditions of the face: (1) Pain, paroxysmal in character, is the only symptom. (2) The pain is confined to the distribution of the trigeminal nerve. (3) The pain is preceded by cutaneous stimuli such as touch, talking, moving the tongue, or even a light breeze blowing against the face. Shaving, brushing the teeth, or even eating becomes impossible for victims in the throes of an attack of tic douloureux. (4) The pain never crosses the midline. Although 1 per cent of patients develop bilateral tic douloureux, the condition rarely occurs simultaneously on both sides of the face. (5) The disorder is subject to exacerbations and remissions. Because of this characteristic, credence has been given to many forms of treatment. However, almost invariably the pain recurs after increasingly short periods of remission, only to persist longer and cause more suffering.

PHYSICAL FINDINGS

During periods of remission, the physical and neurologic examination is normal. The slightest evidence of altered sensation, facial paralysis, or hearing loss should suggest that a neoplasm, vascular anomaly, or compressive lesion may be present. Appropriate diagnostic studies are mandatory.

If examination is conducted during a siege of pain, the face is frequently immobile, hygiene may be disregarded, and the face is protected from any intrusion. If permitted, sensory examination will elicit paroxysms of pain on stimulation of trigger sites, principally around the nose, lips, and eyebrows, even by the most gentle touch. Calibrated testing may demonstrate decreased sensation, a feature that suggests fatigue or metabolic exhaustion of the ganglion cells. Autonomic features such as tearing, rhinorrhea, and redness of the face may accompany attacks of pain in some patients and lead to confusion with cluster or migraine headaches.

Suffering associated with tic douloureux is highly variable. The paroxysmal pain in the early stages is usually mild and is frequently confused with pain of dental origin. This feature leads the victim to seek dental care and, in many circumstances, results in multiple dental extractions, revisions of occlusion, and explorations of the paranasal sinuses. As the attacks become more severe, the pain is variously described as "stabbing," "jabbing," like a hot poker, and even may become constant, as if the face were "on fire." During the attacks of extreme pain, victims may attempt suicide because analgesics and narcotics are ineffective.

NATURAL HISTORY

Remissions and exacerbations are common but spontaneous cure rarely occurs. The disease rarely develops in patients less than 40 years of age. However, we have seen cases in three patients less than 20 years old. There is a predilection for females, the pain is more common on the right side, and familial disposition is recognized. The incidence is approximately 1:25,000 persons.

In time, the condition worsens, often breaks through medical therapy, and recurs after peripheral nerve destruction. It responds to interruption of the nerve proximal to the gasserian ganglion with cure or protracted remission.

LABORATORY DIAGNOSIS

The correct diagnosis of tic douloureux is based almost entirely on the history and observation of the patient during an attack of pain. However, the latter is not necessary since the patients' description of "classic" tic douloureux is seldom misunderstood. Laboratory studies are useful to identify the occasional underlying condition that may cause or mimic idiopathic trigeminal neuralgia.

Skull x-rays will demonstrate basilar impression, osteopetrosis, Paget's disease, or other disorders of the bone that may be associated with compression of the trigeminal nerve. Destruction of the petrous bone, erosion of the internal auditory meatus, or irregular calcification in the lateral aspect of the posterior fossa suggests a tumor.

Computerized tomography of the brain and skull base will effectively demonstrate most brain tumors. Angiography is advisable if a vascular anomaly or aneurysm is suspected. Recently, vascular compression by aberrant or tortuous branches of the arterial system have been implicated as a cause of painful tic. Therefore, angiography may be advisable before a final form of surgical therapy is selected for the patient recalcitrant to medical treatment.

Spinal fluid analysis should be performed if multiple sclerosis is suspected. Selective elevation of the gamma globulin fraction is indicative of multiple sclerosis, whereas elevated total protein is more suggestive of tumor.

Digitalis intoxication is a rare cause of tic-like pain that can be rapidly eliminated by cessation of the drug. Serum digitalis level should be obtained in suspected cases.

DIFFERENTIAL DIAGNOSIS

The differentiation of more obscure forms of facial pain may be quite difficult at times: (1) atypical facial pain, (2) symptomatic lesions, (3) dental neuralgia, (4) cluster migraine, (5) temporomandibular joint disease, (6) multiple sclerosis, (7) other cranial neuralgias.

Atypical facial pain is a descriptive term contrived to catch all the conditions that are not "classic" idiopathic trigeminal neuralgia. This diagnosis is basically one of exclusion; however, there are certain features of the history found in most patients. The pain is gradual in onset, is constant rather than paroxysmal, and often is described as "burning," "boring," or "aching" in character. The pain frequently radiates across the midline and outside the trigeminal distribution. This condition tends to occur in younger persons and to be associated with depression or serious neurosis. Patients with atypical facial pain seldom appear to suffer, frequently rub the face, and rarely, identify trigger points. Unlike tic douloureux, the pain is seldom alleviated by carbamazepine (Tegretol). The physical examination is normal, although the patient with chronic pain may have already been subjected to a series of procedures (nerve destruction,

dental extraction, sinus exploration), to the detriment of his condition. Differentiation is critical because destructive procedures on the nervous system invariably aggravate the pain. Psychotropic drugs and counseling are probably the only effective approaches to this problem.

Symptomatic lesions such as neoplasms, multiple sclerosis, vascular anomalies, and compressive lesions may cause the tic-like pain, but in most instances there are distinguishing features such as constancy of pain or presence of focal neurologic deficits. The appropriate laboratory tests should confirm the diagnosis.

Dental neuralgia is occasionally a perplexing problem since most patients with facial pain have had a considerable number of dental procedures. They may be uncertain which came first, the pain or a dental procedure that may have injured a peripheral nerve and caused a painful neuralgia. Pain of dental origin is more likely constant, burning, limited to distribution of a dental nerve and associated with some sensory deficit in the distribution of that nerve. The pain should be eliminated by local injection with anesthetics but resection of the nerve may fail to provide permanent relief.

Cluster migraine (Horton's cephalgia, red migraine) may be confused with tic douloureux because of its paroxysmal character, radiation into the trigeminal distribution, and association with autonomic phenomena. However, the disorder can be distinguished by familial occurrence, by attacks that are throbbing, constant, and progressive in nature, developing in a crescendo fashion to termination suddenly after 30 to 45 minutes, by the absence of trigger sites, and by provocation by alcohol and certain foods. Interestingly, some patients whose condition cannot be diagnosed with certainty may respond partially to drug treatment and satisfactorily to surgical approach. Their disease has been called by me and my colleagues *cluster tic douloureux*.

Temporomandibular joint disease should never be confused with tic douloureux because the pain caused by malocclusion or arthritis of the temporomandibular joint does not resemble tic pain, is focal in nature, and can be reproduced by manipulation of the jaw. The diagnosis is confirmed by radiographic changes of the temporomandibular joint.

Multiple sclerosis may be associated with painful neuralgia that is indistinguishable from tic douloureux. The physical examination should indicate evidence of neurologic abnormalities such as ataxia, nystagmus, or sensory deficits. The history may indicate previous episodes of neurologic disturbance in an otherwise normal patient. Bilateral tic douloureux in a young woman is a persuasive indicator of multiple sclerosis.

GLOSSOPHARYNGEAL NEURALGIA

Glossopharyngeal neuralgia is a painful condition that emanates from a disorder of the ninth or tenth cranial nerve or both and should properly be called vagoglossopharyngeal neuralgia. The characteristics of the pain are identical to trigeminal neuralgia. Radiation into the pharynx, throat, tonsillar fossa, base of the tongue, and depth of the ear is the distinguishing feature. Occasionally, the two conditions may be confused when the pain radiates into the ear and mastoid region and is provoked by swallowing.

Trigger points are frequently elicited in the tonsillar fossa and pharynx, where application of cocaine may produce immediate cessation of the pain.

An interesting but dangerous feature of the disease is the occasional occurrence of syncope, bradycardia, hypotension, and cardiac arrest.

The reflex that causes this condition is mediated through the nerve of Herring and can be eliminated by local injection of lidocaine (Xylocaine) near the carotid bifurcation. The attacks may be initiated by coughing, swallowing, compression of the neck, or even head turning.

Neuralgia of the ninth and tenth nerves responds to carbamazepine (Tegretol) but may require surgical section of the nerves in intractable circumstances.

GENICULATE NEURALGIA

Geniculate neuralgia is a painful condition similar to trigeminal and glossopharyngeal neuralgia because the pain radiates into or about the ear. The condition is apparently rare but may account for failure of some patients to respond favorably to surgical procedures directed at the fifth, ninth, or tenth nerve. The diagnosis can be proved only by a process of elimination, hopefully by diagnostic nerve blocks rather than by surgical procedures. Fortunately the condition is rare and apparently responds favorably to medical therapy.

EXPANDING INTRASPINAL LESIONS

By MICHAEL POLLAY, M.D.
Oklahoma City, Oklahoma

DEFINITION AND SYNONYMS

Expanding intraspinal lesions are space-occupying masses that are contained within the bony confines of the vertebral canal. These lesions may arise primarily from structures comprising or contained within the bony spinal canal or from more remote sites external to the spine. These lesions adversely affect spinal cord function by direct compression or interference with cord blood supply or both. The major classification of intraspinal lesions is according to their location relative to the spinal cord and its coverings.

1. Extradural. These lesions are located outside of the dura mater but beneath, or within, the bony canal. Examples of lesions in this location are (a) infections, acute (e.g., streptococcus or staphylococcus abscess) and chronic (e.g., tuberculosis or brucellosis), with or without involvement of the vertebrae; (b) herniated or protruded intravertebral discs; (c) metastatic tumors (e.g, lung, breast, bowel, kidney, prostate); (d) some meningiomas (5 to 10 per cent are extradural) and schwannomas (25 to 30 per cent extradural); and (e) epidural bleeding (most common location for intraspinal bleeding). This bleeding may be associated with blood dyscrasias, anticoagulation therapy, trauma, vascular malformation, hypertension, postlumbar puncture, or pneumoencephalography.

2. Intradural Extramedullary. These lesions are within the dural sac but external to the spinal cord or roots. Examples of masses in this location are (a) most of the schwannomas and meningiomas, (b) certain glial tumors (e.g., ependymoma), (c) congenital or embryonic tumors (lipomas, dermoids, epidermoids), and (d) hemorrhage. Hemorrhage in this location has the same causes as listed for epidural hemorrhage but is less common.

3. Intramedullary. These lesions are within the substance of the spinal cord and arise primarily from local cellular elements (e.g., as astrocytes or ependymal cells), although cell rests may lead to the development of lipomas,

dermoids, and epidermoids. Hydromyelia and syringomyelia cavities may also act as expanding intraspinal lesions, the latter alone or in combination with glial spinal tumors.

As a rule, acute intraspinal infection and hemorrhage are most commonly extradural. Extradural tumors are more commonly malignant, whereas intradural tumors are biologically more benign.

SIGNS AND SYMPTOMS

The signs and symptoms related to intraspinal mass lesions vary according to location along the spinal canal, location within the vertebral canal, and biologic activity. Above L2 lesions may involve the spinal cord and/or root, while below this level root dysfunction predominates. Of lesions located within the vertebral canal, extramedullary lesions often give rise to unilateral signs affecting the more external segments of both motor and sensory systems (sacral) first. The opposite usually is true for intramedullary lesions, from which visceral and autonomic dysfunction appears earlier. In the factor of biologic activity, vascular and malignant extradural tumors often have a shorter course after the initial complaints than do benign tumors and chronic infections.

Pain is the most common presenting symptom. Local pain owing to distortion of pain-sensitive structures in the bone or meninges has somewhat less localizing value than radicular pain. Both may be aggravated by increased thoracoabdominal pressure. Sensory complaints such as numbness and paresthesia may follow a distribution in keeping with the structures involved. Irritation of spinal cord tracts gives rise to diffuse sensory complaints below the level of the lesion, whereas those owing to root involvement follow the anatomic (dermatomal) distribution for that root. The findings in extramedullary lesions (intra- or extradural) show a sensory deficit, usually owing to external pressure on the lateral spinothalamic tract, well below the lesion (more than two segments) opposite to the side of cord compression. Radicular sensory loss can be more accurately defined to the side and level of the lesion. Intramedullary sensory loss can affect a distribution closer to the level, with sparing of sensation above and below the lesion.

Motor complaints obviously vary with the level involved and are manifested as weakness or spasticity. Spinal cord involvement gives rise to an upper motor neuron lesion that is characterized by weakness, increased tone, hyperreflexia, and extensor toe response. Lower motor neuron lesions (anterior horn cell and ventral root) may result in weakness, decreased tone, fasciculations, hypo- or areflexia at the level appropriate to the location of the lesions. Above the conus a combination of these two types of lesions is possible; below this level the lower motor neuron findings only are observed.

Dysfunction of the bowel and bladder is seen earlier in intramedullary lesions, and with those above the conus the dysfunction is of the upper motor neuron type. Early complaints of difficulty in initiating urination and dribbling are common. Changes in rectal tone may lead to a complaint of constipation or incontinence.

Skeletal deformity and cutaneous manifestations are more commonly found in the pediatric age groups. The latter findings included hypertrichosis, café au lait spots, angiomas, atrophic skin, and dermal dimple or sinus.

COURSE

The intradural extramedullary lesions tend to be slow growing and the dysfunction often progresses from root complaints and findings to gradual compromise of spinal cord function. Patients with laterally placed lesions may develop a Brown-Séquard syndrome, the major features being ipsilateral upper motor neuron paralysis and contralateral loss of pain and temperature below the level of the lesion. More anteriorly placed lesions in the subdural compartment may affect anterior spinal artery flow to the cord with resulting loss of pain and temperature sensation and motor activity below the level of the lesion. Touch, position, and vibration sensation are relatively preserved.

Extradural lesions are usually malignant and therefore rapidly progress, causing distal motor and sensory loss to a complete sensorimotor loss below the level of the lesion with loss of bowel and bladder function.

Intramedullary lesions are usually slow growing and cause progressive increase in weakness, spasticity, and loss of bowel and bladder function.

COMMON COMPLICATIONS

Total loss of spinal cord function below the level of the lesion is the ultimate and most severe complication of expanding intraspinal lesions. Loss of sensation may lead to breakdown of skin in the denervated areas, as well as the hazards associated with being unable to perceive noxious insults from cutaneous and deep proprioceptive receptors. Poor bladder emptying may lead to ureteral reflux and infection of the kidneys with serious consequences.

Increased tone of muscles can lead to the formation of contractures. Upper cord lesions may affect respiratory activity with secondary development of pulmonary infection and altered gas exchange.

LABORATORY PROCEDURES

All patients should have complete x-rays of the spine and chest. Spine x-rays are necessary to observe destruction or erosion of bone, calcification, or changes in the size of the bony canal. Metastatic tumors may lead to the destruction of body and pedicles, while the more slowly growing intradural and intramedullary tumors may lead to widening of the bony canal and intervertebral foramina. Destruction of intervertebral discs with or without kyphosis or paravertebral masses indicates tuberculosis or brucellosis.

Routine blood chemistry studies such as acid and alkaline phosphatase may reveal changes that indicate the source or extent of the primary disease. The most common and useful test is examination of cerebrospinal fluid (CSF). This test is best accomplished early in the day and with myelography as an accompanying procedure when indicated. The Queckenstedt test, which is less useful now because of the development of sophisticated neuroradiologic procedures, may indicate a complete block of the spinal subarachnoid space owing to an intraspinal lesion and an increase in CSF pressure (secondary to jugular compression) above the lesion is not transmitted to a needle (lumbar) in the subarachnoid space below the lesion. The CSF should be examined for protein (normally below 40 mg per 100 ml), sugar (normally one half to two thirds of blood sugar), cells (<5 cu mm), and electrophoretic pattern. In spinal cord diseases, especially with a complete block, the protein may reach over 1000 mg per 100 ml with coagulation of the fluid on standing (Froin syndrome). Low sugar (as compared with simultaneously drawn blood) may indicate an infectious process or utilization of glucose by leptomeninges infiltrated by metastatic tumor cells. In selected patients a cell block may reveal the source of the metastatic tumor. Immunoelectrophoresis may be useful in ruling out demyelinative diseases.

The most useful laboratory test is the myelogram, performed with oil- or water-soluble contrast media or air with tomography. The upper and lower limits of the lesion can be delineated by a spinal puncture laterally at C1 and posteriorly in the lower lumbar region. The myelogram should be performed at a time and place where definitive surgical therapy can be carried out when indicated.

Spinal cord angiography carries some risk and is not routinely used to diagnose intraspinal disease unless a vascular tumor or malformation is suspected. More recently, computerized tomography of the spine has been used to diagnose intraspinal lesions.

In those patients in whom bladder dysfunction is suspected, a cystometrogram can help distinguish between an upper or lower motor neuron bladder. The functional status of the urinary system can be determined with an intravenous pyelogram and voiding cystogram.

Electromyography is of limited use in diagnosing intraspinal lesions, although denervation caused by root involvement can be detected. Intrinsic non-space-occupying intraspinal disease such as motor neuron disease or extraspinal root and peripheral nerve disease may also be ruled out with this test.

PITFALLS IN DIAGNOSIS

The greatest pitfall in the diagnosis of expanding intraspinal lesions is confusing them with intrinsic spinal cord diseases such as motor neuron disease, multiple sclerosis, arachnoiditis, or combined system disease. Subarachnoid hemorrhage from filum ependymomas or more benign intradural extramedullary tumors such as neurofibromas has been confused with an intracranial cause for such bleeding. In those intraspinal tumors associated with high CSF protein, papilledema has been observed. On occasion this has been wrongly interpreted as indicating an intracranial origin of the observed sensorimotor syndrome. In general, a high index of suspicion and repeated follow-up examination clarify most situations.

IDIOPATHIC POLYNEURITIS

By ELMO F. MASUCCI, M.D.
Chevy Chase, Maryland

SYNONYMS

Guillain-Barré syndrome, Landry-Guillain-Barré-Strohl syndrome, acute idiopathic polyradiculoneuritis, infectious neuronitis, polyneuritis with facial diplegia, infectious polyneuritis, acute polyradiculitis, acute polyradiculoneuropathy, postinfectious polyneuritis, acute inflammatory polyradiculoneuropathy.

DEFINITION

Idiopathic polyneuritis is an acute or subacute, usually progressive, sensorimotor neuropathy initially manifested by muscle weakness or pain, or combinations of motor and sensory disturbances, with variable modes of spread: ascending, descending, or spread only within the confines of extremities initially involved. Bilateral proximal and distal muscle involvement usually is present, and there is an affinity for involvement of particular muscle groups. Deep tendon reflexes are invariably absent or diminished, and cranial nerves may or may not be involved. Cerebrospinal fluid (CSF) protein values are usually elevated and less than 10 mononuclear white cells are present. Occasionally there may be a modest elevation of mononuclear cells or a normal protein level. Complete functional recovery occurs in most but not all patients. Improvement usually occurs within weeks but may extend over months or even years. Severe respiratory, pulmonary, and other complications leading even to death occur in an appreciable number of patients.

The disorder is characterized pathologically by lymphocytic and plasmocytic inflammation and segmental demyelination of roots and nerves. It affects children and adults of all ages and both sexes. It usually occurs as an isolated episode but may be preceded by an upper respiratory or gastrointestinal illness. Less commonly it begins during the phase of abatement of specific viral diseases such as infectious mononucleosis, virus hepatitis, or influenza, and less frequently herpes zoster, varicella, or mumps. Other infections such as scarlet fever, typhoid fever, or pertussis may be the antecedent. Cases have been reported following vaccination against influenza, rabies, swine flu, tetanus, and typhoid-paratyphoid fever. They have also been reported in association with Hodgkin's disease, lymphoma and lupus erythematosus. There have been cases accompanying a variety of other conditions such as allergies and abortions, and following surgical operations. There is increasing evidence that idiopathic polyneuritis may be caused by cell-mediated hyperimmunity; however, the relationship between antecedent or triggering events and subsequent polyneuritis is still undetermined.

PRESENTING SIGNS AND SYMPTOMS

Weakness is usually the most prominent symptom at the onset of the illness. Weakness accompanied by paresthesia is also common. Infrequently the illness may begin with weakness and pain. In about 25 per cent of patients the first symptoms are sensory complaints only, consisting of either pain alone or paresthesia alone. Uncommonly, limb or truncal ataxia may be the presenting sign.

The weakness usually develops acutely or subacutely in the lower extremities. Infrequently it begins in the upper extremities or the cranial nerves. The mode of spread of symptoms is variable. Most common is the ascending variety, in which spread usually occurs from lower to upper limbs to trunk or from lower to upper limbs to cranial nerves. Spread from lower limbs and from four limbs to cranial nerves is less common. Contiguous parts of the body are not always successively involved. Descending spread is not common. Frequently, spread occurs only within the confines of the limbs initially involved. In 15 per cent of patients there is increasing weakness in the limbs involved but no spread.

COURSE

Progression from onset to maximal impairment is usually complete within 2 to 3 weeks. After a stable interval of 1 or 2 weeks, recovery begins. Complete functional recovery within several months occurs in most patients, but not all. Patients with severe involvement may recover slowly over a period of a year or longer. Relapses and recurrences are uncommon. Severe respiratory insufficiency, and pulmonary and other complications leading to death occur in an appreciable number of patients.

PHYSICAL EXAMINATION FINDINGS

Weakness of all four extremities and truncal flaccid weakness is the most common finding. Lower extremity weakness alone occurs in about 20 per cent of patients. Upper extremity weakness alone is uncommon. The predominant type of weakness is combined and equal involvement of the proximal and distal muscles. Less commonly, the weakness may be more pronounced proximally or distally. In about 12 to 15 per cent of patients, proximal weakness only may be present. The degree of weakness may be disproportionately great in selected muscle groups: thigh flexors, hamstring muscles, dorsiflexors of the feet, or wrist extensors. This dissociated muscle weakness occurs commonly in idiopathic polyneuritis and is only rarely present in other types of polyneuropathy or in myopathies. Muscle atrophy may be present in severely involved patients. Fasciculations are uncommon.

Sensory and motor involvement together is most common, but motor manifestations only may occur. Objective sensory disturbances are usually less severe than the motor manifestations but occasionally may be quite marked and may persist for long periods of time. The sensory deficit may involve either superficial or deep sensation or both, and is usually stocking-glove in distribution.

Deep tendon reflexes are invariably absent or diminished and the presence of normal reflexes is most unusual. Superficial abdominal and cremasteric reflexes are frequently absent or diminished.

Cranial nerves may or may not be involved. The seventh nerve is most commonly involved and the ninth and tenth come next. In some patients all the cranial nerves have been involved except the eighth. The third, fourth, and sixth cranial nerves are uncommonly affected. In our own hospital population during the past 15 years there has been a decreasing incidence of cranial neuropathy. This has been significantly correlated with a decrease in the overall severity of the illness (using respiratory insufficiency as a criterion for severe involvement).

Fever, meningeal signs, and headache are rare in this condition. Bilateral Babinski signs and papilledema may be found but are uncommon. Limb and truncal ataxia are present in the Fisher variant (syndrome of ophthalmoplegia, ataxia, and areflexia). Mental manifestations, other than those associated with respiratory insufficiency, are rarely seen.

Manifestations of autonomic nervous system involvement are not uncommon and include hypertension, sinus tachycardia or bradycardia, postural hypotension, urinary and rectal incontinence, paroxysmal facial flushing, chest and abdominal tightness, or profuse diaphoresis.

COMMON COMPLICATIONS

Pulmonary problems are the most common complications. The use of tracheostomy and positive-pressure respirators have resulted in a decrease in pulmonary complications and death; however, respiratory failure, pneumonitis, lobar pneumonia, aspiration pneumonia, and atelectasis still occur. Pulmonary emboli occur in occasional patients and may result in death.

Some patients may improve to the point at which a respirator is no longer necessary, blood gases are within normal range, and respiratory movements and aeration of lung fields appear normal. This period of apparent well-being is then followed by sudden death. Autopsy findings are frequently insufficient to account for these sudden deaths. Other patients may recover from episodes of repiratory distress only to develop sudden irreversible cardiac arrest.

Sudden episodes of hypotension, hyponatremia, and stress ulcers of the stomach or duodenum complicated by severe bleeding or perforation are uncommon complications.

Laboratory Findings

Cerebrospinal fluid (CSF) protein values are usually elevated (greater than 45 mg per 100 ml) but may be within normal limits during the early weeks of the illness and rarely may remain normal for several months. Less than 10 mononuclear white cells are present in the spinal fluid. Modest elevations of the white cell count can occur, with the upper limit for an acceptable number of cells still controversial.

Peripheral blood findings of a mild polymorphonuclear leukocytosis or a mild increase of creatine phosphokinase do occur but are not diagnostically helpful.

Electromyography

Motor nerve conduction velocities performed near the peak time of the illness will show reduced conduction times in most patients. Occasionally, the conduction velocities are normal. When more peripherally determined conduction times are normal, slow F-wave conduction velocities are of value in indicating nerve fiber demyelination in proximal roots or the brachial plexus. Decreased recruitment of motor units and low voltage potentials may be seen. Signs of denervation (fibrillations and positive sharp waves) are not uncommon late in the course of the disease.

Sural Nerve Biopsy

Segmental demyelination combined with lymphocytic inflammatory infiltrates on sural nerve biopsy is diagnostic but is seldom necessary.

Pitfalls in Diagnosis

In the differential diagnosis of idiopathic polyneuritis, one should consider such entities as acute polymyositis, acute intermittent porphyria, infectious mononucleosis, tick paralysis, botulism, paralytic stage of acute poliomyelitis, periodic paralysis, and diphtheritic polyneuropathy.

Idiopathic polyneuritis may be mistakenly diagnosed as acute polymyositis when proximal weakness without sensory manifestations is the presenting sign. Reflexes are usually preserved in polymyositis and the CSF protein levels are not elevated. Electromyography, nerve conduction studies, creatine phosphokinase levels, and muscle biopsy should enable one to distinguish between these two conditions.

Acute intermittent porphyria with peripheral neuropathy may resemble acute idiopathic polyneuritis. However, ascending spread of the weakness or paralysis is rare. The great majority of patients with porphyria have normal CSF proteins, although the level may be increased. Sensory disturbance is uncommon. Abdominal complaints, convulsive seizures, and mental manifestations are frequent. The urine and stool are usually positive for porphobilinogen.

The polyneuritis that accompanies infectious mononucleosis is clinically quite similar to idiopathic polyneuritis. It might be in fact little more than a semantic quibble to separate this out. In most patients the prodromal systemic manifestations permit the diagnosis to be made. The prodrome is usually followed or associated with the onset of the polyneuritis. However, neurologic symptoms may be the only manifestation of the disease. The presence of meningeal signs or encephalitis should suggest the possibility of infectious mononucleosis. A positive heterophile antigen reaction is diagnostic. The fatality rate of this benign disease is considerable when it is complicated by polyneuritis with respiratory involvement. In the few cases of infectious mononucleosis with polyneuritis in which autopsy was performed, the pathologic changes of demyelination and lymphocytic infiltration of roots and nerves are similar to that seen in idiopathic polyneuritis.

Tick paralysis, a reversible disorder of the nervous system, is characterized by weakness of the lower extremities. Within 24 to 48 hours this leads to flaccid paralysis of the extremities, trunk, and bulbar muscles. Death may occur. Removal of the tick results in reversal of symptoms and usually complete recovery. Tendon reflexes are absent and sensation is preserved. There are no abnormalities present in the cerebrospinal fluid. The occurrence of a flaccid paralysis in an individual living close to a tick-infested area should suggest the diagnosis.

Botulism resembles the descending form of idiopathic polyneuritis. Difficulty in converging the eyes followed by ptosis and extraocular muscle paralysis are early manifestations. Weakness of the jaw and difficulty in swallowing are soon followed by weakness of the extremities. Symptoms usually begin 10 to 48 hours after ingestion of contaminated food. Cerebrospinal fluid examination is normal. Repetitive nerve stimulation (30 to 50 per second) will usually show abnormally large potentiation of the evoked muscle potential. The involvement of several members of a family or group with this descending form of weakness and paralysis with or without preceding gastrointestinal complaints should suggest the possibility of botulism. Early recognition and treatment is imperative, since death usually occurs within 4 to 8 days of onset of symptoms when large amounts of toxin are ingested.

The paralytic stage of acute poliomyelitis is usually characterized by asymmetric or spotty weakness of one or more limbs. Symmetrical paresis or paralysis of lower and upper extremities (simulating acute idiopathic polyneuritis) is not common but does occur. Sensory deficits are not found but pain in the muscles is common. Nerve conduction times are normal. In contrast to idiopathic polyneuritis the CSF cell count is almost always increased, with the highest counts in the preparalytic stage. Cell counts less than 10 per cu mm are occasionally seen, even in the preparalytic stage. However, the cells decrease rapidly while the protein rises, so that the spinal fluid in the second week will mimic acute idiopathic polyneuritis. Polio is rarely seen in this country at the present time owing to nationwide vaccination.

Diphtheric polyneuritis is uncommon in the United States as a result of the decreased incidence of faucial diphtheria. It is predominantly a childhood disease. The clinical course might resemble the descending variety of idiopathic polyneuritis in that palatal weakness and blurring of vision owing to paralysis of accommodation are usually the first symptoms. These symptoms usually appear about the third week after the onset of infection. Within the next few days or weeks other cranial nerve and peripheral nerve involvement occurs manifested by paralysis of pharyngeal, facial, external ocular muscles, and extremity muscles. Reflexes are lost early. Stocking-glove sensory deficits may be present. The CSF protein is usually increased. Conduction velocities are reduced. Differential diagnosis may be difficult when the initial infectious phase is slight or not diagnosed. However, palatal and ciliary muscle weakness is rarely seen in idiopathic polyneuritis and should suggest the possibility of diphtheria.

A severe attack of one of the varieties of periodic paralysis lasting for 24 to 48 hours in a patient with no family history and no previous episodes might be mistaken for acute idiopathic polyneuritis. The paresis or paralysis in this condition usually begins distally in the legs and progresses proximally. Legs, arms, trunk, and then neck are commonly involved in that order. However, either the upper or the lower extremities alone may be involved or weakness may be predominantly unilateral. Extensor muscles are more affected than the flexors. The extent of the weakness may vary from a slight focal paresis to paralysis of all muscles of the trunk and extremities. However, the bulbar muscles, diaphragm, and sphincter muscles of the bladder and rectum usually are not involved. Ptosis and blurring of vision may occur. Deep tendon reflexes may be absent or diminished. Superficial abdominal and cremasteric reflexes are usually preserved. Sensory abnormalities are not present. CSF evaluation reveals no changes in dynamics or cell count. A slight increase in protein may accompany a severe attack. The differential diagnosis usually depends upon a history of similar attacks, the history of recurrent episodes in the patient himself, the short duration of the attack (few hours to 24 to 48 hours), the frequent association of attacks with a high carbohydrate meal the evening before the attack, the absence of signs and freedom from symptoms between attacks, and the high or low serum potassium usually associated with most attacks.

MIGRAINE AND ITS VARIANTS

By J. M. S. PEARCE, M.D., F.R.C.P., *and* C. G. CLOUGH, M.R.C.P.

Hull, England

DEFINITION

The word migraine is derived from the term hemicrania first introduced in an account of the disease by Galen (A.D. 131 to 201). It comprises a wide variety of symptoms, the most common being paroxysmal headache. Many diagnostic criteria for migraine have included as necessary elements for diagnosis the occurrence of accompanying neurologic features or the response of headache to ergotamine. Such dogmatism is unwarranted, leading to the elimination of the correct diagnosis for many migraine patients. Vahlquist's definition is one of the more useful: Paroxysmal headaches separated by intervals of freedom from pain plus at least two of the following four points: (1) unilateral headache, (2) nausea, (3) visual or sensorimotor aura, (4) family history.

A distinction is made between common and classic migraine, although many sufferers have both types of attack. Those attacks that have associated visual or cerebral symptoms or signs are termed *classic*; those without focal neurologic disturbance *common* migraine. The second condition is much more frequently encountered. Variants of migraine are listed in Table 1.

CLINICAL FEATURES

Various studies have put the incidence of migraine in the population as between 15 and 25 per cent, females being affected more often than males 3:2. Many patients have infrequent attacks, some three to four in a lifetime. At the other end of the spectrum a minority can have regular attacks, say 5 or 6 per month, and occasional patches when anxiety factors can result in an almost continuous headache. Seventy per cent of patients have a family history, especially those with classic migraine. Migraine is said to affect intelligent people more commonly than others but this may be a false impression; it does seem that sufferers more often than not have obsessional or neurotic personality traits and are prone to anxiety. Indeed, this element is an important factor in precipitation of attacks and a high attendance rate for consultations. The symptoms of a classic attack can be usefully divided into stages.

Prodromal Features. For hours up to a day before the attack, some patients may describe feelings of elation, yawning or euphoria. Others become drowsy and lethargic or even depressed. Clear-cut tension headache may precede migraine attacks and merge into the vascular headache. Weight gain and fluid retention are fairly common.

Aura. This refers to the neurologic warning of the headache that distinguishes classic from common migraine. These symptoms may be due to intracerebral vasoconstriction leading to focal ischemia or to depression of cortical neuronal activity. This results in focal negative or positive phenomena. It is believed that this is followed by a period of vasodilation that produces distension of sensitive pain fibers in the arteries, arterioles, and veins, thus resulting in headache. This is corroborated by the dilation

of extracranial vessels, and relief from headache experienced by many patients on compression of these vessels.

The aura usually occurs before headache and lasts 10 to 40 minutes, although headache sometimes can accompany it. This fact plus the observation that a focal deficit can occur on the same side as headache suggests that vasoconstriction and vasodilation are not mutually exclusive, and may occur in different parts of the brain at the same time. The commonest aura is visual, occurring in up to 30 per cent of migraine patients. Occipital auras frequently take the form of flashing lights or stars (*photopsiae*). These occur in the periphery of the visual field but can expand to involve the central vision or vice versa. They are frequently colored but can be black and white and tend to scintillate. Some patients notice a small paracentral area often described as a filament of a light bulb. Various geometric shapes and zigzag lines known as fortification spectra (*teichopsiae*) may occur in one half of the visual field.

Other more complex hallucinations result from ischemia of the optic radiation in the temporal lobes. These are often bright primary colors and may produce the illusion of a person, animal, or object. Negative effects of ischemia result in scotomas. These can progress to result in complex fragmented or altitudinal visual field defects. Those scotomas involving one eye can be "thrown" by eye movements and are caused by the ischemic retina; indeed, permanent scotomas due to retinal artery occlusion as a complication of migraine have been reported.

Disturbance of parietal lobe function results in disorders of perception (*metamorphopsia*). Objects may appear large (*macropsia*) or small (*micropsia, Lilliputian syndrome*) and the limbs and hands may feel blown up to gigantic size. Visual agnosia is uncommon but can occur so that patients cannot recognize objects or understand their use. Ischemia of the motor and sensory cortex occurs and usually results in feelings of heaviness or vaguely defined numbness and tingling in contralateral limbs. The arm or leg on that side will feel clumsy or useless, although true hemiplegia is rare. When patients first seek medical help, they are understandably alarmed at the symptoms and may think they are developing a stroke. Sensory symptoms such as pins and needles occur most frequently around the mouth and tongue and may spread to the arm and rarely to the leg. If the dominant hemisphere is involved, dysphasia will result. This is usually mild and expressive in type so that patients experience difficulty in getting the right word out. Word blindness and dysgraphia can occur. All these auras disappear in 10 to 60 minutes. Very rarely,

Table 1.　*Migraine and Variants*

Classical — With visual, sensory, or speech disorder
Common — Without such focal neurologic accompaniment
Variants
  1. Cluster headache (periodic, chronic)
  2. Facial migraine (syn. lower half headache)
  3. Ophthalmoplegic migraine
  4. Hemiplegic migraine, including hemisensory attacks
  5. Basilar artery migraine

permanent sequelae betoken infarction that is confirmed by computerized tomographic (CT) scanning.

Headache. Headache may commence during the aura or after. In common migraine, headache may be the only symptom and can occur out of the blue. It is usually unilateral, as the term hemicrania implies. However, it may change sides from attack to attack and can involve both sides at once, spreading to the whole cranium. Headache is described as aching and throbbing like a hammer that is banging inside the head, or the pain can have a burning intensity. It gradually builds up so that it reaches a peak at 1 to 2 hours. It may be just an inconvenience to some, while others have extremely severe prostrating pain with photophobia, resembling a subarachnoid hemorrhage. Most patients have anorexia and nausea; some feel very ill and have marked pallor, sweating, nausea, and vomiting. These last two symptoms occur in 50 per cent of all sufferers and are associated with gastric stasis and slowing of the gastrointestinal motility. Other patients have diarrhea. Polyuria may be noticed, as may tenderness over the scalp or the temporal arteries. The majority of sufferers who cannot work during their attacks will find a quiet darkened room and lie still or sleep until it is over. The slightest noise or movement may make headache worse and some may find normal sounds and smells exaggerated and unpleasant. Headache can last from 1 to 2 hours up to 48 hours and as it dies down many patients are left with a feeling of lifelessness and fatigue: they may be washed out for the next day.

PRECIPITATING FACTORS

Many attacks come for no particular reason. Patients will report many different factors that they believe bring on attacks. Most of these will be casual rather than causal relationships. However, it is worthwhile to record every patient's precipitating factors and to inquire routinely about certain known common precipitants (Table 2).

Table 2. *Precipitants of Migraine*

Common	Less Common
Anxiety states	Alcohol
Relaxation — vacation or weekends	Hunger or fasting
	Dietary idiosyncrasies
Excess or lack of sleep	High humidity
Menstruation, menopause, use of oral contraceptive pill	
Bright lights	
Travel	

The most common precipitating factor is emotional disturbance, and anxiety and stress may result in both tension headache and migraine. Anxiety and depression also result in sleeplessness and fatigue that can trigger attacks, thus initiating a vicious circle that can lead to almost continuous headache — a cross-breed of tension and migraine. Let-down headaches may follow periods of tension, for example, following interviews. This commonly affects the vigorous businessman who, following periods of stress at work, finds his weekends or holidays marred by attacks of headache. As migraine sufferers tend to be obsessional, breaking their fixed routine may well precipitate attacks.

Much emphasis has been placed on diet in causing migraine. Certainly different foodstuffs can provide an attack in susceptible persons; however, this provocation is not as common as once thought. Foods such as cheese and herring that contain tyramine are frequently implicated, as is chocolate, which contains the related amine phenylethylamine. Missing meals or fasting for whatever reason can promote attacks. Sunlight, bright lights, or glare from a reflective surface also provides a trigger, hence many sufferers resort to wearing tinted glasses, although this usually denotes emotional insecurity rather than light-induced migraine. Endocrine factors are certainly important, although the explanations of their effects are somewhat vague. Many women report an association of migraine with menstruation and some a reduced or increased frequency of attacks at the onset of menopause; attacks commonly remit in pregnancy. The approach to this problem should be empirical rather than guided by theoretical considerations.

INVESTIGATIONS

The diagnosis of migraine is made on the basis of history, and this should be confirmed by an absence of findings on clinical examination. Usually no further tests are necessary. Only rarely is it necessary to exclude subarachnoid hemorrhage by lumbar puncture when the patient presents with an acute onset of very severe headache.

Complicated migraine has been extensively investigated by several workers in the past, using carotid angiography. They have seldom found it rewarding, arteriovenous malformations being rarely discovered. Carotid angiography is thus not indicated in the investigation of migraine without clinical signs. If migraine is complicated by focal epilepsy, by fits at the height of an attack, or by subarachnoid hemorrhage, CT scanning and angiography will be necessary. Similarly, the electroencephalogram

(EEG) is a virtually useless diagnostic aid, although it is frequently requested. Associated disorders discovered at clinical examination — for example, hypertension — can be aggravating factors and should be investigated and treated in their own right.

VARIANTS

Cluster Headache. This is known under many synonyms — periodic migrainous neuralgia, histamine headache, ciliary neuralgia, Horton's syndrome, sphenopalatine neuralgia, autonomic facial cephalgia, Harris's neuralgia. Usually it has been regarded as a variant of migraine. However, it is a separate entity and differs in several important aspects. It is important that the condition not be misdiagnosed, as treatment can have a dramatic effect in improving the life of sufferers — this can be an almost unbearable disease. Cluster headache occurs in both sexes; however, it is much more common in men. Age of onset is between 20 and 40 years and there is usually no previous history of migraine or family history of cluster headaches.

As the name implies, headaches occur in clusters or runs typically up to 2 to 3 per day for 1 to 4 months at a time. Remissions then can last for a few months or even years. Classically, paroxysms of headache occur at exactly the same time each day. Patients report they are wakened by headache in the early hours of the morning so regularly that they can set their clocks by it — hence "alarm clock headache." Headaches last 30 minutes to 2 hours and are of a very intense boring, aching, or burning nature. In fact, some consider it the worst pain known to man; some patients contemplate suicide.

This pain is situated around one orbit or supraorbitally and is confined to that orbit for the duration of the cluster, although it may move to the other eye in further bouts. There can be radiation of pain to the nose, cheek, or teeth of the upper jaw, sometimes to the lower jaw and neck.

Commonly, there is watering and redness of the eye on the side of the headache, although these are not invariable signs. The nostril on that side may also be blocked or feel stuffy. The face may appear red and puffy and there may be tenderness over a prominent temporal artery. Autonomic involvement may be signaled by miosis, ptosis, and sweating on the affected side. A Horner's syndrome occurs in 18 per cent of patients and occasionally persists after the attack. Precipitating factors are rare, although alcohol, nitrites, and histamine have been proved to trigger attacks.

The features of this headache are so characteristic that the diagnosis should be made from the history and no further investigation is necessary. The periodicity of attacks, their intense nature, and the associated signs should clearly distinguish this syndrome from tic douloureux and other causes of facial pain. Chronic cluster headache can develop. This is rare and refers to attacks that have become continuous with no periods of remission.

Facial Migraine. This refers to variants of migraine affecting the facial vasculature. It has all the typical features of migraine: periodicity, length of attack and associated features.

Lower-half headache is a unilateral pain affecting the lower face below the ear. There are two maximum sites of pain, one in the orbit and base of nose, the other posterior to the mastoid process in the temporal bone. Its character is dull, bursting, and nagging, and it may sometimes have a throbbing component. Occasionally it may spread to the neck and shoulder and rarely may radiate into the arm.

Other types of facial migraine have similar qualities with deep boring pains in the orbit and cheek; lachrymation and nasal secretion is common, although not an invariable feature. Sometimes the temporal artery is affected with visible swelling and tenderness.

Carotidynia is an episodic throbbing pain in the neck related to a tender carotid artery. Pressure over this causes more pain, but firm pressure may completely relieve symptoms.

Facial migraine is distinguished from trigeminal neuralgia by the short, sharp, lancinating pains of the latter. Facial migraine occurs in younger patients, is seldom confined to the distribution of the trigeminal nerve, and does not have the trigger areas with precipitation of pain by talking and washing so characteristic of trigeminal neuralgia. Atypical or psychogenic facial pain can occur in the maxillary area on one or both sides of the face. It typically affects young women, who will describe the pain as unbearable and yet remain impassive. In highly colored terms the pain will be described as burning, deep, or as if the skin were crawling or being torn from the skull. It is different from that of migraine because it is continuous and sometimes spreads to other areas of the face and neck.

Ophthalmoplegic Migraine. This variant affects both sexes equally and can occur in people who have had previous common or classic migraine, although it often presents in childhood. Headache is of a boring rather than throbbing nature and is periorbital, almost always on the same side. It lasts from 12 to 36 hours and, as it is fading, is accompanied by ptosis and double vision. Headache then disappears and complete closure of the eye can be a sequel. Third-nerve lesions occur in more than 80 per cent of patients. In up to 12 per cent of patients sixth nerve lesions are reported and fourth nerve lesions in a minority. An internal ophthalmoplegia may accompany the external ophthalmoplegia, with a fixed or reacting dilated pupil. The ocular palsy persists for 1 to 4 weeks. Attacks may recur at infrequent intervals.

The differential diagnosis from internal carotid or posterior communicating aneurysms that compress the third nerve can at times be difficult. If the clinical course is not typical, angiography and computerized tomographic (CT) scanning should be performed to exclude a lesion that can be surgically corrected. Angiography is deferred until the attack has resolved, if possible, because complications such as fatal carotid thrombosis have been reported when this is performed during the attack.

Hemiplegic Migraine. Sporadic focal symptoms in migraine are not uncommon. Up to one third of migraine patients will experience hemisensory symptoms or hemiparesis on at least one occasion. This is usually part of the aura and lasts only about an hour. Rarely, symptoms will persist for up to 24 hours and sometimes for a week after the attack. This usually means infarction of cerebral cortex has taken place. Sensory symptoms are commoner, with tingling and "pins and needles" affecting the face, arm, and leg, or characteristically felt around both sides of the tongue and around the lips. Complete hemiplegia is rare; much more frequently feelings of heaviness are present in the arm and rarely the leg.

Familial hemiplegic migraine is a similar but separate entity and is quite rare. In contrast to sporadic hemiplegic migraine, the weakness will always recur on the same side and may outlast the headache. There is always a family history, suggesting an autosomal-dominant inheritance, and within that family hemiplegia always occurs on the same side.

Basilar Migraine. Basilar migraine results from involvement of the basilar artery with ensuing symptoms of brainstem ischemia. Symptoms of brainstem involvement are common in many patients with common or classical migraine. These are described as feelings of dizziness or lightheadedness. Distinguishing features of basilar migraine are vertigo, double vision, dysarthria, and ataxia. These symptoms usually occur as an aura prior to the headache; thus the diagnosis should become clear. Paresthesia may involve the arms and face classically in a perioral fashion. Involvement of the occipital poles results in hemianopia or blindness in both eyes. At the height of an attack of basilar migraine, syncope commonly occurs. Simple vasovagal-initiated syncope can happen to some migraine sufferers because of headache and autonomic disturbance. Prolonged unconsciousness or maintenance of an erect position may even result in an anoxic fit, although this may require investigation on its own account.

Childhood Migraine. Children can present with straightforward migraine and this diagnosis should not be a problem if a history of paroxysmal unilateral headache can be elicited. More often, abdominal symptoms predominate. In the past, these attacks have been labeled by pediatricians as cyclical vomiting, periodic syndrome, or childhood acidosis. If a careful history is taken, more often than not a child will tell you he does have headaches as well as the other more obvious distressing symptoms. Thus it is clear that this is a migraine variant. Attacks may follow exercise. The child appears pale, sweats, and complains of pains in the abdomen. Nausea and vomiting are common accompaniments, and sometimes diarrhea or constipation occurs.

These patients appear to have an acute abdomen and are often suspected of having appendicitis. Fever and leukocytosis can occur, but diagnosis can be made if there is a history of periodic attacks with good health in between, along with a family history of migraine. Attacks tend to be short but may last for 24 hours. Patients appear pale, irritable, and tired. They then become moody or lethargic for the duration of the attack. Childhood migraine has a good prognosis; up to 50 per cent recover completely and have no further problems. Others have attacks of travel sickness or develop symptoms of adult migraine as they reach adolescence.

PITFALLS IN DIAGNOSIS

As stressed, history and examination will establish the diagnosis of migraine in the majority of patients. Difficulty often arises when headache or neurologic deficit presents acutely. In this case other conditions may need to be excluded.

Acute Headaches. *Subarachnoid Hemorrhage.* The onset of headache is more abrupt than in migraine, likened to being "struck on the back of the head or neck with a baseball bat." Loss of consciousness is common, as is associated vomiting. Patients can usually distinguish the severity of this headache from their ordinary headaches; they will be markedly photophobic and have a stiff neck; they will need to lie quietly in a darkened room. Any patient who presents for the first time with such a history should have a lumbar puncture.

Meningitis.   Meningitis is less easily confused. Headache is of gradual onset and is generalized. Pyrexia and neck stiffness usually distinguish these patients.

In patients with chronic or recurring headache, migraine has to be distinguished from other conditions (Table 3).

Recurrent or Chronic Headache. *Tension Headache.* This is the commonest of all headaches. It is produced at times of stress, although this factor may not be apparent. Its character is described as a tight band around the head, as if it were in a vice or a heavy weight were pressing on top of the head. Pain tends to lack the throbbing quality of migraine and is rarely unilateral. Autonomic disturbance can occur, with feelings of nausea and occasional vomiting. It should be remembered that migraine sufferers commonly have tension headaches as well, either separate from or precipitating migraine attacks. In the latter instance, a vicious cycle of tension and migraine headache can arise, with tension precipitating migraine, resulting in more stress and so on. It is important to distinguish the two components in the history and to treat both.

Post-traumatic Headache. This more often follows minor than major head injury. It is seldom seen in sports injuries and is strongly associated with an unsettled compensation claim for injury at work or in road accidents. The pain is at the site of any scar or is diffuse and of the tension type. There are no neurologic signs; it is surprisingly rare as a lasting complaint in those who have been unconscious for 24 hours or more. Although its mechanism is disputed by purists, its recognition is not difficult. Migraine preceding head trauma may be apparently aggravated by it, although probably not by organic mechanisms. Injury to the head is *not a cause* of migraine.

Sinusitis. This can sometimes cause a dull facial pain over the frontal or maxillary sinuses. Local tenderness is present. X-ray may help to confirm the diagnosis. Chronic sinusitis is often implicated in causing recurrent headaches, but this is seldom the case.

Acute Glaucoma. This can produce acute severe orbital pain associated with vomiting and deterioration of vision in that eye. The eye will feel rock hard, with central injection and clouding of the cornea. This can be assessed roughly by digital palpation and by tonometry prior to urgent treatment.

Skull Lesions. Paget's disease of bone or metastases in the skull can cause chronic or recurring headaches of either localized or generalized distribution. Radiology shows the cause.

Temporal Arteritis. Temporal arteritis is not an uncommon cause of headache after the age of 65 years. The onset of headache is gradual. It is constant, can be relieved by simple analgesics, and generally presents with other features such as nocturnal sweating, malaise, and thickened, pulseless, tender temporal arteries. If this diagnosis is suspected, it is a simple matter to check the erythrocyte sedimentation rate (ESR), which will be raised or, if necessary, perform temporal artery biopsy. If this condition is missed, the grave consequences of retinal ischemia can ensue.

Cervical Spondylosis. This can produce headache in the middle-aged, which can aggravate or simulate migraine. It can lead to an occipital ache radiating to the top of the head downward into the shoulder or arms or around into the jaw. Pain can be intermittent and unilateral, although it is rarely associated with systemic upset. On examination one should look for restriction of neck movements or signs and symptoms of root or cord compression. Radiology is seldom helpful, and if both conditions coexist, each may require treatment.

Raised Intracranial Pressure. Raised intracranial pressure due to a tumor or subdural hematoma produces a headache that initially occurs every morning. It has a generalized distribution, may be associated with effortless vomiting, and is made worse by coughing, sneezing, bending, or defecation. Eventually the headaches become constant, and usually at this stage changes of personality, epilepsy, or focal signs supervene, and papilledema may be discovered. A rare cause of episodic headache is intermittent obstructive hydrocephalus secondary to a colloid cyst of the third ventricle or tumors obstructing the fourth ventricle. These

Table 3.   *Pitfalls in Diagnosis*

---

1. Other Acute Headaches
   Subarachnoid hemorrhage
   Acute meningitis
2. Recurrent or Chronic Headaches
   Tension headache
   Post-traumatic headache
   Trigeminal neuralgia
   Atypical facial pain
   Acute sinusitis
   Acute glaucoma (closed angle type)
   Skull lesions: Paget's disease, metastases
   Temporal arteritis
   Cervical spondylosis
   Raised intracranial pressure
      Tumor
      Subdural hematoma
      Hydrocephalus
   Focal cerebral lesions–TIAs
   Paroxysmal or accelerated hypertension
   Cluster headache
   Other migraine variants

---

produce a severe headache and vomiting due to raised intracranial pressure. They will classically be precipitated and relieved by sudden changes of posture. Computerized tomographic (CT) scanning and ventriculography may be required in these rare cases.

Transient Ischemic Attacks. The neurologic symptoms of the aura of migraine can be indistinguishable from transient ischemic attacks. By definition the latter resolve within 24 hours, and they are not usually accompanied by headache, although mild contralateral head pain can occur. The onset of focal neurologic symptoms and signs such as described should always be considered as transient ischemic attacks in older patients who have no previous history of classic migraine or in patients without headache, and investigated accordingly, if necessary with angiography.

Paroxysmal Hypertension. This will produce severe headache that often can mimic migraine. It can be due to a pheochromocytoma, or to a reaction to monoamine oxidase inhibitors, or ingestion of tyramine in cheese. Demonstration of pallor, tachycardia, and a greatly raised blood pressure during an attack will establish the diagnosis.

Headache is not a symptom of uncomplicated hypertension. In malignant or accelerated hypertension (with grade 3 or 4 retinopathy, proteinuria, and diastolic pressure of 130 plus), raised pressure headaches in the mornings, relieved by change of posture and analgesics, do occur in some patients.

EPISODIC VERTIGO

By DAVID D. DeWEESE, M.D.
Portland, Oregon

When a person experiences a disturbance in his normal relationship to space, he complains that he is "dizzy." Subjectively he is indicating that he is not able to orient himself normally with his surroundings. The sensation may be mild or severe and may be more or less continuous or definitely episodic or paroxysmal. The most severe disturbances are usually vertigo, whereas the milder sensations may be only weakness, lightheadedness, giddiness, insecurity, uncertainty, or unsteadiness. It is of utmost importance in establishing a probable diagnosis that the physician learn to differentiate carefully between "dizziness" and "vertigo," as true vertigo usually indicates abnormality of the ear, the eighth cranial nerve, the brainstem, or the central nervous system.

In order to separate vertigo from a less finite symptom, some definition of vertigo is necessary. It is best to assume that *if careful questioning indicates any sense of whirling, falling, or propulsion*, such patients are experiencing vertigo. Once the subjective complaint is definitely identified as whirling, falling, or propulsion, physical examination and diagnostic tests can be concentrated on the ear and the central nervous system.

If the history, however, indicates that vertigo is probably not the complaint, there are still conditions that cause recurrent (not continuous) nonvertiginous dizziness. They must constantly be kept in mind, because there are a moderate number of cases in which even the most careful questioning leaves a reasonable doubt as to whether true vertigo is present. The most common of these conditions are ocular disorders, anemias, labile hypertension, hypoglycemia, migraine equivalents, and the ingestion of alcohol, barbiturates, or other drugs. Although true or whirling vertigo does not occur, each can produce symptoms that may be present for several hours or several days and then may be absent for various periods of time. They are therefore episodic in their natural sequence and can cause confusion if the patient's complaint of "dizziness" is assumed to be vertigo.

When recurrent, or episodic, *vertigo* is the actual complaint, certain guidelines will help to narrow the probabilities.

1. Acute, severe whirling vertigo occurring in separate attacks almost always indicates disease of the labyrinth. Less severe vertigo, manifested usually by true unsteadiness or a feeling of falling or being pushed, *may* also be of labyrinthine origin but is more suggestive of central nervous system disorder.

2. If hearing loss or tinnitus precedes or accompanies an attack of vertigo, the ear or labyrinth is almost certainly the organ involved.

3. If the duration of attacks is of several minutes or hours, labyrinthine disease should be suspected. If attacks last several days, central nervous system disease may be more likely, and careful neurologic examination is indicated.

The most common conditions causing episodic vertigo resulting from disease of the ear are, in approximate order of frequency, acute toxic labyrinthitis (vestibular neuronitis), benign postural vertigo, post-traumatic syndromes, labyrinthine hydrops (Meniere's syndrome), and chronic middle ear disease with or without cholesteatoma. Each has a typical pattern in the majority of patients. Deviations from the usual pattern occur and must be carefully investigated.

Acute toxic labyrinthitis, now most frequently referred to as vestibular neuronitis, is common. It can be caused by viral disease, postinfection toxicity, and various ingested drugs, as well as allergy (usually to food). Acute alcohol intoxication may initiate it. The characteristic sequence of events is a gradual onset of vertigo over 24 to 72 hours, usually leading to prostration, nausea, vomiting, and demonstrable nystagmus. *Neither hearing loss nor tinnitus is present.* After 1 to 3 days the vertigo begins to subside, and stability returns to normal within the next 24 to 48 hours. The only residual symptom may be *postural vertigo,* which may continue, intermittently with decreasing frequency, for 1 to 3 weeks. There is no permanent, subjective residual. When caused by a viral toxicity, recurrence is not expected. If caused by drug toxicity or allergy, recurrence follows a similar pattern.

Benign postural vertigo is usually what its name implies — benign. The patient complains that he suddenly becomes violently dizzy while lying supine in bed and turning to one side or the other or when bending over or turning suddenly. His environment spins, and if standing, he may stagger or fall. If lying down, he feels that the entire bed and room is whirling. The sensation lasts only 10 to 20 seconds and subsides. It may recur each time he repeats a similar motion, or it may reappear erratically. Postural vertigo of this kind may, however, also indicate middle ear disease, or may be a symptom of central nervous system disease. A thorough examination, including a complete examination of the ear, hearing, and labyrinthine function, plus a neurologic examination, is necessary. When no abnormality of the ear is found and the neurologic examination is normal, the symptoms can be properly labeled benign. Any aural or neurologic abnormality must be completely investigated before the symptom can be considered benign. In the absence of demonstrable organic disease the symptom usually subsides in 4 to 6 weeks.

Post-traumatic syndromes are common and difficult to evaluate. After severe head injury, basilar skull fracture, or severe concussion, episodic vertigo of varying forms may continue for weeks or months. Frequently the episodes are brought on by physical exertion, and the person's usual activities are therefore restricted. The fear of being physically incapacitated suggests a functional element to the illness and may confuse the diagnosis. Symptoms may be either recurrent postural vertigo, more or less constant unsteadiness, or periods of several hours or days of unsteadiness. When the labyrinth has been damaged by such injury and is only partially functioning in an abnormal manner (as proved by testing), the symptoms may last for years unless the involved labyrinth is completely destroyed by operation.

Labyrinthine hydrops (Meniere's disease or Meniere's syndrome) is the cause of 3 to 4 per cent of all episodic vertigo. If the physician adheres to the following criteria before making the diagnosis of labyrinthine hydrops, he will not confuse the syndrome with other possible causes of episodic vertigo.

1. There must be paroxysmal attacks of whirling vertigo, usually with acute onset, almost always accompanied by nausea and vomiting, lasting hours, not days — and there must be complete freedom from vertigo between attacks.

2. There must be accompanying perceptive hearing loss, frequently fluctuating, almost always progressive, and usually more severe in one ear.

3. There must be accompanying tinnitus, most commonly persisting between attacks and frequently fluctuating.

Attacks of labyrinthine hydrops are often preceded by an increase in the intensity of the existing tinnitus and a feeling of "fullness" in the involved ear. The vertigo with nausea and vomiting ordinarily reaches its peak in 10 to 20 minutes and may last up to 18 to 20 hours. Most attacks last 1 to 6 hours. Between attacks the hearing loss and tinnitus remain, but there is no vertigo or instability. The frequency of attacks is widely variable — often 6 to 8 months apart and sometimes as often as two to three times a week if the syndrome progresses untreated.

Chronic middle ear disease, particularly cholesteatoma, can cause episodic vertigo. Two types are most common. The first is an intermittent feeling of true vertigo that occurs sporadically with no pattern. This is not violent vertigo but an off-and-on instability with a sense of rotation or tipping of the environment that comes and goes. Second, and more dramatic, is the sudden, uncontrollable violent vertigo that is produced when a "fistula" is present. The symptom is produced when the patient cleans the ear with a swab or, in some other manner, increases or decreases the pressure in the ear by occluding the ear canal with a finger. The reaction is immediate, may throw the patient to the floor, and is gone in seconds. A fistula is suspected by the aforementioned history and can be reproduced by controlled positive or negative pressure to the occluded external auditory canal with a Politzer bag or a rubber syringe (positive fistula test). The proved presence of a fistula requires correction, as there is danger of purulent invasion of the labyrinth or meningitis.

The investigation of the patient with episodic vertigo requires the following:

1. Thorough examination of the ear.
2. Complete hearing testing.
3. Functional tests of labyrinthine activity.
4. Neurologic examination.
5. Roentgenograms of skull and mastoid (internal auditory meati), blood count, serology, or glucose tolerance tests, as indicated by the history and physical examination.

The essential differences between these most common causes of episodic vertigo (or episodic, nonrotational dizziness) can be illustrated in a comparative list of the most common findings (Table 1).

Gradually increasing instability, rather than episodic vertigo, is seen most commonly in posterior fossa tumors (in particular, acoustic neuroma). However, episodic attacks of true vertigo can be caused by cerebellopontine angle tumors. Since unilateral hearing loss and tinnitus are the common signs of tumor in this region, at times careful consideration should be given to this possible diagnosis. "Atypical" types of episodic vertigo, frequently thought to be "Meniere-like" syndromes, should be very carefully studied.

The following special tests are available today and help in specific location of the probable pathology causing episodic vertigo:

1. Complete hearing assessment, including air and bone conduction testing, speech discrimination, tone decay, and short increment sensitivity index (SISI) tests, will aid in localizing pathology to the cochlea or the eighth cranial nerve.
2. Békésy auditory testing may help differentiate cochlear, eighth cranial nerve, or functional complaints.
3. Simple hot and cold caloric testing gives gross information regarding normalcy, hypoactivity, hyperactivity, or absence of function of each labyrinth individually.
4. Electronystagmography can give additional information to caloric testing and also provides a permanent graphic record that can be compared, if necessary, with later similar tests.
5. Routine skull and mastoid x-rays may often have to be supplemented by tomograms or posterior fossa contrast dye studies or arteriography to assist in specific diagnosis and localization of pathology in those patients who do not exhibit clear-cut typical findings.

Table 1

Condition	Physical Findings	Hearing Tests	Labyrinthine Tests	Laboratory Findings	Other
Acute toxic labyrinthitis (vestibular neuronitis)	Nystagmus, vomiting	Normal	Sometimes hypoactive unilaterally	None specific	?Allergy, ? recent medication
Benign postural vertigo	Positional nystagmus	Normal	Usually normal (unless caused by ear disease)	None specific	Normal neurologic
Post-traumatic syndromes	Other neurologic deficits	Normal or sensorineural loss	May be normal or depressed in one ear	None specific	Evidence of skull fracture (?), history — onset after trauma
Labyrinthine hydrops	Nystagmus during attack	Flat, sensorineural loss, unilateral	Hypoactive in one or both ears	None specific	Special hearing tests
Middle ear disease	Perforated tympanic membrane, cholesteatoma	Conductive hearing loss	Positive fistula test in some patients	None specific	Mastoid x-rays, culture
Ocular disorders	Muscle imbalance, refractive errors, glaucoma	Normal	Normal	Normal	—
Anemias	Pallor, weakness	Normal	Normal	Blood count	—
Hypertension	Elevated blood pressure	Normal or high-tone losses	Normal	None specific	Medication being taken
Hypoglycemia	None	Normal	Normal	Abnormal glucose tolerance	Diabetes
Migraine equivalents	None	Normal	Normal	Normal	Family history, menstrual timing ?
Drugs	Usually none	May be diminished	Can be hypoactive or bilateral	None specific	Specific history

In summary, the proper investigation of episodic vertigo requires a thorough systemic history, an attempt to discover typical patterns, and careful examination of the auditory and labyrinthine systems. The investigation may often require thorough neurologic evaluation as well as laboratory tests and roentgenograms to evaluate other possible metabolic and systemic causes of either vertigo or dizziness.

PARKINSON'S DISEASE AND PARKINSONIAN SYNDROMES

By MARGARET M. HOEHN, M.D.
Denver, Colorado

SYNONYMS

Parkinsonism, paralysis agitans, shaking palsy.

DEFINITION

The parkinsonian syndrome is a symptom-complex of disturbed motor functions: tremor, rigidity, slowness and paucity of movement, and disorders of posture and balance. It was named after James Parkinson, who first described the shaking palsy in 1817 as: "Involuntary tremulous motion, with lessened muscular power, in parts not in action and even when supported; with a propensity to bend the trunk forward, and to pass from a walking to a running pace: the senses and intellects being uninjured." Dysfunction of the autonomic nervous system, dementia, and signs attributable to mesencephalic lesions may be part of the syndrome.

Parkinsonism is associated with a wide variety of pathologic processes that involve or damage the basal ganglia and interfere with normal functioning of the extrapyramidal motor system. Decreased dopaminergic activity in the nigrostriatal system has been demonstrated or implicated in several of them, possibly indicating that a single biochemical abnormality may be associated with all. The interchangeable terms *Parkinson's disease, paralysis agitans, shaking palsy, primary parkinsonism,* and *idiopathic parkinsonism* are reserved for that majority of patients in whom the cause of the disease is unknown. *Secondary* or *symptomatic parkinsonism* is associated with a presumptive causative agent: infection (*postencephalitic parkinsonism*), tranquilizers (*drug-induced parkinsonism*), anoxia, carbon monoxide or manganese intoxication, tumor, trauma, and diffuse degenerative or vascular neurologic disease. Patients with secondary parkinsonism usually have neurologic signs indicative of the more diffuse distribution of the pathologic processes involved.

PRESENTING SIGNS AND SYMPTOMS

Parkinson commented in 1817: "So slight and nearly imperceptible are the first inroads of this malady, and so extremely slow is its progress, that it rarely happens that the patient can form any recollection of the precise period of its commencement. The first symptoms perceived are, a slight sense of weakness, with a proneness to trembling in some particular part; sometimes in the head, but most commonly in one of the hands and arms."

Tremor is the presenting complaint of two thirds of the patients. However, in retrospect, mild aching, stiffness, or cramping of muscles, slowness in walking and performing activities of daily living, subtle loss of manual dexterity, focal or generalized fatigability, irritability, and depression have often preceded the tremor by months or years and were at first mistaken for senescence. Less commonly, the initial complaint is difficulty in writing, speech disturbance, drooling, loss of arm swing when walking, paresthesias, or impairment of balance with falling.

When the disease is fully developed, the parkinsonian patient is recognizable on sight by his expressionless face, tremor, paucity and slowness of movement, general attitude of flexion, and slow shuffling gait. Early in its course, and when the syndrome is incomplete, diagnosis can be more difficult. The disease evolves insidiously and may remain confined to one limb for several years, spreading to the other limb on the same side (*hemiparkinsonism*) before finally becoming generalized. The severity of signs and symptoms may fluctuate diurnally and from day to day, week to week. In addition, the sequence in which the signs appear varies, as does the predominance of the different signs. Tremor may be absent or violent and disabling; severe hypokinesia can exist with minimal or no rigidity.

PHYSICAL FINDINGS

Tremor. Tremor has an insidious onset. The patient may feel as though the limb were "going to shake" or were "shaking inside." The tremor may be palpable before it is visible or may appear only sporadically with fatigue or stress. It is produced by fairly regular and rhythmic involuntary sequential contractions of agonistic and antagonistic muscles. The rate seldom is less than 4 or more than 10 per second and is not necessarily the same in all limbs.

Most commonly, tremor starts peripherally in one hand, later spreading to the other limbs. It is more noticeable in distal extremities than in proximal. Jaw, tongue, eyelids (when lightly closed), and lips, but rarely the head, may be involved. The alternating movement between thumb and index finger has been described as *pill rolling, cigarette rolling,* or *coin counting.* Tremor of the thenar muscles and interossei causes movement of the fingers at the metacarpal-phalangeal joints likened to that by which "orientals beat their small drums." The foot may tap the floor while the patient is sitting. The usual flexor-extensor movements sometimes have a lateral component, or there may be pronation-supination. Tremor involving the lips, tongue, and mandible has been described as giving the patient the appearance of "murmuring an interminable litany."

The intensity and amplitude of the tremor vary. Ten to 20 per cent of patients have no tremor at all. Only rarely is it violent and severe enough to be disabling. There are many quiescent periods. Classically, the tremor is present when the limb is at *rest,* fully supported, and as relaxed as possible: the fingers shake while the hand is lying on the lap. The tremor then ceases at the onset of a voluntary movement, allowing the performance of many activities even when resting tremor is severe. There are many exceptions to this classic picture. The tremor may be of even greater amplitude during the continuance of willed activity or during sustained muscular contraction (*sustention tremor*), as when the arms are held outstretched. In many patients tremor appears only in unsupported limbs, as in the hands when walking. Rarely, a tremor present during volitional movement (such as the finger-nose test) increases in amplitude as it approaches target (*intention tremor*) instead of abating, as is usual. Almost always tremor is increased by stress, anxiety, self-consciousness, fatigue, cold, and the performance of tasks with the opposite hand; paradoxically, it may disappear during extreme stress, such as sudden fright. The tremor is absent during deep sleep. Instead of progressing as the disease becomes worse, it may lessen as rigidity supervenes.

On the electromyogram, action potentials appear in short bursts of equal duration, alternating between agonists and antagonists. Amplitude, frequency, duration, and the part involved tend to vary considerably, often from minute to minute.

Rigidity. Rigidity is felt as resistance during passive movement of the part. In contrast to the increased muscular tone of spasticity, rigidity is present in both agonist and antagonist with a fair degree of uniformity throughout the range of motion; because of this uniformity, it has been given names such as *waxy, lead-pipe,* or *plastic rigidity.* However, the uniform resistance may be interrupted by a series of brief jerks, producing a ratchet or *cogwheel* sensation, especially when the passive movement is just begun or when it is rapid. It is not known whether cogwheeling is due to coexistent tremor or to differences in degree of the lengthening and shortening reactions of rival muscles.

Rigidity is most evident around large joints but is widespread, seriously affecting axial and distal musculature as well. The first symptom may be painful muscle cramps and spasms, as in the hand when writing, or in the toes. More commonly, the limb feels stiff, heavy, tired, or aching. When very mild, rigidity can be detected only by comparing the tone of the affected limb with that of the still normal side. Mild rigidity is intensified by varying the speed of passive movement or by the patient's performing tasks, such as tapping the fingers, with the extremity opposite the one being tested. Similarly, mild rigidity of the neck is made more evident by the patient's counting aloud as the head is being passively moved. Rigidity can be so severe as to prevent any movement around a joint; the patient can be moved en bloc: when the head is rocked, the whole trunk follows.

It is difficult to assess the relative contributions of rigidity and akinesia to the impairment of voluntary movement and the postural abnormalities to be discussed, since both can be severe in the absence of rigidity.

The electromyogram, with passive stretch, shows muscle contraction without recruitment; as one motor unit is activated by stretch, a previously active one becomes inactive. The actual mechanism of rigidity, and whether it is caused by decreased or increased activity of the gamma motor system, is still unclear.

Akinesia. There are several abnormalities of the quantity and quality of movement that are considered *akinetic phenomena.* Akinesia makes the parkinsonian patient appear "stiff" and "rigid" even when no resistance to passive movement is present. Therefore the contribution of rigidity to akinesia is unknown. The akinetic phenomena are as follows:

Paucity of Emotional, Voluntary, and Automatic Movement (Hypokinesia). Parkinsonian patients sit and lie motionless for long periods without the little shifts a normal person makes to avert discomfort and stiffness. The arms are seldom folded or the legs crossed. There is little rotary movement of the cervical spine: when the patient looks to the side, the eyes turn first and the head follows slowly, if at all. Few spontaneous gestures are made, and the face is expressionless. Automatic and associated movements, such as swallowing, eye-blinking, and swinging the arms, shoulders, and hips while walking, also are decreased. This poverty of movement has been called by some investigators "decreased impulsion to move" or "decreased activation."

Slowness of Movement (Bradykinesia). Movements become slow, labored, and deliberate. Patients state that they feel "wooden," as though moving "against resistance," and complain of severe fatigue. The time required for all activities of daily living is increased markedly. Execution of repetitive tasks, such as voluntary eye-blinking, forced smiling, tongue protrusion, finger, hand, and foot tapping, and pronation-supination of the forearm, becomes slower and slower and finally stops altogether. This slowness and tendency to fade and stop the performance of movements may be overcome by slight encouragement, but the patient quickly lapses into a slow pace again. Surprisingly, rapid movements requiring considerable exertion often are performed better than slow, less energetic movements *(kinesia paradoxa).* Similarly, with special stimuli, bradykinetic patients sometimes perform with a felicity they are incapable of without the stimulus *(paradoxical response).* Reaction time is reduced. This is due to slowed movement time and, possibly, also to slowed central processing and/or defective auto-evoked phasic arousal or alerting. The latter contribute to the difficulty parkinsonian patients have in initiating movements.

Difficulty Initiating Movements. Delay in the commencement makes each new intended movement a major effort that is easier abandoned; this may account for some of the paucity of movement. Patients have difficulty initiating the first movement necessary to arise from chairs, get out of bed, turn over in bed, walk, speak, and perform manual tasks. The automatic performance of movement patterns seems disturbed. The delay often is mistaken for a failure of comprehension or for apraxia. It may be merely a hesitation. When prolonged, it has been termed *freezing,* leading to helpless, although transient, immobility. Increased effort to move may prolong the freezing, as may certain types of contact, both visual and tactile: a pin or pebble in the path may be an insurmountable obstacle, as may be a narrow doorway or the mechanical attempt to move the patient by grasping the upper arms.

On the other hand, as with bradykinesia, delay in the initiation of movement occasionally can be overcome by an emergency or other unexpected stimulus, or by special techniques: marching in place, lateral rocking, rhythmic music, regular horizontal lines on the pathway, or kicking an object to start walking; light traction of the fingers to help the patient arise from a chair; and provision of a visual image of a manual task, such as finger tapping, for the patient to imitate and follow. This striking variability of performance may be exasperating to the patient's relatives, who cannot understand why he needs so much help with activities he may be able to perform adequately at other times.

Difficulty Continuing Movement. Once started, movements sometimes are carried out with fair rapidity. However, usually they gradually become slower and of lesser amplitude until they quietly stop — a *fading, tapering off,* or *dampening,* of which the patient is scarcely aware. Alternatively, a real or imagined obstacle may stop the activity suddenly. Or the movements may become jerky and irregular, the speed increasing as the amplitude decreases; this stuttering rapidity of minuscule movements terminates with the patient freezing again. The difficulty continuing movements smoothly is evident when the patient is speaking, walking, or performing manual tasks.

Difficulty Performing Synchronous and Consecutive Acts. Each motor act is performed separately by the parkinsonian patient. He seems unable to make the rapid reformulations, corrections, and re-evaluations necessary to integrate two acts (such as speaking and buttoning his shirt at the same time) or to change from one motor pattern to the next in a smooth flow of movement.

These aspects of akinesia may affect all types of motor activity, and their most common manifestations are discussed in detail. The akinetic phenomena, with a variable contribution from rigidity, are very disabling and probably account for "the hand failing to answer with exactness to the dictates of the will," as described by Parkinson. He stated, "The submission of the limbs to the directions of the will can hardly ever be obtained in the performance of the most ordinary offices of life."

Posture and Equilibrium. Especially in postencephalitic parkinsonism and in the advanced stages of idiopathic parkinsonism, abnormalities of posture and equilibrium may be severe and disabling.

Attitude. The general attitude of flexion — the *simian posture* — of the parkinsonian patient can be recognized from a distance. The head is bowed on the shoulders and the trunk inclined forward. (Rarely, the neck may be extended.) In extreme cases, the trunk may be almost horizontal, flexed at a right angle to the legs. Arms are adducted at the shoulders and flexed at the elbows, so that the hands rest over the anterior thighs or lower abdomen. When arms are outstretched, palms down, there is irregular spacing of the fingers. Metacarpal-phalangeal joints are flexed (often to a right angle), interphalangeal joints extended (occasionally to the extent of subluxation), and thumb and fingers adducted and slightly opposed, with slight ulnar deviation, giving the hand a "rheumatoid" appearance. Postural changes are less marked in the legs: thighs adducted, hips and knees slightly flexed, feet inverted. Occasionally, severe deformities occur in the feet, such as talipes equinovarus. Extension of metatarsal-phalangeal joints and flexion of others may produce a claw-like deformity. The postural abnormalities usually are more marked on the side earlier and more severely affected by the akinesia, rigidity, and tremor. The shoulder is lower on that side, and the spine tends to curve, with concavity toward the more affected side. Attitudinal deformities can be overcome temporarily in the early stages by voluntary effort by the patient, but later they may become fixed even to passive manipulation.

Postural Fixation. The normal ability to support a segment of the body on adjoining parts or on the body as a whole is known as *postural fixation*. It is defective in parkinsonism. The abnormal attitude of the patient tends to become worse when he is blindfolded and not consciously correcting it. Forward flexion of the trunk may reach a right angle to the floor when he is walking. When the patient is sitting without stimulation in a chair, the head sags progressively until the chin is resting on the chest. When he sits on the side of the bed, the trunk gradually leans backward until he is lying across the bed. When he is walking, the knees may flex more with each step, and the patient eventually sinks to the floor. When he is asked to hold the arms up while performing a task such as finger tapping, the arms gradually fall. Although able to correct these losses of postural fixation when instructed to do so, the patient is unable to say why he does not correct them spontaneously.

Righting Reflexes. Parkinsonian patients have great difficulty righting the body: arising from the supine or crouched to the upright position, and rolling over from supine to lateral or prone position. Similar defects have been seen in monkeys with bilateral pallidal lesions.

Disorders of Equilibrium. In advanced stages, parkinsonian patients feel insecure, lose their balance easily, and frequently fall. This usually occurs when the trunk is tilted from the vertical, placing the center of gravity, at the first sacral vertebra, outside the narrow support base of the feet — as during turning, when the patient reaches for something, or stumbles. Normally, when posture is unexpectedly dislocated, balance is regained by appropriate and automatic compensatory reflex movements of the arms and legs and by the contraction of truncal muscles. The parkinsonian patient loses these protective reactions and may fall en bloc, like a post, when he starts to tilt. This can be demonstrated during the neurologic examination by a sharp shove to the sternum or midback, or laterally to the upper arms. Before reaching the advanced stage of total loss of protective movements, the parkinsonian patient may break into short stuttering or *festinating* protective steps to save himself; these steps tend to decrease in height and length as they become more rapid, so that he may be unsuccessful in keeping his feet under his shifting center of gravity as his trunk tilts; when he reaches this point he will fall en bloc.

Weakness. Muscle weakness, reflected in the names *shaking palsy* and *paralysis agitans*, was an integral part of the early descriptions of the parkinsonian patient. There is no true paralysis and the patient never loses his ability to innervate his muscles. However, especially in acquired movements of the smaller muscles, such as the interossei, abductor digiti minimi, orbicularis oculi, and tongue, often there is a conspicuous lack of muscle power and poor maintenance of contraction. The strength of a series of contractions almost always is reduced progressively to an abnormal extent; this is especially evident when patients attempt to perform rapid repetitive movements, such as squeezing a dynamometer. They seem incapable of exerting the force necessary to complete many grosser acts, such as arising from a chair. These all may be manifestations of *akinesia*. For example, absence of the normal synergic extension of the wrist may weaken the force of the clenched fist.

Specific Manifestations of Disordered Motility. *Gait.* "Walking becomes a task which cannot be performed without considerable attention. The legs are not raised to that height, or with that promptitude which the will directs, so that the utmost care is necessary to prevent frequent falls" (James Parkinson, 1817).

At first there may be only stiffness of one leg and difficulty raising the foot from the ground, with a tendency to drag it when tired. This is usually on the same side as the semiflexed, nonswinging arm. Locomotion gradually becomes slower, with shorter length of stride and then shuffling. Steps become small and mincing, with the patient having a tendency to walk on the anterior part of the sole. The normal slight lateral and anteroposterior rocking of the trunk is lost, and there is no swing of the shoulders or hips. The appearance has been likened to that of a mechanical toy. As with all parkinsonian manifestations, effort and constant encouragement can produce an almost normal gait, which then gradually reverts, almost without the patient's being aware of the deterioration. Some patients are able to run better than they can walk or can walk backward more easily than forward.

Difficulties initiating locomotion range from slight hesitation to severe *freezing*; patients complain that their feet feel "glued to the floor." Freezing sometimes can be overcome by leaning forward, rocking from side to side, kicking an object on the floor, and marching in place. Uneven ground, small obstacles, passing through doorways, and turning can precipitate the freezing repeatedly.

While the patient is walking, his steps, instead of becoming slower, may become more and more rapid and short, so that eventually the feet are making tiny, irregular, and ineffectual shuffling movements (*festination*); they may then freeze to the ground, the forward momentum of the trunk causing the patient to fall. Or, once started, the pace can involuntarily and inappropriately increase rapidly until the patient breaks into uncontrollable running with short steps, leaning forward, with the center of gravity ahead of the longitudinal axis of the body; the patient is said to be "chasing his center of gravity." This is known as *pulsion* and can occur in any direction when the patient is walking or loses his balance (*propulsion, retropulsion, lateropulsion*). If he does not fall, he may have to run into the wall or other object in order to stop.

Difficulty executing consecutive movements is especially evident when the patient turns. Instead of a smooth pivotal turn on one foot, he hesitates a moment, may freeze, and takes many small steps around the turning point, holding the body stiffly en bloc; he hesitates again and then resumes walking.

Occasionally, loss of postural reflexes causes the patient's knees to flex while walking; he makes progressively deeper genuflexions until he lands on his knees on the floor.

Rhythmical stimuli, such as music or a series of regular lines drawn on the floor across his path, may improve the parkinsonian patient's gait.

Facial Expression. One of the earliest signs of parkinsonism is the expressionless face — *masked facies, starched features, fixed face, wooden face, hypomimia*. It may be remarkably free of wrinkles for the age. The patient appears depressed, anxious, and glum, with little play of expression animating the countenance. Mainly emotional, but also voluntary, movements are slow to develop, of limited amplitude, and usually protracted. The abnormality may be unilateral, with the appearance of a facial weakness. The widened palpebral apertures (Stellwag's sign) and the infrequency of eye blinking produce the *reptilian stare*. At the same time, patients may suffer from repetitive orbicular spasms (*blepharospasms, flickering blepharoclonus*), severe enough to interfere with vision; these may occur spontaneously or may be induced by repetitive voluntary blinking, by a quick thrust of the finger toward the eyes, or by tapping the forehead or bridge of the nose (glabellar reflex, Myerson's sign). A blink may occur each time the eyes are conjugately deviated back and forth laterally. Elevation of the eyebrows in association with upward gaze is lost.

Eyes. There is evidence that bilateral disease of the basal ganglia can be associated with general impairment of conjugate eye movements in all directions. Both voluntary saccadic eye movement and smooth pursuit are impaired. Eye movements may be delayed, slow and feeble, jerky (cogwheel?), and dissociated from head movement. Full deviation often is limited and poorly sustained. Usually the eyes move better on pursuit and still better during head-turning while fixating on a visual target. This *supranuclear palsy* is never as severe as in the disease known as progressive supranuclear palsy, which also has some parkinsonian features.

Impaired conjugate upward gaze and ocular convergence, with decreased pupillary response to accommodation, are common.

Oculogyric crises are a manifestation only of parkinsonism that is secondary to encephalitis lethargica. The eyes are forced upward suddenly, involuntarily, and often violently. This may be so intense that vision is obscured because the pupils are under the lids. Occasionally, the movement is downward, lateral, oblique, in convergence, or even fixed straight ahead. The tonic deviation lasts from minutes to hours, during which time it may temporarily be overcome. It may be accompanied by pain, spasmodic deviation of the head, lid retraction, dilated pupils, sweating, compulsive running, hallucinations, and other psychic disturbances such as marked fear.

Speech. Speech is affected, as are all other motor tasks. Phonation is impaired, and the voice lacks volume and force, fading and "running out of steam," so that sentences often end in a whisper. The lack of variation in pitch and cadence produces a monotonous quality. Enunciation is poor and syllables slurred. There may be hesitation and freezing. Speech may be quite slow. On the other hand, loss of rhythm may result in progressively more rapid, irregular, staccato speech with confluent syllables. The speech is said to festinate, and fades into an unintelligible jumbled mutter.

Palilalia is relatively common in postencephalitic parkinsonism. The term refers to the involuntary, rapid repetition of syllables, words, or short phrases.

Handwriting and Other Manual Tasks. Difficulty in writing is a frequent early symptom; it is laborious, stiff, slow, and sometimes tremulous. The letters become progressively smaller (micrographia), closer together, and bunched up until they may be superimposed upon each other. A type of festination may occur: involuntary small, rapid, ineffectual movements of the hand stutteringly terminate the writing. The ends of lines tend to veer downward or upward.

All other tasks of manual dexterity become slow and clumsy, with apparent decreased power and amplitude. Repetitive movements are progressively dampened and may come to a stop after the first few attempts. Alternatively, as with all attempts at voluntary movement, they may break into rapid, ineffectual festination.

Akathisia. "Harassed by this tormenting round, the patient has recourse to walking, a mode of exercise to which the sufferers from this malady are in general partial; owing to their attention being thereby somewhat diverted from their unpleasant feelings...." (James Parkinson, 1817).

Whether a primary symptom of the disease, or secondary to discomfort, as believed by Parkinson, extreme restlessness is quite common. It is known as *akathisia* or *muscular impatience*. In spite of severe immobility, the patient complains that he is unable to sit still, must get up and walk about, and suffers great discomfort unless his position is changed every few minutes. This presents a serious nursing problem if the patient is no longer independently mobile.

Mental Status. Parkinson specifically stated that there is no deterioration of intellect. However, pneumoencephalographic, pathologic, and psychometric studies indicate a considerably greater incidence of cerebral atrophy and dementia than was formerly believed to exist in parkinsonian patients. Pathologically, there frequently are diffuse neurofibrillary tangles and senile plaques, similar to Alzheimer's disease. In some studies over half of the patients have been found to have impaired memory, especially immediate, and difficulty with abstractions and calculations. Decrements of the Wechsler Adult Intelligence Scale are chiefly in the Performance subtests and those entailing perceptual analysis, organization, and the acquisition of relatively new and unfamiliar material. Occasionally, dementia is severe, and acute confusion may be precipitated by infections, trauma, general anesthesia, or overdose of antiparkinsonian medications.

Perceptual defects have been shown, such as impaired perception of the visual and postural vertical. Reaction time is slowed, and parkinsonian patients perform poorly on various sensorimotor tests. There is some evidence that these defects are not due solely to poor motor performance but to a defect of the central processing of complex material.

Parkinsonian patients often have a decreased range of interest in work, hobbies, social life, and family affairs. Many are anxious, depressed, and irritable. Marked behavioral abnormalities are sequelae of encephalitis lethargica.

Autonomic Dysfunction and Other Disturbances. Symptoms and signs sometimes attributed to autonomic dysfunction are more frequent and severe in postencephalitic parkinsonism than in Parkinson's disease. Low blood pressure and, particularly, orthostatic hypotension are common and have been correlated with Lewy bodies in the sympathetic ganglia. Plasma renin activity may be decreased. Patients sometimes complain of undue sensitivity to heat, hyperhidrosis, and flushing. The skin may be oily with seborrheic dermatitis along the hairline and in the creases of the chin and beside the nose. Ankle edema is often troublesome.

Drooling *(sialorrhea)* is common and probably is due to depression of the automatic process of clearing the throat and swallowing saliva rather than to increased production of saliva.

Constipation is secondary to disturbed autonomic function of the bowel, to inactivity, and to the anticholinergic drugs with which these patients are treated. Bladder function probably is not affected directly. There is difficulty propelling food to the back of the mouth and initiating swallowing. Diffuse esophageal spasm is common. Severe bulbar symptoms occurring early in the disease are not typical of Parkinson's disease. Almost all patients gradually lose weight.

Thoracic expansion is decreased owing to involvement of respiratory muscles. The diaphragm, however, is unaffected. Maximal breathing capacity is diminished, and there is slight retention of carbon dioxide. In postencephalitic parkinsonism, there is some evidence that depressed sensitivity of the respiratory center also contributes to hypoventilation. Coughing may be difficult and ineffective. Pneumonia is the leading cause of death.

Remainder of Neurologic Examination. The remainder of the neurologic examination usually is normal unless the parkinsonism is part of a diffuse neurologic disease involving other systems in addition to the extrapyramidal.

Tics, torticollis, writer's cramp, hyperextension of the great toe, and various dystonic phenomena may occur, especially with parkinsonism secondary to encephalitis lethargica or to use of phenothiazines.

Subjective sensory symptoms are common: aching, drawing, tightening, tingling, heat, and cold. There are, however, no objective abnormalities of the sensory system.

Deep tendon reflexes usually are normal. They may be slightly hyperactive in the early stages; they may be slightly depressed in the presence of severe rigidity. Extensor plantar responses rarely are found. Palmomental reflexes usually are positive; they frequently are asymmetrical, their briskness correlating with the side of the body most severely affected by the disease. Snout and sucking reflexes are only positive when there is severe dementia. As mentioned previously, the glabellar reflex usually is positive.

COURSE

Parkinson's disease is rapidly or slowly, but usually inexorably, progressive. The severity fluctuates diurnally as well as in cycles of longer duration. Acute and severe exacerbations may be precipitated by pneumonia or other infections, general anesthesia, or trauma; patients seldom fully regain their previous functional ability after recovery from the acute episode. In the final stages, there is helpless immobility, with the patient bedridden or confined to a chair. Generalized rigidity, little tremor, severely compromised ability to communicate, and dependence in all activities of daily living are seen. Before the advent of therapy with levodopa (L-dopa), 25 to 30 per cent died or were severely disabled, requiring help with

activities of daily living, by 5 years; 60 per cent by 10 years; and over 80 per cent by 15 years. The prognosis is better now, although parkinsonism shortens life substantially. Before the era of treatment with levodopa, the observed mortality was three times that of the general population of the same age.

The course of secondary parkinsonism depends upon the nature of the causative agent. With the exception of encephalitis lethargica, discrete causative processes, such as carbon monoxide poisoning and the other encephalitides, produce nonprogressive parkinsonism that often improves when the offending agent is removed if damage has not been too severe. Diffuse neurologic diseases usually progress and the parkinsonian manifestations with them.

COMPLICATIONS

The complications of parkinsonism are those of chronic debilitating and immobilizing diseases in the elderly: bronchopneumonia, infections of the urinary system, decubitus ulcers, accidents, pulmonary embolism.

LABORATORY TESTS AND RADIOLOGIC PROCEDURES

There are no specific laboratory tests for parkinsonism. As with many chronic neurologic diseases, some patients have slightly elevated levels of protein (45 to 75 mg per 100 ml) in the cerebrospinal fluid. The electroencephalogram may show mild, diffuse, nonspecific slowing and disorganization, especially if there is dementia. In a certain number of patients, pneumoencephalography and computerized tomography have demonstrated cortical atrophy and enlargement of the ventricles. None of these tests is diagnostic.

PITFALLS IN DIAGNOSIS

Early generalized parkinsonism, especially when mainly akinetic and with onset in the elderly, may be confused with normal senescence. When signs are marked on one side before becoming generalized, the signs may be confused with spastic hemiparesis.

It is important to distinguish between primary and secondary parkinsonism, especially when the latter is potentially curable. The onset of Parkinson's disease, or primary parkinsonism, occurs in the sixth decade in over a third; the course of the disease is progressive, resembling a degenerative process; the patients have no history or other neurologic signs that might suggest that their parkinsonism is a fragment of a more diffuse disease of systems not ordinarily involved in the classic syndrome. If dementia, ocular palsy, dysphagia, or gait disturbance is disproportionately severe compared to akinesia, rigidity, or tremor, it suggests a diffuse neurologic disease other than Parkinson's disease, and one probably not as responsive to therapy.

The parkinsonian syndrome induced by tranquilizing agents is clinically indistinguishable from the idiopathic disease. The diagnosis must be made by a history of ingestion of drugs, such as reserpine, phenothiazines (especially with a chloride or fluoride atom attached to the phenothiazine nucleus), or haloperidol. These drugs produce an absolute or functional decrease in dopaminergic activity by such actions as depleting stores of dopamine or blocking dopamine receptors. The syndrome is most common in older women treated with high dosages for long periods of time, but it may occur at any age and at any dosage. Usually, but not always, the parkinsonian signs disappear when the drug is discontinued. An early diagnosis is therefore important. Alphamethyldopa, used in the treatment of hypertension, also occasionally produces parkinsonism, presumably by interfering with the synthesis of dopamine.

Parkinsonism is a well-known complication of encephalitis lethargica, or Type A encephalitis, described by von Economo, which occurred in epidemic proportions during the 1920s. It began at any age during the acute stage of encephalitis or during recovery; in other patients the onset was delayed for months or years. The classic progressive syndrome was fulminant in many; in most of the patients still alive today, the disease has reached a plateau or progression is slow. Some remained hemiparkinsonian. Postural deformities may be disproportionately severe. Many have other common sequelae of encephalitis lethargica: oculogyric crises, palilalia, oculomotor and other cranial nerve palsies, dystonic phenomena, sleep disturbances, tics, personality changes, and severe autonomic dysfunction.

Postencephalitic parkinsonism has been reported during the acute phase of other viral encephalitides (measles, chickenpox, Japanese B, western equine, coxsackievirus). It usually is associated with other neurologic deficits and may be transient, never progressive. A parkinsonian syndrome may be part of the neurologic picture of central nervous system syphilis. It was *not* a complication of the influenza epidemic that followed World War I.

When parkinsonian signs are part of a more widespread neurologic deficit caused by anoxia, carbon monoxide, manganese, intracerebral tumors, trauma, cerebrovascular disease, calcifi-

cation of the basal ganglia, or other degenerative neurologic diseases, tremor often is absent or inconspicuous,, and the classic syndrome usually is contaminated by neurologic deficits peculiar to the causative agent. Advanced dementia with generalized cortical disease, multifocal cerebral infarctions, and the lacunar state caused by cerebrovascular disease are not always clinically distinguishable. They may present a picture quite similar to Parkinson's disease. However, dementia is severe, there often is evidence of bilateral corticospinal disease (hyperreflexia and extensor plantar responses, and snout, sucking, and rooting reflexes), gait disturbance is disproportionately severe, and there may be other evidence of vascular disease. Passive movements seem actively opposed; this active quality of the increased tone is known as *gegenhalten* and is not true rigidity, even though it is involuntary. In idiopathic orthostatic hypotension (the Shy-Drager syndrome), signs of autonomic dysfunction are more pronounced: orthostatic hypotension and syncope, impotence, nocturnal diuresis, anhidrosis, and severe fatigability. In progressive supranuclear palsy, loss of voluntary and pursuit eye movements is more severe, dystonic head posturing may be marked, and dysarthria and dysphagia are more severe. Early severe gait disturbance, incontinence, and dementia are prominent in normal pressure hydrocephalus. The Parkinson-dementia complex, with or without motor neuron disease, is seen mainly in the Chamorros of Guam. Hepatolenticular degeneration (Wilson's disease), rigid Huntington's disease, and other heredodegenerative diseases of the basal ganglia usually begin at an earlier age and have other signs of extrapyramidal disease, such as dystonia, chorea, or athetosis. Tumors, other space-occupying lesions, and trauma cause generalized retardation of physical activity but rarely the other signs of parkinsonism.

It is important to identify other causes of tremor. Essential (senile, familial, benign) tremor is the most frequently misdiagnosed as parkinsonism. It seldom occurs at rest, usually has a strong intentional component, and more often involves the head and voice. Most importantly, usually it is monosymptomatic, without the disabling akinesia, rigidity, or postural deficits of parkinsonism, although there may be minimal slowing and clumsiness of fine, alternating, and successive movements. Physiologic tremor exaggerated by fatigue or anxiety and tremors caused by systemic conditions, such as hyperthyroidism, alcoholism, electrolyte imbalance, and hypoglycemia, are not present at rest, and usually are finer, more rapid, and unaccompanied by other neurologic deficits.

MULTIPLE SCLEROSIS

By JOHN F. KURTZKE, M.D.
Falls Church, Virginia

Multiple sclerosis (MS) is one of the more common neurologic diseases, particularly of young adults. The name derives from the multiple areas of gliosis (sclerosis) that characterize old lesions within the white matter of the central nervous system; its categorization as a demyelinating disease refects the more essential features of such lesions: loss of myelin sheath and preservation of axons. In size, single lesions or plaques are but a few millimeters in diameter, although they often coalesce into much larger ones. The lesions accrue not only in different areas but also at different times in the course of the illness, and this had led to its description as a disease "scattered in time and space."

DIAGNOSTIC CRITERIA

The diagnosis of MS is a clinical one. There are no pathognomonic laboratory findings, although recent techniques hold some promise (see later discussion). Further, as in most of neurology, there are no pathognomonic signs or symptoms, because the evidences of disturbed neural function will depend upon the location of the lesions and not their cause. The most useful set of criteria for a diagnosis of MS has been that of the Schumacher Committee (Ann. N.Y. Acad. Sci., *122*:552, 1965). In slightly altered format, these criteria are as follows:

1. On neurologic examination there are objective abnormalities attributable to dysfunction of the central nervous system.

2. On examination or by history there is evidence of involvement of two or more separate parts of the central nervous system.

3. The evidence of central nervous system disease must reflect predominantly white matter involvement, that is, fiber tract damage.

4. Involvement of the neuraxis must have followed one of two time patterns: (a) two or more episodes of worsening, each lasting at least 24 hours and at least a month apart; or (b) slow or stepwise progression of signs and symptoms for at least 6 months.

5. At onset the patient should be between 10 and 50 years of age.

6. The signs and symptoms cannot be better explained by some other disease, a decision requiring competence in clinical neurology.

The first three criteria in essence remind us that MS is a white matter disease, with the first one specifying that at some phase at least the examination must reflect the complaints.

The fourth criterion specifies in arbitrary fashion the requirement for disease activity over time. For illness without remissions, the "time" is long enough that most of the tumors masking as MS would likely be manifest. The fifth criterion for age at onset is not without its exceptions on both sides, but when this is the case, one should be especially wary of labeling the patient as having MS. The last criterion merely emphasizes that there *are* indeed other disorders that may affect the same parts of the nervous system, and that also may have not only a progressive but also an exacerbating-remitting course. Regardless of course, if the signs and symptoms can be reasonably attributed to a single locus within the neuraxis, MS should not be given as the diagnosis.

SIGNS AND SYMPTOMS

The most common types of involvement in MS indicate damage to pyramidal tracts, cerebellar systems, brainstem, and sensory systems. Notably less common are evidences of lesions affecting bowel and bladder or visual systems, and least are cerebral (mentation) changes.

The pyramidal tract signs are usually symmetrical with lower limbs more often and severely involved than the uppers. Therefore spastic paraparesis is perhaps the most common single neurologic finding in MS. Hyperreflexia, absent superficial abdominal reflexes, and positive Babinski signs are the hallmarks of the spastic weakness. Fatigability, too, is a very common complaint in MS.

Cerebellar system deficits are almost always symmetrical, and four-limb involvement is not uncommon. The "typical" patient has a spastic-ataxic gait and ataxia of the arms. The signs expected are dysmetria, decomposition of movements, irregular alternating movements, impaired check, intention tremor, and impaired skilled acts.

Brainstem signs reflect lesions of the intramedullary roots or nuclei of the "true" cranial nerves, or of their suprasegmental connections. Nystagmus, dysarthria, and diplopia are the most usual findings. Others not uncommon are vertigo, tinnitus, facial weakness, or facial sensory deficit; dysphagia and deafness are unusual.

The most common sensory signs found at examination are those referable to the posterior columns: vibration and position sense deficits, with decreased graphesthesia. Again symmetry and a predilection for lowers over uppers are usual. Deficits of touch, pain, or temperature, when present, may follow any conceivable pattern, from transverse cord levels to stocking/glove to bizarre-appearing patches. The subjective "numbness" of which many patients complain is often *not* substantiated by "objective" deficits on testing the affected parts—a situation that may lead the unwary to bestow an erroneous label of hysteria.

Bowel and bladder symptoms are uncommon unless there is major involvement in the previous systems. Urinary hesitancy and urgency generally precede the incontinence, and fortunately bowel incontinence is rare, although constipation is not unusual in the severely involved patient. The bladder dysfunction is most often that of the small, spastic bladder, although on occasion a large, flaccid "tabetic" bladder may be found. When sphincter symptoms are present, neurogenic impotence is not unusual.

Clinical involvement of the optic nerve is about as frequent in groups of MS patients as is sphincter involvement, but is far more important, and should be sought aggressively in all patients suspected of having this disease. In this setting, it is the most unequivocal evidence we have of dissemination in the neuraxis. The typical finding is that of a central or cecocentral scotoma with impaired visual acuity and color-vision perception. This may be unilateral or bilateral. In the acute phase these symptoms may reflect optic papillitis with a swollen nerve-head, or retrobulbar neuritis with a normal papilla. Atrophy thereafter of especially the temporal part of the optic nerve-head is common — but the color of the disc alone is *not* a reliable indicator of past or present optic nerve lesions. Lack of small vessels crossing the disc margin is a better clue than the color, but even this is not of itself sufficient to implicate the optic nerve. Other visual field defects may be seen, including even homonymous hemianopsias. Acquired monocular color vision deficit— particularly to red/green—is a very useful bedside sign of optic neuropathy.

Signs of cerebral involvement in the form of demonstrable dementia or "organic brain syndrome" are rare. Euphoria is not common in MS without dementia; in fact depression is more frequent in MS when there is any noteworthy alteration of mood and affect. Seizures are uncommon, although present more often than co-incidence would require; they may be generalized, focal, or psychomotor.

Other neurologic signs may be seen but are unusual. True neurogenic atrophy with fasciculations, extrapyramidal rigidity, and aphasia are quite unexpected phenomena in this disease.

Evidence of dissemination from subclinical lesions can be marshaled at times by the hot-bath test, or by electrophysiologic testing: cortical evoked responses in the visual, somesthetic, or auditory spheres. This last is discussed in succeeding paragraphs. The elevation of body temperature by immersion in a hot bath can be most useful. The "positive" test is one wherein neurologic deficits not previously demonstrable are brought out. Such changes are transient. Aggravation of pre-existing dysfunction has no specificity, and of course a "negative" test does not rule out the disease.

LABORATORY STUDIES

As for the laboratory, for some years elevation of immunoglobulins in the cerebrospinal fluid has been known to be common in MS. This can be measured by IgG levels, or the IgG/albumin ratio, or estimated from oligoclonal bands. Normal spinal fluid does not rule out MS, and abnormalities are not pathognomonic.

Two recent techniques hold promise for a more specific diagnostic test in the future: computerized tomography (CT) of the head and cortical evoked responses (ER). In MS, CT scans may show areas of decreased density compatible with areas of plaques; occasionally, such areas may enhance after intravenous Renografin. The specificity of such changes requires further study, however.

Cortical evoked responses are derived by averaging repetitive stimuli in somesthetic, visual or auditory spheres, and there has been a great deal of work recently to assess their sensitivity and specificity in MS. In my opinion the techniques are not well standardized, and each laboratory must establish its own norms. Lesions in the appropriate neural pathways can be inferred with these tests — but not whether they are lesions of MS, I believe; and the frequency of "false-positives" is, I think, not known. Still, both CT and ER hold great promise as real diagnostic tools in the future. At present, however, I limit the diagnosis of MS to those patients who meet the clinical criteria discussed.

DISEASES OF CENTRAL MYELIN (OTHER THAN MULTIPLE SCLEROSIS)

By AARON MILLER, M.D.,
and LABE SCHEINBERG, M.D.
Bronx, New York

INTRODUCTION

Central nervous system myelin is made up of the compact layers of the oligodendroglial membrane that encircle the axons during myelinogenesis. As a biological tissue it has a relatively active metabolic rate but a slow molecular turnover. The pathologic reactions of myelin are relatively limited, although it responds to a number of insults either to the oligodendroglia or their closely related and interdependent neurons. The central nervous system myelin, once developed, can either swell or break down in response to a variety of injuries. The disorders may be classified as those in which there is a theoretical failure of normal myelin development (dysmyelinating diseases or leukodystrophies and poliodystrophies) or a breakdown of normally developed myelin (demyelinating diseases or leukoencephalopathies) (Table 1). This chapter excludes multiple sclerosis, see p. 932, optic neuritis, see p. 902, and those diseases in which the injury or degeneration primarily affects the neuron (e.g., motor neuron disease) or the primary lesion is elsewhere (uremia, kernicterus, etc.) with secondary demyelination. In some instances the mechanism is poorly understood. This article covers some of the developmental and acquired disorders of myelin.

DEMYELINATING DISORDERS (LEUKOENCEPHALOPATHIES)

ACUTE DISSEMINATED ENCEPHALOMYELITIS

Synonyms. Postinfectious encephalomyelitis, parainfectious encephalomyelitis, allergic encephalomyelitis, hyperergic encephalomyelitis, acute immune-mediated encephalomyelitis, postvaccinal encephalomyelitis, disseminated vasculomyelinopathy.

Table 1. *Disorders of Central Myelin (Other than Multiple Sclerosis)*

Demyelinating Disorders (Leukoencephalopathies)
  Acute disseminated encephalomyelitis
  Transverse myelitis
  Optic neuritis
  Subacute sclerosing panencephalitis
  Progressive multifocal leukoencephalopathy
  Central pontine myelinolysis
  Postanoxic demyelination
  Marchiafava-Bignami disease

Dysmyelinating Disorders (Leukodystrophies)

  Leukodystrophies
    Globoid cell leukodystrophy (Krabbe's disease)
    Metachromatic leukodystrophy
    Pelizaeus-Merzbacher disease
    Spongy sclerosis (Canavan's disease)
    Fibrinoid leukodystrophy (Alexander's disease)
    Adrenoleukodystrophy

  Poliodystrophies
    Gangliosidosis
      Tay-Sachs disease
      Generalized gangliosidosis
      Late infantile GM_1 gangliosidosis
      Juvenile GM_2 gangliosidosis
    Niemann-Pick disease
    Gaucher's disease
    Infantile cerebral atrophy (Alper's disease)
    Juvenile cerebral atrophies
      Bielschowsky-Jansky disease
      Spielmeyer-Vogt disease
      Batten-Mayou disease
      Kufs' disease

Definition. Acute disseminated encephalomyelitis represents a variety of neurologic syndromes, usually temporally related to viral infections or immunizations, in which symptoms reflect inflammatory and demyelinating activity in the central, or occasionally peripheral, nervous system. Irrespective of a relationship to any presumptive precipitating condition, the histologic appearance of the central nervous system is characteristically identical. Inflammatory changes of varying severity and distribution involve both the leptomeninges and parenchyma of the brain and spinal cord. Most striking are perivascular infiltrates concentrated in the white matter around venules and, to a lesser extent, small arteries as well. The cellular infiltrates consist principally of lymphocytes and macrophages, but in severe acute cases polymorphonuclear leukocytes may predominate. Demyelination occurs mainly in perivascular areas of white matter, with scattered lesions at times coalescing into larger plaques.

Presenting Signs and Symptoms. Symptoms most often appear several days to 2 weeks after the clinical appearance of a viral infection or an immunization but may occur during the acute illness. The condition has been reported following many childhood exanthems, most frequently in association with measles. It has also occurred commonly following postexposure immunoprophylaxis for rabies, particularly when the Semple type of vaccine prepared from nervous tissue has been employed. An incidence of neuroparalytic syndromes as high as 1 per 600 persons has been reported following the use of such vaccine. Incidence rates varying from 1 in 2000 to 1 in 70,000 have been reported following primary smallpox vaccination.

The patient most often presents acutely with the symptoms of meningoencephalitis, including headache, fever, and an altered mental status. A wide variety of focal neurologic symptoms and signs appear, reflecting the areas of white matter most prominently affected.

Course. The disease process may be acutely or subacutely progressive, with the outcome difficult to predict. Cases may terminate in death or recovery, with or without neurologic sequelae. The disease seems to be most severe following measles, with a fatal outcome in 20 per cent of patients and major neurologic sequelae in many others.

Physical Examination Findings. Early in the course, evidence of meningeal irritation, such as nuchal rigidity and Kernig and Brudzinski signs, may be present. Weakness ranges from mild hemiparesis to frank hemiplegia, paraplegia, or tetraplegia. Ataxia and other cerebellar signs such as dysmetria and intention tremor may be prominent, particularly in patients following varicella. Brainstem findings, including extraocular muscle palsies, nystagmus, internuclear ophthalmoplegia, or lower cranial nerve palsies may be present and, at times, may predominate. A variety of sensory disturbances may also occur.

Common Complications. During the acute illness itself, complications attendant to an impaired mental status, particularly pneumonia, must be anticipated. After recovery from acute disseminated encephalomyelitis, the patient may be left with neurologic sequelae ranging in severity from very minor to incapacitating. Mental changes run the gamut from mild intellectual dysfunction through definite mental retardation to a persistent vegetative state. Motor and sensory deficits of varying severity may persist. The usual complications of neurologic disability, including pneumonia, urinary tract infection, and decubitus ulcers, may develop.

Laboratory Findings. No specific or diagnostic abnormalities are found. Cerebrospinal fluid (CSF) generally shows mild to moderate pleocytosis with a lymphocytic predominance. Protein may be elevated, but glucose is normal.

Opening pressure may be elevated during the acute illness. The CSF IgG levels are elevated and myelin basic protein may be detected by radioimmunoassay during the acute disease process. Electroencephalography may show focal or generalized slowing, generally consistent with the patient's clinical status. In a minority of patients, radionuclide scans may show focal areas of increased uptake, and computerized tomography may show areas of diminished attenuation with contrast enhancement.

Pitfalls in Diagnosis. The major diagnostic dilemma is in distinguishing between acute disseminated encephalomyelitis (ADE) and an initial episode of multiple sclerosis. The difficulty may be compounded by the fact that a bout of multiple sclerosis (MS) is often precipitated by a febrile illness. Furthermore, ADE may occasionally occur in the absence of an identifiable antecedent infection or immunization. In the absence of discriminating laboratory investigators, in confusing cases only the passage of time will resolve the question. When an encephalomyelitic illness occurs coincident with a viral infection, it may not be possible to distinguish viral invasion of the nervous system from the presumed immunologically mediated ADE. In the absence of specific therapy for either condition, the importance of such differentiation may be moot.

TRANSVERSE MYELITIS

Synonyms. Transverse myelopathy, funicular myelopathy.

Definition. Transverse myelitis is a nonspecific inflammation of the spinal cord, while transverse myelopathy comprises the toxic, metabolic, nutritional, and idiopathic spinal cord diseases. Causes of the primarily infectious myelitides include viral (poliomyelitis, herpes, rabies), bacterial (tuberculosis, spinal abscess), or fungal (actinomycosis, torulosis, etc.); these are covered elsewhere. Many chemical agents such as penicillin, arsenic, anesthetics, and radiographic contrast agents, as well as electrical injury or irradiation, may produce myelopathy. Postinfectious myelitis may occur in relation to exanthems or parotitis or as a postvaccinal complication. Transverse myelitis alone and in association with optic neuritis (neuromyelitis optica or Devic's disease) is usually believed to be part of multiple sclerosis, but sometimes only long follow-up examination may reveal it to be a condition sui generis. This section covers only the last condition.

Presenting Symptoms and Signs. Antecedent viral infection such as an upper respiratory infection, exanthem, or influenza is common.

This is followed by abrupt onset of malaise, fever, and chilly sensation, with a peak of neurologic deficit in 12 to 24 hours, involving usually the thoracic spinal cord. The initial spinal cord symptoms are usually paresthesias of the lower extremities, back and radicular pain, and weakness of the lower extremities. Urinary symptoms (retention or incontinence) are common early.

Physical Examination Findings. Early there is flaccid paraparesis or paraplegia that later may improve or become spastic. Reflexes are depressed early but may become hyperactive, with Babinski signs. Sensory loss of varying degrees below the level of the lesion is common. Autonomic (bowel and bladder symptoms and adynamic ileus) and trophic (pressure sores) changes are common. Low-grade fever may be seen.

Course. The patient may recover with minimal deficit, such as mild spastic paraparesis, or may remain paraplegic. Subsequent course will confirm or exclude multiple sclerosis.

Common Complications. Neurogenic bladder, decubitus ulcers, and contractures may be seen as complications.

Laboratory Findings. Fifty to 100 lymphocytes may be seen in the cerebrospinal fluid (CSF) and elevation of the CSF protein (rarely exceeding 120 mg per 100 ml) may be seen. A mild leukocytosis may be seen in the peripheral blood.

Subacute Sclerosing Panencephalitis

Synonyms. Subacute sclerosing leukoencephalitis, Van Bogaert encephalitis, encephalitis lethargica, Dawson encephalitis, subacute inclusion body encephalitis.

Definition. Subacute sclerosing panencephalitis (SSPE), occurring almost exclusively in children, is a viral disease caused by infection with measles virus (which may exist in modified form). A slowly progressive illness mimicking degenerative disease, it is characterized pathologically by widespread perivascular inflammatory infiltrates in the deep cerebral cortex and subcortical white matter, demyelination, and glial proliferation. Intranuclear Cowdry Type A inclusion bodies are found, but at times with difficulty.

Presenting Signs and Symptoms. SSPE begins insidiously, usually with subtle manifestations such as declining school performance, which are often misinterpreted. Intellectual decline or behavioral changes or both are usually the initial symptoms. The child may complain of headaches and speech may be impaired. At times, the patient may present with other neurologic phenomena such as seizures, intention tremor, dyskinesias, or chorioretinitis.

Course. The clinical course has been divided into four stages, the first of which is described in the preceding paragraph. This is followed several weeks to months later by the second stage, in which major neurologic abnormalities become prominent. Ataxia, dyskinesias, and severe dementia become evident. The child usually has marked visual disturbances caused by either chorioretinitis or subcortical lesions. Myoclonic spikes, either focal or generalized, occurring as often as 4 to 10 times per minute, characterize this stage of SSPE. Although occasional remissions or temporary arrest of the disease occur at this point, most patients pass rapidly into Stage 3, in which they are comatose with opisthotonic, decerebrate, and other abnormal posturing. Autonomic regulation may be impaired. Even from this advanced state, patients may occasionally improve to a variable extent and for an unpredictable period. However, Stage 4 inevitably follows, in which hyperkinesias and rigidity lessen. The patient becomes hypotonic with only startle responses and medullary reflexes present until the illness terminates invariably with death.

Physical Examination Findings. The abnormalities demonstrable on neurologic examination vary with the stage of illness as just described.

Laboratory Findings. Laboratory investigations generally provide diagnostic confirmation in suspected cases of SSPE. Even in the earliest stages of the disease, serum and cerebrospinal fluid show antibody titers against measles that are above those in patients convalescent from acute measles infection or in patients with measles encephalitis. Serum to CSF ratios of measles antibody are markedly reduced from the normal value (approximately 200:1), which reflects the passive transfer of antibody into the CSF, thus indicating the local central nervous system production of antibody in SSPE. In those few instances in which antibody titers may overlap those of controls, electrophoresis of cerebrospinal fluid and serum will show the diagnostic presence of oligoclonal bands in the gamma globulin region. Of course, immunoglobulin levels in the CSF will be markedly elevated as well.

During the second stage of the disease, a characteristic, if not quite pathognomonic, pattern develops on electroencephalography. This is the appearance of synchronous high-amplitude slow waves, "R-complexes," occurring at periodic intervals, coincident with the myoclonic jerks.

Pitfalls in Diagnosis. In the last few years several cases of progressive rubella encephalitis have been described. These cases clinically mimic SSPE almost exactly, although myoclonus is more pronounced in the latter and cerebellar manifestations are more prominent in the former. Most cases have followed congenital rubella. This condition may be distinguished from SSPE by the finding of elevated titers to rubella rather than measles in the serum and CSF.

The early diagnosis of SSPE principally depends on a high index of suspicion. Thus, any child presenting with unexplained deterioration in school performance or behavioral changes should be carefully evaluated and screened for elevations of measles antibody. In cases of SSPE beginning early in childhood, confusion with several lipid storage disorders or myelinoclastic disease (see later discussion) is possible. However, laboratory investigation should readily lead to the correct diagnosis.

The widespread use of attenuated measles virus vaccine has been associated with a significant reduction in the incidence of SSPE in the United States, although cases continue to appear among immunized children.

PROGRESSIVE MULTIFOCAL LEUKOENCEPHALOPATHY

Synonym. PML.

Definition. Progressive multifocal leukoencephalopathy is a rare demyelinating disease of the central nervous system usually occurring in individuals with impaired immunologic responsiveness. It is caused by progressive, destructive papovavirus infection. The disease is most often caused by JC virus, but occasionally by the antigenically different simian virus 40 (SV40–PML).

Because infection with JC virus is quite common — the vast majority of adults show antibody titers against the agent — the pathogenesis of the illness remains unclear. The virus may remain latent after asymptomatic initial infection until, in the setting of depressed immunologic responsiveness, viral activation occurs, with the development of central nervous system lesions. Alternatively, patients with PML may be among those who do not have antibody from earlier infection and first encounter the virus while in an immunologically compromised state, allowing the development of central nervous system invasion and disease.

Presenting Signs and Symptoms. The onset of the disease is frequently insidious, with weakness of a limb or hemiparesis the most common early sign. Impaired alertness or state of consciousness, personality change, intellectual decline, dysarthria, abnormal movements, or visual symptoms may also occur early in the course. The disease usually appears in adults, but recently cases have been reported in children as well. The vast majority of cases have occurred in patients suffering from recognizable causes of immunodeficiency. About half of these have been lymphoproliferative disorders, with the balance including myeloproliferative diseases, non-neoplastic granulomatous disease, and iatrogenic immunosuppression.

Course. The course is almost invariably of subacute progression until death occurs after 3 to 6 months. There may be a more protracted course in those rare cases caused by SV40–PML. Long-term survival has occasionally been reported. The illness is marked by progressive worsening of neurologic signs originally present, as well as the development of signs suggesting additional lesions of cerebral white matter. Eventually coma develops and the patient dies.

Physical Examination Findings. The abnormalities on neurologic examination reflect the corresponding demyelinating lesions that occur most frequently in the cerebral white matter and less commonly in the cerebellum or the brainstem. Spinal cord lesions are rare. Signs often predominate on one side. Corticospinal tract signs such as weakness, spasticity, and extensor plantars are prominent. Visual impairment on a subcortical basis is often seen. Mental impairment and alterations in consciousness are eventually seen in virtually all patients.

Laboratory Findings. Routine laboratory studies reflect the underlying illness. Cerebrospinal fluid is usually normal, although some patients will demonstrate minor elevations in protein and a few will show pleocytosis (usually patients with less severe immunosuppression). The electroencephalogram is usually abnormal with generalized or focal slowing, nonspecific changes. Computerized tomography has not been widely reported but may show single or multiple areas of decreased attenuation.

Definitive intra vitam diagnosis can only be made by brain biopsy, which shows characteristic altered oligodendrocytes with enlarged nuclei devoid of the normal chromatin pattern. Basophilic (or, less frequently, eosinophilic) nuclear inclusion bodies are often seen. Giant astrocytes with pleomorphic, hyperchromatic nuclei resembling malignant glial cells are also observed. Electron microscopy will show the characteristic crystalline array of papovavirions. Furthermore, specific antisera have been developed that permit viral identification by indirect immunofluorescent staining of frozen sections or immune agglutination visible by electron microscopy.

Pitfalls in Diagnosis. The major diagnostic problem lies in distinguishing progressive multifocal leukoencephalopathy (PML) from other neurologic complications of the underlying immunosuppressive disorders. Lymphomatous or granulomatous involvement of the leptomeninges may present with multifocal neurologic abnormalities. Headache and fever, seldom present in PML, are characteristic of such involvement, and, in contrast to PML, the CSF is usually abnormal. Immunosuppressed patients are subject to a wide variety of opportunistic pathogens, particularly fungi, which may cause meningitis or, alternatively, intraparenchymal focal lesions. Again CSF examination and culture will be particularly helpful. Radionuclide scanning and computerized tomography will help to distinguish brain abscess or intracerebral malignancy from PML. Ultimately brain biopsy will be required when the suspicion of PML is high.

CENTRAL PONTINE MYELINOLYSIS

Definition. Central pontine myelinolysis is a demyelinating disease of unknown cause limited to the basis pontis, usually occurring in malnourished and debilitated persons.

Presenting Signs and Symptoms. Since the original description of the condition in alcoholics, many other cases have been described in which this history was lacking, but patients were usually chronically ill and wasted for a variety of other reasons. In many instances the lesions, which are restricted to the basis pontis with minimal encroachment on the medial pontine tegmentum, are clinically silent. However, when a chronically ill patient, particularly an alcoholic, develops the subacute onset of spastic quadriparesis and pseudobulbar palsy, the condition must be strongly suspected.

Course and Physical Findings. Reflecting the pathologic changes in the basis pontis, these patients manifest spastic quadriparesis, dysarthria, dysphagia, and facial weakness. They may progress to the "locked-in" syndrome, a deefferented state in which the patient, although conscious, is able to communicate only by vertical eye movements. Although most cases have been reported after postmortem diagnosis, clinical recovery has now been cited in several instances.

Laboratory Findings. Whereas no specific laboratory abnormalities have been reported, a large majority of patients are hyponatremic.

Pitfalls in Diagnosis. Despite its rarity, central pontine myelinolysis presents a distinctive clinical syndrome that should permit its diagnosis in the setting of a debilitated, hyponatremic patient. Vascular disease affecting the basis pontis usually presents more acutely and generally involves the tegmentum of the pons as well. However, occasionally the onset may be more gradual or stuttering and thus cause confusion.

POSTANOXIC ENCEPHALOPATHY

Definition. An acute demyelinating illness occasionally develops shortly after patients have recovered from an initial, usually severe, hypoxic insult. Most often this phenomenon has followed carbon monoxide or asphyxial gas poisoning, but cases have been reported in which surgical anesthesia, hypoglycemia, or cardiac arrest have provided the original insult.

Presenting Signs and Symptoms. In the typical case, the patient awakens from the antecedent hypoxic insult within 24 to 48 hours and has generally resumed full activity within a few days. Then, after an apparently normal interval of 2 to 21 days, the patient suddenly develops personality change or confusion. The gait often becomes shuffling in quality and diffuse spasticity or rigidity is evident.

Course. Neurologic deterioration often continues to death, but the process may halt at any point. Some patients may go on to a second full recovery. The morbid anatomy of this condition, whose pathogenesis remains an enigma, reveals diffuse, severe bilateral demyelination of the cerebral hemispheres with sparing of the immediate subcortical connecting fibers (U-fibers) and the brainstem. Prediction of this sequela from the original hypoxic insult is not possible.

Laboratory Findings. No laboratory abnormalities other than documentation of the original hypoxic episode are useful.

Pitfalls in Diagnosis. The diagnosis should be made following a history of the initial episode if the physician is aware of the clinical features of this condition.

MARCHIAFAVA-BIGNAMI DISEASE

Definition. Marchiafava-Bignami disease is a demyelinating disease, affecting primarily the medial portion of the corpus callosum, but not infrequently involving other areas of white matter, including the anterior commissure, the subcortical white matter, and the middle cerebellar peduncles.

Bilateral symmetry is always present. The condition was originally described in middle-aged or elderly Italian men who consumed large quantities of red wine. However, cases have now been reported occasionally in non-

Italians, nonalcoholics (or alcoholics not favoring red wine), and, very rarely, in women.

Presenting Signs and Symptoms. The condition is quite difficult to diagnose clinically, as patients may present with the insidious onset of nonspecific dementia or more acutely with impairment of consciousness.

Course and Physical Findings. Patients may also have other neurologic symptoms and signs including seizures, generalized hypertonia, hemiparesis, or language disturbance. The condition has been invariably progressive and fatal.

Laboratory Findings. No specific laboratory abnormalities have been reported. Antemortem diagnosis may be expected more frequently with the widespread availability of computerized tomography, as the demonstration of decreased attenuation in the corpus callosum may be anticipated.

Pitfalls in Diagnosis. Alcoholic patients presenting with nonspecific dementia or more acute impairment of consciousness are much more likely to be suffering from Wernicke-Korsakoff syndrome, acute withdrawal syndrome, or chronic subdural hematoma. These conditions must all be carefully ruled out before serious consideration is given to the diagnosis of Marchiafava-Bignami.

DYSMYELINATING DISORDERS (LEUKODYSTROPHIES)

KRABBE'S DISEASE

Synonym. Globoid cell leukodystrophy.

Definition. Krabbe's disease is a hereditary rare leukodystrophy of childhood characterized by the accumulation of multinucleated globoid cells and widespread dysmyelination in the brain. The enzymatic deficiency has been identified as primarily beta galactosidase. It appears to be transmitted as an autosomal recessive.

Presenting Symptoms and Signs. The onset usually occurs at about 4 months of age with unexplained fevers and hyperirritability to light and noise with tonic spasms.

Course. Rapid motor deterioration with spasticity is seen in the next few months. Later, opisthotonus is frequent; it is accompanied by decorticate posturing, hypertonic fits, and atypical seizures. Excessive salivation, severe optic atrophy, and unresponsiveness are terminal features. Death occurs by the third year.

Physical Examination Findings. These include hyperirritability to noise and light, tonic spasms, motor deterioration, opisthotonic and later decorticate posturing, optic atrophy, unre-

sponsive pupils, atypical seizures, excessive salivation, and pulmonary secretions.

Common Complications. The most common is aspiration pneumonia.

Laboratory Findings. The cerebrospinal fluid protein is usually elevated (100 to 500 mg per 100 ml). Peripheral nerve conduction velocity is reduced, and biopsy shows active and healed segmental demyelination. Deficiency of beta galactosidose activity in serum leukocytes, and the presence of fibroblasts is diagnostic. The tests can be performed to identify heterozygotes or to make prenatal diagnosis using amniotic fluid cells.

Pitfalls in Diagnosis. Spongy sclerosis, amaurotic familial idiocy, and infantile metachromatic leukodystrophy may all be confused early but other features serve to differentiate these disorders.

METACHROMATIC LEUKODYSTROPHY

Synonym. Sulfatide lipidosis.

Definition. This is a hereditary disorder of myelinogenesis occurring at any age and due to deficiency of aryl sulfatase-A, which leads to diminution of sulfatides in the central and peripheral nervous system. It is usually transmitted as an autosomal dominant trait and occurs equally in both sexes and in any race. It may be congenital, late infantile (most common), juvenile, or adult in onset. Its name is derived from the observation that the sulfatide in tissues changes toluidine blue to reddish purple, green, or orange, or crystal violet to brown.

Presenting Symptoms and Signs. Mental regression and motor symptoms such as spastic or flaccid paraplegia, peripheral neuropathy, and optic atrophy are seen most commonly, usually beginning between 1 and 2 years of age.

Course. Progression to decerebrate posture, bulbar paralysis, blindness, deafness, and death by the fourth year are usual. Patients with the juvenile or adult forms may survive much longer.

Physical Examination Findings. These include unsteady gait, flaccid or spastic paraparesis, absent tendon reflexes, muscle atrophy, possibly ataxia, nystagmus and intention tremor, some mental retardation, impaired vision with optic atrophy, nystagmus, strabismus, and, rarely, myoclonus. Cherry-red spots are occasionally seen.

Common Complications. Patients may have pressure sores, urinary tract infections, or pneumonia.

Laboratory Findings. The cerebrospinal fluid protein is almost always elevated and may be over 100 mg per 100 ml.

Other Laboratory Findings. The nitrocatechol sulfate test will show metachromasia in the urine, leukocytes, or cultured fibroblasts. Assay of urinary or leukocyte arylsulfatase A activity shows marked decrease. Biopsy of peripheral nerve or rectal mucosa shows metachromatic inclusions. Nerve conduction velocity is usually diminished. Cholecystography may show a nonfunctioning gallbladder; this condition results from an excess of sulfatide in the wall of the gallbladder.

Pitfalls in Diagnosis. Polyneuropathy, cerebellar tumor, and cerebral palsy are sometimes confused with this as well as any other leukodystrophy, poliodystrophy, or aminoaciduria. Laboratory tests should confirm the diagnosis.

PELIZAEUS-MERZBACHER DISEASE

Definition. Pelizaeus-Merzbacher disease is a rare, usually familial, leukodystrophy with onset in infancy and a slowly progressive course. The disease is characterized primarily by cerebellar symptoms.

Presenting Symptoms and Signs. The onset is usually in infancy or early childhood. Many of the cases are familial and there is a marked predilection for males. The hereditary transmission is not uniform and sporadic cases are reported. Initially, nystagmus, head tremor, and ataxic gait occur. Scanning speech, abnormal involuntary movements, pathologic reflexes, optic atrophy, and mild dementia often develop. Seizures have been reported.

Course. The disease is slowly progressive with death occurring in the second or third decade, but more rapidly progressive cases have been reported.

Physical Examination Findings. The clinical picture is primarily one of "cerebellar findings," with nystagmus, head tremors, intention tremors of the arms, ataxia of gait, scanning speech, early hypotonia, choreoathetoid movements, tics, and, later, spasticity of the extremities with pathologic reflexes. Pallor of the optic discs is common. Mild dementia occurs frequently.

Laboratory Findings. The cerebrospinal fluid is normal.

Pitfalls in Diagnosis. Late-onset cases have been described that could be confused with multiple sclerosis, except there are no remissions. The distinction between this and sudanophilic leukodystrophy is not clear.

SPONGY SCLEROSIS

Synonyms. Spongy degeneration of the central nervous system, Canavan's disease, spongy degeneration of the neuraxis of Van Bogaert and Bertrand.

Definition. Idiopathic spongy sclerosis is a rare genetic disease of obscure pathogenesis that primarily affects infants. The central nervous system is characterized histologically by diffuse vacuolization, particularly in the deep cerebral cortex, and widespread loss of myelin. Most cases appear to follow an autosomal recessive pattern of inheritance and patients have predominantly been Jewish.

Presenting Signs and Symptoms. In the usual infantile case, the baby is normal until several months of age and then suddenly becomes sluggish and hypotonic. Head enlargement is noted by 4 months in the typical case. In the even rarer juvenile form, the child usually presents with signs of cerebellar dysfunction as well as mental deterioration.

Course and Physical Findings. In the infant, definite arrest of psychomotor development is noted by 6 months. Later in the first year episodic attacks of hyperextension resembling decerebrate and decorticate posture appear, often precipitated by visual, auditory, or tactile stimuli. About the same time, the child's vision deteriorates, usually progressing to total blindness by 2 years. During the second year, hypotonia is generally replaced by more persistent hypertonia with spasticity or occasionally rigidity. Choreoathetoid movements and myoclonic seizures are frequently seen. Autonomic disturbances appear terminally and the child inevitably dies, usually about the age of 4.

In the much rarer juvenile form, frequently sporadic and without ethnic selection, no head enlargement develops, in contrast to the usual megalencephaly in the infantile variety. Most of these children develop progressive visual loss with optic atrophy and generalized spasticity. All reported patients have survived to adolescence.

Laboratory Findings. No specific laboratory abnormalities are found, although visual evoked responses will confirm a central basis for the child's blindness. A definitive diagnosis requires cerebral biopsy that will show the characteristic vacuolization, splitting of myelin lamellae, and proliferation of Alzheimer Type II glia. Characteristic of the disease are the markedly swollen astrocytes of the deep cerebral cortex, which often contain giant mitochondria.

Pitfalls in Diagnosis. Because of the rapidly enlarging head circumference, the infants are frequently suspected to be hydrocephalic. However, computerized tomography in the early stages of spongy sclerosis will reveal normal ventricular size. Very similar neuropathologic changes have been described in a large number of aminoacidurias, including phenylketonuria, maple syrup urine disease, and homocystinuria, as well as in hematosidosis (GM_3 gangliosidosis), conditions that must be ruled out by appropriate metabolic studies. The only other leukodystrophy that produces head enlargement in infancy is the even rarer fibrinoid leukodystrophy.

FIBRINOID LEUKODYSTROPHY

Synonym. Alexander's disease.

Definition. Fibrinoid leukodystrophy is an extremely rare disease of infants characterized pathologically by diffuse myelin loss and small, homogeneous, refractile bodies (Rosenthal fibers) in relation to astrocytes in the subpial, subependymal, and perivascular regions.

Presenting Signs and Symptoms. With an average age of onset of 6 months (range from birth to 2 years), affected infants present with psychomotor retardation, head enlargement (megalencephaly and hydrocephalus), spasticity, and seizures. Almost all reported cases have occurred in males.

Course. The illness is inexorably progressive, with an average survival of 2 years and 4 months after onset.

Laboratory Findings. Computerized tomographic findings have not been reported but may be expected to demonstrate ventricular dilatation in some patients and decreased attenuation of cerebral white matter without contrast enhancement.

ADRENOLEUKODYSTROPHY

Synonyms. Sex-linked Schilder's disease, Schaumburg's disease, Addison-Schilder's disease, diffuse sclerosis with adrenal insufficiency, melanodermic leukodystrophy.

Definition. Adrenoleukodystrophy (ALD) is a sex-linked recessive metabolic disorder, most common in juveniles, characterized by a demyelinating process in the central nervous system and evidence of adrenal insufficiency.

Presenting Signs and Symptoms. Adrenoleukodystrophy most frequently presents in boys in the first decade of life. However, several cases have been reported of onset in adult males as old as 53 years. The initial manifestation is most commonly a change in behavior, usually accompanied by deterioration in memory and school performance. Disturbance of gait and loss of vision are often present (20 to 30 per cent) from the onset of symptoms. Less commonly, hearing loss occurs early. Clinical evidence of adrenal insufficiency may precede the development of neurologic abnormalities, but this is exceptional.

Course. Once neurologic symptoms have developed, the patient's condition progressively deteriorates, with death usually occurring in 1 to 5 years. However, the rate of progression of the central nervous system disorder is quite variable and unpredictable. All patients eventually develop spastic quadriparesis and virtually all lose vision. Seizures occur late in the course in many patients but occasionally are an early symptom. Clinical manifestations of adrenal insufficiency, which are not usually severe, may become apparent during the course of the neurologic illness.

Physical Examination Findings. The neurologic examination reflects the pathologic occurrence of loss of central myelin, which commonly proceeds in a posteroanterior direction. Signs of spastic quadriparesis are found in advanced cases and eventually optic atrophy is evident in all patients. Early in the course an asymmetry of findings is common and may be a source of confusion. Darkening of the skin is the most frequent clinical manifestation of adrenal insufficiency, but arterial hypotension may be found in some patients.

Laboratory Findings. Laboratory investigations usually allow a diagnosis to be established during life. The most important study is the ACTH stimulation test, which will show a diminished plasma cortisol response in virtually all patients. This finding in a male with degenerative nervous system disease is diagnostic of ALD. Computerized tomography may demonstrate contrast enhancing lesions because of the marked perivascular inflammatory reaction that accompanies lesions in a certain stage of development. Similarly, radionuclide brain scans may occasionally be positive. The electroencephalogram is often nonspecifically abnormal and cerebrospinal fluid protein is frequently elevated. Brain biopsy is not required for diagnosis and is often misleading.

Biochemical Findings. Evidence for the abnormal metabolism of very long chain fatty acids has been found in ALD. Cultured skin fibroblasts from these patients show an abnormally high ratio of C26 to C22 fatty acids. It has not yet been possible to make a prenatal diagnosis from similar studies of amniotic fluid cells.

Pitfalls in Diagnosis. Once suspected, the diagnosis of ALD should be made easily with the combination of evidence for adrenal cortical failure in a male with diffuse nervous system dysfunction. However, the early presentation of behavioral abnormalities often leads to the mistaken impression of a primary psychiatric condition. The frequent asymmetry early in the course may mislead the clinician to suspect other progressive neurologic conditions, including brain tumor.

POLIODYSTROPHIES

The disorders classified as poliodystrophies include Tay-Sachs disease, Sandhoff's disease, generalized gangliosidosis, late infantile GM_1 gangliosidosis, juvenile GM_2 gangliosidosis, Niemann-Pick disease, Gaucher's disease, juvenile cerebral atrophies, Hallervorden-Spatz disease, and myoclonus epilepsy. Some have as part of the pathology diffuse demyelination because of the neuronal-glial interrelationship. These conditions are discussed elsewhere.

THE NARCOLEPSY SYNDROME

By G. BROWNE GOODE, M.D.
San Francisco, California

SYNONYMS

Narcolepsy–cataplexy syndrome, sleep attacks, REM (rapid eye movement) sleep attacks.

DEFINITION

Narcolepsy Syndrome. A symptom complex with two major conditions, narcolepsy and cataplexy, plus two minor conditions, sleep paralysis and sleep hallucinations.

DESCRIPTION OF SYMPTOMS

Narcolepsy. This condition is characterized by sleep attacks, excessive daytime sleepiness, and automatic behavior. The sleep attacks, usually preceded by overwhelming desire for sleep, last from a few minutes to over half an hour. The settings are most often those conducive to sleep, such as after a meal, during boredom, and while seated in the evening. However, a distinguishing feature of the sleep attacks of narcolepsy is that they sometimes occur in situations inappropriate for sleep, such as while the patient is driving, eating, walking, and talking. The sleep attack often occurs precipitously.

Another feature that distinguishes this condition from other forms of hypersomnolence is that the sleep is often unpreventable. The following question is helpful: "If a loaded pistol were held to your temple while you were sitting in a dimly lit room in the evening after a large meal, and you were told the trigger would be pulled if you closed your eyes, could you remain awake with your eyes open for 2 hours?" Most narcoleptics emphatically reply "no"; most patients with other types of hypersomnolence reply "yes." After the brief sleep period, most narcoleptics are refreshed and "protected" from the need to sleep for variable periods that last minutes to hours. Some patients are not fully alert after their sleep periods and have continuous sleepiness. Those with severe sleepiness may be partly or fully amnesic for periods, during which they may appear awake and perform rote activities, but if mentally challenged are not fully conscious. Nocturnal sleep may be disturbed in narcoleptics but not in any specific or characteristic way helpful in differential diagnosis.

Cataplexy. This condition is characterized by brief episodes of sudden loss of voluntary muscle control that result in partial or complete body collapse, usually induced by laughter or startle or emotional reactions. The duration is usually less than 10 seconds and rarely lasts over half a minute. This condition is rare as an isolated finding and nearly always occurs in association with narcolepsy. Cataplexy, consisting of head or arm drooping or knees buckling for a few seconds, is usually infrequent and mild; if so, the cataplexy is not mentioned by the patient. Occasionally, this symptom is frequent, severe, and even disabling, with the patient falling to the ground immobile for minutes. Within a few years of onset, the majority of patients with narcolepsy syndrome have developed cataplexy; if not, the diagnosis must be seriously doubted.

Sleep Paralysis. This condition consists of brief episodes of inability to move that occur on awakening from sleep or, less commonly, when falling asleep, with preservation of consciousness. Sleep paralysis may be thought of as cataplexy occurring at the beginning or end of a sleep period. The patient hears and may see (but generally does not, because usually the eyes are closed). Breathing is normal. Guttural noises without discernible speech are sometimes made. Great anxiety is usually associated with the episode. If touched, the patient can move immediately. Otherwise, the episode ends spontaneously after a short period that lasts from seconds to a few minutes. Less than half of narcolepsy syndrome patients have sleep paralysis, which also occurs in over 5 per cent of non-narcoleptic groups.

Sleep Hallucinations. In this condition, nightmares that occur during sleep continue with awakening. The patient has brief hallucinations, both visual and auditory, as if dreaming while awake. Many non-narcoleptic groups have this symptom, which occurs in less than half of narcoleptics.

COURSE

The presenting symptom of the narcolepsy syndrome is usually excessive daytime sleepiness, and the sleep attacks usually begin within a few years. The age of onset varies from early childhood to mid-adulthood, but a common time is the early teen years. The symptoms tend to progress in severity until early or mid-adult life and thereafter may improve or at least reach a plateau. Excessive daytime sleepiness and sleep attacks, as the major symptoms for the great majority of cases, account for most of the disability. Cataplexy occasionally precedes or accompanies the onset of narcolepsy but may not begin until years afterward. Rarely is cataplexy a serious problem because of frequency of episodes, social embarrassment, or injury. Sleep paralysis and sleep hallucinations are usually minor and infrequent symptoms.

PHYSICAL EXAMINATION FINDINGS

The physical examination is unremarkable except that the patient sometimes appears sleepy. Ptosis and head nodding may be observed, and the patient may be found asleep in the waiting room or examining room.

LABORATORY EXAMINATION FINDINGS

The only laboratory abnormality identified in the narcolepsy syndrome is in the polygraph recording of sleep onset. In preparation for this test, the patient refrains from any sleep on the day of the test, which is usually done in the early afternoon after the lunch meal. No analeptic drugs are used that day. The polygraph includes the electroencephalogram (EEG), the electrooculogram (EOG) of horizontal eye movements, and an electromyogram (EMG) of an anterior neck muscle. Electrocardiogram (ECG) for rate and rhythm monitor, and respirations (string gauge over chest or abdomen, or both, and thermistor over mouth and nose) are sometimes recorded. The abnormality sometimes found is sleep-onset rapid eye movement (REM) activity. REM activity normally first occurs after 60 to 90 minutes of sleep. Over 90 per cent of patients with narcolepsy plus cataplexy have sleep-onset REM activity. The only other condition associated with sleep-onset REM activity is an alcohol or other drug withdrawal state in some patients. A positive test confirms the diagnosis of narcolepsy syndrome. However, a negative test does not rule it out. Sometimes it may be useful to repeat a negative test, as the characteristic abnormality is not always seen. Ideally, the test should be performed on all patients with suspected narcolepsy.

PROBLEMS IN DIAGNOSIS

Two major concerns exist regarding diagnosis of the narcolepsy syndrome. The first is not to overlook the diagnosis. Many patients with disabling narcolepsy suffer years before the diagnosis is made and proper treatment given. Untreated narcolepsy may lead to lost jobs, physical injuries, and serious problems with interpersonal relationships. The automobile accident rate of untreated narcoleptics is much higher than that of the general population. In order that the physician not overlook the diagnosis, the usual presenting complaint of hypersomnolence must be taken seriously, and carefully evaluated.

The other major concern regarding the narcolepsy syndrome is overdiagnosis. It must be emphasized that not all instances of daytime hypersomnolence are due to narcolepsy. A variety of medications, nocturnal insomnia, and psychologic problems may produce hypersomnolence; treating these conditions as if they were narcolepsy is a disservice to the patient. The combination of sleep attacks and cataplexy is almost diagnostic of the narcolepsy syndrome, and the presence of each should be thought essential for the diagnosis. In doubtful cases, the polygraph sleep recording is particularly important.

A sizable percentage of patients referred to the neurologist with the tentative diagnosis of narcolepsy actually exhibit amphetamine (or other analeptic drug) abuse; the "narcolepsy" either is a mislabel or is fraudulent (malingering). The analeptic drugs are potentially habit forming to anyone, and some patients with non-narcoleptic hypersomnolence inadvertently develop drug dependence through incautious treatment. Other patients who are willful drug abusers use their "narcolepsy" as a ruse to obtain medications.

Cataplexy may be confused with akinetic forms of petit mal seizures in younger patients and with the drop attacks of basilar artery transient ischemic attacks in older patients.

THERAPEUTIC TESTS

Some patients with narcolepsy syndrome can control their hypersomnolence with multiple brief periodic daytime naps. However, a good response is not specific for narcolepsy. A therapeutic trial of medication may be useful when the diagnosis is in doubt, particularly if the polygraph sleep recording is not available. Narcolepsy symptoms are usually controlled by small amounts of analeptic drugs. Methylphenidate hydrochloride, 5 to 10 mg one to three times daily, or dextroamphetamine, 2.5 to 5 mg one to three times daily, gives good symptom relief to most patients. The response to these medications is often dramatic in narcolepsy syndrome cases but does not rule out other forms of hypersomnolence.

Cataplexy, sleep paralysis, and sleep hallucinations are not helped by the analeptic medications. However, the tricyclic antidepressant medications have been found quite helpful. A favorable response to these drugs is fairly specific, so a therapeutic trial at a small to moderate dose of imipramine hydrochloride or related drug may be helpful if the diagnosis is in doubt.

COMPLICATIONS

An infrequent but possibly serious complication of the narcolepsy syndrome is sleep apnea. A small percentage of narcoleptics develop sleep apnea, which may also occur independent of narcolepsy. Sleep apnea is characterized by periods of apnea during sleep, which last from a few seconds to over a minute. The episodes begin suddenly and end with loud stertorous respirations and partial or complete arousal. An observer notes periods of no breathing followed by periods of labored breathing and loud snoring. Over 80 per cent of patients are men. Many are hypertensive and obese, some have polycythemia and right heart enlargement, and a few have heart failure. The condition may be suspected by careful observation of the patient's sleep; the diagnosis can be established by a polygraph sleep record that includes monitoring of nose and mouth and chest and abdomen respiratory movements.

EPILEPSY AND OTHER CONVULSIVE DISORDERS

By B. JOE WILDER, M.D.,
and L. JAMES WILLMORE, M.D.
Gainesville, Florida

INTRODUCTION

Epilepsy should not be considered as a disease entity in itself. It is rather a symptom complex that denotes recurrent episodic central nervous system (CNS) electrical dysfunction that results in convulsions, interference with consciousness, and aberration in ongoing behavior. With few exceptions, the common denominator of epilepsy is recurrent paroxysmal electrical discharge of areas of the cerebral cortex and related subcortical nuclei and brainstem centers or paroxysmal discharge of the cerebral cortex as a whole with or without participation of subcortical and brainstem nuclear centers. The exceptions are rare. Tonic seizures and some clonic attacks may result from paroxysmal electrical burst discharge that may involve only brainstem centers or other subcortical nuclear masses with or without subsequent spread to the cerebral cortex. Different forms of myoclonic spasms may result from the brief cortical or subcortical paroxysmal burst discharge. The international classification of epileptic seizures was published in Epilepsia in 1970 (11:102–113) and is inclusive of most of the epilepsies. This communication will deal primarily with the most prevalent of the epilepsies and other convulsive states.

Partial seizures that may or may not be generalized are properly separated from primary generalized seizures, as shown in Table 1. Partial seizures, whether simple, as in the case of focal motor attacks, or complex, as in temporal lobe seizures, originate from specific areas of the brain and are often quite stereotyped from one attack to the next. Etiologic factors that result in partial seizures can frequently be determined, and pathologic specimens obtained at surgery or postmortem examination often show evidence of focal glial scarring; tumor; vascular malformations; bacterial, fungal, viral, or parasitic infectious processes; infarction or vascular

Table 1. *International Classification of Epileptic Seizures*

I. Partial seizures (seizures beginning locally)
  A. Partial seizures with elementary symptoms (generally without impairment of consciousness)
    1. With motor symptoms (includes jacksonian seizures)
    2. With special sensory or somatosensory symptoms
    3. With autonomic symptoms
    4. Compound forms
  B. Partial seizures with complex symptoms (generally with impairment of consciousness), temporal lobe or psychomotor seizures
    1. With impairment of consciousness only
    2. With cognitive symptoms
    3. With affective symptoms
    4. With "psychosensory" symptoms
    5. With "psychomotor" symptoms
    6. Compound forms
  C. Partial seizures secondarily generalized
II. Generalized seizures (bilaterally symmetric and without local onset)
    1. Absences (petit mal)
    2. Bilateral massive epileptic myoclonus
    3. Infantile spasms
    4. Clonic seizures
    5. Tonic seizures
    6. Tonic-clonic seizures (grand mal)
    7. Atonic seizures
    8. Akinetic seizures
III. Unilateral seizures (or predominantly)
IV. Unclassified seizures (due to incomplete data)

---

insufficiency; vasculitis; or results of old pial intracerebral hemorrhage. The association of such lesions with epilepsy does not imply that basic mechanisms that cause seizures are fully understood. Trauma sustained at birth or during a later epoch, CNS infections, anoxic episodes, and neoplasia are some of the more common causes of partial seizures. Inborn errors of metabolism, CNS storage, and progressive CNS degenerative diseases, although not common, are often accompanied by recurrent partial or generalized convulsions.

Etiologic factors in generalized seizures are less well understood than those in focal or partial seizures. Absence (petit mal) seizures and generalized tonic-clonic (grand mal) seizures, in many instances, have genetic factors involved. Studies indicate that the trait for petit mal and grand mal seizures may be inherited as an autosomal dominant factor. Inheritance plays a role in progressive myoclonic epilepsy. However, specific defects, with the exception of certain of the inborn errors of metabolism — e.g., storage diseases, pyridoxine dependency — have not been identified in generalized seizures. Alcoholic, drug withdrawal, and febrile seizures are not included in a classification of the epilepsies. Hepatic, renal, toxic, and other metabolic encephalopathies result in convulsive attacks and must be considered in diagnosis; however, such states are not included in the classification of epileptic seizures. Likewise, hypocalcemic and hypoglycemic states occur in the neonatal period and are diagnostic considerations but are not properly classified as epilepsy. Conversely, neonatal CNS infections, subdural hematoma, intracerebral hemorrhage, and anoxic episodes are frequent causes of seizures in this age period and often result in recurrent seizures during childhood and later life.

DIAGNOSIS OF GENERALIZED AND PARTIAL EPILEPSY

The aim of diagnosis in convulsive attacks should be to determine etiologic factors whenever possible. As in any disease state, the history is of paramount importance. In children, adolescents, adults, and the elderly, a careful history from both the patient and observers often separates focal or partial from generalized seizures. The examiner should carefully question the patient concerning premonition or aura that may immediately precede the seizure. Such information may establish the cortical site of origin of the partial seizure. Furthermore, in the case of temporal lobe attacks characterized by loss of conscious contact with the environment, the occurrence of an aura will distinguish this form of epilepsy from petit mal absences. However, the examiner should be aware that focal seizures may frequently generalize so rapidly that the patient and even careful observers may not distinguish the focal nature of the seizure. As is often the case, the focal seizure cannot be clinically distinguished from generalized or grand mal seizures until anticonvulsant medication has been started. Anticonvulsant drugs will often prevent generalization of seizures and unmask the clinical signs of focal epilepsy. In our experience, this is often the situation in complex, partial, or temporal lobe seizures.

In obtaining the history, special emphasis should be placed on (1) seizure onset; auras or premonition; (2) seizure duration; (3) seizure content: tonic or clonic convulsive, generalized or focal, or loss of conscious contact with environment; (4) state of consciousness; and (5) postictal state and details of recovery from the seizure.

Clinically, petit mal absences may be difficult to distinguish from certain temporal lobe attacks. However, by history, petit mal often can be distinguished from the temporal lobe absence (loss of consciousness) by onset and recovery. The petit mal patient experiences a rapid onset of loss of awareness of surroundings that is of brief duration followed by rapid return to full awareness. The temporal lobe absence is usually of longer duration, often preceded by an aura and followed by a brief period of postictal confusion.

The review of symptoms, the patient's history, family history, and birth and neonatal history are important in uncovering genetic factors, birth injuries, infectious processes, metabolic abnormalities, or head trauma, any of which may be causative factors in the development of seizures. Inheritance factors are often linked with generalized seizures; however, reliable data have been collected that implicate genetic factors in certain of the partial seizures. Certainly, seizures that accompany inborn errors of metabolism may be associated with positive family histories.

The neurologic and general physical examinations often are unrewarding in the diagnostic work-up of the seizure patient. However, physical examination sometimes reveals characteristic features of patients with certain disorders who often first seek medical aid because of the onset of seizures. Tuberous sclerosis, neurofibromatosis, Sturge-Weber syndrome, and many other examples can be cited.

The neurologic examination becomes critically important when certain specific factors cause convulsions. CNS infections, toxic and metabolic encephalopathies, poisons, subdural hematoma, and alcoholic and drug withdrawal usually can be suspected after careful mental status and neurologic examination. Intracranial mass lesions, including primary brain tumors, metastatic lesions, brain abscess, leukemic infiltrates, and granulomas, often produce gross or subtle neurologic deficits in addition to generalized or partial seizures.

Various etiologic factors, some of which have been mentioned, are of more or less importance, depending on the age of seizure onset. Seizure onset peaks in childhood, drops to its lowest level during the middle adult years, and again rises in the elderly. In the continuum of age, distinct etiologic groupings may be seen and are shown in Table 2.

AIDS TO DIAGNOSIS

Electroencephalography (EEG). The EEG is an indispensable tool in diagnosis and achieves its greatest clinical usefulness in convulsive disorders. It reflects the physiologic activity of the cerebral cortex. Paroxysmal EEG discharge and focal EEG spikes or sharp waves do not confirm the diagnosis of epilepsy but, when coupled with a seizure history, indicate a seizure disorder. An absence of EEG abnormalities does not exclude the presence of a seizure disorder. Approximately 3 to 7 per cent of patients with clinically documented seizures have normal EEG readings, even after serial recordings, sleep recordings, and special activation techniques. EEG spike, spike and wave, sharp, and sharp wave patterns are not invariably associated with specific convulsive disorders; however, strong correlations can be made. Generally, focal EEG abnormalities correlate well with one of the partial seizure disorders, and generalized paroxysmal discharges indicate generalized seizure states. The highest degree of EEG and seizure correspondence occurs in petit mal, with the EEG showing 2½ to 4 cycle per second paroxysmal generalized spike and wave discharge. Focal and generalized EEG abnormalities associated with partial or focal seizures denote brain electrical dysfunction and do not indicate an etiologic factor. However, focal slow wave abnormalities suggest focal damage or a destructive process. Certain of the metabolic encephalopathies accompanied by clinical seizures may present EEG abnormalities characterized by diffuse slowing with disorganization of EEG rhythms.

The EEG evaluation of the seizure patient should be pursued with sleep recording and

Table 2. *Etiology and Age: Epilepsy and Other Convulsive Disorders*

	Newborn	Infancy	Childhood	Adolescence	Young Adult	Old Adult
Severe perinatal injury	———	—				
Metabolic defects	———	—				
Congenital malformation		———	———			
Infection		———	———			
Genetic		———	———	———	———	
Perinatal injury	———	—				
Genetic disease		———	———	———		
Myoclonic syndromes		———	———	———		
Postnatal trauma			———	———	———	———
Brain tumor					———	———
Vascular disease					———	———
Myoclonus epilepsy				———	———	———

activation techniques if routine recordings are normal or inconclusive.

Spinal Puncture. Spinal fluid examination is not necessary in every patient with a convulsive disorder. Findings are usually normal in the patient with uncomplicated epilepsy. Abnormalities of pressure, cells, protein, and sugar (which should be compared with concurrently drawn blood sugar) usually denote CNS disease. Some situations require lumbar puncture and fluid analysis. In patients with febrile convulsions and neurologic signs, CNS infections must be ruled out. In adults with a history of recent seizure onset, spinal fluid examination is indicated; however, neurologic deficit or evidence of increased intracranial pressure may cause the physician to defer the procedure to avoid the possibility of brain herniation. Contrast radiographic studies may be appropriate prior to lumbar puncture.

Radiographic Procedure. Routine skull x-rays are rarely productive except in certain congenital abnormalities or post-trauma states or when intracranial mass lesions contain calcium deposits or produce a shift of a calcified pineal or choroid plexus. Chronically increased intracranial pressure may produce characteristic findings in routine skull films.

Brain scan is a benign procedure that is often positive when intracranial mass lesions are present.

Computerized tomography (CT scan) is a useful noninvasive contrast procedure to visualize the parenchyma of the brain. CT scan is most helpful in children with focal seizures, in patients of suspected mass lesions, and in patients who have adult onset of seizures.

Arteriography and pneumoencephalography should be reserved when a mass lesion or vascular malformation is suspected or in a patient who has adult onset seizures. Contrast studies may be indicated in any epileptic patient who for unknown reasons has an exacerbation of seizures after adequate medical management has been achieved.

FEBRILE CONVULSIONS, NEONATAL SEIZURES, AND INFANTILE SPASMS

Febrile convulsions occur with greatest frequency during the first year of life and generally are self-limiting. In 85 per cent of patients, febrile seizures do not recur. The convulsions develop during the peak of the temperature elevation and, in the absence of other neurologic signs, do not necessitate special neurologic diagnostic procedures. Neonatal convulsions often are associated with hypoglycemia or hypocalcemia. The diagnosis can be confirmed by

appropriate laboratory studies. CNS infection, prenatal or birth brain damage from trauma, and anoxia are considerations that have been mentioned earlier. Inborn errors of metabolism, such as the aminoacidurias, can be diagnosed by appropriate screening procedures.

Infantile spasm describes an epileptic symptom complex of infancy associated with brief severe tonic motor seizures, massive myoclonus, and major and minor motor attacks. No single etiologic factor has been discovered; however, many diverse pathologic processes have been described. The EEG findings have been described as hypsarrhythmia. The diagnosis is made on clinical and EEG findings.

Convulsive disorders, of either a focal or generalized nature, indicate CNS dysfunction, and efforts should be directed to making a specific diagnosis. In many instances, etiologic diagnosis is lifesaving.

HYPERVENTILATION SYNDROME

By DONALD C. ZAVALA, M.D.

Iowa City, Iowa

DEFINITION

Hyperventilation is defined as increased alveolar ventilation that leads to hypocapnia and acute alkalosis.

ETIOLOGY

It is a common manifestation of anxiety, especially in nervous young women, and may be acute or chronic. Other causes are listed in Table 1.

SIGNS AND SYMPTOMS

Symptoms characteristic of the hyperventilation syndrome are dizziness, lightheadedness; sense of unreality; air hunger; deep sighing; blurred vision; palpitations; premature beats; rapid pulse; discomfort in the throat, precordium, or epigastrium; numbness of the hands, feet, and perioral region; and apprehension. Usually the patients are not aware of their overventilation, even if it is obvious to others. Sometimes the overbreathing occurs so quietly

Table 1. *Causes of Hyperventilation*

1. Functional: psychogenic
2. Physiologic: exercise, high altitude, pregnancy, mechanical overventilation
3. Pathologic
   a. Pulmonary: embolization, interstitial pneumonia, fibrosing alveolitis, pneumothorax, atelectasis, severe chest wall deformity, etc.
   b. Cardiac: mitral stenosis, left ventricular failure, etc.
   c. Metabolic acidosis: diabetes, renal failure, chronic diarrhea, methyl alcohol, ethylene glycol
   d. Neurogenic: pontine or lower midbrain lesion, meningitis, encephalitis, cerebral hemorrhage, trauma
   e. Drugs: salicylates, doxapram
   f. Hormones: epinephrine, progesterone
   g. Hypermetabolism: hyperthyroidism, fever, gram-negative septicemia
   h. Pain
   i. Hypotension

that no one takes notice. Cold extremities and aerophagia are common. The attacks vary in length, but those lasting several hours are often attended by carpopedal spasm. Tetany is rare. Occasionally there is loss of consciousness, similar to the common faint, followed by post-syncopal confusion, headache, and weakness.

PATHOPHYSIOLOGY

Hyperventilation rapidly causes a decrease in the alveolar P_{CO_2}, but adds little to the arterial O_2 saturation under normal conditions. The hypocapnia may produce a reduction in the cerebral blood flow with changes in the electroencephalogram. Bronchoconstriction, when present, increases the work of breathing. Alkalosis may bring about migration of intracellular potassium, decrease in ionized calcium, and alteration of cell membrane potential, as reflected in the electrocardiogram.

LABORATORY FINDINGS

Characteristically, the Pa_{CO_2} is reduced to approximately 20 to 30 mm Hg, the arterial pH is raised to 7.5 to 7.65, slow wave activity is seen in the electroencephalogram (EEG), and nonspecific ST-T wave changes appear in the electrocardiogram (ECG), which reverse promptly when the attack ends. Pulmonary function studies, serum calcium, potassium, sodium, magnesium, glucose, blood urea nitrogen (BUN), and creatinine are within a normal range. During prolonged hyperventilation the serum inorganic phosphorus is often decreased.

RESPIRATORY ALKALOSIS

Acute respiratory alkalosis is produced by the lungs "blowing off" large quantities of CO_2, thereby lowering the level of carbonic acid (H_2CO_3), which is almost entirely in the form of dissolved CO_2. A rise in the pH or a fall in the hydrogen-ion concentration (H^+) occurs, with a "relative" bicarbonate (HCO_3^-) overload. If the hyperventilation is continuous, as it may be in physiologic or pathologic overbreathing, then in 2 to 3 days the pH is "compensated" to or toward the normal range (7.4 ± 0.04) by renal excretion of bicarbonate and re-establishment of the $(HCO_3^-):(H_2CO_3)$ ratio to 20:1 (Table 2). In simple, chronic respiratory alkalosis each mm Hg decrement of P_{CO_2} causes a 0.4 to 0.5 mEq per liter reduction in the concentration of HCO_3.

In functional hyperventilation the attacks often are of relatively short duration. Even if symptoms are severe and prolonged, the patient's breathing characteristically reverts to a normal pattern during sleep. Thus the arterial pH and P_{CO_2} values return to normal until the next attack.

In patients requiring assisted ventilation for respiratory failure, mechanical hyperventilation will rapidly reduce an elevated arterial P_{CO_2} without allowing enough time for the kidneys to excrete the bicarbonate overload. The result is an unbalanced $(HCO_3^-):(H_2CO_3)$ ratio, which may produce a severe, life-threatening respiratory alkalosis. Therapy must be directed toward correcting the P_{CO_2} by adjustment of the ventilator or adding dead space. Also, serum electrolyte deficiencies must be corrected, as the kidneys will not unload $NaHCO_3$ if the serum chloride is low or there is a strong stimulus to conserve sodium.

Table 2. *The Henderson-Hasselbalch Equation*

$$pH = pK + \log \frac{HCO_3^-}{H_2CO_3}$$

Where:
(1) pK = 6.1 (log of dissociation constant)
(2) $\dfrac{HCO_3^-}{H_2CO_3} = \dfrac{\text{bicarbonate } CO_2 \text{ (kidney)}}{\text{dissolved } CO_2 \text{ (lung)}} = \dfrac{20}{1}$
ratio
(3) Solubility coefficient of CO_2 = 0.03
(4) $[H_2CO_3] = 0.03 \times P_{CO_2}$

Then,

$$pH = 6.1 + \log \frac{[HCO_3^-]}{0.03 \times P_{CO_2}}$$

DIAGNOSIS AND PITFALLS

Usually a diagnosis of the hyperventilation syndrome is made with assurance after a careful history and physical examination. Nevertheless, the physician must be alert for the unusual or unexpected. For example, breathlessness may be a manifestation of "silent" pulmonary emboli, fibrosing alveolitis, spontaneous pneumothorax, atelectasis, or mitral stenosis. The presence of hypoxemia (PaO_2 less than 80 mm Hg), pulmonary hypertension, abnormal pulmonary or cardiac signs, or an abnormal chest x-ray should prevent the misdiagnosis of "functional" overbreathing.

It is not unusual for tense patients with breathlessness and precordial discomfort to undergo a cardiac evaluation. T-wave inversion and ST-segment depression secondary to hyperventilation may resemble the ECG changes seen in coronary insufficiency. A helpful diagnostic maneuver is to obtain two ECGs for comparison, one during voluntary hyperventilation and the other during standard exercise. An abnormal tracing with exercise but not with hyperventilation is considered to be positive evidence for coronary artery disease. An abnormal ECG during rapid, deep breathing but not with exercise is consistent with hyperventilation. Similar, abnormal results in both tracings favor the diagnosis of hyperventilation but are not diagnostic, as both conditions could coexist.

PROVOCATIVE TEST

Generally, the diagnosis can be confirmed by having the patient voluntarily hyperventilate for 2 to 3 minutes while sitting. Since many patients somewhat resist the idea of breathing rapidly at command, cooperation frequently can be obtained by first showing the patient how to hyperventilate and then getting him to breathe fast for several minutes while a stethoscope is placed on his chest. In such a manner the "attack" often can be reproduced and then aborted by having the patient rebreathe into a paper bag. The build-up of alveolar and arterial PCO_2 that occurs by rebreathing into a closed system will shortly terminate the symptoms.

A WORD OF CAUTION

Voluntary hyperventilation commonly seen in children is harmless unless the child should be injured by falling. Hyperventilation performed by swimmers prior to diving (to stay under the water longer) is a dangerous practice to be condemned! With vigorous underwater activity there is a rapid drop in the arterial PO_2 so that unconsciousness can occur from cerebral hypoxia before the submerged swimmer has an urge to breathe.

HYSTERICAL NEUROSIS

By HERBERT S. RIPLEY, M.D.
Seattle, Washington

SYNONYMS

Hysterical neurosis, conversion type or dissociative type; hysteria; conversion reaction; Briquet's syndrome.

DEFINITION

Hysterial neurosis is a disorder characterized by involuntary psychogenic alterations in (1) the conversion type of sensory or motor functions and in (2) the dissociative type of the state of consciousness or identity. The symptoms occur without any structural lesion but simulate those caused by anatomic or physiologic pathology. Intrapsychic conflicts and the anxiety associated with them are repressed and converted into symptoms that have psychologic meaning.

The choice of the symptom is influenced by the nature of the conflict and the ability of the organ chosen to symbolize the unconscious content. For example, a typist who wished to attack a hated employer developed a paralysis of her right arm that interfered with both carrying out her duties and striking her boss. She also had to endure self-punishment for the distorted partial gratification of her wishes by the limitations that the symptom placed upon her daily living. The symbolic meaning and protective value of the symptom is evident in such cases as those of an unhappy housewife who developed disabling muscle spasms and of an army private who became mute when he desired to curse his sergeant. A young woman with sexual conflicts and the desire for a child, who had hysterical urinary retention, remarked that had she not resisted the sexual advances of an aggressive man, the swelling in her abdomen "would be due to something else."

The symptom may also be determined by a part of the body that has previously been the site of disease or by imitation of a symptom in another person. For example, one patient who had made a good recovery from a head injury developed headaches and another whose close friend has died of cancer of the throat had hysterical difficulty in swallowing.

PRESENTING SIGNS AND SYMPTOMS

The symptoms may be consistent or vary at different examinations. Common motor manifestations are paralysis, paresis, ataxia, akinesia, and dyskinesia. Sensory disturbances include blindness, deafness, loss of sense of taste or smell, anesthesia, hypesthesia, hyperesthesia, and paresthesia. The most common visceral symptoms are vomiting, bulimia, difficulty in swallowing, hiccups, hyperventilation, and urinary retention.

In the dissociative type such symptoms as amnesia, somnambulism, fugue, and multiple personality may occur. Frequently the patient displays an emotional apathy and lack of concern about the disturbance, which was termed *la belle indifférence* by Janet. However, in some patients, especially those in whom the hysterical symptoms may not be sufficiently expressed to give protection against disturbing emotions, anxiety or depression or both may be present as well. It is not uncommon to have a mixture of neurotic symptoms with the presence of two or more of the following: hysterical, phobic, compulsive, obsessive, neurasthenic, and hypochondriacal. Although in the past hysteria, which is a Greek word meaning wandering uterus, was considered a disorder of women, it is often found in men.

COURSE

The onset is usually in late adolescence or early adulthood. It may be acute and of short duration but recurrences are common when there are repeated stresses and when the attacks result in gratification of personal needs. Factors favoring a good prognosis are a relatively well-integrated personality, a history of stable relationships with others, good adjustment to school and work, and symptoms of short duration resulting from severe rather than mild environmental stresses. A variety of conflicts can be responsible for the condition, but situations involving dangers, resentments, and sexual maladjustment are especially common causes. The historic formulation of Breuer and Freud states that when fears and guilt over sexual desires or trauma are denied and re-pressed, they are relieved by conversion into hysterical symptoms. However, it has subsequently been considered that this basic mechanism of conversion may be initiated by any serious emotional trauma. Generally there is a favorable response to psychotherapeutic measures, but in some patients the illness becomes chronic.

PHYSICAL EXAMINATION FINDINGS

No evidence of anatomic or physiologic disease is found. However, the diagnosis should not be based on exclusion but rather on positive findings. Inconsistencies in the symptoms are the rule.

Some examples of common findings are given. Weakness tends to vary with the effort of the examiner testing the strength of the muscles. The patient may contract antagonist muscles in order to prove weakness in the protagonist muscles. When surprised by pain due to stimuli, the affected muscles may be used to withdraw. Gait disturbances are bizarre and exaggerated. Sensory impairment does not conform to the anatomic nerve distribution. For example, glove and stocking anesthesias are found and sensory changes are sharply defined at the midline. Reflexes are usually normal and equal on both sides. Hearing loss is most often bilateral and complete. However, the patient may respond to sudden loud or unpleasant sounds and makes no effort to read lips. Hysterical blindness is usually associated with tubular vision.

Convulsions occur in the presence of others and are not accompanied by complete loss of consciousness, biting of the tongue, and loss of sphincter control. The patient resists attempts to open his eyes and withdraws on putting pressure on the supraorbital notch. The movements are often similar to those occurring during coitus.

In contrast with the generalized difficulty in thinking in the patient with organic memory loss, the patient with hysterical amnesia is usually in excellent contact with the surroundings and has a selective loss of memory for stressful situations.

COMMON COMPLICATIONS

Organic disease may be complicated by an overlay of hysterical symptoms. The complaints are then often exaggerated and dramatized. With the relaxation brought about by hypnosis or intravenous sodium amobarbital (Amytal), the hysterical symptoms are usually dispelled. These procedures are of great diagnostic value in that with them psychogenic symptoms disappear or are greatly ameliorated, whereas symptoms due to malingering or organic disease are unchanged or intensified.

Hypnoanalysis and narcoanalysis are useful in revealing repressed emotions and conflicts and establishing a positive relationship between them and the symptoms. Failure to distinguish between seizures and hysterical fits may lead to the prolonged inappropriate use of anticonvulsive medications. Hysterical pain that is often vague but at times closely resembles organic lesions, especially abdominal pathology, may result in surgical intervention followed by recurrences of pain and further surgery and eventual "operation addiction." Prolongation of hysterical symptoms can be accompanied by irreversible organic changes as occurs in muscle paralysis with wasting and contractures or in severe anorexia with widespread deterioration of bodily tissues. In cases in which monetary compensation is pending or being given, the secondary gain is so powerful an influence that there seldom is symptomatic improvement.

TEST PROCEDURES

Personality tests such as the Minnesota Multiphasic Personality Inventory and indices such as the Cornell Medical Index have value in helping to make or confirm the diagnosis of hysterical neurosis. However, chief reliance should be placed on a careful medical work-up with an evaluation of (1) the onset, character, and exacerbation of the symptoms and their relationship to life situations and traumatic experiences and (2) the findings on physical examination.

PITFALLS IN DIAGNOSIS

Hysterical neurosis needs to be distinguished from central nervous system diseases, especially those such as multiple sclerosis in which the early symptoms may be transitory and not clearly defined. Other organic conditions that are difficult to diagnose, such as pancreatitis, cortical blindness, and the urinary retention of cauda equina compression, may be erroneously termed psychogenic. Hysterical neurosis is sometimes confused with hypochondriacal neurosis, in which the complaints center around presumed diseases of organs of the body and do not involve actual losses or distortions of function. In the conscious feigning of symptoms of malingering there is more overt evidence for secondary gain through monetary compensation in contrast with more frequent need in neurosis to gain attention, sympathy and changes in the

conduct of others, or, as in war time, escape from danger.

Although in pure hysterical neurosis the symptoms are completely instigated by unconscious mechanisms, frequently there is conscious exaggeration. Hysterical symptoms may be the first signs of a schizophrenic illness and for a time appear to ward off the development of a full-blown psychosis. They also may occur in patients with recognized schizophrenia. The autism of schizophrenia is often mistaken for hysterical dissociation. Hysterical hallucinations are usually visual and represent realistic scenes, whereas schizophrenic hallucinations are most often auditory and are vague and bizarre.

SCHIZOPHRENIA

By ROBERT G. HEATH, M.D.
New Orleans, Louisiana

Schizophrenia is the name Eugen Bleuler applied in 1911 to a specific diagnostic entity that Emil Kraepelin had first described and categorized in 1899 under the heading dementia praecox. Known to mankind for many centuries, schizophrenia has essentially the same incidence in all countries and among all cultures, an estimated 4 to 5 million new cases of schizophrenia appearing in the world each year. Whereas its incidence in the United States is generally accepted to be about 0.3 per cent, some estimates are three times that, based on the assumption that for every hospitalized schizophrenic patient, there are three living in the community who do not require hospitalization. About 60 per cent of all psychiatric hospital beds in the United States are used by patients being treated for this devastating disease.

DEFINITION

In the Diagnostic and Statistical Manual (DSM-II) on Mental Disorders of the American Psychiatric Association, schizophrenia is described as "a group of disorders manifested by characteristic disturbances in mood and behavior." Schizophrenia, fundamentally a disease affecting the nervous system, is manifested principally by behavioral aberrations.

SIGNS AND SYMPTOMS

The symptoms of schizophrenia can be classified as primary and secondary. Principal symptoms are usually present before and between episodes of secondary symptoms. Secondary symptoms are blatant and, in most cases, intermittent. Earliest symptoms are changes in feelings and self-awareness. A consistent feature is an impaired ability to integrate pleasurable feelings. Beyond this, symptoms vary widely in type and intensity. Schizophrenia is the commonest cause of psychotic signs and symptoms, and many authorities agree on a diagnosis of schizophrenia only when psychotic symptoms are apparent.

Primary Symptoms. Among the most common signs and symptoms are thought deprivation (disappearance of thoughts, with consequent blocking of speech and illogical statements or defects in association); autism, that is, a tendency to daydream excessively; disturbances in affect or feelings that make it difficult for others to empathize with the patient; and absence of pleasurable feelings often associated with a preponderance of adversive emotional feelings, such as anxiety and rage. This emotional state and consequent behavioral defenses, often resulting in a clinical picture resembling the neuroses, has led to introduction of the term pseudoneurotic schizophrenia to categorize the incipient symptoms. The more severe manifestations are those of psychosis, and the classic symptoms of schizophrenia are those seen when the patient is fully psychotic.

Secondary Symptoms. Principal features of psychotic behavior are disturbances in thinking and changes in sensory perception. Disturbances in thinking are manifested by changes in concept formation, which may lead to misinterpretation of reality and, in more severe form, to delusions (false ideas). Sensory perceptive disturbances (hallucinations) usually occur in the auditory sphere, the most common involving imaginary voices. Disturbances in body image (proprioception) are also common. Less frequent are visual hallucinations and somatosensory disturbances, such as bizarre pains and paresthesias. Usually, there is also reduced psychologic awareness, the patient appearing dazed or in a dreamlike state. Most profound is the stuporous state of the catatonic patient. Motor retardation is also a characteristic, most pronounced in the stuporous patient.

SUBCATEGORIES OF SCHIZOPHRENIA

Conventionally, schizophrenic patients are subclassified according to the signs and symptoms that are predominant when they are psychotic. Textbook subcategories are:

Simple. Characteristics are social withdrawal, disordered thinking, and flat affect.

Hebephrenic. Behavior is grossly inappropriate, usually "silly," and mood is extremely labile.

Catatonic. Two labels are used: (1) retarded, indicating immobility and mute waxy flexibility; and (2) excited, indicating a constant state of extreme agitation.

Paranoiac. Characteristics are ideas of reference, overt delusions of persecution, and auditory accusatory hallucinations evolving into delusions of grandeur.

Schizoaffective. Primarily a schizophrenic thought disorder (differentiated from manic depressive), but with a strong affective component, usually depression.

COURSE

In schizophrenic patients with psychotic signs and symptoms, the spontaneous course is characteristically one of remission and relapse, but there is considerable variability. About 30 per cent have remittance and remain healthy after the first break and one or a few subsequent psychotic episodes. Another 30 to 40 per cent have spontaneous remissions and relapses, the relapses recurring more frequently and the remissions becoming briefer. Another 30 per cent of patients with schizophrenia tend to remain ill, some with fluctuating signs and symptoms and others never having a clear remission.

With the advent of electroconvulsive therapy, the number of patients whose signs and symptoms remitted increased notably. Over a 5 year follow-up period, however, the percentage of remissions was not significantly greater than those occurring spontaneously. In contrast, the introduction of neuroleptic medications has strikingly altered the characteristic course of schizophrenia; the percentage of patients who remain chronically hospitalized has been reduced more than 50 per cent. But those patients with the poorest prognosis for spontaneous remission, the "hard-core" 30 per cent, have failed to benefit sufficiently from medications to allow their re-entry into society, and they continue to require chronic hospitalization.

Significant change in the course of the disease has occurred in patients who had frequent remissions and relapses. Whereas long-term hospitalization is usually unnecessary, the ability of these patients to function on drugs varies. The majority retain some degree of emotional blunting and thought disturbance, of imprecision in sensory perception, and of inefficient performance in interpersonal relationships, as well as a continued deficit in ability to integrate pleasurable feelings and obtain maximal gratification in life.

PHYSICAL EXAMINATION FINDINGS

The general physical examination and the neurologic examination are essentially negative in the schizophrenic. A careful general physical examination is nevertheless important because many endocrinologic conditions can induce a syndrome of psychosis that quite closely simulates the schizophrenic psychosis. A careful neurologic examination is similarly important because certain subtle neurologic findings can often reveal a structural brain lesion as the cause of symptoms.

DIAGNOSTIC TEST PROCEDURES

No current physiologic or biochemical laboratory procedures are specific for the diagnosis of schizophrenia. Laboratory tests are, however, important in ruling out other causes for psychosis, since psychoses of other origins can produce essentially the same clinical picture as schizophrenia. The following laboratory tests are an integral part of establishing diagnosis.

Electroencephalogram. The electroencephalogram of the schizophrenic patient is usually normal. Certain forms of epilepsy with a pattern similar to schizophrenia are associated with electroencephalographic changes, usually over the temporal lobe.

Brainstem (Auditory) Evoked Responses. Evoked responses of the schizophrenic patient are usually normal; they are abnormal in many drug-induced psychoses and in some forms of epilepsy.

Body Fluid Toxicologic Studies. While yielding normal results in schizophrenic patients, thin-layer chromatography is helpful in ruling out drug-induced psychosis, and gas chromatography–mass spectrophotometry is required to rule out the possibility of psychosis induced by phencyclidine (angel dust), which often mimics schizophrenic psychosis.

Computerized Tomography (CT Scan). This practical, noninvasive diagnostic procedure is of great value in ruling out structural disorders that can resemble schizophrenic psychosis. Recent studies suggest that a significantly high percentage of patients diagnosed and treated as schizophrenics have demonstrable structural lesions as revealed by the CT scan. A site frequently involved is the vermis of the cerebellum.

Psychologic Testing. Some psychologic tests are of value in establishing diagnosis. In particular, projective tests such as the Rorschach and the thematic apperception test (TAT) complement the clinical interview. These tests, however, like the clinical mental status examination, often do not elucidate the underlying cause.

ETIOLOGY AND PATHOGENESIS

The etiology of schizophrenia is not known, but there is some evidence to suggest a genetic transmission.

In contrast to the paucity of specific clinical diagnostic tests, research laboratory findings provide some understanding of the pathogenesis of schizophrenia. Laboratory data and therapeutic research studies in human subjects, with use of deep and surface brain electrodes, have shown a consistent correlation between abnormal recording activity through specific subcortical circuits and psychotic behavior. The psychotic syndrome is present, regardless of its cause, when the characteristic dysrhythmia appears. The aberrant brain activity has been demonstrated in association with a wide variety of disorders of the brain, including tumor, infection, nutritional deficiency, toxic state (endogenous and exogenous), and trauma. It is also present in the psychotic schizophrenic patient. In schizophrenia, there are no structural changes in the brain, and no other causative factor has been proved. A logical assumption, currently under active investigation, is that the brain dysrhythmia in schizophrenia, in the absence of structural change or demonstrable toxin, is caused by a quantitative or qualitative aberration in the chemical transmitter at the intact synapse. Because the neuroleptic drugs that are most effective in reducing psychotic symptoms are known to block dopamine receptors, it is currently speculated that dopamine excess at certain brain sites is responsible for the dysrhythmia and consequent psychotic signs and symptoms.

PITFALLS IN DIAGNOSIS

Psychosis is a syndrome — not a disease. Schizophrenia is only one of many causes of this symptom complex. Establishing the correct diagnosis is critical if proper treatment is to be instituted.

It is less difficult to establish diagnosis when overt psychotic symptoms are present, in contrast with earlier stages of schizophrenia when only basic or primary signs and symptoms, often mimicking neurotic behavioral disturbances, are present. One should suspect the possibility of incipient or "schizotypal" behavior when the patient's neurotic symptoms border on the bizarre, when an empathic relationship is difficult, when an inability to integrate pleasurable feelings is foremost, and especially when progressive psychologic deterioration frustrates therapeutic efforts. In such patients, additional psychiatric consultation and projective psychologic testing is of value in establishing a definite diagnosis of incipient schizophrenia (schizotypal behavior).

DEPRESSION

By WILLIAM P. WILSON, M.D.
Durham, North Carolina

The literature of the 1920s and the late 1960s is replete with articles that attempt to clarify the nature of "depression." Still there exists considerable confusion as to its mechanisms and possible causes. Contributing to the confusion that has so long existed was the development of the concept of manic depression by Kraepelin, which tended to suggest that only two emotions would be exaggerated in the disease, i.e., joy (mania) and sorrow (depression). He noted that there were two dimensions to the disease of manic depression: intensity and duration. It was therefore necessary, when the concept of neurosis was being developed more fully, that some attention be given to the factors that differentiate neurotic depression from manic-depressive illnesses of the depressed type. The writings of the English school in the 1920s again focused on the dimensions of intensity and duration but also included as a differentiating factor the way the illness began. Finally, it has long been recognized that most persons with exaggerated emotional states have developed their symptoms as a result of a stress from either external or internal sources. Thus when we have considered depression nosologically, we have tried to do so from the standpoints of whether it was precipitated (endogenous vs. exogenous), its degree of severity (psychotic vs. neurotic) and its duration (stress reaction, grief reaction, or catastrophic reactions vs. neurosis or psychosis). Unfortunately these factors vary in each illness, and it is only by carefully assessing the natural history of the disease that an accurate diagnosis can be reached.

NAME AND DEFINITION

Depression is a variety of illnesses that occur with a primary disturbance manifested by an exaggerated emotion of sorrow in which the sorrow or depression is more or less continuously felt. Most often one may find that other emotions are also exaggerated periodically throughout the illness; thus one may see fear (anxiety), shame, confusion, disgust, emptiness, or even anger (irritability) occurring with increased intensity for brief periods. Nevertheless the pervasive disturbance of depression will predominate. Associated with this will be alterations in thinking characterized commonly by feelings of unworthiness, hopelessness, inferiority, sinfulness or guilt, obsessional thinking, and phobias. Biologic changes involving sexual function, appetite, sleep, and psychomotor activity commonly occur. *Thus we can define depression as several disease states of different causes manifested by a pervasive depressed mood associated with ideational distortions compatible with the altered mood, and with alterations in basic biologic functions.*

SYNONYMS

Depressive neurosis; psychotic depressive reaction; manic-depressive illness, depressed type; manic-depressive illness, circular type, depressed; schizophrenia, schizoaffective type, depressed; transient situational disturbance; adjustment reaction of adult life.

These terms may also refer to depression: unipolar manic-depressive illness, depressed type; bipolar manic-depressive illness, depressed type; catastrophic reaction; endogenous depression; and reactive depression.

PRESENTING SIGNS AND SYMPTOMS

The depressed patient usually comes to the attention of his family, friends, or pastor, priest, or rabbi because of a lack of interest in previously enjoyed pursuits or increased inability to function adequately. He may contact his family physician because of the changes that have occurred in his biologic functions. Indigestion, weight loss, insomnia, or fatigue results in physical examination and not infrequently — when there is little ideational distortion — in the diagnosis of hypoglycemia, hypothyroidism, anemia, "ulcers," or hiatal hernia when minor changes in accessory clinical findings suggest these diagnoses. Vague aches and pains in the head, chest, abdomen, pelvis, and anal area often will lead to an extensive medical examination. It must be noted that depressive pains are generally periaxial and not clearly localized anatomically, or vary significantly from the expected pain of organic disease. Only if the precipitating event was physical trauma, either accidental or iatrogenic (usually surgical intervention), or was related to some physical disease, will the pain closely resemble that which was present at the time of the trauma or disease. In these patients it is necessary for one to look beyond the physical symptomatology into the psychologic areas of function.

When carefully interrogated, the depressed patient will admit to his depression. The terminology he uses to describe his symptoms will be socioculturally influenced. Thus if asked if he is depressed he may say "no," but he may admit to being low, melancholy, blue, sad, downhearted, empty, or hopeless. Many times he blames these feelings on his physical symptoms, especially if he has pain. He will then describe his feelings of hopelessness, and the worries that he has about money, family, his physical well-being, his religious life, his adequacy as a person, and especially how he "suffers." He will sometimes describe, if asked, diurnal variation in mood, usually feeling worse in the morning than the evening, although the change may be the opposite or variable.

Sleep, appetite, and sexual functions will usually be altered to some degree. These will most often be decreased. The hours of sleep will be shortened because of difficulties in going to sleep or remaining asleep, or because of early awakening. Appetite can be decreased, sometimes associated with early morning nausea and degrees of weight loss. Sexual desire and ability may both be decreased, or there may be a decrease in one of these only. Thus some patients will describe a decrease in desire but no loss of function or vice versa. It must be made clear that a few patients will have no change or an increase in these biologic functions rather than a decrease. Thus one may see hypersomnia, bulimia, or increased sex desire and function.

Psychomotor activity is almost always altered. Motor activity may be decreased or increased. Decreases are manifested by slowed movements or at times by almost complete cessation of motor activity, as can be seen in depressive stupors. On the other hand, excessive increases result in marked restlessness or in the extreme restlessness called agitation. Sighing, respirations, wringing of the hands, or picking at the fingernails, hands, or face may be manifestations of moderate to severe agitation. Mild changes in motor activity are less obvious, although mild decreases or increases in activity

may be apparent to relatives or friends and will result in complaints of lack of energy or easy fatigability. Changes in psychic activity will be expressed as difficulties in concentration, subjective memory problems, slowed thinking, and an inability to respond affectively to environmental stimuli. The patient's attention is difficult to obtain and hold. He can often easily be irritated and may cry for no reason, especially when efforts are made to stimulate him out of his unhappiness.

Observation of the patient will often reveal a depressed facies; he will become tearful on occasion when talking about his family, feelings of guilt, or the hopelessness of his imagined physical or mental state. There may be delay in answering questions, and his attention will sometimes wander; he may sigh on occasion or become anxious and will have an increased pulse rate and diaphoresis. The patient will often take several seconds to respond to questions and will walk slowly. All movements can be slowed. If one monitors his nocturnal activity, he will be found to have shortened hours of sleep. Inspection of meal trays reveals much uneaten food. In mild depression there may be little to observe; in such a situation, all one has for diagnosis is the subjective reports of the patient.

COURSE

Almost all depression that arises as a response to insoluble real-life conflict or as a response to catastrophic loss will be initially acute, with varying degrees of severity of symptomatology. The symptoms usually ameliorate over a 1 to 12 week period if the conflict is resolved, and except for the stress of readjustment the patient will show little residual change.

Neuroses usually begin early in life and tend to be chronic. In these illnesses the patient is usually responding to an increase in extrapsychic or intrapsychic stress that may be mild but which, because of his conflicts, becomes the source of manifest symptoms. Because of the chronicity and tendency for symptoms to decrease in severity or to be relieved when stress decreases or is no longer present, one must carefully correlate the relationship of stress to the occurrence or remission of symptoms. Usually one can find adequate stress and trauma in early life to explain the patient's over-responsiveness to mild to moderately severe "normal" conflicts. These illnesses tend to be chronic and recurrent with exacerbations and remissions.

Manic-depressive disorders usually begin with an acute stress. These stresses most often are the loss of a loved one, the birth of a child, occupational problems, illness, trauma, or social adjustment problems. The patient will have symptoms temporarily related to the event, with the symptoms appearing within 6 weeks of the stress if it is acute, after longer periods, or even when there is relief of the stress if it is a chronic stress. The illness may last from 6 months to 3 years (mean, 18 months) if untreated and will spontaneously remit. Manic depression of the depressed type may begin with a short episode of mania (elation) and/or end with such an episode. Patients with previous attacks and intervening periods of good life adjustment are diagnosed manic-depressive. These are commonly referred to as unipolar illnesses. When attacks of both depression and elation occur, they are called bipolar. A strong family history of similar illnesses can often be obtained in these cases.

PHYSICAL EXAMINATION FINDINGS

Careful physical examination of patients with depression will occasionally elicit evidences of conversion phenomenon. Pain on movement, tenderness, tactile sensory defects, and disturbances of motor function such as weakness, posture, or gait are the most common. It must be noted that in contrast to the *belle indifférence* of hysterical conversion neurosis the hysterical symptoms of depression are accompanied by suffering, although not always directed toward the symptoms. Evidence of weight loss will be present when the suffering has been profound. Patients with concomitant anxiety may have tachycardia and diaphoresis of the palms and axillae.

The remainder of the findings will be those of depression. As stated previously, there are postural changes, agitation, or restlessness. The voice is hollow, and the patient's speech, which conveys so much of his feelings, has a cadence and inflection pattern that dramatize his feelings of depression. The content of his complaints will often be constricted and relate to his somatic complaints or preoccupations with his past and future life. Patients with milder disease will be preoccupied with career, marriage, family and physical health. Patients who are grieving will be preoccupied with their loss.

It must be pointed out that careful attention must be given in the physical examination to the presence of signs of hypothyroidism, pernicious anemia, adrenal dysfunction, and frontal lobe brain disease, as all of these problems may be accompanied by significant secondary depression.

COMMON COMPLICATIONS

Suicide is by far the most common complication of depression. Depression does not account for all suicides but it does account for a lion's share. The suicide rate in the United States is 11.1 per 100,000, and approximately 40 per cent of the suicides are persons with depression.

Alcoholism and drug abuse can complicate the illness. It is common for the patient with depression to seek some chemical relief of his symptoms. As both alcohol and sedative drugs tend to relieve the suffering, the patient will increase his intake of these substances. Patients who are abstinent prior to the illness rarely seek chemical relief.

Fecal impaction may occur in patients with profound retardation, especially the older patient. Anemia and inanition can occur if there is a prolonged decrease in food intake, and in some patients a sudden shift to mania can occur.

Finally, the illness can produce occupational, marital, family, and economic crisis. Many times patients will resign positions or sell a business that they believe to be responsible for their illness only to find on recovery that this had been an unwise decision. Less often they will leave or desert their families, but they may do so if they believe that these relationships have contributed to their unhappiness.

LABORATORY FINDINGS

In uncomplicated illnesses no changes are observed in the results of the standard laboratory tests. The desirability of obtaining these tests must be emphasized. A complete hematologic and blood chemical battery should be performed, as well as tests for thyroid function, when patients have a history of gradual onset of symptoms with no apparent precipitating stress. An electroencephalogram and/or brain or computerized tomography (CT) scan should be done if there is any suspicion that a brain tumor might be the cause of the patient's illness.

Psychologic testing may be of considerable help when the patient is using denial as a mechanism for dealing with his illness. Brief self-administered tests such as the Zung Self-Rating Depression Scale can be administered with ease and provide a quantitative aspect to the examination. The MMPI, Rorschach, and Thematic Apperception Test all may be used but require administration by a person trained in psychologic test administration and interpretation.

PITFALLS IN DIAGNOSIS

No disease process is as commonly misdiagnosed or ignored as is depression. Because all persons suffer periodically from depressed moods, there is a natural tendency for the harried, often depressed physician to ask himself: So what? everyone gets depressed! There is also the chronic problem of treating the symptoms and not looking for the cause.

Because some physicians feel inadequate in dealing with psychiatric disease, they are likely to ignore the more subtle symptoms of depression and instead prescribe iron and vitamins, a high protein diet, or thyroid hormone instead of evaluating the problem psychiatrically. It is tragic, too, that some physicians do not take the time to explore adequately the possibilities for organic disease in patients with what seem to be purely psychiatric complaints; thus many depressed patients "muddle" along for months or years with no relief when referral for counseling or appropriate medical treatment for their psychiatric illness could have brought about a rapid amelioration of symptoms.

It is necessary therefore that patients with vague ill-defined pains, with fatigue, or with alterations in sleep, sexual function, and appetite be considered potential cases of depression and that some inquiry be made concerning their mood. As the most common depressive illnesses are the result of problems of living, of neurosis, and of manic-depressive disorders, and as all these have as symptoms a pervasive disturbance of mood, ideational changes, and biologic change, it behooves the diagnostician to learn how to elicit these symptoms and to correlate his findings with his negative physical findings and arrive at an appropriate diagnosis.

Depression is archetypal suffering. No emotional pain is more agonizing than depression. It is important then that we learn to diagnose these diseases in order that appropriate treatment can be instituted to relieve the suffering.

Section 14

DISORDERS OF THE LOCOMOTOR SYSTEM

BURSITIS AND TENDINITIS

By DAVID H. NEUSTADT, M.D.
Louisville, Kentucky

The designations bursitis and tendinitis are frequently used loosely and imprecisely (by physicians and laity alike) to describe a variety of regional musculoskeletal conditions, characterized chiefly by pain and associated disability, often in the shoulder region. Many diverse conditions can masquerade under the guise of these wastebasket terms. In some instances, the "diagnosis" even offers a certain respectability to those incomprehensible and ill-defined soft tissue pain problems that often appear to be devoid of any organic basis. "The doctor said I have bursitis or tendinitis" is the satisfying refrain. However, for purposes of this discussion, in consideration of making an accurate diagnosis, the terms will be reserved for relatively well-defined or specific clinical entities.

DEFINITIONS AND ANATOMIC CONSIDERATIONS

Bursae are subcutaneous spaces or sacs, lined with modified synovial lining cells; they are provided by nature to facilitate the gliding motion of tendons and muscles, especially over bony prominences or across other tendons and muscles, between opposing surfaces. There are approximately 78 bursae in each side of the body. The normal bursal wall is as cellophane thin as the peritoneum, but when subacutely or chronically inflamed, the surface may become 1 to 2 mm thick. Direct trauma, infection, crystal deposition, or chronic friction may cause an inflammatory process of the bursa or bursal wall. Adventitial bursae may form at sites subjected to chronic irritation, such as the "bunion" over a hallux valgus. Involvement of the synovial tissue of tendon sheaths and bursae may also result from underlying disease such as ankylosing spondylitis, rheumatoid arthritis, and gout. The commonest bursal lesions in these systemic arthropathies involve the olecranon region, but smaller bursae, especially those at the Achilles tendon, may be involved. In addition, tendon sheaths at the hands, wrists, and ankles may be affected by chronic or acute infections such as tuberculosis or gonorrhea.

Tendinitis is a useful term employed to describe nonspecific low-grade inflammatory reaction in tendons and their sheaths (*tenosynovitis*). Calcareous (or calcific) tendinitis of the shoulder is involvement of one of the rotator (musculotendinous) cuff tendons, associated with a calcific deposit in and about the tendon (often the supraspinatus). The supraspinatus, infraspinatus, teres minor, and subscapularis muscles insert as the conjoined tendon into the greater tuberosity of the humerus.

The primary pathologic process is considered the calcific deposit within the substance of one or more of the rotator tendons. The process has been likened to a chemical furuncle ("calcium boil"). Release of the pressure from the fluid with rupture into the contiguous bursa (subacromial) gives prompt relief. Calcific tendinitis may be classified as hyperacute or acute, subacute, and chronic.

CLASSIFICATION

Bursitis and tendinitis embrace a variety of conditions that may be grouped together on a regional basis for the sake of simplicity and convenience (Table 1).

SITES OF INVOLVEMENT AND CLINICAL DISORDERS

Elbow. *Radiohumeral bursitis* occurs at the juncture of the radial head and lateral epicondyle of the elbow. It is most often found in combination with lateral humeral epicondylitis ("tennis elbow"). The symptoms are similar to epicondylitis with pain in the elbow, but tenderness is localized over the site of the radiohumeral groove. A clinical sign supporting the diagnosis of "tennis elbow" is the provocation

Table 1. *Classification of Bursitis and Tendinitis by Location*

Upper Extremity Disorders
Elbow
  Radiohumeral bursitis, tendinitis, olecranon bursitis
Shoulder
  Bicipital tenosynovitis, calcareous tendinitis (subacromial, subdeltoid bursitis), supraspinatus (rotator cuff) tendinitis
Wrist and Hand
  Stenosing tenosynovitis ("trigger finger")
  de Quervain's syndrome (tenovaginitis of thumb)

Lower Extremity Disorders
Hip bursae
  Ischiogluteal, trochanteric, iliopectineal
Knee bursae
  Supra-, infra-, and prepatellar, anserine
Heel bursae
  Achillocalcaneal, retrocalcaneal, and subcalcaneal

---

of pain when the patient attempts dorsiflexion (elevation) of the middle finger against resistance with the wrist and elbow held in extension (Maudsley's test). Pain produced on forced ulnar deviation at the wrist with the elbow in extension is an additional confirmatory test (Mill's sign).

Olecranon bursitis ("student's elbow" or "miner's elbow") is apparent when the elbow is inspected and palpated during flexion and extension. In rheumatoid arthritis and gout, nodules or tophi may be readily palpated within the bursa. Idiopathic or traumatic olecranon bursitis is most often painless unless there has been bleeding into the bursa or the swelling is extremely tense.

Fluid may be aspirated for synovioanalysis to help distinguish noninflammatory bursitis from an inflammatory disorder. The most commonly involved olecranon bursae lies between the skin and the olecranon process. Flexion and extension at the elbow joint remain full and painless unless there is associated elbow joint involvement.

Shoulder. Pain associated with restricted motion may result from any of the common intrinsic shoulder syndromes, including calcific tendinitis, bicipital tendinitis, and subdeltoid and subacromial bursitis. Numerous synonyms exist, such as calcific bursitis, calcareous tendinitis, and rotator cuff (supraspinatus) tendinitis or tenosynovitis.

Bicipital tendinitis (tenosynovitis) is a low-grade, nonspecific inflammation of the long head of the biceps tendon sheath. The tendon courses through the joint and along the so-called bicipital (intertubercular) groove. Pain develops at the shoulder region, accompanied by disturbed range of motion. Efforts to elevate the shoulder or reach the hip pocket, hook a bra, or pull a back zipper all cause an increase in pain. "Flipping" or rolling the bicipital tendon, especially with the patient's arm in external rotation, produces localized tenderness (Lipmann's test). Yergason's sign is a useful clinical test in which the patient is asked to supinate the forearm against resistance applied by the examiner, while holding the flexed elbow at a 90-degree angle against the side of the body. A positive test provokes or intensifies pain along the bicipital tendon or groove. In Ludington's test, pain is elicited in the involved biceps when the patient grasps both hands above his head. X-rays disclose no abnormality.

Calcific tendinitis, subacromial bursitis and *rotator cuff tendinitis without calcification* are so closely related that their symptoms and signs can be easily discussed together. It is especially difficult to dissociate supraspinatus tendinitis from subacromial bursitis. The acute irritative inflammatory phenomenon of the bursa usually is a secondary reaction produced by the calcific tendinitis of the supraspinatus or one of the other rotator cuff tendons. After the offending calcific material escapes into the subdeltoid bursa, it is absorbed and spontaneous clinical recovery usually ensues within a few days or weeks. Tenderness, which may be diffusely perihumeral or localized to the greater tuberosity, just distal to the tip of the acromion, varies with the stage of the disorder. During the hyperacute or acute stage, the anguished patient characteristically holds the affected arm against the chest wall. The pain may be incapacitating and the tenderness excruciating. All ranges of motion are restricted, with internal rotation the first to go and the last to return. When calcium is visualized on x-ray, the shadow has a "hazy" appearance with "lightening" at the margins due to a ring of inflammatory edema. Night pain may be intolerable.

In the subacute or chronic stages the loss of motion is frequently associated with a "painful arc." This is demonstrated by passively abducting the arm; pain is evoked as the arm passes the horizontal line but is absent before and after that point is reached. When "positive," this sign indicates a "pinching" mechanism of the involved tissue between the greater tuberosity and the acromion process.

Acute or hyperacute (calcific) tendinitis is most often a self-limiting disease. Tendinitis involving the infraspinatus, teres minor, or subscapularis may cause pain at the posterior region of the shoulder. Constitutional symptoms are rare, but occasionally in the hyperacute form, swelling may be visible and there may be slight fever and an accelerated sedimentation rate. When complete resolution does not occur, progression to the subacute and chronic stages may develop.

Wrist and Digits. *De Quervain's disease* is a tenosynovitis of the long abductor and short extensor tendons of the thumb. The disorder occurs more commonly in women, often following repetitive activities of the involved hand, especially a wringing motion. In the past the syndrome was called "washerwoman's sprain." The patient complains of pain in the wrist and tenderness is elicited just distal to the ulnar radial styloid. A useful clinical sign is Finklestein's test. The thumb is adducted into the palm of the hand, clenched by the flexed fingers and then forcible ulnar deviation at the wrist is carried out, provoking severe pain at the site of the involved tendon sheaths.

Stenosing tenosynovitis of digital flexor tendons ("trigger" or "snapping" finger). The tendon usually catches at a point in the tendon sheath on the flexor surface of the finger over the base of the metacarpal head. Characteristically, tenderness is confined to this site. In rheumatoid arthritis, if the synovitis is abundant, a springy crepitus is palpable in the line of the flexor tendon sheath (tendovaginitis crepitans). Locking usually occurs when the offending finger is in flexion, and is especially bothersome when the patient rises in the morning.

The Hip Region. *Trochanteric bursitis* may simulate hip joint disease and sciatica. The bursa is between the gluteus maximus muscle and the posterolateral surface of the greater trochanter. Pain is usually near the greater trochanter and radiates down the lateral or posterolateral aspect of the thigh. Pain may begin after lying on the side of the hip and can be provoked by stepping from curbs or descending steps. A so-called gluteal limp may be present. Tenderness is in the trochanter region. Lying on the opposite (uninvolved) side and abducting the affected limb usually intensifies the symptoms. Although abduction and internal rotation may be uncomfortable, usually a complete passive range of motion is present, in contrast with the situation in which there is true hip involvement. X-ray may demonstrate a calcific deposit adjacent to the trochanter.

Ischiogluteal bursitis ("weaver's bottom") is characterized by pain over the center of the buttocks. The bursa is adjacent to the ischial tuberosity, overlying the sciatic nerve and the posterior femoral cutaneous nerve. Pain has been thought to be produced by sitting on hard benches. Frequently, night pain disturbs sleep. Tenderness is elicited with pressure over the ischial tuberosity when the patient is examined in a prone position.

Iliopectineal bursitis (psoas) is a rarely described condition with relatively vague and poorly localized symptoms. The bursa is considered the largest synovial bursa in the body, situated between the deep surface of the iliopsoas muscle and the anterior surface of the hip joint. The clinical picture includes hip or groin pain with difficulty in walking due to the painful extremity. The extremity is held in flexion and moderate external rotation. Point tenderness may be present just inferior to Poupart's ligament.

Knee. Although there are numerous bursae in the region of the knee, only certain of these require consideration in the differential diagnosis of knee pain.

Prepatellar bursitis ("housemaid's knee"), manifested by swelling and effusion of the superficial bursa overlying the patella, is usually an obvious abnormality. Direct trauma as from a fall rarely may cause an acute bursitis, but the chronic bursal reaction usually occurs from repetitive activity or pressure, such as kneeling on a firm surface ("nun's knee"). Pain is usually minimal except during extreme knee flexion or by direct pressure. Passive flexion and extension are fully preserved.

Suprapatellar bursitis is associated usually with synovitis of the knee. Occasionally when the suprapatellar bursa or pouch is largely separated developmentally from the knee cavity with only a slight communication, effusion is especially prominent at the suprapatellar region.

Gastrocnemiosemimembranosus bursitis (posterior bursitis) when distended with fluid is termed a Baker's or popliteal cyst. In an adult a significant popliteal cyst is almost invariably rheumatoid in origin. The fullness in the popliteal space causes an inability to fully extend the knee, interfering with walking. If the cyst ruptures, the fluid may leak out and dissect into the calf, producing a clinical picture mimicking thrombophlebitis.

Deep infrapatellar bursitis is a rarely recognized problem. The bursa is well protected by the patella and underlying fat pad, and involvement usually results from repeated overuse with friction against the upper tibia. Clinical findings include tenderness confined to the area behind the infrapatellar tendon, and pain provoked in the same region at the extremes of forced flexion and extension of the knee.

Anserine bursitis ("cavalryman's disease") now mainly occurs in obese women with disproportionately heavy legs. The anserine bursa is located on the anteromedial surface of the tibia just below the joint line of the knee, at the insertion of the conjoined tendon of the sartorius, semitendinosus, and gracilis, and superficial to the medial collateral ligament. Clinical features include knee pain, palpable swelling, and tenderness over the site of the bursa. The lesion may simulate or coexist with osteoarthritis of the knee. An increase in knee discomfort or development of angular knee deformity in an obese woman with or without degenerative changes should suggest the possibility of this easily overlooked entity.

Ankle, Foot, and Heel. *Ankle tendinitis* is a relatively uncommon condition. The entity is differentiated from underlying ankle joint involvement by the lack of pain and restricted motion during passive flexion and extension of the ankle. However, actively flexing and extending the toes does provoke pain. Local tenderness is elicited along the flexor or extensor tendons. Crepitant and enlarged tendon sheaths at the ankles occurs not uncommonly in rheumatoid arthritis.

Painful heels may be caused by Achilles tendinitis, calcaneal bursitis, or plantar fasciitis. The bursae around the heel that are of potential clinical significance include the bursa between the skin and Achilles tendon, the retrocalcaneal bursa (between Achilles tendon and calcaneous), and the subcalcaneal bursa (between the skin and the calcaneous). The intimate relationship of the anatomy of the heel region may make precise differential diagnosis impossible. Achilles tendinitis or bursitis is associated with tenderness and swelling of the back of the heel. Subcutaneous involvement is frequently traumatic in origin, whereas inflammation of the deeper bursa, between the calcaneous and Achilles tendon, is more apt to represent a systemic disease such as rheumatoid arthritis. Calcaneal bursitis ("policeman's heel" or "soldier's heel") is frequently associated with a calcaneal bony spur. The spur may or may not be a factor in the production of symptoms. X-ray may demonstrate large asymptomatic spurs. Fluffy exuberant spurs associated with erosions may be found in Reiter's disorder or ankylosing spondylitis. Plantar fasciitis is manifested by pain and tenderness beneath the posteromedial border of the heel. X-rays may show a bony spur at the attachment of the plantar fascia to the calcaneous. Occasionally an adventitious bursa may form around the bony spur.

SEPTIC BURSITIS

Recently, attention has been called to an increased occurrence rate of septic bursitis. Predisposing factors include trauma or occupational-related pressure, steroid therapy, uremia, or diabetes mellitus. Superficial bursae, such as the olecranon and prepatellar, are the most commonly affected. The infected bursa is usually hot, red, and exquisitely tender. Aspiration with culture of a few drops of the fluid will suffice to establish an absolute diagnosis.

SEPTIC ARTHRITIS

By VICTOR G. BALBONI, M.D.

Boston, Massachusetts

SYNONYMS

Septic arthritis, acute infectious or bacterial arthritis, purulent arthritis, pyogenic arthritis, suppurative arthritis, pyoarthritis.

DEFINITION

Septic arthritis denotes an intra-articular infection with pyogenic organisms.

PATHOGENESIS

Pyogenic organisms reach the joint by the following routes: (1) via the bloodstream from focal infection elsewhere in the body, (2) by direct extension from a neighboring area of infection, (3) by penetrating wounds, and (4) by contaminated surgical procedures of the joint. In blood-borne infection the original focus frequently is never found.

PRESENTING SIGNS AND SYMPTOMS

Severe joint pain and limitation of motion of the painful joint are the usual presenting symptoms. Septic arthritis characteristically begins suddenly and progresses rapidly. The four cardinal signs of local infection are customarily present: pain, swelling, heat, and often redness of the skin overlying the joint, and fever. Chills often occur early in the course of septic arthritis during bloodstream dissemination of the infecting organism and when present are a most important diagnostic symptom, because they rarely, if ever, occur in other forms of arthritis. Occasionally a migratory phase may be seen in which there are mild pains in multiple joints for a few days before the bacteria settle in a joint (rarely more than two joints) and a true septic arthritis develops. *This early migratory phase is seen most often in meningococcal and in gonococcal arthritis.*

It must be remembered that in tuberculous and mycotic infections of joints the systemic symptoms may be minimal. The affected joint is painful and boggy to palpation (a cold abscess) but not hot as in the usual bacterial infection.

When a joint has been damaged by prior disease a superimposed infection may be less obvious; the physician may not easily appreciate that a new process has developed. Patients with rheumatoid arthritis and other forms of arthritis may develop infection in their joints. When this occurs, the infected joint may become lost among the other painful swollen joints. This is especially true when the patient has been receiving steroid hormones that may act to lessen the usual inflammatory and febrile responses. However, if the possibility of septic arthritis is always considered, careful questioning of the patient usually reveals that the infected joint has become more inflamed than it was previously. The expected signs of inflammation may also be muted in joints remote from the skin surface, such as in hip or spinal joints.

Radionuclide scanning can be helpful in localizing the process in joints not readily palpable from the skin surface.

CLINICAL COURSE

Septic arthritis is a curable disease if diagnosis is prompt and treatment adequate. However, it is always a serious illness. Its course depends on the virulence of the invading bacteria and the resistance of the host and may vary from a mild transient synovitis to a virulent infection that destroys the joint and leads to death from spreading sepsis. If the typical case were allowed to run its course untreated or inadequately treated, total or partial loss of motion of the affected joint could be expected.

PREDISPOSING FACTORS

Any local infection, however mild, may be the source from which a septic arthritis is seeded via the bloodstream. Those illnesses in which septicemia commonly occurs, such as pneumococcal pneumonia, meningococcal meningitis, bacterial endocarditis, and salmonella infections, are always likely to produce metastatic foci of infection. Streptococci, staphylococci and *Escherichia coli* are other common causes of septic arthritis. The aged, the very young, and those with chronic debilitating diseases are especially susceptible. This is true of patients with chronic rheumatoid arthritis; any such patient who shows a sudden deterioration of condition with increased pain and swelling of one joint, especially if chills and fever occur, should be suspected of having developed a septic arthritis, and this may be superimposed on a rheumatoid joint.

Infants under 1 year of age, and especially premature infants, have an increased incidence of septic arthritis. This may develop in any joint, but it is prone to occur in the hip joint, where its recognition may be difficult. Pain and swelling of the thigh often are found. Although this pain may be minimal, fever is almost invariably present. The hip is held in partial flexion and motion is restricted, especially extension and abduction.

All the steroid hormones decrease resistance to infection so that patients receiving them should be watched carefully for infection. The development in such patients of a swollen joint, even though only mildly painful, should raise the question of septic arthritis, for in patients receiving these hormones the usual local signs of infection may be minimal and the systemic effects mild or absent. Steroid hormones given intra-articularly reduce resistance to infection locally. If in the first 24 hours after an intra-articular injection of steroid the joint becomes more painful rather than less painful, the possibility that sepsis has been introduced into the joint by the arthrocentesis should be seriously considered.

DIAGNOSIS

The most important factor in diagnosis is an awareness of the possibility of septic arthritis in any acute arthritis or in any sudden change for the worse and/or development of fever in a chronic arthritic.

Arthritic disorders that have an acute onset may be mistakenly diagnosed as being septic arthritis. These include gout and pseudogout, rheumatic fever, rheumatoid arthritis, trauma, and particularly monoarticular rheumatoid arthritis in children. Constitutional symptoms such as fever, marked leukocytosis, and chills are uncommon in these conditions, and, if present, suggest a septic arthritis. In all such patients an examination of the joint fluid should be performed to substantiate the diagnosis of an infectious process or rule it out.

A complete history and physical examination is essential. Attention should be paid to possible portals of entry for infection, including the paranasal sinuses, the ears, the lungs, the skin, the urethra, and pelvic areas. Gonorrhea is a common, if not the most common, cause of septic arthritis.

In septic arthritis the initial laboratory studies usually reveal leukocytosis in the peripheral blood with a shift to immature leukocytes in the differential count. Absence of leukocytosis does not rule out septic arthritis, especially in aged or debilitated patients.

If the initial findings support a diagnosis of septic arthritis and especially if fever is present, the blood should be cultured in an effort to identify a bacterial organism. In many instances it is easier to grow and identify the offending organisms from the blood than from the joint itself, although the diagnosis is most probable when the organism is recovered from both the blood and joint fluid. Two blood cultures for both aerobic and anaerobic organisms should be done within several hours. Two blood cultures containing the same organism practically rules out contamination. Cultures should also be made of any exudate or secretions at a site of suspected portal of entry for infection.

X-ray Studies. Roentgenographic examination is of little aid in the diagnosis of acute septic arthritis because changes that can be seen by x-ray require 2 weeks or more to develop. The first abnormality to be seen in the x-rays is a general rarefaction of subchondral bone, unless, of course, the infection has spread from an adjacent area of osteomyelitis, which would be visible even earlier. The stage of subchondral bone atrophy is followed by the development of areas of erosion of the articular ends of the adjacent bone, and finally by narrowing of the joint space owing to destruction of articular cartilage.

Even during the first 2 weeks when conventional x-rays and even tomograms do not reveal bone or joint abnormalities, with radionuclide imaging after injection of a polyphosphonate compound tagged with radioactive technetium definite lesions can be identified and their extent delineated clearly. Since many other types of injury to the joint or bone may produce similar findings, the method lacks specificity. Its application lies in revealing the presence of an abnormality, particularly in deepseated joints of the spine, sacroiliac, hip, and shoulder joints. Radionuclide imaging may have its greatest usefulness for the early detection of bone and joint sepsis in children in whom history and physical findings may be minimal.

Joint Fluid Examination. A diagnosis of septic arthritis is confirmed by a study of the joint fluid of the affected joint and the culture of bacteria from it. The joint tap, or arthrocentesis, is the most important diagnostic procedure. Strict asepsis is essential in the arthrocentesis. The overlying skin is thoroughly washed with an antibacterial soapless skin cleaner (pHisoHex), scrubbed with iodine, and then washed with 70 per cent isopropyl alcohol. While equipment for the aspiration is being readied for use, a moist alcohol sponge should be kept on the skin at the site of the proposed aspiration. Purulent fluid may be difficult to aspirate through a small-bore needle, so if possible use of an 18-gauge needle is advised, although in smaller joints a needle of 20 or 21 gauge may be as large as one can use. Equipment available at the bedside should include several sterile tubes for culture and clot examination as well as tubes for sugar determination and cell counts. (The latter should contain either heparin or ethylenediamine tetraacetic acid (EDTA) to prevent clot formation.) A small amount of fluid is aspirated and promptly inoculated into the sterile tube for culture and Gram stain and then into the heparin or EDTA tube for cell count. This must be promptly shaken to ensure mixing of the aspirate with heparin. Additional fluid, if obtained, is put in tubes for sugar and for clot determination. Whenever possible, the joint aspiration should be done after the patient has fasted at least 4 hours to allow equilibration of glucose between blood and joint fluid.

The importance of aspirating a joint and studying the synovial fluid when septic arthritis is suspected cannot be too strongly emphasized. Simultaneously a blood sugar should be drawn for comparison with the joint fluid sugar. Minimal studies of the joint fluid should include a Gram stain, aerobic and anaerobic cultures, total and differential leukocyte counts, and a fasting joint fluid and blood sugar. If the Gram stain is negative, a Ziehl-Neelsen stain for tuberculosis and a Wright stain for mycoses should be made.

In septic arthritis the joint fluid always shows a leukocytosis and 90 per cent or more of the cells are polymorphonuclear leukocytes. Initial cell counts on septic joint fluid may vary from 25,000 to 250,000 or more per cu mm, and average in the vicinity of 100,000. This cell count makes the fluid turbid. The sugar content of the joint fluid is reduced in nearly all instances in septic arthritis. For a joint fluid sugar test to be reliable it is important that the joint tap be done after the patient has fasted for 4 or more hours. In a healthy patient in a fasting state, the joint fluid sugar approximates that found in the serum. In septic arthritis the joint

Table 1. *Synovial Fluid Findings in Acute Pyogenic Arthritis*

Joint Fluid Examination	Noninflammatory Fluids	Inflammatory Fluids Noninfectious	Infectious
Color	Colorless, pale yellow	Yellow	Yellow
Turbidity	Clear, slightly turbid	Turbid	Turbid, purulent
Viscosity	Not reduced	Reduced	Reduced
Mucin clot	Tight clot	Friable	Friable
Cell count (per mm³)	200–1,000	1,000–>10,000	10,000–>100,000
Cell type	Mononuclear	PMN°	PMN°
Synovial fluid/blood glucose ratio	0.8–1.0	0.5–0.8	<0.5
Gram stain for organisms	None	None	Positive†
Culture	Negative	Negative	Positive†

°PMN = polymorphonuclear leukocyte.

†In some cases, especially with the gonococcus, no organisms may be demonstrated.

From Arthritis and Allied Conditions, 9th edition, edited by Daniel J. McCarty. Chapter on Principles of Diagnosis and Treatment of Infectious Arthritis by Frank R. Schmid. Philadelphia, Lea and Febiger, 1979.

fluid sugar will usually vary from 25 to 115 mg below the blood sugar. *A difference of 40 mg or more between the synovial fluid and blood sugar is considered highly suggestive of bactterial invasion of the synovial fluid (septic arthritis).*

A negative joint fluid culture may be obtained when the bacteria have invaded the periarticular tissues but are not free in the synovial cavity. A more common cause for a negative culture is the prior administration of antibiotics or chemotherapeutic agents. Infecting bacteria may often be obtained by blood culture, and, in cases of meningitis, by culture of the spinal fluid. Although confirmation of the diagnosis may have to wait for reports of the joint fluid and blood cultures, a presumptive diagnosis should be made and treatment started on the basis of the history, the clinical findings, the cell count of the joint fluid, and the Gram stain of the joint fluid. If bacteria are found in the Gram stain of the joint fluid, the diagnosis of septic arthritis is correct. Morphologic study of the bacteria and their reaction to the Gram stain are most helpful in selecting the initial antibiotic therapy. If no organisms are isolated by Gram stain and culture and if the Ziehl-Neelsen stain for tuberculosis and Wright stain for fungi are negative, and still the joint fluid and clinical picture indicate a bacterial infection, counterimmunoelectrophoresis may aid in determining its bacterial cause.

JUVENILE RHEUMATOID ARTHRITIS

By BRAM BERNSTEIN, M.D.,
Los Angeles, California

and THOMAS J. A. LEHMAN, M.D.
San Diego, California

INTRODUCTION

Juvenile rheumatoid arthritis (JRA) is a major cause of chronic disability in childhood. It is currently estimated to affect 250,000 children in the United States. The clinical manifestations of JRA are varied and, in the absence of known cause, JRA may actually represent several different diseases. However, the common patho-logic picture of chronic inflammatory synovitis, and the occurrence of many common symptoms in all of the subtypes, make it useful to consider JRA as a single disease at the present time.

The diagnosis of definite JRA is based upon the presence of persisting arthritis in a child under 16 years of age for at least 6 weeks with exclusion of other diseases (Table 1). In recent years, three clinical onset patterns of JRA have been distinguished: *systemic*, *polyarticular*, and *pauciarticular*. These subtypes are based on the pattern of disease during the first 6 months of illness and vary in their relative frequency, sex ratio, and mean age of onset (Table 2). Their recognition permits more accurate diagnosis, clearer prediction of disease course, and more appropriate selection of therapeutic modalities.

SYSTEMIC JRA

The hallmark of systemic JRA is the occurrence of intermittent fever spikes to greater than 38.5 C (101.4 F). In a typical case, the patient will have a single fever spike in the late afternoon or early evening, with temperatures dropping to normal or subnormal at other times. Occasionally, patients will manifest a biphasic fever curve, but prolonged fever elevation is not characteristic of JRA. While febrile, children may appear toxic, but they frequently seem much better when the fever has resolved. Preliminary criteria from the American Rheumatism Association for systemic JRA require that these fevers be present for at least a 2-week period. The fevers characteristically occur at the onset of disease and may continue for long periods. Fever occurring for the first time later in the course of childhood arthritis should be thoroughly investigated.

Most children with systemic JRA develop a characteristic rash. The rash, which consists of small erythematous macules or maculopapules, is found predominantly on the trunk and proximal extremities, with accentuation in pressure areas. A striking aspect of the rash is its evanescence. Typically, the rash becomes prominent as the child's temperature rises and disappears as the fever subsides. Stroking or scratching the skin may be sufficient to provoke development of the rash (Koebner's phenomenon).

Lymphadenopathy may be prominent in systemic JRA. These children frequently have palpable nodes larger than 0.5 cm in diameter and involving not only the cervical and inguinal nodes but the axillary and epitrochlear nodes as well. The extreme size of the lymph nodes may suggest underlying malignancy. In JRA, however, the histology is nonspecific, with reactive hyperplasia and prominent germinal centers.

Table 1. *Differential Diagnosis of Arthritis in Childhood*[*]

1. Connective tissue diseases
   a. Rheumatoid arthritis
   b. Rheumatic fever
   c. Systemic lupus erythematosus
   d. Anaphylactoid purpura
   e. Systemic vasculitis
   f. Erythema nodosum
   g. Dermatomyositis
   h. Scleroderma
   i. Mixed connective tissue disease
   j. Ankylosing spondylitis
   k. Rheumatoid nodules sine arthritis
   l. Related conditions
      (1) Ulcerative colitis
      (2) Regional enteritis
      (3) Psoriasis
      (4) Sarcoid
      (5) Reiter's syndrome
      (6) Stevens-Johnson syndrome
      (7) Behçet's syndrome
      (8) Sjögren's syndrome
   m. Polyarteritis nodosa

2. Septic arthritis and virus related
   a. Septic
      (1) Staphylococcus
      (2) Other common pyogens
      (3) Gonococcus
      (4) Mycobacteria
   b. Virus related
      (1) Rubella
      (2) Hepatitis
      (3) Mumps
      (4) Other

3. Osteomyelitis

4. Neoplastic diseases
   a. Leukemia
   b. Lymphoma
   c. Neuroblastoma

5. Heritable disorders
   a. Sickle cell disease
   b. Marfan's syndrome
   c. Familial Mediterranean fever
   d. Hereditary multicentric osteolysis
   e. Mucopolysaccharidoses
   f. Mucolipidoses
   g. Fabry's disease
   h. Weill-Marchesani syndrome
   i. Farber's disease
   j. Epiphyseal dysplasia
   k. Ehlers-Danlos syndrome
   l. Homocystinuria
   m. Hemophilia
   n. Immune deficiency syndromes

6. Metabolic-endocrine
   a. Gout
   b. Pseudogout
   c. Hypothyroidism
   d. Hypoparathyroidism
   e. Progeria
   f. Other

7. Miscellaneous
   a. Transient synovitis
   b. Palindromic rheumatism
   c. Traumatic arthritis
   d. Popliteal cysts
   e. Villonodular synovitis
   f. Osteochondritis syndromes
   g. Hypertrophic osteoarthropathy
   h. Osteoid osteoma
   i. Tietze's syndrome
   j. Short bowel syndrome
   k. Periodic fever
   l. Histiocytoses
   m. Juvenile osteoporosis
   n. Reflex neurovascular dystrophy
   o. Psychogenic rheumatism
   p. Arthromyalgia

[*]From Hanson, V.: Introduction to the First ARA Conference on the Rheumatic Diseases of Childhood. Arthritis Rheum. *20*:156, 1977 (Suppl.).

Internal organ involvement is commonly present in systemic JRA. The most serious is cardiac involvement. Pericardial effusions may be detected in the majority of patients with active systemic disease if sought by echocardiography, but only a minority of patients have electrocardiographic changes or cardiomegaly. A small percentage of patients may develop a pericardial friction rub and chest pain, but the risk of pericardial tamponade or later constrictive pericarditis is small. Myocarditis is infrequent but does occur and should always be

Table 2. *The Subtypes of Juvenile Rheumatoid Arthritis*

	Systemic	Polyarticular	Pauciarticular
Number of joints	Variable	>4	≤4
Relative frequency	20%	40%	40%
Males:Females	1:1	4:1	4:1
Mean age of onset	6 years	10 years	4 years
Fever	100%	Low grade, variably present	Absent
Visceral involvement	Common	Occasional	Absent
Iridocyclitis	<5%	5–10%	30%
ANA	10%	40%	40%
RF	5%	60%	<5%

considered to be a potentially life-threatening complication. In contrast to the carditis of acute rheumatic fever, valvular disease is rarely if ever associated with JRA.

Pulmonary involvement in systemic JRA may consist of pleuritis, pneumonitis, or both. Pleural effusions and thickening may be apparent on chest roentgenograms, and an interstitial pneumonitis may appear. Although the pleuritis and pneumonitis may be associated with chest pain, cough, or dyspnea, some patients remain asymptomatic.

Enlargement of both the liver and the spleen is often present. Although the hepatic involvement is usually moderate, instances of massive hepatomegaly have been observed. Serum transaminase levels are generally normal but may be mildly elevated even in the absence of salicylate therapy. Liver biopsies reveal a mild mononuclear cell infiltrate in the portal areas without evidence of hepatocellular necrosis or scarring. Splenomegaly is typically not marked, but extremely large spleens are occasionally noted.

For a definite diagnosis of JRA to be made, involvement of joints must be present. Frank arthritis may or may not be present at the onset of symptoms and may not develop until weeks or months into the illness. Arthralgias, however, are frequently present early. The pattern of joint involvement is highly variable, but large joints are usually affected. Neck pain with limited extension and rotation due to involvement of the cervical spine is frequent. Hip joint involvement is common and may be a source of severe functional disability in the child with systemic JRA. X-ray changes, with the exception of soft tissue swelling and osteoporosis, are usually late findings. In the cervical spine, however, there may be early x-ray evidence of apophyseal joint narrowing or fusion.

POLYARTICULAR JRA

Polyarticular JRA is defined as arthritis in more than four joints persisting for at least 6 weeks. This subtype of JRA is the form most similar to adult-onset rheumatoid arthritis. Children with polyarticular disease may have low-grade fevers and mild constitutional symptoms, but internal organ involvement is rare. Polyarticular disease occurs most frequently in females around puberty and, like adult rheumatoid arthritis, may be associated with the presence of rheumatoid factor. Painless movable subcutaneous rheumatoid nodules may develop. They characteristically occur over "pressure points" such as the elbows, knuckles, heels, or toes and may be attached to the deep fascia. They are usually associated with a high titer of rheumatoid factor, but small nodules are seen in some seronegative children. Unlike systemic-onset disease, polyarticular disease tends to be indolent but slowly progressive, with infrequent remissions. Despite this, the majority of patients are able to maintain satisfactory joint function for many years.

The pattern of joint involvement is similar to that of adult-onset rheumatoid arthritis but is usually not as symmetrical. There is also a tendency for more large joint involvement in children. The distal interphalangeal joints, which are only rarely involved in adult rheumatoid disease, are frequently affected in children. As with systemic disease, there is frequently involvement of the cervical spine. Temporomandibular joint disease is a striking feature in many of these children, which may lead to marked undergrowth of the mandible and a characteristic facies. Hip involvement bears special emphasis because of its potential for causing severe functional disability. It may occur early in the course of disease and may vary in its pattern according to the age of the child. Subluxation and persistent coxa valga are seen in children with onset of disease at a younger age, whereas protrusio acetabulae is more likely to develop in patients whose hips become affected in the teenage years.

PAUCIARTICULAR JRA

A child is considered to have pauciarticular disease if there is involvement of four or fewer joints during the first 6 months of disease and systemic manifestations are absent. Initial monoarticular disease is common and must be differentiated from septic arthritis. Pauciarticular JRA is most commonly seen in young females. It is a relatively mild form of disease with a favorable prognosis in up to 70 per cent of patients. Since only a few joints are involved, it is unlikely to result in serious functional impairment. Large joints, particularly the knees, are frequently affected, and prolonged synovitis may result in bony overgrowth and a longer extremity on the affected side.

A potentially disabling complication of pauciarticular disease that develops in 25 to 30 per cent of patients is chronic iridocyclitis. The iridocyclitis of JRA is an insidious and chronic process that may develop in the total absence of ocular symptoms or signs observed by the parents or in the absence of abnormality detected by routine ophthalmoscopy. There may be no correlation between the activity of the joint disease and the ocular inflammation. Iridocyclitis has developed prior to the onset of the arthritis in some children and long after remission of arthritis in others. The risks of iridocyclitis include band keratopathy and the formation of anterior synechiae, which may lead to narrow-angle glaucoma and blindness. Ninety per cent of these patients are seropositive for antinuclear antibodies. Thus, all children with JRA should have an initial slit-lamp examination. Children with pauciarticular disease whose sera are positive for antinuclear antibodies should have routine slit-lamp examinations thereafter at 3-month intervals. Even more frequent slit-lamp examinations should be performed in those children who have had previous episodes of iridocyclitis.

Laboratory Findings

Although no single test is diagnostic of juvenile rheumatoid arthritis, there are characteristic constellations of laboratory findings associated with each of the clinical presentations. Recognition of the typical pattern of laboratory abnormalities for each onset subgroup will aid the clinician in establishing the diagnosis of JRA and excluding other causes of arthritis in childhood.

The most striking laboratory abnormalities are associated with systemic JRA. The clinical manifestations of these children are usually accompanied by marked leukocytosis, anemia, and an elevated sedimentation rate. The total white blood cell count often exceeds 20,000 per cu mm and may exceed 50,000 per cu mm. Many of these children are initially thought to have leukemia. Thrombocytosis is a helpful finding in this regard, as it commonly occurs in children with systemic JRA, while children with leukemia are most often thrombocytopenic. Absolute differentiation is not always possible, however, and if leukemia is suspected, a bone marrow aspiration should be performed. The child with systemic JRA typically has a hyperplastic marrow with increased cellular elements despite the anemia.

The combination of fever, anemia, and leukocytosis also suggests an infectious process, and appropriate cultures should be obtained. Leukopenia in a child with high spiking fevers who is not septic should prompt a careful search for underlying malignancy. Felty's syndrome is rare in childhood. If antinuclear antibodies are present in conjunction with leukopenia, systemic lupus erythematosus must be strongly suspected.

Children with systemic JRA often have a hypochromic microcytic anemia despite normal marrow iron stores. A defect in reticuloendothelial cell iron release has been hypothesized, but poor oral intake and occult blood loss from the gastrointestinal tract may also contribute to the anemia.

The elevated erythrocyte sedimentation rate is the result of increased production of acute phase reactants. Most such reactants have been measured in JRA and found to parallel the sedimentation rate without adding information of diagnostic significance. The newer "zeta sed rates" are elevated in JRA as they are in other diseases that elevate the Westergren sedimentation rate. In children with systemic JRA, hypergammaglobulinemia may be marked, with reversal of the normal albumin-globulin ratio. Mild elevations of the febrile agglutinins as a result of this hypergammaglobulinemia may lead to diagnostic confusion. Levels of antistreptococcal antibodies may also be mildly elevated as a result of the hypergammaglobulinemia and the frequency of streptococcal infections in childhood, but these levels are lower than those seen in acute rheumatic fever.

Children with pauciarticular disease have the lowest incidence of laboratory abnormalities. Although patients may have elevated sedimentation rates it is not uncommon for a patient with pauciarticular JRA to have a normal sedimentation rate. A markedly elevated sedimentation rate in a child with monoarticular arthritis, although compatible with rheumatoid disease, should prompt a thorough search for infection, including synovial fluid analysis.

A laboratory abnormality of great clinical importance in a child with pauciarticular JRA is the presence of antinuclear antibodies. This is because of the strong association between antinuclear antibodies and chronic iridocyclitis in children with JRA. The chronic iridocyclitis of JRA is seen almost exclusively in children whose sera contains antinuclear antibodies.

The laboratory abnormalities found in children with polyarticular JRA are similar to those found in adults with rheumatoid arthritis. Although "hidden rheumatoid factor" is being reported in JRA with increasing frequency, rheumatoid factor as detected by latex fixation and other conventional techniques is uncommon in young children with JRA. In older children it is more common, occurring in about 75 per cent of children with onset over age 12 years. Antinuclear antibodies may also be seen with polyarticular disease and should prompt careful follow-up for chronic iridocyclitis.

Diagnostic Pitfalls

Although JRA is the most common cause of noninfectious arthritis in childhood, more than 40 additional causes have been described in children (Table 1). Despite this multitude of possible causes, the correct diagnosis can usually be established after a careful history and physical examination, followed by judicious use of laboratory and radiographic procedures. The primary consideration in evaluating a child with joint symptoms must always be the exclusion of infection, malignancy, or orthopedic disease before the diagnosis of JRA is accepted. Failure to exclude one of these entities is the greatest pitfall in the evaluation of children with possible joint disease.

In evaluating a child with high spiking fevers, sepsis must always be excluded. Every child presenting with fever should have appropriate cultures and a tuberculin test. Although rare, both malaria and brucellosis are causes of arthralgias and relapsing fevers that will not be detected by routine blood cultures. They should be suspected if a history of travel to endemic areas is obtained. Another infectious cause of arthritis that is not detected by routine blood cultures is hepatitis. During the anicteric prodromal period the patient may have severe joint pain, stiffness, and swelling associated with fever. Although children with JRA may have elevated liver enzymes secondary to salicylate therapy, the enzymes are otherwise unlikely to be markedly elevated. Testing for hepatitis-associated antigens should clarify any confusion.

Most children with malignancy will have symptoms localized to one or few joints unless they have a superimposed infection. Children with acute leukemia, however, may present with high spiking fevers and diffuse, severe joint pain. Although the pain is generally due to leukemic infiltration, true arthritis may occur. Roentgenograms of the involved joints will frequently demonstrate metaphyseal lucent lines, *leukemic lines*, but if there is uncertainty, a bone marrow examination should be performed. Infrequently, we have seen patients with joint pains and a normal marrow examination initially that subsequently became abnormal.

Although systemic lupus erythematosus may begin with arthritis or arthralgias without malar rash or renal involvement, the diagnosis should be suspected in patients with high titers of antinuclear antibodies and leukopenia. Polyarteritis nodosa may be difficult to exclude, but the majority of children with polyarteritis will have urinary abnormalities and hypertension. Most of the other rheumatic diseases that occur in childhood can be eliminated on clinical grounds. The self-limiting nature of serum sickness and a history of an inciting agent make its exclusion easy.

Kawasaki's disease (mucocutaneous lymph node syndrome) may be mistaken for JRA. The combination of fever, dry cracked red lips, and conjunctivitis, followed by characteristic peeling of the skin of the digits, should suggest this diagnosis. These children are plagued by painful swelling of the hands and feet that may be accompanied by frank arthritis, but this is usually transient. Sarcoid may present with fevers, arthritis, or arthralgias, and erythema nodosum. It can be diagnosed by biopsy or measurement of the level of angiotensin-converting enzyme.

Gonococcal disease is currently epidemic in this country and is the most common cause of fever with arthritis in adolescent females. It may involve one or several joints. All females with fever and arthritis should be questioned carefully for a history of sexual contact and appropriate cervical cultures obtained if the history is suggestive. In the male, questioning should also include a sexual history, and evidence of urethral discharge should be sought. Reiter's syndrome must be considered if diarrhea or conjunctivitis is present.

The child with polyarticular arthritis has essentially the same differential diagnosis as the child with systemic symptoms. Although in the absence of fever sepsis is less likely, osteomyelitis, gonococcal infection, hepatitis, and malignancy all may present as polyarticular joint pains without fever. In the adolescent female with polyarticular disease and antinuclear antibodies, consideration must be given to the possibility of systemic lupus erythematosus, but in the absence of multisystem involvement this is unlikely. Appropriate testing for double-stranded DNA antibodies is helpful because these are rarely present in JRA.

Acute rheumatic fever without carditis is often considered in the evaluation of a child with JRA who has involvement of several joints and evidence of a recent streptococcal infection. However, rheumatic fever is increasingly rare in the United States. Although differentiation may not be possible at the time the child first is brought for medical help, the tendency of the arthritis to migrate and its short duration are both in sharp contrast to the persistence of the arthritis of JRA.

The disorder in a child with arthritis of one or few joints is the most difficult to diagnose with certainty. Infection of the joint space by gonococci, streptococci, staphylococci, hemophilus, or mycobacteria may occur without fever. Involvement of several joints does not exclude the possibility of osteomyelitis; both secondary infection and "sympathetic" arthritis may occur. A markedly elevated sedimentation rate is a useful indicator because this is uncommon in pauciarticular disease, but its absence does not exclude infection.

Orthopedic entities such as chondromalacia patellae, aseptic necrosis, or chondrolysis of the hip can usually be excluded by appropriate x-rays. In the absence of radiologic findings, the child with monoarticular arthritis may require a synovial biopsy in order to exclude with certainty diseases such as villonodular synovitis. An additional entity is plant thorn synovitis. Small children presenting with swelling and stiffness of a single knee may not recall falling on a plant thorn several weeks earlier. In such cases the diagnosis is possible only after appropriate histologic examination of the synovium. Relief requires synovectomy.

Few other rheumatic diseases that occur in childhood present with monoarticular symptomatology. Primary gout is extremely rare in childhood, and the mildly elevated uric acid levels seen in sick children should not be interpreted as indicating this diagnosis. Toxic synovitis is an important form of arthritis in childhood but may be distinguished by its predilection for the hip — a rare site of isolated symptomatology in JRA. In childhood, ankylosing spondylitis and other seronegative spondyloarthropathies may begin with peripheral arthritis, often predominating in the lower extremities. Therefore juvenile ankylosing spondylitis should be suspected in HLA B27 antigen–positive children with peripheral arthritis, even in the absence of sacroiliac and spine symptoms or x-ray changes. A positive family history for back symptoms is often present in such patients. Since HLA B27 antigen is present in 9 per cent of the Caucasian population, however, its presence or absence in an individual patient cannot absolutely be used to distinguish between JRA and juvenile ankylosing spondylitis.

RHEUMATOID ARTHRITIS

By RONALD ANDERSON, M.D.

Boston, Massachusetts

DEFINITION

Rheumatoid arthritis (RA) is a chronic inflammatory disease of unknown cause primarily involving the joints. Although it may occur in either sex or at any age, its predilection is for the middle years and it affects women two to three times more frequently than men. The disease is prevalent in roughly 2 per cent of the population and is found with apparent equal frequency among all races and in all climates.

Genetic factors do not appear to play a major causative role.

The hallmark of the disease is a chronic sterile synovitis that, pathologically, is marked by edema and hyperplasia of the synovial membrane. There is usually an outpouring of excessive synovial fluid with an increase in the number of leukocytes in the fluid. The degree of inflammation varies with time and has the ability to completely resolve. On the other hand, if persistent, the developing synovial pannus has the ability to erode articular cartilage and create a mechanical lesion resulting from cartilage loss. Unlike bone, articular cartilage does not regenerate, and the mechanical lesion of the cartilage persists. After many years, bony ankylosis may occur across the joint.

PRESENTATION

Rheumatoid arthritis usually presents as a systemic disorder in which the patient, in addition to having involvement of the joints, is "sick." Frequently a flu-like illness, respiratory in nature, heralds the onset. Generalized fatigue is the most common systemic complaint, and frequently patients will note this prior to the onset of arthritis. Initially the arthritis may be monoarticular or asymmetrical and follows a somewhat migratory course. Although an intermittent, palindromic course may continue for several months, eventually (usually within 1 to 2 months) the illness becomes established and a more typical symmetrical polyarthritis becomes apparent.

A unique feature of rheumatoid arthritis and its variants (ankylosing spondylitis and psoriatic arthritis) is morning stiffness. All arthritic conditions, including a sprained ankle, are worse upon arising, but in other states the morning stiffness subsides after 5 to 10 minutes of activity. In RA, the stiffness is pervasive, often involving areas not obviously involved with disease, and persists for 2 or more hours. The duration of morning stiffness seems to correlate well with the activity of the disease and therefore is a critical parameter to be used in continued evaluation of the patient. Because of this, an attempt should be made to quantitate the duration of stiffness as accurately as possible. By phrasing the question in a manner such as: "How much time does it take until you are as good as you'll ever be during a day?", one is able to determine reproducibly a measurement of this symptom.

Other symptoms, not obviously arthritic in nature, are a sore throat with associated hoarseness caused by involvement of the cricoarytenoid joint. The pain is felt directly over the larynx, and both the discomfort and hoarseness are most dominant in the first few hours after arising. Sjögren's syndrome may also occur simultaneously with the onset of arthritis. In this condition, any mucous membrane (e.g., vaginal oral, ocular) may be involved. The eye symptoms of keratoconjunctivitis sicca are variable, and in fact the patient may complain of increased tearing, secondary to constant irritation of the conjunctivae.

COURSE

The course of RA is highly variable, in both its pattern and its severity. Approximately 10 per cent of the patients will undergo a complete remission. This usually occurs within the first 6 months of the disease. Furthermore, if a remission has not occurred within the first 2 years, it is highly unlikely that it will ever occur.

A comment should be made here about the concept of "burned out" rheumatoid arthritis. This term is usually used in describing a severely crippled patient whose joints do not demonstrate obvious signs of inflammation. On closer examination, however, these patients have significantly prolonged morning stiffness and laboratory findings of an elevated sedimentation rate (ESR) and an anemia consistent with active disease. The explanation lies in the fact that immobilization of any inflamed joint leads to a diminution of the obvious signs of inflammation. This finding is also seen in other inflammatory forms of arthritis.

The activity of the disease tends to fluctuate greatly, with the rate of change being measured in terms of weeks and months. It is highly unusual, however, for its course to follow an abruptly changing pattern with intervals of complete inactivity. Although the severity of the inflammation fluctuates, the inflammation in the specific joints involved tends to remain static after the first year of the disease. In other words, joints that have been spared from inflammation after a period of 1 to 2 years will rarely become involved in the future.

Prognosis is difficult in RA. In general, latex positivity, nodules, and systemic toxicity carry a poor prognosis. On the other hand, approximately 50 per cent of the patients treated with salicylates are static in regard to functional status when examined 10 years after the initial diagnosis, and only 10 per cent of these patients are crippled at this time.

PHYSICAL EXAMINATION

Fever is occasionally seen in the early stages of rheumatoid arthritis in patients with marked systemic involvement. As a general rule, the extent of fever is directly proportional to the apparent severity of the evident synovitis. It is rarely seen in the later stages of the disease, except when there is an associated vasculitis or abrupt decrease of a steroid dosage. In juvenile rheumatoid arthritis (JRA), fever may occur as an isolated finding without evidence of synovitis or other organ involvement. In this situation the fever frequently antedates the advent of the arthritis by a month or more and presents a diagnostic dilemma. The diagnosis in this situation is made by the characteristic clinical picture, particularly if a transient, macular truncal rash occurs. In the adult form of RA the rheumatoid nodule, found in approximately a third of the patients, is the most specific diagnostic finding. These nodules usually occur abruptly with an obvious inflammatory response. Over a few months, the inflammation subsides and the nodule becomes firmer, often freely movable, and occasionally may disappear completely. The most common site for their occurrence is over the olecranon, but other "pressure points" (the occiput, sacrum, and palm) may frequently develop nodules. On physical examination the olecranon nodule may be indistinguishable from a gouty tophus that also has a predilection for this site (but not for the occiput or sacrum). The following points are useful in differentiating between the two: *Tophi* develop gradually and seldom are seen until the disease has been active for at least 5 years. On the other hand, rheumatoid nodules often occur early in the course of the disease and develop explosively and characteristically become smaller after their development, whereas tophi become larger. When there is doubt, the tophi can be identified by either biopsy or needle aspiration, followed by identification of urate crystals by polarized light microscopy. The rheumatoid nodule can be identified by a biopsy showing a characteristic histology.

The joint examination discloses a synovitis that is usually symmetrical and can involve essentially any joint in the body with the exception of the thoracolumbar spine and the sacroiliac joint. The appearance of deformities within nonweight-bearing joints (e.g., elbow, wrists, metacarpophalangeals) is indicative of synovitis as opposed to osteoarthritis, which occurs almost exclusively in weight-bearing joints. Involvement of the temporomandibular joint is common in RA and is never seen in gout, a differentiating point. A record should be made in regard to the following findings in each joint.:

1. Is it tender? In synovitis, the entire joint should be tender, and localized tenderness suggests a local mechanical or inflammatory condition (e.g., tendinitis).

2. Is it swollen? In synovitis, the swelling is of the soft tissue, which distinguishes it from the bony hypertrophy of osteoarthritis.

3. What is the range of motion? Certain joints, such as the spine and hips, are sufficiently "buried" so that the detection of effusions, warmth, and synovial thickening is impossible. In these joints, the diagnosis of involvement rests upon the demonstration of limited motion. In addition, an examination should be made to detect joints in which passive motion exceeds active motions. The rheumatoid pannus, which has the ability to erode cartilage, may also erode tendons or compress peripheral nerves and thus limit active motion.

Splenomegaly and lymphadenopathy occur in about 5 per cent of rheumatoids. When leukopenia coexists, the patient is categorized as having Felty's syndrome. Infiltrates within the mucous membranes are pathognomonic of Sjögren's syndrome. This can be identified most easily by performing a Schirmer test, in which tear production is measured by the extent to which the tears moisten a piece of filter paper placed under the lower lid. If less than 15 mm of the filter paper becomes moist in 5 minutes, the test is abnormal. Involvement of the pleura, pericardium, and peripheral nerves may also occur; needless to say, the patient requires a complete physical examination.

LABORATORY FINDINGS

With the exception of a positive biopsy of a rheumatoid nodule, the diagnosis of rheumatoid arthritis cannot be made by means of the laboratory. The tests to be mentioned are entirely nonspecific and neither substantiate nor rule out the diagnosis.

The latex fixation test is a serologic test for the presence of rheumatoid factor, an antibody (usually of the IgM class) against aggregated gamma globulin that has been coated over latex particles. It is positive in approximately 80 per cent of patients with rheumatoid arthritis, 20 to 40 per cent of patients with other collagen diseases or chronic inflammatory diseases such as subacute bacterial endocarditis, and 5 to 15 per cent of normal controls. As the incidence of rheumatoid arthritis is approximately 2 per cent, it can be realized that only about one fifth of patients who are latex positive will have rheumatoid arthritis.

Other serologic abnormalities are a diffuse hypergammaglobulinemia, hypoalbuminemia (which usually parallels the severity of the disease), and positive antinuclear antibodies in close to 25 per cent of patients with the disease.

The sedimentation rate is usually elevated during periods of disease activity. It is entirely nonspecific and is elevated in any other inflammatory condition such as gout or septic arthritis. Its major value is to measure the degree of inflammation rather than to make a specific diagnosis.

Hematologic findings are nonspecific and usually reveal a mild anemia in the 30 to 35 per cent hematocrit range, which is either normochromic or slightly hypochromic. Leukopenia and occasionally thrombocytopenia may be seen with associated splenomegaly (Felty's syndrome). Isolated thrombocytosis occasionally may also be seen.

X-rays are of no diagnostic value in establishing a diagnosis in the early phases of RA, as radiologic techniques essentially demonstrate bone and the primary lesion of this disease involves the synovium. It is only after the process has eroded into the bone that the characteristic picture of the disease becomes apparent. Essentially all inflammatory conditions involving the joints look alike initially, and it is only when progression to bony erosion occurs that a more specific diagnosis may be made based upon the pattern of involvement, rate of destruction, and characteristic response of the juxta-articular bone.

Examination of the synovial fluid demonstrates a sterile inflammatory picture with a leukocyte count, primarily polymorphonuclear, of between 3000 and 15,000 per cu mm. Wide variations may occur; although the white blood cell count (WBC) seldom exceeds 25,000 per cu mm in adult RA, it may approach 100,000 per cu mm in juvenile rheumatoid arthritis. The mucin clot is poor, but this is a nonspecific finding that essentially correlates with the extent of inflammation. The aforementioned findings overlap with the "rheumatoid variants," frequently with gout, and occasionally with the infectious arthritides.

The synovial biopsy in RA shows a nonspecific synovitis containing a predominantly mononuclear infiltrate. This does not distinguish it from other sterile inflammatory conditions, with the probable exceptions of gout and hemochromatosis, which have a specific histopathology. Synovial biopsy is of greatest value in excluding the diagnosis of tuberculosis.

In conclusion, mention should be made of the American Rheumatism Association criteria for the diagnosis of rheumatoid arthritis. These criteria are of value primarily in clinical and epidemiologic studies and are of little value in making a diagnosis in the individual patient. Essentially, rheumatoid arthritis is diagnosed on clinical grounds entirely, the diagnosis must be individualized, and a biopsy of a rheumatoid nodule is the only specific diagnostic technique.

ANKYLOSING SPONDYLITIS

By ERSKINE M. CAPERTON, M.D., *and* PAUL J. BILKA, M.D.
Minneapolis, Minnesota

SYNONYMS

Rheumatoid spondylitis, Marie-Strümpell disease, von Bechterew's disease, spondylitis deformans, pelvospondylitis ossificans, spondylitis ankylopoietica, spondylitis ossificans ligamentosa, atrophic spondylitis, Pierre Marie's syndrome, and spondylose rhizomelique.

DEFINITION

Ankylosing spondylitis is a chronic progressive form of arthritis affecting primarily the central skeleton, including the sacroiliac joints, the spinal apophyseal (synovial) joints, and the paravertebral soft tissues. Although the specific cause is unknown, genetic predisposition is well established as a single autosomal factor. Approximately 90 per cent of the clinical cases are in men, and the disease is generally more severe in males than in females.

PRESENTING SIGNS AND SYMPTOMS

The onset is usually in patients 15 to 30 years of age but may occur in childhood, and is more often insidious with pain or stiffness in the lower back. Backache is usually lumbosacral and often is worse in bed at night. In about 10 per cent of patients, especially in the early stages, pain may radiate in the sciatic nerve distribution, often alternating sides, but neurologic findings are rare. Stiffness is noted after a period of rest so that the patient complains most on awakening in the morning and attempting to rise.

The initial manifestation may be peripheral in approximately 20 per cent of patients, partic- ularly in children and adolescents, beginning as an asymmetrical polyarthritis in large joints such as the hips and knees. Other, less usual initial modes of presentation include recurrent attacks of iritis, heel pain, acute back pain with fever (often associated with major trauma), and chest pain related to costosternal joint involvement.

Systemic symptoms are unusual at onset, although in severe illness, fever, fatigue, anorexia, and weight loss may accompany the initial symptoms.

COURSE

Ankylosing spondylitis follows a highly variable course from patient to patient. At the one extreme are patients who never had symptoms, the diagnosis being discovered serendipitously when x-ray reveals fused sacroiliac joints. At the other extreme, a rare patient presents with explosive onset of back pain and progresses to advanced stages with a nearly immobile axial skeleton in but a few months.

In the majority of patients the disease follows a course of exacerbations and remissions with episodic lower back pain of variable intensity, nocturnal pain that awakens the patient from sleep, and persistent spinal stiffness relieved only by movement and exercise. The disease, beginning in the sacroiliac joints, characteristically progresses cephalad, progressively involving the lumbar, thoracic, and cervical vertebral areas. With costovertebral involvement, chest expansion becomes limited and may be associated with dyspnea. Approximately half of the patients will exhibit signs and symptoms of involvement of joints other than those of the spine at some time in the course of their disease; this peripheral joint involvement, particularly affecting the shoulders, hips, and knees, may be chronic.

The majority of patients remain active, and with proper management are usually able to lead active, productive lives. Rapid, often dramatic improvement of symptoms after therapy with a nonsteroidal anti-inflammatory drug is often of diagnostic importance.

PHYSICAL EXAMINATION

The physical signs of ankylosing spondylitis vary with the mode of onset and the stage of disease. Early, stiffness of the lower back and tenderness over the sacroiliac joints are observed, although in mild early disease the physical examination may be normal. Inability to flex the lower back is a hallmark of the disease; this gets progressively worse with time. With progression, paravertebral muscle spasm leads to loss of the normal lumbar curvature, and involvement of the thoracic spine produces an exaggerated kyphosis. Tenderness may be elicited on palpation and percussion over the vertebral spinous processes. With involvement of the costovertebral joints, chest expansion becomes very limited; this is a relatively late development in the majority of patients. Later still, cervical involvement leads to forward flexion of the neck and severe loss of motion of the neck.

Peripheral joint involvement may lead to synovial hypertrophy and effusions, and may be difficult to differentiate from rheumatoid arthritis. Loss of motion of the shoulders and hips and effusions in the knees are the most common findings, although occasionally swelling of the small joints of the hands and feet may be observed. Subcutaneous nodules do not develop.

COMMON COMPLICATIONS

The three major complications of ankylosing spondylitis are iritis, cardiac involvement, and pulmonary complications. Iritis occurs in approximately 20 per cent of patients and may be the presenting feature. The iritis is usually unilateral. Aortic incompetence is the most severe cardiac complication, occurring in approximately 2 per cent of patients. Conduction defects occur in 10 per cent, first-degree A-V block being most common; complete A-V block may occur. Cardiomegaly and pericarditis are also observed. Dyspnea may be related to cardiac disease, to a lack of chest expansion secondary to costovertebral and costosternal joint involvement, and to pulmonary fibrotic changes. The pulmonary fibrotic changes affect the upper lobes and are seen as spotty irregular opacities in the upper lobes of both lungs on x-ray.

Rare complications include neurologic signs secondary to cervical vertebral involvement, particularly with subluxation of the cervical vertebrae. Amyloidosis, although reported, is rarely of clinical importance.

LABORATORY FEATURES

Ankylosing spondylitis is a genetic disease; the genetic predisposition to developing ankylosing spondylitis is closely associated with the genes that code for cell surface antigens, the HLA antigens. Specifically, ankylosing spondylitis is associated with HLA antigen B27 (formerly W27). Ninety to 95 per cent of patients with ankylosing spondylitis have HLA antigen B27 on their cells, whereas this antigen is present in less than 8 per cent of the general population.

Radiologic findings, when present, are diagnostic of ankylosing spondylitis, but they may take years to develop. Prior to the development of HLA B27 testing, which allows earlier confirmation of the disease, the demonstration of bilateral sacroiliitis was (and according to most authorities remains) the sine qua non for the diagnosis. The characteristic changes in the sacroiliac joints are generalized osteoporosis with increased periarticular bone density, followed by erosion of the joint margins and finally bony ankylosis of the joint — virtual disappearance of the joint margins. With involvement of the vertebral column, other changes may be seen on x-ray, including "squaring" of the vertebral bodies; calcification of the paraspinous ligaments and anulus fibrosis of the intervertebral discs, producing typical smooth syndesmophytes and leading in advanced cases to the "bamboo spine"; and erosions and subsequent fusion of the apophyseal joints. In addition, diffuse narrowing with erosions of the hips and shoulders and erosions at the margins of the symphysis pubis may occur. Periostitis may be noted on the ischial bones and lesser trochanter, and spurs are common on the heel.

Other laboratory studies are either normal or undependable. Blood studies are nonspecific. The erythrocyte sedimentation rate is elevated in about 80 per cent of patients, but may be normal. Rheumatoid factor, although usually negative, may be positive in 5 to 10 per cent. Muscle enzymes, liver function studies, and serum protein are normal, the minimal gamma globulin elevation sometimes observed being no different from that seen in other chronic diseases.

DIFFERENTIAL DIAGNOSIS

The diagnosis of ankylosing spondylitis is obvious in a young man with back pain, spinal stiffness, HLA B27, elevated sedimentation rate, and radiologic evidence of sacroiliitis; the presence of any of these features or iritis should prompt a search for the others. When any two of these features are lacking, the diagnosis may be difficult. The disease is often confused with other entities, especially rheumatoid arthritis, Reiter's syndrome, and psychoneurosis.

Rheumatoid arthritis does not affect the lower back, has a predilection for symmetrical involvement of the small joints of the hands and feet in addition to the large peripheral joints occasionally affected by ankylosing spondylitis, and is not associated with HLA antigen B27. Rheumatoid arthritis is more common in females; 80 per cent of patients have rheumatoid factor.

Reiter's disease can usually be excluded by the absence of the other features characteristic of Reiter's disease, including urethritis, conjunctivitis, and mucocutaneous eruptions. However, Reiter's disease does affect the lower back and large peripheral joints and is associated with HLA B27, so that the distinguishing features must be searched for.

Psychoneurosis in a young man presenting with back pain may be very difficult to distinguish from early mild ankylosing spondylitis; however, true back stiffness and tenderness localized specifically to the sacroiliac joints are rarely found in neurotics. Test for HLA B27 is helpful in these situations.

Other conditions one must consider in the differential diagnosis of ankylosing spondylitis, and which can usually be distinguished by specific features, include psoriatic arthritis, in which the rash is characteristic; spondylitis associated with inflammatory bowel disease, in which episodes of diarrhea and crampy abdominal pain are prominent; degenerative disease of the back, distinguished by its later onset and characteristic radiographic appearance; anatomic back deformity (e.g., spondylolisthesis, spina bifida), again recognized by the radiologic appearance without sacroiliac involvement; mechanical lower back strain, characterized by muscle spasm, often unilateral, without sacroiliac tenderness; and osteitis condensans ilii, a disease primarily of young mothers and characterized on x-ray by sclerosis of the ilium at the margin of the sacroiliac joint. Sacroiliitis affecting a single sacroiliac joint radiologically should suggest the diagnosis of infectious arthritis, particularly tuberculosis. The other inflammatory diseases, such as gout, pyogenic infection, and rheumatic fever, and the connective tissue diseases associated with arthritis, such as systemic lupus erythematosus, polymyositis, and scleroderma, are all easily distinguished by their characteristic manifestations and lack of lower back involvement.

OSTEOARTHRITIS

By JAMES B. PETER, M.D.
Santa Monica, California

Osteoarthritis, a disease of synovial (diarthrodial) joints, is characterized by degeneration of hyaline articular cartilage with abnormal remodeling of subchondral bone. The remodeling probably leads to progressive damage and ultimate loss of cartilage and certainly is part of the eburnation of the bone ends and marginal proliferation of bone (osteophyte formation) that are characteristic of osteoarthritis.

The disease is considered *primary or idiopathic* when no causes are apparent. *Secondary osteoarthritis* may reflect causation or acceleration by metabolic, inflammatory, physical, developmental, or other factors. Whether the fundamental abnormality in primary osteoarthritis lies in cartilage, bone, or elsewhere is unknown.

The term "osteoarthrosis" emphasizes the contention of some that the inflammatory features of osteoarthritis are an epiphenomenon of no significance to the progress of the disease. This point is debatable, but the term "osteoarthrosis" may have definite merit, because as Hench said: "Arthritis is not a designation to bandy about promiscuously. To all but the most phlegmatic patient it comes as a prophecy of real trouble ahead, a threat of long illness and perhaps of slow, painful retirement." Such prophecy is certainly unjustified, and the physician rendering a diagnosis of osteoarthritis will greatly benefit his patient with words of reassurance in this regard. Osteoarthrosis as a diagnosis has little merit when applied to those patients whose osteoarthritis of the interphalangeal joints of the hands is associated with synovitis of variable but sometimes incapacitating severity.

The term "degenerative joint disease" is recommended by the American Rheumatism Association for reasons that are not compelling except that its use does avoid the term "arthritis." There is ample evidence that degenerative joint disease is not a necessary consequence of senescence or of hard, traumatic work.

HIP

Pain is invariably the problem for which these patients seek relief. The source of the pain is characteristically obvious except for osteoarthritis (OA) of the hip. These patients early in the course have aching diffuse pain over the posterolateral aspect of the ipsilateral buttock. Only when the disease is far advanced is the pain felt in the inguinal area. In the early stages the pain is rarely well localized. In these situations it is usually lateral over the greater trochanter and reflects greater trochanteric bursitis that sometimes accompanies OA of the hip but more often occurs alone. At other times there is confusion with bursitis of the ischial-gluteal bursa (weaver's bottom), which is characterized by pain on sitting and localized tenderness over the ischial tuberosity.

The patient with OA of a large joint does not have the long-lasting morning stiffness (1 hour or more) that characterizes rheumatoid arthritis and some other diseases with flagrant inflammatory synovitis. Rather, the morning stiffness is short lived and is often noticeable only during the first few steps taken in the morning. The pain is worsened by activity, and the short-lived stiffness recurs during the day when a period of rest follows activity. Patients complain that they move very stiffly across a room from a chair in which they have rested for 30 minutes or more after walking or exercise.

Not all patients with OA of the hip have an inexorable course to inguinal pain, joint destruction, loss of motion (especially abduction), and audible, painful crepitus. Spontaneous resolution of symptoms compatible with osteoarthritis is recognized, as is excellent relief when anti-inflammatory agents are given.

In OA of the hip, pain on full internal rotation or, less frequently, on abduction is a frequent early finding and may be present long before the discomfort is felt in the inguinal area with walking. Crepitus is common, and abduction is grossly compromised as the disease progresses. Occasionally, pain originating in the hip will be felt near the knee, usually the lateral aspect, and knee pain may be the presenting complaint.

Roentgen studies show loss of cartilage, subchondral sclerosis, osteophytosis, and other bone remodeling that leads to a thick buttress of bone at the medial aspect of the femoral neck. The latter may be present quite early in the disease; this observation is consistent with the notion that bony stiffness arising from remodeling is an important aspect of the progressive cartilage damage of osteoarthritis. Perhaps we shall someday be able to investigate the possibility that separate genetic factors predispose to cartilage damage and to bony remodeling and that both are necessary for the development of classic advanced osteoarthritis.

Aside from synovial fluid analysis (see later discussion), laboratory studies are of no direct help in the diagnosis of any type of primary OA. In secondary OA, diagnosis of the underlying or predisposing disease necessitates laboratory evaluation of inflammatory causes (sedimentation rate and rheumatoid factors in RA), endocrine disturbances (diabetes mellitus, acromegaly), and metabolic abnormalities (ochronosis, hemochromatosis, gout, Paget's disease, and chondrocalcinosis), among other less frequent causes of secondary osteoarthritis.

Osteoarthritis of the hip is said to be a characteristic component of *primary generalized osteoarthritis*. This is a syndrome described by Kellgren and Moore as a polyarticular form of osteoarthritis involving the hips; knees; distal interphalangeal finger joints; first carpometacarpal, first tarsometatarsal, and first metatarsophalangeal joints; and the interfacetal joints of the spine. An important unresolved question is whether *Kellgren's disease* reflects the presence of true generalized osteoarthritis or the aggregation in some persons of the factors that might separately predispose to the development of OA of the knees, hips, or hands.

KNEES

Osteoarthritis of the knees presents with symptoms similar to OA of the hips, including short-lived or absent morning stiffness, exercise-induced exacerbation of the pain, stiffness on initial movements after rest following exercise, synovial effusions in the early stages, and varus or valgus deformities.

The location of the pain is lateral, medial, or bilateral at the tibial plateaus, depending on the major site of damage. Early in the wet phase when effusions are present, the pain may be more generalized and even be prominent posteriorly with fluid distention of the capsule and distention of Baker's cysts, giving rise to the patient's discomfort and complaint that squatting (or other full-flexion) maneuvers are difficult and painful, with a feeling of tightness.

Osteoarthritis of the knee, especially when most prominent in the medial compartment, often is first manifested by localized pain at the medial joint line. Tenderness and palpable swelling may also occur over the pes anserina bursa, which lies on the anteromedial aspect of the tibial plateau superficial to the tibial collateral ligament and deep to the tendons of the sartorius, gracilis, and semimembranosus. This presenting manifestation of inflammation of the knee is more frequent in obese women, is most often accompanied by roentgenographically demonstrable OA of the same knee, and should be suspected when OA of the knees suddenly worsens with pain in the area of the anserine bursa.

Secondary OA of the knee often reflects damage to one compartment of the joint, with trauma, fractures, meniscal tears, or surgery for torn meniscus. A common and sometimes vexing problem is pain over the knee laterally or medially with grating and perhaps sensation of locking pain at extreme range of motion against resistance. These patients, frequently thought to have torn meniscus, are often found at surgery to have osteoarthritis. This problem, sometimes referred to as the "meniscus trap," should be suspected when signs of meniscal tear are atypical and when signs of torn meniscus come on gradually in an elderly patient. In such patients x-ray studies are often particularly valuable, including weight-bearing anteroposterior views and arthrography.

Findings on physical examination vary with the stage of the disease. Early there is almost always minor synovial thickening with synovial effusion, with fullness both anteriorly and in the popliteal fossa. Mediolateral instability is usually obvious in contrast to anteroposterior stability. Osteophytes are palpable at the tibial plateaus. Patellofemoral crepitus is generally of little significance. Later in the course of OA of the knees the joints are relatively fluid free and there are increased instability, large palpable osteophytes, and valgus or varus deformity.

Synovial fluid analysis shows a Class I non-inflammatory fluid with less than 1000 white blood cells (WBC) per cu mm. The cells are largely lymphocytes, and the quality of the mucin clot and the fluid viscosity is characteristically good but may be only fair even though the WBC count is less than 200. The ratio of hemolytic complement activity (CH 50) in synovial fluid to that of serum is said to be above 55 per cent in osteoarthritis (OA) and below 35 per cent in rheumatoid arthritis (RA). As might be expected, the histopathology of the synovium reflects the stage of the disease, with infiltration of round cells and synovial cell changes more prominent in the early phases of osteoarthritis. Synovial biopsy is generally not diagnostic and often is not useful in limiting the diagnostic possibilities.

Roentgenographic studies of the knees show loss of cartilage, subchondral sclerosis, osteophytosis, sharpening of the tibial spines, and variable degrees of varus and valgus. Early in the disease weight-bearing anteroposterior views of the knees are particularly helpful in showing the juxtaposition of femoral condyle and tibial plateau to a distance of less than 3 mm, as is characteristic of cartilage loss. In some patients weight-bearing views in about 15-degree flexion can show narrowing, which is otherwise inapparent. Occasionally, stress views with the joint forced into varus or valgus are helpful.

Arthrography is of special benefit with double contrast. In osteoarthritis the menisci are often ground up. Such a picture suggests the diagnosis of osteoarthritis in a patient suspected of having meniscus syndrome; loss of cartilage can be defined by double contrast arthrography. Such studies generally allow confident prediction of whether meniscectomy will benefit such patients or if joint replacement is necessary.

HANDS

Osteoarthritis of the interphalangeal joints of the hands is very common in women. Heberden's and Bouchard's nodes, seen in these patients, are characteristically painless, bony enlargements that have developed without discomfort over the years. In some patients the nodes develop rapidly in association with variable degrees of painful inflammation, with soft tissue swelling, mild warmth, and erythema.

Of patients with Heberden's nodes, some 25 per cent will also have Bouchard's nodes (osteophytes at the proximal interphalangeal finger joints). It is in these patients during the inflammatory phase of osteoarthritis that the diagnosis of rheumatoid arthritis is too often rendered. The term "erosive osteoarthritis" was coined some years ago to emphasize the bone destruction and synovitis that occur in some of these middle-aged patients during the formation of these nodes. Not infrequently there is a history of similar disease in these joints in other women of the family, but the degree of inflammation is quite variable.

The natural history of erosive osteoarthritis has not been fully defined. In some patients the inflammation, which is greatly benefited by use of nonsteroidal anti-inflammatory drugs, subsides after several years and the patient is left with static deformities that are not very painful or disabling. The disease, although it may be intensely inflammatory in some patients and result in severe destruction, does not become generalized. It appears that erosive osteoarthritis does not antedate rheumatoid arthritis more than would be expected from the occasional, coincidental association of two common diseases.

Findings on physical examination in erosive osteoarthritis, like the pathology of the synovium, reflect the stage of the disease. Early there is synovitis with palpable synovial thickening in several distal interphalangeal and proximal interphalangeal joints, the interphalangeal joints of the thumbs, and occasionally at the second and even more infrequently at the third metacarpal-phalangeal joints. Osteophytes are typically present and palpable at the distal interphalangeal joints very early in the course of the erosive osteoarthritis.

In erosive osteoarthritis, like other forms of primary osteoarthritis, tests for rheumatoid factors and the other commonly assayed autoantibodies are characteristically negative. An occasional patient may have borderline titers of rheumatoid factors, but such a result by itself should not lead to a change of diagnosis if the patient otherwise has typical erosive osteoarthritis. The erythrocyte sedimentation rate is also normal or only slightly elevated.

Synovial biopsies in erosive osteoarthritis reveal synovitis and synoviocyte hypertrophy and hyperplasia in the inflammatory (early) phases of the disease. Later these changes regress spontaneously in parallel with decreased inflammation clinically.

Roentgenographic features of erosive osteoarthritis include loss of cartilage, subchondral sclerosis, osteophytosis, and erosions that, although typically marginal, may sometimes be central and even occasionally resemble the sawtooth pattern seen in psoriatic arthritis. Even in the early, acute inflammatory phase of erosive osteoarthritis there is not much periarticular osteoporosis. This feature, sparing of the metacarpal joints by the erosive process, and the lack of erosions of the ulnar styloid allow easy roentgenographic distinction from rheumatoid arthritis.

WRIST

Osteoarthritis in the wrist is generally confined to the radial side. Involvement of the first carpometacarpal joints accounts for the vast majority of problems, with isolated osteoarthritis of the trapezioscaphoid joint being a distant second.

These patients complain of pain in the hand on grasping, pinching, and especially wringing movements. As with other forms of osteoarthritis, the pain, swelling, and stiffness are increased by use and relieved by rest. Patients commonly have difficulty localizing the pain, which is often thought to arise in the first metacarpal joint, a quite uncommon site of symptomatic osteoarthritis of the hand. Prolonged morning stiffness is not a problem, and as with all forms of osteoarthritis the discomfort is worse with repeated use. Later in the course of osteoarthritis of the first carpometacarpal joint there is a tendency to radial subluxation of the base of the first metacarpal, with a resultant squared appearance of the hand.

Osteoarthritis in these joints is disabling in certain occupations such as in supermarket checkout personnel, who must repetitively move heavy objects with a wide grip. These patients perform a powerful pincer movement not by approximating the tips of the thumb and index finger in the usual position of great power with the thumb and index finger forming an "O" shape; rather the thumb pad is approximated near the distal interphalangeal joint of the index finger. This position avoids abduction of the thumb, a maneuver that maximizes contact between the base of the metacarpal and the transverse hollow of the trapezium, especially at its medial aspect where the osteoarthritis is first manifest.

Physical examination in the early, inflammatory stages reveals thickening and point tenderness at the dorsolateral aspect of the joint. With the wrist fixed the examiner can elicit crepitus and pain in the joint by forcefully rotating the first metacarpal at its head while immobilizing the first metacarpal-phalangeal joint. This clearly localizes the pain to the first carpometacarpal joint and the patient immediately identifies it as "my pain" and recognizes its source. Atrophy of the thenar muscles is commonly seen, but its mechanism is not well defined. Peter, Marmor, and others described a special position of the hand for roentgenograms that can show very early changes in the first carpometacarpal joint.

Osteoarthritis of the trapezioscaphoid (greater multangular-navicular) joint occasionally accompanies that of the first carpometacarpal joint (trapeziometacarpal) and much less frequently occurs alone. As an isolated problem the symptoms are similar to those at the first carpometacarpal joint. Sometimes, however, there is also ganglion-like swelling at the radial volar wrist that usually reflects communication between the space around the flexor carpi radialis tendon and the trapezioscaphoid joint.

Median neuropathy caused by *carpal tunnel syndrome* is an infrequently recognized but common accompaniment of osteoarthritis of the wrist. The symptoms are generally less profound than in rheumatoid arthritis. Atrophy of the thenar muscles contributes to the squared appearance of the affected hand.

SPINE

The term "osteoarthritis of the spine" should, as Collins pointed out, be restricted to disease of the apophyseal (interfacetal) joints. It is not synonymous with disc disease and its accompanying osteophytosis and disc space narrowing, which are best referred to as spondylosis. Some use the term "spondylosis" to include disc degeneration, osteophytosis, and osteoarthritis of the apophyseal joints, but there is little merit to this because the pathogenetic mechanisms of disc degeneration and apophyseal osteoarthritis are probably different and there is no evidence that disc deterioration causes osteoarthritis of the apophyseal (interfacetal) joints. Cervical osteoarthritis refers to degenerative disease of the apophyseal joints.

Cervical Spondylosis and Osteoarthritis. Spondylosis at C5–6 and C6–7 is present in more than 50 per cent of the population over 40 years of age. These radiographic changes increase in frequency and severity with age. The discrepancy between such changes and appropriate clinical symptoms is well known, as is the converse. The relevance of the radiographic findings to the clinical problem must be analyzed critically, with special attention to (1) correspondence of the neurologic level with the level of radiographic abnormality, (2) the exclusion of other lesions, and (3) the possibility of a recent lesion that is not apparent on the films. In general, cervical spondylosis presents with radicular findings, myelopathy, neck pain, headache, or insufficiency of the vertebral-basilar system. Radicular pain other than C6 or C7 in distribution necessitates special attention to other diagnostic possibilities.

In contrast to cervical spondylosis, cervical apophyseal osteoarthritis is more common at C3–4 and C4–5. Oblique views taken about 12 degrees from true lateral show the profiles of the apophyseal joints at a given level, and this demonstrates whether the OA is unilateral or bilateral.

When neck pain, limitation of motion, muscle spasm, and crepitus are the major clinical problems, it is likely that there is an inflammatory component to the spondylosis and osteoarthritis and that response to indomethacin or another anti-inflammatory compound can be expected.

Lumbar Spondylosis and Osteoarthritis. The problems of lumbar disc disease and herniated nucleus pulposus with radicular findings are well known. Osteoarthritis of the lumbar apophyseal joints, like the spondylosis, is more common at L4–5 and L5–S1.

Lumbar Stenosis Syndrome. A syndrome less well recognized is lumbar stenosis with multiple neurologic abnormalities caused by severe lumbar spondylosis. This problem is especially confusing when it presents with so-called pseudoclaudication, the symptom of buttock and variable lower extremity pain, which is accentuated in the erect position and sometimes worsened with walking.

Ischemic neuropathy of the lumbosacral plexus, an unusual problem, is often manifested at night. In the elderly, careful auscultation of the abdominal aorta and its branches as well as evaluation of the patient's glucose tolerance will sometimes allow proper diagnosis as opposed to easy but unjustifiable attribution of the symptoms to lumbar disc disease in the elderly.

It is useful to remember that isolated, surgically curable herniated nucleus pulposus is uncommon after middle age. The clinical syndromes resultant from disc disease of the cervical and lumbar spines are well defined and characteristically accompanied by definite neurologic signs that correspond exactly to the defect(s) outlined by myelography. In the absence of these definitive, precisely corresponding clinical and myelographic abnormalities, surgery should be recommended with great

hesitancy. Finally, the undisputed presence of degenerative disease in the elderly (or young) does not relieve the physician of responsibility for excluding other complicating problems.

OSTEOPOROSIS

By C. CONRAD JOHNSTON, Jr., M.D.
Indianapolis, Indiana

SYNONYMS

Postmenopausal osteoporosis, senile osteoporosis, idiopathic osteoporosis.

DEFINITION

Osteoporosis is a condition characterized by decreased mass of bone in the skeleton, leading to structural failure with fracture. The bone present is of normal quality with a normal mineral-to-matrix ratio, but is simply decreased in quantity. There may be abnormalities of skeletal remodeling present in this disease.

PRESENTING SIGNS AND SYMPTOMS

The morbid event in osteoporosis is the development of fractures. These occur most commonly in vertebrae and in the proximal femora and distal radii. Vertebral collapse fractures may develop gradually and may be asymptomatic. The patient notes loss of height with anterior wedging of the dorsal vertebrae and increasing kyphosis. The "dowager's hump" is an early sign of anterior wedging.

Pain is the principal symptom of the fracture. These fractures characteristically occur with little trauma. When vertebral collapse occurs acutely, the pain is usually severe and is localized to the area of the collapse, with some lateral radiation. This pain is aggravated by movement. There may be associated paravertebral muscle spasm and consequent pain. Cord compression and neurologic signs are extremely rare and, if present, suggest another cause of collapse. This severe pain usually dissipates over a period of several weeks, but a milder, more chronic pain may persist for several months. When numerous collapse fractures have occurred, chronic postural back pain may result.

COURSE

There is an accelerated rate of bone loss that begins in women in the fifth decade and slows in the seventh decade. Men begin to lose somewhat later, and the rate of loss is slower. Fractures of the vertebrae may occur in clusters of several at one time, and then the patient may have no more fractures for some years, if ever. Current methods of measurements of bone mass do not allow accurate prediction of that patient who is most subject to the development of fractures.

PHYSICAL EXAMINATION FINDINGS

Findings are not specific for osteoporosis. The "dowager's hump" and increasing dorsal kyphosis may be early findings. With increasing kyphosis and loss of height, prominent skinfolds may be apparent over the lower anterior chest and abdomen. The lower rib margins may actually impinge on the anterior iliac crest. When acute vertebral collapse develops, there may be localized tenderness and paravertebral muscle spasm in the area of the fracture.

LABORATORY FINDINGS

Serum and urinary calcium, serum phosphorus, alkaline phosphatase, and serum protein electrophoresis are within normal limits.

X-rays reveal the presence of fractures or the deformity of vertebrae or both. Prior to the development of the fracture, x-rays show demineralization (decreased radiographic density), but standard roentgenograms are notoriously poor for estimating the mass of bone present. It has been estimated that greater than 30 per cent of the bone present must be lost before it can be detected by x-ray examination. Early signs of spinal osteoporosis include accentuation of end-plates and vertical striations and ballooning of the intervertebral discs. Such findings are not diagnostic and can be produced artifactually. The finding of demineralization by x-ray is *not* specific for osteoporosis.

Newer methods for quantitation of skeletal mass, such as photon absorptiometry or measurement of total body calcium by neutron activation, are promising for the future but currently remain investigative tools.

PITFALLS IN DIAGNOSIS

Osteoporosis may occur as a secondary finding in other systemic diseases, and these must be considered in the differential diagnosis.

Cushing's disease and the administration of exogenous glucocorticoids are associated with excessive bone loss and fractures. Hyperthyroidism also produces excessive bone loss in some instances and can produce osteoporosis.

Hyperparathyroidism may be associated with generalized demineralization of the skeleton, and the classic radiologic findings of subperiosteal bone resorption and cyst formation may be absent. In this disease, serum calcium is characteristically elevated.

A more difficult diagnostic dilemma is posed by the problem of malignancy. Some tumors elaborate a substance immunologically similar to parathyroid hormone that can produce demineralization. In addition, metastases to the spine can produce collapse fractures that might be mistaken for osteoporotic collapse fractures. Metastatic disease more often involves a single vertebra, whereas several fractures are commonly found in osteoporosis. Nevertheless, bone biopsy may be necessary in some instances to rule out the presence of malignancy. Multiple myeloma should be carefully looked for as it may be associated with generalized demineralization rather than the classic punched-out lesions of the bone. In most patients, abnormalities are found by serum protein electrophoresis in this disease.

Osteomalacia must always be considered in the differential diagnosis of osteoporosis, particularly because it is more readily amenable to therapy. Today, in the United States, osteomalacia is usually found in patients with various forms of malabsorption or renal tubular acidosis. A relatively high incidence of this disease has been found in the elderly population in Great Britain and is responsible in part for the increased incidence of fractures in that age group. The incidence of osteomalacia in the elderly population within the United States has not been clearly delineated, and thus this disease should always be considered in the differential diagnosis. The pain of osteomalacia is usually more generalized and is often associated with proximal muscle weakness. There is usually a decrease in the serum calcium level, a decrease in serum phosphorus, and an increase in serum alkaline phosphatase. In severe disease, the characteristic pseudofractures of osteomalacia are found on x-ray examination. The disease can perhaps best be diagnosed by a study of undecalcified bone samples taken by needle biopsy. At present this technique is available at only a few centers, but it should become more readily available in the near future. Such a biopsy should be considered in the more difficult-to-diagnose cases.

ANTERIOR HORN CELL DISEASE OF INFANCY AND CHILDHOOD AND THE PROGRESSIVE MUSCULAR DYSTROPHIES

By J. R. MENDELL, M.D.,
and E. W. JOHNSON, M.D.
Columbus, Ohio

A motor unit is composed of one anterior horn cell of the spinal cord, its long cytoplasmic process or axon that courses through the peripheral nerve, and all muscle fibers innervated by the terminal arborizations of the axon. Diseases affecting this anatomic and physiologic unit of the nervous system have long puzzled the clinician because of their great overlap in clinical presentation. Although the pathogenesis of neuromuscular disorders remains an enigma in most cases, our skill in diagnosis has been greatly enhanced in the past two decades. This can be attributed to the accessibility of a combination of diagnostic tools available to the clinician.

SERUM ENZYMES

The simplest of these tools is estimation of the serum levels of creatinine phosphokinase (CPK), aldolase, lactic dehydrogenase (LDH), glutamic oxaloacetic transaminase (GOT), and glutamic pyruvic transaminase (GPT). These enzymes are found in the muscle cell, and when there is a breakdown in the integrity of the muscle cell membrane, as in necrosis of muscle fibers, they are released into the serum in excess quantities.

ELECTRODIAGNOSIS

Electromyography (EMG) offers a relatively rapid assessment of the physiologic state of the motor unit and can be used to differentiate between muscle weakness of nerve or muscle origin. In diseases affecting the anterior horn cell or peripheral nerve, spontaneous activity in the resting muscle in the form of fibrillation and fasciculation potentials and positive sharp waves may be seen. In addition there may be motor unit potentials of increased size and duration, particularly in anterior horn cell disease, early perhaps as synchronous recruitment and later as a result of collateral sprouting of axons. These large potentials are frequently polyphasic. During voluntary activity in neurogenic weakness, there is a decreased number of motor unit potentials as compared with strength of contraction. In disease processes affecting primarily the peripheral nerves, especially those that impair Schwann cell function, there is a slowing of the conduction velocity of the nerve.

In diseases in which the muscle fibers are undergoing a degenerative change, we find motor unit potentials of small size and short duration. During voluntary activity there is an increase in the number of motor unit potentials recruited as compared to strength of contraction and an increased proportion of polyphasic potentials of normal or reduced duration. In some disorders of muscle, presumably involving the membrane, insertion or movement of the EMG needle results in the appearance of bursts of high-frequency, short-duration potentials lasting several seconds and accompanied by a sound similar to that made by an old-fashioned dive bomber (*myotonia*). This characteristic sound is the result of high-frequency discharges, varying in both frequency and amplitude. In diseases such as myasthenia gravis in which there is a defect in neuromuscular transmission, repetitive supramaximal stimulation of the nerve, with surface recording electrodes over the appropriate muscle, shows a decline in the amplitude of the muscle action potential.

MUSCLE BIOPSY

Advances in histochemical staining techniques on fresh frozen skeletal muscle also provide us with a readily available tool for distinguishing between neurogenic and myopathic disorders. We now know that the most frequently biopsied human muscles are composed of two basic muscle fiber types, forming a mosaic pattern. Type I fibers contain higher amounts of oxidative enzymes and neutral fat droplets and lesser amounts of glycogen and phosphorylase than type II fibers. Furthermore, myofibrillar ATPase activity (at pH 9.4) is greater in type II fibers than in type I. Recent studies in both animals and man suggest that each motor unit is composed of a uniform histochemical fiber type.

Neurogenic disorders result in a combination of abnormalities easily recognized on muscle biopsy. The earliest observable change is the presence of small angular fibers scattered throughout the biopsy specimen. As the disease progresses we see groups of small angular fibers, most commonly affecting both histochemical fiber types. These small angular fibers often appear darker than normal with oxidative enzyme stains. Target fibers are one of the hallmarks of denervation and are characterized by a central area of diminished staining for oxidative enzymes, phosphorylase, and myofibrillar ATPase. In the more chronic forms of denervation, in which there has been reinnervation of muscle fibers by collateral sprouting of axons, we see large groups of fibers of the same histochemical fiber type; this is known as type grouping.

Varying degrees of necrosis, phagocytosis, and regeneration of muscle fibers are the hallmarks of myopathic disorders. Internal nuclei and proliferation of endomysial connective tissue around individual muscle fibers are also characteristic.

ANTERIOR HORN CELL DISEASES OF INFANCY AND CHILDHOOD

INFANTILE SPINAL MUSCULAR ATROPHY

Infantile spinal muscular atrophy (ISMA), or Werdnig-Hoffmann disease, is a progressive anterior horn cell disease of infancy. It is most commonly inherited as an autosomal recessive trait and rarely as an autosomal dominant trait.

Much confusion still surrounds the terms "amyotonia congenita," or Oppenheim's disease. In 1900 Oppenheim briefly described what he called myatonia congenita, later called amyotonia congenita by Collier and Wilson (1908). As originally described it referred to a nonfamilial form of muscle weakness and hypotonia present at birth that tended to improve slowly but steadily. Subsequent follow-up of Oppenheim's original six patients revealed at least two separate conditions; thus, it described only a syndrome of a "floppy" infant at birth, whose prognosis could not be accurately predicted. It appears now that this terminology is confusing and should be avoided since it adds little to our understanding.

CLINICAL FEATURES

The onset of ISMA may occur at any time during the first 2 years of life. Onset at birth or during the first 2 months results in a hypotonic infant who fails to achieve motor skills such as head control or the ability to turn over, sit, or stand. These infants have severe proximal limb weakness that often results in a "frog-leg position," in which the legs are abducted at the hips and flexed at the knees. The shoulders may also be abducted with flexion at the elbows. Spontaneous movements are limited to distal muscles of the arms and legs. Tongue fasciculations are common. Diaphragmatic breathing with flaring of the lower ribs and an associated pectus excavatum is commonly encountered. Other important signs include absent or depressed deep tendon reflexes and a normal sensory examination. Fasciculations are not characteristically present in the limb muscles by clinical observation because of the excess subcutaneous fat in infancy. In these children life expectancy is rarely beyond 3 years of age owing to complications, such as pulmonary infection.

Patients with the onset of the disease after the first 12 months usually exhibit a less fulminating course with slow progression similar to juvenile spinal muscular atrophy, as discussed in a later section of this article. The distribution of weakness is similar but less severe than that described with early onset, and their lower extremities are weaker than their upper extremities. Some of these children acquire the ability to stand with assistance, and some can learn to walk.

LABORATORY FINDINGS

Serum enzyme values are usually not elevated in this disease. Electrodiagnostic studies reveal fibrillation and fasciculation potentials with a reduced number of motor unit potentials as compared to strength of contraction.

Muscle biopsy with histochemical staining may show a characteristic pattern with hypertrophy of type I muscle fibers as well as atrophy preferentially affecting type I fibers with type II fibers remaining about normal in size. In other areas entire fascicles of muscle fibers may appear atrophic.

PITFALLS IN DIAGNOSIS

The clinician is presented with a variety of diseases in infancy characterized by hypotonia, or "floppiness," that may be confused with ISMA. Many children with a diffuse cerebral encephalopathy from such causes as cerebral birth injury and developmental and degenerative brain disorders may be hypotonic. In these cases, careful examination may reveal signs of cerebral dysfunction such as persistence of a Moro reflex or clenched fists with adduction of the thumbs after 3 months of age. The presence of a tonic neck reflex beyond 6 months of age carries the same significance. Hyperactive deep tendon reflexes are also indicative of upper motor neuron involvement, although reflexes may be normal or even depressed with cerebral hypotonia. One further helpful clue may be Förster's sign, which is flexion of hips when the infant is vertically suspended. Other conditions involving "floppy" infants should also be kept in mind, including a variety of diseases affecting the motor unit. Peripheral neuropathies in the infantile age group are rare, but some polyradiculopathies have been seen. Prolonged nerve conduction velocities may help distinguish this group.

Neonatal myasthenia gravis or transient myasthenia gravis in an infant born to a myasthenic mother should be considered. A decrementing response on repetitive nerve stimulation or a positive edrophonium (Tensilon) test will identify this group. Some diseases of muscle, such as myotonic dystrophy or the glycogen storage disease acid maltase deficiency (Pompe's disease), may present early in infancy. The presence of cardiomegaly and an enlarged liver will help differentiate the latter. In both conditions the EMG shows marked insertional activity. Furthermore, a relatively new group of neuromuscular disorders, sometimes referred to as the "congenital myopathies," may be confused with ISMA. These disorders include central core disease, rod myopathy (nemaline myopathy), myotubular myopathy (centronuclear myopathy), and also congenital fiber type disproportion. Muscle biopsy must be used to distinguish these neuromuscular disorders from ISMA.

JUVENILE SPINAL MUSCULAR ATROPHY

Juvenile spinal muscular atrophy (JSMA), or the Wohlfart-Kugelberg-Welander disease, is also a progressive anterior horn cell disease but appears at a later age than ISMA; the mean age of onset is about 9 years. Patients have been described with onset as early as age 2 years or as late as age 17. It is inherited most frequently as an autosomal recessive trait, but there have been occasional reports of autosomal dominant inheritance.

CLINICAL FEATURES

The most striking feature of this disease is the marked proximal muscle weakness, with greater involvement of the legs. This leads to an early waddling gait; difficulties in running, jumping, and climbing stairs; and the presence of Gowers' sign on examination, which is characterized by the patient climbing up his own legs when rising from the floor. The proximal upper extremity muscles may also be involved,

occurring later in the course of the disease, resulting in atrophy of the shoulder girdle muscles and difficulty in holding the arms above the head. Weakness of muscles innervated by cranial nerves is not a prominent part of the clinical picture, although occasional patients are seen with fasciculations of tongue and sternocleidomastoid muscle weakness. Rare examples of extraocular muscle weakness have been reported. Deep tendon reflexes are usually reduced or absent. No sensory abnormalities are found on examination.

The disease is one in which symptoms progress very slowly. In general the patients continue to ambulate for many years after the onset of their illness.

LABORATORY FINDINGS

Despite the rather typical pathologic alterations of the anterior horn cells shown to exist in this disease by postmortem observation, laboratory evaluation may reveal signs of muscle involvement. Elevations of CPK and other serum enzymes are frequently encountered but never reach the magnitude seen in Duchenne muscular dystrophy.

Electrodiagnostic studies are extremely helpful and show very large amplitude motor unit potentials of increased size and duration, typical of anterior horn cell disease. Fasciculation potentials are also frequently encountered. Conduction velocities are normal.

On muscle biopsy the signs of denervation predominate, but some myopathic features are also seen. These features include occasional fibers undergoing necrosis and phagocytosis and some fibers with internal nuclei. This finding appears to correlate with elevated serum enzymes.

PITFALLS IN DIAGNOSIS

Owing to the distribution of weakness observed in these patients — that is, a proximal distribution, which is generally considered atypical of neuropathic disease — these patients are frequently confused with those having progressive forms of muscular dystrophy. JSMA with an early onset must be differentiated from Duchenne muscular dystrophy, and that which appears later must be differentiated from the more chronic form of X-linked recessive muscular dystrophy described by Becker or from limb-girdle dystrophy. The most reliable means of differentiation are electromyography and muscle biopsy. The two varieties of anterior horn cell disease described here (ISMA and JSMA) may form a continuum of disease with overlap between the late onset of ISMA and the early onset of JSMA.

PROGRESSIVE MUSCULAR DYSTROPHIES

The progressive muscular dystrophies are often discussed together as a group of related disorders. This is somewhat misleading, since they are quite distinct, and this should not suggest that they are related etiologically. The only justification for considering these diseases together is that they are hereditary conditions characterized by progressive muscle weakness of unknown cause. The major forms of muscular dystrophy are now separated by their clinical presentation and genetic modes of inheritance.

DUCHENNE MUSCULAR DYSTROPHY

Duchenne muscular dystrophy (DMD) is a progressive disease of skeletal muscle transmitted as an X-linked recessive trait. It is also called X-linked pseudohypertrophic muscular dystrophy, although pseudohypertrophy is not limited to or diagnostic of DMD. The mutation rate is among the highest of known genes, and about one third of new cases are thought to be mutations. Some recent studies suggest that more sensitive methods of carrier detection provide evidence that new mutations are much less common than previously estimated.

CLINICAL FEATURES

The clinical recognition of the disease is made early in the first decade of life, usually by age 3 to 4 years. Subtle manifestations of the disease, however, are often present prior to this time, with careful histories revealing a delay in developmental milestones. The first muscles affected are the hip extensors (glutei maximi) followed by involvement of hip abductors (glutei medii). This distribution of weakness results in lumbar lordosis and a "waddling" gait. As the weakness progresses the child has difficulty in climbing stairs and in most cases never develops the ability to run normally. Joint muscle tightness represents an early manifestation of the disease and may be prominent by age 6. Muscle groups showing early tightness include tensor fascia lata and gastrocnemius-soleus. As the disease progresses, weakness of muscles of the upper extremity becomes prominent.

A positive Gowers' sign is commonly seen. Another frequently observed sign is enlargement of the calf muscles, which are often said to feel "rubbery." Weakness in cranial nerve distribution is not common. Reflexes are usually difficult to elicit from biceps, triceps, and quadriceps, but ankle jerks are characteristically preserved until late in the course of the disease. Ultimately, muscle weakness leads to wheelchair confinement, usually by age 10.

A significant percentage of DMD children, estimated at 30 per cent, have IQ's below 75. This is not related to environmental factors. No consistent morphologic substrate for mental subnormality has been observed in the brain. DMD patients also have frequent changes on electrocardiograms consisting of tall right precordial R waves and deep Q waves in limb or left precordial leads. Late in the disease a variety of cardiac arrhythmias, of both atrial and ventricular origin, may be observed.

A more chronic form of X-linked recessive muscular dystrophy was originally described by Becker. It is characterized by a later onset with much slower progression. In this form of muscular dystrophy ability to walk is preserved much longer than in DMD. The distribution of weakness mimics that observed in Duchenne dystrophy, and calf enlargement is also seen.

LABORATORY FINDINGS

Serum enzyme elevations in DMD reach extremely high levels, particularly during the early and middle stages of the disease. In the late stage of the disease when the muscle mass has been severely reduced, serum enzyme levels may be only minimally elevated.

Electromyography shows a myopathic pattern as described, but fibrillation potentials and positive waves are usually seen early in the course of the disease. The histologic changes on muscle biopsy early in the disease show rather characteristic focal groups of muscle fibers undergoing necrosis, phagocytosis, and regeneration. In addition there is variability in fiber size, internal nuclei, and proliferation of endomysial connective tissue. Late in the disease, the biopsy will show rather marked connective proliferation and fatty infiltration.

PITFALLS IN DIAGNOSIS

In the typical clinical presentation with a positive family history, DMD is not difficult to diagnose. In other instances, however, the condition may be extremely difficult to differentiate clinically from JSMA, since the distribution of the weakness is similar in these two disorders. An early clue that should alert the physician to the possibility that a disease other than DMD may be at hand will be a minimally elevated CPK. The EMG and muscle biopsy will differentiate these disorders.

Another disease entity that presents with a clinical picture similar to DMD is the glycogen storage disease, late infantile or juvenile acid maltase deficiency. In acid maltase deficiency disease no involvement of visceral organs is seen as in the infantile form, and skeletal muscle weakness may be the only manifestation. A clue to the presence of this glycogen storage disease may be a patulous anal sphincter on physical examination. On EMG, high-frequency discharges are seen in addition to the usual features of a myopathy. The muscle biopsy will show a vacuolar myopathy with excess glycogen.

FACIOSCAPULOHUMERAL DYSTROPHY

Facioscapulohumeral dystrophy (FSH) is a distinct form of muscular dystrophy affecting primarily the facial and shoulder girdle muscles. It is inherited as an autosomal dominant trait with variable expressivity. It is also called Landouzy-Dejerine dystrophy.

CLINICAL FEATURES

In its typical form the onset of clear-cut clinical weakness is usually not seen until the second decade of life, when shoulder girdle weakness becomes apparent. Careful history taking, however, will often reveal the presence of facial weakness as early as age 6 to 7 years. This is manifested as an inability to develop a full smile or difficulty in sucking through a straw. The trapezius muscle weakness and atrophy result in prominence of bony protuberances around the shoulders, especially of the clavicles and scapulae. Winging and elevation of the scapulae are observed, and the patient has difficulty raising the arms above the head. A loss of muscle bulk and mild weakness of biceps and triceps may be present, but distal upper extremity strength is well preserved. In the lower extremities, the first muscles affected are usually the anterior tibials, leading to foot drop. Less commonly, weakness of the proximal lower extremities and trunk may be observed.

In the distribution of cranial nerves, facial muscle weakness is commonly encountered, particularly of the orbicularis oris, resulting in a transverse smile. Orbicularis oculi weakness produces inability to close the eyes tightly. The extraocular muscles are not involved.

Of all the progressive muscular dystrophies, the degree of limb muscle weakness in FSH may be the most asymmetric, especially early in the course. It should also be noted that a variable expression of the disease is common, and several family members may be affected to different degrees. Often after identification of a propositus, examination of an affected parent or sibling may reveal a mild degree of facial weakness or asymmetrical shoulder girdle involvement.

The disease is characterized by its usual slow progression and long insidious course. Severe disability and wheelchair confinement are unusual. The major exception to this is an accelerated form of the disease in which weakness begins in early childhood. In these patients severe proximal weakness of the lower extremities can result in wheelchair confinement at 10 to 15 years of age. Cardiac involvement is usually not seen as an accompaniment to this form of muscular dystrophy.

LABORATORY FINDINGS

Serum enzyme levels may be normal or slightly elevated. Electromyography reveals a pattern typical of muscle degeneration. In the muscle biopsy, isolated, single scattered fibers undergoing necrosis and phagocytosis are seen. In some cases a biopsy picture indistinguishable from inflammatory myopathy may be present. Despite this histologic picture, these patients do not have polymyositis in the usual sense and do not have significant clinical benefit from steroid therapy.

PITFALLS IN DIAGNOSIS

It has been increasingly emphasized that patients with weakness in the facioscapulohumeral distribution may represent a heterogeneous group of clinical disorders. One should always consider other diagnostic possibilities in patients with this clinical syndrome. A rare congenital myopathy, such as rod myopathy, as well as limited forms of spinal muscular atrophy secondary to anterior horn cell disease, may reproduce the clinical picture. In addition, one should always be on the lookout for true polymyositis, which rarely may produce an overlapping clinical presentation. In order for the physician to avoid mistaken diagnoses, a careful diagnostic work-up is recommended for patients with weakness in a facioscapulohumeral distribution, particularly if there is no family history. Additionally, electrodiagnostic studies and muscle biopsy should be performed. A clinical dilemma may ensue in a patient whose case has occurred sporadically with inflammatory changes on biopsy: distinction from a collagen vascular disease is virtually impossible. In this instance careful review of the clinical course and examination of other family members may be necessary to arrive at the correct diagnosis.

LIMB-GIRDLE DYSTROPHY

The term limb-girdle dystrophy refers to a less distinct, clinically heterogeneous group of patients with progressive muscle weakness inherited as an autosomal recessive trait. Sporadic cases are common.

It should be recognized that at present this category of muscular dystrophy is the least well defined and probably represents several distinct etiologic groups. The term limb-girdle is merely descriptive of the distribution of weakness.

The onset of this disease is usually in the second and third decades of life or even later. It is characterized by weakness in the shoulder or pelvic girdles and proximal muscles. The exact distribution of weakness and the rate of progression depend upon the individual case. Weakness in the upper extremities produces difficulty in raising the arms above the head, and proximal lower extremity weakness results in difficulty climbing stairs or rising from chairs. Gowers' sign may also be observed. Varying degrees of trunk and neck muscle weakness can be seen, but cranial nerve muscles are rarely affected. In general the disease is one of insidious slow progression with variable prognosis.

LABORATORY FINDINGS

Minimal to moderate elevations of serum enzymes are usually seen. The electromyogram and muscle biopsy show the nonspecific changes of a primary muscle disease as previously described.

PITFALLS IN DIAGNOSIS

Continued investigation of neuromuscular disorders has demonstrated that the syndrome of limb-girdle dystrophy can be simulated by a variety of diseases affecting the motor unit. As discussed, JSMA may produce a similar clinical picture and can be differentiated by EMG and muscle biopsy. Furthermore, the late onset of rod myopathy and various forms of glycogen storage disease (acid maltase deficiency, phosphorylase deficiency, and debrancher enzyme deficiency) and lipid storage disease (carnitine deficiency) can also simulate the picture of limb-girdle dystrophy. These observations illustrate our continued need for histologic diagnosis in this group of patients.

MYOTONIC MUSCULAR DYSTROPHY

Myotonic muscular dystrophy is a slowly progressive disease of skeletal muscle characterized by ptosis, facial, neck, and distal limb muscle weakness associated with myotonia, an abnormal persistence of muscle contraction with inability to relax. Involvement of other organ systems is common in myotonic dystrophy. The disease is transmitted as an autosomal dominant trait. Synonyms for this syndrome include myotonia atrophica and dystrophia myotonica.

CLINICAL FEATURES

The onset is usually late in the first decade or in the second decade of life. Either myotonia or weakness may be the initial manifestation. If myotonia is the presenting complaint, the patients may have difficulty with hand grip, particularly in opening jars, or they may complain of "stiffness" in the muscles. These symptoms are accentuated by cold weather. If the complaints are primarily those of weakness, the distribution is distal in the limb muscles involving the hands or the dorsiflexors of the feet. As the patients are seen they often present a rather characteristic clinical picture. Frontal baldness in males may be quite apparent, as is atrophy of the temporalis muscle and bilateral ptosis. Lack of facial expression due to weakness of facial muscles is common, and palatal weakness may lead to a nasal speech. Neck muscle weakness, particularly involving the flexors and sternocleidomastoids, may result in the appearance of a "swan neck" deformity. In the limbs, loss of strength and atrophy, as mentioned, are mainly distal. Myotonia can be elicited by percussion in several areas including the tongue, forearm muscles, and thenar eminence. In each site, striking the muscle with the reflex hammer results in a sustained muscle contraction. In the tongue this may be seen by holding the tongue between two tongue depressors. Gentle percussion then results in a sustained contraction on the lateral aspects.

It should be emphasized that this disease is associated with various systemic abnormalities. Early frontal baldness is frequently observed, as are posterior subcapsular cataracts, which are most easily identified by slit-lamp examination. In approximately one fourth of the patients cataracts may be severe enough to impair vision. In males testicular atrophy is common, and females may have irregular menses. Skull x-rays may show hyperostosis frontalis interna, large paranasal sinuses, and a sella turcica that appears small but has a normal volume. The serum protein electrophoresis may show low gamma globulin, which is due to hypercatabolism of immunoglobulin G (IgG). Abnormal electrocardiograms due to disturbances of intraventricular conduction may be seen. Another common manifestation of the disease is mental subnormality.

In most cases this is a very slowly progressive disease. An important aspect of this syndrome is its variable expressivity, and many patients will not exhibit all of the features described.

Exceptions to the usual presentation are patients who present during infancy or in the neonatal period with difficulties in swallowing and sucking, facial diplegia, ptosis, and hypotonia. These infants, usually born to affected mothers, may have delayed motor milestones.

LABORATORY FINDINGS

Serum enzymes are usually normal or minimally elevated. The EMG provides a valuable tool in the diagnosis of this disorder because electrical myotonia may be present when other manifestations of the disease are subtle. The EMG may also show motor unit potentials of small size and short duration with increased recruitment, depending on the degree of involvement. The muscle biopsy is characterized early by mild atrophy of muscle fibers with frequent preference for type I fibers, although both types may be involved. Later in the course of the disease the muscle shows more variability in fiber size with some atrophic fibers, nuclear clumps, and many internal nuclei. It should be emphasized that necrosis, phagocytosis, and marked connective tissue proliferation, as seen in DMD, are not prominent, although ring fibers and sarcoplasmic masses may be seen in severely affected patients.

PITFALLS IN DIAGNOSIS

Because of the characteristic appearance of these patients, there is no problem in making the diagnosis. Early in the course, however, before weakness is present, it may be quite difficult to differentiate from myotonia congenita (Thomsen's disease). In the latter disease the outstanding features are generalized myotonia and muscle stiffness. The patients often exhibit striking muscle hypertrophy, but no weakness is found on examination if the patients are given adequate time to "warm up." The systemic abnormalities described are not part of myotonia congenita. It should also be recognized that the clinical phenomenon of myotonia can be seen in hyperkalemic periodic paralysis and also rarely in hypokalemic periodic paralysis. A very rare disorder called paramyotonia congenita is characterized by clinical myotonia with attacks of generalized weakness that are induced by cold. Paramyotonia congenita, however, is probably more closely related to hyperkalemic periodic paralysis than to myotonic dystrophy or myotonia congenita.

OCULAR INVOLVEMENT IN "MUSCULAR DYSTROPHY"

A group of patients exists who present with a clinical syndrome characterized chiefly by ptosis and progressive external ophthalmoplegia (PEO) associated with varying degrees of dysphagia and limb muscle weakness. The disease in these patients can perhaps be best separated into two classifications. One type, known as *oculopharyngeal muscular dystrophy,* is particularly rare. The disorder is characterized by autosomal dominant inheritance in persons of French-Canadian descent. More recently it has also been described in Spanish-American families in the southwestern United States. The disease usually begins in the third or fourth decade with ptosis that may be associated with or followed by pharyngeal and limb weakness. Significant debilitation may occur, with severe loss of swallowing resulting in marked weight loss. The disease is usually one of slow progression over many years.

The other group of PEO patients has a rather widespread multisystem disorder. The disorder is often referred to as *oculocraniosomatic neuromuscular disease with ragged-red fibers.* The term "ragged-red fibers" is derived from a characteristic change in limb skeletal muscle shown on biopsy. In these biopsies approximately 3 to 20 per cent of muscle fibers show accumulation of abnormal mitochondria often associated with excessive lipid droplets. These abnormal fibers appear "ragged red" in the modified trichrome stain. Ragged-red fibers may be present in a clinically normal limb muscle.

Despite this change in the limb muscles, the cause of the extraocular muscle weakness is still a matter of speculation. While some authors have claimed that the eye muscles also show ragged-red fibers, this has not been clearly established. The disease may be inherited as an autosomal dominant trait but many cases occur sporadically. The muscle changes may be associated with a wide range of central and peripheral nervous system involvement that is variable from patient to patient. Abnormalities may include hearing loss of mixed conductive and sensorineural type, abnormal caloric responses on vestibular testing, electroencephalographic abnormalities, slowing of nerve conduction velocities, cerebellar ataxia, corticospinal tract involvement, and mental subnormality. Cerebrospinal fluid protein elevation is common.

Involvement of other organ systems has also been seen in association with this syndrome. These include cardiac conduction defects, retinal pigmentary degeneration, growth retardation, and decreased hydroxycorticoid and 17-ketosteroid excretion. The description of this disease should make it somewhat clear why there has been reluctance to call it a form of muscular dystrophy.

Section 15

OBSTETRICS AND GYNECOLOGY

BREAST LESIONS

By DAVID W. KINNE, M.D.,
and GUY F. ROBBINS, M.D.

New York, New York

The failure of women to seek medical attention concerning significant changes in their breasts continues to be a major deterrent in diagnosing and treating breast carcinoma, precancerous lesions, and the many benign entities that are sometimes thought to be carcinomas until they are studied histologically. The physician's armamentarium for detecting significant breast abnormalities has been enhanced by low-dose mammography or xerography for careful physical examination of the breasts. The routine use of conventional mammography or xerography when lumps or thickenings exist not only gives important information as to the type of clinical mass under observation but also frequently demonstrates suspicious areas elsewhere that are not detectable by palpation. Currently, the definitive diagnosis of breast lesions must be made by histologic study of involved tissues.

THE WOMAN'S RESPONSIBILITY

Although many women have learned how to examine their breasts regularly, surveys have demonstrated that this form of detection is not utilized by most women. This is especially true of women of minority groups. Unfortunately, some women who do detect postmenstrual thickenings, well-circumscribed masses, bloody nipple discharge, or persistent (over 1 month) postmenopausal thickenings do not seek immediate medical advice. Many procrastinate for weeks, months, or even years before they are examined by a physician.

THE PHYSICIAN'S RESPONSIBILITY

Physicians must become more involved in teaching their patients to do breast self-examination. The American Cancer Society and the National Cancer Institute have excellent publications on breast self-examination that are available at no cost to physicians for distribution to their patients. Physicians are aware that persistent postmenstrual and postmenopausal thickenings may well be caused by small breast cancers. Certainly most of these will prove to be benign, but mammograms and clinical palpation have a recognized error rate of 20 to 40 per cent. Therefore histologic study of these lesions by a pathologist is currently the only way of making the definitive diagnosis.

Other diagnostic tests, such as thermography, sonography, and computed tomography, are being evaluated. Biologic markers, to date, have proved less accurate than palpation and mammography. We and many others have little faith in cytologic examination of serous or bloody nipple discharge or nonbloody fluid aspirated from a cyst. Bloody fluid aspirated from a cyst may prove on cytologic examination to be from a carcinoma. Bloody or serous nipple discharge is an indication for major duct excision. Overall, about 10 per cent of women with this symptom prove to have carcinoma, but the figure is higher in older patients. Many others will have atypical papillomatosis, a condition considered to be a precancerous lesion.

Fortunately, many masses palpated in the breasts of women prove to be gross cysts that can be diagnosed and treated definitively by needle aspiration. If bloody fluid is obtained, or if the mass does not completely subside after aspiration, we advise surgical excision. In any event, a mammogram after aspiration is advisable to determine whether or not suspicious nonpalpable lesions exist in either breast.

Physicians should plan careful follow-up for patients in groups at high risk for developing breast carcinoma, such as patients with positive family histories and those who have had breast cancer on one side or biopsy of a precancerous lesion. Such patients should be examined frequently (every 3 to 6 months), with mammography done periodically.

BIOPSY PROCEDURES

The object of taking a specimen for breast biopsy is to give the pathologist enough material to make a diagnosis and for the surgeon to remove all the suspicious area from the breast.

Outpatient Biopsy. At our institution, this procedure, done under local anesthesia, is reserved for superficial, well-circumscribed lesions thought to be benign, such as fibroadenomas in young women. However, with an increase across the country in outpatient surgery under general anesthesia, many definitive breast biopsies are being done in this manner.

Aspiration Biopsy. Large carcinomas of the breast can frequently be diagnosed by aspiration preoperatively under local anesthesia. Our pathologist prefers cytologic examination of such smears to needle aspiration in which a core of tissue is removed. Aspiration is done with a large-bore needle and a large syringe, with enough cellular material and blood drawn out to prepare at least four slides.

Incisional Biopsy. If aspiration biopsy of a clinical carcinoma does not establish the diagnosis with certainty, incisional wedge biopsy under general anesthesia becomes the preferred way of doing this. Minimal dissection and handling of the cancer is required, as well as minimal interference with tissue planes to be developed during mastectomy. In this situation, with a large cancer that is apparent clinically, there is no role for the so-called two-stage procedure, in our opinion. The patient should be brought to the operating room after complete diagnostic evaluation has been carried out and should be prepared to undergo mastectomy following the biopsy.

Excisional Biopsy. Benign and precancerous lesions, as well as small carcinomas, should be completely excised under general anesthesia. A rim of surrounding breast tissue that appears normal is often included with suspicious lesions to be examined for extension of carcinoma and for accurate measurement of its size. The skin incision may be circumareolar or curvilinear if the lesion is considered to be benign, but no incision should be placed in such a way as to interfere with possible subsequent mastectomy.

For nonpalpable lesions discovered by mammography, preoperative localization of the area by mammogram is often helpful. The patient is brought to the x-ray suite a few hours before surgery, and a needle under x-ray control is placed near the lesion. Then a small amount of radiopaque dye mixed with methylene blue is injected near the lesion. Continued injection as the needle is withdrawn may allow the surgeon to dissect the needle tract and easily remove the suspicious area. Most often, because these lesions are areas of fine calcifications, specimen mammography is required to ensure complete removal.

Opposite Breast Biopsy. In patients with carcinoma of one breast, biopsy of the other breast is indicated if any suspicious areas are present on physical examination or mammography. Although the role of blind, mirror image biopsy remains to be determined, it is indicated for lesions that commonly are bilateral (such as lobular carcinoma) or if multicentric lesions are present on the primary side. A yield of 10 to 15 per cent of carcinoma in the second breast may be expected with this procedure.

OVARIAN TUMORS

By HERBERT J. BUCHSBAUM, M.D.,
and J. PETER FORNEY, III, M.D.
Dallas, Texas

The ovary is a complex organ with endocrine and reproductive function. It can be the site of a host of functional and neoplastic tumors. These tumors can be solid or cystic, endocrine active or inactive, benign or malignant.

Cystic tumors are generally benign; solid tumors are far more likely to be malignant. The most critical factor in evaluating an ovarian tumor is to determine whether it is benign or malignant. The poor prognosis in ovarian carcinoma is related to advanced stage at diagnosis. Fully two thirds of patients have intraperitoneal dissemination when the diagnosis is first established.

FUNCTIONAL CYSTS

Follicle and corpus lutein cysts are found only in ovulating women. Germinal inclusion cysts occur in postmenopausal women and rarely exceed 3 to 4 cm in diameter. During pregnancy, and more commonly with hydatidiform mole, the ovaries may contain theca-lutein cysts. These can reach enormous size but regress spontaneously with decline in human chorionic gonadotropin (HCG). Hirsute and anovulatory women (Stein-Leventhal disease) may have bilaterally enlarged polycystic ovaries.

All of these functional tumors are self-limiting and cause serious problems only when the pedicle undergoes torsion and infarction, or when they rupture.

NEOPLASTIC TUMORS

Neoplastic tumors can arise from any of the varied ovarian tissues: the celomic epithelium, the supporting stroma, or the germ cells. An appropriate classification of ovarian neoplasms is that based on tissue of origin (Table 1). Tumors arising from the celomic epithelium are by far the most common, accounting for 85 to 90 per cent of all neoplasms. These tumors are most common in perimenopausal and postmenopausal women. Tumors arising from germ cells occur most commonly in children and adolescents. Gonadal stromal tumors can be found in

Table 1. *Histologic Classification of Ovarian Tumors*

1. Epithelial tumors
   a. Serous
   b. Mucinous
   c. Endometrioid
   d. Clear cell
   e. Brenner
2. Sex cord-stromal tumors
   a. Granulosa cell
   b. Thecoma
   c. Fibroma
   d. Androblastomas (Sertoli-Leydig tumors)
   e. Gynandroblastoma
3. Germ cell tumors
   a. Dysgerminoma
   b. Endodermal sinus tumor
   c. Embryonal carcinoma
   d. Polyembryoma
   e. Choriocarcinoma
   f. Teratomas
      (1) Immature
      (2) Mature
      (3) Monodermal (e.g., struma ovarii)
   g. Mixed forms

any age group and can be hormone-producing.

The malignant tumors arise in their benign counterparts, e.g., mucinous cystadenocarcinomas arise in mucinous cystadenomas. Recently, a histologically intermediate form has been identified: *borderline tumors.* These tumors appear histologically to be of low malignant potential and may metastasize, but they have a very good prognosis.

There are nearly 20,000 new cases of ovarian carcinoma diagnosed annually in this country and approximately 11,000 deaths due to this disease. One in 70 females born will develop ovarian carcinoma during her lifetime; during the fifth and sixth decades of life, one in 100 women will die of ovarian carcinoma.

There are no well-defined epidemiologic characteristics for women at risk; however, epithelial malignancies develop more commonly in white women of low parity.

The ovary can also be the site of metastatic tumors, usually arising from a primary tumor in the endometrium, breast, or bowel.

HISTORY

A complete medical history can give valuable clues as to the nature of an ovarian tumor. Follicle and corpus luteum cysts occur only in ovulating women; germinal inclusion cysts usually in postmenopausal women. Granulosa-theca cell tumors may be estrogen-producing and cause postmenopausal bleeding in elderly women or premature sexual development in youngsters. Virilization with hirsutism and deepening voice accompany androgen-secreting tumors.

SYMPTOMS

Symptoms from ovarian tumors are a reflection of tumor size and generally relate to pressure on the bladder, rectum, or other abdominal viscera. Torsion of the infundibulopelvic ligament with infarction or rupture of a cystic tumor causes sharp pain.

In ovarian carcinoma, abdominal distention resulting from ascites, and shortness of breath, are the most common presenting symptoms. Upper abdominal metastases may produce bloating, heartburn, and nausea simulating primary gastrointestinal disease.

PHYSICAL EXAMINATION

In evaluating an ovarian tumor a complete physical examination must be carried out, with particular attention directed to the abdominal and pelvic examinations.

The finding of ascites is an ominous sign, suggestive of malignant ovarian neoplasm. On pelvic examination, mobile and unilateral cystic lesions are generally benign, while solid, fixed, and bilateral tumors and cul-de-sac nodularity found on rectovaginal examination are suggestive of malignant neoplasm. Size of an ovarian tumor gives no clue as to its histologic character; the largest are usually mucinous cystadenomas.

LABORATORY STUDIES

Unfortunately, the clinical laboratory is of little use in the diagnosis of ovarian tumors. In early ovarian neoplasia there are no demonstrable chemical, hematologic, or enzymatic derangements; in advanced disease, anemia, hypoalbuminemia, and an elevation of lactic dehydrogenase may be present.

With gonadal stromal tumors and clinical evidence of endocrine activity, there may be an elevation in serum testosterone or estradiol. Virilized women with a normal 24-hour urine 17-ketosteroid determination (<15 mg per 24 hours) but an elevated serum testosterone (>1 nanogram per ml) are assumed to have an ovarian stromal tumor until proven otherwise.

Radioimmunoassay for specific tumor markers, while the most promising diagnostic tool for detection of asymptomatic ovarian neoplasms, is at present not sufficiently sensitive or specific enough for clinical use. Radioimmunoassay for HCG in ovarian choriocarcinoma and for alpha-feto protein in endodermal sinus tumors, however, is of utility in both diagnosis and follow-up of patients with these rare germ cell tumors.

X-Rays

Ovarian tumors will produce nonspecific soft tissue densities on scout films of the pelvis. Only rarely will specific patterns of calcification in an ovarian teratoma or a myoma be seen. Gastrointestinal contrast studies can be helpful in eliminating primary bowel neoplasms from the differential diagnosis and in identifying the size and site of the ovarian tumor by demonstrating displacement of the large and small bowel.

A chest x-ray should be performed to exclude pulmonary metastases or pleural effusion. An intravenous pyelogram may disclose urinary tract obstruction or an ectopic kidney.

Lymphangiography, venography, and arteriography have no proven value in the evaluation of ovarian tumors.

Scans

Isotope scans have no role in the delineation of ovarian tumors. Computerized tomography has had only limited application in the diagnosis of benign and malignant tumors. The cost is still too high and the experience with this technique too limited to suggest its use in evaluating ovarian tumors.

Ultrasonography

Pelvic ultrasonography has been used extensively in the assessment of ovarian tumors. It is a noninvasive and painless method for examination of pelvic tumors in three dimensions. While ultrasound does not establish a histologic diagnosis, it can give useful clues as to the nature of pelvic masses and it allows for accurate assessment of dimensions and consistency. Unilocular cysts are likely to be benign, while multicystic and solid tumors are commonly malignant. Additionally, ascites not apparent on clinical examination can be identified by sonography.

Cytology

Occasionally, cells exfoliated from an ovarian neoplasm may be transported via the fallopian tube and uterus to be detected by cervicovaginal cytology (Papanicolaou smear). Generally, the Pap smear is positive only if ovarian malignancy has metastasized to the uterine cavity or vagina. More rewarding than cytology is biopsy of any vaginal lesions and endometrial sampling. Hyperplastic endometrium and carcinoma are not infrequent findings in women with estrogen-producing tumors of stromal origin or in celomic epithelial tumors with luteinized gonadal stroma.

Advanced ovarian carcinoma is often associated with ascites, with malignant cells in the fluid. Diagnostic paracentesis is rarely indicated. Paracentesis should be performed only after ultrasonography has demonstrated that the abdominal distention is a result of ascites and not a result of a large fluid-filled cyst.

Laparoscopy

While laparoscopy may verify the presence of a suspected pelvic tumor, rarely can visual examination alone determine its clinical significance. Laparoscopically directed cyst aspiration or biopsy, in most situations, is contraindicated because of the risks involved with spillage of malignant cells and inadequate sampling of the ovarian tumors. Furthermore, it is impossible to estimate the resectability of a tumor by laparoscopic examination alone: examination of the abdominal contents is limited and the retroperitoneal areas are inaccessible.

Celiotomy

Exploratory celiotomy (laparotomy) is the final and definitive diagnostic procedure in assessing ovarian tumors. In benign tumors and in early ovarian carcinoma it allows for complete extirpation. In more advanced ovarian carcinoma it allows the surgeon to explore adequately and stage the disease and to obtain biopsies of representative tissue for histologic examination, and it allows for the performance of reduction surgery. In addition to local, hematologic, and lymphatic spread, ovarian carcinoma can involve intraperitoneal structures through implantation metastases. No serosal surface is immune. Malignant cells exfoliated by the neoplasm are borne in a clockwise current that runs from the left upper quadrant to the right upper quadrant. The current is maintained by the respiratory movement of the diaphragms, the bowel peristalsis, and the visceral suspensory ligaments.

For these reasons, a complete staging celiotomy should include visual or digital examination, or both, of the inferior surface of the diaphragms, both surfaces of the liver, serosal surface of small and large bowel and their mesenteries, the paracolonic gutters, and the para-aortic lymph nodes. The pelvic viscera and parietal peritoneum should be carefully examined and any suspicious areas biopsied. All fluid present in the abdomen should be aspirated for cytologic examination. If no fluid is found in the peritoneal cavity, washings should be obtained separately from the pelvis and the paracolonic gutters, and from above the liver.

SECOND-LOOK SURGERY

If surgery, chemotherapy and/or radiation therapy in advanced ovarian carcinoma should result in a complete clinical remission, it is becoming increasingly popular to perform a "second-look" operation. This is most often a diagnostic procedure to confirm remission. If no evidence of disease is found, it will allow the physician to discontinue chemotherapy. Rarely, a single site of tumor will be found that can be completely resected. Additionally, when residual disease is found, a new form of therapy can be instituted.

BENIGN UTERINE TUMORS

By THOMAS R. BRYANT, M.D.
Oklahoma City, Oklahoma

Benign tumors of the uterus are commonly seen in clinical practice. This discussion concentrates on the types of tumors that the practicing physician is most likely to encounter. For simplification, the tumors are grouped anatomically according to their location in the uterus: those occurring in the cervix and those occurring in the uterine corpus.

CERVIX

Condylomata Acuminata (Venereal Warts). These verrucous growths may occur solely on the cervix, although they are more commonly seen in association with lesions of the vulva and vagina. They are usually asymptomatic. Diagnosis may be confirmed by biopsy.

Cervical Papillomas. These friable papillary excrescences on the surface of the cervix may cause irregular spotting or bleeding, particularly with irritation such as coitus. They are seen most often in pregnancy and tend to regress after the pregnancy has ended. Since such lesions are uncommon in the nonpregnant female, they should probably be biopsied in these women to confirm the diagnosis.

Nabothian Cysts. Although not true tumors, these white or pink cysts are frequently seen on the cervices of parous women. They cause no symptoms and have no clinical significance.

Cervical Polyps. These are formed from a hyperplastic area of cervical tissue that subsequently becomes pedunculated. They are usually quite vascular and are most commonly covered with a single layer of endocervical columnar epithelium. For this reason, they are a common cause of intermenstrual or postcoital bleeding. They can usually be seen readily on examination, appearing as a red velvety mass protruding from the cervical os.

CORPUS UTERI

Leiomyomas (Fibromyomas, Fibroids). These benign tumors of smooth muscle and fibrous tissue are the most common pelvic tumors in women. They may occur at any age, although they are most common during the fourth and fifth decades of life. They are somewhat more common in black women than in white women. Myomas are frequently asymptomatic; but when symptoms occur, they are usually related to the location of the tumors.

Submucous myomas occur just beneath the endometrium. They may cause hypermenorrhea or, less commonly, intermenstrual bleeding. The uterus may or may not be enlarged on examination. Occasionally, submucous fibroids become pedunculated, and cramping may occur as the uterus tries to rid itself of the tumor. In these cases, the tumor may be visible in the cervical os. In most cases, however, the diagnosis depends on uterine curettage, both to rule out endometrial pathology and to confirm the presence of irregularities of the uterine cavity.

Intramural myomas are the most common and occur within the muscular wall of the uterus. Symptoms of pelvic pressure and urinary frequency may be present with large tumors. Crampy or constant pelvic pain may be seen with degeneration of the tumors. Dysmenorrhea may be associated. Uterine enlargement is usually noted on examination. In the case of a large, solitary intramural fibroid, the uterus may be symmetrically enlarged and may simulate a gravid uterus. If examination and pregnancy test are inconclusive, ultrasound is a valuable tool in differentiating these conditions.

Subserous myomas occur just beneath the uterine serosa and are usually encountered on examination as the characteristic firm, "knobby," enlarged uterus. Symptoms, if present, are usually related to increasing size or to degeneration, as described with intramural tumors. If the fibroids grow between the leaves of the broad ligament, they are known as *interligamentous* myomas. On intravenous pyelography these may account for deviation of the distal ureter, or, in rare cases, partial or complete obstruction with hydroureter and hydronephrosis.

Subserous myomas may occasionally become pedunculated. If torsion of the pedicle occurs, infarction of the tumor may cause sudden pain, fever, leukocytosis, nausea, and signs of peritoneal irritation. In the absence of torsion, a pedunculated fibroid is usually found as an adnexal mass on examination. Ultrasound may be helpful in differentiating these from cystic ovarian tumors; but in cases in which doubt exists, and particularly in postmenopausal patients, surgical evaluation is indicated.

Myomas in any location tend to enlarge during pregnancy or with the administration of exogenous estrogen. The tumors usually shrink following the menopause. Malignancy, although rare, should be suspected in any fibroid that initially arises or enlarges after menopause, or that enlarges rapidly at any age. This diagnosis can be confirmed only by surgical removal, with microscopic examination of the tumor.

Adenomyosis. This is a condition in which the endometrial glands and stroma grow within the muscular wall of the uterus. A triad of enlarged uterus, hypermenorrhea, and dysmenorrhea has been described with adenomyosis. However, the condition is often encountered as an incidental pathologic finding in uteri removed for other reasons. The true clinical significance therefore remains unclear.

Endometrial Hyperplasia and Polyps. Hyperplasia and polyps of the endometrium may cause no symptoms, or they may be responsible for irregular uterine bleeding. Usually, there are no specific physical findings. Diagnosis is dependent upon uterine curettage, which may be therapeutic as well.

Endolymphatic Stromal Myosis (Stromal Endometriosis). In this unusual condition, islands of endometrial stroma (but no glands) are found in the myometrium, occasionally even in the lumina of blood and lymphatic vessels. The uterus may be enlarged, and irregular bleeding may be seen. However, the main dilemma is for the pathologist, as it is frequently difficult to distinguish this from endometrial sarcoma or mixed Müllerian tumor.

Rare Benign Tumors. Hemangiomas, lymphangiomas, hemangiopericytomas, and lipomas rarely occur within the uterus. They may cause uterine enlargement and irregular bleeding, thus simulating other, more common uterine abnormalities. The correct diagnosis is usually made by the pathologist following hysterectomy.

ENDOMETRIOSIS

By MASON C. ANDREWS, M.D.
Norfolk, Virginia

Endometriosis is one of the most common gynecologic disorders and may produce the symptoms and signs of most others. Early diagnosis and treatment may abort its inherently destructive course.

The lesion consists of endometrial tissue growing outside the uterine cavity. When this occurs in the wall of the uterus (adenomyosis), it produces a somewhat different specific clinical entity and is best considered separately. The inappropriately located foci of endometrium respond to the ovarian hormone cycle with proliferation, multiplication of the number of foci, and local bleeding. This produces local irritation and an attempt by the surrounding tissues to encase the invader with fibrous tissue and to absorb it with macrophages. The success of this host resistance varies greatly; some patients live comfortably with endometriosis with little or no progress, whereas in others the process is rapidly progressive and destructive of surrounding tissues through the production of scar tissue and accumulations of old blood.

When the menstrual cycle ceases, the ectopic endometrium becomes atrophic, the host healing prevails, and signs and symptoms disappear almost invariably. During pregnancy, the cessation of cyclic stimulation of the ectopic endometrium is accompanied by absence of local bleeding and a change to decidua, permitting the host to arrest progress of the endometriosis at least temporarily and sometimes permanently. Similar results can be achieved by estrogen-progestogen medication (birth control pills) continuously for 7 months in appropriate doses, but these benefits tend to be temporary. Also, the ectopic endometrium may be rendered atrophic for host resorption through systemic medication with danazol (Danocrine), a gonadotropin inhibitor, used in a 7- to 8-month period.

This promises results superior to pseudopregnancy because of the prompt endometrial atrophy and the minimum systemic effects. The duration of beneficial effect still must be determined.

The location of endometriosis seems to follow the path predicted for spread by retrograde menstruation: ovaries (80 per cent); cul-de-sac–uterosacral ligaments (50 per cent); serosa of the uterus, bladder, rectal wall, or pelvic peritoneum (30 per cent). It may also occupy locations that must represent induction by direct implantation: laparotomy or cesarean section scar, episiotomy, or cervix; and locations achieved through lymphatic transmission (umbilicus, pelvic lymph nodes) or embolism (arms, lungs, mouth). Endometriosis may penetrate into and through the wall of the bladder, rectum, or small intestine. It may involve the ureter to the extent of partial or complete occlusion of its lumen.

In most locations the foci form nodular 2- to 10-mm scars that grossly contain purple or brown spots and sometimes trap small pockets of chocolate-colored material formed from old blood. When the ovary is involved, the first result is adhesions; as the process progresses, increasing amounts of old blood accumulate in the ovary, destroying its tissue and causing cysts of various size, usually in the 6- to 8-cm range but up to 15 or more cm on occasion.

Signs and Symptoms

Pain associated with menses, particularly acquired, progressively increasing pain, is considered to be the cardinal symptom of endometriosis and is present in 80 per cent of patients who come to operation. Earlier diagnosis will reduce this figure. It commonly begins in patients in their late 20s or early 30s. It occurs at or just before menses and is characteristically a dull aching low abdominal and back pain. As involvement becomes more extensive, pain precedes menses increasingly. Sterility is present in about 50 per cent of patients found to have endometriosis. With the widespread use of laparoscopy for investigation of infertility patients, unsuspected endometriosis is being found in many more patients. Earlier treatment made possible thereby will improve results in regard to fertility and also reduce the need for more extensive pelvic surgery.

The menstrual flow is increased in amount and duration in about a fourth of patients having endometriosis, and 10 per cent have menometrorrhagia. Possibly, the invasive process in the ovary distorts its ability to produce precisely the necessary ovarian steroids.

Dyspareunia is not usually the symptom for which the patient seeks advice, but is present in about one fourth of all patients, its frequency varying with the extent of the disease. Severity increases near menstruation as well as with the extent of the disease into the cul-de-sac, uterosacral ligaments, and rectosigmoid.

Sudden, severe abdominal pain may result from intra-abdominal leakage or rupture of an endometrial cyst. Because the accumulations of old blood in an endometrial cyst are merely trapped in or next to the ovary with no specific cyst wall, they tend to leak occasionally. The urinary tract is involved in 2 per cent of all patients, with 40 per cent of these patients reporting frequency of urination. In partial ureteral obstruction, costovertebral angle tenderness and repeated urinary tract infections may help to identify the correctable lesion in time to save the kidney.

Adenomyosis tends to present at a later age, in the late 30s or 40s. Typically, it produces increasingly painful periods after years of painless menstruation. Abnormal bleeding is common. The uterus tends to be slightly enlarged and globular.

Physical Findings

The most typical, and usually reliable, physical indicators are uterosacral nodules (one or more) of about 2 to 8 mm that become increasingly tender near a menstrual period.

Involved ovaries may be of normal size and adherent only to the uterus or pelvic wall. These may increase in size to large, tender, fixed cysts. Six to 8 cm is a common size, although they may be much larger and are frequently smaller.

Although the uterus is retroverted in less than a third of the patients, the most typical patient has a tender fixed retroverted uterus, uterosacral nodules, and fixed ovaries. Combined rectovaginal examination helps to evaluate involvement of the cul-de-sac.

Periodic painful enlargement of small nodules in abdominal scars, groin (round ligament), episiotomy scar, or umbilicus corresponding to the menstrual cycle may well signal endometriosis.

Associated Pelvic Pathology

Uterine myomas are found in conjunction with endometriosis in about one fifth of the patients and may make the diagnosis more difficult. Pelvic adhesions of ovaries, uterus, sigmoid, ileum, and omentum are common.

Neoplastic cysts and solid tumors of the ovary

are relatively common in association with endometriosis. Endometrial cancer in endometriosis occurs in about 1 per cent of patients, and this possibility adds to the importance of accurate diagnosis and treatment.

Congenital malformations of the vagina or uterus that prevent egress of menstrual flow greatly increase the risk of endometriosis and damage therefrom. These include imperforate hymen, vaginal atresia, cervical atresia, and noncommunicating horn of a bicornuate uterus. There is great importance in making the diagnosis promptly in girls in their early teens to save future reproductive potential. Cyclic severe pain in a sexually mature amenorrheic girl should lead to examination and correct diagnosis in all but the patient with noncommunicating horn. In such a patient the severity of pain and the examination should lead to a hysterosalpingogram and diagnosis.

DIFFERENTIAL DIAGNOSIS

Any woman between the ages of 20 and 50 years complaining of increasing pain with periods should be strongly suspected of harboring endometriosis or adenomyosis. The presence of tender uterosacral nodules with or without fixed enlarging tender ovaries tends to differentiate this from pelvic inflammatory disease and ectopic pregnancy.

Ovarian or sigmoid neoplasms may produce very similar findings, as may diverticulitis from the colon. The history of increasing cyclic pain should assist in this distinction. After the menopause, appearance of a uterosacral nodule or other signs characteristic of endometriosis at other ages are far more likely to be due to malignancy or diverticulitis.

The direct visualization of the pelvis through the laparoscope can now be so easily performed that the slightest suspicion should be confirmed or dismissed in this way. Also it is possible to find and treat the process much earlier, preserving reproductive potential. Endometriosis has not infrequently caused extensive damage to pelvic organs during a time of physician observation because the signs and symptoms were not severe or definitive enough. Earlier laparoscopy is certainly reducing the number of such cases. The mere finding of isolated small spots of endometriosis may not justify immediate surgery, but precise visual diagnosis makes the management much more reliable. This may include medical suppression or observation.

FUNCTIONAL MENSTRUAL DISORDERS

By PAUL F. BRENNER, M.D.,
and DANIEL R. MISHELL, JR., M.D.
Los Angeles, California

Abnormal uterine bleeding is a common clinical problem. Although determining the correct cause of this symptom is at times difficult, failure to do so may be life-threatening.

The differential diagnosis of abnormal uterine bleeding encompasses many gynecologic pathologic entities as well as many diseases that originate in organs other than the pelvic organs. If an organic cause cannot be found to explain the abnormal bleeding, the condition is categorized as *dysfunctional uterine bleeding*, also referred to as functional uterine bleeding, anovulatory bleeding, and, in the older literature, as metropathia hemorrhagica. Therefore the diagnosis of dysfunctional uterine bleeding is one derived by exclusion. In order to establish the diagnosis of dysfunctional uterine bleeding, the clinician must first eliminate the organic causes of abnormal uterine bleeding by utilizing the appropriate diagnostic aids. There is no symptom complex, clinical sign, or adjunctive diagnostic procedure that is pathognomonic of functional uterine bleeding.

For accurate diagnosis of aberrations of the menstrual cycle, the variations of the normal menstrual cycle should be understood. Menarche normally occurs between the ages of 9 and 16.5 years. Menses normally last 1 to 7 days. The duration of each menstrual cycle normally varies between 21 to 35 days. Total blood loss during menses is normally less than 80 ml with an average of 35 ml.

ABNORMAL UTERINE BLEEDING: INCREASE

Excessive uterine bleeding may be defined as either menstrual cycles shorter than 21 days, menses lasting longer than 7 days, total blood loss greater than 80 ml, or any combination of these. For a specific individual, excessive bleeding may be defined as menses lasting 2 or more days longer than normal or a menstrual flow that requires the use of 2 or more sanitary napkins than usual.

Although it may seem superfluous to mention, it must be stated that abnormal uterine bleeding as perceived by the patient is not always derived from the pelvic organs. Blood seen on a sanitary napkin or in the lavatory may be coming from either the urinary or the gastrointestinal system. If any doubt exists as to the anatomic source of the blood, urinalysis and stool guaiac test should be performed.

When the blood is coming from the reproductive organs, the differential diagnosis includes organic gynecologic disease, systemic disease, blood dyscrasia, iatrogenic source, trauma, and functional uterine bleeding. Again, the last diagnosis can be established only by excluding all the other possibilities.

Eighty per cent or more of patients with dysfunctional uterine bleeding have anovulatory menstrual cycles. Anovulation occurs as the result of a delay in the maturation or alterations in the neuroendocrine regulation of the hypothalamic–pituitary–ovarian axis. Women with dysfunctional uterine bleeding who do not ovulate fail to form a corpus luteum. Their ovaries secrete estrogen but do not produce progesterone. The constant stimulation of the endometrium by estrogen unopposed by progesterone results in the abnormal uterine bleeding.

Organic gynecologic disease includes complications of pregnancy, tumors, and infections. A major principle of obstetrics and gynecology is that abnormal uterine bleeding in a woman of childbearing age is most likely due to a complication of pregnancy, until proven otherwise. Complications of pregnancy refer to abortion, ectopic pregnancy, and trophoblastic disease. A high index of suspicion of problems of pregnancy is warranted for all women in their reproductive years who manifest abnormal uterine bleeding. The history and examination must include a reference to the presence or absence of the symptoms or signs of pregnancy. The use of a pregnancy test is necessary. The clinical reliability will depend upon the sensitivity and specificity of the test chosen.

The 2-minute latex agglutination inhibition slide test has a sensitivity of 1500 to 3000 IU human chorionic gonadotropin (HCG) per liter and the 2-hour hemagglutination inhibition tube tests have a sensitivity of about 750 IU HCG per liter. Radioimmunoassay for the beta subunit of HCG is highly specific with a sensitivity of less than 10 milli-international units (mIU) HCG per milliliter. However, this test is impractical for rapid clinical use because several days are required to obtain the results. A new radioreceptor assay has a sensitivity of 200 mIU HCG per ml and may be completed in 2 hours but requires the use of isotopic counting equipment. This assay is not specific for HCG because it detects luteinizing hormone (LH) also; however, it is a valuable aid in the diagnosis of threatened abortion and ectopic pregnancy.

When the clinical signs and symptoms suggest the possibility of an *ectopic pregnancy,* a culdocentesis is an important diagnostic procedure. If nonclotting blood is obtained, the diagnosis of hemoperitoneum is evident. A hematocrit should be performed on the sanguineous fluid obtained by culdocentesis. If the hematocrit of the specimen is more than 15 per cent, there is a high probability that the specimen has come from lysed blood clots. If the hematocrit is less than 15 per cent, particularly if the peripheral hematocrit is substantially greater, the specimen most likely originates from blood-tinged fluid, for example, from a ruptured ovarian cyst.

Tumors of any of the pelvic organs, but particularly those from the endometrium, may have as their only clinical manifestation abnormal uterine bleeding. Another important principle of obstetrics and gynecology is that perimenopausal and postmenopausal bleeding indicates malignancy until proven otherwise. This is not to imply that the most common cause of abnormal bleeding among women of this age is cancer. Approximately 10 per cent of abnormal perimenopausal bleeding is due to malignancy and although this incidence increases to 25 per cent in the postmenopausal woman, malignancy is still not the most common cause of postmenopausal bleeding. In the United States, exogenous estrogen administration is the most common cause. The use of the Papanicolaou smear in diagnosing cervical cancer as well as its limitations in the detection of endometrial cancer is well known. The incidence of endometrial carcinoma is known to increase with the advancement of age.

One must decide when the frequency of this tumor is great enough to necessitate performing a dilation and curettage (D&C) to rule out the diagnosis. After the age of 35 years it is recommended that all women with abnormal uterine bleeding have an adequate sampling of the lining of the uterus. If an endometrial biopsy or aspirate does not reveal the cause of the bleeding, a dilation and curettage should be performed. Some women present with a menstrual history suggestive of many years of oligoovulatory or anovulatory cycles. They are known to be at greater risk for developing carcinoma of the endometrium, and should abnormal uterine bleeding occur in these women, the endometrium must be adequately investigated before they reach the age of 35.

Submucous leiomyomas usually cause a heavy and/or prolonged but regular menstrual flow, referred to as *menorrhagia.* Pedunculated leiomyomas and endometrial polyps usually produce intermenstrual spotting or bleeding. An unusual but extremely serious problem occurs when the young patient who has not yet completed her family develops recurrent episodes of severe uterine bleeding at the time of menses. The bleeding should be stopped by a surgical curettage. This history strongly suggests the existence of a submucous leiomyoma. If a defect in the endometrial cavity is not detected, the interior of the endometrial cavity should be outlined by hysterosalpingography or directly visualized by hysteroscopy shortly after the bleeding has ceased.

Infections anywhere in the reproductive tract, such as vaginitis, cervicitis, endometritis, and salpingitis, may be the cause of abnormal uterine bleeding. Nonspecific tests including temperature, white count, differential count, and sedimentation rate, particularly if normal, would indicate that an inflammatory process is probably not present, whereas abnormal results are consistent with infection but do not localize the involved organs. A cervical culture for gonorrhea should be performed and possibly other aerobic and anaerobic cultures, depending upon the facts obtained in the history, including those related to instrumentation or pregnancy. When the possibility of pelvic inflammatory disease is high, examination of a Gram stain of the cervical secretions is quite helpful.

Systemic diseases not directly involving the pelvic organs may also be a cause of abnormal uterine bleeding. Hypothyroidism and advanced liver disease are the two most common. The patient with obvious myxedema usually has no menses, but less pronounced hypofunction of the thyroid gland is associated with increased uterine bleeding. A history with symptoms of weight gain, marked fatigue, cold hands and feet, and a failure to perspire in warm weather is suggestive of hypothyroidism. Elevated serum thyroid-stimulating hormone (TSH) is the most sensitive laboratory parameter to establish the diagnosis of hypothyroidism. TSH may be elevated in the presence of a normal T_3 and T_4. Marked liver disease may result in the failure of estrogens to be conjugated and inactivated in the liver. The resulting increase of circulating free estrogen may produce abnormal uterine bleeding. A history of liver disease, excessive alcohol intake, and the physical findings of jaundice, hepatomegaly, spider hemangiomata, palmar erythema, and ascites indicate the need for a liver profile.

It is rare for a *blood dyscrasia* to become initially manifested clinically as abnormal uterine bleeding. Although uncommon, idiopathic thrombocytopenic purpura, leukemia, aplastic anemia, and Minot-von Willebrand syndrome may first present clinically as abnormal pelvic bleeding. Petechial hemorrhages or ecchymoses, excessive bleeding from any site, a history of easy bleeding or bruising, a family history of a bleeding disorder, and excessive bleeding associated with minor trauma, minor surgery, or dental surgery will usually identify those individuals with a blood dyscrasia. Blood studies are indicated when the history suggests an individual who is at particular risk or when the abnormal bleeding continues to be resistant to therapy and is undiagnosed. These studies include a platelet count, examination of the stained blood smear, and tests of bleeding time and partial thromboplastin time.

Iatrogenic sources have become an increasingly common cause of abnormal uterine bleeding. The bleeding problems associated with oral contraceptives and intrauterine devices are well known. Synthetic estrogens and gestagens are not the only steroids to be associated with uterine bleeding problems. Corticosteroids, androgens, and anabolic agents are also associated with menstrual aberrations. Nonsteroidal agents, including hypothalamic depressants and anticholinergic drugs acting on the reproductive axis at the level of the central nervous system, may result in abnormal menstrual patterns. Other pharmaceutical agents with potential for a similar clinical result include digitalis and anticoagulants. There is no pathognomonic laboratory test for the diagnosis of an iatrogenic cause of abnormal uterine bleeding and a careful history is essential for the correct diagnosis.

Trauma to the pelvis may result in injury to the reproductive organs and abnormal uterine bleeding. History and examination are important in establishing the diagnosis.

ABNORMAL UTERINE BLEEDING: DECREASE

Abnormal uterine bleeding may also occur when there is a reduction in the amount of normal menses. A patient who develops a marked decrease in the menstrual flow or a reduction in the number of days of menses does not warrant diagnostic evaluation as long as the menstrual cycles occur with a regular cyclicity. The fact that menstruation occurs indicates that there remains a normal amount of estrogen being presented to the endometrium.

OLIGOMENORRHEA — SECONDARY AMENORRHEA

Before the development of radioimmunoassays for protein and steroid hormones, some rationale may have existed for considering amenorrhea as a possible functional menstrual disorder. This is no longer true. Patients with this problem must be properly evaluated so that the physician can exclude pituitary adenomas and prognosticate future fertility, as well as determine therapeutic management. When menstrual cycles spontaneously occur at an interval greater than every 35 days, an evaluation is warranted. The patient has either secondary amenorrhea or oligomenorrhea. *Secondary amenorrhea* is defined as the sudden cessation of menses for at least 6 months or the cessation of menses for 1 year that has been preceded by an interval of irregular menstrual cycles. *Oligomenorrhea* is defined as a time interval between menses that exceeds 35 days but is less than the period necessary to be classified as secondary amenorrhea. Pregnancy, thyroid disease, and diabetes mellitus should be ruled out in all patients with oligomenorrhea and secondary amenorrhea by a pregnancy test and evaluations of TSH, T_3, T_4, and fasting blood sugar.

A patient presenting with only oligomenorrhea or secondary amenorrhea needs to have a progesterone withdrawal, or challenge, test. Progesterone, 100 mg in oil, is administered in a single dose intramuscularly. The challenge must be with progesterone in oil, not with aqueous progesterone, which is rapidly conjugated. Medroxyprogesterone acetate (Depo-Provera) is not the same agent and is totally inappropriate for this test. The amount of uterine bleeding may vary from minimal dark-brown spotting to a normal menstrual flow. If the patient fails to have withdrawal bleeding in the next 14 days following administration of 100 mg of progesterone in oil, a 200-mg dose should be administered before the patient is classified as having a negative progesterone challenge test.

Patients who have uterine bleeding following the intramuscular administration of progesterone should next have serum LH concentration measured. A serum LH level exceeding 30 mIU per ml in an anovulatory woman with a positive response to progesterone is diagnostic of polycystic ovarian disease. Patients who have withdrawal bleeding after progesterone and have a normal LH concentration have hypothalamic-pituitary dysfunction. In these patients a serum prolactin concentration should be measured. An elevated serum prolactin is an indication that the patient should have radiologic studies of the sella turcica to exclude the presence of a pituitary tumor.

If the patient should fail to have withdrawal bleeding following progesterone administration, the diagnostic possibilities are indeed more serious. Ovarian failure may be distinguished from hypothalamic-pituitary failure by a serum FSH determination. An elevated FSH concentration indicates ovarian failure. Some patients with premature ovarian failure may have an autoimmune disease that affects multiple glands. Therefore patients with premature ovarian failure should have adrenal and thyroid function studies. A normal or low FSH concentration after the patient has failed to have progesterone-induced withdrawal bleeding indicates hypothalamic-pituitary failure. The underlying disease process for these patients may be a pituitary tumor. Patients with hypothalamic-pituitary failure should have a pituitary evaluation that includes a serum prolactin measurement and anteroposterior and lateral cone views of the sella turcica. If these x-ray studies are normal, polytomographic studies of the sella turcica are necessary to exclude the presence of a tumor if prolactin levels are elevated. Patients with abnormal x-ray studies should have a visual field examination, computed tomography scan, and a test of ACTH reserve.

When oligomenorrhea or secondary amenorrhea is part of a symptom complex in which galactorrhea, androgen excess, cortisol excess, or an end-organ defect is present, a specific evaluation is required in each of these instances.

Galactorrhea may be the first sign of a pituitary adenoma. The breasts must be carefully palpated in any patient with oligomenorrhea or secondary amenorrhea. The serum prolactin assay and polytomographic studies of the sella turcica are recent methodologic advancements that aid in the diagnosis of pituitary adenomas. The presence of galactorrhea or an elevation in serum prolactin or both is an indication that the patient should have a pituitary evaluation to exclude the presence of a tumor.

Signs and symptoms of hirsutism, increased muscle mass, clitoromegaly, temporal balding, and deepening of the voice all suggest the presence of *androgen excess*. When they occur concomitantly with increasingly longer intervals between menses, the source of the androgen excess must be determined. A pelvic examination to search for a unilaterally enlarged ovary, followed by measurements of serum testosterone and either urinary 17-ketosteroids or serum dehydroepiandrosterone sulfate, is all that is necessary in the vast majority of patients. If the urinary excretion of 17-ketosteroids is less than 25 mg per day or the serum dehydroepiandrosterone sulfate concentration is less than 5000 nanograms per ml and the serum testosterone concentration is less than 150 nanograms per 100 ml, the patient has

either idiopathic hirsutism or polycystic ovarian disease. When these results are abnormally elevated, the patient should have a further diagnostic evaluation to rule out the possibility of several rare but potentially life-threatening processes.

Patients may present with various combinations of the following symptoms: amenorrhea, centripetal obesity, thinning of the skin with facial flushing, supraclavicular and dorsal neck fat pads, purple striae, muscle wasting and weakness, increase of fine hair on the face and extremities, easy bruisability, ecchymoses, osteoporosis, hypertension, and diabetes. The possibility of *cortisol excess*, Cushing's syndrome, must be excluded. The most efficient and practical means for both the patient and physician to rule out cortisol excess is the overnight dexamethasone suppression test. The patient is instructed to take 1.0 mg of dexamethasone at 11 P.M. on the night before and at 8 A.M. on the next morning she reports for a plasma sample to be obtained. If the cortisol concentration in this sample is less than 5 micrograms per 100 ml the patient does not have Cushing's syndrome. If normal suppression does not occur, further evaluation and hospitalization are necessary.

The characteristic history of an *end-organ defect*, Asherman's syndrome, is one of intrauterine manipulation associated with a pregnancy or a complication of a pregnancy. The most likely candidate to develop this syndrome is a woman who has undergone curettage in the second to fourth week postpartum. Synechiae may be detected with a uterine sound, hysterogram, or hysteroscopy. If one of four consecutive weekly serum progesterone concentrations exceeds 3 nanograms per ml, ovulation has occurred; this test is a valuable indicator of an end-organ defect.

If the signs or symptoms of galactorrhea, androgen excess, cortisol excess, and end-organ defect are not present, evaluation of urinary 17-ketosteroids, 17-ketogenic steroids, 17-hydroxycorticosteroids, and pregnanetriol is not necessary. Neither are serum testosterone, estradiol, progesterone, 17 α-hydroxyprogesterone nor cortisol tests indicated. If laboratory tests are ordered in a logical, sequential fashion, it will be necessary to utilize a very few, usually four or less, for any one patient with a reproductive endocrinologic problem.

Functional uterine bleeding is a common gynecologic problem for which considerable controversy exists as to definition, diagnostic procedures, and management. There should be no argument against the fact that each patient should be properly interviewed and examined as to all the possible disease entities mentioned. When the history and physical examination point out specific diagnostic possibilities, appropriate adjunctive laboratory aids should be ordered to exclude other possibilities and to confirm the diagnosis.

INFLAMMATION AND INFECTION OF THE FEMALE GENITAL TRACT

By GREGORY C. BOLTON, M.D.
Philadelphia, Pennsylvania

Of the many problems facing the practicing physician, none is more perplexing than the diagnosis and therapeutic management of vulvovaginal diseases, which account for a sizeable number of patient visits. The art of diagnosing these diseases is often bypassed in our formal training, and often our treatment goes the way of therapeutic trials and gross mismanagement. This review attempts to cover the diagnosis of these inflammatory and infectious diseases of the female genital tract, beginning with the common vulvovaginitis, continuing through the various vulvar infectious and dermatologic disorders, and ending with the vulvar dystrophies.

Because of similarities in gross appearance and a vast array of differential diagnoses, the vulvovaginal infection lookalikes necessitate the use of several techniques that are readily available in the office setting. Careful evaluation by history seems to correlate well with improved diagnostic efficiency. The presence of other systemic disorders, coital involvement, use of contraceptives (e.g., pill, foam, jelly), use of other medications (e.g., steroids or antibiotics), and even a conception history all aid in increasing diagnostic efficiency. The physical examination, concentrating on palpation and careful visualization, is paramount in making an accurate diagnosis of vulvovaginal disease. The availability of an adequate light source along with a low power magnifying lens provides excellent visibility of the vulva and eliminates the necessity for use of a colposcope. Photogra-

phy and chart diagrams facilitate diagnosis, as do second opinions, patient education, and follow-up. Other simple techniques include Collins' dye (toluidine blue dye), Papanicolaou smears of specific lesions, cultures, and serologic tests. One should not overlook, however, the very rapid, simple and relatively painless and benign office biopsy. This can be employed for definitive diagnosis or when specific areas are highlighted by the nuclear stain.

VULVOVAGINITIS

Because the sensory nerve endings for pain in the vagina are few in number, most vaginal infections are not noticed until the discharge reaches the external vulvar area, where it is perceived as itching, burning, or pain. The normal healthy vaginal ecosystem revolves around the careful balance of the normal flora, glycogen content, and vaginal pH. The normal flora consists mainly of lactobacilli, corynebacteria, and Candida species. The relationship between these bacteria, vaginal pH, and glycogen content allows for their growth but inhibits other aerobic and anaerobic organisms, present but in small numbers, from proliferating.

CANDIDIASIS

The Candida species (*Candida albicans*) ranks as one of the most common causes of vaginitis (about 50 per cent). Because of its presence in normal vaginal flora and presence in the human gastrointestinal tract, a breakdown in the normal symbiotic relationship in the vagina allows this opportunistic organism to overgrow. This breakdown often occurs during a pregnancy, with oral contraceptive use, with long-term antibiotic use, in diabetics, and in patients undergoing steroid therapy. The major complaint is usually an intense vulvar pruritus (80 to 90 per cent of cases) associated with a white curd-like discharge. The discharge begins premenstrually secondary to increased vaginal glycogen content.

On speculum examination, erythematous vaginal walls occasionally are seen to be marked with small reddish macules, the so-called "satellite lesions." These are covered by classic lard-like patches (thrush patches) loosely adherent to the mucosal walls. This material is easily scraped off; on examination by wet smear with 10 per cent KOH solution the spores and filaments characteristic of fungal infection are revealed. One should also look at the saline smear for evidence of trichomonads, which accompany the candidal infection in 5 to 10 per cent of the patients. Culturing of Candida from vaginal swabs is possible using thioglycollate broth and Sabouraud's agar. Growth is moderately rapid and appears in 2 to 3 days.

TRICHOMONAS VAGINALIS

Trichomoniasis is the second most common vaginitis. *Trichomonas vaginalis* is a tetraflagellate protozoan with a prominent axostyle and an undulating membrane. It is present in the lower genitourinary tract, including Bartholin's glands, bladder, and Skene's glands in women, and the prostate, seminal vesicles, and epididymis in men. Transmission of this organism is believed to be venereal in nature. Presenting symptoms include a profuse, frothy, gray, and often malodorous discharge associated with pruritus, redness, swelling, and dyspareunia. Vaginal examination reveals mild to moderate erythema and edema, along with a mild cervicitis. The classic patchy inflammation or punctate submucosal hemorrhage (strawberry vagina or cervix) is not very common. Roughly 70 per cent of women harboring these organisms and more than 90 per cent of male carriers are asymptomatic. Examination of the KOH smear is often unrevealing. However, the actively motile organisms on saline smear are easily seen, and diagnosis is relatively simple. Often, both in severe infections and in asymptomatic males, no obvious motility is noted, and one must rely on cultures (Feinberg-Whittington or Kupferberg media) or Papanicolaou smears to make the diagnosis. Admittedly, Pap smears are often not as reliable, but they are important in view of the 30 to 40 per cent of abnormal cytologic diagnoses associated with *T. vaginalis*. Examination of smears should be repeated after adequate therapy.

HEMOPHILUS VAGINALIS

This relatively common cause of vaginitis (40 per cent) used to be listed as a "catch-all" in diagnosis of nonspecific vaginitis to explain any unusual vaginal discharge having no identifiable trichomonads or fungal organisms. This organism is a surface parasite that does not invade the vaginal wall. Consequently, relatively few patients present with irritable pruritus or burning; instead they complain of a discharge and malodor. The discharge is gray-white and homogenous in consistency. Diagnosis can be made with certainty when one observes stratified squamous epithelial cells with a granular appearance (clue cells) on saline wet smear. Laboratory confirmation is available by culturing on Casman broth treated with defibrinated sheep blood and incubated under CO_2. Sexual intercourse seems to be the means of transmission; the bacteria can be found in a high percentage of the consorts of infected patients. It is important to treat the men as well to avoid reinfection.

VULVAR PARASITES

Included among the vulvar infections or infestations are the two human parasites: pubic lice (*Phthirus pubis*) and scabies (*Sarcoptes scabiei*). Pediculosis pubis is caused by the pubic or crab louse, which is an obligate parasite whose specific host is man. It is usually confined to the hair-bearing regions, where it pierces the skin and secretes a noxious substance that produces severe pubic and vulvar pruritis. The disease can be spread venereally but also by infected bedding and linen. The pale-gray adult forms are almost transparent, but when they are blood-filled, the alimentary tract is visible under the microscope. The presenting symptoms of intense pruritus of the mons and labia, in the absence of a vaginitis, should lead one to suspect pubic lice, although the differential diagnoses include Fox-Fordyce disease. Careful inspection of the skin, looking for the characteristic rusty spots close to hairshafts and nits attached to the hairshaft, aids in making the diagnosis.

Scabies is caused by the female itch mite *Sarcoptes* (*Acarus*) *scabiei*. Again intense pruritus, often worse at night, leads the patient to seek help. The diagnosis can be made by obtaining the Acarus from the skin burrows with a needle and identifying it under the microscope. Other skin appendages can be affected — sides of fingers, palms, axillae, and wrist flexures.

SEXUALLY TRANSMITTED DISEASES

Many infections and inflammatory lesions of the female genital tract are transmitted to the vulva and perineum by sexual contact.

Condylomata accuminatum is a disease state in which multiple papillary lesions (genital warts) involve the labia, vagina, cervix, and perirectal area. These lesions, although viral in cause (papovavirus), could also be classified as benign solid vulvar tumors because of their solid nature and proliferative growth during pregnancy. The association of the papovavirus, the prevalence during sexually active years, and the findings of penile warts in sexual partners lend weight to the premise that this is a sexually transmitted disease.

Physical examination reveals an immense range in multicentricity and size of these papillomatous lesions, from small discrete papillary growths to large cauliflower-like lesions. Histologic identification is based on hyperplasia of the squamous epithelium with parakeratosis and acanthosis, as well as marked convoluting of papillary processes. Biopsy is necessary in this disease to rule out condylomata lata or verrucous carcinoma. One should also search for coexisting causes of secondary vulvitis such as trichomonas, and for other venereal disease such as syphilis. In general, a so-called venereal disease alert should be instituted to check for gonorrhea, herpes, molluscum, and lice.

Molluscum contagiosum is another of the sexually transmitted diseases of the vulva that has a viral cause. The lesions are small, elevated, well-circumscribed pearly papules that increase in size. As they mature, the lesions become round and form central dimples. The lesions may persist for months and even years. The diagnosis is readily made by unroofing the papule from the central core. Electron microscopy has shown the cytoplasmic molluscum (Henderson-Patterson) bodies to be composed of aggregates of DNA virus presumed to be in the poxvirus group. Definitive diagnosis must be made by biopsy in order to distinguish this from other similar lesions of systemic importance, such as granuloma.

Herpes progenitalis, perhaps the most common and most important of the many viral infections of the vulva, is caused by the herpes simplex virus. Herpetic vulvovaginitis due to the Herpesvirus hominis type II (10 per cent due to type I) is found almost exclusively in the female cervix, vagina, and vulva. Close personal contact (venereal transmission) and local tissue trauma are important aspects in the establishment of the herpetic infection and lesions. Approximately 50 to 80 per cent of females coming in contact with the virus develop clinical disease.

Clinical diagnosis by virtue of the appearance of the very typical vesicles 2 to 7 days following exposure, associated with increasing vaginal discharge, fever, pain, and inguinal lymphadenopathy, is relatively easy. The initial vesicles often rupture and become secondarily infected and ulcerated in appearance. Unlike the RNA virus, the DNA makeup of this viral infection prevents immune elimination. Because of this and the ability of the virus to persist in host cells in a repressed state (latency in sensory sacral nerve ganglia), recurrent flare-ups of the disease are relatively common.

The major concerns about herpes genitalis in man are several. One of these is neonatal disease — a threefold increase in the rate of spontaneous abortion in early pregnancy when mothers contract a primary infection. Neonatal infection immediately postpartum results in a mortality rate higher than 60 per cent and neurologic damage in 50 per cent of the survivors. Another concern is related to the close association of genital herpes and other venereal diseases, as well as the possible incrimination of herpes type II as an oncologic agent for cervical carcinoma.

Patients with cervical carcinoma (80 per cent) have positive serologic evidence of type II infection. Definitive diagnosis can be documented by Papanicolaou smear or biopsy showing the presence of multinucleated cells with intranuclear inclusion bodies. Viral cultures that permit identification in 1 to 3 days, as well as special serologic tests that can differentiate primary from recurrent infection, are available.

For completeness one should include among the other viruses known to infect the female genitalia the varicella-herpes zoster and vaccinia. Varicella-zoster (VZ) represents an endogenous reactivation of VZ virus acquired as a consequence of a previous attack of varicella (chickenpox). Although a rare lesion of the vulva, VZ infection can present as a unilateral lesion of grouped vesicles almost always limited to the labia. It occurs with equal frequency throughout the year and has a higher prevalence in individuals receiving immunosuppressive therapy or corticosteroids, and patients with Hodgkin's disease whose cell-mediated responses have been inactivated. Vaccinia usually is contracted after close personal contact by an unvaccinated child or in an adult through contact with a recently vaccinated person. The lesions very closely follow the pattern of a smallpox vaccination, that is, papular to vesicular, then pustular, in appearance.

Granuloma inguinale, lymphogranuloma venereum, and chancroid are relatively rare infections of the vulva. However, because of the communicability, disabling consequences, and availability of therapy, they are of considerable importance to practicing physicians.

Granuloma inguinale (Donovanosis) is a chronic cutaneous granulomatous reaction involving the external genitalia and surrounding skin. Despite our inability to fulfill Koch's postulations, the causative organism appears to be *Calymmatobacterium granulomatis*, a gram-negative bacteria common to the gastrointestinal tract and related antigenically to members of the Enterobacteriaceae, e.g., Klebsiella.

The prevalence of lesions in the genital area and the 25 to 50 per cent association of sexual partners having evidence of the infection lends credence to the presumption that transmission is via sexual intercourse. Initial lesions occur on the genitalia in about 90 per cent of patients, especially on the perirectal skin, inguinal area, and mouth in 10 per cent of the cases. It usually begins as a reddish-brown papule that erodes in the center. After several papules appear, ulcerate, and coalesce, the overall outline is serpiginous in appearance. The borders are well defined and scrolled, with some undermining of the skin. The lesion usually has a predilection for the fourchette; even when it has developed into chronic granulomatous ulceration, the ulcer is painless and relatively nondestructive. However, in its later stages, genital elephantiasis may occur. Often vaginal or cervical lesions feature gross local swelling that is hard and knobby secondary to closure of efferent lymphatics. Because of its close resemblance to carcinoma, regardless of the location, biopsy should be performed. The diagnosis is invariably made on the identification of classic Donovan bodies. These are clusters of small rod-shaped intracellular organisms found in the foamy cytoplasm of large mononuclear cells. They are more readily demonstrated with Giemsa stain.

Lymphogranuloma venereum (lymphopathia venereum) is a venereally transmitted disease produced by *Chlamydia trachomatis*, formally known as Miyagawanella lymphogranulomatosis. This member of the group Bedsoniae is an obligate parasite that possesses bacteria-like susceptibility to antibiotics. It is more common in tropical countries and has a mode of transmission through coitus as well as autoinnoculation. Along with chills, fever, headache, malaise, and anorexia as presenting signs, lymphogranuloma venereum may occur as one of two syndromes: either inguinal or genitorectal.

Following an incubation period of 1 to 4 weeks, the initial genital lesion — a small transient herpetiform erosion involving the fourchette — develops and may pass unnoticed. This is followed by a necrotizing granulomatous inflammation of the regional lymph nodes that may perforate and drain through the matted adherent overlying skin. The inflammatory changes cause a prominent lymphangitis throughout the pudendal connective tissue. The external scarring that follows here and in the lymph nodes obstructs lymphatics, causing lymphedema, and produces strictures. The confluent foci of necrosis produces "stellate abscesses." Rectal involvement, initially a proctolitis, is characterized by a mucopurulent discharge and bloody diarrhea. If not treated, the rectal and perirectal inflammation can result in strictures, elephantiasis-esthiomene, vulvar lesions, and rectovaginal fistulas. Late sequelae include stricture or loss of the urethra, notching of the labia, and stenosis of the vagina.

Diagnosis of the lymphadenopathy of lymphogranuloma venereum includes a differentiation of many chronic inflammatory diseases and even lymphoma, gonococcal proctitis, and ulcerative colitis. Confirmation is best achieved through a complement-fixation test, but the antigen reacts with serum from patients with other chlamydial infections. Therefore only in the presence of a fourfold rise in titer can a definitive diagnosis be made. Biopsy of nodes, although helpful, is not specific enough, and the skin test antigen (Frei test) lacks sensitivity and is difficult to obtain in the United States. Other laboratory tests that point to the diagnosis are hyperglobulinemia, reversal of albumin/globulin ratio, and culture of the virus from lymph node aspirates.

Chancroid is a superficial ulcerating disease of the female external genitalia that appears to be venereally transmitted and caused by a gram-negative bacteria *Hemophilus ducreyi*. Following sexual contact (within 3 to 14 days) the coital lesion appears. This is at first 1 to 2 cm macular area that rapidly becomes vesicular and pustular in appearance. This then rapidly forms a painful irregularly bordered ulcer with a granulating base, often covered by a necrotic grayish exudate. About 50 per cent of infected patients develop a unilateral inguinal lymphadenitis that can progress to a draining sinus but rarely becomes as destructive as granuloma inguinale or lymphogranuloma venereum. Although often confused with herpes genitalis, the ulcer is different in appearance and is not known to be recurrent. Definitive diagnosis is usually confirmed by biopsy, which by exclusion eliminates the diagnoses of granuloma inguinale, syphilitic chancre, and the herpes ulcer. On Gram or Wright stain a classic pattern of gram-negative rods with a "school of fish" appearance is noted. As with all of the venereally related vulvar diseases, concomitant testing for syphilis and other diseases should be performed.

DERMATOLOGIC DISORDERS AND VULVAR DYSTROPHY

Because of the close similarity of the vulva to normal skin elsewhere on the body, there are many diseases of the vulva that are also a result of infection, irritation, and allergic response. They are often present as inflammatory lesions or as white lesions of the vulva or combinations of the two. The definitive diagnosis of these lesions is essential because of the ever-present possibility of underlying malignancy.

CUTANEOUS INFLAMMATION

Contact dermatitis is a term that encompasses lesions caused by plants, chemicals, and many allergens. The normal cutaneous reaction to the causative agent is redness, inflammation, and weeping of the contact or exposure areas. Contact dermatitis of the vulva is almost always secondary to the application of external agents to skin areas or even to the wearing of certain clothing. A careful history and notation of patterns of vulvar involvement often gives one a clue to the diagnosis as well as the cause.

Pyodermas are the infections of the vulvar skin that result from any breakdown of the skin that allows entry of bacteria or a decrease in host resistance by corticosteroids or other disease states. The basic pattern is erythema, pustules, ulcers, and abscess formation. Culture and sensitivity studies are required for appropriate diagnosis. The main causative agents are the staphylococcus and the beta-hemolytic streptococcus or a mixture of the two.

Erythrasma is usually found in the pubic, axillary, and genitocrural areas, and presents as a macerated or inflamed dry, scaly and slow-spreading macular patch.

Differentiation between tinea cruris, seborrheic dermatitis, and tinea versicolor is made by identification of *Corynebacterium minutissima* by culture or microscopically. Using Gram stain, one sees gram-positive rod-like, filamentous organisms. The orange to coral red fluorescence of the lesion under the Wood's light is diagnostic.

Seborrheic dermatitis or chronic reactive vulvitis usually is recurrent and found in areas of high sebaceous gland activity. The skin eruptions are usually red, often greasy, with a fine, scaly covering. The symptom of pruritus and a past history of similar attacks help in making the diagnosis.

Neurodermatitis is often the result of an established itch-scratch cycle, stimulated by insect bites, contact dermatitis, or seborrheic dermatitis. The clinical presentation of neurodermatitis (lichen simplex chronicus) reveals a localized dry, scaly lesion with some excoriation and crusting. The vulva and perianal areas are favored sites in women for this dermatitis. Scratching and rubbing often lead to secondary bacterial infection. The lesion is also confused with psoriasis and contact dermatitis.

Psoriasis, a relatively common skin disorder, has specific predilection for certain areas of the skin, including the scalp, anogenital area, elbows, and knees. A typical lesion is a well-circumscribed plaque that is red in color and has scales. These scales have a characteristic "silver sheen" and flake easily. Pitting of the fingernails is often a telling diagnostic point. If the scales are scratched off, fine bleeding points are noted (Auspitz' sign), and rubbing or scratching can cause formation of new lesions (Koebner phenomenon). Biopsy of the lesion reveals intradermal abscesses of Munro as well as parakeratosis. These plaques also respond with toluidine blue dye retention.

VULVAR DYSTROPHY

The remaining lesions of the vulva and female genitalia have historically been set apart as a group: the so-called white lesions of the vulva. Because of the past (and present) confusion in various terminologies and classifications, unnecessary delays in diagnosis and treatment of these lesions was common.

Currently the International Society for the Study of Vulvar Diseases has proposed the term "vulvar dystrophies" for these lesions with white surface changes. These are subgrouped into three classes on the basis of easily recognizable histologic changes. The main factors that account for the overall white appearance are keratin formation, depigmentation, and avascularity.

Lichen sclerosis et atrophicus clinically presents as a pruritic, thin, parchment-like lesion with characteristic atrophic introital stenosis. Histologically the tissue is thin with loss of rete pegs and a subepithelial homogenous zone with deep inflammatory infiltrate.

Hyperplastic dystrophies clinically are pruritic, thick, gray or white plaques that microscopically show thickened epithelium, acanthosis, hyperkeratosis, and inflammatory infiltrates.

Mixed dystrophies have clinical and histologic areas compatible with both forms at the same time.

The clinical features of vulvar skin that possesses white, gray, or simply pale coloring along with surface architecture compatible with one of these groups gives a tentative clinical diagnosis. However, the lesions should all be biopsied to support this impression and to aid in choosing the appropriate treatments. Staining with 1 per cent toluidine blue dye and rinsing with 1 per cent acetic acid aids in pinpointing areas that need to be biopsied.

THE MENOPAUSE

By JOHN STUDD, M.D.
London, England

In the latter part of the twentieth century women will live approximately one third of their lives after the cessation of reproductive potential. Far from being a welcome relief from fertility, these years are considered by doctors and patients alike as something more than a manifestation of the natural aging process. Current medical opinion clearly accepts that the postmenopausal woman is suffering a chronic endocrinopathy associated with varied symptomatic and degenerative changes that may be greatly affected by her sociocultural background. The symptoms in 25 per cent of women are severe enough to warrant specific replacement therapy. Fifty per cent of women have minimal symptoms that last for a few months, and the remainder seem to be untouched by any characteristic climacteric problems.

The menopause occurs on average at age 50 and simply refers to the cessation of menstruation. This well-defined point in life may occur abruptly or after cycles of increasing length with decreasing menstrual flow. Heavy, frequent, or irregular periods at this time are not part of the normal approach to the menopause and should be investigated. Ovarian failure begins many years, perhaps as many as 10, before periods cease as the number of oocytes in the ovary diminish in number by a progressive process of atresia. This prolonged time of failure of ovulation and the decreasing output of ovarian hormones is known as the climacteric. This may last for as long as 20 years, taking the woman through decreasing fertility, the menopause, and the atrophies of prolonged estrogen lack. The long-term effect of the climacteric may be particularly severe after oophorectomy in younger women or in those women who suffer a premature menopause.

PATHOLOGIC CHANGES

Pelvic tissues are the principal target organs for the sex steroids, and the changes are most readily observable in the vagina. The vaginal skin atrophies and loses its glycogen and protective acidic environment, allowing infection with commensal organisms. Vaginal cytology will show a preponderance of basal and parabasal cells with few mature, superficial cornified cells. Atrophic vaginitis may be obvious on examination. The uterus and fallopian tubes also involute, and the tiny cervix becomes flush with a narrowed vaginal vault. The labia and clitoris atrophy and become less sexually responsive. The bladder mucosa may show atrophic trigonitis, and the urethral tone decreases with resultant loss of urinary control. Estrogen deprivation leads to a negative nitrogen balance with a reduction in muscular strength as muscles become invaded with fibroblasts. The epidermis becomes thinner, and the subcutaneous fat atrophies with loss of elasticity and turgor. Similar changes occur in the breasts, causing them to lose contour. The ligaments surrounding joints lose their tone, giving rise to joint pain.

There are two important metabolic effects of estrogen deficiency, namely coronary thrombosis and postmenopausal osteoporosis. After ovarian failure the plasma levels of cholesterol, triglyceride, and β-lipoproteins rise. These are factors in the complex pathogenesis of coronary thrombosis, because before the menopause nonsmoking women have a virtual immunity from coronary heart disease, but subsequently the incidence of myocardial infarction approaches that of men. The age at which the menopause occurs is significant, as epidemiologic studies in women who have suffered an early myocardial infarction demonstrate that an early menopause is a considerable risk factor, occurring in 18 per cent of the study population, compared with 3 per cent of controls.

Similarly, menopausal bone disease in the form of osteoporosis, with an increased incidence of fracture of the lower radius or neck of femur and crush fractures of the vertebrae, is now recognized as a hazard of estrogen deprivation. Estrogens act as an antiparathormone, being anticatabolic to bone formation. With ovarian failure, demineralization of the bone occurs to the extent of 1 to 3 per cent of body calcium per year, with a demonstrable increase in plasma calcium and alkaline phosphatase and an increased urinary calcium loss.

HORMONAL CHANGES

In the premenopausal woman the source of most estrone and estradiol is from direct ovarian secretion. The remainder is an insignificant amount from peripheral conversion of androstenedione and testosterone. Estrone and estradiol are interconvertible. On the other hand, there is virtually no ovarian production of steroids after menopause; estrone is produced by the peripheral conversion of adrenal androstenedione, and estradiol results from the conversion of estrone, testosterone, and androstenedione. Estrone and estradiol values fall to 20 and 30 per cent, respectively, of normal proliferative phase values. Testosterone levels remain essentially unchanged in the 30 years after the menopause, but androstenedione values fall to 40 per cent of normal values. The pituitary gonadotropins — follicle-stimulating hormone (FSH) and luteinizing hormone (LH) — are secreted in increased amounts in a vain attempt to stimulate ovulation even before the periods cease. The peak climacteric values are found 2 to 3 years after the menopause, with FSH being 13 times the levels of the proliferative phase and LH being three times the proliferative phase levels. However, the climacteric levels of LH never reach those of the periovulatory surge found in the reproductive phase of life. Consequently, an LH assay cannot be used as a simple diagnostic test of ovarian failure.

Symptoms

The symptomatic response to the menopause will depend on the amount and rate of estrogen depletion, the inherited and acquired ability of the woman to succumb to or withstand the natural aging process, and, above all, the individual psychologic impact of the emotional implications of the change of life. The classic symptoms of the climacteric are those of vasomotor instability and vaginal atrophy. The hot flushes (or flashes) and sweats, particularly at night, tension or migrainous headaches, and palpitations are distressing symptoms that may antedate the menopause by several years. Disturbed sleep may lead to fatigue and loss of concentration. Dyspareunia, lack of lubrication, itching, and bleeding may follow the vaginal changes. Loss of libido, sometimes resulting from these local changes, may also be a manifestation of systemic decreases in estradiol and androgen levels in women who do not complain of a dry, uncomfortable vagina during intercourse.

Depression associated with low levels of free tryptophan is an integral part of the protean symptomatology, as is bone, joint and muscle pain. Certainly these symptoms have a multifactorial cause, and the stressful social environment of the middle-aged woman should not be underestimated; but if these problems occur for the first time during middle age, it is likely that they are a direct result of loss of ovarian hormones. The bladder, urethra, and genital tract have a common embryologic origin, and the atrophy of the trigone and the periurethral vascular tissues is a cause of many cases of urinary frequency, urgency, and urge-incontinence that are commonplace in women of this age group.

In 1969 the International Health Foundation undertook a survey by questionnaire of 2000 women between the ages of 46 and 55 in several European countries. It emerged that the symptoms most commonly experienced were flushes (55 per cent), tiredness (43 per cent), nervousness (41 per cent), sweating (39 per cent), headaches (38 per cent), insomnia (32 per cent), depression (30 per cent), irritability (29 per cent), joint and muscle pain (25 per cent), dizziness (24 per cent), palpitations (24 per cent), and pins and needles (22 per cent). However, *the order of symptoms complained of* was very different, the patients being worried most by depression, sexual difficulties, and faulty memory.

Diagnosis

The diagnosis in a woman whose periods have ceased for a year or more should be straightforward. She is postmenopausal and will be estrogen deficient, although in some patients, particularly the obese, extraovarian conversion of adrenal androstenedione in the body fat and muscle may be responsible for considerable amounts of estrone. The symptoms outlined, if occurring close to the menopause, should be adequate for diagnosis without the need of any hormone assays. Cytologic studies of the cornification of vaginal cells may show an estrogen-deficient smear but, unless read by an expert cytologist, are useful only in those patients in whom the diagnosis is obvious without laboratory tests.

The difficulty in diagnosis occurs in the premenopausal woman and those who have previously had a hysterectomy with ovarian conservation. In the former the cycles may be anovulatory; in the other group progressive ovarian failure may occur unnoticed. The diagnosis, if suspected, can usually be made by a careful history eliciting mood change, dry vagina during intercourse, and recent loss of libido. It is important to establish that these are new symptoms, as psychologic problems abound at this age and one must be cautious of the chronic hypochondriacal psychoneurotic patient attempting to cure her long-term ills with estrogen therapy. The appearance of hot flushes and sweats should virtually clinch the diagnosis. If diagnostic proof is required, a single elevated plasma FSH result, a simpler assay than estradiol, or simply a trial of estrogen therapy should be sufficient.

Differential Diagnosis

It is possible in a state of therapeutic enthusiasm to ascribe spurious symptoms to the climacteric syndrome. Long-standing foibles of behavior or mood, reactive depression, and the domestic frustrations of middle age are not part of a deficiency state. Similarly arthritis, backache, and headache may have other causes and require careful investigation. Hyperthyroidism may produce disorders of temperature response identical to those of vasomotor instability of the climacteric. Nevertheless, "common things occur commonly," and many debilitating symptoms occurring in women for the first time at about the time of the menopause are directly the result of the local and metabolic effects of estrogen loss.

PREGNANCY

By RICHARD A. KOPHER, M.D.,
and GEORGE E. TAGATZ, M.D.

Minneapolis, Minnesota

Pregnancy is defined as the condition of a woman who is carrying a developing fetus in the uterus. Indeed, normal pregnancy has its inception with fertilization, extends through implantation, growth, and development of the fetus in utero, and terminates with delivery of the infant.

The diagnosis of early pregnancy must be considered in any female patient during her reproductive years. Subjective symptoms such as fatigue, malaise, sensitivity to odors, nausea, retching, vomiting, hyperphagia, anorexia, constipation, breast fullness and tenderness, and urinary frequency are notoriously nonspecific and involve many organ systems. Diagnoses of psychosomatic, gastrointestinal, and urinary tract disorders are not infrequently entertained. Diagnostic x-rays are particularly worrisome during organogenesis and should be scrupulously avoided until either the diagnosis of pregnancy is excluded, or the suspected disease justifies performance of diagnostic procedures despite the possible coexistence of pregnancy.

The diagnostic signs of pregnancy are more specific than the ofttimes confusing array of symptoms, but findings are often equivocal and when present are at best presumptive. Pregnancy is the most common cause of secondary amenorrhea during the reproductive years; delayed or missed menses mandates a search for pregnancy. On rare occasion, an adolescent has become pregnant when ovulation preceded her first menses, thus presenting with primary amenorrhea. However, amenorrhea is not an invariable concomitant of pregnancy; uterine bleeding occurs in about half of early pregnancies.

The occasional patient who is taking basal body temperatures can provide further presumptive evidence of pregnancy. The increased concentrations of progesterone during the luteal phase and early pregnancy have a thermogenic effect on the hypothalamus that is reflected in a rise of 0.5 to 1 F in the basal body temperature (BBT). Pregnancy can be presumed if the BBT remains elevated for 20 or more days. However, since the temperature rise is caused by progesterone, infrequent ovarian disorders that are unrelated to stimulation by human chorionic gonadotropin (HCG), such as persistent corpus luteum and theca luteinization, will also induce a prolonged thermogenic effect.

Physical examination as often as not provides little further information. Classic presumptive signs are firm, hyperpigmented breasts; congested, bluish vagina and cervix; shoftening of the uterus at the implantation site; and discernible enlargement of the uterus. Enlargement of the uterus is subtle in early pregnancy and often detectable only if related to the uterine size at a prior examination.

If the diagnosis is equivocal, the passage of time permitting uterine growth and fetal development will eventually clarify the condition. However, the possibility of pregnancy-related complications and the patient's desires often necessitate further immediate diagnostic efforts.

The progesterone provocative test is mentioned to be condemned. Failure to exhibit withdrawal bleeding following the administration of intramuscular progesterone or oral progestins is not diagnostic of pregnancy. The administration of progestins during pregnancy has recently been associated with an increased incidence of congenital heart disease and the rare devastating syndrome of multiple congenital anomalies termed VACTERL (vertebral anal cardiac tracheoesophageal renal limb).

Pregnancy tests are designed to detect the presence of the placental hormone HCG in maternal urine or blood. Bioassays of HCG are no longer used for routine pregnancy diagnosis. Unfortunately, with the exception of the reliable radioimmunoassay for the beta subunit of HCG, commonly available tests are deficient in both sensitivity and specificity. Placental HCG shares a molecular subunit with pituitary luteinizing hormone (LH), which is termed the alpha subunit. Because of this similarity, LH and HCG cross react in assays designed to detect the complete molecule of either LH or HCG. When interpreting HCG-pregnancy assays, the physician is obliged to exclude the possibility of ovarian failure and menopause or the possibility that a sample was obtained at the time of the maximal LH surge at midcycle. Conversely, LH assays will be falsely elevated in the presence of placental HCG. When confusion arises from an LH assay, it is important to recall that FSH is low during pregnancy but is usually elevated to levels higher than LH in the presence of ovarian failure. Since HCG production in early pregnancy is significantly greater than that of LH in the ovulating or menopausal woman, commonly used pregnancy tests are intentionally designed to be less sensitive to reduce the incidence of cross reaction with LH.

Immunologic tests utilize one of two designs: direct agglutination or agglutination inhibition. In *direct agglutination*, HCG in pregnancy urine agglutinates visible particles coated with anti-HCG antibodies. In *agglutination inhibition*, HCG antibody is added to pregnancy urine. Then HCG-coated sheep erythrocytes or latex particles are added. If HCG is present in urine, HCG antibodies are bound to the maternal HCG and are not available to agglutinate the visible particles; when agglutination fails to occur, the test is positive for the presence of HCG in the urine. If HCG is not present in the urine, the HCG antibodies will be free to agglutinate the added particles (negative test). At least nine commercial pregnancy tests are available. Sensitivity is such that the tests are positive about 90 per cent of the time at 5 weeks' menstrual age (3 weeks' gestational age). False-positive reactions have occurred in the presence of proteinuria, with the protein mimicking the presence of the glycoprotein HCG. For each assay utilized, the sensitivity and specificity should be carefully determined from the manufacturer's description.

A recently developed radioreceptor assay (RRA) is highly sensitive but has the limitation of also detecting LH. Since the radioisotope ^{125}I and a gamma counter are required for the performance of this assay, its application will be limited. The test becomes positive one week after conception (i.e., day 21 in a 28-day cycle) and is invariably positive at the time of the next expected menses. When ectopic pregnancy is present, the RRA is usually positive, whereas conventional pregnancy tests are positive less than half the time.

Instruments utilizing ultrasound are increasingly useful. Display scanners allow the expert to detect the gestational sac as early as 5 weeks' menstrual age. The embryo can be visualized at 7 to 8 weeks. The image of the gestational sac is transiently lost at 10 to 11 weeks, when the amniotic sac expands to fuse with the chorion. The fetal heartbeat can be heard with ultrasound devices as early as 10 weeks' gestation and reliably by 16 weeks' gestation. Real time ultrasound techniques allow detection of motion of the fetal heart as early as 8 to 9 weeks' gestation. Detection of the fetal heartbeat with the conventional fetoscope is usually not reliable until 20 weeks' gestation.

As pregnancy progresses, the breasts enlarge, become hyperpigmented, and contain expressible milk. The uterus can be palpated abdominally by 12 weeks' gestation and grows upward from the symphysis at a rate of approximately 1 cm per week after 16 weeks' gestation. The auscultated fetal heart rate of 120 to 160 per minute is readily differentiated by simultaneously palpating the maternal pulse.

DIFFERENTIAL DIAGNOSIS

1. Pregnancy-related complications

   a. *Ectopic pregnancy*
   Tubal, abdominal, characterized by abnormal bleeding and abdominal pains, often with palpable adnexal mass. Intra-abdominal bleeding following rupture may lead to hypovolemic shock and death. Culdocentesis may reveal unrecognized intra-abdominal bleeding. Laparoscopy indicated if findings suggest this diagnosis.

   b. *Trophoblastic disease (hydatidiform mole; choriocarcinoma)*
   Characterized by abnormal bleeding and often rapid enlargement of uterus suggesting multiple pregnancy. HCG titers extraordinarily high. Ultrasound or direct intrauterine injection of diatrizoate sodium (Hypaque) is indicated for early diagnosis.

   c. *Threatened abortion*
   Characterized by bleeding and uterine cramps. HCG and placental assays remain positive after fetal demise. Dilatation of internal os and expulsion of fetal parts justify intervention.

   d. *Missed abortion*
   Failure of uterine growth, reversion of pregnancy tests to negative, absence or loss of fetal heartbeat, possibly radiologic signs of fetal death. Danger of developing DIC if dead fetus retained for prolonged period.

2. False pregnancy (pseudocyesis)
   Symptoms mimic pregnancy. Breast engorge-

ment common. However, no evidence of uterine growth or fetal presence. May have hyperprolactinemia. Pregnancy tests negative.

3. Uterine enlargement
   Exclude leiomyofibromata and sarcoma.

4. Positive pregnancy tests
   All positive pregnancy tests do not indicate normal pregnancy. Trophoblastic, ovarian, and other neoplasias may secrete HCG. Pregnancy tests may be falsely positive because of interfering substances such as urinary protein and, occasionally, drug metabolites.

ECTOPIC PREGNANCY

By JAMES A. O'LEARY, M.D.
Mobile, Alabama

SYNONYM

Tubal pregnancy.

DEFINITION

A pregnancy located outside the uterus.

SYMPTOMS AND SIGNS

Amenorrhea, usually irregular light vaginal bleeding, followed by the onset of abdominal pain of any degree that may be lower abdominal or unilateral, is a common finding. If the structure containing the conceptus ruptures, symptoms of shock develop. The presence of a unilateral pelvic mass is frequently mentioned, but usually a mass cannot be felt because of the tenderness. Shoulder pain indicates intra-abdominal bleeding.

COURSE

The natural history of a tubal or ovarian pregnancy is for the structure involved to rupture. This is a dramatic event. Intra-abdominal bleeding may precede rupture. On rare occasions the conceptus may be aborted out of the distal end of the tube. This is called a *tubal abortion* and may be followed by cessation of bleeding.

A chronic ectopic pregnancy may result from clotting of blood and adhesion formation. Ultimately a soft, tender mass can be felt in the cul-de-sac.

DIFFERENTIAL DIAGNOSIS

Hemorrhage into an ovarian cyst, rupture or torsion of an ovarian cyst, pelvic inflammatory disease, and incomplete or threatened abortion must all be considered in the differential diagnosis.

COMMON COMPLICATIONS

The most serious complications following tubal rupture are hemorrhage, shock, and death. Thrombophlebitis and pulmonary embolus are rare. Postoperative morbidity is frequent, probably from blood left in the abdominal cavity. Long-term complications include pelvic adhesions, recurrent tubal pregnancy, and decreased fertility.

LABORATORY FINDINGS

Complete blood counts and sedimentation rate are not helpful. The same is true for biochemical tests. The only good test is the very sensitive radioimmunoassay for the beta subunit of HCG (human chorionic gonadotropin). It will be positive soon after ovulation when all other tests are negative. It is a uniquely accurate test and will not cross-react with other hormones.

THERAPEUTIC TESTS

Ultrasound can be helpful. It can identify a gestational sac and an empty uterus. There are no harmful effects as can happen with x-rays. X-rays are not helpful and hysterosalpingography may be dangerous.

Culdocentesis is most helpful but occasionally overlooked. Some physicians do not use it because of the slight pain associated with the procedure. It is a very simple matter to puncture the posterior cul-de-sac with a 16-gauge needle. The presence of nonclotting blood is diagnostic of a hemoperitoneum.

Papanicolaou smears really have no place in the diagnosis of ectopic pregnancy. Laparoscopy is being utilized more frequently in suspected ectopic pregnancy. Early definitive diagnosis is easily accomplished with the laparoscope.

PITFALLS IN DIAGNOSIS

The most common pitfall is a low index of suspicion and hence a delay in diagnosis.

Reliance on standard pregnancy tests is a pitfall because this type of test is of no value, whether positive or negative.

Lastly, failure to administer Rh_0 (D) immune globulin (human) (Rhogam) to an Rh negative woman is a most serious oversight.

VAGINAL BLEEDING IN PREGNANCY

By CHRISTOPHER J. JOLLES, M.D., *and* LARRY COUSINS, M.D.

San Diego, California

Vaginal bleeding occurs in 20 per cent of pregnancies. Conditions that cause bleeding contribute significantly to both maternal and perinatal morbidity.

Physiologic bleeding, usually described as far less than a menstrual period, occurs at the time of ovum implantation in approximately 1 in 10 pregnancies. The major consequence of implantation bleeding is the confusion generated regarding gestational age. The diagnosis is usually made in retrospect when suggested by other gestational age indicators, e.g., positive pregnancy test, uterine size, quickening, the time that fetal heart tones are first heard, and sonogram.

Patients with coagulopathy may experience vaginal bleeding at any stage of pregnancy, and this may be detected by history and appropriate laboratory parameters. Pathologic causes of vaginal bleeding may be divided into uterine and extrauterine causes. Of the *extrauterine types of bleeding,* vaginal trauma is usually suggested by history and constitutes a rare cause of bleeding in pregnancy. Bleeding from the cervix is most commonly caused by inflammation. The incidence of such bleeding increases with progression of pregnancy and is caused by the great increase in vascularity, stromal softening, and exposure of the delicate columnar epithelium to infection and trauma in the vagina. Endocervical epithelial hyperplasia, often seen in pregnancy, may result in polyp formation and bleeding. Rarely, carcinoma of the cervix presents as a complication of pregnancy with vaginal bleeding, and this must be excluded by cytology and appropriate biopsy of gross lesions.

The cornerstone of diagnosis of all extrauterine types of vaginal bleeding is a careful speculum examination. However, if the diagnosis of placenta previa is suspected (see later discussion), it is prudent to defer speculum examination until placenta previa is ruled out.

The causes of pathologic *uterine bleeding* may be divided into those presenting in the first and second halves of pregnancy.

FIRST HALF OF PREGNANCY

Vaginal bleeding in the first half of pregnancy is termed abortion. *Threatened abortion* is uterine bleeding in the first half of pregnancy without passage of tissue. It is most common before 15 weeks' gestation. One half of patients with threatened abortion continue their pregnancy well into the third trimester with no further complications and one half will continue to bleed and subsequently abort. Approximately one third of spontaneous abortions will involve a fetus with karyotypic abnormalities, many of which consist of trisomy. Inevitable abortion is defined as vaginal bleeding with cervical dilation. Incomplete abortion is defined as passage of a portion of the products of conception. Missed abortion is prolonged retention of the conceptus after death of the fetus.

The diagnosis of *ectopic pregnancy* must be considered in all patients with vaginal bleeding, because this constitutes the most common life-threatening cause of bleeding in the first half of pregnancy. Ectopic pregnancy presents with vaginal bleeding in approximately 1 of every 150 pregnancies. The bleeding is usually described as dark spotting, although profuse hemorrhage is seen in approximately 5 per cent of patients. A history of amenorrhea suggestive of pregnancy is absent in one quarter to one half of patients. The temperature is rarely higher than 101 F (38.3 C). Hypotension is present in 10 per cent of patients. Abdominal tenderness ranging from mild lower quadrant tenderness to a pattern of severe peritonitis is seen in three quarters of patients. The pelvic examination reveals tenderness, especially on cervical motion. Cervical softening suggestive of pregnancy is present in 75 per cent of patients. The uterus is often enlarged appropriately for menstrual dates in first trimester ectopic gestation. A painful adnexal mass, usually of spongy consistency, is noted in approximately one third of the patients. The leukocyte count is normal in 50 per cent and mild anemia is usually found.

Return of nonclotting blood on culdocentesis is helpful because false-positive results are rare.

The conventional latex agglutination pregnancy test is positive in approximately 50 per cent of patients; however, the recently developed, more sensitive radioreceptor assay (RRA) holds promise for the earlier diagnosis of ectopic gestation. Endometrial biopsy is of limited value in that true decidua is obtained in only 20 per cent of patients. Early laparoscopy of the patient with a suspected ectopic pregnancy is essential and avoids unnecessary laparotomy in patients with corpus luteum cysts in whom bleeding has ceased.

Gestational trophoblastic disease is found in 1 in 2000 deliveries in the United States. Molar pregnancies may present with painless bleeding late in the first half of pregnancy. Signs and symptoms of toxemia appearing in the first half of pregnancy should suggest trophoblastic disease and are present in more than 20 per cent of such patients. Severe hyperemesis gravidarum is seen in a somewhat larger proportion of patients. The diagnosis is supported by 24-hour urinary chorionic gonadotropins greater than 500,000 IU. This level may also occasionally be seen with multiple gestation. Sonography usually reveals characteristic intrauterine echoes. If the sonogram is not diagnostic or not available, amniography may be performed.

SECOND HALF OF PREGNANCY

Selected causes of vaginal bleeding early in pregnancy may initially present in the second half. These include coagulopathy, cervicitis, premature cervical dilation, ectopic gestation, cervical cancer, and gestational trophoblastic disease. The two most significant and common causes of bleeding late in pregnancy are abruptio placenta and placenta previa; however, less than half of bleeding patients can be definitely diagnosed as having either of these. Abruption is present in 0.75 to 1.5 per cent of all deliveries. Predispositions to abruption include a history of severe previous abruption, hypertension, and multiparity. The disease in both its mild and severe forms may appear at any time in the second half of pregnancy. In addition to vaginal bleeding, the diagnosis is suggested by uterine contractions, irritability, and tenderness. Uterine pain and irritability may be absent in cases of abruption with posterior placental implantation.

The triad of vaginal bleeding, painful uterine contractions, and absent fetal heart tones is particularly suggestive of severe *abruptio placenta* and must be borne in mind, as the demise implies a greater degree of abruption and there-

fore a higher risk of disseminated intravascular coagulation.

Clinically detectable coagulopathy secondary to abruption is rare in mild cases but can be found in one third of cases of sufficient severity to produce fetal demise. Consumption of coagulation factors, overt renal failure, and shock disproportionate to the degree of demonstrable hemorrhage may be seen, especially in the concealed type of abruption.

Diagnostic tests to detect coagulopathy are indicated in all patients with vaginal bleeding in which placental abruption is suspected. These include observation of a tube of blood for clot formation and subsequent fibrinolysis, examination of a stained blood smear, and formal coagulation parameters. The most sensitive parameters are plasma fibrinogen and platelet count. Decreased fibrinogen levels are seen in 10 to 30 per cent of patients. Frequent measurements of the fundal height may disclose a progressively enlarging uterus, suggestive of abruption with an enlarging retroplacental clot.

Sonography may disclose the presence of a retroplacental clot suggesting abruption. Not infrequently, the sonographic demonstration of a fundal placenta can be made, excluding the diagnosis of placenta previa except in the case of a succenturiate lobe.

The syndrome of separation of the marginal placental sinus that presents as an abruption without the associated signs and symptoms of persistent uterine irritability, pain, coagulopathy, shock, and fetal compromise is believed by many to be a forme fruste of abruption.

Placenta previa's hallmark is *painless*, bright red vaginal bleeding in the mid to late second half of pregnancy and complicates 0.25 to 0.5 per cent of pregnancies. The diagnosis must be made by indirect means because injudicious direct cervical examination may result in maternal and fetal death. Uterine contractions and tenderness are generally absent. The diagnosis may be supported by a floating or high presenting part and by an abnormal presentation.

The clinical course of placenta previa is often dependent on the exact relationship between the internal cervical os and the placental implantation site. Hemorrhage with total or central placenta previa occurs earlier in gestation, the extent of hemorrhage is often greater, and delivery becomes necessary earlier than with lesser degrees of previa. The time course from the first hemorrhage to delivery is shorter in total placenta previa than with partial or marginal placental implantation.

An expectant course of management (no vaginal or rectal examinations) is urged because more than 90 per cent of first episodes of third trimester bleeding cease after one day of observation and any cervical manipulation may precipitate life-threatening hemorrhage.

The diagnosis of third trimester bleeding is entirely based on the clinical presentation and course followed by the patient. Regardless of diagnostic findings, if bleeding is severe or progressive in nature, the cause of hemorrhage does not guide clinical management.

Several diagnostic tests aimed at placental localization to detect implantation over the internal cervical os have been developed to aid in the diagnosis of third trimester bleeding. These screening tests must be timed appropriately because the majority of patients with placenta previa in the second trimester, even those with symptoms, will not have a persistent placenta previa at the time of delivery. An apparent change in the site of placental implantation can be found well into the third trimester.

The most commonly used method of placental localization currently is sonography using gray scale techniques in the bistable mode. Maneuvers should be applied to decrease the incidence of false sonographic diagnoses, including the gentle application of pressure to the fetal presenting part to move it in closer apposition to the posterior uterine wall, scans in multiple orientations, and appropriate positioning of the patient to elevate the presenting part out of the bony pelvis. The ultrasound method of placental localization is largely limited by the lack of a reliable marker for the position of the internal cervical os. A helpful diagnostic sign is the presence of a step-like configuration of the placenta as it crosses the cervix. Sonographic accuracy in placental localization is greater than 95 per cent.

Other methods of placentography with varying degrees of accuracy may still be applicable when sonography is not available. These include radioisotope placentography and radiographic techniques. Radiographic placental localization may be enhanced with intra-amniotic contrast agents.

Vaginal bleeding in pregnancy may infrequently be entirely fetal in origin and result from rupture of *vasa previa*. The rapid progression to intractable fetal distress should suggest this diagnosis and usually precludes delivery of a viable infant, even by emergency cesarean section, except in unusual circumstances. The Apt test for fetal hemoglobin may be rapidly performed as a bedside diagnostic technique; it relies on the instability of fetal hemoglobin in the presence of strong alkali. The Kleihauer-Betke technique for staining a blood smear may also be used to estimate the degree of admixture of fetal blood in maternal vaginal bleeding.

ABORTION

By KAIGHN SMITH, M.D.

Philadelphia, Pennsylvania

The diagnosis of abortion should be considered at any time a normally menstruating woman complains of abnormal bleeding. The time-honored medical adage "the commonest cause of amenorrhea is pregnancy" might be extended to "abnormal bleeding in women of childbearing age should be considered related to pregnancy until this cause is firmly ruled out."

DEFINITION

Abortion may be classified as *early abortion,* i.e., interruption of any pregnancy of less than 12 weeks' duration, or *late abortion,* i.e., interruption of pregnancy between 12 and 20 weeks. If a pregnancy terminates after 20 weeks' gestation, it should be considered as premature labor, rather than abortion, as viability of the infant becomes a remote possibility.

A further description of abortion must include a definition of types.

Spontaneous Abortion. This is termination of pregnancy before 20 weeks without medical interference.

Therapeutic Abortion. This is defined as termination of pregnancy for medical or socioeconomic reasons before 20 weeks by a licensed physician.

Criminal Abortion. This is termination of pregnancy by means of instrumentation or aspiration by an unlicensed individual. Since legalization of abortion in the United States, criminal abortion has markedly decreased with a concomitant decrease in maternal mortality resulting from such practices.

Spontaneous abortion has been further described according to the symptoms and physical findings of the patient.

Threatened Abortion. Uterine bleeding occurring in pregnancy without cervical dilatation or decrease in uterine size and with no history of the patient having passed tissue may be defined as "threatened."

Incomplete Abortion. When there is indication that parts, but not all, of the products of conception have already been passed, the diagnosis "incomplete abortion" should be made.

Inevitable Abortion. Uterine bleeding in pregnancy associated with severe cramping resulting from uterine contractions and dilatation or effacement of the cervix yields the diagnosis of "inevitable abortion." Generally, the membranes will be seen bulging through the cervix, placental tissue will be located here, or bleeding will be profuse.

Missed Abortion. When the uterus no longer is growing but no tissue or significant bleeding has passed, the diagnosis of "missed abortion" must be entertained. Such abortions are not uncommon in patients treated with large doses of progestins for an earlier threatened abortion.

Septic Abortion. If there is evidence of infection in any of the aforementioned conditions, the diagnosis of "septic abortion" must be made. The range of possibilities runs from infected products of conception to the most severe forms of septic abortion, leading to endotoxic shock.

Habitual Abortion. The patient who has had three consecutive spontaneous abortions may be called a "habitual aborter."

DIAGNOSIS

In order to make the diagnosis of abortion, one must first attempt the diagnosis of pregnancy, as any abnormal bleeding in a female of childbearing age may in reality be an abortion.

HISTORY

A period of amenorrhea of 6 weeks or longer, followed by any bleeding, should immediately raise the suspicion of abortion. Even a scant menstrual period at the regular time may indicate pregnancy. Other symptoms such as breast fullness, nausea, urinary frequency, and constipation can be absent. This may be because the products of conception are defective and have an inadequate hormone output.

PHYSICAL EXAMINATION

Uterine size is not always commensurate with the period of amenorrhea in abortion, particularly if a missed or incomplete abortion is present. Softening, blueness, and congestion of the uterine cervix are often telltale signs. Pulsations of the uterine vessels felt along the lower uterine segment are often prominent in pregnancy and should make one suspicious. Occasionally, a corpus luteum may cause moderate enlargement of one ovary, although if such a mass is tender, ectopic pregnancy must always be considered.

LABORATORY TESTS

The pregnancy test is still the most reliable method of determining the presence of chorionic tissue, and each laboratory must have one or more of these tests available. The Aschheim-Zondek and Friedman tests have been replaced by other modern immunologic techniques, which are better than 90 per cent reliable. Newer quick immunologic tests that are very reliable are now available to patients and physicians. One must remember that the pregnancy test is often negative in early pregnancy (less than 2 weeks after a missed period) or in a late missed abortion. If suspicion of an early ectopic pregnancy exists, a sophisticated laboratory test for the beta subunit of the chorionic hormone is available that gives results even before a period is missed.

CONCLUSION

Any bleeding in early pregnancy must be considered at least a threatened abortion. Of the 25 or 30 per cent of women who experience vaginal bleeding in the first trimester, only one half will ultimately abort. It is important to make the diagnosis between threatened and inevitable abortion, because a hands-off policy is obvious in the former condition.

Watchful waiting will often differentiate a minor threat to the conceptus from a developing incomplete or inevitable abortion.

The patient presenting with abortion and shock must be carefully evaluated for sepsis resulting from bacterial endotoxin and for ectopic pregnancy. These two pitfalls in diagnosis can be critical to the patient's life.

HYPERTENSIVE STATES IN PREGNANCY

By FRANK A. FINNERTY, JR., M.D.
Washington, D.C.

The finding of an elevated blood pressure in a pregnant patient always suggests toxemia. It must be emphasized at the outset, however, that toxemia has always served as a wastebasket term for a variety of disease states characterized

$$\text{TOXEMIA} \Longleftarrow \begin{array}{l} \text{ELEVATED B.P.} \\ \text{ALBUMINURIA} \\ \text{EDEMA} \end{array}$$

	OPHTHALMOSCOPIC EXAMINATION		URINALYSIS		
	Arterial Spasm	Retinopathy and A.V. Nicking	Alb.	W.B.C.	R.B.C.
PURE TOXEMIA	√	O	√	O	O
H.V.D.	O	√	±	O	O
H.V.D. + TOXEMIA	√	√	√	O	O
PYELONEPHRITIS	O	O	√	√	O
GLOMERULO- NEPHRITIS	√	O	√	√	√

Figure 1. Differential diagnosis of toxemia. B.P.: blood pressure; H.V.D.: hypertensive vascular disease; A.V.: arterio-venous; Alb.: albumin; W.B.C.: white blood cells; R.B.C.: red blood cells.

by an increased arterial pressure, edema, and albuminuria (Fig. 1). Although this triad is consistent with the diagnosis of toxemia, it is not diagnostic. These abnormalities may be found in pregnant patients with hypertensive vascular disease, pyelonephritis, glomerulonephritis, or any combination of these.

During a 2-year period, 4273 patients were studied in our toxemia clinic (Table 1). Although 95 per cent of these patients were originally diagnosed by the obstetricians as having toxemia, it is interesting to note the frequency of hypertensive vascular disease and pyelonephritis and the relative rarity of true toxemia. Differentiation of these disease states has more than academic interest. The finding of definite hypertensive changes and the absence of retinal artery spasm in a pregnant patient with an elevated arterial pressure are reassuring to the physician (Fig. 1). These patients are not toxemic — they are patients with hypertensive

Table 1. *Diagnosis in 4273 Patients, 1961–1963*

Pure toxemia	167	4%
Toxemia and hypertensive vascular disease	42	6%
Toxemia and pyelonephritis	67	
Pyelonephritis	704	25%
Pyelonephritis and hypertensive vascular disease	287	
Hypertensive vascular disease	804	
Glomerulonephritis	84	
Nonrelated medical disease (anemia, heart disease, etc.)	214	
Edema without disease	387	
Asymptomatic bacteriuria	469	
No disease	944	
Questionable diagnosis	104	
	4273	

vascular disease who happen to be pregnant. The indications for hypotensive therapy should be the same as though the patient were not pregnant — e.g., vascular damage; cerebral, cardiac, or renal impairment; and/or a rising diastolic pressure. A single elevated blood pressure reading or even several elevated office blood pressure readings are not indications for hypotensive therapy or immediate hospitalization, nor do they indicate toxemia of pregnancy.

HYPERTENSIVE VASCULAR DISEASE

During the past 20 years we have followed 2000 hypertensive patients throughout pregnancy. Most of them had a known history of hypertension prior to pregnancy, In a third of these patients, the blood pressure remained essentially unchanged; in one third, the blood pressure increased; and in one third, the blood pressure became normotensive or hypotensive. In the group of patients whose arterial pressure increased, there was usually evidence of superimposed toxemia, e.g., periorbital edema or albuminuria or both. In the group of patients whose blood pressure became normotensive or hypotensive, the fall in arterial pressure was noted during the first trimester and remained low or normal throughout pregnancy. Immediately after delivery the blood pressure in these patients would again become hypertensive (higher than the usual level in the nonpregnant state) and would then fall in several days to its usual hypertensive level before pregnancy.

It has always been our impression that the majority of the immediate postpartum rises in blood pressure are a result of the routine administration of oxytocic agents to hypertensive patients who have become normotensive during pregnancy. It seems logical therefore to check the patient's past record and examine the retinal vessels before routinely administering oxytocic agents.

Ophthalmologically these hypertensive patients could be divided into 704 patients with normal fundi and 1296 patients with abnormal fundi. In the group showing abnormal fundi, 591 showed Grade I changes (increased light striping and tortuosity); 692 showed Grade II changes (more pronounced Grade I changes plus arteriovenous nicking); and 13 showed hemorrhages or exudates.

Except perhaps for their age, the group of hypertensive patients with normal fundi differs in no way from the large number of nonpregnant hypertensive patients seen routinely by the internist. The symptoms, if any, are related to anxiety and not to the arterial pressure. These are patients without evidence of vascular disease except for the high blood pressure reading. This state therefore might better be called "a high blood pressure reading" than hypertensive vascular disease. As with the nonpregnant patient, there is no relation between the severity of the disease and the blood pressure reading. These patients with normal fundi present no problem medically or obstetrically. They respond well to diuretics or mild sedation, and their pregnancy is in no way affected by the high blood pressure reading.

The overwhelming numbers of black patients in our clinic (all except 19 were black) may explain, in part at least, the prominence of hypertension in this group, because hypertension is known to develop earlier in the black. Without examination of the retina, however, many of these patients, particularly the group under 20 years of age, would be classified as having toxemia, the severity of the toxemia judged by the height of the arterial pressure.

On the other hand, failure to examine the retina in the group of hypertensive patients whose blood pressure went down during pregnancy would account for a diagnosis of "normal pregnancy." Recognition of the abnormal fundi in this group forewarns the physician of the possible postpartum rise in blood pressure, which might or might not be significant. Although described by Dieckmann and Teel, the frequency of this phenomenon has not been appreciated.

Work-Up of the Hypertensive Patient

Even though the majority of pregnancy patients with hypertension are usually under 35 years of age, most of them have essential hypertension. This generalization is even more valid in blacks, who rarely develop renovascular hypertension. Since the telltale signs and symptoms of the secondary types of hypertension are usually evident from a careful history, physical examination, and standard laboratory procedures, an exhaustive search in every patient seems hardly warranted, particularly during pregnancy when certain x-ray procedures may be harmful to the fetus. Indeed, determinations of renin activity, urinary catecholamines, and the like should certainly not be part of a routine work-up in an asymptomatic patient, whether she is pregnant or not.

In addition to the history and physical examination, the only routine laboratory procedures indicated are blood for potassium, glucose, creatinine, cholesterol, and uric acid. An elevated cholesterol level is not only an independent risk factor but also may suggest chronic renal disease; whereas an elevated uric acid level in a pregnant patient not on thiazide diuretic would indicate the presence of superimposed toxemia.

A complete urinalysis and urine culture should be part of the routine work-up of every pregnant patient in order to document the presence of asymptomatic genitourinary tract infection. The obstructive uropathy associated with normal pregnancy not only may aggravate already existing disease, but unsuspected and therefore untreated genitourinary tract infection may contribute to fetal prematurity and mortality. In this regard, our experience would indicate that the finding of albuminuria in a pregnant patient should be considered as a sign of genitourinary tract infection until proved otherwise and makes a urine culture mandatory.

Although an intravenous pyelogram (IVP) might well be routine in the work-up of a young hypertensive female who is not pregnant, particularly when albuminuria is present, such a procedure is contraindicated in the pregnant patient unless absolutely necessary because of danger to the fetus. The only indications for IVP would be in the patient with obstructive uropathy in whom imminent surgery is planned. It should also be emphasized that it is not practical to perform an IVP in the pregnant patient or in the patient immediately postpartum, because the ureteral dilatation normally associated with pregnancy (which may be confused with obstruction) takes 6 weeks to subside.

Pyelonephritis

Many studies have emphasized (1) the high incidence of genitourinary tract infection in pregnancy, (2) its asymptomatic nature, (3) the fact that it may manifest itself as toxemia of pregnancy, and (4) the relationship between unsuspected genitourinary tract infection and prematurity. Studies in our laboratory have demonstrated a 13 to 14 per cent incidence of significant genitourinary tract infection (colony count in excess of 100,000 [10^5] per ml) in normal pregnant patients and a 25 per cent incidence of significant bacteriuria in patients with albuminuria who were suspected of having toxemia.

The majority of pregnant patients with proteinuria are usually considered by their obstetricians to have toxemia, whereas in actuality less than half of them have toxemia by our criteria. Clinical experience has attested to the fact that proteinuria is usually the last sign to occur in toxemia, appearing long after the rise in arterial pressure and the occurrence of edema. It is our opinion therefore that the finding of proteinuria in a pregnant patient with or without a rise in arterial pressure or edema should suggest pyelonephritis and make bacteriologic studies of the urine mandatory. If genitourinary tract infection is not to be overlooked, a urine culture and colony count should be performed on every pregnant patient and should be repeated on every patient with proteinuria. In our experience, the most common cause of proteinuria in the pregnant patient is genitourinary tract infection.

POSTPARTUM HYPERTENSION

Studies from our clinic have demonstrated that the 2- to 17-week postpartum period (usually 4 to 6 weeks) may be associated with a pressor phenomenon. In 1 per cent of 10,000 postpartum patients, the first elevation of arterial pressure occurred during this period. These patients had an entirely normal past history, pregnancy, delivery, and immediate postpartum period. Of 2311 patients with a history of hypertension or toxemia, the highest level of arterial pressure occurred during this same postpartum period. In other words, 20 per cent of the patients who exhibited any pressor phenomenon in relation to pregnancy showed the highest level of arterial pressure during the postpartum period. As these patients are asymptomatic and as this is a self-limiting state, one would have great difficulty in evaluating the effectiveness of any type of therapy. Unless other obvious signs of end-organ damage or any evidence of the accelerated phase exists, it would seem that no definitive antihypertensive therapy would be required at this time. Monthly follow-up is essential until the patient becomes normotensive.

POSTPARTUM COMPLICATIONS

By JOHN F. J. CLARK, M.D., and ERNEST LOYD HOPKINS, M.D. Washington, D.C.

The postpartum period begins at the end of labor. It is a part of the puerperium. The puerperium is defined as that period from the end of labor up to 6 weeks after birth, during which time the tissues are returning to the prepregnant state.

The postpartum period is defined for this discussion as that period from the end of labor up to 2 weeks after delivery. During this period all the complications to be discussed will have become symptomatic. It should be clear that the incidence, severity, and end result of postpartum complications are a byproduct of many preceding factors: interconceptional health status of the mother, antepartum care, intrapartum management, and many factors during the aforementioned periods that positively or negatively influence the well-being of the mother or the fetus.

The major alterations that occur are within the cardiovascular, pulmonary, hematopoietic, gastrointestinal, renal, musculoskeletal, neurological, and psychologic systems. During pregnancy these variations pose a great challenge to our diagnostic skill because the complications we are called upon to define and evaluate are occurring within a period of dynamic change. At this time tissues are attempting to return to the prepregnant state.

The postpartum complications may occur either early or late. By early postpartum complications we refer to those occurring within the first seconds after the end of labor up to the first 24 hours. The late events are those that occur after 24 hours with onset of diagnosable symptoms and signs within the first 2 weeks after labor.

RETAINED PLACENTA

The placenta that remains within the uterus 30 minutes after the delivery of the single newborn is considered retained. Often the placenta is partially separated, and the introduction of a gloved finger into the vagina will reveal the presence of the placenta in the lower segment. When the placenta is partially separated, there is often bleeding from the implantation site. From this location the placenta can be easily removed. When the placenta is not partially separated, manual exploration of the uterus is done to make a proper diagnosis. In the majority of patients a normally implanted placenta will be encountered and can be easily removed. In many instances patients will bleed heavily because of the retention of a small volume of placental fragments and membranes. This may not be detected in the placental examination. The diagnosis is established when the fragments are removed at exploration of the uterus and the bleeding stops.

It is imperative that the responsible physician familiarize himself with the palpable findings of an empty uterine implantation site in the early postpartum period.

CHORIONIC VILLOUS INVASION OF THE MYOMETRIUM (PLACENTA ACCRETA, INCRETA, AND PERCRETA)

In this condition, there is an absence of a cleavage plane between the maternal surface of the placenta and the decidua basalis of the uterus. This condition may vary from the placenta accreta, in which there is slight invasion of the chorionic villi into the decidua basalis, to the placenta percreta, which is characterized by complete infiltration of the chorionic villi into the myometrium, and through the serosa of the uterus. When there is massive fixation of the placenta to the myometrium, vigorous attempts to separate the placenta from the uterus will result in alarming hemorrhage. There is an intermediate condition called placenta increta in which the chorionic villi invade to various depths of the myometrium. Except for mildest accreta, manual removal attempts are associated with massive hemorrhage. This diagnosis is made by palpation of the implantation site. The laboratory findings will depend upon the volume of bleeding and the general status of the patient in a given case.

LACERATIONS OF THE PERINEUM, VAGINA, AND CERVIX

The most common maternal injury in pregnancy is the laceration of the perineum. The least significant but most frequent tear is first degree perineal tear. In this tear, vaginal and perineal skin are injured but the perineal muscles are intact. In second degree tear the posterior commissure is torn down to the anal sphincter. The vaginal tear may extend up both sides of the vagina, from a perineal laceration or episiotomy to the posterior and lateral fornices. In third degree tear the entire anal sphincter is torn apart. This is characterized by a retraction of the sphincter muscles. This injury leaves the patient with incontinence of stool if the tear is not repaired.

Laceration of the cervix usually follows precipitate labor and sometimes follows forceps deliveries. Annular cervical laceration should be suspected when a mass of tissue with a central opening is found in the vagina.

The arterial blood supply to the cervix and upper third of the vagina is the cervical-vaginal branch of the uterine artery. The middle third of the vagina is supplied by branches of the middle hemorrhoidal artery and the vaginal branches of the internal pudendal artery. The perineum and vulva are supplied by the perineal branches of the internal pudendal artery. It should be remembered, as pointed out by William Goddard, that the vessels supplying the vaginal wall course medially and downward toward the vaginal opening just before entering the wall. Vessels supplying the perineum course medially and upward toward the clitoris.

The symptoms of laceration of perineum, vagina, and cervix are related to maternal hemorrhage. Usually the bleeding will not reach a maximum level of severity until the postpartum period. Careful inspection of the perineum, vagina, and cervix must be done in every patient. Elevation of anterior and posterior lips of the cervix with a ring forceps is mandatory so that visualization of the cervix in its entirety will be possible. Concomitant with cervix inspection should be careful visualization of lateral and posterior fornices and the entire length of the vaginal wall, including the periurethral areas.

The diagnosis is established when evidence of laceration is visualized. Highly saturated arterial blood from the vagina should alert the operator to the possibility of a laceration with arterial bleeding. These evaluations should be made in the presence of a well-contracted uterus. Bleeding from the large vascular channels at the placental implantation site can be confused with arterial bleeding from a uterine vessel.

At the onset of heavy bleeding, coagulation studies should be obtained. Bleeding time, fibrinogen, partial thromboplastin, prothrombin time, split fibrin products, and complete blood count (CBC) may be obtained, but in the absence of a blood volume measurement the estimated blood loss from tape weights and suction volume should be the index for transfusion, along with the clinical condition of the patient. In instances of acute blood loss the hemoglobin and hematocrit may subtly increase as the patient is losing more blood.

VULVAR, PERINEAL, AND INTRA-ABDOMINAL HEMATOMAS

Hematomas follow pressure injuries to the vulva and perineal area during childbirth. The incidence is greater in multiparous patients who have extensive vulvar and perineal varicosities. They may occur, however, in patients who do not have venous incompetency. The major injury is occasioned by the effusion of blood from injured submucosal vessels, resulting in a blood mass that becomes more and more confined to the alveolar and connective tissue spaces surrounding injured blood vessels.

Hematomas found in the tissues below the pelvic fascia usually remain vulvar. Those found in the tissue lateral to the cervix above the pelvic fascia dissect upward into the leaves of the broad ligament and may reach the level of the round ligament. This intra-abdominal extension of a pelvic hematoma results in massive blood loss. The patient may be in shock from blood loss without visible evidence of active bleeding.

The diagnosis is made by vaginal abdominal examination, revealing an expanding mass that can be followed from the vagina up to the upper abdomen. Hypertension, elevated pulse, pallor, and anemia, as indicated by falling hemoglobin and hematocrit, are usual findings. Fortunately, most of the hematomas are recognizable as a purplish asymmetry of the vulvar-perineal area that presents soon after injury. Prompt diagnosis of the extent and severity of the injury and appropriate treatment will usually avert the most serious sequelae described.

POSTPARTUM HEMORRHAGE DUE TO UTERINE MYOMETRIAL DYSFUNCTION

Charles Hendricks and others have demonstrated that after the delivery of the newborn and the placenta, the uterine contractility proceeds in a coordinated fashion. The intrauterine pressure increases several times to levels of 200 to 210 mm Hg, and this facilitates the compression of the major vascular sinuses at the placental site. There are a number of conditions during pregnancy that predispose to the existence of uncoordinated uterine contractility postpartum. When the uterine contractility is not coordinated, the uterine contractions are ineffective, the uterus is flaccid, and serious bleeding ensues. This is postpartum hemorrhage resulting from uterine myometrial dysfunction when the blood loss is 500 ml or more. The following conditions in pregnancy are associated with an increased incidence of postpartum hemorrhage:

uterine anomalies, multiple gestation, uterine myomas, polyhydramnios, multiparity, prolonged labor, and myometrial dysfunction during labor.

The incidence of this type of hemorrhage is about 4 per cent of all deliveries. The diagnosis is made when heavy bleeding ensues in the presence of a relaxed noncontracted uterus. The important differential diagnosis is from lacerations of the cervix that sometimes bleed massively. It should be borne in mind that the seriousness of heavy bleeding associated with this condition may not be reflected by the patient's vital signs and level of consciousness.

Patients may lose 1500 to 2000 ml of whole blood and retain average blood pressure and pulse readings. Suddenly there is a precipitous drop in blood pressure, with an increase in the pulse rate to 130 to 140 beats per minute, associated with shortness of breath, tachypnea, and anxiety. Even in the presence of shock these patients will remain quite lucid and conscious. Whenever this condition can be anticipated, the availability of a large bore 16-gauge needle and several units of typed and crossmatched packed cells will provide the necessary preparation to assure a safe outcome for the patients.

UTERINE RUPTURE

Uterine rupture refers to separation of the uterine wall and rupture of the membranes with continuity between the uterine and peritoneal cavities. Extrusion of the products of conception, pain, and bleeding are inevitable sequelae.

This is to be differentiated from "dehiscence" or occult rupture, in which the membranes are not ruptured and in which most often there is no pain. This condition may not be diagnosed until the uterus is explored during or after the third stage of labor.

The incidence of uterine rupture is 1:1000 to 1:1500 pregnancies. Eastman classifies uterine rupture in the following three categories: (1) rupture of previous uterine scar, (2) spontaneous rupture of the intact uterus, and (3) traumatic rupture of the intact uterus.

Rupture of the previous uterine scar occurs in less than 5 per cent of all cesarean section deliveries. The perinatal mortality for uterine rupture newborns is very close to 50 per cent. Traumatic rupture of the bladder is a possible secondary event that must be anticipated.

Spontaneous rupture of the intact uterus is significantly more frequent than rupture of a previous uterine scar. In our experience, gravid-ity of four or more appears to be the signal for possible spontaneous rupture. Traumatic rupture of the intact uterus, after the period of viability, is invariably associated with some obstetric manipulations. Versions of various types, total breech extraction, and fundal pressure with patient-initiated Valsalva maneuver are all indicated factors associated with traumatic rupture.

The primary causative factor in uterine rupture appears to be excessive thinning of the lower uterine segment with development of a pathologic retraction ring.

When the uterus ruptures during labor without anesthesia, there is the onset of severe pain and the patient describes a tearing sensation. This is followed by a feeling of relief. The presenting part cannot be palpated vaginally, and there is marked anterior abdominal tenderness. Within the first few minutes after rupture the uterus may be felt distinctly and separately from the fetus. After bleeding has proceeded, the abdomen becomes distended and generalized rebound tenderness with rigidity of the abdomen rapidly follows.

Blood pressure, pulse, and respirations deteriorate rapidly with hypotension, tachycardia, tachypnea, pallor, and diaphoresis following. Heavy genital bleeding associated with shock and semiconsciousness follows closely. At the time of marked prostration, abdominal signs may be misleading, as the abdomen may be distended, but the patient may not respond with rebound tenderness and evidence of peritoneal irritation as before. Catheterization of the bladder with retrieval of blood supports the diagnosis of rupture. Vaginal exploration of the uterus confirms the diagnosis. Under anesthesia the first indication of rupture may be the presence of unsaturated blood with a generalized shock-like state. Vaginal-abdominal compression may result in temporary improvement as laparotomy preparation proceeds. Rapid transfusion along with preparation for immediate laparotomy is life-saving. Complete blood count and coagulation studies are helpful. Once the diagnosis is established, particularly in the complete rupture, stabilization of the patient's condition may be possible only by ligation of the bleeding vessels.

Uterine Inversion

Uterine inversion is a condition in which the uterus becomes inverted incompletely or completely. In the complete variety the uterine protrusion through the external os is apparent. This entity is very rare but is still seen in the United States. The admonition "Never perform a Credé maneuver on a relaxed uterine fundus" will completely eliminate this complication from obstetric practice. It is interesting to note that of the patients reported in the literature more than 50 per cent were primigravidas. The incomplete variety offers the greatest challenge to diagnosis. The mortality is increased as the failure to diagnose the condition increases to 48 hours. The characteristic finding in the incomplete variety is a crater-like depression in the area where the fundus is expected suprapubically. Abdominal-vaginal examination confirms the diagnosis.

Postpartum Eclampsia

Postpartum eclampsia is a rare complicating variant of toxemia of pregnancy in which the first convulsion occurs during the first 24 hours after delivery, although in a few patients it has occurred several days after delivery. If a first convulsion occurs after 24 hours postpartum, the patient must be carefully evaluated for evidence of cerebrovascular dysfunction, intracerebral mass, or thrombosis of the major cerebral sinuses. All postpartum eclampsia patients have a history of preeclampsia during the last trimester of pregnancy. The diagnosis is one of exclusion, and recovery from this condition is without permanent sequelae.

Postpartum Cardiovascular Accidents

Patients who are pregnant may present with signs of neurologic decompensation postpartum. Intracerebral hemorrhage resulting from ruptured congenital aneurysms, thrombosis of major arterial or venous cerebral channels, and cerebral vascular spasm with edema may produce symptoms and signs initially in the postpartum period.

Patients with intracerebral hemorrhage may have changing neurologic signs and varying degrees of consciousness. Inequality of pupils and evidence of motor weakness with flaccid or spastic paralysis of one or more extremities may occur. The patient with cerebral thrombosis may have weakness and paralysis associated with anisocoria. Loss of consciousness is not as frequent as that found in patients with intracerebral hemorrhage. In cerebrovascular spasm transient loss of consciousness and convulsion with weakness and transient spastic paralysis occur. These patients always present a marked elevation in blood pressure with diastolic pressures above 110 mm Hg. A careful neurologic examination, including a funduscopic examination, is mandatory in these patients. If there is no evidence of increased intracranial pressure, an examination of the cerebrospinal fluid will be helpful. The fluid should be evaluated for pressure, color, cell count, protein, glucose, and bacterial content. The opening and closing pressure should be recorded, and the presence or absence of trauma during the procedure should be carefully documented. Immediate neurologic and neurosurgical evaluation and treatment in these patients are life-saving.

AMNIOTIC FLUID INFUSION

This condition is associated with the entry of amniotic fluid into the maternal circulation. The association of ruptured membranes, intravenous oxytocin stimulation, and hypertonic uterine contractions has been implicated as partially causative in this condition. Small amounts of amniotic fluid that gain access to many organs, including the lungs and the brain, are identifiable as a cluster of squamous cells of fetal origin in these organs. The clinical picture is that of convulsions and profuse genital bleeding. The partial thromboplastin time is increased. Split fibrin products are significantly increased within the maternal blood, and the clot retraction is poor. This condition is often fatal, with only a small amount of fluid and cellular debris being demonstrated in the maternal circulation. The best results are obtained from early diagnosis and immediate treatment.

PULMONARY EMBOLISM

The intravascular dissemination of clots from the pelvic veins is a major threat in multiparous patients. Because of chronic intracaval increase in venous pressure, there is a less dynamic circulatory return as pregnancy progresses. In multiparous patients who have significant varicosities there is venous valvular incompetency and significant stasis of blood. The presence of puerperal infection increases the incidence of pelvic venous clotting. The complication of pulmonary embolism is a dangerous progression of pelvic thrombophlebitis. The condition is associated with the sudden onset of chest pain, with or without hemoptysis, shortness of breath and tachypnea, increased pulse rate significant beyond expectation, and a shift toward right axis deviation in the electrocardiogram (ECG). The acute onset of P pulmonale waves on ECG is often found. Anterior and lateral lung scans are often diagnostic. The best outcome for patients is found in the prompt treatment of the first signs of pelvic infection and pelvic thrombophlebitis.

POSTPARTUM THROMBOPHLEBITIS

Pelvic thrombophlebitis must be suspected in any patient with pelvic puerperal infection in whom there is a persistent fever with pelvic tenderness, a persistent elevation of the pulse rate, and evidence of hypermetabolism. Cultures from the cervix and the vagina and blood cultures will often help to identify the offending organism. Because of the frequency with which the condition may progress to pulmonary embolization, a baseline electrocardiogram, bleeding time, partial thromboplastin and prothrombin times, and fibrinogen should be obtained very early during the course of therapy.

CARDIAC ARREST

A most unfortunate and highly fatal complication of the postpartum period is circulatory collapse and cardiac arrest. Marked blood loss during delivery of the newborn and the placenta, uterine rupture, deep anesthesia or any condition that results in maternal hypotension, and loss of effective circulating volume may be the cause in this condition. During delivery, whether vaginal or abdominal, constant observation of the color of the blood as an index of oxygen saturation of hemoglobin is a helpful marker of cardiovascular dysfunction. Teamwork between the obstetrician and the anesthesia person, or other support persons in attendance after delivery, may avert this most serious complication. An accurate estimate of blood loss, a careful documentation of the status of the patient before labor, and prompt replacement of volume deficits as they occur must be performed. Prompt consultative correction of any serious alteration from the normally expected physiology of the patient should be instituted before it has proceeded to the point of irreversibility. The average obstetric patient is young and has a reserve distinctly above that of the average patient. This reserve serves her well in the resolution of complicated states.

PUERPERAL INFECTION (PUERPERAL SEPSIS, CHILDBED FEVER)

Any infection developing in the genital tract after the period of viability as a consequence of labor and delivery is referred to as puerperal infection. Puerperal morbidity has been defined as a temperature elevation above 100.4 F (38 C) on any 2 of the first 10 postpartum days, exclusive of the first 24 hours. The temperature should be recorded orally every 4 hours for a minimum of four times during a 24-hour period.

About 65 per cent of the puerperal infections are caused by the anaerobic streptococcus. The infections caused by these organisms are usually mild. These organisms can often be cultured from the vagina and uterus of a perfectly asymptomatic puerperal female. The remainder of the infections are caused by beta-hemolytic streptococci, gonococci, *Escherichia coli, Clostridium welchii, Clostridium tetani,* and pneumococci. Gonococci rarely cause puerperal infections even though they may be present in the cervix. When *Clostridium welchii, Clostridium tetani,* and pneumococci cause puerperal infection, it is very serious and often lethal.

The ultimate tissue involvement in this condition is dependent upon the local tissue resistance, the overall health of the mother, the virulence of the organisms involved, and the particular site of bacterial inoculation. The bacteria invade the tissues from a site in the cervix or endometrium, spreading laterally to involve the myometrium by direct extension and the uterine veins and lymphatics through which they are transported to the parametrial areas surrounding the cervix and lower uterine segment. They invade loose areola tissue and connective tissue between the leaves of the broad ligament and the subperitoneal tissue surrounding the tubes and ovaries, resulting in an extensive cellulitis.

The obvious difference here is that the involvement in relationship to the pelvic organs, such as the tubes and ovaries, is at the peritoneal covering and the serosal surface. Involvement of the deep-seated mucosa of the fallopian tube very rarely occurs in this condition.

The diagnosis is established from the pelvic findings. Laboratory studies should include complete blood count, urinalysis (microscopic and culture), and cultures from the vagina and cervix. Serial blood cultures should be obtained. The cultures should be both aerobic and anaerobic, and the minimum inhibitory concentration as found on the sensitivity studies should be used as an aid in adjustment of the antibiotic dose. Blood volume and gastrointestinal function should be evaluated. Any deviation from the normal expected findings should be corrected promptly.

Postpartum Mastitis

Postpartum mastitis often proceeds to abscess formation and is common in women who are nursing or attempting to nurse their babies.

The peak time of incidence is 2 weeks after delivery. Trauma to the maternal nipple seems to provide the portal of entry for organisms. The symptom complex involves painful, tender breasts with fever and regional lymphadenopathy and pain. Treatment is largely preventive, and nursing should be prohibited in women with cracked and reddened nipples.

COMPLICATIONS OF OBSTETRIC ANESTHESIA

Intravenous Anesthesia

Inadvertent Intra-arterial Injection of Barbiturates. This dramatic complication occurs most often when the antecubital fossa is used for intravenous anesthesia. Often the needle is pushed through the vein into the artery that accompanies it. When the alkaline barbiturate solution is induced, patients complain of excruciating pain that is pathognomonic of intra-arterial injections. The injection should be discontinued and the needle left in place, with intravenous heparin and lidocaine to follow.

Regional Anesthesia

Epidural Anesthesia. *Subarachnoid Injection.* The inadvertent subarachnoid injection occurs when the needle is pushed through the ligamentum flavum and through the peridural space, into and through the subarachnoid membrane. This results in massive spinal blockage unless a very small test dose of the anesthesia is given. If a small dose of the anesthetic is given, the key to subarachnoid injection is to be found in the type of blockage which ensues.

With subarachnoid injection, the block is complete — sympathetic, sensory, and motor. With peridural injection, a small test dose will provide sympathetic blockade, minimal sensory blockade, and very minimal motor effect.

Intraspinal Injection. This complication should never occur. It arises from injections into the spinal nerves. This complication is associated with excruciating pain. Injection of an anesthetic should never be continued in the presence of pain resulting from the injection. The spinal cord ends at L1; injections made at L2 or below reduce the probability of spinal cord injury.

Aseptic Meningitis from Powder or Iodine Particles. Powder or iodine particles on the skin or hands of the operator may be driven into the peridural space by the needle, giving rise in susceptible patients to an aseptic meningitis. This disease process is seldom fatal but is associated with considerable patient morbidity. The use of highly powdered gloves and iodine-containing solutions should be carefully controlled when regional anesthesia is used.

Caudal Anesthesia. *Inadvertent Intravenous Injection.* The peridural space in the region of the sacrococcygeal membrane has a rich distribution of venous channels. In passing the needle carefully into the peridural space at this level it is often impossible to prevent minimal capillary damage. Prior to injection into this area an attempt to aspirate blood or fluid should always be carried out. The injection should be slow and without significant resistance. Intravascular absorption of the anesthetic gives varied symptoms, depending upon the agent being used, but generally the patient has a jittery, highly nervous sensation with general symptoms related to cerebral irritability.

Convulsions are not uncommon, and they may respond immediately to oxygen administration.

Inadvertent intravascular absorption of epinephrine-containing agents causes, in addition to the other manifestations indicated, increased blood pressure, increased pulse rate, and fetal tachycardia with irregularity of the fetal heart rate.

An additional complication of the use of epinephrine solutions may be a reduction in the coordination of uterine contractility. Another complication of caudal anesthesia is perianal or perirectal hematomas. Inadvertent misdirection of the injecting needle will result in trauma to the vascular plexus around the rectum or the perirectal area, causing oozing and hematoma formation in these areas.

Inadvertent injury to the fetal head or scalp is another complication. When the presenting part is very low in the perineum and caudal anesthesia is attempted with misdirection of the needle, injury to the presenting fetal part may occur.

Transrectal puncture with infection and perirectal abscess formation is a possibility. This can be avoided by careful orientation of the pathway of the needle to prevent injury to the rectum and contamination.

Total blockade or clavicular anesthesia is possible but most infrequently found with the reduction of anesthetic dosage used in most maternity settings today.

Supine hypotension, which occurs in approximately 15 per cent of pregnant patients and may be intimately related to inadequate vertebral venous collateral circulation, may contribute to hypotension caused by anesthetic agents. Increasing the venous return by changing the posture of the patient from supine to lateral, along with intravenous infusion as indicated, appears to be the treatment of choice. The use of vasopressors must be reserved for the individual patient after consideration of all factors.

The period of time in which the complication of hypotension occurs after peridural injection cannot be predicted. It is not safe to assume that after any given period of time the likelihood of hypotension is less, as it is clear that hypotension can occur any time during the life of the anesthetic agent.

SPINAL ANESTHESIA

The most frightening complication of spinal anesthesia is high or total spinal. This complication can be produced by inappropriate or careless movement of a patient under spinal anesthesia, who has received an otherwise satisfactory and well-managed spinal blockade.

The first indication of impending spinal blockade is often a change in the voice of the patient much before the drop in blood pressure occurs. The patient complains of a change in voice or difficulty in speaking. Often the first indication may be a complaint of chest tightness or labored breathing. If oxygen is administered by mask immediately and respirations are assisted, very often hypotension can be prevented. However, a vasopressor agent should be immediately available for circulatory stimulation under these circumstances. It is axiomatic that before anesthesia is started a large needle be well placed within a vein and intravenous fluids be infusing well.

Assisted respiration, circulatory support if needed, and careful monitoring of the patient until the effect of the anesthetic wears off will result in 100 per cent salvage of this patient group. However, if oxygen-assisted respiration and circulatory support are not forthcoming as they become indicated, mortality is likely to result.

GENERAL ANESTHESIA

Aseptic necrosis of the condyles of the mandible results from inadvertent prolonged pressure in the region of the condyles of the mandible while the patient is under anesthesia. The best treatment is prevention.

Other complications of general anesthesia are (1) teeth fractured during induction of anesthesia, (2) atelectasis caused by undetected intratracheal loss of tooth fragments broken during induction of anesthesia, (3) aspiration of gastric contents during the induction of anesthesia, (4) aspiration of stomach contents or solid food particles during induction of anesthesia, and (5) mixed polarizing or depolarizing blocks from relaxants administered during anesthesia.

LOCAL ANESTHESIA

Pudendal Block. Hematomas of the pelvis resulting from inadvertent injection of pudendal vessels may occur. Pudendal nerve neuritis resulting from direct injection into the pudendal nerve may also occur.

Paracervical Block. Complications that may occur with paracervical block are paracervical hematomas, injury to the presenting part of the fetus, unexplained fetal bradycardia and tachycardia, or cardiac irregularities associated with this type of anesthesia.

POSTSPINAL HEADACHES

Postspinal headaches occur in approximately 5 per cent of the anesthetized patients. The incidence can be reduced by limiting the size of the needle used to pierce the dura. The headache usually begins on the second or third postpartum day. The pain is severe and prevents any movement of the head without pain. The cephalalgia may be accompanied by visual disturbance and dizziness. The differential diagnosis includes sinusitis with headache, meningitis, arachnoiditis, and severe migraine cephalalgia.

Section 16

DISORDERS OF THE NEWBORN, INFANTS, AND CHILDREN

BLEEDING DISORDERS IN THE NEWBORN

By MARGARET W. HILGARTNER, M.D.
New York, New York

Bleeding disorders in the neonate can be divided into the same categories as for the older child: (1) those due to congenital deficiencies of the clotting proteins, (2) those due to acquired deficiencies, (3) those due to quantitative or qualitative platelet disorders, and (4) those due to vessel disease. The clotting mechanism of the neonate has been described as essentially the same as that known for the adult, although a consistent array of deficits relative to the adult values exists in the screening tests of prothrombin time (PT), partial thromboplastin time (PTT), and thrombin time, (TT) and activities of certain coagulation factors and platelet function in the neonate. These deficits may vary, depending on the gestational age and state of health of the infant. For proper interpretation of results, an understanding of the "physiologic" deficiencies and the variations caused by the state of health of the patient is necessary.

The term "physiologic deficiency" was originally applied to those lowered levels of the clotting factor activities of Factors II, VII, IX, and X found in cord blood. Today the term may be extended to those levels found in the preterm infant as well as the term infant. The best data concerning these levels and the results on the usual hemostatic screening tests are shown in Tables 1 and 2. This deficiency is due to an immaturity of the liver enzyme system, which produces all of the clotting factors except Factor VIII, and to a relative deficiency of vitamin K, which does not cross the placenta. The protein precursors are present in the infant's plasma and require vitamin K for acetylation and conversion into the clotting factor activity. It is well to remember that the levels of the vitamin K–dependent factors—Factors II, VII, IX, and X—may fall lower within the first 3 days of life in the continued absence of vitamin K; therefore the necessity exists for the intramuscular administration of vitamin K (1.0 mg in aqueous solution) at delivery for adequate synthesis of these factors. Levels should rise within 4 hours of administration of vitamin K in the full-term infant to reach near normal adult levels within 24 hours. The full-term infant may not achieve full adult levels for Factor IX for as long as 9 months; Factors XI, XII, and XIII may be low at birth and not reach adult levels for 2 to 24 weeks, and "fetal" fibrinogen, the term given to a functionally different form of fibrinogen, may be present for 3 to 6 weeks after delivery. The remaining Factors, V and VIII, as well as total fibrinogen are present in adult levels.

The preterm infant however has a greater deficiency of the precursor moieties of Factors II, VII, IX, and X and may not respond to the administration of vitamin K because of liver immaturity and inability to utilize the vitamin K. The levels for Factors V and VIII may also be low in the very small preterm infant for reasons that are not understood as yet (Table 2).

Low levels of the clotting factors are reflected in prolonged normal levels of the screening tests for clotting function (Table 1). However, a bleeding diathesis is not necessarily present unless these screening test limits are exceeded. Concentrations of 20 to 25 per cent of vitamin K–dependent factors are critical values below which a potential hemorrhagic state exists, although bleeding does not occur unless two or more of these factors are below the critical hemostatic level.

The "sick" infant with problems relating to the superimposed illness may present even greater difficulty in producing clotting factors. This infant may have a consumption coagulopathy present due to sepsis or hyaline membrane disease. With the acidosis often associated with hyaline membrane disease there may also be decreased production of the clotting factor activity, probably because of pH changes and tissue anoxia in the liver.

Platelets should be present in the normal numbers found in older children and adults,

Table 1. *Neonatal Screening Tests*

| | | Preterm | | |
	Normal Adult	27–31 wks	32–36 wks	Term
Prothrombin time (sec)	< 13.0	23	17 (12–21)	16 (13–20)
Activated PTT (sec)	< 40.0	–	70	55 ± 10
Thrombin time (sec)	< 20.0	–	14 (11–17)	12 (10–16)
Bleeding time (min)	4 ± 1.5	–	4 ± 1.5	4 ± 1.5
Platelet count /mm³	300 ± 50	275 ± 60	290 ± 70	310 ± 68

Table 2. Neonatal Coagulation Data

	Normal Adult	Preterm 27–31 wks	Preterm 32–36 wks	Term
Fibrinogen mg/ml	315 ± 60	270 ± 140	226 ± 70	246 ± 55
Factor				
II (%)	100	30 ± 10	35 ± 12	45 ± 15
V (%)	100	72 ± 25	91 ± 23	98 ± 40
VII + X (%)	100	32 ± 15	39 ± 14	56 ± 16
VIII (%)	100	70 ± 30	98 ± 40	105 ± 35
IX (%)	100	27 ± 10	–	28 ± 8
XI (%)	100	–	–	30
XII (%)	100	–	30	51
XIII (%)	100	100	100	100
Plasminogen %	100	25	40	43
Euglobulin lysis time (min)	140	95	95	84
FSP μg/ml	0–7	0–10	0–7	0–7
Antithrombin III %	100	–	48	55

with slightly lower levels in the premature infant. The function of these platelets, however, may be abnormal with decreased aggregation in response to adenosine diphosphate (ADP) and collagen, and increased dysfunction produced by exaggerated susceptibility to maternally ingested drugs such as aspirin and promethazine. However, the bleeding time should be normal in both full-term and preterm infants.

Vessel fragility should be normal in the full-term infant. It increases with decreasing gestational age but is rarely ever implicated in a bleeding diathesis in the newborn and will not be discussed further.

CONGENITAL DISORDERS

The congenital disorders of the coagulation proteins infrequently are the cause of bleeding in the newborn period, although the deficiencies of Factor VIII and IX (classical hemophilia and Christmas disease, respectively) may be the cause of bleeding with excessive trauma at delivery and with the surgical trauma of circumcision. The deficiency of Factor XIII can invariably be linked with bleeding from the cord. The other inherited coagulation deficiencies are rarely the cause of difficulty at this age.

Acquired deficiencies are usually seen in "sick" infants and are related to the secondary illness, as previously mentioned. These are associated with liver failure and subsequent lack of production of the clotting factors II, V, VII, IX, and X as seen with sepsis or other infections of the liver, such as cytomegalovirus (CMV), hepatitis B infection, and rubella. Disseminated intravascular coagulation (DIC), when seen with bacterial sepsis, other viral infections, or hyaline membrane disease, may cause a generalized bleeding tendency owing to consumption of platelets and coagulation factors. An acquired deficiency in a well infant presenting as an exaggerated vitamin K deficiency with marked decrease in Factors II, VII, and X may occur secondary to maternal ingestion of anticonvulsants. The problem is usually seen with phenytoin but may be present with primidone and phenobarbital. Competitive binding, with albumin inhibiting the transport of vitamin K, is thought to be the cause.

PLATELET DISORDERS

By far the most common cause of a bleeding disorder with purpura in the neonatal period is the thrombocytopenias, which are immune in origin. The passive-induced disorders due to diseases in the mother are immune thrombocytopenia purpura or systemic lupus erythematosus (SLE), with passive transfer of the antibody across the placenta that may affect the infant. This may occur even when the mother's condition appears stable and well compensated with her disease. Active disease may occur with isoimmunization in the infant because of a difference in platelet type between mother and infant, similar to the isoimmunization that happens with different red cell types in mother and infant. However, difficulties may occur in the first pregnancy of a mother whose platelet type is dissimilar to those of the infant and the infant's father.

The less common hereditary thrombocytopenias that may present with purpura at birth are the TAR syndrome (thrombocytopenia with absent radii), possibly Fanconi's disease (although this usually does not become apparent until later on in life), and the disorders of hereditary thrombocytopenia, which may be dominant or recessive in transmission. Both the TAR syndrome and Fanconi's disease are associated with skeletal anomalies.

Rare disorders occurring with purpura in the newborn period are the hereditary platelet functional disorders such as Glanzmann's thrombasthenia, Bernard-Soulier syndrome, von Willebrand's disease, and defects such as those associated with aspirin-like defects. All of these disorders are extremely rare and, with the exception of von Willebrand's disease, should not cause a great deal of difficulty for the newly born.

DIAGNOSTIC TOOLS

The common laboratory tests available in most clinical pathology laboratories are listed in Table 1. These are all relatively simple tests and should be done on a venous sample to avoid error. Care must be taken to have the correct plasma/anticoagulant ratio, and if the hematocrit is above 50 or below 30, the appropriate amount of citrate must be subtracted or added to the collecting tube. Inappropriate ratio of citrate to plasma may give false values to these screening tests, as will inappropriate venipuncture or collection from a line contaminated with heparin.

The prothrombin time (PT) and partial thromboplastin time (PTT) measure the clotting proteins of the extrinsic and intrinsic pathways of coagulation and are quite adequate as screening tests. In some laboratories the term "activated PTT" (activated partial thromboplastin time) is used and merely implies the use of an additional activator along with the lipid platelet substitute that is used to shorten the clotting time of the platelet-poor plasma with no increase in sensitivity implied.

The thrombin time (TT) is a measure of the presence of fibrin split products, afibrinogenemia or dysfibrinogenemia, and the presence of heparin. The TT should correct to normal when mixed with normal plasma if a state of dysfibrinogenemia or afibrinogenemia is present. If it does not correct to normal on mixing, proteolysis of fibrinogen and the presence of fibrin split products should be suspected. In the presence of a prolonged PT and PTT, heparin contamination of the sample should be suspected. For the latter, reptilase should be used in the place of thrombin to rule out the presence of fibrin split products.

LABORATORY EVALUATION

When an infant has bleeding in the newborn period, the course that is followed in the workup will be the same, whether the child is well or sick. The interpreter of the laboratory results, however, must take into consideration the status of the child's gestational age and whether there may be associated illness.

When the screening tests are done, if a prolongation is *not* present, a Factor XIII deficiency may be suspected and could be confirmed by monochloracetic acid screening test for clot stability, or a platelet function abnormality should be suspected. Confirmation of platelet abnormalities may be difficult in the newborn period because of the quantities of blood required to isolate platelets for study, and frequently must wait until the child is older.

If all of the screening tests are grossly abnormal, either severe DIC or dysfibrinogenemia is present, and either may be confirmed by subsequent factor assays. Heparin contamination of the sample may confuse the interpretation of these results and require use of reptilase in the thrombin time .

If the PT is more prolonged than the PTT, an additional dose of vitamin K may be given. Subsequent assays for Factors II, V, VII, and X should then be done to learn whether vitamin K was inadequate or whether a congenital deficiency exists.

Should the PTT alone be excessively long, a congenital deficiency of Factor VIII, IX, or XI should be suspected and confirmed by appropriate assay.

In summary, the diagnostic endeavors utilized for this bleeding infant are the same as those for the older child. They require only a careful maternal and perinatal history and adequate laboratory methodology, scaled for the small sample. Those involved in testing should be cognizant of the differences in plasma volume of the newborn and should provide knowledgeable interpretation of the results, considering the physiologic differences of the age.

HEMOLYTIC DISEASE OF THE NEWBORN

By JOHN M. BOWMAN, M.D.
Winnipeg, Manitoba, Canada

SYNONYM

Erythroblastosis fetalis.

DEFINITION

Hemolytic disease of the newborn is a disease of the fetus and newborn infant characterized by red blood cell destruction, anemia, and extramedullary erythropoiesis. Universal edema (hydrops fetalis) with fetal or neonatal death occurs in the most severe cases. Jaundice (icterus gravis neonatorum) after birth with risk of brain damage (kernicterus) if the infant is not properly treated is a hazard in less severe cases.

PRESENTING SIGNS AND SYMPTOMS

The Infant. Presenting signs and symptoms vary from none at all to sudden fetal death as early as 20 to 22 weeks' gestation. In 40 to 50 per cent of infants with Rh erythroblastosis (90 to 95 per cent with ABO erythroblastosis), the baby appears clinically normal at birth. In the intermediate 25 to 30 per cent (5 to 10 per cent with ABO erythroblastosis), hepatosplenomegaly, varying degrees of pallor due to anemia, and jaundice are present. Contrary to the usual reports, the jaundice may be visible at birth if looked for carefully. In the most severely affected group, 20 to 25 per cent of Rh erythroblastotic infants (no ABO erythroblastotic infants), the disease is so severe that ascites and generalized edema develop in utero (hydrops fetalis). Fetal death usually occurs. At delivery, maceration is frequently so marked that the diagnosis of hydrops cannot be made. Live-born infants with hydrops fetalis are waterlogged, as the name implies. They are extremely edematous; ascites is very marked; the liver and spleen are greatly enlarged; the placenta is very bulky and pale. The infant is extremely pale and usually dies of respiratory failure after birth.

The Mother. In most pregnancies the isoimmunized mother experiences no untoward symptoms. Polyhydramnios is common in the presence of hydrops fetalis. It is probably due to the inability of the edematous infant to swallow amniotic fluid. Some women with severely affected prehydropic or hydropic fetuses will have excessive weight gain with some degree of edema and albuminuria. These signs disappear after delivery or following amelioration of fetal disease due to successful intrauterine fetal transfusions. Although some women report diminution of fetal movement in the presence of severe erythroblastosis, others do not note any apparent diminution until just before fetal death.

COURSE OF THE DISEASE

Classification of severity of erythroblastosis is outlined in Table 1. The mildly affected infants develop minimal to moderate jaundice during their first few days of life. The jaundice is differentiated from "physiologic" jaundice of the newborn with difficulty. It fades promptly. The baby remains neurologically intact and sucks well. He may develop mild anemia in the first 4 to 6 weeks of life from which he recovers spontaneously. He does very well without treatment, as his counterpart did prior to 1940 when no treatment was available because the cause of erythroblastosis fetalis was unknown.

The babies in the moderately affected group appear jaundiced within the first 24 hours (often at birth). There are varying degrees of associated pallor. If left untreated, the jaundice deepens (icterus gravis). On the second to fifth day of life, depending upon the rapidity of increase in the degree of jaundice, the untreated infant, now yellow with a serum indirect bilirubin level usually in excess of 25 mg per 100 ml (lower if he is premature or acidotic or has been given competitive albumin-binding drugs), becomes lethargic. He stops sucking. His temperature falls. He becomes spastic and lies in a position of opisthotonus. He may convulse. Finally in the majority of such cases apnea supervenes and the baby dies. At postmortem exami-

Table 1. *Classification of Severity of Erythroblastosis*

Degree of Severity	Incidence
1. Mild: no treatment needed; indirect bilirubin does not exceed 16 to 20 mg. per 100 ml; no anemia	45–50%
2. Moderate: fetal hydrops will not develop; anemia is moderate; severe jaundice and risk of kernicterus unless treated after birth	25–30%
3. Severe: fetal hydrops will develop in utero; before 33 weeks' gestation, 8 to 10 per cent; after 33 weeks' gestation, 12 to 15 per cent	20–25%

nation certain areas of the brain — the basal ganglia, cerebellum, hippocampus, medulla, and the eighth cranial nerve nuclei particularly — are stained a bright yellow. In the past the case of death was attributed to "kernicterus," which simply means yellow staining of the brain.

In about 10 to 20 per cent of these unfortunate infants after a few days the jaundice fades, the lethargy disappears, the spasticity appears to be less, and the infant starts sucking. He may appear quite normal for 2 to to 3 months. As he grows older, however, he fails to respond to sound and shows signs of neuromuscular damage (choreoathetosis with increased spasticity). Varying degrees of intellectual retardation (ofter surprisingly mild) are found in association with deafness (usually profound) and cerebral palsy (usually very severe). Some other jaundiced infants who do not develop the full-blown signs of kernicterus just described have been noted in later childhood to have minor degrees of proprioceptive and fine motor coordinative defects with normal intelligence. These children have the mildest degree of brain damage due to jaundice. Kernicterus is now completely preventable with the use of exchange transfusion and ancillary treatment measures such as phototherapy and serum albumin administration.

Rarely, a baby in the intermediate moderately affected group will develop minimal or no jaundice but will become severely anemic in the first 7 to 14 days of life (anemia neonatorum). Hemoglobin levels may drop below 2 grams per 100 ml, and the child may die unless he is given a transfusion.

The most severely affected group, those with hydrops fetalis, until recently followed a brief and uniform course. The majority died suddenly in utero. Most of the remainder died within a few minutes of birth. Recently a few of these babies have been salvaged with expert neonatal intensive care management. Much more promising is the ability to forestall hydrops through early delivery or intrauterine fetal transfusion and early delivery. Indeed, 50 per cent of fetuses with hydrops fetalis (gross ascites) may be salvaged with multiple intrauterine transfusions and the use of diuretics and digoxin.

The live-born severely affected erythroblastotic infant born prematurely, with or without preceding intrauterine transfusion, faces several potential risks that may influence the course of his disease. Since, until recently, delivery as early as 32 to 34 weeks of gestation carried the best hope of salvage, all the complications of prematurity, particularly the respiratory distress syndrome, were serious hazards. With reduction in the risks of fetal transfusion, the risks of prematurity are less because only rarely are these fetuses now deliberately delivered before 35 weeks' gestation. Spontaneous early delivery, however, occurs in about 20 per cent of fetuses after intrauterine transfusion.

Thrombocytopenia is frequently present in the severely affected baby. Although partially a result of exchange transfusion, it is predominantly caused by a reduction of marrow megakaryocytes as a result of excess erythropoiesis. If left untreated, there is a high risk of intracranial, intrapulmonary, and gastrointestinal bleeding.

Severely affected erythroblastotic babies have transient hepatocellular damage that interferes with transfer of conjugated bilirubin across the hepatic cell into the biliary canaliculi. Because islets of extramedullary erythropoiesis enlarge and deform the liver, the canaliculi themselves may be partially obstructed. Direct as well as indirect bilirubin levels rise. In this situation cord bilirubin levels may be in excess of 10 mg per 100 ml (of which one third to two thirds is direct-acting bilirubin). Peak bilirubin levels may climb, despite treatment, into the 30 mg per 100 ml range (of which two thirds is direct-acting bilirubin). Although Dunn has reported a considerable mortality in babies with this complication, in our experience it is generally benign. The jaundice and hyperbilirubinemia disappear over a 3-week to 3-month period. Babies with this complication have a bronzed muddy green appearance quite different from the bright yellow or orange-yellow hue of the baby with indirect hyperbilirubinemia.

Two major complications of exchange transfusion may also alter the course of the infant with erythroblastosis. In the past, cardiac fibrillation was a hazard. This complication was related to faulty exchange transfusion techniques, donor blood more than 4 days old with high potassium levels, or hypocalcemia due to chelation of ionized calcium with citrate. With proper techniques, the use of fresh blood, and calcium replacement, this hazard has vanished. The development of postexchange transfusion necrotizing enterocolitis with attendant peritonitis, bowel infarction, intestinal perforation, stenosis, and bowel obstruction is the major hazard associated with exchange transfusion today. Lethargy, abdominal distention, and melena are the usual presenting symptoms. This complication carries with it considerable mortality. The underlying mechanism is unknown. The primary cause may be viral or bacterial, but the disorder appears to be confined to sick infants whose intestinal circulation may be compromised by anoxia or possibly by mesenteric vascular spasm, thrombosis, or embolization brought about by a poorly understood factor at exchange transfusion.

HISTORY

Diagnosis and prediction of severity of hemolytic disease were possible only after the discovery of the Rh blood group system. Although hydrops and icterus gravis were described as early as 1609, it was not until 1932 that it was demonstrated that they were varying degrees of the same disease and that erythroblastosis was common to them both. In 1938 Darrow postulated that the cause of erythroblastosis was fetal red blood cell destruction by immune bodies produced in the mother in response to the passage of fetal red blood cells across the placenta. In 1940 Landsteiner and Wiener and Levine and Stetson proved that Darrow's postulation was correct.

The pregnant woman (usually Rh negative), in response to exposure to a red blood cell antigen that she does not possess (usually Rh antigen), produces an antibody to the antigen. The antibody traverses the placenta, and if the red blood cells of the fetus are positive for the antigen, they are coated by the antibody and destroyed.

BLOOD GROUPS AND ISOIMMUNIZATION

ABO System. Many essential components of the red blood cell membrane are antigenic. A and B (the ABO system) discovered by Landsteiner in 1900 are complex polysaccharides. They are ubiquitous in nature. Individuals missing these antigens are exposed to them early in life. By 6 to 9 months of age they have produced corresponding isohemagglutinins (anti-A and B if they are group O, anti-B if group A, anti-A if group B). The group O individual produces more anti-B than the group A, and more anti-A than the group B person. He is also capable of producing more immune (IgG) anti-A and anti-B. So-called naturally occurring anti-A and anti-B are for the most part IgM (molecular weight 900,000) and do not cross the placenta. However, in about 50 per cent of group O individuals there is a small but significant amount of IgG anti-A and anti-B that can traverse the placenta. Since A and B antigens are present in other tissues and secretions, only a small proportion of the anti-A or anti-B that crosses the placenta adheres to the corresponding antigen in the red blood cell membrane. These two facts — (1) very little anti-A or anti-B crosses the placenta and (2) most of the antibody that does cross combines with A or B antigen in secretions and tissues other than that on the red blood cell membrane — explain why ABO hemolytic disease of the newborn is usually very mild. Twenty per cent of newborn babies are ABO incompatible with their mothers (i.e., they are A or B and their mother O). One third to one half of them will show serologic evidence of erythroblastosis, but fewer than 10 per cent will have increased jaundice, and fewer than 1 per cent, with modern ancillary treatment measures such as phototherapy and albumin administration will require exchange transfusion. Hydrops fetalis probably never occurs as a result of ABO incompatibility.

The Rh System. Incompatibility in the Rh system is the most common cause of clinical hemolytic disease of the newborn. Knowledge of the Rh system has been advanced since Landsteiner and Wiener's original 1940 Rhesus monkey experiments. There is a family of inherited Rh antigens. Nomenclature and basic genetic concepts are controversial. Although Wiener's concept of a single locus occupied by a pair of complex antigens may be correct, and Rosenfield's numerical system the most logical, the nomenclature and theories of inheritance proposed by Fisher and Race are simple and easy to understand, and work well in clinical practice.

According to Fisher and Race, there are six genetically determined antigens grouped in three sets: Cc, Dd, and Ee. It is the presence or absence of D that determines whether an individual is Rh positive or negative. Since no antibody of the specificity anti-d has been discovered, it remains hypothetical. D is the most potent antigen in the Rh system, and it is the most common cause of clinical erythroblastosis.

The antigens are inherited in two sets of three, each parent contributing one set. Two Rh positive sets CDe (R^1) and cDE (R^2) and one Rh negative set cde (r) are the most common. However, all the other possible combinations occur. Cde (r'), cdE (r'') and cDe (R^0) are not rare.

Since an Rh positive man may receive a D-containing set of antigens from one or both parents, he may be either heterozygous or homozygous for D. His zygosity for D is important if he is married to an Rh negative woman. If he is homozygous, all his offspring will be Rh positive; if heterozygous, there is a 50 per cent chance that each child will be Rh negative and an equal chance that it will be Rh positive. Since only Rh positive fetuses will be affected by anti-D, the zygosity of an isoimmunized Rh negative woman's husband for D is of crucial importance.

Table 2.   *Zygosity for Rh(D) of D + Husband*

Antigens Present in Husband	A Most Likely Rh Genotype	B Less Likely Rh Genotype	C Least Likely Rh Genotype
1. CDe	$CDe \cdot CDe(R^1R^1)$ Homozygous	$CDe \cdot Cde(R^1r')$ Heterozygous	
2. CDce	$CDe \cdot cde(R^1r)$ Heterozygous	$CDe \cdot cDe(R^1R^0)$ Homozygous	$Cde \cdot cDe(r'R^0)$ Heterozygous
3. CDEce	$CDe \cdot cDE(R^1R^2)$ Homozygous	$Cde \cdot cDE(r'R^2)$ $CDe \cdot cdE(R^1r'')$ $CDE \cdot cde(R^2r)$ Heterozygous	$CDE \cdot cDe(R^2R^0)$ Homozygous
4. DEc	$cDE \cdot cDE(R^2R^2)$ Homozygous	$cDE \cdot cdE(R^2r'')$ Heterozygous	
5. DEce	$cDE \cdot cde(R^2r)$ Heterozygous	$cDE \cdot cDe(R^2R^0)$ Homozygous	$cdE \cdot cDe(r''R^0)$ Heterozygous
6. Dce	$cDe \cdot cde(R^0r)$ Heterozygous	$cDe \cdot cDe(R^0R^0)$ Homozygous	

Genotypes 1A and 4A can never be proved, because the baby will be of only one paternal genotype (CDe in 1A and cDE in 4A).

The remainder of the husband's possible genotypes can be proved only if he produces children of two different genotypes.

Because anti-d has never been found, the zygosity for D of an Rh positive husband cannot be determined unless he produces two infants who have inherited two different combinations of Rh antigens from him. However, since certain combinations are more common than others (Table 2), the determination of the other Rh antigens present may indicate the likely zygosity of the husband.

The chemical constitution of the Rh antigens is unknown. D appears to be a protein or a complex polypeptide with one or more sulfhydryl groups. Unlike A and B, the Rh antigens are found only in the red blood cell membrane. Their presence is essential to the normal function of the membrane. The rare individuals with no Rh antigens (Rh null) have defective red blood cell membranes and have some degree of hemolytic anemia.

Antigens Producing Atypical Antibodies. Other antigens of the Rh system (c, D, E, e) and antigens outside the Rh system (Kell, Duffy, etc.) are, on occasion, capable of producing isoimmunization (atypical antibodies). They are relatively less antigenic, and the incidence of isoimmunization is lower than it is for D. However, once isoimmunization is produced, anti-c and Kell and less commonly anti-E are quite capable of producing very severe erythroblastosis in fetuses positive for the corresponding antigens. In contradistinction to anti-A and anti-B that always develop and anti-D that usually develops in the absence of blood transfusion, atypical antibodies are usually transfusion induced.

So-called "compatible" blood is only compatible in the ABO system and for D in the Rh system. Therefore every blood transfusion is incompatible for many other antigens. Fortunately, most of them are not good antibody producers. Nevertheless, 1 to 2 per cent of transfused individuals will be isoimmunized. Although most of the antibodies produced (Le^a, P, M, N, etc.) will not cause erythroblastosis, c, Kell, and some others will do so. The responsible physician will transfuse patients, particularly girls and women in their childbearing years, only when the indications are absolute.

PATHOGENESIS OF RH ISOIMMUNIZATION

Although transplacental passage of fetal red blood cells was postulated as the cause of Rh isoimmunization as early as 1948, it was not until 1954 that the theory was proved. An Rh negative primigravida after giving birth to an anemic Rh positive infant was shown by differential agglutination and adult hemoglobin denaturation techniques to have 5 per cent fetal Rh positive red blood cells. Within 20 days of delivery she had developed a strong Rh antibody.

Following the development in 1956 by Kleihauer, Braun, and Betke of a technique for differential fetal red blood cell staining (acid

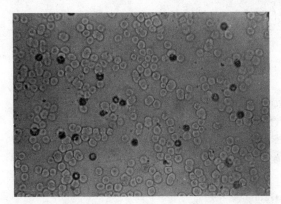

Figure 1. Acid elution technique of Kleihauer. Fetal red blood cells stain with eosin (appear dark), adult red blood cells do not stain (appear as ghosts). This maternal blood smear contained 11.2 per cent fetal red blood cells representing a transplacental hemorrhage of about 450 ml. of blood.

elution technique, Fig. 1), it became possible to determine with great accuracy the incidence and size of fetal transplacental hemorrhage and the attendant risk of isoimmunization.

About one half of all pregnant women show small numbers of fetal red blood cells in their circulations at some time during pregnancy or at delivery. The incidence is halved if the fetus is ABO incompatible. Over 50 per cent of women who have fetal cells in their circulation always have less than 0.1 ml. Less than 1 per cent of pregnant women have more than 5 ml; less than 0.3 per cent have more than 30 ml in their circulations.

Obstetric factors such as cesarean section and manual removal of the placenta materially increase the incidence of transplacental hemorrhage greater than 0.1 ml, as does amniocentesis. For some unknown reason toxemia of pregnancy also increases the size and incidence of transplacental hemorrhage. During a normal pregnancy the incidence and size of transplacental hemorrhages increases as pregnancy advances, reaching a peak at the time of delivery. Abortions, particularly therapeutic abortions, are associated with a significant risk of transplacental hemorrhage (15 per cent).

An Rh negative woman with an Rh positive ABO compatible fetus has a 16 per cent chance of becoming isoimmunized (Table 3). The incidence is 2.0 per cent by the time of delivery; a further 7.0 per cent by 6 months after delivery; and another 7.0 per cent, not detectable during or after delivery, but demonstrating a secondary immune response by the middle of a subsequent Rh positive pregnancy. The risk is much lower if the fetus is Rh positive ABO incompatible (about 2 per cent) and is about 2 to 3 per cent if the Rh negative woman aborts.

Table 3. *Approximate Risk of Rh Isoimmunization*

	Risk
1. Husband D-negative, baby D-negative	0
2. Husband D-positive homozygous, ABO compatible	16%
3. Husband D-positive homozygous, ABO incompatible, ABO of baby unknown	7%
4. Baby D-positive, ABO incompatible	2%
5. Husband D-positive heterozygous, ABO compatible	8%
6. Husband D-positive heterozygous, ABO incompatible—ABO and Rh of baby unknown	3.5%

If no fetal cells have been demonstrated at any time during pregnancy or delivery, the risk that the Rh negative woman with an ABO compatible Rh positive baby will become Rh immunized drops to about 3 per cent; if greater than 5 ml bleeding has occurred, the risk rises to 50 to 65 per cent.

The type of antibody produced and its strength will influence the severity of erythroblastosis. The initial (primary response) antibody is characteristically slow to develop and weak. It is predominantly IgM and may only be demonstrable by sensitive manual enzyme or AutoAnalyzer techniques. As it increases in strength, if it remains primarily IgM, it will produce agglutination of Rh positive red blood cells suspended in saline. Since IgM anti-D does not cross the placenta, this antibody does not cause fetal erythroblastosis. Unfortunately, in most Rh negative women this phase is short. Following a second antigenic stimulus, either at the end of the same pregnancy or during a subsequent Rh positive pregnancy, a secondary immune response occurs. This response is usually very rapid in onset with production of large amounts of IgG anti-D. Because of its small molecular size (molecular weight 160,000), IgG anti-D cannot produce agglutination of Rh positive red blood cells suspended in saline. They must be suspended in a thicker medium such as albumin. This antibody (called albumin anti-D because of this property) traverses the placenta. It coats the fetal Rh positive red blood cell destroying it. Red blood cell destruction caused by anti-D is extravascular and occurs primarily in the spleen.

The Anti-Human Globulin (Coombs') Test. The coating and destruction of the Rh positive red blood cells start the chain of events that produce all the pathologic changes of hemolytic disease of the newborn. At the same time the coating of the red blood cell with Rh and antibody (gamma globulin) is the basis for a simple and accurate test for erythroblastosis.

Anti-human globulin produced in other species (rabbits, goats, etc.) by the injection of human serum or purified human IgG will produce agglutination of antibody-coated red blood cells. A positive test in the newborn is diagnostic of erythroblastosis fetalis.

With the exception of ABO erythroblastosis, the anti-human globulin test, frequently called the Coombs' test after its discoverer, is almost never negative in erythroblastotic infants. The baby with ABO erythroblastosis frequently has so few molecules of anti-A or anti-B adhering to his red blood cell membrane that the test is negative. However, if cord blood is tested and a sensitive Coombs' method (capillary) is used, the anti-human globulin test is usually positive even in ABO hemolytic disease. The test is much weaker than in other forms of erythroblastosis, including Rh.

The indirect anti-human globulin method can be used for screening pregnant women for Rh and other blood antibodies and for titering the strength of these antibodies. It is not as sensitive as manual enzyme or AutoAnalyzer methods for the demonstration of very weak antibodies. Since the indirect Coombs' technique is somewhat more sensitive than albumin methods for titration of the strength of Rh antibodies, it is important that the clinician be aware of this in assessing fetal hazards in his isoimmunized patient. (In most laboratories there is a one or two tube difference, i.e., an indirect antiglobulin titer of 1:160 is equivalent to an albumin titer of 1:32 to 1:64.)

PATHOGENESIS OF ERYTHROBLASTOSIS FETALIS

Degree of severity of erythroblastosis is determined by the amount of anti-D IgG the mother has produced, its avidity for the fetal red blood cell Rh antigen, i.e., "binding constant," and the ability of the fetus to replace the red blood cells that are being destroyed.

Icterus Gravis and Kernicterus. In moderately affected offspring fetal erythropoiesis keeps up with red blood cell hemolysis and the infant is born in reasonably good condition. The products of hemolysis pose no problems for the fetus, since they traverse the placenta and are metabolized by the mother. After delivery, when the fetus has to rely on his resources, indirect bilirubin, the toxic metabolite of hemoglobin, cannot be adequately conjugated to bilirubin diglucuronide. The liver of the newborn infant is deficient in both the hepatic mitochondrial conjugating enzyme glucuronyl transferase and one of the intracellular transport proteins. As indirect bilirubin, which is lipid-soluble and water-insoluble, accumulates, it ultimately reaches a level (unless reduced by exchange transfusion, phototherapy, etc.) at which the binding capacity of its plasma carrier, albumin, is exceeded. Plasma albumin-binding capacity may be reduced by the presence of competitive binding ions such as sulfa, salicylates, or unesterified free fatty acids. In the presence of acidosis (pH 7.1) the ability of albumin to bind bilirubin is halved. Once the albumin-binding capacity of the plasma is exceeded, further indirect bilirubin produced cannot be bound. Since it is fat-soluble, it migrates into fatty areas. Whereas albumin-bound indirect bilirubin and conjugated bilirubin diglucuronide do not cross cell membranes, free indirect bilirubin readily does so. It penetrates the neuron membrane, interfering with vital oxidative functions causing swelling and ballooning of the mitochondria and cell death (i.e., kernicterus).

Hydrops Fetalis. Hydrops fetalis was originally thought to be due to failure of fetal erythropoiesis to keep up with hemolysis, with progressive anemia, hypervolemia, heart failure, and anasarca. Although cardiac failure is almost certain to occur in the hydropic neonate if he lives long enough, the primary cause of hydrops fetalis is now thought to be hepatic failure. In the most severe degrees of hemolytic disease extramedullary erythropoiesis, particularly in the liver, is extreme. Hepatosplenomegaly develops with portal and umbilical venous hypertension. Ascites develops. Placental perfusion diminishes. Replacement and distortion of hepatic cell cords and reduced circulation to remaining hepatic cells reduce the synthesizing capacity of the liver. Hypoalbuminemia develops. As hypoproteinemia increases, ascites becomes more severe and generalized edema develops. In the final stage of hydrops, hydrothorax, compression hypoplasia of the lung, and pulmonary edema make postdelivery respiratory exchange impossible. The aforementioned outline explains the variable relation of hydrops to hemoglobin concentrations. Because hydrops fetalis is due to hepatic dysfunction, not anemia, some fetuses become hydropic with hemoglobin levels of 7 or 8 grams per 100 ml. Others are not hydropic with hemoglobin levels of 3 or 4 grams per 100 ml. Sixty per cent of fetuses destined to become hydropic will do so between 34 and 40 weeks' gestation and may be salvaged with early delivery. The remaining 40 per cent become hydropic between 20 and 33 weeks' gestation. Their only hope of survival is with intrauterine transfusions and early delivery.

THE DIAGNOSIS OF THE RH NEGATIVE WOMAN AT RISK

The clinician must know which of his patients is at risk. Such knowledge can be obtained only if blood samples are sent for Rh blood grouping and antibody screening from every patient at her first prenatal visit. This should be done no matter what screening tests have shown in previous pregnancies. It is quite possible that an Rh negative woman may have been incorrectly typed in the past. Also, if an Rh positive woman has been transfused in the past, she may have developed dangerous atypical antibodies (anti-c, Kell, etc.). The antibody screening tests used by the referral laboratory must be sensitive enough to detect very weak Rh antibodies. This is particularly important now that there is a method of prevention of Rh isoimmunization available (administration of Rh_0 [D] immune globulin to the unimmunized Rh negative woman who has delivered an Rh positive infant). Insensitive screening tests that fail to detect early Rh immunization are responsible for most reported failures of Rh prevention (i.e., the woman was already weakly Rh immunized by the time the material was given). The indirect antiglobulin test is not adequate for Rh antibody screening. The more sensitive manual enzyme-treated red blood cell techniques and AutoAnalyzer methods (bromelin and low ionic Polybrene) are much better screening tests. Using these sensitive methods it can be shown that 1.8 per cent of Rh negative women at risk will already be Rh immunized by the time of delivery and will not be protected by postdelivery Rh immune globulin. The remaining 14 per cent of these destined to become Rh immunized will be protected by postdelivery Rh immune globulin, with the exception of one third of the 0.23 per cent with transplacental hemorrhages of greater than 30 ml of blood. In these cases the amount of Rh antigen is too great for a single prophylactic dose (300 μg of anti-D) to be completely protective. If Kleihauer tests are done routinely after delivery, transplacental hemorrhages greater than 30 ml may be detected and adequate amounts of Rh immune globulin given.

If the husband of the Rh negative unimmunized woman is Rh positive (85 per cent will be), her blood should be rechecked at monthly intervals until delivery. If screening tests remain negative and her infant is Rh positive, she should be given Rh immune globulin within 72 hours of delivery. Although the infant's cord red cells usually will be direct Coombs' negative, a weakly positive direct Coombs' test in the presence of ABO incompatibility should not preclude administration of the globulin.

DIAGNOSIS OF SEVERITY OF RH IMMUNIZATION IN UTERO

When Rh antibody screening tests indicate that his Rh negative pregnant patient is isoimmunized, the physician, in order to carry out optimal management, must be able to diagnose the degree of severity of disease in the fetus. This will vary from (1) no treatment of the Rh negative or mildly affected Rh positive infant, (2) management of hyperbilirubinemia in the moderately affected term infant, (3) early delivery of the infant destined to be hydropic after 33 weeks' gestation to (4) intrauterine transfusion and early delivery of the infant doomed to become hydropic before 33 weeks' gestation. Failure to diagnose the degree of disease in utero accurately may lead to loss of an unaffected or mildly affected infant due to too early delivery or conversely to development of hydrops fetalis because of failure to transfuse in utero and/or deliver early enough.

Criteria for Assessment (Table 4). *Past History.* The disease in subsequent fetuses tends to be as severe as or more severe than in earlier affected fetuses. If a previously affected sibling required exchange transfusion or died in utero of erythroblastosis, there is a significant risk of stillbirth in a succeeding affected fetus (90 per cent if the previous pregnancy ended in fetal death). History is of no value in the first affected pregnancy in which the risk of stillbirth is 8 to 10 per cent. History of a past stillbirth does not allow prediction of the gestation of a subsequent stillbirth (treatment necessary to prevent fetal death at 25 weeks differs greatly from that at 37 weeks' gestation).

Maternal Antibody Titer. Despite many statements to the contrary, serial Rh antibody titers carried out in good laboratories do allow some prediction of severity of disease. Since techniques and methods vary from laboratory to laboratory, the significance of specific titers must be ascertained for each laboratory. In our laboratory an albumin titration of less than 1:16, in the absence of a history of affected siblings,

Table 4. *Prediction of Severity of Erythroblastosis Fetalis Criteria*

1. History of degree of disease in affected siblings
2. Maternal Rh antibody titers
3. Amniotic fluid examination
   a. Spectrophotometry
   b. Quantitative bilirubin levels
   c. Chloroform extraction
   d. Bilirubin-albumin ratio
   e. Hemopexin-albumin ratios
   f. Amniotic fluid Rh antibody titers
   g. Amniotic fluid and urinary estriol levels

stillborn or requiring exchange transfusion, carries with it no risk of hydrops fetalis developing before term. Titers of 1:16, 1:32, 1:64, and 1:128 carry stillbirth risks of 10, 25, 50, and 75 per cent, respectively. However, titers in the high-risk range do not tell which fetus will die and at what gestation.

Amniotic Fluid Examination. History and titer combined allow only 62 per cent accuracy of prediction of severity of fetal erythroblastosis. Amniotic fluid spectrophotometric examination increases the accuracy of prediction to 95 per cent. Many different methods have been described, none of which is more accurate than any other. More important than the method is the experience of the laboratory carrying out the test and that of the laboratory director in interpreting the results of the test to the clinician. The method of Liley is undoubtedly the most popular (Fig. 2). The optical density deviation from linearity at 450 mμ (the OD rise at 450 mμ), the wavelength at which bilirubin absorbs light, is directly related to severity of disease. However, gestation at the time of the amniocentesis must be known, as bilirubin is normally present in amniotic fluid in early pregnancy, reaching a peak at about 24 weeks' gestation and diminishing thereafter. As a result the same optical density rise value indicates more severe disease as pregnancy advances.

Liley was able to divide his optical density rise graph into three zones (Fig. 3). Zone 1 indicates either a mildly affected or an Rh negative fetus (Fig. 4), zone 3, a severely affected fetus either hydropic at the time of amniocentesis or destined to become hydropic within 7 days of the amniocentesis (Fig. 3). Zone 2 is an intermediate zone with disease becoming progressively more severe as the optical density rise approaches the zone 3 boundary.

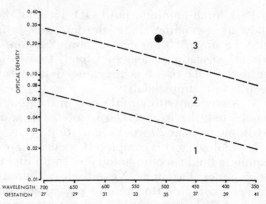

Figure 3. Plotting the 450 mμ optical density rise according to gestation. As gestation advances, the same 450 mμ OD rise indicates progressively more severe disease.

Hydrops fetalis may develop as early as 20 to 22 weeks' gestation, and in our experience successful fetal transfusions can be carried out as early as 22 weeks' gestation. Therefore initial amniocenteses when indicated should be carried out at 20 to 21 weeks' gestation. At this period of gestation the three zones are poorly delineated. Waiting for an OD rise to reach zone 3 frequently results in a hydropic fetus. Conversely, an OD 450 mμ rise of 0.200 zone 3 and of very serious significance at 29 to 30 weeks' gestation may, at 21 to 22 weeks, be associated with an unaffected fetus. Serial amniotic fluid examinations at 7- to 28-day intervals are of greater prognostic value. The following general observations are based upon 2823 amniotic fluid examinations carried out in 997 isoimmunized pregnancies:

1. A single amniotic fluid optical density rise of 0.400 or higher at any stage of gestation is associated with hydrops fetalis at the time of amniocentesis in 65 per cent of cases.

2. Hydrops may be associated with 450 mμ OD rises as low as 0.250 at 28 weeks' gestation (0.180 on one occasion).

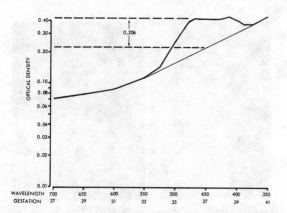

Figure 2. Spectrophotometric curve of amniotic fluid from a severely affected erythroblastotic fetus. Note the deviation from linearity of the curve at 450 mμ. The degree of deviation (i.e., optical density rise at 450 mμ), 0.206 in this figure, is directly related to severity of erythroblastosis.

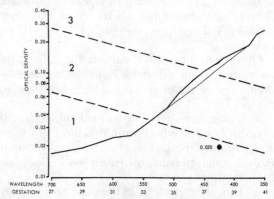

Figure 4. Spectrophotometric curve of amniotic fluid from an unaffected fetus. Amniotic fluid 450 mμ optical density rise (0.020) is in the lowest zone (zone 1).

3. If serial amniotic fluid OD 450 mμ rises show an ascending slope, the final one rising into the upper 80 per cent of zone 2 before 28 weeks' gestation, delaying fetal transfusion until the OD rise reaches zone 3 frequently results in hydrops fetalis.

4. A woman with an OD rise of 0.240 at 27 weeks may have an OD rise of 0.370 and a hydropic fetus at 29 weeks' gestation.

No biologic test is completely accurate. Serial amniotic fluid spectrophotometry in Rh disease is 95 per cent accurate. Nevertheless, there is a 2.0 per cent life-threatening inaccuracy rate. Four of 263 fetuses subjected to intrauterine transfusion in Winnipeg were subsequently shown to be negative for the antigen to which the mother was sensitized (three Rh [D], one Kell).

Amniocentesis, although benign as far as the mother is concerned, carries a definite hazard to the fetus. Unless preceded by placental localization 10 per cent of amniocenteses will be associated with placental trauma and transplacental hemorrhage. In at least half of the 10 per cent there will be a rise in maternal antibody titer and increased severity of fetal erythroblastosis. Placental localization by ultrasound or radioisotope technique is mandatory prior to initial amniocentesis. Even with placental localization the risk of transplacental hemorrhage, although much less, is not entirely removed.

Amniocentesis therefore should be limited to women who by history (previous stillborn or exchanged baby) or titer (1:16 in albumin or higher in our laboratory) are at risk of having stillborn babies. Using these criteria, 50 per cent of the fetuses of Rh immunized women will be spared the hazards of amniocentesis.

There are certain sources of error in amniotic fluid examination. These are heavily meconium- or bloodstained amniotic fluid (Fig. 5) and inadvertent exposure to light that destroys amniotic fluid bilirubin. Congenital anomalies of the fetus such as tracheoesophageal fistula, gastrointestinal obstruction, and anencephaly will produce false high 450 mμ OD values.

Other amniotic fluid parameters have been measured in an effort to improve accuracy of diagnosis of severity of fetal erythroblastosis (Table 4):

a. Chloroform extraction of bilirubin (Brazie) may be helpful when amniotic fluid is moderately bloodstained. However, if heavily contaminated, fetal plasma bilirubin will give false high readings.

b. Bilirubin protein ratios do not improve accuracy of prognosis over simple amniotic fluid spectrophotometry.

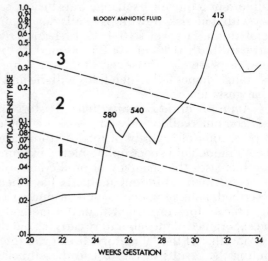

Figure 5. Spectrophotometric curve (Liley method) of amniotic fluid grossly contaminated with blood. Note sharp peaks at 580, 540, and 413 mμ which obscure the 450 mμ rise.

c. The hemopexin-albumin ratio (Muller-Eberhard and Bashore) decreases as fetal erythroblastosis becomes more severe and may on occasion increase prognostic accuracy.

d. Amniotic fluid Rh antibody titers in some laboratories are of value in predicting severity of disease.

e. Amniotic fluid and urinary estriol levels are not of prognostic help until the fetus is moribund and past salvaging.

Diagnosis of Hydrops Fetalis in Utero. The presence of hydrops fetalis may be suspected if the amniotic fluid 450 mμ OD rise is greater than 0.400. It may be established with certainty radiologically either at amniogram (fetal scalp edema and limb extension) or at fetal transfusion when injection of radiopaque dye intraperitoneally reveals gross ascites (Fig. 6). Although

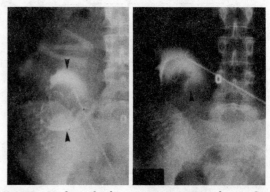

Figure 6. Hydrops fetalis at intrauterine transfusion. Gross ascites (arrows) present at both transfusions at 28 and 29½ weeks' gestation. The fetus, hydropic at birth, with a cord hemoglobin of 9.0 grams per 100 ml. (all donor red blood cells), survived.

some authors advise against intrauterine transfusion if hydrops is present, 50 per cent of fetuses with gross ascites are salvageable with fetal transfusion, diuretics, and digoxin in the author's series.

DIAGNOSIS OF ERYTHROBLASTOSIS IN THE NEWBORN INFANT

Presenting signs and symptoms of erythroblastosis fetalis have been described earlier in this article. Jaundice developing within the first 24 hours of life or becoming more than moderately severe in the first few days of life must be considered to be erythroblastosis until proved otherwise and investigated accordingly. Not all jaundice in the newborn period is due to erythroblastosis (Table 5). Sepsis must always be considered in the differential diagnosis and appropriately investigated and treated.

Cord Blood Findings. The cord blood direct Coombs' test is invariably positive in the erythroblastotic infant with, as already noted, the exception of some cases of ABO erythroblastosis. Cord blood Coombs' tests should be part of the routine examination of every infant shortly after birth. A negative Coombs' test is valuable evidence against the diagnosis of erythroblastosis other than ABO. If the Coombs' test is positive and maternal blood group and antibody status unknown (indicative of inadequte prenatal care), the ABO and Rh of both baby and mother should be determined and the mother's serum screened for Rh or atypical antibodies. If exchange transfusion is being considered, the blood used should be cross-matched with maternal serum and be ABO compatible with her blood, ensuring that there will be no passive maternal antibodies in the infant that will destroy the tranfused red blood cells.

About 60 per cent of infants born after intrauterine transfusion will appear to be Coombs' negative Rh negative because all their circulating red blood cells are donor cells. One should not be lulled into a false sense of security, as there usually is very marked continuing erythropoiesis with rapidly rising bilirubin levels.

Cord hemoglobin and bilirubin levels give an indication of the degree of severity of erythroblastosis and the need for early therapy (exchange transfusion). As a rule a cord hemoglobin of less than 14 grams per 100 ml indicates some degree of hemolysis, although there is no indication for immediate treatment unless the cord hemoglobin level is below 11 grams per 100 ml.

Cord bilirubin levels above 2.5 mg per 100 ml are abnormal and indicative of hemolysis. However, again there is no indication for immediate treatment unless the cord bilirubin level is above 4.0 mg per 100 ml (3.5 grams per ml in the premature infant). With the use of phototherapy many mature babies with cord bilirubin levels of 4.5 mg per 100 ml do not require exchange transfusion.

The leukocyte count is of no value in the diagnosis of erythroblastosis. Recticulocyte counts, normally 5 to 10 per cent, may be markedly elevated in the erythroblastotic infant (up to 25 to 50 per cent in severe cases). Reticulocytosis is simply a reflection of hemolysis, as is the finding of nucleated red blood cells in great profusion and variety in the cord blood (Fig. 7). Although a few normoblasts may be seen in normal cord or newborn blood smears, circulating erythroblasts are indicative of either severe hemolysis (usually erythroblastosis) or chronic severe blood loss (chronic gross transplacental hemorrhage).

Peripheral Blood. Serial hemoglobin and bilirubin estimations at 8- to 12-hour intervals are valuable in predicting the course of erythroblastosis, the risk of kernicterus, and the need for active treatment. A serum indirect bilirubin rise of >0.5 mg per hour usually indicates the need for prompt therapy. In the past an indirect bilirubin level of 20 mg per 100 ml was considered hazardous (10 per cent risk of kernicterus) and exchange transfusion was advised. Phototherapy has reduced indirect bilirubin levels, and administration of serum albumin has lowered the risk of kernicterus by

Table 5. *Neonatal Jaundice Due to Causes Other Than Isoimmunization*

1. Conjugation defects
   a. "Physiologic"
   b. Prematurity and anoxia
   c. Maternal diabetes
   d. Breast milk transferase inhibitor
   e. Transient familial nonhemolytic icterus (serum factor)
   f. Crigler-Najjar syndrome
2. Increased bilirubin production
   a. Hereditary spherocytosis
   b. Red blood cell enzymatic defects (G-6-PD, pyruvate kinase, etc.)
   c. Excessive vitamin K
   d. Extravascular extravasation (cephalohematoma, etc.)
3. Infections
   a. Bacterial sepsis
   b. Rubella
   c. Neonatal hepatitis
   d. Cytomegalic inclusion disease
   e. Congenital syphilis
   f. Toxoplasmosis
   g. Neonatal herpes simplex
4. Hepatic damage (noninfectious)
   a. Galactosemia
   b. Biliary atresia
   c. Choledochal cyst

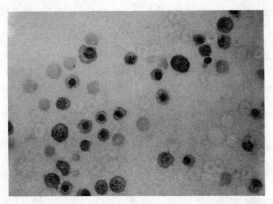

Figure 7. Photomicrograph of cord blood of baby with severe Rh erythroblastosis fetalis who required multiple fetal transfusions and exchange transfusions. Smear treated by Kleihauer technique and Wright's stain. Note adult donor ghost red blood cells, dark fetal red blood cells, and early fetal erythroid series from erythroblasts through to normoblasts.

increasing the plasma albumin-binding capacity of the jaundiced infant.

Albumin-Binding Capacity. Different methods of measuring the reserve albumin-binding capacity of the affected infant's serum have been developed in an attempt to increase the accuracy of determination of the risk of kernicterus. Those in use are: (1) the salicylate saturation index, (2) Sephadex G–25 gel filtration, (3) hydroxybenzeneazo benzoic acid (HBABA) colorimetry, (4) fluorescent yellow dye binding, and (5) horseradish peroxidase oxidation. All have certain drawbacks. Although gel filtration and fluorescent yellow appear to be the most accurate, gel filtration gives a false reading in the presence of direct bilirubin (as does the peroxidase method) and fluorescent yellow is extremely light and time sensitive. Salicylate saturation appears to be the least helpful.

Although HBABA binds not only to bilirubin albumin binding sites but also to other albumin-binding sites, it is rapid and easy to carry out. If its limitations are borne in mind, it can be helpful in determining the risk of kernicterus and modifying the need for exchange transfusion. A reserve albumin-binding capacity greater than 50 per cent by the HBABA method, provided that the infant is mature and not acidotic, indicates little or no risk of kernicterus and the absence of any need for exchange transfusion unless the indirect bilirubin level rises into the 23 to 24 mg per 100 ml range.

Platelet Count. The platelet count of the normal infant is always above 100,000 per cu mm. In severe erythroblastosis fetalis platelet counts below 40,000 per cu mm are not uncommon. They carry with them a considerable risk

of spontaneous hemorrhage unless appropriate treatment is undertaken.

PITFALLS IN DIAGNOSIS

Pitfalls in diagnosis are as follows:

1. Failure to recognize that a pregnant woman is isoimmunized because of failure to send prenatal blood samples for blood grouping and antibody screening tests.

2. Failure to recognize the significance of history and Rh antibody titers in the Rh negative pregnant woman and failure to carry out diagnostic amniocentesis preceded by placental localization early enough to enable therapeutic measures to prevent the development of hydrops fetalis.

3. Failure to recognize the significance of early jaundice in the newborn infant and failure to carry out appropriate investigative and therapeutic measures before kernicterus develops.

NEONATAL PULMONARY DISORDERS

By N. R. C. ROBERTON, M.A., M.B., F.R.C.P.

Cambridge, England

RESPIRATORY DISORDERS PRESENTING IN THE FIRST 4 HOURS OF LIFE

Respiratory distress syndrome (RDS)– Hyaline membrane disease (HMD); transient tachypnea of the newborn; pneumothorax, pneumomediastinum; pneumonia; massive pulmonary hemorrhage; aftermath of birth asphyxia; meconium aspiration; congenital malformations–congenital heart disease, diaphragmatic hernia, pulmonary hypoplasia, other lung abnormalities; miscellanea.

All these conditions may present within 4 hours of delivery, and with the exception of pneumonia, congenital heart disease, and some of the other congenital disorders, rarely develop de novo after this age. Several of the conditions may develop at any age as a complication of therapy, particularly in infants with severe RDS who are being treated with intermittent positive pressure ventilation (IPPV).

RESPIRATORY DISTRESS SYNDROME (RDS)-HYALINE MEMBRANE DISEASE (HMD)

This is the commonest form of respiratory disease in the neonate. Not only that, but Table 1 shows that it was one of the commonest causes of neonatal death and also of all deaths in childhood in England and Wales in 1976. In addition, many of the infants whose deaths were attributed to asphyxia, extreme prematurity, and multiple pregnancy probably died of RDS.

RDS is due to a lack of surfactant in the alveoli of premature infants. This may be because the premature infant is born before enough surfactant had been synthesized, or because he lacks a specific subunit of surfactant such as phosphatidylglycerol, which is deficient in infants of diabetic mothers. In any infant with low surfactant stores, perinatal asphyxia will further decrease surfactant levels and increase the likelihood of postnatal RDS.

DEFINITION

RDS presents within 4 hours of birth; the signs are sternal retraction and intercostal and subcostal recession, an expiratory grunt, and tachypnea greater than 60 per minute. Since the signs may be transient in some infants without true RDS, the definition of RDS usually includes some statement of the duration of symptoms. However, common to all definitions of the disease, the signs should be present *before* 4 hours of age, should still be there *at* 4 hours of age, and should persist for some period *beyond* 4 hours of age. If the last criterion is of long duration, say 24 hours, then respiratory illness that may be due to mild and transient surfactant deficiency will be excluded.

Table 1. *Leading Causes of Death in Children 0–14 Years, England and Wales 1976*

	Total (11,986)	Neonatal (0–28 days) (5681)
Malformations	2536	1456
Respiratory infections and asthma	1515	208
Accidents	1401	47
RDS/HMD	966	963
Extreme prematurity	676	676
Cancer including leukemia	665	12
Crib death	513	43
Multiple pregnancy	316	312

Infants who show the aforementioned clinical picture have respiratory distress. Various causes of respiratory distress present by 4 hours of age (Table 2), but if these can be excluded, which is usually comparatively easy on the basis of history, clinical signs, and chest x-ray, the infant is said to have respiratory distress syndrome (RDS). Histologically the lesion that is present in the lungs of these infants is that of hyaline membrane disease (HMD). Strictly speaking, one should use the term HMD only if one has histologic (i.e., postmortem) proof of the diagnosis. In this article, therefore, the term RDS will be used with the understanding that if a lung biopsy should be taken (!), it would show HMD caused by surfactant deficiency.

CLINICAL SIGNS OF RDS

The infant is premature and may have the signs of RDS from the moment of delivery or they may evolve gradually over the first 4 hours of life. If the infant is not given supplementary oxygen he will be cyanosed. (Cyanosis is not a sign of RDS but is a sign that the RDS is being badly managed.) On auscultation of the chest, the most striking finding is the extremely poor air entry; occasionally a few sticky crepitations are heard. The pulse rate is often quite regular and steady at around 120 per minute, and the infant may be mildly hypotensive with a blood pressure of 35 to 40/20 mm Hg. Profound hypotension down to levels around 20/12 is sometimes seen in severe cases and requires immediate correction. The infant is inactive and tends to lie in the frog position. A moderate degree of generalized subcutaneous edema develops because of the increased capillary leakiness that occurs in this disease. The infant passes only small amounts of urine, and the passage of meconium is delayed often until the second or third day of life.

Generally speaking, the quicker the signs of respiratory difficulty appear, the more severe the disease. The two major determinants of prognosis are birth weight and whether or not the infant requires intermittent positive pressure ventilation (IPPV) from the moment of birth. Death from RDS should now be rare in infants weighing more than 1500 grams at birth and unusual in those who are able to sustain some period of spontaneous respiration after delivery.

The assessment of the severity of RDS is done most accurately by measuring the blood gases and noting the infant's oxygen requirements. Infants less than 1500 grams body weight who require 40 per cent or more oxygen to keep their PaO_2 60 mm Hg or higher and infants of more than 1500 grams body weight who need 60 per cent or greater oxygen to keep their PaO$_2$ above this level have severe disease and often need some form of respiratory assistance.

In uncomplicated RDS, surfactant begins to appear in the lungs (and laryngeal aspirate) at 36 to 48 hours of age. The illness in a given infant therefore gradually becomes worse over the first 24 to 36 hours as he gets progressively tired by the efforts of breathing. His condition then stabilizes for 24 hours, and from 60 to 72 hours of age he steadily improves. By the end of the first week he has usually recovered. The natural history of the disease is much longer if assisted ventilation of any type is required, because of the increased severity of the disease as well as the side effects of the techniques used.

RADIOLOGY

The typical x-ray shows a reticulogranular pattern that represents the atelectasis, and, because of the atelectasis, air-filled major airways stand out as radiolucent areas — the so-called "air bronchogram." In the most severe cases the lung becomes so atelectatic that it cannot be clearly separated from the cardiac border. To some extent, the severity of the x-ray changes reflects the severity of the disease, but if assisted ventilation or continuous positive airway pressure (CPAP) is being used, the purpose is to reverse the atelectasis, and the chest x-ray changes may look surprisingly mild.

DIFFERENTIAL DIAGNOSIS OF RDS

Differential diagnosis (Table 2) is usually quite easily made on the basis of the history,

Table 2. *Differential Diagnosis of RDS*

Condition	Gestation	Clinical Signs	History	X-ray
RDS	Prem ≫ Mature	Dyspnea	Prem delivery asphyxia	Reticulogranular; air bronchogram
Meconium aspiration	Mature	Distended chest; meconium-stained skin, nails, cord	Meconium-stained liquor; birth asphyxia; meconium in trachea at resuscitation	Streaky atelectasis; over-expanded lung
Postperinatal asphyxia; other aspiration–liquor amnii, blood	Mature	Usually dyspnea only; neurologic abnormalities	Perinatal asphyxia	Slightly streaky only
Transient tachypnea of newborn	Mature ≫ Prem	Tachypnea ++; little grunting	NAD	Wet lungs
Massive pulmonary hemorrhage	Mature > Prem	Blood welling up trachea or ETT	Usually severe birth asphyxia; fluid overload; hypothermia	++ opacity, white-out
Congenital pneumonia	Any•	May be T° ↑ or ↓ WBC may be ++ ↓ Hypotonia, early jaundice	Infection in mother, prolonged rupture of membranes; malodorous liquor amnii	Usually more blotchy than RDS but may have a bronchogram
Congenital malformation				
1. Diaphragmatic hernia	Mature > Prem	Scaphoid abdomen	NAD	Diagnostic
2. Potter's syndrome	Usually < term	Potter's facies, oligohydramnios, amnion nodosum	NAD	White-out, very small lungs
3. Other malformations	Usually mature	Dyspnea	NAD	Diagnostic changes (cysts, emphysema, agenesis)
4. Hydrops with pleural effusions	Any	Hydrops obvious	Variable	Clinically obvious; effusions may appear as white-out
Pneumothorax	Usually mature if < 4 hours	Hyperresonant, swollen abdomen; transillumination	May be birth asphyxia → IPPV	Diagnostic
Congenital heart disease	Usually mature if < 4 hours	Other signs CCF–enlarged liver, heart; slate-gray cyanosis; odd ECG; murmur	NAD	Enlarged heart; oligemia or hyperemic lungs
Persistent transitional circulation	Usually mature	None of heart disease; profound cyanosis	Often mild asphyxia	Chest x-ray often surprisingly normal

simple clinical examination, the chest x-ray, and the fact that most of the other problems are seen primarily in mature infants. It should be emphasized that a chest x-ray must be done in all dyspneic newborn infants because of the paucity of physical signs that differentiate one cause of dyspnea from another.

It is most difficult to differentiate RDS from congenital pneumonia. Although this may be possible on the basis of the maternal history or the findings in the infant, in some patients one is left with no alternative but to give antibiotics until cultures are known to be negative.

Problems in the differentiation of RDS from cyanotic congenital heart disease are rare. Any baby with congenital heart disease in trouble in the first hours of life usually has a major defect and will have grossly abnormal physical findings and a very abnormal electrocardiogram (ECG). The chest x-ray virtually always shows a large heart and either oligemic or hyperemic lung fields.

Much more of a diagnostic problem is persistence of the transitional circulation. These infants clinically resemble those with cyanotic congenital heart disease — they are deeply cyanosed with a low or normal $PaCO_2$. They are only mildly or moderately dyspneic, their chest x-ray and ECG look normal, and they often have no murmurs. The echocardiogram is normal. This combination is sufficiently diagnostic to justify a test infusion of tolazoline, which usually causes a rise in the infant's PaO_2 if he has persistent transitional circulation. It will have no effect on the PaO_2 in congenital heart disease and none of the other conditions listed in Table 2 will be adversely affected by this procedure; some, indeed, may be improved.

The most effective way of differentiating RDS from most of the conditions in Table 2 is to assess the amount of surfactant present in a laryngeal or gastric aspirate. It has been shown that this correlates closely with the amount of surfactant present in the alveoli and with the incidence of RDS. The surfactant is usually measured chromatographically as the ratio of lecithin (the major component of surfactant) to sphingomyelin (a lipid present in all the fluids tested whose concentration is unaffected by the degree of pulmonary maturity). If the lecithin/sphingomyelin (L/S) ratio is equal to or less than 1.5:1, the infant has RDS. If it is equal to or more than 2:1, then some other cause of neonatal dyspnea is present except in infants of diabetic mothers. However, one still must deal with the possible coexistence in ill premature infants of infection and RDS.

TRANSIENT TACHYPNEA OF THE NEWBORN

Transient tachypnea of the newborn (TTN) is a condition that affects mature infants but can occur occasionally in those born prematurely. It has been attributed to delayed clearing of the fetal lung fluid after the onset of respiration. We do not yet know why affected infants have less efficient clearing of their pulmonary fluid than do others, suffering from what is in effect mild pulmonary edema. The disease is not due to surfactant deficiency, and the presence of a mature L/S ratio on laryngeal aspirates can be used to differentiate this condition from RDS.

CLINICAL SIGNS

The infant, after an uneventful pregnancy and labor and with little or no birth asphyxia, develops symptoms within an hour or so of delivery. Most commonly he has mild grunting and little sternal intercostal or subcostal recession. However, the respiratory rate is usually at least 100 and may be more. On auscultation the chest sounds normal with good air entry; there are no rales. Cyanosis may be present while the infant is breathing air but is relieved by the administration of 30 to 40 per cent oxygen. Another group of infants who probably have the same disease show a different clinical picture. Their body temperatures often drop to around 35 C (95 F). They breathe quite slowly, have varying degrees of recession, but grunt loudly. When their body temperature rises to normal, they have conversion to the more typical clinical pattern of TTN.

The illness lasts 24 to 48 hours and has a uniformly benign course. The differential diagnosis on presentation is from other causes of dyspnea in the first few hours (Table 2), and is usually easily made on the basis of the mild nature of the illness, the absence of adverse factors in the perinatal history, and the chest x-ray that shows "wet lungs" with prominent vascular markings and fluid in the lung fissures.

PNEUMOTHORAX AND PNEUMOMEDIASTINUM

CLINICAL SIGNS

Pneumothorax. A small pneumothorax that is not under tension may produce very few signs: mild respiratory difficulty may be present in an infant immediately after birth or may develop in a previously asymptomatic infant. Slight deterioration may be noted in an infant receiving IPPV. Radiologic surveys of whole neonatal populations have shown an incidence of pneumothorax of 1.0 to 1.5 per cent, with most of the infants affected being asymptomatic.

Tension pneumothorax presents much more dramatically because ventilation is severely compromised, with the lung collapsed on the side of the lesion and the mediastinal shift compressing the contralateral lung. This mediastinal shift, by distortion of the great vessels as they come through the diaphragm, may sometimes impair arterial perfusion to the lower half of the body or dam back the venous return from the lower half. With impaired venous return the cardiac output will be markedly reduced. These vascular effects may result in the infant being differentially perfused, with striking color differences between the top and bottom halves of the body.

The infant often becomes apneic or shows severe dyspnea, and he is pale and cyanosed. Although on auscultation air entry may sound surprisingly good on both sides, the affected side will have a hyperresonant percussion note. This side will also transilluminate with an appropriate bright light source. The abdomen may be distended and appear rigid as a result of the tension pneumothorax pushing the diaphragm down and compressing the abdominal contents.

Pneumomediastinum. This may occur in isolation or in association with a pneumothorax and is commonly asymptomatic. However, in addition to mild to moderate dyspnea, there may be other physical signs, including anterior bowing of the sternum and distant heart sounds.

RADIOLOGY

The aforementioned conditions are all diagnosed by appropriate chest x-ray. In addition to the usual anteroposterior chest x-ray, it is essential to obtain a lateral horizontal beam film of the chest. This is the only satisfactory way of demonstrating a pneumomediastinum, in which, with the infant lying supine, the air collects under the sternum. A similar view is also essential for assessing the size of the pneumothorax in RDS, in which there is always a major degree of lung collapse, even without tension developing. In such cases the AP chest x-ray taken with the infant supine may show only a comparatively small rim of air between the lung edge and the chest wall. However, the horizontal beam lateral x-ray will show that the collapsed lung is lying on the posterior wall of the chest with a large pneumothorax anterior to it.

DIFFERENTIAL DIAGNOSIS

There is rarely any difficulty with the differential diagnosis once the x-ray is taken; the problem is remembering to exclude a pneumothorax by x-ray in any infant with dyspnea or when dyspnea in a pre-existing illness has suddenly become more marked.

PNEUMONIA

In the first few hours of life pneumonia is a diagnosis that is reasonably easy to be certain about, but virtually impossible to exclude with certainty. Because of the rapid progression and the dissemination of all infections in the neonatal period, especially the fulminating form of group B streptococcal sepsis in which the mean age at death is 12 to 18 hours, many neonatologists now give routine antistreptococcal therapy to all dyspneic newborns until cultures are known to be negative.

The clinical, laboratory, and radiologic findings listed in Table 3 suggest infection. The more of them that are present, the more likely is infection — pulmonary or generalized — to be the cause of the infant's early neonatal respiratory illness.

MASSIVE PULMONARY HEMORRHAGE

This commonly occurs in association with other severe neonatal disorders, including severe birth asphyxia, hypothermia, rhesus hemolytic (Rh) disease, vascular overload, oxygen toxicity, and hemostatic failure. The unifying concept for all these factors is that in them left-sided heart failure may be combined with damage to the pulmonary capillaries. If both of these are bad enough, not only will there be pulmonary edema but red cells will leak out of capillaries as well. In support of this theory, in most cases of massive pulmonary hemorrhage the hematocrit of the fluid produced is less than 10 per cent — that is, it is a hemorrhagic pulmonary edema.

CLINICAL SIGNS

The condition of the infant, already severely ill with one of the aforementioned conditions, suddenly deteriorates, and he becomes pale, cyanosed, and limp, often over a 2 to 5 minute period. If the infant is being ventilated, bloody fluid will be found welling up the endotracheal tube. If not, he will usually become apneic or develop an irregular breathing pattern and at laryngoscopy bloody fluid will be seen welling up the trachea.

Table 3. Features Suggesting Infection as Cause of Neonatal Respiratory Distress

Respiratory illness in mature infant

Delivery through potentially infected birth canal
1. Rupture of membranes > 24 hours
2. Maternal pyrexia in labor
3. Maternal symptoms of infectious disease
4. Purulent vaginal discharge; malodorous liquor amnii
5. Poor maternal antenatal care

Atypical clinical course of RDS at any gestation

Unusually hypotonic, hypotensive, or underperfused infant

Pyrexia > 38 C (100.5 F) or hypothermia < 35 C (95 F) in an infant in the absence of other identifiable cause of temperature instability, usually environmental

Early onset jaundice

Early onset apneic attacks

Coarse crepitations, localized or generalized

Unusually severe acidemia: marked hypoxemia without hypercapnia

Total WBC < 6400/cu mm or polymorphs < 2800/cu mm in first 24 hours or polymorphs > 8000/cu mm beyond 48 hours

Bacteria identified on Gram stain of gastric aspirate or of swab from external auditory meatus

Chest x-ray showing patchy consolidation, coarse generalized mottling, anything unlike the typical air bronchogram of RDS

Normal L/S ratio — excluding RDS — on liquor amnii obtained antenatally, or on pharyngeal or gastric aspirate collected after delivery

In the acute phase the x-ray usually shows homogeneously opaque lungs with some cardiac enlargement.

AFTER-EFFECTS OF SEVERE PERINATAL ASPHYXIA

Infants who are born prematurely and suffer severe perinatal asphyxia will develop RDS. In those who are born at term however postnatal dyspnea may develop for the following reasons: (1) persisting metabolic acidemia with or without brain damage, (2) heart failure and pulmonary edema due to transient myocardial ischemia of the neonate, (3) amniotic fluid aspiration, (4) massive pulmonary hemorrhage, (5) persistent transitional circulation, (6) meconium aspiration syndrome, and (7) tension pneumothorax.

These infants are readily identifiable by the fact that they were in poor condition at birth and have required active resuscitation with IPPV and perhaps parenteral base, glucose, or opiate antagonists.

CLINICAL SIGNS

The signs of those with pulmonary hemorrhage, meconium aspiration, pneumothorax, and transitional circulation are described elsewhere. However, even in the absence of these conditions, some full-term infants following resuscitation from perinatal asphyxia remain dyspneic, because of various combinations of the first three reasons listed.

Auscultation of the chest is usually normal and the infants rarely require more than 40 per cent oxygen to stay pink. They are often pale, with a tachypnea of more than 160 per minute, and may be hypotensive or hypertensive, depending on their blood volume and the degree of myocardial involvement as a result of the asphyxia. In the small number of infants with ischemic myocardial injury, heart failure with hepatosplenomegaly and pulmonary edema with crepitations may develop.

Neurologically they may be wide-eyed and jittery, and either hypotonic or hypertonic. Their fontanels may be tense, usually due to cerebral edema rather than intracranial hemorrhage, and they may convulse. The head circumference should always be measured for future reference.

INVESTIGATIONS

These are (1) hemoglobin (or hematocrit) to exclude blood loss causing or resulting from perinatal asphyxia, (2) blood gases to exclude metabolic acidemia, (3) blood glucose to exclude hypoglycemia, (4) electrolytes and serum calcium, (5) urinalysis and fluid balance to exclude acute renal damage, (6) chest x-ray, (7) electrocardiogram, and (8) lumbar puncture.

Urine should be collected from these infants to ensure that there is urinary output following a severe asphyxial episode that may have caused renal damage and to check for renal damage. The presence of blood or numerous epithelial cells in the urine suggests that renal damage has occurred. Daily electrolytes and plasma and urinary osmolarity should be obtained if there is any suspicion that the infant is developing renal failure or inappropriate ADH secretions.

Chest x-ray is usually unremarkable in the absence of pneumothorax or meconium aspiration, although some streaky shadows may be present if there has been aspiration. The x-ray may show a large heart, and the ECG may show

ST segment depression and deep Q waves if there is myocardial damage as a result of the perinatal asphyxia.

I do not believe that lumbar puncture should be carried out routinely in such infants. However, if the neurologic condition remains poor or if fits or fever develop, a lumbar puncture should be done to exclude intracranial hemorrhage or early-onset meningitis.

MECONIUM ASPIRATION

This condition is limited to mature infants, since premature infants virtually never pass meconium in utero, no matter how severely they are asphyxiated. Any meconium in an infant's mouth or pharynx will be inhaled when he gasps and this is particularly likely to happen in the few seconds after delivery. The meconium causes airways obstruction, which is more marked in expiration and leads to air trapping and overdistension of the lungs with a considerable risk of pneumomediastinum and pneumothorax. The irritant properties of meconium also cause a chemical pneumonitis, and the presence of inhaled organic material predisposes to bacterial colonization of the lungs.

CLINICAL SIGNS

The infant is often postmature with wrinkled green meconium-impregnated skin, nails, and umbilical cord. Meconium may be present in the pharynx and trachea at birth. In this case the infant's trachea should be sucked clear under direct vision. This is not only therapeutic but also establishes the diagnosis.

If, despite these maneuvers, meconium is inhaled beyond the reach of direct suction, the infant will develop respiratory distress soon after birth. This may be quite severe, with a tachypnea of more than 100 per minute. The air trapping caused by the meconium gives the infant an overdistended chest, marked anterior bowing of the sternum, and an increased anteroposterior diameter to the chest. On auscultation, there are widespread added sounds with rhonchi and both fine and sticky crepitations. The infant's condition may steadily deteriorate over the first 24 hours of life if chemical pneumonitis and secondary infection develop, and depending on the severity of the disease the infant may take a week or more to recover. Differential diagnosis is rarely a problem (Table 2), but other conditions may coexist, particularly pneumothorax and pneumonia.

INVESTIGATIONS

The severity of the disease is best assessed by a blood gas analysis. Infants with severe cases will be profoundly hypoxic even in 90 to 95 per cent oxygen due to right to left intrapulmonary shunting, but most infants hyperventilate sufficiently to keep their $PaCO_2$ normal. However, a progressively rising $PaCO_2$ is an indication of severe disease with plugging of the airways with meconium or of the development of a secondary pneumonia.

The tests that are used for the evaluation of the severely asphyxiated infant should also be carried out in infants suffering from meconium aspiration.

X-ray shows overexpanded lungs with multiple streaky areas of atelectasis. As the disease progresses the lungs may become more diffusely opaque owing to the chemical pneumonitis or bacterial superinfection. AP and lateral x-rays should be repeated whenever the infant's condition deteriorates, because of the high risk of pneumothorax, which can be impossible to detect clinically.

CONGENITAL MALFORMATIONS

CONGENITAL HEART DISEASE

If this presents in the first 4 to 6 hours, there is usually some major malformation. The signs are usually gross, with profound cyanosis, severe heart failure, or both. If the malformation is of the type causing cyanotic heart disease, the infant, usually mature, in addition to having cyanosis, has only mild or moderate dyspnea. The cyanosis has a characteristic slate-gray tinge. It is impossible to raise the PaO_2 above 40 to 50 mm Hg despite administration of 100 per cent oxygen.

If the presentation is with heart failure, there will be marked hepatomegaly, splenomegaly, and pulmonary edema. Murmurs and tachycardia are usually present but may be absent in infants with cyanotic heart disease. The femoral pulses may be reduced or absent with aortic abnormalities. All the pulses may be reduced with systemic hypotension, with major structural abnormalities of the left side of the heart, or in advanced heart failure. With a large left-to-right shunt, the pulses are characteristically bounding.

The chest x-ray and ECG will be clearly abnormal in virtually all patients, with the changes depending on the underlying malformation. The differential diagnosis of these conditions is shown in Table 2.

DIAPHRAGMATIC HERNIA

The dyspnea caused by this condition in the neonatal period is more related to the underlying pulmonary hypoplasia than to the displacement of the thoracic contents by the bowel herniated through the diaphragmatic defect.

Symptoms and Signs. At birth the infant has great difficulty in establishing adequate respiration. Despite the fact that one hemithorax — usually the left — is full of bowel, physical signs in the chest are remarkably unhelpful and the diagnostic clue comes from the scaphoid abdomen. The chest x-ray early on shows an opaque hemithorax, since in the very ill infant it may take 2 to 3 hours for gas to get into the intrathoracic bowel. The clinical picture is so characteristic that barium studies are almost never necessary. Such infants, with pulmonary hypoplasia, have severely compromised gas exchange with a low PaO_2 and high $PaCO_2$, despite 90 to 95 per cent oxygen and IPPV at pressure exceeding 35/5 cm H_2O. They have a high mortality rate.

The condition in infants with diaphragmatic hernia with lesser degrees of pulmonary hypoplasia may present at any time during the early neonatal period as the intrathoracic bowel fills with gas (or food) and further reduces lung volume.

Such infants, may have mild dyspnea with or without cyanosis. The abdomen in these infants may be scaphoid and bowel sounds can often be heard over the relevant hemithorax. X-ray confirms the diagnosis, and blood gas abnormalities are mild. Once the diagnosis is confirmed, no further evaluation is required prior to surgery.

PULMONARY HYPOPLASIA

As well as occurring in association with diaphragmatic hernia, this condition is found in cases of Potter's syndrome. These infants at birth have severe respiratory failure. They are usually anephric or virtually so and never pass urine. Other diagnostic clues are oligohydramnios, amnion nodosum, squashed facial appearance, deficient ear cartilages, large floppy hands, and postural abnormalities in the limbs. The condition is fatal.

OTHER INTRATHORACIC MALFORMATIONS

These include congenital lobar emphysema, congenital adenomatoid malformation, space-occupying lesions such as mediastinal tumors and neurenteric cysts, accessory or sequestrated lobes, and eventration of the diaphragm. These cause dyspnea and may occur at any time in the neonatal period or beyond. No specific diagnostic clues are present, and the diagnosis is made from x-ray.

MISCELLANEA

PLEURAL EFFUSIONS

These are rare in the neonatal period and are usually found in association with other obvious abnormalities, e.g., hydrops fetalis from any cause, gross congestive cardiac failure, or pulmonary lymphangiectasia. Isolated pleural effusions present as dyspnea and are usually due to "idiopathic" chylothorax. On clinical examination large effusions may be detected by decreased percussion notes and air entry. These signs are difficult to elicit in the sick neonate and are absent with small effusions.

Radiology. Neonates are usually x-rayed in the supine position so that a fluid level is not seen, although it may be picked up on a horizontal beam decubitus film. A complete "whiteout" in one hemithorax or a diffuse loss of definition should cause the investigator to suspect that fluid is present. Appropriate x-ray views should then be taken. A diagnostic tap should always be carried out to differentiate serous, chylous, and bloody effusions; chyle will appear in an effusion only after a fat-containing feeding has been taken. Following aspiration, underlying lung pathology may be revealed. If a hemothorax is found, clotting studies should be carried out to exclude a bleeding diathesis.

NEONATAL POLYCYTHEMIA

Infants with a hematocrit of more than 75 per cent may become dyspneic. A hematocrit should always be included in the diagnostic evaluation of a dyspneic neonate. Caution should be exercised in attributing neonatal respiratory symptoms to this condition alone.

The response to a small dilutional exchange transfusion can be evaluated — exchanging 20 to 30 ml per kg with plasma. If the infant becomes asymptomatic, the diagnosis is made; if not, another diagnosis must be sought.

OTHER RARE CAUSES OF NEONATAL RESPIRATORY PROBLEMS

These may present either as respiratory failure, apnea, or respiratory distress. These include congenital or acquired brain abnormality causing dyspnea, hyperpnea, or apnea; primary muscle disorders, e.g., dystrophia myotonica; Werdnig-Hoffmann disease; myasthenia gravis; neonatal poliomyelitis; Erb's palsy with diaphragmatic involvement; and metabolic acidemia due to drugs, inborn errors of metabolism, and so forth.

DETERIORATING RESPIRATORY FUNCTION IN INFANTS WITH RDS OR OTHER CONDITIONS REQUIRING IPPV

PNEUMOTHORAX

Following any unexplained deterioration in the condition of an infant on a ventilator, pneumothorax must be excluded. Although the aforementioned physical signs may be present, in many cases the diagnosis can only be established radiologically.

Massive pulmonary hemorrhage is discussed under a previous heading.

PNEUMONIA

Many infants are already receiving antibiotics by the time they are placed on the ventilator. In those who are not, infection appears as a gradual clinical deterioration over a period of hours. This is shown by some combination of the following features: increase in lethargy, decrease in peripheral perfusion, mottled skin; increase in jaundice; nasogastric feeds no longer tolerated, with occurrence of vomiting and abdominal distention; increase in thick (purulent) secretions up the endotracheal tube, with positive culture from these secretions; temperature instability, (hypothermia or pyrexia); x-ray changes that are patchy, suggesting pneumonia; localized or generalized crepitations on auscultation; and a raised white count and a rise in neutrophils to more than 8000 per cu mm. Most of these findings are compatible with simple deterioration of the RDS, but they could also mean infection. Since to be wrong is so serious, after appropriate cultures and a white count in these infants, antibiotics should be started.

PULMONARY EDEMA WITH PATENT DUCTUS ARTERIOSUS

SYMPTOMS AND SIGNS

On the fifth to sixth day in an infant with RDS who had begun to improve on IPPV, the blood gases deteriorate, with a fall in PaO_2 and a rise in $PaCO_2$. Crepitations are heard in both lung fields, the heart rate is over 150 to 160 beats per minute with characteristically hyperdynamic pulses, and a loud systolic murmur is heard maximally over the base with occasional extension of the murmur into diastole. Signs of congestive cardiac failure are absent. X-ray shows the perihilar haze of pulmonary edema with resolution of the changes of RDS, and ECG rarely shows any abnormality. Echocardiog-

raphy demonstrates a left atrium/aortic route ratio of over 1:1.

These findings are sufficient to establish the diagnosis of patent ductus in such infants, but the diagnosis can be confirmed at cardiac catheterization by demonstration of a large left-to-right shunt at the ductus level or by angiocardiography.

BRONCHOPULMONARY DYSPLASIA

This condition is the end result of prolonged IPPV using high inflating pressures, but the condition may also be contributed to by the original lung pathology, oxygen toxicity, infection, and retention of secretions below an endotracheal tube. The disease is very unusual, irrespective of the duration of oxygen therapy, in infants who have only breathed spontaneously, or infants who have only received continuous positive airway pressure (CPAP) or *negative* pressure ventilation.

SYMPTOMS AND SIGNS

The condition occurs as a failure to maintain progress after 2 to 3 weeks on the ventilator. $PaCO_2$ remains elevated at 50 to 60 mm Hg, the oxygen requirements stabilize often at 50 to 60 per cent, and the inflating pressures of the ventilator usually must be kept above 25 cm H_2O. There are no specific physical signs. The diagnosis is made on the basis of this clinical picture plus the x-ray, which shows widespread fibrosis and scarring of the lung, often with areas of compensatory emphysema or large loculations of interstitial air.

In some infants it is possible to lower gradually the inflating pressures and inspired oxygen concentrations over a period of weeks and months and wean them off IPPV. However, in infants who develop this more severe form of the condition, mild hypoxemia and hypercapnia may persist up to a year of age, with increased airways resistance and increased functional residual capacity and reduced lung compliance.

In a small number of infants the bronchopulmonary dysplasia gets progressively worse on the ventilator until the infant dies aged 2 to 3 months from respiratory failure or cor pulmonale.

RESPIRATORY ILLNESS PRESENTING AFTER 4 HOURS OF AGE IN PREVIOUSLY WELL INFANTS

The causes are pneumonia, congenital heart disease, pneumothorax, and congenital malformations. All these conditions involve dyspnea, problems with feeding, and either cyanotic attacks or persisting cyanosis. It is, nevertheless, unusual for previously well term infants to develop signs of respiratory distress beyond 4 to 6 hours of age. With pneumothorax and congenital malformations excluded by immediate x-ray, the differential diagnosis lies between heart failure or chest infection, and this is usually straightforward. The premature infant, however, because of his increased susceptibility to infection, is more prone to pneumonia than the term infant. In addition, late-onset respiratory disease in premature infants may be due to one of the chronic noninfectious lung diseases to be described in later paragraphs.

PNEUMONIA

Pneumonia should be detected on the basis of the rather subtle signs of infection in the neonatal period listed in Table 3. If these are combined with tachypnea of 60 per minute or more, pneumonia is the likely cause of the lung disease. If pneumonia is recognized only when the infant shows severe respiratory difficulties, cyanosis, and signs of septicemia, this suggests that earlier diagnostic clues have passed unrecognized. Cough is a rare symptom in neonates, and sputum is not produced. On examination there may be localized or generalized creptitations. The presenting signs can be confirmed.

The common organisms responsible for pneumonia in the neonate are those of the group B streptococcus, coliforms, and *Staphylococcus aureus*. All can disseminate rapidly and cause death within 24 hours of presentation. For this reason, a clinical suspicion of lung infection should always be followed by appropriate antibiotic therapy after cultures are taken.

INVESTIGATION

Cultures of nose and throat should be taken; a blood culture is essential, and a differential white count should be done. Beyond 48 hours of age, a count of more than 8000 WBC per cu mm, a left shift in the morphology of the neutrophil population, or toxic granulation of the neutrophils is strong evidence of infection.

A chest x-ray should always be done in any febrile infant, even one without tachypnea. If parenchymal lung infection is present, there may be either localized or general patchy infiltrates, or more rarely, collapse and consolidation of one lobe or segment. However, the absence of findings on x-ray should not deter one from a diagnosis of pneumonia in the presence of fever plus clinical signs of lung disease. Since sys-temic dissemination of infection is so rapid in the neonatal period, a lumbar puncture should always be considered if there is any doubt as to whether the pulmonary disease is responsible for all the symptoms, or whether there might be coexisting meningitis.

CONGENITAL HEART DISEASE

This may masquerade as lung disease by causing either cyanosis or dyspnea, the latter often being the result of pulmonary edema of left ventricular failure, which in the premature infant is often due to a patent ductus arteriosus.

The presentation of congenital heart disease beyond 4 hours of age differs from presentations before this age mainly in the speed at which the abnormal physical signs develop. This speed is in turn related to the severity of the underlying defect. For the differential diagnosis see Table 2.

PNEUMOTHORAX

This rarely presents after 6 hours of age in spontaneously breathing infants. However, it must always be excluded by x-ray in any infant with dyspnea or cyanosis.

CONGENITAL MALFORMATIONS

These may cause symptoms at any time in the neonatal period, although usually symptoms occur early. Malformations must be excluded by x-ray in all dyspneic neonates.

CHRONIC RESPIRATORY PROBLEMS OF THE PREMATURE NEONATE

WILSON-MIKITY SYNDROME

This is a disease of very low birth weight (less than 1200 gram) infants who characteristically have not had any previous serious respiratory disease.

ETIOLOGY

The cause is not fully understood, but it has been suggested that the disorder is caused by the trapping of air behind the highly compliant and therefore collapsible lung airways in very low birth weight infants. The trapped air caused alveolar distention, rupture, and fibrosis. Pulmonary function studies confirm an increased thoracic gas volume (TGV) and airways resistance.

CLINICAL FEATURES

A previously healthy low birth weight baby becomes progressively dyspneic during the second and third weeks of life and requires supplementary oxygen. There may be a few fine crepitations in the lungs. Blood gases initially show hypoxemia and mild carbon dioxide retention.

In most infants spontaneous recovery begins by the sixth to eighth week of life, and they are asymptomatic by the age of 3 months. For some unknown reason, however, a small percentage develop progressive disease with more and more profound hypoxia and severe hypercapnia, culminating in death from respiratory failure and cor pulmonale by 3 to 4 months.

RADIOLOGY

The chest x-ray characteristically shows a honeycomb appearance with coarse interstitial fibrosis outlining areas of hyperaeration. These changes are most prominent in the upper lobes and may take over 12 months to clear.

CHRONIC PULMONARY INSUFFICIENCY OF PREMATURITY

Many low birth weight infants who may or may not have had RDS become mildly dyspneic around 2 to 4 weeks of life, with an increased frequency of apneic attacks. They require an increased inspired oxygen concentration to keep their PaO_2 at 60 to 90 mm Hg.

Clinically they behave similarly to infants with Wilson-Mikity syndrome. Radiologically, however, they show a diffusely hazy x-ray. Pulmonary function studies show a decreased functional residual capacity and thoracic gas volume, and normal airways resistance.

The condition, which has been attributed to transient postnatal surfactant deficiency, runs a benign course over 2 to 3 weeks before oxygen therapy can be discontinued.

APNEIC ATTACKS

Many otherwise entirely normal premature infants breathe irregularly or may show periodic breathing in which regular bursts of 3 to 6 breaths are separated by periods of apnea lasting less than 10 seconds. As a matter of definition, apneic attacks last longer than 10 seconds. During them, the infant may develop cyanosis, bradycardia, and hypertension, followed by hypotension if the apnea is prolonged.

Table 4. *Causes of Apnea in Newborn Infants*

RDS — deteriorating or undiagnosed
Massive pulmonary hemorrhage
Other lung disease, e.g., Wilson-Mikity, pneumothorax
Septicemia, meningitis, pneumonia
Hypocalcemia
Hypoglycemia
Heart failure — especially pulmonary edema with a patent ductus arteriosus (PDA)
Intracranial hemorrhage especially intraventricular hemorrhage (IVH)
Convulsions
Respiratory depression by drugs
Aspiration and inhalation of a feed
Rare metabolic disease, e.g., methylmalonic acidemia — consider only if the infant has other appropriate signs

SYMPTOMATIC APNEA

The development of apneic attacks in an infant who is already unwell is commonly a sign of deterioration of his condition, whereas in the previously asymptomatic infant, it may be the first indication of serious underlying disease. For this reason, whenever an infant develops apneic attacks the conditions in Table 4 should be excluded clinically or by laboratory investigation.

The final common pathway for many of these conditions is hypoxia, which may depress respiration in normal neonates as well as in those who are ill. In some of the other conditions, circulating toxins or metabolic disturbance will cause apnea by direct effect on the central nervous system.

In addition to these illnesses, an infant's tendency to periodic breathing or apnea can be aggravated by the conditions listed in Table 5. As with the pathologic causes of apnea, the final common pathway in many of these conditions is hypoxia.

Reflex apnea is a particularly interesting phenomenon in neonatal animals who have upper airways receptors that, when stimulated, produce apnea that persists until the stimulus is withdrawn. Any liquid in the airway other than species-specific milk, saline, or liquor amnii may induce apnea. Upper airway reflexes may

Table 5. *Factors That Increase the Incidence of Apnea, Particularly in Low Birth Weight Infants*

Reflexes from upper airway receptors
Anemia; (PCV < 35–40%)
Surges in incubator temperature
Feeding
Physical handling
Airways obstruction, e.g., nasogastric tube, neck flexion

also be important in the development of apnea following transient obstruction of the airways. The apnea of temperature surges is probably the reverse of the reflex response by which a draft of cold air on the face of normal infants initiates respiration after birth.

Apnea following feeding can be particularly exasperating in otherwise healthy infants (< 1200 gm) and may necessitate drip feeding, nasojejunal feeding, or even a period of intravenous feeding. Part of the problem in such infants may be apnea from airways obstruction by the indwelling nasogastric tube in addition to the hypoxia induced by feeding.

RECURRENT APNEA OF PREMATURITY

A group of otherwise entirely healthy infants may develop apneic attacks. The condition is almost confined to those less than 1500 gm and fewer than 32 weeks' gestation. Characteristically these attacks develop on the fifth to sixth day of life and are more likely to occur in the presence of the aggravating factors listed in Table 5. Between attacks the infant shows no clinical abnormalities, and in particular there is no dyspnea and no abnormal signs in the chest. Other than excluding the conditions in Table 4 by appropriate blood tests and a chest x-ray no further investigation is required.

INNOCENT HEART MURMURS IN CHILDREN

By HERBERT S. HARNED, JR., M.D.
Chapel Hill, North Carolina

Several common cardiac murmurs occur in healthy children with no evidence of heart disease. To avoid ambiguity, most cardiologists prefer to call such murmurs "innocent" rather than "functional." The latter term has been applied to murmurs observed in normal persons but is also applied to murmurs generated as a result of such general states as anemia, fever, nervousness, exercise, hyperthyroidism, and pregnancy. Also, use of the term "innocent" in explaining the murmur to children and their parents offers reassurance. It is very necessary for the physician, confronted with a child with a heart murmur, to define the condition as precisely as possible in his own mind, so that he is in a position to inform the parents of its implications, including recommendations relating to the patient's physical activities and need for additional diagnostic studies or medical follow-up. Since most innocent murmurs of childhood have characteristics that distinguish them from organic murmurs, knowledge of these features will enable the physician to avoid unnecessary procedures and referrals and will permit him to allay the anxiety that is so frequently evident in the parents and the child.

The innocent murmurs of childhood can be classified conveniently in relation to their timing in the cardiac cycle (Fig. 1).

EARLY AND MIDSYSTOLIC MURMURS

Vibratory or Musical Murmur. This murmur is particularly noted in the preschool and early schoolage periods and is usually located best at the lower left sternal border. Radiation to the apex and upper left sternal border may occur and rarely the murmur appears to be most prominent at the apex. The vibratory quality of the murmur has captured the imagination of physicians since Still's early description emphasized its musical character. Other descriptive adjectives such as "twanging string," "groaning," and "honking" emphasize its harmonic nature. Phonocardiography usually reveals a symmetric sine wave pattern originating after the first heart sound, increasing in intensity usually before midsystole, and then fading before the second heart sound. The frequency of 70 to 160 cycles results in its low-pitched sound.

The origin of this murmur is really not known. Various authors have suggested that it might originate from vibrations generated by the heart muscle itself, the pulmonic valve, outflow portion of the right ventricle, pericardial or extracardial structures, or even the aortic valve. Estimates of its occurrence in all children range from 15 to 60 per cent; these estimates vary because of the overlap in auscultatory findings between some of these vibratory murmurs and some of the pulmonic systolic ejection murmurs to be described later.

The innocent vibratory murmur, when it is located at the apex, may be difficult to differentiate from the soft murmur of mitral regurgitation. Helpful in the differential diagnosis is the blowing quality found in the latter (actually often a "swishing" sound), its holosystolic timing, and its referral to the axilla. Also, the

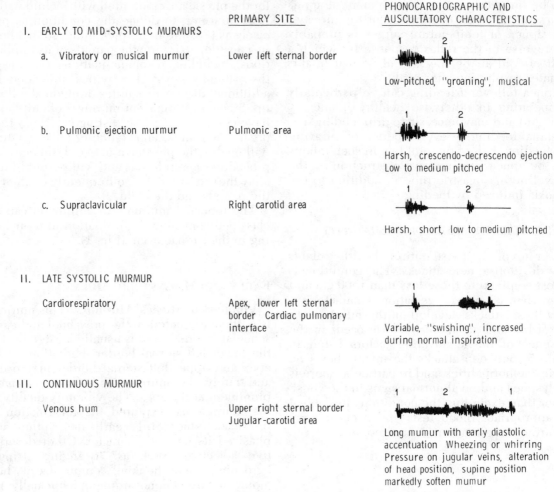

	PRIMARY SITE	PHONOCARDIOGRAPHIC AND AUSCULTATORY CHARACTERISTICS

I. EARLY TO MID-SYSTOLIC MURMURS

a. Vibratory or musical murmur — Lower left sternal border

Low-pitched, "groaning", musical

b. Pulmonic ejection murmur — Pulmonic area

Harsh, crescendo-decrescendo ejection
Low to medium pitched

c. Supraclavicular — Right carotid area

Harsh, short, low to medium pitched

II. LATE SYSTOLIC MURMUR

Cardiorespiratory — Apex, lower left sternal border Cardiac pulmonary interface

Variable, "swishing", increased during normal inspiration

III. CONTINUOUS MURMUR

Venous hum — Upper right sternal border Jugular-carotid area

Long mumur with early diastolic accentuation Wheezing or whirring Pressure on jugular veins, alteration of head position, supine position markedly soften mumur

Figure 1. Classification and characteristics of innocent heart murmurs of childhood.

innocent vibratory murmur may be difficult to distinguish from that due to ventricular septal defect, especially if the organic murmur originates from a muscular defect. In this instance, the usual holosystolic timing may not be observed, probably because of diminution in late systolic flow through the defect. The innocent vibratory murmur may usually be distinguished from the murmurs of pulmonic and aortic stenosis by their higher locations and transmissions, but in the older child with idiopathic hypertrophic subaortic stenosis, a murmur with qualities simulating this innocent murmur may occur.

The innocent vibratory murmur is louder in the supine than in the sitting subject, may vary from examination to examination, and is usually aggravated by exercise. It is not associated with a thrill, another useful finding in its delineation from the organic murmurs.

Pulmonic Ejection Murmur. A harsh, crescendo-decrescendo ejection murmur, heard best in the pulmonic region, is perhaps more

common than the vibratory murmur but has a peak incidence in schoolage children. Its characteristics are identical to those of the pulmonic flow murmur detected in atrial septal defect, and indeed, the innocent pulmonic murmur has been shown by intracardiac phonocardiography to be generated by flow through a pulmonic valve. This murmur is also loudest when the subject is recumbent and usually is increased by exercise. In young children, it may be transmitted posteriorly to the left scapular region.

The phonocardiogram will reveal that this innocent murmur originates shortly after the first sound, has a relative frequency usually between 90 and 130 cycles per second, is less harmonic than the vibratory innocent murmur, and occupies one fourth to three fourths of the systolic interval. It varies in intensity on auscultation from grades 1 to 3 (grading 1 to 6), is not associated with a thrill, and shows considerable variability from one examination to the next.

Because this murmur results from flow

through the pulmonic valve, general factors increasing right ventricular output, such as fever, exercise, anemia, and anxiety, will intensify it, and the physician should consider these factors in the physical examination. Since the murmur is identical to that observed in atrial septal defect, the important additional findings in the latter condition should be searched for specifically. The key observations of fixed splitting of the second sound and the increased intensity of the second component of the second sound, which may produce audible splitting of the second sound at the apex, may indicate that an atrial septal defect is present. Also, if such a defect is quite large, an early diastolic rumbling murmur, representing increased tricuspid flow, may be detected at the left sternal border. Mild valvular pulmonic stenosis may result in an ejection murmur similar to this innocent murmur, but often the murmur of pulmonic stenosis is much louder and harsher and is associated with a thrill in the pulmonic area and with posterior transmittal of a degree greater than that from the innocent murmur. The early systolic click, often found in pulmonic stenosis, also serves as a differential feature. Idiopathic pulmonary dilatation, peripheral pulmonic stenosis, infundibular pulmonic stenosis, coarctation of the aorta, and aortic stenosis can produce ejection murmurs that may mimic the innocent pulmonic flow murmur.

Although the primary location of such flow murmurs is in the pulmonic region, on other occasions systolic ejection murmurs may be heard well in the aortic region. Intra-arterial phonocardiographic studies indicate that in many normal children, systolic ejection murmurs may be generated by flow past the aortic valve. Such innocent aortic ejection murmurs can mimic serious cardiac disorders, such as aortic stenosis and idiopathic hypertrophic subaortic stenosis. This differential diagnosis is particularly difficult in the teenage boy, presenting in an anxious state during an examination that may determine his participating in athletics, in whom a systolic ejection murmur is heard at the aortic region. Before such patients can be cleared for active competition, they must be examined carefully for the telltale organic signs such as an early systolic ejection click or thrills over the aortic and suprasternal regions. These patients may require additional noninvasive studies that may be useful in identifying the various types of aortic stenosis. In addition to chest x-rays, electrocardiograms, and vectoreardiograms, the use of phonocardiograms with carotid pulse tracings and echocardiograms is particularly helpful in this situation. Usually, these studies will be sufficiently specific, but

occasionally left-sided heart catheterization will be needed. Also, many of these patients should undergo periodic profiling during their adolescent growth spurt to identify changing features of the aortic murmurs.

Pulmonary systolic ejection murmurs are also noted frequently in the straight-back syndrome, in which the AP diameter of the chest is relatively small. In this disorder, the heart is "pancaked" in the narrow space between the spine and sternum and on PA x-ray may appear somewhat enlarged. Loud closure of the tricuspid valve, exaggerated splitting of the second sound during inspiration, and a palpable left parasternal impulse are also features of the straight-back syndrome, but the heart is structurally normal. One can readily see the controversy in semantics over whether the systolic ejection murmur in this syndrome can indeed be labeled "innocent."

Supraclavicular Arterial Bruit. A short systolic ejection bruit may be detected in approximately 30 per cent of children in the supraclavicular areas, most frequently over the right carotid area. This murmur is affected by the pressure applied by the stethoscope, intensifying with increased pressure or partial occlusion of the carotid artery and lengthening then in duration. With increased occlusion of the carotid artery, the bruit may vanish. This murmur usually is soft, but has been described as being as intense as grade 4 (grading 1 to 6). Often, it is associated with a venous hum and is aggravated by exercise and anemia, but not by changes in position or by altering respiration.

The origin of this murmur is believed to be from the great arterial vessels in the neck, but an aortic valve origin has also been proposed, The murmur may usually be distinguished from that of aortic stenosis by absence of a thrill, by absence of a systolic ejection click, and by the short duration in early systole of the innocent bruit, as well as by its lack of localization in the aortic region of the precordium.

LATE SYSTOLIC MURMURS

Cardiorespiratory Murmur. Bizarre timing and variability are characteristics of the so-called "cardiorespiratory" or "cardiopulmonary" murmur. Generally this unusual murmur is heard in mid to late systole, may have a "swishing" or "whiffing" quality, and is loudest in a localized region, usually over a heart-lung interface such as the apex or the left sternal border areas. The murmur may be soft or moderately loud, is often intensified during normal inspiration, and may disappear during held expiration. Its intensity varies with changes in position of the subject, and exercise may accentuate the murmur. The origin of this type of murmur is obscure, but it may result from the systolic impact of the heart on adjacent lung, causing intrapulmonic movement of air.

At times this murmur may be confused with late systolic murmurs caused by organic lesions such as mitral regurgitation, ventricular septal defect, idiopathic hypertrophic subaortic stenosis, Marfan's syndrome, and pleural and pericardial adhesions.

MITRAL VALVE PROLAPSE SYNDROME

A murmur, formerly believed to be innocent, was described occurring in mid systole to late systole and not showing the variable features of the cardiorespiratory murmur. Recent studies have shown that late systolic murmurs of this type usually result from insufficiency of the posterior leaflet of the mitral valve; they have been categorized as representing the mitral valve prolapse syndrome. Such murmurs are often associated with a click occurring soon after the murmur starts in midsystole, and which is believed to be related to a ballooning of the valve leaflet. Electrocardiographic changes, including inversion of T waves in the left precordial leads, may suggest a localized disorder of myocardial function that may be noted angiographically by an inactive left ventricular segment, perhaps interfering with papillary muscle function. This condition appears to be benign in childhood except that it is occasionally associated with dysrhythmias, but in the adult it may also be associated with symptoms of myocardial ischemia or with subacute bacterial endocarditis. The echocardiogram is very valuable in identifying the abnormal ballooning valve.

Another murmur that may be confused with innocent late systolic murmurs is the systolic "whoop," which has a harmonic quality and may be extremely loud. At times, these whoops may be noted in patients with the mitral valve prolapse syndrome. In certain cases, they may be projected from the patient and even heard many feet away.

The milder variety of late systolic murmur, noted most frequently in females, is very common and usually but not always can be related to a late mitral valve prolapse shown on echocardiogram. Again one can see the problem in defining this as a truly organic condition, since most individuals with this murmur have no other signs or symptoms of cardiac disease.

Other organic conditions may also be associated with late systolic murmurs, including chronic pericardial adhesions or inflammation, ventricular septal defect, coarctation of the aorta, idiopathic hypertrophic subaortic stenosis, and Marfan's syndrome. It is thus obvious that to label the late systolic murmur as "innocent," the physician has to carefully eliminate those organic disorders.

CONTINUOUS MURMURS

Venous Hum. Probably the most common innocent murmur of childhood is the venous hum, which may be detected in nearly all children under the proper circumstances. The term "hum" is a misnomer, because the murmur usually has a "wheezing" quality, resembling the breath sounds.

It is heard well in the supraclavicular area over the jugular veins and also in the parasternal regions, immediately below these areas. It is usually considerably louder on the right side. Phonocardiography reveals that the venous hum may continue throughout most of the cardiac cycle and is particularly accentuated in early diastole. It is heard best with the patient in the sitting position. The precordial diastolic component disappears when the patient lies supine.

This bruit is clearly attributable to venous flow through the jugular veins because it may be modified markedly by external pressure over the veins. The diastolic component may be eliminated by this maneuver. Positioning of the head also modifies the intensity of the murmur; turning the head away from the side being auscultated tends to intensify the bruit.

Usually this murmur is easy to distinguish from the continuous murmur of patent ductus arteriosus, which is maximal at the pulmonic area and is not modified by the maneuvers described. The ductal murmur usually reaches its greatest intensity in late systole or at the time of the second heart sound. The alterability of the venous hum also aids in distinguishing it from organic murmurs caused by such disorders as peripheral pulmonic stenosis, aorticopulmonary window, ventricular septal defect with aortic regurgitation, anomalous pulmonary venous drainage, and A-V fistulas.

Continuous carotid bruits, presumably originating from carotid arterial vessels, have been described that may not disappear entirely with pressure over the jugular region. Several patients with such murmurs have been studied by carotid angiography with entirely negative results.

With the exception of the diastolic accentuation observed with the venous hum, very few instances of innocent diastolic murmurs have been observed. However, a cardiorespiratory murmur may occur in early diastole. Also, the third heart sound, a normal finding in many children, may be prolonged in duration. Then, its sound characteristics may be very similar to those of the early diastolic rumbles generated from excessive flow past the tricuspid valve (as in atrial septal defect) or mitral valve (as in ventricular septal defect or patent ductus). The additional systolic murmur detected in these organic conditions usually will aid in the differential diagnosis.

For purposes of defining the innocent murmurs, they have been described separately, but very often several are audible in the same healthy child. Not rarely, a vibratory murmur, a pulmonic ejection murmur, a supraclavicular arterial bruit, and a venous hum may be heard in the same patient. Also, the physician should be aware that one or more of these murmurs may also be detected in a patient who has an additional murmur indicating organic disease.

INNOCENT MURMURS IN THE NEWBORN

During the first few hours after birth, a late systolic crescendo or a continuous murmur may be audible over the pulmonic region, presumably originating in the ductus arteriosus. This murmur should vanish by 10 to 15 hours of age when arteriovenous ductal flow ceases. Early systolic murmurs have been noted, often associated with systolic ejection clicks, and may be analogous to the pulmonic ejection murmurs that develop later in childhood. These systolic murmurs are often transmitted quite well to the posterior chest and may persist for several months. This type of murmur is especially frequent in the 2- to 3-month-old infant who was born prematurely and may be anemic at the time of examination. Vibratory murmurs similar to those heard in older children may also be noted in the newborn.

INTERPRETATION OF INNOCENT MURMURS

Because of the characteristic features of the innocent murmurs of childhood, most of these can be diagnosed by auscultation alone, without resort to chest films and electrocardiography. In borderline situations, however, these procedures can contribute vitally to the correct diagnosis by revealing presence or absence of enlargement of specific cardiac chambers or great vessels. The physician must realize that a negative chest film and electrocardiogram do not necessarily rule out organic disease, a fact that emphasizes the need to be able to identify murmurs by their auscultatory characteristics. If

an innocent murmur is detected, the physician must weight the desirability of discussing this finding with the child and his parents, but in any event should make careful note of its characteristics on the patient's record. If the family is informed, a careful discussion of what is meant by the term "innocent murmur" can usually put the finding in proper perspective. Indeed, the "art of medicine" is especially important in interpreting heart murmurs to children and their parents and, when practiced properly, can favorably influence their attitudes concerning health and activities for years to come.

CYSTIC FIBROSIS*

By RALPH W. RUCKER, M.D.
Orange, California

SYNONYMS AND DEFINITION

Cystic fibrosis of the pancreas, hitherto unrecognized, was first established and named as a separate entity in 1938. The condition has subsequently been defined over the years as a complex disorder of abnormalities of the mucus-secreting glands. Other designations have been used, such as "mucosis" and "mucoviscidosis," which emphasize the mucus abnormalities, or "pancreatic achylia", "fibrocystic disease of the pancreas," and "pancreatic fibrosis," which center on only one organ system. These fail to emphasize the multiple system involvement of this disorder. Although the name cystic fibrosis (CF) is not a perfect designation, this shortened form of the original name, cystic fibrosis of the pancreas, remains the name of choice.

Cystic fibrosis is a genetic disease of unknown cause of infants, young children, and young adults that affects most organ systems in the body. With an incidence of 1 in 1500 to 2000 Caucasian births and a carrier rate of approximately 5 per cent of the population, it remains the most common and lethal inherited disease among Caucasians. Much less seen in blacks (1:17,000), it is almost never found in orientals.

*This work was supported in part by a Center Grant from the Cystic Fibrosis Foundation.

It is a chronic progressive illness in which, although no therapy is known for the exact cause, early diagnosis and amelioration of the symptoms and complications can lead to a much reduced morbidity and increased longevity.

Presenting Signs and Symptoms

The initial suspicion of cystic fibrosis in an infant should be derived from a review of the family history. Cystic fibrosis is perpetuated as an autosomal recessive trait, and therefore would be expected in a ratio of approximately 25 per cent if a previous sibling is affected with cystic fibrosis. If other relatives have the diagnosis of cystic fibrosis, the likelihood of the disease in the present patient is also increased. For example, if a cousin of the infant has CF, the risk in this pregnancy would be 1:120 (N.E.J. Med. 294:937, 1976). There is, as yet, no known test to detect the presence of cystic fibrosis from amniotic fluid or to detect whether the mother or the father is a carrier.

The earliest detectable problem in the infant is that of meconium ileus, which may be detected in utero if the bowel has ruptured, leading to calcific meconium peritonitis. Meconium ileus presents, however, usually with ileal obstruction in the newborn period, with thick, tenacious meconium obstructing the lumen. Volvulus, perforation, or atresia can be associated. The infant presents with abdominal distention, failure to pass normal meconium, and vomiting with inability to tolerate feedings. The x-ray picture in this entity may be characteristic, with calcific densities throughout the abdomen, because the intestinal tract may have ruptured earlier, leading to calcific peritonitis. At surgery, ileal obstruction with thick, tenacious meconium is found.

Meconium ileus occurs in 15 per cent of cystic fibrosis patients and therefore it is an early sign that must not be ignored. Although meconium ileus is similar to other intestinal obstructions in the initial presentation, at surgery the findings are characteristic and invariably indicate a patient with cystic fibrosis. Another intestinal variation in newborns, the passage of a meconium plug, has also been reported to occur in patients later diagnosed to have CF.

The classic presentation of cystic fibrosis in early infancy is *failure to thrive.* This is the result of pancreatic insufficiency in these babies, present in approximately 85 per cent of CF patients. These babies have excessive appetites, distended abdomens, and very thin muscle and soft tissue development, especially in the thighs and buttocks. They fail to grow primarily in weight, and height is also affected.

The stools in these children are always abnormal. The abnormality may take many forms, with occasionally only diarrhea seen; the stools range in color from yellow to green. Some babies have considerable variation in stools, with solid stools seen sometimes and very abnormal stools at other times. Classically, the stool of a cystic fibrosis patient is bulky and bubbly and tan to light yellow in color. It is very malodorous, appears greasy on the diaper, and floats in the toilet bowl. Only when the stool pattern is quite characteristic does it aid much in the recognition of the disease itself.

The baby with malnutrition can also present with rectal prolapse. This dramatic and somewhat startling entity occurs in from 7 to 22 per cent of the children with CF. It is believed to be due to large bulky stools and lack of muscular support of the anal sphincter; the incidence lessens when the stools and the nutrition are improved. Some infants have this symptom for a prolonged period. Any baby with rectal prolapse should be considered to have cystic fibrosis until proved otherwise.

Another presentation related to failure to thrive is the symptom complex of edema and hypoproteinemia. This is related to poor absorption of protein because of the pancreatic insufficiency and is a recently recognized early sign of this condition. This is aggravated by breast milk or soy feedings. In addition, the malabsorption can result in a severe vitamin K depletion with hypoprothrombinemia and bleeding. It is a rare condition, but CF should be considered in any infant or child with an unexplained bleeding diathesis.

Cystic fibrosis patients have an elevated sodium and chloride concentration in their sweat. This is the reason for the sweat test. A salty taste on the skin of these infants is occasionally the first indication of the diagnosis. It is the basis for a successful early detection program directed to the public, the so-called "Kiss your baby" campaign, in which parents are urged to kiss their infants to check for the salty taste. In addition, this phenomenon of cystic fibrosis is responsible for one of the other occasionally occurring signs, that of salt depletion in infants and young children during extremely hot weather. This can present as cardiovascular collapse because of the tremendous sodium loss. Another presentation, that of persistent metabolic alkalosis, is also related to excessive loss of sodium and chloride in the sweat.

Repeated attacks of respiratory disease in young children is one of the major indications of cystic fibrosis. Repeated attacks of bronchiolitis, repeated wheezing episodes of unknown cause, bronchopneumonia, or lobar pneumonia can be the presentation. These conditions usually do not clear without specific therapy. The wheezing occurs with the early manifestation of cystic fibrosis of narrowing and plugging of the small airways in a generalized pattern throughout the lungs. Early diagnosis of cystic fibrosis in these children is imperative. If early diagnosis is not made, repeated lung infections can permanently injure the lung with scarring and other complications to be described, thereby shortening the life expectancy sharply. Any infant with a respiratory infection in the first year of life, especially one that is manifested by wheezing and/or one that requires hospitalization for pneumonia, should have the other diagnostic tests such as a sweat test to rule out or confirm the diagnosis. Some children may not present in early infancy with this but may present much later with asthma-like symptoms, x-ray diagnosis of streaky infiltrates, and/or hyperinflation. A history of repeated cough and sputum production, usually presenting from an earlier age, should alert the observer to the possible diagnosis of CF.

Another presentation (10 to 15 per cent) in later childhood is that of recurrent polyposis of the nasal passages, as well as chronic pansinusitis. In numerous adolescents and young adults the diagnosis of cystic fibrosis has been made primarily on the finding of a minor lung infection with a history of recurrent polyposis in earlier childhood. Many of these children do not proceed to the other manifestations such as malabsorption or repeated respiratory infections or both but instead have the disease primarily confined to the nasal and sinus area.

COURSE

Untreated cystic fibrosis has an extremely high mortality at a very early age. The children suffer from severe malabsorption, repeated respiratory infections, multiple complications from these infections, and early respiratory death. Unless a cure or control is found, cystic fibrosis must continue to be known as a fatal disease; i.e., the patient's death will usually be caused by its complications. The course is usually one of stabilization of the marginal nutritional abnormalities, repeated lung infections, and development of chronic obstructive pulmonary disease. The rate of progression and the severity of respiratory complications are the absolute determinants of longevity or early demise. No other parameters, e.g., a sibling's course and the presence of meconium ileus at birth, imply necessarily that an irreversibly severe form of CF is present. Some of the patients will succumb as young children to aggressive and relentless bronchopulmonary infection. Others will die in mid adolescence, with an average 50 per cent mortality at about 20 years.

This mortality seems to be related to early diagnosis and the course of the lung disease in the first year after diagnosis. During the child's life, the course can be monitored by a variety of means, the most common one being the Shwachman-Kulczycki score, which, although quite subjective, evaluates many of the important features of the child's physical and laboratory findings. In addition, a separate scoring system, the NIH Scoring System, places 75 per cent of the evaluation on the pulmonary system. It can be used effectively in many of the older patients because of their ability to perform pulmonary function tests.

Close evaluation of the pulmonary function tests is mandatory because the progression is that of obstructive pulmonary disease with a gradual increase in the total lung capacity, functional residual capacity, and ratio of residual volume to total lung capacity. In addition, the vital capacity is lowered, especially with the onset of more extensive and progressive lung disease. There appears to be approximately an 8 to 10 per cent decrease per year in the maximal expiratory flow rate (MEFR) in females and less of a decrease in males, paralleling the observed increased longevity of CF males. Most of the therapeutic measures center around improving nutrition and lung function with repeated hospitalizations, up to six to eight per year. Terminally, the children develop respiratory insufficiency as well as other pulmonary complications of the disease.

These long-term evaluations of patient progress as well as care are best developed and continued through established cystic fibrosis centers. There are 120 of these established throughout the United States, receiving support from the Cystic Fibrosis Foundation, to monitor effectively the care of these children and help direct their therapy. Through these centers, the prognosis of children with cystic fibrosis has vastly improved over the years, with a doubling of the average age of survival in the past 11 years. All children with the diagnosis of cystic fibrosis should be referred to one of these centers for consultation or management or both.

PHYSICAL EXAMINATION FINDINGS

The physical findings and evaluation of the young child with cystic fibrosis are centered primarily around the nutritional status and the pulmonary system. Classically these children are very thin and lack subcutaneous tissue and muscle mass. This is most prominent in the thighs and buttocks and the large muscle groups but may also be present in many other muscle areas. Prominence of the ribs and wasted intercostal musculature may be evident. The weight and height are usually below percentiles for age. The skin of the children is often quite pale, reflecting the anemia caused by malabsorption of protein that is not uncommon, and the skin may taste salty, consistent with high salt content of the sweat. Ear, nose, and throat findings more commonly seen in cystic fibrosis patients than others include antral polyposis and evidence of pansinusitis. The discoloration of the teeth, long considered a hallmark of cystic fibrosis in children, is unequivocably the result of tetracycline administration in the first 8 years of life, and is rarely seen in the younger patients.

The pulmonary pathology is manifested by a barrel-shaped chest, with a sharp increase in the anterior-posterior diameter and a considerable number of rales and rhonchi throughout both lung fields. The lung findings are often symmetrical in the upper lobes but may be in all areas. Continued coughing and sputum production is not uncommon, with paroxysms of cough typical of cystic fibrosis being both described and observed. Tachypnea, as well as clubbing of the fingertips and toes, may be observed. Cyanosis may occur, usually not seen on early examination, and usually indicating much more extensive involvement of the lungs. The cardiovascular examination is usually normal. Many times the children will have a very bloated abdomen, sometimes presenting with umbilical hernias and even a rectal prolapse. Rarely is any hepatosplenomegaly present, but in children with far advanced disease, especially those with hyperinflation of the chest pushing the liver down and/or primary liver disease from the cystic fibrosis, the liver edge may be felt below the right costal margin.

COMPLICATIONS

Major life-threatening complications in the patient with cystic fibrosis are centered around the pulmonary system. Initially presenting as a distal small airway obstruction, *concurrent infection* results in bronchiolitis. Later this can develop into bronchitis, and with extended infection, airway destruction leading to severe bronchiectasis may develop. Bacteria causing these infections are usually *Pseudomonas aeruginosa, Staphylococcus aureus, Hemophilus influenzae,* and other pathogens. The CF lung has the additional peculiarity of harboring the mucoid variant of pseudomonas, which may coexist with the non-mucoid variety. Once established, this pathogen is rarely eradicated from the respiratory tract. Intercurrent pneumonias can

hasten the process of gradual lung destruction, leading finally to respiratory insufficiency. This respiratory insufficiency is manifested first by hypoxia in room air and later by hypoxia with added oxygen as well as an initially compensated but later uncompensated respiratory acidosis. The development of this sequence usually takes years and can be retarded with close monitoring in an aggressive treatment program. Intercurrent hospitalizations for the therapy of these manifestations may be necessary.

In addition to infection, one of the most distressing complications of cystic fibrosis is *hemoptysis*. This can be continuous and of no major consequence in many of the children with chronic bronchiectasis and purulent secretions. In other children, however, or at other times in the same child, the hemoptysis can be massive, resulting in the need for blood transfusions, immediate hospitalization, or even bronchoscopy.

Another major complication is *pneumothorax*. This usually occurs in the older children during the course of an acute infection but occasionally occurs when the infection is deemed under control. The patients suffer from acute lateralizing chest pain as well as acute dyspnea, and this may be a cause for sudden demise. This not uncommon complication can be insignificant and asymptomatic in approximately 15 per cent of the episodes but can recur in some patients, leading to the need for some type of pleural abrasion procedure. Related to the pulmonary system is the inevitable cor pulmonale that develops in these children. This is the result of the chronic obstructive pulmonary disease, as well as the hypoxemia. Hypoxemia out of proportion to the lung disease is one of the distinguishing features of this complication, as the physical findings of an abnormal second heart sound may be obscured by the overlying emphysematous lung. Rarely, cardiomegaly is seen. X-ray, electrocardiogram (ECG) and echocardiogram are helpful but not consistently diagnostic. It appears that a vital capacity less than 60 per cent predicted and PaO_2 less than 50 mm Hg are the best indicators of its presence.

The abdominal complications of cystic fibrosis are many. Untreated, the pancreatic insufficiency results in severe malabsorption and malnutrition with subsequent inanition and inability to handle stress or infection. Hypoproteinemia, depletion of vitamins A, E, and K, and malabsorption of vitamin B_{12} can develop. A fair number of the children develop an entity called *meconium ileus equivalent;* partial intestinal obstruction occurs as a result of the thick tenacious stool obstructing the small bowel. This can look and act exactly like small bowel obstruction on an anatomic basis, and although usually treated with conservative measures, may require laparatomy. This may mimic the presence of intussusception, common in CF patients. Other children present with mid abdominal pain and have pancreatitis, both acute and recurrent. Other abdominal complications include the development of hepatic disease with biliary cirrhosis (4 to 6 per cent), portal hypertension, and esophageal varices. This is uncommon but is extremely difficult to treat once established. Liver failure is rare. Cholestasis may occur, usually in the older child, and the presentation is that of cholecystitis with the findings of cholelithiasis by x-ray examination. One of the most distressing complications of this disease is that of a glucose intolerance as the child grows. A large number of the young adults can be shown to have glucose intolerance by chemical testing and a smaller number require insulin for the management of this manifestation of pancreatic endocrine insufficiency. Diabetic ketoacidosis is extremely rare.

Infertility in the young male with cystic fibrosis has recently been recognized as an almost invariable (97 per cent) complication of the disease. This is the result of developmental defects in the wolffian duct structures such as the vas deferens, epididymis, and seminal vesicle, the abnormalities of which are as diagnostic of CF as are those of any other organ. Males may also suffer hernias or testicular vascular accidents or both in an undue proportion. The onset of puberty and menses may be delayed. Females with this disease have reduced fertility, and complications of recurrent vaginitis and abnormal menstrual periods are not uncommon.

Another complication is multiple antral polyposis, requiring frequent surgery. Digital clubbing is a common sequela and pulmonary osteoarthropathy an uncommon one of the pulmonary disease. Complications secondary to medications commonly used in cystic fibrosis include hyperuricemia secondary to large doses of pancreatic enzyme supplementations, optic and peripheral neuritis or depression of the red cell series secondary to chronic chloramphenicol use, dental staining with early tetracyline use, goiter with iodide therapy, and occasional auditory or renal difficulty or both with the use of high dose aminoglycosides.

LABORATORY FINDINGS

The diagnosis of cystic fibrosis rests primarily on the proper performance and interpretation of the *sweat test*, the quantitative determination of

the level of the sweat chlorides. This is a very difficult test to do correctly consistently, but the chloride level is invariably elevated in cystic fibrosis. The sweat defect is present at birth, but testing should be delayed for 2 to 3 months to get the most accurate readings. In adults as well, the sweat test is a highly accurate determinant of the presence of cystic fibrosis and is the procedure of choice for diagnosis. The test is based upon iontophoresis with pilocarpine to produce the necessary 50 to 100 mg of sweat. The sample must be collected by a skilled operator who must manage the problem of evaporation, and the results then must be quantitatively determined. In some patients with diabetes insipidus, glycogen storage disease, or adrenal insufficiency, a positive sweat test has been reported, but these conditions should be excluded by their signs and symptoms.

Most laboratories in general hospitals throughout the United States cannot perform this test with accuracy. In cystic fibrosis centers, however, where this test is done repeatedly and professional guidance over the testing system is constantly applied, the test has a high accuracy rate. In most laboratories a sweat chloride determination greater than 60 mEq per liter is deemed to be positive for cystic fibrosis. For a reliable diagnosis, however, a repeat sweat test should be done, and the patient should have one or more of the presenting signs and symptoms of the disease. Marginal sweat tests, in the 30 to 60 mEq per liter range, usually indicate allergic lung disease and not cystic fibrosis, with the vast majority of cystic fibrosis patients having about 90 to 100 mEq per liter of chloride. The sweat chloride mean normally is about 20 mEq per liter during childhood and approximately 35 mEq per liter during adulthood, and, although there is a greater standard deviation as age increases, the value of the sweat test for diagnosis in CF in adulthood is certainly well established. The level of the sweat chloride does not determine the severity of the disease; the affected patient has a very constant level of his own sweat on repeated testings. The sweat test is normal in obligate heterozygotes (parents) and siblings. It is not to be used as a test for the carrier state. *In summary, the basic diagnosis of cystic fibrosis is established with a positive quantitative sweat chloride test and evidence of either a chronic infective and obstructive pulmonary process or nutritional abnormalities with evidence of pancreatic insufficiency.*

Other tests have been devised to ascertain the presence or absence of pancreatic insufficiency in this disease in order to help with the diagnosis. Based on the presence of pancreatic insufficiency and the inability of the infant with cystic fibrosis to absorb adequately proteins in meconium, the meconium strip test (Boehringer–Mannheim) was devised. This test indicates cystic fibrosis if an albumin concentration of over 20 mg per gram of meconium is present. For effective screening of all newborns, this test has been shown not to be useful, giving far too many false-negative results. However, the quantitative determination of albumin in first meconium samples may be of help in ascertaining the likelihood of a sibling of a cystic fibrosis patient having the disease. Other tests, such as a 72-hour fecal fat and a duodenal aspiration for trypsin, amylase, and lipase activity, can be done, although they are not of real practical use in clinical medicine. Since CF accounts for nearly all cases of pancreatic deficiency in children, these tests would be of use only if the sweat test were equivocal. Analysis of hair and nails has been done but again has not proved of practical use.

Laboratory evaluation of complications includes a chest x-ray to detect many pulmonary complications, such as lobar atelectasis, severe bronchiectasis, pneumothorax, cardiomegaly, and pneumonia. Sinus x-rays are necessary in patients with cystic fibrosis to ascertain the extent of the sinusitis. Experience has shown that almost no cystic patient over the age of 8 years has development of frontal sinuses seen on the plain sinus films. The presence of frontal sinuses or the absence of sinusitis or both should lead one to question seriously the diagnosis of cystic fibrosis.

The complication of cor pulmonale must be confirmed by laboratory evidence, with the ECG occasionally showing right ventricular hypertrophy and the echocardiogram showing a thickened right ventricular wall. Pulmonary function tests with a sharp increase in residual volume and other major manifestations of obstructive lung disease are invariably obtained. This airway obstruction tends to be progressive over the years and must be serially evaluated. Other pulmonary tests, such as arterial blood gases and sputum cultures, are necessary. The growing realization that fungi can colonize the respiratory tract of cystic fibrosis patients has led to further studies to try to delineate these organisms, with fungal cultures and serum precipitins to various strains of aspergillus and candida occasionally necessary. In addition, other tests to evaluate the CF complications are helpful, such as sperm count on a young adult male, as well as glucose tolerance tests, urinalyses, and blood sugars to ascertain the pres-

ence or absence of the diabetic-like state in the older children. Liver function tests, cholecystograms, serum amylase evaluations, and abdominal films may occasionally be necessary to judge the presence or course or both of these complications.

PITFALLS IN DIAGNOSIS

Missing the early diagnosis of cystic fibrosis is usually the result of the physician not including it in his differential. "Failure to thrive" work-ups involving the cardiac, renal, or hormonal systems are often done before someone thinks of doing a sweat chloride test to confirm this most common cause of malnutrition in children. The oft-heard expression "he doesn't look like a cystic fibrosis child" may be a reflection that up to 15 per cent of cystic fibrosis children have no major pancreatic defect and therefore do not show the effects of severe malabsorption. The diagnosis in many little children with recurrent wheezes is carried as asthma or recurrent viral bronchitis, when in reality these patients have small airway obstruction from cystic fibrosis. Any child with more than *one* not fully explained lower respiratory illness in the first year of life should certainly have a sweat chloride determination. It has commonly been the case that recurrent wheezing was the only early manifestation of this disease.

One of the most common problems in the overdiagnosis of cystic fibrosis is the inaccuracy of sweat test determinations in most general hospitals. Skin galvanometry, evaporative concentration of chloride, and inaccurate quantitative measurements are just three of the common errors that lead to a considerable amount of parental frustration and anxiety. Once a physician thinks of cystic fibrosis and orders a sweat chloride, he is not usually satisfied with a normal reading in the presence of major symptoms. Usually the patient is then referred to a CF center and the test done by quantitative measurement to confirm the diagnosis. In addition, no child should be labeled as having CF without a second sweat chloride test being performed to confirm the accuracy of the first elevation. Early work-ups, accurate diagnoses, and aggressive therapy over a long period of time through organized regional centers is the way to manage the disease at this time. Further studies of its causes and more effective therapeutic modalities will lead us to better understanding and therapy of this most devastating genetic childhood illness.

GLYCOGEN STORAGE DISEASE*

By GEORGE HUG, M.D.
Cincinnati, Ohio

Glycogen storage disease (GSD) exists if concentration or molecular structure or both of glycogen are abnormal anywhere in the body. At present, we distinguish 12 types of GSD. This classification is based on enzymatic defects and clinical presentation (Fig. 1, Table 1).

CLINICAL PRESENTATION

GSD may be present if the patient has disease of liver, heart, skeletal muscle, kidney, bones or brain.

Liver.　Hepatomegaly can be minimal or se-

*This work was supported by NIH Grants RR005535 and RR00123 and by the Children's Hospital Research Foundation, Cincinnati, Ohio.

vere. It may be asymptomatic or associated with hypoglycemia, acidosis, gout, short stature, hypotonia, and increased serum concentration of lactic acid, transaminases, lipids, and uric acid. Ascites is present only in GSD IV. Splenomegaly is rare. Jaundice or elevation of serum bilirubin has not been observed in more than 150 patients treated by me and my colleagues. Asymptomatic hypoglycemia (of as little as 10 mg of glucose per 100 ml of blood) is typical for GSD I; however, if it is corrected by nocturnal continuous feeding and this treatment is discontinued, renewed hypoglycemia may be accompanied by convulsion. The patient has lost the hypoglycemic tolerance during treatment.

Heart.　Clinical signs of cardiac involvement, such as exists in GSD III, can be difficult to detect. The absence of cardiac disease in GSD IIb may explain the survival of these patients to adulthood. Marked cardiomegaly and severe hypotonia in an infant who was normal at birth are suggestive of GSD IIa. The electrocardiogram (ECG) is less useful, except perhaps for the differential diagnosis between GSD IIa and aberrant coronary artery.

Muscle.　GSD IIa results in a "floppy infant" with marked cardiomegaly and death, often·

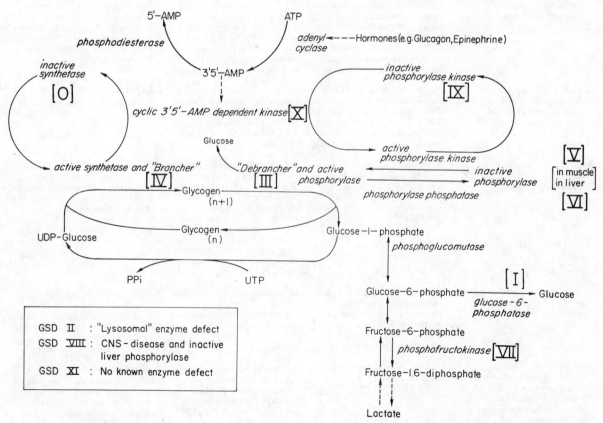

Figure 1.　Enzymatic cascade for activation and deactivation of glycogen synthetase and phosphorylase; pathway of anaerobic glycolysis. Defects therein may result in GSD; the respective type is identified by roman numeral in brackets next to the affected enzyme.

Table 1. *The 12 Types of Glycogen Storage Disease (GSD 0–XI)*

Type, Enzyme Affected	Tissue Distribution	Clinical Symptoms	Alternate Names, Comments
Type 0 Glycogen synthetase	Liver but not muscle, hepatic glycogen synthetase less than 2% of normal, but some hepatic glycogen (< 2% demonstrable).	Fasting hypoglycemia, prolonged hyperglycemia after glucose administration; mental retardation follows hypoglycemic convulsions; when these are avoided by frequent protein-rich meals, psychomotor development can be normal.	Aglycogenosis; defect convincingly demonstrated in 2 unrelated families; early diagnosis and dietary treatment important for prevention of hypoglycemia, mental retardation; some children with "ketotic hypoglycemia" have GSD 0.
Type I Glucose-6-phosphatase	Liver, kidney, intestine; frequent intranuclear glycogen seen in these organs not diagnostic; continuous nighttime feeding by tube and pump may alleviate clinical symptoms; portacaval shunt risky, clinically disappointing; treatment with phenytoin or phenobarbital ineffective.	Enlarged liver and kidney; "doll face," stunted growth; normal mental development; tendency to hypoglycemia, lactic acidosis, hyperlipidemia, hyperuricacidemia, gout; bleeding; IV galactose or fructose not converted to glucose (caution: these tests may precipitate acidosis.) Abortive or no rise in blood glucose after IV glucagon; prognosis fair to good.	Von Gierke disease, hepatorenal glycogenosis; no involvement of skeletal or cardiac muscle, of leukocytes or cultured skin fibroblasts (glucose-6-phosphatase not normally present in these tissues); prenatal diagnosis not feasible and not indicated.
Pseudo Type I (in vitro activity of glucose-6-phosphatase is normal)	Despite normal glucose-6-phosphatase activity, liver glycogen concentration is increased.	Symptoms are those of GSD I.	Normal in vitro activity of glucose-6-phosphatase that is perhaps not operational in vivo.
Types IIa and IIb Lysosomal acid alpha-glucosidase (deficient activity of acid α-1.4- and of α-1.6-glucosidase; the latter could be considered "lysosomal glycogen debrancher")	In the fatal infantile classic form (GSD IIa), glycogen concentration excessive in all organs examined; acid α-glucosidase deficiency was generalized in 1 patient, in others normal renal acid α-glucosidase; amniotic *fluid* (in contrast to cultured amniotic fluid *cells*) contains acid α-glucosidase activity even if fetus has the disease.	GSD IIa: clinically normal at birth, though minimal cardiomegaly, abnormal ECG, increased tissue glycogen, abnormal lysosomes in liver and skin, and acid α-glucosidase deficiency demonstrable at birth; within a few months marked hypotonia, severe cardiomegaly; normal mental development; death usually in infancy.	Pompe disease, generalized glycogenosis, cardiac glycogenosis; prenatal diagnosis within a few days after amniocentesis by electron microscopic demonstration of abnormal lysosomes in uncultured amniotic fluid cells; for prenatal diagnosis by enzyme analysis cultured amniotic fluid cells required, which also show the abnormal lysosomes.
In GSD IIa, alpha glucosidase seems structurally altered; in GSD IIb the enzyme seems structurally normal but reduced in amount	In the adult form (GSD IIb) cardiac muscle was normal clinically and morphologically but deficient in α-glucosidase activity, although cardiac glycogen concentration is normal.	GSD IIb: involvement of muscle and liver but without cardiomegaly described in children and adults (GSD IIb), normal blood glucose response to glucagon	GSD IIa: infantile fatal form. GSD IIb: late juvenile adult form.
Type III Amylo-1,6-glycosidase "debrancher enzyme"	Liver, muscle, heart, etc. in various combinations designated types IIIA through D; cultured amniotic fluid cells have diagnostic biochemical abnormality.	Moderate to marked hepatomegaly; none to moderate hypotonia; none to moderate cardiomegaly; ECG rarely abnormal; no acidosis or hypoglycemia; no hyperlipidemia; glucagon produces a normal rise in blood glucose after a meal but not after fasting; normal mental development; prognosis fair to good.	Limit dextrinosis, debrancher glycogenosis, Cori disease, Forbes disease; prenatal diagnosis by enzyme assay of cultured amniotic fluid cells feasible but unnecessary owing to the usual benign course.
Type IV Amylo-1,4→1,6-transglucosidase, "brancher enzyme"	Generalized (?); low to normal levels of abnormally structured glycogen (amylopectin-like molecules) with fewer branch points than in animal glycogen.	Hepatosplenomegaly, ascites cirrhosis, liver failure; normal mental development, death in early childhood.	Amylopectinosis, brancher glycogenosis, Andersen's disease; prenatal diagnosis of this incurable disease may be feasible and indicated by enzyme analysis of cultured amniotic fluid cells.
Type V Muscle phosphorylase (congenital absence of skeletal muscle phosphorylase; phosphorylase activating system intact)	Skeletal muscle, liver, myometrium normal.	Temporary weakness, cramping of skeletal muscle after exercise, no rise in blood lactate during ischemic exercise; symptoms like type VII glycogenosis; normal mental development; myoglobinuria in later life; fair to good prognosis.	McArdle syndrome; liver and smooth muscle phosphorylase not affected; cardiac muscle phosphorylase not examined; prenatal diagnosis not feasible or indicated.

Table 1. *The 12 Types of Glycogen Storage Disease (GSD 0–XI)* (Continued)

Type, Enzyme Affected	Tissue Distribution	Clinical Symptoms	Alternate Names, Comments
Type VI Liver phosphorylase (phosphorylase-activating system intact)	Liver; skeletal muscle normal; leukocytes unsatisfactory for diagnosis.	Marked hepatomegaly, no splenomegaly; no hypoglycemia; no acidosis, no hyperlipemia; no rise of blood glucose after glucagon; normal mental development; good prognosis.	Lack of glucagon-induced hyperglycemia distinguishes GSD VI from GSD IX; the latter shows a normal glucagon response; prenatal diagnosis not feasible or indicated.
Type VII Phosphofructokinase	Skeletal muscle, erythrocytes (in initial report other tissue not examined).	Temporary weakness, cramping of skeletal muscle after exercise; no rise in blood lactate during ischemic exercise; normal mental development; symptoms identical to those of type V glycogenosis; good prognosis.	Reduction of phosphofructokinase activity severe in skeletal muscle, mild in erythrocytes, not established in other tissues; not known whether cultured amniotic fluid cells are affected but prenatal diagnosis not indicated.
Type VIII No enzymatic deficiency demonstrated. Total liver phosphorylase normal; most of it is in inactive form although the phosphorylase activating system is intact. This reflects loss of (? cerebral) control over the degree of hepatic phosphorylase activation.	Liver, brain, skeletal muscle normal; cerebral glycogen increased; electron microscopy shows some cerebral glycogen in form of giant α-particles within axon cylinders and synapses.	Occasional hepatomegaly, truncal ataxia, nystagmus, "dancing eyes;" neurologic deterioration progressing to spasticity, decerebration, and death; urinary epinephrine and norepinephrine increased during acute phase of disease but not stationary end phase.	Predominant clinical problem of 3 patients with this presumptive diagnosis was progressive degenerative disease of brain. Addition of ATP and MgCl to liver homogenate results in full activation of the endogenous (deactivated) phosphorylase.
Types IXa and IXb Liver phosphorylase kinase. Total liver phosphorylase normal but most of it is in the inactive form because of deficient endogenous kinase.	Liver, muscle tissue normal biochemically and microscopically; D-thyroxin-induced liver phosphorylase kinase activity and corrected the other biochemical, clinical and morphologic defects in 1 patient but not in 2 others of a different family.	Marked hepatomegaly, no splenomegaly; no hypoglycemia or acidosis; normal rise in blood glucagon; prognosis good; treatment may be unnecessary. "Benign hepatomegaly" may disappear in early adulthood, although enzymatic defect persists.	Liver phosphorylase can be activated in vitro by addition of exogenous kinase to homogenate; not the human counterpart of muscle phosphorylase kinase deficiency in mice; normal glucagon response is a distinguishing feature vs GSD VI GSD IXa: autosomal recessive. GSD IXb: X-linked recessive; prenatal diagnosis not demonstrated or indicated.
Type X Loss of activity of cyclic-3'5'-AMP dependent kinase in muscle and presumably liver. (Total phosphorylase content of liver and skeletal muscle normal but the enzyme completely deactivated in both organs; phosphorylase kinase activity 50% of normal, possibly owing to loss of 3'5'-AMP dependent kinase activity).	Liver and muscle (other organs not tested); identical biochemical findings in muscle biopsy specimens obtained 6 years apart.	Marked hepatomegaly; patient otherwise clinically healthy initially but 6 years after diagnosis mild recurrent muscle pain; no cardiomegaly or hypoglycemia; no rise in blood glucose after IV glucagon; the only person known to have this condition is not incapacitated at 12 years of age.	In vitro activation of this patient's phosphorylase occurs (1) under assay conditions not requiring 3'5'-AMP dependent kinase, or (2) after the patient's muscle homogenate has been fortified with phosphorylase kinase deficient mouse muscle that supplied 3'5'-AMP dependent kinase; postulated defect restricted to the activity of the cyclic 3'5'-AMP dependent kinase that phosphorylates phosphorylase kinase; other cyclic 3'5'-AMP dependent phosphorylations are intact.
Type XI All enzymatic activities measured to date are normal (e.g., adenyl cyclase, 3'5'-AMP dependent kinase, phosphorylase, debrancher, brancher, glucose-6-phosphatase).	Liver, or liver and kidney.	Tendency for acidosis; markedly stunted growth; vitamin D-resistant rickets (may be cured with high-dose vitamin D, oral supplementation of phosphate); hyperlipidemia, generalized aminoaciduria, galactosuria, glucosuria, phosphaturia, normal renal size; no rise in blood glucose after IV glucagon.	Muscle usually not affected; GSD XI may include patients with glycogenoses of different enzymatic defects.

before 1 year of age. GSD IIb patients exhibit similar morphologic and biochemical abnormalities, but size and function of heart remain normal and the muscle disease progresses at a rate less than that of GSD IIa. I know of a 12-year-old boy with abnormalities typical of GSD IIb in liver and muscle who is clinically symptom free. Patients with GSD V and VII exhibit normal or somewhat bulky contour of skeletal muscle. Here the characteristic complaints are intermittent muscle cramps and pain after exercise, relieved by rest. These symptoms appear unmistakably in the patient but not the control during the ischemic exercise test, to be described later in this article. In GSD IX the muscle is normal. Muscle with increased glycogen and deactivated phosphorylase is indicative of GSD X.

Kidney. Slight renal enlargement is consistent with GSD I but not with GSD III. Renal stones may occur in GSD I together with hyperuricemia and gout. GSD XI is associated with the Fanconi syndrome (i.e., excessive urinary excretion of glucose, phosphate, and amino acids).

Bone. Shortness of stature can be present in GSD I. It is marked in GSD XI when the patient at 14 years of age is the size of a 6-year-old child. Evidence of rickets is missing in GSD I but is present in GSD XI on clinical, radiologic, and serum examination. Healing of the rickets can be effected by phosphate supplementation and high doses of vitamin D.

Brain. In GSD VIII, symptoms of cerebral involvement may begin in the first year; they include delay in mental and motor development, nystagmus, "dancing eyes," ataxia, hypotonia, and inability to swallow, followed by increasing spasticity, decerebrate rigidity, and death. The other 11 types of GSD do not involve signs of brain disease. Psychomotor retardation in GSD 0 can be avoided by prompt recognition and treatment of the hypoglycemia. None of our 32 patients with GSD IIa has shown evidence of mental retardation.

Such clinical findings may indicate glycogen storage disease involving liver, heart, skeletal muscle, kidney, bones or brain. The lack of abnormal findings does not exclude involvement of the "mute" organ when the diagnosis is based on abnormal findings in another organ system.

CLINICAL, BIOCHEMICAL, AND MORPHOLOGIC EVALUATION

Clinical Evaluation. Routine laboratory tests on serum, blood cells, or urine are not diagnostic for GSD. Abnormalities of liver function tests are not impressive. Acidosis, hypoglycemia, hyperlipidemia, and acetonuria are consistent with, but not diagnostic of, GSD I. In fact, the acute appearance of hypoglycemic symptoms and of ketoacidosis within 12 hours after a meal is so suggestive of GSD 0 that it is necessary to exclude the existence of this disease. Urinary chromatography for amino acids and sugars is indicated, as are x-ray examinations for size of heart and kidney and for rachitic changes. The ECG may be suggestive of GSD IIa and electromyogram (EMG) of primary myopathy.

Carbohydrate tolerance tests with glucose or insulin are not informative. Epinephrine test is not necessary, since glucagon injection gives similar answers with fewer side effects. We give crystalline glucagon intravenously in a single dose of 0.7 mg per square meter of body surface, 2 to 3 hours after the completion of a substantial meal. Blood sugars are obtained 15 minutes before the glucagon injection and again immediately before the injection, and thereafter at 15, 30, 45, 60, 90, and 120 minutes. The magnitude of the rise of blood glucose depends on the status of hepatic glycogen stores and liver enzymes that catalyze the conversion of glycogen into glucose (Fig. 1). A rise of 50 or more mg of glucose per 100 ml of blood 30 minutes after the glucagon administration may be accepted as normal. After a patient with GSD has a meal, flat glucagon tolerance curves are obtained in GSD 0 (because of decreased glycogen stores), in GSD I (for lack of glucose production from glucose-6-phosphate), in GSD VI (for lack of glycogen degradation), and in GSD XI (for unknown reasons). Patients with GSD IX exhibit *normal* glucose response to glucagon, and this type is thereby separable clinically from GSD VI. In GSD III the normal rise of blood glucose is abolished if the glucagon is given after food has been withheld overnight. In our experience, glucagon has no ill effects and provides more information than do fructose and galactose. Tolerance tests with these sugars may precipitate acidosis. They are best avoided.

In patients suspected of having GSD VIII, 24-hour urine for determination of catecholamine excretion is collected into bottles kept on ice, containing 10 ml of 6 N HC1.

When GSD V is suspected, the ischemic exercise test should be performed as follows: A blood pressure cuff is applied to the upper arm and inflated above the arterial pressure for the duration of the test. The patient is requested to pump a rubber bulb with the hand of the same arm about once every second. A healthy person will easily pump 70 to 100 times with some discomfort but without cramping of the musculature or objective residual symptoms after release of the blood pressure cuff. In GSD V, muscle cramps may result in involuntary arrest of the hand after 20 to 30 pumping movements. When the cuff is released, these cramps will persist, with a tetanic position of the hand (bent wrist, stretched fingers) that cannot be corrected by the patient or by the examiner. After several minutes, there is a gradual release of the cramp. The pain may persist for 1 to 2 days. *In theory*, in the healthy person, blood samples taken from the antecubital vein of the ischemic arm during the exercise will show a rise in serum lactate that does not occur in GSD V, indicative of the inability of the muscle to produce lactate from glycogen. *In fact*, blood samples are difficult to obtain during the exercise; thus lactates are inaccurate. They are also unnecessary because of the impressive tetanic response if GSD V is present.

Biochemical and Morphologic Evaluation. Tissue analysis is indispensable for the diagnosis of GSD. If the analytical methods are not locally available, the biopsy material may be shipped to a laboratory with a special interest in GSD. Handling and shipping should be as follows to assure adequate tissue diagnosis. In every case of open liver biopsy, muscle tissue should also be obtained from the abdominal wall, since the diagnosis is strengthened always by the combined analysis of liver *and* muscle. Within seconds after removal of the specimens, 6 to 8 cubes not larger than 1 cu mm in size should be sliced from the material (with a surgical blade). These cubes are gently transferred into a vial containing about 2 ml of a solution of 3 per cent glutaraldehyde in 0.1 M phosphate buffer, pH 7.2 to 7.4. *The vials must not be frozen.* They are tightly capped and are sent in an ordinary cardboard mailer, without refrigeration, to the cooperating laboratory for electron microscopy. Do not send these vials attached to the dry ice–containing box; they will likely freeze. This renders the tissue useless for electron microscopy.

The rest of the biopsy specimens must not be contaminated with the glutaraldehyde. An additional small specimen is obtained for routine light microscopy. The remainder of the biopsy that optimally should weigh about 1 gram is immediately frozen between two blocks of solid dry ice. (Do *not* use solutions of such fluid as acetone to expedite freezing.) The handling of the tissue to the time of freezing should require not more than 30 to 60 seconds after the surgeon has removed the tissue. The frozen specimens are wrapped tightly in aluminum foil and put into small, precooled glass containers (e.g., standard vials used for scintillation counting).

These are labeled clearly, capped, put immediately into a generous amount of dry ice (between 15 and 20 pounds), and packed in a shipping container of a construction (e.g., Styrofoam insulated) that will guarantee preservation of the dry ice for at least 48 to 72 hours The samples are assigned, *prepaid,* to a national air freight company that will ask for the completion of a simple federal form for dry ice shipments. The cooperating laboratory is advised by telephone or telegram of the date and time of shipment, the name of the freight company, and the air bill number so that the package can be traced. If these rules are followed, one may expect that the tissues will be preserved adequately. For an intelligent, diagnostic interpretation of analytical results, it is mandatory that the tissues arrive with a reasonably complete clinical summary of the patient.

Analysis of frozen tissue is sometimes not sufficient for investigating unknown aspects of glycogen storage disease and certain possibilities for adequate treatment. As part of the Clinical Research Center program of the National Institutes of Health, patients may be hospitalized for study without cost to them. Their physicians may consider entering into a cooperative study with centers investigating the disease by sending the patient (accompanied by parents) to the cooperating center. We have found that this approach is effective and is in the best interest of the patient with GSD.

ADDITIONAL CONSIDERATIONS

GSD IIa, IV, and VIII are fatal. Diagnosis of the remaining types that are compatible with life is important for the exclusion of other diseases mimicking GSD but requiring specific therapy, such as hepatomegaly in neuroblastoma. Moreover, typing of GSD is important for the avoidance of unnecessary procedures such as portacaval shunt or attempts at enzyme induction with phenytoin (Dilantin) and phenobarbital. During diagnostic procedures one must remember the tendency for bleeding in GSD I and that for pneumonia in GSD III. GSD VIII can be diagnosed by the demonstration of increased glycogen and reduced phosphorylase activity of liver in the presence of hepatomegaly and progressive brain disease. Patients with central nervous system disease and enlarged liver should thus be considered candidates for hepatic biopsy, possibly with the Menghini needle. Whereas blood cells in my experience are diagnostically not reliable (possibly because of the time and manipulations required for their isolation), I have found that the diagnosis of GSD IIa or IIb can be made by demonstrating electron microscopically the abnormal lyso-somes typical for the disease in a superficial skin biopsy specimen obtained without bleeding or anesthesia and within seconds by using sharp, curved, sterile scissors.

Prenatal diagnosis is not indicated in our judgment regardless of technical feasibility in those types of GSD that are compatible with normal life (Table 1). Prenatal diagnosis is of practical importance in GSD IV and in GSD IIa. In GSD IV it can be done using the assay of brancher enzyme in cultured amniotic fluid cells. Regarding GSD IIa, more than 20 women with high-risk pregnancies who had the history of previous children with GSD IIa were examined. I found that the electron microscopic demonstration of membrane surrounded glycogen accumulation within the uncultured amniotic fluid cells allows the unequivocal diagnosis of GSD IIa 1 day after the amniocentesis. Again, for this ultrastructural assay to be successful, the amniotic fluid specimens must be handled as previously described.

GENETIC DEFECTS OF AMINO ACID METABOLISM AND TRANSPORT*

By IRVIN A. KAUFMAN, M.D.,
and WILLIAM L. NYHAN, M.D.

San Diego, California

Disorders of amino acid metabolism and transport are hereditary conditions all but one of which described to date are transmitted as autosomal recessive traits. Parents of affected children are asymptomatic heterozygous carriers of the mutant gene. In most populations the frequency of the carrier state is relatively high, whereas the chance that two nonconsanguineous carriers will mate is small. In any pregnancy the chance is one in four that two carriers will produce an affected child. For the most part, these disorders result from a defect in a single enzyme. Thus they are classic inborn

*Supported by a grant from Maternal and Child Health Services MCT-000274.

errors of metabolism as first described by Garrod, the founder of the science of modern biochemical genetics.

These disorders include conditions in which the metabolic defect is generalized throughout the body and those in which the abnormality is specific to a single tissue or transport function. Aminoaciduria is the hallmark of most of these disorders. However, in some, such as albinism, the defect is so localized that there is no evidence of altered metabolism in urine or blood. Aminoaciduria can result from inefficient metabolism of amino acids, leading to elevated levels in the blood, which then exceed the renal capacity for reabsorption and overflow into the urine. Alternatively, aminoaciduria can be the result of defects in renal tubular transport. In these conditions, plasma concentrations of amino acids are normal or low. There are also the no-threshold aminoacidurias, such as argininosuccinicaciduria. In these situations the compound is excreted so efficiently or reabsorbed so inefficiently that elevated concentrations are not found in blood even though the basic mechanism for the aminoaciduria is a defect of cellular metabolism.

The clinical manifestations of these disorders vary widely (Table 1). Some are biochemical abnormalities in which there are no clinical consequences at all, whereas in others life-threatening illnesses many manifest themselves from the moment of birth. With few exceptions, the manifestations of these diseases are not specific. Many interfere with the development of the central nervous system, causing mental retardation. Seizures may occur with or without other neurologic signs. Many of the disorders of amino acid metabolism and transport have been discovered by screening populations of retarded individuals.

An increasing number of disorders of amino acid metabolism are recognized to produce severe illness and death in early life. They should be considered in very ill newborns with unexplained acidosis, hyperammonemia, convulsions, coma, or hypotonia. Early recognition and diagnosis are important, as these diseases that present with overwhelming illness in the newborn period do not necessarily cause mental retardation.

When large populations of patients with established symptoms—for instance, populations with mental retardation—are screened for aminoaciduria, the incidence of positives is small, approximately 0.2 per cent. Screening is nevertheless important, because the recognition of an affected child alerts the physician to the possibility of further cases in a family. Many of these disorders are susceptible to programs of

Table 1. *Inborn Errors of Amino Acid Metabolism*

Disorder	Enzyme Defect	Manifestations
Phenylketonuria	Phenylalanine-hydroxylase	Blond hair, blue eyes, eczema, FeCl₃,MR° Urinary reducing substance
Tyrosinosis (Medes) Tyrosinosis	p-Hydroxyphenylpyruvic acid oxidase	Hepatic cirrhosis, renal Fanconi syndrome
Alkaptonuria	Homogentisic acid oxidase	Dark, urine, reducing substance; ochronosis; arthritis
Albinism	Tyrosinase (melanocyte granules)	Lack of pigment, local or universal—skin, hair, and eyes
Histidinemia	Histidase	Speech retardation, FeCl₃ may have MR°
Maple syrup urine disease	Branched-chain keto acid decarboxylase	Urinary odor, coma, flaccidity, opisthotonus, death,† MR°
Hypervalinemia	Valine transaminase	Death,† MR°
Isovaleric acidemia		Odor, convulsions, coma, MR,° death†
α-Methyl-β-hydroxybutyric acidemia	α-Methylacetoacetyl CoA thiolase	Intermittent acidosis, ketosis, MR°
β-Methylcrotonylglycinuria	β-Methylcrotonyl CoA carboxylase	Failure to thrive, dermatosis, ketosis, acidosis, death†
Methylmalonic acidemia	Methylmalonyl CoA mutase	Recurrent vomiting, ketosis, coma, failure to thrive, pancytopenia, death,† MR°
Nonketotic hyperglycinemia		Convulsions, cerebral palsy, MR,° death†
Oxalosis	Glyoxylate carboligase	Renal calculi, renal failure
Hyperprolinemia	Proline oxidase, Δ-pyrroline-5-carboxylic acid dehydrogenase	Nephropathy, deafness, MR,° may be normal
Hyperhydroxyprolinemia	Hydroxyproline oxidase	Small kidneys, hematuria, MR,° may be normal
Propionic acidemia	Propionyl CoA carboxylase	Recurrent vomiting and ketosis, thrombocytopenia, neutropenia, osteoporosis, death,† MR°
Pyroglutamic acidemia		Chronic acidosis, ataxia, MR°
Argininosuccinic aciduria	Argininosuccinase	Trichorrhexis nodosa, seizures, hyperammonemia, MR°
Citrullinemia	Argininosuccinate synthase	Mental retardation, hyperammonemia death†
Hyperammonemia	Carbamylphosphate synthetase, ornithine transcarbamylase	Episodic coma, MR
Hyperlysinemia	Lysine α-ketoglutarate reductase	Convulsions, hypotonia, growth retardation
Cystathioninuria	Cystathionase	Mental retardation; may be normal
Homocystinuria	Cystathionine synthase	Ectopia lentis, thromboembolism, failure to thrive, MR°
Hypersarcosinemia		MR,° vomiting, failure to thrive

In each instance it is recognized that there may be heterogeneity in which multiple forms of a defective enzyme may lead to different phenotypic manifestations. For instance, in the decarboxylation of the branched-chain keto acids a complete deficiency leads to classic maple syrup urine disease; a different level of defect leads to a milder disease known as branched chain ketoaciduria. In this table only one form has been listed.

°MR indicates mental retardation.

†The disorders designated as causing death are those in which a rapid fulminating course often complicates early infancy.

prenatal diagnosis and carrier detection once an index case has been diagnosed.

Because some of these disorders are associated with no obvious abnormality of development or intelligence, it is possible that other inborn errors of metabolism occur in populations of children who have never been screened. With current technology and the growing recognition that the metabolic screening of newborns is a worthwhile public health measure, it is likely that we will be able to establish the true incidence and significance of many more inborn disorders of metabolism.

PHENYLKETONURIA

Phenylketonuria is the result of a metabolic defect in which phenylalanine cannot be converted to tyrosine and phenylpyruvic acid is excreted in the urine. With the advent of large-scale screening of newborn infants, it has become evident that a variety of phenylalaninemias exist in addition to what has come to be known as classic phenylketonuria.

The most important clinical characteristic in classic phenylketonuria is mental retardation. Most untreated patients have a severe degree of mental deficiency, with intelligence quotients under 30. However, a few untreated phenylketonuric patients have been reported with borderline intelligence. Phenylketonuric infants appear normal at birth. Symptoms occur in over half of them early in life. Vomiting has been severe enough to lead to surgery for pyloric stenosis. Irritability, an eczematoid rash, or a peculiar odor may also be present in the early months. General physical development is usually normal. These children are fair-haired, fair-skinned, and blue-eyed in over 90 per cent of the cases. However, dark skin, hair, or irides do not exclude the diagnosis. Minor anomalies such as epicanthal folds may be seen in an appreciable number of patients with this disorder or with other inborn errors of metabolism.

Neurologic findings are not prominent. A third of the patients have none, whereas minimal signs, such as hyperactivity of deep tendon reflexes or mildly hypertonic muscles, occur in another third. More severely involved patients may have manifestations of spastic cerebral palsy. Seizures occur in about a fourth of the patients, usually those most severely retarded. Electroencephalographic abnormalities have been described in approximately 80 per cent of patients, and pneumoencephalograms may reveal cortical atrophy.

Autopsy reports on affected children show lack of myelinization in the central nervous system. The absence of these findings in patients studied after 21 years of age suggests that the formation of myelin is delayed or inhibited by the chemical abnormality and is consistent with the idea that the manifestations of phenylketonuria are those of an intoxication.

Phenylalanine is normally converted to tyrosine in the first step of its oxidative metabolism. The tyrosine formed is then oxidized, ultimately forming acetoacetate and fumarate, which are readily converted to carbon dioxide and water. The fundamental defect in phenylketonuria is the absence of phenylalanine hydroxylase. With a block in phenylketonuria hydroxylase, tyrosine becomes an essential amino acid and alternate pathways are used to metabolize phenylalanine, which along with its metabolic products accumulates in body fluids. These compounds are normal metabolites present in abnormal amounts. Plasma concentrations of phenylalanine range from 6 to 80 mg per 100 ml in patients with phenylketonuria, in contrast to values approximating 1 mg per 100 ml in controls. Most patients with classic phenylketonuria have concentrations well over 30 mg per 100 ml throughout infancy. There is a roughly linear relation between levels of phenylalanine in the blood and the urinary excretion of phenylpyruvic acid.

The disease occurs in 1 out of every 10,000 to 20,000 persons. It is an autosomal recessive character, equally represented in both sexes. Many heterozygotes may be recognized by the measurement of plasma concentrations of phenylalanine and tyrosine after oral loading with phenylalanine, but there is overlap with the normal population and a normal phenylalanine tolerance curve does not exclude heterozygosity.

Successful prevention of the clinical manifestations of the disease by restriction of the dietary intake of phenylalanine has provided strong support for the concept that the clinical disease represents an intoxication produced by the abnormal chemical milieu in which these patients must live and develop. Palatable preparations such as Lofenolac (Mead Johnson) make long-term treatment economically feasible. Dietary therapy readily lowers levels of phenylalanine in the blood, and concomitantly phenylpyruvic acid and its metabolic products disappear. Clinical improvement in neurologic findings, in behavior, and in the electroencephalogram is observed. Eczematoid lesions heal and increase in pigmentation occurs. Patients tolerate the diet well, but the management of an infant on a low phenylalanine diet is not easy. Phenylketonuric infants often vomit or refuse feedings. Infections may complicate their metabolic state. Management should be under the direction of an experienced physician with the laboratory facilities for the routine accurate determination of the serum concentration of phenylalanine. All infants, including those with phenylketonuria, require a certain amount of phenylalanine. These minimal essential quantities are known and should be employed in management.

The major criterion for undertaking dietary therapy is its effect on mental capacity. In general, the diet is effective in preventing mental deficiency and neurologic abnormalities, if started in the first weeks of life. A loss of 5 IQ units for each 10 weeks that treatment is delayed has been calculated. This figure is certainly only approximate, but it provides a strong argument for early diagnosis and the early institution of dietary therapy. Treatment of patients for the first time after the age of 3 years is without effect on mental development. Therapy may be of use in the clinical management of older patients because of beneficial effects on eczema, seizures, or uncontrollable behavior even in the absence of effects on intelligence.

It has now become routine in the United States and most of the developed countries of the world to test all newborn infants in the population in order to recognize patients with phenylketonuria as early as possible. Urine tests are of limited value for this purpose, for phenylpyruvic acid is not detected until plasma phenylalanine levels exceed 15 to 20 mg per 100 ml and may be absent from the urine of phenylketonuric patients for 1 to 2 months. Current screening procedures employ an assay for the concentration of phenylalanine in a drop of blood spotted on a piece of filter paper. Levels of phenylalanine above 6 mg per 100 ml are considered positive. Once the physician is confronted with a positive screening test, he must then make a diagnosis.

The first step in diagnosis is the quantitative analysis of the concentrations of phenylalanine and tyrosine in the blood. Most infants turned up in the screening programs simply have a delayed maturation of amino acid metabolizing enzymes, and their tyrosine concentrations are very high. These infants can then be excluded and followed expectantly. On a normal diet the patient with classic phenylketonuria generally has a very rapid rise in the serum concentration of phenylalanine to levels well over 30 mg per 100 ml, whereas the concentration of tyrosine is low. We like to admit infants with elevations of serum phenylalanine without tyrosine to the hospital to study them while they are receiving known daily intake of phenylalanine. We initiate dietary therapy in patients who have high concentrations of phenylalanine in the blood and excrete its metabolites in urine.

When the baby is 3 to 4 months old we readmit to the hospital and challenge with a 3-day phenylalanine load. An infant with classic PKU will experience a steady rise in serum phenylalanine concentration to a level over 30 mg per 100 ml. Metabolites will appear in the urine. These methods reliably distinguish patients with hyper-phenylalaninemia who do not need dietary treatment from patients with PKU who do.

A number of patients have recently been described with hyper-phenylalaninemia and normal phenylalanine hydroxylase activity. These patients have presented with progressive cerebral symptoms in spite of adequate dietary treatment, with serum phenylalanine levels maintained in a range usually associated with a good prognosis. They have been found to have defects in the synthesis of tetrahydrobiopterin, the cofactor for phenylalanine hydroxylase or in the enzyme dihydropteridine reductase, which regenerates tetrahydrobiopterin from the quinonoid dihydrobiopterin that results from the phenylalanine hydroxylase reaction. Thus, each of these newly described defects results in the inability to convert phenylalanine to tyrosine, even though the phenylalanine hydroxylase apoenzyme is normal.

Tetrahydrobiopterin is also the cofactor for the hydroxylation of tryptophan and tyrosine. Thus its deficiency should interfere with the synthesis of serotonin, dihydroxyphenylalanine (dopa), and norepinephrine. Data have been obtained that indicate that this is the case, since levels of 5-hydroxyindoleacetic acids, vanillylmandelic acids, and homovanillic acid in the urine were considerably lower than normal.

Involved patients have had marked hypotonia, as well as spasticity and dystonic posturing. Some have seizures, myoclonus, and electroencephalographic abnormalities. Drooling is common. The delay in psychomotor development is usually profound.

The diagnosis of dihydropteridine reductase deficiency can be confirmed by assay of the enzyme in biopsied liver or cultured fibroblasts. The defective biosynthesis of tetrahydrobiopterin can be made by assay of the pattern of excretion of pterins in the urine. It can also be made by quantitative assay of tetrahydrobiopterin in the plasma, especially after the administration of a phenylalanine load. Phenylalanine leads to a dramatic increase in the level of tetrahydrobiopterin in normal individuals and in those with PKU or with dihydropteridine reductase deficiency, but there is no change in patients with defective biopterin synthesis.

The administration of tetrahydrobiopterin, which is currently available from investigators in Switzerland, leads to a prompt decrease to normal of serum concentrations of phenylalanine in patients with reductase and synthesis defects while the patient is receiving a normal diet. However, there is some question from animal experiments as to whether any administered tetrahydrobiopterin can get into the brain. Thus it is recommended that patients with these abnormalities be treated with biogenic amine precursors, such as 5-hydroxytryptophan and dopa, that do not require hydroxylation.

TYROSINOSIS

Tyrosinemias are much more common than phenylalaninemias. In addition to the tyrosinemias that result from delayed maturation of tyrosine metabolizing enzymes and are particularly common in premature infants, tyrosinemia occurs in scurvy and many forms of liver disease. There are three disorders known as tyrosinosis.

In the form first described, tyrosinosis is an extremely rare metabolic disorder characterized by the excretion of p-hydroxyphenylpyruvic acid in the urine. There are probably no clinical manifestations of this metabolic abnormality, although the patient initially described had myasthenia gravis. These patients have a reducing reaction to the urine, which is due to the excretion of p-hydroxyphenylpyruvic acid. Patients with liver disease excrete abnormal quantities of this keto acid, but levels found in tyrosinosis were nearly 10 times the highest values observed in liver disease. The metabolic abnormaltiy of tyrosinosis could result from a deficiency of p-hydroxyphenylpyruvic acid oxidase. Exogenously administered, homogentisic acid is metabolized normally.

A much more common form of tyrosinosis is manifested by abnormalities in hepatic and renal function. Symptoms may begin early in infancy with an acute rapid course to demise or may progress more chronically. Although the disease has been described in two forms, acute and chronic, both have occurred in the same family, suggesting that a single disease is involved. Most patients have presented with failure to thrive and hepatosplenomegaly. The livers of these patients are cirrhotic, and icterus, ascites, and hemorrhage often ensue. They also develop a renal tubular acidosis of the Fanconi type, with glycosuria, hyperphosphaturia, and generalized amino-aciduria. Clinical rickets and typical roentgenographic changes may develop.

Biochemical alterations include elevated plasma concentrations of tyrosine, usually in the range of 3 to 12 mg per 100 ml, and the excretion of tyrosyl compounds in the urine. Methionine concentrations in the plasma are also usually elevated. Hypoglycemia may occur with liver failure. Coagulation defects are common. Study of the enzymes of liver obtained at biopsy has indicated a deficiency of p-hydroxyphenylpyruvic acid oxidase, but it has not been established that this is the primary expression of the abnormal gene.

Genetic transmission appears to be that of an autosomal recessive. A particularly high frequency (0.67 per 1000 births) has been observed in a French-Canadian isolate. Frequency data are not available for other populations.

Treatment has been undertaken with diets low in both phenylalanine and tyrosine. Some patients have responded quite favorably in both the clinical and chemical features of the disease. Others have not.

Another form of tyrosinemia has been described in which the activity of tyrosine aminotransferase is deficient in the soluble cytoplasm of the liver. None of the patients with this disorder have had any evidence of hepatic or renal damage. One patient described in detail had multiple congenital anomalies, severe mental retardation, and self-mutilative behavior. He had corneal ulcers early in life and erythematous papular lesions on the palms and soles. Plasma concentrations of tyrosine ranged from 20 to 60 mg per 100 ml.

Five other patients have been reported. All of them have had marked retardation of mental development. A number have had corneal ulcers and lesions on the palms and soles that were either erythematous or keratotic.

Tyrosine aminotransferase is found in the mitochondria and in the cytoplasm. Only the cytoplasmic enzyme is deficient.

ALKAPTONURIA

Alkaptonuria results from a defect in the enzyme homogentisic acid oxidase. It is characterized by a dark color of the urine.

In this disorder fresh urine appears normal, but, on standing and particularly after alkalinization, oxidation of homogentisic acid proceeds and a dark brown or black pigment appears in the urine. This permits the condition to be recognized very early in life. However, the diagnosis is usually first made in adult life through routine urinalysis or in the investigation of arthritis. The urine also gives a positive test for reducing substance and a positive ferric chloride test. Testing for glucose with glucose oxidase sticks is negative.

Persons with this condition are usually asymptomatic in childhood. After the third decade, deposition of brownish or bluish pigment is seen, particularly in the ears and sclerae. The deposition of pigment, which may be extensive in fibrous tissues, is referred to as ochronosis. Ochronotic arthritis occurs later. Symptoms may resemble those of rheumatoid arthritis or osteoarthritis. Some degree of limitation of motion is usually seen, and complete ankylosis is not uncommon. Degeneration in the intervertebral discs may be striking. The condition is inherited as an autosomal recessive character.

Although homogentisic acid is excreted in large quantities in the urine, blood levels of the compound are not detectable. This disorder is a classic example of the no-threshold metabolic disorders.

The original suggestion of Garrod that the disorder resulted from an absence of the enzyme in the liver that catalyzed the oxidation of homogentisic acid was confirmed by La Du and colleagues, who found the enzyme catalyzing the conversion of homogentisic acid to maleylacetoacetate to be absent in biopsied liver from an alkaptonuric patient.

ALBINISM

Albinism is an inherited metabolic defect confined to the melanocyte, in which this cell cannot form melanin.

Albinism occurs in all races of man. Universal albinism, in which melanin is absent from the pigment cells of the skin, hair, and retina, is readily recognized. A variety of localized forms occur in which the defect is confined to an area of skin, the eyes, or a white forelock of hair. The skin in universal albinism is milk-white; the hair is white or yellow and, in Caucasians, very fine. The iris is generally blue. The pupil is red in children, but usually becomes black in adulthood. Photophobia and horizontal nystagmus are characteristic, and visual acuity is nearly always decreased. The skin is very sensitive to sunlight, and these patients have a propensity to develop skin cancers.

Universal albinism is inherited as an autosomal recessive character, although more than one gene produces the disorder. Normally pigmented children have occurred in a family in which both parents were albinos. Localized forms of albinism may be inherited as dominant, recessive, or — as in the case of ocular albinism — sex-linked characters.

A few patients have been reported in whom universal albinism has been associated with prolonged bleeding time and peculiarly pigmented reticuloendothelial cells in the marrow, lymph nodes, and liver.

Melanin is a polymer that exists in nature in high molecular weight. It is a brown or black insoluble material contained in the melanin granules of the melanocytes, where the entire transformation from tyrosine takes place. These granules can be demonstrated with the electron microscope and have been shown to be present, but without melanin, in albinism. The enzyme tyrosinase is a copper-containing oxidase that catalyzes the first two steps in the conversion of tyrosine to melanin. The first step, the conversion of tyrosine to 3,4-dihydroxyphenylalanine, is the limiting step, for the second step and most of the rest of melanogenesis may proceed nonenzymatically. Tyrosinase has been demonstrated in tissues radioautographically, and shown to be absent in the usual form of albinism.

Tyrosinase can be demonstrated by incubating hair roots with tyrosine. It is now clear that there are tyrosinase positive as well as tyrosinase negative forms of universal albinism. The tyrosinase-positive patients have creamy rather than milk-white skin; the hair may be yellow and tends to darken with age. These patients have severe visual defects, but less so than the tyrosinase negative albinos, most of whom ultimately become legally blind.

HISTIDINEMIA

Histidinemia is a disorder of metabolism in which large amounts of histidine are found in blood and urine. The condition must be included in the differential diagnosis of phenylketonuria, for the urine is positive when examined with ferric chloride.

The condition may occur without clinical manifestations, but more than half of reported patients have had speech retardation. Mental deficiency and growth retardation have also been observed in individual patients. Relatively fair hair and blue eyes have been common.

In histidinemia elevated concentrations of histidine have been demonstrated in the plasma, urine, and cerebrospinal fluid. Imidazolepyruvic acid is excreted in the urine, and is responsible for the positive ferric chloride test. Many patients also have elevations of alanine in the plasma.

Deficiency of histidase has been demonstrated by direct assay of the enzyme in skin. When histidine cannot be converted to urocanic acid, it is converted to imidazolepyruvic acid and its derivatives, much as phenylalanine is metabolized in phenylketonuria.

MAPLE SYRUP URINE DISEASE: BRANCHED-CHAIN KETOACIDURIA

In this syndrome major cerebral symptoms appear very rapidly in the newborn period, and there is an odor in the urine reminiscent of maple syrup. The branched-chain amino acids, leucine, isoleucine, and valine, are present in high concentration in the blood and urine, and the keto acid analogues are found in the urine.

Infants with maple syrup urine disease appear well at birth. In the typical case, symptoms begin at 3 to 5 days of life and progress rapidly to death. Early manifestations include feeding difficulty, vomiting, and irregular respirations. The infant then develops progressive neurologic symptoms, including convulsions, opisthotonos, and generalized muscular rigidity with or without flaccidity.

Severe hypoglycemia has occasionally been observed. Slight cortical atrophy has been seen on pneumoencephalography. In patients surviving past the first year, defective myelinization similar to that of phenylketonuria has been reported.

A few patients have been described in whom milder forms of the disease have occurred with characteristic biochemical abnormalities. The conditions in these patients are known as intermittent or variant branched-chain aminoaciduria and appear to represent distinct alterations at the same locus as that of classic maple syrup urine disease. Ataxia and repeated episodes of lethargy progressive to coma have been seen without mental retardation. These episodes have been induced by infection and by surgery with anesthesia, and they have responded to the removal of milk from the diet and the substitution of parenteral fluid therapy.

A disorder of branched-chain keto acid decarboxylation has been described by Scriver and colleagues in which the abnormal accumulation of amino acids in blood was completely reversed by the administration of thiamine. The patient described was retarded and had an abnormal electroencephalogram, but had not had any of the life-threatening crises typical of maple syrup urine disease. The therapeutic dose of thiamine hydrochloride was 10 mg per day.

The characteristic that permits any form of branched-chain ketoaciduria to be distinguished from other cerebral degenerative diseases of infancy is the characteristic odor of maple syrup to the urine, skin, or hair. The odor may become evident after 1 or 2 days of life and persist thereafter, but considerable variation in intensity has been observed, and in some specimens the odor cannot be detected. Freezing the urine intensifies the odor in an oil at the top of the specimen. Keto acids may be recognized in the urine by the yellow precipitate that forms on the addition of 2,4-dinitrophenylhydrazine.

The branched-chain ketoacidurias all appear to be transmitted as autosomal recessives.

Maple syrup urine disease is an abnormality in the metabolism of the branched-chain amino acids, resulting in increased quantities of leucine, isoleucine, and valine in the plasma and urine.

The catabolism of leucine and the other branched-chain amino acids is initiated by transamination to form the keto acids, α-ketoisocaproic acid, and the corresponding derivatives of isoleucine and valine. This is followed by decarboxylation to coenzyme A derivatives.

The presence of the keto acid derivatives of leucine, isoleucine, and valine in the urine and the absence of the decarboxylation products suggested a block in the oxidative decarboxylation of the keto acids. This can be demonstrated both in leukocytes and in fibroblasts in culture.

In patients with intermittent branched-chain ketoaciduria there is a partial defect in this decarboxylation reaction. In thiamine-responsive patients, treatment with thiamine permits oxidative decarboxylation of leucine at a rate 40 per cent of normal.

Experience has now been accumulated in the dietary therapy of maple syrup urine disease, using a synthetic diet made up of individual amino acids, in which the intake of leucine, isoleucine, and valine is closely controlled. Plasma concentrations of the branched-chain amino acids can in this way be maintained within normal limits. Therapy is very difficult and may require prolonged hospitalization; most patients have had permanent brain damage before treatment was started. Experience with siblings or previous cases, in whom very early diagnosis is possible, and with at least one patient detected by a neonatal screening program, indicates that a normal IQ may be achieved.

HYPERVALINEMIA

Hypervalinemia has been described in a single patient who was both mentally and physically retarded. Vomiting and difficulty with feeding were prominent findings early in infancy. He was treated with a diet low in valine, with concomitant lowering of the plasma concentration of valine, improvement in weight gain, and reduction of vomiting and hyperactivity.

The plasma concentration of valine was as high as 10 mg per 100 ml, and there was increased excretion in the urine. A defect has been documented in the leukocyte in the transamination of valine.

PROPIONIC ACIDEMIA

Propionic acidemia is a disorder of branched-chain amino acid metabolism in which elevated concentrations of propionate are found in body fluids. These patients also have elevated concentrations of glycine. A number of disorders of amino acid metabolism present with abnormal concentrations of glycine in body fluids. These include nonketotic hyperglycinemia, propionic acidemia, and methylmalonic aciduria. Isovaleric acidemia may also present with hyperglycinemia. All these disorders present clinically with overwhelming illness in early infancy. Patients with propionic acidemia and methylmalonic acidemia have what has been called the ketotic hyperglycinemia syndrome.

This syndrome is characterized by recurrent episodes of metabolic acidosis and massive ketosis, similar to that observed in diabetic coma. These patients may also have neutropenia, thrombocytopenia, and osteoporosis severe enough to lead to pathologic fracture. Mental retardation occurs except in cases in which there are early diagnosis and effective dietary therapy. Symptoms have begun as early as 18 hours after birth, with vomiting, acidosis, and ketonuria. Death has occurred with intractable acidosis, and it seems probable that other patients may have died unrecognized early in life. Convulsions and electroencephalographic abnormalities may be found.

The disease is transmitted as an autosomal recessive.

The diagnosis can be suspected clinically. It should be documented chemically. In our hands the most useful determination in the initial documentation of the diagnosis is the detection of methylcitric acid in the urine. This unique metabolite is found only in the presence of disorders of propionate metabolism, such as propionic acidemia and methylmalonic acidemia. It is present in large amounts and is quite stable; thus it is suitable for the diagnosis in a specialized laboratory distant from the patient. Propionic acid, by contrast, is highly volatile. It should be measured in the blood, but it is not the most reliable approach to the initial diagnosis. The danger is that the propionic acid may disappear from the blood after the blood has been removed from the patient. The chemical diagnosis may be suggested by the detection of elevated concentrations of glycine in the blood or urine. Examination of the urine by paper chromatography may be helpful and is often the first test that suggests the diagnosis. However, the amounts of glycine excreted in normal urine are large, and a prominent glycine spot is so commonly encountered that it is easy to miss a hyperglycinuria with the methods usually employed in screening the urine for amino acids. The plasma concentrations of glycine are nearly always elevated, often approximating 10 times those of controls. However, a normal concentration of glycine, especially in a very sick infant, does not rule out a diagnosis of propionic acidemia. We have recently been able to detect propionic acidemic fetuses in utero by the identification of methylcitrate by gas chromatography-mass spectrometry in the amniotic fluid. Restriction of the dietary intake of protein in these patients was found to reduce the frequency and severity of attacks of ketosis and acidosis. Ketosis could be produced by the administration of leucine, isoleucine, threonine, valine, or methionine, as well as by natural stresses such

as infection. The metabolic defect is in the enzyme propionyl CoA carboxylase, which catalyzes the formation of methylmalonyl CoA from propionyl CoA.

This defect explains the intolerance of these patients to isoleucine, methionine, valine, and threonine, for they are all metabolized through this pathway. The defect can be demonstrated in leukocytes and in cultured fibroblasts and amniotic fluid cells.

Diets in which the amounts of the amino acids listed above are restricted are tolerated by patients with the disease. At least two infants have now been diagnosed early in infancy and raised with these dietary principles in mind. Both have reached the age of 15 years and appear to have normal intelligence.

METHYLMALONIC ACIDEMIA

At least three different disorders present with methylmalonic acidemia. They have similar clinical manifestations to those of the ketotic hyperglycinemia syndrome. Episodes of ketoacidosis may begin very early in life and lead to coma and death. Neutropenia, thrombocytopenia, and osteoporosis are prominent manifestations. Mental retardation has been observed in surviving patients.

Infections are common and may precipitate life-threatening ketoacidosis. Some patients have had chronic monilial infection. The bone marrow is not megaloblastic. Growth retardation is striking.

Methylmalonic acid is normally formed from methylmalonyl CoA, which is the product of the propionyl CoA carboxylase reaction. Methylmalonyl CoA is converted by methylmalonyl CoA mutase to succinyl CoA, which can then be metabolized through the citric acid cycle. The amino acids isoleucine, valine, methionine, and threonine are catabolized along this pathway, and they are all precursors of methylmalonic acid in man. The mutase enzyme has a B_{12} coenzyme. Patients have been treated with vitamin B_{12} in large doses. Some have responded and some have not, thus delineating two forms of the disease. Patients who do not respond to B_{12} may be successfully treated with diets low in threonine, isoleucine, valine, and methionine. In a third form of methylmalonic acidemia, increased quantities of homocystine and cystathionine were found in the urine. In this condition there is a defect in the activity of tetrahydrofolate methyltransferase and a defect in the accumulation of coenzymatically active derivatives of vitamin B_{12}. The B_{12} responsive individuals who have no problem with sulfur amino acid metabolism have a defect in the conversion of B_{12} to deoxyadenosyl B_{12}.

BETA-METHYLCROTONYLGLYCINURIA

Two patients have been described in whom large amounts of beta-methylcrotonylglycine and beta-hydroxyisovaleric acid have been found in the urine. In the patient described by Eldjarn and colleagues, the parents were first cousins. The patient had feeding difficulties from the second week of life and developed hypotonia and retardation.

The patient described by Gompertz and colleagues had persistent vomiting, ketosis, and acidosis. An erythematous rash was resistant to topical therapy. This patient had a dramatic clinical response to therapy with biotin. The skin lesions disappeared, as did the abnormal compounds in the urine. With time the latter returned, but the clinical manifestations did not.

This patient of Gompertz appears to have defects in the carboxylation of both beta-methylcrotonyl coenzyme (CoA) and propionyl CoA. This and the clinical response in the patient suggest the possibility of a defect in the metabolism of biotin.

ALPHA-METHYL-BETA-HYDROXYBUTYRIC ACIDURIA

This disorder of isoleucine metabolism has been reported in four patients. The patient of Daum and colleagues was first admitted in coma after an upper respiratory infection and was found to have severe metabolic acidosis. Thereafter he had multiple episodes of recurrent ketosis and acidosis. The second patient was studied at 4 years of age because of vomiting and ketonuria. Her sister had died at 12 months of age in a similar episode. The patient had normal intelligence, but an older brother who had the same disease was retarded.

These patients were all typical examples of the ketotic hyperglycinemia syndrome. However, the concentration of glycine in the blood was never elevated. In contrast, the patient of Keating and colleagues had the ketotic hyperglycinemia syndrome in its complete expression. In addition to recurrent episodes of ketosis and acidosis, this patient was operated on for pyloric stenosis. She also had neutropenia, thrombocytopenia, and osteoporosis. Large amounts of glycine were found in the blood and urine.

Alpha-methyl-beta-hydroxybutyric acid and alpha-methylacetoacetic acid were found in the urine of these patients. Isoleucine was converted imperfectly to carbon dioxide, whereas labeled propionate and methylmalonate were oxidized normally. These observations suggest that the defect in these patients is in the betaketothiolase that converts alphamethylacetoacetyl CoA to propionyl CoA and acetyl CoA.

NONKETOTIC HYPERGLYCINEMIA

Patients with nonketotic hyperglycinemia have all had severe seizure disorders. Convulsions or lethargy have been observed from birth. One patient had almost continuous status epilepticus for his first year of life. This disease also can produce overwhelming illness in the neonatal period, and death in the first year of life is common.

Most patients have had very severe mental retardation in which there was little functional cortical activity. Two had irritability and microcephaly. Hypertonicity and hypotonicity have been observed, often in the same patient. Hyperreflexia is the rule. Porencephaly and ventricular dilatation have been seen on pneumoencephalography. Electoencephalograms were very abnormal.

Plasma concentrations of glycine were elevated in a range of about 5 to 12 mg per 100 ml. The amounts of glycine in the urine were also increased, and the glycine content of the cerebrospinal fluid and its ratio to that of the plasma in this disorder appear to exceed those of any other condition. Neutropenia has been observed in only one patient.

A defect has been found in vivo in the conversion of carbon 1 of glycine to CO_2 and of carbon 2 of glycine to carbon 3 of serine. This would be consistent with a defect in an enzyme catalyzing the conversion of glycine to CO_2 and hydroxymethyl-tetrahydrofolic acid. This is known as the glycine cleavage enzyme.

SARCOSINEMIA

Sarcosine is the N-methyl derivative of glycine. It is formed from dimethylglycine, which may be a product of betaine or choline. Although sarcosine is not normally present in blood or urine in amounts sufficient to be detected, sarcosinuria is occasionally found after the ingestion of lobster or other foods.

Seven patients have been reported with sarcosinemia. Three had subnormal intelligence. The others had shortness of stature. Sarcosine concentrations in the blood ranged from 0.5 to 6.8 mg per 100 ml. Urinary excretion of sarcosine was as high as 168 mg per 24 hours in a patient less than 1 year of age and 500 mg per 24 hours in a 2 year old. A deficiency of hepatic sarcosine dehydrogenase has been postulated.

HYPEROXALURIA AND OXALOSIS

Primary hyperoxaluria is a metabolic disorder in which large amounts of oxalate are excreted in the urine, leading to calcium oxalate lithiasis and nephrocalcinosis. When extrarenal deposits of calcium oxalate ensue, the condition is known as oxalosis.

There are reports of 20 to 30 patients, in most of whom the diagnosis was not established during life. An early onset of symptoms of urolithiasis, hematuria, passage of calculi, and colic, as well as nephrocalcinosis, urinary tract infections, and extrarenal deposits, is sufficiently characteristic to warrant investigation for the presence of oxalate in the urine. Renal failure is common, and the mean age at death in 16 cases was 4 years. Attempts at treatment have not been effective.

The disorder is caused by a rare recessive gene.

Oxalic acid is a dicarboxylic acid that forms a calcium salt of very low solubility. It may be formed from glyoxylic acid, which may be formed from glycine, or glycolic acid. It may also be a metabolite of ascorbic acid. In hyperoxaluria, levels of oxalate excretion may reach 30 times those of control subjects. The site of the defect appears to be the metabolism of glyoxylic acid, in a carboligase enzyme which catalyzes the reaction of glyoxylate and α-ketoglutarate to α-hydroxy-β-ketoadipate.

HYPERPROLINEMIA, HYDROXYPROLINEMIA

Hyperprolinemia was first recognized in a family in which cerebral dysfunction, renal anomalies, nephropathy, and deafness occurred in various members. The initial patient presented at 2 years with congenital renal hypoplasia, deafness, convulsions, and mental retardation. He was found to have hyperprolinemia, as were three female siblings, all of whom had electroencephalographic abnormalities. Another of the siblings had renal hypoplasia, nerve deafness, hematuria, and electroencephalographic abnormalities. Neither her proline levels nor those of the father were abnormal. Hematuria and deafness occurred frequently in the mother's family in a pattern suggesting dominant inheritance.

In affected persons plasma concentrations of proline were between 7.9 and 20.1 mg per 100 ml. Proline was not elevated in the cerebrospinal fluid. In the urine, proline and hydroxyproline, which are not found in the urine after the neonatal period, were prominent, and in some instances glycine excretion was increased.

The infusion of proline into normal adults produced a hydroxyprolinuria and glycinuria as well as prolinuria, indicating that the urinary findings are secondary to the basic defect in the metabolism of proline.

Hydroxyprolinemia has been described in a mentally retarded girl who also had increased numbers of leukocytes and erythrocytes in the urine and roentgenographically small kidneys. Shortness of stature was also observed. Her mother was also mentally retarded, but had no hydroxyproline abnormality.

Thus both hyperprolinemia and hydroxyprolinemia have been associated with mental deficiency and nephropathy. In involved families, members with the metabolic abnormality have had no clinical defect and vice versa. Therefore it is probable that these abnormalities of amino acid metabolism are simply biochemical phenotypes without clinical disease.

It is now known that there are two forms of hyperprolinemia: type I, in which there is a deficiency of proline oxidase, and type II, in which the next enzyme on the degradative pathway, Δ'-pyrroline-5-carboxylic acid dehydrogenase, is deficient. In hydroxyprolinuria a defect in hydroxyprolin oxidase has been reported.

CYSTATHIONINURIA

Cystathioninuria was first reported in two adults with mental deficiency. It has also been observed in patients with thrombocytopenia and endocrinopathy, as well as in persons with no disease. It is possible that the biochemical defect is coincidental, yet most patients have had some clinical abnormality. The first patients were 64 and 44 years of age when the disease was recognized. Developmental retardation was present from birth. One was otherwise normal except for talipes calcaneovalgus. The other had acromegaly, small ears, deafness, and facial clefts. The abnormal aminoaciduria has generally been found in the course of routine screening. Cystathioninuria also occurs in a secondary fashion in patients with neuroblastoma, hepatoma, galactosemia, or other forms of hepatocellular disease.

Cystathionine is an intermediate in the formation of cysteine and homoserine from methionine and serine. Cystathionine is normally cleaved to form cysteine and α-ketobutyrate. The compound is not usually found in the urine, but in patients as much as 500 to 1300 mg is excreted each day. Cystathionine is not usually detected in the blood. Pyridoxine (vitamin B_6) administration may lead to a decrease in cystathionine excretion. High doses of B_6 have been used to maintain urine concentrations of cystathionine near zero.

The enzyme cystathionase has been found to be defective in the liver of patients with cystathioninuria, and the in vitro addition of large amounts of pyridoxine corrected the defect.

The disorder is transmitted as an autosomal recessive trait.

HOMOCYSTINURIA

Homocystinuria is a disorder of the metabolism of the sulfur-containing amino acids. Homocystinuria is especially prevalent in Ireland, where a frequency of 0.7 per 100,000 population has been estimated.

Most patients described have been mentally retarded. Many have had marked failure to thrive. They have been thin and hypertonic. Some had died before a year of age. Less severely affected patients have had mental deficiency without systemic disease. Ectopia lentis is the most characteristic feature of the disease, and may be the only manifestation. Cataracts and glaucoma have also been seen. The hair is usually fair and sparse, the complexion fair, and the eyes blue. A malar flush and livedo reticularis are characteristic. Most patients have had skeletal abnormalities, such as genu valgum, pes cavus, or pectus excavatum or carinatum. Osteoporosis is common, and patients are frail and thin. They are frequently mistaken for patients with the Marfan syndrome and vice versa. In homocystinuria the joints tend to be limited in mobility rather than hypermobile.

Spontaneous thromboembolic phenomena are prominent in homocystinuria and often the cause of death in the disease. Occlusion of coronary, renal, or cerebral arteries or veins may lead to major complications such as hemiplegia or renal hypertension as well as death. Pulmonary embolism is a frequent terminal complication. Many patients have convulsions, and the electroencephalogram is usually abnormal. Classic tests of clotting function have been normal, but platelets from these patients have shown unusual adhesiveness. Furthermore, the addition of homocystine to normal blood causes the platelets to become sticky.

Homocystine is an intermediate in the metabolism of methionine. After the conversion of methionine to S-adenosylmethionine, demethylation yields S-adenosylhomocysteine, which is cleaved to homocysteine. This compound is normally combined with serine in the presence of cystathionine synthase to form cystathionine. Free homocysteine condenses to form the disulfide homocystine, as cysteine does to form cystine.

The presence of homocystine in the urine may be the only readily detectable abnormality in these patients, but the compound should be detectable in the blood and levels of methionine are usually elevated. The amounts of homocystine excreted in the urine of these patients usually exceed 20 mg per day and can be increased by the oral administration of methionine. The mixed disulfide of cysteine and homocysteine is also present in the urine. Screening of urine for the presence of homocystine can be carried out by the addition of cyanide and nitroprusside.

The enzymatic defect in the most common form of homocystinuria is in cystathionine synthase. The enzyme defect can be demonstrated using biopsied liver or cultured fibroblasts or amniotic fluid cells. The disorder is transmitted as an autosomal recessive trait. Heterozygotes have reduced levels of activity of cystathionine synthase.

Experience with treatment provided the first evidence of genetic heterogeneity in homocystinuria, for some patients respond to the administration of large doses (100 to 500 mg per day) of pyridoxine and some do not. Patients who respond to pyridoxine should be treated with this vitamin. Those who do not respond to pyridoxine may be treated with a diet in which methionine is restricted and a supplement of cystine is added. There is accumulating evidence for clinical benefit from each of these forms of therapy.

Homocystinuria may result from defects other than that of cystathionine synthase. The disorder in which homocystinuria coexists with cystathioninuria and methylmalonic aciduria tends to lead to overwhelming illness and death early in life, as does the usual form of methylmalonic aciduria. Enzyme assay in these patients reveals abnormally low activity of N^5-methyl-tetrahydrofolate-homocysteine methyl transferase. In this reaction 5-methyltetrahydrofolate is demethylated to tetrahydrofolate, yielding the methyl group for the conversion of homocysteine to methionine. The defect is not in the apoenzyme of the methyltransferase; it is in the conversion of hydroxy B_{12} and deoxy-adenosyl B_{12} that serves as cofactor for methyl-malonyl-CoA mutase. The underlying defect is probably in the uptake or reduction of B_{12}.

A different form of aberrant B_{12} metabolism leads to homocystinuria because of the role of B_{12} in the activity of methyltransferase. These patients have a familial selective B_{12} malabsorption, with a megaloblastic anemia. They excrete methylmalonic acid as well as homocystine, and all these findings disappear on treatment with parenteral B_{12}.

Three patients have been described in whom homocystinuria was due to deficiency of $N^{5, 10}$-methylene tetrahydrofolate reductase. These patients had 10 times normal concentrations of methionine and normal concentrations of B_{12}. They did not have methylmalonic aciduria. The defect in $N^{5, 10}$-methylene tetrahydrofolate reductase leads to a deficiency in methyltetrahydrofolate, which is the methyl donor in the methyl transferase reaction that converts homocysteine to methionine.

ARGININOSUCCINICACIDURIA

Argininosuccinicaciduria is one of a group of metabolic defects involving enzymes of the urea cycle.

Twenty-five patients have been reported and two clinical forms have been distinguished. One is an overwhelming neonatal illness that leads to early death. Two patients with this disease have been reported. The late onset form of the disease is marked by severe mental deficiency, generalized seizures, electroencephalographic abnormalities, and ataxia. Hepatomegaly is common. A certain number of patients have short, brittle hair that seldom needs cutting, diagnosed as trichorrhexis nodosa. The biochemical findings of this disease may be found in patients in whom mild mental deficiency is the only clinical abnormality.

Argininosuccinic acid is formed from citrulline and aspartic acid and is not normally found in body fluids. Argininosuccinic aciduria represents a failure in the cleavage of this compound to arginine and fumaric acid, which is catalyzed by argininosuccinase. This enzyme is defective in argininosuccinic aciduria. Correlation of the severity of the clinical disease and molecular abnormality has not yet been made.

Low plasma concentrations of argininosuccinic acid and its very high urinary excretion in this condition are consistent with very efficient renal clearance. Thus this disorder is among the no-threshold aminoacidurias. High concentrations of argininosuccinic acid are found in the cerebrospinal fluid. Therefore it has been suggested that the enzyme defect is present in the brain and that argininosuccinic acid produced in the brain may produce cerebral symptoms. These patients develop postprandial elevation of blood ammonia and signs of ammonia toxicity. Dietary protein restriction has been employed in treatment.

CITRULLINEMIA

Citrullinemia is a disorder of urea cycle metabolism that was originally recognized through screening survey of the urine of mentally retarded children for amino acids. It is now apparent that there are at least three forms of citrullinemia, and there is a good correlation between the severity of the clinical disease and the nature of the molecular defect.

The acute neonatal form of citrullinemia has been reported in five patients, and we have seen two more. Of these seven patients, all but one died at less than a week of age. Most diseases which present with acute overwhelming illness in the neonatal period are probably much more common than reports in the literature would suggest. The picture is that of death in coma with respiratory arrest. Blood concentrations of ammonia are very high.

Patients with the second form of citrullinemia have episodic vomiting and postabsorptive elevation in blood ammonia. Severe vomiting, coma, and seizures may develop. Microcephaly with severe mental deficiency is the rule.

The third form of citrullinemia has been reported in only one patient, a boy who may be clinically normal. He was admitted to the hospital because of aspiration and tachypnea, and he was found to have citrullinemia on a routine screen. No hyperammonemia was demonstrated, even postprandially.

The metabolic block in this disease is in the formation of argininosuccinic acid from citrulline. Argininosuccinic acid synthase has been found to be deficient in liver and in fibroblasts cultured from the skin. The disorder is inherited as an autosomal recessive trait. Molecular heterogeneity is evident in the levels of activity of argininosuccinic acid synthase, virtually absent in patients with the acute neonatal form, and considerably greater in the third or benign form.

The acute hyperammonemic episodes that characterize the neonatal forms of citrullinemia and ornithine transcarbamylase deficiency, and occur in some argininosuccinic aciduria and carbamylphosphate synthetase deficiency, may be treated successfully with exchange transfusion or peritoneal dialysis. More long-term therapy has been developed using a mixture of the keto acids or hydroxy acids of a number of essential amino acids. This form of treatment has been successful in bringing ammonia levels to normal and permitting the intake of sufficient quantities of protein to permit normal growth and development. More experience is required before the effects of treatment on long-term survival may be assessed for the usually lethal forms of citrullinemia and ornithine transcarbamylase deficiency.

CARBAMYL PHOSPHATE SYNTHETASE DEFICIENCY

The first step at which a defect in the urea cycle leads to hyperammonemia is that of carbamyl phosphate synthetase. This enzyme catalyzes the formation of carbamyl phosphate from NH_4^+, and HCO_3^-, and thus provides a branch point to pyrimidine biosynthesis as well as urea synthesis. Clinical manifestations are those of ammonia intoxication. Episodic vomiting, lethargy, and stupor or coma may be seen as early as 10 days of age. Most patients described have been mentally retarded. Convulsions have been reported, and elevated concentrations of ammonia are found. Assay of the enzyme requires liver tissue.

ORNITHINE TRANSCARBAMYLASE DEFICIENCY

Carbamyl phosphate reacts with ornithine in the presence of ornithine transcarbamylase to form citrulline. Assay of this enzyme also requires liver.

A number of patients have been described with deficiency of this enzyme. The gene is on the X chromosome. Involved males have usually died in the newborn period. Symptoms have begun with vomiting and lethargy, progressing to coma. Activity of the enzyme in liver was less than 2 per cent of normal. Female patients have had a more indolent course. Mental deficiency, episodic vomiting, hypotonia, and lethargy have been prominent. Some patients have had seizures. Concentrations of ammonia were elevated. Increased amounts of orotic acid are found in the urine in this condition and in citrullinemia.

ARGININEMIA

A small number of patients with argininemia have been described. They presented, like other patients with hyperammonemia, with vomiting and retarded mental and motor development. One had a spastic quadriparesis. Two had seizures, and one had an abnormal electroencephalogram. Hepatomegaly with abnormal liver function tests was observed.

The blood ammonia was markedly elevated both in the fasting state and postprandially. There was a pattern in the urine similar to that seen in cystinuria, with increased excretion of cystine, lysine, and ornithine, as well as arginine. Citrulline was also excreted in abnormal quantities. The concentration of arginine in the plasma was elevated 6 to 15 times, and the cerebrospinal fluid concentration was also increased. Arginase assays were performed on the erythrocytes of the patients, and the activity was greatly reduced or unmeasurable.

ORNITHINEMIA

Two types of ornithinemia have been reported. In the first, mental retardation, prolonged icterus, and electroencephalographic abnormalities were associated with increased concentrations of ornithine in the blood. There was a generalized aminoaciduria but not hyperammonemia or homocitrullinuria. The activity of hepatic ornithine-keto acid transaminase (OKT) was deficient.

In the second, there were mental retardation, ataxia, and hyperammonemia, along with homocitrullinuria. The activity of OKT in the patient's fibroblasts was normal.

HYPERLYSINEMIA

A number of different inborn errors of metabolism present with elevated concentrations of lysine in the blood. One of these is due to a deficiency of lysine: α-ketoglutarate reductase. The first child described with this disorder had mental retardation and delayed physical development, but two subsequent children were mentally and physically normal. Consanguinity has been observed. Concentrations of lysine were elevated in the blood, with levels generally exceeding 10 mg per 100 ml. The product of the reductase enzyme is saccharopine. This pathway is the major route of lysine catabolism. The enzyme defect is demonstrable in cultured fibroblasts.

Saccharopinuria has been found in two patients as a result of routine screening of mentally retarded individuals. Plasma lysine was elevated in both. This abnormality is due to a defect in saccharopine dehydrogenase.

An alternate pathway for the catabolism of lysine is through pipecolic acid. A patient has been described who appeared to have a defect in this pathway because large amounts of pipecolic acid were found in the plasma and urine. Concentrations of lysine were not elevated. This child died of a progressive neurologic disease associated with hepatomegaly.

Another disorder has been described under the heading of lysine intolerance in which there is episodic ammonia intoxication and coma. Such a patient would be clinically indistinguishable from those described under hyperammonemia. Patients described from Finland as having "familial protein intolerance" all had hyperammonemia and hyperlysinuria.

HYPER-β-ALANINEMIA AND CARNOSINEMIA

Hyper-β-alaninemia has been reported in a single infant who died very early in life. Symptoms were those of somnolence, hypotonia, and intermittent seizures, which could not be controlled with the usual anticonvulsant therapy. Deep tendon reflexes were depressed.

β-Alanine was found to be elevated in the blood, urine, and cerebrospinal fluid. Large amounts of taurine and β-aminoisobutyric acid were also found in the urine. γ-aminobutyric acid was present in the plasma, urine and cerebrospinal fluid. The concentration of γ-aminobutyric acid in brain tissue obtained post mortem was markedly increased.

Carnosine is the dipeptide of β-alanine and histidine. It is normally present in high concentrations in muscle and thus is a common dietary constituent. It is not normally found in the blood. Seven patients have been reported with carnosinemia. Five had progressive neurologic degeneration with onset early in infancy. They also had seizures and electroencephalographic abnormalities. However, two persons have been described in whom the biochemical abnormality was present without detectable clinical manifestations. Carnosinase activity, normally present in the serum, is absent in patients with carnosinemia.

Carnosinemia should be distinguished from normal dietary carnosinuria. Patients with carnosinemia have persistent carnosinuria while receiving a carnosine-free diet. They do not have 1-methylhistidine in the urine. Normal persons receiving a meal rich in protein such as white meat of chicken excrete anserine, β-alanyl-1-methylhistidine, and the urine always contains 1-methylhistidine.

PYROGLUTAMIC ACIDEMIA

Pyroglutamic acidemia was first described by Eldjarn and colleagues in Norway in 1970. A second patient was observed in Sweden. Metabolic acidosis is a consistent feature of this disorder. The first patient with this disorder was mentally retarded and ataxic. At the age of 16 years he began to have episodes of violent vomiting. His metabolic acidosis was first noted when he was admitted to the hospital for repair of a hiatal hernia, and it became life threatening in the postoperative period. Over a 3-year period of study he was admitted to a hospital five times, always revealing a chronic acidosis without acute exacerbations. It is not clear that any of his clinical manifestations were related to his pyroglutamic acidemia. The second patient developed a severe metabolic acidosis on the third day of life. This was correctable with NaHCO$_3$, but she had exacerbations of acidosis whenever alkali therapy was discontinued. This patient had no other abnormalities, and at 14 months of age her physical and intellectual development were normal.

Pyroglutamic acid is 2-pyrrolidone-5-carboxylic acid. Glutamine cyclizes readily to pyroglutamic acid in aqueous solutions at physiologic pH. The compound does not react with ninhydrin. Therefore it is not detectable using routine methods of screening the urine for amino acids. It has been found using gas liquid chromatography.

The first patient excreted 30 to 40 grams of pyroglutamate in the urine in 24 hours. Serum concentrations were as high as 50 to 60 mg per 100 ml or 4 to 5 mEq per liter. This would account for the acidosis. In the second patient 6 to 7 grams of pyroglutamate was excreted each day in the urine.

The kidney appears to be the site of formation of pyroglutamate. A relationship has been suspected between renal ammonia production and pyroglutamate formation. It is generally accepted that the amide nitrogen of glutamine is the source of renal NH$_4^+$. Spontaneous deamination of glutamine in aqueous solutions yields predominantly pyroglutamate, not glutamate. Furthermore, there is generally a close parallel in patients with pyroglutamic aciduria between the amounts of pyroglutamate and ammonia in the urine. Pyroglutamate can be formed in the enzymatic hydrolysis of gamma-glutamyl peptides.

DISORDERS OF AMINO ACID TRANSPORT

HARTNUP DISEASE

Hartnup disease is an unusual disorder in which the transport of certain amino acids, particularly tryptophan, is abnormal in the intestine and in the renal tubule. It was named for the first family described, in which four of the eight children of parents who were first cousins were affected. The constant feature of the disease is the aminoaciduria.

Clinical characteristics are intermittent and variable. Patients may develop a pellagra-like, photosensitive, red, scaly eruption on the exposed skin. In addition, they have cerebellar ataxia occurring in attacks of variable severity, which are completely reversible. Other patients have had psychiatric abnormalities similar to those observed in pellagra. Mental retardation is common but not uniform. Attacks have been precipitated by infection. Transmission is as an autosomal recessive character.

Patients may be recognized even in the absence of symptomatology by the aminoaciduria. It is renal in type, with plasma concentrations of amino acids normal or decreased. The following amino acids are excreted in five to ten times the usual amounts: threonine, serine, asparagine, glutamine, alanine, valine, isoleucine, leucine, tyrosine, phenylalanine, histidine, and tryptophan. This is a large group of amino acids, but the pattern is striking. It differs from the commonly encountered generalized aminoaciduria in that the excretion of glycine, glutamic acid, and lysine are normal, and that there is no free proline or hydroxyproline in the urine. The urine in this condition is also characterized by the presence of a number of indolic derivatives of tryptophan, including indican. These patients respond to an oral load of tryptophan with increased excretion of indican and indolic acids. Tryptophan loading after sterilization of the intestinal flora with antibiotics resulted in no increase in indole excretion, and unabsorbed tryptophan accumulated in the feces. These observations indicate that there is a defect in the absorption of tryptophan in the cells of the intestine as well as in the kidney. The indoles found in the urine in this disease are secondary to the action of intestinal bacteria on unabsorbed tryptophan.

Most patients have been treated with nicotinamide. It is not certain that improvements observed in cutaneous and neurologic manifestations with treatment were not spontaneous, but treatment is recommended.

CYSTINURIA

Cystinuria is an inherited defect in renal tubular function in which the reabsorption of cystine, lysine, arginine, and ornithine is impaired. The abnormality is of clinical significance because of the insolubility of cystine which can form stones when present in the urine in high concentration. The excretion of the other three amino acids does not influence the health of the patient.

Patients with cystinuria generally develop calculi some time before the age of 30 years. Some have large numbers of calculi requiring surgical removal for relief of colic or obstruction. Repeated infections of the urinary tract and renal failure are common. The stones represent aggregations of cystine varying from tiny sands of gravel to staghorn calculi filling the renal pelvis or huge calculi of the bladder. Pure cystine crystals are radiolucent, but variable contents of calcium make stones opaque. This disorder should be distinguished from cystinosis or the Lignac-de Toni-Fanconi syndrome, in which glycosuria, generalized aminoaciduria, phosphaturia, and renal rickets are associated with deposits of cystine in tissues. Such patients do not have abnormal amounts of cystine in the urine.

In cystinuria the concentrations of cystine and the other amino acids in the blood are not elevated. The clearance of cystine, lysine, arginine, and ornithine is markedly elevated. There is also a disorder of intestinal absorption, in some patients with cystinuria, involving the amino acids cystine, lysine, arginine, and ornithine. Inefficiently absorbed lysine, arginine, and ornithine are converted by intestinal bacteria to the diamines, cadaverine and putrescine, which may be detected in the urine.

Genetic studies indicate that there are at least three forms of cystinuria in which the homozygotes are clinically indistinguishable. They are now designated types I, II, and III. In type I the heterozygotes are detectable only by studies of the intestinal transport of cystine or the dibasic amino acids. This is the most common form, accounting for almost two thirds of all carriers. Type I homozygotes, of course, also have the intestinal transport defect. In types II and III the heterozygotes excrete increased amounts of cystine and lysine in the urine. Type II differs from type III in that in the former an oral load of cystine appears not to be absorbed into the blood and lysine transport is altered in intestinal cells in vitro. The three genes are allelic, and double heterozygotes have been observed who carry two different abnormal genes and thus have clinical manifestations of homozygous cystinuria.

Cystinuria is relatively common, occurring about once in every 20,000 live births. The condition can be screened for, using the simple cyanide nitroprusside test. Confirmation of the diagnosis requires a quantitative assay of cystine content of the urine.

Treatment of cystinuria is aimed at the prevention of urinary lithiasis. Crystallization and stone formation can be minimized by increasing urine volumes or by increasing cystine solubility. However, very large amounts of oral fluids are required, and in practice very few adults and almost no children will drink enough to prevent stones. Alkalinization sufficient to promote the solubility of cystine requires a urine pH of over 7.6, which is not achievable physiologically. Penicillamine therapy has therefore brought about a real advance in the management of this disease. Penicillamine forms a mixed disulfide with cystine that is considerably more soluble than cystine. Oral administration of penicillamine to cystinuric patients can reduce the cystine content in the urine to levels at which stones do not form.

Two conditions related to cystinuria are hyperdibasic aminoaciduria and hypercystinuria. In the former, the dibasic amino acids, lysine, ornithine, and arginine, are excreted in large amounts because of a renal tubular absorptive defect, but cystine excretion is normal. Lysine transport in the intestine appears also to be abnormal. The trait is inherited as a dominant and appears to have no clinical manifestations. In hypercystinuria, cystine is excreted in the urine in increased amounts because of a specific tubular transport defect, whereas the excretion of the dibasic amino acids is normal. The amounts of cystine in the urine in this condition are only 25 per cent of those found in cystinuria. Clinical manifestations have not been observed, but the disorder has been observed in only one family. The existence of these two conditions indicates that more than one transport system is involved in the excretion of cystine and the dibasic amino acids.

IMINOGLYCINURIA

Renal iminoglycinuria appears to be a benign chemical abnormality in which there is no clinical abnormality. There is selective impairment in the shared transport system for proline, hydroxyproline, and glycine. Net renal tubular reabsorption of the amino acids is about 80 per cent of normal and that of glycine is about 60 per cent of normal. An intestinal transport defect for the same amino acids has been observed in some families but not in others.

In most heterozygotes there is impaired renal tubular transport of glycine. Thus these individuals may present with tubular hyperglycinuria. It is thought that this accounts for patients with glycinuria reported as having a dominantly inherited condition. On the other hand, some heterozygotes may have no glycinuria. These observations and those on intestinal transport suggest that there is more than one allelic mutation responsible for iminoglycinuria.

ERRORS OF CARBOHYDRATE METABOLISM IN INFANTS AND CHILDREN

By JOHN FERNANDES, M.D.
Groningen, The Netherlands

Pyruvate is an important substrate in carbohydrate metabolism, as it is the end point of glycolysis and the starting point of gluconeogenesis. Furthermore, pyruvate is an important contributor to the citric acid cycle by its oxidative decarboxylation into acetyl coenzyme A. For this conversion the multienzyme pyruvate dehydrogenase complex is involved. Several enzyme defects of gluconeogenesis and pyruvate dehydrogenase, although very different biochemically, entail metabolic abnormalities, some of which are similar, and clinical syndromes, which are more or less homogeneous.

Common metabolic abnormalities are accumulation of pyruvate, lactate, and alanine, which equilibrate with each other. High concentrations of these metabolites in serum and urine are due to overflow proximal to the enzyme defect in disorders of gluconeogenesis and in pyruvate dehydrogenase deficiency. Low concentrations of glucose is by the same token related to deficiency of "end-products" distal to the enzyme defect.

Clinical signs, which are more or less homogeneous, are of cerebral origin, such as mental and motor retardation, convulsions, ataxia, hypotonia, and, ultimately, hypertonia. Abnormalities of the eyes and enlargement of the liver are frequently observed. During stress, such as febrile infections, and after changes of the diet, latent metabolic abnormalities may become manifest and rapidly lead to metabolic acidosis, coma, and a fatal outcome.

The cases described in many reports in the older literature under the common designation "lactic acidosis in infancy" may have been due to a deficiency of one of the key enzymes of gluconeogenesis or of the pyruvate dehydrogenase complex.

ERRORS OF GLUCONEOGENESIS

Deficiencies of each of four one-way enzymes involved in gluconeogenesis (Fig. 1) have been described. These enzymes are pyruvate carboxylase, phosphoenolpyruvate carboxykinase, fructose-1,6-diphosphatase, and glucose-6-phosphatase. Deficiency of the last enzyme is not further dealt with here, as it is discussed in the article Glycogen Storage Disease.

PYRUVATE CARBOXYLASE DEFICIENCY

Pyruvate carboxylase (PC) is the first one-way enzyme of gluconeogenesis that converts pyruvate to oxaloacetate. It is a mitochondrial enzyme, mainly localized in the liver.

CLINICAL SIGNS AND SYMPTOMS

Some patients with PC deficiency show neurologic abnormalities such as convulsions, muscular hypotonia, ataxia, nystagmus, oculomotoric palsy, and psychomotoric retardation. The clinical course is usually rapidly fatal. In rare instances a milder protracted course or intermittent episodes of hyperventilation and ataxia are observed. Metabolic abnormalities directly related to the enzyme defect are elevated blood levels of pyruvate, lactate, and alanine, and decreased concentrations of glucose. Further abnormalities are hyperketonemia and hyperammonemia. These metabolic perturbations may be precipitated by infections, fasting, and during a high-protein, high-fat diet. At autopsy widespread symmetrical demyelinization and periventricular cavities have been found in

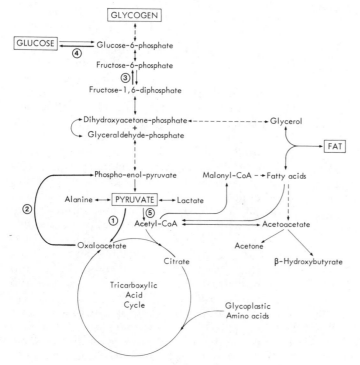

Figure 1.   Glycolysis and gluconeogenesis.

① Pyruvate-carboxylase

② Phospho-enol-pyruvate-carboxykinase

③ Fructose-1,6-diphosphatase

④ Glucose-6-phosphatase

⑤ Pyruvate-dehydrogenase-complex

some patients, and subacute necrotizing encephalomyelopathy as described by Leigh in others. A similar wide spectrum of abnormalities has been found in patients with other enzyme defects of gluconeogenesis and the pyruvate dehydrogenase complex.

DIAGNOSIS AND MANAGEMENT

The diagnosis can be made by enzyme assay of liver tissue and cultured skin fibroblasts. The enzyme defect is also present in the brain.

No beneficial effect of biotin, a co-enzyme for pyruvate carboxylase, has yet been described. Exacerbations of lactic acidosis are difficult to manage even with high doses of glucose and sodium bicarbonate intravenously and simultaneous restriction of the protein and fat intake.

PHOSPHOENOLPYRUVATE CARBOXYKINASE DEFICIENCY

Phosphoenolpyruvate carboxykinase (PEPCK) is the second one-way enzyme of gluconeogenesis that phosphorylates oxaloacetate to phosphoenolpyruvate. In man 80 per cent of PEPCK activity is localized in the mitochondria. The disorder is very rare.

CLINICAL SIGNS AND SYMPTOMS

These are convulsions, hypotonia, mental and motor retardation, enlarged liver and tongue, hypoglycemia, and icterus. The fatal outcome is preceded by coma and severe hypoglycemia. Chemical findings are metabolic acidosis, elevated serum transaminases, lactate dehydrogenase, alkaline phosphatase, hypercholesterolemia, and hypertriglyceridemia. Lactate, pyruvate, β-hydroxybutyrate and acetoacetate were within normal limits in one patient.

DIAGNOSIS

The diagnosis has been made by enzyme assay of fresh frozen liver tissue, obtained postmortem. Generalized fat storage has been found in the liver, muscles, and other organs, but not in the central nervous system.

FRUCTOSE-1,6-DIPHOSPHATASE DEFICIENCY

Fructose-1,6-diphosphatase (FDPase) is the third one-way enzyme of gluconeogenesis, which dephosphorylates fructose-1,6-diphosphate to fructose-6-phosphate.

CLINICAL SIGNS AND SYMPTOMS

These develop soon after birth or later when the infant is weaned from breast feeding to sugar-containing baby foods. The main symptoms are hyperventilation due to lactic acidosis, muscular hypotonia, hepatomegaly, jaundice, failure to thrive, diarrhea, and, ultimately, convulsions and coma. Mild obesity may be present. Chemical findings are markedly increased levels of pyruvate, lactate, and alanine in serum and urine. Hypoglycemia occurs during fasting and infections. Secondary abnormalities are tyrosyluria, tyrosinemia, and hyperuricemia during exacerbations. The course may be severe and rapidly fatal or episodic with exacerbations during infections or without apparent reason. Regression of symptoms — even of hepatomegaly and of fatty changes of the liver — suppression of metabolic abnormalities, and restoration of normal mental and motor development may occur after timely dietary treatment.

SPECIAL TESTS

Tolerance tests with alanine, fructose, dihydroxyacetone, glycerol, and a fasting test may be carried out for a tentative diagnosis and before performing the enzyme essay. It is mandatory to perform any of these tests under close clinical supervision with continuous monitoring of blood glucose and acid-base equilibrium, as hypoglycemia and lactic acidosis may develop precipitously.

L-alanine, the main glucoplastic aminoacid, can be administered intravenously or orally to investigate gluconeogenesis. A marked drop of blood glucose and a concomitant rise of blood lactate and pyruvate point to a deficiency of one of the four key enzymes. A fasting test can be used instead of the alanine tolerance test. Finally, a tolerance test with either fructose or dihydroxyacetone or glycerol can be of help to localize the presumed block in gluconeogenesis. All these substrates enter this pathway at the level of the trioses, between phosphoenolpyruvate and fructose-1,6-diphosphate (Fig. 1). The results of two or three of these tests may allow the differentiation between pyruvate carboxylase and phosphoenolpyruvate carboxykinase deficiency on the one hand and fructose-1,6-diphosphatase and glucose-6-phosphatase deficiency on the other hand. The latter two enzyme defects can be differentiated by means of a glucagon test after a short fast. In FDPase deficiency, glucose rises normally; in glucose-6-phosphatase deficiency, blood glucose fails to rise or even drops.

DIAGNOSIS AND MANAGEMENT

The diagnosis can be made by enzyme assay of liver tissue or leukocytes. Because FDPase deficiency is normally not present in cultured fibroblasts, prenatal diagnosis of this autosomal recessively inherited enzyme defect is not possible.

Dietary restriction of protein, fructose, sucrose, and sorbitol appear to be of value for long-term management of this potentially fatal error of gluconeogenesis. Prolonged fasting has to be prevented and the timely administration of glucose intravenously may be necessary to suppress metabolic deviations during infections.

DEFICIENCY OF THE PYRUVATE DEHYDROGENASE COMPLEX

Pyruvate dehydrogenase (PDH) is an enzyme complex, consisting of five enzymes. The combined and sequential action of this multienzyme promotes the oxidative decarboxylation of pyruvate into acetyl coenzyme A. The enzyme complex is thus very important for channeling the end product of glycolysis (pyruvate) into the citric acid cycle and eventually to fatty acid synthesis (liponeogenesis). The third enzyme of the PDH complex is also a component of the α-ketoglutarate dehydrogenase complex. Deficiency of this enzyme, which is required for the conversion of α-ketoglutarate to succinyl coenzyme A in the tricarboxylic acid cycle, thus evokes more complicated metabolic abnormalities.

CLINICAL SIGNS AND SYMPTOMS

These are too variable to be diagnostic. Some children were mentally retarded and had seizures and other neurologic abnormalities. They had chronic metabolic acidosis associated with elevated blood and urine levels of lactate, pyruvate, and alanine, while α-ketoglutaric acid excretion in the urine was increased. Hypoglycemia occurred with fasting. In other patients the symptoms were milder or intermittent. Weakness, a wide-based ataxic gait, dysmetria during rapid alternating movements, slurring and explosive speech, irregular wandering eye movements without true nystagmus, and rapid breathing were the most prominent symptoms. These symptoms tended to become more marked later in the day. Metabolic abnormalities were not detectable in the "silent" phase of the illness of these patients, but after a febrile illness or other stress situation, deterioration of the neurologic abnormalities and lactic acidosis occurred with elevated levels of lactate, pyruvate, and alanine in serum and urine. Some patients became hypoglycemic after a short fast; others could withstand fasting remarkably well. It is clear that the variable symptomatology is in some respects similar to that of errors of gluconeogenesis.

DIAGNOSIS AND MANAGEMENT

As some patients are intolerant of a high carbohydrate intake, a glucose-pyruvate or a glucose-lactate test has been recommended for a tentative diagnosis. Serum lactate and pyruvate rise to abnormally high levels during the oral glucose tolerance test. The patient needs close supervision during the test, as one of my patients subsequently developed lactic acidosis.

Enzyme assays of the enzymes of the PDH complex have been performed in liver, muscles, brain, kidney, leukocytes, and cultured fibroblasts. In case of deficient activity of the total PDH complex, assays of separate enzymes of the multienzyme have to be carried out in leukocytes, fibroblasts, or liver tissue. As enzyme defects of PDH can be demonstrated in fibroblasts, antenatal detection of this autosomal recessive seems feasible.

The episodic nature of the clinical course makes the assessment of therapeutic measures difficult. Symptomatic treatment with sodium bicarbonate is necessary. Carbohydrate restriction and a high fat intake improved the clinical course in some patients. Other patients seemed to benefit from extra glucose. Administration of thiamine and other coenzymes of the PDH complex was without effect or of questionable effect.

ERRORS OF GALACTOSE METABOLISM

Three errors of galactose metabolism occur in which the galactose blood level rises abnormally high as soon as the child ingests lactose or galactose. The accumulation of galactose is due to enzyme defects of one of the first three steps of galactose conversion, as shown in Table 1. Because the clinical and biochemical abnormalities of the disorders caused by these enzyme defects differ considerably, they will be discussed separately.

GALACTOKINASE DEFICIENCY

Galactokinase (abbreviated as kinase) is the first enzyme of galactose metabolism, which

Table 1. *Errors of Galactose Metabolism*

(1) Galactose + ATP	→ galactose-1-phosphate + ADP
(2) Galactose-1-phosphate ⇌ UDP galactose + glucose-1- + UDP glucose	phosphate
(3) UDP galactose	⇌ UDP glucose
(4) Galactose	→ galactitol

Enzymes: (1) galactokinase, (2) galactose-1-phosphate-uridyltransferase, (3) UDP-galactose-4-epimerase, (4) aldoreductase.

catalyzes the conversion of galactose to galactose-1-phosphate (Table 1). Kinase deficiency causes increased galactose levels in blood and urine as soon as the child consumes lactose-containing milk, such as human milk, cow's milk, or a cow's milk adapted formula. The accumulated galactose is not only excreted in the urine but also small amounts of it are converted to galactitol in various organs (Table 1, reaction 4). Galactitol is very noxious for the crystalline lens of the eye, in which its accumulation causes cataract.

CLINICAL SIGNS AND SYMPTOMS

There are no abnormalities except for nuclear cataracts, which appear during the first weeks of life. Early treatment will prevent the cataracts or arrest their further increase. Hepatosplenomegaly was found to be a reversible abnormality in the newborn period in few patients. Besides the cataracts, galactokinase deficiency thus appears to be a benign disorder.

DIAGNOSIS

After ingestion of lactose-containing milk, the newborn's urine has to be screened for reducing sugars by Clinitest or an equivalent test. Specific glucose tests are inadequate for screening the urine of newborns for sugars other than glucose. A positive Clinitest has to be followed by enzymatic or chromatographic assay of galactose and other sugars in urine and blood. In some countries all newborns are screened for the presence of elevated blood levels of galactose by means of a blood spot test. In case of doubt a direct assay of the erythrocytes for galactokinase and galactose-1-phosphate-uridyltransferase has to be performed.

GENETICS

Kinase deficiency is transmitted as an autosomal recessive. The incidence is approximately 1:50,000. The presence of the enzyme in cultured fibroblasts allows antenatal detection of an affected fetus. It is important to investigate all first and second degree relatives of a kinase-deficient patient, because cataract has been found even in heterozygotes.

A lactose-free and galactose-free diet is indicated. The prescription of such a diet has to be considered even for heterozygotes, in order to prevent cataract at a later age.

GALACTOSE-1-PHOSPHATE URIDYLTRANSFERASE DEFICIENCY

Synonyms are galactosemia and galactose intolerance.

Galactose-1-phosphate uridyltransferase (abbreviated as transferase) is the second enzyme of galactose metabolism catalyzing the conversion of galactose-1-phosphate to UDP galactose. Deficiency of this enzyme is followed by accumulation of galactose and galactose-1-phosphate as soon as the newborn is fed a lactose-containing milk. Excess of galactose-1-phosphate is the main cause of the severity of the disease, as this substrate is very toxic for cell function. Its adverse influence on gluconeogenesis and glycogenolysis and its damaging effect on various tissues is very complex.

CLINICAL SIGNS AND SYMPTOMS

The newborn's illness becomes usually manifest a few days after a lactose-containing milk diet is started. Failure to thrive, vomiting, jaundice, hepatomegaly, hypoglycemia, convulsions, edema, ascites, and cataract are the main features. Serum bilirubin is often of the unconjugated type. Failure to form clotting factors may be the cause of purpura.

Renal tubular damage is reflected by glucosuria, proteinuria, and hyperaminoaciduria. A fulminant course may lead to the death of the infant within the first weeks of life. In some children the illness is less serious and the detection of cataract due to galactitol accumulation in the lens may be the first clue to the diagnosis. A milder course of the disease has been described in variant forms of the transferase defect. Cataract may, on the other hand, be the only symptom even before the lactose-containing feeding is given.

The liver and kidney damage is usually reversible, if lactose and galactose elimination from the diet has not been initiated too late. Some degree of mental retardation and behavioral changes are, however, permanent sequelae in children whose disease is discovered late.

DIAGNOSIS

In some countries all newborns are screened for galactose or for transferase activity, either from cord blood or from heelprick blood. In countries without such a screening the diagnosis depends on the rapid interpretation of the first clinical abnormalities and the finding of a reducing sugar or galactose or both in the urine. In case of doubt a galactose tolerance test is not indicated, as toxic symptoms may be precipitated by the test. Direct enzyme assay in the erythrocytes has to be performed in all patients suspected of having galactosemia or in families with affected siblings. Variants of transferase deficiency may be missed, because the enzyme activity of these patients' erythrocytes may be in the range for heterozygotes. Further study of the abnormal enzyme is indicated in these cases.

GENETICS

Transferase deficiency is transmitted as an autosomal recessive. The incidence is approximately 1:50,000. Partial deficiency states and variant forms are probably more common. The presence of the enzyme in cultured fibroblasts allows antenatal detection and appropriate dietary treatment during gestation (see later discussion).

MANAGEMENT

The timely institution of a lactose-free and galactose-free diet can be a life-saving procedure for the patient. Prevention or arrest of all or some abnormalities or restoration of function is related to the duration of the damaging effect of lactose-containing feeding before institution of the appropriate diet. A heterozygous mother must be treated with a lactose-restricted diet during pregnancy to prevent fetal damage in case that the fetus is a transferase-deficient homozygote. The diet has to be continued until term, unless antenatal diagnosis reveals the fetus to be normal or heterozygote.

UDP-GALACTOSE-4-EPIMERASE DEFICIENCY

This rare biochemical defect was detected by Gitzelmann in a screening program for errors in galactose metabolism in newborns. Accumulation of galactose and galactose-1-phosphate was found in the erythrocytes only, and hypergalactosemia and galactosuria were absent. There were no clinical manifestations of this apparently benign error of galactose metabolism. The diagnosis was established by assaying UDP-galactose-4-epimerase in red blood cells.

ERRORS OF FRUCTOSE METABOLISM

Two errors of fructose metabolism occur in which the fructose concentration in blood and urine rises abnormally high as soon as the child ingests sucrose or fructose.

FRUCTOKINASE DEFICIENCY

Synonyms are essential fructosuria and benign fructosuria.

Fructokinase is the first enzyme of fructose metabolism, phosphorylating fructose to fructose-1-phosphate in liver, intestine, and kidneys. Affected persons therefore cannot retain the fructose absorbed from their intestine. Clinical signs and symptoms are absent in this benign error of fructose metabolism.

Fructokinase is transmitted as an autosomal recessive. The incidence is approximately 1:130,000.

DIAGNOSIS

After ingestion of fructose-containing or sucrose-containing food the urine contains fructose, which gives a positive reduction test, does not react with glucose oxidase reagents, and can be identified by chromatography. In case of doubt an intravenous fructose tolerance test can be carried out. Marked fructosemia and fructosuria are the only abnormalities during the test; other metabolic perturbations are not present. A direct enzyme assay of fructokinase in liver tissue is not indicated in this harmless condition.

FRUCTOSE-1-PHOSPHATE ALDOLASE DEFICIENCY

Synonyms are fructosemia and fructose intolerance.

Fructose-1-phosphate aldolase (abbreviated as aldolase) is the second enzyme of fructose metabolism. The aldolases are present as the A, B, and C isoenzymes, each of which has specific properties and tissue localization. In fructose intolerance, aldolase B is deficient. This enzyme, which is localized in liver, intestine, and kidneys, cleaves the phosphorylated hexoses fructose-1-phosphate (F-1-P) and fructose-1,6-diphosphate (FDP) into the trioses dihydroxy-acetone-phosphate and glyceraldehyde (-phosphate). The phosphorylated trioses equilibrate into each other and are condensed to FDP by the reversed action of aldolase B. Inherited deficiency of aldolase B results in complete or near-complete inactivity of the enzyme with F-1-P and a smaller reduction in activity with FDP. As soon as the child ingests fructose,

F-1-P accumulates in the cells and a secondary inhibition of fructokinase accounts for the high blood levels of fructose. Excess of F-1-P is the main cause for the severity of the disease, as this substrate is very toxic for cell function.

Not only does F-1-P accumulate after fructose ingestion, but depletion of adenosine-triphosphate (ATP) also ensues. This high-energy nucleotide, consumed by phosphorylation of fructose to F-1-P, is not regenerated from adenosine-di-phosphate (ADP). ADP is degraded to AMP instead and the end-product uric acid is liberated in excess from the liver. Accumulation of F-1-P and depletion of ATP entail several metabolic abnormalities, such as impaired glycolysis and gluconeogenesis.

CLINICAL SIGNS AND SYMPTOMS

As soon as fructose-containing or sucrose-containing nutrients are introduced in the infant's diet, symptoms of intolerance develop. Acute symptoms are vomiting, drowsiness, seizures, coma, and other manifestations of hypoglycemia. In older children diarrhea and abdominal pain follow fructose ingestion. With continued fructose feeding, anorexia, failure to thrive, jaundice, hepatomegaly, splenomegaly, and ascites develop. Serum transaminases are increased, and serum albumen and fibrinogen are decreased. Hemorrhagic manifestations are due to abnormalities in coagulation factors. These symptoms reflect progression of the disease to cirrhosis of the liver. Fructosuria, albuminuria, and aminoaciduria (especially tyrosine and methionine) are usual findings. The aminoaciduria is a reflection of renal tubular damage.

Aversion to sweets develops early in life and by avoiding sweetened foods, most patients protect themselves from the toxic effects of fructose. Preservation of the teeth in a caries-free condition is a remarkable result. The distaste for anything sweet should be a marker for the diagnosis. Variability in symptoms and differences in clinical course from mild to fatal may reflect differences in fructose intake or heterogeneity of the enzyme defect.

All clinical and all abnormal laboratory findings may be reversible after timely exclusion of fructose from the diet.

DIAGNOSIS

The striking aversion to sweets and the identification of fructose in the urine after ingestion of fructose-containing or sucrose-containing food are highly suggestive of the diagnosis. In case of doubt, an intravenous fructose tolerance test should be carried out. Characteristic abnor-

malities are a precipitous drop of blood glucose and inorganic phosphate and an increase of blood urate and magnesium. A moderate fructose dose (0.25 gram per kg), by the intravenous (not oral) route and close supervision of the patient are prerequisites of the test. For confirmation of the diagnosis, biochemical investigation of a liver biopsy may be carried out. The activity of aldolase B with F-1-P as substrate is markedly reduced, with FDP only slightly or moderately. Thus the ratio of aldolase activities, utilizing these substrates, is different from normal.

GENETICS

Aldolase B deficiency is transmitted as an autosomal recessive. The incidence is approximately 1:30,000. Incidentally, symptoms have been found in one parent and one or more of this parent's children. This may be due to dominant or pseudodominant inheritance (symptoms in both the homozygous affected child and *one* heterozygous parent). Antenatal detection is not possible, because aldolase B activity is normally not present in cultured fibroblasts.

MANAGEMENT

The timely institution of a fructose-free and sucrose-free diet can prevent or arrest all or most abnormalities and restore function. Attention to details is necessary for strict fructose elimination, because the fructose content of some nutrients depends on their harvesting, cooking, or storing (potatoes). The intravenous administration of invert sugar, sorbitol, or fructose-containing fluid may precipitate profound illness.

MUCOPOLYSAC-CHARIDOSES

By ALLEN HORWITZ, M.D.
Chicago, Illinois

The mucopolysaccharidoses are a group of inherited storage diseases resulting from abnormalities of mucopolysaccharide (glycosaminoglycan) metabolism. Biochemically, they are characterized by excessive amounts of mucopo-

Table 1. *The Mucopolysaccharidoses:*
Synonyms

Disorder	Synonyms
Hurler syndrome	MPS I, MPS IH, gargoylism
Hunter syndrome	MPS II
Sanfilippo syndrome types A and B	MPS III A and MPS III B polydystrophic oligophrenia
Morquio syndrome	MPS IV, Morquio-Ullrich, Brailsford syndrome
Maroteaux-Lamy syndrome	MPS VI, polydystrophic dwarfism
Scheie syndrome	MPS IS, MPS V
Hurler-Scheie compound	MPS IH/S
β-glucuronidase deficiency	MPS VII
N-acetylglucosamine 6-sulfate sulfatase deficiency	MPS VIII

lysaccharides in tissues and urine. The clinical syndromes resulting from these biochemical abnormalities involve various combinations of mental retardation, hepatosplenomegaly, and malformations of connective tissues. The various terms that have been applied to these syndromes are listed in Table 1.

CLINICAL MANIFESTATIONS

The diagnosis of mucopolysaccharidosis should be considered in a patient who develops progressive dysmorphic features such as coarse facies, skeletal disorder with dwarfism, and hepatosplenomegaly — especially in association with mental retardation. The progressive nature results from an ongoing accumulation of mucopolysaccharides, so that by 12 to 18 months of age many of the clinical manifestations are obvious in these patients. A summary of the clinical features of the mucopolysaccharidoses is shown in Table 1. The order of discussion of the individual syndromes is approximately in the order of frequency of occurrence.

HURLER SYNDROME

Hurler syndrome has the most severe manifestations among the mucopolysaccharidoses. Children with this disease have coarse facies and thick skin with abundant hairs. Patients have a prominent forehead, depressed nasal bridge, hypertelorism, thick lips, and low hair-line. The teeth are peg-like and there is noisy mouth breathing along with chronic rhinorrhea. Corneal clouding is seen by age 2.

Patients often present with heart murmurs resulting from various degrees of mitral insufficiency or aortic regurgitation or both. The abdomen is protuberant with hepatosplenomegaly, and hernias often occur. The skeletal changes are manifested as "cat back" gibbus, broad claw-like hands, and stiff joints with moderate contractures at the elbows and the knees.

Mental retardation is noted by age 1 year as a progressive slowing of the acquisition of developmental milestones. Regression with loss of skills occurs so that speech is often lost. Progressive deafness is common in these children. Death occurs in the first decade, most commonly from respiratory infection complicating heart failure.

The x-ray findings of Hurler syndrome are most apparent on the lateral spine film, which shows deformities of the vertebral bodies with anterior beak-like projections, especially in the upper lumbar vertebrae. The skull shows an enlarged boot-shaped sella turcica, and the ribs are wide and spatula-like.

The mucopolysaccharides in the urine will flocculate albumin at an acid pH that is the basis for a turbidity screening test. Likewise, the excessive mucopolysaccharides will show a purple metachromasia when spotted on a commercially available toluidine blue filter paper. Analysis of the urine shows excess dermatan sulfate and haparan sulfate. Leukocytes or cultured skin fibroblasts are deficient in L-α-iduronidase. The diagnosis of Hurler syndrome in a patient with compatible clinical manifestations is confirmed by the deficiency of L-α-iduronidase in leukocytes or cultured skin fibroblasts.

HUNTER SYNDROME

This disorder is sex-linked and thus to be considered in males, especially when male relatives have been affected. The patients often present with either delay in mental development or signs of coarse features. Among the constant physical findings are: thickened skin, often with a pebbly texture; coarse facies; stiff joints with a clawhand deformity; and hepatosplenomegaly. Hernias are common and most patients have progressive deafness. X-ray findings resemble those of Hurler syndrome, but they are less severe; significant gibbus is not seen. Lack of corneal clouding helps to differentiate Hunter syndrome from Hurler syndrome. In general, the progress of disease is slower than in Hurler syndrome.

There may be two clinical types of Hunter

syndrome: *type A* involves mental retardation and more severe somatic changes and *type B*, a mild form, produces little or no mental retardation. Laboratory findings include mucopolysacchariduria with increases of dermatan and heparan sulfates. The diagnosis is confirmed by the absence of iduronosulfate sulfatase in serum or cultured skin fibroblasts.

SANFILIPPO SYNDROMES

Sanfilippo syndromes type A and type B are phenotypically indistinguishable, although they are caused by different enzyme defects (Table 2). They are noted for the severity of progressive mental retardation that includes behavior management problems; these problems often lead to institutionalization. The somatic changes are mild and of late onset. Moderately coarse features, somewhat thickened skin with hirsutism, and minimal visceral changes are noted. There is no corneal clouding. X-ray findings of an ovoid dysplasia of vertebral bodies may be seen.

Screening tests for mucopolysacchariduria may be weakly positive. The biochemical ab-

normality is the excessive accumulation and excretion of heparan sulfate. The diagnosis is confirmed by the demonstration of deficiencies of heparan N-sulfatase (type A) or α-N-acetylglucosaminidase in leukocytes and serum.

MORQUIO SYNDROME

Patients with Morquio syndrome usually first present in the second year of life with a prominence of the lower ribs and dwarfism. The major manifestations are related to the skeletal dysplasia that results in a barrel-shaped chest, knock-knees, short neck, loose joints, and progressively severe dwarfism. The face shows a broad mouth with prominent maxilla. Mental development is normal. Due to hypoplasia of the odontoid process of the C2 vertebra, atlantoaxial subluxation leads to cervical myelopathy. Patients may show subtle neurologic signs but occasionally develop acute quadriplegia or die suddenly. Corneas slowly become clouded. X-ray shows spondyloepiphyseal dysplasia with striking platyspondly. Patients commonly die in their third or fourth decade

Table 2. *The Mucopolysaccharidoses*

Syndrome	Clinical Manifestations	Mucopolysac-chariduria	Deficient Enzyme
Hurler	Severe mental retardation; hepatosplenomegaly; corneal clouding; skeletal deformities; autosomal recessive	Heparan sulfate Dermatan sulfate	L-α-iduronidase
Hunter	Mental retardation; hepatosplenomegaly; skeletal deformities; no corneal clouding; mild and severe forms; X-linked recessive	Heparan sulfate Dermatan sulfate	Iduronosulfate sulfatase
Sanfilippo types A and B	Severe mental retardation; mild skeletal changes; no corneal clouding; both types clinically identical and autosomal recessive	Heparan sulfate	A: Sulfamidase B: α-N-acetylglucos-aminidase
Morquio	Severe dysplastic skeletal deformities; no mental retardation; corneal opacities; autosomal recessive	Keratan sulfate	N-acetylgalactosamine 6-sulfate sulfatase
Maroteaux-Lamy	Severe skeletal deformities; corneal clouding; normal intelligence; autosomal recessive; may be mild and severe forms	Dermatan sulfate	N-acetylgalactosamine 4-sulfate sulfatase (arylsulfatase B)
Scheie	Normal intelligence; corneal clouding; claw hand and stiff skin, minimal skeletal changes	Dermatan sulfate Heparan sulfate	L-α-iduronidase
Hurler-Scheie compound	Mental retardation and somatic changes intermediate between Hurler and Scheie	Dermatan sulfate Heparan sulfate	L-α-iduronidase
β-glucuronidase deficiency	Mental retardation variable; features and skeletal changes resemble Hurler; autosomal recessive	Dermatan sulfate Heparan sulfate	β-glucuronidase
N-acetylglucosamine 6-sulfate sulfatase deficiency	Mental retardation; skeletal dysplasias	Keratan sulfate Heparan sulfate	N-acetylglucosamine 6-sulfate sulfatase

because of respiratory complications of myelopathy or thoracic deformities or both. The screening tests for mucopolysaccharides may be only weakly positive, especially in the older patient. Keratan sulfate in the urine suggests the diagnosis and the deficiency of N-acetylgalactosamine 6-sulfate sulfatase is confirmatory. A variant in which β-galactosidase is lacking has been described. These patients are not otherwise distinguishable from other patients with Morquio syndrome.

MAROTEAUX-LAMY SYNDROME

The somatic changes in this disorder resemble those of Hurler syndrome, but mental retardation is absent. Symptoms of hydrocephalus may appear and atlantoaxial subluxation may cause neurologic complications. Hepatosplenomegaly and corneal opacities are usual. Skeletal changes include kyphosis, joint contractures, and hip dysplasias evident on x-ray. Mild forms resulting in little functional disability have been noted. The urinary excretion of dermatan sulfate only helps to distinguish this disorder from Hurler syndrome. Diagnosis is confirmed by demonstration of absence of N-acetylgalactosamine 6-sulfatase also known as arylsulfatase B.

SCHEIE SYNDROME AND HURLER-SCHEIE COMPOUND

Scheie syndrome produces the mildest effects of the mucopolysaccharidoses, although corneal clouding may be severe. Patients have normal intelligence, stature, and life span. Claw hands and joint stiffness are most common. Carpal tunnel syndrome is a common complication. The urine has excessive amounts of dermatan sulfate and heparan sulfate, and cells have a deficiency of L-α-iduronidase. The disease thus seems to be a mild allele of Hurler syndrome.

Patients demonstrating abnormalities with severity intermediate between Hurler and Scheie syndrome are believed to have a compound of the Hurler and Scheie genes. They have similar biochemical abnormalities and also lack L-α-iduronidase. Survival is to the mid twenties, but with eventual skeletal and visceral abnormalities with mental retardation.

β-GLUCURONIDASE DEFICIENCY AND N-ACETYLGLUCOSAMINE 6-SULFATE SULFATASE DEFICIENCY

Most patients with β-glucuronidase deficiency have had somatic changes similar to those of Hurler disease, but the severities of clinical manifestations have been variable. Coarse facies and hepatosplenomegaly have been constantly noted, but only some patients have had other visceral changes or delay in mental development. Elevation of urinary mucopolysaccharides may be mild, with increases in dermatan sulfate and heparan sulfate. The diagnosis rests mainly on absence of β-glucuronidase in leukocytes or cultured fibroblasts.

Two patients have been described who had skeletal dysplasia similar to that of a mild form of Morquio syndrome, but who also had mental retardation. Hepatosplenomegaly was noted, along with short stature. This condition has been determined to be a new type of mucopolysaccharidosis, on the basis of the finding of both keratan sulfate and heparan sulfate in the urine and the absence of N-acetylglucosamine 6-sulfate sulfatase in the patients' cells.

DIFFERENTIAL DIAGNOSIS

Since these disorders are progressive, it may be difficult to differentiate one syndrome from another on clinical grounds when the patient is very young. The pattern of urinary mucopolysaccharides is useful but often inconclusive. For example it may be difficult to distinguish Hurler syndrome from Hunter syndrome in a male below the age of 18 months. The determination of the specific enzyme deficiency in serum, leukocytes, or fibroblasts grown from a skin biopsy make the diagnosis conclusive. The Hurler, Scheie, and Hurler-Scheie compound all lack L-α-iduronidase and thus must be differentiated by the clinical course, which should be obvious by the second or third year.

There are a number of other disorders including other storage diseases that may share one or more clinical effects with the mucopolysaccharidoses, such as dysmorphic features, hepatosplenomegaly, skeletal dysplasias, and mental retardation. They are distinguished by a lack of mucopolysacchariduria and by the presence of the biochemical abnormalities and enzymic deficiencies noted in Table 3.

Spondyloepiphyseal dysplasia resembles Morquio syndrome clinically, but patients lack urinary mucopolysaccharides or the specific enzymic deficiency. The Kniest syndrome has some indications that resemble those of the Morquio syndrome, including keratan sulfate in the urine, but again patients with Kniest syndrome do not have the specific enzyme deficiency. A clear pattern of dominant inheritance in Kniest syndrome will aid in the differential diagnosis.

Table 3. *Diseases Resembling the Mucopolysaccharidoses*

Disorder	Diagnostic Biochemical Abnormalities
G_{M1} gangliosidosis	G_{M1} ganglioside and glycoprotein in tissues and urine; β-galactoside deficiency
Mannosidosis	Glycoprotein in urine; α-mannosidase deficiency
Fucosidosis	Glycolipids and glycoproteins in urine and tissues; α-fucosidase deficiency
Mucolipidosis II and mucolipidosis III	Increased lysosomal hydrolases in serum; deficiencies of multiple hydrolases in cells
Multiple sulfatase deficiency	Sulfatides and mucopolysaccharides in tissues; deficient in many sulfatases
Kniest syndrome	Keratan sulfate in urine; no known enzyme deficiency
Spondyloepiphyseal dysplasia	No specific biochemical abnormalities

HETEROZYGOTE DETECTION AND PRENATAL DIAGNOSIS

Heterozygotes for the various mucopolysaccharidoses have cellular levels of the affected enzymes intermediate between those of normal and affected homozygotes. Thus, heterozygotes can often be detected in families of patients having one of the syndromes. Techniques are under development in specialized laboratories to detect female carriers of Hunter syndrome by testing cloned fibroblasts or clonally derived cells present in hair root bulbs.

Cells obtained by amniocentesis during the early second trimester of pregnancy can be cultured and assayed for each of the enzymes involved in the mucopolysaccharidoses. Prenatal diagnosis thus can be done in pregnancies at risk for all of the mucopolysaccharidoses and has been accomplished in a number of cases.

THE NOONAN SYNDROME AND ABNORMALITIES OF THE SEX CHROMOSOMES

By ROBERT L. SUMMITT, M.D.
Memphis, Tennessee

THE NOONAN SYNDROME

SYNONYMS

Male Turner syndrome, female Turner syndrome with normal XX sex karyotype, female pseudo-Turner syndrome, Turner phenotype with normal karyotype, Ullrich syndrome, Ullrich-Noonan syndrome.

DEFINITION

In 1944 Flavell reported a young man who was short of stature and had a webbed neck, cubitus valgus, and evidence to suggest hypogonadism. Flavell was the first to describe this phenotype as the "male Turner syndrome." Similar patients were subsequently reported, and it became obvious that the same phenotype occurred in the female. Following the advent of cytogenetic techniques, patients with this phenotype, both males and females, were found to have sex karyotypes in keeping with their clinical sexual phenotypes. This was in contrast to phenotypic females with the Turner syndrome, in which a sex chromosome abnormality is invariably present.

In 1963, Noonan and Ehmke reported six males and three females with valvular pulmonic stenosis, short stature, hypertelorism, mild mental retardation, ptosis of the eyelids, skeletal anomalies, and, in affected males, cryptorchidism. These children, although manifesting some features in common with the Turner syndrome, were clearly different. None had a chromosome abnormality. Opitz had worked with Noonan during some of her observations and suggested that this phenotype be designated "the Noonan syndrome." We have favored the designation "Noonan syndrome" for several reasons. First, when the name "Turner" is in any way used in the designation of a syndrome, the reader immediately thinks of a sex chromosome abnormality. No sex chromosome abnormality is found in patients with the Noonan syndrome, and avoidance of the eponym "Turner" lessens confusion as to nosology.

Second, when the "Turner" eponym is used, the reader immediately focuses on the clinical features of the Turner syndrome. This is misleading, as it emphasizes only those features of the Noonan syndrome that are in common with the Turner syndrome, and ignores a number of other features that characterize the Noonan syndrome. Third, the Noonan syndrome is heritable, and once a case is identified in a family, a definite recurrence risk applies. In the Turner syndrome, the recurrence risk within a family is virtually zero. Thus the differences between these two conditions must be clearly understood if an accurate diagnosis is to be made and if accurate genetic counseling is to be provided.

The exact frequency of the Noonan syndrome is not known, but it appears to be much more common than the Turner syndrome.

CLINICAL MANIFESTATIONS

The Noonan syndrome is necessarily a clinical entity, as no laboratory test is available to substantiate its diagnosis. Thus its signs and symptoms are based upon clinical observation only and may be somewhat arbitrarily assigned. The diagnosis may be suspected as early as the newborn period in the fully developed phenotype. Shortness of stature is common, occurring in over 70 per cent of those affected. This shortness has been shown to be unassociated with a specific hormone deficiency. Mental retardation is apparent in at least 50 per cent of patients. This is in most instances mild, but IQ scores below 40 have been observed. Convulsive seizures have been observed in 6 of 25 patients in one series. The facies is quite characteristic (Fig. 1), with excessively folded auricular helices in 84 per cent of cases, ears that appear to be low-set in 62 per cent, ocular hypertelorism in 84 per cent, inner epicanthal folds in 58 per cent, ptosis of the eyelids in 50 per cent, downward slanting palpebral fissures in 83 per cent, narrow or high palatal arch in 65 per cent, dental malocclusion or other anomalies of dentition in 52 per cent, and micrognathia in 70 per cent. Scalp defects have been observed, and the hair is often curly and light in color, extending low on the posterior aspect of the neck in 81 per cent of persons affected.

The neck is webbed in 78 per cent of patients and is broad, short, or thick in others. The thorax is malformed in over 75 per cent of

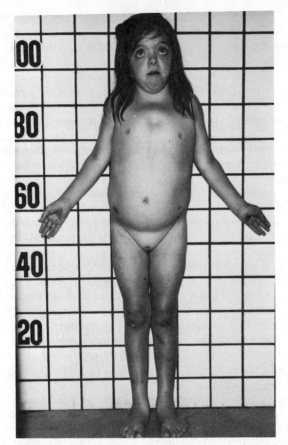

Figure 1. Female child with the Noonan syndrome.

patients, with a peculiar combination of proximal pectus carinatum and distal pectus excavatum. The nipples have been described often as widely spaced, but recent evidence by Collins indicates that this is only an illusion. A "shield chest" is often mentioned. Congenital cardiac defects are encountered in approximately 55 per cent of cases, the most common single defect being pulmonary valvular or infundibular stenosis. Other lesions include atrial septal defect, peripheral pulmonary artery stenosis, patent ductus arteriosus, anomalous pulmonary venous return, and tetralogy of Fallot. In contrast to the Turner syndrome, in which most cardiovascular lesions involve the left side of the heart or the aorta, lesions in the Noonan syndrome characteristically (80 per cent) affect the right side of the heart. Cubitus valgus, or increased carrying angle at the elbow, is seen in 85 per cent of patients, but other limb anomalies are uncommon. No characteristic dermatoglyphic features are known. Renal anomalies are found in about 27 per cent of patients. These include hydronephrosis due to obstructive uropathy, duplication of the collecting systems, and renal hypoplasia. Peripheral lymphedema occurs at some time in life in about 35 per

cent of patients. Unilateral or bilateral cryptorchidism occurs in 70 per cent of affected males. Gonadal function may vary from rare agonadism on one extreme to the completely normal state on the other. Most patients do manifest normal or near normal gonadal function with reproductive potential in females in contrast to the complete absence of gonadal function in the vast majority of persons with the Turner syndrome.

COURSE

The clinical spectrum of severity in the Noonan syndrome is quite variable. In general, some degree of correlation can be drawn between the severity of the somatic phenotype and the degree of mental retardation. However, no such correlation exists regarding the degree of gonadal dysfunction. Every adolescent female under our observation has undergone normal sexual development and has regular menses, although pubescence and menarche have been delayed in some. A few reported females have, on the other hand, had primary or early secondary amenorrhea. Fertility is the rule in affected females. Affected mother and son and/or daughter have been reported and are not uncommon. Affected males most often have normal gonadal function, but seminiferous tubular dysgenesis has been noted along with poor differentiation of Leydig or Sertoli cells. Father-to-son transmission of the Noonan syndrome has now been undeniably documented. The mode of inheritance is probably autosomal dominant. Life span is normal unless shortened by complications related to congenital heart disease.

LABORATORY AND OTHER DIAGNOSTIC TESTS

The primary feature that marks laboratory diagnostic tests in the Noonan syndrome is the fact that they produce normal results. The buccal smear shows that the X- and Y-chromatin patterns are in keeping with the phenotypic sex. Analysis of chromosomes reveals a karyotype appropriate for the phenotypic sex: 46,XX for the affected female, 46,XY for the affected male. These criteria are necessary for a diagnosis of the Noonan syndrome.

No characteristic roentgen findings are known. Bone age may be slightly delayed. The frequency of urinary tract anomalies occurrence is a firm indication that an intravenous urogram should be obtained on every patient with the Noonan syndrome. Electroencephalographic abnormalities are not uncommon, and a peculiar electrocardiographic abnormality has been found not only in affected patients but also in apparently unaffected first-degree relatives. This involves a pronounced left-axis deviation of the QRS complex in the frontal plane. Intelligence testing may reveal deficiency or normal function.

Testicular histologic abnormalities are uncommon and have already been mentioned. No consistent abnormalities have been found in specific tests for endocrine function, including those for pituitary gonadotropins and growth hormone and those which assess target gland function.

Pitfalls in Diagnosis

Since diagnosis of the Noonan syndrome is based solely upon its clinical phenotype, the most common confusion occurs when one is confronted by a prepubertal female and involves the question of whether the patient has the Turner syndrome or the Noonan syndrome. In most cases, familiarity with the complete somatic phenotype of each will allow the correct diagnosis. This can be confirmed by chromosome analysis.

The Noonan syndrome is similar in some ways to the multiple lentigines syndrome. Both appear to be inherited in an autosomal dominant manner. However, the profound deafness so common in the multiple lentigines syndrome, as well as the common occurrence of hypospadias, and the presence of multiple lentigines, should serve to differentiate the multiple lentigines syndrome from the Noonan syndrome.

THE TURNER SYNDROME

Synonyms

Ullrich-Turner syndrome, Bonnevie-Ullrich syndrome, ovarian aplasia or gonadal dysgenesis with associated somatic anomalies, XO syndrome.

Definition

In 1938 H. H. Turner described seven adult phenotypic females with shortness of stature, sexual infantilism, webbed neck, and cubitus valgus. He did not know the etiology of this phenotype that subsequently acquired his name, but he suggested that it was the result of deficiency of pituitary trophic hormones. Several years later exploratory surgery revealed that such patients lacked ovaries, and the term ovarian agenesis, or aplasia, was applied to the condition. Still, the etiology was not known

until 1959, when Ford and co-workers showed that cells cultured from patients with the Turner syndrome contained only one sex chromosome, an X. Such a karyotype is designated 45,X. As a result of this discovery, it became obvious that the clinical spectrum of the Turner syndrome was much broader than previously presumed. It also was found that some patients previously thought to have the Turner syndrome had no demonstrable chromosome abnormality. Such patients are now known to have the Noonan syndrome. In addition, a number of chromosome abnormalities other than 45,X were found to be associated with the clinical phenotype of the Turner syndrome. Nevertheless, all still had one thing in common — the absence of part of the second sex chromosome. As a result of this accumulated knowledge, we have adopted and recommended, for the sake of nosologic clarity, the definition of the Turner syndrome as that spectrum of features that is the result of complete or partial monosomy for the short arm of the X chromosome. Complete monosomy X is the 45,X karyotype, appearing as the only chromosome complement in 57 per cent of patients with the Turner syndrome. Partial monosomy X may result from absence in all cells of part but not all of a second X chromosome due to a structural abnormality, or may result from mosaicism, a situation in which some of the patient's cells are normal but some lack a second X chromosome or part thereof. Rarely, the Turner syndrome may result from the presence of a severely deleted Y chromosome along with a normal X.

The Turner syndrome has an incidence of about 1 in 10,000 live-born females. A much higher incidence at conception is indicated by chromosome studies performed on the products of spontaneous abortion. Recent studies have suggested that only 1 in 300 to 1 in 500 conceptions with a 45,X karyotype survive pregnancy. This means that the 45,X abnormality is a highly lethal situation.

Clinical Manifestations and Course

In only a small percentage of persons affected is the diagnosis of the Turner syndrome made in the newborn period. Only if prominent webbing of the neck or lymphedema of the limbs or both are present at birth is the Turner syndrome suspected. The presence of shortness of stature at birth in the absence of these somatic anomalies ordinarily goes unnoticed, and only later when the patient falls obviously behind her peers in growth rate does the shortness stimulate concern on the part of the parents. Adult shortness is a constant feature, the height range being 114 to 147 cm with a mean of 140.8 cm. The growth rate is not altered by the administration of growth hormone. Lymphedema, present in early infancy, may abate later in childhood only to return in some cases in the second decade of life, with or without estrogen therapy.

Craniofacial features (Fig. 2) include external ears that are longer and narrower than normal and that may have hypoplastic superior helices, hypertelorism, inner epicanthal folds, ptosis of the eyelids, maxillary and mandibular hypoplasia, highly and narrowly arched palate, micrognathia, and dental malocclusion. Although some of these features are also seen in the Noonan syndrome, the total facial phenotypes of the two conditions are quite different (Figs. 1 and 2). The neck is webbed in approximately 50 percent of cases, or it may be short and broad. The hairline extends lower than normal on the posterior aspect of the neck in 73 per cent of patients.

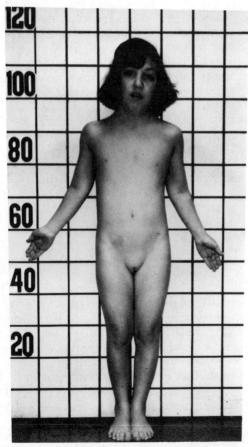

Figure 2. Female child with the Turner syndrome. (From Summitt, R. L.: Endocrine and metabolic disturbances—sex determination, differentiation, and development. *In* Hughes, J. G.: Synopsis of Pediatrics, 3rd ed. St. Louis, The C. V. Mosby Co., 1971.)

Skeletal abnormalities include cubitus valgus (56 per cent of patients) and metacarpal or metatarsal shortening (44 per cent of patients). This shortness most often involves the fourth and fifth metacarpals and metatarsals. Fingernails and toenails are hypoplastic and hyperconvex in 73 per cent of patients. Lymphedema of the dorsa of the hands and feet increases the prominence of the usual dimples overlying the metacarpophalangeal and interphalangeal joints.

The commonly mentioned "shield chest" deformity is apparent in 60 per cent of patients and results from the presence of a rather broad thorax, pectus excavatum in some cases, the appearance of widely spaced nipples, and hypoplasia of the nipples. Congenital heart disease occurs in 15 per cent of patients. Cardiac lesions involve primarily the left side of the heart or aorta and include aortic stenosis and coarctation of the aorta. However, other defects, such as ASD and VSD, do occur. Idiopathic medial necrosis and aneurysm of the aorta are encountered less frequently. Left-sided cardiac lesions are uncommon in the normal female, being limited ordinarily to the male. Renal anomalies occur in 38 per cent of patients and include horseshoe kidney, rotational anomalies, duplication of the collecting systems, and unilateral renal agenesis. Even in the absence of renal anomalies unexplained hypertension occurs in about 25 per cent of patients. Numerous pigmented nevi are notable in 60 per cent of cases. Dermatoglyphic features include distal displacement of the axial triradii, an A main line that extends to the radial base of the thenar region, increased incidence of hypothenar patterns and of third and fourth interdigital patterns, and a high digital ridge count.

While mental retardation has not been considered a feature of the Turner syndrome, 16 per cent of 223 patients in four series of patients with a 45,X karyotype were found to be mentally subnormal. Adult patients may manifest defective space and form perception, diminished mathematical ability, and difficulty with word association. It appears that the incidence of mental subnormality in the Turner syndrome is significantly increased over that in the general population.

Sexual infantilism is part of the syndrome, and only rarely does sex development occur. Because of the absence of functional ovaries, primary amenorrhea occurs with rare exception; in a few cases spontaneous ovarian function has occurred. Ninety-six per cent of 271 patients in four tabulated series of patients with the Turner syndrome had primary amenorrhea, and most of the remaining 4 per cent experienced early secondary amenorrhea. Failure of sex development at puberty, attributable to gonadal dysgenesis, occurs in 94 per cent of patients with the 45,X karyotype. More than 99 per cent of affected females are sterile. However, pubertal feminization, menses, and fertility have been encountered in the Turner syndrome. Thirteen pregnancies have been reported in 10 women with nonmosaic 45,X Turner syndrome. Of these pregnancies, seven infants were normal, two were stillborn, and one had Down syndrome; three pregnancies resulted in spontaneous abortions. Forty-three pregnancies have been reported in women with mosaicism which includes a 45,X cell line in combination with a 46,XX cell line or a 47,XXX cell line or both. Outcomes of these pregnancies included 16 spontaneous abortions, three therapeutic abortions, two stillbirths, two neonatal deaths, 11 infants with congenital anomalies, and nine normal infants. Eight of those with congenital anomalies had chromosome abnormalities; five had mosaic Turner syndrome and three had Down syndrome.

In infancy and childhood a patient with the Turner syndrome may present for one of the following reasons: (1) The Bonnevie-Ullrich phenotype of webbed neck and lymphedema in infancy. (2) Significant prepubertal shortness of stature. When the physician encounters any female child who is short of stature, the Turner syndrome should always be a prominent consideration and proper diagnostic tests should be undertaken. (3) A left-sided congenital heart or aortic lesion. Any female child with such an anomaly has the Turner syndrome until proved otherwise. (4) In the second decade of life, the most common presenting problem is sexual infantilism and primary amenorrhea.

COURSE AND COMPLICATIONS

The course relative to sexual function has been described. Compromised renal function may lead to hypertension, or hypertension may occur even in the absence of renal disease or other demonstrable cause. Victims of the Turner syndrome may live to the fifth or sixth decade of life. Some investigators have reported an increased incidence of thyroid disease and diabetes mellitus in the Turner syndrome. With the exception of patients with 45,X/46,XY mosaicism, gonadal dysgenesis does not apparently predispose to gonadal neoplasia.

LABORATORY DIAGNOSTIC TESTS

In consideration of the definition of the Turner syndrome just set forth, the diagnosis necessarily depends upon the demonstration,

by chromosome analysis, of partial or complete monosomy of the short arm of X. Since 45,X cells bear only one X chromosome, interphase cells from affected patients (obtained most often from a buccal smear) contain no X-chromatin mass. Thus a buccal smear is a useful screening technique in suspected cases of the Turner syndrome. It must be emphasized, however, that it is *only* a screening test, and ultimate diagnosis must depend upon chromosome analysis. In most laboratories, 20 to 50 per cent of buccal mucosal cells from a normal 46,XX female contain an X-chromatin mass (Fig. 3). The presence of an X-chromatin mass in a few but less than 20 per cent of cells suggests sex chromosome mosaicism in which some cells bear two X chromosomes and some only one. If an X-chromatin positive buccal smear is found in a patient who clinically bears a strong resemblance to the phenotype of the Turner syndrome, analysis often demonstrates one normal X chromosome but a structural abnormality of the second X chromosome, such as an isochromosome of the long arm of X [46,X,i(Xq)], deletion of the short arm of X [46,XXp-], 45,X plus fragment that may be of X or Y origin, or a ring-X chromosome [46,X,r(X)]. In such cases chromosome analysis may also reveal mosaicism including a normal cell line and an X-monosomic cell line (45,X/46,XX), or mosaicism involving a structurally abnormal X. Approximately two thirds of patients with the Turner syndrome are X-chromatin negative; one third are X-chromatin positive.

Elevated levels of urinary gonadotropins are found after the expected age of pubescence. Bone age is usually not significantly delayed. Skeletal roentgenograms demonstrate osteoporosis, particularly in untreated adults.

PITFALLS IN DIAGNOSIS

If the previously described modes of presentation are kept in mind, the main diagnostic pitfalls can be avoided. In addition, it should be re-emphasized that the buccal smear is no more than a screening procedure, and if confronted by an X-chromatin positive buccal smear in the presence of a phenotype nevertheless suggestive of the Turner syndrome, the physician must not stop short of analysis of chromosomes. However, a buccal smear should be performed on every patient with Turner syndrome or suspected to have it. Occasionally, analysis of chromosomes from cells from multiple tissues reveals only a 45,X karyotype, while a buccal smear is unequivocally X-chromatin positive. In such an event, the X-chromatin positive buccal smear, if properly documented, indicates the presence of

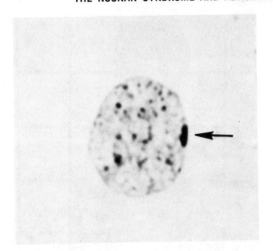

Figure 3. Buccal mucosal cell stained with Fuelgen reaction, demonstrating presence in nucleus, adjacent to nuclear membrane, of densely stained X-chromatin mass or Barr body.

a cell line containing two X chromosomes — thus the presence of mosaicism.

A clinical and cytogenetic variant of the Turner syndrome may occur in the presence of 45,X/46,XY mosaicism. This will be discussed under the heading of 45,X/46,XY mosaicism. Gonadal dysgenesis can occur without the somatic features of the Turner syndrome in an XX female and in an XY individual with a female phenotype. Such patients have primary amenorrhea and sexual infantilism. These instances of so-called XX or XY gonadal dysgenesis are not caused by a sex chromosome abnormality but are the result of a single gene mutation. I would like to emphasize that these patients do *not* have the Turner syndrome. Patients with pseudohypoparathyroidism or pseudopseudohypoparathyroidism (Albright hereditary osteodystrophy) may resemble those with the Turner syndrome because of their shortness of stature, facial phenotype, and skeletal malformations, but they do not have gonadal dysgenesis and do not have a chromosome abnormality. Confusion with the Noonan syndrome has already been discussed.

THE KLINEFELTER SYNDROME

SYNONYMS

True Klinefelter syndrome, seminiferous tubule dysgenesis, primary microorchidism, XXY syndrome.

DEFINITION

The original report of the Klinefelter syndrome by Klinefelter, Reifenstein, and Albright in 1942 described males with testicular hypoplasia, aspermatogenesis, underdevelopment of secondary sex characteristics, gynecomastia, and increased urinary excretion of gonadotropins. However, the etiology was not elucidated until 1959 when Jacobs and Strong found 47 chromosomes in cells from a patient with the Klinefelter syndrome and suggested an XXY sex karyotype. This was subsequently confirmed by others, and other sex chromosome abnormalities have been described. These facts have led us to define the Klinefelter syndrome as the spectrum of features occurring as the result of a sex chromosome complement including two or more X chromosomes in the presence of one or more Y chromosomes. Thus in the absence of such a chromosome abnormality, the Klinefelter syndrome does not exist. The incidence of the Klinefelter syndrome is about 1 in 1000 liveborn males. Significant prenatal mortality has not been documented in the Klinefelter syndrome.

CLINICAL MANIFESTATIONS AND COURSE

Only rarely is a diagnosis of the Klinefelter syndrome made prior to puberty. The prepubertal patient has no characteristic phenotype. However, because mental retardation is a part of the Klinefelter syndrome in about 5 per cent of cases, a child with the condition may be investigated because of mental retardation. If chromosome analysis is a part of that investigation, then the diagnosis of the Klinefelter syndrome can be made. In addition, the testes of patients with the Klinefelter syndrome are abnormally small even prior to puberty. The finding of small testicles in the physical examination of an otherwise normal prepubertal male should alert the examiner to the possibility of the Klinefelter syndrome.

While the prepubertal appearance of patients is not characteristic, several minor anomalies, not limited to and not diagnostic of the Klinefelter syndrome, may be found. These include brachycephaly, minor anomalies of the ears, radioulnar synostosis, and clinodactyly of the fifth finger. Simian palmar creases are more frequent than normal and dermatoglyphic findings include distal displacement of the palmar axial triradius, the presence of hypothenar patterns, and a low digital ridge count.

Ordinarily the symptoms and signs that lead to medical attention are noted only at the time of puberty or thereafter. Hypogonadism is the primary problem at this time. The upper body segment is shorter than the lower, whereas arm span is usually no greater than height and may be shorter. Hypogonadism may lead to a delay in the appearance of secondary sex characteristics or their incomplete development or both. The penis is usually of normal size, but testicles are always very small and insensitive, and pubic hair may have a female distribution. Hyalinization and fibrosis of seminiferous tubules make sterility a constant feature of the Klinefelter syndrome. Progression of these testicular changes may also interfere with testicular endocrine function, leading to reduced libido and impotence. Osteoporosis may be a result of hypogonadism. Truncal obesity may develop, and gynecomastia occurs in approximately 50 per cent of cases.

As mentioned previously, we know that a number of patients with the Klinefelter syndrome are mentally retarded. In addition, personality defects, behavioral problems, minor criminal offenses, and frank psychosis are seen with increased frequency. Approximately 1 per cent of male residents of institutions for the mentally retarded have the Klinefelter syndrome, and the incidence in men in psychiatric institutions is about 0.6 per cent. Life span in the Klinefelter syndrome is normal.

The aforementioned findings describe the so-called "classic" case of the Klinefelter syndrome. In the affected adult population, excluding those with mental retardation, the primary presenting complaint is infertility. Many patients are well developed with no other obvious clinical evidence of hypogonadism. The Klinefelter syndrome affects approximately 10 to 20 per cent of men attending infertility clinics. Thus the Klinefelter syndrome should be kept in mind as an important cause of sterility in men.

The foregoing discussion has dealt primarily with the 47,XXY form of the Klinefelter syndrome. However, other karyotypes are found, including 48,XXXY, 49,XXXXY, 48,XXYY and a 49,XXXYY. As a general rule, the greater the number of X chromosomes, the more severe the phenotypic alteration. All 48,XXXY and 49,XXXXY patients are mentally retarded. All persons with karyotypes more complex than 47,XXY are sterile, and most have more complex congenital anomalies than the 47,XXY patient. Cryptorchidism, although uncommon in the 47,XXY patient, is frequently encountered in the 48,XXXY and 49,XXXXY patients, as is shortness of stature. Skeletal anomalies are more common in those with 48 or 49 chromosomes. A characteristic facial phenotype has been described for the 48,XXXY and 49,XXXXY patients and includes (Fig. 4) minor ear anomalies; epicanthal folds; widely spaced, upward slanting eyes; strabismus; a broad, flat nose; a wide mouth; a short maxilla; and prog-

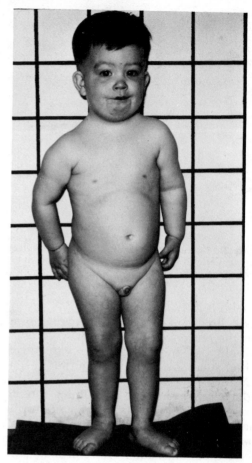

Figure 4.   Male child with karyotype 48,XXXY.

nathism. In the 49,XXXXY patients pes planus is common, and skeletal abnormalities include limitation of flexion at the elbow (caused in about half of patients by radioulnar synostosis); elongation of the distal ulna; metacarpal pseudoepiphyses; clinodactyly of fingers; coxa valga; a short, wide distal phalanx of the great toe; and a thick or abnormally segmented sternum. Dermatoglyphic features include an increased frequency of low arch patterns on the fingertips and the occasional presence of simian creases. Other occasional features include microcephaly, congenital heart disease, cleft palate, clubfoot, small peg-shaped teeth, Brushfield spots in the irides, myopia, inguinal hernia, and hypotonia.

Patients with the 48,XXYY Klinefelter syndrome, although resembling those with the XXY Klinefelter syndrome in the pattern of sexual development, testicular size, and histologic changes, differ in that they are generally taller and more commonly mentally retarded. Other features include short fingers, clinodactyly, cubitus valgus, kyphoscoliosis, varicose veins, and problems with social adjustment such as aggressive or delinquent behavior.

Some investigators have included males with a 46,XX karyotype under the term Klinefelter syndrome. We have preferred the term "XX male." The XX male may be the result of a single gene mutation. However, recent evidence has identified a specific antigen, the HY antigen, as a product of the Y-borne gene that induces male sex determination or of a gene linked closely thereto. This antigen is absent in XX females and in the presence of all other karyotypes that do not include a Y chromosome. This HY antigen, on the other hand, has been detected in some XX males, leading to the suggestion that the male determining segment of the Y chromosome is in fact present in the XX male, translocated to an autosome or to an X chromosome. Such a translocation has, however, not been demonstrated cytologically.

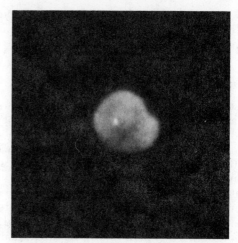

Figure 5. Buccal mucosal cell stained with quinacrine mustard and photographed in fluorescence microscope, demonstrating presence of brightly fluorescent point or Y-chromatin mass within nucleus.

COMPLICATIONS

Complications are in general related to mental retardation and aberrant social adjustment in all forms of Klinefelter syndrome. Early onset of peripheral vascular disease seems to occur not only in the 48,XXYY form but in other forms as well. Vertebral collapse may result from osteoporosis. Gonadal neoplasia does not seem to be a problem.

LABORATORY AND OTHER DIAGNOSTIC TESTS

By definition the Klinefelter syndrome involves an abnormality of chromosomes, the most common karyotypic abnormality being 47,XXY. The presence in cells of two X chromosomes (as in the normal female) makes the determination of the presence of the X-chromatin mass in such cells as those from the buccal mucosa a useful screening procedure for the detection of 47,XXY and more complex Klinefelter karyotypes. The buccal smear in all forms of the Klinefelter syndrome is invariably X-chromatin positive. If the karyotype is 48,XXXY, the buccal mucosal cells may contain two X-chromatin masses, and the 49,XXXXY form may contain three X-chromatin masses. The maximum number of X-chromatin masses visible in a cell is one less than the number of X chromosomes in that cell. The use of fluorescence techniques for evaluating buccal mucosal cells allows determination of the number of Y chromosomes in those cells. A Y chromosome is demonstrated by the presence, in interphase cells stained with quinacrine mustard or a similar compound and examined in the fluorescence

microscope, of a brightly fluorescent mass of chromatin within the nucleus (Fig. 5). The number of such brightly fluorescent masses within a nucleus bears a 1:1 ratio to the number of Y chromosomes within that nucleus. Thus cells from a patient with the 48,XXYY Klinefelter syndrome would contain a maximum of one X-chromatin mass by ordinary techniques and a maximum of two Y chromatin masses by the fluorescence technique.

Any abnormality demonstrated in a buccal smear must be confirmed by chromosome analysis. In addition to the 47,XXY, 48,XXXY, 49,XXXXY, and 48,XXYY abnormalities already discussed, karyotypes in the Klinefelter syndrome have included 46,XY/47,XXY or 46,XX/47,XXY mosaicism. Although the presence of mosaicism may be suggested by buccal smear findings, it is elucidated only by chromosome analysis.

Investigation is indicated for any male with sterility or other evidence of hypogonadism, any male who is mentally retarded, and any male with gynecomastia or other somatic features encountered in the Klinefelter syndrome.

In pubertal and postpubertal patients, urinary excretion of gonadotropins is excessive, and if endocrine gonadal function is compromised, urinary excretion of 17-ketosteroids is deficient. Roentgenograms are indicated to elucidate suspected skeletal anomalies such as radioulnar synostosis. Testicular biopsy prior to puberty reveals little, but close scrutiny may demonstrate a deficiency of germ cells. Changes occurring after puberty include hyalinization, fibrosis, and atrophy of seminiferous tubules. Some tubules may be lined only by Sertoli cells. Leydig cells, even if present in increased numbers, may be histologically abnormal.

PITFALLS IN DIAGNOSIS

A diagnosis of the Klinefelter syndrome should not be made in the absence of one of the sex chromosome abnormalities previously discussed. Some authors still include X-chromatin negative, karyotypically normal patients with seminiferous tubule dysgenesis within the scope of the Klinefelter syndrome. In view of current knowledge of the cytogenetic nature of the Klinefelter syndrome, such cases should not be included. The X-chromatin negative, karyotypically normal form of hypogonadism and seminiferous tubule dysgenesis, which resembles clinically the Klinefelter syndrome, represents a nosologically heterogeneous group of conditions that may include the del Castillo syndrome, the Kallmann syndrome of hypogonadism and anosmia, the "fertile eunuch" syndrome, and other conditions, some of which are determined by a single gene mutation. Awareness of the phenotypic features of the Klinefelter syndrome and its variants and proper utilization and interpretation of diagnostic tests should prevent diagnostic errors.

THE POLYSOMY-X CONDITIONS

SYNONYMS

Triple-X female, XXX female, "superfemale"; four-X female, XXXX female, tetra-X female; five-X female, XXXXX female, penta-X female; X-polysomy.

DEFINITION

The term "polysomy-X" is used here to describe any phenotypic female whose cells contain more than two X chromosomes. The first triple-X (47,XXX) female was reported in 1959 by Jacobs and coworkers in a 17-year-old "superfemale" with secondary amenorrhea. Subsequent reports have dealt with triple-X females ascertained primarily in institutions for the mentally retarded or mentally ill. Other affected persons have been mentally normal. The current estimate of the frequency of the triple-X female, based upon population surveys, approximates 1 per 1000 live female births. However, the rate in mentally ill females is 1 in 420, and in mentally retarded females may be as high as 1 in 220.

In contrast to the triple-X female, the tetra-X and penta-X conditions are rare. The 48,XXXX karyotype has been reported in 21 females and the 49,XXXXX karyotype, without mosaicism, in only 9.

CLINICAL FINDINGS AND COURSE

In the triple-X female no characteristic phenotype has been formulated on the basis of numerous case reports. Although most reported patients are mentally retarded or mentally ill, this is a reflection of the fact that these patients were ascertained through surveys of institutions for the mentally retarded and mentally ill. It is now apparent that although some triple-X females are retarded, have personality deviations, manifest ovarian dysfunction, and exhibit various congenital anomalies, many others have normal mental and gonadal function, are fertile, and are physically normal. Recent studies of 11 XXX females discovered at birth and followed for 9 years have revealed that about two thirds are intellectually normal and well adjusted, whereas one third have exhibited delay in early motor development and speech, a mild intellectual deficit, and disturbance in interpersonal relationships. Reported abnormalities include infertility, early secondary amenorrhea, underdeveloped breasts, cretinism, strabismus, nystagmus, congenital heart defect, and skeletal malformations. Again, however, these features occur irregularly, and no pattern has evolved. Ordinarily life span is not affected.

On the basis of the finding in the Klinefelter syndrome that more severe phenotypic alteration accompanies the presence of more than two X chromosomes, early predictions were made that higher grades of X-polysomy would also result in more severe phenotypic alterations. The small number of cases of tetra-X and penta-X females does not allow firm conclusions, but even the few reports available indicate that the phenotypic variability in the tetra-X and penta-X females is probably as wide as in the triple-X female. Although most affected patients are mentally retarded or mentally ill, the majority of them have been found in surveys of mental institutions. No characteristic phenotype has evolved. Normal intelligence has been reported in at least one patient each with a 48,XXXX and a 49,XXXXX karyotype.

The one phenotypic feature that does characterize all forms of X-polysomy is a decrease in the digital dermal ridge count on the fingertips. This is similar to that associated with extra X chromosomes in the Klinefelter male.

LABORATORY AND OTHER DIAGNOSTIC TESTS

A decreased number of primordial follicles has been reported in the ovaries of a few triple-

X females. However, ovarian function is normal in most and most are fertile. No consistent biochemical abnormalities, including hormonal, have been found. Electroencephalographic abnormalities have been described in the triple-X, tetra-X, and penta-X female. IQ determinations have revealed subnormal intelligence in many, and tests for personality have commonly revealed deviations such as paranoid or schizoid personality and inability to form meaningful interpersonal relationships. However, none of these features is characteristic of or diagnostic of X-polysomy.

X-chromatin study is an effective screening procedure for X-polysomy, because as many as two X-chromatin masses may be found in cells of a triple-X female. It should be kept in mind that not all X-chromatin-bearing cells contain the maximum number, but cells containing the maximum number are ordinarily abundant enough that they can be confirmed in the evaluation of 100 to 200 cells.

The ultimate diagnosis of X-polysomy depends upon the demonstration by chromosome analysis of cells with karyotypes 47,XXX, 48,XXXX, 49,XXXXX, or mosaicism involving these cell lines.

PITFALLS IN DIAGNOSIS

The primary diagnostic pitfall in the poly-X conditions is the failure to obtain X-chromatin determination and chromosome analysis in females with mental retardation or mental illness. A buccal smear is a simple and inexpensive screening technique. The evaluation of every female with mental retardation, frank mental illness, or behavioral deviation should include a buccal smear for X-chromatin evaluation.

THE XYY ABNORMALITY

SYNONYMS

XYY male, YY male, "supermale."

DEFINITION

Since the original description of a male with a 47,XYY karyotype by Sandberg and coworkers in 1961, this chromosome abnormality has stimulated great interest among cytogeneticists, psychiatrists and psychologists, attorneys, and criminal investigators. The terms XYY male and XYY abnormality are self-explanatory and need no further definition. The XYY condition is probably one of the most common chromosome abnormalities in man, with an estimated frequency of 1 in 1000 live-born males.

CLINICAL FINDINGS AND COURSE

Following the original description of an XYY male, a considerable number of cases were found in surveys of institutions for mentally defective or mentally ill criminals. Phenotypes associated with a 47,XYY karyotype have included male pseudohermaphroditism with female phenotype (probably coincident testicular feminization) or intersex genitalia; tall males with normal genitalia but with behavioral aberrations; radioulnar synostosis; pachydermoperiostosis; and phenotypes suggesting the action of simple autosomal gene mutations such as the Marfan syndrome. On the other hand, some XYY males have no abnormalities.

Based upon the consensus of available information, the primary phenotypic features, although by no means constant, include increased stature and an increased risk of aberrant behavior. This behavioral aberration is characterized by immaturity of personality, a passive, dependent personality, and the inability to control impulses. Otherwise the only frequent finding is a decreased digital ridge count. Affected patients are fertile, and despite the presence of an extra Y chromosome in a father, offspring of XYY men with three exceptions have been karyotypically normal. The first reported XYY male was the father of a child with (47,XX,+21) Down syndrome, and one XYY man has fathered a 47,XYY son. In addition, an XYY son of a mosaic 46,XY/47,XYY father has been reported.

LABORATORY DIAGNOSTIC TESTS

Plasma testosterone levels have been elevated in some series, and normal or even low in other cases. Urinary excretion of testosterone and gonadotropins has also been quite variable. Bone age is normal.

X-chromatin determination of the conventional variety used in the investigation of deficiency or excess of X chromosomes is of no value in the investigation of the XYY abnormality. However, two fluorescent Y-chromatin masses are visible in interphase cells from the buccal mucosa that have been stained with a quinacrine compound. Still, ultimate diagnosis depends upon the demonstration by analysis of a 47,XYY karyotype.

PITFALLS IN DIAGNOSIS

The primary problem is probably the clinical overdiagnosis of this abnormality. Because of its publicized association with tall stature and tendency to criminal behavior, the search for XYY males has been biased in this direction. There can be no doubt that the frequency of the

47,XYY karyotype is increased in such populations as compared with the frequency in the general population. On the other hand, tall stature in a male with criminal tendencies does not per se indicate the presence of a 47,XYY karyotype, and doubtlessly the 47,XYY karyotype is commonly associated with phenotypic normality.

45,X/46,XY MOSAICISM

SYNONYMS

Mixed gonadal dysgenesis, asymmetric gonadal dysgenesis, mosaic male pseudohermaphroditism, male hermaphroditism due to X-chromosomal defects, XO/XY mosaicism, gonosomal intersexuality.

DEFINITION

The term "mixed gonadal dysgenesis," coined by Sohval in 1964, describes patients, most but not all of whom had intersex genitalia, with an undifferentiated gonadal streak on one side and an intra-abdominal testis on the other side. Such patients have been found to have a chromosome abnormality with 45,X/46,XY mosaicism. Opitz has thus preferred the designation gonosomal intersexuality. Accordingly, gonosomal intersexuality is defined as that spectrum of features associated with a 45,X/46,XY mosaic karyotype.

CLINICAL FINDINGS AND COURSE

The 45,X/46,XY chromosome abnormality is interesting in that it is associated with a wide variety of sexual phenotypes. On one extreme of the spectrum is the phenotypic female with somatic and gonadal features of the Turner syndrome. In some such patients with somatic features of the Turner syndrome, clitoral enlargement and other signs of virilization may occur. On the other extreme of the phenotypic spectrum is the male without somatic, genital, or reproductive abnormality. Between these extremes are several varieties of intersex, including those involving an apparently otherwise normal male phenotype with hypospadias, a hypoplastic or cleft scrotum, and varying degrees of labial fusion with enlarged clitoris and perineal urogenital orifice. Gonadal development varies from the presence of bilateral streak gonads on one extreme to bilateral apparently normal testicles on the other. Some patients have, as in Sohval's original reports, a streak gonad on one side and a normal or dysgenetic

testicle on the other. Some streak gonads contain mesonephric hilar remnants, and hilus cells in these areas are apparently capable of stimulating genital virilization.

The possibility of 45,X/46,XY mosaicism should be considered in any patient with the Turner syndrome, especially if that patient has clitoral enlargement, in any patient with intersex genitalia, and in any male with apparently isolated hypospadias. A proper karyotypic diagnosis is important, because in those patients with 45,X/46,XY mosaicism an increased risk of gonadal neoplastic change exists, and in such cases streak gonads or hypodysplastic testes should be removed.

Life span is normal in this condition unless shortened by cardiac or urinary tract abnormalities or complicated by a malignant gonadal neoplasm.

LABORATORY DIAGNOSTIC TESTS

Gonadal histology usually reveals more or less dysplasia, although histologically normal testes are possible. A testis may envelop a neoplasm such as a gonadoblastoma or seminoma, or may reveal seminiferous tubule dysplasia with absence of germ cells. Streak gonads may be typical of the type seen in the 45,X Turner syndrome, may contain mesonephric hilar remnants, or may contain neoplastic cells.

The buccal smear stained by conventional techniques is invariably X-chromatin negative. However, cells stained with quinacrine, depending upon the percentage of 46,XY cells within the cell population investigated, contain a brightly fluorescent Y chromatin mass. Ultimate diagnosis of 45,X/46,XY mosaicism depends upon its demonstration by chromosome analysis. The demonstration of this mosaicism may require analysis of cells from multiple tissues such as blood, skin, fascia, and even gonad. We have studied one patient with the Turner syndrome and clitoral enlargement in whom cells from blood and skin were 46,XY, and 45,X/46,XY mosaicism was demonstrable only by analysis of cells from a streak gonad.

PITFALLS IN DIAGNOSIS

45,X/46,XY mosaicism emphasizes the need for adequate cytogenetic investigation of all patients with evidence of intersex genitalia, of males with apparently isolated hypospadias (probably excluding glandular hypospadias), and of patients with features of the Turner syndrome, especially those with clitoral enlargement. "Adequate cytogenetic investigation" in this sense means the analysis of cells cultured from multiple tissues if necessary to demonstrate 45,X/46,XY mosaicism.

COMMENT ON PRENATAL DIAGNOSIS

Current techniques for the culture of cells from amniotic fluid allow chromosome analysis of fetal cells. Thus any sex chromosome abnormality can be diagnosed in the fetus at 15 to 16 weeks' gestation. However, this technique does not now have the importance in these conditions that it has in certain autosomal abnormalities. In the case of some autosomal abnormalities, the risk of an affected child is a definite indication for offering to parents the possibility of prenatal diagnosis. However, at this time the low risk in most pregnancies of a sex chromosomally abnormal product, and questions surrounding indications for therapeutic abortion in sex chromosome abnormalities, the phenotypes of which are so variable, give these conditions a low priority rating in consideration of prenatal diagnosis.

COMMON SURGICAL DISEASES OF THE NEWBORN

By DAVID L. COLLINS, M.D.
San Diego, California

BIRTH TRAUMA

FRACTURES

The commonest bone to be fractured at birth is the clavicle. Signs are not usually apparent immediately, but during the second week a lump will be noticed due to excess callus formation. Depressed fractures of the skull are usually of the Ping-Pong ball variety and are diagnosed by simple palpation.

INJURIES OF PERIPHERAL NERVES

Injury to the brachial plexus (Erb's palsy) is caused by mild to severe tears of the roots of the brachial plexus. The Moro reflex will be absent on the affected side. The arm will not move spontaneously, but passive movements are normal. C5 and C6 roots are commonly injured, resulting in extension of the upper arm with medial rotation and adduction. Injury of the phrenic nerve roots and paralysis of the diaphragm may also be observed.

INJURY TO INTRA-ABDOMINAL ORGANS

Rupture of the liver or spleen may cause intra-abdominal bleeding with shock and abdominal distension. If the processus vaginalis is patent, scrotal discoloration may be observed. Rupture of the adrenal or kidney may cause retroperitoneal hemorrhage with a bulging flank on the affected side.

CEPHALHEMATOMA

This is a large, fluctuant swelling that is limited by the periostial attachments of one of the cranial bones, usually parietal. A ridge is commonly felt around the periphery of the hematoma, which, to the uninitiated, feels like a depressed fracture. It is to be distinguished from caput succedaneum, which is simply postpartum scalp edema and which is not confined to the surface of one cranial bone.

TUMORS OF THE HEAD AND NECK

CYSTIC HYGROMA

Most hygromas are evident at birth and present as a swelling in the neck that usually transilluminates brilliantly but, following trauma, may contain blood. They may also be located in the axilla or groin, or they may extend into the mediastinum. There is usually no airway obstruction immediately unless there is extension into the pharynx or upper trachea. Chest x-rays should always be taken to determine the presence of mediastinal extension.

CERVICAL TERATOMA

These lesions may be confused with cystic hygroma but are solid, lumpy and pendulous. They do not transilluminate and are usually centrally located in the neck.

CONGENITAL CLEFTS

A cleft lip is usually obvious to gross inspection and may be unilateral or bilateral, and may or may not be associated with a cleft palate.

There is a minor form of cleft lip in which the skin and lip itself are intact but in which there is a gap in the underlying tissues and a widened nostril on the affected side.

Clefts of the palate usually present as an inability to suck properly and may be displayed with a tongue depressor and flashlight, taking care to get complete exposure back to the tip of the uvula.

A cleft palate associated with micrognathia, or Pierre Robin syndrome, results in moderate to severe airway obstruction when the baby is supine owing to the tongue falling back through the cleft and obstructing the airway. The condition is usually promptly corrected by nursing the baby in a prone position.

CHOANAL ATRESIA

This is a dangerous condition in the newborn that, if bilateral, demands early diagnosis. This is because the newborn baby breathes through his nose; mouth breathing is learned in later life. Thus, a baby with bilateral choanal atresia may asphyxiate. The diagnosis is suggested by noting that a baby who has adequate ventilation when he is crying, and hence mouth breathing, is unable to breathe and has severe retraction and cyanosis when he is quiet. The diagnosis is established if a catheter cannot be passed through one or both nostrils into the pharynx. It will also be noted that the respiratory distress may be relieved by opening the mouth with a tongue depressor or laryngoscope. Radiologic confirmation is obtained by filling the nostrils with barium and taking lateral x-rays in the supine position.

CONGENITAL DIAPHRAGMATIC HERNIA

POSTEROLATERAL (FORAMEN OF BOCHDALEK)

The signs and symptoms of this condition vary greatly according to the magnitude of the hernia. It is believed that well over half of these hernias are so massive that they cause stillbirth or death very shortly after birth, before diagnosis can be made.

Patients with the very large hernias who do survive long enough to permit diagnosis present with severe respiratory distress, tachypnea, and cyanosis at birth. One of the most helpful diagnostic signs is a flat abdominal wall caused by the absence of abdominal organs from their normal location. Auscultation of the chest usually reveals displacement of the heart sounds away from the affected side. Absence of breath sounds on the side of the hernia may be more difficult to determine. Bowel sounds in the chest are not usually heard in the severe neonatal variety of hernia but may be helpful in milder cases diagnosed in older babies and children.

The diagnosis is confirmed by plain chest roentgenograms, which usually show a bowel gas pattern in the chest. In a very young baby, during the first hour or so of life and before much air has been swallowed, the herniated viscera may be largely airless, and diagnosis can be made by noting mediastinal shift and compression of the opposite lung.

The use of contrast media is usually unnecessary and may be dangerous. However, in doubtful cases, particularly less severe cases in older children, it may be helpful.

Radiologically, the main condition to be differentiated is cystic adenomatoid malformation of the lung. In this condition the intact diaphragm and the normal distribution of abdominal viscera may be seen on x-ray. Less severe degrees of posterolateral diaphragmatic hernia may cause mild to moderate respiratory symptoms in the infant at a few days of age or even later. This condition in the occasional patient may go undiagnosed until late childhood or even adult life.

ANTERIOR DIAPHRAGMATIC HERNIA (FORAMEN OF MORGAGNI)

Mild symptoms of respiratory distress may be present. A lateral roentgenogram of the chest may be most helpful in demonstrating passage of small bowel in front of the liver and into the anterior mediastinum. The use of contrast media in the intestine is frequently helpful; the contrast medium may be given either by enema or by mouth. It has been suggested that there may be an association between this condition and mental retardation, especially Down's syndrome.

EVENTRATION OF THE DIAPHRAGM

This consists of a congenital weakness and elevation affecting the *entire* diaphragm and is to be distinguished from congenital diaphragmatic hernia by the presence of a sac in which part of the diaphragm is normal and only part is attenuated. It is also to be distinguished from paralysis of the diaphragm due to nerve or muscle disease.

Respiratory symptoms may be mild or severe. The diagnosis is made radiologically by noting a smooth elevation of the entire hemidiaphragm.

HIATAL HERNIA AND GASTROESOPHAGEAL REFLUX

In the newborn the most prominent symptom is vomiting, which may start in the first few days of life and result in poor weight gain or aspiration or both. An upper gastrointestinal series using barium will usually indicate the diagnosis by demonstrating free gastroesophageal reflux with or without the presence of hiatal hernia.

ESOPHAGEAL ATRESIA

Atresia of the esophagus may be associated with tracheoesophageal fistula, most commonly from the lower esophagus to the trachea, or from the upper trachea, which is quite rare, or there may be no fistula at all. Maternal hydramnios is present in 85 per cent of babies with esophageal atresia owing to the inability of the infant to swallow amniotic fluid.

The first symptom is inability of the infant to swallow saliva. The presence of large quantities of saliva in the mouth will be noted early by the alert nurse. The diagnosis may be confirmed clinically by the fact that a stout rubber catheter cannot be passed into the stomach. It is important not to use a flimsy feeding tube, which may curl up in the upper esophagus and give the erroneous impression that it is passing into the stomach. A No. 12 urethral catheter, well lubricated, is passed in through the mouth. If esophageal atresia is present, the catheter will pass only a distance of approximately 11 cm down from the lips.

The diagnosis may be confirmed radiologically simply by taking an x-ray of an opaque catheter curled in the upper esophagus, or by the injection of a few drops of barium into the upper esophagus, with care taken not to cause aspiration of barium into the lungs.

CONGENITAL TRACHEOESOPHAGEAL FISTULA WITHOUT ATRESIA

This lesion often escapes diagnosis during the neonatal period, since there is no obstruction to swallowing. The major symptom is coughing and cyanosis, present only during feeding, with frequent attacks of pneumonia. The fistula may be seen by upper gastrointestinal series but is most readily diagnosed by bronchoscopy using the Hopkins lens system, which makes it possible to see the orifice of the fistula on the back of the trachea and to cannulate it with a ureteral or small Fogarty catheter. Passage of the catheter into the esophagus is then confirmed by esophagoscopy.

SPACE-OCCUPYING LESIONS OF THE CHEST

PNEUMOTHORAX

This condition may be spontaneous or may be associated with vigorous attempts at resuscitation. The major symptom is usually severe respiratory distress with cyanosis. Breath sounds may be diminished, although in the newborn infant this is difficult to determine because of transmission of normal breath sounds from the opposite side. Shift of the trachea is also difficult to determine. Whenever the condition is suspected, chest x-ray should be obtained immediately. If the baby is in extremis and immediate x-rays are unobtainable, a diagnostic thoracentesis should be done using a 14-gauge plastic intravenous cannula over a needle and withdrawing the needle part as soon as possible to prevent injury to the underlying lung. The plastic cannula will also serve as a temporary treatment while awaiting x-rays; it may be connected to an intravenous set, with the other end put under water.

PLEURAL EFFUSION

Congenital pleural effusion is uncommon but causes mild to moderate respiratory distress. Plain roentgenograms of the chest are usually diagnostic, and the diagnosis is confirmed by aspiration of the fluid through a plastic cannula of the type just mentioned.

CYSTIC ADENOMATOID MALFORMATION OF THE LUNG

This condition also causes mild to moderate respiratory distress. X-rays of this condition may be mistakenly believed to show congenital diaphragmatic hernia, since the gas pattern sometimes resembles that of the gastrointestinal tract. However, the presence of a normal diaphragm and a normal distribution of abdominal organs should suggest the correct diagnosis. If necessary, a barium series may be done.

CONGENITAL LOBAR EMPHYSEMA

This condition may present in the newborn as an emergency but usually comes on gradually at 2 or 3 weeks of age. The symptoms are those of respiratory distress. Plain roentgenograms are usually diagnostic, indicating overdistension of either an upper or right middle lobe, but almost never a lower lobe.

DISORDERS OF THE ABDOMINAL WALL

INGUINAL HERNIA

This lesion is not usually an emergency in the newborn, and its diagnosis is usually comparatively simple at a later age. However, occasionally a newborn baby will be noticed to have a hard mass at the external inguinal ring that may demand immediate treatment. In a boy, the main differential is between incarcerated inguinal hernia and encysted hydrocele of the cord. If the mass has been present for a day or more and the baby shows no symptoms of bowel obstruction, the diagnosis is hydrocele. Transillumination is not of much help in differentiating the two. In the infant, it is frequently possible to make the correct diagnosis by means of a rectal examination. The examining finger is passed up into the sigmoid colon and the inguinal area is examined from the back. If the lesion is an incarcerated hernia containing intestine, comparison of the two sides will lead to the discovery of the bowel mesentery stretched taut and passing down into the internal ring.

In difficult cases x-rays may show gas-filled intestine in the scrotal or inguinal area, together with evidence of small bowel obstruction.

While the bowel is rarely infarcted in an incarcerated hernia in an infant, the testicle frequently is, and immediate treatment is therefore necessary.

A small, mobile mass situated in an inguinal hernia in a girl is most likely ovary. Although frequently it is irreducible, there is rarely any vascular embarrassment. This has been reported, however, and it is probably desirable to operate on these hernias without delay if there is any doubt.

OMPHALOCELE

The diagnosis of the condition is usually quite obvious. In the intact form of omphalocele a mass of protruding viscera of varying size will be present, covered by a sac composed of an inner layer of peritoneum and an outer layer of amnion. Small omphaloceles, however, may be missed and may simply look like a thickening of the base of the cord. This condition is dangerous in that the cord may be amputated close to the abdominal wall with resulting injury to the omphalocele contents.

There is a type of omphalocele in which the sac is absent and the intestines may be thickened and matted, because they have been bathed in amniotic fluid for a variable period of time. This lesion is commonly called gastroschisis. The opening may appear to be to one side of the midline but this is more apparent than real and is due to the insertion of the umbilical cord structures at the edge of the defect, usually on the baby's left side.

Omphalocele may be part of a syndrome associated with macroglossia, low blood sugar, and other anomalies described by Beckwith. It also may be associated with cleft of the sternum, anterior diaphragmatic hernia, cardiac diverticulum, and intracardiac anomaly (pentology).

PATENT OMPHALOMESENTERIC DUCT

Presence of a communication between the umbilicus and the ileum may be first disclosed by the passage of meconium or gas. A potentially serious complication of the condition is prolapse of the bowel to form a typical ram's horn lesion with a single stem and two curved arms composed of everted ileum, which may result in intestinal obstruction and strangulation. For this reason, early treatment of a patent omphalomesenteric duct is necessary.

URACHAL REMNANTS

There may be a complete communication between the umbilicus and the bladder, allowing urine to leak from the umbilicus. More commonly, a cystic remnant of the urachus is sealed off in the abdominal wall; this may produce a subumbilical mass or infection, usually in later life.

GASTROINTESTINAL OBSTRUCTION

HYPERTROPHIC PYLORIC STENOSIS

The chief symptom of this condition is vomiting, which usually does not begin at birth but at 2 to 3 weeks of age. The vomiting becomes forceful and projectile, and is never bile-stained. The infant is typically hungry immediately after vomiting. Observation of the epigastrium in a suitable light may reveal peristaltic waves passing from left to right. The most important diagnostic sign is palpation of the hypertrophied pylorus. This may be facilitated by emptying the stomach with a No. 10 plastic catheter with extra holes cut near its end, inserted through the nose. This catheter should be left in the stomach and the baby given some glucose water to drink via a nipple. With the stomach empty, the pylorus will be felt in the midline, just above the umbilicus. It is most helpful for the examiner to relax the rectus abdominus muscles by flexing the baby's hips and lumbar spine, with the feet held in his right hand while he feels for the pylorus with his left index finger.

While in obscure cases a barium upper gastrointestinal series may be helpful, it should be remembered that spasm of the gastric antrum can produce all the radiologic signs of hypertrophic pyloric stenosis. Operation should not be undertaken until the pylorus has been definitely felt.

INTESTINAL OBSTRUCTION

A family history of cystic fibrosis of the pancreas or Hirschsprung's disease and the presence of hydramnios or Down's syndrome should suggest the possibility of congenital intestinal obstruction. The three cardinal clinical findings in intestinal obstruction are as follows: (1) Vomiting. This is copious and usually bile-stained unless the obstruction is in the supra-ampullary duodenum. (2) Abdominal distension. This is more marked the lower the site of obstruction and may be absent in cases of duodenal obstruction. (3) Absence of bowel movements. In high intestinal obstruction there may be one or two bowel movements after birth, composed of pre-existing meconium. The absence of a bowel movement in the first 24 hours of life in itself is an indication for further investigation and should direct attention particularly to the possibility of Hirschsprung's disease.

The diagnosis of intestinal obstruction can usually be made by simple x-rays of the abdomen taken in upright, supine, and lateral views. In obscure cases, the administration of contrast media may be helpful. X-rays may also suggest the cause of the obstruction. For example, large masses of meconium giving a ground glass appearance will suggest the diagnosis of meconium ileus associated with cystic fibrosis of the pancreas. A barium enema is frequently helpful. A microcolon indicates simply that the colon has never been used and the congenital small bowel obstruction is present. Typical findings of Hirschsprung's disease may not be demonstrable by barium enema in infancy. The outlining and subsequent passage of a meconium plug may be aided by barium enema and should raise the possibility of Hirschsprung's disease. The diagnosis of Hirschsprung's disease may be established definitely by rectal biopsy. If an experienced pediatric pathologist is available, a suction biopsy of mucosa alone, as described by Noblett, is adequate.

It is especially important to make an early diagnosis of volvulus of the small bowel, which, in the newborn, is associated with incomplete rotation and may progress to gangrene. This diagnosis is suggested by the onset of vomiting, either at birth or a few days or weeks later. Plain x-rays may demonstrate obstruction at the ligament of Treitz, usually without gross duodenal distension, which serves to differentiate this condition from duodenal atresia. The passage of blood per rectum is a late sign, indicating impairment of blood supply to the bowel.

Because of the possibility of volvulus, all cases of duodenal obstruction in the newborn demand immediate urgent operation or a barium enema to rule out malrotation.

NECROTIZING ENTEROCOLITIS

This condition has become more common in recent years, probably due to the ability of the neonatologist to keep small, sick, premature babies alive. It is this portion of the neonatal population that usually develops necrotizing enterocolitis. The condition seems to be caused by vascular insufficiency to the intestine, resulting in partial or complete infarction. It is often associated with periods of anoxia, respiratory distress, or shock. It is characterized by abdominal distension, passage of bloody diarrhea, vomiting, and circulatory collapse. Abdominal x-rays may demonstrate only distended bowel. However, the pathognomonic radiologic findings are gas in the intestinal wall or gas in the hepatic portal vein or both.

BILIARY ATRESIA

This condition was formerly thought to consist of a congenital atresia of the bile duct analogous to intestinal atresia and was distinguished from neonatal hepatitis. These two conditions are now believed to be different stages of the same process. Neonatal hepatitis is an inflammatory condition of the liver resulting in obstruction at the small bile duct level. This may apparently progress down the biliary tree and cause inflammatory obstruction, stenosis, and atresia of the major bile ducts. Babies with biliary atresia typically become jaundiced at a week of age. The elevation of bilirubin seldom exceeds 15 mg per 100 ml and is almost entirely of the direct-acting variety. Physical examination may reveal an enlarged, hard liver, although this is not always the case. Many attempts have been made to distinguish biliary atresia from neonatal hepatitis by means of such tests as radioactive rose bengal administration and its subsequent measurement in the stools and urine and its localization in the abdomen by means of radionuclide scanning.

However, the definitive diagnosis still must be made surgically by means of an operative cholangiogram and liver biopsy. It is possible to perform these procedures via the laparoscope, but most surgeons prefer to do it by means of a laparotomy.

IMPERFORATE ANUS

This condition is usually obvious if the perineum is carefully inspected in a good light at birth. However, this is often not done and the diagnosis may not be made until a nurse attempts to take a rectal temperature. A fistula may be present to the perineum in males or females, or to the urinary tract in males, or to the vestibule or vagina in females. It is important to determine the presence of such a fistula. A fistula that is not obvious immediately at birth may show itself 24 hours or more later by the presence of a drop of meconium. For this reason, injudicious early colostomy is to be avoided. Careful inspection of the perineum with a hand lens is often helpful.

There is a rare variant of imperforate anus (rectal atresia) in which the anus itself appears normal but in which there is an obstruction in the midportion of the rectum. This diagnosis may be made by digital rectal examination and confirmed by barium enema. It is important to do the barium enema, because to the inexperienced examiner all babies may appear on palpation to have a high atresia of the rectum due to characteristic narrowness of the rectosigmoid junction.

Demonstration of the site of the fistula in a male may often be made by means of retrograde urethrogram. If no fistula to the perineum or genitourinary tract can be demonstrated, it is possible to inject diatrizoate sodium (Hypaque) directly into the rectum. A No. 14 plastic cannula over a sharp needle is introduced through the anal dimple, and with guidance via an image intensifier with the baby in the lateral position, the tip of the needle is guided up the curve of the sacrum and into the rectal pouch. The needle is then withdrawn and the plastic cannula irrigated with saline. The recovery of meconium-stained fluid proves the location of the cannula in the rectum. The rectal pouch may then be outlined by the injection of diatrizoate sodium (Hypaque). This method is much superior to the upside down x-ray, which is notorious for its inaccuracy in demonstrating the end of the rectal pouch.

ABDOMINAL TUMORS

RENAL MASSES

The commonest renal tumor in the neonate is not the classic Wilms' tumor of older childhood, but a benign variant that may be called congenital mesoblastic nephroma. This lesion is quite benign and has an excellent prognosis. It presents as a firm flank mass in the neonate. Intravenous pyelography shows deformity of the collecting system.

Cystic renal lesions such as hydronephrosis or multicystic kidney are usually distinguished clinically because of the consistency of the swelling. A large cystic lesion may occasionally be transilluminated in a newborn. In these lesions intravenous pyelography will often show nonfunction.

NEUROBLASTOMA

Neuroblastoma in the newborn may arise in the adrenal medulla anywhere along the sympathetic chain in the abdomen or chest. X-rays will show a large, soft tissue tumor often containing calcification. Elevated levels of urinary catecholamines will strongly suggest diagnosis of neuroblastoma.

Infantile neuroblastoma may be associated with multiple subcutaneous metastases. The metastatic nodules are blue and may be surrounded by a blanched area of skin, owing to their production of catecholamines. This condition is called "blueberry muffin" syndrome.

OVARIAN TUMORS

These are most commonly non-neoplastic in the newborn girl and are commonly large unilocular cysts arising either from the follicle or corpus luteum. Torsion may occur if the cyst is not removed promptly.

UROGENITAL ANOMALIES

EXSTROPHY OF THE BLADDER

This unfortunate condition is immediately obvious at birth. The everted bladder extends from the low-placed umbilicus down to the site of the urethra. The ureteral orifices may be visualized in the trigone.

There is a variant of this lesion called exstrophy of the cloaca, which is associated with an imperforate anus and a fistula between the intestine and the bladder. This condition is often associated with short gut and has a high mortality.

AMBIGUOUS GENITALIA

Grossly ambiguous genitalia constitute a neonatal surgical emergency. It is essential to establish the sex of rearing before the baby leaves the hospital. Adrenogenital syndrome may be associated with the inability to retain salt and may be diagnosed by analysis of the serum electrolytes demonstrating a low sodium and elevated potassium. In addition, complete endocrinologic analysis will be necessary to establish the exact type of this syndrome. Another helpful study in many cases of this type is the retrograde "urethrogram," which may demonstrate that the urethra is actually a urogenital sinus or vagina. Chromosome analysis will also be necessary in many of these patients and can now be done rapidly using cells from the bone marrow. The services of an experienced dysmorphologist and pediatric endocrinologist are often invaluable.

HYPOSPADIAS

In this condition the urethral opening is located at varying points on the underside of the penis instead of at the tip. It is associated with a chordee or ventral curvature of the shaft. In a simple hypospadias with normally located testes no further investigation is necessary. However, if a hypospadias is associated with either unilateral or bilateral undescended testis, then complete evaluation to establish sex is indicated.

EPISPADIAS

In this condition the penile shaft is foreshortened and the opening is located on the dorsal surface. It is a minor degree of exstrophy of the bladder and, if the opening is located far enough back, will be associated with diastasis pubis and urinary incontinence.

UNDESCENDED TESTIS

It is normal for the testes to be undescended in smaller premature babies, born at 7 months gestation or less. Such testes may be expected to descend spontaneously. In full-term babies, testicular descent may also occur up to the age of 9 months. After this time, however, it has been established that spontaneous descent almost never takes place.

SACROCOCCYGEAL TERATOMA

This tumor is thought to arise from totipotent cells of Hensen's node, which is situated in the sacrococcygeal area. The tumor may be quite small or as large as the baby's head. It is usually external but may be internal, pushing the rectum forward and partially or completely obstructing it. The incidence of malignancy in neonatal sacrococcygeal teratoma is approximately 7 per cent. This rises with the age of diagnosis up to 50 per cent at the age of 2 years. The main clinical differentiation to be made is between sacrococcygeal teratoma and low sacral myelomeningocele. In the latter, paralysis and anesthesia of the perineum or lower extremities are to be expected. Teratomas tend to displace the anus forward. Pressure on a myelomeningocele may produce increased tension in a fontanel.

LOWER URINARY TRACT OBSTRUCTION IN CHILDREN

By STEPHEN P. SMITH, M.D., and JOHN P. SMITH, M.D.
Columbus, Ohio

SYNONYMS

Bladder neck contracture, spasm of bladder neck, bladder sphincter dyssynergia, bladder neck hypertrophy, median bar, outlet obstruction, Marion's disease (congenital bladder neck obstruction), ectopic ureteroceles, posterior urethral valves, prostatic sarcoma, urethral stenosis, urethral stricture, urethral valves, urethral diverticula, meatal stenosis, hymenal veil or ring, and urogenital sinus with obstruction. (Lyon's ring may in some circumstances be included in this group as well as other less frequently encountered obstructive conditions.)

DEFINITION

Bladder neck obstruction, in contrast with ureteral obstruction, over the years has been deemed less important in urinary tract disorders in the pediatric age group. A spectrum of conditions occur in children, of which outlet (lower urinary tract) obstruction or resistance is a component. These related conditions interfere with normal voiding patterns and perpetuate the overlying symptom complex of obstruction. This causes bladder distention which leads to reflux or ureteral outflow resistance. If the condition goes untreated, dilatation of the ureters and renal pelvis will result, with retained urine and possible concomitant infection. Both the abnormal intraluminal pressures and infection contribute to reduction or eventual permanent loss of renal function.

Presenting Signs and Symptoms

The age of which clinical manifestations of lower urinary tract obstruction appear may depend upon the severity and degree of obstruction. Symptoms may become manifest at birth, in the neonatal period, in early childhood, or during adolescence. The pathophysiology of the obstructive lesions involved must be considered, since they range from congenital abnormalities to acquired progressive lesions. The most severe lesions are usually recognized in the immediate neonatal period. These include sepsis, pyuria, hematuria, abdominal distension, neonatal ascites, flank masses, and electrolyte disturbances. Less severe obstructive disorders may present clinically as failure to thrive, abnormal renal function, abnormal voiding patterns, abdominal pain, and nausea and vomiting. Acquired lesions, neurogenic disorders, and extrinsic obstructive lesions are often first noted in a change in the voiding pattern or with the symptoms of a urinary tract infection, such as urgency, frequency, dribbling, burning, enuresis, retention, or voluntary infrequency. In boys, a change in the caliber of stream may be noted.

Course

The severity of the lesion is often associated with symptom duration before diagnosis. Severe upper tract deterioration is uncommon except in patients with posterior urethral valves, ectopic ureteroceles, prune belly syndrome, and hydrometrocolpos. The major damaging factors are the degree of the obstruction and the chronicity of the lesion. Lower tract obstruction leads to increased bladder pressure and incomplete bladder emptying. Subsequent bladder hypertrophy, bladder diverticula, ureteral reflux, hydroureteronephrosis, recurrent cystitis, and pyelonephritis may be the result.

The diagnosis should lead to treatment to assure adequate drainage and to lessen the intraluminal pressures. It should also decrease urinary stasis.

Physical Examination

The physical findings may be totally diagnostic or may be unrevealing. Inspection of the external genitalia is essential. In males, retraction of the foreskin with inspection of the meatus and palpation of the urethra may reveal phimosis, paraphimosis, meatal stenosis or inflammation, urethral diverticula, and anterior urethral valve and urethral strictures (especially in the acquired lesions of the perineum secondary to straddle injuries of the bulbous urethra). In females, by gentle lifting of the labia upward and outward, the urethral meatus and vaginal introitus are nearly always excellently exposed. Prolapsed urethrocele, paraurethral cysts, hydrometrocolpos, labial fusion, or sarcoma botryoides may be seen.

Whenever it is possible, observation of voiding can prove invaluable to detect narrow-caliber stream, spraying, dribbling, straining, and intermittency, all of which are suggestive of obstruction of the lower urinary tract.

Rectal examination for sphincter tone may be helpful in detecting neurogenic lesions. The presence of constipation may be associated with neurologic lesions or voluntary voiding disorders. Inspection of the lower spine might reveal signs of spinal dysrhaphia or lipoma associated with neurologic defects.

Abdominal palpation should be done for suprapubic masses and bladder distention. Renal palpation is rarely useful unless severe decompensation has already resulted.

Common Complications

The most severe problems are usually seen in the neonatal age groups and are associated with severe obstruction. Ascites, uremia, electrolyte imbalance, as well as dehydration and associated infection, may be seen. More commonly cystitis and pyelonephritis are the initial complications. These complications usually lead to diagnosis before progressive renal damage occurs.

Laboratory Findings

Abnormal urinalysis and positive urine cultures are very helpful. Abnormal results in blood studies such as blood urea nitrogen (BUN), creatinine, calcium, phosphorus and electrolytes reflect severe renal impairment and are useful only in diagnosis of the more severe obstructive lesions. Specific gravity change may be an early indication of neonatal urinary obstruction.

Radiography is usually the most definitive diagnostic adjunct in these lesions. The intravenous pyelogram reveals the status of the upper tract and the size and shape of the bladder. Trabeculation, diverticula, ureteroceles, and tumors such as rhabdomyosarcomas can be outlined. Voiding studies are diagnostic of posterior urethral valves. Urethral strictures, diverticula, and anterior urethral valves are also defined with the aid of a retrograde urethrogram. Cinefluoroscopy may be useful in the more subtle voiding disorders. Barium enemas and vaginograms are indicated when extrinsic lesions are present.

Cystoscopic examination can confirm a radiologic diagnosis and help in evaluating the extent of bladder hypertrophy.

Nuclear imaging techniques are now proving useful in assessment not only of renal function but also of bladder function. The nuclear cystogram with simultaneous pressure monitoring can provide accurate information, including the presence of reflux, pressure at time of reflux, bladder volume, and residual volume.

Increasing sophistication of micturition urodynamic flow studies has improved our record of diagnosis of neurologic voiding disorders. Noninvasive techniques, with the use of skin electrodes to assess the sphincter activity, are helping in the diagnosis of the more subtle disorders of voiding. Measure of the flow rate and urethral pressure profilimetry are methods of urodynamic evaluation that are useful in diagnosing non-neurologic obstructive lesions.

THERAPEUTIC TESTS

Insertion of suprapubic Intracath as a form of temporary diversion in cases of severe renal impairment may prove or disprove the existence of associated bladder outlet obstruction.

PITFALLS IN DIAGNOSIS

Rapid response in urinary tract infections to therapy may be misleading. High urinary concentration levels of antibiotics can often obliterate a urinary infection without relieving obstruction or urinary stasis.

Obstruction may be relative and present with constant dribbling or "overflow incontinence." In these instances the constant voiding may mislead the practitioner into missing this diagnosis.

Failure to thrive, dehydration, nausea and vomiting, and fever of unknown origin must also arouse suspicion of conditions of urinary tract involvement.

DOWN'S SYNDROME*

By FRANK J. MENOLASCINO, M.D.
Omaha, Nebraska

SYNONYMS

Mongolism, trisomy 21, congenital acromicria.

DEFINITION

Down's syndrome is the most common recognizable cause of serious mental retardation. It is caused by the presence of an extra number 21 chromosome within the normal chromosome complement. Besides mental retardation, Down's syndrome is associated with many physical stigmata and a variety of congenital malformations. The incidence among live-born infants ranges between 1.0 and 1.5 per 1000. The prevalence of Down's syndrome at all ages is on the order of 0.35 to 0.50 per 1000.

CLINICAL DIAGNOSIS

In recent years the importance of the clinical diagnosis of Down's syndrome has been somewhat overshadowed by the relative ease of cytologic diagnostic confirmation. Yet clinical diagnosis is of particular importance to the parents, who usually can be informed of the clinical test results as early as 24 hours after birth, long before the results of standard chromosomal studies are available.

The diagnosis of Down's syndrome is usually straightforward in older children and adults. In the newborn it is more difficult, since isolated signs of Down's syndrome may also be found in normal newborns. However, there are certain signs on physical examination, x-rays, and dermatoglyphics that may be used to confirm a clinical impression of Down's syndrome.

*Support of this review was provided by the Mental Health Project of the UNICO National.

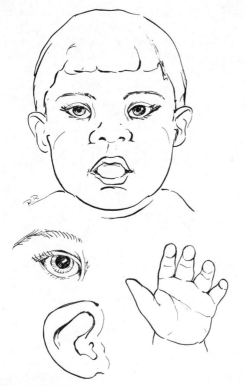

Figure 1. Clinical signs in the facies, eye, hand, and ear in Down's syndrome.

The most common presentation of the newborn with Down's syndrome is a small, slightly premature infant displaying marked generalized hypotonia. The incidence of prematurity is increased 20 per cent compared to the 6 per cent of normal neonates, and birth weight averages 400 grams less than that of term infants. Other pertinent signs are evident in the head and extremities. The skull is brachycephalic (shortened in the anteroposterior diameter) with a flattened occipital protuberance. The anterior fontanel may be enlarged and a sagittal fontanel is frequently found 1 to 2 cm anterior to the occipital fontanel. The typical flattened facies is secondary to poorly developed nasal bones. The palate is narrow and high-arched in configuration. Four major eye signs are associated with Down's syndrome: oblique palpebral fissures, epicanthic folds, Brushfield spots (densely packed stromal fibers on the iris appearing as white or light-colored specks), and hypoplasia, or thinning, of the peripheral third of the iris. Recently, the "purse-string" sign has been described, in which the eyelids of crying infants appear pursed up with vertical wrinkling of the eyebrows. The ears of Down's syndrome infants are often small and dysplastic, with changes in the helix (i.e., overlapping or rectangular configuration), and are often comma-

shaped in appearance. An excess of skin on the back of the neck, while difficult to quantify, is another common physical finding.

Additional diagnostic signs are found in the hands and feet. The hands are small and spade-like in shape. There is often a single transverse palmar crease (simian line) and the fifth finger may be curved inward (clinodactyly) secondary to dysplasia of the middle phalanx. Abnormalities seen in the feet include a wide space between the first and second toe (the "sandal gap") and an adjacent plantar furrow.

Significant radiologic findings include dysplasia of the middle phalanx of the fifth finger and characteristic changes in the pelvis. Caffey and Ross originally described two main diagnostic pelvic features: the first is bilateral flattening of the lower edges of the iliums, measured as the acetabular angle, and the second is bilateral widening and flaring of the iliac wings, which is measured as the iliac angle. The sum of both acetabular angles and both iliac angles divided by 2 is the iliac index or Caffey's index.

A number of diagnostic indices for Down's syndrome have been constructed, using dermal configurations. Perhaps the easiest and most widely used configuration is the *atd angle*. The angle is formed by lines drawn from the palmar triradius (t) to the triradius proximal to the base of the index finger (a), and from (t) to the triradius proximal to the base of the fifth finger (d). In normal infants, the palmar triradius is at the base of the palm and the atd angle is usually less than 45 degrees. In Down's syndrome infants, the palmar triradius is often at or near the center of the palm, so that the atd angle is usually greater than 80 degrees.

A number of checklists have been compiled to aid in diagnosis. Table 1 synopsizes the 10 cardinal signs; the presence of six or more of

Table 1. *The 10 Most Characteristic Physical Features of Down's Syndrome in Infants and Children*

Physical Feature	Percentage Affected
Flat facies, brachycephalic skull	95
Oblique palpebral fissures, epicanthal folds	88
Lack of Moro reflex, muscular hypotonia	88
Hyperflexibility of joints	85
Abnormal teeth; malocclusion	75
Dysplastic pelvis (x-ray)	75
Narrow and high-arched palate	75
Dysplastic ears	72
Short, curved 4th finger (dysplastic middle phalanx on x-ray); short, broad hands	72
Transverse palmar crease	67

these signs in infants and children is considered diagnostic of Down's syndrome. However, diagnostic difficulties may arise because normal premature newborns and young infants may display stigmata that make a clinical differentiation from Down's syndrome very difficult. Whenever the diagnosis is in doubt, a chromosome analysis is indicated. If the complement of chromosomes is normal, Down's syndrome is almost certainly excluded.

MEDICAL COMPLICATIONS

The Down's syndrome patient is at risk for many medical complications. The neonatal period is a particularly critical time for the appearance of cardiovascular and gastrointestinal malformations. The increased incidence of congenital heart disease in Down's syndrome over the general population is about 40 times, with estimations ranging between 28 and 56 per cent. Approximately one third of these defects is atrioventricularis communis while another third is composed of isolated ventricular septal defects. Common major congenital abnormalities of the gastrointestinal tract include tracheoesophageal fistula or stenosis, duodenal obstruction, congenital megacolon, and imperforate anus. Also found are relative in-

creases in the frequency of cleft palate and bifid uvula.

The most significant hematologic aberration associated with Down's syndrome is acute leukemia of childhood. There are also a number of other congenital hematologic disorders seen with Down's syndrome, the most common of which is the leukemoid reaction of white cells. Transient leukemoid reactions can resemble leukemia, and occur not infrequently in Down's syndrome children.

The ocular signs seen in the newborn are not harmful. Yet, as these children age, a number of ocular complications arise, such as lens opacities, strabismus (usually convergent), nystagmus, and keratoconus.

Difficulties with dentition are also characteristic of Down's syndrome. Eruption of deciduous and permanent teeth is delayed and irregular. Congenital absence or fusion of both deciduous and permanent teeth is not unusual. The teeth are commonly microdentic or malformed. Significant malocclusions are seen in the majority of older patients. Interestingly, the incidence of dental caries is relatively low in those having Down's syndrome.

In Down's syndrome, there is an increased incidence of infections, particularly those of the upper respiratory tract. Down's syndrome has also been frequently associated with hepatitis.

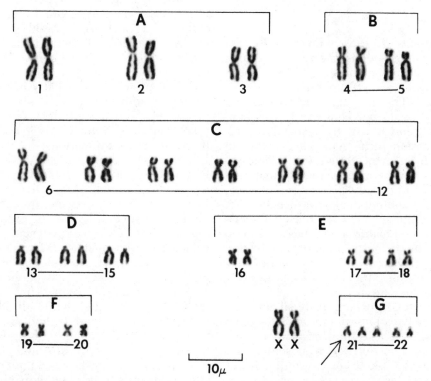

Figure 2. Karyotype of two-month-old girl with Down's syndrome illustrating the most common chromosomal finding: trisomy of the G(21–22) group.

In institutions, the frequency of Australian antigen is 10 times greater in Down's syndrome residents than in other residents. The presence of this antigen leads to a chronic anicteric hepatitis characterized by persistent abnormal liver chemistries.

In almost all Down's syndrome adults over 40 years of age there is evidence of microscopic and histochemical changes in the brain identical to those in Alzheimer's disease (e.g., characteristic neurofibrils). Yet only 35 per cent of these persons over age 40 demonstrate any clinical evidence of this condition.

INTELLIGENCE AND DEVELOPMENT

Mental retardation is the most consistent clinical feature in Down's syndrome. The majority of persons with Down's syndrome have an IQ between 35 and 54, with about 10 per cent having an IQ greater than 55 and 10 per cent having one below 35. Developmental attainments are behind those of normal children. (Most Down's syndrome infants are not able to sit up unaided until after age 12 months or walk without assistance until after 24 months.) Important differences in rates of development are seen when comparing persons with Down's syndrome raised at home and in institutions; those raised at home consistently show a superiority in rate of development.

CYTOGENETICS

It was Lejeune in 1959 who initially described 47 chromosomes in the tissue cultures of Down's syndrome persons. Since then, three categories of the trisomy 21 phenomenon have been described. The first, standard trisomy 21, is found in 94 to 95 per cent of Down's syndrome persons and is usually associated with primary disjunction during meiosis, resulting in a gamete with an extra chromosome. The incidence of trisomy 21 with respect to maternal age is biomodal in distribution; young mothers are affected, and another peak is associated with increased maternal age. This increased association with advanced maternal age has long been thought to be due to faulty oogenesis; however, recent studies have shown that the father may be the source of the extra chromosome in up to 30 per cent of the cases.

The second category of chromosomal phenomena is the translocations found in 3 to 4 per cent of the cases. These translocations usually involve another acrocentric chromosome, such as the D-group (13, 14, 15) or G-group (21, 22), and are referred to as D/G or G/G translocations. In Down's syndrome, about one half are D/G and one half are G/G. This is not dependent on maternal age and no phenotypic differences exist between standard trisomy 21 and translocation trisomy 21. Fifty per cent of the D/G and 90 per cent of the G/G translocations are sporadic or de novo translocations in which the parents have normal chromosomal complements. The remainder are the results of one of the parents having a "balanced" translocation. Female carriers of a balanced D/G translocation have a 10 to 15 per cent chance of producing offspring with Down's syndrome, while male carriers have a 4 to 5 per cent chance. Risks for 21/22 balanced carriers having affected offspring is 6 per cent for females and less than 3 per cent for males. All offspring of 21/21 translocations are affected.

Lastly, chromosomal mosaicism accounts for 1 to 2 per cent of Down's syndrome cases. Phenotypically, mosaics range from being indistinguishable from typical Down's syndrome to being clinically normal.

Indicated for chromosome analysis is any infant suspected of having Down's syndrome clinically, especially if the clinical diagnosis is not clear-cut. Chromosome analysis for parents is reserved for those whose infants karyotypically show translocation.

LABORATORY STUDIES

In the neonate with Down's syndrome, there is a greater than expected frequency of polycythemia as well as elevated bilirubin levels. Other hematologic findings include macrocytosis, reticulocytosis and, later, acute leukemia of childhood.

Serum proteins are usually in the lower normal range with decreased levels of albumin and increased gamma globulin. This could be a reflection of nutritional deficiencies and the increased rate of infections.

Increased serum uric acid levels have been found. This could be due to rapid turnover of leukocytes, which may also explain why Down's syndrome persons generally show an increase of several leukocytic enzymes, including alkaline phosphatase, acid phosphatase, galactose-1-phosphate, uridyl transferase, and glucose-6-phosphate dehydrogenase. Two erythrocytic enzymes, phosphohexokinase and serum glutamic oxaloacetic transaminase (SGOT), are elevated, while all other enzymes in erythrocytes, platelets, and fibroblasts seem to be unaltered. Currently, the relationship between alpha-1-antitrypsin and Down's syndrome is unclear. Although a high percentage of young Down's syndrome persons have been found to have elevated enzyme levels, adults with the syndrome show normal serum concentrations.

Earlier studies on oral tryptophan loading noted decreased urinary excretion of xanthuremic acid and indoacetic acid. Since these findings suggested a disorder of tryptophan metabolism in Down's syndrome, treatment with oral 5-hydroxytryptophan has been utilized to improve developmental progress. To date, neither the general developmental progress nor global intellectual levels have been appreciably or consistently improved.

ENDOCRINE FUNCTION

Mean fasting blood sugar, glucose tolerance tests, and fasting insulin levels in children with Down's syndrome are within normal limits, although there have been reports of significantly increased frequency of diabetes mellitus in Down's syndrome patients under 20 years of age.

Infants and young children with Down's syndrome are almost always euthyroid clinically and have normal laboratory assessment of thyroid function despite increased levels of thyroid antibodies in this population. Recently it has been shown that a large percentage of the adult population with Down's syndrome have abnormal thyroid function tests.

AMNIOCENTESIS

Amniocentesis for the prenatal diagnosis of Down's syndrome is done between 14 and 16 weeks of gestation. Consultation with a center that provides this service, and also genetic counseling, is to be recommended. Indications for amniocentesis are:

1. Chromosomal signs in the parents. This includes D/G, 21/22, 21/21 balanced carrier states, mosaicism with trisomic 21 cell line, and maternal standard trisomy 21.

2. Maternal age. Women 35 years or older should be offered the option of amniocentesis.

3. Family history of Down's syndrome. With the birth previously of an infant with Down's syndrome, the risk that a subsequent infant will have Down's syndrome is 1 to 2 per cent, regardless of maternal age.

A recent large study by the National Institute of Child Health and Human Development found no increase in fetal loss due to midtrimester amniocentesis and a diagnostic accuracy of 99.4 per cent. A new experimental procedure, whose safety and efficacy has not yet been determined, involves obtaining a transvaginal sample of the trophoblast at 6 to 8 weeks of gestation. This would result in earlier studies that, if positive, would allow for suction curettage rather than intra-amniotic injection of an abortifacient agent.

Currently, social and religious points of view have seriously questioned the morality of this prenatal approach to diagnosis. An often forgotten point is that amniocentesis most frequently eventuates in a comforting (negative) diagnosis for the parents. At all times, pastoral or personal counseling or both should be offered to the prospective parents.

CONCLUSION

It would be remiss not to underscore that a confirmative clinical diagnosis should be followed by supportive counseling for the parents. Focus on explanation, guidance as to developmental expectations, and emotional support are extremely helpful. It is to be noted that the modern long-term management of these youngsters within their family and home setting has proven to be most beneficial in furthering the extent of their ultimate developmental attainments. Citizen and professional advocacy groups, such as the National Association for Retarded Citizens, have been very supportive of the modern community-based approach to providing services and help for these handicapped citizens and their parents.

Section 17

DISEASES OF CONNECTIVE TISSUE (THE COLLAGEN DISEASES)

SYSTEMIC LUPUS ERYTHEMATOSUS

By CAROLYN M. BRUNNER, M.D.,
and JOHN S. DAVIS, IV, M.D.
Charlottesville, Virginia

SYNONYMS

SLE, "lupus," disseminated lupus erythematosus.

DEFINITION

Systemic lupus erythematosus (SLE) is a multisystem, episodic disease of unknown cause but associated with an altered immune reactivity. Its outstanding pathologic feature is inflammation of small blood vessels. Proliferative changes of the vascular endothelium are noted in some patients, while in others, especially those who have central nervous system manifestations, no significant microscopic abnormalities are found. The disease predominantly affects females, in whom the peak incidence occurs between the second and fourth decades of life. The incidence of SLE in males remains constant throughout life.

The American Rheumatism Association has proposed the following "preliminary" criteria for a diagnosis of SLE. If four or more are present, serially or simultaneously, a patient is said to have the disease: (1) butterfly rash, (2) discoid lupus, (3) Raynaud's phenomenon, (4) alopecia, (5) photosensitivity, (6) oral or nasopharyngeal ulceration, (7) arthritis without deformity, (8) LE cells, (9) chronic false-positive serologic test for syphilis, (10) profuse proteinuria, (11) cellular casts, (12) pleuritis or pericarditis, (13) psychosis or convulsions in the absence of uremia or offending drugs, and (14) hemolytic anemia or leukopenia or thrombocytopenia. These criteria have been found to be most useful for classification of lupus patients in clinical studies. In the individual patient, fewer than four of the criteria may exist at time of presentation to the physician, or, as will be detailed, symptoms and signs *not* included in the criteria list may be predominant.

PRESENTING SIGNS AND SYMPTOMS

The onset of SLE can be insidious, manifested by vague constitutional symptoms such as low-grade fever and easy fatigability, or explosive, with several systems actively involved. Since each system can be part of the illness, it is probably best to review the spectrum of alterations within each.

Over 90 per cent of patients have some type of rash. A violaceous erythema over the malar eminence resembling a butterfly shape is considered the "classic" rash. The discoid lupus lesion, prominent on the helix of the ear and over the upper trunk, is distinctive because of the hyperkeratosis and depigmentation that develop in the healing phase. (The latter is responsible for the name *lupus*, Latin for wolf. The skin lesion is suggestive of the wolf's bite.) A variety of other skin changes — urticaria, generalized erythematous maculopapules, periungual erythema or telangiectasia or both, bullae, discrete vasculitic macules, and ulcerations — are nonspecific. Photosensitivity is characteristic but does not occur in all patients. Mucous membrane lesions include ulcerations in the nose and oropharynx, the latter usually on the palate and tongue rather than on the buccal mucosa.

Alopecia, or excessive hair loss, is frequently frontal but may be patchy (alopecia areata). Rarely, there is total loss of hair.

Musculoskeletal involvement may be manifested by joint pain (arthralgia) or objective joint heat, swelling, and tenderness, which can progress to deformity in the form of contractures and subluxations, especially in digits. This arthritis is distinguished from rheumatoid arthritis radiographically by being nonerosive. Muscular pain and tenderness can be related to an inflammatory myopathy; rarely, muscle weakness is secondary to a syndrome resembling myasthenia gravis.

The most common form of pulmonary change is pleurisy, but parenchymal involvement ranges from acute pneumonitis ("lupus pneumonia") to chronic interstitial fibrosis; both are characterized by dyspnea. Vascular inflammation can produce pulmonary hypertension, as well as pulmonary hemorrhage and secondary hemoptysis. Pericarditis is the most frequently encountered cardiac symptom; myocarditis is suggested by cardiomegaly and congestive heart failure or arrhythmias or both. Although verrucous endocarditis (Libman-Sacks disease), suspected because of a murmur, is generally not hemodynamically significant, acute aortic and mitral regurgitation can occur as a result of valvular perforation. Coronary insufficiency is most likely related to premature atherosclerosis as a complication of steroid therapy but can be secondary to arteritis. Arterial instability is most commonly recognized as Raynaud's phenomenon.

Hepatosplenomegaly is very common in children with SLE but is unusual in affected adults.

Although mild liver function abnormality may be detected, striking derangement of hepatic enzymes is usually related to salicylate ingestion. Perforations of the small and large intestines have been reported. Lupus peritonitis can be difficult to distinguish from appendicitis or pancreatitis.

The true incidence of renal involvement in patients with SLE is unknown but probably ranges between 75 and 100 per cent. Urine sediment and urinary protein can suggest glomerulonephritis, but these do not appear to be an accurate indicator of the type of renal lesion (see later discussion). Recently, interstitial nephritis has been recognized in some patients; however, it has no distinctive clinical pattern.

The frequency of neuropsychiatric involvement has gained attention during recent years. Seizures and organic brain syndromes are most common; hemiparesis, transverse myelitis, chorea, headaches, and cranial nerve and peripheral neuropathies also occur.

COURSE

Characteristic of the disease is the variability of its course, as well as a tendency to remit and exacerbate independent of therapy. Involvement of certain systems, such as renal and neurologic, is more predictable and tends to have a worse prognosis. Generally in the individual patient flares of disease activity are mimetic; patterns of system involvement tend to recur. New manifestations may evolve but are usually not dominant.

PHYSICAL EXAMINATION FINDINGS

The alterations on physical examination will depend on the system and extent to which it is involved. In mild or early disease, no abnormalities may be found. The only typical findings are related to the skin when malar erythema or "discoid" lupus lesions are present. Thinning of hair and mucosal ulceration tend to parallel disease activity. Swelling and tenderness of peripheral joints, especially proximal interphalangeal and metacarpal phalangeal joints of the hands, will occasionally progress to easily reducible swan-neck deformities. A rub confirms pleuritis or pericarditis. Adenopathy and hepatosplenomegaly may be found. Muscle weakness may be demonstrated. There is some indication that retinal cytoid bodies (whitish exudates) correlate with neurologic involvement.

COMMON COMPLICATIONS

Many of the complications during the course of SLE are related to therapy and may be difficult to distinguish from disease activity. Although patients with the disease may be prone to infections, the addition of high-dose corticosteroids or immunosuppressive drugs or both increases the probability of infection, especially by fungi and unusual bacterial or viral organisms. The appearance of fever must be approached as infection rather than disease activity until infection has been ruled out. Common symptoms such as headache may be the first indication of cryptococcal meningitis.

Posterior subcapsular cataracts, excessive weight gain, gastrointestinal bleeding, and osteoporosis are frequent side effects of corticosteroid use; corticosteroids also aggravate hypertension and lead to premature atherosclerosis. Aseptic necrosis of bone is being recognized increasingly as the cause of joint pain, especially in weight-bearing joints such as hips and knees. (Aseptic necrosis can also occur during the course of SLE, in the absence of corticosteroids.)

LABORATORY FINDINGS

Since the patient with SLE often presents with multiple nonspecific complaints that are easily confused with many other disorders, the laboratory holds a strong position in the patient's evaluation. The most valuable tests for the diagnosis of SLE are those that detect serum antibodies to nuclear materials (ANA). Since refinements in technique and antigenic purification are occurring so rapidly, it is difficult to recommend a "one best approach." However, an immunofluorescence screening test is the first step: the absence of antinuclear antibody (ANA) virtually excludes a diagnosis of SLE. An outline of selected ANA characteristics is shown in Table 1.

Historically, the LE cell phenomenon was the first diagnostic test for the disease, and while it continues to be relatively specific for SLE, it is positive in only 60 to 70 per cent of patients at any given time. Almost all patients with active SLE, however, will demonstrate a positive ANA, and most patients will still have demonstrable antibody during periods of remission. But a positive ANA may be found in many other conditions, so for this reason additional assays must be performed. The finding of either anti-DNA (native or double stranded) or anti-Sm antibody is considered strong evidence for a diagnosis of SLE.

Mild normochromic, normocytic anemia is present in most SLE patients; it is clearly hemo-

Table 1. *Characteristics of Antinuclear Antibodies (ANA, Antinuclear Factors, ANF)*

Antibody	Methods of Detection	Properties	Significance
Anti-nucleoprotein (LE cell factor)	Immunofluorescence (whole tissue sections)	Homogeneous pattern, very sensitive	Most SLE patients, many other diseases (RA, hepatitis, drug-induced SLE)
Anti-DNA (anti-deoxyribonucleic acid)	Farr technique (radiolabeled double-stranded DNA as antigen); filtering assay (nitrocellulose membrane); immunofluorescence (Crithidia luciliae, a trypanosome, as substrate); counterimmunoelectrophoresis (CIE)	1st 2 require radiolabeled DNA; CIE is less sensitive than the others but simple to perform	Specific for SLE, rarely found in other conditions (JRA, hepatitis) Various methods of detection differ greatly in sensitivity; lack of close correlation among these tests suggests that they identify different subsets of anti-DNA
Anti-ENA (anti-extractable nuclear antigen)	Immunofluorescence (whole tissue sections)	Rim (peripheral) pattern	
	Immunofluorescence (screening) (whole tissue sections)	Speckled pattern	Go on to further studies
1. Anti-RNP (anti-ribonucleoprotein)	Hemagglutination; gel diffusion; CIE	Reactivity abolished by RNAse digestion	High titers in mixed connective tissue disease (MCTD)
2. Anti-Sm (named after a patient, Smith)	Same as (1), after enzyme digestion of RNP	Requires reference antiserum	Specific for SLE (but only detected in 1/3 of patients)
3. Anti-SS-B (the "B" antigen of Sjögren's syndrome) = anti-Ha	Gel diffusion; complement fixation; immunofluorescence	Requires reference antiserum	13% SLE patients
4. Anti-PM-1 (anti-polymyositis antigen)	Gel diffusion; complement fixation inhibition	Requires reference antiserum	Found almost exclusively in patients with polymyositis
Anti-RNA (anti-ribonucleic acid)	Hemagglutination	Requires purified antigens	Limited usefulness in diagnosis; found often in asymptomatic relatives of patients with SLE
Anti-cytoplasmic antigens (anti-La, anti-Ro)	Gel diffusion	Requires reference antisera	May be markers for SLE in ANA-negative patients; may cross-react with nuclear antigens

lytic with a positive Coombs' test in less than 10 per cent. Leukopenia (WBC less than 4,000 cells per cu mm) is very common and is an extremely important finding in differential diagnosis (e.g., a patient with SLE *and* pneumococcal pneumonia rarely achieves a WBC greater than 10,000 per cu mm). A lymphopenia (less than 1,000 per cu mm) is often striking and appears to correlate with disease activity. Differentiation between disease and drug effects is sometimes difficult.

A low platelet count (less than 100,000 platelets per cu mm) is relatively frequent, although it is usually not associated with purpura. Thrombocytopenia may be the presenting laboratory abnormality.

The erythrocyte sedimentation rate is frequently elevated, even during periods of apparent disease remission. There appears to be a close association between a high ESR and the degree of hypergammaglobulinemia.

Determination of serum complement activity is very useful, both diagnostically and for following disease activity. A low level of total hemolytic complement is found in about 75 per cent of all patients with active SLE and in almost all of those with active kidney disease. Total hemolytic complement levels are especially helpful, since they reflect diminution of any rate-limiting factors. Detection of C3 (BIC) or C4 by immunodiffusion is easier and, although it is less sensitive, the method has practical value. More recently, antisera have become available for detection of complement breakdown products (e.g., C3d). The finding of *high* levels of such activation products may be especially useful.

Recently, a wide variety of tests have been introduced for the detection of circulating immune complexes (IC). Since such complexes are a fundamental feature of SLE, their detection would seem to have special significance. To date no single test has emerged that reliably detects IC in all patients with SLE. Cryoglobulins, detected after placing serum of SLE patients at 4 C for 2 or 3 days, are found in about 50 per cent of active SLE patients. (This test is clearly the easiest!) Other methods currently in vogue include the C1q binding assay, the conglutinin-binding test, the monoclonal rheumatoid factor binding assay, and the Raji cell assay. All of these tests require purified radiolabeled reagents or cells grown in tissue culture or both; such materials are primarily available in research laboratories. Until there is an improved standardization of methods, results should be interpreted with caution.

Rheumatoid factors may be found in about 20 per cent of patients with SLE; usually the titers are low and evanescent. They are most frequently found in patients over the age of 50.

There are a variety of nonspecific blood abnormalities in some patients with SLE. Hypergammaglobulinemia has already been noted. Hypoalbuminemia and hyper-alpha-2-macroglobulinemia are common. In the patient with kidney disease, findings of renal failure (increased urea, creatinine, uric acid, phosphate, etc.) and the nephrotic syndrome may be noted. In the patient with myositis, evidence of muscle injury (elevated creatine phosphokinase, aldolase, and transaminase) may be found. Various clotting abnormalities are occasionally discovered, suggesting the presence of antibodies to specific clotting factors. The presence of the "lupus anticoagulant" is suggested by a prolongation of the prothrombin time and the partial thromboplastin time. Elevation of liver enzymes may be due to salicylate therapy as opposed to a disease effect per se. A false-positive test for syphilis (VDRL) reflects the general overproduction of autoantibodies. The fluorescein treponemia antibody test (FTA) can be used to distinguish between a true and a false positive.

Serial urinalyses are important since the kidney is likely to be involved in over half of the patients; nephritis (and also central nervous system disease) often has a poor prognosis and usually requires aggressive therapy. The finding of white cells, red cells, and a wide range of cellular remnants and casts (a "telescoped" sediment) supports the diagnosis of SLE nephritis. Proteinuria of mild or extensive degree is the most common urinary abnormality, but it is nonspecific, especially when found in small amounts. A careful creatinine clearance is often helpful in the discovery for early renal insufficiency and should be obtained as a baseline reference in every patient with SLE. (Incomplete collections are a major problem, even when the patients are being evaluated in the hospital.) Consistent abnormalities in any of the aforementioned tests may suggest the need for a renal biopsy to determine the severity and type of kidney involvement (e.g., mesangial, focal, membranous, diffuse proliferative).

Synovial fluid may be helpful in the differential diagnosis of SLE arthritis. Usually the synovial fluid leukocytes number less than 2,000 per cu mm, in sharp contrast to the high counts found in patients with most other inflammatory arthritis. The percentage of neutrophils may be low. Sometimes the protein level is low (less than 3 grams per dl [100 ml]), but this is inconsistent. Complement levels are also relatively low in synovial fluid, but this is also observed in synovial fluid of patients with rheumatoid arthritis.

Findings in pleural and pericardial fluid are similar to those in joint fluid. Particularly unhelpful are cerebrospinal fluid findings; often there is a modest elevation of protein and cellular elements in the cerebrospinal fluid (CSF), but no currently available tests establish the diagnosis of SLE with central nervous system involvement. One must look carefully for infectious organisms and carry out additional studies such as electroencephalograms, brain scans, and occasionally computerized tomography (CT scans) to rule out other causes of the central nervous system findings. Complement determinations on CSF have not proved useful.

X-rays of the chest are often useful in detecting pleural or pericardial effusions, atelectasis, or pneumonitis. Patchy and transient infiltrates are typical of SLE pneumonitis but are often difficult to distinguish from infiltrates caused by infectious agents; both may be present simultaneously. Roentgenograms of the joints are sometimes useful, since the lack of destruction helps rule out rheumatoid arthritis or infectious arthritis; occasionally, aseptic necrosis of bone is discovered.

Biopsies

Occasionally a biopsy of skin is useful in the diagnosis of SLE. Deposits of immunoglobulin and complement (detected by immunofluorescence) are found in a distinctive pattern at the dermal-epidermal junction in skin obtained from discoid and SLE lesions. About 50 per cent of patients with SLE will also exhibit these changes in *uninvolved* skin, usually obtained from areas not exposed to light, such as the buttocks. These abnormalities have also been reported in a few patients with mixed connective tissue disease and with rheumatoid arthritis and high titers of ANA.

Renal biopsy is not used to make the diagnosis of SLE; rather, the tissue can document the presence or extent or both of renal involvement. Such information can be helpful in determining prognosis and making a decision for vigorous therapy. Renal biopsy should be performed in consultation with a qualified specialist. Immunofluorescence and electron microscopy are important adjuncts to the light microscopic study of the tissue.

Pitfalls in Diagnosis

A lupus-like syndrome can be induced by a large number of drugs, the most common ones being procainamide, hydralazine, isoniazid (INH), phenytoin, and the phenothiazines. The symptoms — pleurisy, pericarditis, arthralgias and arthritis, weakness, rash — are indistinguishable from idiopathic SLE, but it is rare to have renal or central nervous system involvement. Laboratory abnormalities can include anemia, leukopenia, thrombocytopenia, hypergammaglobulinemia, and an elevated Westergren sedimentation rate. All patients have a positive ANA but lack antibodies to dsDNA (antibodies to ssDNA are frequently present) and complement levels are normal. Usually the symptoms subside after discontinuation of the offending drug, although some patients do require therapy with anti-inflammatory drugs. The ANA may persist for several years.

Because a positive ANA can be found in patients with many other rheumatic diseases, such as rheumatoid arthritis, polymyositis, progressive systemic sclerosis, and juvenile rheumatoid arthritis, and early in the course the clinical features may be poorly defined, it is important to consider diagnostic possibilities carefully before deciding on a diagnosis of SLE. This may require a period of observation and repeated clinical and laboratory evaluations.

Although fever can occur as part of the symptom complex and SLE should be included in any work-up for fever of unknown origin, it is always necessary to rule out the presence of a superimposed infection. Also, as ANA may appear during the course of viral infections such as those secondary to cytomegalovirus, it is important *not* to make the diagnosis of SLE on the basis of laboratory data alone. Chronic active hepatitis is also associated with hypergammaglobulinemia and positive ANA and must be distinguished from the hepatitis secondary to salicylate ingestion in SLE.

The variety of the aforementioned central nervous system syndromes, especially seizures and psychoses, emphasizes the need to entertain the diagnosis of SLE in any young person who presents with a central nervous system lesion that has no readily apparent cause.

Although discoid lupus is usually localized to the skin, a small group of patients have arthralgias and leukopenia or a positive ANA or both. Rarely, these patients will have progression to the systemic form of the disease, but they should be followed at regular intervals during the early years after diagnosis to confirm the limited nature of their disease.

DERMATOMYOSITIS

By STEPHEN A. ESTES, M.D.,
and GEORGE W. HAMBRICK, JR., M.D.

Cincinnati, Ohio

DEFINITION

Dermatomyositis is a rare connective tissue disease characterized by a nonsuppurative inflammation of the skin and striated muscle. A combination of diagnostic criteria based on the patient's skin eruption, pattern of muscle weakness, serum enzyme levels, electromyographic findings, and muscle histopathology serve to delineate clearly dermatomyositis from other entities. Polymyositis presents identical findings but lacks a characteristic skin eruption. Dermatomyositis appears in children and adults with a slight female preponderance. The adult form may or may not be associated with malignancy.

Although the pathogenesis of dermatomyositis is unknown, bacterial and viral infections, drug reactions, or immunizations have been reported as possible initiating factors in some cases. The association on occasion with scleroderma, systemic lupus erythematosus, rheumatoid arthritis, or internal malignancy suggests an autoimmune pathogenesis.

SIGNS AND SYMPTOMS

The two most common presenting symptoms in the childhood and adult forms of dermatomyositis are muscle weakness and skin rash. Malaise, weight loss, anorexia, myalgias, arthralgias, fever, dysphagia, dyspnea, and photosensitivity represent other less frequently encountered symptoms.

Early in the course of the disease, patients frequently demonstrate difficulty rising from a chair, walking up stairs, and combing their hair. This notable weakness develops over a period of weeks to months. Later, difficulty chewing and swallowing food, as well as in breathing, occurs.

On examination, the muscle weakness is characteristically symmetrical and involves the shoulder and pelvic musculature more severely. The proximal muscles are more involved than the distal ones and the extensors tend to be more affected than the flexors, as do the abductors over the adductors. The muscles may appear swollen initially and be tender. The deep tendon reflexes are usually intact.

The skin findings in dermatomyositis are nu-merous and varied. The most characteristic rash consists of a symmetrical, scaly, erythematous to violaceous maculopapular eruption involving the face, neck, shoulders, upper torso, and distal arms with similar lesions over the knuckles, interphalangeal joint areas, elbows, and knees. Flat-topped violaceous papules over the interphalangeal joint areas, called *Gottron's papules*, are thought to be a pathognomonic sign of dermatomyositis. A dusky erythema or lilac discoloration of the eyelids with edema described as heliotrope is characteristic. Periungual erythema and telangiectasia with thick, hard, hyperkeratotic cuticles are frequently seen, along with palmar erythema and scaling. Some patients develop a finely speckled, irregular hyperpigmented and hypopigmented eruption in the seborrheic areas that may extend to involve the entire body. This mottled pigmentation is known as *poikiloderma*.

Hypertrichosis, although rare, at times may be dramatic. Tender necrotic areas may also develop in patients with severe cutaneous vasculitis. Painful cutaneous calcinosis also occurs frequently in the childhood form. Raynaud's phenomenon and sclerodactyly also may occur.

Fever, when present, is usually low grade, intermittent, and appears after the development of muscle weakness.

LABORATORY FINDINGS

Elevated serum enzyme levels are helpful in making the diagnosis and monitoring therapy. Muscle enzymes that are released as a result of the destructive myopathy include creatine phosphokinase (CPK), serum glutamic oxaloacetic transaminase (SGOT), serum glutamic-pyruvic transaminase (SGPT), aldolase and lactic dehydrogenase (LDH). While the CPK is considered to be the most sensitive and reliable of the serum enzymes, it is best to order a complete "battery" of enzymes. Serial determinations, when clinically indicated, are appropriate. The serum enzymes are not infallible. A few patients with active myositis have been reported with normal serum enzyme levels. It is important to recognize that other motor-neuron diseases, dystrophies, infections, endocrinopathies, and metabolic disorders may elevate these enzyme levels. Muscle enzymes usually fall 3 to 4 weeks before clinical improvement in muscle strength occurs and rise 5 to 6 weeks before clinical relapse.

Other blood findings that may be abnormal include a leukocytosis, elevated sedimentation rate, increased gamma globulins, positive latex fixation titer for rheumatoid factor, and, occasionally, a positive antinuclear factor.

The electromyogram is useful for diagnosing polymyositis-dermatomyositis, for excluding disorders of denervation, and for selecting the appropriate muscle group for biopsy. The characteristic triad of findings for the electromyography (EMG) includes (1) polyphasic, short, small motor unit potentials; (2) fibrillation, positive sharp moves, and increased insertional irritability (membrane irritability); and (3) bizarre, high-frequency repetitive discharges. The electromyogram needle may produce myopathic histologic changes; thus the tested site should not be biopsied.

The muscle biopsy is a fundamental investigational step in making the diagnosis of dermatomyositis. The features seen on biopsy include (1) primary focal or extensive degeneration of muscle fibers, sometimes with vacuolation; (2) evidence of regeneration, demonstrated by sarcoplasmic basophilia and the presence of large vesicular nuclei and prominent nucleoli; (3) necrosis of a part or the whole of one or more fibers with phagocytosis; (4) interstitial infiltrates of chronic inflammatory cells focally or diffusely and usually with perivascular components; (5) variation in individual cross-sectional fiber size; and (6) interstitial fibrosis. In the childhood type of dermatomyositis more dramatic vasculitis pathology has been noted, consisting of endothelial cell prominence without hyperplasia, intimal hyperplasia, thrombus formation, and infarction. The most severe changes in muscle biopsies are seen in the childhood type and in the adult type associated with malignancy.

The histologic changes in skin are not specific and are sometimes indistinguishable from those seen in systemic lupus erythematosus. Epidermal atrophy, basal cell layer degeneration, dermal edema with a scattered mononuclear infiltrate, and fibrinoid deposits at the dermal-epidermal junction and around blood vessels occur. Older cutaneous lesions mimic those of poikiloderma atrophicans vasculare, with a band-like mononuclear infiltrate beneath an atrophic epidermis. Vasculitis, panniculitis, and later calcification in the subcutis may also be seen.

The direct immunofluorescence test on a frozen skin specimen usually helps to differentiate dermatomyositis from systemic lupus erythematosus by the absence of immunoglobulin deposition at the dermal-epidermal junction.

A 24-hour urine creatinine and creatine collection can also be used to substantiate and quantitate the amount of ongoing muscle destruction. The creatinine is decreased and the creatine increased. Albumin and myoglobulin may also be formed in the urine.

COURSE AND COMPLICATIONS

Adult patients with dermatomyositis should be evaluated for an associated internal malignancy. Most patients with this association are 30 to 80 years old. Patients in whom the diagnosis of dermatomyositis was made initially demonstrate their malignancy within the next 24 months. Malignancies of all types have been reported in association with dermatomyositis. Adequate treatment of the malignant disease may cause a remission of the dermatomyositis.

The course of dermatomyositis that is not associated with malignancy is variable. It can be acute and fulminant with death occurring within months, or polyphasic with exacerbations and remissions, or slowly progressive over years, and it may be uniphasic with complete remission. Children may have a slightly better prognosis, but the more severe angiopathy frequently results in more morbidity. At this time there are no clear-cut prognostic factors other than the presence of internal malignancy.

Complications of dermatomyositis include atrophy, contractures, calcinosis, disturbances in gastrointestinal motility, bowel perforation, renal failure, livedo reticularis with cutaneous infarctions and ulcerations, and chronic weakness. Severe muscle weakness involving the swallowing and respiratory muscles is responsible for aspiration pneumonia, a frequently lethal event.

Iatrogenic complications are significant in this disease, with the use of corticosteroids and other immunosuppressive agents. Cushing's syndrome, diabetes mellitus, peptic ulceration, growth retardation, and infections are examples of these.

DIFFERENTIAL DIAGNOSIS

Numerous diseases of several different etiologies may mimic polymyositis. Relatively few diseases present a differential diagnosis problem with dermatomyositis since most lack cutaneous findings. From a dermatologic standpoint, systemic lupus erythematosus (SLE), mixed connective tissue disease, scleroderma, trichinosis, poikiloderma vasculare atrophicans, photosensitivity eruptions, pellagra, eczematous processes, and drug eruptions may have some features in common with dermatomyositis. Historical, clinical histiologic immunofluorescence pathology findings, and other laboratory features usually make this differential easy to resolve.

Other connective tissue diseases with a myositis component may present some difficulty. Progressive systemic sclerosis, SLE, mixed connective tissue disease, rheumatoid arthritis, polyarteritis, polymyalgia rheumatica, polymyositis and Sjögren's syndrome may have overlapping features with dermatomyositis. Hereditary C_2 deficiency has been reported to cause a syndrome similar to SLE or dermatomyositis. These entities are usually separated on clinical and laboratory data.

Several disease processes may give rise to weakness that mimics the muscle findings in dermatomyositis. These are: neurologic and myopathic processes such as limb-girdle dystrophy, myasthenia gravis, and muscular dystrophy; infectious diseases such as hepatitis B, echovirus 24, toxoplasmosis, schistosomiasis, cysticercosis, and trichinosis; endocrine disease such as hyperthyroidism, hypothyroidism, hyperparathyroidism, and hyperadrenocorticism; metabolic diseases such as McArdle's syndrome, central core disease, hypocalcemia and potassium depletion; drug or toxic diseases induced by alcohol, penicillamine, clofibrate, steroids, chloroquine, penicillin, emetine, and azathioprine; and diseases such as amyloid, sarcoid, and carcinomatous myopathy. All those may produce muscle impairment clinically similar to the muscle findings found in dermatomyositis.

PERIARTERITIS NODOSA

By DANIEL E. FURST, M.D.,
and CARL M. PEARSON, M.D.

Los Angeles, California

In 1755 Michaelis and Matanni published a paper describing the lesions of diffuse vasculitis. In 1866 Kussmaul and Maier described what is now considered to be classic periarteritis nodosa (PAN). Between then and the 1950s, however, a great deal of confusion arose as to what truly defined the disease. Even now there is a proliferation of names to describe this entity, including polyarteritis nodosa (PAN), necrotizing angiitis, hypersensitivity angiitis, and nodular vasculitis. In children it may be called infantile periarteritis nodosa, Kawasaki's disease, or fatal mucocutaneous lymph node syndrome.

DEFINITION

For the purpose of this article, the classic definition of Kussmaul and Maier appears most appropriate. They described PAN as a segmental, necrotizing vasculitis of the small and medium-sized muscular arteries, with a predilection for bifurcations. Lesions tend to spread distally from these to involve arterioles and even, occasionally, adjacent veins. Histologically, vascular lesions in all stages of development are found with (1) acute polymorphonuclear infiltrates throughout all layers of vascular walls in early lesions, followed later by mononuclear infiltrates; and (2) vascular wall degeneration, fibrinoid necrosis, thrombosis, and intimal proliferation. All occur in varying degrees, depending on the age and severity of the lesion. As opposed to allergic granulomatosis and angiitis (also called Churg-Strauss syndrome), eosinophilia and granulomas are not characteristically seen, nor is there major splenic involvement. The inclusion of lung involvement, it should be noted, is a source of confusion, for Rose and Spencer incorporated PAN with lung involvement as a subset of PAN. Today many would call this entity Churg-Strauss syndrome and separate it from classic PAN. Furthermore, there exists a syndrome that appears clinically to be PAN but that on histological study predominantly involves small vessels and has lung involvement and eosinophilia. This syndrome, called "overlap" by Fauci, is an example of the problems inherent in the classification of the vasculitides in general.

In view of the widespread nature of this histologic picture, it is not surprising that PAN is a disease with many and varied manifestations.

PATHOGENESIS

The pathogenesis of PAN, as for most vasculitic syndromes, is believed to be closely associated with immune complex deposition. Circulating immune complexes are thought to become trapped in vessel walls as a result of vasodilatation. The vasodilatation, in turn, results from the release of platelet and basophil-derived vasoactive amines. Next, complement is activated, calling forth polymorphonuclear leukocytes that release their lysosomal enzymes and initiate vascular damage and necrosis. From this arises amplification of the inflammatory response and eventual thrombosis and healing with fibrosis. PAN associated with hepatitis B surface antigen (HB_sAg) is thought to result from just such a mechanism.

DEMOGRAPHY

Prevalence figures are remarkably scarce, although Shulman and Harvey reported that 1 in 137 autopsies demonstrated PAN, in a study between 1936 and 1944. Others estimate an incidence of two cases per million per year. The disease is one of male predominance, with two to three men affected for every woman. Peak incidence is between 40 and 60 years, although PAN has been diagnosed in both infants and 78-year-olds. There is no racial predisposition, nor is there any apparent genetic predisposition.

SIGNS, SYMPTOMS, AND COMMON COMPLICATIONS

As would be expected from the histopathology and pathogenesis just outlined, periarteritis presents in any of a large variety of ways. Table 1 gives a general view of the incidence and type of organ involvement. The first column details overall involvement in four series of patients, while the second column has a clinical overview of the initial organ involvement from a study of 130 patients with PAN. It is clear from the table that nearly any organ may be involved at any point in the course of PAN, making the task of outlining characteristic patterns of presentation and course of disease very difficult.

Although they are infrequent signs, subcutaneous nodules, mononeuritis multiplex, and myocardial infarction in a young man as well as sudden renal failure and progressive hypertension in a middle-aged man should all make the physician suspect PAN.

Constitutional symptoms are a frequent clue to diagnosis. The fever found in PAN has no characteristic pattern, although it is common at some point in the disease. Weight loss and malaise are among the most common presenting symptoms and may be out of proportion to the initial clinical examination.

Tender subcutaneous nodules, which are characteristic of PAN, occur in only about 15 per cent of cases, although petechiae, purpura, ulcerations, urticaria or nonspecific maculopapular rashes, in aggregate, occur more frequently (25 to 35 per cent).

Neurologic involvement includes both central and peripheral signs and symptoms. Central nervous system symptoms may be relatively nonspecific, such as confusion, disorientation, or delirium. On the other hand, blurred vision, transient blindness, hemiplegia, aphasia, head-

Table 1. *Clinical Signs and Symptoms Plus Selected Laboratory Findings From 377 Cases in 4 Literature Series*

	Overall Incidence (%)	Initial Findings
Constitutional		71
Fever	75	
Weight loss, malaise	67	
Skin		58
Purpura	33	
Rash	28	
Subcutaneous nodules	16	
Urticaria	3	
Neurological		55
Peripheral neuropathy (including mononeuritis multiplex)	50	
CNS (including confusion, visual loss, aphasia, subarachnoid hemorrhage)	11	
Cardiovascular		28
Edema or ascites	33	
Congestive heart failure	12	
Myocarditis	3	
Phlebitis	6	
ECG abnormalities or cardiomegaly on x-ray	50	
Gastrointestinal		40
Abdominal pain and diarrhea	65	
Bleeding or abdominal catastrophy	12	
Hepatomegaly	50	
Renal		8
Proteinuria, hematuria	66	
Azotemia (≥ 40 BUN)	24	
Hypertension	36	
Musculoskeletal		55
Arthralgias or arthritis	66	
Muscular pain and weakness	26	
Laboratory		
Anemia	67	
Elevated ESR	89	
Leukocytosis	54	
HB_sAg	20–50	
Lung		38
Asthma	13	
Pneumonia or pleurisy	33	
Eosinophilia	31	

ache, convulsions, and subarachnoid hemorrhages have been reported — not necessarily associated with hypertension or preterminal events. Of the peripheral neuropathies, mononeuritis multiplex is the most distinctive, although a symmetrical, sensory, or sensorimotor neuropathy is more common, occurring in upwards of 30 per cent of patients.

Cardiovascular signs and symptoms (excluding hypertension, which will be mentioned under renal disease) are also frequent (up to 50 per cent) although they may be as nonspecific as disproportionate tachycardia. Symptoms include those associated with congestive heart failure, myocarditis, or even myocardial infarction. Cardiomegaly may be seen on chest x-ray, while electrocardiographic signs can include nonspecific ST-T wave changes, arrhythmias, or heart block.

Gastrointestinal manifestations range from nonspecific abdominal pain and diarrhea to massive hepatic or gastrointestinal infarction. The abdominal pain may be severe enough to require laparotomy. Bowel infarction, ulcers, and hemorrhagic infarction of the pancreas (with acquired diabetes mellitus) have been seen. Approximately half of reported massive liver infarctions are due to PAN. Since the reports of HB$_s$Ag-associated PAN, liver function test abnormalities and hepatomegaly have been reported frequently, but an overall incidence of these findings is difficult to ascertain. Earlier autopsy reports mentioned 50 per cent hepatic involvement, while recent clinical series range from 5 to 40 per cent hepatomegaly, jaundice, or abnormal liver function tests. Jaundice may be an early sign in a few patients.

Abnormal *urinary findings* are extremely common, with proteinuria and hematuria in 60 to 70 per cent of most series at some time in the disease course. Glomerulonephritis is the most frequent pathologic finding, although renal arteritis is occasionally seen. Azotemia (BUN more than 40 mg per dl [100 ml]) is usually a late finding and heralds a poor prognosis. Hypertension was the initial finding in 25 per cent of one series and should alert the physician to possible PAN in young males.

Musculoskeletal symptoms may be found in approximately 60 per cent of patients in most series. Arthralgias and myalgias are most common. Both tend to be transient and migratory, although they may be very severe. Arthritis, with objective swelling, has been reported in 8 to 27 per cent of patients. It can affect large or small joints, either symmetrically or asymmetrically. Large joints, such as knees and wrists, are most commonly affected. The arthritis is usually of short duration, lasting days to weeks, but may occasionally last years. Tender muscles, muscular atrophy, and weakness on physical examination occur in 20 to 30 per cent of patients with PAN.

If *pulmonary involvement* is considered part of PAN, then the definition of Rose and Spencer can be considered. By their definition: (1) asthma, pneumonia or chronic bronchitis, and (2) eosinophilia, in addition to the usual findings in PAN, define the clinical subgroup of PAN with lung involvement. Pneumonia, bronchitis, and asthma were seen by them in 13 to 33 per cent of patients in the series quoted in Table 1, although both higher and lower estimates may be found. Eosinophilia occurred in approximately 30 per cent of patients in a larger series. Symptoms include dyspnea, wheezing, hemoptysis, and pleuritic pain. X-rays may show fibrosis, and pulmonary function tests may show obstructive or restrictive disease.

All these protean manifestations point out the large variety of clinical signs and symptoms associated with PAN. They again emphasize the need to consider PAN in any patient with an unexplained multisystem disorder, particularly when associated with fever, malaise, and weight loss.

LABORATORY FINDINGS

In most series the erythrocyte sedimentation rate (ESR) is elevated in more than 90 per cent of patients. In one series of 124 patients, the average initial ESR was 75 mm per hour. Anemia (hemoglobin less than 14 grams per dl in males and less than 12 grams per dl in females) is as common in some series as an elevated ESR, although in the combined series of 377 patients used here, it occurred in 67 per cent. Leukocytosis (greater than 10,000 per cu mm) occurred in over 50 per cent. Eosinophilia of more than 1500 per cu mm has been mentioned, especially with respect to pulmonary findings.

A number of immunologic parameters are abnormal in various series, but this occurrence may depend on the associated disease. Thus the rheumatoid factor or ANA may be positive, but these results are seen most often in the presence of rheumatoid arthritis, systemic lupus erythematosus, or liver disease. Other findings include hyperglobulinemia and elevated cryoglobulins. Serum complement has been normal or elevated in most series, although a recent study of PAN associated with hepatitis B demonstrated decreased C_3 or C_4 in about 50 per cent of patients. HB$_s$Ag is noted in 30 to 50 per cent of patients with PAN, although the presence of HB$_s$Ag does not correlate with PAN disease activity. If one screens for both HB antigen and antibody, this percentage increases. Liver function tests are abnormal in 70 to 100 per cent of HB$_s$Ag-positive PAN patients and may be abnormal even without such a positive test.

IgG immune complexes, assayed by the polyethylene glycol (PEG) method, were elevated in about 60 per cent of a group of 23 clinically severely ill patients with PAN, 38 per cent of whom were also HB$_s$Ag positive. In other studies in which *most* patients were HB$_s$Ag positive, no immune complexes were found, although only the C1q method for assessment of immune complexes was utilized. Of interest is the finding that positive IgG immune complexes are able to predict disease activity correctly 82 per cent of the time and also correctly predicted lack of disease activity 79 per cent of the time. C1q immune complexes are much less reliably found.

Urinary findings have already been outlined. Some emphasis should be placed on the fact that with renal disease, PAN patients may have glomerulonephritis, therefore the urinary findings may include not only hematuria and proteinuria but also pyuria and red and white cell casts.

Diagnosis

Given the protean clinical manifestations of PAN and the generally nonspecific nature of the laboratory findings, the diagnosis may be extremely difficult to make.

Recently, abdominal angiography, used in searching for multiple aneurysms, has been utilized as a diagnostic tool. Of a group of 17 patients with clinically diagnosed PAN, intra-abdominal arteriography (usually including renal, hepatic, and mesenteric circulations) yielded signs of definite, multiple aneurysms in 60 per cent of the patients. Sixty per cent sensitivity is better than most other diagnostic techniques in PAN, but still leaves 40 per cent negative by this test. The specificity of this technique is excellent, but not 100 per cent, since multiple aneurysms occurred occasionally in other diseases involving vasculitis (e.g., Wegener's granulomatosis, systemic lupus erythematosus, Churg-Strauss syndrome, thrombotic thrombocytopenic purpura, and drug abuse-related PAN) and may reflect the intensity of the vasculitis rather than their etiopathogenesis.

Definitive diagnosis can be made by means of biopsy of tissue specimens. An important point in terms of biopsies is that the diagnostic usefulness of this procedure depends on obtaining specimens from *clinically and pathologically affected tissues*. Thus only 13 to 32 per cent of blind muscle biopsies without localization of muscle symptoms in patients suspected of the disease are positive for PAN. Only an estimated 22 per cent of blind testicular biopsies can be expected to be positive. Although testicular tenderness or swelling is relatively unusual (20 per cent in one series), the diagnostic yield of testicular biopsies in a group of patients with this feature would be expected to be higher than 22 per cent. The same would be true of the 15 per cent of patients with subcutaneous nodules, although biopsies of nonspecific rashes would have lower positive yields. If biopsies of nonspecific rashes are taken, they must at least be deep enough (deep dermis and panniculus) to obtain specimens of muscular arteries or arterioles. Many organs (e.g., the kidneys) often reveal only nonspecific changes and may not be diagnostic. In general only 20 to 30 per cent of antemortem biopsies, unless taken from clinically involved tissue, will be diagnostic. Furthermore, immunofluorescent studies will only occasionally be helpful, for the IgG and C3 deposition found in the vessels of PAN patients are not specific for that disease.

With the aid of these diagnostic tools and the use of a combination of nonspecific (therefore nondiagnostic) clinical and laboratory findings, the diagnosis can be made.

Although the usual considerations relating to ruling out infection, malignancies, allergic reactions, and other connective tissue diseases must be heeded, particular attention with respect to PAN should be paid to patients with : (1) Unexplained prominent fever, weight loss, and myalgias with elevated ESR, particularly those who are in their 40's and 50's and who are male. (2) Unexplained multi-system disease, particularly when involving the central nervous system, peripheral nerves, and kidneys, or associated with abdominal catastrophies. (3) Myocardial infarctions or disease in the very young. (4) Unexplained sudden onset of hypertension and renal failure, particularly in middle-aged males.

Course and Prognosis

In adults, the prognosis of periarteritis nodosa has changed over the years. In 1938, the 1-year survival rate in a study of 152 patients was 13 per cent, most patients dying of renal failure. By 1967, with the use of corticosteroids, the 5-year survival was 50 to 60 per cent in most series. Most recently, with the combined use of steroids and immunosuppressives, the 5-year survival statistic is 80 per cent.

The course of PAN shows the highest mortality in the first 3 to 6 months (when 20 to 25 per cent of patients die), with hypertension and renal disease being the worst prognostic signs.

The most recent data relating to PAN in children intimate that this disease may often be remarkably benign, with a single, possibly severe flare. After this the child may recover completely, with the disease leaving no clinical or laboratory evidence of its presence. As in adults, however, it occasionally is devastating, as it appears to have a predilection for the coronary arteries in the young.

SCLERODERMA

By VICTORIA L. BECKETT, M.D.,
and DOYT L. CONN, M.D.
Rochester, Minnesota

SYNONYMS

Systemic sclerosis or progressive systemic sclerosis (PSS).
1. Diffuse or generalized scleroderma
2. CREST syndrome
3. Mixed connective tissue disease variant
Localized or focal scleroderma
1. Morphea
2. Linear scleroderma

DEFINITION

Scleroderma, or systemic sclerosis, is a disease characterized by obliteration of capillary beds, sclerosis of small arteries, and collagen deposition and fibrosis primarily in the skin but also in the gut, lung, heart, and kidney. The initial stage may be inflammatory, followed by fibrous and degenerative changes. It is the vascular insufficiency, tissue infiltration, and atrophy that produce the clinical picture. The disease is more common in females and the cause is unknown.

There is a spectrum of involvement, both clinically and pathologically. Not all patients develop extensive skin effects or significant visceral involvement. The disease may progress to a point, stop, and remain limited.

When there is limited skin involvement (often confined to hands and face) and relatively confined internal involvement, it may be termed the CREST syndrome (Calcinosis, Raynaud's phenomenon, Esophageal dysfunction, Sclerodactyly, Telangiectasia). These features may be present in various combinations, but indicate chronic and generally limited disease.

Many patients have an antinuclear antibody with a speckled pattern, and in some cases this antibody is directed toward an extractable nuclear antigen (ENA) containing primarily ribonuclear protein (RNP). In this situation, the disease is called *mixed connective tissue disease* when there are overlapping clinical features of systemic lupus erythematosus or polymyositis or both. These patients may evolve into a more typical clinical picture of scleroderma.

There are localized (focal) forms of scleroderma limited to the skin. Single or multiple sclerotic plaques characterize "morphea" and linear atrophic bands can occur on the trunk, extremities, face, or scalp.

PRESENTING SIGNS AND SYMPTOMS

The initial complaint is usually Raynaud's phenomenon, which often occurs shortly before the onset of swelling and thickening of the skin of the fingers and hands. Occasionally, it may antedate other symptoms by many years. The patients may present with polyarthralgias or polyarthritis mimicking rheumatoid arthritis. The condition in still another group starts with inflammatory features of myositis or lupus-like picture accompanied by systemic symptoms. Finally, the disease in a small group begins with visceral involvement alone (PSS sine scleroderma) before any evidence is seen of skin changes.

Localized scleroderma develops insidiously as indurated plaques or linear lesions on the trunk, extremities, scalp, or face.

COURSE

Individual patients with systemic sclerosis show a wide variety of involvement of tissues or organs or both and rate of progression. The disease may be limited to relatively localized skin effects, and in these patients the life span is unchanged. Others have gradual or rapid progression of skin, muscle, and joint effects, resulting in a wooden stick-like body frame and disabling flexion contractures. Alternatively, they may have visceral changes resulting in pulmonary or cardiac insufficiency or both, renal insufficiency with hypertension, or intestinal malabsorption or obstipation. These latter conditions have a poor prognosis and may proceed to death.

Localized (focal) scleroderma involves only skin and muscle, resulting in thickening or atrophy of strictly confined areas without progression.

CLINICAL FEATURES AND PHYSICAL FINDINGS

The hallmark of systemic sclerosis is skin involvement with acrosclerosis. This can be appreciated by observing and palpating the thickened skin of the fingers, which later become tethered to the underlying tissue. Functionally, there is limitation of extension and abduction of the fingers. Skin changes may progress up the arms and include the face, portions of the trunk, and, less commonly, the legs and feet. The face gives a tight appearance with lack of normal skin folds. The nose appears pinched and the mouth puckered and limited in opening. Pigmentation and spotty depigmentation occurs in areas of involved skin. Telangiectasia, which is a vascular lesion formed of dilated capillary loops, may emerge on fingertips, face, and lips, giving a pink, spotty appearance. Chronicity can produce subcutaneous calcification. These most often occur in areas of increased trauma, such as fingers and elbows. With time, the skin may actually become slightly more pliable owing to final atrophic changes.

Raynaud's phenomenon is due to vasospasm of the digitial arteries secondary to cold exposure. Toes and tongue may also be involved. Typically on cold exposure, fingers turn dead-white; this is followed by a bluish tinge and then erythema as they become warm again. Fingertip ischemic ulcerations may occur. When anoxia is severe, gangrene supervenes, often causing much pain.

Diffuse polyarthralgias with joint stiffness involving the fingers, wrists, shoulders, knees, and ankles occur frequently. Joint swelling may occur and an adhesive tendinitis may develop, leading to a unique leathery crepitus over involved joints on motion. Mild muscle weakness, representing mild muscle inflammation (myositis), is a frequent accompanying feature in the early stages of disease. Later, striking muscle mass decrease may occur because of fibrous replacement and atrophy.

Neurologic features are rare. Trigeminal neuropathy does occur with primarily mild decreased sensation along the second or third division of the trigeminal nerve, frequently with associated feeling of burning and tingling around the mouth and in the oral cavity. This feature of disease is unique to scleroderma and the mixed connective tissue disease variant.

Visceral involvement, insidious and subtle in the early stages, may lead to death in some patients. Decreased esophageal motility in the lower esophagus often causes no dysphagia initially. However, it may proceed to esophagitis with reflux and stricture formation. About 90 per cent of patients have esophageal involvement. A smaller percentage of patients develop small intestine and large bowel changes. Small bowel involvement may be manifested by symptoms of bloating, and later a picture of pseudo-obstruction owing to atonic dilated loops of bowel. Malabsorption with diarrhea secondary to bacterial overgrowth may occur. The large bowel sacculations noted on barium enema rarely give rise to symptoms other than obstipation.

A majority of patients have pulmonary interstitial fibrosis, causing a little exertional dyspnea at first; crackling rales are noted on auscultation. This sometimes progresses to cor pulmonale and right heart failure. Cardiac involvement, often accompanying later stages of pulmonary disease, is that of cardiomyopathy secondary to myocardial fibrosis. Pericardial effusion may be associated. Symptoms of progressive dyspnea and intractable cardiac failure are unusual.

Finally, the most ominous development is that of renal scleroderma. This may or may not be associated with hypertension. The hypertension may be malignant, with rapid progression to oliguria and renal failure. Death may occur within days or a few weeks. Small artery involvement with cortical infarction may be seen on autopsy.

The prognosis, therefore, depends on degree of involvement of heart, lungs, and kidneys. One rare malignant "complication" of this disease is alveolar cell carcinoma in patients with severe pulmonary disease. Only a few cases have been reported. This may occur in a setting of pneumoconiosis. Other associated immune conditions, such as primary biliary cirrhosis and Sjögren's syndrome, have been reported in patients with scleroderma. Hashimoto's thyroiditis may also occur.

LABORATORY STUDIES

The laboratory abnormalities are often nonspecific. In patients with little inflammation, the erythrocyte sedimentation rate is normal. Those with more inflammation and systemic symptoms often have an elevated erythrocyte sedimentation rate, anemia, hypoalbuminemia, and elevated serum gamma globulins. The antinuclear antibody test is positive with a speckled pattern in 60 per cent of patients. The antibody may be directed toward a unique nuclear antigen as yet incompletely characterized. In the mixed connective tissue disease variant, the antibody is directed to nuclear ribonuclear protein, and is often in high titers. Elevated antibody titer to native DNA, a positive LE cell test, and low serum complement are usually not present. The serum creatine kinase may be elevated moderately when there is muscle inflammation (myositis) but is usually not strikingly elevated as in the case of polymyositis without scleroderma.

Skin biopsy may be consistent with scleroderma in the later stages of disease but often is unhelpful in earlier stages. Esophageal motility studies may be positive when esophageal x-rays appear normal. Pulmonary function studies may depict diminished carbon monoxide diffusing capacity when chest x-ray may be negative or show only basilar fibrosis.

Hand x-rays can be diagnostic. Absorption of terminal tufts and subcutaneous calcinosis around the fingers is a combination of findings seen in no other condition. This generally occurs in the chronic stage of this disease.

Intestinal involvement is best studied with x-rays. Typical decreased motility or dilatation of the lower esophagus is characteristic. Also, the dilated duodenum "loop sign" and large-mouth saccular diverticula of the colon are unique in this disease. Stool studies positive for fat and depressed serum carotene may be found in malabsorption secondary to bacterial overgrowth.

Advanced pulmonary involvement can show diffuse honeycombing on chest x-ray. Pulmonary function studies show a restrictive pattern with decreased vital capacity. Cardiac arrhythmia may be documented on electrocardiogram, and heart block might indicate a cardiomyopathy. Echocardiogram is helpful to document pericardial effusion. Otherwise, the cardiac finding in advanced disease is frequently that of left and right ventricular enlargement.

Renal disease is evidenced by proteinuria, an elevated serum creatinine, low creatinine clearance or iodothalamate clearance test. An elevated peripheral venous renin activity may antedate renal insufficiency and may augment renal and peripheral vasospasm and hypertension. A microangiopathic peripheral blood smear with burr cells may be seen in patients with sclerodermatous renal vascular disease.

It is important to define the type and extent of clinical involvement because this will determine the management approach. The proper course would be to continue treating the patient with the reassurance that the disease may stop at any stage, and treat symptoms as they occur.

Section 18

DISEASES OF
UNKNOWN CAUSE

SARCOIDOSIS

By HAROLD L. ISRAEL, M.D.
Philadelphia, Pennsylvania

and ROBERT A. GOLDSTEIN, M.D.
Bethesda, Maryland

DEFINITION

Sarcoidosis is a systemic granulomatosis, still known as Besnier-Boeck-Schaumann disease in Europe. A definition is proposed by Scadding: "Sarcoidosis is a disease characterized by the presence in all of several affected organs or tissues of epithelial cell tubercles, without caseation though some fibrinoid necrosis may be present at the centres of a few tubercles, proceeding either to resolution or to conversion of the epithelioid cell tubercles into avascular hyaline fibrous tissue." This is based on the concept that the disorder may have a variety of causes.

Most investigators consider sarcoidosis to be an entity separable from other granulomatous diseases that resemble it pathologically, and prefer a looser definition adopted at the 6th International Conference on Sarcoidosis: "Sarcoidosis is a multisystem granulomatous disorder of unknown etiology, most commonly affecting young adults and presenting most frequently with bilateral hilar lymphadenopathy, pulmonary infiltration, skin or eye lesions. The diagnosis is established most securely when clinicoradiographic findings are supported by histological evidence of widespread noncaseating epithelioid-cell granulomas in more than one organ or a positive Kveim-Siltzbach skin test. Immunological features are depression of delayed-type hypersensitivity suggesting impaired cell-mediated immunity and raised or abnormal immunoglobulins. There may also be hypercalciuria, with or without hypercalcemia. The course and prognosis may correlate with the mode of onset: An acute onset with erythema nodosum heralds a self-limiting course and spontaneous resolution, whereas an insidious onset may be followed by relentless, progressive fibrosis. Corticosteroids relieve symptoms and suppress inflammation and granuloma formation."

Although atypical cases occur in which experts disagree about the diagnosis, such instances are infrequent. For both clinical and investigative purposes the term sarcoidosis represents a generally accepted diagnostic categorization. In our experience the diagnosis of sarcoidosis is more accurate than would be anticipated in a disease whose causative agent cannot be demonstrated. Patients referred because of suspicion of this disease only rarely prove to have mycobacterial or fungal disease, lymphoma, or extrinsic alveolitis. In contrast, tuberculosis, which is precisely defined, is more often overdiagnosed as a result of roentgenologic, pathologic, or microbiologic errors.

PRESENTING SIGNS AND SYMPTOMS

The clinical manifestations and sarcoidosis vary according to the site and severity of tissue involvement. Although the frequency of involvement may differ in specialized medical centers, Table 1 indicates the general experience with system or organ involvement. In the United States, blacks are affected 10 to 12 times more often than whites; the disease is also common among white North Europeans. The incidence is greatest among women in the third and fourth decades of life; sarcoidosis is quite rare before 20 and after 50 years of age. Many intrathoracic lesions that spontaneously resolve are asymptomatic and may escape detection. On the other hand, some patients may have high fever and be subjected to protracted investigation before the diagnosis of sarcoidosis is accepted.

COMMON MANIFESTATIONS OF SARCOIDOSIS

Thoracic involvement is the major source of disability and death in this disease, and the patients are commonly grouped according to the appearance of their chest roentgenogram: I —adenopathy alone; II — adenopathy with pulmonary lesions; III — pulmonary lesions

Table 1. *Clinical Varieties of Sarcoidosis*

Common
  1. Mediastinal and hilar adenopathy
  2. Pulmonary infiltration
  3. Cutaneous sarcoids
  4. Ocular
  5. Febrile arthralgia and erythema nodosum
Occasional
  6. Peripheral adenopathy
  7. Bones, joints, and skeletal muscles
  8. Nervous system
  9. Liver
  10. Heart
  11. Upper respiratory tract
Rare
  12. Parotid and lacrimal glands
  13. Spleen
  14. Kidneys
  15. Endocrine glands
  16. Gastrointestinal tract
  17. Genitourinary tract

without adenopathy; O — normal chest. It should be emphasized that these are not stages through which all patients progress, and that classification of patients by radiologic appearance alone provides an incomplete assessment of the clinical status in an individual patient.

Mediastinal and Hilar Adenopathy. Although it is often considered that hilar/mediastinal lymphadenopathy is an early stage of sarcoidosis, the fact is that massive adenopathy may be of many years' duration when discovered. Some patients present with pulmonary infiltration without evidence of prior adenopathy, and in 10 per cent the chest roentgenogram is normal. Bilateral hilar and right paratracheal lymphadenopathy is the hallmark of sarcoidosis, but unilateral hilar adenopathy occurs in 5 per cent of patients. Calcification of sarcoidal hilar lymph nodes occurs in a few patients in the absence of complicating mycobacterial or fungal infection.

Pulmonary Lesions. The most common form of pulmonary involvement is a diffuse reticular nodular interstitial pattern, especially in upper lung fields. Occasionally fluffy, confluent lesions with air bronchograms simulating alveolar exudate or neoplastic masses are noted. Chronic pulmonary sarcoidosis is often complicated by apical bullae, bronchiectatic dilatations, and even thick-walled cavities simulating those of tuberculosis. Fungus balls caused by aspergillus frequently develop in such cavities. Sarcoidal pleural effusions occur more often than was previously realized.

Skin and Mucous Membranes. Small nonpruritic raised facial nodules near the nose, eyes, and mouth, or on the back of the neck and of the extremities, are the most common cutaneous manifestation of sarcoidosis. Patients with recent sarcoidosis may exhibit extensive erythematous lesions of the extremities or trunk. Cutaneous involvement is more common in black patients and is an indication of chronic and widespread disease. Old scars and tattoos may become inflamed when sarcoidosis develops or recurs.

Ocular Involvement. Eye involvement occurs in approximately 15 per cent of patients, most commonly as granulomatous uveitis. Acute or subacute uveitis or iridocyclitis presents with watering, redness, and photophobia. Chronic uveitis is more insidious and may produce glaucoma and blindness. Phlyctenular or nonspecific conjunctivitis may occur; if millet seed nodules are seen, they provide a source for biopsy. Rarely, lacrimal gland dysfunction may cause dry eyes with corneal scarring. Slit lamp examination is essential, as ocular sarcoidosis requires prompt corticosteroid treatment.

Erythema Nodosum. Erythema nodosum, which appears as red raised nodules on the legs varying in size from 1 to 5 cm, associated with painful arthralgia, is a frequent feature of sarcoidosis in Northern Europe, where it is known as Löfgren's syndrome.

Peripheral Lymphadenopathy. Massive lymphadenopathy is an infrequent presenting symptom, but careful physical examination will reveal enlarged cervical, inguinal, epitrochlear, or axillary lymph nodes in many patients; even small nodes provide a safe and productive source for biopsy.

Bones, Joints, and Skeletal Muscles. Asymptomatic punched-out lesions in the distal phalanges of hands and feet may be demonstrable on roentgenographic examination but occur only in patients with obvious widespread chronic sarcoidosis, and such roentgenograms are useless as a diagnostic procedure in investigation of suspected sarcoidosis. Arthralgia may be an early prominent feature with or without erythema nodosum. In the United States, periarticular inflammation of the ankle and hilar adenopathy frequently occur without erythema nodosum, probably representing an incomplete form of Löfgren's syndrome. Rarely, arthritis may develop during the course of chronic sarcoidosis with clinical and roentgenographic changes stimulating rheumatoid arthritis. Gastrocnemius muscle biopsy may reveal granulomas in patients with erythema nodosum and arthralgias, but rarely otherwise. Chronic myopathy is an infrequent but distressing manifestation that mimics muscular dystrophy.

Nervous System. Cranial nerve palsies, especially seventh facial nerve palsy (Bell's), as well as peripheral neuropathies are the most frequent abnormality. These manifestations are usually seen among patients whose disease is of recent onset, and are often transient. In contrast, central nervous system involvement typically occurs later in the course of the disease. Central nervous system involvement may become manifest as granulomatous meningitis, localized tumor-like lesions, diffuse disease simulating multiple sclerosis, or pituitary involvement producing loss of vision or endocrine syndromes. Nervous system involvement in sarcoidosis is suspected when neurologic abnormalities appear during the course of disease; however, emphasis should be placed upon the exclusion of infectious complications of sarcoidosis. For example, the spinal fluid abnormalities described in sarcoidal leptomeningitis — including elevated protein, pleocytosis with lymphocytic cell predominance, and lowered glucose — are similar to those of tuberculous and fungal meningitis.

Liver. Although the liver is palpable in less than 15 per cent of patients, liver biopsy demonstrates granulomas in 70 per cent of sarcoidosis patients, irrespective of laboratory abnormalities. Fever higher than 101 F (38 C), which may be seen in as many as 35 to 40 per cent of patients, is commonly associated with hepatic infiltration. Granulomatous liver infiltration in sarcoidosis rarely progresses to hepatic insufficiency and portal hypertension. When the chest roentgenogram is normal, there is often uncertainty about whether febrile hepatic granulomatosis represents a manifestation of systemic sarcoidosis; it is often possible to support the diagnosis of sarcoidosis by biopsy demonstrations of granulomas elsewhere.

Salivary Glands. Nontender and firm enlargement of parotid and other salivary glands has been noted. The combination of fever, uveitis, and lacrimal and salivary gland enlargement (uveoparotid fever) is occasionally seen.

Spleen. The spleen, palpable in 5 per cent of patients, may occasionally produce hypersplenism.

Kidneys. Sustained hypercalcemia is rare but is an important and preventable cause of renal damage. Granulomatous renal involvement is equally infrequent.

Heart. Abnormalities ranging from sinus tachycardia to multiple premature ventricular contractions are not infrequent if electrocardiograms are routinely made. Myocardial sarcoidosis is a significant feature in 1 per cent, showing most commonly conduction disturbances (A-V), arrhythmias (especially ventricular), or diffuse cardiomyopathy causing congestive failure. Pericardial and valvular involvement are extremely rare. Cor pulmonale is a common complication of severe pulmonary fibrosis.

Gastrointestinal Tract. Sarcoidosis of the esophagus, intestines, and peritoneum is extremely rare. Involvement of the stomach and mesenteric adenopathy are more frequent but rarely are a cause of clinical manifestations.

Endocrine System. The pituitary gland and hypothalamus may be invaded by sarcoid granulomas causing the clinical syndrome of diabetes insipidus and panhypopituitarism. Thyroid, adrenal, and ovarian involvement are rare, but associated hyperthyroidism or myxedema may occur.

Upper Respiratory Tract. Nasal involvement in sarcoidosis is an uncommon but extremely annoying manifestation. The epiglottis, larynx and trachea, and paranasal sinuses may also be affected.

Lower Genitourinary Tract and Reproductive System. The rarity with which the female reproductive tract is involved is remarkable, as surgical specimens are so frequently examined in women with this disease. There is no evidence that sarcoidosis diminishes fertility. Sarcoidosis often regresses during pregnancy only to relapse postpartum.

LABORATORY FINDINGS

Hematologic. Leukopenia with lymphopenia is the most constant feature; slight eosinophilia (4 to 6 per cent) and elevated erythrocyte sedimentation rates are occasionally encountered. When splenomegaly is present, thrombocytopenia and purpura may be observed.

Chemical. Hypercalcemia and hypercalciuria were in the past reported to be common manifestations of sarcoidosis. Recent studies demonstrated persistent elevation of serum calcium in less than 3 per cent of patients, who almost invariably have severe and extensive sarcoidosis. Hypercalciuria is dependent to a large extent on dietary intake of calcium; when this is controlled, increased urinary excretion of calcium is rare. Serum urate levels may be slightly elevated, but gout is rare. Elevation of serum alkaline phosphatase is frequent, usually reflecting hepatic involvement. Other liver function tests are rarely abnormal. Recently attention has been directed to increased serum lysozyme and angiotensin converting enzyme levels in active sarcoidosis. The elevations are, however, not of practical diagnostic value.

Angiotensin-converting enzymes are elevated in about 60 per cent of patients with active sarcoidosis but are frequently raised in patients with miliary tuberculosis, asbestosis, pneumoconiosis, and lymphoma. Serum lysozyme levels are increased both in sarcoidosis and tuberculosis. Gallium scans usually show uptake in the mediastinal nodes or lungs of patients with active sarcoidosis, but are also nonspecific and cannot be relied upon to distinguish sarcoidosis from other granulomatous diseases and neoplasms.

IMMUNOLOGIC

Humoral. Hypergammaglobulinemia is a significant feature chiefly among black patients with chronic forms of sarcoidosis, and serum immunoglobulin A, G, and M levels are often increased; serum immunoglobulin D and E levels are not significantly altered in sarcoidosis. Serum protein electrophoresis has proved to be of little diagnostic value. Rheumatoid factor and antibodies to a variety of viral agents are often increased, but offer little diagnostic help. Antimitochondrial antibodies are usually negative in sarcoidosis, and may aid in distinguishing biliary cirrhosis from sarcoidosis. Measurement of antibodies to detect aspergillus infection is often important. Serologic studies to detect histoplasmosis or coccidioidomycosis as well as hypersensitivity pneumonitis may be useful in some areas of the country.

Cell-Mediated Hypersensitivity. Although diminished cell-mediated immunity is characteristic of sarcoidosis, study of this defect has little diagnostic value. Application of a battery of skin test antigens reveals that 50 per cent of patients react to at least one antigen, and the demonstration of anergy adds little support to the diagnosis. Although impairment of delayed hypersensitivity might be expected to impair the clinical usefulness of the tuberculin test in sarcoidosis, our experience has been that all patients who develop tuberculosis react to 5 TU or 250 TU. When tuberculosis complicates sarcoidosis there is sufficient antigenic stimulation to evoke a tuberculin reaction.

In vitro studies of lymphocyte function have failed to show features diagnostic of sarcoidosis. Depressed responses to nonspecific mitogenic stimulation of lymphocytes appear not only in patients with sarcoidosis but also in a wide variety of other clinical disorders.

The Kveim test has not proved valuable as a specific test in patients who present a diagnostic problem. Usually positive in typical cases of sarcoidosis with massive adenopathy or erythema nodosum in which the diagnosis is already quite secure on a clinical basis, the Kveim reaction is usually negative in pulmonary and extrathoracic forms without adenopathy. False-positive reactions occur with some batches, and a positive test with a single antigen is not as a consequence reliable. It is in the diagnosis of atypical forms of sarcoidosis that a specific biologic test would be most helpful, but in these circumstances the Kveim test is usually negative. Kveim test materials are unavailable for clinical use in the United States and are not likely to be adequately standardized for commercial distribution until a soluble antigen is isolated.

Investigators have utilized Kveim materials in assays of lymphocyte function in an effort to develop an in vitro diagnostic test for sarcoidosis, with little success.

PULMONARY FUNCTION TESTS

Pulmonary function tests commonly demonstrate restriction, decreased compliance, and loss of effective diffusing surface. There is often a striking discrepancy between physiologic and radiographic changes. As a rule pulmonary function is not significantly impaired when there is no roentgenographic evidence of infiltrate. When infiltration is present, even if scant, physiologic changes may be marked or slight. The course of the disease is adequately followed by serial spirograms in most instances.

SELECTION OF BIOPSY PROCEDURES

There is growing acceptance of the concept that the diagnosis of sarcoidosis is basically a clinical one. In the past the constant concern was distinguishing tuberculosis from sarcoidosis, and it was this difficulty that led to the emphasis on the importance of biopsies to exclude caseation. The present rarity of glandular tuberculosis and the recognition that the tuberculin test is reliable in patients with sarcoidosis for the exclusion of tuberculosis have made confusion of these diseases rare.

As the presence of epithelioid granulomas in tissue specimens is properly reported by the pathologist as "compatible with sarcoidosis," it is clear that the histologic appearance does not *prove* the diagnosis of sarcoidosis. The demonstration of epithelioid granulomas in biopsy samples does not satisfactorily exclude Hodgkin's disease. Five per cent of liver biopsies in this disease show granulomas typical of those seen in sarcoidosis, and mediastinal lymph nodes in patients with lymphoma may show sarcoid tubercles.

Absence of symptoms and a negative physical examination provide strong evidence that mediastinal adenopathy is not due to lymphoma. Although it is unnecessary to hospitalize patients with asymptomatic hilar adenopathy, biopsies should be secured when this can easily be accomplished. The safest and most rewarding sites are the accessible ones: palpable lymph nodes, cutaneous lesions, visible conjunctival lesions, or enlarged parotid or lacrimal glands. In the absence of visible or palpable abnormalities, a variety of other techniques have been utilized (Table 2). Mediastinoscopy and open lung biopsy provide close to 100 per cent yield but require general anesthesia and

Table 2. *Biopsy Procedures*

When physical examination demonstrates abnormalities accessible to biopsy:
    Peripheral adenopathy (epitrochlear, cervical, axillary or inguinal), subcutaneous nodules
    Cutaneous, conjunctival, palatal, or nasal lesions
When physical examination is normal:
    Fiberoptic bronchoscopy and transbronchial biopsy
    Mediastinoscopy or mediastinostomy
    Percutaneous liver biopsy
    Biopsy of normal conjunctiva
    Surgical biopsy of lung

are not without hazard. The greater yield from mediastinoscopy has made performance of scalene node biopsy obsolete. Percutaneous lung puncture is productive but has been abandoned in most centers because of the frequency of hemorrhage and air leaks. Transbronchial lung biopsy by means of the fiberoptic bronchoscope provides a yield of more than 60 per cent and is growing in popularity.

Percutaneous needle biopsy of the liver reveals granulomas in 70 per cent of patients with sarcoidosis, but this approach should not be used in ill or febrile patients, because similar granulomas may be present in Hodgkin's disease and miliary tuberculosis. Other tissue sources such as bone marrow and bronchial, palatal, or conjunctival mucosa occasionally demonstrate granulomas, but the yield is too low to encourage routine application of these procedures. Although some investigators have argued that lung tissue is more "specific" than other tissues obtained in support of a diagnosis of sarcoidosis, the demonstration of noncaseating granulomas, with or without giant cells, Schaumann bodies, or asteroid inclusions, is not "specific" for the disease sarcoidosis irrespective of site. The use of special stains in an effort to demonstrate acid-fast bacteria (AFB) and fungi is a desirable routine in the study of granulomas, but organisms are rarely found in the absence of caseation necrosis.

Multiple biopsies are needed for the diagnosis of sarcoidosis only in order to demonstrate generalized involvement in atypical cases. Patients with the usual manifestations of sarcoidosis should not be subjected to multiple biopsy procedures.

PATHOLOGIC DIAGNOSIS

Large numbers of well-defined hard tubercles of the same age are readily recognized by all pathologists as characteristic of sarcoidosis. When only a single granuloma is found or when vasculitis or necrosis is prominent, however, there may be significant variation in interpretation.

Giant cells of the Langhans type and inclusion bodies are frequently seen, but are not diagnostic of sarcoidosis. Distinction between these features and those found in other infectious or hypersensitivity granulomatous disorders depends upon demonstration of organisms by special staining, mineral analysis, and search for foreign particles.

COURSE

In the United States approximately one third of the patients make a complete recovery and an additional third recover with minimal roentgenographic residuals. From 5 to 10 per cent of sarcoidosis patients ultimately die from their disease, and 25 per cent have significant morbidity or disability. A third of the patients require corticosteroid therapy.

Patients whose sarcoidosis begins with erythema nodosum or acute arthralgia have a remarkably favorable outcome, usually obtaining complete recovery within 2 years. The more systems involved by the disease, the worse the prognosis. Cutaneous sarcoids usually indicate chronic and disseminated involvement, and the prognosis is worse among persons so afflicted. Although anterior uveitis may be evanescent, posterior uveitis is often associated with a chronic course and a worse prognosis.

Persons who present with pulmonary disease are less likely to recover than those who have adenopathy alone. The prognosis is worse among American blacks than in whites.

The most common causes of death in sarcoidosis are cardiorespiratory insufficiency and aspergillomas, which frequently cause hemorrhage.

PITFALLS IN DIAGNOSIS

An excess of diagnostic zeal resulting from unwarranted concern about the possibility of lymphoma is frequently responsible for the recommendation of thoracotomy in persons with mediastinal adenopathy. If careful questioning elicits no symptoms and if careful examination reveals no nodes, such patients can safely be observed, as the adenopathy in these circumstances is often transient.

On the other hand, an excessive reliance on histologic diagnosis may result in error, as when a diagnosis of sarcoidosis is based on granulomatous changes in lymph nodes or liver in a patient who has intermittent fever or pruritus.

Patients with extensive pulmonary damage from sarcoidosis are prone to develop secondary infection with aspergillosis. Not infrequently such infections, characterized by hemoptysis, purulent sputum, and fluid-containing cavities, are mistakenly identified as tuberculosis. Utilization of second-strength tuberculin tests and precipitin tests for aspergillosis should prevent errors of this type.

Perplexing diagnostic problems may be present in patients in whom there may be reason to suspect beryllium disease and extrinsic alveolitis caused by fungal, protein, or drug hypersensitivity. These disorders are principally pulmonary reactions, but sarcoidosis is, as a rule, a systemic reaction. If histologic study of lung tissue leaves the diagnosis in doubt, the demonstration of numerous typical granulomas in distant tissues should establish the diagnosis of sarcoidosis. Similarly, when localized masses of epithelioid granulomas are encountered in bones, liver, kidneys, or other organs, the most convincing evidence that systemic granulomas are present even when the chest roentgenogram is normal can be obtained by use of mediastinoscopy or transbronchial biopsy.

The diagnostic pitfall that was most emphasized in the past — namely, confusion between sarcoidosis and tuberculosis — is rarely a problem at present. Prolonged observation of 300 patients with sarcoidosis in our clinic in the past decade disclosed the development of tuberculosis in only one instance, readily signaled by conversion of the tuberculin reaction. Even massive pleural effusions, common in tuberculosis and infrequent in sarcoidosis, can be accepted as a manifestation of the latter disease when the second strength tuberculin test is negative.

SJÖGREN'S SYNDROME

By LARRY G. ANDERSON, M.D.
Portland, Maine

SYNONYMS

Sicca syndrome, Mikulicz's disease, benign lymphoepithelial lesion.

DEFINITION

The complete Sjögren's syndrome is a triad of (1) keratoconjunctivitis sicca (dry eyes), (2) xerostomia (dry mouth), and (3) a connective tissue disease (usually rheumatoid arthritis). The presence of any two of these components establishes the diagnosis. Nearly half the patients have just the incomplete syndrome of keratoconjunctivitis sicca and xerostomia, also called the sicca complex. Other connective tissue diseases fulfilling the third criterion include systemic lupus erythematosus, polymyositis, and scleroderma. The sicca complex may also be associated with immunologic liver disease such as chronic active hepatitis and primary biliary cirrhosis.

The diagnosis of Mikulicz's disease applies nonspecifically to lacrimal and parotid gland swelling of varied causes, including Sjögren's syndrome. Benign lymphoepithelial lesion is the descriptive histopathologic diagnosis of the lymphocytic infiltration of lacrimal and salivary glandular tissue in Sjögren's syndrome.

PRESENTING SIGNS AND SYMPTOMS

Most patients with Sjögren's syndrome are postmenopausal women, but the condition can exist in men and at any age, including adolescence. The patient with keratoconjunctivitis sicca complains of eye irritation, grittiness, foreign body sensation, morning crusting, and, infrequently, inability to produce tears while weeping. The annoying symptoms of xerostomia include mouth dryness and parched sensation, with difficulty in chewing and swallowing food because of deficient saliva. Prolonged speaking is an effort. Many patients require several glasses of liquid to complete a meal, and some keep a glass of water at the bedside at night. Another presentation of Sjögren's syndrome is acute or chronic salivary gland swelling, which may be painful. Glandular involvement elsewhere in the body may result in chronic bronchitic cough or vaginal dryness.

The presenting problems of Sjögren's syndrome may be those of the associated connective tissue disease. The diagnosis is usually readily apparent when eye and mouth dryness develop in the patient with long-standing rheumatoid arthritis. The most severe sicca problems may be associated with advanced and destructive joint disease.

The diagnosis is more elusive in the patient presenting with sicca complex overshadowed by serious "extraglandular" features of Sjögren's syndrome. Patients may be systemically ill with fatigue and weight loss. Cough, dyspnea, or abnormal chest x-ray may herald lymphoproliferative lung disease, which may be benign or malignant. Other features of "pseudolymphoma" or benign extraglandular lymphoproliferation include lower extremity purpura or necrotizing cutaneous vasculitis, lymphadenopathy, hepatosplenomegaly, and renal involvement with renal tubular acidosis, concentrating defects, and even renal insufficiency. Unfortunately, some patients have an associated malignant lymphoproliferative disease when Sjögren's syndrome is first recognized.

COURSE

The course of Sjögren's syndrome is variable and unpredictable. Some patients report waxing and waning in intensity of sicca symptoms, and rare patients even note remission of dryness. However, most experience an insidiously progressive worsening over the years. Often the sicca problems are secondary in importance to the course of progressive arthritis or other multisystem connective tissue disease.

PHYSICAL EXAMINATION FINDINGS

Routine eye examination is usually normal, but the examiner may detect gross conjunctival dryness or injection, lacrimal gland swelling, or gross corneal defects or ulcerations. A simple bedside diagnostic procedure to be included in the physical examination is Schirmer's test, which measures tear production by the degree of wetting of filter paper strips draped over the lower eyelids for 5 minutes. The Schirmer filter paper strips, which are available commercially, show greater than 15 mm wetting over 5 minutes in normal persons. Most patients with keratoconjunctivitis sicca have less than 5 mm wetting. Diagnostic physical findings require a slit lamp, with demonstration by rose bengal staining of tear film disruption, corneal defects, and filamentary keratitis.

Oral examination findings in patients with xerostomia vary from grossly normal to severely dried and cracked mucous membranes. Parotid or submandibular glands may be enlarged or tender. A complete careful physical examination is essential, with special search for chest abnormalities, skin lesions, enlargement of lymph nodes, liver, or spleen, joint deformity or synovitis, and signs of peripheral neuropathy.

COMMON COMPLICATIONS

The glandular deficiencies of Sjögren's syndrome are annoying and bothersome but rarely lead to serious local complications such as corneal ulceration. Dental caries may be a problem with xerostomia. Some patients regard chronic parotid swelling as a major cosmetic problem.

Vasculitis or extraglandular lymphoproliferation in Sjögren's syndrome can lead to serious complications, such as disfiguring cutaneous vasculitis, peripheral neuropathy, pulmonary insufficiency, renal tubular acidosis, or renal insufficiency. A major concern is the potential in some patients with pseudolymphoma or benign lymphoproliferative disease for progression to true lymphoproliferative malignancy such as lymphoma or reticulum cell sarcoma.

LABORATORY FINDINGS

Many patients with Sjögren's syndrome have nonspecific laboratory abnormalities consistent with active connective tissue disease, such as moderate anemia (hematocrit in low or mid 30's), elevated erythrocyte sedimentation rate, low serum albumin, and elevated gamma globulins. There is a high incidence of autoantibodies such as rheumatoid factor and antinuclear antibody, with lesser frequency of anti-DNA and antithyroid antibodies. The antisalivary duct antibody is not specific for Sjögren's syndrome and to date has not proved to be of practical clinical value in diagnosis. Urinalysis may show hyposthenuria, hematuria, and pyuria, and the urine may not show an appropriate low pH in response to an acid load.

OTHER DIAGNOSTIC PROCEDURES

Documentation of salivary gland function is achieved by sequential salivary scintigraphy, a simple, sensitive, and noninvasive technique that can distinguish significant xerostomia by abnormal uptake, concentration, and secretion of technetium. Salivary flow rates provide useful information but are somewhat tedious and require special equipment and expertise. Contrast radiography with sialography provides limited information about gland function.

An attempt at biopsy documentation of disease is indicated in patients under consideration for steroid or immunosuppressive therapy because of extraglandular spread of lymphoproliferation. Minor salivary glands are readily accessible by simple biopsy of the lower lip, and lymphocytic infiltration and possible acinar destruction may be seen in the tissue. Material obtained from lung biopsies in Sjögren's syndrome may show infiltration by lymphocytes, plasma cells, histiocytes, or malignant lymphoreticular cells. Renal involvement is characterized by an interstitial nephritis with similar round cell response. Lymph node tissue obtained by biopsy may show hyperplasia or true malignancy.

PITFALLS IN DIAGNOSIS

In Sjögren's syndrome, acute painful parotid swelling with accompanying fever and toxicity may be mistakenly diagnosed and treated as suppurative bacterial parotitis. A more serious error is unnecessary surgical excision of major salivary glands because of the misdiagnosis of neoplasm in patients with chronic firm glandular swelling. Lip biopsy should help identify patients with sarcoidosis, which may also cause keratoconjunctivitis sicca, xerostomia, and lacrimal and salivary gland swelling.

The most important clinical diagnosis regarding Sjögren's syndrome is the recognition and documentation of pseudolymphoma or benign lymphoproliferation in organs such as lungs, liver, kidneys, or lymph nodes. Patients with such multisystem disease have caused problems in diagnosis because the sicca complex was not prominent. Early and effective treatment with steroids or immunosuppressive agents may prevent progression to malignant lymphoproliferative disease unresponsive to any treatment.

REITER'S SYNDROME

By DENYS K. FORD
Vancouver, British Columbia, Canada

SYNONYMS

Reiter's syndrome may be referred to as Reiter's disease, postdysenteric arthritis, or the Fiessinger-Leroy-Reiter syndrome.

DEFINITION

"Reiter's syndrome" applies to the triad of conjunctivitis, urethritis, and arthritis; other characteristic manifestations include circinate balanitis, keratodermia blennorrhagica, and superficial erosions on the palate or dorsum of the tongue or both. Often the syndrome does not occur in its classic form and combinations of any two or more of the conditions listed may exist without the triad. Almost all cases encountered in North America occur in men.

PRESENTING SIGNS AND SYMPTOMS

In North America, urethritis is usually the presenting symptom. Less often cystitis initiates the triad, and, occasionally, diarrhea precedes or occurs with the urethral discharge or dysuria. In the parts of the world where dysentery is common, an attack of typical Shigella dysentery may be followed by "postdysenteric Reiter's syndrome." The syndrome occasionally follows Salmonella or Yersinia infections.

COURSE

The course is variable. The urethritis or cystitis may be mild and usually clears either spontaneously in 1 to 4 weeks or more rapidly with tetracycline therapy. The conjunctivitis is usually transient over a few days. The arthritis may affect a single joint such as one knee or may involve several joints, often asymmetrical —the knees, ankles, feet, and sacroiliac joints being favored. Maximal spread of the arthritis usually develops within the first 2 weeks. The arthritis may continue for periods varying from 2 weeks to over a year, but improvement usually begins within 2 to 6 weeks, so that the duration of the arthritis is commonly from 1 to 4 months. Pain in the feet, heels, and sacroiliac joints tends to persist longer than elsewhere.

Recurrence is common and up to eight attacks have been recorded in some patients. Recurrences may take the form of "complete" or "incomplete" syndromes.

PHYSICAL EXAMINATION FINDINGS

General. A variable, usually mild fever may be present; only in unusually severe cases is the patient toxic or debilitated.

Head and Neck. Conjunctivitis ranging from mild and unilateral to severe and bilateral may be present. Evidence of recent or old iritis may be found. Superficial erythematous erosions on the palate and dorsum of the tongue occur commonly.

Joints. Signs of acute or subacute inflammation will be found in a single joint, several joints, or many joints, and in the lower extremities particularly. Extremely acute attacks may resemble gout or septic arthritis. Involvement of several joints acutely may resemble rheumatic fever, while a subacute onset may simulate rheumatoid arthritis. Sacroiliac tenderness, localized periostitis unrelated to affected joints, and painful heels may be present.

Genitalia. The urethral meatus and mucosa are usually somewhat reddened and show a grayish or white mucoid semipurulent discharge. This may be minimal and apparent only in the early morning after the urethra has been stripped.

Circinate balanitis may present as small red spots, grayish thickened mucosal patches, or superficial ulcerations on the glans penis or less often on the coronal sulcus.

Skin. Usually the skin lesions of keratodermia blennorrhagica are confined to the soles of the feet, where they appear as small red spots that progress to small flat pustules and later to hyperkeratotic lesions. Occasionally the skin elsewhere shows hyperkeratotic and crusted papules and the fingernails may show changes resembling those of psoriasis.

COMPLICATIONS

Iritis may develop in the later stages of an episode or after recurrent episodes, and ankylosing spondylitis may also be a sequela to recurrent attacks. Rarely, in severe cases there may be electrocardiographic abnormalities with prolongation of the P-R interval and ST-T wave abnormalities; very rarely, aortic incompetence has been a sequela.

LABORATORY FINDINGS

Laboratory and x-ray findings are not helpful, apart for excluding other forms of arthritis.

An elevated sedimentation rate will be found with or without a slight to moderate blood leukocytosis. The synovial fluid contains from 5000 to 50,000 cells, of which over 90 per cent are polymorphonuclear leukocytes. Microbiological studies of exudates and biopsy tissue have not yet revealed any causative agent. Chlamydia agents and mycoplasmas may be cultured from the genital tract but have not been isolated consistently from synovial fluid or tissue and their significance is therefore still debated. The presence of gonococci in urethral exudate may indicate only that gonorrhea and Reiter's syndrome coexist.

X-rays of joints that have been persistently affected may show periosteal proliferation near the joint and, with chronic heel pain, characteristic calcanean spurs. Sacroiliitis or the changes of spondylitis may be found after recurrent or chronic Reiter's syndrome.

Histocompatibility typing shows the presence of HLA B27 in about 80 per cent of patients, but this test is not needed for diagnosis.

PITFALLS IN DIAGNOSIS

The diagnosis may be missed because the patient is reticent about his urethritis or because he overlooked the mild urethral exudate. The diagnosis depends on the history and demonstration of characteristic physical findings.

MYASTHENIA GRAVIS

By RONALD A. YOUMANS, M.D.

Kansas City, Missouri

SYNONYMS

Goldflam's disease, myasthenia gravis pseudoparalytica.

DEFINITION

Myasthenia gravis is an immunologic disease in which the patient produces antibody to acetylcholine receptor protein of the striated muscle fiber; not all receptors are affected equally. In nearly 90 per cent of patients, significant levels of antibody to acetylcholine receptor protein can be demonstrated in the serum. Clinically, myasthenia gravis is manifest by fluctuating muscle weakness, which is exacerbated by exercise, emotional stress, and physiologic or endocrine stress such as menstruation or infection. Strength is improved by rest. Pharmacologically, strength and endurance are improved by use of anticholinesterase medications, although not to normal.

PRESENTING SIGNS AND SYMPTOMS

Weakness may develop so slowly as to not be recognized as a problem, being present only in the evening or after unusual exercise. It may be accepted initially by the patient as unusual fatigue and exhaustion. Unilateral ptosis or mild, transient diplopia may develop, but any striated muscle may be affected. Clinical distress is more apparent if bulbar functions such as chewing, swallowing, or breathing are involved. Proximal muscles of the shoulder or pelvic girdle are commonly weak, usually asymmetrically. Over a few weeks the relative weakness of various muscle groups may change.

Urgent assistance is needed if onset is abrupt. Often within a few hours minor problems can become critical, particularly if muscles of respiration are involved. Dysphagia may produce choking. The patient discovers that effective coughing is not possible, and there is dysarthria so severe that the patient's speech cannot be understood.

Onset may be recognized from the time the patient begins falling while walking or climbing stairs or when the patient loses the ability to do housework because knees buckle. Often mild transient weakness has been present, but its significance has been minimized by the patient. Repetitive use of the arms and hands may demonstrate the weakness. Stretching arms above head level or lifting and moving objects is difficult because of grip and arm weakness. A man who has done heavy work may find his hip and leg muscles too weak to perform. A child at school may be observed to fall when running or climbing stairs, and to support his head with his hands because of neck muscle weakness or tilt it to correct fluctuating diplopia. The face may appear expressionless. Sometimes a child will be found holding his eyes open because the ptosis covers the pupil.

Myasthenia gravis can occur at any age. In the 20 to 40 year group women affected outnumber men 3:1. In the 50 to 70 year group men outnumber women. A myasthenic mother may deliver a baby with transient myasthenia. This condition may threaten the infant's life unless it is promptly given appropriate medication and respiratory care. Such neonatal myasthenia usually resolves spontaneously in 4 to 8 weeks; the baby may not have myasthenia later. According to the current theory of cause, placental transfer of the mother's IgG antibody is probably the mechanism of neonatal myasthenia.

Rarely, a baby of a nonmyasthenic mother may show evidence of weakness and improve when given small amounts of anticholinesterase medication. Since good response to anticholinesterase medication is part of the definition of myasthenia, this is regarded as congenital myasthenia, although the physiologic mechanism may not be identical with juvenile-onset or adult-onset myasthenia. Sometimes anticholinesterase medication will produce improved strength in persons with muscular dystrophy, myositis, motor neuron disease, or other processes that have unrelated pathophysiology.

CLINICAL COURSE

The natural course of this fluctuating muscle weakness is variable. It is suspected that many cases are so mild and transient that diagnosis is not established. Often in the adult with obvious disease a history of transient juvenile weakness can be elicited, such as clumsiness, falling or poor endurance in athletic endeavors for a few days without apparent illness. The disability demands diagnosis when the weakness is moderately severe, the patient being unable to lift dishes, books, or household objects, or falling when climbing stairs with slipping or tripping. Double vision that precludes reading or driving is an urgent complaint. An infant with ineffective coughing, weak cry, or weak sucking response may not be so easily identified. A young lady with situational stresses who stumbles on stairs or has trouble using her hands to fix her hair may feel that she is being neurotic. One has to be aware of myasthenia gravis to suspect this physiologic weakness in the school child with dull and expressionless face who may drool or use his hands to support his head during afternoon class. The elderly man with feeble gait, expressionless face, and drooling may have myasthenia gravis rather than vascular disease, senility, or extrapyramidal disease.

If symptoms remain confined to eye movement and ptosis for 2 years, generalized myasthenia is unlikely to develop.

If symptoms are minimal and adequately controlled on anticholinesterase medication, this may be adequate management. Obviously, the clinical status should be reviewed regularly and chest x-rays obtained.

If respiratory reserve is affected, very close observation is advisable, preferably in an intensive care unit while evaluation is progressing. If anticholinesterase medication is not adequate, high doses of prednisone may be given daily. Some neurologists may prefer intravenous ACTH. Some clinical worsening is usual for the first 4 days, and intubation with respiratory assistance may be necessary. As the patient's strength improves in the next 2 to 3 weeks, the physician may consider giving single-dose prednisone on alternate days. In these critical cases of myasthenia gravis, plasmapheresis may be performed, usually 3 to 4 times a week for several weeks, mechanically removing circulating antibody to the acetylcholine receptor protein.

Before the use of anticholinesterase medications, much clinical disability persisted in fluctuating severity with premature death related to pulmonary infection from aspiration, ventilatory insufficiency, hypoxia, or malnutrition from inability to chew and swallow well; the mortality rate of recognized myasthenia gravis was probably 90 per cent in the first year. Acute fulminating cases still carry high mortality unless complications can be avoided by respiratory assistance, plasmapheresis, and appropriate medication program.

With current programs, including early diagnosis, much less physical disability and suffering can be expected, with a mortality of less than 5 per cent.

The clinical correlation of myasthenia gravis and thymus pathology has long been recognized. In theory, thymectomy may help stabilize the course and allow gradual clinical improvement in less than 2 years, although many post-thymectomy patients still require anticholinesterase medication and have less than optimal strength. If a thymic tumor can be identified on lateral chest film, tomograms, computed tomography (CT) scan or isotope studies, it should be removed. Some thymic tumors are malignant. More commonly, a diffusely enlarged thymic shadow may be found in about 25 per cent of myasthenics, with increased numbers of germinal centers reported by the pathologist.

PHYSICAL EXAMINATION

General. Depending on degree of clinical involvement, the patient may appear perfectly normal until exercise is performed. Nutrition is generally adequate unless dysphagia has been a problem. If respiratory compensation is marginal, the myasthenic may appear mildly cyanotic and anxious, with tachycardia and perhaps mildly elevated blood pressure.

Head and Neck. Ptosis of either or both eyelids may be present or may be induced by squinting the eyes closed for 30 seconds, or by elevating the eye position for 30 seconds. Pupillary size and responses continue to be normal despite ptosis. Testing extraocular eye movements may demonstrate dysconjugate positioning not attributable to specific nerve dysfunction. Obviously, a history of eye injury or familial lazy eye should be considered. The face may be expressionless, with sardonic smile, weakness of eye closure, and difficulty blowing forcefully. Masseter weakness may be demonstrated by asking the patient to chew gum. Submandibular muscle weakness may be demonstrated by asking the patient to open his mouth against resistance. Observe the ease with which he quickly drinks a glass of water.

Extremities. Variable objective weakness can be demonstrated by exercise of various muscle groups. A hand dynamometer or ergograph may quantitate the muscle fatigability. Grip testing can be done with a rolled blood pressure cuff; the pressure is noted initially and again after 15 and 30 squeezes.

The physician should test how long the arms can be held extended. With the patient sitting, hip flexion strength and quadriceps strength can easily be estimated. The patient can be asked to do 5 knee bends, to hop 10 times on either foot, and to do sit ups. During these exercises, the physician should observe for weakness carefully and should document the number of exercises performed.

Other Organs. The heart is generally normal. Lungs are normal, but ventilatory muscles may readily fatigue. Vital capacity before and after exercise may demonstrate weakness. The physician should test how far the patient can count on a single breath. Observe for changes in enunciation as well as how long breath can be held. Abdomen is normal.

Neurologic Examination. Other than motor fatigability and weakness, this may be normal. Reflexes may be hypoactive, especially after appropriate exercise. Sensory examination is normal. Coordination is not affected except by weakness. Sensory cranial nerve functions are normal. Anxiety and apprehension are added to normal orientation and psychiatric survey.

THEORY OF PATHOPHYSIOLOGY

Current thinking implies a change in muscle cell metabolism that may allow atypical muscle receptor protein to be produced; or changes in T cell "self-recognition" may occur. The immune system produces antiacetylcholine muscle receptor protein antibodies. The thymus and T cell immunoregulatory system is primarily involved, although B cell and helper-cell systems are probably involved.

The discovery that bungarotoxin specifically binds muscle receptor protein led to experimental autoimmune myasthenia gravis, which seems to be a good animal model for the clinical disease. Similar antibodies are produced. Infusion of appropriate IgG creates the symptoms by passive transfer, and a neonatal form has been identified. The distortion of end-plate anatomy resembles the changes in myasthenia gravis.

Antimyoid antibodies are often present. The receptor protein antibody may be involved with thymic antibody in crossed reactions. HL-A typing indicates that a genetic predisposition is present statistically although not exclusively. Antimuscle antibodies are present in 30 per cent of myasthenics. Serum complement level C3 drops as clinical worsening occurs. Statistically, higher levels of antiparietal cell antibody, antithyroid antibody, and antinuclear antibody are present in myasthenics than in the general population.

Historically, myasthenia has been recognized as a "neuromuscular transmission defect." Acetylcholine is appropriately released from the nerve endings; it should function briefly in stimulating the receptor protein, and be destroyed promptly by acetylcholinesterase. Medications can be used to destroy the esterase, allowing acetylcholine to be effective longer. Such medication is helpful but may improve only to 30 to 90 per cent of expected strength. Such medications in common use include neostigmine (Prostigmin) with duration of action of 2 to 3 hours; pyridostigmine (Mestinon) with duration of action of 4 to 6 hours; edrophonium (Tensilon) with brief duration of action of per-

haps 3 to 5 minutes. Appropriate timing and dosage must be considered in prescribing. Overdosage may cause weakness with increased gastrointestinal motility, increased sweating, salivation, and tearing.

COMMON COMPLICATIONS

Intercurrent infection and secondary worsening of the myasthenia is perhaps the most threatening problem.

Several medications and antibiotics (e.g., streptomycin and others) may worsen neuromuscular transmission and should be used cautiously.

Occasionally, persons with undiagnosed mild myasthenia may be given general anesthesia for unrelated surgery. Because myasthenics are very sensitive to small amounts of curare-like agents, the neuromuscular function may be more effectively blocked for a much longer time than expected if the patient is given a usual dosage, calculated on body weight. Ventilatory assistance may be needed until the effect clears.

Using one thirtieth to one tenth the usual curare dosage has been devised as a clinical diagnostic test. It may provide helpful information but is not specific for myasthenia. Smaller amounts used in a "regional curare test" in an arm may be safer, but such testing may also require intubation and ventilatory assistance.

Since gradually increasing the dosage of anticholinesterase medication can produce weakness, the question frequently arises as to whether more medication is likely to be helpful. Edrophonium (Tensilon) given in very small dosage, 1 to 2 mg, may give a brief test to help the physician with this decision.

DIAGNOSTIC PROCEDURES

A careful history, general physical examination, and basic laboratory survey should be done to exclude hematologic reasons for weakness and metabolic problems including diabetes, thyroid dysfunction, renal disease, electrolyte disturbance, and liver disease. Also an immunologic survey should be carried out for antimuscle receptor protein, antithyroid, antimyoid, and antinuclear antibodies. Chest x-ray, including lateral view, should be done, and computed tomography (CT) scan of the anterior mediastinum may be performed.

Much information can be obtained by electrical repetitive nerve stimulation, and the recording of the amplitude of the muscle action potential. In myasthenia gravis, stimulation at three per second produces prompt loss of amplitude in 2 to 3 seconds. A myasthenia-like syndrome related to neoplasm has been described by Eaton and Lambert. In the Eaton-Lambert syndrome, stimulation at 20 per second will augment the amplitude within a few seconds. Although a patient with Eaton-Lambert syndrome may present with weakness, the syndrome should be specifically distinguished because of significant clinical correlation and better response to other medication.

Muscle biopsy with appropriate enzymatic stains may be helpful. Muscles affected with myasthenia may have lymphocyte clusters called *lymphorrhages*. Other diseases causing muscle weakness may be identified.

PHARMACOLOGIC DIAGNOSTIC PROCEDURES

Edrophonium is usually preferred for testing because of prompt onset of effect in 1 to 2 minutes and brief duration of effect. If the patient has not been on anticholinesterase medication, up to 10 mg may be given slowly intravenously with reasonable safety. The 10 mg edrophonium should be given from a 1 ml syringe to allow greater accuracy of administration and should be given slowly, about 0.1 ml (1 mg edrophonium) every 15 seconds. The injection should be stopped when clinical information is obtained. Only 3 to 4 mg may be required to correct ptosis, increase facial strength for a smile, obviously increase grip strength, or improve enunciation. Nausea, abdominal cramping, and some twitching fasciculation may develop if clinical tolerance is exceeded.

If clinical deficit is minimal, or if psychoneurosis is suspect, placebo injection may be tried initially, perhaps followed by 0.4 mg of atropine, then followed in a few minutes by the edrophonium. Atropine can be a very helpful medication in controlling the nicotinic muscular effects of the anticholinesterase medications.

In infants use of neostigmine, 0.125 to 0.25 mg intramuscularly, may be an easier test. The infant should be observed for strength changes for an hour, including limb movement, head support, and strength of crying and sucking. In adults 1.5 mg of neostigmine can be given intramuscularly, alone, or with 0.4 mg atropine. Observe for strength changes for an hour. Neo-

stigmine 0.5 mg may be given slowly intravenously (timed for 1 minute) for more prompt effect.

An oral clinical trial with neostigmine or pyridostigmine can be helpful with some alert patients who can objectively quantitate their mild symptoms. The clinician should still do comprehensive laboratory and edrophonium testing to help distinguish psychogenic changes from physiologic changes.

PITFALLS IN DIAGNOSIS

Development in the immunologic testing field is new, and not necessarily specific. Surely new refinements in the antiacetylcholine receptor antibody testing will be developed. Studies of experimental autoimmune myasthenia gravis have provided a major advance in understanding this disease.

The causes of clinical weakness are myriad. Objective testing and documentation is to be encouraged. An informed patient and family is crucial for satisfactory management. Anxiety neurosis or subtle depression can cause functional "fatigue," but these conditions need other specific management. Hypoglycemia and other metabolic disorders belong in the differential diagnosis. A careful history for toxic exposure may give other reasons for neuropathy, or myopathy allowing nonmyasthenic weakness.

The response to anticholinesterase medication is not specific. It may give minor clinical improvement in bulbar palsy syndrome of amyotrophic lateral sclerosis, myopathy and polymyositis, and post-poliomyelitis. Other autoimmune diseases including vasculitis and hyperthyroidism may coexist with myasthenia gravis.

Toxins from *C. botulinum* can produce clinical weakness, dyspnea, dysphagia and diplopia, usually with severe nausea and vomiting. This can present a respiratory emergency before clinical distinctions are made.

Appropriate diagnosis includes a thorough history of onset and exploration of other factors that may contribute to clinical weakness. Also included are appropriate pharmacologic testing, chest x-ray, electrical testing, and immunologic antibody survey.

Section 19

LABORATORY
REFERENCE VALUES
OF CLINICAL IMPORTANCE

LABORATORY REFERENCE VALUES OF CLINICAL IMPORTANCE

Prepared by
REX B. CONN, M.D.

Atlanta, Georgia

THE INTERNATIONAL SYSTEM OF UNITS FOR LABORATORY MEASUREMENTS (LE SYSTÈME INTERNATIONAL D'UNITÉS)

Physicians are accustomed to receiving laboratory reports with measurements expressed in metric units such as the gram, liter, or milliliter; however, an extensive modification of the metric system has been adopted by clinical laboratories in many countries, and plans are being formulated to make a similar change in the United States. This adaptation is the International System of Units (Le Système International d'Unités), usually abbreviated S.I. Units. Whereas the metric system utilizes the centimeter, the gram, and the second as basic units, the International System uses the meter, the kilogram, and the second as well as four other basic units.

The overriding consideration for adopting the International System is that it will provide a common language among the various scientific disciplines throughout the world for unambiguous communication regarding all types of measurements. In the medical field, the advantages of conversion are that chemical relationships between various substances will become more readily apparent and there will be an international uniformity in laboratory reporting. The most serious disadvantage in making this conversion is that physicians will have to become accustomed to a new set of figures for almost all laboratory measurements. Because of this inconvenience, as well as a potential for serious misinterpretation of laboratory data, the conversion must be undertaken cautiously and only after a logical plan has been formulated and discussed. There appears to be little question, however, that the International System will be adopted in this country. Clinical laboratories in most western European countries, Canada, and Australia are already using S.I. Units, and American medical journals are adopting the practice of expressing measurements in both conventional and S.I. Units.

The International System

The International System is a coherent approach to all types of measurement which utilizes seven dimensionally independent basic quantities: mass, length, time, thermodynamic temperature, electric current, luminous intensity, and amount of substance. Each of these quantities is expressed in a clearly defined *basic unit* (Table 1).

Two or more basic units may be combined to provide *derived units* (Table 2) for expressing other measurements such as mass concentration (kilograms per cubic meter) and velocity (meters per second). Standardized prefixes (Table 3) for basic and derived units are used to express fractions or multiples of the basic units so that any measurement can be expressed in a value between 0.001 and 1000.

Medical Applications

The most profound change in laboratory reports will result from expressing concentration as amount per volume (moles per liter) rather than mass per volume (milligrams per 100 milliliters). The advantages in the former expression can be seen in the following:

Conventional Units

1.0 gram of hemoglobin
    Combines with 1.37 ml. of oxygen
    Contains 3.4 mg. of iron
    Forms 34.9 mg. of bilirubin

S.I. Units

1.0 mmol of hemoglobin
    Combines with 4.0 mmol of oxygen
    Contains 4.0 mmol of iron
    Forms 4.0 mmol of bilirubin

Chemical relationships between lactic acid and pyruvic acid and the glucose from which both are derived, as well as the relationship between bilirubin and the binding capacity of albumin, are other examples of chemical relationships that will be clarified by using the new system.

There are a number of laboratory and other medical measurements for which the S.I. Units appear to offer little advantage, and some which

TABLE 1. **Basic Units**

PROPERTY	BASIC UNIT	SYMBOL
Length	metre	m
Mass	kilogram	kg
Amount of substance	mole	mol
Time	second	s
Thermodynamic temperature	kelvin	K
Electric current	ampere	A
Luminous intensity	candela	cd

TABLE 2. **Derived Units**

DERIVED PROPERTY	DERIVED UNIT	SYMBOL
Area	square metre	m^2
Volume	cubic metre	m^3
	litre	l
Mass concentration	kilogram/cubic metre	kg/m^3
	gram/litre	g/l
Substance concentration	mole/cubic metre	mol/m^3
	mole/litre	mol/l
Temperature	degree Celsius	$C = K - 273.15$

are disadvantageous because the change would require replacement or revision of instruments such as the sphygmomanometer. The cubic meter is the derived unit for volume; however, it is inappropriately large for medical measurements and the liter has been retained. Thermodynamic temperature expressed in kelvins is not more informative for medical measurements. Since the Celsius degree is the same as the Kelvin degree, the Celsius scale will be used. Celsius rather than centigrade is the preferred term.

Selection of units for expressing enzyme activity presents certain difficulties. Literally dozens of different units have been used in expressing enzyme activity, and interlaboratory comparison of enzyme results is impossible unless the assay system is precisely defined. In 1964 the International Union of Biochemistry attempted to remedy the situation by proposing the International Unit for enzymes. This unit was defined as the amount of enzyme that will catalyze the conversion of 1 micromole of substrate per minute under standard conditions. Difficulties remain, however, as enzyme activity is affected by the temperature, pH, the type and amount of substrate, the presence of inhibitors, and other factors. Enzyme activity can be expressed in S.I. Units, and the katal has been proposed to express activities of all catalysts, including enzymes. The katal is that amount of enzyme which catalyzes a reaction rate of 1 mole per second. Thus adoption of the katal as the unit of enzyme activity would provide no

TABLE 3. **Standard Prefixes**

PREFIX	MULTIPLICATION FACTOR	SYMBOL
atto	10^{-18}	a
femto	10^{-15}	f
pico	10^{-12}	p
nano	10^{-9}	n
micro	10^{-6}	μ
milli	10^{-3}	m
centi	10^{-2}	c
deci	10^{-1}	d
deca	10^1	da
hecto	10^2	h
kilo	10^3	k
mega	10^6	M
giga	10^9	G
tera	10^{12}	T

more information than is obtained when results are expressed in International Units.

Hydrogen ion concentration in blood is customarily expressed as pH, but in S.I. Units it would be expressed in nanomoles per liter. It appears unlikely that the very useful pH scale will be discarded.

Pressure measures, such as blood pressure and partial pressures of blood gases, would be expressed in S.I. Units, using the Pascal, a unit that can be derived from the basic units for mass, length, and time. This change probably will not be adopted in the early phases of the conversion to S.I. Units. Similarly, a proposed change in expressing osmolality in terms of the depression of freezing point is inappropriate, because osmolality may be calculated from vapor pressure as well as freezing point measurement.

Conventions

A number of conventions have been adopted to standardize usage of S.I. Units:

1. No periods are used after the symbol for a unit (kg not kg.), and it remains unchanged when used in the plural (70 kg not 70 kgs).

2. A half space rather than a comma is used to divide large numbers into groups of three (5 400 000 not 5,400,000).

3. Compound prefixes should be avoided (nanometer not millimicrometer).

4. Multiples and submultiples are used in steps of 10^3 or 10^{-3}.

5. The degree sign for the temperature scales is omitted (38 C not 38°C).

6. The preferred spelling is metre not meter, litre not liter.

7. Report of a measurement should include information on the system, the component, the kind of quantity, the numerical value, and the unit. For example: *System,* serum. *Component,* glucose. *Kind of quantity,* substance concentration. *Value,* 5.10. *Unit,* mmol/l.

8. The name of the component should be unambiguous; for example, "serum bilirubin" might refer to unconjugated bilirubin or to total bilirubin. For acids and bases, the maximally ionized form is used in naming the component; for example, lactate or urate rather than lactic acid or uric acid.

Tables of Reference Values

Tables accompanying this article indicate "normal values" for most of the commonly performed laboratory tests. The title of the tables has been changed from the "normal values" of previous years to "reference values" to conform to current usage. The reference value is given in conventional units, the conversion factor is indicated when appropriate, and the value in S.I. Units is calculated from these figures. Notes (pp. 1171 and 1172) are used to provide additional information.

REFERENCE VALUES IN HEMATOLOGY

	CONVENTIONAL UNITS		FACTOR	S.I. UNITS	NOTES
Acid hemolysis test (Ham)	No hemolysis		—	No hemolysis	
Alkaline phosphatase, leukocyte	Total score 14–100		—	Total score 14–100	
Carboxyhemoglobin	Up to 5% of total		0.01	0.05 of total	a
Cell counts					
Erythrocytes					
Males	4.6–6.2 million/cu. mm.		10^6	$4.6–6.2 \times 10^{12}/l$	
Females	4.2–5.4 million/cu. mm.			$4.2–5.4 \times 10^{12}/l$	
Children (varies with age)	4.5–5.1 million/cu. mm.			$4.5–5.1 \times 10^{12}/l$	
Leukocytes					
Total	4500–11,000/cu. mm.		10^6	$4.5–11.0 \times 10^9/l$	
Differential	*Percentage*	*Absolute*	10^6		
Myelocytes	0	0/cu. mm.		0/1	b
Band neutrophils	3–5	150–400/cu. mm.		$150–400 \times 10^6/l$	
Segmented neutrophils	54–62	3000–5800/cu. mm.		$3000–5800 \times 10^6/l$	
Lymphocytes	25–33	1500–3000/cu. mm.		$1500–3000 \times 10^6/l$	
Monocytes	3–7	300–500/cu. mm.		$300–500 \times 10^6/l$	
Eosinophils	1–3	50–250/cu. mm.		$50–250 \times 10^6/l$	
Basophils	0–0.75	15–50/cu. mm.		$15–50 \times 10^6/l$	
Platelets	150,000–350,000/cu. mm.		10^6	$150–350 \times 10^9/l$	b
Reticulocytes	25,000–75,000/cu. mm. 0.5–1.5% of erythrocytes		10^6	$25–75 \times 10^9/l$	
Coagulation tests					
Bleeding time (Duke)	1–5 min.		—	1–5 min	
Bleeding time (Ivy)	Less than 5 min.		—	Less than 5 min	
Clot retraction, qualitative	Begins in 30–60 min. Complete in 24 hrs.		—	Begins in 30–60 min Complete in 24 h	
Coagulation time (Lee-White)	5–15 min. (glass tubes) 19–60 min. (siliconized tubes)		—	5–15 min (glass tubes) 19–60 min (siliconized tubes)	
Euglobulin lysis time	2–6 hr. at 37 C		—	2–6 h at 37 C	
Factor VIII and other coagulation factors	50–150% of normal		—	0.50–1.5 of normal	a
Fibrin split products (Thrombo-Wellco test)	Negative at 1:4 dilution		—	Negative at 1:4 dilution	
Fibrinogen	200–400 mg./100 ml.		0.0293	5.9–11.7 μmol/l	c
Fibrinolysins	0		—	0	
Partial thromboplastin time, activated (APTT)	35–45 sec.		—	35–45 s	
Prothrombin consumption	Over 80% consumed in 1 hr.		0.01	Over 0.80 consumed in 1 h	
Prothrombin content	100% (calculated from prothrombin time)		0.01	1.0 (calculated from prothrombin time)	a
Prothrombin time (one stage)	12.0–14.0 sec.		—	12.0–14.0 s	
Thromboplastin generation test	Compared to normal control		—	Compared to normal control	
Tourniquet test	Ten or fewer petechiae in a 2.5 cm. circle after 5 min.		—	Ten or fewer petechiae in a 2.5 cm circle after 5 min	a
Cold hemolysin test (Donath-Landsteiner)	No hemolysis		—	No hemolysis	
Coombs test					
Direct	Negative		—	Negative	
Indirect	Negative		—	Negative	

	Conventional	Factor	SI	Ref
Corpuscular values of erythrocytes (values are for adults; in children, values vary with age)				
M.C.H. (mean corpuscular hemoglobin)	27–31 picogm.	0.0155	0.42–0.48 fmol	d
M.C.V. (mean corpuscular volume)	80–105 cu. micra	1.0	80–105 fl	a
M.C.H.C. (mean corpuscular hemoglobin concentration)	32–36%	0.01	0.32–0.36	
Haptoglobin (as hemoglobin binding capacity)	100–200 mg./100 ml.	0.155	16–31 µmol/l	d
Hematocrit				
Males	40–54 ml./100 ml.	0.01	0.40–0.54	a
Females	37–47 ml./100 ml.		0.37–0.47	
Newborn	49–54 ml./100 ml.		0.49–0.54	
Children (varies with age)	35–49 ml./100 ml.		0.35–0.49	
Hemoglobin				
Males	14.0–18.0 grams/100 ml.	0.155	2.17–2.79 mmol/l	d
Females	12.0–16.0 grams/100 ml.		1.86–2.48 mmol/l	
Newborn	16.5–19.5 grams/100 ml.		2.56–3.02 mmol/l	
Children (varies with age)	11.2–16.5 grams/100 ml.		1.74–2.56 mmol/l	
Hemoglobin, fetal	Less than 1% of total	0.01	Less than 0.01 of total	a
Hemoglobin A_{1c}	3–5% of total	0.01	0.03–0.05 of total	a
Hemoglobin A_2	1.5–3.0% of total	0.01	0.015–0.03 of total	a
Hemoglobin, plasma	0–5.0 mg./100 ml.	0.155	0–0.8 µmol/l	d
Methemoglobin	0–5.0 mg./100 ml.	171	4.7–20 µmol/l	e
Osmotic fragility of erythrocytes	Begins in 0.45–0.39% NaCl		Begins in 77–67 mmol/l NaCl	
	Complete in 0.33–0.30% NaCl		Complete in 56–51 mmol/l NaCl	
Sedimentation rate				
Wintrobe: Males	0–5 mm. in 1 hr.	—	0–5 mm/h	
Females	0–15 mm. in 1 hr.	—	0–15 mm/h	
Westergren: Males	0–15 mm. in 1 hr.	—	0–15 mm/h	
Females	0–20 mm. in 1 hr.	—	0–20 mm/h	
(May be slightly higher in children and during pregnancy)				
Bone marrow, differential cell count		0.01		a

	Conventional Range	Conventional Average	SI Range	SI Average
Myeloblasts	0.3–5.0%	2.0%	0.003–0.05	0.02
Promyelocytes	1.0–8.0%	5.0%	0.01–0.08	0.05
Myelocytes: Neutrophilic	5.0–19.0%	12.0%	0.05–0.19	0.12
Eosinophilic	0.5–3.0%	1.5%	0.005–0.03	0.015
Basophilic	0.0–0.5%	0.3%	0.00–0.005	0.003
Metamyelocytes	13.0–32.0%	22.0%	0.13–0.32	0.22
Polymorphonuclear neutrophils	7.0–30.0%	20.0%	0.07–0.30	0.20
Polymorphonuclear eosinophils	0.5–4.0%	2.0%	0.005–0.04	0.02
Polymorphonuclear basophils	0.0–0.7%	0.2%	0.00–0.007	0.002
Lymphocytes	3.0–17.0%	10.0%	0.03–0.17	0.10
Plasma cells	0.0–2.0%	0.4%	0.00–0.02	0.004
Monocytes	0.5–5.0%	2.0%	0.005–0.05	0.02
Reticulum cells	0.1–2.0%	0.2%	0.001–0.02	0.002
Megakaryocytes	0.3–3.0%	0.4%	0.003–0.03	0.004
Pronormoblasts	1.0–8.0%	4.0%	0.01–0.08	0.04
Normoblasts	7.0–32.0%	18.0%	0.07–0.32	0.18

REFERENCE VALUES FOR BLOOD, PLASMA AND SERUM

(For some procedures the reference values may vary depending upon the method used)

	CONVENTIONAL UNITS	FACTOR	S.I. UNITS	NOTES
Acetoacetate plus acetone, serum				
Qualitative	Negative	—	Negative	
Quantitative	0.3–2.0 mg./100 ml.	10	3–20 mg/l	
Adrenocorticotropin (ACTH), plasma	10–80 picogm./ml.	1.0	10–80 ng/l	
Aldolase, serum	0–11 milliunits/ml. (I.U.) (30 C)	1.0	0–11 units/l (30 C)	f
Alpha amino nitrogen, serum	3.0–5.5 mg./100 ml.	0.714	2.1–3.9 mmol/l	
Ammonia, plasma	20–120 mcg./100 ml.	0.554	11–67 μmol/l	
Amylase, serum	Less than 160 Caraway units/100 ml.	—	Less than 160 Caraway units/dl	f
Anion gap	8–16 mEq./liter	1.0	8–16 mmol/l	
Ascorbic acid, blood	0.4–1.5 mg./100 ml.	56.8	23–85 μmol/l	
Base excess, blood	0 ± 2 mEq./liter	1.0	0 ± 2 mmol/l	
Bicarbonate, serum	23–29 mEq./liter	1.0	23–29 mmol/l	
Bile acids, serum	0.3–3.0 mg./dl.	10	3.0–30.0 mg/l	
Bilirubin, serum				
Direct (conjugated)	0.1–0.4 mg./100 ml.	17.1	1.7–6.8 μmol/l	
Indirect (unconjugated)	0.2–0.7 mg./100 ml. (Total minus direct)	17.1	3.4–12 μmol/l (Total minus direct)	
Total	0.3–1.1 mg./100 ml.	17.1	5.1–19 μmol/l	
Bromsulphalein (BSP) (Inject 5 mg./kg. body weight, draw sample at 45 min.)	Less than 5%	0.01	Less than 0.05	a
Calcium, serum	4.5–5.5 mEq./liter	0.50	2.25–2.75 mmol/l	
	9.0–11.0 mg./100 ml.	0.25	2.25–2.75 mmol/l	
	(Slightly higher in children)		(Slightly higher in children)	
	(Varies with protein concentration)		(Varies with protein concentration)	
Calcium, ionized, serum	2.1–2.6 mEq./liter	0.50	1.05–1.30 mmol/l	
	4.25–5.25 mg./100 ml.	0.25	1.05–1.30 mmol/l	
Carbon dioxide content, serum				
Adults	24–30 mEq./liter	1.0	24–30 mmol/l	
Infants	20–28 mEq./liter	1.0	20–28 mmol/l	
Carbon dioxide tension (Pco_2), blood	35–45 mm. Hg	—	35–45 mm Hg	
Carotene, serum	50–300 mcg./100 ml.	0.0186	0.93–5.58 μmol/l	
Ceruloplasmin, serum	23–44 mg./100 ml.	0.0662	1.5–2.9 μmol/l	g
Chloride, serum	96–106 mEq./liter	1.0	96–106 mmol/l	h
Cholesterol, serum				
Total	150–250 mg./100 ml.	0.0259	3.9–6.5 mmol/l	
Esters	68–76% of total cholesterol	0.01	0.68–0.76 of total cholesterol	a
Cholinesterase				
Serum	0.5–1.3 pH units	—	0.5–1.3 pH units	f
Erythrocytes	0.5–1.0 pH unit	—	0.5–1.0 pH unit	f
Copper, serum				
Males	70–140 mcg./100 ml.	0.157	11–22 μmol/l	
Females	85–155 mcg./100 ml.	0.157	13–24 μmol/l	
Cortisol, plasma (8 A.M.)	6–23 mcg./100 ml.	27.6	170–635 nmol/l	

Analyte	Conventional	Factor	SI	Ref.
Creatine kinase, serum				
Males	0–50 milliunits/ml. (I.U.) (30°) (Oliver-Rosalki)	1.0	0–50 units/l (30 C) (Oliver-Rosalki)	f
Females	0–30 milliunits/ml. (I.U.) (30°) (Oliver-Rosalki)	1.0	0–30 units/l (30 C) (Oliver-Rosalki)	f
Creatine kinase isoenzymes, serum				
CK-MM	Present	—	Present	
CK-MB	Absent	—	Absent	
CK-BB	Absent	—	Absent	
Creatinine, serum	0.7–1.5 mg./100 ml.	88.4	62–133 µmol/l	
Cryoglobulins, serum	0	—	0	
Fatty acids, total, serum	190–420 mg./100 ml.	0.0352	7–15 mmol/l	i
Ferritin, serum	20–200 nanogm./ml.	1.0	20–200 µg/l	
Fibrinogen, plasma	200–400 mg./100 ml.	0.0293	5.9–11.7 µmol/l	c
Folate, serum	>2.3 nanogm./ml.	2.27	>5.2 nmol/l	
Erythrocytes	>140 nanogm./ml.	2.27	>318 nmol/l	
Follicle-stimulating hormone (FSH), plasma				
Males	4–25 milliunits/ml. (I.U.)	1.0	4–25 IU/l	
Females	4–30 milliunits/ml. (I.U.)		4–30 IU/l	
Postmenopausal	40–250 milliunits/ml. (I.U.)		40–250 IU/l	
Gamma glutamyltransferase				
Males	6–32 milliunits/ml. (I.U.) (30°)	1.0	6–32 units/l (30 C)	f
Females	4–18 milliunits/ml. (I.U.) (30°)	1.0	4–18 units/l (30 C)	f
Gastrin, serum	0–200 picogm./ml.	1.0	0–200 ng/l	
Glucose (fasting)				
Blood	60–100 mg./100 ml.	0.0555	3.33–5.55 mmol/l	
Plasma or serum	70–115 mg./100 ml.	0.0555	3.89–6.38 mmol/l	
Growth hormone, serum	0–10 nanogm./ml.	1.0	0–10 µg/l	
Haptoglobin, serum	100–200 mg./100 ml. (As hemoglobin binding capacity)	0.155	16–31 µmol/l (As hemoglobin binding capacity)	d
Hydroxybutyric dehydrogenase, serum	0–180 milliunits/ml. (I.U.) (30°) (Rosalki-Wilkinson)	1.0	0–180 units/l (30 C) (Rosalki-Wilkinson)	f
17-Hydroxycorticosteroids, plasma	114–290 units/ml. (Wroblewski)	—	114–290 units/ml (Wroblewski)	f
	8–18 mg/100 ml.	0.0276	0.22–0.50 µmol/l	j
Immunoglobulins, serum				
IgG	550–1900 mg./100 ml.	0.01	5.5–19.0 g/l	
IgA	60–333 mg./100 ml.	0.01	0.60–3.3 g/l	
IgM	45–145 mg./100 ml.	0.01	0.45–1.5 g/l	
IgD	0.5–3.0 mg./dl.	10	5–30 mg/l	
IgE	<500 nanogm./ml.	1	<500 µg/l	
Insulin, plasma (fasting)	(Varies with age in children) 5–25 microunits/ml.	1.0	(Varies with age in children) 5–25 milliunits/l	k
Iodine, protein bound, serum	3.5–8.0 mcg./100 ml.	0.0788	0.28–0.63 µmol/l	
Iron, serum	75–175 mcg./100 ml.	0.179	13–31 µmol/l	
Iron binding capacity, serum				
Total	250–410 mcg./100 ml.	0.179	45–73 µmol/l	
Saturation	20–55%	0.01	0.20–0.55	a
17-Ketosteroids, plasma	25–125 mcg./100 ml.	0.0347	0.87–4.34 µmol/l	l
Lactate, blood, venous	0.6–1.8 mEq./liter	1.0	0.6–1.8 mmol/l	
Lactate dehydrogenase, serum	0–300 milliunits/ml. (I.U.) (30°) (Wroblewski modified)	1.0	0–300 units/l (30 C) (Wroblewski modified)	f
	150–450 units/ml. (Wroblewski)	—	150–450 units/ml (Wroblewski)	
	80–120 units/ml. (Wacker)	—	80–120 units/ml (Wacker)	

Table continued on the following page

REFERENCE VALUES FOR BLOOD, PLASMA AND SERUM (Continued)

(For some procedures the reference values may vary depending upon the method used)

	CONVENTIONAL UNITS	FACTOR	S.I. UNITS	NOTES
Lactate dehydrogenase isoenzymes, serum				
LDH_1	22–37% of total	0.01	0.22–0.37 of total	a
LDH_2	30–46% of total		0.30–0.46 of total	
LDH_3	14–29% of total		0.14–0.29 of total	
LDH_4	5–11% of total		0.05–0.11 of total	
LDH_5	2–11% of total		0.02–0.11 of total	
Leucine aminopeptidase, serum	14–40 milliunits/ml. (I.U.) (30°)	1.0	14–40 units/l (30 C)	f
Lipase, serum	0–1.5 units (Cherry-Crandall)	—	0–1.5 units (Cherry-Crandall)	f
Lipids, total, serum	450–850 mg./100 ml.	0.01	4.5–8.5 g/l	m
Lipoprotein cholesterol, serum				
LDL cholesterol	60–180 mg./100 ml.	10	600–1800 mg/l	
HDL cholesterol	30–80 mg./100 ml.	10	300–800 mg/l	
Luteinizing hormone (LH), serum				
Males	6–18 milliunits/ml. (I.U.)	1.0	6–18 IU/l	
Females, premenopausal	5–22 milliunits/ml. (I.U.)	1.0	5–22 IU/l	
midcycle	3 times baseline	—	3 times baseline	
postmenopausal	Greater than 30 milliunits/ml. (I.U.)	1.0	Greater than 30 IU/l	
Magnesium, serum	1.5–2.5 mEq./liter	0.50	0.75–1.25 mmol/l	
	1.8–3.0 mg./100 ml.	0.411		
5'-Nucleotidase, serum	Less than 1.6 milliunits/ml. (I.U.) (30°)	1.0	Less than 1.6 units/l (30 C)	f
Nitrogen, nonprotein, serum	15–35 mg./100 ml.	0.714	10.7–25.0 mmol/l	
Osmolality, serum	285–295 mOsm./kg. serum water	—	285–295 mmol/kg serum water	n
Oxygen, blood				
Capacity	16–24 vol.% (varies with hemoglobin)	0.446	7.14–10.7 mmol/l (varies with hemoglobin)	o
Content Arterial	15–23 vol.%	0.446	6.69–10.3 mmol/l	o
Venous	10–16 vol.%	0.446	4.46–7.14 mmol/l	o
Saturation Arterial	94–100% of capacity	0.01	0.94–1.00 of capacity	a
Venous	60–85% of capacity	0.01	0.60–0.85 of capacity	a
Tension, pO_2 Arterial	75–100 mm. Hg	—	75–100 mm Hg	g
P_{50}, blood	26–27 mm. Hg	—	26–27 mm. Hg	g
pH, arterial, blood	7.35–7.45	—	7.35–7.45	p
Phenylalanine, serum	Less than 3 mg./100 ml.	0.0605	Less than 0.18 mmol/l	
Phosphatase, acid, serum	0–7.0 milliunits/ml. (I.U.) (30°)	1.0	0–7.0 units/l (30 C)	f
	1.0–5.0 units (King-Armstrong)	—	1.0–5.0 units (King-Armstrong)	
Phosphatase, alkaline, serum	10–32 milliunits/ml. (I.U.) (30°)	1.0	10–32 units/l (30 C)	f
	5.0–13.0 units (King-Armstrong) (Values are higher in children)	—	5.0–13.0 units (King-Armstrong) (Values are higher in children)	
Phosphate, inorganic, serum				
Adults	3.0–4.5 mg./100 ml.	0.323	1.0–1.5 mmol/l	
Children	4.0–7.0 mg./100 ml.		1.3–2.3 mmol/l	
Phospholipids, serum	6–12 mg./100 ml. (As lipid phosphorus)	0.323	1.9–3.9 mmol/l (As lipid phosphorus)	
Potassium, serum	3.5–5.0 mEq./liter	1.0	3.5–5.0 mmol/l	
Protein, serum				
Total	6.0–8.0 grams/100 ml.	10	60–80 g/l	m
Albumin	3.5–5.5 grams/100 ml.	10	35–55 g/l	
		0.154	0.54–0.85 mmol/l	q

Test	Conventional value	Factor	SI value	Ref
Electrophoresis				
Albumin	3.5–5.5 grams/100 ml.	10	35–55 g/l	q
	52–68% of total	0.01	0.52–0.68 of total	a
Globulin				
Alpha$_1$	0.2–0.4 gram/100 ml.	10	2–4 g/l	m
	2–5% of total	0.01	0.02–0.05 of total	a
Alpha$_2$	0.5–0.9 gram/100 ml.	10	5–9 g/l	m
	7–14% of total	0.01	0.07–0.14 of total	a
Beta	0.6–1.1 grams/100 ml.	10	6–11 g/l	m
	9–15% of total	0.01	0.09–0.15 of total	a
Gamma	0.7–1.7 grams/100 ml.	10	7–17 g/l	m
	11–21% of total	0.01	0.11–0.21 of total	a
Protoporphyrin, erythrocyte	27–61 mcg./100 ml. packed RBC	0.0178	0.48–1.09 μmol/l packed RBC	k
Pyruvate, blood	0.01–0.11 mEq./liter	1.0	0.01–0.11 mmol/l	
Sodium, serum	136–145 mEq./liter	1.0	136–145 mmol/l	
Sulfates, inorganic, serum	0.8–1.2 mg./100 ml.	104	83–125 μmol/l	
Testosterone, plasma				
Males	275–875 nanogm./100 ml.	0.0347	9.5–30 nmol/l	
Females	23–75 nanogm./100 ml.	0.0347	0.8–2.6 nmol/l	
Pregnant	38–190 nanogm./100 ml.	0.0347	1.3–6.6 nmol/l	
Thyroid stimulating hormone (TSH), serum	0–7 microunits/ml.	1.0	0–7 milliunits/l	
Thyroxine, free, serum	1.0–2.1 nanogm./100 ml.	12.9	13–27 pmol/l	k
Thyroxine (T$_4$), serum	4–11 mcg./100 ml.	12.9	52–142 nmol/l	
Thyroxine binding globulin (TBG), serum (as thyroxine)	10–26 mcg./100 ml.	12.9	129–335 nmol/l	
Thyroxine iodine, serum	2.9–6.4 mcg./100 ml.	78.8	229–504 nmol/l	a
Tri-iodothyronine (T$_3$), serum	150–250 nanogm./100 ml.	0.0154	2.3–3.9 nmol/l	
Tri-iodothyronine (T$_3$) uptake, resin (T$_3$RU)	25–38%	0.01	0.25–0.38 uptake	
Transaminase, serum				
SGOT (aspartate aminotransferase)	0–19 millunits/ml. (I.U.) (30°) (Karmen modified)	1.0	0–19 units/l (30 C) (Karmen modified)	f
	15–40 units/ml. (Karmen)		15–40 units/ml (Karmen)	
	18–40 units/ml. (Reitman-Frankel)		18–40 units/ml (Reitman-Frankel)	
SGPT (alanine aminotransferase)	0–17 millunits/ml. (I.U.) (30°) (Karmen modified)	1.0	0–17 units/l (30 C) (Karmen modified)	f
	6–35 units/ml. (Karmen)		6–35 units/ml (Karmen)	
	5–35 units/ml. (Reitman-Frankel)		5–35 units/ml (Reitman-Frankel)	
Triglycerides, serum	40–150 mg./100 ml.	0.01	0.4–1.5 g/l	
		0.0114	0.45–1.71 mmol/l	r
Urate (serum)				
Males	2.5–8.0 mg./100 ml.	0.0595	0.15–0.48 mmol/l	
Females	1.5–7.0 mg./100 ml.	0.0595	0.09–0.42 mmol/l	
Urea				
Blood	21–43 mg./100 ml.	0.167	3.5–7.2 mmol/l	
Plasma or serum	24–49 mg./100 ml.	0.167	4.0–8.2 mmol/l	
Urea nitrogen				
Blood	10–20 mg./100 ml.	0.714	7.1–14.3 mmol/l	
Plasma or serum	11–23 mg./100 ml.	0.714	7.9–16.4 mmol/l	
Viscosity, serum	1.4–1.8 times water	—	1.4–1.8 times water	
Vitamin A, serum	20–80 mcg./100 ml.	0.0349	0.70–2.8 μmol/l	
Vitamin B$_{12}$, serum	180–900 picogm./ml.	0.738	133–664 pmol/l	k

REFERENCE VALUES FOR URINE

(For some procedures the reference values may vary depending upon the method used)

	CONVENTIONAL UNITS	FACTOR	S.I. UNITS	NOTES
Acetone and acetoacetate, qualitative	Negative	—	Negative	
Addis count				
Erythrocytes	0–130,000/24 hrs.	—	0–130 000/24 h	
Leukocytes	0–650,000/24 hrs.	—	0–650 000/24 h	
Casts (hyaline)	0–2000/24 hrs.	—	0–2000/24 h	
Albumin				
Qualitative	Negative		Negative	
Quantitative	10–100 mg./24 hrs.	—	10–100 mg/24 h	q
Aldosterone	3–20 mcg./24 hrs.	0.0154	0.15–1.5 μmol/24 h	
Alpha amino nitrogen	50–200 mg./24 hrs.	2.77	8.3–55 nmol/24 h	
Ammonia nitrogen	20–70 mEq./24 hrs.	0.0714	3.6–14.3 mmol/24 h	
Amylase	35–260 Caraway units/hr.	1.0	20–70 mmol/24 h	
Bilirubin, qualitative	Negative	—	35–260 Caraway units/h	f
			Negative	
Calcium				
Low Ca diet	Less than 150 mg./24 hrs.	0.025	Less than 3.8 mmol/24 h	
Usual diet	Less than 250 mg./24 hrs.	0.025	Less than 6.3 mmol/24 h	
Catecholamines				
Epinephrine	Less than 10 mcg./24 hrs.	5.46	Less than 55 nmol/24 h	s
Norepinephrine	Less than 100 mcg./24 hrs.	5.91	Less than 590 nmol/24 h	t
Total free catecholamines	4–126 mcg./24 hrs.	5.91	24–745 nmol/24 h	
Total metanephrines	0.1–1.6 mg./24 hrs.	5.07	0.5–8.1 μmol/24 h	
Chloride	110–250 mEq./24 hrs.	1.0	110–250 mmol/24 h	
	(Varies with intake)		(Varies with intake)	
Chorionic gonadotropin	0	—	0	
Copper	0–50 mcg./24 hrs.	0.0157	0–0.80 μmol/24 h	
Creatine				
Males	0–40 mg./24 hrs.	0.00762	0–0.30 mmol/24 h	
Females	0–100 mg./24 hrs.	0.00762	0–0.76 mmol/24 h	
	(Higher in children and during pregnancy)		(Higher in children and during pregnancy)	
Creatinine	15–25 mg./kg. body weight/24 hrs.	0.00884	0.13–0.22 mmol·kg⁻¹ body weight/24 h	
Creatinine clearance				
Males	110–150 ml./min.	—	110–150 ml/min	
Females	105–132 ml./min. (1.73 sq. meter surface area)	—	105–132 ml/min (1.73 m² surface area)	
Cystine or cysteine, qualitative	Negative	—	Negative	
Dehydroepiandrosterone	Less than 15% of total 17-keto-steroids	0.01	Less than 0.15 of total 17-keto-steroids	a
Delta aminolevulinic acid	1.3–7.0 mg./24 hrs.	7.63	10–53 μmol/24 h	

Test	Conventional	Factor	SI	
Estrogens				
Males				
Estrone	3–8 μg./24 hrs.	3.70	11–30 nmol/24 h	
Estradiol	0–6 μg./24 hrs.	3.67	0–22 nmol/24 h	
Estriol	1–11 μg./24 hrs.	3.47	3–38 nmol/24 h	
Total	4–25 μg./24 hrs.	3.60	14–90 nmol/24 h	u
Females				
Estrone	4–31 μg./24 hrs.	3.70	15–115 nmol/24 h	
Estradiol	0–14 μg./24 hrs.	3.67	0–51 nmol/24 h	
Estriol	0–72 μg./24 hrs.	3.47	0–250 nmol/24 h	
Total	5–100 μg./24 hrs.	3.60	18–360 nmol/24 h	u
	(Markedly increased during pregnancy)		(Markedly increased during pregnancy)	
Glucose (as reducing substance)	Less than 250 mg./24 hrs.	—	Less than 250 mg/24 h	
Gonadotropins, pituitary	10–50 mouse units/24 hrs.	—	10–50 mouse units/24 h	
Hemoglobin and myoglobin, qualitative	Negative	—	Negative	
Homogentisic acid, qualitative	Negative	—	Negative	
17-Hydroxycorticosteroids				
Males	3–9 mg./24 hrs.	2.76	8.3–25 μmol/24 h	
Females	2–8 mg./24 hrs.		5.5–22 μmol/24 h	j
5-Hydroxyindoleacetic acid				
Qualitative	Negative	—	Negative	
Quantitative	Less than 9 mg./24 hrs.	5.23	Less than 47 μmol/24 h	
17-Ketosteroids				
Males	6–18 mg./24 hrs.	3.47	21–62 μmol/24 h	
Females	4–13 mg./24 hrs.		14–45 μmol/24 h	l
	(Varies with age)		(Varies with age)	
Magnesium	6.0–8.5 mEq./24 hrs.	0.5	3.0–4.3 mmol/24 h	
Metanephrines (see Catecholamines)				
Osmolality	38–1400 mOsm./kg. water	—	38–1400 mmol/kg water	n
pH	4.6–8.0, average 6.0	—	4.6–8.0, average 6.0	p
	(Depends on diet)		(Depends on diet)	
Phenolsulfonphthalein excretion (PSP)	25% or more in 15 min.	0.01	0.25 or more in 15 min	
	40% or more in 30 min.		0.40 or more in 30 min	
	55% or more in 2 hrs.		0.55 or more in 2 h	
	(After injection of 1 ml PSP intravenously)		(After injection of 1 ml PSP intravenously)	a
Phenylpyruvic acid, qualitative	Negative	—	Negative	
Phosphorus	0.9–1.3 gm./24 hrs.	32.3	29–42 mmol/24 h	
Porphobilinogen				
Qualitative	Negative	—	Negative	
Quantitative	0–0.2 mg./100 ml.	4.42	0–0.9 μmol/l	
	Less than 2.0 mg./24 hrs.		Less than 9 μmol/24 h	
Porphyrins				
Coproporphyrin	50–250 mcg./24 hrs.	1.53	77–380 nmol/24 h	
Uroporphyrin	10–30 mcg./24 hrs.	1.20	12–36 nmol/24 h	
Potassium	25–100 mEq./24 hrs.	1.0	25–100 mmol/24 h	
	(Varies with intake)		(Varies with intake)	

Table continued on the following page

REFERENCE VALUES FOR URINE (Continued)

(For some procedures the reference values may vary depending upon the method used)

	CONVENTIONAL UNITS	FACTOR	S.I. UNITS	NOTES
Pregnanediol				
Males	0.4–1.4 mg./24 hrs.	3.12	1.2–4.4 μmol/24 h	
Females				
Proliferative phase	0.5–1.5 mg./24 hrs.		1.6–4.7 μmol/24 h	
Luteal phase	2.0–7.0 mg./24 hrs.		6.2–22 μmol/24 h	
Postmenopausal phase	0.2–1.0 mg./24 hrs.		0.6–3.1 μmol/24 h	
Pregnanetriol	Less than 2.5 mg./24 hrs. in adults	2.97	Less than 7.4 μmol/24 h in adults	
Protein				
Qualitative	Negative	—	Negative	
Quantitative	10–150 mg./24 hrs.		10–150 mg/24 h	
Sodium	130–260 mEq./24 hrs.	1.0	130–260 mmol/24 h	m
	(Varies with intake)		(Varies with intake)	
Specific gravity	1.003–1.030	—	1.003–1.030	
Titratable acidity	20–40 mEq./24 hrs.	1.0	20–40 mmol/24 h	
Urate	200–500 mg./24 hrs.	0.00595	1.2–3.0 mmol/24 h	
	(With normal diet)		(With normal diet)	
Urobilinogen	Up to 1.0 Ehrlich unit/2 hrs.	—	Up to 1.0 Ehrlich unit/2 h	
	(1–3 P.M.)		(1–3 P.M.)	
	0–4.0 mg./24 hrs.		0–4.0 mg/24 h	
Vanillylmandelic acid (VMA)	1–8 mg./24 hrs.	5.05	5–40 μmol/24 h	
(4-hydroxy-3-methoxymandelic acid)				

REFERENCE VALUES FOR THERAPEUTIC DRUG MONITORING

	CONVENTIONAL UNITS	FACTOR	S.I. UNITS	NOTES
Carbamazepine, serum	0	4.23	0	
(Tegretol)	Therapeutic levels:		Therapeutic levels:	
	5.0–14.0 mg./liter		21–59 μmol/l	
Digoxin, serum	0	1.28	0	
With dose of 0.25 mg. per day	Therapeutic levels:		Therapeutic levels:	
	0.8–1.6 mcg./liter		1.0–2.3 nmol/l	

	Conventional Value	Conversion Factor	SI Value
With dose of 0.5 mg. per day (Sample obtained 12 to 24 hrs. after last dose)	0.9–2.4 mcg./liter		1.2–3.1 nmol/l
Ethosuximide, serum (Zarontin)	0 Therapeutic levels: 40–80 mg./liter	7.08	0 Therapeutic levels: 283–566 μmol/l
Lithium, serum	0 Therapeutic levels: 0.8–1.5 mEq./liter Toxic level: Above 2 mEq./liter	1.0	0 Therapeutic levels: 0.8–1.5 mmol/l Toxic level: Above 2 mmol/l
Phenobarbital, serum	0 Therapeutic levels: 10.0–25.0 mg./liter Toxic levels: Vary widely because of developed tolerance	4.31	0 Therapeutic levels: 43–108 μmol/l Toxic levels: Vary widely because of developed tolerance
Phenytoin, serum (diphenylhydantoin, Dilantin)	0 Therapeutic levels: 10–20 mg./liter Toxic levels: Above 20 mg./liter	3.65	0 Therapeutic levels: 37–73 μmol/l Toxic levels: Above 73 μmol/l
Primidone, serum (Mysoline)	0 Therapeutic levels: 4.0–10.0 mg./liter	4.58	0 Therapeutic levels: 18–46 μmol/l
Procainamide, serum (Pronestyl)	0 Therapeutic levels: 4.0–8.0 mg./liter	4.24	0 Therapeutic levels: 17–34 μmol/l
Quinidine, serum	0 Therapeutic levels: 2.0–5.0 mg./liter Toxic levels: Over 10 mg./liter	3.08	0 Therapeutic levels: 6.2–15 μmol/l Toxic levels: Over 31 μmol/l
Salicylate, plasma	0 Therapeutic levels: 20–25 mg./100 ml. Toxic levels: Over 30 mg./100 ml. Death 45–75 mg./100 ml.	0.0555	0 Therapeutic levels: 1.0–1.4 mmol/l Toxic levels: Over 1.7 mmol/l Death 2.5–4.2 mmol/l
Theophylline, serum	0 Therapeutic levels: 5.0–20.0 mg./liter Toxic levels: Above 30.0 mg./liter	5.55	0 Therapeutic levels: 28–111 μmol/l Toxic levels: Above 167 μmol/l
Thiocyanate, serum (Metabolite of sodium nitroprusside)	0 Therapeutic levels: 80–120 mg./liter	0.0169	0 Therapeutic levels: 1.4–2.0 mmol/l

REFERENCE VALUES IN TOXICOLOGY

	CONVENTIONAL UNITS	FACTOR	S.I. UNITS	NOTES
Arsenic, blood	3.5–7.2 mcg./100 ml.	0.133	0.47–0.96 μmol/l	
Arsenic, urine	Less than 100 mcg./24 hrs.	0.0133	Less than 1.3 μmol/24 h	
Bromides, serum	0	1.0	0	
Carbon monoxide, blood	Toxic levels:		Toxic levels:	a
	Above 17 mEq./liter		Above 17 mmol/l	
	Up to 5% saturation	—	Up to 0.05 saturation	
	Symptoms occur with 20% saturation		Symptoms occur with 0.20 saturation	
Ethanol, blood	Less than 0.005%	217	Less than 1 mmol/l	
Marked intoxication	0.3–0.4%		65–87 mmol/l	
Alcoholic stupor	0.4–0.5%		87–109 mmol/l	
Coma	Above 0.5%		Above 109 mmol/l	
Lead, blood	0–40 mcg./100 ml.	0.0483	0–2 μmol/l	
Lead, urine	Less than 100 mcg./24 hrs.	0.00483	Less than 0.48 μmol/24 h	
Mercury, urine	Less than 10 mcg./24 hrs.	4.98	Less than 50 nmol/24 h	

REFERENCE VALUES FOR CEREBROSPINAL FLUID

	CONVENTIONAL UNITS	FACTOR	S.I. UNITS	NOTES
Cells	Fewer than 5/cu. mm.; all mononuclear	—	Fewer than 5/μl; all mononuclear	
Chloride	120–130 mEq./liter	1.0	120–130 mmol/l	
	(20 mEq./liter higher than serum)		(20 mmol/l higher than serum)	
Electrophoresis	Predominantly albumin		Predominantly albumin	
Glucose	50–75 mg./100 ml.	0.0555	2.8–4.2 mmol/l	
	(20 mg./100 ml. less than serum)		(1.1 mmol/l less than serum)	
IgG				
Children under 14	Less than 8% of total protein	—	Less than 0.08 of total protein	a,m
Adults	Less than 14% of total protein		Less than 0.14 of total protein	
Pressure	70–180 mm. water		70–180 mm water	g
Protein, total	15–45 mg./100 ml.	0.01	0.150–0.450 g/l	m
	(Higher, up to 70 mg./100 mL., in elderly adults and children)		(Higher, up to 0.70 g/l, in elderly adults and children)	

REFERENCE VALUES FOR GASTRIC ANALYSIS

	CONVENTIONAL UNITS	FACTOR	S.I. UNITS	NOTES
Basal gastric secretion (1 hour)				
Concentration	(Mean ± 1 S.D.)		(Mean ± 1 S.D.)	
Males	25.8 ± 1.8 mEq./liter	1.0	25.8 ± 1.8 mmol/l	
Females	20.3 ± 3.0 mEq./liter		20.3 ± 3.0 mmol/l	
Output	(Mean ± 1 S.D.)		(Mean ± 1 S.D.)	
Males	2.57 ± 0.16 mEq./hr.	1.0	2.57 ± 0.16 mmol/h	
Females	1.61 ± 0.18 mEq./hr.		1.61 ± 0.18 mmol/h	
After histamine stimulation				
Normal	Mean output 11.8 mEq./hr.	1.0	Mean output 11.8 mmol/h	
Duodenal ulcer	Mean output 15.2 mEq./hr.		Mean output 15.2 mmol/h	
After maximal histamine stimulation				
Normal	Mean output 22.6 mEq./hr.	1.0	Mean output 22.6 mmol/h	
Duodenal ulcer	Mean output 44.6 mEq./hr.		Mean output 44.6 mmol/h	
Diagnex blue (Squibb): Anacidity	0–0.3 mg. in 2 hrs.	1.0	0–0.3 mg in 2 h	
Doubtful	0.3–0.6 mg. in 2 hrs.		0.3–0.6 mg in 2 h	
Normal	Greater than 0.6 mg. in 2 hrs.	—	Greater than 0.6 mg in 2 h	
Volume, fasting stomach content	50–100 ml.	—	0.05–0.1 l	
Emptying time	3–6 hrs.	—	3–6 h	
Color	Opalescent or colorless	—	Opalescent or colorless	
Specific gravity	1.006–1.009	—	1.006–1.009	
pH (adults)	0.9–1.5	—	0.9–1.5	p

PANCREATIC (ISLET) FUNCTION TESTS

Glucose tolerance tests

Oral

Patient should be on a diet containing 300 grams of carbohydrate per day for 3 days prior to test. After ingestion of 100 grams of glucose or 1.75 grams glucose/kg. body weight, blood glucose is not more than 160 mg./100 ml. after 60 minutes, 140 mg./100 ml. after 90 minutes, and 120 mg./100 ml. after 120 minutes. Values are for blood; serum measurements are approximately 15% higher.

Intravenous

Blood glucose does not exceed 200 mg./100 ml. after infusion of 0.5 gram of glucose/kg. body weight over 30 minutes. Glucose concentration falls below initial level at 2 hours and returns to preinfusion levels in 3 or 4 hours. Values are for blood; serum measurements are approximately 15% higher.

Cortisone-glucose tolerance test

The patient should be on a diet containing 300 grams of carbohydrate per day for 3 days prior to test. At 8½ and again 2 hours prior to glucose load patient is given cortisone acetate by mouth (50 mg. if patient's ideal weight is less than 160 lb., 62.5 mg. if ideal weight is greater than 160 lb.). An oral dose of glucose, 1.75 grams/kg. body weight, is given and blood samples are taken at 0, 30, 60, 90, and 120 minutes. Test is considered positive if true blood glucose exceeds 160 mg./100 ml. at 60 minutes, 140 mg./100 ml. at 90 minutes, and 120 mg./100 ml. at 120 minutes. Values are for blood; serum measurements are approximately 15% higher.

GASTROINTESTINAL ABSORPTION TESTS

	CONVENTIONAL UNITS	FACTOR	S.I. UNITS	NOTES
d-Xylose absorption test	After an 8 hour fast, 10 ml./kg. body weight of a 0.05 solution of d-xylose is given by mouth. Nothing further by mouth is given until the test has been completed. All urine voided during the following 5 hours is pooled, and blood samples are taken at 0, 60, and 120 minutes. Normally 0.26 (range 0.16–0.33) of ingested xylose is excreted within 5 hours, and the serum xylose reaches a level between 25 and 40 mg./100 ml. after 1 hour and is maintained at this level for another 60 minutes.		No change	
Vitamin A absorption	A fasting blood specimen is obtained and 200,000 units of vitamin A in oil is given by mouth. Serum vitamin A level should rise to twice fasting level in 3 to 5 hours.		No change	

REFERENCE VALUES FOR FECES

	CONVENTIONAL UNITS	FACTOR	S.I. UNITS	NOTES
Bulk	100–200 grams/24 hrs.	—	100–200 g/24 h	
Dry matter	23–32 grams/24 hrs.	—	23–32 g/24 h	
Fat, total	Less than 6.0 grams/24 hrs.	—	Less than 6.0 g/24 h	
Nitrogen, total	Less than 2.0 grams/24 hrs.	—	Less than 2.0 g/24 h	
Urobilinogen	40–280 mg./24 hrs.	—	40–280 mg/24 h	
Water	Approximately 65%	0.01	Approximately 0.65	a

REFERENCE VALUES FOR SEMEN ANALYSIS

	CONVENTIONAL UNITS	FACTOR	S.I. UNITS	NOTES
Volume	2–5 ml.; usually 3–4 ml.	—	2–5 ml; usually 3–4 ml	
Liquefaction	Complete in 15 min.	—	Complete in 15 min	
pH	7.2–8.0; average 7.8	—	7.2–8.0; average 7.8	p
Leukocytes	Occasional or absent	—	Occasional or absent	
Count	60–150 million/ml.	—	60–150 million/ml	
	Below 60 million/ml. is abnormal	—	Below 60 million/ml is abnormal	a
Motility	80% or more motile	—	0.80 or more motile	a
Morphology	80–90% normal forms	—	0.80–0.90 normal forms	a

REFERENCE VALUES FOR IMMUNOLOGIC PROCEDURES

	CONVENTIONAL UNITS	FACTOR	S.I. UNITS	NOTES
Syphilis serology (RPR and VDRL)	Negative		No change	
Mono screen	Negative		No change	
R.A. test (latex)	1:40 Negative		No change	
	1:80–1:160 Doubtful			
	1:320 Positive			
Rose test	1:10 Negative		No change	
	1:20–1:40 Doubtful			
	1:80 Positive			
Anti-streptolysin O titer	Normal up to 1:128. Single test usually has little significance. Rise in titer or persistently elevated titer is significant.		No change	
Anti-hyaluronidase titer	Less than 1:200. Significant if rising titer can be demonstrated at weekly intervals.		No change	
C-reactive protein	Negative		No change	
Anti-nuclear antibody	One specimen is sufficient, unless the result is inconsistent with the clinical impression. Most patients with active lupus have high ANA titers (160 or greater); some have lower titers (20–40). Patients with inactive lupus may have a negative test. Antinuclear antibodies are occasionally present in patients with no evidence of systemic lupus, usually in lower titers (20–40).		No change	
Febrile agglutinins	Titers of 1:80 or greater may be significant, particularly if subsequent samples show rise in titer.		No change	
Tularemia agglutinins	1:80 Negative		No change	
	1:160 Doubtful			
	1:320 Positive			
Proteus OX-19 agglutinins	Titers of 1:80 or greater may be significant, particularly if subsequent samples show rise in titer.		No change	
Complement fixation tests	Titers of 1:8 or less are usually not significant. Paired sera showing rise in titer of more than two tubes are usually considered significant.		No change	
C3 Test	80–140 mg./100 ml.	0.01	0.80–1.40 g/l	q
C4 Test	11–75 mg./100 ml.	0.01	0.11–0.75 g/l	

NOTES

a. Percentage is expressed as a decimal fraction.

b. Percentage may be expressed as a decimal fraction; however, when the result expressed is itself a variable fraction of another variable, the absolute value is more meaningful. There is no reason, other than custom, for expressing reticulocyte counts and differential leukocyte counts in percentages or decimal fractions rather than in absolute numbers.

c. Molecular weight of fibrinogen = 341,000 daltons.

d. Molecular weight of hemoglobin = 64,500 daltons. Because of disagreement as to whether the monomer or tetramer of hemoglobin should be used in the conversion, it has been recommended that the conventional grams per deciliter be retained. The tetramer is used in the table; values given should be multiplied by 4 to obtain concentration of the monomer.

e. Molecular weight of methemoglobin = 64,500 daltons. See note d above.

f. Enzyme units have not been changed in these tables because the proposed enzyme unit, the katal, has not been universally adopted (1 International Unit = 16.7 nkat).

g. It has been proposed that pressure be expressed in the Pascal (1 mm Hg = 0.133 kPa); however, this convention has not been universally accepted.

h. Molecular weight of ceruloplasmin = 151,000 daltons.

i. "Fatty acids" includes a mixture of different aliphatic acids of varying molecular weight. A mean molecular weight of 284 daltons has been assumed in calculating the conversion factor.

j. Based upon molecular weight of cortisol 362.47 daltons.

k. The practice of expressing concentration of an organic molecule in terms of one of its constituent elements originated when measurements included a heterogeneous class of compounds (nonprotein nitrogenous compounds, iodine-containing compounds bound to serum proteins). It was carried over to expressing measurements of specific substances (urea, thyroxine), but the practice should be discarded. For iodine and nitrogen 1 mole is taken as the monoatomic form, although they occur as diatomic molecules.

l. Based upon molecular weight of dehydroepiandrosterone 288.41 daltons.

m. Weight per volume is retained as the unit because of the heterogeneous nature of the material measured.

n. The proposal that osmolality be reported as freezing point depression using the millikelvin as the unit has not been received with universal enthusiasm. The milliosmole is not an S.I. unit, and the unit used here is the millimole.

o. Volumes per cent might be converted to a decimal fraction; however, this would not permit direct correlation with hemoglobin content, which is possible when oxygen content and capacity are expressed in molar quantities. One millimole of hemoglobin combines with 4 millimoles of oxygen.

p. Hydrogen ion concentration in S.I. units would be expressed in nanomoles per liter; however, this change has not received general approval. Conversion can be calculated as antilog (−pH).

q. Albumin is expressed in grams per liter to be consistent with units used for other proteins. Concentration of albumin may be expressed in mmol/l also, an expression that permits assessment of binding capacity of albumin for substances such as bilirubin. Molecular weight of albumin is 65,000 daltons.

r. Most techniques for quantitating triglycerides measure the glycerol moiety, and the total mass is calculated using an average molecular weight. The factor given assumes a mean molecular weight of 875 daltons for triglycerides.

s. Calculated as norepinephrine, molecular weight 169.18 daltons.

t. Calculated as metanephrine, molecular weight 197.23 daltons.

u. Conversion factor calculated from molecular weights of estrone, estradiol, and estriol in proportions of 2:1:2 daltons.

REFERENCES

1. Baron, D. N., Broughton, P. M. G., Cohen, M., Lansley, T. S., Lewis, S. M., and Shinton, N. K.: J. Clin. Path., 27:590, 1974.

2. Dawson, R. M. C., Elliott, D. C., Elliott, W. H., and Jones, K. M.: Data for Biochemical Research, 2nd ed. New York and Oxford, Oxford University Press, 1969.

3. Dybkaer, R.: Amer. J. Clin. Path., 52:637, 1969.

4. Henry, J. B.: Clinical Diagnosis and Management by Laboratory Methods, 16th ed. Philadelphia, W. B. Saunders Co., 1979.

5. Henry, R. J., Cannon, D. C., and Winkleman, J. W.: Clinical Chemistry—Principles and Techniques, 2nd ed. New York, Harper & Row, 1974.

6. International Committee for Standardization in Hematology, International Federation of Clinical Chemistry and World Association of Pathology Societies: Clin. Chem., 19:135, 1973.

7. Lehmann, H. P.: Amer. J. Clin. Path., 65:2, 1976.

8. Miale, J. B.: Laboratory Medicine—Hematology, 5th ed. St. Louis, C. V. Mosby, 1977.

9. Page, C. H., and Vigoureux, P.: The International System of Units (S.I.). U.S. Department of Commerce, National Bureau of Standards, Special Publication 330, 1974.

10. Scully, R. E., McNeely, B. U., and Galdabini, J. J.: New Engl. J. Med., 302:37, 1980.

11. Tietz, N. W.: Fundamentals of Clinical Chemistry, 2nd ed. Philadelphia, W. B. Saunders Co., 1976.

12. Wintrobe, M. D., Lee, G. R., Boggs, D. R., Bithell, T. C., Athens, J. W., and Foerster, J.: Clinical Hematology, 7th ed. Philadelphia, Lea & Febiger, 1974.

13. Young, D. S.: New Engl. J. Med., 292:795, 1975.

INDEX